The Oxford Handbook of Sleep and Sleep Disorders

OXFORD LIBRARY OF PSYCHOLOGY

AREA EDITORS:

Clinical Psychology
David H. Barlow

Cognitive Neuroscience
Kevin N. Ochsner and Stephen M. Kosslyn

Cognitive Psychology
Daniel Reisberg

Counseling Psychology
Elizabeth M. Altmaier and Jo-Ida C. Hansen

Developmental Psychology
Philip David Zelazo

Health Psychology
Howard S. Friedman

History of Psychology
David B. Baker

Methods and Measurement
Todd D. Little

Neuropsychology
Kenneth M. Adams

Organizational Psychology
Steve W.J. Kozlowski

Personality and Social Psychology
Kay Deaux and Mark Snyder

OXFORD LIBRARY OF PSYCHOLOGY

The Oxford Handbook of Sleep and Sleep Disorders

SECOND EDITION

Edited by

Colin A. Espie,

Phyllis C. Zee,

Charles M. Morin

OXFORD
UNIVERSITY PRESS

OXFORD
UNIVERSITY PRESS

Oxford University Press is a department of the University of Oxford.
It furthers the University's objective of excellence in research, scholarship,
and education by publishing worldwide. Oxford is a registered trade mark of
Oxford University Press in the UK and certain other countries.

Published in the United States of America by Oxford University Press
198 Madison Avenue, New York, NY 10016, United States of America.

Library of Congress Cataloging-in-Publication Data
Names: Espie, Colin A., editor. | Zee, Phyllis C., 1954– editor. |
Morin, Charles M., editor.
Title: The Oxford handbook of sleep and sleep disorders /
[edited by] Colin A. Espie, Phyllis C. Zee, Charles M. Morin.
Other titles: Handbook of sleep and sleep disorders |
Oxford library of psychology.
Description: 2nd edition. | New York, NY : Oxford University Press, [2025] |
Series: Oxford library of psychology series |
Includes bibliographical references and index.
Identifiers: LCCN 2024024062 (print) | LCCN 2024024063 (ebook) |
ISBN 9780197602751 (hardback) | ISBN 9780197602775 (epub) |
ISBN 9780197602782 (digital online)
Subjects: MESH: Sleep | Sleep Wake Disorders
Classification: LCC RC547 (print) | LCC RC547 (ebook) |
NLM WL 108 | DDC 616.8/498—dc23/eng/20241101
LC record available at https://lccn.loc.gov/2024024062
LC ebook record available at https://lccn.loc.gov/2024024063

DOI: 10.1093/oxfordhb/9780197602751.001.0001

Printed by Integrated Books International, United States of America

MIX
Paper
FSC FSC® C183721

CONTENTS

Section 6 • Disorders of Sleep and Circadian Function: Life Span Issues and Special Populations

FIGURES

TABLES

CONTRIBUTORS

Valentina Alfonsi
Sapienza University of Rome, Italy
Ali Amidi
Aarhus Univsrsity, Denmark
Sonia Ancoli-Israel
University of California, San Diego, USA
Thomas Andrillon
Paris Brain Institute, Sorbonne Université, Inserm-CNRS, France
J. Todd Arnedt
University of Michigan, Ann Arbor, USA
Arturo Arrona-Palacios
Brigham and Women's Hospital and Harvard Medical School, Boston, USA
Daniel Baena
University of Ottawa, Canada
Chiara Baglioni
University G. Marconi, Rome, Italy
Fiona C. Baker
SRI International, Menlo Park, California, USA
Erik N. T. P. Bakker
Amsterdam University Medical Center, The Netherlands
Bilgay Izci Balserak
University of Illinois, Chicago, USA
Lucie Barateau
National Reference Center for Narcolepsy and Rare Hypersomnia, University Hospital of Montpellier, France
Célyne H. Bastien
Université Laval, Quebec City, Canada
Simon Beaulieu-Bonneau
Université Laval, Quebec City, Canada
Bjørn Bjorvatn
University of Bergen, Norway
Tormod Bøe
University of Bergen, Norway
Diane B. Boivin
Douglas Mental Health University Institute, McGill University, Montreal, Canada
Michel A. Cramer Bornemann
Minnesota Regional Sleep Disorders Center, Hennepin County Medical Center, Minneapolis, USA
Philippe Boudreau
Douglas Research Centre, Montreal, Canada
Yosef Bronsteyn
University of Michigan, Ann Arbor, USA
Oliviero Bruni
Sapienza University of Rome, Italy
Orfeu M. Buxton
Pennsylvania State University, USA
Daniel J. Buysse
University of Pittsburgh, Pennsylvania, USA
M. Elizabeth Cardoni
University of Michigan, Ann Arbor, USA
Anne-Marie Chang
Pennsylvania State University, USA

Lindsey Clark
University of Pennsylvania, Philadelphia, USA
Rachel P. K. Conlon
University of Pittsburgh, PA, USA
Megan Crawford
University of Strathclyde, Scotland, UK
Yves Dauvilliers
University of Montpellier and Gui de Chauliac Hospital, Montpelier, France
Luigi De Gennaro
Sapienza University of Rome, Italy
Joseph De Koninck
University of Ottawa, Canada
Christopher M. Depner
University of Utah, Salt Lake City, USA
Jessica R. Dietch
Oregon State University, Corvallis, USA
Derk-Jan Dijk
University of Surrey, England, UK
Innessa Donskoy
Advocate Children's Hospital, Illinois, USA
Helen S. Driver
Kingston Health Sciences Centre and Queen's University, Ontario, Canada
Jeanne F. Duffy
Brigham and Women's Hospital and Harvard Medical School, Boston, USA
Danny J. Eckert
Flinders University, Adelaide, Australia
Jack D. Edinger
National Jewish Health, Denver, Colorado
Jason G. Ellis
Northumbria University, Newcastle upon Tyne, England, UK
Alexander J. Erickson
VA Greater Los Angeles Health Care System, California, USA
Colin A. Espie
University of Oxford, England, UK
Ingo Fietze
Charité – Universitätsmedizin Berlin, Germany
Ana I. Fins
Nova Southeastern University, Florida, USA
Samantha Fisher-Hicks
Swansea University and Swansea Bay University Health Board, Wales, UK
Leanne Fleming
UUniversity of Strathclyde, Scotland, UK
Stuart M. Fogel
University of Ottawa, Canada
Elisa Gamo
Hospital Puerta de Hierro, Madrid, Spain
Alba García
Sleep Research Institute, Madrid, Spain
Diego García-Borreguero
Sleep Research Institute, Madrid, Spain
Celia García-Malo
Sleep and Neuroscience Center CISNe, Madrid and Barcelona, Spain
Elham Garmroudinezhad-Rostami
Université Laval, Quebec City, Canada
Philip Gehrman
Perelman School of Medicine, University of Pennsylvania, Philadelphia, USA
Martin Glos
Charité – Universitätsmedizin Berlin, Germany
Michael Gradisar
Sleep Cycle, Adelaide, Australia

Mandilyn Graham
University of Michigan, Ann Arbor, USA
Nicole B. Gumport
Stanford University, California, USA
Marquis S. Hawkins
University of Pittsburgh, Pennsylvania, USA
H. Craig Heller
Stanford University, California, USA
Alejandro Herrero
Hospital 12 de Octubre, Madrid, Spain
Joel Hordijk
University of Ottawa, Canada
Mari Hysing
University of Bergen, Norway
Christopher C. Imes
University of Pittsburgh School of Nursing, Pennsylvania, USA
Alex Iranzo
Hospital Clinic de Barcelona, Spain
James B. Jaggard
Stanford University, California, USA
Michal Kahn
Tel Aviv University, Israel
Praneet C. Kaki
Sidney Kimmel Medical College, Thomas Jefferson University, Philadelphia, USA
Monica R. Kelly
University of California, Los Angeles and VA Greater Los Angeles Healthcare System, USA
Bhanu Prakash Kolla
Mayo Clinic, Rochester, Minnesota, USA
Courtney A. Kurinec
Washington State University, Pullman, USA
Simon D. Kyle
University of Oxford, England, UK
Leon C. Lack
Flinders University, Adelaide, Australia
Florence Lambert-Beaudet
Université Laval, Quebec City, Canada
Alpar S. Lazar
University of East Anglia, Norwich, England, UK
Kathryn Aldrich Lee
University of California, San Francisco, USA
Nicole Lovato
Flinders University, Adelaide, Australia
Jeanne E. Maglione
University of California, San Diego, USA
Rachel Manber
Stanford University, California, USA
Bethany Martin
University of Strathclyde, Scotland, UK
Jennifer L. Martin
University of California, Los Angeles and VA Greater Los Angeles Healthcare System, USA
Raquel Martín
Hospital Universitario Puerta de Hierro-Majadahonda, Madrid, Spain
Monica Martoni
University of Bologna, Italy
Debora Meneo
University G. Marconi, Rome, Italy
Gorica Micic
Flinders University, Adelaide, Australia
Charles M. Morin
Université Laval, Quebec City, Canada
Philippe Mourrain
Stanford University, California, USA
Keri J. Ngo
Stanford University, California, USA

Christoph Nissen
Geneva University Hospitals, Switzerland
Jason C. Ong
Nox Health, Dallas, Texas, USA
Marie-Christine Ouellet
Université Laval, Quebec City, Canada
Temitayo Oyegbile-Chidi
University of California Davis, USA
Mhairi Patience
University of Strathclyde, Scotland, UK
Philippe Peigneux
Université Libre de Bruxelles, Belgium
Thomas Penzel
Charité – Universitätsmedizin Berlin, Germany
Michael Perlis
Perelman School of Medicine, University of Pennsylvania, Philadelphia, USA
Alyssa Pozzobon
University of Ottawa, Canada
Laura B. Ray
University of Ottawa, Canada
Dieter Riemann
Freiburg University Medical Center, Germany
Sofía Romero
Sleep Research Institute, Madrid, Spain
Liliia Roshchupkina
Université Libre de Bruxelles, Belgium
Lisa Rosenblum
Charité – Universitätsmedizin Berlin, Germany
Alexandre Rudziavic Provençal
Université Laval, Quebec City, Canada
Bruno Saconi
Geisinger, Phoenix, Arizona, USA
Matthew Salanitro
Charité – Universitätsmedizin Berlin, Germany
Amy M. Sawyer
University of Pennsylvania, Philadelphia, USA
Serena Scarpelli
Sapienza University of Rome, Italy
Carlos H. Schenck
University of Minnesota Medical School, Minneapolis, USA
Hannah Scott
Flinders University, Adelaide, Australia
Holly Scott
University of Glasgow, Scotland, UK
Jonah A. Scott
George Fox University, Newberg, Oregon, USA
Francesca Siclari
Netherlands Institute for Neuroscience, Amsterdam
Norah Simpson
Stanford University, California, USA
Børge Sivertsen
Norwegian Institute of Public Health, Oslo, Norway
Pamela Song
Inje University College of Medicine, Ilsan Paik Hospital, Ilsan, Republic of Korea
Kai Spiegelhalder
Freiburg University Medical Center, Germany
Katie Stone
California Pacific Medical Center Research Institute, San Francisco, USA
Caitlan A. Tighe
Providence College, Rhode Island, USA
Liat Tikotzky
Ben-Gurion University of the Negev, Israel
Charline Urbain
Université Libre de Bruxelles, Belgium

Ysbrand D. van der Werf
Amsterdam University Medical Centre, The Netherlands
Hans P. A. van Dongen
Washington State University, Pullman, USA
Eva M. van Heese
Amsterdam University Medical Centre, The Netherlands
Vladyslav V. Vyazovskiy
University of Oxford, England, UK
Siri Waage
Haukeland University Hospital, Bergen, Norway
Meredith L. Wallace
University of Pittsburgh, Pennsylvania, USA
Rena Wang
SSM Health Saint Mary's Hospital, St Louis, Missouri, USA
Alexa J. Watach
University of Pennsylvania, Philadelphia, USA
Emerson M. Wickwire
University of Maryland School of Medicine, Baltimore, USA
Luci D. Wiggs
Oxford Brookes University, England, UK
Heather Cleland Woods
University of Glasgow, Scotland, UK
Lisa M. Wu
Reykjavik University, Iceland
James K. Wyatt
Rush Medical College/Rush University Medical Center, Chicago, USA
Qian Xiao
The University of Texas Health Science Center at Houston, USA
Nathaniel Yuan
University of California, Los Angeles, USA
Robin K. Yuan
Brigham and Women's Hospital and Harvard Medical School, Boston, USA
Antonio Zadra
Université de Montréal, Quebec, Canada
Phyllis C. Zee
Northwestern University Feinberg School of Medicine, Chicago, Illinois, USA

HISTORICAL LANDMARKS AND CURRENT STATUS OF SLEEP SCIENCE AND SLEEP MEDICINE: AN INTRODUCTION TO THE SECOND EDITION OF THE HANDBOOK

Colin A. Espie, Phyllis C. Zee, *and* Charles M. Morin

History and Landmarks

We all sleep, and we all must sleep. Indeed, sleep is by no means an exclusive feature of human physiology and behavior. All other mammals sleep too, albeit in some cases with adaptations. For example, prey species may have to delay sleep for periods of time to avoid being eaten, and the blind Indus dolphin sleeps in very short bursts to ensure safe navigation. Insects like the fruit fly also display sleep- and wake-like states. Indeed, it is fair to say that when defined more broadly as rest/activity, sleep in some form is essential for survival. Nearly all organisms, from bacteria to plants to humans, have an endogenous time-keeping, circadian clock mechanism that synchronizes the internal biological processes with the daily changes in light and darkness. Not least because of these universal imperatives, the study of sleep and circadian processes and of sleep and circadian rhythm sleep–wake disorders is accelerating.

An Early History of Sleep

Of course, we know relatively little about sleep in primitive times, but we can deduce enough to be certain that sleep is no modern invention. For example, it has been suggested that Neanderthals (70,000 to 40,000 BC) may have represented a transitional stage between the nonhuman primate pattern, which was polyphasic (multiple rest–activity cycles in a 24-hour period) and the monophasic pattern (sleep at night, awake by day) that we are familiar with. Monophasic sleep is thought to have become dominant in the Neolithic period (ca. 10,000 years ago). By the time we come to the early civilizations of Mesopotamia, India, Egypt, and China, people appear to have been aware of the importance of sleep and dreams, with documented remedies ranging from divination and chanting to bloodletting, and the use of medicinal plants to promote sleep or wakefulness. Indeed, the yin-yang symbol attributed to the ancient Chinese (ca. 2900 BC) was adopted by the American Sleep Disorders Association (now the American Academy of Sleep Medicine) as its emblem.

Likewise, there are many references to sleep in ancient literature. The Bible, for example, refers to sleep being associated with contentment and hard work but also with laziness, and dreaming is seen as a means of communication between God and humans in many religions. The Greek philosopher Hippocrates (born ca. 460 BC, died ca. 375 BC) suggested that sleep resulted from blood moving from the limbs to be warmed in the "inner regions" of the body. Aristotle in the fourth century BC believed that dreams were portents of the future but also suggested that the ingestion of food indirectly induced sleepiness by taking heat away from the brain. Sleep was also used as a synonym for death in ancient Rome and Greece by poets such as Homer and Ovid.

Moving on to more recent times, by the end of the first millennium the scientific influence had become more dominant, reducing the previous emphasis on philosophy and mysticism. The use of medicinal plants continued, but behavioral recommendations also began to emerge. For example, the Jewish philosopher Maimonides in the 12th century stated that "the day and night consist of 24 hours. It is sufficient for a person to sleep one third thereof, which is 8 hours. These should be at the end of the night so that from the beginning of sleep until the rising of the sun will be 8 hours. Thus, he will arise from bed before the sun rises." A theory on sleep mechanisms was proposed by René Descartes in the 17th century. His hydraulic model of sleep suggested that the pineal gland helped to maintain alertness and that the "loss of animal spirit" from the pineal gland caused the ventricles to collapse, thereby inducing sleep. Thomas Willis and Thomas Sydenham, a little later, first developed what might be seen as the emergent clinical neurology of sleep, with work including the first references to restless legs syndrome and contributions on nightmares and insomnia.

Some Modern Landmarks in Our Understanding of Sleep

Some of these latter insights are suggested by the sleep pioneer William Dement to have occurred too early to be exploited by the as-yet-unborn field of sleep medicine. In this context he also mentions other scientific landmarks such as the demonstration of the persistence of circadian rhythms in the absence of environmental cues by De Mairan (1729) and Gellineau's publication of a description of the narcolepsy syndrome in 1880. Likewise, Caton demonstrated electrical rhythm in the brains of animals in 1875, and Hans Berger's early descriptions of the differences between brain wave patterns in awake and sleeping brains continued the perspective that sleep was essentially the brain turned off, the so-called passive process theory.

Since the early 1950s, discoveries about sleep seem to have increased almost exponentially, revealing that sleep is a varied, complex, and active arrangement of processes. Starting with the "discovery" of rapid-eye-movement (REM) sleep in 1952 by Aserinsky and Kleitman, the relationship between eye movements and dream activity was reported by Dement, who later also demonstrated the effects of sleep deprivation upon REM sleep in 1960. At around the same time, Jouvet showed that, during REM sleep, the voluntary muscle groups are essentially paralyzed; and by the mid-1960s the essential features of sleep had become established to the extent that a standardized manual for the scoring of human sleep had been published by Rechtschaffen and Kales. In parallel to the growing recognition of the importance of "homeostatic regulation"—sleep deprivation leads to growing sleep debt and increased pressure to sleep—seminal work was being carried out looking at circadian influences relating to sleep and wake timing: the so-called body clock. As early as 1938, Kleitman and his graduate student had conducted heroic personal experiments on circadian function by sleeping for a month in the depths of Mammoth Cave (Kentucky). They were trying to find out if our 24-hour rhythm is simply a reaction to environmental circumstances. However, it was not until the 1960s that Aschoff described the complexity of the cyclic sleep–wake pattern. In 1982 Borbély would later publish his "two-process model" of sleep regulation, demonstrating the interaction between homeostatic and circadian functions. The discipline of chronobiology was now born.

Extending from the work of Konopka and Benzer on fruit flies in the early 1970s, other researchers have since provided clear evidence of specific "clock genes," with the cloning of the first mammalian clock gene by Takahashi in 1997 and Hall, Rosbash, and Young jointly being awarded the 2017 Nobel Prize in Physiology or Medicine for their discoveries of molecular mechanisms controlling the circadian rhythm. Likewise, the predictions of von Economo in the 1920s were developed into a testable model of the hypothalamic control of sleep and wakefulness: the sleep (flip-flop) switch by the turn of the 21st century (e.g., Saper, Chou, Scammell). Importantly our understanding of sleep in relation to neuronal assemblies and the emergence of the notion of "local sleep" (e.g., Krueger, Vyazovskiy) is now proving very influential.

Despite the fact that we live in a 24-hour world, it is of considerable interest that the human biological clock appears to be set slightly longer than 24 hours. The discovery that people who are retinally blind would naturally follow what is called a "free-running period," with progressive delay in the timing of the sleep/wake and other physiological rhythms, led to the realization that we need our eyes for our sense of time as well as our sense of sight. Entrainment of the circadian sleep–wake rhythm to a 24-hour schedule requires daily exposure to zeitgebers (time givers), of which daylight is the most powerful. In humans, the circadian hormone melatonin plays a crucial role in the timing of sleep and wakefulness propensity. The interaction of the sleep homeostat with circadian timing mechanisms is now recognized as a mutual feedback process (e.g., Czeisler, Dijk), and productive laboratory studies have gone on to demonstrate a relationship between circadian physiology, sleepiness, and human performance.

Interest in the phenomenon of sleepiness has evolved from distinctive scientific and clinical areas of enquiry—from those who were interested in the essential nature of sleepiness, its causes, and its consequences (e.g., Dinges) to those who became particularly interested in the risks associated with undertaking waking tasks while sleepy (not least driving; e.g., Phillips, Akerstedt, Mitler) and those who were interested in sleep disorders where excessive daytime sleepiness was a hallmark feature. Sleep apnea was reported independently by two research groups in France and Germany in 1965, following Lugaresi's recognition of the relationship between hypersomnia and periodic breathing. The most important development in the treatment of obstructive sleep apnea (OSA), however, came from Australia in the 1980s, where Sullivan developed a novel but simple preventive treatment that has become known as continuous positive airway pressure (CPAP).

Excessive daytime sleepiness is also the cardinal feature of central hypersomnias, such as narcolepsy. As previously mentioned, clinical descriptions of narcolepsy have been available for a very long time, but it was not until the early 1970s that canine narcolepsy provided a unique animal model in which to study the disorder. The discovery of a hypocretin/orexin mutation in narcoleptic Doberman pinschers (by Mitler) and an orexin deficiency in narcoleptic mice (by Yanagisawa, De Lecea) led to the observation that narcolepsy is associated with HLA-DR2 and the hypothesis that narcolepsy may result from an autoimmune insult to the central nervous system. It is now known that complex HLA-DR and DQ interactions confer risk of the narcolepsy with cataplexy syndrome (e.g., Mignot).

Excellent and very readable overviews of such early influential times have been published by William Dement (*The Promise of Sleep*, 1999) and Peretz Lavie (*The Enchanted World of Sleep*, 1996), and these books are recommended to the reader. Those interested in sleep through the ages will also find fascinating insights in Michael Thorpy's (1991) *A History of Sleep in Man*, and there are many other more recent resources including *The Science of Sleep* (Mendelson, 2017), *Dreaming: A Very Short Introduction* (Hobson, 2008), *When Brains Dream* (Zadra and Stickgold, 2021), and *Why We Sleep* (Walker, 2017).

Indeed, consideration of the functions of sleep has been of great interest both before and since Rechtschaffen's famous statement, first made at the University of Chicago Sleep Laboratory in 1978: "if sleep does not serve an absolutely vital function, then it is the biggest mistake the evolutionary process ever made." Candidate areas now include cellular homeostasis and growth (e.g., Cirelli and Tononi, van Cauter), immune signaling and infection control (e.g., Redwine, Besedovsky), neurotoxic waste clearance (e.g., Hardy and Selkoe, Nedergaard), brain plasticity and cognitive functioning (e.g., Maquet, Van Dongen, Rasch and Born), emotion regulation (e.g., Yoo and Walker, Palmer and Alfano), as well as energy conservation (e.g., Berger and Philips). These reasons for why we sleep are, of course, not incompatible; and there are almost certainly species-specific functions of mammalian sleep (e.g., Spiegel, Tobler).

The Emergence of Sleep Medicine

We have already referred to several disorders of sleep and wakefulness, and these are currently classified across three diagnostic systems (the *Diagnostic and Statistical Manual of Mental Disorders*, fifth edition, 2013, with a text revision in 2022; the *International Classification of Diseases*, 11th revision, 2022; the *International Classification of Sleep Disorders*, third edition, 2014, with text revision, 2023) into six categories, namely sleep-related breathing disorders (SRBDs), sleep-related movement disorders (SRMDs), circadian rhythm sleep–wake disorders, insomnia disorders, parasomnias, and central disorders of hypersomnia. There are some differences in nomenclature across the nosologies; however, what the diagnostic systems represent is the need for a comprehensive approach to the practice of what has become known as sleep medicine, not least because the disorders tend to fall within the ambit of different professional groups, for example, SRBDs (respiratory medicine/pulmonology), insomnia disorders (clinical psychology, psychiatry), SRMDs and hypersomnia (neurology).

There are numerous ways in which sleep continuity, sleep architecture, and sleep–wake schedules can become disturbed; and daytime sequelae to personal functioning and cognitive performance are integral to the diagnoses. Excessive daytime sleepiness, to which we have alluded above, is particularly marked in disorders of hypersomnia and in SRBDs and may be an important feature also of the other sleep disorders. Progress in understanding the etiology and pathophysiology of specific sleep problems and the emergence of effective therapeutics have been notable in recent years. Treatment guidelines have been developed and updated, often under the auspices of now well-established professional sleep societies. For example, in the interval 2020–2024, the Sleep Research Society issued a white paper on circadian rhythm sleep–wake disorders (lead author Duffy); the American Academy of Sleep Medicine (AASM) and the European Sleep Research Society (ESRS) issued practice guidelines on insomnia disorder (Edinger, Sateia [AASM]; Riemann [ESRS]); the National Institute for Health and Care excellence provided guidelines on CPAP and mandibular advancement for OSA; the AASM published referral guidelines for patients with OSA requiring surgical consultation (Kent) and practice guidelines for REM sleep behavior disorder (Howell); AASM guidelines on the treatment of restless legs syndrome (RLS) and periodic limb movement disorder are due; and European guidelines (supported by the ESRS, the European Academy of Neurology, and the European Narcolepsy Network) on the management of narcolepsy in adults and children were published (Bassetti). In parallel there are practice parameter guidelines for the appraisal of sleep disorders. Examples, again for the period 2020–2024, include the AASM position statement on home sleep apnea testing (Rosen), AASM protocols for using the Multiple Sleep Latency Test and Maintenance of Wakefulness Test (Krahn), and the Restless Legs Syndrome Foundation's updated algorithm for appraising RLS (Silber).

One example of change in understanding and clinical practice is our approach to the most common sleep disorder of all, insomnia. Historically regarded as a symptom problem most likely resulting from or secondary to "something else" (e.g., depression, pain, physical illness), insomnia has emerged as a disorder in its own right, which should be actively treated whenever it presents, whether or not there are comorbid conditions also present. Moreover, insomnia was typically managed using sedative pharmacotherapy, an approach which is now regarded as suboptimal when insomnia becomes chronic. Following the work of early pioneers (e.g., Bootzin, Spielman, Hauri), the burgeoning evidence base for cognitive behavioral therapy (CBT), delivered in person or digitally, has resulted in all guidelines recommending CBT as first-line care. The still emerging "behavioral sleep medicine" approach also now extends to supporting management of most other sleep disorders too.

Sleep medicine is in every domain a fast-growing field, and in recent decades it has been supported by tremendous growth in journals and journal outputs. The journal *Sleep* was first published in 1978. There are now a dozen or more scientific journals dedicated to sleep and circadian research that have an impact index >1.00, and the standard text for the field, the *Principles and Practice of Sleep Medicine*, which was first published in 1989, had its seventh edition published in 2021. The vast literature on sleep also continues to grow year upon year. A PubMed search on the term *sleep* revealed that 60,701 articles were published in the 50-year period 1950–1999, compared with 235,328 in the 24-year period 2000–2023. Indeed, the annual rate of publication at the time of writing (2024) is about 24,000, an approximate 10-fold increase since the year 2000. It is impossible therefore to mention by name even the most influential of the contemporary figures in the field because there are so many outstanding contributors—although many of these are authors in this handbook! In keeping with this growth, we have seen bigger national and international scientific and clinical meetings, a growth in the membership of existing sleep societies and more professional societies being established, and increasing demand for and provision of training in sleep and circadian medicine. Moreover, there is recognition that population-level sleep health is every bit as important as the absence of sleep disorder. Indeed, sleep itself is the medicine that nature provides for everyday health, function, well-being, and quality of life.

Aims and Scope of This Handbook

Having considered some of the historical landmarks in the field of sleep research and practice and having also outlined the current status of sleep medicine, we hope that we have persuaded you of the timeliness of the second edition of our handbook. Our vision has been to compile a resource that will meet the needs of the many professionals who have an interest in sleep and sleep disorders. To achieve this, we are thrilled that each chapter in the handbook is authored by eminent international figures. If the handbook works as a source of educational, clinical, and indeed inspirational material, it is largely to their credit.

The handbook is divided into six sections covering a total of 46 chapters: Section 1: The Fundamentals of Sleep and Circadian Processes; Section 2: The Roles and Functions of Sleep; Section 3: Societal Factors Influencing Sleep; Section 4: Disorders of Sleep and Circadian Function: Epidemiology, Classification, and Assessment; Section 5: Disorders of Sleep and Circadian Function: Management and Treatment; and Section 6: Disorders of Sleep and Circadian Function: Life Span Issues and Special Populations.

Section 1: The Fundamentals of Sleep and Circadian Processes comprises Chapters 1 to 6, respectively, "Sleep and the Brain" (Liliia Roshchupkina, Charline Urbain, and Philippe Peigneux), "The Regulation of Human Sleep and Wakefulness: Sleep Homeostasis and Circadian Rhythmicity" (Alpar S. Lazar and Derk-Jan Dijk), "Sleep and Circadian Development in the Early and Developing Years" (Innessa Donskoy and Temitayo Oyegbile-Chidi), "Sleep and Circadian Development in Adults and Older Adults" (Jeanne F. Duffy, Arturo Arrona-Palacios, and Pamela Song), "The Genetics of Sleep" (James B. Jaggard, Keri J. Ngo, and Philippe Mourrain), and "Local Sleep" (Vladyslav V. Vyazovskiy and Thomas Andrillon).

Section 2: The Roles and Functions of Sleep comprises Chapters 7 to 13, respectively, "Why We Sleep" (H. Craig Heller), "Brain Clearance, Sleep, and Circadian Rhythms: Implications for Brain Health" (Eva M. van Heese, Erik N. T. P. Bakker, and Ysbrand D. van der Werf), "Sleep and Circadian Rhythms and Metabolism" (Anne-Marie Chang, Praneet C. Kaki, Robin K. Yuan, Christopher M. Depner, and Orfeu M. Buxton), "Sleep, Neurocognitive Function, Learning, and Memory" (Daniel Baena, Alyssa Pozzobon, Joel Hordijk, Laura B. Ray, and Stuart M. Fogel), "Sleep and Human Performance" (Courtney A. Kurinec, Jonah A. Scott, and Hans P. A. Van Dongen), "Sleep and Emotion Regulation" (Debora Meneo, Monica Martoni, and Chiara Baglioni), and "Sleep, Dreams, and Dreaming" (Joseph De Koninck).

We then turn in Section 3 to Societal Factors Influencing Sleep, which are considered over the course of a further six contributions in Chapters 14 to 19. These are "Multidimensional Sleep Health: An Emerging Framework for Understanding Sleep in Relation to Multiple Health Outcomes" (Caitlan A. Tighe, Meredith L. Wallace, Rachel P. K. Conlon, Marquis S. Hawkins, Christopher C. Imes, and Daniel J. Buysse), "Sleep, Social Inequalities, and Societal Costs" (Mari Hysing, Tormod Bøe, and Børge Sivertsen), "Sleep, Health, and Shift Work" (Siri Waage and Bjørn Bjorvatn), "Sex Differences in Sleep" (Fiona C. Baker, Rena Wang, and Helen S. Driver), "The Impact of Prescription and Recreational Drugs on Sleep" (Kai Spiegelhalder, Christoph Nissen, and Dieter Riemann), and "Bedtime Social Media Use and Sleep: A New Understanding of Social, Emotional, and Cognitive Processes" (Holly Scott and Heather Cleland Woods).

In Section 4: Disorders of Sleep and Circadian Function: Epidemiology, Classification, and Assessment we address clinical matters across Chapters 20 to 25. These comprise "Epidemiology of Sleep and Circadian Health" (Qian Xiao and Katie Stone), "Sleep Disorders: Classification and Diagnosis" (Jack D. Edinger, Ana I. Fins, and Charles M. Morin), "Value-Based Clinical Sleep Medicine: Health Economic Considerations Regarding Insomnia and Obstructive Sleep Apnea" (Emerson M. Wickwire), "Clinical Assessment of Sleep–Wake Complaints" (Jason C. Ong, Colin A. Espie, and James K. Wyatt), "Actigraphy and Behavioral Assessments of Sleep and Circadian Disorders"

(Monica R. Kelly, Nathaniel Yuan, Alexander J. Erickson, and Jennifer L. Martin), and "Polysomnography and Emerging Technologies to Evaluate Sleep Disorders" (Thomas Penzel, Ingo Fietze, Martin Glos, Lisa Rosenblum, and Matthew Salanitro).

Section 5: Disorders of Sleep and Circadian Function: Management and Treatment comprises 12 chapters (Chapters 26 to 37). These cover the range of sleep disorders, specifically: "Insomnia I: Conceptualization and Etiology" (Hannah Scott, Philip Gehrman, and Michael Perlis), "Insomnia II: Behavioral and Physiological Assessment" (Célyne H. Bastien, Jason G. Ellis, Florence Lambert-Beaudet, Alexandre Rudziavic Provençal, and Elham Garmroudinezhad-Rostami), "Cognitive Behavioral Therapies for Insomnia: Current Status and Challenges Ahead" (Charles M. Morin and Simon D. Kyle), "Parasomnias I: Nightmares" (Serena Scarpelli, Valentina Alfonsi, and Luigi De Gennaro), "Parasomnias II: Rapid-Eye-Movement Sleep Behavior Disorder (Alex Iranzo), "Parasomnias III: Sleep Terrors and Somnambulism" (Antonio Zadra and Francesca Siclari), "Circadian Rhythm Sleep–Wake Disorders I: Advanced and Delayed Phase Disorders" (Leon C. Lack, Gorica Micic, and Nicole Lovato), "Circadian Rhythm Sleep–Wake Disorders II: Shift Work, Irregular, and Non-24-Hour Sleep–Wake Rhythm Disorders (Diane B. Boivin and Philippe Boudreau), "Sleep-Related Breathing Disorders I: Physiology and Etiology" (Danny J. Eckert), "Sleep-Related Breathing Disorders II: Clinical Management" (Amy M. Sawyer, Alexa J. Watach, Bruno Saconi, and Lindsey Clark), "Narcolepsies and Other Central Hypersomnolence Disorders" (Yves Dauvilliers and Lucie Barateau), and "Restless Legs Syndrome and Periodic Limb Movement Disorder" (Raquel Martín, Celia García-Malo, Elisa Gamo, Alejandro Herrero, Sofía Romero, Alba García, and Diego García-Borreguero).

The handbook concludes with Section 6: Disorders of Sleep and Circadian Function: Life Span Issues and Special Populations. These final chapters (38 to 46) comprise "Sleep-Related Problems in Childhood and Adolescence" (Liat Tikotzky, Michal Kahn, Michael Gradisar, and Oliviero Bruni), "Sleep Disorders in the Elderly" (Ali Amidi, Sonia Ancoli-Israel, Jeanne E. Maglione, and Lisa M. Wu), "Sleep and Psychiatric Disorders" (Rachel Manber, Jessica R. Dietch, Nicole B. Gumport, and Norah Simpson), "Women's Sleep and Circadian Rhythms From Puberty to Menopausal Transition" (Bilgay Izci Balserak and Kathryn Aldrich Lee), "Sleep and Medical Disorders" (Leanne Fleming, Megan Crawford, Bethany Martin, Mhairi Patience, and Samantha Fisher-Hicks), "Sleep in Patients With Substance Use Disorders" (M. Elizabeth Cardoni, Bhanu Prakash Kolla, Mandilyn Graham, Yosef Bronsteyn, and J. Todd Arnedt), "Sleep–Wake Disturbances in Individuals with Traumatic Brain Injury" (Marie-Christine Ouellet, Simon Beaulieu-Bonneau, and Charles M. Morin), "Sleep in People with Intellectual Disabilities" (Luci D. Wiggs), and "Sexsomnia and Sexual Assault: The Role of the Sleep Forensics Investigator in Court" (Michel A. Cramer Bornemann and Carlos H. Schenck).

Conclusion

In the 1980s the importance of diet and exercise to health and well-being was barely acknowledged in mainstream science or clinical practice. At some level everyone knew of their importance, but they were lifestyle factors, lifestyle choices, were they not? How much has changed since then. Now they are major health policy drivers and cost headings. Their influence on health and health outcomes is highlighted in every medical and health professional course, they are routinely measured by various indices, and they are actively promoted and their adverse consequences treated in every community and on every hospital campus.

So the story goes for sleep, and sleep's time has come! From ancient times to the present day, the importance of sleep has seldom been disputed, but it has never had top billing. The combined critical mass of research evidence, the needs of the population, and the shifting weight of professional interest, however, are now pushing sleep onto center stage. We hope this handbook will be helpful to you as together we seek to understand the enchanted world of sleep and to manage sleep and circadian disorders more effectively.

SECTION 1

The Fundamentals of Sleep and Circadian Processes

CHAPTER

1 Sleep and the Brain

Liliia Roshchupkina, Charline Urbain, *and* Philippe Peigneux

Abstract

The questions "why" and "how" do we sleep have been investigated and discussed by scientists across the globe for a century. Available evidence shows that sleep is much more complicated than a simple switch mechanism shutting off the neurophysiological processes associated with an active and costly wake state of vigilance. Rather, it is a complex, multidimensional, and active brain state. In this chapter, the authors review wakefulness and sleep as dynamic states viewed from behavioral, neurobiological, neurophysiological, and functional neuroanatomical perspectives. Due to the universality of sleep and/or sleep-like phenomena across animal species, the authors also review sleep phylogenesis from the simplest living organisms to humans.

Key Words: NREM, REM, SWS, neurobiology, neurophysiology, phylogenesis, EEG, PET, fMRI, MEG

Sleep Overview

Sleep is a complex, cyclical phenomenon that most living organisms experience in one form or another. Even though significant research advances have been achieved over the last decades, sleep functions are still debated. Among others, inactivity/adaptive, energy conservation, restoration, and brain plasticity theories have emerged in an attempt to reveal why we sleep (Bodizs, 2021). In a nutshell, the *inactivity/adaptive theory* is grounded on the idea that inactivity at night is beneficial and creates an evolutionary and reproductive advantage, partly because the chances of being injured or attacked in the darkness are reduced (at least if in a protected environment, e.g., a burrow). The *energy conservation theory* claims that a function of sleep is to decrease the organism's energetic needs (since the metabolic rate significantly decreases during sleep) through part of the day/night when it is least able to search for food (Schmidt, 2014). The *restorative theory* posits that sleep provides the necessary conditions for the body to rest, repair, enhance the immune response, detoxify, and avoid the deleterious effects of sleep deprivation (Freiberg, 2020). Finally, the *brain plasticity theory* states that sleep is necessary for neural growth and reorganization, supporting the brain's structure and function. These theories are certainly not exclusive or exhaustive. Instead, they highlight the utmost value of sleep and the variety of functions it may support. This chapter will review sleep and its defining features, viewed from behavioral, neurobiological, neurophysiological, and functional neuroanatomical perspectives.

At the behavioral level, sleep has definite features that humans share with most animal species. Sleep is a state of physical quiescence, characterized by closure of the eyes, reduction of movements or immobility, and stereotypic body posture (e.g., in humans, lying down; in horses, standing or lying; in bats, hanging upside down). The rapid reversibility between states distinguishes sleep from other specific states of altered vigilance like coma, hypothermia, or hibernation as the sleeper can wake up when stimulated or when the need for sleep is fulfilled. Nonetheless, it is challenging to ensure from the behavioral observation that an individual genuinely sleeps or rather merely experiences other vigilance states such as relaxed eye-closed wakefulness or drowsiness. Most importantly, behavioral observations alone cannot reveal the dramatic changes in brain activity from wakefulness to sleep and the different sleep stages alternating in a night of sleep. Introduced by Hans Berger (1931), the recording of brain's electrical activity (i.e., electroencephalography [EEG]) enabled the study of brain activity patterns across various states of vigilance. Berger described different EEG oscillation patterns in the brain and already noticed a slowing down in the frequency of EEG oscillations during sleep as compared to wakefulness. Davis et al. (1937) further contributed sleep research by dividing sleep into five levels (A–E) featuring the spectrum of changing frequencies from waking to non-rapid-eye-movement (NREM) deep Sleep Stages 1–4 (now reorganized into three stages, N3 encompassing prior Stages 3 and 4 or slow oscillations). Finally, Aserinsky and Kleitman (1953) evidenced a distinct sleep stage characterized by rapid low-voltage oscillations in brain activity and rapid ocular movements, which they named *rapid-eye-movement* (REM) sleep; the state was discovered in parallel under the name of *paradoxical sleep* by Jouvet et al. (1959), who highlighted the characteristic muscular atonia in this stage. Based on these findings, Rechtschaffen and Kales's *Manual of Standardized Terminology, Techniques and Scoring System for Sleep Stages of Human Subjects* (1968) became the first reference manual on how human sleep should be recorded and scored for clinical and research purposes. Despite technological advances and the development of innovative methods for the analysis of sleep neurophysiology, the classification and main rules for the clinical identification of sleep patterns remain essentially similar to the original proposal, based on visual then computerized inspection of 30-second polysomnographic epochs of EEG, electro-oculographic, and electromyographic (EMG) signals (see Berry et al., 2020, for recent information on international consensus guidelines).

As mentioned above, sleep features two main physiological stages: NREM and paradoxical or REM sleep. In humans, NREM sleep consists of three distinct stages according to sleep depth and the slowing frequency of the brain oscillations, from the intermediate Stage N1 sleep (drowsiness and sleep onset) to light Stage N2 sleep to the deepest Stage

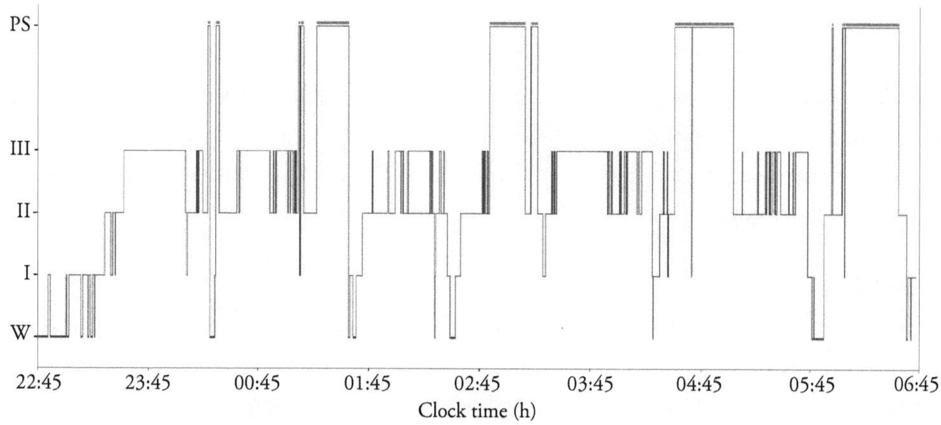

Figure 1.1 Typical hypnogram of a healthy adult participant
Note. W = wakefulness; I–III = non–rapid-eye-movement Sleep Stages 1–3; PS = paradoxical (rapid-eye-movement) sleep. Scoring window = 30 seconds.

N3 sleep, also known as slow-wave sleep (SWS) (Figure 1.1). In turn, REM sleep is characterized by the occurrence of rapid eye movements (REMs) and low-voltage desynchronized brain waves (similar to wakefulness).

Typically, NREM always precedes REM sleep within an ultradian cycle lasting on average 90 minutes and repeating itself several times over the night (Figure 1.2c). Furthermore, sleep is a process rigorously regulated by both a homeostatic drive and the endogenous circadian rhythm (Figure 1.2b), as proposed by Borbely's two-process sleep model (Borbely, 1982, 2016). Basically, the two-process model postulates that sleep pressure accumulates in the course of the day, likely due to gradually increasing sleep-inducing substances in the brain. This triggers a sleep drive and a need to sleep after a certain time of being awake. The process is homeostatic in that the longer one stays awake, the more sleep pressure is accumulated, and restorative sleep is needed. In the case of extended wakefulness (i.e., above normal levels of a day's work, as when deprived of sleep for 36 hours), sleep debt is created, eventually leading to higher sleep duration than usual (i.e., a rebound) on a subsequent night. However, the gradual accumulation in homeostatic sleep pressure is moderated by the circadian process, that is, the nearly 24-hour endogenous oscillatory variation in alertness and sleep propensity. Globally speaking, the circadian signal for sleep/alertness is high/low in the early hours and low/high in the evening. The consequence is that homeostatic and circadian processes actually work in opposition during the day as the circadian signal for alertness increases in parallel with mounting sleep pressure but cooperates at night as there is high sleep pressure and increasing circadian sleep propensity/reducing alertness, ensuring consolidated periods of wakefulness and sleep. Slow-wave activity (SWA; <1 Hz) in SWS is the sleep marker of accumulated sleep pressure, and therefore, the first half of the night is particularly rich in N3 sleep SWA (about 80% of the time). In parallel, the length of REM periods increases with each next sleep cycle, whereas SWS length and depth decrease in the second half of the night with the diminution of accumulated sleep pressure (Figure 1.2c). The amount of Stage N2 sleep remains stable overnight. Before diving into the phylogeny and physiology of sleep, we will briefly describe more precisely the different stages of sleep with their behavioral and electrophysiological features.

Wakefulness

Wakefulness can be described as a state of full consciousness, alertness, and awareness, which allows effective interaction with the environment. The waking EEG in humans is characterized by a so-called desynchronized neuronal firing pattern, reflected in the EEG by rapid, high-frequency (beta range, 14–40 Hz), low-amplitude (10–30 μV) waves, as well as high muscular tonus as reflected by the EMG (see Table 1.1). In a quiet, relaxed

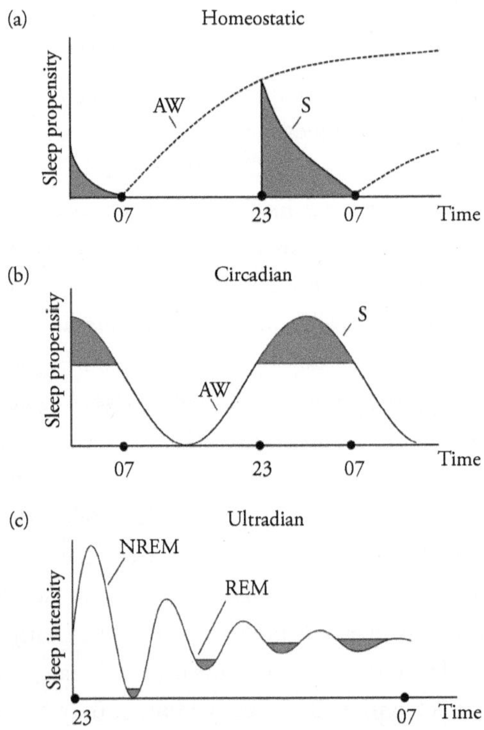

Figure 1.2 Schematic representation of the three main processes of sleep regulation

Note. Panel a: The homeostatic process maintains sleep propensity (duration and intensity of sleep), which builds up during wakefulness and releases during sleep. Panel b: The circadian process is a nearly 24-hour endogenous oscillatory variation that determines the timing of the propensity to sleep. Panel c: The ultradian mechanisms underlie the non–rapid-eye-movement (NREM)—rapid-eye-movement (REM) sleep cycle. As the sleep episode progresses, the intensity of NREM sleep declines, and the duration of successive REM sleep intervals increases. AW = awake state; S = sleep. Adapted from Borbély et al. (2000).

Table 1.1 Summary of the main features of sleep stages

Stages	EEG (frequency, Hz)	Amplitude (μV)	Waveform type	Characteristics
Wakefulness	14–40	10–30	β	State of full consciousness characterized by a desynchronized EEG low-amplitude pattern of high–beta frequency waves. EOG is characterized by sharp eye movements and blinks. EMG is high.
N1 (drowsiness)	4–7	50–100	θ	Transition period with little or no body movements characterized by the diminution of alpha waves and the appearance of theta waves, slower in frequency and greater in amplitude than alpha waves. EOG may show slow sinusoidal eye movements. EMG is lower than during wakefulness.
N2 (light sleep)	11–16	50–150	Occurrence of sleep spindles (σ) and K-complexes, slow waves	Basal oscillations below 5 Hz are called *slow waves*, with periodically superimposed sleep spindles (short-lasting, waxing and waning oscillations in the 11–16-Hz frequency range) and K-complexes (negative sharp waves immediately followed by a positive component standing out from the background EEG with a total duration at least equal to 0.5 seconds). EMG is relatively low.
N3 (SWS)	0.5–2	<75–>140	Slow waves ++	The deepest possible state of physical rest. SWS is characterized by slow, high-amplitude oscillations in the 0.5–2-Hz frequency range, which are maximally expressed at frontal locations. Slow oscillations (<1 Hz). Spindles and K-complexes are also possible. Eye movements are not typically seen, and EMG remains low.
REM (paradoxical sleep)	15–30	<50	Occasional sawtooth waves	Desynchronized EEG activity is close to that recorded during wakefulness, characterized by low-amplitude/mixed frequency EEG background in total muscular atonia, except for oculomotor activity responsible for rapid eye movements.

Note. EEG = electroencephalography; EMG = electromyographic; EOG = electro-oculographic; REM = rapid eye movement; SWS = slow-wave sleep.

state or resting, especially with eyes closed, EEG recorded from the posterior part of the brain (mostly at occipital locations) depicts patterns of alpha or Berger waves of lower frequency (8–12 Hz) and an increased amplitude (20–40 μV; Figure 1.3), reflecting increased synchrony of underlying neural activity (Borbély et al., 2000), which disappears with opening the eyes.

NREM Sleep

In humans, NREM sleep stages are characterized by decreasing muscular tonus together with a gradual slowing down of the EEG activity (Figure 1.3). The amplitude of the EEG waves steadily increases from Stage N1 (drowsiness) to N2 (light sleep) and then N3 (deep SWS), reflecting the progressive synchronization of brain activity within and between neuronal populations. Additionally, spectral analysis reveals a background pattern of SWA below 1 Hz (Achermann & Borbély, 1997), which is not visually apparent in the EEG recording but has important physiological implications (Steriade et al., 1993). Superimposed on slow rhythmic activities are transient events, mainly K-complexes and

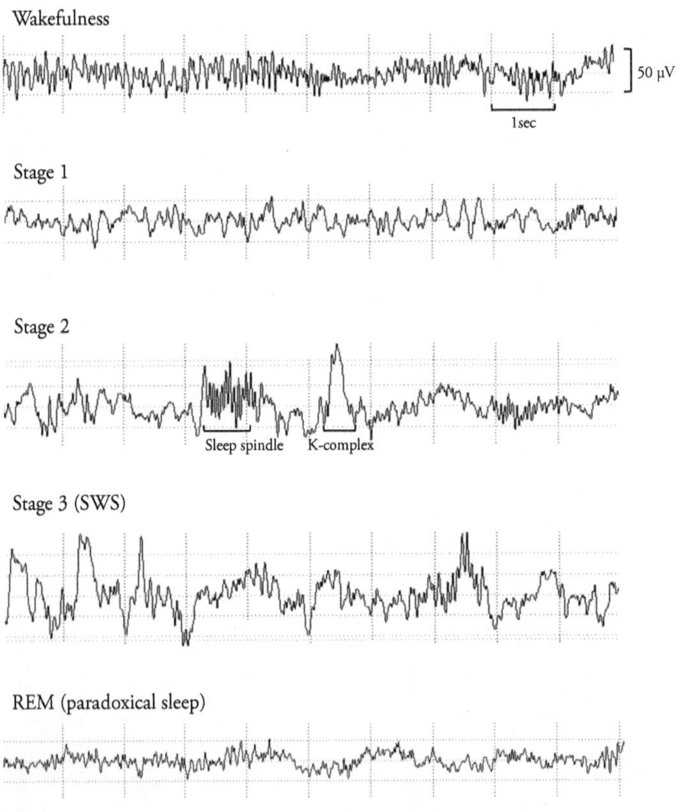

Figure 1.3 Typical electroencephalographic patterns of wakefulness and sleep stages
Note. REM = rapid eye movement; SWS = slow-wave sleep.

sleep spindles in N2, whose recurrence (every 3–10 seconds) is regulated by the underlying SWA (Steriade & Amzica, 1998).

NREM SLEEP STAGE N1

The transition period between wakefulness and sleep is the NREM Sleep Stage N1, representing drowsiness. At the behavioral level, subjects start failing to respond at the presentation of auditory tones, although awakening thresholds remain low, to the point that subjects awoken during this stage may often report not having been asleep at all. The EEG features the occurrence of theta waves, slower in frequency (4–8 Hz) and greater in amplitude (50–100 μV) than alpha waves. At the same time, muscular activity decreases, and typical slow-rolling eye movements appear. A valid electrophysiological marker of sleep onset is the attenuation of the alpha rhythm, most prominent at the occipital EEG derivations, which signals the transition from relaxed wakefulness to Stage N1.

NREM SLEEP STAGE N2

Drowsiness continues into the next NREM Sleep Stage N2, known as light NREM sleep. At this stage, the eye movements cease, the heart rate slows down, and body temperature decreases, preparing the body to enter deep sleep. Background EEG oscillations continue to slow down and enter the delta range (1–4 Hz). The distinctive features of the N2 sleep stage are sleep spindles and K-complexes, which are superimposed on slow oscillations (Figure 1.3). Spindles are short-lasting (0.5–3 seconds), waxing and waning oscillations in the sigma range (11–16 Hz), whose maximal amplitude is mainly found over central regions (De Gennaro et al., 2000). Furthermore, there is functional differentiation and there are distinct neuroanatomical bases for slow (11–13 Hz) and fast (13–15 Hz) spindles (Fernandez & Lüthi, 2020). In turn, the K-complexes are distinct waveforms with a negative sharp wave of high amplitude, immediately followed by a positive component standing out from the background EEG, lasting at least 0.5 seconds. K-complexes are optimally recorded at frontal electrodes (e.g., F4 or Fz).

NREM SLEEP STAGE N3

A further decrease in muscle tone, pulse, and breathing rate characterizes the deepest stage of NREM sleep. The arousal thresholds are very high, with a more extended period of sleep inertia after awakening. This stage is also called SWS due to the high prevalence of slow EEG waves in the 0.5–2-Hz frequency range. The onset of the N3 stage is scored when slow waves represent at least 20% of the 30-second EEG epoch. Usually, slow waves are maximally expressed at frontal sites (Happe et al., 2002), as well as K-complexes.

REM Sleep Stage

Five main features determine REM sleep: REMs, muscular atonia, irregular breath, body temperature fluctuations, and a low-amplitude/mixed-frequency (15–30 Hz, <50 μV)

EEG background. REMs are conjugate, irregular, and sharply peaked eye movements with an initial deflection usually lasting less than 500 milliseconds. The background EEG signals are desynchronized, low-amplitude, and rapid, visually close to those recorded during wakefulness; hence, REM sleep is also called "paradoxical" sleep (Jouvet et al., 1959). The presence of sawtooth waves (bursts of frontocentral slow oscillations) and transient muscle activity (phasic twitches) are traits of this stage, enabling the scoring of REM when one or more primary features are equivocal.

The Phylogenesis of Sleep

The alternation between periods of activity and sleep/resting states has been found across all studied animal species, indicating a vital role of the sleep/sleep-like rest state. However, physiological and neurophysiological characteristics may widely differ within the animal kingdom. Even though sleep appears to be a universal phenomenon, the appearance of REM sleep, typical of mammalians and birds, is not present or at least cannot be convincingly disclosed in the lower taxa (e.g., insects, amphibians, and reptiles), raising supplementary questions about the role of sleep in evolution. Further in this section, we cover sleep and sleep-like states across the animal kingdom.

Sleep-Like State of Invertebrates (Hydra, Insects, and Spiders)

There is increasing evidence for the presence of activity/sleep-like states even in the simplest organisms. For instance, cnidarians (medusae and sessile polyps), which lack a centralized nervous system (CNS; and, therefore, are considered brainless creatures), demonstrate a daily periodic quiescence. As well, soft corals display 24-hour pulsation–rest rhythms in their tentacle movements (Kremien et al., 2013), and the upside-down jellyfish *Cassiopea* exhibits sleep-like behaviors (Nath et al., 2017) that are comparable to those observed in other animals with a well-defined CNS. These findings support the hypothesis that the phylogenetic origin of sleep preceded the evolution of a CNS. In insects, evidence of a close-to-sleep state has long been primarily behavioral. However, recent findings suggest a discrete deep-sleep stage in the fruit fly *Drosophila melanogaster*, named *proboscis extension sleep* and characterized by repeated stereotyped proboscis extensions and retractions (van Alphen et al., 2022). Interestingly, the authors showed that sleep deprivation in fruit flies reduces waste clearance, a function linked to the deep-sleep stage; it suggests that waste clearance is a core and ancient function of deep sleep. Honeybees (*Apis mellifera*) exhibit three relatively immobile states: S1, characterized by swaying motions of the antennae; S2, marked by minute twitching of the antennae; and S3, the deep-sleep state, defined by complete antennal immobility and the highest reaction thresholds (Eban-Rothschild & Bloch, 2008; Klein et al., 2008). Moreover, exposing bees during the deep-sleep stage to the same odor adorned during a prior learning episode improves memory performance on the following day (Zwaka et al., 2015), like in humans, suggesting similar sleep effects on memory consolidation in insects and mammals. It was also assumed for a long time that REM sleep only occurs in terrestrial vertebrates (primarily birds and mammals), an assumption recently challenged in a study on sleep in spiders. The most salient indicator of REM sleep is eye movements, yet movable eyes feature a limited number of lineages and are absent in insects and most terrestrial arthropods. However, this is not the case with jumping spiders (*Evarcha arcuata*), which possess movable retinal tubes to redirect their gaze. In newly born and not fully mature spiderlings, these movements can be directly observed through their temporarily translucent exoskeleton (Rößler et al., 2022). In their study, the researchers observed consistent movement bouts of the spiders' retinal tubes, with quite regular durations and intervals, increasing over the night. These are features of REM sleep–like behaviors that exist in a highly visual, long-diverged animal lineage. Further comparisons across lineages likely could resolve questions about the origin, evolution, and function of REM sleep.

Activity/Inactivity States in Poikilothermic Vertebrates

FISH

Due to the difficulties in recording brain activity underwater, little is known about sleep in cartilaginous fishes. Sharks and rays facilitate respiration by lowering and raising the floor of the buccal cavity and thus can remain stationary for extended periods. However, species using ram ventilation have to move forward to push oxygenated water into the mouth and over the gills, making these animals obligate swimmers (Kelly et al., 2019). It has been shown that buccal sharks and rays express a circadian rhythm (some may be active during the day and rest at night and vice versa). The rest/sleep-like periods are characterized by immobilization and lowered responsiveness. In turn, activity pattern changes are much more moderate in obligatory swimmers, even though they express circadian rhythmicity. As there is a lack of studies looking at sleep homeostasis or sleep/wake recordings of brain activity in cartilaginous fish, it remains unclear whether extensive periods of restfulness in buccal-pumping sharks and rays can be considered sleep or simply quiet wakefulness. In the case of the bony fish, research suggests the presence of well-established behavioral criteria such as the exhibition of circadian-regulated periods of reversible immobility associated with an increased arousal threshold (Yokogawa et al., 2007) as well as sleep rebound in response to sleep deprivation (Aho et al., 2017; Appelbaum et al., 2009; Tobler & Borbély, 1985). In order to find neuronal sleep signatures in a teleost fish brain, researchers examined the dorsal pallium, considered to be a homolog of the neocortex (Mueller et al., 2011). Neuronal sleep signatures in the best-studied teleost fish, zebrafish (*Danio rerio*), revealed slow, synchronous oscillations in the dorsal pallium (the slow bursting sleep state) and a sleep state initiated with propagating waves, both of which occur in an overall background of reduced brain activity (Leung et al., 2019). The dynamics of these two sleep states share many commonalities with those of SWS and REM, respectively.

AMPHIBIANS

The amphibians are of interest because they represent the basal stock from which evolved land vertebrates (Fields, 1968). Available data on sleep in amphibians is scarce (for a review, see Hartse, 2011). Some species maintain constant vigilance levels during behavioral rest (e.g., the bullfrog), whereas reactivity to sensorial stimulations decreases in others (e.g., the tree-dwelling frog). Salamanders (*Ambystoma tigrinum*) display rhythmic behavioral activity with a 4-hour rest–activity cycle (Libourel & Herrel, 2016), and EEG analysis reveals decreased frequency and amplitude during prolonged resting periods. The absence of clear neck atonia and distinct eye movements precludes the unambiguous identification of any state analogous to mammalian active sleep.

REPTILES

Sleep has been more extensively studied in reptiles than in most nonmammalian species. Behavioral quiescence associated with high-amplitude electrical activity that disappears with behavioral waking was reported in snakes, *Python saebe* (Peyrethon & Dusan-Peyrethon, 1969); caiman, *Caiman sclerops* (Flanigan et al., 1973); and turtles (Flanigan et al., 1974), with spikes and a rebound following enforced wakefulness. It was hypothesized that high amplitude, spikes, and sharp waves define a reptilian sleep state functionally homologous to the mammalian and avian SWS (Hartse, 1994). Indeed, EEG spikes are associated with the presence of a behavioral sleep state in reptilians, and their density increases after sleep deprivation in chelonian (Flanigan et al., 1974), iguanid (Flanigan, 1973), and crocodilian (Flanigan et al., 1973) reptiles, suggesting homeostatic regulation. Still, no conclusive evidence of REM sleep exists in any examined reptile species. However, recent recordings from the brain of a lizard, the Australian dragon (*Pogona vitticeps*), disclosed clear SWS and REM sleep patterns that oscillate continuously for 6–10 hours with a period of ~80 seconds (Shein-Idelson et al., 2016). Interestingly, lizard slow-wave dynamics closely resemble those observed in rodent hippocampal CA1, although they originate from the dorsal ventricular ridge, which has no apparent hodological similarity with the mammalian hippocampus. The study was replicated with similar results (Libourel et al., 2018). Still, those two sleep states are not entirely matched to classical mammalian sleep in terms of the number of sleep cycles (the lizard sleep rhythm is faster and more frequent, resulting in hundreds of short cycles), the speed and number of eye movements, and the absence of a wake-like EEG for lizards compared to mammalian REM sleep. Therefore, more research is needed to complete the sleep picture in reptiles.

NREM and REM Sleep in Homeothermic Vertebrates (Birds, Mammals)

In contrast to invertebrates and "cold-blooded" vertebrates, sleep in birds and mammals has been extensively studied (for reviews, see Rattenborg & Martinez-Gonzalez, 2015, and Jha & Jha, 2020). Birds evolved from the stem reptiles and exhibit two distinct phases of sleep, NREM sleep and REM sleep (Low et al., 2008), like mammals, even though birds are devoid of a neocortex (Rattenborg, 2006). The electrical signals recorded as EEG in birds are high-frequency waves having low amplitude during wakefulness and REM sleep and prominent SWA with high amplitude in the range of 1–4 Hz during NREM sleep (Jones et al., 2008). Nevertheless, it is essential to remember that not all aspects of birds' sleep are comparable to mammals' sleep (Rattenborg & Martinez-Gonzalez, 2015).

ADAPTATIVE SLEEP IN BIRDS

Birds have developed the ability to sleep with one eye open, enabling the contralateral hemisphere to be awake to overcome the problem of sleeping in specific situations. Spooner and Winters (1965) were the first to observe an association between unilateral eye closure and unihemispheric SWS (USWS) in young chickens (*Gallus gallus domesticus*). They observed that the hemisphere contralateral to the open eye showed EEG activity typical of wakefulness, whereas, in the other hemisphere, EEG activity was specific to SWS. The fact that birds can control which hemisphere sleeps in response to anticipated risks suggests that USWS and unilateral eye closure may serve a predator-detection function. Rattenborg and colleagues (1999) demonstrated that mallard ducks (*Anas platyrhynchos*) positioned at the edge of the group during rest (a position perceived by the animals as dangerous) exhibit a 150% increase in USWS and a strong preference for directing the open eye toward the potential source of danger. In contrast, the ducks positioned safely in the center of the group display bihemispheric sleep. But what about the diverse array of birds, including swifts (Liechti et al., 2013), sandpipers (Klaassen et al., 2011), songbirds (Bairlein et al., 2012; DeLuca et al., 2015), and seabirds (Weimerskirch et al., 2016), engaged in non-stop flights for several days, weeks, or longer? Rattenborg and colleagues (2016) showed that frigate birds (*Fregata minor*) could sleep in flight with one hemisphere at a time or both together while flying over the ocean for up to 10 days. Brain activity recordings revealed that despite frigate birds engaging in both types of sleep on the wing, sleep in flight is more asymmetric than on land. Frigate birds can sleep mostly while circling in rising air currents; however, they keep the eye connected to the awake hemisphere facing the direction of flight, suggesting that they use unihemispheric sleep for observing where they are going. Nevertheless, when compared with sleep on land, flying frigate birds sleep very little, in shorter bouts, and less deeply, implying that frigate birds face ecological demands for attention that usually cannot be met through sleeping unihemispherically. Another function of unihemispheric sleep was described in polygynous male pectoral sandpipers (*Calidris melanotos*; Lesku et al., 2012). These birds breed under the constant light of the Arctic summer. This is the time for male–male competition for access to fertile females, and some males sleep very little for 3 weeks. Interestingly, the males that slept the least sired the most offspring. These results have challenged the view that decreased performance is an inescapable outcome of sleep loss. Hence, unihemispheric sleep in birds serves various functions, such as constant monitoring of the environment, predator detection, breeding, etc.

SLEEP IN MAMMALS

Even though mammals represent a small fraction of living species, they have been the most thoroughly investigated.

Archaic Sleep in Monotremes

Most studies investigating mammalian sleep have been performed on eutherians (placental mammals) or marsupials (pouched mammals), the two main subclasses of mammals. However, there is the third subclass, monotremes (egg-laying mammals), whose two living species are echidna (*Tachyglossus aculeatus*) and platypus (*Ornithorhynchus anatinus*). Fossil and genetic evidence indicates that monotremes diverged from other mammalian lines about 150 million years ago and that both echidna and platypus are derived from a platypus-like ancestor (Edwards & Westerman, 1992) and gave rise to eutherians and marsupials (Siegel, 2022). That is why these living fossil mammals are of specific interest as they may inform us about the evolution of sleep. Early studies suggested that echidna lacks REM sleep (Allison et al., 1972) because no typical REM sleep low-voltage EEG pattern is observed at the cortical level like in eutherian and marsupial mammals. Nevertheless, a subsequent sleep study in the short-beaked echidna demonstrated that despite the high-voltage cortical EEG signals typical for NREM sleep, the brainstem reticular formation shows burst–pause patterns of neuronal activity, resembling the patterns seen in REM sleep throughout the echidna's sleep period (Siegel et al., 1996). Sleep recordings in the platypus (Siegel et al., 1999) revealed REM sleep during most of the sleep period; however, similarly to echidna's sleep patterns, it often occurred within high-voltage cortical EEG patterns featuring the NREM sleep in placental and marsupial mammals and birds. Interestingly, these EEG patterns are similar to those of many newborn placental mammals (including humans; Siegel, 2022). The patterns of high-voltage cortical EEGs are seen during the so-called active sleep, which is the developmental precursor to REM sleep. The platypus has more REM sleep than any other animal, accompanied by eye movements and vigorous jaw and head twitching, akin to movements occurring in placental mammals during REM sleep. These results in monotremes suggest that low-voltage EEG and cortical desynchronization are more recently evolved features of mammalian REM sleep, which may have had its precursor state in reptilian species (Siegel et al., 1999).

Adaptive Sleep in Marine Mammals

Marine air-breathing animals sleeping in water must deal with many challenges, determined by the nature of their environment. Thus, they must surface regularly for breathing, watch for possible predators, and thermoregulate their bodies to prevent heat loss or overheating; and immobilization during sleep would endanger them (Lyamin & Siegel, 2019). Cetaceans are the order of fully aquatic marine mammals whose sleep is the most studied. All cetaceans studied during sleep displayed unihemispheric sleep (similar to that found in birds), allowing one-half of the brain to sleep while the other half remains awake (Lyamin et al., 2008). In this case, high-voltage slow waves rarely occur in both hemispheres simultaneously, and an animal keeps a contralateral eye closed while the other eye remains open (Lyamin & Siegel, 2019; Lyamin et al., 2004). Notably, USWS is a core feature of cetaceans' sleep regardless of the specific experimental conditions, including when the animals were lying in stretchers, swimming in shallow pools while connected to recording equipment with low-noise cables, or freely swimming in spacious pools or enclosures when the EEG was recorded via portable data loggers attached to the animals (Lyamin et al., 2008). Moreover, USWS in cetaceans represents the most extreme case of interhemispheric EEG asymmetry recorded in mammals and birds. In different cetaceans, USWS represented 70%–90% of the total sleep time, making USWS the major sleep state. Contrastingly, there are also no reliable recordings of REM sleep in cetaceans. Only one published study reported EEG features of REM sleep with marked loss of tonus of the trunk muscle in a pilot whale but for no more than 6 minutes and one time only out of three non-consecutive nights (Shurley et al., 1969). This can be explained by the fact that the criteria used to identify and score REM sleep in land mammals are not designed to detect short REM sleep episodes lasting for only several seconds (which might be the case for cetaceans; Lyamin & Siegel, 2019). Nevertheless, some typical behavioral features of REM sleep in land mammals (such as muscle jerks, body twitches, and REMs) have been recorded in resting cetaceans of six species (Lyamin et al., 2008). However, without substantial neural correlates, behavioral manifestations are not sufficient proof for the presence or absence of REM sleep in cetaceans. As most land mammals express the most extended duration of REM sleep shortly after birth, it was proposed that newborn dolphins might express REM sleep, which would align with the hypothesis of the essential role of REM in neural development. Still, experiments including newborn dolphins and killer whales (*Orcinus orca*), which are the largest species of the dolphin family, did not provide evidence for the presence of REM sleep; instead, they showed that the calves do not sleep at all for several weeks after birth (Lyamin et al., 2005). Usually, mothers and calves migrate from their birthing area to the feeding "fields" for thousands of miles. The migration requires maximal alertness as the calves could be attacked by sharks and other killer whales, meaning that the mother and calf must stay together and be responsive to threats. Hence, based on available data, we currently cannot exclude or confirm REM sleep in cetaceans. This is in opposition to what we know of fur seals (*Callorhinus ursinus*; Lyamin et al., 2018). Indeed, fur seals have about 80 minutes of REM and approximately 5–6 hours of NREM sleep per day while sleeping on land. Yet, once they go to the water, where they live for around 7 months of the year, they switch to unihemispheric high-voltage activity, like that seen in the cetacean species. Interestingly, REM sleep fades when the seals are in the water. Furthermore, upon returning to land, they do not show a rebound in NREM or REM sleep, in contrast to terrestrial mammals. These results provide evidence of adaptation mechanisms developed by marine mammals driven by the physical and contextual properties of the aquatic environment.

Neurobiology of Sleep in Humans

Initiation and control of sleep–wake cycles and alternation between sleep states are regulated by the activity of specific neuronal populations located in different brain structures. Before we consider the physiological mechanism maintaining the wake–sleep cycle, it is worth understanding the neurochemical systems supporting this cycle.

Wakefulness

During wakefulness, multiple neurochemical systems subtend the activated cortical state. Several of them belong to the ascending reticular activating system (Figure 1.4). Within the brainstem, serotonergic neurons are primarily localized in the dorsal raphe nucleus, noradrenergic neurons in the locus coeruleus (LC), and cholinergic neurons in

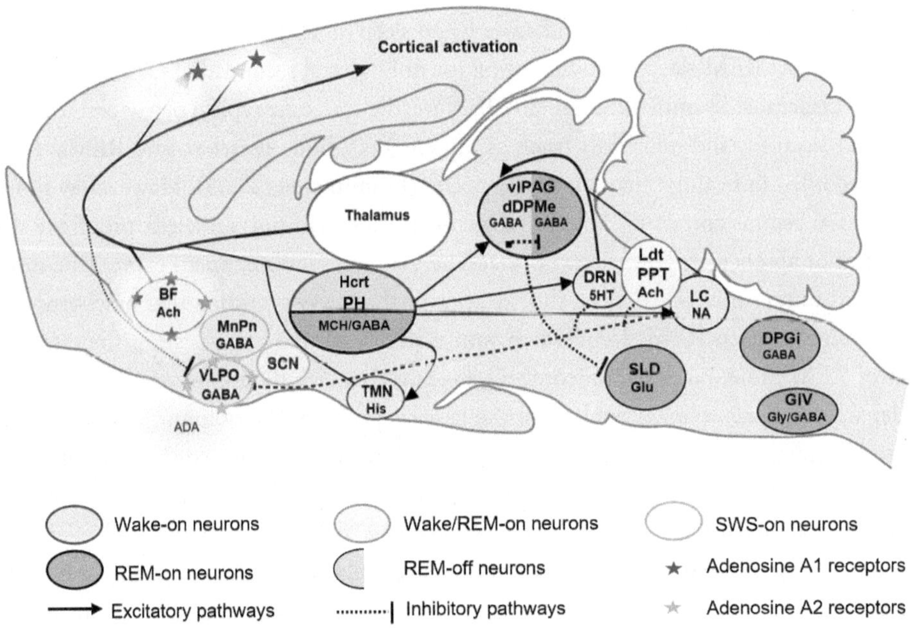

Figure 1.4 Neuronal networks subtending wakefulness

Note. During sleep–wake transitions, the hypocretin neurons start firing, exciting all the other waking systems (histaminergic, monoaminergic, cholinergic). Then waking systems activate the thalamus and/or the cortex and inhibit the GABAergic slow-wave sleep active neurons within the median preoptic nucleus and ventrolateral preoptic nucleus. Ach =acetylcholine; ADA = adenosine; BF =basal forebrain; dDPMe = deep mesencephalic reticular nucleus; DPGi = dorsal paragigantocellular reticular nucleus; DRN = dorsal raphe nucleus; GABA = gamma-aminobutyric acid; GIV = ventral gigantocellular reticular nucleus; Glu = glutamate; Gly = glycine; Hcrt = hypocretin (orexin)–containing neurons; His = histamine; 5HT = 5-hydroxytryptamine (serotonin); LC = locus coeruleus; Ldt = laterodorsal tegmental nucleus; MCH = melanin-concentrating hormone; MnPn = median preoptic nucleus; NA = noradrenaline; PH = posterior hypothalamus; PPT = pedunculopontine tegmental nucleus; REM = rapid eye movement; SCN = suprachiasmatic nucleus; SLD = sublaterodorsal nucleus; SWS = slow-wave sleep; TMN = tuberomammillary nucleus; vlPAG = ventrolateral periaqueductal gray; VLPO = ventrolateral preoptic nucleus. Adapted from Adamantidis and Fort (2021).

the pontine tegmentum (Adamantidis & Fort, 2021). The rostrally located systems in the basal forebrain include the cholinergic neurons, the histaminergic neurons within the tuberomammillary nucleus (TMN), and the hypocretins/orexins system in the lateral hypothalamus (Fort et al., 2009). Wakefulness and arousal are controlled by the activation of these systems through brain-wide projections, reaching the basal forebrain, thalamus, and neocortex. A recent model of neuronal networks responsible for waking (Adamantidis & Fort, 2021) suggests that the first link in a chain reaction for the sleep–wake transition would be hypocretin neurons firing, which will excite all the other waking systems (histaminergic, monoaminergic, and cholinergic). Consecutively, these waking systems would activate the thalamus and/or the cortex, leading to inhibition of the gamma-aminobutyric acid-ergic (GABAergic) SWS neurons of the ventrolateral preoptic nucleus (VLPO) and median preoptic nucleus (MnPn), described in detail below.

Generation and Maintenance of NREM Sleep

Over recent decades, our understanding of the neural mechanisms underlying NREM sleep significantly progressed, although its brain-wide organization in space and time remains unclear. Recent studies identified multiple cell populations whose activity strongly correlates with NREM sleep in several brain areas, suggesting multiple origins of NREM sleep onset. On the one hand, sleep initiation results from the decreasing power of wake-promoting brain neurons. On the other hand, NREM sleep generation and maintenance depend on the implication of four molecules: adenosine, prostaglandin, cytokine, and, most importantly, inhibitory amino acid (GABA). Already in 1930, Economo demonstrated the existence of a sleep-promoting area in the brain by showing a correlation between severe insomnia and damage to the anterior hypothalamus. A few decades later, GABAergic neurons were detected in the hypothalamic VLPO area. GABAergic cells became of specific interest due to their maximal activation during NREM sleep, decreased activity in REM sleep, and minimal activation during wakefulness (Siegel, 2004; Szymusiak et al., 2001). In this respect, these neurons may be viewed as the most potent sleep-promoting component of the brain. Additionally, the bursting activity of GABAergic cells in the VLPO abolishes transmission of incoming signals to the cortex by inhibiting the serotonergic and noradrenergic activity of the brainstem but also in histaminergic and cholinergic systems, two major arousal systems in the brain. In this way, continuous GABA release suppresses activity in wake-promoting areas and activates NREM sleep (Datta & Maclean, 2007; Siegel, 2005). Immunohistochemistry in rats provided evidence that activity in the VLPO and the MnPn of the preoptic area positively correlates with sleep quantity and consolidation, as well as with sleep deprivation during wakefulness (Alam et al., 2014; Gvilia, Xu, et al., 2006). Also, MnPn neurons often fire before sleep onset, suggesting a role in accumulating sleep pressure. This hypothesis was strengthened by evidence that MnPn neurons become active during sleep deprivation, while VLPO neurons increase their activity during sleep (Gvilia, Turner, et al., 2006).

Moreover, the MnPn provides a major input to the VLPO (Chou et al., 2002; Uschakov et al., 2007), which enables driving of VLPO activity; and activation of GABAergic cells in the preoptic area leads to a reduction of neuronal activity in wake-promoting brain regions, which in turn induces SWS. The GABAergic inhibitory function is facilitated by increased synthesis of the growth hormone–releasing hormone, which also increases the depth and duration of SWS (Krueger & Obal, 2003). These results suggest that VLPO and MnPn neurons are responsible for sleep induction and homeostatic regulation. Still, animal studies showed that rats with large VLPO lesions sleep about 50% as much as intact animals. Thus it is likely that the sleep-promoting system in the brain is distributed and, in addition to the VLPO and MnPn, contributes to the inhibition of the arousal systems during sleep (Saper et al., 2010). Saper and colleagues (2010) proposed the "flip-flop switch" model, suggesting that transitions from wake to sleep and vice versa are similar to the electrical switch incorporated into electrical circuits. The model states that neurons on each side of the circuit inhibit those on the other side and, in a case of a small advantage of one side, turn the neurons off on the other side, thus causing a rapid collapse in activity and a state-switching. In contrast to an electronic flip-flop switch which has just one element on either side and acts almost instantly, in the brain, the mutual antagonism among large neuronal populations, which may also be responding to other inputs, may last from seconds to minutes (varying across species), resulting in clearcut changes in behavioral and electrophysiological states. As soon as the boundary of one state is crossed, the firing of the counterbalanced population is suppressed. Practically, this "switch" should enable a stable wake/sleep state, preventing an individual from falling asleep during quiet wakefulness or rest or waking up from a slight noise during the night. Therefore, a variety of other sleep-promoting factors that are accumulated during wakefulness represent homeostatic regulators that are crucial for triggering sleep. Among those are prostaglandin (PG) D2 and adenosine. PGD2 circulates in the cerebrospinal fluid as a sleep hormone and stimulates basal forebrain (BF) cells to release adenosine, a signaling molecule to promote sleep (Cherasse et al., 2018). In turn, adenosine activates adenosine A2A sleep-active neurons in the BF and the VLPO area. The latter downregulates wake-active neurons in the TMN through GABAergic or galaninergic inhibitory signals to the TMN, which promotes arousal through histamine H1 receptors. These findings suggest that the VLPO and TMN regulate sleep and wakefulness by a "flip-flop" mechanism during sleep/wake state transitions. Despite the recent discoveries in NREM sleep onset and regulation, the exact pathways, the cellular mechanisms, and the variety of interactions among them are still to be investigated. The most up-to-date comprehensive model of NREM sleep is illustrated in Figure 1.5.

As described above, there is a progressive change in how neuronal populations fire from wakefulness to NREM sleep. Thus, corticothalamic oscillations (often called *thalamocortical*, even though axons are way more numerous in the descending pathway than in the ascending pathway; White & Keller, 1989) enable synchronous low-frequency,

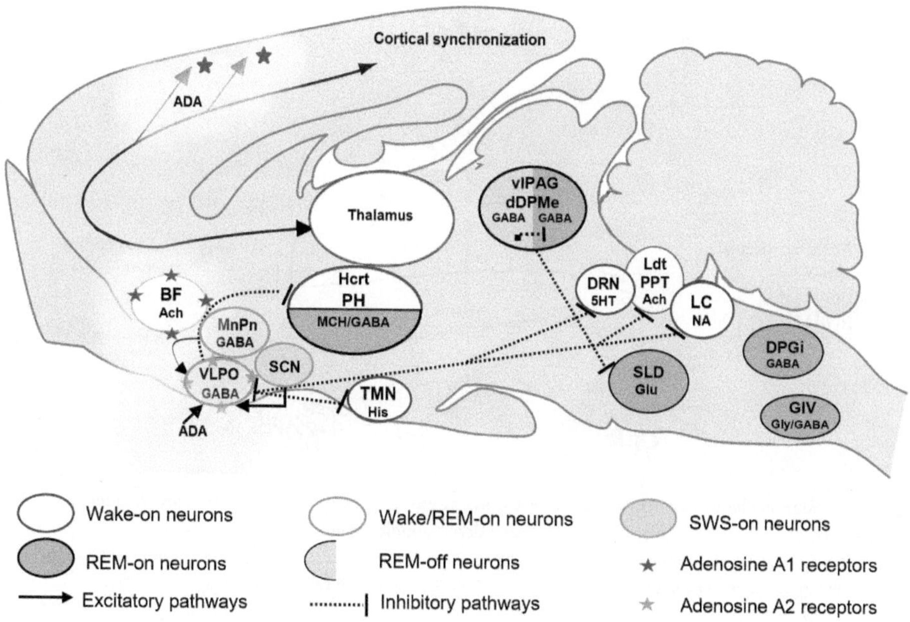

Figure 1.5 Neuronal networks subtending slow-wave sleep

Note. At first, ventrolateral preoptic nucleus (VLPO) and median preoptic nucleus (MnPn) GABAergic start firing at sleep onset (drowsiness) under excitatory, homeostatic (adenosine), and circadian drives (suprachiasmatic input). This neuronal activation together with the reciprocal GABAergic inhibition of wake-promoting systems would be in a position to suddenly unbalance the "flip-flop" network, which is essential for switching from waking (drowsiness) to a progression of slow-wave sleep. Contrariwise, the gradual removal of excitatory influences would result in a progressive firing decrease of MnPn and VLPO, leading to wake-promoting systems activation and wakefulness. Ach =acetylcholine; ADA = adenosine; BF =basal forebrain; dDPMe = deep mesencephalic reticular nucleus; DPGi = dorsal paragigantocellular reticular nucleus; DRN = dorsal raphe nucleus; GABA = gamma-aminobutyric acid; GIV = ventral gigantocellular reticular nucleus; Glu = glutamate; Gly = glycine; Hcrt = hypocretin (orexin)–containing neurons; His = histamine; 5HT = 5-hydroxytryptamine (serotonin); LC = locus coeruleus; Ldt = laterodorsal tegmental nucleus; MCH = melanin-concentrating hormone; NA = noradrenaline; PH = posterior hypothalamus; PPT = pedunculopontine tegmental nucleus; REM = rapid eye movement; SCN = suprachiasmatic nucleus; SLD = sublaterodorsal nucleus; SWS = slow-wave sleep; TMN = tuberomammillary nucleus; vlPAG = ventrolateral periaqueductal gray. Adapted from Adamantidis and Fort (2021).

high-amplitude EEG typical of NREM sleep. Figure 1.6 illustrates three interconnected neuronal populations involved in the generation of NREM sleep oscillations: (i) cortico-thalamic neurons (neurons A) that have excitatory synapses on thalamocortical neurons and thalamic reticular neurons; (ii) thalamocortical relay neurons (neurons B), with their cell bodies in the thalamus and axons making excitatory synapses on pyramidal neurons in the cerebral cortex and on neurons in the thalamic reticular nucleus; and (iii) thalamic reticular neurons (neurons C), located in the reticular thalamic nuclei and forming inhibitory synapses on thalamocortical neurons. Neurons A and B are excitatory glutamatergic neurons, whereas neurons C are GABAergic inhibitory neurons. The resulting loops into the corticothalamocortical network are involved in different ways in the generation of

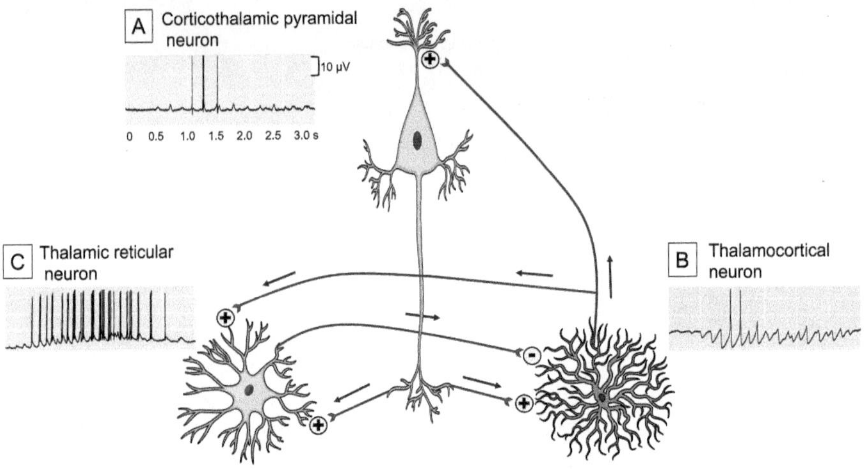

Figure 1.6 Neuronal loops in corticothalamic networks engaged in generating the coherent low-frequency oscillations characteristic of non–rapid-eye-movement sleep (spindles, delta, and slow oscillations)
Note. Panel A: Corticothalamic neurons. Panel B: Thalamocortical relay neurons. Panel C: Thalamic reticular neurons. + = excitatory and – = inhibitory connections within the loop. Adapted from Borbély et al. (2000) and Purves and Williams (2001).

spindles and delta waves, which in turn are organized by cortically generated slow oscillations (<1 Hz; Steriade et al., 1993). Altogether, these rhythms are produced by a "unified oscillatory machine" encompassing thalamic and cortical structures under the control of brainstem and forebrain modulatory systems and are coalescent within specific time windows corresponding to the depolarizing phase ("up"-state) of the slow oscillations (Steriade, 2006).

NEURAL CORRELATES OF NREM SLEEP

Early neuroimaging studies mostly investigated sleep in healthy humans and were dedicated to highlighting differences in brain activity between various sleep stages and wakefulness (for review, see Dang-Vu et al., 2010). These studies were mainly performed using positron emission tomography (PET), which uses positron-emitting isotopes to label the neural distribution of compounds and provides information about either regional brain glucose metabolism or regional cerebral blood flow (CBF) depending on the type of isotope. PET studies have consistently reported decreased regional CBF and oxygen consumption during NREM sleep, as compared to wakefulness or REM sleep, in a set of subcortical and cortical regions encompassing the dorsal pons and the mesencephalon, cerebellum, thalamus, basal ganglia, BF, anterior hypothalamus, neocortical prefrontal and anterior cingulate cortices, and precuneus and mesial parts of the temporal lobe (Andersson et al., 1998; Kajimura et al., 1999; Maquet et al., 2000). The relationship between the depth of NREM sleep and decreased regional CBF was thought to reflect increased synchronization. This assumption was further confirmed by correlations between increased EEG spectral power for slow oscillations in the delta (1–4 Hz) range and decreased regional CBF in most of the cortical regions reported above, particularly in medial prefrontal regions where the response to homeostatic sleep pressure is prominent (Dang-Vu et al., 2005). The PET technique has a high spatial resolution (a few millimeters) but a poor temporal resolution (up to several minutes). Further studies used techniques providing higher temporal resolution, such as functional magnetic resonance imaging (fMRI), which like PET can measure blood oxygen–dependent level (BOLD) and hemodynamic changes induced by regional changes in neuronal activity at the scale of the second, and EEG and magnetoencephalography (MEG), measuring the neuronal electrical or magnetic activity with exquisite temporal resolution (milliseconds), though with a slightly poorer spatial resolution (i.e., a few millimeters to 1 centimeter; Gosseries et al., 2008). To overcome the limitations of one neuroimaging technique, researchers often use a combination of different methods (e.g., fMRI/EEG), optimally combining high temporal and spatial resolutions. For instance, transient changes in regional cerebral activity specifically associated with slow (<1 Hz, >140 μV) and delta waves (0.5–4 Hz, 75–140 μV) during NREM sleep were highlighted utilizing simultaneous fMRI and EEG recordings (Dang-Vu et al., 2008). Using an endogenous event-related approach, these authors searched for brain regions where changes in activity (i.e., BOLD responses in fMRI) were coincident with the active depolarized ("up") state of these oscillations, as indexed by peak negativity in the EEG. Results showed increased cerebral activity associated with both slow and delta waves in several cortical areas, including the inferior frontal and medial prefrontal cortices and the precuneus and posterior cingulate areas. Besides these commonalities, however, slow oscillations were linked to increased activity in the parahippocampal gyrus, the cerebellum, and the brainstem, whereas delta waves were specifically associated with increased activity in frontal areas. Additionally, Dang-Vu and colleagues (2008) found increased activity related to slow oscillations in the midbrain and the pontine tegmentum, a region that includes critical structures involved in regulating sleep and wakefulness, the activation encompassing the noradrenergic LC. This result suggests that these structures are active in phase with slow oscillations, perhaps allowing the brain to periodically restore microwake-like activity patterns to facilitate neuronal interactions. Taken together, these results suggest that SWS is not, as may have been thought, a state of brain quiescence but genuinely is an active state during which phasic increases in brain activity are synchronized to slow oscillations. An fMRI/EEG study looking at sleep signatures in brain hemodynamic activity (Song et al., 2022) showed that at the transition from wake to sleep, activity progresses from a mixed-frequency pattern to one featuring two distinct oscillations: a low-frequency (<0.1 Hz) oscillation correlated with the occurrence of spindles and a high-frequency oscillation (>0.1 Hz) detected in deep sleep, correlated with the occurrence of slow waves. Interestingly, within drowsiness, the low-frequency oscillation first emerges in the thalamus, then in the posterior cortex, and lastly, the frontal cortex. In turn, the high-frequency oscillation first appears in the midbrain, next within the frontal cortex, and eventually in the posterior cortex. During the waking-up process, both oscillations disappear, first from the thalamus, then the frontal cortex, and lastly, the posterior cortex. Based on these findings, the authors assumed this might reflect the order in which brain regions fall asleep and wake up.

Another approach to look at brain neural dynamics during NREM sleep was introduced by Stevner and colleagues (2019), using a Markovian data-driven analysis of continuous fMRI/EEG neuroimaging data. The hidden Markov model (HMM) is a data-driven approach that infers unique spatiotemporal patterns of activity (band-limited amplitude fluctuations) rapidly reoccurring (every tens to hundreds milliseconds) at different points in time (within the whole lengths of the signal) and identifies them as distinct HMM states (Rezek & Roberts, 2005). This method allows investigation of the dynamic choreography between different whole-brain networks across the wake–NREM sleep cycle at a fine temporal resolution (i.e., at the sub-second scale). The researchers inferred 19 HMM states and compared the temporal evolution of the HMM-derived whole-brain network states with the EEG-based polysomnographic (PSG) scoring. Results showed that wakefulness corresponds to a collection of whole-brain network states, while N2 and N3 are only dominated by two and one HMM whole-brain states, respectively, demonstrating good correspondence with the PSG score. In contrast, no specific HMM states were found in the N1 transition sleep. Notably, wakefulness before and after sleep was represented in the transition map (a probabilistic map representing transitions among the HMM states) as two different modules with different repertoires of large-scale brain networks, although it is treated similarly in PSG staging. It suggests that falling asleep and waking up are two asymmetric processes, which may lead to two separated transition modules of whole-brain network states during wakefulness, with one more likely to occur after consolidated sleep. Additionally, HMM identified transitions occurring among wakefulness, N2, and N3—represented by whole-brain states characterized by subcortical–cortical decoupling, which is in line with intracortical evidence of brain activity during sleep onset (Magnin et al., 2010). Altogether, these results demonstrate the complexity of NREM sleep and suggest a global interplay among various brain regions supporting numerous neural networks involved in the sleep/wake cycle.

SLEEP SPINDLES

As mentioned above, spindles are short-lasting (0.5–3 seconds) waxing and waning oscillations in the sigma range (11–16 Hz) during NREM sleep, especially during Stage N2. Spindles are affected by a series of factors (for a comprehensive review, see Fernandez & Lüthi, 2020), including circadian modulation (Bódizs et al., 2021), age (Clawson et al., 2016; Crowley et al., 2002), menstrual cycle (Alonso et al., 2021; Genzel et al., 2012; Plamberger et al., 2021), and drugs (Ayoub et al., 2013; Leong et al., 2022). Spindles have been shown to be under both circadian and homeostatic control (De Gennaro & Ferrara, 2003). Spindle density is decreased in early sleep stages in an inverse homeostatic relationship to slow waves. The same is observed after sleep deprivation, when the spindle amplitude increases while the intraspindle frequency variability drops, indicating a higher level of synchronization in corticothalamic cells under increased sleep pressure. Two types of mechanisms underlying spindle rhythm generation have been proposed: those producing the electrical sources of spindles recorded on EEG/MEG and those responsible for triggering, spreading, synchronizing, and stopping this rhythm (Urakami et al., 2012). The spindle rhythm is paced from the thalamus as it disappears after thalamotomy. The spindle frequency is determined by an interplay between the bilaterally interconnected GABAergic inhibitory neurons in the reticular nucleus of the thalamus (RT) and the corticothalamic neurons, their intrinsic properties, and their influence by cortical as well as brainstem ascending inputs. The electrical generators of spindles were identified with intracranial EEG recordings. These are superficial and deeper frontal cortical sources as well as the ventrobasal thalamus, which are usually but not necessarily synchronous with scalp EEG recordings (Schomer et al., 2010). Cortical excitation of RT neurons is also found to be instrumental in the spreading and synchronizing of spindles through corticothalamic and corticocortical excitations. The frequency of occurrence of spindles is reported to peak at 0.2–0.3 Hz (Achermann & Borbély, 1997). The association of spindles with the slow cortical oscillation (~0.75 Hz; Steriade, 2006) is proposed to be causative in the sense that this oscillation (supposedly generated within neocortical networks) synchronizes neuronal activity into generalized down-states (hyperpolarization) of global neuronal silence and subsequent up-states (depolarization) of increased wake-like neuronal firing. With the beginning of the latter, corticothalamic volleys are proposed to drive the generation of spindle activity. The different slow (11–13 Hz) and fast (14–16 Hz) spectra are proposed to depend on distinct anatomical substrates (various thalamic rhythm generators and varying distances from the cortical electrical generators). It has been proposed that corticothalamic neurons in anteroventral and anteromedial nuclei, connecting limbic structures with cingulate and prefrontal areas, do not receive inhibition from the RT but are suppressed by other regions and, thus, do not fire in coherence with other corticothalamic neurons during spindles (Paré et al., 1987; Ueda et al., 2001). Moreover, the two types of spindle activity express different maturational courses (De Gennaro & Ferrara, 2003), suggesting functional differences. In line with this assumption, neuroimaging (EEG-fMRI) data showed that spindle occurrence is associated with transient increases in regional brain activity in thalamic and paralimbic areas (anterior cingulate and insular cortices) and the superior temporal gyrus (Schabus et al., 2007). In particular, slow spindles elicited additional increased activity in the frontal gyrus, while fast spindles were associated with activations in a large set of cortical regions involved in sensorimotor processing, as well as in the orbital and mesial prefrontal cortex, hippocampus, and anterior insula, further supporting the hypothesis that generation of fast and slow spindles relies upon two functionally separated systems. Currently, it is thought that brain oscillations are structured by a functional hierarchy orchestrating communication in distributed neural networks on broad spatial and spectral scales (Buzsáki, 2006; Engel et al., 2013). MEG/EEG findings (Klinzing et al., 2016) support previous results showing that the slow oscillation phase temporally organizes fast and slow spindles. Fast spindle activity was found most prominent during the slow oscillation "up"-states, whereas slow spindle activity occurred mainly during the up- to down-state transition of the slow oscillation. For a better understanding of the interactions between SWS elements as well as their role in cognition, we refer the reader to Fernandez and Lüthi (2020) and Rasch and Born (2013).

Generation and Maintenance of REM Sleep

In normal circumstances, REM sleep does not appear during wakefulness or immediately after going to sleep but systematically follows a period of NREM sleep. In humans, the duration and number of REM sleep episodes increase with the progress of sleep cycles through the night. To explain the mechanisms of REM sleep, Hobson et al. proposed the *reciprocal interaction model* in 1975, positing that REM sleep generation and maintenance depend on reciprocal interactions between so-called REM-promoting (*REM-on*) and REM-suppressing (*REM-off*) groups of cells. In a nutshell, this model suggests that REM-off neurons (monoaminergic [serotonergic and noradrenergic] neurons located in the LC) are inhibitory to REM-on neurons (reticular cholinergic cells located in the pedunculopontine tegmentum [PPT] and lateral dorsal tegmentum of the brainstem) and to themselves. In turn, the REM-on neurons are excitatory to the REM-off ones and themselves. Thus, according to the model, the inactivation of putative monoaminergic REM-off neurons plays a critical role in generating and maintaining REM sleep. In the *mutual inhibitory model* proposed by Sakai (1988), REM sleep can appear either by excitation of the REM-on neurons or by inhibition of the REM-off neurons. This hypothesis seems to imply that cholinergic neurons directly inhibit norepinephrinergic REM-off neurons for the generation of REM sleep. However, later findings (Fuller et al., 2007) revealed the presence of noncholinergic and nonmonoaminergic mutually inhibitory REM-off and REM-on areas in the mesopontine tegmentum that may form the neuroanatomical basis of the switching circuitry for REM sleep. These findings suggest a *REM switching circuitry model* analogous to an electronic "flip-flop" switch (similar to the one described for NREM sleep). In a nutshell, the "flip-flop" switch model suggests that the REM-off neural activity gradually decreases during NREM sleep until the critical switch point is achieved, where REM-on neurons become active and REM sleep takes place. In this framework, during wakefulness, REM-off GABAergic neurons within the ventrolateral periaqueductal gray matter (vlPAG) and dorsal deep mesencephalic reticular nucleus (dDPMe) tonically inhibit sublaterodorsal nucleus (SLD) glutamatergic neurons (Figure 1.7; Luppi et al., 2021). These REM-off GABAergic neurons receive excitation from monoaminergic and hypocretin neurons. Wake-on neurons can activate the cortex directly or via a relay within the intralaminar thalamic nuclei. REM sleep onset and

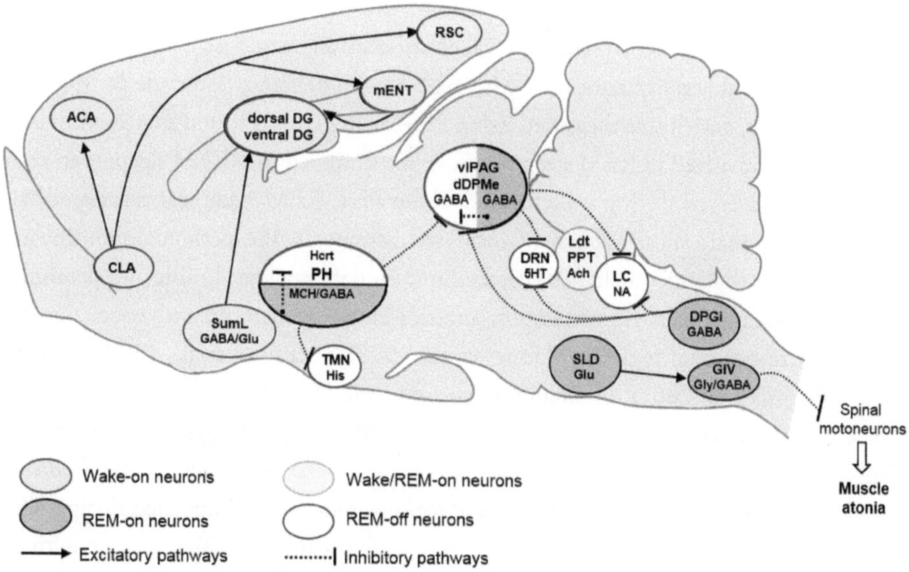

Figure 1.7 The onset and maintenance of REM sleep is under the intrinsic "clock-like" activation of GABAergic and glutamatergic neurons localized in the posterior hypothalamus (part of them containing also MCH), the vlPAG/dDPMe, and the DPGi

Note. These neurons inhibit all wakefulness-promoting neurons and the REM-off GABAergic neurons of the vlPAG and dDPMe. Then SLD glutamatergic neurons are disinhibited and provoke muscle atonia via excitation of glycinergic/GABAergic neurons of the GIV, which in turn hyperpolarize spinal and cranial motoneurons. Ach =acetylcholine; ACA = anterior cingulate cortex; CLA = claustrum; dDPMe = deep mesencephalic reticular nucleus; DG = dentate gyrus; DPGi = dorsal paragigantocellular reticular nucleus; DRN = dorsal raphe nucleus; GABA = gamma-aminobutyric acid; GIV = ventral gigantocellular reticular nucleus; Glu = glutamate; Gly = glycine; Hcrt = hypocretin (orexin)–containing neurons; His = histamine; 5HT = 5-hydroxytryptamine (serotonin); LC = locus coeruleus; LdT = laterodorsal tegmental nucleus; MCH = melanin-concentrating hormone–containing neurons; mENT = medial entorhinal cortex; NA = noradrenaline; PH = posterior hypothalamus; PPT = pedunculopontine tegmental nucleus; REM = rapid eye movement; RSC = retrosplenial cortex; SLD = sublaterodorsal nucleus; SumL = lateral supramammillary nucleus; TMN = tuberomammillary nucleus; vlPAG = ventrolateral periaqueductal gray. Adapted from Luppi et al. (2021).

maintenance occur due to the intrinsic "clock-like" activation of GABAergic and glutamatergic neurons in the posterior hypothalamus (a part of these neurons contains melanin-concentrating hormone [MCH], which also modulates REM sleep), vlPAG/dDPMe, and the dorsal paragigantocellular reticular nucleus (DPGi). The posterior hypothalamus neurons inhibit wakefulness and the REM-off GABAergic neurons in the vlPAG and dDPMe. Then glutamatergic REM-on neurons in the SLD become disinhibited and start generating muscle atonia via excitation of glycinergic/GABAergic neurons of the ventral gigantocellular reticular nucleus, which in turn hyperpolarizes spinal and cranial motoneurons. The timing of REM sleep is under the control of GABAergic neuron activity in the vlPAG and DPGi as well as hypothalamic MCH neurons and cholinergic cells in the laterodorsal tegmental nucleus and PPT in the brainstem (Fraigne et al., 2015).

NEURAL CORRELATES OF REM SLEEP

At variance with NREM, REM sleep and wakefulness are characterized by sustained, desynchronized neuronal activity associated with high energy demands (Steriade & McCarley, 1990). Therefore, activity, as measured using PET or fMRI, was found increased in brain regions actively involved in REM sleep processes as compared to NREM sleep, even above activity levels observed during wakefulness. Using PET, REM sleep was associated with a specific neuroanatomical pattern of increased activity in the pedunculopontine tegmentum (PPT), thalamic nuclei, BF, cerebellum, caudate nucleus, limbic and paralimbic structures (e.g., amygdala, hippocampus, anterior cingulate cortex), and associative posterior temporo-occipital regions (Maquet et al., 1996; Nofzinger et al., 1997; Peigneux, Laureys, Fuchs, et al., 2001). In parallel, decreased regional CBF was found in frontal and parietal regions (dorsolateral prefrontal cortex, posterior cingulate gyrus, precuneus, and inferior parietal cortex), as well as in primary sensory areas (Braun et al., 1997; Maquet et al., 2005), indicating that activity in these regions is strongly diminished during REM sleep. Increased regional CBF activity in the PPT, thalamus, and BF is in line with the neurobiological literature, indicating that REM-on neurons and other cellular populations responsible for REM sleep induction are located in these regions and mediate widespread cortical activation through innervations in the thalamus and BF (Capece et al., 1997; Datta, 1997). Also, increased activity in amygdaloid complexes involved in the generation of REM sleep reflects their potential role in the modulation of regional activation/deactivation patterns during REM sleep (Amaral & Price, 1984). Indeed, most activated areas during REM sleep are regions receiving numerous amygdalar projections, whereas deactivated frontal and parietal cortices are practically devoid of amygdalar afferents (Aggleton, 1993; Amaral & Price, 1984). Additional animal data showed that electrical stimulation of the central nucleus of amygdaloid complexes increases phasic ponto-genicular-occipital activity (Calvo et al., 1987), one of the most distinguishing features of REM sleep. REM sleep is also the sleep stage during which dreams are the most prominent, and it was proposed to interpret functional brain mapping in REM sleep in the light of dreaming phenomenology (Banks, 2009; Barrett & McNamara, 2007).

PHASIC AND TONIC REM SLEEP

REM sleep is composed of two distinguishable microstates. *Phasic REM sleep* is characterized by bursts of eye movements linked to ponto-genicular-occipital waves (Ioannides et al., 2004), sawtooth waves, myoclonic twitches of skeletal muscles, and irregular cardiac and respiratory activity (Dickerson et al., 1993). *Tonic REM sleep* comprises longer and quieter segments (without eye movements) amid periods of phasic activity. These two states significantly differ with regard to external information processing. During tonic REM sleep, alertness and environmental processing are partially preserved, resembling a wake-like state, while in phasic periods, external information processing is attenuated (Takahara et al., 2002, 2006). Early studies suggested that intense dream experiences are subtended by phasic periods due to intense eye movements and involvement in sensorimotor activity (Berger & Oswald, 1962). Accordingly, individuals awakened from phasic REM periods reported more movement and self-participation in their dream, in contrast to more thought-like experiences when awakened from tonic states (Pivik, 1991). In the same line, a more recent study showed that suppressing REMs by acoustic stimulation facilitated the transition to tonic REM sleep and decreased the rate of visual imagery reports collected after awakening (Stuart & Conduit, 2009). The duration of phasic REM sleep increases toward the end of the night, together with the decrease in homeostatic sleep pressure (Marzano et al., 2011), suggesting a potential homeostatic component in REM sleep regulation (besides the well-known circadian drive). The functional roles of phasic and tonic REM sleep components are still debated. Simor and colleagues (2020) proposed a framework in which phasic states are considered as an offline mode, promoting sleep stability and internal processing, whereas tonic periods represent an online mode, facilitating environmental alertness and responsiveness to external inputs. It has been speculated that the dynamic alternations of phasic and tonic REM periods not only regulate sleep and arousability but also play a role in facilitating learning and memory and affect regulation through processes of exaptation and secondary adaptation.

Relevance of NREM/REM Cycles

Among the multiple functions of sleep, its role in memory systems has attracted particular attention. During sleep, new and "fragile" memories encoded during wakefulness become more stable (consolidated) and undergo integration into preexisting long-term memory networks (for review, see Rasch & Born, 2013). On the one hand, the *dual processes hypothesis* assumes that different sleep stages enable the consolidation of different types of memories (Gais & Born, 2004; Rauchs et al., 2005). Specifically, it has been assumed that declarative memory, which consists of facts and events that can be consciously recalled, profits from SWS. In contrast, the consolidation of procedural memory involved in the performance of different actions and skills is supported by REM sleep. However, this somehow simplistic distinction has long been challenged (Peigneux, Laureys, Delbeuck, & Maquet, 2001) and is not supported by current literature (see Rasch & Born, 2013). On the other hand, the *sequential hypothesis* stresses the importance of the cyclic succession of SWS (or NREM sleep) and REM sleep episodes for memory formation, with sleep stages serving complementary functions. In the first processing step during SWS, nonadaptive (i.e., irrelevant) memories are weakened, and adaptive (useful) responses are strengthened, while during the second processing step occurring in REM sleep, the adaptive memories are integrated and stored in preexisting knowledge networks (Ambrosini & Giuditta, 2001; Ngo et al., 2015). Supporting evidence for the sequential hypothesis was found in narcoleptic patients who often start sleeping directly in the REM state. In this study, consolidation-related spindles were correlated with oversleep performance changes only in naps in which the physiological order of sleep stages was respected, that is, NREM then REM sleep (Strauss et al., 2022). Finally, the *active system consolidation framework* integrates aspects of both the abovementioned hypotheses (Born & Wilhelm, 2012). The central idea of this hypothesis is that during wakefulness, experienced episodes are encoded within neocortical networks, and some parts of the newly formed memory traces are stored in the medial temporal lobe, especially in the hippocampus. During SWS, reactivation of recent memories in hippocampal networks promotes the activation of cortical memory parts, thereby successively strengthening corticocortical connections. This process mediates the redistribution of the temporarily stored memory representations (in the hippocampus) to long-term storage sites (neocortex), where they undergo integration into preexisting long-term memories (Buzsáki, 1998). Due to limited resources available during SWS for the strengthening of the synaptic connections, SWS memory reactivations might only tag the involved cortical synapses for later strengthening during subsequent REM sleep, in line with the sequential hypothesis (Ribeiro et al., 2007).

Besides consolidation, reorganization, and subsequent integration of new memories into existing knowledge networks, sleep was also shown to promote generalization (e.g., abstracting regularities from specific examples to apply in future situations). History tells us that great scientists woke up from sleep with the solution for problems they were trying to solve, for example, Albert Einstein's equations and comforting folk psychology that advises us to sleep on a problem to solve it. Experimental studies indicate a facilitating role of sleep in extracting rules and generalizing knowledge. For instance, in one study (Wagner et al., 2004), participants were trained in a problem-solving numerical task where a sequence of operations had to be applied to reach the solution. Results showed that participants exposed to the task and then allowed to sleep got the insight for this hidden rule two times faster than participants who did not sleep, suggesting that sleep facilitates insight and problem-solving. Similarly, sleep benefits have been reported for rule-dependent memory tasks using probabilistic learning (Fischer et al., 2006; Peigneux et al., 2003), musical sequences (Durrant et al., 2011), and language acquisition (Batterink et al., 2014). Altogether, these results suggest a facilitating role of sleep in abstracting and generalizing information. Thus, it allows accessing general rules and shortcuts, leading to solving problems rehearsed during wakefulness. In this respect, sleep-dependent generalization processes may positively affect other cognitive activities, such as inferential judgments and decision-making.

Sleep/Wake Interplay

Typically, sleep is considered as a global phenomenon that affects the whole brain uniformly and simultaneously. In the same vein, sleep and wakefulness are generally treated as two mutually exclusive behavioral states—aka an all-or-none model. However, the view of sleep as a global state has been recently challenged by intracranial findings of topographically local sleep and local wakefulness states (Siclari & Tononi, 2017). An animal study demonstrated that individual neurons display brief periods of SWA in wakefulness, accompanied by transient behavioral impairments (Vyazovskiy et al., 2011). Additionally, human studies revealed subsets of brain regions showing wake-like activity (Nobili et al., 2011) within deep NREM sleep, tentatively associated with dreaming activity (Siclari et al., 2017). These findings stress the fact that sleep-like and wakefulness-like states are not mutually exclusive but rather can occur simultaneously in the brain, with some neuronal populations exhibiting one state and the rest the other. In this respect, the *local use-dependent sleep theory* proposes that sleep and wakefulness might coexist at the same time and in different areas of the brain (Krueger et al., 2008; Siclari & Tononi, 2017). The notion that sleep and wakefulness might be considered dynamic processes that unfold through local brain changes from full wakefulness to global sleep and vice versa is supported by a growing amount of data (Ferrara & De Gennaro, 2011; Marzano et al., 2013; Sarasso et al. 2013). It has been proposed that during extended waking periods, the progressive slowing of brain rhythms was due to local use-dependent sleep (Hung et al., 2013; Nir et al., 2017), namely a type of sleep that occurs locally as the homeostatic consequence of sustained use of neuronal circuits (Krueger et al., 2013). Prolonged waking experiments (>24 hours) disclosed local task-dependent EEG power changes in the 5–9-Hz range within task-related brain regions, linked to a worsening in performance (Bernardi et al., 2015; Hung et al., 2013). Using high-density EEG recordings, Quercia and colleagues (2018) showed that brain regions involved in learning spatial navigation tasks during wakefulness exhibit higher delta activity and are behaviorally correlated with increased error rates in the task. By contrast, the intensive use of the same task-related circuits in a control experiment (in which no learning was required) induced neither behavioral performance nor local sleep in wakefulness. These findings suggest that sustained usage of learning-related neuronal circuits initiates local sleep, which might reflect local recovery and learning-related cortical plasticity.

Conclusion

In summary, this chapter guided the reader beyond the concept of a cessation of waking activity during sleep. We have seen that despite evolutionary adaptations and divergences among species, sleep is a universal phenomenon whose generation and maintenance are under the control of complex regulatory physiological mechanisms. Most importantly, we have learned that sleep is not a uniform but rather a dynamic state. Sleep-related changes in brain activity can be observed at neurobiological, neurophysiological, and neuroanatomical levels, including, among others, cellular and molecular interactions, re-equilibration of the neurotransmitter balance, and changes in functional neuroanatomical patterns resulting in different sleep stages and the variety of their characteristics. We saw the importance of sleep stages as well as wake/sleep interplay for memory and cognitive functioning. Thus, our exponentially growing understanding of the sleeping brain should bring us closer to the answers to the fundamental questions of "how" and "why" we sleep.

Acknowledgments

L. R. is a research fellow supported by the Fonds de la Recherche Scientifique (FRS-FNRS, Brussels, Belgium) and PhD research grant "Mini-ARC" from the Université Libre de Bruxelles, Belgium.

References

Achermann, P., & Borbély, A. A. (1997). Low-frequency (<1 Hz) oscillations in the human sleep electroencephalogram. *Neuroscience, 81*(1), 213–222. https://doi.org/10.1016/s0306-4522(97)00186-3

Adamantidis, A., & Fort, P. (2021). The neurophysiology and neurobiology of wakefulness and non-rapid eye movement (NREM) sleep. In C. Bassetti, W. McNicholas, T. Paunio, & P. Peigneux (Eds.), *European sleep medicine textbook* (2nd ed., pp. 7–25). European Sleep Research Society.

Aggleton, J. P. (1993). The contribution of the amygdala to normal and abnormal emotional states. *Trends in Neurosciences, 16*(8), 328–333. https://doi.org/10.1016/0166-2236(93)90110-8

Aho, V., Vainikka, M., Puttonen, H. A. J., Ikonen, H. M. K., Salminen, T., Panula, P., Porkka-Heiskanen, T., & Wigren, H.-K. (2017). Homeostatic response to sleep/rest deprivation by constant water flow in larval zebrafish in both dark and light conditions. *Journal of Sleep Research, 26*(3), 394–400. https://doi.org/10.1111/jsr.12508

Alam, M. A., Kumar, S., McGinty, D., Alam, M. N., & Szymusiak, R. (2014). Neuronal activity in the preoptic hypothalamus during sleep deprivation and recovery sleep. *Journal of Neurophysiology, 111*(2), 287–299. https://doi.org/10.1152/jn.00504.2013

Allison, T., Van Twyver, H., & Goff, W. R. (1972). Electrophysiological studies of the echidna, *Tachyglossus aculeatus*. I. Waking and sleep. *Archives Italiennes de Biologie, 110*(2), 145–184.

Alonso, A., Genzel, L., & Gomez, A. (2021). Sex and menstrual phase influences on sleep and memory. *Current Sleep Medicine Reports, 7*(1), 1–14. https://doi.org/10.1007/s40675-020-00201-y

Amaral, D. G., & Price, J. L. (1984). Amygdalo-cortical projections in the monkey (*Macaca fascicularis*). *Journal of Comparative Neurology, 230*(4), 465–496. https://doi.org/10.1002/cne.902300402

Ambrosini, M. V., & Giuditta, A. (2001). Learning and sleep: The sequential hypothesis. *Sleep Medicine Reviews, 5*(6), 477–490. https://doi.org/10.1053/smrv.2001.0180

Andersson, J. L., Onoe, H., Hetta, J., Lidström, K., Valind, S., Lilja, A., Sundin, A., Fasth, K.-J., Westerberg, G., Broman, J.-E., Watanabe, Y., & Långström, B. (1998). Brain networks affected by synchronized sleep visualized by positron emission tomography. *Journal of Cerebral Blood Flow & Metabolism, 18*(7), 701–715. https://doi.org/10.1097/00004647-199807000-00001

Appelbaum, L., Wang, G. X., Maro, G. S., & Mourrain, P. (2009). Sleep–wake regulation and hypocretin–melatonin interaction in zebrafish. *Proceedings of the National Academy of Sciences of the United States of America, 106*(51), 21942–21947. https://doi.org/10.1073/pnas.906637106

Aserinski, E., & Kleitman, N. (1953). Regularly occurring periods of eye motility, and concomitant phenomena, during sleep. *Science, 118*(3062), 273–274. https://doi.org/10.1126/science.118.3062.273

Ayoub, A., Aumann, D., Hörschelmann, A., Kouchekmanesch, A., Paul, P., Born, J., & Marshall, L. (2013). Differential effects on fast and slow spindle activity, and the sleep slow oscillation in humans with carbamazepine and flunarizine to antagonize voltage-dependent Na^{+} and Ca^{2+} channel activity. *Sleep, 36*(6), 905–911. https://doi.org/10.5665/sleep.2722

Bairlein, F., Norris, D. R., Nagel, R., Bulte, M., Voigt, C. C., Fox, J. W., Hussell, D. J. T., & Schmaljohann, H. (2012). Cross-hemisphere migration of a 25 g songbird. *Biology Letters, 8*(4), 505–507. https://doi.org/10.1098/rsbl.2011.1223

Banks, W. P. (2009). *Encyclopedia of consciousness*. Academic Press.

Barrett, D., & McNamara, P. (2007). *The new science of dreaming*. Praeger.

Batterink, L. J., Oudiette, D., Reber, P. J., & Paller, K. A. (2014). Sleep facilitates learning a new linguistic rule. *Neuropsychologia, 65*, 169–179. https://doi.org/10.1016/j.neuropsychologia.2014.10.024

Berger, H. (1931). Über das elektrenkephalogramm des menschen—Dritte mitteilung. *Archiv für Psychiatrie und Nervenkrankheiten, 94*(1), 16–60. https://doi.org/10.1007/BF01835097

Berger, R. J., & Oswald, I. (1962). Eye movements during active and passive dreams. *Science, 137*(3530), 601. https://doi.org/10.1126/science.137.3530.601.a

Bernardi, G., Siclari, F., Yu, X., Zennig, C., Bellesi, M., Ricciardi, E., Cirelli, C., Ghilardi, M. F., Pietrini, P., & Tononi, G. (2015). Neural and behavioral correlates of extended training during sleep deprivation in humans: Evidence for local, task-specific effects. *Journal of Neuroscience, 35*(11), 4487–4500 https://doi.org/10.1523/JNEUROSCI.4567-14.2015

Berry, R. B., Quan, S., & Abreu, A.(2020). *The AASM manual for the scoring of sleep and associated events: Rules, terminology and technical specifications* (Version 2.6). American Academy of Sleep Medicine.

Bodizs, R. (2021). Theories on the functions of sleep. In C. Bassetti, W. McNicholas, T. Paunio, & P. Peigneux (Eds.), *Sleep medicine textbook* (2nd ed., 41–56). European Sleep Research Society.

Bódizs, R., Horváth, C. G., Szalárdy, O., Ujma, P. P., Simor, P., Gombos, F., Kovács, I., Genzel, L., & Dresler, M. (2021). Circadian modulation of human sleep spindle frequency. bioRxiv. https://doi.org/10.1101/2021.06.28.450146

Borbely, A. A. (1982). A two-process model of sleep regulation. *Human Neurobiology, 1*(3), 195–204.

Borbély, A. A., Daan, S., Wirz-Justice, A., & Deboer, T. (2016). The two-process model of sleep regulation: A reappraisal. *Journal of Sleep Research, 25*(2), 131–143. https://doi.org/10.1111/jsr.12371

Borbély, A. A., Hayaishi, O., Sejnowski, T. J., & Atman, J. S. (Eds.). (2000). *The regulation of sleep*. Human Frontier.

Born, J., & Wilhelm, I. (2012). System consolidation of memory during sleep. *Psychological Research, 76*(2), 192–203. https://doi.org/10.1007/s00426-011-0335-6

Braun, A. R., Balkin, T. J., Wesenten, N. J., Carson, R. E., Varga, M., Baldwin, P., Selbie, S., Belenky, G., & Herscovitch, P. (1997). Regional cerebral blood flow throughout the sleep–wake cycle. An H2(15)O PET study. *Brain, 120*(Pt. 7), 1173–1197. https://doi.org/10.1093/brain/120.7.1173

Buzsáki, G. (1998). Memory consolidation during sleep: A neurophysiological perspective. *Journal of Sleep Research*, 7(S1), 17–23. https://doi.org/10.1046/j.1365-2869.7.s1.3.x

Buzsáki, G. (2006). *Rhythms of the brain*. Oxford University Press. https://doi.org/10.1093/acprof:oso/9780195301069.001.0001

Calvo, J. M., Badillo, S., Morales-Ramirez, M., & Palacios-Salas, P. (1987). The role of the temporal lobe amygdala in ponto-geniculo-occipital activity and sleep organization in cats. *Brain Research, 403*(1), 22–30. https://doi.org/10.1016/0006-8993(87)90118-1

Capece, M. L., Efange, S. M., & Lydic, R. (1997). Vesicular acetylcholine transport inhibitor suppresses REM sleep. *Neuroreport, 8*(2), 481–484. https://doi.org/10.1097/00001756-199701200-00021

Cherasse, Y., Aritake, K., Oishi, Y., Kaushik, M. K., Korkutata, M., & Urade, Y. (2018). The leptomeninges produce prostaglandin D2 involved in sleep regulation in mice. *Frontiers in Cellular Neuroscience, 12*, Article 357. https://www.frontiersin.org/articles/10.3389/fncel.2018.00357

Chou, T. C., Bjorkum, A. A., Gaus, S. E., Lu, J., Scammell, T. E., & Saper, C. B. (2002). Afferents to the ventrolateral preoptic nucleus. *Journal of Neuroscience, 22*(3), 977–990. https://doi.org/10.1523/JNEUROSCI.22-03-00977.2002

Clawson, B. C., Durkin, J., & Aton, S. J. (2016). Form and function of sleep spindles across the lifespan. *Neural Plasticity, 2016*, Article 6936381. https://doi.org/10.1155/2016/6936381

Crowley, K., Trinder, J., Kim, Y., Carrington, M., & Colrain, I. M. (2002). The effects of normal aging on sleep spindle and K-complex production. *Clinical Neurophysiology, 113*(10), 1615–1622. https://doi.org/10.1016/S1388-2457(02)00237-7

Dang-Vu, T. T., Desseilles, M., Laureys, S., Degueldre, C., Perrin, F., Phillips, C., Maquet, P., & Peigneaux, P. (2005). Cerebral correlates of delta waves during non-REM sleep revisited. *NeuroImage, 28*(1), 14–21. https://doi.org/10.1016/j.neuroimage.2005.05.028

Dang-Vu, T. T., Schabus, M., Desseilles, M., Albouy, G., Boly, M., Darsaud, A., Gais, S., Rauchs, G., Sterpenich, V., Vandewalle, G., Carrier, J., Moonen, G., Balteau, E., Degueldre, C., Luxen, A., Phillips, C., & Maquet, P. (2008). Spontaneous neural activity during human slow wave sleep. *Proceedings of the National Academy of Sciences of the United States of America, 105*(39), 15160–15165. https://doi.org/10.1073/pnas.0801819105

Dang-Vu, T. T., Schabus, M., Desseilles, M., Sterpenich, V., Bonjean, M., & Maquet, P. (2010). Functional neuroimaging insights into the physiology of human sleep. *Sleep, 33*(12), 1589–1603. https://doi.org/10.1093/sleep/33.12.1589

Datta, S. (1997). Cellular basis of pontine ponto-geniculo-occipital wave generation and modulation. *Cellular and Molecular Neurobiology, 17*(3), 341–365. https://doi.org/10.1023/a:1026398402985

Datta, S., & Maclean, R. R. (2007). Neurobiological mechanisms for the regulation of mammalian sleep–wake behavior: Reinterpretation of historical evidence and inclusion of contemporary cellular and molecular evidence. *Neuroscience & Biobehavioral Reviews, 31*(5), 775–824. https://doi.org/10.1016/j.neubiorev.2007.02.004

Davis, H., Davis, P. A., Loomis, A. L., Harvey, E. N., & Hobart, G. (1937). Changes in human brain potentials during the onset of sleep. *Science, 86*(2237), 448–50. https://doi.org/10.1126/science.86.2237.448

De Gennaro, L., & Ferrara, M. (2003). Sleep spindles: An overview. *Sleep Medicine Reviews, 7*(5), 423–440. https://doi.org/10.1053/smrv.2002.0252

De Gennaro, L., Ferrara, M., & Bertini, M. (2000). Topographical distribution of spindles: Variations between and within NREM sleep cycles. *Sleep Research Online, 3*(4), 155–160.

DeLuca, W. V., Woodworth, B. K., Rimmer, C. C., Marra, P. P., Taylor, P. D., McFarland, K. P., Mackenzie, S. A., & Norris, D. R. (2015). Transoceanic migration by a 12 g songbird. *Biology Letters, 11*(4), Article 20141045. https://doi.org/10.1098/rsbl.2014.1045

Dickerson, L. W., Huang, A. H., Thumher, M. M., Nearing, B. D., & Verrier, R. L. (1993). Relationship between coronary hemodynamic changes and the phasic events of rapid eye movement sleep. *Sleep, 16*(6), 550–557. https://doi.org/10.1093/sleep/16.6.550

Durrant, S. J., Taylor, C., Cairney, S., & Lewis, P. A. (2011). Sleep-dependent consolidation of statistical learning. *Neuropsychologia, 49*(5), 1322–1331. https://doi.org/10.1016/j.neuropsychologia.2011.02.015

Eban-Rothschild, A. D., & Bloch, G. (2008). Differences in the sleep architecture of forager and young honeybees (*Apis mellifera*). *Journal of Experimental Biology, 211*(15), 2408–2416. https://doi.org/10.1242/jeb.016915

Economo, C. V. (1930). Sleep as a problem of localization. *Journal of Nervous and Mental Disease, 71*(3), 300–302. https://journals.lww.com/jonmd/Fulltext/1930/03000/SLEEP_AS_A_PROBLEM_OF_LOCALIZATION.1.aspx

Edwards, D., & Westerman, M. (1992). DNA–DNA hybridization and the position of leadbeater possum (*Gymnobelideus-leadbeateri* Mccoy) in the family Petauridae (Marsupialia, Diprotodontia). *Australian Journal of Zoology, 40*(6), 563–571. https://doi.org/10.1071/ZO9920563

Engel, A. K., Gerloff, C., Hilgetag, C. C., & Nolte, G. (2013). Intrinsic coupling modes: Multiscale interactions in ongoing brain activity. *Neuron, 80*(4), 867–886. https://doi.org/10.1016/j.neuron.2013.09.038

Fernandez, L. M. J., & Lüthi, A. (2020). Sleep spindles: Mechanisms and functions. *Physiological Reviews, 100*(2), 805–868. https://doi.org/10.1152/physrev.00042.2018

Ferrara, M., & De Gennaro, L. (2011). Going local: Insights from EEG and stereo-EEG studies of the human sleep–wake cycle. *Current Topics in Medicinal Chemistry, 11*(19), 2423–2437. https://doi.org/10.2174/156802611797470268

Fields, R. W. (1968). Vertebrate paleontology. *Journal of Mammalogy, 49*(1), 165–166. https://doi.org/10.2307/1377759

Fischer, S., Drosopoulos, S., Tsen, J., & Born, J. (2006). Implicit learning–explicit knowing: A role for sleep in memory system interaction. *Journal of Cognitive Neuroscience, 18*(3), 311–319.

Flanigan, W. F. J. (1973). Sleep and wakefulness in iguanid lizards, *Ctenosaura pectinata* and *Iguana iguana. Brain, Behavior and Evolution, 8*(6), 401–436. https://doi.org/10.1159/000124366

Flanigan, W. F. J., Knight, C. P., Hartse, K. M., & Rechtschaffen, A. (1974). Sleep and wakefulness in chelonian reptiles. I. The box turtle, *Terrapene carolina. Archives Italiennes de Biologie, 112*(3), 227–252.

Flanigan, W. F. J., Wilcox, R. H., & Rechtschaffen, A. (1973). The EEG and behavioral continuum of the crocodilian, *Caiman sclerops. Electroencephalography and Clinical Neurophysiology, 34*(5), 521–538. https://doi.org/10.1016/0013-4694(73)90069-2

Fort, P., Bassetti, C. L., & Luppi, P.-H. (2009). Alternating vigilance states: New insights regarding neuronal networks and mechanisms. *European Journal of Neuroscience, 29*(9), 1741–1753. https://doi.org/10.1111/j.1460-9568.2009.06722.x

Fraigne, J. J., Torontali, Z. A., Snow, M. B., & Peever, J. (2015). REM sleep at its core—Circuits, neurotransmitters, and pathophysiology. *Frontiers in Neurology*, 6, Article 123.

Freiberg, A. S. (2020). Why we sleep: A hypothesis for an ultimate or evolutionary origin for sleep and other physiological rhythms. *Journal of Circadian Rhythms, 18*(1), 1–5. https://doi.org/10.5334/jcr.189

Fuller, P. M., Saper, C. B., & Lu, J. (2007). The pontine REM switch: Past and present. *Journal of Physiology, 584*(3), 735–741. https://doi.org/10.1113/jphysiol.2007.140160

Gais, S., & Born, J. (2004). Declarative memory consolidation: Mechanisms acting during human sleep. *Learning & Memory, 11*(6), 679–685. https://doi.org/10.1101/lm.80504

Genzel, L., Kiefer, T., Renner, L., Wehrle, R., Kluge, M., Grözinger, M., Steiger, A., & Dresler, M. (2012). Sex and modulatory menstrual cycle effects on sleep related memory consolidation. *Psychoneuroendocrinology, 37*(7), 987–998. https://doi.org/10.1016/j.psyneuen.2011.11.006

Gosseries, O., Demertzi, A., Noirhomme, Q., Tshibanda, J., Boly, M., Op de Beeck, M., Hustinx, R., Maquet, P., Salmon, E., Moonen, G., Luxen, A., Laureys, S., & De Tiège, X. (2008). Functional neuroimaging (fMRI, PET and MEG): What do we measure? *Revue Medicale de Liege, 63*(5–6), 231–237.

Gvilia, I., Turner, A., McGinty, D., & Szymusiak, R. (2006). Preoptic area neurons and the homeostatic regulation of rapid eye movement sleep. *Journal of Neuroscience, 26*(11), 3037–3044. https://doi.org/10.1523/JNEUROSCI.4827-05.2006

Gvilia, I., Xu, F., McGinty, D., & Szymusiak, R. (2006). Homeostatic regulation of sleep: A role for preoptic area neurons. *Journal of Neuroscience, 26*(37), 9426–9433. https://doi.org/10.1523/JNEUROSCI.2012-06.2006

Happe, S., Anderer, P., Gruber, G., Klösch, G., Saletu, B., & Zeitlhofer, J. (2002). Scalp topography of the spontaneous K-complex and of delta-waves in human sleep. *Brain Topography, 15*(1), 43–49. https://doi.org/10.1023/A:1019992523246

Hartse, K. M. (1994). Sleep in insects and nonmammalian vertebrates. In M. H. Kryger, T. Roth, & W. C. Dement (Eds.), *Principles and practice of sleep medicine* (pp. 95–104). W. B. Saunders.

Hartse, K. M. (2011). *The phylogeny of sleep* (3rd ed.). Elsevier.

Hobson, J. A., McCarley, R. W., & Wyzinski, P. W. (1975). Sleep cycle oscillation: Reciprocal discharge by two brainstem neuronal groups. *Science, 189*(4196), 55–58. https://doi.org/10.1126/science.1094539

Hung, C.-S., Sarasso, S., Ferrarelli, F., Riedner, B., Ghilardi, M. F., Cirelli, C., & Tononi, G. (2013). Local experience-dependent changes in the wake EEG after prolonged wakefulness. *Sleep, 36*(1), 59–72. https://doi.org/10.5665/sleep.2302

Ioannides, A. A., Corsi-Cabrera, M., Fenwick, P. B. C., del Rio Portilla, Y., Laskaris, N. A., Khurshudyan, A., Theofilou, D., Shibata, T., Uchida, S., Nakabayashi, T., & Kostopoulos, G. K. (2004). MEG tomography of human cortex and brainstem activity in waking and REM sleep saccades. *Cerebral Cortex, 14*(1), 56–72. https://doi.org/10.1093/cercor/bhg091

Jha, V. M., & Jha, S. K. (2020). Sleep: Evolutionary and adaptive changes in birds and mammals. In V. M. Jha & S. K. Jha (Eds.), *Sleep: Evolution and functions* (pp. 37–59). Springer.

Jones, S. G., Vyazovskiy, V. V., Cirelli, C., Tononi, G., & Benca, R. M. (2008). Homeostatic regulation of sleep in the white-crowned sparrow (*Zonotrichia leucophrys gambelii*). *BMC Neuroscience, 9*(1), Article 47. https://doi.org/10.1186/1471-2202-9-47

Jouvet, M., Michel, F., & Courjon, J. (1959). On a stage of rapid cerebral electrical activity in the course of physiological sleep. *Comptes Rendus des Seances de la Société de Biologie et de ses Filiales, 153*, 1024–1028.

Kajimura, N., Uchiyama, M., Takayama, Y., Uchida, S., Uema, T., Kato, M., Sekimoto, M., Watanabe, T., Nakajima, T., Horikoshi, S., Ogawa, K., Nishikawa, M., Hiroki, M., Kudo, Y., Matsuda, H., Okawa, M., & Takahashi, K. (1999). Activity of midbrain reticular formation and neocortex during the progression of human non-rapid eye movement sleep. *Journal of Neuroscience, 19*(22), 10065–10073. https://doi.org/10.1523/JNEUROSCI.19-22-10065.1999

Kelly, M. L., Collin, S. P., Hemmi, J. M., & Lesku, J. A. (2019). Evidence for sleep in sharks and rays: Behavioural, physiological, and evolutionary considerations. *Brain, Behavior and Evolution, 94*(1–4), 37–50. https://doi.org/10.1159/000504123

Klaassen, R. H. G., Alerstam, T., Carlsson, P., Fox, J. W., & Lindström, A. (2011). Great flights by great snipes: Long and fast non-stop migration over benign habitats. *Biology Letters, 7*(6), 833–835. https://doi.org/10.1098/rsbl.2011.0343

Klein, B. A., Olzsowy, K. M., Klein, A., Saunders, K. M., & Seeley, T. D. (2008). Caste-dependent sleep of worker honey bees. *Journal of Experimental Biology, 211*, 3028–3040.

Klinzing, J. G., Mölle, M., Weber, F., Supp, G., Hipp, J. F., Engel, A. K., & Born, J. (2016). Spindle activity phase-locked to sleep slow oscillations. *NeuroImage, 134*, 607–616. https://doi.org/10.1016/j.neuroimage.2016.04.031

Kremien, M., Shavit, U., Mass, T., & Genin, A. (2013). Benefit of pulsation in soft corals. *Proceedings of the National Academy of Sciences of the United States of America, 110*(22), 8978–8983. https://doi.org/10.1073/pnas.1301826110

Krueger, J. M., Huang, Y. H., Rector, D. M., & Buysse, D. J. (2013). Sleep: A synchrony of cell activity-driven small network states. *European Journal of Neuroscience*, *38*(2), 2199–2209. https://doi.org/10.1111/ejn.12238

Krueger, J. M., & Obal, F. J. (2003). Sleep function. *Frontiers in Bioscience*, *8*, 511–519. https://doi.org/10.2741/1031

Krueger, J. M., Rector, D. M., Roy, S., Van Dongen, H., Belenky, G., & Panksepp, J. (2008). Sleep as a fundamental property of neuronal assemblies. *Nature Reviews Neuroscience*, *9*(12), 910–919.

Leong, C. W. Y., Leow, J. W. S., Grunstein, R. R., Naismith, S. L., Teh, J. Z., D'Rozario, A. L., & Saini, B. (2022). A systematic scoping review of the effects of central nervous system active drugs on sleep spindles and sleep-dependent memory consolidation. *Sleep Medicine Reviews*, *62*, Article 101605. https://doi.org/10.1016/j.smrv.2022.101605

Lesku, J. A., Rattenborg, N. C., Valcu, M., Vyssotski, A. L., Kuhn, S., Kuemmeth, F., Heidrich, W., & Kempenaers, B. (2012). Adaptive sleep loss in polygynous pectoral sandpipers. *Science*, *337*(6102), 1654–1658. https://doi.org/10.1126/science.1220939

Leung, L. C., Wang, G. X., Madelaine, R., Skariah, G., Kawakami, K., Deisseroth, K., Urban, A. E., & Mourrain, P. (2019). Neural signatures of sleep in zebrafish. *Nature*, *571*(7764), 198–204. https://doi.org/10.1038/s41586-019-1336-7

Libourel, P.-A., Barrillot, B., Arthaud, S., Massot, B., Morel, A.-L., Beuf, O., Herrel, A., & Luppi, P.-H. (2018). Partial homologies between sleep states in lizards, mammals, and birds suggest a complex evolution of sleep states in amniotes. *PLOS Biology*, *16*(10), Article e2005982. https://doi.org/10.1371/journal.pbio.2005982

Libourel, P.-A., & Herrel, A. (2016). Sleep in amphibians and reptiles: A review and a preliminary analysis of evolutionary patterns. *Biological Reviews*, *91*(3), 833–866. https://doi.org/10.1111/brv.12197

Liechti, F., Witvliet, W., Weber, R., & Bächler, E. (2013). First evidence of a 200-day non-stop flight in a bird. *Nature Communications*, *4*(1), Article 2554. https://doi.org/10.1038/ncomms3554

Low, P. S., Shank, S. S., Sejnowski, T. J., & Margoliash, D. (2008). Mammalian-like features of sleep structure in zebra finches. *Proceedings of the National Academy of Sciences of the United States of America*, *105*(26), 9081–9086. https://doi.org/10.1073/pnas.0703452105

Luppi, P.-H., Adamantidis, A., & Fort, P. (2021). The neurophysiology and neurobiology of paradoxical (REM) sleep. In C. Bassetti, W. McNicholas, T. Paunio, & P. Peigneux (Eds.), *European sleep medicine textbook* (2nd ed., pp. 15–27). European Sleep Research Society.

Lyamin, O., Pryaslova, J., Lance, V., & Siegel, J. (2005). Continuous activity in cetaceans after birth. *Nature*, *435*(7046), Article 1177. https://doi.org/10.1038/4351177a

Lyamin, O. I., Kosenko, P. O., Korneva, S. M., Vyssotski, A. L., Mukhametov, L. M., & Siegel, J. M. (2018). Fur seals suppress REM sleep for very long periods without subsequent rebound. *Current Biology*, *28*(12), 2000–2005.e2. https://doi.org/10.1016/j.cub.2018.05.022

Lyamin, O. I., Manger, P. R., Ridgway, S. H., Mukhametov, L. M., & Siegel, J. M. (2008). Cetacean sleep: An unusual form of mammalian sleep. *Neuroscience & Biobehavioral Reviews*, *32*(8), 1451–1484. https://doi.org/10.1016/j.neubiorev.2008.05.023

Lyamin, O. I., Mukhametov, L. M., & Siegel, J. M. (2004). Relationship between sleep and eye state in cetaceans and pinnipeds. *Archives Italiennes de Biologie*, 142(4), 557–568.

Lyamin, O. I., & Siegel, J. M. (2019). Sleep in aquatic mammals. *Handbook of Behavioral Neuroscience*, *30*, 375–393. https://doi.org/10.1016/b978-0-12-813743-7.00025-6

Magnin, M., Rey, M., Bastuji, H., Guillemant, P., Mauguière, F., & Garcia-Larrea, L. (2010). Thalamic deactivation at sleep onset precedes that of the cerebral cortex in humans. *Proceedings of the National Academy of Sciences of the United States of America*, *107*(8), 3829–3833. https://doi.org/10.1073/pnas.0909710107

Maquet, P., Laureys, S., Peigneux, P., Fuchs, S., Petiau, C., Phillips, C., Aerts, J., Del Fiore, G., Degueldre, C., Meulemans, T., Luxen, A., Franck, G., Van Der Linden, M., Smith, C., & Cleeremans, A. (2000). Experience-dependent changes in cerebral activation during human REM sleep. *Nature Neuroscience*, 3(8), 831–836. https://doi.org/10.1038/77744

Maquet, P., Péters, J.-M., Aerts, J., Delfiore, G., Degueldre, C., Luxen, A., & Franck, G. (1996). Functional neuroanatomy of human rapid-eye-movement sleep and dreaming. *Nature*, *383*(6596), 163–166. https://doi.org/10.1038/383163a0

Maquet, P., Ruby, P., Maudoux, A., Albouy, G., Sterpenich, V., Dang-Vu, T., Desseilles, M., Boly, M., Perrin, F., Peigneux, P., & Laureys, S. (2005). Human cognition during REM sleep and the activity profile within frontal and parietal cortices: a reappraisal of functional neuroimaging data. *Progress in Brain Research, 150*, 219–227. https://doi.org/10.1016/S0079-6123(05)50016-5

Marzano, C., De Simoni, E., Tempesta, D., Ferrara, M., & De Gennaro, L. (2011). Sleep deprivation suppresses the increase of rapid eye movement density across sleep cycles. *Journal of Sleep Research, 20*(3), 386–394. https://doi.org/10.1111/j.1365-2869.2010.00886.x

Marzano, C., Moroni, F., Gorgoni, M., Nobili, L., Ferrara, M., & De Gennaro, L. (2013). How we fall asleep: Regional and temporal differences in electroencephalographic synchronization at sleep onset. *Sleep Medicine, 14*(11), 1112–1122. https://doi.org/10.1016/j.sleep.2013.05.021

Mueller, T., Dong, Z., Berberoglu, M. A., & Guo, S. (2011). The dorsal pallium in zebrafish, *Danio rerio* (Cyprinidae, Teleostei). *Brain Research, 1381*, 95–105. https://doi.org/10.1016/j.brainres.2010.12.089

Nath, R. D., Bedbrook, C. N., Abrams, M. J., Basinger, T., Bois, J. S., Prober, D. A., Sternberg, P. W., Gradinaru, V., & Goentoro, L. (2017). The jellyfish *Cassiopea* exhibits a sleep-like state. *Current Biology, 27*(19), 2984–2990.e3. https://doi.org/10.1016/j.cub.2017.08.014

Ngo, H. V. V., Miedema, A., Faude, I., Martinetz, T., Mölle, M., & Born, J. (2015). Driving sleep slow oscillations by auditory closed-loop stimulation—A self-limiting process. *Journal of Neuroscience, 35*(17), 6630–6638. https://doi.org/10.1523/JNEUROSCI.3133-14.2015

Nir, Y., Andrillon, T., Marmelshtein, A., Suthana, N., Cirelli, C., Tononi, G., & Fried, I. (2017). Selective neuronal lapses precede human cognitive lapses following sleep deprivation. *Nature Medicine, 23*(12), 1474–1480. https://doi.org/10.1038/nm.4433

Nobili, L., Ferrara, M., Moroni, F., De Gennaro, L., Lo Russo, G., Campus, C., Cardinale, F., & De Carli, F. (2011). Dissociated wake-like and sleep-like electro-cortical activity during sleep. *NeuroImage, 58*(2), 612–619. https://doi.org/10.1016/j.neuroimage.2011.06.032

Nofzinger, E. A., Mintun, M. A., Wiseman, M., Kupfer, D. J., & Moore, R. Y. (1997). Forebrain activation in REM sleep: An FDG PET study. *Brain Research, 770*(1–2), 192–201. https://doi.org/10.1016/s0006-8993(97)00807-x

Paré, D., Steriade, M., Deschênes, M., & Oakson, G. (1987). Physiological characteristics of anterior thalamic nuclei, a group devoid of inputs from reticular thalamic nucleus. *Journal of Neurophysiology, 57*(6), 1669–1685. https://doi.org/10.1152/jn.1987.57.6.1669

Peigneux, P., Laureys, S., Delbeuck, X., & Maquet, P. (2001). Sleeping brain, learning brain: The role of sleep for memory systems. *NeuroReport, 12*, A111–A124. https://doi.org/10.1097/00001756-200112210-00001

Peigneux, P., Laureys, S., Fuchs, S., Delbeuck, X., Degueldre, C., Aerts, J., Delfiore, G., Luxen, A., & Maquet, P. (2001). Generation of rapid eye movements during paradoxical sleep in humans. *NeuroImage, 14*(3), 701–708. https://doi.org/10.1006/nimg.2001.0874

Peigneux, P., Laureys, S., Fuchs, S., Destrebecqz, A., Collette, F., Delbeuck, X., Phillips, C., Aerts, J., Del Fiore, G., Degueldre, C., Luxen, A., Cleeremans, A., & Maquet, P. (2003). Learned material content and acquisition level modulate cerebral reactivation during posttraining rapid-eye-movements sleep. *NeuroImage, 20*(1), 125–134. https://doi.org/10.1016/s1053-8119(03)00278-7

Peyrethon, J., & Dusan-Peyrethon, D. (1969). Etude polygraphique due cycle veille—Sommeil chez trois genres de reptiles. *Comptes Rendus des Séances de la Société de Biologie, 163*, 181–186.

Pivik, R. T. (1991). Tonic states and phasic events in relation to sleep mentation. In A. M. Arkin, J. S. Antrobus, & S. J. Ellman (Eds.), *The mind in sleep: Psychology and psychophysiology* (2nd ed., pp. 214–247). John Wiley & Sons.

Plamberger, C. P., Van Weijk, H. E., Kerschbaum, H., Pletzer, B. A., Gruber, G., Oberascher, K., Dresler, M., Hahn, M. A., & Hoedlmoser, K. (2021). Impact of menstrual cycle phase and oral contraceptives on sleep and overnight memory consolidation. *Journal of Sleep Research, 30*(4), Article e13239. https://doi.org/10.1111/jsr.13239

Purves, D., & Williams, S. M. (2001). *Neuroscience* (2nd ed.). Sinauer Associates.

Quercia, A., Zappasodi, F., Committeri, G., & Ferrara, M. (2018). Local use-dependent sleep in wakefulness links performance errors to learning. *Frontiers in Human Neuroscience*, 12, Article 122. https://doi.org/10.3389/fnhum.2018.00122

Rasch, B., & Born, J. (2013). About sleep's role in memory. *Physiological Reviews, 93*, 681–766. https://doi.org/10.1152/physrev.00032.2012

Rattenborg, N. C. (2006). Evolution of slow-wave sleep and palliopallial connectivity in mammals and birds: A hypothesis. *Brain Research Bulletin, 69*(1), 20–29. https://doi.org/10.1016/j.brainresbull.2005.11.002

Rattenborg, N. C., Lima, S. L., & Amlaner, C. J. (1999). Facultative control of avian unihemispheric sleep under the risk of predation. *Behavioural Brain Research, 105*(2), 163–172. https://doi.org/10.1016/s0166-4328(99)00070-4

Rattenborg, N. C., & Martinez-Gonzalez, D. (2015). Avian versus mammalian sleep: The fruits of comparing apples and oranges. *Current Sleep Medicine Reports, 1*(1), 55–63. https://doi.org/10.1007/s40675-014-0001-9

Rattenborg, N. C., Voirin, B., Cruz, S. M., Tisdale, R., Dell'Omo, G., Lipp, H.-P., Wikelski, M., & Vyssotski, A. L. (2016). Evidence that birds sleep in mid-flight. *Nature Communications, 7*(1), Article 12468. https://doi.org/10.1038/ncomms12468

Rauchs, G., Desgranges, B., Foret, J., & Eustache, F. (2005). The relationships between memory systems and sleep stages. *Journal of Sleep Research, 14*(2), 123–140. https://doi.org/10.1111/j.1365-2869.2005.00450.x

Rechtschaffen, A., & Kales, A. (Eds.). (1968). *A manual of standardized terminology, techniques and scoring system for sleep stages of human subjects.* US National Institute of Neurological Diseases and Blindness, Neurological Information Network.

Rezek, I., & Roberts, S. (2005). Ensemble hidden Markov models with extended observation densities for biosignal analysis. In D. Husmeier, R. Dybowski, & S. Roberts (Eds.), *Probabilistic modeling in bioinformatics and medical informatics. Advanced information and knowledge processing* (pp. 419–450). Springer.

Ribeiro, S., Shi, X., Engelhard, M., Zhou, Y., Zhang, H., Gervasoni, D., Lin, S.-C., Wada, K., Lemos, N. A. M., & Nicolelis, M. A. L. (2007). Novel experience induces persistent sleep-dependent plasticity in the cortex but not in the hippocampus. *Frontiers in Neuroscience, 1*, 43–55. https://www.frontiersin.org/articles/10.3389/neuro.01.1.1.003.2007

Rößler, D. C., Kim, K., De Agrò, M., Jordan, A., Galizia, C. G., & Shamble, P. S. (2022). Regularly occurring bouts of retinal movements suggest an REM sleep–like state in jumping spiders. *Proceedings of the National Academy of Sciences of the United States of America, 119*(33), Article e2204754119. https://doi.org/10.1073/pnas.2204754119

Sakai, K. (1988). Executive mechanisms of paradoxical sleep. *Archives Italiennes de Biologie, 126*(4), 239–257.

Saper, C. B., Fuller, P. M., Pedersen, N. P., Lu, J., & Scammell, T. E. (2010). Sleep state switching. *Neuron, 68*(6), 1023–1042. https://doi.org/10.1016/j.neuron.2010.11.032

Sarasso, S., Proserpio, P., Pigorini, A., Moroni, F., Ferrara, M., De Gennaro, L., De Carli, F., Lo Russo, G., Massimini, M., & Nobili, L. (2014). Hippocampal sleep spindles preceding neocortical sleep onset in humans. *NeuroImage, 86*, 425–432. https://doi.org/10.1016/j.neuroimage.2013.10.031

Schabus, M., Dang-Vu, T. T., Albouy, G., Balteau, E., Boly, M., Carrier, J., Darsaud, A., Degueldre, C., Desseilles, M., Gais, S., Phillips, C., Rauchs, G., Schnakers, C., Sterpenich, V., Vandewalle, G., Luxen, A., & Maquet, P. (2007). Hemodynamic cerebral correlates of sleep spindles during human non-rapid eye movement sleep," *Proceedings of the National Academy of Sciences of the United States of America, 104*(32), 13164–13169. https://doi.org/10.1073/pnas.0703084104

Schmidt, M. H. (2014). The energy allocation function of sleep: A unifying theory of sleep, torpor, and continuous wakefulness. *Neuroscience & Biobehavioral Reviews, 47*, 122–153. https://doi.org/10.1016/j.neubiorev.2014.08.001

Schomer, D. L., Lopes da Silva, F. H., & Niedermeyer, E. (2010). *Electroencephalography: Basic principles, clinical applications, and related fields.* Lippincott.

Shein-Idelson, M., Ondracek, J. M., Liaw, H.-P., Reiter, S., & Laurent, G. (2016). Slow waves, sharp waves, ripples, and REM in sleeping dragons. *Science, 352*(6285), 590–595. https://doi.org/10.1126/science.aaf3621

Shurley, T. G., Serafetinides, E. A., Brooks, R. E., Elsner, R., & Kenney, D. W. (1969). Sleep in cetaceans: I. The pilot whale, *Globicephala scammoni. Psychophysiology, 6*, 230.

Siclari, F., Baird, B., Perogamvros, L., Bernardi, G., LaRocque, J. J., Riedner, B., Boly, M., Postle, B. R., & Tononi, G. (2017). The neural correlates of dreaming. *Nature Neuroscience, 20*(6), 872–878. https://doi.org/10.1038/nn.4545

Siclari, F., & Tononi, G. (2017). Local aspects of sleep and wakefulness. *Current Opinion in Neurobiology, 44*, 222–227. https://doi.org/10.1016/j.conb.2017.05.008

Siegel, J. M. (2004). The neurotransmitters of sleep. *Journal of Clinical Psychiatry, 65*(S16), 4–7.

Siegel, J. M. (2005). Clues to the functions of mammalian sleep. *Nature, 437*(7063), 1264–1271. https://doi.org/10.1038/nature04285

Siegel, J. M. (2022). Sleep function: An evolutionary perspective. *Lancet Neurology*, *21*(10), 937–946. https://doi.org/10.1016/S1474-4422(22)00210-1

Siegel, J. M., Manger, P. R., Nienhuis, R., Fahringer, H. M., & Pettigrew, J. D. (1996). The echidna *Tachyglossus aculeatus* combines REM and non-REM aspects in a single sleep state: Implications for the evolution of sleep. *Journal of Neuroscience*, *16*(10), 3500–3506. https://doi.org/10.1523/JNEUROSCI.16-10-03500.1996

Siegel, J. M., Manger, P. R., Nienhuis, R., Fahringer, H. M., Shalita, T., & Pettigrew, J. D. (1999). Sleep in the platypus. *Neuroscience*, *91*(1), 391–400. https://doi.org/10.1016/s0306-4522(98)00588-0

Simor, P., van der Wijk, G., Nobili, L., & Peigneux, P. (2020). The microstructure of REM sleep: Why phasic and tonic? *Sleep Medicine Reviews*, *52*, Article 101305. https://doi.org/10.1016/j.smrv.2020.101305

Song, C., Boly, M., Tagliazucchi, E., Laufs, H., & Tononi, G. (2022). fMRI spectral signatures of sleep. *Proceedings of the National Academy of Sciences of the United States of America*, *119*(30), Article e2016732119. https://doi.org/10.1073/pnas.2016732119

Spooner, C. E., & Winters, W. D. (1965). Evidence for a direct action of monamines on the chick central nervous system. *Experientia*, *21*(5), 256–258. https://doi.org/10.1007/BF02297010

Steriade, M. (2006). Grouping of brain rhythms in corticothalamic systems. *Neuroscience*, *137*(4), 1087–1106. https://doi.org/10.1016/j.neuroscience.2005.10.029

Steriade, M., & Amzica, F. (1998). Coalescence of sleep rhythms and their chronology in corticothalamic networks. *Sleep Research Online*, *1*(1), 1–10.

Steriade, M., Contreras, D., Curró Dossi, R., & Nuñez, A. (1993). The slow (<1 Hz) oscillation in reticular thalamic and thalamocortical neurons: Scenario of sleep rhythm generation in interacting thalamic and neocortical networks. *Journal of Neuroscience*, *13*(8), 3284–3299. https://doi.org/10.1523/JNEUROSCI.13-08-03284.1993

Steriade, M., & McCarley, R. W. (1990). *Brainstem control of wakefulness and sleep*. Springer.

Stevner, A. B., Vidaurre, D., Cabral, J., Rapuano, K., Nielsen, S. F. V., Tagliazucchi, E., Laufs, H., Vuust, P., Deco, G., Woolrich, M. W., Van Someren, E., & Kringelbach, M. L. (2019). Discovery of key whole-brain transitions and dynamics during human wakefulness and non-REM sleep. *Nature Communications*, *10*(1), Article 1035. https://doi.org/10.1038/s41467-019-08934-3

Strauss, M., Griffon, L., Van Beers, P., Elbaz, M., Bouziotis, J., Sauvet, F., Chennaoui, M., Léger, D., & Peigneux, P. (2022). Order matters: Sleep spindles contribute to memory consolidation only when followed by rapid-eye-movement sleep. *Sleep*, *45*(4), Article zsac022. https://doi.org/10.1093/sleep/zsac022

Stuart, K., & Conduit, R. (2009). Auditory inhibition of rapid eye movements and dream recall from REM sleep. *Sleep*, *32*(3), 399–408. https://doi.org/10.1093/sleep/32.3.399

Szymusiak, R., Steininger, T., Alam, N., & McGinty, D. (2001). Preoptic area sleep-regulating mechanisms. *Archives Italiennes de Biologie*, *139*(1–2), 77–92.

Takahara, M., Nittono, H., & Hori, T. (2002). Comparison of the event-related potentials between tonic and phasic periods of rapid eye movement sleep. *Psychiatry and Clinical Neurosciences*, *56*(3), 257–258. https://doi.org/10.1046/j.1440-1819.2002.00999.x

Takahara, M., Nittono, H., & Hori, T. (2006). Effect of voluntary attention on auditory processing during REM sleep. *Sleep*, *29*(7), 975–982. https://doi.org/10.1093/sleep/29.7.975

Tobler, I., & Borbély, A. A. (1985). Effect of rest deprivation on motor activity of fish. *Journal of Comparative Physiology A*, *157*(6), 817–822. https://doi.org/10.1007/BF01350078

Ueda, K., Nittono, H., Hayashi, M., & Hori, T. (2001). Spatiotemporal changes of slow wave activities before and after 14 Hz/12 Hz sleep spindles during stage 2 sleep. *Psychiatry and Clinical Neurosciences*, *55*(3), 183–184. https://doi.org/10.1046/j.1440-1819.2001.00817.x

Urakami, Y., Ioannides, A. A., & Kostopoulos, G. K. (2012). Sleep spindles—As a biomarker of brain function and plasticity. In I. M. Ajeena (Ed.), *Advances in clinical neurophysiology* (chap. 4). IntechOpen.

Uschakov, A., Gong, H., McGinty, D., & Szymusiak, R. (2007). Efferent projections from the median preoptic nucleus to sleep- and arousal-regulatory nuclei in the rat brain. *Neuroanatomy*, *150*(1), 104–120. https://doi.org/10.1016/j.neuroscience.2007.05.055

van Alphen, B., Semenza, E. R., Yap, M., van Swinderen, B., & Allada, R. (2022). A deep sleep stage in *Drosophila* with a functional role in waste clearance. *Science Advances*, 7(4), Article eabc2999. https://doi.org/10.1126/sciadv.abc2999

Vyazovskiy, V. V., Olcese, U., Hanlon, E. C., Nir, Y., Cirelli, C., & Tononi, G. (2011). Local sleep in awake rats. *Nature*, *472*(7344), 443–447.

Wagner, U., Gais, S., Haider, H., Verleger, R., & Born, J. (2004). Sleep inspires insight. *Nature, 427*(6972), 352–355. https://doi.org/10.1038/nature02223

Weimerskirch, H., Bishop, C., Jeanniard-du-Dot, T., Prudor, A., & Sachs, G. (2016). Frigate birds track atmospheric conditions over months-long transoceanic flights. *Science, 353*(6294), 74–78. https://doi.org/10.1126/science.aaf4374

White, E. L., & Keller, A. (1989). *Cortical circuits: Synaptic organization of the cerebral cortex—Structure, function, and theory*. Springer.

Yokogawa, T., Marin, W., Faraco, J., Pézeron, G., Appelbaum, L., Zhang, J., Rosa, F., Mourrain, P., & Mignot, E. (2007). Characterization of sleep in zebrafish and insomnia in hypocretin receptor mutants. *PLOS Biology, 5*(10), Article e277. https://doi.org/10.1371/journal.pbio.0050277

Zwaka, H., Bartels, R., Gora, J., Franck, V., Culo, A., Götsch, M., & Menzel, R. (2015). Context odor presentation during sleep enhances memory in honeybees. *Current Biology, 25*(21), 2869–2874. https://doi.org/10.1016/j.cub.2015.09.069

CHAPTER

2

The Regulation of Human Sleep and Wakefulness: Sleep Homeostasis and Circadian Rhythmicity

Alpar S. Lazar *and* Derk-Jan Dijk

Abstract

The alternation of sleep and wakefulness is a major determinant of the structure and quality of life. The sleep–wake cycle is regulated by a fine-tuned balance between two physiological processes: sleep homeostasis, which measures sleep debt, and circadian rhythmicity, which determines the optimal internal (biological) time for sleep and wakefulness. Sleep homeostasis and circadian rhythmicity together influence many aspects of sleep, such as the time it takes to fall asleep, the timing of awakening and the interruptions of sleep, as well as the duration of rapid-eye-movement sleep, slow-wave sleep, and specific brainwaves during sleep, such as sleep spindles. Alterations in the balance between sleep homeostasis and circadian rhythmicity contribute to sleep phenotypes such as morningness–eveningness and short–long sleepers as well as sleep disturbances. Emerging insights into the environmental, behavioral, physiological, neurochemical, and molecular-genetic determinants of sleep homeostasis and circadian rhythmicity provide new avenues for the understanding and improvement of the sleep–wake cycle.

Key Words: sleep physiology, circadian rhythmicity, sleep homeostasis, slow-wave sleep, REM sleep, sleep spindle, sleep deprivation, melatonin, photoreception, chronotype

Assessment of Sleep Physiology

The regular alternation of sleep and wakefulness is a defining characteristic of our daily lives. We regain consciousness when we wake up in the morning, go about our work and social activities, and then retire for sleep, during which we are unconscious for most of the time except for when we dream. Most of us will have no serious complaints about our sleep–wake cycle, except maybe that we don't get enough sleep, have the occasional bad night's sleep, or wish there were more hours in the day. We attribute functions to sleep when we blame the bad mood, lack of concentration, or an embarrassing lapse of memory on insufficient sleep during the previous night but probably do not subscribe to any comprehensive theory on sleep's contribution to brain function. Sleep physiologists have provided a detailed description of the changes in brain activity as well as changes in hormones and peripheral physiology during sleep. Sleep and circadian physiologists have uncovered some of the mechanisms underlying the alternation of sleep and wakefulness and provided clues about the functions of sleep—for the brain and the body. These insights on the mechanisms underlying normal sleep–wake regulation have also provided indications about the putative mechanisms underlying sleep disorders.

Within the context of the regulation of the sleep–wake cycle, nocturnal sleep is not viewed in isolation, but it is rather viewed within the context of circadian rhythmicity, that is, all the rhythms that characterize human physiology and are synchronized to the rhythms in the environment. Nocturnal sleep is also viewed as part of the 24-hour day. It can be seen as a response to the duration and experiences of the previous wake period. Finally, nocturnal sleep can be viewed within the context of the subsequent wake episode. Nocturnal sleep may affect our behavior the next day, and the demands of the next waking period may also affect the quality and duration of our sleep. We will first provide an overview of the phenomenology of sleep and wakefulness.

The Three Vigilance States (Wakefulness, Non–Rapid-Eye-Movement Sleep, Rapid-Eye-Movement Sleep)

The physiology of sleep can be assessed by polysomnography (PSG), which is the simultaneous recording of many physiological variables. Recordings of the patterns of electrical activity of the brain by placing electrodes at the surface of the scalp (electroencephalogram), recordings of the tone of muscles (electromyogram [EMG]), recordings of the movements of the eyes (electrooculogram), respiration, and the electrocardiogram reveal the changes that take place in the brain and body when we transition from wakefulness to sleep. During wakefulness, the eyes are open and show fast saccadic movements while tracking objects. When we lie down and close our eyes, these rapid eye movements give way to slow, rolling eye movements, indicating the lack of focus on objects in the visual field. At the same time, the tone of skeletal muscles drops and high-frequency, low-amplitude EEG oscillations give way to EEG oscillations that are characteristic for drowsiness and sleep. Beta waves (20–40-Hz oscillations) subside, and alpha waves (8–12-Hz oscillations) appear. These then give way to theta waves (4.5–8 Hz); K-complexes, which are isolated sharp, negative EEG deflections; sleep spindles (12–15-Hz, 0.5–2-second-long spindle trains); and slow waves (0–4-Hz, large-amplitude oscillations, also called *slow-wave activity* [SWA]; see Figure 2.1).

The EEG becomes more and more dominated by slow waves, and throughout these periods of sleep the eyes are not moving. This phase of sleep is referred to as *non-rapid-eye-movement* (NREM) sleep, during which EEG activity transits from superficial N1 and N2 stages to N3 or slow-wave sleep (SWS). In adults, depending on their age (Ohayon et al., 2004), after an average of 60–90 minutes, the EEG reverts abruptly to a pattern similar to the transition stage between wakefulness and sleep. Low-amplitude theta-like waves with the occasional alpha train now make up the EEG trace. Muscle tone remains but is

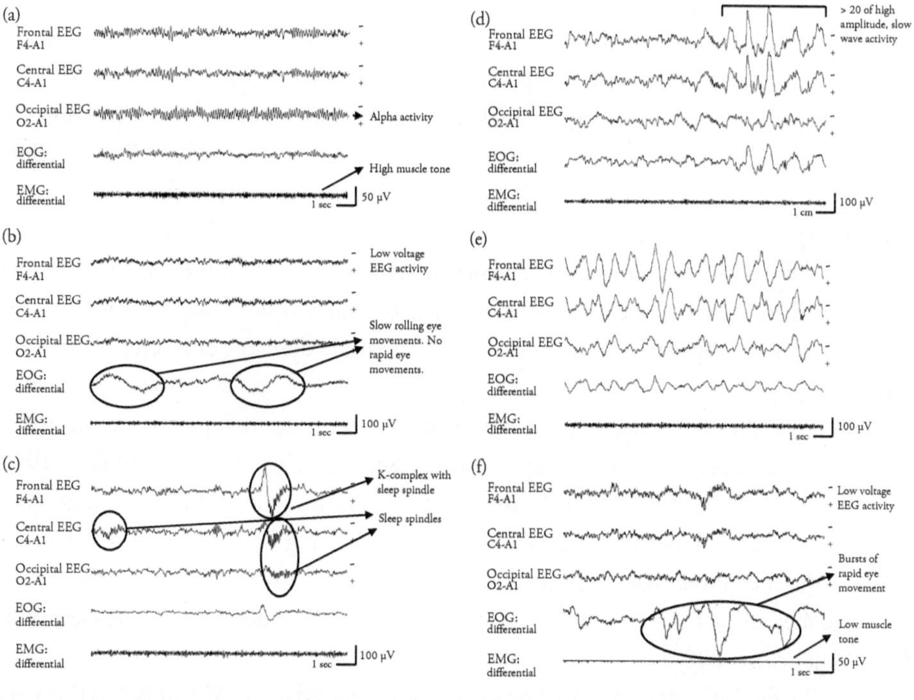

Figure 2.1 Polysomnographic recordings of wakefulness and the stages of sleep

Note. Panel A: Wakefulness. Panel B: Non-rapid-eye-movement (NREM) Stage 1 (N1). Panel C: NREM Stage 2 (N2). Panels D and E: Slow-wave sleep (N3). Panel F: REM sleep. Recordings were made in a 23-year-old healthy female. EEG = electroencephalogram; EMG = electromyogram. EOG = electro-oculogram.

very low—virtually absent. The eyes now display rapid eye movements, and this is why this sleep stage is referred to as *rapid eye movement* (REM). It is also referred to as *paradoxical sleep* to indicate that while the EEG patterns appear activated similar to wake, the individual is asleep. Characterization of NREM, REM, and wakefulness by the analysis of numerous physiological variables and their interrelations indicates that these are truly different states; and they are sometimes referred to as the *three vigilance states* or the *three states of being*. Coma and anesthesia are also considered states that are different from the normal physiological states and will not be considered here. Understanding the alternation between wakefulness, NREM, and REM sleep and their regulation in response to changes in the time allowed for any of them (i.e., sleep deprivation and extension, as well as the interaction with endogenous circadian rhythmicity, clocks that continue to tick even in the absence of external time cues or behavioral cycles) has been the aim of many scientific investigations. In these investigations, sleep is quantified in a standard manner, which we will describe next.

Characteristics of Sleep in Good Sleepers

The progression in the changes of the EEG and sleep stages in the course of a sleep episode can be quantified by visual inspection of consecutive 30-second epochs of these PSG traces or by computer-assisted signal analyses such as the fast Fourier transform or other methods. This latter method will return the EEG power spectral density, allowing estimation of the amount of EEG signal for each frequency bin. For example, the dominant spectral peak in the delta range (0.5–4 Hz) for SWS, in the alpha range (8–10 Hz) for wake, and in the sigma or sleep spindle range (11–16 Hz) for NREM 2 (Figure 2.2A). The distribution of EEG power along the frequency scale changes throughout the night. A graph of sleep stages and a spectrogram reveal the dynamic character of sleep (see Figure 2.2B).

After the lights are turned off, it takes the good sleeper on average 10–15 minutes to reach Stage 1 and several more minutes to reach Stage 2 (Carskadon & Dement, 1996; Ohayon et al., 2004). When asked in the morning how long it took to fall asleep, good sleepers will report an average of 15–30 minutes, suggesting that the onset of Stage 2 is related to the subjective onset of sleep, although wide discrepancies between objective and subjective measures of sleep latency have also been reported in good sleepers (Baker et al., 1999; Majer et al., 2007).

After the first episode dominated by slow waves, referred to as SWS or N3, REM sleep occurs. The interval between sleep onset (usually defined as the first occurrence of Stage 1 or 2) and REM sleep is referred to as *latency to REM sleep* and in healthy young sleepers averages 70–100 minutes. The first REM episode is generally short. Together, the first NREM and first REM episode constitute the first NREM–REM cycle (see Figure 2.2B).

A prototypical 8-hour sleep episode contains four or five of these NREM–REM cycles. Whereas the duration of the entire cycle doesn't change much in the course of a sleep episode, the duration of NREM and REM episodes does. At the beginning of a nocturnal sleep episode the REM episodes are short and the NREM episodes are long. In the course of a nocturnal sleep episode REM episodes become longer and NREM episodes become shorter (Feinberg & Floyd, 1979). This periodic recurrence of the NREM–REM cycles during the sleep episode follows a clock-like ultradian rhythmicity.

According to the scoring criteria for human sleep, a good sleeper will return to wakefulness (i.e., at least one 30-second PSG epoch scored as W) as often as 15–20 times per night. Many of these awakenings will occur at the transitions between NREM and REM sleep and in association with adjustments of body position. These awakenings last only 30–60 seconds or so and will not be remembered in the morning. In fact, good sleepers, when asked in the morning, will report an average of only one to three awakenings.

Quantification of the time course of slow waves and sleep spindle activity reveals more of the dynamic characteristics of sleep. Whereas in the first NREM episode SWA rises fast and high levels of SWA are observed, the rise rate of SWA and maximum levels attained within an NREM episode decline gradually as the night progresses. It should

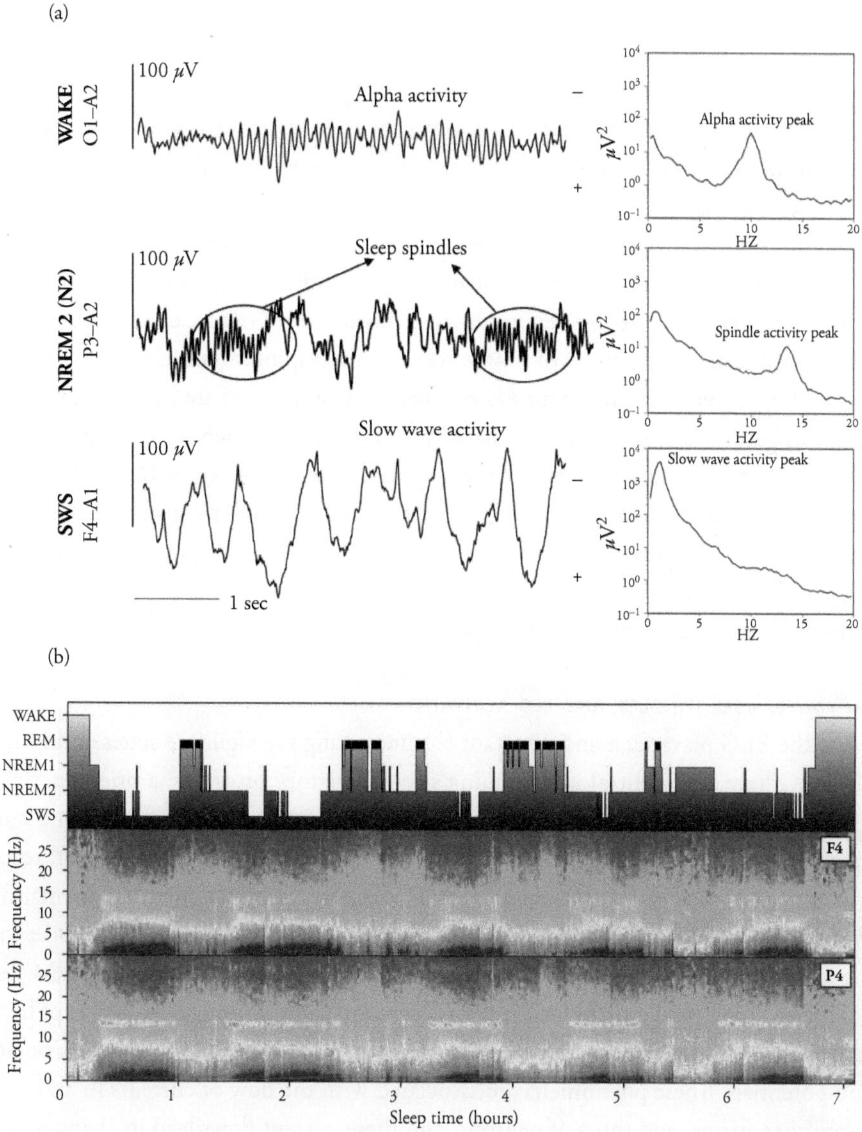

Figure 2.2 The frequency characteristics of the human electroencephalography signal across different vigilance states

Note. Panel A: Electroencephalographic (EEG) traces during wakefulness, NREM Stage 2 (N2), and slow-wave sleep and corresponding power spectral density plots. Panel B: Time course of EEG power spectral density during a whole-night-sleep episode of a young adult over the right fontal (F4) and parietal (P4) channels. Warmer colors represent higher power (logarithmic scale). NREM = non–rapid eye movement; SWS = slow-wave sleep.

be noted that even though the latter part of sleep consists primarily of Stage 2 (N2) and REM sleep, this stage will still contain some slow waves.

In contrast to SWA, the maximum values of sleep spindle activity do not change much in the course of sleep, except for a minor increase toward the end of the sleep episode. Within each NREM episode, neither SWA nor sleep spindle activity is constant, but instead they display a typical dynamic. SWA rises gradually to reach its highest levels in the middle and last part of the episode before it drops suddenly just prior to the onset of REM sleep. In contrast, the time course of sleep spindle activity resembles a U-shaped pattern with high levels at the beginning and end of each NREM episode (Dijk et al., 1993). Analyses of the dynamics of slow waves and sleep spindles based on the simultaneous recording of hundreds of electrodes revealed that slow waves are dominant in frontal derivations and, to a large extent, originate in frontal areas and behave as a traveling wave with other (temporal and parietal) cortical areas as their destination (Massimini et al., 2004). Sleep spindles are most prominent along the midline derivations and differ in their frequency between frontal and more posterior derivations (De Gennaro & Ferrara, 2003). Thus, slow waves and sleep spindles display dynamics within and across NREM episodes, and these dynamics also exhibit topographical specificity.

SLOW WAVES, SLEEP SPINDLES, AND EEG ACTIVATION

Because the EEG plays such an important role in scoring the vigilance states and changes in the EEG have been central in describing sleep regulatory processes, a brief description of the underlying mechanisms is provided. The EEG patterns as derived from a single scalp electrode reflect the behavior of thousands of cortical neurons. Intracranial recording in animals and in a few studies in human subjects, usually epileptic patients, have demonstrated that the firing patterns of cortical neurons change from a single spike tonic firing mode to a burst–pause pattern at the transition from wakefulness to NREM sleep. In the latter mode, single neurons display the slow oscillation, in which a phase of hyperpolarization of the membrane potential is followed by a depolarization and a burst of action potentials. These phenomena are associated with the flow of currents in and out of the dendrites, axons, and soma of neurons; and these current flows lead to changes in the local field potential. The synchronization of the slow oscillation (~1Hz) in thousands of neurons leads to the appearance of slow waves in the surface EEG. The occurrence of slow oscillations and their synchronization depend on both the dissipation of activating inputs from noradrenergic, serotonergic, histaminergic, and cholinergic modulatory systems as well as the local connectivity in cortical networks. Sleep spindles are observed in the cortex and in the thalamus and are strongly dependent on the nucleus reticularis of the thalamus (Crunelli & Hughes, 2009; Esser et al., 2007; Steriade, 2003). The cortically generated slow oscillations and sleep spindles and/or sleep spindle–like oscillations generated in the thalamus are phase-coupled with each other. That is, thalamic sleep spindles coincide with the up-state (depolarization) of slow oscillations (Mak-McCully et al., 2017). Recently it has been reported that spindle activity and the corresponding EEG sigma (10–15 Hz) power exhibits infraslow oscillations with a period of 50 seconds particularly over the centro-parieto-occipital regions and the second half of the night (Z. I. Lazar et al., 2019; Lecci et al., 2017).

Body, Skin, and Brain Temperature During Sleep

Sleep is associated with changes not only in the EEG but also in many other physiological variables, which may contribute to the sleep process and our experience of it. Core body temperature drops at the onset of sleep and reaches its lowest levels in the last part of the nocturnal sleep episode. This drop in core body temperature reflects the combined influences of sleep and associated changes in activity and body posture, as well as the influence of endogenous circadian rhythmicity. In the absence of sleep and under constant routine conditions (i.e., when a volunteer is kept awake in a constant posture and in dim light), core body temperature will continue to oscillate, reaching its circadian nadir approximately 1–3 hours before habitual wake time and its crest 2–4 hours before habitual bedtime. In the presence of sleep, the amplitude of the rhythm in core body temperature is much greater. One important contributor to the drop in temperature during sleep is the change from the upright to the supine posture, which normally precedes sleep onset. A drop in core body temperature is to a large extent a consequence of the dissipation of body heat. This dissipation of body heat is associated with a rise in skin temperature, in particular in the extremities. Highest skin temperatures are observed at sleep onset due to vasodilatation in the hands and feet. This heat loss is closely associated with the time it takes to fall asleep, suggesting that temperature regulation and sleep initiation are closely interrelated (Krauchi, 2007). For the remainder of the sleep episode, the associations between temperature and sleep are unremarkable. In humans, core body temperature and skin temperature are not substantially modulated by the NREM–REM cycle, even though animal studies have clearly documented that brain temperature is affected by the NREM–REM cycle.

Respiration, Heart Rate, and Blood Pressure During Sleep

In healthy sleepers, respiratory rhythms continue uninterrupted during sleep in an autonomous way. Respiratory rates in general drop during NREM sleep, and respiration can become irregular and shallow during REM sleep. Challenge studies have indicated a reduced responsiveness to CO_2 and reduced muscle tone during sleep, and REM sleep in particular may contribute to the occasional collapse of the upper airway and cessation of airflow in the presence of respiratory effort (Krimsky & Leiter, 2005).

Heart rate drops at sleep onset, and heart rate is modulated considerably by the NREM–REM cycle. Heart rate reaches its lowest levels during NREM sleep, and this is in part due to a shift in the sympathovagal balance, from sympathetic to parasympathetic dominance. During REM sleep, heart rate increases, and analyses of its variability indicate a much stronger sympathetic input to the heart (Jurysta et al., 2003). In healthy sleepers, blood pressure drops during sleep at night, and studies in which subjects are kept awake at night indicate that these nocturnal changes in heart rate and blood pressure, as well as respiration, are to a large extent sleep-dependent (i.e., the amplitude of the nocturnal changes in the absence of sleep is only minimal).

Hormone Release During Sleep

When sleep occurs at night, it occurs in a particular endocrine environment. The plasma concentrations of melatonin, the hormone secreted by the pineal gland, will have started to rise 1–2 hours before habitual bedtime. It will maintain high levels throughout the nocturnal sleep episode, but during the waking day levels are very low. The rhythm of melatonin will persist in the absence of sleep provided light levels are modest, and we now know that its rhythm is driven by the suprachiasmatic nucleus (SCN), locus of the circadian pacemaker in humans and other mammals through a well-characterized polysynaptic pathway. When we go to sleep at night, plasma concentrations of the hormone cortisol, synthesized and secreted by the adrenal cortex, are very low; and they will continue to rise throughout the sleep episode, to reach their daily peak levels, at around habitual wake time. The rhythm of this hormone is also nearly sleep-independent (i.e., it persists in the absence of sleep). Sleep only slightly inhibits cortisol. It is a connection from the circadian clock which resides in the SCN of the hypothalamus to the paraventricular nucleus of the hypothalamus that drives the release of cortisol-releasing factor, which in turn drives adrenocorticotropic hormone release from the anterior pituitary in the general circulation, which then drives cortisol synthesis from the adrenal cortex.

At sleep onset, and during SWS in particular, the anterior pituitary will release a surge of growth hormone. In the absence of sleep, the nocturnal surge of growth hormone is not observed, indicating that this hormone is very much sleep-dependent. Other hormones in which the release is sleep-dependent include prolactin and thyroid-stimulating hormone as well as the appetite-regulating hormones ghrelin and leptin (Czeisler & Klerman, 1999; Spiegel et al., 2004).

Assessment of Wakefulness

Sleep and Wake Propensity

Analysis of sleep within a 24-hour context requires that we quantify both sleep and wakefulness. Within the context of sleep regulation, wakefulness is mostly viewed as the absence of sleep, the absence of sleepiness, and the ability to perform behaviors typical for wakefulness. Subjective assessment of sleepiness while people are conducting their daily activities reveals that immediately upon awakening we are still somewhat sleepy and that this sleepiness/fatigue then dissipates to a minimum later in the morning and early afternoon and then increases again (Kahneman et al., 2004).

Assessment of the ability to fall asleep in the laboratory as measured by PSG in the Multiple Sleep Latency Test (MSLT) yielded patterns of sleep propensity, in which the longest latency to sleep is present when first assessed approximately 2 hours after habitual sleep onset. This is followed by a reduction in sleep latency to reach a minimum at approximately 2:00–4:00 p.m., and thereafter sleep latencies increase again (Carskadon & Dement, 1982). The time course of theta activity in the waking EEG, which is often considered an electrophysiological marker of sleepiness, increases during the day. This increase continues during sleep deprivation, albeit modulated by a circadian phase so that in the evening hours levels are somewhat lower (Finelli et al., 2000). Thus, the diurnal patterns of both subjective sleepiness/fatigue or objective sleepiness do not reflect a simple progressive increase with time awake but instead show non-monotonic and somewhat counterintuitive patterns. Variation in MSLT values within and between individuals have been reported. Several studies show that within a narrow age cohort of a healthy good sleeper, short habitual nocturnal sleep duration is associated with increased daytime sleepiness; that is, shorter MSLT values and higher subjective sleepiness and extension of sleep lead to a reduction of daytime sleepiness (Arand et al., 2005; Kamdar et al., 2004).

Performance

When sleep is viewed as a recovery process maintaining the integrity of brain function, the assessment of our ability to perform during wakefulness becomes relevant for sleep research and the evaluation of sleep quality. Assessment of the diurnal patterns of performance on a variety of tasks demonstrates that immediately upon awakening, performance is impaired; and this phenomenon is referred to as *sleep inertia* (Scheer et al., 2008). Performance then recovers and remains fairly constant over most of the waking day. Minor variations in performance are observed, and these variations depend on factors such as workload, task difficulty, etc. The often mentioned mid-afternoon increase in sleep propensity is in general not accompanied by a major decline in performance. Thus, a healthy individual can uphold performance throughout a normal waking day. Sleep restriction will, however, lead to an impairment of waking performance (Banks & Dinges, 2007). A stable level of performance during the day and lack of sleepiness are indicators of sufficient sleep.

Sleep Homeostasis

The description of the phenomenology of the sleep–wake cycle in good sleepers begs the question of which factors underlie its regulation and how various aspects of its phenomenology interrelate. Do we go to sleep because we have been awake for 14–17 hours, and do we wake up because we have slept enough; or is the sleep–wake cycle governed by a simple clock that keeps track of only time and not of sleep need? If we use an alarm clock, does this imply that we override our internal sleep-timing mechanisms and have not had enough sleep?

As described, the phenomenology of a nocturnal sleep episode is complex: After the lights are turned off, sleep onset occurs after 10–15 minutes; SWS is high at the beginning of the nocturnal sleep episode, REM sleep is abundant at the end of the nocturnal sleep episode, and then we wake up. What underlies this phenomenology? Is it determined by time-of-day/clock-like influences on sleep propensity and structure, or do sleep propensity and the changes in sleep physiology simply reflect a response to the duration and characteristics of the previous wake episode and the progression of the sleep process? To answer these questions, sleep scientists have manipulated the sleep–wake cycles of good sleepers in many different ways, and sleep deprivation has been among the most popular approaches. This approach is inspired by the concept of homeostasis, which in the context of sleep regulation, implies that sleep occurs when certain variables/parameters deviate from a set point or reference level and that sleep restores these variables/parameters to this reference level (see Figure 2.3). The deviations are in general thought to be a consequence of the duration of wakefulness, but specific conditions, such as infections, could also lead to a greater sleep need.

Total Sleep Deprivation

Staying awake for one night and the next day and then going to sleep at a habitual bedtime represents one night of total sleep deprivation. In a young adult it entails losing 8 hours of sleep—2 hours of REM sleep, 2 hours of SWS, and another 4 hours of Stages 2 and 1 sleep. At the same time, wakefulness preceding sleep increases from 16 hours to 40 hours or so. What are the characteristics of recovery sleep from total sleep deprivation? Not all of the lost sleep is immediately recouped, and recovery sleep is indeed not 16 hours in duration. Unfortunately, in most studies the time allowed for a recovery sleep episode was restricted. Therefore, not much information on the duration of recovery sleep after total sleep deprivation under unlimited sleep opportunity conditions is available. In one such study in which subjects were in bed for 24 hours, subjects slept approximately 5 hours more after one night of sleep deprivation compared to no sleep deprivation (Rosenthal et al., 1991). When we consider the sleep deprivation studies in which recovery sleep was restricted, we find that the 2 hours of lost REM sleep are not regained. In fact, in young adults, REM sleep during recovery sleep from total sleep deprivation may be somewhat below baseline. The rhythmicity of the NREM–REM cycle is also not much affected, illustrating its ultradian clock-like regulation, which is unperturbed by total sleep loss. The lost time in Stages 2 and 1 sleep is not recovered, but indeed less time is spent in these stages than at baseline. The main differences between recovery sleep and baseline sleep are the reduced latency to sleep onset, the reduced number of awakenings, and the increased contribution of SWS/SWA (Borbély et al., 1981). These findings have been interpreted as evidence for the predominance and importance of SWS. Quantitative analyses of the EEG and its dynamics have shown that after sleep deprivation the transition of spindle-dominated to slow wave–dominated EEG occurs at a more rapid rate. These analyses have

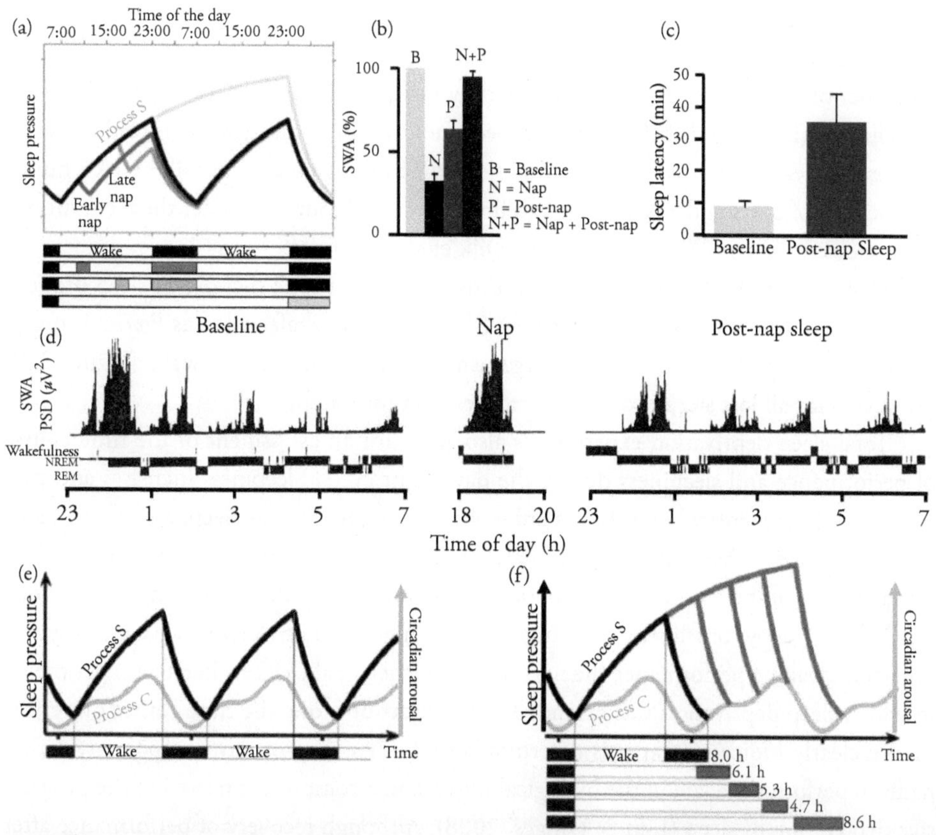

Figure 2.3 Sleep–wake homeostasis and the two-process model of sleep–wake regulation

Note. Panel A: Simulation of the time course of Process S (i.e., homeostatic sleep pressure) during a 16-hour wake/8-hour sleep cycle (black line), during a 40-hour sleep deprivation (gray line), and during an early nap or a late nap is much lower than baseline and lower than after an early nap. Modified with permission from Werth E, et al. *Am J Physiol Regulatory Integrative Comp Physiol* 1996; 271:501–510. Panel B: Effect of an early evening nap on slow-wave activity (SWA) during the subsequent nocturnal sleep. SWA at baseline = 100%. The early evening nap already contains a considerable amount of SWA. During the nap sleep debt dissipates, and the interval between the end of the nap and the beginning of the nocturnal sleep episode is not sufficient to increase the pressure of SWA to baseline level. The sum of SWA in the nap and post-nap sleep is close to 100%. Panel C: Effect of an early evening nap on sleep latency in the subsequent nocturnal sleep. Average sleep latency at baseline and during post-nap sleep. Panel D: Time course of SWA spectral power during baseline sleep, the nap, and post-nap sleep in an individual. Panel E: The two-process model of sleep–wake regulation. During a normal sleep–wake cycle, the homeostatic sleep pressure (indicated by Process S) increases during time awake and decreases during sleep, as shown in black. The circadian arousal signal (indicated by Process C) is a clock-like process, not affected by sleep history (i.e., Process S), which projects an arousal signal modeled as the sum of a sine wake with a period of 24 hours and one of 12 hours (gray). During the day circadian wake propensity is high, and during the night it is low. The switching between wake and sleep occurs at threshold modulated by Process C. The timing of sleep is indicated by the black horizontal bars. Panel F: When bedtime is delayed from 16 hours up to 28 hours, the duration of recovery sleep becomes successively shorter despite the increasing homeostatic sleep pressure (Process S) due to the modulatory effect of awakening by Process C. Only when bedtime is delayed to 32 hours is an increase in sleep duration observed. NREM = non–rapid eye movement.

also revealed that the increase in SWA is short-lived. At the end of an 8-hour recovery sleep episode, SWA is indistinguishable from baseline. A more detailed picture of the dynamics of recovery sleep can be obtained by initiating recovery sleep after 36 hours of wakefulness (i.e., 4 hours before habitual bedtime). If subjects are also instructed to stay in bed until at least noon the next day, total sleep time (TST) on average will be 13.5 hours. An increase of SWS and SWA above baseline is observed, but also under these conditions the increase in SWS/SWA is short-lived (Dijk et al., 1990).

In summary, total sleep deprivation leads to an asymptotic increase in sleep propensity, sleep consolidation, and enhanced SWS/SWA, which is referred to as *Process S*, marking the homeostatic response of the organism's brain to time spent awake (Figure 2.3). However, not all lost sleep is or can be recovered immediately.

Total sleep deprivation experiments also allow for an assessment of the time course of performance and sleepiness during the day–night cycle. Sleepiness increases and performance deteriorates when subjects enter the first night without sleep, and a first nadir in performance is observed at approximately 6:00–9:00 a.m., the exact timing depending on the nature of the task. Hereafter, performance improves somewhat during the next day but remains below baseline, indicating that one night of lost sleep will have a negative impact on waking performance the next day (Cajochen et al., 1999). In a few experiments in which sleep deprivation was extended to 64 hours or more, the time course of performance clearly indicates that it is determined by both a time-of-day component, with a nadir in performance late in the biological night, and a component related to the progressive deprivation of sleep (Lim & Dinges, 2008). Although recovery of performance after sleep loss hasn't been studied in great detail, the available data shows that some aspects of performance when assessed during the daytime recover almost immediately after one recovery sleep period, although other aspects may take more time to recover (Belenky et al., 2003).

Partial Sleep Deprivation

Partial sleep deprivation, in which sleep is restricted to 6, 4, or fewer hours, is probably a more ecologically valid model of sleep deprivation, or at least one to which we can more easily relate. In principle, partial sleep deprivation can be achieved by either postponing sleep onset, advancing sleep end, or a combination of the two. As far as its effects on the type of sleep lost are concerned, the results are equivocal. This is because SWS will always dominate the beginning of sleep, and partial sleep restriction therefore leads primarily to a reduction in Stage 2 and Stage 1 as well as REM sleep. Partial sleep deprivation will lead to an increase in sleep propensity as measured by sleep onset latencies at the beginning of the nocturnal sleep episode and a reduced number of nocturnal awakenings. It will also lead to an enhancement of SWS, even though very little SWS, but some SWA, is lost. The dynamics of the response to a partial-sleep-deprivation regime has been described in studies in which the regime is maintained for 4–7 days or so (Akerstedt et al., 2009;

Brunner et al., 1993). The increase of SWA levels off at approximately 120% after only a few days, sleep efficiency is as high as 96%, and REM sleep will constitute nearly 30% of TST. Alpha/theta activity in REM sleep progressively declines. The effects of chronic partial sleep deprivation are not restricted to sleep. Daytime sleep propensity as assessed by the MSLT increases in the course of a sleep restriction period (Carskadon & Dement, 1981). Waking performance is also affected in a negative way. For example, lapses on a psychomotor vigilance task will increase dramatically. Unlike the increase in SWA and subjective sleepiness, which level off after a few days, performance continues to deteriorate progressively in the course of the chronic partial sleep restriction (Dinges et al., 1997). Performance during the daytime, however, appears to recover swiftly after one or two nights of 8–10 hours of sleep.

Selective Sleep Deprivation

The question of whether deprivation of either SWS or REM sleep leads to a differential effect on sleep and waking performance has been addressed in selective sleep deprivation experiments. Stimuli delivered when slow waves appear in the EEG can prevent the subject from entering deep SWS (Agnew et al., 1967). Hundreds of very loud acoustic stimuli (up to 100 dB) are required for successful SWS deprivation, which will lead to arousals but will hardly affect TST, REM sleep, or the NREM–REM cycle and primarily replace SWS by Stage 2 and Stage 1 sleep. If the SWS deprivation is terminated after a few hours, an intra-night rebound of SWS/SWA will occur. Thus, the decline in SWS/SWA normally observed in a sleep episode appears to be dependent not only on the time asleep but also on how much SWS/SWA was obtained (Dijk, Beersma, et al., 1987). If the SWS/SWA deprivation is continued throughout the sleep episode and no daytime naps are allowed, SWS will be enhanced in the next undisturbed sleep episode (Ferrara et al., 1999). Thus, the SWS deficit incurred during the SWS deprivation is carried over the intervening wake episode to be expressed in the next recovery sleep episode. Consequences of SWS deprivation for daytime functioning have also been studied. They include increases in daytime sleep propensity and some decrements in performance, although the question of whether these effects are specific to SWS lost are related to the increased number of arousals has not been answered definitely (Bonnet, 1986; Walsh et al., 1994). SWS deprivation also has consequences for metabolic function and glucose regulation (Tasali et al., 2008). Two recent studies indicate that SWS deprivation may affect consolidation of perceptual learning and visuomotor learning (Aeschbach et al., 2008; Landsness et al., 2009).

Selective deprivation of REM sleep cannot be accomplished without awakenings, unless pharmacological tools are used. As soon as the first signs of REM sleep appear in the PSG, the subject is awakened (Agnew et al., 1967). After a few minutes, return to sleep is allowed, but this will nearly always be a return to NREM sleep. By repeating this procedure whenever signs of REM sleep appear, REM sleep can be almost completely abolished without major changes in TST or SWS, although some changes in sleep structure occur. In the course of one night or several nights of REM sleep deprivation, more and more awakenings are required, which has been taken as evidence for the accumulation of a REM sleep deficit. Indeed, recovery sleep after several nights of REM sleep deprivation is characterized by an increase in REM sleep, demonstrating also that REM sleep is to some extent under homeostatic control (Endo et al., 1998). This homeostatic control can already be observed within one night of REM sleep deprivation (Beersma et al., 1990).

Extra Sleep: Naps and Sleep Extension

The manipulation opposite to restriction/deprivation is extension of the sleep opportunity, and these extension studies have also provided insight into the homeostatic regulation of sleep. Scheduling naps either in the morning or in the afternoon/early evening, extending the nocturnal sleep episode by a few hours, and scheduling people to be in bed in darkness for up to 16 hours per 24 hours for several days are among the approaches used.

Nap studies have demonstrated that most young adults can initiate sleep during the day and that the sleep structure of the naps varies in a predictable way. Early morning naps contain little SWS and consist primarily of Stage 2 and REM sleep. Afternoon and evening naps contain more SWS and less REM sleep (Dijk, Beersma, & Daan, 1987; Karacan et al., 1970). These changes in sleep structure are particularly clear when only one nap per day is taken and a nap in the afternoon is thereby preceded by a longer wake period than a morning nap. In fact, both SWS and SWA in the initial part of naps increase monotonically with the duration of wakefulness (Dijk, Beersma, & Daan, 1987; Figure 2.3A). The influence of naps on subsequent nocturnal sleep has also been studied. Whereas early morning naps were shown to have little effect on subsequent nocturnal sleep, naps in the afternoon or early evening led to profound effects. In one study it was reported that following an early evening nap SWS was reduced from 81 to 52 minutes and EEG-assessed sleep latency increased from less than 10 to more than 35 minutes. Subjective sleep latency increased from less than 15 minutes to more than 45 minutes (Werth et al., 1996; see Figure 2.3B–D). An evening nap can turn a good sleeper into a sleeper with sleep onset problems! The differential effects of morning and afternoon sleep can be understood based on the very different sleep structure contents of these naps and can also be understood within the context of the two-process model of sleep regulation and the time course of the sleep homeostatic process.

Early studies indicated that extending sleep for one night has only minor effects on the subsequent nocturnal sleep structure. Fundamental questions about sleep regulation can be addressed by extending sleep opportunities to 10, 14, or 16 hours or so for many nights (Klerman & Dijk, 2005, 2008; Roehrs et al., 1996; Wehr, 1991). These studies have shown that TST is initially well above our habitual sleep time by as much as 4 or 5 hours, but after a few days on this extended sleep opportunity schedule, TST becomes smaller, although in general it remains above baseline. For young adult good sleepers, estimation of the asymptotic sleep durations (i.e., the maximal capacity for sleep when given ample opportunity for many days) averages approximately 8.9 hours, with an average of 2 hours of REM sleep (Klerman & Dijk, 2008). Please note that whereas TST remains above baseline, sleep efficiency, which is TST divided by the duration of the sleep opportunity, will fall well below baseline. Thus sleep, although longer, becomes also less consolidated. At the same time, daytime sleepiness and performance are improved (Kamdar et al., 2004; Roehrs et al., 1996).

Models and Physiology of Sleep Homeostasis

TIME COURSE/TIME CONSTANTS OF HOMEOSTASIS

The data summarized above provide strong evidence that sleep is not just an optional behavior but rather a state regulated in response to the sleep–wake history. Sleep loss leads to changes in daytime sleepiness and decrements in performance. Sleep loss and sleep extension also lead to changes in the consolidation and structure of subsequent sleep. The regulation of the various aspects of sleep varies with respect to the precision and the time course of the compensatory responses. TST and REM sleep duration respond slowly to deficits, and clear dose–response relations have not always been obtained. In contrast, deficits in SWS/SWA are almost immediately recovered and in a very precise way. Quantitative models of the homeostatic regulation of sleep and its underlying neurochemistry are almost entirely based on the regulation of SWS/SWA. Both human and animal data shows that SWA behaves like an hourglass oscillator (Borbély & Achermann, 1999). The propensity for SWA increases in a saturating exponential way during wakefulness and, when averaged per NREM episode, declines exponentially during sleep (Dijk, Beersma, & Daan, 1987a; Dijk et al., 1990). More detailed models, which incorporate the NREM–REM cycle, allow for a description of the dynamics of SWA across a nocturnal sleep episode in great detail (Achermann et al., 1993). More recent models allow for a description of the changes in NREM EEG power spectra in the course of a sleep episode (Esser et al., 2007). The essential assumptions of these recent models (Krueger et al., 2008; Tononi & Cirelli, 2006) are that during wakefulness, changes in connectivity of cortical networks or neurochemical changes occur, which ultimately lead to the initiation of SWS, during which these changes are reversed. The accurate regulation of SWS should not be taken as evidence that TST is not an important determinant of the recovery aspect of sleep. In fact, the chronic partial sleep deprivation experiments during which very little SWS is lost but a substantial part of TST is lost lead to significant performance decrements. Nevertheless, the precise regulation of SWS has inspired much research into the underlying mechanisms.

USE-DEPENDENT CHANGES IN NEURAL NETWORKS AND SWS HOMEOSTASIS

During wakefulness, cortical neurons fire in the typical phasic single action potential mode, while we are engaged in multiple behaviors and diverse experiences. These activity patterns and experiences are thought to lead to increases in synaptic strength of neural networks. These changes in synaptic strength are similar to those involved in long-term potentiation and reflect plasticity of the brain in response to experiences during wakefulness. This increased connectivity will lead to an increased likelihood of synchronized oscillatory behavior, which during sleep is expressed as SWS/SWA. Evidence for this scenario includes the observation that sleep regulation in humans also displays local aspects. Networks in most brain areas will be used extensively, and in the course of the waking day, overall synaptic strength will increase. Some areas, however, may be used more extensively than others; and indeed, local activation of, for example, the left somatosensory cortex through vibration of the right hand for 6 hours prior to sleep will lead to slightly more SWA in this particular brain region (Kattler et al., 1994). Likewise, constraining an arm during wakefulness will lead to a reduction in SWA (Huber et al., 2006). During SWA the strength of the synapses is downscaled, and this downscaling is necessary because of space and energy limitations (Tononi & Cirelli, 2006, 2014). This scenario provides a link between the concept of sleep homeostasis and changes in neural networks, plasticity, and even memory consolidation. At a neurophysiological level synaptic strength has been shown to be reliably expressed in the slope of the slow waves. This is because slow waves represent synchronized oscillation of neural networks between depolarized (up-state) and hyperpolarized states, and the steeper the slope is the faster and larger is the transition between neural down-state to up-state. As such, the slope of slow waves has been suggested as a surrogate marker of homeostatic sleep propensity (Esser et al., 2007; Riedner et al., 2007; Vyazovskiy et al., 2007, 2009).

ADENOSINE AND OTHER NEUROCHEMICAL CORRELATES OF SLEEP HOMEOSTASIS

The neural activity patterns during wakefulness are also accompanied by neurotransmitter release and high levels of energy metabolism to sustain firing rates and the required repolarization of membrane potentials. The associated neurochemical processes could provide a basis for SWS homeostasis. The neurochemical that has received the most attention is adenosine, which is a by-product of energy metabolism. It is assumed that the wake-dependent increase in adenosine concentration, through its effects on adenosine receptors, leads to either activation of sleep active neurons in the ventrolateral preoptic area, changes in neuronal potassium currents, or global cortical disfacilitation (Landolt, 2008). The direct relevance for sleep–wake regulation in humans relates to the effects of caffeine. Caffeine acts as an antagonist at adenosine receptors and, by blocking the effects of adenosine, can counter the sleep deprivation–associated decrements in performance, even during wake periods that are as long as 28 hours (Wyatt et al., 2004). Genetically determined differences in adenosine deaminase as well as polymorphism in the gene coding for the adenosine receptor have been shown to predict differences in SWS. Many other neurochemical changes may contribute to SWS homeostasis and individual differences therein (Krueger et al., 2008). They may include cytokines as well as classical neurotransmitter systems such as dopamine and serotonin.

Circadian Rhythmicity

Many behaviors and physiological variables continue to oscillate within a near 24-hour period when animals are kept under constant environmental conditions. This includes the rest–activity and sleep–wake cycles. Thus, when kept in constant darkness for many months, the activity pattern of a rat or mouse will display an alternation of an episode of high levels of activity with an episode of low levels of activity, and the total duration of these two periods is approximately 24 hours. A perturbation of the rest–activity cycle by, for example, a 6- or 12-hour sleep deprivation does not abolish this rhythm and does not lead to a 6- to 12-hour shift of the rhythm. Similar observations have also been made in diurnal species, including squirrel monkeys and humans; and this has led to the recognition that self-sustained biological oscillators, the molecular mechanisms that have been described in some detail, govern the timing of behavior. In mammals, the SCN of the hypothalamus is the locus of the circadian pacemaker, imposing rhythmicity on the rest of the brain and the body (see Figure 2.4). From a sleep regulation perspective, we consider

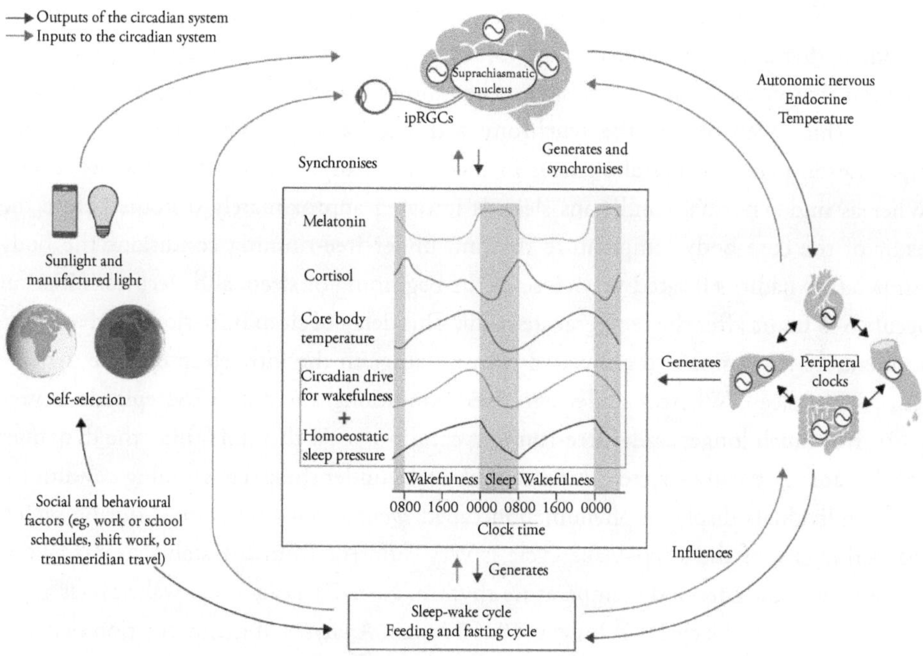

Figure 2.4 The human circadian timekeeping system

Note. Comprising a network of hierarchically organized cell-autonomous oscillators, the circadian system modulates the timing of most physiological functions and behavior. The circadian wake-promoting signal interacts with the homeostatic sleep propensity (i.e., Process S) to generate the sleep–wake cycle. The master clock located in the suprachiasmatic nucleus (SCN) is synchronized with environmental time cues primarily by light as transduced by the intrinsically photosensitive retinal ganglionic cells. Importantly, social and behavioral factors, including sleep–wake and feeding behavior, and light exposure cycles also feed back to the circadian clock and modulate circadian phase. Peripheral clocks are synchronized by the SCN via signals transmitted through the autonomic nervous and endocrine systems and periodic changes in body temperature but also by feeding behavior independently of the master clock. ipRGCs = intrinsically photosensitive retinal ganglionic cells. From Meyer et al. (2022).

the circadian clock to be self-sustaining not only because it does not require rhythmic input from the environment but also because it continues to oscillate in the absence of sleep–wake behavior. Does this imply that we go to sleep and wake up in the morning because our biological clock tells us to do so? To investigate this question, sleep scientists have studied humans under conditions very similar to those the animals were subjected to by circadian biologists (i.e., free-running conditions). Human circadian biologists have also used protocols to assess the extent to which the sleep–wake cycle leads to rhythmic variation in other variables and the extent to which circadian rhythmicity in these variables persists in the absence of a sleep–wake cycle.

Evidence for Endogenous Circadian Rhythmicity in Humans from Free-Running Studies

Early approaches to the study of the circadian regulation of sleep in humans involved underground windowless bunkers, caves, and hospital basements in which volunteers were studied for many weeks or months while in social isolation (for review, see Czeisler and Dijk, 2001). The volunteers had no access to time-of-day information, and the light–dark cycle was under the control of the subjects and thereby was also devoid of time-of-day information. From these experiments, several key characteristics of human circadian rhythmicity emerged. Most importantly, the sleep–wake cycle persists with a period that varies from 24 hours, and the ratio of wakefulness to sleep remains close to 2:1. Thus, even though the synchrony with the 24-hour cycle is lost, the internal organization persists. Several changes in the internal organization do, however, occur. Whereas under normal conditions sleep is initiated approximately 6 hours before the nadir of the core body temperature rhythm, under free-running conditions the body temperature nadir is located very close to the beginning of sleep, and sleep termination occurs 6–8 hours after the temperature nadir. This delay of sleep initiation relative to the temperature rhythm is also associated with a change in the intra-sleep episode dynamics of REM sleep. Whereas under entrained conditions, the first REM episode is very short. It is much longer under free-running conditions. At the same time, the dynamics of SWS are not greatly affected. After several weeks under these free-running conditions, many individuals display a phenomenon called *spontaneous desynchrony*, during which the periodicity of the sleep–wake cycle is very different from the stable near-24-hour periodicity of the core body temperature rhythm. Near-24-hour sleep–wake cycles alternate with sleep–wake cycles as long as 40–50 hours. Analyses of the interaction between the sleep–wake oscillator and the temperature oscillator have revealed a number of regularities (Czeisler, Weitzman, et al., 1980; Zulley et al., 1981). When sleep is initiated on the rising limb of the core body temperature rhythm, its duration can be as short as 5 hours, whereas sleep episodes initiated a few hours before the crest of the core body temperature rhythm can be very long, up to 18 hours or so. Considering the duration of the wake episode preceding these sleep episodes did not reveal a major contribution of "sleep homeostasis" (Strogatz et al., 1986). Interestingly, PSG recording of sleep has demonstrated that SWS declined in the course of the sleep episode, whether it occurred on the rising or falling limb of the core body temperature rhythm (Weitzman et al., 1980). In contrast, REM sleep was linked to the core body temperature rhythm. This data was interpreted as evidence for the regulation of the sleep–wake cycle by two oscillators: a deep stabile circadian oscillator driving the core body temperature rhythm and a labile sleep–wake oscillator linked to SWS. Forty years after the first description of this phenomenon of spontaneous internal desynchronization, the brain basis of it remains unknown. The recognition that besides the SCN multiple circadian oscillators exist in various brain structures in other mammals as well makes the phenomenon less exotic or specifically human, although not better understood. Research subsequent to the discovery of human circadian rhythmicity internal desynchrony has focused on understanding the characteristics of the deep circadian oscillator, entrainment of the oscillator to the 24-hour day, and the interaction between the sleep–wake oscillator and the deep circadian oscillator (Czeisler & Gooley, 2007). The sleep–wake oscillator is often considered synonymous with the hourglass process underlying SWS/SWA regulation, and the deep oscillator is thought to be identical to the circadian oscillator located in the suprachiasmatic oscillator. Although definite evidence for either assertion is currently lacking, much progress in the understanding of human sleep–wake regulation has been made by quantifying the parameters of these two separate processes.

Evidence for Endogenous Circadian Rhythmicity from Constant Routine Protocols

Another approach to assess endogenous circadian rhythmicity is to observe multiple physiological and behavioral variables in subjects who are kept awake for 40 hours or so under constant conditions. In this context, constant conditions imply constant dim light, a constant posture, and a constant vigilance state (i.e., wakefulness). Events such as large meals, which may induce apparent rhythmicity in hormones such as insulin, are avoided; and food intake is distributed uniformly across the 40-hour wake period by providing hourly snacks. This approach, referred to as a *constant routine protocol*, allows for the assessment of the timing and amplitude of rhythms in many variables, within a relatively short period of time. Application of this method is less labor-intensive than free-running or forced desynchrony studies, although still quite involved. This demonstrates that it is indeed not easy to assess endogenous circadian rhythmicity. The constant routine approach has revealed rhythmicity in nearly every variable ever studied. It also has revealed, by comparing the observed rhythmicity in the presence of a sleep–wake cycle to rhythmicity under constant routine conditions, that the presence of a sleep–wake cycle induces and adds to endogenous circadian rhythmicity (Duffy & Dijk, 2002).

Entrainment of the Human Circadian Clock

Given that endogenous circadian rhythmicity has been established in humans, a first question concerns the environmental variables that mediate synchronization of the human deep circadian pacemaker, which also influences sleep timing, to the 24-hour cycles of the rotating Earth. At first glance this question could be answered by sequentially removing all known rhythmic environmental variables until desynchrony is observed. In the real world, answering this question has, however, not been that easy.

LIGHT AND CIRCADIAN PHOTORECEPTION

Animal research has established that circadian pacemakers are located close to, or are well connected to, photoreceptive systems. Severing the connection between the photoreceptors and the circadian pacemaker will result in loss of synchrony between the behavioral and physiological rhythm and the 24-hour light–dark cycle. In mammals, including humans, the circadian pacemaker is located in the SCN, which is connected to retinal ganglion cells by a monosynaptic pathway. It is now well established that it is indeed the light–dark cycle that is the main synchronizer of the circadian clock in humans as well (Figure 2.4). The evidence comes from many different approaches. These include laboratory experiments of exposure to light pulses and subsequent assessment of the timing of variables, such as core body temperature and melatonin, that are considered reliable markers of the circadian pacemaker. These experiments have demonstrated that the timing of these physiological rhythms can be shifted by light exposure. The effects of the light pulses depend on the timing, duration, and intensity of the light. Light in the morning and afternoon hours (i.e., during the approximately 10-hour period following the core body temperature nadir) will advance the timing of rhythms. This means that on the days subsequent to a morning light pulse, melatonin will rise earlier. The advances are greatest for light pulses administered during the first 4 hours following the temperature nadir. Light pulses administered in the evening and nighttime hours before the core body temperature nadir will lead to a delay of these rhythms. This data can be summarized in phase–response curves, and it has been established that all variables that are known to be under circadian control, including sleep propensity, can be shifted by light exposure. The magnitude of the phase shift depends on the intensity of the light in a logarithmic manner. Room light with an intensity of 100–200 lux, or even candlelight (i.e. a few lux), may already have a significant effect; but the effect of bright (1,000–2,000 lux) or daylight (50,000–100,000 lux) is two to three times greater. Phase shifts of up to 12 hours can be accomplished by 6 hours of timed light exposure for about 3 days (Duffy & Wright, 2005).

Despite the fact that laboratory experiments have indicated that light is considered the most important synchronizer of human circadian rhythmicity, the demonstration of the importance of light for sleep–wake regulation in the real world has not been straightforward. For example, in many blind individuals living in society, the sleep–wake rhythm does cycle with a 25-hour period, as observed in free-running experiments where participants have no access to the natural 24-h light–dark cycle (please see below, "Intrinsic Period"). This is in part because the sleep–wake rhythm is determined not only by internal clock factors but also by social factors, and many of these blind individuals attempt to adhere to a socially dictated 24-hour sleep–wake cycle. Such a self-imposed sleep–wake cycle will induce apparent 24-hour rhythmicity in many variables—for example, in the core body temperature rhythm. It is only by long-term recordings of physiological variables such as core body temperature and sleep that it can be demonstrated that in these blind individuals physiological variables driven by the circadian clock are not synchronized to the Earth's rotation. Long-term recordings of subjective and objective sleep patterns have demonstrated that in many of these blind individuals, nocturnal sleep is periodically disrupted, and during these periods daytime naps occur frequently (Lockley et al., 1997, 2008). Simultaneous recordings of physiological markers of the circadian clock indicate that these periods of sleep disruption coincide with periods during which melatonin is secreted during the day rather than during the night. Whereas the sleep–wake patterns of these blind individuals confirm the importance of the light–dark cycle for entrainment, there is another group of blind individuals in whom the sleep–wake cycle and the melatonin rhythms are synchronized to the 24-hour day. In one group of blind individuals, this may be because the period of the circadian clock is sufficiently close to 24 hours to be synchronized by the weak synchronizing effects of the self-imposed 24-hour sleep–wake cycle. In another group of blind individuals, light may actually still reach the circadian clock, despite the lack of vision. This is because the effects of light on circadian rhythms are mediated in part by retinal ganglion cells that express the photopigment melanopsin. These ganglion cells, which project to the SCN, are directly sensitive to light and light of approximately 460–480 nm (i.e., blue light in particular). Thus, in some blind individuals light can still shift the timing of circadian rhythms and can still acutely suppress the secretion of melatonin. It should be noted that these intrinsically photosensitive retinal ganglion cells project not only to the SCN but also to the ventrolateral preoptic area in the anterior hypothalamus, which contains sleep active neurons; and it is through this projection that light, and blue light in particular, is thought to exert its well-known alerting and performance-enhancing effects (Cajochen et al., 2005). Thus, the timing, intensity, and spectral composition of light shape our sleep–wake propensity rhythm through its effects on the timing of circadian rhythm and through its direct activating effects. These direct activating effects of light demonstrate that apparent sleep propensity is modulated by both internal factors, such as circadian phase and sleep debt, and environmental factors, such as the intensity and spectral composition of light. The direct activating effects of light extend beyond alerting effects and include effects on functional magnetic resonance imaging (fMRI) and positron emission tomography–assessed brain response to cognitive tasks (Vandewalle, Maquet, & Dijk, 2009).

Intrinsic Period

We have discussed synchronization of the human circadian pacemaker and mentioned that under free-running conditions its period deviates from 24 hours. How much does it deviate? How stable is this intrinsic period, and do individual differences in intrinsic period predict individual characteristics of sleep timing? A first question related to the deep oscillator is how its self-sustained oscillation can be best characterized. How stable is its period? Is it genetically determined? Does it change with age, and does it predict interindividual differences in sleep–wake timing? Addressing these questions requires protocols that allow for an assessment of period that is not confounded by factors that are distinct from the deep circadian oscillator. Initial observations in healthy sighted individuals under classical free-running conditions in which the volunteers could choose when to go to sleep and had control over the light–dark cycle yielded estimates near 25 hours. It has since been recognized that given its sensitivity to light, assessment of the intrinsic period of the circadian clock should ideally be conducted in constant darkness, but this is not acceptable to sighted subjects. There are two alternative approaches. The first approach is to quantify the period of the circadian rhythms of blind individuals who are non-entrained, while living in society. The estimate of intrinsic period in this population is somewhat less than 25 hours. It has been argued that this estimate in not entirely unconfounded because the average does not include the periods of those subjects who are entrained, and it may be that these periods are closer to 24 hours than the periods of the free-running group. This estimate may also be confounded by feedback from the self-imposed 24-hour sleep–wake cycle and associated factors such as caffeine consumption. The second alternative approach is to minimize the confounding effects of light by distributing the effects over the circadian cycle. We have learned that light in the morning advances the clock (i.e., speeds it up) and that light in the evening delays the clock (i.e., slows it down). By scheduling the sleep–wake cycle and associated (dim) light–dark cycle to a period far away from the circadian range (e.g., 20 or 28 hours), uniform distribution of light across the circadian cycle can be achieved. This is because the intrinsic period of the circadian clock is too close to 24 hours and too robust to follow these non-circadian sleep–wake schedules. Estimates of intrinsic period from these forced desynchrony protocols are on average 24.2 hours (Czeisler et al., 1999). Estimates from various physiological variables (e.g., melatonin, cortisol, and core body temperature) are very similar and highly correlated, suggesting that one circadian pacemaker is driving all these rhythms. Several genes involved in the generation of circadian rhythmicity have been identified in mouse studies in particular. These genes include the *PERIOD* genes, *CLOCK, NPAS2, BMAL1*, and the *CRY* genes; and their involvement in sleep and other physiological processes is under intense investigation (Takahashi, 2017; Takahashi et al., 2008).

A first question about the circadian clock and sleep is, how does the intrinsic period of the circadian clock relate to sleep–wake timing?

Entrained Phase

In healthy good sleepers living their normal lives, the circadian clock will not be free-running but synchronized, or entrained, to the 24-hour day–night cycle.

Entrainment theory assumes that the difference between the intrinsic period and the 24-hour period is compensated for on a daily basis by light exposure in particular. Theoretically, the stable, synchronized (entrained) timing of the endogenous rhythms relative to the light–dark cycle depend on the magnitude of the mismatch as well as the strength of the light–dark cycle. Thus, in an individual in which the intrinsic period is 24.2 hours, the timing of the melatonin rhythm will be later when the subject is exposed to a weak light–dark cycle compared to a strong light–dark cycle. Furthermore, when two individuals are exposed to an identical light–dark cycle but the second subject's intrinsic period is 24.5 hours, entrainment theory predicts that the entrained melatonin rhythm, even though synchronized to the 24-hour light–dark cycle, will be phased later. A final prediction is that when the deviation of the intrinsic period from 24 hours is greater than the maximal achievable daily adjustment, the subject's circadian clock will not be synchronized to the 24-hour light–dark cycle. Assessment of intrinsic period is labor-intensive and expensive, and in only a few subjects has data on intrinsic period and entrained phase been obtained. As mentioned, entrained phase relates to the timing of endogenous circadian rhythms, such as the melatonin rhythm, relative to the light–dark cycle. In humans, light exposure consists of the natural light–dark cycle and artificial light. We will turn artificial lights on and off in synchrony with our sleep–wake cycle, and a first estimate of the timing of the light–dark cycle can be obtained from the habitual sleep–wake cycle. It turns out that the timing of the rise of plasma melatonin in the evening relative to the onset of sleep is remarkably tightly associated with the intrinsic period as assessed under desynchronized conditions. Please note that for the assessment of the endogenous rise of melatonin, subjects need to be studied in dim light conditions because light acutely suppresses melatonin. Data collected under these controlled conditions also shows that minor differences in intrinsic period lead to considerable changes in entrained phase. Thus, a difference in intrinsic period of as little as 15 minutes leads to a difference in the phase angle of the melatonin rhythm and habitual sleep time by as much as 1 hour (Gronfier et al., 2007).

Evidence that entrained phase is also determined by light exposure has also been obtained. Direct measurements of the light–dark cycle to which subjects are exposed have shown differences between early risers and late raisers, although it is not possible to identify the direction of the causality, that is, if an early wake time causes an early light exposure or the other way around (Goulet et al., 2007). Additional evidence for the role of light in determining entrained phase, or at least the timing of wake time, comes from large survey studies. The timing of sleep in people living in rural areas appears to be more closely linked to the natural light–dark cycle than that of people living in large cities. This suggests that also in the real world, light is a determinant of entrained phase (Roenneberg et al., 2007).

Sleep–Wake Regulation: Interaction of Circadian Rhythmicity and Sleep Homeostasis

Our current thinking about sleep–wake regulation has been influenced to a considerable extent by the two-process model of sleep regulation (Borbély, 1982; Daan et al., 1984). In essence, it posits that sleep duration and sleep structure are governed by sleep homeostasis (Process S), allowing for recovery of lost sleep, as well as being influenced by circadian clocks (Process C; see Figures 2.3 and 2.4). What is the evidence that both of these processes contribute simultaneously to sleep timing and sleep structure?

Sleep Displacement and the Two-Process Model of Sleep Regulation

One approach to studying the interaction of sleep homeostasis and circadian rhythmicity consists of extension of wakefulness with recovery sleep initiated at other than habitual bedtimes. In one early experiment, wakefulness was extended from 16 to 20, 24, 28, 32, 36, or 40 hours with bedtimes at 11 p.m., 3 a.m., 7 a.m., 11 a.m., 3 p.m., 7 p.m., and 11 p.m. (Åkerstedt & Gillberg, 1981). A key feature of the design of this influential study was that recovery sleep was not restricted and the subjects decided when to get up. Homeostatic regulation of sleep duration predicts a progressive increase in sleep duration when wake duration preceding sleep is extended from 16 to 40 hours. If sleep termination were governed solely by a circadian clock, then one may predict sleep to always terminate at 7:00 a.m. independent of the duration of wakefulness. The data shows a complex pattern, with an initial reduction in sleep duration for the first four conditions followed by a sudden increase when sleep is initiated at or after 15 hours. Now, how do we understand this data?

Borbély and colleagues proposed a model for the contribution of sleep homeostasis and circadian rhythmicity to explain this sleep displacement data as well as the sleep patterns observed during free-running conditions, including spontaneous desynchrony. In essence, it assumes that sleep pressure (i.e., Process S) builds up during wakefulness and dissipates during sleep. The time course of this homeostatic sleep pressure was derived from measurement of SWA during baseline sleep and recovery sleep from 40 hours of sleep loss. The model assumes that sleep is terminated when this sleep pressure hits a lower threshold, which is modulated by the circadian pacemaker (see Figure 2.3E). This threshold is higher during the biological day than the biological night, and as a consequence, daytime sleep duration is short even when wake duration is relatively long. This model and its successors have generated many research questions. Are all aspects of sleep, such as SWS, REM sleep, and sleep spindles, influenced by sleep homeostasis and circadian rhythmicity? What does the circadian sleep propensity rhythm look like, and what is the relative contribution of sleep homeostasis and circadian rhythmicity to sleep propensity? Does the circadian clock influence sleep homeostasis, or does sleep homeostasis influence the clock? How can we investigate the separate contributions of these two sleep regulatory processes?

Forced Desynchrony of the Sleep–Wake Cycle and Circadian Rhythmicity

Quantifying the contribution of sleep homeostasis and circadian rhythmicity to aspects of sleep regulation requires that sleep occurs at all circadian phases and that at the same time homeostatic sleep pressure at sleep onset can be quantified. This can be achieved in a variety of protocols, an essential feature of which is that the period of the sleep–wake cycle is much shorter or much longer than 24 hours. Weitzman and colleagues (1974) used 3-hour sleep–wake cycles; Carskadon and others (Carskadon & Dement, 1977) used very short 90-minute "days." More recently, 20, 28, and 42.85 hours have been used (see Figure 2.5A). Because in these protocols the ratio of wakefulness to sleep in general is kept to 2:1, sleep episode duration varied from 0.5 to 14 hours or so. Whereas the short sleep episodes allow an assessment of the circadian variation of the ability to initiate sleep, long sleep episodes are required to study the dynamics of the sleep process at all circadian phases. When the sleep episodes are sufficiently long, it is also possible to study the relative contribution of sleep-dependent and circadian processes. The analysis of the circadian influence on data collected in these protocols requires that each observation is assigned a circadian phase. This requires the assessment of reliable circadian markers such as core body temperature or melatonin. The analysis of sleep–wake homeostasis on the data collected requires that each observation is assigned a homeostat coordinate. This is accomplished by determining the duration of wakefulness or sleep preceding the time point at which an observation was made.

TIME COURSE OF SWS/SWA: HOMEOSTATIC AND CIRCADIAN ASPECTS

SWS/SWA are considered markers of the sleep homeostat (i.e., Process S) driven by the sleep–wake cycle independent of the circadian cycle. It is therefore predicted that SWS/SWA decline during all sleep episodes and that the level of SWS/SWA is high at the beginning of sleep and at similar levels independent of circadian phase provided that wakefulness preceding sleep for these sleep episodes is similar. This prediction has been confirmed by PSG analyses in sleep-displacement studies, spontaneous desynchrony studies, and forced desynchrony studies (see Figure 2.5B). The latter data indicates that there is a minor circadian modulation of SWA at the beginning of sleep, but when comparing the sleep-dependent and circadian component, the predominance of the homeostatic component is very evident (Dijk & Czeisler, 1995; see Figure 2.5B). The implication is that both the buildup of homeostatic sleep pressure during wakefulness and its expression as SWA during sleep are not markedly affected by a circadian process. A detailed analysis of the individual slow waves that represent the oscillatory basis of SWA shows that the incidence and the amplitude of slow waves are indeed almost entirely driven by the sleep homeostat without much circadian modulation. Other features such as the slope of slow waves, shown to reflect synaptic strength, are to a great extent under circadian regulation that can even exceed the sleep-homeostat effect over the central brain regions (A. S. Lazar et al., 2015). While there is a clear decrease in the slope of slow waves during the sleep

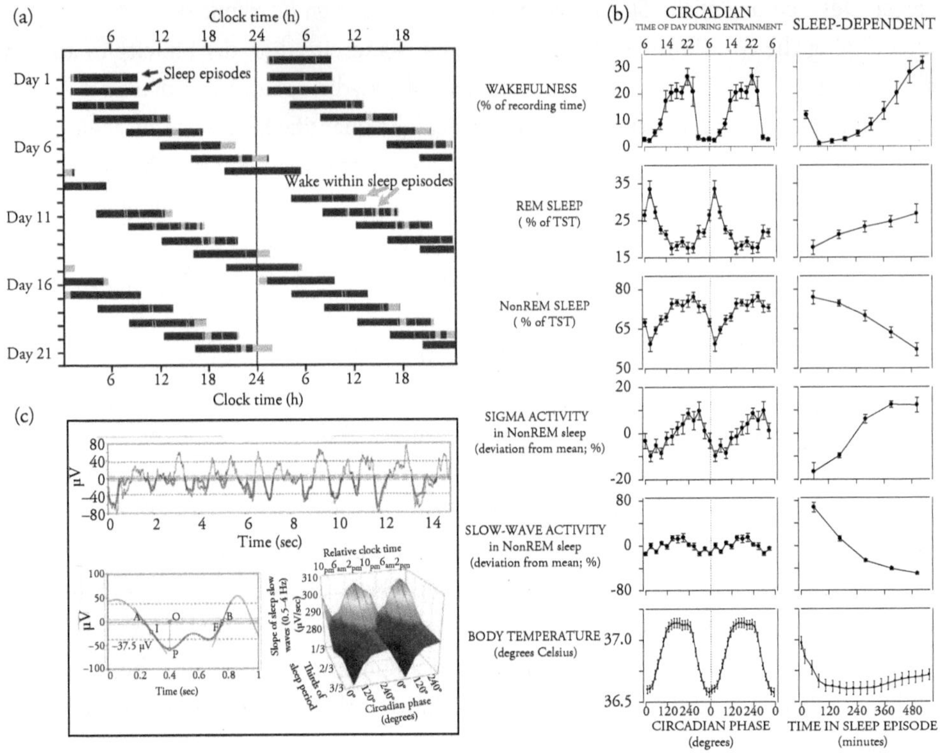

Figure 2.5 A forced desynchrony between the sleep–wake cycle and endogenous circadian rhythmicity in a healthy adult

Note. Panel A: Data are presented in double raster plot format in which consecutive days are plotted both next to and below each other. After 3 baseline days with sleep (dark blue horizontal bars) scheduled at the subject's habitual sleep time, the subject was scheduled to a 28-hour sleep–wake cycle while in dim light. Light blue areas within sleep episode represent polysomnography-determined wakefulness. The experimental protocol allows for measuring and estimating the independent effect of sleep history (Process S) and circadian phase (Process S) on the brain and the body. Adapted from Dijk DJ, Duffy JF, Riel E, Shanahan TL, Czeisler CA. Ageing and the circadian and homeostatic regulation of human sleep during forced desynchrony of rest, melatonin and temperature rhythms. *J Physiol (London), 1999; 516.2*: 611–627. Panel B: Circadian and sleep-dependent modulation of wakefulness, rapid-eye-movement (REM) sleep, non-REM sleep, sigma activity, slow wave activity and body temperature. From DJ Dijk and CA Czeisler, Contribution of the circadian pacemaker and the sleep homeostat to sleep propensity, sleep structure, electroencephalographic slow waves, and sleep spindle activity in humans, *J Neuroscience 1995 15*(5 Pt 1):3526–38. doi: 10.1523/JNEUROSCI.15-05-03526.1995 with permission. Panel C: Slow-wave detection, slope analysis, and the circadian and homeostatic regulation of the slope of the slow waves. Adapted from Lazar AS, Lazar ZI, Dijk DJ. Circadian regulation of slow waves in human sleep: Topographical aspects. *Neuroimage. 2015 Aug 1;116*:123–34. doi: 10.1016/j.neuroimage.2015.05.012. Epub 2015 May 12. PMID: 25979664; PMCID: PMC4503801.

episode, there is independent circadian modulation, with peak values during the second part of the day and a nadir during the circadian night (see Figure 2.5C). This has implications for the contribution of the circadian pacemaker to synaptic plasticity and cognition (Frank, 2016).

Please note that when we consider the duration of NREM sleep (i.e., the duration of the sum of Stages 1, 2, 3, and 4, expressed as a percentage of TST), in addition to a sleep-dependent modulation, a circadian modulation becomes apparent. The crest of the circadian modulation is located at a circadian phase corresponding to approximately 10:00 p.m. and the minimum at 8:00 a.m.

CIRCADIAN MODULATION OF SLEEP SPINDLES

Given the different neurophysiological basis of slow waves and sleep spindles, it may not be surprising that their circadian and sleep-dependent regulation differs to a considerable extent. In contrast to slow waves, sleep spindles are to a considerable extent under circadian control (Dijk & Czeisler, 1995). Quantification of both total EEG activity in the frequency range of sleep spindles as well as of parameters of sleep spindles—such as their density, amplitude, and frequency—has revealed a crest in spindle activity during the circadian night, in close association with the melatonin peak and the falling limb of the temperature rhythm (Dijk & Czeisler, 1995; Dijk et al., 1997; Wei et al., 1999). During sleep at night the frequency of sleep spindles is lower; that is, the average frequency shifts from approximately 13.25 Hz when sleep occurs during the biological day to 12.75 Hz during the biological night. At the same time, the duration of spindles increases, the number of spindles increases, and their amplitude is greater. Sleep spindle characteristics also show a sleep-dependent regulation. Spindles become faster and longer as sleep progresses. Sleep spindles are of interest because they have been implicated in the consolidation of memory, in particular on procedural tasks but also on declarative memories. Sleep spindles have been implicated in blocking the transfer of sensory information at the level of the thalamic relay nuclei, thereby contributing to the consolidation of sleep. It is also of interest that sleep spindles decline with age and are enhanced by hypnotics that interact with the gamma-aminobutyric acid A–benzodiazepine receptor complex, and it has been argued that the circadian modulation of sleep spindles represents an endogenous circadian hypnotic signal (Dijk et al., 1997; Knoblauch et al., 2003).

CIRCADIAN MODULATION OF REM SLEEP: A GATE TO AND FROM WAKEFULNESS?

In contrast to SWS, REM sleep is under strong circadian control (see Figure 2.5B). Evidence for this has been derived from PSG analyses of sleep during free-running studies, spontaneous desynchrony studies, and forced desynchrony studies. The crest of the REM sleep propensity rhythm, assessed as REM sleep expressed as a percentage of TST, is located 1–2 hours after the core body temperature nadir. REM sleep propensity can also be assessed by measuring the latency to REM sleep. The distribution of REM latency is bimodal, with a first peak in the distribution for latencies around 20 minutes and a second peak around 50–110 minutes. REM latencies belonging to the first peak in the distribution are referred to as *sleep-onset REM episode*. When sleep is initiated around the core body temperature nadir, sleep-onset REM episodes are very frequent (Czeisler,

Zimmerman, et al., 1980). Sleep-dependent regulation of REM sleep is characterized by what has been coined *sleep-dependent disinhibition*. REM sleep appears somewhat inhibited at the beginning of sleep, particularly in young individuals who have much SWS; and then its propensity increases as sleep progresses (Dijk et al., 1999). The sleep-dependent disinhibition is also observed in phasic events, such as the density of rapid eye movements (Khalsa et al., 2002). Because of the predominance of the circadian regulation of REM sleep, the time course of REM sleep in the course of a sleep episode very much depends on the circadian phase of sleep onset. REM sleep declines as sleep progresses when sleep is initiated on the rising limb of the core body temperature rhythm. In contrast, REM sleep increases as sleep progresses when sleep is initiated on the falling limb, as is the case during entrainment. This polarity is of interest because most spontaneous awakenings occur from REM sleep and because the combination of the sleep-dependent and circadian regulation of REM sleep results in a sharp peak in REM sleep propensity at habitual wake time. REM sleep indeed has been considered a gate to wakefulness (Lavie, 1986), and awakening from REM sleep leads to less sleep inertia than awakening from Stage 2 sleep (Silva & Duffy, 2008). Paradoxically, it is also at this circadian phase that circadian sleep propensity is greatest; and, maybe, REM sleep should be considered both a gate from and to sleep.

SLEEP INITIATION AND SLEEP TERMINATION: A PARADOXICAL RHYTHM OF CIRCADIAN SLEEP—WAKE PROPENSITY

The circadian and homeostatic regulation of sleep structure occurs within a sleep episode, the initiation and duration of which is also under the control of these two processes. During spontaneous desynchrony, sleep termination occurs almost exclusively on the rising limb of the core body temperature (CBT) rhythm. Sleep initiation preferentially occurs on the falling limb of the CBT rhythm or on the middle part of the rising limb. In the latter case, sleep episodes can be very long—up to 18 hours. Interestingly, sleep is rarely initiated in the early evening hours, and this phase has been referred to as the *wake maintenance zone* (Strogatz et al., 1987) or the *forbidden zone for sleep* (Lavie, 1986). Please note that during spontaneous desynchrony, the very long sleep episodes that are initiated on the rising limb will continue throughout this wake maintenance zone. Thus, it may be more appropriate to consider this phase as a time during which it is difficult to initiate sleep. During spontaneous desynchrony, the assessment of the circadian sleep propensity rhythm is confounded by the variation in wake duration preceding sleep. Assessments of the circadian sleep propensity rhythm in forced desynchrony are less affected by this confound. The circadian rhythm of sleep propensity as assessed by sleep initiation is very pronounced, with peak (i.e., shortest sleep latencies) at approximately 0–2 hours after the temperature nadir. Longest sleep latencies are observed 10–8 hours before the temperature nadir. Under conditions of entrainment, these circadian phases correspond to a maximum propensity to initiate sleep at 6:00–8:00 a.m. and a minimum likelihood to initiate sleep at 8:00–10:00 p.m. In other words, the circadian drive for sleep is greatest around habitual wake time, and the circadian drive for wakefulness is greatest around bedtime. Assessment of the circadian rhythm of the propensity to terminate sleep can be derived on the basis of TST as well as assessment of wakefulness (i.e., sleep disruption) in the last part of the sleep opportunity (see Figure 2.5B). The waveform of the propensity to terminate sleep is just the opposite of the waveform of sleep initiation. In other words, the circadian drive for wakefulness as assessed by disruption of sleep consolidation is greatest in the wake maintenance zone. The circadian drive for sleep as assessed by the continued consolidation of sleep is greatest near the crest of propensity to initiate sleep. Thus, there is no apparent need to postulate separate circadian drives for sleep initiation and sleep termination (Dijk & Czeisler, 1994).

We are still left with the paradoxical observation that the circadian drive for wakefulness is greatest near sleep onset and the circadian drive for sleep is greatest at the end of the habitual sleep episode. Review of relevant data from many different protocols confirms the consistency of this rhythm, provided that the homeostatic drive for sleep is controlled.

CONSOLIDATION OF SLEEP AND WAKEFULNESS THROUGH INTERACTION OF PROCESSES S AND C

The paradoxical phase relationship between the timing of the habitual sleep–wake cycle and the circadian sleep propensity rhythm can be understood when we consider that both the sleep homeostat and the circadian pacemaker contribute to sleep timing and sleep continuity. When sleep consolidation is plotted as a simultaneous function of circadian phase and time since the start of the sleep episode, it becomes clear that a full 8 hours of sleep consolidation can be accomplished only when sleep is initiated just after the wake maintenance zone. Homeostatic sleep pressure dissipates as sleep progresses, but this does not lead to sleep interruption because the circadian drive for wake dissipates and turns into a circadian drive for sleep. It is only at the inflection point of the circadian sleep–wake propensity rhythm that sleep is terminated. In contrast, when sleep is initiated just after habitual wake time, initially sleep consolidation is high because of the high homeostatic sleep pressure; but as soon as this dissipates, sleep is interrupted because the circadian drive for wakefulness increases. Thus, a precise alignment of the sleep–wake homeostat (i.e., Process S) and circadian rhythms (i.e., Process C) is essential for sleep consolidation. If the circadian wake maintenance zone occurs too late, the strong circadian arousal signal may prevent sleep initiation at socially accepted times, and the subject may postpone bedtimes. And indeed, the shorter interval distance between the wake maintenance zone measured by the onset of the melatonin rhythm in dim light and the habitual sleep time is associated with increased latency to persistent sleep and insomnia complaints (A. S. Lazar et al., 2015). If the homeostatic drive for sleep is too weak, both sleep initiation and consolidation may be compromised. A precise alignment and well-balanced contribution of the sleep–wake homeostat and circadian sleep–wake propensity rhythm is essential not only for sleep consolidation but also for wake consolidation (Dijk et al., 1992; Dijk &

Czeisler, 1994; Wyatt et al., 1997, 1999). In the opposing process model of sleep regulation, which can be considered a variation of the two-process model, a primary role of the circadian arousal signal is to consolidate the wake episode in the presence of the buildup of homeostatic sleep pressure (Edgar et al., 1993). Indeed, when the SCN is lesioned, as can be done experimentally in squirrel monkeys, and the circadian arousal signal is no longer present, the wake episodes become highly fragmented. In humans, the contribution of the circadian arousal signal to sleep propensity and waking performance has been analyzed in forced desynchrony protocols. The laboratory data shows that performance and alertness can be maintained only throughout a 16- to 18-hour wake episode if the alignment with the circadian rhythm of arousal is under entrained conditions (Wyatt et al., 1999). Otherwise, as evidenced by forced desynchrony protocols, performance and alertness present a clear circadian pattern, with lowest values in early morning and highest values in the evening hours. Interestingly, sex has been shown to modulate the circadian modulation of cognition, with greater impact of adverse circadian phase (i.e., early morning hours) on performance across multiple cognitive domains in women (Santhi et al., 2016).

When we extrapolate these findings to the real world, the following scenarios emerge. The day-shift worker will wake along a trajectory on which the circadian drive for wakefulness opposes the increase in homeostatic sleep pressure during the working period and for most of the leisure period. In contrast, alertness and performance in the night-shift worker, waking up in the afternoon, will initially be supported by the circadian drive for wakefulness. As the night shift starts, the already considerable homeostatic sleep pressure will no longer be opposed by the circadian arousal rhythm, and performance will be compromised. In fact, at approximately 7:00 or 8:00 a.m., coinciding with the end of the night shift/commute home, the combination of high homeostatic sleep pressure and lack of circadian drive for wakefulness is such that performance is most compromised. Evidence that the interaction between circadian rhythmicity and sleep homeostasis determines performance and alertness in individuals living in their habitual environment has been obtained in blind individuals (Lockley et al., 2008).

CONTRIBUTION OF MELATONIN TO CIRCADIAN REGULATION OF SLEEP–WAKEFULNESS: PHASE SHIFTING AND SILENCING OF WAKE-PROMOTING CIRCADIAN SIGNALS

Both core body temperature and plasma melatonin have been used extensively as markers of circadian phase, and the circadian sleep–wake propensity rhythm displays a close temporal association with both. To what extent these physiological variables and underlying processes play a causal role in circadian sleep–wake regulation has been investigated, particularly for melatonin (see Figure 2.6A). Melatonin's role in circadian sleep–wake regulation has been related to its direct sleep-inducing/-facilitating effects and its effects on shifting the timing of circadian rhythm (Arendt, 2006; Srinivasan et al., 2009). The latter role is relevant in

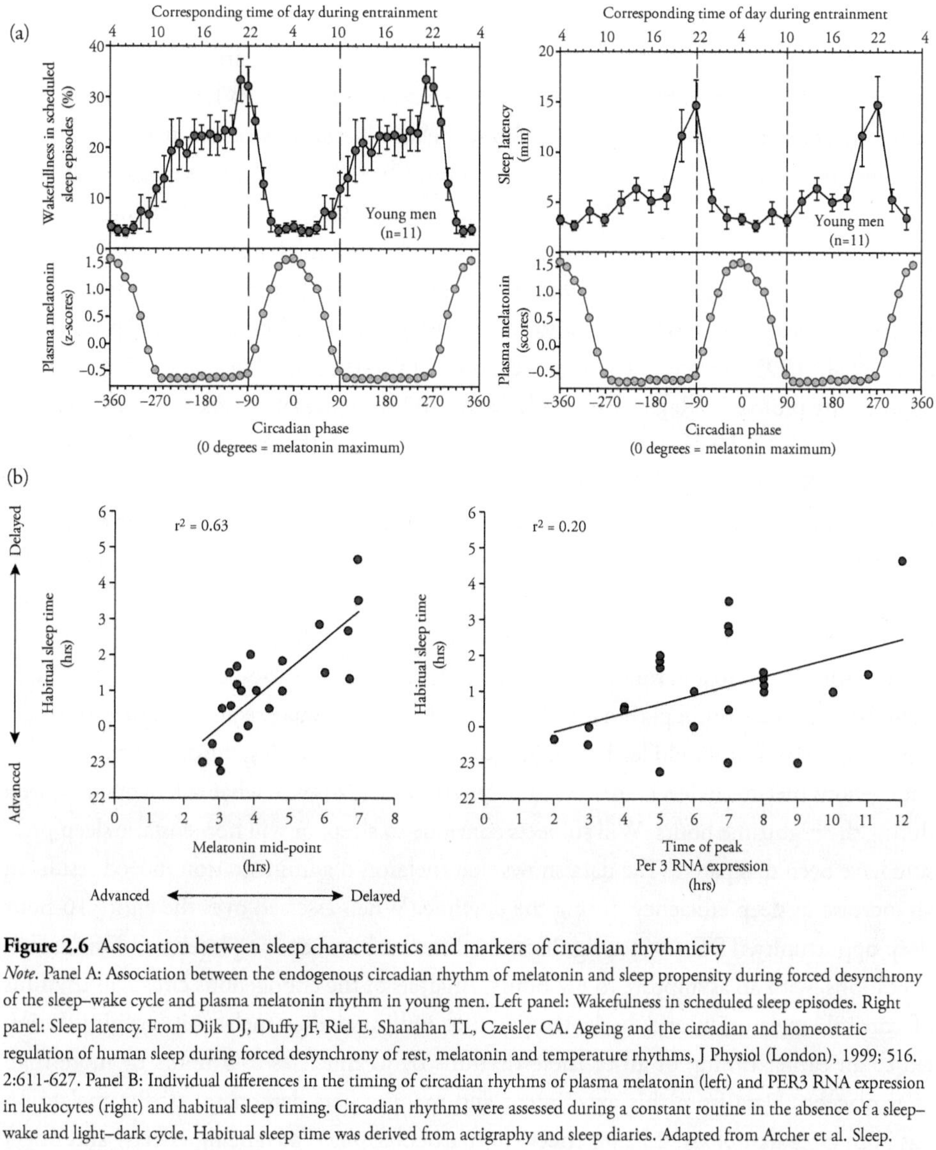

Figure 2.6 Association between sleep characteristics and markers of circadian rhythmicity

Note. Panel A: Association between the endogenous circadian rhythm of melatonin and sleep propensity during forced desynchrony of the sleep–wake cycle and plasma melatonin rhythm in young men. Left panel: Wakefulness in scheduled sleep episodes. Right panel: Sleep latency. From Dijk DJ, Duffy JF, Riel E, Shanahan TL, Czeisler CA. Ageing and the circadian and homeostatic regulation of human sleep during forced desynchrony of rest, melatonin and temperature rhythms, J Physiol (London), 1999; 516. 2:611-627. Panel B: Individual differences in the timing of circadian rhythms of plasma melatonin (left) and PER3 RNA expression in leukocytes (right) and habitual sleep timing. Circadian rhythms were assessed during a constant routine in the absence of a sleep–wake and light–dark cycle. Habitual sleep time was derived from actigraphy and sleep diaries. Adapted from Archer et al. Sleep. 2008;31:608–17.

the context of the question of whether the human circadian pacemaker is synchronized by 24-hour cycles of pharmacological or non-pharmacological manipulations other than light. An answer to this question is obviously relevant to the traveler who frequently crosses multiple time zones, the shift worker, and the non-entrained blind individuals. To date, the only known manipulation for which this has been established unequivocally in humans is the timed administration of exogenous melatonin. Similar to light, a phase–response curve for melatonin has been established. There are important differences between the effects of light and melatonin. Whereas light exposure in the evening delays circadian rhythms, melatonin administration in the evening advances circadian rhythms. Whereas light exposure in the morning advances circadian rhythms, melatonin administration at this time does not seem to substantially delay circadian rhythms. Overall, the effects of melatonin which are presumably mediated by melatonin receptors in the SCN, are much more modest than the effects of light. The effects of melatonin are not limited to phase-shifting effects. Just as with the direct alerting effects of light, melatonin has direct sleep-facilitating effects. These effects have been demonstrated in a variety of protocols including daytime nap protocols (Nave et al., 1995), forced desynchrony protocols (Wyatt et al., 2006), and extended sleep opportunity protocols (Rajaratnam et al., 2003, 2004). In the latter protocols subjects were instructed to be in bed for 16 hours per 24-hour period with lights out at 4:00 p.m. and lights on at 8:00 a.m. This bedtime starts well before the endogenous rise of the melatonin rhythm. Subjects were exposed to this extended sleep schedule for 9 days on two occasions. On one occasion, melatonin was administered at lights-out of all extended sleep episodes except the last one. In the other condition, placebo was administered at lights-out of all extended sleep episodes, and sleep was recorded throughout the protocol. In addition, constant routines prior to and following this schedule were used to assess endogenous circadian rhythmicity. If melatonin plays a physiological role in sleep–wake regulation, then administration of melatonin should lead to an improvement of sleep during the daytime (i.e., when endogenous melatonin levels are low). The question then arises of what will happen to sleep during the nighttime hours. Will subjects continue to sleep, or will homeostatic sleep pressure have been dissipated? The data shows that melatonin administration indeed results in an increase in sleep efficiency during the daytime. When assessed over the entire 16-hour sleep opportunity, TST was not significantly different between the placebo and melatonin conditions, with an asymptote to 8.7 hours. Analysis of the endogenous circadian rhythms of cortisol, melatonin, and body temperature indicated that melatonin administration led to an earlier timing of all of these rhythms by as much as 2–3 hours or more than after placebo. Data from this experiment and many others demonstrates that melatonin has both circadian phase-shifting effects (in particular phase-advancing effects) and direct sleep-facilitating effects. The effects are thought to be mediated by melatonin receptors in the SCN, the locus of the biological clock in humans. The direct sleep-facilitating effects have been interpreted as a silencing of the wake-promoting signal from the biological clock. It is the combination of phase-shifting and sleep-facilitating effects that makes melatonin useful in the treatment of sleep timing disorders in, for example, blind individuals but also in delayed sleep-phase syndrome.

CONTRIBUTION OF OREXIN TO CIRCADIAN REGULATION OF SLEEP–WAKEFULNESS

The peptide orexin, also referred to as *hypocretin*, was discovered by looking for transcripts that were selectively expressed in the hypothalamus, the brain area essential to the maintenance of homeostasis and circadian rhythmicity. Hypocretin neurons are located in the lateral hypothalamus and project to numerous brain areas, including brainstem nuclei that play a key role in sleep–wake regulation. It is an activating neurotransmitter system thought to play an important role in the consolidation of vigilance states and maintenance of wakefulness in particular. In the squirrel monkey, concentrations of orexin in cerebrospinal fluid increase in the course of the waking day, and this increase is thought to be driven by the SCN and motor activity. Deficiencies in orexin are associated with excessive sleepiness and cataplexy, typical for the sleep disorder narcolepsy (Fronczek et al., 2009).

Individual Differences in Homeostatic and Circadian Regulation of Sleep–Wake Cycles in Healthy Men and Women: Physiology and Genes

The concept of sleep–wake regulation through interaction of circadian and homeostatic processes provided a powerful framework for the study of sleep at both the group and individual levels. The multiple phenotypic aspects of sleep vary between individuals, and many of these individual differences are stable over time and across conditions. Such stable, trait-like differences often (but not always) have a genetic basis, and the study of individual differences may provide new insights into the mechanisms underlying normal and pathological variation in sleep. In recent years, some of the individual differences in sleep have been studied in some detail, and in a few cases some of the interindividual differences have been linked to variations in specific genes.

Deep Sleep/Shallow Sleep: Slow Waves and Other EEG Oscillations

The EEG plays an important role in sleep research. Marked differences in EEG characteristics exist between individuals, and it was recognized early on that the EEG is among the most heritable characteristics. SWS and slow oscillations differ between individuals, and these differences are very stable across conditions in which sleep regulatory systems are differentially activated, for example, baseline sleep and recovery from sleep deprivation. The magnitude of these interindividual differences is considerable. In fact, the interindividual differences in SWS are much greater than the differences induced by sleep deprivation (Tucker et al., 2007). Some of these interindividual differences in SWS are attributable to known factors such as the age and sex of the subject. Starting during adolescence, SWS and SWA exhibit a marked decline throughout the life span, and throughout the life span women have more SWS/SWA than men (Carrier et al., 2001). But even within a relatively narrow age group of only men or women, differences in SWS and SWA persist. Some of these differences have been related to variation in genes. Thus, a polymorphism in the gene coding for adenosine deaminase, which leads to reduced breakdown of adenosine, has been linked to increased SWS and SWA. Furthermore, a polymorphism in a gene coding for the adenosine 2A receptor has also been shown to associate with changes in SWS and SWA (Landolt, 2008). These associations are consistent with our current views on a role for adenosine in sleep regulation. SWS and SWA are also affected by a polymorphism in *PER3*, which is one of the genes involved in circadian rhythmicity (see below, "Early Sleep/Late Sleep: Chrono- or Homeotypes?").

Individual differences in the EEG are not limited to slow waves but have also been reported for sleep spindles and higher-frequency activities such as beta activity, for which the estimated heritability is 96% (De Gennaro et al., 2008). For most of these individual differences, associations with variations in specific genes have not been identified. A polymorphism in the gene coding for the enzyme catechol-*O*-methyltransferase, which plays a significant role in dopamine metabolism, leads to changes in alpha activity in the EEG during sleep (Bodenmann et al., 2009).

One key question in the research on interindividual differences in sleep regulation, including SWS and the EEG, is how these differences relate to differences in sleep regulatory processes. For example, do differences related to either genes or age in SWS simply reflect differences in EEG generating mechanisms with no link to sleep homeostasis, or do these differences indeed imply differences in sleep intensity and sleep need? To answer these questions, individuals who differ with respect to these sleep characteristics will have to be studied under conditions in which the sleep regulatory processes are challenged and correlations between these heritable characteristics and outcome measures such as sleep quality, sleep depth, and waking performance are assessed.

Long Sleep/Short Sleep

The notion that some of us are short sleepers and others are long sleepers is widespread, and the statement that we sleep for 8 hours or so after 16 hours of wakefulness is certainly not true of the population of good sleepers in general.

Several studies on the distribution of sleep duration show that reported sleep duration is 7.0 hours with a standard deviation of 1.5 hours (Groeger et al., 2004). This normal distribution implies that many factors (genes) contribute to sleep duration and that indeed some of us fall within the extremes on either end of the distribution. Age is again a major contributor to this variation, with children, adolescents, and young adults sleeping considerably longer than middle-aged and healthy older adults. Within the age group of young adults, short and long sleepers have been studied in the laboratory. A consistent finding across these studies is that SWS is preserved in short sleepers or may even be slightly enhanced. REM sleep is curtailed. The response to sleep deprivation differs between short and long sleepers, such that long sleepers show more of an increase in SWS/SWA than short sleepers. Quantification of this response to sleep deprivation suggests that this may be related to a lower level of SWS at baseline in long sleepers, which leaves them more room for an increase (Aeschbach et al., 1996). Short or long sleep is also associated with changes in circadian organization. In the absence of the sleep–wake and light–dark cycles (i.e., during constant routine conditions), the biological night, indexed by the rhythm of melatonin and other physiological markers, is shorter in short sleepers than in long sleepers (Aeschbach et al., 1996, 2003). Whether this circadian difference causes the differences in sleep duration or is a consequence of the short period of darkness and longer period of light short sleepers have exposed their circadian system to remains unclear. Recently, two short sleepers were shown to carry a point mutation in yet another circadian gene, *DEC2*. When this genetic variation was introduced in mice and fruit flies, somewhat shorter sleep duration was observed in these species as well, suggesting that this mutation in a circadian gene could contribute to the regulation of sleep duration (He et al., 2009). One major question in the study of short and long sleepers is to what extent short sleepers are better at tolerating the increases in sleep pressure associated with wakefulness or whether there is a slower buildup of homeostatic sleep pressure in short sleepers. Much of the evidence to date favors the former interpretation. Thus, short sleepers display more EEG signs of drowsiness during wakefulness (i.e., more theta activity). When habitual sleep duration is quantified through actigraphy and sleep diaries and sleep propensity is then assessed in the laboratory by assessment of daytime sleep latencies or TST in extended sleep opportunities, short sleepers show signs of a sleep debt (i.e., their sleep latencies are shorter, and the rebound in TST is greater). Thus, the endophenotype of short and long sleepers may be more complicated than just a difference in sleep need. The data shows that adequate phenotyping of individuals who differ with respect to reported sleep characteristics is essential for identifying the sleep regulatory processes that are affected. As such, better phenotyping is also required to interpret age-related changes in sleep structure, sleep propensity, and sleep duration. Whereas healthy older people sleep less at baseline, with less SWS and reduced sleep consolidation, this does not lead to an increase in daytime sleep propensity. In fact, older people are less sleepy than young adults, and when given 16 hours of sleep opportunity per 24 hours for several days, older people sleep only 7.5 hours, whereas young adults sleep 8.9 hours (Klerman & Dijk, 2008). Thus, age-related reduction in sleep duration indeed appears to reflect a reduction in sleep need, in contrast to the reduction in habitual sleep duration experienced by many young adults, which most likely reflects sleep restriction.

Early Sleep/Late Sleep: Chrono- or Homeotypes?

Another phenotype that attracts much attention is the owl versus the lark phenotype. Variation in sleep timing is considerable indeed. Some of us go to sleep when others wake up. Just like for some of the other individual differences we discussed, aging is a major explanatory variable. Whereas teenagers and young adults sleep late, older people sleep and wake early. Furthermore, there are sex differences as far as sleep timing is concerned. Women tend to wake slightly earlier than men. As with the previously discussed characteristics of sleep, variation in the preferred timing for sleep and waking activities, also referred to as *chronotype*, differs even within a narrow age range. Laboratory studies have shown that early sleepers are also characterized by earlier rhythms of body temperature and melatonin as well as earlier timed cycles of the expression of clock genes in leukocytes (Archer et al., 2008; Duffy et al., 1999; Mongrain et al., 2004, 2006a; see Figure 2.6B).

In addition, assessment of endogenous circadian period in forced desynchrony protocols has shown that ratings on morningness–eveningness questionnaires indeed correlate with entrained phase and intrinsic period of circadian rhythms (Duffy et al., 2001). The clock runs fast in early birds. Whereas these associations are in full agreement with the prevailing view of the role of circadian rhythmicity in sleep timing, analysis of PSG-recorded sleep has shown that aspects other than the timing of sleep are also affected by chronotype. It has been reported repeatedly that morning types have more SWS and SWA, in particular in the first NREM cycle, and a faster decline of SWA during sleep (Kerkhof, 1991; Mongrain et al., 2006b). Furthermore, increases in signs of drowsiness in the EEG during wakefulness appear to be faster in morning types (Taillard et al., 2003). Within the conceptual framework of the homeostatic and circadian regulation of sleep, you may go to sleep and wake early because your clock is set early or the buildup and dissipation of sleep pressure are fast. The data indicates that both pathways contribute to the observed phenotypes. Clock genes are obvious candidates to contribute to variation in chronotype. So far, the clock genes *PERIOD2* as well as *CK1δ*, genes coding for enzymes involved in phosphorylation of clock proteins, have been implicated in abnormally early sleep (Toh et al., 2001; Xu et al., 2005). Variation in the clock gene *CLOCK* and *PER3* has been associated with variation in chronotype (Archer et al., 2003; A. S. Lazar et al., 2012). The contribution of the variable number tandem repeat polymorphism in PER3 to circadian rhythmicity and sleep physiology has been investigated in a prospective study in which subjects were selected only on the basis of their genotype, independent of chronotype or any other sleep characteristic (Viola et al., 2007). It was found that whereas the polymorphism did not affect circadian phase, it did affect SWS, SWA, and the increase of theta activity during wakefulness. Furthermore, cognitive decline during sleep deprivation, and in particular during the early morning hours, was much more severe in the subjects homozygous for the allele previously associated with morningness. A subsequent fMRI study revealed that the gene predicted an altered dynamic in the brain responses during an executive task in the course of a normal sleep–wake cycle and a night of sleep deprivation (Vandewalle, Archer, et al., 2009). The data demonstrates that the effects of polymorphisms in clock genes associated with individual differences in sleep timing are associated with changes that go well beyond changes in the timing of rhythms and affect many aspects of sleep physiology (Dijk & Archer, 2009).

Homeostatic and Circadian Regulation of Sleep: Summary and Implications for the Understanding of Sleep Disorders

It is well established that sleep is regulated through a fine-tuned interaction of circadian and homeostatic processes. These two processes emerge from and affect multiple physiological and molecular processes and concern many aspects of sleep and wakefulness. Disruption of the phase relationship between the homeostatic and circadian process as well as changes in the strength of homeostatic sleep pressure and circadian drive for wakefulness and sleep lead to disturbance in sleep and alertness and other aspects of physiology. Sleep homeostatic mechanisms and circadian processes can be manipulated by a variety of behavioral, environmental, and pharmacological interventions and may be used to improve sleep and wakefulness. Emerging knowledge about interindividual differences in sleep–wake regulation and the identification of the underlying genomic variation provides for new avenues in sleep research and holds promise for the development of individualized treatment paradigms.

References

Achermann, P., Dijk, D.-J., Brunner, D. P., & Borbély, A. A. (1993). A model of human sleep homeostasis based on EEG slow-wave activity: Quantitative comparison of data and simulations. *Brain Research Bulletin, 31*, 97–113.

Aeschbach, D., Cajochen, C., Landolt, H.-P., & Borbély, A. A. (1996). Homeostatic sleep regulation in habitual short sleepers and long sleepers. *American Journal of Physiology: Regulatory, Integrative and Comparative Physiology, 270*, R41–R53.

Aeschbach, D., Cutler, A. J., & Ronda, J. M. (2008). A role for non-rapid-eye-movement sleep homeostasis in perceptual learning. *Journal of Neuroscience, 28*, 2766–2772.

Aeschbach, D., Sher, L., Postolache, T. T., Matthews, J. R., Jackson, M. A., & Wehr, T. A. (2003). A longer biological night in long sleepers than in short sleepers. *Journal of Clinical Endocrinology and Metabolism, 88*, 26–30.

Agnew, H. W., Jr., Webb, W. B., & Williams, R. L. (1967). Comparison of stage four and 1-REM sleep deprivation. *Perceptual and Motor Skills, 24*, 851–858.

Åkerstedt, T., & Gillberg, M. (1981). The circadian variation of experimentally displaced sleep. *Sleep, 4*, 159–169.

Akerstedt, T., Kecklund, G., Ingre, M., Lekander, M., & Axelsson, J. (2009). Sleep homeostasis during repeated sleep restriction and recovery: Support from EEG dynamics. *Sleep, 32*, 217–222.

Arand, D., Bonnet, M., Hurwitz, T., Mitler, M., Rosa, R., & Sangal, R. B. (2005). The clinical use of the MSLT and MWT. *Sleep, 28*, 123–144.

Archer, S. N., Robilliard, D. L., Skene, D. J., Smits, M., Williams, A., Arendt, J., & von Schantz, M. (2003). A length polymorphism in the circadian clock gene Per3 is linked to delayed sleep phase syndrome and extreme diurnal preference. *Sleep, 26*, 413–415.

Archer, S. N., Viola, A. U., Kyriakopoulou, V., von Schantz, M., & Dijk, D.-J. (2008). Inter-individual differences in habitual sleep timing and entrained phase of endogenous circadian rhythms of BMAL1, PER2 and PER3 mRNA in human leukocytes. *Sleep, 31*, 608–617.

Arendt, J. (2006). Melatonin and human rhythms. *Chronobiology International, 23*, 21–37.

Baker, F. C., Maloney, S., & Driver, H. S. (1999). A comparison of subjective estimates of sleep with objective polysomnographic data in healthy men and women. *Journal of Psychosomatic Research, 47*, 335–341.

Banks, S., & Dinges, D. F. (2007). Behavioral and physiological consequences of sleep restriction. *Journal of Clinical Sleep Medicine, 3*, 519–528.

Beersma, D. G. M., Dijk, D.-J., Blok, C. G. H., & Everhardus, I. (1990). REM sleep deprivation during 5 hours leads to an immediate REM sleep rebound and to suppression of non-REM sleep intensity. *Electroencephalography and Clinical Neurophysiology, 76*, 114–122.

Belenky, G., Wesensten, N. J., Thorne, D. R., Thomas, M. L., Sing, H. C., Redmond, D. P., Russo, M. B., & Balkin, T. J. (2003). Patterns of performance degradation and restoration during sleep restriction and subsequent recovery: A sleep dose–response study. *Journal of Sleep Research, 12*, 1–12.

Bodenmann, S., Rusterholz, T., Durr, R., Stoll, C., Bachmann, V., Geissler, E., Jaggi-Schwarz, K., & Landolt, H. P. (2009). The functional Val158Met polymorphism of COMT predicts interindividual differences in brain alpha oscillations in young men. *Journal of Neuroscience, 29*, 10855–10862.

Bonnet, M. H. (1986). Performance and sleepiness following moderate sleep disruption and slow wave sleep deprivation. *Physiology & Behavior, 37*, 915–918.

Borbély, A. A. (1982). A two process model of sleep regulation. *Human Neurobiology, 1*, 195–204.

Borbély, A. A., & Achermann, P. (1999). Sleep homeostasis and models of sleep regulation. *Journal of Biological Rhythms, 14*, 557–568.
Borbély, A. A., Baumann, F., Brandeis, D., Strauch, I., & Lehmann, D. (1981). Sleep deprivation: Effect of sleep stages and EEG power density in man. *Electroencephalography and Clinical Neurophysiology, 51*, 483–493.
Brunner, D. P., Dijk, D.-J., & Borbély, A. A. (1993). Repeated partial sleep deprivation progressively changes the EEG during sleep and wakefulness. *Sleep, 16*, 100–113.
Cajochen, C., Khalsa, S. B. S., Wyatt, J. K., Czeisler, C. A., & Dijk, D.-J. (1999). EEG and ocular correlates of circadian melatonin phase and human performance decrements during sleep loss. *American Journal of Physiology, 277*, R640–R649.
Cajochen, C., Munch, M., Kobialka, S., Krauchi, K., Steiner, R., Oelhafen, P., Orgul, S., & Wirz-Justice, A. (2005). High sensitivity of human melatonin, alertness, thermoregulation, and heart rate to short wavelength light. *Journal of Clinical Endocrinology and Metabolism, 90*, 1311–1316.
Carrier, J., Land, S., Buysse, D. J., Kupfer, D. J., & Monk, T. H. (2001). The effects of age and gender on sleep EEG power spectral density in the middle years of life (ages 20–60 years old). *Psychophysiology, 38*, 232–242.
Carskadon, M. A., & Dement, W. C. (1981). Cumulative effects of sleep restriction on daytime sleepiness. *Psychophysiology, 18*, 107–113.
Carskadon, M. A., & Dement, W. C. (1982). The Multiple Sleep Latency Test: What does it measure? *Sleep, 5*, S67–S72.
Carskadon, M. A., & Dement, W. C. (1996). Normal human sleep: An overview. In M. H. Kryger, T. Roth, & W. C. Dement (Eds.), *Principles and practice of sleep medicine* (pp. 16–25). Saunders.
Carskadon, M. A., & Dement, W. C. (1977). Sleepiness and sleep state on a 90-min schedule. *Psychophysiology, 14*(2), 127–133.
Crunelli, V., & Hughes, S. W. (2009). The slow (<1 Hz) rhythm of non-REM sleep: A dialogue between three cardinal oscillators. *Nature Neuroscience, 13*, 9–17.
Czeisler, C. A., & Dijk, D.-J. (2001). Human circadian physiology and sleep–wake regulation. In J. S. Takahashi, F. W. Turek, & R. Y. Moore (Eds.), *Circadian clocks* (pp. 531–569). Kluwer Academic/Plenum Publishers.
Czeisler, C. A., Duffy, J. F., Shanahan, T. L., Brown, E. N., Mitchell, J. F., Rimmer, D. W., Ronda, J. M., Silva, E. J., Allan, J. S., Emens, J. S., Dijk, D.-J., & Kronauer, R. E. (1999). Stability, precision, and near-24-hour period of the human circadian pacemaker. *Science, 284*, 2177–2181.
Czeisler, C. A., & Gooley, J. J. (2007). Sleep and circadian rhythms in humans. *Cold Spring Harbor Symposia on Quantitative Biology, 72*, 579–597.
Czeisler, C. A., & Klerman, E. B. (1999). Circadian and sleep-dependent regulation of hormone release in humans. *Recent Progress in Hormone Research, 54*, 97–132.
Czeisler, C. A., Weitzman, E. D., Moore-Ede, M. C., Zimmerman, J. C., & Knauer, R. S. (1980). Human sleep: Its duration and organization depend on its circadian phase. *Science, 210*, 1264–1267.
Czeisler, C. A., Zimmerman, J. C., Ronda, J. M., Moore-Ede, M. C., & Weitzman, E. D. (1980). Timing of REM sleep is coupled to the circadian rhythm of body temperature in man. *Sleep, 2*, 329–346.
Daan, S., Beersma, D. G. M., & Borbély, A. A. (1984). Timing of human sleep: Recovery process gated by a circadian pacemaker. *American Journal of Physiology, 246*, R161–R178.
De Gennaro, L., & Ferrara, M. (2003). Sleep spindles: An overview. *Sleep Medicine Reviews, 7*, 423–440.
De Gennaro, L., Marzano, C., Fratello, F., Moroni, F., Pellicciari, M. C., Ferlazzo, F., Costa, S., Couyoumdjian, A., Curcio, G., Sforza, E., Malafosse, A., Finelli, L. A., Pasqualetti, P., Ferrara, M., Bertini, M., & Rossini, P. M. (2008). The electroencephalographic fingerprint of sleep is genetically determined: A twin study. *Annals of Neurology, 64*, 455–460.
Dijk, D.-J., & Archer, S. N. (2009). PERIOD3, circadian phenotypes, and sleep homeostasis. *Sleep Medicine Reviews, 14*, 151–160.
Dijk, D.-J., Beersma, D. G. M., & Daan, S. (1987). EEG power density during nap sleep: Reflection of an hourglass measuring the duration of prior wakefulness. *Journal of Biological Rhythms, 2*, 207–219.
Dijk, D.-J., Beersma, D. G. M., Daan, S., Bloem, G. M., & van den Hoofdakker, R. H. (1987). Quantitative analysis of the effects of slow wave sleep deprivation during the first 3 h of sleep on subsequent EEG power density. *European Archives of Psychiatry and Neurological Sciences, 236*, 323–328.

Dijk, D.-J., Brunner, D. P., & Borbély, A. A. (1990). Time course of EEG power density during long sleep in humans. *American Journal of Physiology: Regulatory, Integrative and Comparative Physiology, 258*, R650–R661.

Dijk, D.-J., & Czeisler, C. A. (1994). Paradoxical timing of the circadian rhythm of sleep propensity serves to consolidate sleep and wakefulness in humans. *Neuroscience Letters, 166*, 63–68.

Dijk, D.-J., & Czeisler, C. A. (1995). Contribution of the circadian pacemaker and the sleep homeostat to sleep propensity, sleep structure, electroencephalographic slow waves and sleep spindle activity in humans. *Journal of Neuroscience, 15*, 3526–3538.

Dijk, D.-J., Duffy, J. F., & Czeisler, C. A. (1992). Circadian and sleep/wake dependent aspects of subjective alertness and cognitive performance. *Journal of Sleep Research, 1*, 112–117.

Dijk, D.-J., Duffy, J. F., Riel, E., Shanahan, T. L., & Czeisler, C. A. (1999). Ageing and the circadian and homeostatic regulation of human sleep during forced desynchrony of rest, melatonin and temperature rhythms. *Journal of Physiology, 516*(Pt. 2), 611–627.

Dijk, D.-J., Hayes, B., & Czeisler, C. A. (1993). Dynamics of electroencephalographic sleep spindles and slow wave activity in men: Effect of sleep deprivation. *Brain Research, 626*, 190–199.

Dijk, D.-J., Shanahan, T. L., Duffy, J. F., Ronda, J. M., & Czeisler, C. A. (1997). Variation of electroencephalographic activity during non-rapid eye movement and rapid eye movement sleep with phase of circadian melatonin rhythm in humans. *Journal of Physiology, 505*(Pt. 3), 851–858.

Dinges, D. F., Pack, F., Williams, K., Gillen, K. A., Powell, J. W., Ott, G. E., Aptowicz, C., & Pack, A. I. (1997). Cumulative sleepiness, mood disturbance, and psychomotor vigilance performance decrements during a week of sleep restricted to 4–5 hours per night. *Sleep, 20*, 267–277.

Duffy, J. F., & Dijk, D. J. (2002). Getting through to circadian oscillators: Why use constant routines? *Journal of Biological Rhythms, 17*, 4–13.

Duffy, J. F., Dijk, D.-J., Hall, E. F., & Czeisler, C. A. (1999). Relationship of endogenous circadian melatonin and temperature rhythms to self-reported preference for morning or evening activity in young and older people. *Journal of Investigative Medicine, 47*, 141–150.

Duffy, J. F., Rimmer, D. W., & Czeisler, C. A. (2001). Association of intrinsic circadian period with morningness–eveningness, usual wake time, and circadian phase. *Behavioral Neuroscience, 115*, 895–899.

Duffy, J. F., & Wright, K. P., Jr. (2005). Entrainment of the human circadian system by light. *Journal of Biological Rhythms, 20*, 326–338.

Edgar, D. M., Dement, W. C., & Fuller, C. A. (1993). Effect of SCN lesions on sleep in squirrel monkeys: Evidence for opponent processes in sleep-wake regulation. *Journal of Neuroscience, 13*(3), 1065–1079.

Endo, T., Roth, C., Landolt, H. P., Werth, E., Aeschbach, D., Achermann, P., & Borbely, A. A. (1998). Selective REM sleep deprivation in humans: Effects on sleep and sleep EEG. *American Journal of Physiology: Regulatory, Integrative and Comparative Physiology, 274*, R1186–R1194.

Esser, S. K., Hill, S. L., & Tononi, G. (2007). Sleep homeostasis and cortical synchronization: I. Modeling the effects of synaptic strength on sleep slow waves. *Sleep, 30*, 1617–1630.

Feinberg, I., & Floyd, T. C. (1979). Systematic trends across the night in human sleep cycles. *Psychophysiology, 16*, 283–291.

Ferrara, M., De Gennaro, L., & Bertini, M. (1999). Selective slow-wave sleep (SWS) deprivation and SWS rebound: Do we need a fixed SWS amount per night? *Sleep Research Online, 2*, 15–19.

Finelli, L. A., Baumann, H., Borbely, A. A., & Achermann, P. (2000). Dual electroencephalogram markers of human sleep homeostasis: Correlation between theta activity in waking and slow-wave activity in sleep. *Neuroscience, 101*, 523–529.

Frank, M. G. (2016). Circadian regulation of synaptic plasticity. *Biology (Basel), 5*(3), Article 31.

Fronczek, R., Baumann, C. R., Lammers, G. J., Bassetti, C. L., & Overeem, S. (2009). Hypocretin/orexin disturbances in neurological disorders. *Sleep Medicine Reviews, 13*, 9–22.

Goulet, G., Mongrain, V., Desrosiers, C., Paquet, J., & Dumont, M. (2007). Daily light exposure in morning-type and evening-type individuals. *Journal of Biological Rhythms, 22*, 151–158.

Groeger, J. A., Zijlstra, F. R., & Dijk, D.-J. (2004). Sleep quantity, sleep difficulties and their perceived consequences in a representative sample of some 2000 British adults. *Journal of Sleep Research, 13*, 359–371.

Gronfier, C., Wright, K. P., Jr., Kronauer, R. E., & Czeisler, C. A. (2007). Entrainment of the human circadian pacemaker to longer-than-24-h days. *Proceedings of the National Academy of Sciences of the United States of America, 104*, 9081–9086.

He, Y., Jones, C. R., Fujiki, N., Xu, Y., Guo, B., Holder, J. L., Jr., Rossner, M. J., Nishino, S., & Fu, Y. H. (2009). The transcriptional repressor DEC2 regulates sleep length in mammals. *Science, 325*, 866–870.

Huber, R., Ghilardi, M. F., Massimini, M., Ferrarelli, F., Riedner, B. A., Peterson, M. J., & Tononi, G. (2006). Arm immobilization causes cortical plastic changes and locally decreases sleep slow wave activity. *Nature Neuroscience, 9*, 1169–1176.

Jurysta, F., van de Borne, P., Migeotte, P. F., Dumont, M., Lanquart, J. P., Degaute, J. P., & Linkowski, P. (2003). A study of the dynamic interactions between sleep EEG and heart rate variability in healthy young men. *Clinical Neurophysiology, 114*, 2146–2155.

Kahneman, D., Krueger, A. B., Schkade, D. A., Schwarz, N., & Stone, A. A. (2004). A survey method for characterizing daily life experience: The day reconstruction method. *Science, 306*, 1776–1780.

Kamdar, B. B., Kaplan, K. A., Kezirian, E. J., & Dement, W. C. (2004). The impact of extended sleep on daytime alertness, vigilance, and mood. *Sleep Medicine, 5*, 441–448.

Karacan, I., Williams, R. L., Finley, W. W., & Hursch, C. J. (1970). The effects of naps on nocturnal sleep: Influence on the need for stage 1 REM and stage 4 sleep. *Biological Psychiatry, 2*, 391–399.

Kattler, H., Dijk, D.-J., & Borbély, A. A. (1994). Effect of unilateral somatosensory stimulation prior to sleep on the sleep EEG in humans. *Journal of Sleep Research, 3*, 159–164.

Kerkhof, G. A. (1991). Differences between morning-types and evening-types in the dynamics of EEG slow wave activity during night sleep. *Electroencephalography and Clinical Neurophysiology, 78*, 197–202.

Khalsa, S. B. S., Conroy, D. A., Duffy, J. F., Czeisler, C. A., & Dijk, D.-J. (2002). Sleep- and circadian-dependent modulation of REM density. *Journal of Sleep Research, 11*, 53–59.

Klerman, E. B., & Dijk, D.-J. (2005). Interindividual variation in sleep duration and its association with sleep debt in young adults. *Sleep, 28*, 1253–1259.

Klerman, E. B., & Dijk, D.-J. (2008). Age-related reduction in the maximal capacity for sleep—Implications for insomnia. *Current Biology, 18*, 1118–1123.

Knoblauch, V., Martens, W. L. J., Wirz-Justice, A., Krauchi, K., & Cajochen, C. (2003). Regional differences in the circadian modulation of human sleep spindle characteristics. *European Journal of Neuroscience, 18*, 155–163.

Krauchi, K. (2007). The thermophysiological cascade leading to sleep initiation in relation to phase of entrainment. *Sleep Medicine Reviews, 11*, 439–451.

Krimsky, W. R., & Leiter, J. C. (2005). Physiology of breathing and respiratory control during sleep. *Seminars in Respiratory and Critical Care Medicine, 26*, 5–12.

Krueger, J. M., Rector, D. M., Roy, S., Van Dongen, H. P., Belenky, G., & Panksepp, J. (2008). Sleep as a fundamental property of neuronal assemblies. *Nature Reviews Neuroscience, 9*, 910–919.

Landolt, H. P. (2008). Sleep homeostasis: A role for adenosine in humans? *Biochemical Pharmacology, 75*, 2070–2079.

Landsness, E. C., Crupi, D., Hulse, B. K., Peterson, M. J., Huber, R., Ansari, H., Coen, M., Cirelli, C., Benca, R. M., Ghilardi, M. F., & Tononi, G. (2009). Sleep-dependent improvement in visuomotor learning: A causal role for slow waves. *Sleep, 32*, 1273–1284.

Lavie, P. (1986). Ultrashort sleep–waking schedule III. “Gates” and “forbidden zones” for sleep. *Electroencephalography and Clinical Neurophysiology, 63*, 414–425.

Lazar, A. S., Lazar, Z. I., & Dijk, D. J. (2015). Circadian regulation of slow waves in human sleep: Topographical aspects. *Neuroimage, 116*, 123–134.

Lazar, A. S., Slak, A., Lo, J. C., Santhi, N., von Schantz, M., Archer, S. N., Groeger, J. A., & Dijk, D.-J. (2012). Sleep, diurnal preference, health and psychological well-being: A prospective single-allelic-variation study. *Chronobiology International, 29*(2), 131–146.

Lazar, Z. I., Dijk, D. J., & Lazar, A. S. (2019). Infraslow oscillations in human sleep spindle activity. *Journal of Neuroscience Methods, 316*, 22–34.

Lecci, S., Fernandez, L. M., Weber, F. D., Cardis, R., Chatton, J. Y., Born, J., & Luthi, A. (2017). Coordinated infraslow neural and cardiac oscillations mark fragility and offline periods in mammalian sleep. *Science Advances, 3*(2), Article e1602026. https://doi.org/10.1126/sciadv.1602026

Lim, J., & Dinges, D. F. (2008). Sleep deprivation and vigilant attention. *Annals of the New York Academy of Sciences, 1129*, 305–322.

Lockley, S. W., Dijk, D.-J., Kosti, O., Skene, D. J., & Arendt, J. (2008). Alertness, mood and performance rhythm disturbances associated with circadian sleep disorders in the blind. *Journal of Sleep Research, 17*, 207–216.

Lockley, S. W., Skene, D. J., Arendt, J., Tabandeh, H., Bird, A. C., & Defrance, R. (1997). Relationship between melatonin rhythms and visual loss in the blind. *Journal of Clinical Endocrinology and Metabolism*, *82*, 3763–3770.

Majer, M., Jones, J. F., Unger, E. R., Youngblood, L. S., Decker, M. J., Gurbaxani, B., Heim, C., & Reeves, W. C. (2007). Perception versus polysomnographic assessment of sleep in CFS and non-fatigued control subjects: Results from a population-based study. *BMC Neurology*, *7*, Article 40.

Mak-McCully, R. A., Rolland, M., Sargsyan, A., Gonzalez, C., Magnin, M., Chauvel, P., Rey, M., Bastuji, H., & Halgren, E. (2017). Coordination of cortical and thalamic activity during non-REM sleep in humans. *Nature Communications*, *8*, Article 15499.

Massimini, M., Huber, R., Ferrarelli, F., Hill, S., & Tononi, G. (2004). The sleep slow oscillation as a traveling wave. *Journal of Neuroscience*, *24*, 6862–6870.

Meyer, N., Harvey, A. G., Lockley, S. W., & Dijk, D. J. (2022). Circadian rhythms and disorders of the timing of sleep. *Lancet*, *400*(10357), 1061–1078.

Mongrain, V., Carrier, J., & Dumont, M. (2006a). Circadian and homeostatic sleep regulation in morningness–eveningness. *Journal of Sleep Research*, *15*, 162–166.

Mongrain, V., Carrier, J., & Dumont, M. (2006b). Difference in sleep regulation between morning and evening circadian types as indexed by antero-posterior analyses of the sleep EEG. *European Journal of Neuroscience*, *23*, 497–504.

Mongrain, V., Lavoie, S., Selmaoui, B., Paquet, J., & Dumont, M. (2004). Phase relationships between sleep–wake cycle and underlying circadian rhythms in morningness–eveningness. *Journal of Biological Rhythms*, *19*, 248–257.

Nave, R., Peled, R., & Lavie, P. (1995). Melatonin improves evening napping. *European Journal of Pharmacology*, *275*, 213–216.

Ohayon, M. M., Carskadon, M. A., Guilleminault, C., & Vitiello, M. V. (2004). Meta-analysis of quantitative sleep parameters from childhood to old age in healthy individuals: Developing normative sleep values across the human lifespan. *Sleep*, *27*, 1255–1273.

Rajaratnam, S. M., Dijk, D.-J., Middleton, B., Stone, B. M., & Arendt, J. (2003). Melatonin phase-shifts human circadian rhythms with no evidence of changes in the duration of endogenous melatonin secretion or the 24-hour production of reproductive hormones. *Journal of Clinical Endocrinology and Metabolism*, *88*, 4303–4309.

Rajaratnam, S. M., Middleton, B., Stone, B. M., Arendt, J., & Dijk, D.-J. (2004). Melatonin advances the circadian timing of EEG sleep and directly facilitates sleep without altering its duration in extended sleep opportunities in humans. *Journal of Physiology*, *561*, 339–351.

Riedner, B. A., Vyazovskiy, V. V., Huber, R., Massimini, M., Esser, S. K., Murphy, M., & Tononi, G. (2007). Sleep homeostasis and cortical synchronization: III. A high-density EEG study of sleep slow waves in humans. *Sleep*, *30*(12), 1643–1657.

Roehrs, T., Shore, E., Papineau, K., Rosenthal, L., & Roth, T. (1996). A two-week sleep extension in sleepy normals. *Sleep*, *19*, 576–582.

Roenneberg, T., Kumar, C. J., & Merrow, M. (2007). The human circadian clock entrains to sun time. *Current Biology*, *17*, R44–R45.

Rosenthal, L., Merlotti, L., Roehrs, T. A., & Roth, T. (1991). Enforced 24-hour recovery following sleep deprivation. *Sleep*, *14*, 448–453.

Santhi, N., Lazar, A. S., McCabe, P. J., Lo, J. C., Groeger, J. A., & Dijk, D. J. (2016). Sex differences in the circadian regulation of sleep and waking cognition in humans. *Proceedings of the National Academy of Sciences of the United States of America*, *113*(19), E2730–2739.

Scheer, F. A., Shea, T. J., Hilton, M. F., & Shea, S. A. (2008). An endogenous circadian rhythm in sleep inertia results in greatest cognitive impairment upon awakening during the biological night. *Journal of Biological Rhythms*, *23*, 353–361.

Silva, E. J., & Duffy, J. F. (2008). Sleep inertia varies with circadian phase and sleep stage in older adults. *Behavioral Neuroscience*, *122*, 928–935.

Spiegel, K., Tasali, E., Penev, P., & Van Cauter, E. (2004). Brief communication: Sleep curtailment in healthy young men is associated with decreased leptin levels, elevated ghrelin levels, and increased hunger and appetite. *Annals of Internal Medicine*, *141*, 846–850.

Srinivasan, V., Pandi-Perumal, S. R., Trahkt, I., Spence, D. W., Poeggeler, B., Hardeland, R., & Cardinali, D. P. (2009). Melatonin and melatonergic drugs on sleep: Possible mechanisms of action. *International Journal of Neuroscience*, *119*, 821–846.

Steriade, M. (2003). The corticothalamic system in sleep. *Frontiers in Bioscience, 8*, d878–d899.
Strogatz, S. H., Kronauer, R. E., & Czeisler, C. A. (1986). Circadian regulation dominates homeostatic control of sleep length and prior wake length in humans. *Sleep, 9*, 353–364.
Strogatz, S. H., Kronauer, R. E., & Czeisler, C. A. (1987). Circadian pacemaker interferes with sleep onset at specific times each day: Role in insomnia. *American Journal of Physiology, 253*, R172–R178.
Taillard, J., Philip, P., Coste, O., Sagaspe, P., & Bioulac, B. (2003). The circadian and homeostatic modulation of sleep pressure during wakefulness differs between morning and evening chronotypes. *Journal of Sleep Research, 12*, 275–282.
Takahashi, J. S. (2017). Transcriptional architecture of the mammalian circadian clock. *Nature Reviews Genetics, 18*(3), 164–179.
Takahashi, J. S., Hong, H. K., Ko, C. H., & McDearmon, E. L. (2008). The genetics of mammalian circadian order and disorder: Implications for physiology and disease. *Nature Reviews Genetics, 9*, 764–775.
Tasali, E., Leproult, R., Ehrmann, D. A., & Van Cauter, E. (2008). Slow wave sleep and the risk of type 2 diabetes in humans. *Proceedings of the National Academy of Sciences of the United States of America, 105*, 1044–1049.
Toh, K. L., Jones, C. R., He, Y., Eide, E. J., Hinz, W. A., Virshup, D. M., Ptacek, L. J., & Fu, Y. H. (2001). An hPer2 phosphorylation site mutation in familial advanced sleep phase syndrome. *Science, 291*, 1040–1043.
Tononi, G., & Cirelli, C. (2006). Sleep function and synaptic homeostasis. *Sleep Medicine Reviews, 10*, 49–62.
Tononi, G., & Cirelli, C. (2014). Sleep and the price of plasticity: From synaptic and cellular homeostasis to memory consolidation and integration. *Neuron, 81*(1), 12–34.
Tucker, A. M., Dinges, D. F., & Van Dongen, H. P. (2007). Trait interindividual differences in the sleep physiology of healthy young adults. *Journal of Sleep Research, 16*, 170–180.
Vandewalle, G., Archer, S. N., Wuillaume, C., Balteau, E., Degueldre, C., Luxen, A., Maquet, P., & Dijk, D.-J. (2009). Functional MRI assessed brain responses during an executive task depend on interaction of sleep homeostasis, circadian phase, and PER3 genotype. *Journal of Neuroscience, 29*, 7948–7956.
Vandewalle, G., Maquet, P., & Dijk, D.-J. (2009). Light as a modulator of cognitive brain function. *Trends in Cognitive Sciences, 13*, 429–438.
Viola, A. U., Archer, S. N., James, L. M., Groeger, J. A., Lo, J. C., Skene, D. J., von Schantz, M., & Dijk, D.-J. (2007). PER3 polymorphism predicts sleep structure and waking performance. *Current Biology, 17*, 613–618.
Vyazovskiy, V. V., Olcese, U., Lazimy, Y. M., Faraguna, U., Esser, S. K., Williams, J. C., Cirelli, C., & Tononi, G. (2009). Cortical firing and sleep homeostasis. *Neuron, 63*, 865–878.
Vyazovskiy, V. V., Riedner, B. A., Cirelli, C., & Tononi, G. (2007). Sleep homeostasis and cortical synchronization: II. A local field potential study of sleep slow waves in the rat. *Sleep, 30*(12), 1631–1642.
Walsh, J. K., Hartman, P. G., & Schweitzer, P. K. (1994). Slow-wave sleep deprivation and waking function. *Journal of Sleep Research, 3*, 16–25.
Wehr, T. A. (1991). The durations of human melatonin secretion and sleep respond to changes in daylength (photoperiod). *Journal of Clinical Endocrinology and Metabolism, 73*, 1276–1280.
Wei, H. G., Riel, E., Czeisler, C. A., & Dijk, D.-J. (1999). Attenuated amplitude of circadian and sleep-dependent modulation of electroencephalographic sleep spindle characteristics in elderly human subjects. *Neuroscience Letters, 260*, 29–32.
Weitzman, E. D., Czeisler, C. A., Zimmerman, J. C., & Ronda, J. M. (1980). Timing of REM and stages 3 and 4 sleep during temporal isolation in man. *Sleep, 2*, 391–407.
Weitzman, E. D., Nogeire, C., Perlow, M. J., Fukushima, D. K., Sassin, J. F., McGregor, P. A., Gallagher, T. F., & Hellman, L. (1974). Effects of a prolonged 3-hour sleep-wake cycle on sleep stages, plasma cortisol, growth hormone and body temperature in man. *The Journal of Clinical Endocrinology and Metabolism, 38*(6), 1018–1030.
Werth, E., Dijk, D.-J., Achermann, P., & Borbély, A. A. (1996). Dynamics of the sleep EEG after an early evening nap: Experimental data and simulations. *American Journal of Physiology: Regulatory, Integrative and Comparative Physiology, 271*, R501–R510.
Wyatt, J. K., Cajochen, C., Ritz-De Cecco, A., Czeisler, C. A., & Dijk, D.-J. (2004). Low dose, repeated caffeine administration for circadian-phase dependent performance degradation during extended wakefulness. *Sleep, 27*, 374–381.
Wyatt, J. K., Dijk, D.-J., Ritz-de Cecco, A., Ronda, J. M., & Czeisler, C. A. (2006). Sleep-facilitating effect of exogenous melatonin in healthy young men and women is circadian-phase dependent. *Sleep, 29*, 609–618.

Wyatt, J. K., Ritz-De Cecco, A., Czeisler, C. A., & Dijk, D.-J. (1999). Circadian temperature and melatonin rhythms, sleep, and neurobehavioral function in humans living on a 20-h day. *American Journal of Physiology: Regulatory, Integrative and Comparative Physiology*, *277*, R1152–R1163.

Xu, Y., Padiath, Q. S., Shapiro, R. E., Jones, C. R., Wu, S. C., Saigoh, N., Saigoh, K., Ptacek, L. J., & Fu, Y. H. (2005). Functional consequences of a CKIdelta mutation causing familial advanced sleep phase syndrome. *Nature*, *434*, 640–644.

Zulley, J., Wever, R., & Aschoff, J. (1981). The dependence of onset and duration of sleep on the circadian rhythm of rectal temperature. *Pflügers Archiv*, *391*, 314–318.

CHAPTER 3

Sleep and Circadian Development in the Early and Developing Years

Innessa Donskoy *and* Temitayo Oyegbile-Chidi

Abstract

The human circadian rhythm begins to develop during the fetal period and becomes more robust and refined through infancy, childhood, and adolescence. While the fetus heavily relies on maternal circadian control, the infant and child largely respond to their own endogenous and exogenous circadian cues. Sleep architecture and staging also change with age, maturing to familiar adult landmarks in late childhood. Adolescence brings significant delays in the sleep–wake phase from both endogenous and exogenous cues, and this issue has the magnitude to influence legislative decisions on appropriate school start times. Sleep disorders that present in early life may linger and continue to negatively impact sleep quality in the future. Continued translational research on pediatric sleep and circadian physiology is critical in order to raise a generation of optimal sleepers who move forward into adulthood efficiently getting their required sleep, which ultimately enhances mental and physical health.

Key Words: circadian, sleep, fetal, infant, children, adolescent, school start time, social jet lag

Introduction

Sleep patterns vary throughout the life span. From conception through adolescence, the pediatric period encompasses the early development, continued cultivation, and maturation of the circadian rhythm. This rhythm plays an integral role in controlling sleep patterns as well as other body processes. An aspect of circadian control can be seen in almost all organ systems of the human body as well as across a multitude of species. The so-called master clock of the human body resides in the suprachiasmatic nucleus (SCN) and is controlled by an elegant feedback loop. The most potent influence upon this master clock is the presence of light, often referred to as a *zeitgeber* (time giver), aligning an individual's internal time zone to match that of the light/dark cycle to which they are exposed. The eye has a cluster of designated retinal ganglion cells (RGCs) that respond to light, with increased sensitivity to the blue wavelength of visible light (400–490 nm) (Tosini et al., 2016), which is a separate system from the rod and cone cells that control vision. Upon exposure to light, a compound called *melanopsin* within these photosensitive RGCs is activated and sends this time-of-day signal to the hypothalamus through the retinohypothalamic tract (RHT). Within the hypothalamus, there is a structure designated as the SCN. It is comprised of an inner core of neurons expressing vasoactive intestinal polypeptide (VIP) and an outer lining of neurons expressing the neuropeptide arginine vasopressin (AVP) (Abrahamson & Moore, 2001). The SCN receives light information through the RHT, which prompts the expression of several key circadian genes. In the presence of light, which represents the traditional human "day," the genes *BMAL* (brain and muscle Arnt-like factor) and *CLOCK* (circadian locomotor output cycle kaput) are transcribed and translated, and their final protein products dimerize in the nucleus. The duo then binds to the promoter region of the genes *PER* (period) and *CRY* (cryptochrome) to allow for their expression in the cellular cytoplasm. During the "night," PER and CRY associate with other proteins (including casein kinase 1) and are trafficked back into the nucleus to inhibit the BMAL:CLOCK dimer's activity, effectively turning off further PER and CRY expression (Aryal et al., 2017). There are other known factors at play, including casein kinase 1 mediating PER's degradation and CLOCK:BMAL1's transcription of *Rorα* (retinoic acid receptor–related orphan receptor α, which activates BMAL's transcription) and *Rev-Erbα* (reverse erythroblastosis virus α, which inhibits BMAL's transcription) (Buhr & Takahashi et al., 2013; Meng et al., 2008). These feedback loops allow for the self-contained control of an approximately 24-hour process. *PER* gene expression within the neurons of the SCN can be seen even when the cells are maintained in vitro for over 30 days (Yamazaki et al., 2000). While the SCN houses the primary central control of an organism's day and night, it also communicates with other tissues exhibiting circadian gene expression, termed *peripheral oscillators*, such as in heart, adrenal, and liver tissue (Brown et al., 2019). These peripheral clocks do not self-maintain as robust of a circadian rhythm and in vitro lose their cycling pattern within approximately 7 days (Yamazaki et al., 2000).

In discussing the function of the SCN, it is imperative to understand that its endogenous cycle is not exactly 24 hours but rather closer to 24.2 hours. Therefore, external light input in the "morning/day" is critical to prevent the slow drifting forward of the internal clock. One well-known hormone under circadian control is melatonin. The SCN neurons project to the superior cervical ganglion, which signals to the pineal gland to promote the production of melatonin during the human dark/night phase. Endogenous melatonin levels begin to rise prior to sleep onset, reach their peak in the middle of the night, and then decrease by the end of the night. Upon exposure to light, melatonin production is halted (Wong et al., 2022). Melatonin receptors such as MT1 and MT2 are expressed in numerous tissues, including the retina and SCN, contributing to the elegance of this feedback loop (Dubocovich, 2007). It is the interplay of intrinsic circadian processes and extrinsic factors (light, food, socialization, medication, and physical and psychological stress) that influences the timing of sleep and myriad other processes under circadian control. Any of these factors can cause the circadian rhythm and secondary sleep to go awry. From the initial development of the fetal brain and structures that will house and control central and peripheral circadian control to birth, infancy, childhood development, and through adolescence, the circadian rhythm continues to develop. Endogenous and exogenous factors can positively or negatively impact internal rhythmicity. This chapter will explore all these aspects throughout the pediatric period.

Sleep in the Developing Fetus

Circadian Development

Sleep begins as early signs of life and development become apparent in utero. As the growing fetus develops its own RHT, a mature hypothalamus with an SCN, and a pineal gland, it is largely maternal external activity and internal processes which entrain the fetus to the timing of its outer world (McCarthy et al., 2019; Wong et al., 2022). The maternal clock appears to communicate with the fetal clock through melatonin as a primary zeitgeber. It influences the development of the fetal circadian rhythm similar to the entrainment of other peripheral maternal clocks (skin tissue, intestinal tissue, etc.) (Lam et al., 2003). In embryonic mice, *CLOCK* gene expression is noted in the SCN (Honma, 2020). In humans, SCN development can already be detected prior to the halfway point of a full gestation (Swaab et al., 1990). Fetal squirrel models suggest that the SCN is functional and can control peripheral clocks such as glucose regulators prior to birth (Reppert & Schwartz, 1984). In capuchin monkeys at 90% gestation, there is already circadian gene expression of *BMAL1* and *Per2* and specific receptors for melatonin (Reppert & Schwartz, 1984). In the human fetus, the presence of a typically developed brain with an intact SCN is not only a luxury but a necessity for developing a diurnal rhythm following maternal signaling (Lunshof et al., 1997). Mutations in specific genes such as *Per*, *Cry*, and *CLOCK* as noted above have been implicated in familial cases of circadian rhythm disorders (Mainieri et al., 2021). Although the fetal SCN is present and continues to develop, maternal central and peripheral clocks control the fetal rhythm (Reppert & Schwartz, 1984). For example, the fetal adrenal gland may continue to produce cortisol in the presence of maternal adrenal input, even without maternal SCN input (Valenzuela et al., 2008). Maternal feeding times also play a key role in fetal circadian entrainment, even if at odds with maternal rest/activity times (Ohta et al., 2008). There is likely an intended level of redundancy to prioritize fetal circadian development, and this continues to be an evolving area of study.

Circadian Disruption

While the mother's central and peripheral clocks directly influence fetal circadian development, there are also several key changes during pregnancy to these clocks. There is a loss of rhythmicity in metabolism and an early onset of decreased daily activity, presumably to allow for nutrient delivery to the growing fetus to be prioritized (McCarthy et al., 2019). Maternal melatonin production naturally shifts in pregnancy, with a decrease in the first two trimesters and an increase in the final trimester, from maternal and placental sources (Nakamura et al., 2001). Placental melatonin, endogenous maternal melatonin, as well as melatonin consumed by the mother have been shown to pass to the fetus (McCarthy et al., 2019; Okatani et al., 1998; Wong et al., 2022). As early as 18 weeks' gestation, the expression of melatonin receptors can be seen in the fetal SCN and other peripheral tissues, although fetal melatonin production does not begin until after birth (Kennaway et al., 1992; Reppert et al., 1988). This reinforces the developing fetus's dependence on maternal circadian control. In animal models, when mothers are exposed to continuous light conditions throughout pregnancy or have a nonfunctioning SCN, both limiting normal circadian cycling to differing degrees, their offspring can have diminished rhythmicity at birth (Bellavia et al., 2006; Torres-Farfan et al., 2004). This has a profound real-world impact today, with frequent shift work or late-night electronic device use. Shift work disorder has been well described in association with increased rates of spontaneous abortions, premature delivery, and low birth weights (Abeysena et al., 2009; Aspholm et al., 1999; Zhu et al., 2004). Animal models of continued maternal circadian disruption demonstrate blunted or altered clock gene expression as well as macronutrient breakdown, which can directly impact the fetus which is entirely reliant on these maternal cues (Serón-Ferré et al., 2013). Disrupters of fetal circadian development can have short-term impacts on prenatal outcomes and delivery as well as lasting impacts on the long-term physical and psychological health of the child (Chaves et al., 2019; Galdames et al., 2014; Mendez et al., 2016; Varcoe et al., 2011; Zhang et al., 2017). In animal models, decreased maternal melatonin appears to decrease the expression of certain clock genes (*BMAL1* and *PER2*) in the fetal SCN and is associated with dysregulation of important circadian-controlled processes such as activity and temperature control after birth (Reppert & Schwartz et al., 1984; Serón-Ferré et al., 2013). This can be corrected with the administration of exogenous melatonin (Serón-Ferré et al., 2013). These resounding effects speak to the lack of clear distinction between "endogenous" and "exogenous" sources of circadian development in the fetus. Until the moment of birth, the fetal internal clock is primarily and secondarily influenced by the phase of the maternal clocks and any misalignment that may come the mother's way.

Sleep Development

Sleep is a pertinent and prominent outcome of circadian development. Early oscillations of rest and activity are noted in utero, suggestive of the beginning of sleep (Rivkees & Hao, 2000; Sheldon, 2012). At approximately 10 to 12 weeks' gestation, spontaneous fetal movements can be identified. At 20 weeks, signs of rhythmic cycling of rest and activity can be clinically noted (Escobar et al., 2021). A lack of consistent cycling between rest and activity between 20 and 24 weeks is concerning and warrants further clinical investigation (Kintraia et al., 2005). Both pre- and postnatally, an infant's activity is classified as wake, active sleep (later to be known as REM, or rapid-eye-movement, sleep), quiet sleep (non-REM), or transitional sleep when it is not clear (Berry et al., 2017; Mulder et al., 1987). Even after birth, behavioral observations such as having one's eyes closed, few versus many movements, and "squirming, sucking, grimacing" are integral to the official scoring of infant sleep on polysomnography (Berry et al., 2017; Mulder et al., 1987). Around 24 weeks' gestation, physiologic electroencephalogram (EEG) activity becomes recognizable (although this should be interpreted with caution as it is recorded from infants born prematurely and already exposed to the extrauterine environment) (Rivkees & Hao, 2000; Sheldon, 2012). Also, in premature infants, at 32 weeks, body movements are absent in 50% of 20-second epochs in 2–3-hour recordings, suggestive of rest/sleep (Sheldon, 2012). Fetal studies have also shown increasing quiet sleep between 32 and 40 weeks' gestation (Bennet et al., 2018), leading to the 50% expected in the full-term infant (Visser et al., 2021).

Sleep Disruption

While the signs of sleep can be seen early, the full 40-week gestation period is critical for the development of an aligned circadian rhythm and robust sleep landmarks as prematurity is correlated with alterations in total sleep time, sleep efficiency, and sleep architecture in infancy and later childhood (Erickson et al., 2021; Visser et al., 2021). Infants born prematurely have different EEG findings noted on sleep staging and can take up to a corrected gestational age of 40 weeks to exhibit mature sleep landmarks, as seen in Table 3.1. Prematurity can be associated with immature respiratory control, including "apnea of prematurity," a form of central sleep apnea with prolonged pauses, bradycardia, and hypoxia, often resolving as an infant nears full term (Bourjeily et al., 2017).

Table 3.1 Neonatal EEG background evolution in different behavioral states

Conceptional age	Awake (eyes open)	Active sleep (eyes closed)	Quiet sleep (eyes closed)
24–29 weeks	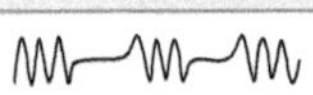	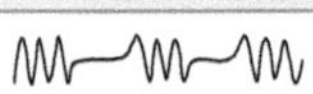	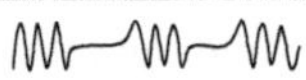
30–34 weeks	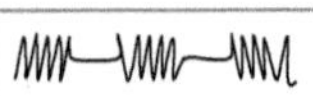	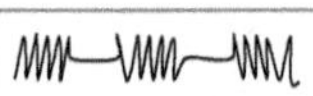	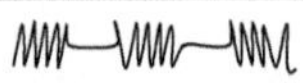
35–36 weeks	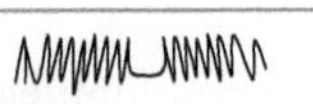	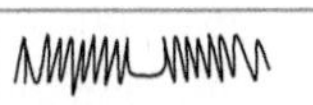	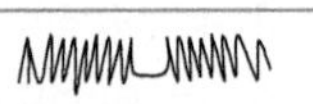
37–40 weeks	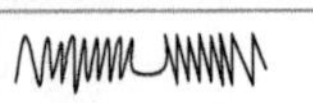	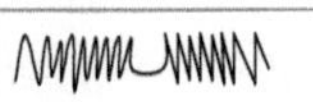	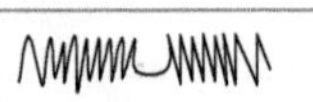
40–44 weeks	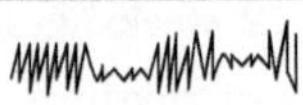	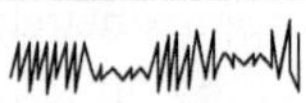	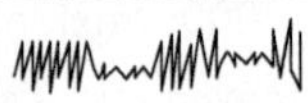
44–46 weeks	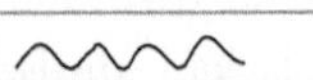	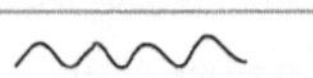	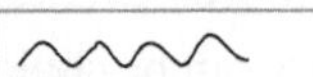

Note. CSWS = continuous slow wave sleep; EEG = electroencephalogram; TA = trace alternans; TD = trace discontinue. Reprinted from Britton JW, Frey LC, Hopp JL et al., authors; St. Louis EK, Frey LC, editors. Electroencephalography (EEG): An Introductory Text and Atlas of Normal and Abnormal Findings in Adults, Children, and Infants [Internet]. Chicago: American Epilepsy Society; 2016. The Developmental EEG: Premature, Neonatal, Infant, and Children.

There are myriad physical and psychosocial causes of premature birth, but a prominent maternal sleep disorder that has finally garnered ample attention is maternal (established and perinatal) obstructive sleep apnea (OSA). OSA in the peripartum period is significantly associated with not only prematurity but also other significant infant morbidity and mortality outcomes (Sánchez-Sánchez et al., 2022). Achieving healthy infant outcomes for overall well-being, as well as sleep, must begin with prioritizing the maternal timing, quantity, and quality of sleep.

Sleep in the Infant

Prior to birth, the infant has a sleep–wake pattern and circadian rhythm connected to the mother. After birth, the sleep pattern and circadian rhythm become weakly associated with the mother's (exogenous) sleep/circadian patterns, while the infant's endogenous sleep and circadian systems begin to undergo significant developmental changes from the neonatal to the infancy period, as overarchingly seen in Figure 3.1. This sleep/circadian

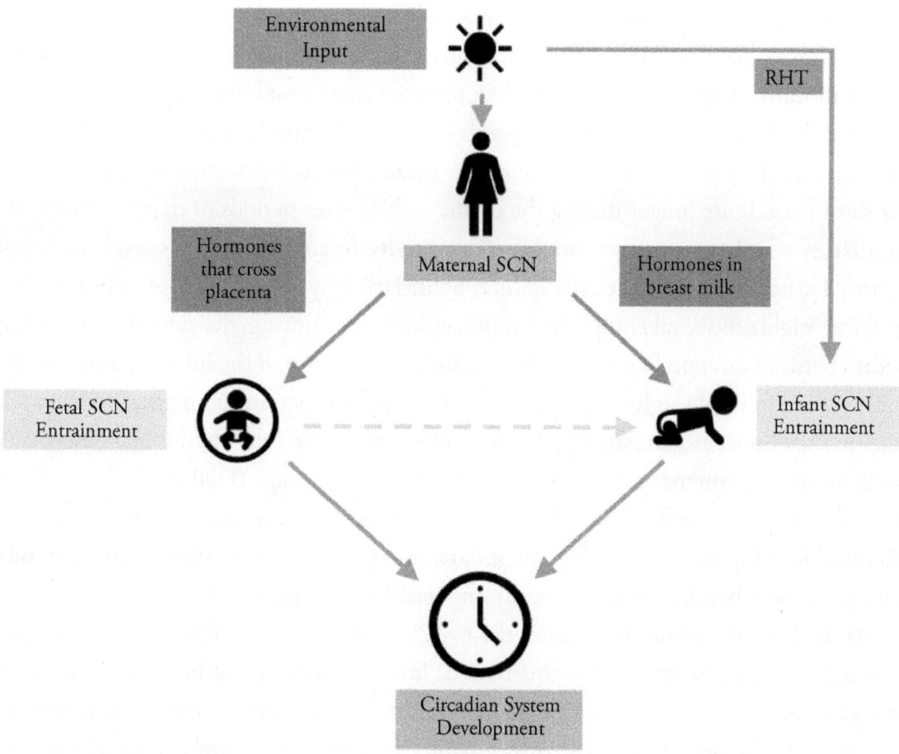

Figure 3.1 Influential factors for fetal and infant circadian development

Note. RHT = retinohypothalamic tract; SCN = suprachiasmatic nucleus. Reprinted from Wong SD, Wright KP Jr, Spencer RL, et al. Development of the circadian system in early life: Maternal and environmental factors. *J Physiol Anthropol. 2022;41*(1):22. Published 2022 May 16. doi:10.1186/s40101-022-00294-0. Reproduced under a Creative Commons Attribution 4.0 International License.

development involves a complex multifactorial process influenced by genetics, environment, as well as familial and individual differences such as temperament and health status. As a result, this is a key period in sleep and circadian development as the foundations of healthy sleep habits are established at this time, serving the child well throughout life. Quality and quantity of sleep during infancy can also be very impactful on a child's overall growth and development. Consequently, adequate sleep is crucial for memory consolidation, emotion regulation, language acquisition, and nervous system development.

Developmental Stages

In the neonatal period, neonates sleep up to 70% of the day (16–17 hours within a 24-hour period) and sleep no more than 4 hours continuously, due to immature sleep and circadian rhythm patterns. Infants show a very irregular sleep–wake pattern with poorly consolidated sleep periods lasting only several minutes to several hours scattered irregularly throughout the 24-hour period. In the newborn period, the sleep–wake pattern is primarily influenced by physiological needs including hunger (feeding). At this stage, infants have a very weak connection between their internal biological clock and external environmental cues such as light/dark and noise patterns as the master circadian clock, the SCN in the hypothalamus, is poorly developed. By the first month of life, infants sleep about 14–17 hours per day. By 3–6 months of age, sleep and circadian patterns show notable change. Infants at this age begin sleeping about 13–15 hours per day with more consolidated sleep episodes. The circadian and sleep advancement manifests as more predictable sleep–wake patterns such that sleep periods are longer during the night, with shorter periods of daytime sleep. The circadian system begins to show increased sensitivity to environmental cues, resulting in improved synchronization with the natural light/dark (day/night) cycle. As a result, there are fewer nighttime awakenings and more wakefulness during the daytime. Circadian rhythm patterns develop in a more robust fashion at this stage, if the infant receives consistent exposure to bright light during the day and low-light patterns at night. On the other hand, less robust circadian patterns develop at this stage when the child is exposed to only low light levels throughout the day at this developmental stage (Hall et al., 2017; Yates, 2018). In addition, consistency in bedtime routines and associations (e.g., sleep blankets, crib toys), keeping the sleep environment dark and quiet, as well as avoiding overstimulation right before bedtime assist in promoting healthy sleep pattern development.

As the baby continues to mature, the 6–12-month period establishes a much richer sleep and circadian array. During this period, infants naturally fall into a regular sleep–wake schedule with clear stability in their circadian rhythms. This is also when infants are more likely to develop poor sleep pattern habits resulting from unrelated developmental changes such as teething, more independence from new milestones (e.g., crawling, walking, and running), and more exposure to microbes, leading to increased illness. By 12 months, sleep lasts 10–12 hours at night with one or two naps during the day. Genetic factors may also account for up to 40% of the variance in infant sleep timing and duration.

Feeding times, parenting style, parental behavior/stress, and parental/maternal depression can also strongly influence infant sleep/circadian patterns, resulting in a wide range of variation in sleep at this developmental stage (Lam et al., 2003; Swaab et al., 1994).

Development of Sleep Markers on EEG

In the neonatal period, sleep stages are classified as quiet and active sleep (Berry et al., 2017; Mulder et al., 1987). There are brisk shifts between sleep stages. Active sleep is analogous to adult REM sleep and can occur over longer periods, up to 50% of total sleep. These prolonged periods of active/REM sleep are thought to be essential for adequate brain development and cognitive function at this time. At 3 months, the posterior dominant amplitude gradient becomes prominent during wakefulness and quiet sleep. In addition, an immature form of sleep spindles begins to appear over the vertex with varying interhemispheric synchrony and symmetry. Over the next 2 months, sleep patterns begin to mature and rapidly emulate adult sleep EEG patterns by 12 months of age. Figure 3.2 highlights these and further EEG landmarks which develop with progressing age.

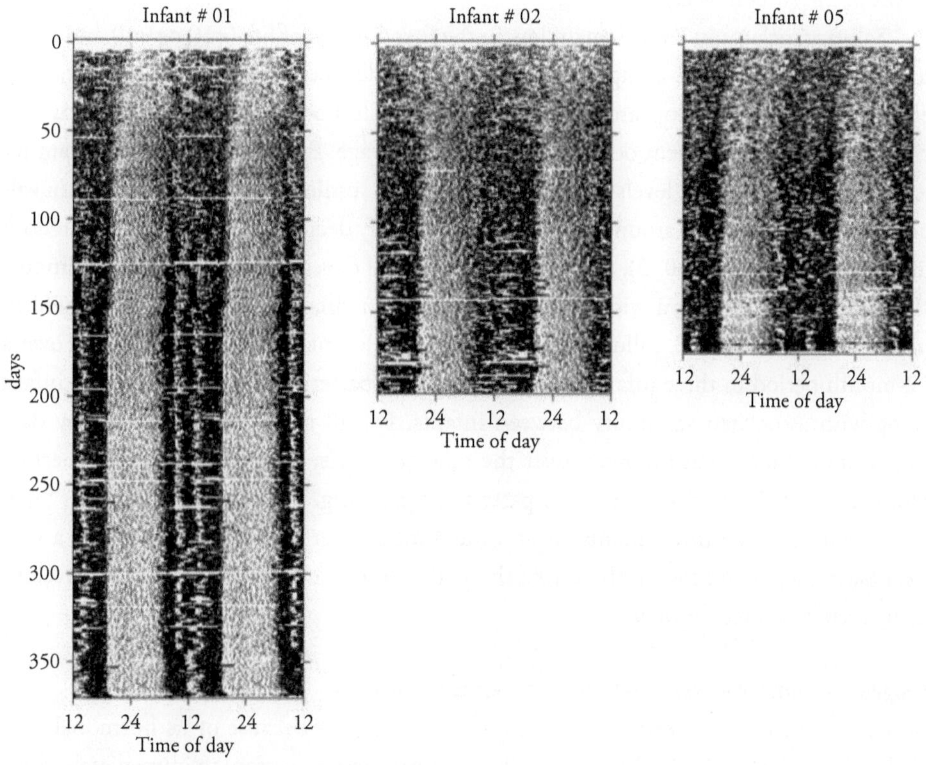

Figure 3.2 Variable infant circadian pattern development
Note. Reprinted from "Development of the 24-h rest-activity pattern in human infants," by O. G. Jenni, T. Doboer, and P. Achermann, 2006, *Infant Behavior & Development, 29*, p. 143–152. Adapted with permission from Elsevier.

Development of Circadian Phase Markers

Circadian rhythm patterns are poorly developed in the neonatal period, as a result of an immature nervous system, specifically the SCN. As a result, the ability to differentiate between day and night is limited. The SCN contains only about 13% of the adult number of AVP- and VIP-expressing neurons at this stage (Brooks & Canal, 2013). The rapid development of the SCN leads to adult levels of neurons by 24–36 months of life. Weak cues such as feeding and specific components in the breast milk (see section "Exogenous Phase Marker Development—Chrononutrition") can begin to provide exogenous timing and hormonal circadian signals that function as early circadian markers prior to the complete establishment of the infant's natural endogenous circadian rhythm.

Endogenous Phase Marker Development

In the newborn stage, circadian rhythms begin to develop as light enters the eye and is detected by the retina. Information is relayed through the RHT to the SCN. From the SCN, output signals reach other parts of the brain and body to synchronize the circadian rhythm. Circadian phase markers, including melatonin, cortisol, body temperature, movement, blood pressure, digestion, and consolidated sleep, synchronize over the first 12 weeks of life (McGraw et al., 1999).

Salivary melatonin levels remain low in the first 6 weeks of life (<10 pg/ml) and begin to increase by 8–9 weeks along with cortisol (Caba-Flores et al., 2022). As a result, sleep efficiency patterns develop around 9–10 weeks, while body temperature rhythms and circadian gene development occur by 11–12 weeks of age. By 6 months of age, melatonin levels have reached adult levels (>110 pg/ml). Indeed, studies indicate that melatonin values peak during infancy (around 12 months) and slowly decrease from infancy throughout life (Caba-Flores et al., 2022). In spite of these general development patterns, it is important to note that there is a wide range of variability in circadian pattern development in infancy. Indeed, Figure 3.2 illustrates this variability elegantly with actigraphy data over a 12-month period in three infants, showing circadian pattern development in each infant along with associated variability between infants. For all three infants, actigraphy data shows limited circadian influence over the infants' activity during the newborn period. However, by 2–3 months of age, clear patterns are forming. The variability becomes more prominent across all three infants around the 3-month period as Infant #1 shows a very clear pattern by 3 months and Infant #2 shows the least clear pattern of circadian development even by 6 months of age.

Exogenous Phase Marker Development—Chrononutrition

Breast milk serves as an excellent exogenous phase marker because of its hormonal cues (Caba-Flores et al., 2022). This form of chrononutrition is necessary to immediately commence entrainment of the circadian clock during the newborn stage. Breast milk is known to contain higher levels of cortisol when expressed during the day and higher levels of melatonin when expressed at night. As a result, breastfed newborns exhibit higher levels of melatonin, higher sleep efficiency, less sleep fragmentation, longer sleep duration, and lower levels of infant colic. Similar patterns have been noted in association with breast milk cortisol, which regulates infant peripheral clocks.

Potential Disruptions to Sleep and Circadian Pattern Development During Infancy

Behavioral Sleep Issues

There is a growing concern about adverse health impacts on excessive light exposure at night from the newborn period through adulthood. Night light exposure has rapidly increased since the invention of the light bulb (Yates, 2018). Newborns require well-defined dark and light periods for adequate circadian entrainment. Nocturnal light exposure changes the pathways involved in SCN development and affects genes associated with peripheral circadian clocks in the heart, lungs, and spleen as the child reaches adulthood. Peripheral circadian gene alterations have been associated with hypertension, airway inflammation, and aberrant immune responses. In a mouse model, constant exposure to night light, even at dim levels, was associated with the development of anxiety-like behaviors (Borniger et al., 2014) and bipolar disorder in humans. Studies have posited that cancers, metabolic disorders, and sudden infant death syndrome may also be a result of poor circadian entrainment (Bauer et al., 2015; Cornwell & Feigenbaum, 2006; Lewis & Erren, 2017).

Sleep Disorders

Sleep disruption and sleep disorders can develop during infancy and can be prevalent and persistent. As many as 10%–46% of infants aged 6–18 months show symptoms such as bedtime fussiness, difficulty falling asleep, and frequent and prolonged nighttime awakenings (Wong et al., 2022). Such sleep problems are posited to occur secondarily to a constant misalignment between environmental cues and endogenous biological circadian rhythms during the postnatal, and possibly prenatal, periods. These should be treated as soon as possible because studies indicate that the persistence of poor sleep habits and sleep disorders is associated with childhood psychosocial issues including aggression, attention problems, anxiety, mood problems, and hyperactivity. Poorer cognitive performance and poor school performance can also be associated with sleep disruption and deprivation. Sleep and circadian pattern development can also be affected by maternal depression and poor parental health.

Sleep in the Growing Child

As children move out of infancy and through the toddler (1–2 years old), preschool (3–5 years old), and school-age (6–13 years old) years, their sleep needs decrease and consolidate. According to a consensus statement from the National Sleep Foundation, most school-age children will sleep an average of 9–11 hours a night (Hillard, 2015). In addition, by approximately 5 years of age, many children will stop napping in the daytime. In the absence of this nap, a child can effectively build sleep pressure throughout the day and have nightly sleep onset at a more predictable time, one that is revealing of their circadian sleep–wake rhythm. Younger children tend to have more of an advanced sleep–wake time and maintain it well (Wickersham, 2006), at times to the chagrin of a sleep-deprived caregiver on a weekend.

Development of Sleep Markers on EEG

By this point in development, most of the EEG findings noted in sleep are similar to those of the adult brain. The exception is the posterior dominant rhythm (PDR). In younger children (3–7 years old) this rhythm is in the theta frequency (4–8 Hz) and then increases through childhood and adolescence toward alpha (8–12 Hz) (Berry et al., 2017; Hillard, 2015). These varying frequencies of neural oscillation play an important role in the primary work performed by the central nervous system at each age. There is research to suggest that the slower theta rhythm (when seen in the frontal region of adult EEGs) may be indicative of situations where there is a need for greater cognitive control (Cavanagh & Frank, 2014), while the faster alpha rhythm is thought to play a role in inhibiting or suppressing distracting input (Foxe & Snyder, 2011). While vastly oversimplified and gathered from adults, this data highlights the different neuronal processes most pertinent to the child's current stage of development. While younger children may still be learning the fine art of falling asleep (and doing so independently), in contrast, adolescents have the challenging task of putting their day away for sleep onset.

Development of Sleep and Circadian Phase Markers

While early sleep onset and offset times are frequently seen in younger children, advanced sleep–wake phase disorder is rare. However, an important exception to this is in children with a history of prematurity (Hibbs et al., 2014). While increasingly common in adolescents, delayed sleep–wake phase disorder is also rare in younger children. Research on pediatric circadian rhythms often relies heavily on questionnaires of habitual sleep/wake times, while the gold standard for circadian research utilizes a highly invasive collection of other classic circadian markers (core body temperature, serum cortisol, etc.). Salivary melatonin collected hourly in dim light conditions can generate a peak concentration at what is referred to as the *DLMO* (dim light melatonin onset). This is considered a less invasive mechanism to understand the timing of an individual's melatonin rise. The time between the DLMO and sleep onset is referred to as a *phase angle*, and there can be notable variation between individuals. In toddlers and younger children, phase angles may be very small (LeBourgeois et al., 2013). In older children and those nearing adolescence, the phase angle widens (Crowley et al., 2014). This may be seen with the same melatonin onset timing, which poses questions about what influences sleep onset in addition to circadian readiness. The delay in falling asleep may have more to do with autonomy around evening activities and bedtime than how ready for sleep a child's central clock may be.

There is also data suggesting that reported sleep onset and offset times do not predict DLMO well in younger children (5–8 years old) compared to older children (9–17 years old) (Moreno et al., 2022). This estimation improves with objectively measured actigraphy. Further research is needed to understand the unique circadian model of a younger child, with consideration of a continuously developing circadian neural network, pupillary changes in sensitivity to light (Higuchi et al., 2014), and social pressure on caregivers for an "earlier bedtime," which may create negative associations around sleep and ironically foster possible sleep onset challenges.

Potential Disruptions to Sleep and Circadian Pattern During Childhood

Many sleep disorders that arise in infancy can persist into preschool and later childhood (Byars et al., 2012; Lam et al., 2003). Unaddressed sleep onset associations and lagging skills necessary for independent sleep will result in a child who awakens each ultradian cycle. A youngster spending time in bed far earlier than when ready for sleep onset may also develop a chronic insomnia disorder that persists into later childhood. They may even perceive themselves as a "bad sleeper." A young child with potentially unrecognized adenotonsillar hypertrophy may be waking from OSA and then sleeping later in the morning hours in recovery. Another child with an overweight body habitus may have a different driver for OSA. These nuances may impact sleep onset and maintenance independent of a particular sleep–wake phase or in tandem with a circadian rhythm disorder. Consultation with a knowledgeable pediatric sleep specialist is critical for identifying all the possible diagnoses and necessary next steps in the management of a particular child's sleep challenges. Circadian rhythm disorders, such as delayed sleep–wake phase disorder, can be very effectively treated with low-dose, well-timed melatonin (van Geijlswijk et al., 2010). However, when the cause of difficulty with falling asleep, and even more so staying asleep, is not circadian in origin, melatonin may fail. While beyond the scope of this chapter, there are groups looking at melatonin use for insomnia in children with particular neurodevelopmental challenges such as autism spectrum disorder (Zisapel, 2022) and attention deficit hyperactivity disorder (Punja et al., 2016). However, there is yet to be a clear consensus that melatonin is an effective treatment for chronic insomnia (Sateia et al., 2017) or that it is a safe and reliable compound to be used over the counter (Erland & Saxena, 2017). While some aspects of the behavioral treatments for chronic insomnia and circadian sleep–wake phase disorder may overlap, their pathophysiology is different; and accurate diagnosis is invaluable for supporting the child and family.

As children participate in school with early start times and take on extracurricular activities late into the evening, this may behaviorally impede their ability to get the sleep they need. This exogenous impact on circadian rhythm is not to be underestimated. A well-meaning parent allowing their child to awaken later or nap on weekends to "catch up" on sleep may be taking the first steps in fostering a delay or irregularity of a sleep–wake rhythm. Even 1 or 2 days per week with later exposure to light in the morning, our strongest zeitgeber, can make an impact. This can begin the process of a circadian delay even without a genetic predisposition. It can also precipitate social jet lag on weekdays, with the child suddenly unable to fall asleep or awaken at reasonable times for school. Consultation with a competent sleep provider can start the important work of entraining the child back to the schedule they need. This will set them up for success as they transition to adolescence.

Sleep in the Adolescent

Adolescence heralds a period of rapid sleep and circadian rhythm change and development. This developmental stage marks a crucial transition from childhood into adulthood associated with rapid intellectual and physical maturation largely secondary to significant hormonal changes. As a result, notable hormone-related brain maturation, especially within the frontal lobe, occurs. Simultaneously, sleep patterns and circadian patterns make a sharp shift in baseline, often with both biological and environmental influences. In adolescence, a natural tendency to delay sleep until later at night and to sleep in later in the morning (delayed sleep phase patterns) can be quite prevalent. A delay in melatonin release, secreted by the pineal gland, is thought to be responsible for this adolescent circadian pattern (Carskadon, 2011). Stress and anxiety can have a significant impact on sleep and circadian rhythms during this developmental stage of life. In addition, environmental factors such as increased light and noise exposure (e.g., from TV/phone/tablet screens) in the evening can adversely affect sleep and circadian patterns by delaying melatonin production and release. Despite required early wake times among adolescents attending school, a tendency to sleep later into the night prevails. Social factors such as evening work shifts, extended screen time, or social/sports-related events may play a role in these patterns. However, it is clear that these distracting environmental evening wakefulness cues do not fully account for all the patterns we see. Even when well rested, adolescents have less propensity to fall asleep during evening hours and an increased propensity for sleepiness during midday hours (Taylor et al., 2005). Adolescents tend to fall back to delayed patterns even after adequate circadian entrainment therapy to get on regulated schedules in both laboratory and real-world settings.

Sex Differences

Sex differences are notable in sleep and circadian patterns at this developmental stage of life, which may be associated with sex differences in pubertal onset times (Hagenauer et al., 2009). Girls begin to exhibit a delay in sleep times about a year earlier than boys, paralleling their younger pubertal onset. In addition, the age at which delay in sleep and circadian phase is highest in females (age 19 years) occurs about a year earlier than in their male counterparts (age 20 years) (Roenneberg et al., 2004). Notably, this delayed circadian phase pattern correlates directly with secondary sex development (Tanner Stage 5) and not with early/primary sex development (Tanner Stages 1 and 2). This provides evidence that a neurobiological component is associated with adolescent sleep and circadian patterns. Furthermore, there are many animal studies corroborating a propensity for delay in adolescent circadian and sleep patterns, including primate and rodent species (Hagenauer et al., 2009).

Development of Sleep Markers on EEG

At this stage, sleep EEG patterns mimic adult sleep EEG patterns. As such, the PDR and awake beta activity fall into a higher frequency range, similar to adult ranges (Hagenauer et al., 2009). Sleep Stages N1, N2, and N3 are clearly delineated along with well-defined REM sleep patterns at this developmental stage.

Development of Sleep and Circadian Phase Markers

During this stage of development, the two primary endogenous components to sleep and sleep timing—homeostatic drive (Process S) and circadian timing (Process C)—follow an adult pattern.

Process S

Sleep pressure (also known as *homeostatic drive* or *Process S*) describes the pressure to sleep that builds up throughout the daytime/awakening period and dissipates over time as an individual sleeps. Slow wave activity (SWA) on EEG can serve as a physiological marker of sleep pressure. As sleep pressure builds, SWA begins to intrude into the wake EEG pattern at higher rates, congruent with the level of sleep pressure. As a consequence, SWA is highest at the beginning of the night right before sleep, declines exponentially with successive episodes of non-REM sleep, and is lowest upon awakening the next morning. This general pattern exhibited in children and adults differs among adolescents. Adolescents are less likely to exhibit an accumulation of SWA (a marker of homeostatic drive on sleep EEG), indicating a slower buildup of sleep pressure throughout the day compared to prepubertal children and adults (Crowley et al., 2007). Alternatively, adolescents may develop a resistance to sleep pressure, further allowing them to tolerate longer wake periods. However, they exhibit similar sleep pressure dissipation rates compared to preadolescents, suggesting that the sleep recovery process remains stable and comparable to other developmental stages during this period.

Process C

The circadian pattern (Process C) follows environmental (zeitgebers) and innate cues, resulting in promoting sleepiness in the evening and wakefulness in the morning. The circadian pattern among adolescents becomes relatively delayed, which keeps them awake later in the evening and allows them to sleep through the early morning. Older adolescents (Tanner Stage 5) are significantly less sensitive to dim light exposure in the morning compared to early adolescents (Tanner Stages 1 and 2), suggesting that the shape of the phase response curve changes during puberty, akin to how much impact light has on shifting (Crowley et al., 2007). (The phase response curve measures how well input from light shifts the circadian phase in an individual.) In spite of these findings, DLMO patterns over a 24-hour period only minimally change in puberty, suggesting that there may be a blunting of sensitivity to the advancing phase mechanisms within the brain. In fact, it has been demonstrated that adolescents have an internal clock that interprets environmental time cues differently from adults. This indicates that circadian mechanisms develop in a very dynamic pattern from infancy to adulthood (Foxe & Snyder, 2011).

Potential Disruptions to Sleep and Circadian Pattern Development During Adolescence

Sleep Deprivation and the COVID-19 Pandemic

The COVID-19 pandemic has affected sleep globally. The new "work from home" and "school from home" arrangements over a prolonged period have changed the ability of adults and adolescents alike to maintain their daily structured schedules as daytime and nighttime activities were suddenly all performed in the same location. Consequently, daily routines became chaotic as a result of changes in school schedules, social isolation, increased screen time, and reduced physical activity. Sleep pattern disruptions soared, with increased insomnia and daytime sleepiness compared to prepandemic levels. Adolescents particularly reported further delay in their sleep onset patterns, poor sleep quality, nightmares, and shorter sleep duration (Blume et al., 2020). Anxiety and stress also increased in this population, worsening sleep problems (Giri et al., 2013).

School Start Times

Awareness of the physiologic delays in adolescent sleep–wake patterns has prompted the development of the delayed school start times movement, an initiative to allow adolescents to get the sleep they need by waking close to their natural timing (Adolescent Sleep Working Group et al., 2014). While adolescents have a naturally delayed sleep and circadian pattern, school start times can be as early as 6:40 a.m. The National Sleep Foundation notes that 45% of adolescents in the United States have inadequate sleep (National Sleep Foundation Sleep and Teens Task Force, 2000). The resulting insufficient sleep negatively impacts academic performance, focus and attention (increased motor vehicle accidents), decision-making, mental health, and overall global health. Studies have shown that among schools with later start times (after 8:30 a.m.), adolescents experience increases in sleep duration and improved academic performance (Dunster et al., 2018; Nahmod et al., 2017). Delaying school start times by just 30 minutes can improve adolescent sleep duration, mood, and alertness.

Unfortunately, this movement has received significant scrutiny from policymakers and lobbyists. Despite decades of discussion on this topic, implementation changes have remained a challenge due to the numerous associated logistical and practical factors that would be affected—parental schedules, teachers' schedules, sports and extracurricular scheduling, and even school bus schedules. Another opposing standpoint indicates that delaying school start times may simply promote even further delayed adolescent bedtimes, resulting in zero net gain in sleep benefits and significant disruption to the school system and infrastructure (Rhie & Chae, 2018).

Media Use

Electronic devices (e.g., TV, tablets, and smartphones) have been shown in the literature to have a negative impact on adolescents and their sleep. The blue light emitted from these devices interferes with sleep by delaying melatonin release, leading to difficulty falling asleep and overall shorter sleep duration. In addition, stimulation from the device content can delay relaxation, which leads to a shorter sleep latency. As a result, insufficient sleep, poor sleep quality, and excessive daytime sleepiness are common in this population.

Conclusion

The ever-evolving neural network of the human brain undergoes the most change from the early fetal period through adolescence. Nestled within this powerhouse is the central clock and controller of the human circadian rhythm, along for the ride of tremendous growth and development. Less than halfway through the fetal period, early signs of circadian control are observed, largely maternally driven. The fetus acts like a peripheral clock in response to the mother's "central" control. After birth, the infant's SCN begins to harness input from zeitgebers, such as light and feeding, to foster its own early measurable rhythms. It also begins to influence its own peripheral clocks for necessary bodily processes. As sleep consolidates into a sole nocturnal period in early childhood, the day/night rhythm to which a child is entrained will reinforce itself through consistent exposure to light and other key social cues. Through later childhood, endogenous factors such as genetics and exogenous inputs from the environment continue to influence the developing rhythm. The impact of these factors has a great deal of individual variation. The massive shifts in tolerance of homeostatic pressure and social expectations which come with pubertal onset also promote changes in the circadian rhythm, often delays, in adolescence. Attention to drivers of internal rhythms is key at every stage of the pediatric period. A lack of understanding of key circadian players and processes may also lead to the misdiagnosis of discrete sleep issues. Difficulties with sleep onset or excessive daytime sleepiness may be incorrectly labeled as insomnia or narcolepsy, while there may simply be profound social jet lag. Misaligned rhythms or inconsistencies in schedules may create problems early on that can continue into adulthood. Awareness of and education on the power of central and peripheral clocks are key. Appropriate prenatal guidance, infant sleep guidelines, early childhood initiatives, and adolescent legislation can all set up children for circadian success. Children with fine-tuned internal clocks can grow into adults who are programmed to be well rested.

Questions/Future Directions

1. Could prenatal care with an emphasis on sleep/circadian well-being result in improved infant morbidity/mortality outcomes?
2. Why does evening light exposure affect the circadian rhythm of specific pediatric groups differently?
3. What is the full pathophysiologic mechanism behind the sleep–wake delay that occurs in adolescence?

References

Abeysena, C., Jayawardana, P., & De A Seneviratne, R. (2009). Maternal sleep deprivation is a risk factor for small for gestational age: A cohort study. *The Australian & New Zealand Journal of Obstetrics & Gynaecology, 49*(4), 382–387. https://doi.org/10.1111/j.1479-828X.2009.01010.x

Abrahamson, E. E., & Moore, R. Y. (2001). Suprachiasmatic nucleus in the mouse: Retinal innervation, intrinsic organization and efferent projections. *Brain Research, 916*(1–2), 172–191. https://doi.org/10.1016/s0006-8993(01)02890-6

Adolescent Sleep Working Group, Committee on Adolescence, Council on School Health; Au, R., Carskadon, M., Millman, R., Wolfson, A., Braverman, P. K., Adelman, W. P., Breuner, C. C., Levine, D. A., Marcell, A. V., Murray, P. J., O'Brien, R. F., Devore, C. D., Allison, M., Ancona, R., Barnett, S. E., Gunther, R., . . . Young, T. (2014). School start times for adolescents. *Pediatrics, 134*(3), 642–649. https://doi.org/10.1542/peds.2014-1697

Aryal, R. P., Kwak, P. B., Tamayo, A. G., Gebert, M., Chiu, P. L., Walz, T., & Weitz, C. J. (2017). Macromolecular assemblies of the mammalian circadian clock. *Molecular Cell, 67*(5), 770–782.e6. https://doi.org/10.1016/j.molcel.2017.07.017

Aspholm, R., Lindbohm, M. L., Paakkulainen, H., Taskinen, H., Nurminen, T., & Tiitinen, A. (1999). Spontaneous abortions among Finnish flight attendants. *Journal of Occupational and Environmental Medicine, 41*(6), 486–491. https://doi.org/10.1097/00043764-199906000-00015

Bauer, M., Glenn, T., Alda, M., Andreassen, O. A., Angelopoulos, E., Ardau, R., Baethge, C., Bauer, R., Baune, B. T., Bellivier, F., Belmaker, R. H., Berk, M., Bjella, T. D., Bossini, L., Bersudsky, Y., Wo Cheung, E. Y., Conell, J., Del Zompo, M., Dodd, S., . . . Whybrow, P. C. (2015). Influence of light exposure during early life on the age of onset of bipolar disorder. *Journal of Psychiatric Research, 64*, 1–8. https://doi.org/10.1016/j.jpsychires.2015.03.013

Bellavía, S. L., Carpentieri, A. R., Vaqué, A. M., Macchione, A. F., & Vermouth, N. T. (2006). Pup circadian rhythm entrainment—Effect of maternal ganglionectomy or pinealectomy. *Physiology & Behavior, 89*(3), 342–349. https://doi.org/10.1016/j.physbeh.2006.06.018

Bennet, L., Walker, D. W., & Horne, R. S. C. (2018). Waking up too early—The consequences of preterm birth on sleep development. *The Journal of Physiology, 596*(23), 5687–5708. https://doi.org/10.1113/JP274950

Berry, R. B., Brooks, R., Gamaldo, C., Harding, S. M., Lloyd, R. M., Quan, S. F., Troester, M. T., & Vaughn, B. V. (2017). AASM Scoring Manual Updates for 2017 (Version 2.4). *Journal of Clinical Sleep Medicine, 13*(5), 665–666. https://doi.org/10.5664/jcsm.6576

Blume, C., Schmidt, M. H., & Cajochen, C. (2020). Effects of the COVID-19 lockdown on human sleep and rest-activity rhythms. *Current Biology, 30*(14), R795–R797. https://doi.org/10.1016/j.cub.2020.06.021

Borniger, J. C., McHenry, Z. D., Abi Salloum, B. A., & Nelson, R. J. (2014). Exposure to dim light at night during early development increases adult anxiety-like responses. *Physiology & Behavior, 133*, 99–106. https://doi.org/10.1016/j.physbeh.2014.05.012

Bourjeily, G., Danilack, V. A., Bublitz, M. H., Lipkind, H., Muri, J., Caldwell, D., Tong, I., & Rosene-Montella, K. (2017). Obstructive sleep apnea in pregnancy is associated with adverse maternal outcomes: A national cohort. *Sleep Medicine, 38*, 50–57. https://doi.org/10.1016/j.sleep.2017.06.035

Brooks, E., & Canal, M. M. (2013). Development of circadian rhythms: Role of postnatal light environment. *Neuroscience & Biobehavioral Reviews, 37*(4), 551–560. https://doi.org/10.1016/j.neubiorev.2013.02.012

Brown, A. J., Pendergast, J. S., & Yamazaki, S. (2019). Peripheral circadian oscillators. *The Yale Journal of Biology and Medicine, 92*(2), 327–335.

Buhr, E. D., & Takahashi, J. S. (2013). Molecular components of the mammalian circadian clock. In A. Kramer & M. Merrow (Eds.), *Circadian clocks. Handbook of experimental pharmacology* (Vol. 217, pp. 3–27). Springer. https://doi.org/10.1007/978-3-642-25950-0_1

Byars, K. C., Yolton, K., Rausch, J., Lanphear, B., & Beebe, D. W. (2012). Prevalence, patterns, and persistence of sleep problems in the first 3 years of life. *Pediatrics, 129*(2), e276–e284. https://doi.org/10.1542/peds.2011-0372

Caba-Flores, M. D., Ramos-Ligonio, A., Camacho-Morales, A., Martínez-Valenzuela, C., Viveros-Contreras, R., & Caba, M. (2022). Breast milk and the importance of chrononutrition. *Frontiers in Nutrition, 9*, Article 867507. https://doi.org/10.3389/fnut.2022.867507

Carskadon, M. A. (2011). Sleep in adolescents: The perfect storm. *Pediatric Clinics of North America, 58*(3), 637–647. https://doi.org/10.1016/j.pcl.2011.03.003

Cavanagh, J. F., & Frank, M. J. (2014). Frontal theta as a mechanism for cognitive control. *Trends in Cognitive Sciences, 18*(8), 414–421. https://doi.org/10.1016/j.tics.2014.04.012

Chaves, I., van der Eerden, B., Boers, R., Boers, J., Streng, A. A., Ridwan, Y., Schreuders-Koedam, M., Vermeulen, M., van der Pluijm, I., Essers, J., Gribnau, J., Reiss, I. K. M., & van der Horst, G. T. J. (2019). Gestational jet lag predisposes to later-life skeletal and cardiac disease. *Chronobiology International, 36*(5), 657–671. https://doi.org/10.1080/07420528.2019.1579734

Cornwell, A. C., & Feigenbaum, P. (2006). Sleep biological rhythms in normal infants and those at high risk for SIDS. *Chronobiology International, 23*(5), 935–961. https://doi.org/10.1080/07420520600921070

Crowley, S. J., Acebo, C., & Carskadon, M. A. (2007). Sleep, circadian rhythms, and delayed phase in adolescence. *Sleep Medicine, 8*(6), 602–612. https://doi.org/10.1016/j.sleep.2006.12.002

Crowley, S. J., Van Reen, E., LeBourgeois, M. K., Acebo, C., Tarokh, L., Seifer, R., Barker, D. H., & Carskadon, M. A. (2014). A longitudinal assessment of sleep timing, circadian phase, and phase angle of entrainment across human adolescence. *PLOS ONE, 9*(11), Article e112199. https://doi.org/10.1371/journal.pone.0112199

Dubocovich, M. L. (2007). Melatonin receptors: Role on sleep and circadian rhythm regulation. *Sleep Medicine, 8*(S3), 34–42. https://doi.org/10.1016/j.sleep.2007.10.007

Dunster, G. P., de la Iglesia, L., Ben-Hamo, M., Nave, C., Fleischer, J. G., Panda, S., & de la Iglesia, H. O. (2018). Sleepmore in Seattle: Later school start times are associated with more sleep and better performance in high school students. *Science Advances, 4*(12), Article eaau6200. https://doi.org/10.1126/sciadv.aau6200

Erickson, G., Dobson, N. R., & Hunt, C. E. (2021). Immature control of breathing and apnea of prematurity: The known and unknown. *Journal of Perinatology, 41*(9), 2111–2123. https://doi.org/10.1038/s41372-021-01010-z

Erland, L. A., & Saxena, P. K. (2017). Melatonin natural health products and supplements: Presence of serotonin and significant variability of melatonin content. *Journal of Clinical Sleep Medicine, 13*(2), 275–281. https://doi.org/10.5664/jcsm.6462

Escobar, C., Rojas-Granados, A., & Angeles-Castellanos, M. (2021). Development of the circadian system and relevance of periodic signals for neonatal development. In D. F. Swaab, F. Kreier, P. J. Lucassen, A. Salehi, & R. M. Buijs (Eds.), *The human hypothalamus: Anterior region. Handbook of clinical neurology* (Vol. 179, pp. 249–258). https://doi.org/10.1016/B978-0-12-819975-6.00015-7

Foxe, J. J., & Snyder, A. C. (2011). The role of alpha-band brain oscillations as a sensory suppression mechanism during selective attention. *Frontiers in Psychology, 2*, Article 154. https://doi.org/10.3389/fpsyg.2011.00154

Galdames, H. A., Torres-Farfan, C., Spichiger, C., Mendez, N., Abarzua-Catalan, L., Alonso-Vazquez, P., & Richter, H. G. (2014). Impact of gestational chronodisruption on fetal cardiac genomics. *Journal of Molecular and Cellular Cardiology, 66*, 1–11. https://doi.org/10.1016/j.yjmcc.2013.10.020

Giri, P., Baviskar, M., & Phalke, D. (2013). Study of sleep habits and sleep problems among medical students of Pravara Institute of Medical Sciences Loni, Western Maharashtra, India. *Annals of Medical and Health Sciences Research*, *3*(1), 51–54. https://doi.org/10.4103/2141-9248.109488

Hagenauer, M. H., Perryman, J. I., Lee, T. M., & Carskadon, M. A. (2009). Adolescent changes in the homeostatic and circadian regulation of sleep. *Developmental Neuroscience*, *31*(4), 276–284. https://doi.org/10.1159/000216538

Hall, W. A., Moynihan, M., Bhagat, R., & Wooldridge, J. (2017). Relationships between parental sleep quality, fatigue, cognitions about infant sleep, and parental depression pre and post-intervention for infant behavioral sleep problems. *BMC Pregnancy and Childbirth*, *17*(1), Article 104. https://doi.org/10.1186/s12884-017-1284-x

Hibbs, A. M., Storfer-Isser, A., Rosen, C., Ievers-Landis, C. E., Taveras, E. M., & Redline, S. (2014). Advanced sleep phase in adolescents born preterm. *Behavioral Sleep Medicine*, *12*(5), 412–424. https://doi.org/10.1080/15402002.2013.825838

Higuchi, S., Nagafuchi, Y., Lee, S. I., & Harada, T. (2014). Influence of light at night on melatonin suppression in children. *The Journal of Clinical Endocrinology and Metabolism*, *99*(9), 3298–3303. https://doi.org/10.1210/jc.2014-1629

Hillard, P. J. (2015). National Sleep Foundation's sleep time duration recommendations: Methodology and results summary. *Sleep Health*, *1*(1), 40–43. https://doi.org/10.1016/j.sleh.2014.12.010

Honma, S. (2020). Development of the mammalian circadian clock. *European Journal of Neuroscience*, *51*(1), 182–193. https://doi.org/10.1111/ejn.14318

Kennaway, D. J., Stamp, G. E., & Goble, F. C. (1992). Development of melatonin production in infants and the impact of prematurity. *The Journal of Clinical Endocrinology and Metabolism*, *75*(2), 367–369. https://doi.org/10.1210/jcem.75.2.1639937

Kintraia, P. I., Zarnadze, M. G., Kintraia, N. P., & Kashakashvili, I. G. (2005). Development of daily rhythmicity in heart rate and locomotor activity in the human fetus. *Journal of Circadian Rhythms*, *3*(1), Article 5. https://doi.org/10.1186/1740-3391-3-5

Lam, P., Hiscock, H., & Wake, M. (2003). Outcomes of infant sleep problems: A longitudinal study of sleep, behavior, and maternal well-being. *Pediatrics*, *111*(3), e203–e207. https://doi.org/10.1542/peds.111.3.e203

LeBourgeois, M. K., Carskadon, M. A., Akacem, L. D., Simpkin, C. T., Wright, K. P., Jr., Achermann, P., & Jenni, O. G. (2013). Circadian phase and its relationship to nighttime sleep in toddlers. *Journal of Biological Rhythms*, *28*(5), 322–331. https://doi.org/10.1177/0748730413506543

Lewis, P., & Erren, T. C. (2017). Perinatal light imprinting of circadian clocks and systems (PLICCS): The PLICCS and cancer hypothesis. *Frontiers in Oncology*, *7*, Article 44. https://doi.org/10.3389/fonc.2017.00044

Lunshof, S., Boer, K., van Hoffen, G., Wolf, H., & Mirmiran, M. (1997). The diurnal rhythm in fetal heart rate in a twin pregnancy with discordant anencephaly: Comparison with three normal twin pregnancies. *Early Human Development*, *48*(1–2), 47–57. https://doi.org/10.1016/s0378-3782(96)01802-6

Mainieri, G., Montini, A., Nicotera, A., Di Rosa, G., Provini, F., & Loddo, G. (2021). The genetics of sleep disorders in children: A narrative review. *Brain Sciences*, *11*(10), Article 1259. https://doi.org/10.3390/brainsci11101259

McCarthy, R., Jungheim, E. S., Fay, J. C., Bates, K., Herzog, E. D., & England, S. K. (2019). Riding the rhythm of melatonin through pregnancy to deliver on time. *Frontiers in Endocrinology*, *10*, Article 616. https://doi.org/10.3389/fendo.2019.00616

McGraw, K., Hoffmann, R., Harker, C., & Herman, J. H. (1999). The development of circadian rhythms in a human infant. *Sleep*, *22*(3), 303–310. https://doi.org/10.1093/sleep/22.3.303

Mendez, N., Halabi, D., Spichiger, C., Salazar, E. R., Vergara, K., Alonso-Vasquez, P., Carmona, P., Sarmiento, J. M., Richter, H. G., Seron-Ferre, M., & Torres-Farfan, C. (2016). Gestational chronodisruption impairs circadian physiology in rat male offspring, increasing the risk of chronic disease. *Endocrinology*, *157*(12), 4654–4668. https://doi.org/10.1210/en.2016-1282

Meng, Q. J., Logunova, L., Maywood, E. S., Gallego, M., Lebiecki, J., Brown, T. M., Sládek, M., Semikhodskii, A. S., Glossop, N. R. J., Piggins, H. D., Chesham, J. E., Bechtold, D. A., Yoo, S. H., Takahashi, J. S., Virshup, D. M., Boot-Handford, R. P., Hastings, M. H., & Loudon, A. S. I. (2008). Setting clock speed in mammals: The CK1 epsilon tau mutation in mice accelerates circadian pacemakers by selectively destabilizing PERIOD proteins. *Neuron*, *58*(1), 78–88. https://doi.org/10.1016/j.neuron.2008.01.019

Moreno, J. P., Hannay, K. M., Walch, O., Dadabhoy, H., Christian, J., Puyau, M., El-Mubasher, A., Bacha, F., Grant, S. R., Park, R. J., & Cheng, P. (2022). Estimating circadian phase in elementary school children: Leveraging advances in physiologically informed models of circadian entrainment and wearable devices. *Sleep, 45*(6), Article zsac061. https://doi.org/10.1093/sleep/zsac061

Mulder, E. J., Visser, G. H., Bekedam, D. J., & Prechtl, H. F. (1987). Emergence of behavioural states in fetuses of type-1-diabetic women. *Early Human Development, 15*(4), 231–251. https://doi.org/10.1016/0378-3782(87)90082-x

Nahmod, N. G., Lee, S., Buxton, O. M., Chang, A. M., & Hale, L. (2017). High school start times after 8:30 am are associated with later wake times and longer time in bed among teens in a national urban cohort study. *Sleep Health, 3*(6), 444–450. https://doi.org/10.1016/j.sleh.2017.09.004

Nakamura, Y., Tamura, H., Kashida, S., Takayama, H., Yamagata, Y., Karube, A., Sugino, N., & Kato, H. (2001). Changes of serum melatonin level and its relationship to feto-placental unit during pregnancy. *Journal of Pineal Research, 30*(1), 29–33. https://doi.org/10.1034/j.1600-079x.2001.300104.x

National Sleep Foundation Sleep and Teens Task Force. (2000). *Adolescent sleep needs and patterns: Research report and resource guide.*

Ohta, H., Xu, S., Moriya, T., Iigo, M., Watanabe, T., Nakahata, N., Chisaka, H., Hanita, T., Matsuda, T., Ohura, T., Kimura, Y., Yaegashi, N., Tsuchiya, S., Tei, H., & Okamura, K. (2008). Maternal feeding controls fetal biological clock. *PLOS ONE, 3*(7), Article e2601. https://doi.org/10.1371/journal.pone.0002601

Okatani, Y., Okamoto, K., Hayashi, K., Wakatsuki, A., Tamura, S., & Sagara, Y. (1998). Maternal–fetal transfer of melatonin in pregnant women near term. *Journal of Pineal Research, 25*(3), 129–134. https://doi.org/10.1111/j.1600-079x.1998.tb00550.x

Punja, S., Nikles, C. J., Senior, H., Mitchell, G., Schmid, C. H., Heussler, H., Witmans, M., & Vohra, S. (2016). Melatonin in youth: N-of-1 trials in a stimulant-treated ADHD population (MYNAP): Study protocol for a randomized controlled trial. *Trials, 17*, Article 375. https://doi.org/10.1186/s13063-016-1499-6

Reppert, S. M., & Schwartz, W. J. (1984). Functional activity of the suprachiasmatic nuclei in the fetal primate. *Neuroscience Letters, 46*(2), 145–149. https://doi.org/10.1016/0304-3940(84)90432-4

Reppert, S. M., Weaver, D. R., Rivkees, S. A., & Stopa, E. G. (1988). Putative melatonin receptors in a human biological clock. *Science, 242*(4875), 78–81. https://doi.org/10.1126/science.2845576

Rhie, S., & Chae, K. Y. (2018). Effects of school time on sleep duration and sleepiness in adolescents. *PLOS ONE, 13*(9), Article e0203318. https://doi.org/10.1371/journal.pone.0203318

Rivkees, S. A., & Hao, H. (2000). Developing circadian rhythmicity. *Seminars in Perinatology, 24*(4), 232–242. https://doi.org/10.1053/sper.2000.8598

Roenneberg, T., Kuehnle, T., Pramstaller, P. P., Ricken, J., Havel, M., Guth, A., & Merrow, M. (2004). A marker for the end of adolescence. *Current Biology, 14*(24), R1038–R1039. https://doi.org/10.1016/j.cub.2004.11.039

Sánchez-Sánchez, M., García, T. L., Heredia, D., Reséndiz, I., Cruz, L., Santiago, J., Rojas-Granados, A., Ubaldo-Reyes, L., Pérez-Campos-Mayoral, L., Pérez-Campos, E., Vásquez, G. S., Moguel, J. M., Zarate, R., García, O., Sánchez, L., Torres, F., Paz, A., Elizarraras-Rivas, J., Hernández-Huerta, M. T., & Angeles-Castellanos, M. (2022). Effect of a light–darkness cycle on the body weight gain of preterm infants admitted to the neonatal intensive care unit. *Scientific Reports, 12*(1), Article 17569. https://doi.org/10.1038/s41598-022-22533-1

Sateia, M. J., Buysse, D. J., Krystal, A. D., Neubauer, D. N., & Heald, J. L. (2017). Clinical practice guideline for the pharmacologic treatment of chronic insomnia in adults: An American Academy of Sleep Medicine clinical practice guideline. *Journal of Clinical Sleep Medicine, 13*(2), 307–349. https://doi.org/10.5664/jcsm.6470

Serón-Ferré, M., Forcelledo, M. L., Torres-Farfan, C., Valenzuela, F. J., Rojas, A., Vergara, M., Rojas-Garcia, P. P., Recabarren, M. P., & Valenzuela, G. J. (2013). Impact of chronodisruption during primate pregnancy on the maternal and newborn temperature rhythms. *PLOS ONE, 8*(2), Article e57710. https://doi.org/10.1371/journal.pone.0057710

Sheldon, S. (2012). Development of sleep in infants and children. In S. H. Sheldon, R. Ferber, M. H. Kryger, & D. Gozal (Eds.), *Principles and practice of pediatric sleep medicine* (2nd ed., pp. 17–23). Elsevier Saunders. https://doi.org/10.1016/B978-1-4557-0318-0.00003-6

Swaab, D. F., Hofman, M. A., & Honnebier, M. B. (1990). Development of vasopressin neurons in the human suprachiasmatic nucleus in relation to birth. *Developmental Brain Research, 52*(1–2), 289–293. https://doi.org/10.1016/0165-3806(90)90247-v

Swaab, D. F., Zhou, J. N., Ehlhart, T., & Hofman, M. A. (1994). Development of vasoactive intestinal polypeptide neurons in the human suprachiasmatic nucleus in relation to birth and sex. *Developmental Brain Research, 79*(2), 249–259. https://doi.org/10.1016/0165-3806(94)90129-5

Taylor, D. J., Jenni, O. G., Acebo, C., & Carskadon, M. A. (2005). Sleep tendency during extended wakefulness: Insights into adolescent sleep regulation and behavior. *Journal of Sleep Research, 14*(3), 239–244. https://doi.org/10.1111/j.1365-2869.2005.00467.x

Torres-Farfan, C., Richter, H. G., Germain, A. M., Valenzuela, G. J., Campino, C., Rojas-García, P., Forcelledo, M. L., Torrealba, F., & Serón-Ferré, M. (2004). Maternal melatonin selectively inhibits cortisol production in the primate fetal adrenal gland. *The Journal of Physiology, 554*(Pt. 3), 841–856. https://doi.org/10.1113/jphysiol.2003.056465

Tosini, G., Ferguson, I., & Tsubota, K. (2016). Effects of blue light on the circadian system and eye physiology. *Molecular Vision, 22*, 61–72.

Valenzuela, F. J., Torres-Farfan, C., Richter, H. G., Mendez, N., Campino, C., Torrealba, F., Valenzuela, G. J., & Serón-Ferré, M. (2008). Clock gene expression in adult primate suprachiasmatic nuclei and adrenal: Is the adrenal a peripheral clock responsive to melatonin? *Endocrinology, 149*(4), 1454–1461. https://doi.org/10.1210/en.2007-1518

van Geijlswijk, I. M., van der Heijden, K. B., Egberts, A. C., Korzilius, H. P., & Smits, M. G. (2010). Dose finding of melatonin for chronic idiopathic childhood sleep onset insomnia: An RCT. *Psychopharmacology, 212*(3), 379–391. https://doi.org/10.1007/s00213-010-1962-0

Varcoe, T. J., Wight, N., Voultsios, A., Salkeld, M. D., & Kennaway, D. J. (2011). Chronic phase shifts of the photoperiod throughout pregnancy programs glucose intolerance and insulin resistance in the rat. *PLOS ONE, 6*(4), Article e18504. https://doi.org/10.1371/journal.pone.0018504

Visser, S. S. M., van Diemen, W. J. M., Kervezee, L., van den Hoogen, A., Verschuren, O., Pillen, S., Benders, M. J. N. L., & Dudink, J. (2021). The relationship between preterm birth and sleep in children at school age: A systematic review. *Sleep Medicine Reviews, 57*, Article 101447. https://doi.org/10.1016/j.smrv.2021.101447

Wickersham, L. (2006). Time-of-day preference for preschool-aged children. *Chrestomathy, 5*, 259–268.

Wong, S. D., Wright, K. P., Jr., Spencer, R. L., Vetter, C., Hicks, L. M., Jenni, O. G., & LeBourgeois, M. K. (2022). Development of the circadian system in early life: Maternal and environmental factors. *Journal of Physiological Anthropology, 41*(1), Article 22. https://doi.org/10.1186/s40101-022-00294-0

Yamazaki, S., Numano, R., Abe, M., Hida, A., Takahashi, R., Ueda, M., Block, G. D., Sakaki, Y., Menaker, M., & Tei, H. (2000). Resetting central and peripheral circadian oscillators in transgenic rats. *Science, 288*(5466), 682–685. https://doi.org/10.1126/science.288.5466.682

Yates, J. (2018). The long-term effects of light exposure on establishment of newborn circadian rhythm. *Journal of Clinical Sleep Medicine, 14*(10), 1829–1830. https://doi.org/10.5664/jcsm.7426

Zhang, P., Li, G., Li, H., Tan, X., & Cheng, H. M. (2017). Environmental perturbation of the circadian clock during pregnancy leads to transgenerational mood disorder-like behaviors in mice. *Scientific Reports, 7*(1), Article 12641. https://doi.org/10.1038/s41598-017-13067-y

Zhu, J. L., Hjollund, N. H., Andersen, A. M., & Olsen, J. (2004). Shift work, job stress, and late fetal loss: The National Birth Cohort in Denmark. *Journal of Occupational and Environmental Medicine, 46*(11), 1144–1149. https://doi.org/10.1097/01.jom.0000145168.21614.21

Zisapel, N. (2022). Assessing the potential for drug interactions and long term safety of melatonin for the treatment of insomnia in children with autism spectrum disorder. *Expert Review of Clinical Pharmacology, 15*(2), 175–185. https://doi.org/10.1080/17512433.2022.2053520

CHAPTER

4 Sleep and Circadian Development in Adults and Older Adults

Jeanne F. Duffy, Arturo Arrona-Palacios, *and* Pamela Song

Abstract

This chapter reviews age-related changes in sleep, circadian rhythms, and sleep disorders in adults and older adults. With advancing age there are major changes in sleep, including sleep timing, the amount of slow-wave sleep, the number of nocturnal awakenings, sleep consolidation, and total sleep time. There are also changes in circadian rhythmicity with aging, including a reduced amplitude of some circadian rhythms and some evidence for reduced sensitivity to light. The interaction between the sleep and circadian regulatory systems also changes with age, resulting in greater difficulty sleeping during the biological daytime, the nocturnal sleep episode occurring at earlier circadian phases than in young adults, and a reduced ability to obtain a long and consolidated sleep episode. In addition to these general changes in sleep and circadian rhythmicity with aging, the sleep of many older people is impacted by a higher prevalence of specific sleep disorders, including obstructive sleep apnea, periodic limb movements of sleep, and rapid-eye-movement behavior disorder; and they are also more likely to have chronic medical problems that interfere with sleep and to take medications that either disrupt nighttime sleep or impact daytime alertness.

Key Words: aging, sleep timing, melatonin, synchronization, peripheral oscillator, suprachiasmatic nucleus

Introduction

While the specific purpose and function of sleep are sometimes a topic of debate, there is general consensus that sleep is an essential restorative process that provides the body, and especially the brain, time to recover from the activities occurring during waking hours.

Two major physiological regulatory systems interact to allow adults to have a long and consolidated wake episode during the daytime and a consolidated sleep episode at night. The first is a sleep–wake homeostatic process by which the longer one is awake, the greater the amount of sleep pressure they accumulate; and that sleep pressure is then reduced during sleep. If wake duration is not excessive and sleep duration and quality are adequate, each night will bring sleep pressure back to baseline and the individual begins the next day refreshed and alert. The second regulatory system is the circadian timing system. This system regulates cycles of sleep and wake promotion across the 24-hour day, strongly promoting sleep at certain times and strongly promoting wake at other times. There are major changes in sleep across development from infancy to adulthood, reviewed in other chapters. Here, we review how these two systems interact in adults, how each of the processes and their interaction change with age, and how this may contribute to specific age-related sleep problems.

Human sleep is divided into two major types, non-rapid-eye-movement (NREM) sleep and rapid-eye-movement (REM; Sewell et al., 2021) sleep; and these alternate several times across the night. NREM, which composes the majority of the night, is further subdivided into three stages: N1, N2, and N3 (Berry et al., 2017). N1 is a transitional stage between wake and sleep during which the individual still usually has some awareness of their environment and is easily aroused. As the sleeper enters N2 they are usually no longer aware of their environment, and N3 is the deepest stage of sleep, sometimes called *slow-wave sleep* (SWS) due to the high-amplitude, slow-frequency electroencephalographic (EEG) waves that characterize it. In all stages of NREM sleep, typical homeostatic mechanisms for breathing, cardiovascular, gastrointestinal, and thermoregulatory functions that are present during waking still operate, although typically at a slower/lower level. In contrast, REM sleep is a unique physiological state characterized by variations and instability in cardiopulmonary function and instability or lack of thermoregulatory control. First described by Aserinsky and Kleitman (1953), REM sleep is named for the rapid eye movements that occur during this state, and it is associated with vivid dreams. REM sleep has both tonic and phasic components (Eugene & Masiak, 2015), the phasic part identified as a sympathetically driven state and characterized by rapid eye movements as well as respiratory variability and muscle twitches (Tsoukalas, 2012). Tonic REM sleep consists of parasympathetic activity and no eye movements. There is a general skeletal muscle atonia (sparing only the diaphragm and intercostal muscles involved in breathing) during REM sleep, thought to be protective so that we do not "act out" our dreams. The sleep cycle typically begins with an NREM bout and is then followed by a REM bout (Carskadon & Dement, 1994). During an ~8-hour sleep episode the brain goes through these NREM–REM cycles about four to five times, with the deepest NREM occurring in the first (and second) NREM cycle and the REM bouts getting longer as the night progresses.

The term *sleep architecture* refers to the distribution of sleep stages across the night. Overall sleep architecture is dependent upon stage of development and age (Ohayon et al., 2004). For instance, infants generally spend up to 50% of the night in REM sleep and often have a bout of REM sleep prior to NREM sleep. In addition, the duration of the NREM–REM cycle is 60 minutes through most of childhood (Ohayon et al., 2004). By the time children reach primary school age, REM sleep is reduced to around 20% of sleep time and there is a lot of SWS. With the onset of puberty, SWS and slow-wave activity (SWA; Evans et al., 2021) start declining in parallel with synaptic density in cortical layers, with a 65% decrease in SWA observed between the ages of 11 and 17 years (Feinberg

& Campbell, 2010). This decline of SWS/SWA somewhat levels off during young adulthood but then declines again throughout middle age, with decreases varying in magnitude depending on sex (Carrier et al., 2001). A continued decline in the amount of SWS/SWA is seen for older adults but at a slower rate (Skeldon et al., 2016). This reduction in SWS across adulthood may help to explain the increased number of nighttime awakenings as people age, particularly given that those awakenings are most likely to occur from NREM sleep (Dijk et al., 2001).

In addition to the changes in sleep architecture that occur with development and aging, total sleep time (TST) changes. Numerous surveys and research studies have found that average sleep duration of ~10 hours during middle childhood decreases during adolescence (Wolfson et al., 2003). The decrease in sleep duration from childhood to adolescence reflects a shift in sleep/wake patterns that begins during puberty and is marked by later bedtimes (Crowley et al., 2018). When accompanied by early wake times to attend school, this results in shortened sleep on school nights. While societal demands such as school start times play a significant role in the shift of sleep/wake timing and the shortening of TST in adolescence, these are accompanied by developmental changes in sleep and the circadian system that also contribute to later sleep timing (Crowley et al., 2018). Most evidence suggests that sleep needs do not change dramatically between late childhood and into adolescence (Carskadon, 2011). However, adolescents get considerably less sleep than their younger counterparts.

In young adulthood, the overall discrepancy between sleep need and actual sleep duration persists for many individuals. Laboratory-based studies suggest that most young adults need approximately 8–8.5 hours of sleep each night (Klerman & Dijk, 2005; Roehrs et al., 1996; Wehr, 1991), whereas most adults report getting substantially less than that (Ohayon et al., 2004). Survey studies show gradual reductions in sleep duration across adulthood and middle age (Ohayon et al., 2004), and more recent large-scale studies of sleep duration estimated from activity monitors confirm that (Su et al., 2022). There is some discrepancy in whether sleep duration continues to decline or instead plateaus or even increases in older age. Ohayon and colleagues (2004) found that after age 60, TST plateaus. However, a Scandinavian study found that TST increased from age 60–64 years and then reached a plateau from the age of 70–74 years (Sivertsen et al., 2021). The increase in sleep time in the early 60s may be due to more opportunity to sleep resulting from retirement from work (for a review, see Myllyntausta & Stenholm, 2018). A nationwide survey study in Mexico among adults aged 20–95 years found that after plateauing, TST increased around age 80, especially in women living in rural areas in central Mexico (Arrona-Palacios & Gradisar, 2021). A study examining more than 11,000 accelerometer recordings in US individuals ranging from age 6 to 80 found a U-shaped curve of sleep duration across the life span, with sleep duration decreasing significantly from age 10 to age 50, before slightly increasing again in the older age groups (Su et al., 2022). It is not clear whether the increase in sleep duration among the oldest age groups represents a change in normal sleep physiology or is instead a result of age-associated increases in undiagnosed sleep disorders, increased medical burden, and/or medication use. Long sleep duration has been associated with cardiometabolic disease and depression (Knutson, 2010), as well as an increased risk of dying, falls, and frailty (da Silva et al., 2016; Mesas et al., 2011).

A study by Klerman and Dijk (2008) comparing sleep capacity in healthy young and older adults found that the maximal capacity for sleep in older adults was about 1.5 hours shorter than in young adults (7.4 vs. 8.9 hours), and the older adults showed less daytime sleep propensity on multiple sleep latency tests. Studies of acute sleep deprivation in healthy older adults show that they are able to maintain their vigilance while sleep-deprived to a greater extent than younger adults (Adam et al., 2006; Bonnet & Rosa, 1987; Buysse et al., 1993; Duffy et al., 2009), and similar results have been reported in response to chronic sleep loss (Bliese et al., 2006; Stenuit & Kerkhofs, 2005; Zitting et al., 2018). Some have interpreted these findings as evidence that older adults need less sleep than young adults, whereas others have suggested that the *ability* to sleep is what changes with age. Supporting the latter interpretation is evidence from rats demonstrating that while levels of adenosine in the basal forebrain are higher in older animals at baseline and in response to sleep loss, the adenosine receptors are less sensitive (Murillo-Rodriguez et al., 2004).

In addition to sleep duration, sleep timing is impacted by aging. After a delay in sleep timing in late adolescence, sleep timing is generally stable through young adulthood (Fischer et al., 2017; Su et al., 2022). Beginning in middle age, however, bedtimes and wake times move earlier (Carrier et al., 2002; Duffy et al., 1998; Fischer et al., 2017; Roenneberg et al., 2007; Su et al., 2022; Taillard et al., 2021), and individuals are more likely to rate themselves as "morning" types (Carrier et al., 1997; Duffy et al., 1999).

When it comes to sleep efficiency, studies have indicated that overall it remains largely unchanged from childhood to adolescence and then starts decreasing in adulthood, continuing to decline slowly with advancing age (Bliwise, 2005; Ohayon et al., 2004). Recent meta-analysis and population-based studies have corroborated the suggestion of a linear decline of sleep efficiency with increasing age (Evans et al., 2021; J. Li et al., 2018).

Overall, compared to healthy people in their 20s, healthy older people go to bed earlier, wake up earlier, have shorter sleep that contains a greater percentage of light NREM sleep and a decreased percentage of deep NREM sleep (Ohayon et al., 2004; Skeldon et al., 2016).

Circadian Rhythms in Adults

The circadian system regulates the timing of physiology and behavior within the 24-hour day. It plays a key role in sleep–wake regulation in humans by generating daily rhythms in sleepiness and alertness, as well as a rhythm in REM sleep propensity. The circadian system provides an adaptive mechanism for organisms to coordinate their cellular processes, physiological functions, and behaviors with the predictable 24-hour cycle of light and darkness on Earth (Partch et al., 2014). In humans, like in other mammals, the suprachiasmatic nucleus (SCN) of the hypothalamus is the central pacemaker for the generation and/or expression of circadian rhythms (Moore & Eichler, 1972; Ralph et al., 1990; Stephan & Zucker, 1972). In constant conditions, the period (cycle length) of rhythms driven by the circadian system is close to, but not exactly, 24 hours, hence the name "circadian" (*circa* = approximately, *diem* = day).

In humans, the average circadian period in healthy sighted adults is approximately 24.15 hours (Czeisler et al., 1999). This means that, on average, the system must be set 9 minutes earlier each day to remain synchronized to the external world. Under typical conditions, the near-24-hour circadian system is synchronized to the 24-hour day by signals from the environment (called *zeitgeber*, German for "time giver"), a process called *entrainment*. The range of periods observed in healthy sighted humans is from about 23.5 to 24.7 hours (Crowley & Eastman, 2018; Duffy et al., 2011). Thus, while the circadian system of the average adult must be reset by 9 minutes each day in order for them to remain entrained, some individuals require 30 minutes or more. These individual differences in circadian period contribute to differences in sleep timing, morningness–eveningness, and susceptibility to circadian rhythm sleep disorders (Crowley & Eastman, 2018; Duffy et al., 2011). There is evidence that period differs by sex, with women having periods that average 6 minutes shorter than men, and significantly more women (~35%) having a period shorter than 24 hours than men (~14%; Duffy et al., 2011).

In most mammals, including humans, light exposure is considered to be the dominant time cue for entraining circadian rhythms. Light has a phase-dependent impact on the circadian system (Daan & Pittendrigh, 1976). This means that for a given light signal, the phase (or time within the 24-hour circadian cycle) at which light is given will influence the magnitude and direction of the response. Light exposure in the late day/early evening will shift the rhythms later, light exposure in the late night/early morning will shift the rhythms earlier, and light exposure in mid-day will produce smaller shifts in rhythm timing (Khalsa et al., 2003). Thus, the average adult with a longer than 24-hour period requires morning light exposure to remain entrained, whereas individuals whose periods are shorter than 24 hours require evening light to remain entrained.

There are centrally driven circadian rhythms that can be easily measured, and thus are used to determine the status of the human circadian system, including rhythms in plasma cortisol and melatonin levels and the rhythm in core body temperature. Robust circadian rhythms can also be detected in peripheral tissues (Davidson et al., 2004, 2005), with about 10% of the genes being rhythmic, and often specific to an organ system; however, the rhythmic expression of these genes is controlled by a molecular clock machinery that is common among organ systems (e.g., liver, heart, lungs, muscle, kidney; Ruben et al., 2018). At the cellular level, circadian rhythms in mammals are generated and sustained by a cell-autonomous circadian clock comprised of a core group of genes (activators and repressors) which regulate their own transcription and translation over 24 hours via a series of interacting transcription–translation feedback loops. Within a given organ, the molecular clocks of individual cells are synchronized with each other to achieve coordinated activity. The organ systems of the body are synchronized with each other (internal synchronization) and with the timing of the external environment (external synchronization) via signals from the central pacemaker. In this way, the central pacemaker coordinates the rhythmic activity of the cells, tissues, and organs to achieve maximum efficiency with respect to the external environment that the organism is living in.

Epidemiological and laboratory studies have provided evidence that disruption of the circadian system can be associated with adverse health effects, including immune dysfunction, cardiometabolic disorders, and cancers (Antunes et al., 2010; Castanon-Cervantes et al., 2010; Morris, Purvis, Hu, & Scheer, 2016; Morris, Purvis, Mistretta, & Scheer, 2016; Resuehr et al., 2019). Clock disruption is strongly associated with chronic diseases, as well as deregulation of acute responses such as inflammation. One of the mechanisms of these adverse effects is loss of synchronization: either internal, that is, between the timing of peripheral clocks or between the timing of the central and peripheral clocks, or external, that is, between internal clocks and external cycles such sleep/wake, light/dark, and meal timing. Another source of circadian disruption can be the weakening of rhythms, that is, damped oscillations characterized by a reduction in the amplitude (Kervezee et al., 2018). Both underlying causes of circadian disruption are in turn associated with increased risk of metabolic disorders (Ando et al., 2009; Dibner & Schibler, 2015; Mantele et al., 2012; Sohail et al., 2015). Common everyday situations such as shift work, irregular sleeping and eating patterns, jetlag, or irregular light exposure patterns can disrupt circadian rhythms. Emerging evidence indicates that chronic exposure to internal desynchrony (misalignment of the central and peripheral clocks) increases the risk of developing obesity, diabetes, hypertension, impaired glucose regulation, and dyslipidemia in shift workers (Antunes et al., 2010; Kervezee et al., 2020; Morris, Purvis, Mistretta, & Scheer, 2016).

Changes in Circadian Rhythmicity in Older Adults

By 2050, the number of Americans aged 65 and older is projected to be more than 82 million, more than double the number in 2010 (Mather & Scommegna, 2024). Aging affects all aspects of physiology and behaviors, including the circadian system. These age-related changes (reviewed in Duffy et al., 2015; Hood & Amir, 2017) include changes in sleep timing and architecture (Bliwise, 2005; Carrier et al., 1997; Czeisler et al., 1992; Duffy et al., 1998), diurnal preference shifting from eveningness to morningness (Carrier et al., 1997; Duffy et al., 1999; Roenneberg et al., 2007), and the circadian phase of centrally controlled rhythms of core temperature, melatonin, and cortisol moving to earlier clock times with age (Carrier et al., 2002; Czeisler et al., 1992; Duffy et al., 1998, 2002; Sharma et al., 1989; Sherman et al., 1985; Tozawa et al., 2003; Van Cauter et al., 1996; Weitzman et al., 1982). In addition to changes in sleep timing and circadian rhythm timing, the phase relationship between sleep and circadian rhythm timing changes with age such that older adults go to bed and wake at an earlier clock time and at an earlier internal rhythm timing. Another common age-related feature of the circadian system is the dampening of many rhythms (i.e., reduced peak-to-trough amplitude), including those of core temperature, melatonin, and cortisol (Carrier et al., 1996; Czeisler et al., 1992; Van Coevorden et al., 1991; Weitzman et al., 1982; Zeitzer et al., 1999).

The ability of the circadian system to adjust to abrupt changes in the light–dark schedule (e.g., the changes associated with jetlag and rotating shift work) has also been reported to be reduced with age (Duffy et al., 2015; Hood & Amir, 2017; Klerman et al., 2001; Monk, 2005). Moreover, evidence from both human and animal studies suggests that there are structural and functional changes in the aging SCN. These age-related changes include decreased SCN volume and cell number in older compared to younger adults (Swaab et al., 1985) and in older compared to younger rats (Tsukahara et al., 2005; Zhou & Swaab, 1999), reduced expression of arginine vasopressin and vasoactive intestinal polypeptide in the shell and core of the SCN in older humans and rodents compared to younger (Chee et al., 1988; Hofman & Swaab, 1994; Roozendaal et al., 1987; Zhou et al., 1995), and reduced amplitude and loss of coherence in SCN firing patterns (Nakamura et al., 2011, 2016; Satinoff et al., 1993; Watanabe et al., 1995). Other compelling evidence for age-related changes in the SCN comes from transplant experiments in which fetal SCN tissue was transferred into the brain of older animals, which then restored dampened rhythms of activity, temperature, drinking, and corticotrophin-releasing hormone in the brain (Cai et al., 1997; Hurd et al., 1995; H. Li & Satinoff, 1998).

Peripheral metabolic clocks are entrained primarily by autonomic innervation, glucocorticoid hormones, and body temperature (Reddy & Maywood, 2007). A dampening of rhythmic output from the central clock with age may lead to desynchronization between central and peripheral oscillators and consequently to misalignment between peripheral oscillators and external temporal cues (Hood & Amir, 2017). Indirect evidence for weaker control by the central clock over the peripheral oscillators comes from phase-shifting studies in which sleep, activity, and temperature rhythms in older humans and animals take longer to re-entrain to a light/dark cycle after a phase advance (Monk et al., 1993; Valentinuzzi et al., 1997). Additional support for desynchronization within and/or between central and peripheral oscillators with age comes from studies showing that imposing and/or strengthening external temporal cues such as temperature and meal timing (to better align peripheral rhythms with the central clock) can improve behavioral rhythms in aged animals and with neurodegenerative disorders (Luo et al., 2012; Walcott & Tate, 1996). Related evidence in humans has shown that strengthening the light–dark cycle can improve sleep (Brown et al., 2022).

Sleep Disruption and Disorders in Adults

There is a general consensus that adults require 7–9 hours of proper sleep each night for optimal physical and mental health (Watson et al., 2015). Unfortunately, there is extensive evidence that a majority of adults do not obtain optimal sleep, for a variety of reasons. In many cases, the sleep deficiency is behavioral in nature, meaning that the individual does not spend enough time in bed each night. This may be due to working long hours, child- or elder-care responsibilities, choosing to forgo sleep for social or leisure activities, or lack of an adequate environment for sleep.

In addition to behavioral sleep restriction, there are a variety of sleep disorders that impact sleep quality, sleep duration, or both; and several of these sleep disorders are more prevalent with age. Insomnia, obstructive sleep apnea (OSA), restless legs syndrome (RLS), periodic limb movements during sleep (PLMS), REM behavior disorder (RBD), and advanced sleep–wake phase disorder (ASWPD) all are more common among older adults than younger individuals. A brief description of each of these disorders, and their impact on the sleep of older adults, follows.

Insomnia

Insomnia is the most common sleep disturbance in the adult and older population (Foley et al., 1995; Morin & Benca, 2012). The reported prevalence of insomnia ranges from 6% to 10%, it increases with age, and it is more prevalent in women than men (Morin et al., 2006; Ohayon, 2002; Ohayon & Reynolds, 2009). Those with insomnia can have difficulty with sleep initiation, maintenance of sleep, or early morning awakening, accompanied by daytime symptoms of sleepiness and fatigue (Sateia, 2014). The pathophysiological mechanisms underlying insomnia are not clear, but there is evidence that people who experience insomnia show hyperarousal brain activity when asleep, which may then result in insufficient sleep quality or quantity (Bonnet & Arand, 2010; Riemann et al., 2010). There is also evidence that the hyperarousal may be present during waking as well as sleep (Pillai et al., 2016). When untreated and unresolved, insomnia is a risk factor for mental disorders, most commonly depression (Baglioni et al., 2011), as well as metabolic syndrome (Troxel et al., 2010), hypertension (Vgontzas et al., 2009), and coronary heart disease (Laugsand et al., 2011). There is general consensus that cognitive-behavioral therapy for insomnia (CBT-I) is the most effective treatment (Mitchell et al., 2012). While originally constructed as six to eight intervention sessions over 6–10 weeks, and including sleep restriction, stimulus control, relaxation, cognitive strategies, and sleep hygiene education, methods using shortened, online, and virtual delivery of CBT-I have also been shown to be effective (Alimoradi et al., 2022; Arnedt et al., 2021; Drake et al., 2019; Edinger et al., 2021; Gehrman et al., 2021). While hypnotic medications are often prescribed together with CBT-I at the start of treatment, over the long term they are not as effective as CBT-I. Typical pharmacological treatments for insomnia include benzodiazepines, benzodiazepine receptor agonists (BzRAs), dual orexin receptor antagonists, antihistamines, tricyclic antidepressants, melatonin receptor agonists, sedating antidepressants, antipsychotics, and anticonvulsants (Benca, 2005). The mainstay of insomnia treatment are the BzRAs, although benzodiazepines are generally recommended only for short-term use as long-term use may result in adverse events such as residual sedation in the morning, impaired motor and cognitive function, falls, and fractures (Madari et al., 2021), especially in the older patient (Sys et al., 2020).

OSA

OSA is repetitive complete (apnea) or partial (hypopnea) upper airway obstruction during sleep. It is diagnosed from overnight polysomnography during which respiratory effort, nasal pressure, and oxygen saturation are recorded in order to document the number of apneas and hypopneas per hour of sleep, the Apnea/Hypopnea Index (AHI; Bonakis et al., 2009). While a few (fewer than five) apneas are not uncommon, when the AHI is ≥10, especially when accompanied with oxygen desaturations and complaints about sleep quality or daytime sleepiness, treatment is warranted (Sateia, 2014). While once thought to be fairly rare (Young et al., 1993), it is now recognized that OSA is common and impacts older men and women to the same extent (Moreno-Tamayo et al., 2021; Pavlova et al., 2008). Risk factors for OSA are older age, male sex (until menopause, when women's rates of OSA are similar to men's), obesity, craniofacial and upper airway abnormalities, and neurologic disorders (Jennum & Riha, 2009; Tufik et al., 2010; Young et al., 2004, 2009). There are a few contributing factors known to increase the risk of OSA, including structural changes in pharyngeal anatomy that promote easy collapsibility (Edwards et al., 2014; Eikermann et al., 2007), a less sensitive respiratory control system (Kronenberg & Drage, 1973), and a lower arousal threshold (Eikermann et al., 2007). Untreated OSA is associated with a significant increase in cardiovascular disease due to the intermittent hypoxemia, hemodynamic changes, increase in sympathetic activity, inflammation, and metabolic effects associated with OSA (Bradley & Floras, 2009; Seif et al., 2013). The standard treatment for OSA is continuous positive airway pressure therapy (Jordan et al., 2014), in which air is delivered into the airway of the patient during sleep to maintain enough positive pressure to prevent airway collapse (Giles et al., 2006; McDaid et al., 2009; McEvoy et al., 2016; Walia et al., 2019).

RLS and PLMS

RLS presents during waking, with uncomfortable and unpleasant sensations typically in the lower legs, and the symptoms worsen during rest, are relieved by movement, and typically occur in the evening (Sateia, 2014). The prevalence of RLS has been estimated to be 5%–10%, increasing to 9%–20% with age (Ohayon et al., 2012; Ohayon & Roth, 2002; Yeh et al., 2012). RLS is classified as primary or secondary, in association with precipitating disorders: iron deficiency, pregnancy, chronic renal failure, certain medications, electrolyte imbalances, and prolonged immobility (Manconi et al., 2021).

PLMS is periodic dorsiflexion of the ankle and/or flexion of the knee that occurs rhythmically during sleep. PLMS is diagnosed by electromyography on both tibialis anterior muscles throughout sleep to determine the number of leg movements per hour of sleep (the periodic limb movement index). In addition, the number of periodic limb movements (PLMs) that trigger EEG arousals is also often quantified. The prevalence of PLMs increases with age (Ohayon & Roth, 2002; Youngstedt et al., 1998). PLMs have been reported in at least 80% of patients with RLS (Allen, Picchietti, et al., 2014; Garcia-Borreguero et al., 2014). Treatment for PLMS is considered when there are many arousals associated with the leg movements and when patients complain of poor sleep quality and/or daytime sleepiness. The treatment options for managing symptoms of RLS include $\alpha 2\delta$ ligands such as gabapentin, pregabalin, and gabapentin enacarbil (Allen, Chen, et al., 2014) along with opioids (Silber et al., 2018; Silver et al., 2011). The dopaminergic drugs were initially the primary treatment for symptoms of RLS (Winkelman et al., 2016). However, standard use of these medications is now advised against due to accumulating evidence indicating a risk of augmentation (Winkelman et al., 2024). If RLS symptoms are accompanied by low (<75 μg/l) ferritin levels and transferrin saturation <20% to 45%, iron therapy is also indicated (Allen et al., 2018; Winkelman et al., 2024).

Circadian Rhythm Sleep–Wake Disorders

Circadian rhythm sleep-wake disorders (CRSWDs) are caused by a misalignment between the timing of the endogenous biological clock with the exogenous 24-hour environmental time. As discussed above, under normal entrained sleep–wake conditions, the timing of the endogenous biological rhythm of sleep–wake propensity interacts with a sleep homeostatic process to allow adults to remain awake for an extended duration each day and similarly to remain asleep for an extended duration each night. When this interaction is altered, a CRSWD can develop, not necessarily because there is anything wrong with sleep but because of the internal biological time at which sleep is attempted (Duffy et al., 2021). One characteristic of the CRSWDs is that if patients are allowed to sleep at times of their choosing, they are able to initiate and consolidate sleep for a normal duration.

There are six types of CRSWD according to the International Classification of Sleep Disorders: delayed sleep-wake phase disorder (DSWPD), in which the timing of sleep is later than desired; advanced sleep-wake phase disorder (ASWPD), in which the timing of sleep is earlier than desired; irregular sleep–wake rhythm disorder (ISWD); non-24-hour sleep–wake rhythm disorder (N24SWD); shift work disorder; and jet lag disorder (American Academy of Sleep Medicine, 2014).

To diagnose CRSWDs, the misalignment of endogenous circadian rhythm in relation to the external environment needs to be evaluated. The sleep–wake timing can be documented by sleep logs (Carney et al., 2012) and actigraphy (Fekedulegn et al., 2020) and should be followed for at least two weeks, including both weekdays (when there are work or school obligations) and weekends or free days. In order to determine whether an abnormality of circadian timing is a cause of the abnormal sleep timing, some measure of circadian phase timing should be collected (Duffy et al., 2021). While not used routinely in sleep clinics, some specialized circadian clinics assess the timing of the salivary dim light melatonin onset to measure circadian timing. While DSWPD is more common in young adults, ASWPD is more common in older adults. ASWPD is characterized by excessive sleepiness in the early evening, leading to an early bedtime and a corresponding early morning wake time. This is frustrating for the affected patient because they are too sleepy to be able to socialize with friends and family in the evening and then are awake when no one else is in the early morning. Evening bright light therapy is the typical treatment for ASWPD, sometimes combined with reduction in light exposure in the morning. The bright evening light acts to shift the timing of the internal circadian system later (Czeisler et al., 1986).

RBD

REM sleep is normally accompanied by skeletal muscle atonia, via a pathway from the brainstem through the spinal cord (Arrigoni et al., 2016). RBD is characterized by dream enactment during sleep, usually presenting with complex motor behaviors and/or vocalization (Sateia, 2014). The dreams are often violent or unpleasant, thus leading to aggressive behaviors that can include shouting, swearing, screaming, as well as punching and kicking the bed partner, running away from the threat, and other behaviors consist with the dream content (Boeve, 2010). The actions of the patient with RBD can lead to injury to themselves or their bed partner. The pathophysiology of RBD is linked to the neural network disruption in physiologic REM sleep atonia control, mainly located in the pons (Boeve et al., 2007). RBD presents differently among older (≥50 years) adults as compared with younger (<50 years) adults. RBD in older adults is more common in men and is highly associated with future development of neurodegenerative diseases, especially α-synuclein pathologies such as Parkinson's disease, multiple systemic atrophy, and dementia with Lewy bodies. In fact, RBD is now considered a marker for this neurodegenerative syndrome, for it typically precedes the core features of the neurodegenerative syndrome by a decade or more (Boeve et al., 2003, 2007; Claassen et al., 2010; Iranzo et al., 2006). The conversion rates average up to 73.5% to 91% after a 12- to 14-year follow-up (Postuma et al., 2019; Schenck et al., 2013). RBD among younger adults has similar distribution for men and women, is commonly comorbid with narcolepsy, is related to antidepressant use, and has a higher prevalence of isolated RBD (Bonakis et al., 2009; Teman et al., 2009). The treatment for RBD is aimed at decreasing the frequency and severity of violent behavior to avoid injury to the patient and bed partner (Boeve et al., 2003; Ittner & Götz, 2011).

Shift Work

Shift-work disorder occurs when the work schedule overlaps with the usual time for sleep overnight and then the corresponding sleep time occurs during the daytime hours.

Common symptoms are insomnia during desired sleep time (typically an inability to remain asleep) and excessive sleepiness during work hours. Older shift workers experience more sleep disturbances than younger ones (Åkerstedt & Torsvall, 1981; Duffy, 2003; Folkard, 2008; Luckhaupt, 2012; Marquié & Foret, 1999; Reid & Dawson, 2001; Torsvall et al., 1981). Laboratory studies have shown that the sleep of older adults is much more sensitive to the circadian time at which it occurs than is the sleep of young adults (Dijk et al., 1999), thus making older adults more vulnerable to shift-work disorder (Folkard & Tucker, 2003; Härmä et al., 1998; Marquié & Foret, 1999). Studies in which the circadian time of sleep is systematically manipulated have revealed that there may be an age-related reduction in the amplitude of the circadian rhythm of sleep–wake propensity that not only makes consolidation of an extended nighttime sleep episode more difficult but also makes it more difficult to sleep at an adverse circadian time, as is required when working at night and sleeping during the day (Dijk et al., 1999; Klerman et al., 2004).

Sleep and Alzheimer's Disease

Alzheimer's disease (AD) is a prevalent neurodegenerative disorder. The pathogenesis is the accumulation of amyloid plaque and neurofibrillary tangles which eventually cause neuronal death (Ittner & Götz, 2011). The characteristic symptom of AD is cognitive impairment, which includes memory, language, visuospatial function, and executive function; but it may vary between individuals (Knopman et al., 2021). Sleep disturbances are reported in nearly a quarter of AD patients and are known to be associated with behavioral symptoms (Moran et al., 2005). The sleep disturbances in AD are sometimes considered as circadian rhythm disturbances, while normal age-related sleep disturbances are considered to be consequences of sleep homeostatic changes (Buysse et al., 1993; Duffy et al., 1998). The pathological changes as AD progresses in relation to specific sleep symptoms are not clear, but sleep symptoms often present before the cognitive changes in AD and can be considered a "preclinical symptom" of AD (Musiek et al., 2018; van Someren et al., 1996). The sleep complaints are associated with pathologic brain alterations as assessed by "Braak staging," suggesting a direct effect of AD on the sleep symptoms (Harper et al., 2004). As AD progresses, there is evidence of specific pathologic changes in sleep structures in the brain. In severe AD patients, the SCN (the central circadian pacemaker) was noted to have deposition of neurofibrillary tangles but not amyloid plaque (Stopa et al., 1999). Other structures that are part of the circadian system, intrinsically photosensitive retinal ganglion cells, are reported to show cell loss and amyloid deposition in moderate to severe AD patients (La Morgia et al., 2016). Research using actigraphy and core body temperature to evaluate circadian rhythms in AD patients found phase variations in the timing of circadian rhythms throughout the clinical continuum of AD. The actigraphy studies suggest that early AD is not associated with changes in rhythm timing (Musiek et al., 2018), mild cognitive impairment (MCI) is associated with a phase advance (Naismith et al., 2014; Ortiz-Tudela et al., 2014), and symptomatic AD is associated with a phase delay (Harper et al., 2001, 2004; Wang et al., 2015). Similarly, studies that examined the phase of the core body temperature rhythm in AD patients found a phase advance in MCI (Ortiz-Tudela et al., 2014) but a phase delay in AD (Abulafia et al., 2017). Although there is still much that is not understood about changes in sleep and circadian rhythms in AD, there is now evidence for typical pathologic abnormalities in sleep structures and evidence that circadian rhythms may be impacted due to pathologic changes in circadian structures.

Conclusion

Aging is associated with major changes in sleep, including its timing, duration, consolidation, and stage distribution. The circadian timing system similarly undergoes age-related changes, including a reduction in amplitude of some rhythms and changes in light sensitivity. The interaction between the sleep and circadian regulatory systems also changes with age, resulting in greater difficulty sleeping during the biological daytime, the nocturnal sleep episode occurring at earlier circadian phases than in young adults, and a reduced ability to obtain a long and consolidated sleep episode. With advancing age there is also a greater likelihood of developing a sleep disorder, having a chronic medical problem that interferes with sleep, and taking medications that either disrupt nighttime sleep or impact daytime alertness. Thus, sleep problems can have a major impact on health, safety, and quality of life of the older adult. With rapidly aging populations in most countries, over the next few decades the number of people over age 60 will double from approximately one billion in 2020 to 2.1 billion in 2050, and those over age 80 will triple during the same time frame, reaching 426 million (World Health Organization, 2022). Thus, understanding how sleep changes with age and addressing sleep problems with age-appropriate treatments are critical for a healthy society.

Future Direction

While much is known about sleep and circadian rhythms in adults and how those systems change with age, there are a number of outstanding questions that remain to be answered. As mentioned above, the conflicting evidence whereby healthy older adults are able to perform better than young adults under acute or chronic sleep deprivation conditions even though they show worse sleep quality has raised the still unanswered question of whether older people need less sleep. There are numerous outstanding issues related to how lifetime sleep, sleep disorders, or circadian disruption may contribute to AD and other neurodegenerative disorders and whether interventions designed to strengthen circadian rhythms or those aimed at improving sleep duration and quality can impact the cognitive symptoms or trajectory of cognitive decline. As we identify more types of peripheral circadian rhythms, understanding how they are impacted by light exposure, food intake, sleep, activity, and other behaviors will be important for being able to detect changes or abnormalities that may lead to long-term adverse health outcomes.

References

Abulafia, C., Duarte-Abritta, B., Villarreal, M. F., Ladrón-de-Guevara, M. S., García, C., Sequeyra, G., Sevlever, G., Fiorentini, L., Bär, K.-J., Gustafson, D. R., Vigo, D. E., & Guinjoan, S. M. (2017). Relationship between cognitive and sleep–wake variables in asymptomatic offspring of patients with late-onset Alzheimer's disease. *Frontiers in Aging Neuroscience, 9*, Article 93.

Adam, M., Rétey, J. V., Khatami, R., & Landolt, H.-P. (2006). Age-related changes in the time course of vigilant attention during 40 hours without sleep in men. *Sleep, 29*(1), 55–57.

Åkerstedt, T., & Torsvall, L. (1981). Age, sleep and adjustment to shiftwork. In W. P. Koella (Ed.), *Sleep 1980* (pp. 190–195). S. Karger.

Alimoradi, Z., Jafari, E., Broström, A., Ohayon, M. M., Lin, C.-Y., Griffiths, M. D., Blom, K., Jernelöv, S., Kaldo, V., & Pakpour, A. H. (2022). Effects of cognitive behavioral therapy for insomnia (CBT-I) on quality of life: A systematic review and meta-analysis. *Sleep Medicine Reviews, 64*, Article 101646.

Allen, R. P., Chen, C., Garcia-Borreguero, D., Polo, O., DuBrava, S., Miceli, J., Knapp, L., & Winkelman, J. W. (2014). Comparison of pregabalin with pramipexole for restless legs syndrome. *New England Journal of Medicine, 370*(7), 621–631.

Allen, R. P., Picchietti, D. L., Auerbach, M., Cho, Y. W., Connor, J. R., Earley, C. J., Garcia-Borreguero, D., Kotagal, S., Manconi, M., Ondo, W., Ulfberg, J., & Winkelman, J. W.; International Restless Legs Syndrome Study Group. (2018). Evidence-based and consensus clinical practice guidelines for the iron treatment of restless legs syndrome/Willis-Ekbom disease in adults and children: An IRLSSG task force report. *Sleep Medicine, 41*, 27–44.

Allen, R. P., Picchietti, D. L., Garcia-Borreguero, D., Ondo, W. G., Walters, A. S., Winkelman, J. W., Zucconi, M., Ferri, R., Trenkwalder, C., & Lee, H. B.; International Restless Legs Syndrome Study Group. (2014). Restless legs syndrome/Willis-Ekbom disease diagnostic criteria: Updated International Restless Legs Syndrome Study Group (IRLSSG) consensus criteria—History, rationale, description, and significance. *Sleep Medicine, 15*(8), 860–873.

American Academy of Sleep Medicine. (2014). *International classification of sleep disorders* (3rd ed.).

Ando, H., Takamura, T., Matsuzawa-Nagata, N., Shima, K. R., Eto, T., Misu, H., Shiramoto, M., Tsuru, T., Irie, S., Fujimura, A., & Kaneko, S. (2009). Clock gene expression in peripheral leucocytes of patients with type 2 diabetes. *Diabetologia, 52*(2), 329–335.

Antunes, L. C., Levandovski, R., Dantas, G., Caumo, W., & Hidalgo, M. P. (2010). Obesity and shift work: Chronobiological aspects. *Nutrition Research Reviews, 23*(1), 155–168.

Arnedt, J. T., Conroy, D. A., Mooney, A., Furgal, A., Sen, A., & Eisenberg, D. (2021). Telemedicine versus face-to-face delivery of cognitive behavioral therapy for insomnia: A randomized controlled noninferiority trial. *Sleep, 44*(1), Article zsaa136.

Arrigoni, E., Chen, M. C., & Fuller, P. M. (2016). The anatomical, cellular and synaptic basis of motor atonia during rapid eye movement sleep. *Journal of Physiology, 594*(19), 5391–5414.

Arrona-Palacios, A., & Gradisar, M. (2021). Self-reported sleep duration, sleep quality and sleep problems in Mexicans adults: Results of the 2016 Mexican National Halfway Health and Nutrition Survey. *Sleep Health, 7*(2), 246–253.

Aserinsky, E., & Kleitman, N. (1953). Regularly occurring periods of eye motility, and concomitant phenomena, during sleep. *Science, 118*, 273–274.

Baglioni, C., Battagliese, G., Feige, B., Spiegelhalder, K., Nissen, C., Voderholzer, U., Lombardo, C., & Riemann, D. (2011). Insomnia as a predictor of depression: A meta-analytic evaluation of longitudinal epidemiological studies. *Journal of Affective Disorders, 135*(1–3), 10–19.

Benca, R. M. (2005). Diagnosis and treatment of chronic insomnia: A review. *Psychiatric Services, 56*(3), 332–343.

Berry, R. B., Brooks, R., Gamaldo, C., Harding, S. M., Lloyd, R. M., Quan, S. F., Troester, M. T., & Vaughn, B. V. (2017). AASM Scoring Manual updates for 2017. *Journal of Clinical Sleep Medicine, 13*(5), 665–666.

Bliese, P. D., Wesensten, N. J., & Balkin, T. J. (2006). Age and individual variability in performance during sleep restriction. *Journal of Sleep Research, 15*(4), 376–385.

Bliwise, D. L. (2005). Normal aging. In M. H. Kryger, T. Roth, & W. C. Dement (Eds.), *Principles and practice of sleep medicine* (4th ed., pp. 24–38). Elsevier Saunders.

Boeve, B. F. (2010). REM sleep behavior disorder: Updated review of the core features, the REM sleep behavior disorder–neurodegenerative disease association, evolving concepts, controversies, and future directions. *Annals of the New York Academy of Sciences, 1184*, 15–54.

Boeve, B. F., Silber, M. H., & Ferman, T. J. (2003). Melatonin for treatment of REM sleep behavior disorder in neurologic disorders: Results in 14 patients. *Sleep Medicine, 4*(4), 281–284.

Boeve, B. F., Silber, M. H., Saper, C. B., Ferman, T. J., Dickson, D. W., Parisi, J. E., Benarroch, E. E., Ahlskog, J. E., Smith, G. E., Caselli, R. C., Tippman-Peikert, M., Olson, E. J., Lin, S.-C., Young, T., Wszolek, Z., Schenk, C. H., Mahowald, M. W., Castillo, P. R., Del Tredici, K., & Braak, H. (2007). Pathophysiology of REM sleep behaviour disorder and relevance to neurodegenerative disease. *Brain, 130*(Pt. 11), 2770–2788.

Bonakis, A., Howard, R. S., Ebrahim, I. O., Merritt, S., & Williams, A. (2009). REM sleep behaviour disorder (RBD) and its associations in young patients. *Sleep Medicine, 10*(6), 641–645.

Bonnet, M. H., & Arand, D. L. (2010). Hyperarousal and insomnia: State of the science. *Sleep Medicine Reviews, 14*(1), 9–15.

Bonnet, M. H., & Rosa, R. R. (1987). Sleep and performance in young adults and older normals and insomniacs during acute sleep loss and recovery. *Biological Psychology, 25*(2), 153–172.

Bradley, T. D., & Floras, J. S. (2009). Obstructive sleep apnoea and its cardiovascular consequences. *Lancet, 373*(9657), 82–93.

Brown, T. M., Brainard, G. C., Cajochen, C., Czeisler, C. A., Hanifin, J. P., Lockley, S. W., Lucas, R. J., Münch, M., O'Hagan, J. B., Peirson, S. N., Price. L. L. A., Roenneberg, T., Schlangen, L. J. M., Skene, D. J., Spitschan, M., Vetter, C., Zee, P. C., & Wright, K. P., Jr. (2022). Recommendations for daytime, evening, and nighttime indoor light exposure to best support physiology, sleep, and wakefulness in healthy adults. *PLOS Biology, 20*(3), Article e3001571.

Buysse, D. J., Monk, T. H., Reynolds, C. F., 3rd, Mesiano, D., Houck, P. R., & Kupfer, D. J. (1993). Patterns of sleep episodes in young and elderly adults during a 36-hour constant routine. *Sleep, 16*(7), 632–637.

Cai, A., Scarbrough, K., Hinkle, D. A., & Wise, P. M. (1997). Fetal grafts containing suprachiasmatic nuclei restore the diurnal rhythm of CRH and POMC mRNA in aging rats. *American Journal of Physiology, 273*(5 Pt. 2), R1764–R1770.

Carney, C. E., Buysse, D. J., Ancoli-Israel, S., Edinger, J. D., Krystal, A. D., Lichstein, K. L., & Morin, C. M. (2012). The consensus sleep diary: Standardizing prospective sleep self-monitoring. *Sleep, 35*(2), 287–302.

Carrier, J., Land, S., Buysse, D. J., Kupfer, D. J., & Monk, T. H. (2001). The effects of age and gender on sleep EEG power spectral density in the middle years of life (ages 20–60 years old). *Psychophysiology, 38*(2), 232–242.

Carrier, J., Monk, T. H., Buysse, D. J., & Kupfer, D. (1996). Amplitude reduction of the circadian temperature and sleep rhythms in the elderly. *Chronobiology International, 13*(5), 373–386.

Carrier, J., Monk, T. H., Buysse, D. J., & Kupfer, D. J. (1997). Sleep and morningness–eveningness in the "middle" years of life (20–59y). *Journal of Sleep Research, 6*, 230–237.

Carrier, J., Paquet, J., Morettini, J., & Touchette, E. (2002). Phase advance of sleep and temperature circadian rhythms in the middle years of life in humans. *Neuroscience Letters, 320*, 1–4.

Carskadon, M. A. (2011). Sleep in adolescents: The perfect storm. *Pediatric Clinics of North America, 58*(3), 637–647.

Carskadon, M. A., & Dement, W. C. (1994). Normal human sleep: An overview. In M. H. Kryger, T. Roth, & W. C. Dement (Eds.), *Principles and practice of sleep medicine* (2nd ed., pp. 16–25). Saunders.

Castanon-Cervantes, O., Wu, M., Ehlen, J. C., Paul, K., Gamble, K. L., Johnson, R. L., Besing, R. C., Menaker, M., Gewirtz, A. T., & Davidson, A. J. (2010). Dysregulation of inflammatory responses by chronic circadian disruption. *Journal of Immunology, 185*(10), 5796–5805.

Chee, C. A., Roozendaal, B., Swaab, D. F., Goudsmit, E., & Mirmiran, M. (1988). Vasoactive intestinal polypeptide neuron changes in the senile rat suprachiasmatic nucleus. *Neurobiology of Aging, 9*, 307–312.

Claassen, D. O., Josephs, K. A., Ahlskog, J. E., Silber, M. H., Tippmann-Peikert, M., & Boeve, B. F. (2010). REM sleep behavior disorder preceding other aspects of synucleinopathies by up to half a century. *Neurology, 75*(6), 494–499.

Crowley, S. J., & Eastman, C. I. (2018). Free-running circadian period in adolescents and adults. *Journal of Sleep Research, 27*(5), Article e12678.

Crowley, S. J., Wolfson, A. R., Tarokh, L., & Carskadon, M. A. (2018). An update on adolescent sleep: New evidence informing the perfect storm model. *Journal of Adolescence, 67*, 55–65.

Czeisler, C. A., Allan, J. S., Strogatz, S. H., Ronda, J. M., Sánchez, R., Ríos, C. D., Freitag, W. O., Richardson, G. S., & Kronauer, R. E. (1986). Bright light resets the human circadian pacemaker independent of the timing of the sleep–wake cycle. *Science, 233*, 667–671.

Czeisler, C. A., Duffy, J. F., Shanahan, T. L., Brown, E. N., Mitchell, J. F., Rimmer, D. W., Ronda, J. M., Silva, E. J., Allan, J. S., Emens, J. S., Dijk, D. J., & Kronauer, R. E. (1999). Stability, precision, and near-24-hour period of the human circadian pacemaker. *Science, 284*, 2177–2181.

Czeisler, C. A., Dumont, M., Duffy, J. F., Steinberg, J. D., Richardson, G. S., Brown, E. N., Sánchez, R., Ríos, C. D., & Ronda, J. M. (1992). Association of sleep–wake habits in older people with changes in output of circadian pacemaker. *Lancet, 340*, 933–936.

Daan, S., & Pittendrigh, C. S. (1976). A functional analysis of circadian pacemakers in nocturnal rodents. II. The variability of phase response curves. *Journal of Comparative Physiology A, 106*, 253–266.

da Silva, A. A., de Mello, R. G. B., Schaan, C. W., Fuchs, F. D., Redline, S., & Fuchs, S. C. (2016). Sleep duration and mortality in the elderly: A systematic review with meta-analysis. *BMJ Open, 6*(2), Article e008119.

Davidson, A. J., Castanon-Cervantes, O., & Stephan, F. K. (2004). Daily oscillations in liver function: Diurnal vs circadian rhythmicity. *Liver International, 24*(3), 179–186.

Davidson, A. J., London, B., Block, G. D., & Menaker, M. (2005). Cardiovascular tissues contain independent circadian clocks. *Clinical and Experimental Hypertension, 27*(2–3), 307–311.

Dibner, C., & Schibler, U. (2015). Circadian timing of metabolism in animal models and humans. *Journal of Internal Medicine, 277*(5), 513–527.

Dijk, D.-J., Duffy, J. F., & Czeisler, C. A. (2001). Age-related increase in awakenings: Impaired consolidation of nonREM sleep at all circadian phases. *Sleep, 24*(5), 565–577.

Dijk, D. J., Duffy, J. F., Riel, E., Shanahan, T. L., & Czeisler, C. A. (1999). Ageing and the circadian and homeostatic regulation of human sleep during forced desynchrony of rest, melatonin and temperature rhythms. *Journal of Physiology, 516*(2), 611–627.

Drake, C. L., Kalmbach, D. A., Arnedt, J. T., Cheng, P., Tonnu, C. V., Cuamatzi-Castelan, A., & Fellman-Couture, C. (2019). Treating chronic insomnia in postmenopausal women: A randomized clinical trial comparing cognitive-behavioral therapy for insomnia, sleep restriction therapy, and sleep hygiene education. *Sleep, 42*(2), Article zsy217.

Duffy, J. F. (2003). Shift work and aging: Roles of sleep and circadian rhythms. *Clinics in Occupational and Environmental Medicine, 3*, 311–332.

Duffy, J. F., Abbott, S. M., Burgess, H. J., Crowley, S. J., Emens, J. S., Epstein, L. J., Gamble, K. L., Hasler, B. P., Kristo, D. A., Malkani, R. G., Rahman, S. A., Thomas, S. J., Wyatt, J. K., Zee, P. C., & Klerman, E. B. (2021). Workshop report. Circadian rhythm sleep–wake disorders: Gaps and opportunities. *Sleep, 44*(5), Article zsaa281.

Duffy, J. F., Cain, S. W., Chang, A. M., Phillips, A. J. K., Munch, M. Y., Gronfier, C., Wyatt, J. K. Dijk, D.-J., Wright, K. P., Jr., & Czeisler, C. A. (2011). Sex difference in the near-24-hour intrinsic period of the human circadian timing system. *Proceedings of the National Academy of Sciences of the United States of America, 108*(S3), 15602–15608.

Duffy, J. F., Dijk, D. J., Hall, E. F., & Czeisler, C. A. (1999). Relationship of endogenous circadian melatonin and temperature rhythms to self-reported preference for morning or evening activity in young and older people. *Journal of Investigative Medicine, 47*, 141–150.

Duffy, J. F., Dijk, D. J., Klerman, E. B., & Czeisler, C. A. (1998). Later endogenous circadian temperature nadir relative to an earlier wake time in older people. *American Journal of Physiology, 275*(5 Pt. 2), R1478–R1487.

Duffy, J. F., Willson, H. J., Wang, W., & Czeisler, C. A. (2009). Healthy older adults better tolerate sleep deprivation than young adults. *Journal of the American Geriatric Society, 57*(7), 1245–1251.

Duffy, J. F., Zeitzer, J. M., Rimmer, D. W., Klerman, E. B., Dijk, D. J., & Czeisler, C. A. (2002). Peak of circadian melatonin rhythm occurs later within the sleep of older subjects. *American Journal of Physiology, 282*(2), E297–E303.

Duffy, J. F., Zitting, K. M., & Chinoy, E. D. (2015). Aging and circadian rhythms. *Sleep Medicine Clinics, 10*(4), 423–434.

Edinger, J. D., Arnedt, J. T., Bertisch, S. M., Carney, C. E., Harrington, J. J., Lichstein, K. L., Sateia, M. J., Troxel, W. M., Zhou, E. S., Kazmi, U., Heald, J. L., & Martin, J. L. (2021). Behavioral and psychological treatments for chronic insomnia disorder in adults: An American Academy of Sleep Medicine clinical practice guideline. *Journal of Clinical Sleep Medicine, 17*(2), 255–262.

Edwards, B. A., Wellman, A., Sands, S. A., Owens, R. L., Eckert, D. J., White, D. P., & Malhotra, A. (2014). Obstructive sleep apnea in older adults is a distinctly different physiological phenotype. *Sleep, 37*(7), 1227–1236.

Eikermann, M., Jordan, A. S., Chamberlin, N. L., Gautam, S., Wellman, A., Lo, Y. L., White, D. P., & Malhotra, A. (2007). The influence of aging on pharyngeal collapsibility during sleep. *Chest, 131*(6), 1702–1709.
Eugene, A. R., & Masiak, J. (2015). The neuroprotective aspects of sleep. *MEDtube Science, 3*(1), 35–40.
Evans, M. A., Buysse, D. J., Marsland, A. L., Wright, A. G., Foust, J., Carroll, L. W., Kohli, N., Mehra, R., Jasper, A., Srinivasan, S., & Hall, M. H. (2021). Meta-analysis of age and actigraphy-assessed sleep characteristics across the lifespan. *Sleep, 44*(9), Article zsab088.
Feinberg, I., & Campbell, I. G. (2010). Sleep EEG changes during adolescence: An index of a fundamental brain reorganization. *Brain and Cognition, 72*(1), 56–65.
Fekedulegn, D., Andrew, M. E., Shi, M., Violanti, J. M., Knox, S., & Innes, K. E. (2020). Actigraphy-based assessment of sleep parameters. *Annals of Work Exposure and Health, 64*(4), 350–367.
Fischer, D., Lombardi, D. A., Marucci-Wellman, H., & Roenneberg, T. (2017). Chronotypes in the US—Influence of age and sex. *PLOS ONE, 12*(6), Article e0178782.
Foley, D. J., Monjan, A. A., Brown, S. L., Simonsick, E. M., Wallace, R. B., & Blazer, D. G. (1995). Sleep complaints among elderly persons: An epidemiologic study of three communities. *Sleep, 18*(6), 425–432.
Folkard, S. (2008). Shift work, safety, and aging. *Chronobiology International, 25*(2), 183–198.
Folkard, S., & Tucker, P. (2003). Shift work, safety and productivity. *Occupational Medicine (London), 53*(2), 95–101.
Garcia-Borreguero, D., Patrick, J., DuBrava, S., Becker, P. M., Lankford, A., Chen, C., Miceli, J., Knapp, L., & Allen, R. P. (2014). Pregabalin versus pramipexole: Effects on sleep disturbance in restless legs syndrome. *Sleep, 37*(4), 635–643.
Gehrman, P., Gunter, P., Findley, J., Frasso, R., Weljie, A. M., Kuna, S. T., & Kayser, M. S. (2021). Randomized noninferiority trial of telehealth delivery of cognitive behavioral treatment of insomnia compared to in-person care. *Journal of Clinical Psychiatry, 82*(5), Article 20m13723.
Giles, T. L., Lasserson, T. J., Smith, B. J., White, J., Wright, J., & Cates, C. J. (2006). Continuous positive airways pressure for obstructive sleep apnoea in adults. *Cochrane Database of Systematic Reviews*, (1), Article CD001106.
Härmä, M., Tenkanen, L., Sjöblom, T., Alikoski, T., & Heinsalni, P. (1998). Combined effects of shift work and life-style on the prevalence of insomnia, sleep deprivation and daytime sleepiness. *Scandinavian Journal of Work, Environment and Health, 24*, 300–307.
Harper, D. G., Stopa, E. G., McKee, A. C., Satlin, A., Fish, D., & Volicer, L. (2004). Dementia severity and Lewy bodies affect circadian rhythms in Alzheimer disease. *Neurobiology of Aging, 25*(6), 771–781.
Harper, D. G., Stopa, E. G., McKee, A. C., Satlin, A., Harlan, P. C., Goldstein, R., & Volicer, L. (2001). Differential circadian rhythm disturbances in men with Alzheimer disease and frontotemporal degeneration. *Archives of General Psychiatry, 58*(4), 353–360.
Hofman, M. A., & Swaab, D. F. (1994). Alterations in circadian rhythmicity of the vasopressin-producing neurons of the human suprachiasmatic nucleus (SCN) with aging. *Brain Research, 651*(1–2), 134–142.
Hood, S., & Amir, S. (2017). The aging clock: Circadian rhythms and later life. *Journal of Clinical Investigation, 127*(2), 437–446.
Hurd, M. W., Zimmer, K. A., Lehman, M. N., & Ralph, M. R. (1995). Circadian locomotor rhythms in aged hamsters following suprachiasmatic transplant. *American Journal of Physiology, 269*, R958–R968.
Iranzo, A., Molinuevo, J. L., Santamaria, J., Serradell, M., Marti, M. J., Valldeoriola, F., & Tolosa, E. (2006). Rapid-eye-movement sleep behaviour disorder as an early marker for a neurodegenerative disorder: A descriptive study. *Lancet Neurology, 5*(7), 572–577.
Ittner, L. M., & Götz, J. (2011). Amyloid-β and tau—A toxic pas de deux in Alzheimer's disease. *Nature Reviews: Neuroscience, 12*(2), 65–72.
Jennum, P., & Riha, R. L. (2009). Epidemiology of sleep apnoea/hypopnoea syndrome and sleep-disordered breathing. *European Respiratory Journal, 33*(4), 907–914.
Jordan, A. S., McSharry, D. G., & Malhotra, A. (2014). Adult obstructive sleep apnoea. *Lancet, 383*(9918), 736–747.
Kervezee, L., Cuesta, M., Cermakian, N., & Boivin, D. B. (2018). Simulated night shift work induces circadian misalignment of the human peripheral blood mononuclear cell transcriptome. *Proceedings of the National Academy of Sciences of the United States of America, 115*(21), 5540–5545.
Kervezee, L., Kosmadopoulos, A., & Boivin, D. B. (2020). Metabolic and cardiovascular consequences of shift work: The role of circadian disruption and sleep disturbances. *European Journal of Neuroscience, 51*(1), 396–412.

Khalsa, S. B. S., Jewett, M. E., Cajochen, C., & Czeisler, C. A. (2003). A phase response curve to single bright light pulses in human subjects. *Journal of Physiology (London)*, *549*(Pt. 3), 945–952.

Klerman, E. B., Davis, J. B., Duffy, J. F., Dijk, D. J., & Kronauer, R. E. (2004). Older people awaken more frequently but fall back asleep at the same rate as younger people. *Sleep*, *27*, 793–797.

Klerman, E. B., & Dijk, D. J. (2005). Interindividual variation in sleep duration and its association with sleep debt in young adults. *Sleep*, *28*, 1253–1259.

Klerman, E. B., & Dijk, D. J. (2008). Age-related reduction in the maximal capacity for sleep—Implications for insomnia. *Current Biology*, *18*(15), 1118–1123.

Klerman, E. B., Duffy, J. F., Dijk, D. J., & Czeisler, C. A. (2001). Circadian phase resetting in older people by ocular bright light exposure. *Journal of Investigative Medicine*, *49*(1), 30–40.

Knopman, D. S., Amieva, H., Petersen, R. C., Chételat, G., Holtzman, D. M., Hyman, B. T., Nixon, R. A., & Jones, D. T. (2021). Alzheimer disease. *Nature Reviews: Disease Primers*, *7*(1), Article 33.

Knutson, K. L. (2010). Sleep duration and cardiometabolic risk: A review of the epidemiologic evidence. *Best Practice & Research. Clinical Endocrinology & Metabolism*, *24*(5), 731–743.

Kronenberg, R. S., & Drage, C. W. (1973). Attenuation of the ventilatory and heart rate responses to hypoxia and hypercapnia with aging in normal men. *Journal of Clinical Investigation*, *52*(8), 1812–1819.

La Morgia, C., Ross-Cisneros, F. N., Koronyo, Y., Hannibal, J., Gallassi, R., Cantalupo, G., Sambati, L., Pan, B. X., Tozer, K. R., Barboni, P., Provini, F., Avanzini, P., Carbonelli, M., Pelosi, A., Chui, H., Liguori, R., Baruzzi, A., Karonyo-Hamaoui, M., Sadun, A. A., & Carelli, V. (2016). Melanopsin retinal ganglion cell loss in Alzheimer disease. *Annals of Neurology*, *79*(1), 90–109.

Laugsand, L. E., Vatten, L. J., Platou, C., & Janszky, I. (2011). Insomnia and the risk of acute myocardial infarction: A population study. *Circulation*, *124*(19), 2073–2081.

Li, H., & Satinoff, E. (1998). Fetal tissue containing the suprachiasmatic nucleus restores multiple circadian rhythms in old rats. *American Journal of Physiology*, *275*, R1735–R1744.

Li, J., Vitiello, M. V., & Gooneratne, N. S. (2018). Sleep in normal aging. *Sleep Medicine Clinics*, *13*(1), 1–11.

Luckhaupt, S. E. (2012). Short sleep duration among workers—United States 2010. *Morbidity and Mortality Weekly Report*, *61*(16), 281–285.

Luo, W., Chen, W. F., Yue, Z., Chen, D., Sowcik, M., Sehgal, A., & Zheng, X. (2012). Old flies have a robust central oscillator but weaker behavioral rhythms that can be improved by genetic and environmental manipulations. *Aging Cell*, *11*(3), 428–438.

Madari, S., Golebiowski, R., Mansukhani, M. P., & Kolla, B. P. (2021). Pharmacological management of insomnia. *Neurotherapeutics*, *18*(1), 44–52.

Manconi, M., Garcia-Borreguero, D., Schormair, B., Videnovic, A., Berger, K., Ferri, R., & Dauvilliers, Y. (2021). Restless legs syndrome. *Nature Reviews: Disease Primers*, *7*(1), Article 80.

Mantele, S., Otway, D. T., Middleton, B., Bretschneider, S., Wright, J., Robertson, M. D., Skene, D. J., & Johnston, J. D. (2012). Daily rhythms of plasma melatonin, but not plasma leptin or leptin mRNA, vary between lean, obese and Type 2 diabetic men. *PLOS ONE*, *7*(5), Article e37123.

Marquié, J. C., & Foret, J. (1999). Sleep, age, and shiftwork experience. *Journal of Sleep Research*, *8*, 297–304.

Mather, M., & Scommegna, P. (2024). *Fact Sheet: Aging in the United States*. Population Reference Bureau, Washington, DC.

McDaid, C., Griffin, S., Weatherly, H., Durée, K., van der Burgt, M., van Hout, S., Akers, J., Davies, R. J. O., Sculpher, M., & Westwood, M. (2009). Continuous positive airway pressure devices for the treatment of obstructive sleep apnoea–hypopnoea syndrome: A systematic review and economic analysis. *Health Technology Assessment*, *13*(4), 1–142.

McEvoy, R. D., Antic, N. A., Heeley, E., Luo, Y., Ou, Q., Zhang, X., Mediano, O., Chen, R., Drager, L. F., Liu, Z., Chen, G., Du, B., McArdle, N., Mukherjee, S., Tripathi, M., Billot, L., Li, Q., Lorenzi-Filho, G., Barbe, F., . . . Anderson, C. S. (2016). CPAP for prevention of cardiovascular events in obstructive sleep apnea. *New England Journal of Medicine*, *375*(10), 919–931.

Mesas, A. E., López-García, E., & Rodríguez-Artalejo, F. (2011). Self-reported sleep duration and falls in older adults. *Journal of Sleep Research*, *20*(1 Pt. 1), 21–27.

Mitchell, M. D., Gehrman, P., Perlis, M., & Umscheid, C. A. (2012). Comparative effectiveness of cognitive behavioral therapy for insomnia: A systematic review. *BMC Family Practice*, *13*, Article 40.

Monk, T. H. (2005). Aging human circadian rhythms: Conventional wisdom may not always be right. *Journal of Biological Rhythms*, *20*(4), 366–374.

Monk, T. H., Buysse, D. J., Reynolds, C. F., III, & Kupfer, D. J. (1993). Inducing jet lag in older people: Adjusting to a 6-hour phase advance in routine. *Experimental Gerontology, 28*, 119–133.

Moore, R. Y., & Eichler, V. B. (1972). Loss of a circadian adrenal corticosterone rhythm following suprachiasmatic lesions in the rat. *Brain Research, 42*, 201–206.

Moran, M., Lynch, C. A., Walsh, C., Coen, R., Coakley, D., & Lawlor, B. A. (2005). Sleep disturbance in mild to moderate Alzheimer's disease. *Sleep Medicine, 6*(4), 347–352.

Moreno-Tamayo, K., Manrique-Espinoza, B., Guerrero-Zúñiga, S., Ramírez-García, E., & Sánchez-García, S. (2021). Sex differences in the association between risk of obstructive sleep apnea, insomnia, and frailty in older adults. *Nature and Science of Sleep, 13*, 1461–1472.

Morin, C. M., & Benca, R. (2012). Chronic insomnia. *Lancet, 379*(9821), 1129–1141.

Morin, C. M., LeBlanc, M., Daley, M., Gregoire, J. P., & Mérette, C. (2006). Epidemiology of insomnia: Prevalence, self-help treatments, consultations, and determinants of help-seeking behaviors. *Sleep Medicine, 7*(2), 123–130.

Morris, C. J., Purvis, T. E., Hu, K., & Scheer, F. A. (2016). Circadian misalignment increases cardiovascular disease risk factors in humans. *Proceedings of the National Academy of Sciences of the United States of America, 113*(10), E1402–E1411.

Morris, C. J., Purvis, T. E., Mistretta, J., & Scheer, F. A. (2016). Effects of the internal circadian system and circadian misalignment on glucose tolerance in chronic shift workers. *Journal of Clinical Endocrinology and Metabolism, 101*(3), 1066–1074.

Murillo-Rodriguez, E., Blanco-Centurion, C., Gerashchenko, D., Salin-Pascual, R. J., & Shiromani, P. J. (2004). The diurnal rhythm of adenosine levels in the basal forebrain of young and old rats. *Neuroscience, 123*(2), 361–370.

Musiek, E. S., Bhimasani, M., Zangrilli, M. A., Morris, J. C., Holtzman, D. M., & Ju, Y. S. (2018). Circadian rest–activity pattern changes in aging and preclinical Alzheimer disease. *JAMA Neurology, 75*(5), 582–590.

Myllyntausta, S., & Stenholm, S. (2018). Sleep before and after retirement. *Current Sleep Medicine Reports, 4*(4), 278–283.

Naismith, S. L., Hickie, I. B., Terpening, Z., Rajaratnam, S. M., Hodges, J. R., Bolitho, S., Rogers, N. L., & Lewis, S. J. (2014). Circadian misalignment and sleep disruption in mild cognitive impairment. *Journal of Alzheimer's Disease, 38*(4), 857–866.

Nakamura, T. J., Nakamura, W., Yamazaki, S., Kudo, T., Cutler, T., Colwell, C. S., & Block, G. D. (2011). Age-related decline in circadian output. *Journal of Neuroscience, 31*(28), 10201–10205.

Nakamura, T. J., Takasu, N. N., & Nakamura, W. (2016). The suprachiasmatic nucleus: Age-related decline in biological rhythms. *Journal of Physiological Sciences, 66*(5), 367–374.

Ohayon, M. M. (2002). Epidemiology of insomnia: What we know and what we still need to learn. *Sleep Medicine Reviews, 6*(2), 97–111.

Ohayon, M. M., Carskadon, M. A., Guilleminault, C., & Vitiello, M. V. (2004). Meta-analysis of quantitative sleep parameters from childhood to old age in healthy individuals: Developing normative sleep values across the human lifespan. *Sleep, 27*(7), 1255–1273.

Ohayon, M. M., O'Hara, R., & Vitiello, M. V. (2012). Epidemiology of restless legs syndrome: A synthesis of the literature. *Sleep Medicine Reviews, 16*(4), 283–295.

Ohayon, M. M., & Reynolds, C. F., 3rd. (2009). Epidemiological and clinical relevance of insomnia diagnosis algorithms according to the DSM-IV and the International Classification of Sleep Disorders (ICSD). *Sleep Medicine, 10*(9), 952–960.

Ohayon, M. M., & Roth, T. (2002). Prevalence of restless legs syndrome and periodic limb movement disorder in the general population. *Journal of Psychosomatic Research, 53*(1), 547–554.

Ortiz-Tudela, E., Martinez-Nicolas, A., Díaz-Mardomingo, C., García-Herranz, S., Pereda-Pérez, I., Valencia, A., Peraita, H., Venero, C., Madrid, J. A., & Rol, M. A. (2014). The characterization of biological rhythms in mild cognitive impairment. *BioMed Research International, 2014*, Article 524971.

Partch, C. L., Green, C. B., & Takahashi, J. S. (2014). Molecular architecture of the mammalian circadian clock. *Trends in Cell Biology, 24*(2), 90–99.

Pavlova, M. K., Duffy, J. F., & Shea, S. A. (2008). Polysomnographic respiratory abnormalities in asymptomatic individuals. *Sleep, 31*(2), 241–248.

Pillai, V., Cheng, P., Kalmbach, D. A., Roehrs, T., Roth, T., & Drake, C. L. (2016). Prevalence and predictors of prescription sleep aid use among individuals with DSM-5 insomnia: The role of hyperarousal. *Sleep, 39*(4), 825–832.

Postuma, R. B., Iranzo, A., Hu, M., Hogl, B., Boeve, B. F., Manni, R., Oertel, W. H., Arnulf, I., Ferini-Strambi, L., Puligheddu, M., Antelmi, E., De Cock, V. C., Arnaldi, D., Mollenhauer, B., Videnovic, A., Sonka, K., Jung, K.-Y., Kunz, D., Dauvilliers, Y., . . . Pelletier, A. (2019). Risk and predictors of dementia and parkinsonism in idiopathic REM sleep behaviour disorder: A multicentre study. *Brain, 142*(3), 744–759.

Ralph, M. R., Foster, R. F., Davis, F. C., & Menaker, M. (1990). Transplanted suprachiasmatic nucleus determines circadian period. *Science, 247*(4945), 975–978.

Reddy, A. B., & Maywood, E. S. (2007). Circadian rhythms: Per2bations in the liver clock. *Current Biology, 17*(8), R292–R294.

Reid, K., & Dawson, D. (2001). Comparing performance on a simulated 12 hour shift rotation in young and older subjects. *Occupational and Environmental Medicine, 58*(1), 58–62.

Resuehr, D., Wu, G., Johnson, R. L., Jr., Young, M. E., Hogenesch, J. B., & Gamble, K. L. (2019). Shift work disrupts circadian regulation of the transcriptome in hospital nurses. *Journal of Biological Rhythms, 34*(2), 167–177.

Riemann, D., Spiegelhalder, K., Feige, B., Voderholzer, U., Berger, M., Perlis, M., & Nissen, C. (2010). The hyperarousal model of insomnia: A review of the concept and its evidence. *Sleep Medicine Reviews, 14*(1), 19–31.

Roehrs, T., Shore, E., Papineau, K., Rosenthal, L., & Roth, T. (1996). A two-week sleep extension in sleepy normals. *Sleep, 19*(7), 576–582.

Roenneberg, T., Kuehnle, T., Juda, M., Kantermann, T., Allebrandt, K., Gordijn, M., & Merrow, M. (2007). Epidemiology of the human circadian clock. *Sleep Medicine Reviews, 11*(6), 429–438.

Roozendaal, B., van Gool, W. A., Swaab, D. F., Hoogendijk, J. E., & Mirmiran, M. (1987). Changes in vasopressin cells of the rat suprachiasmatic nucleus with aging. *Brain Research, 409*, 259–264.

Ruben, M. D., Wu, G., Smith, D. F., Schmidt, R. E., Francey, L. J., Lee, Y. Y., Anafi, R. C., & Hogenesch, J. B. (2018). A database of tissue-specific rhythmically expressed human genes has potential applications in circadian medicine. *Science Translational Medicine, 10*(458), Article eaat8806.

Sateia, M. J. (2014). International Classification of Sleep Disorders–third edition: Highlights and modifications. *Chest, 146*(5), 1387–1394.

Satinoff, E., Li, H., Tcheng, T. K., Liu, C., McArthur, A. J., Medanic, M., & Gillette, M. U. (1993). Do the suprachiasmatic nuclei oscillate in old rats as they do in young ones? *American Journal of Physiology, 265*, R1216–R1222.

Schenck, C. H., Boeve, B. F., & Mahowald, M. W. (2013). Delayed emergence of a Parkinsonian disorder or dementia in 81% of older men initially diagnosed with idiopathic rapid eye movement sleep behavior disorder: A 16-year update on a previously reported series. *Sleep Medicine, 14*(8), 744–748.

Seif, F., Patel, S. R., Walia, H., Rueschman, M., Bhatt, D. L., Gottlieb, D. J., Lewis, E. F., Patil, S. P., Punjabi, N. M., Babineau, D. C., Redline, S., & Mehra, R. (2013). Association between obstructive sleep apnea severity and endothelial dysfunction in an increased background of cardiovascular burden. *Journal of Sleep Research, 22*(4), 443–451.

Sewell, K. R., Erickson, K. I., Rainey-Smith, S. R., Peiffer, J. J., Sohrabi, H. R., & Brown, B. M. (2021). Relationships between physical activity, sleep and cognitive function: A narrative review. *Neuroscience and Biobehavioral Reviews, 130*, 369–378.

Sharma, M., Palacios-Bois, J., Schwartz, G., Iskandar, H., Thakur, M., Quirion, R., & Nair, N. P. V. (1989). Circadian rhythms of melatonin and cortisol in aging. *Biological Psychiatry, 25*, 305–319.

Sherman, B., Wysham, C., & Pfohl, B. (1985). Age-related changes in the circadian rhythm of plasma cortisol in man. *Journal of Clinical Endocrinology and Metabolism, 61*, 439–443.

Silber, M. H., Becker, P. M., Buchfuhrer, M. J., Earley, C. J., Ondo, W. G., Walters, A. S., & Winkelman, J. W. (2018). The appropriate use of opioids in the treatment of refractory restless legs syndrome. *Mayo Clinic Proceedings, 93*(1), 59–67.

Silver, N., Allen, R. P., Senerth, J., & Earley, C. J. (2011). A 10-year, longitudinal assessment of dopamine agonists and methadone in the treatment of restless legs syndrome. *Sleep Medicine, 12*(5), 440–444.

Sivertsen, B., Pallesen, S., Friborg, O., Nilsen, K. B., Bakke, Ø. K., Goll, J. B., & Hopstock, L. A. (2021). Sleep patterns and insomnia in a large population-based study of middle-aged and older adults: The Tromsø study 2015–2016. *Journal of Sleep Research, 30*(1), Article e13095.

Skeldon, A. C., Derks, G., & Dijk, D.-J. (2016). Modelling changes in sleep timing and duration across the lifespan: Changes in circadian rhythmicity or sleep homeostasis? *Sleep Medicine Reviews, 28*, 96–107.

Sohail, S., Yu, L., Bennett, D. A., Buchman, A. S., & Lim, A. S. (2015). Irregular 24-hour activity rhythms and the metabolic syndrome in older adults. *Chronobiology International, 32*(6), 802–813.
Stenuit, P., & Kerkhofs, M. (2005). Age modulates the effects of sleep restriction in women. *Sleep, 28*(10), 1283–1288.
Stephan, F. K., & Zucker, I. (1972). Circadian rhythms in drinking behavior and locomotor activity of rats are eliminated by hypothalamic lesions. *Proceedings of the National Academy of Sciences of the United States of America, 69*(6), 1583–1586.
Stopa, E. G., Volicer, L., Kuo-Leblanc, V., Harper, D., Lathi, D., Tate, B., & Satlin, A. (1999). Pathologic evaluation of the human suprachiasmatic nucleus in severe dementia. *Journal of Neuropathology and Experimental Neurology, 58*(1), 29–39.
Su, S., Li, X., Xu, Y., McCall, W. V., & Wang, X. (2022). Epidemiology of accelerometer-based sleep parameters in US school-aged children and adults: NHANES 2011–2014. *Scientific Reports, 12*(1), 1–8.
Swaab, D. F., Fliers, E., & Partiman, T. S. (1985). The suprachiasmatic nucleus of the human brain in relation to sex, age and senile dementia. *Brain Research, 342*, 37–44.
Sys, J., Van Cleynenbreugel, S., Deschodt, M., Van der Linden, L., & Tournoy, J. (2020). Efficacy and safety of non-benzodiazepine and non-Z-drug hypnotic medication for insomnia in older people: A systematic literature review. *European Journal of Clinical Pharmacology, 76*(3), 363–381.
Taillard, J., Gronfier, C., Bioulac, S., Philip, P., & Sagaspe, P. (2021). Sleep in normal aging, homeostatic and circadian regulation and vulnerability to sleep deprivation. *Brain Sciences, 11*(8), Article 1003.
Teman, P. T., Tippmann-Peikert, M., Silber, M. H., Slocumb, N. L., & Auger, R. R. (2009). Idiopathic rapid-eye-movement sleep disorder: Associations with antidepressants, psychiatric diagnoses, and other factors, in relation to age of onset. *Sleep Medicine, 10*(1), 60–65.
Torsvall, L., Åkerstedt, T., & Gillberg, M. (1981). Age, sleep and irregular workhours: A field study with electroencephalographic recordings, catecholamine excretion and self-ratings. *Scandinavian Journal of Work, Environment and Health, 7*, 196–203.
Tozawa, T., Mishima, K., Satoh, K., Echizenya, M., Shimizu, T., & Hishikawa, Y. (2003). Stability of sleep timing against the melatonin secretion rhythm with advancing age: Clinical implications. *Journal of Clinical Endocrinology and Metabolism, 88*(10), 4689–4695.
Troxel, W. M., Buysse, D. J., Matthews, K. A., Kip, K. E., Strollo, P. J., Hall, M., Drumheller, O., & Reis, S. E. (2010). Sleep symptoms predict the development of the metabolic syndrome. *Sleep, 33*(12), 1633–1640.
Tsoukalas, I. (2012). The origin of REM sleep: A hypothesis. *Dreaming, 22*(4), 253–283.
Tsukahara, S., Tanaka, S., Ishida, K., Hoshi, N., & Kitagawa, H. (2005). Age-related change and its sex differences in histoarchitecture of the hypothalamic suprachiasmatic nucleus of F344/N rats. *Experimental Gerontology, 40*(3), 147–155.
Tufik, S., Santos-Silva, R., Taddei, J. A., & Bittencourt, L. R. (2010). Obstructive sleep apnea syndrome in the Sao Paulo Epidemiologic Sleep Study. *Sleep Medicine, 11*(5), 441–446.
Valentinuzzi, V. S., Scarbrough, K., Takahashi, J. S., & Turek, F. W. (1997). Effects of aging on the circadian rhythm of wheel-running activity in C57BL/6 mice. *American Journal of Physiology, 273*(6 Pt. 2), R1957–R1964.
Van Cauter, E., Leproult, R., & Kupfer, D. J. (1996). Effects of gender and age on the levels and circadian rhythmicity of plasma cortisol. *Journal of Clinical Endocrinology and Metabolism, 81*(7), 2468–2473.
Van Coevorden, A., Mockel, J., Laurent, E., Kerkhofs, M., L'Hermite-Balériaux, M., Decoster, C., Nève, P., & Van Cauter, E. (1991). Neuroendocrine rhythms and sleep in aging men. *American Journal of Physiology, 260*, E651–E661.
van Someren, E. J., Hagebeuk, E. E., Lijzenga, C., Scheltens, P., de Rooij, S. E., Jonker, C., Pot, A. M., Mirmiran, M., & Swaab, D. F. (1996). Circadian rest–activity rhythm disturbances in Alzheimer's disease. *Biological Psychiatry, 40*(4), 259–270.
Vgontzas, A. N., Liao, D., Bixler, E. O., Chrousos, G. P., & Vela-Bueno, A. (2009). Insomnia with objective short sleep duration is associated with a high risk for hypertension. *Sleep, 32*(4), 491–497.
Walcott, E. C., & Tate, B. A. (1996). Entrainment of aged, dysrhythmic rats to a restricted feeding schedule. *Physiology and Behavior, 60*(5), 1205–1208.
Walia, H. K., Thompson, N. R., Pascoe, M., Faisal, M., Moul, D. E., Katzan, I., Mehra, R., & Foldvary-Schaefer, N. (2019). Effect of positive airway pressure therapy on drowsy driving in a large clinic-based obstructive sleep apnea cohort. *Journal of Clinical Sleep Medicine, 15*(11), 1613–1620.

Wang, K., Wu, Y., Yang, Y., Chen, J., Zhang, D., Hu, Y., Liu, Z., Xu, J., Shen, Q., Zhang, N., Mao, X., & Liu, C. (2015). The associations of bedtime, nocturnal, and daytime sleep duration with bone mineral density in pre- and post-menopausal women. *Endocrine, 49*(2), 538–548.

Watanabe, A., Shibata, S., & Watanabe, S. (1995). Circadian rhythm of spontaneous neuronal activity in the suprachiasmatic nucleus of old hamster in vitro. *Brain Research, 695*, 237–239.

Watson, N. F., Badr, M. S., Belenky, G., Bliwise, D. L., Buxton, O. M., Buysse, D., Dinges, D. F., Gangwisch, J., Grandner, M. A., Kushida, C., Malhotra, R. K., Martin, J. L., Patel, S. R., Quan, S. F., & Tasali, E. (2015). Recommended amount of sleep for a healthy adult: A joint consensus statement of the American Academy of Sleep Medicine and Sleep Research Society. *Sleep, 38*(6), 843–844.

Wehr, T. A. (1991). The durations of human melatonin secretion and sleep respond to changes in daylength (photoperiod). *Journal of Clinical Endocrinology and Metabolism, 73*(6), 1276–1280.

Weitzman, E. D., Moline, M. L., Czeisler, C. A., & Zimmerman, J. C. (1982). Chronobiology of aging: Temperature, sleep–wake rhythms and entrainment. *Neurobiology of Aging, 3*, 299–309.

Winkelman, J. W., Armstrong, M. J., Allen, R. P., Chaudhuri, K. R., Ondo, W., Trenkwalder, C., Zee, P. C., Gronseth, G. S., Gloss, D., & Zesiewicz, T. (2016). Practice guideline summary: Treatment of restless legs syndrome in adults: Report of the Guideline Development, Dissemination, and Implementation Subcommittee of the American Academy of Neurology. *Neurology, 87*(24), 2585–2593.

Winkelman, J. W., Berkowski, J. A., DelRosso, L. M., Koo, B. B., Scharf, M. T., Sharon, D., Zak, R. S., Kazmi, U., Carandang, G., Falck-Ytter, Y., Shelgikar, A. V., Trotti, L. M., & Walter, A. S. (in press, 2024). Treatment of restless legs syndrome and periodic limb movement disorder: An American Academy of Sleep Medicine clinical practice guideline. *Journal of Clinical Sleep Medicine.*

Wolfson, A. R., Carskadon, M. A., Acebo, C., Seifer, R., Fallone, G., Labyak, S. E., & Martin, J. L. (2003). Evidence for the validity of a sleep habits survey for adolescents. *Sleep, 26*(2), 213–216.

World Health Organization. (2022). *Ageing and health fact sheet.* https://www.who.int/news-room/fact-sheets/detail/ageing-and-health

Yeh, P., Walters, A. S., & Tsuang, J. W. (2012). Restless legs syndrome: A comprehensive overview on its epidemiology, risk factors, and treatment. *Sleep & Breathing, 16*(4), 987–1007.

Young, T., Palta, M., Dempsey, J., Peppard, P. E., Nieto, F. J., & Hla, K. M. (2009). Burden of sleep apnea: Rationale, design, and major findings of the Wisconsin Sleep Cohort study. *WMJ, 108*(5), 246–249.

Young, T., Palta, M., Dempsey, J., Skatrud, J., Weber, S., & Badr, S. (1993). The occurrence of sleep-disordered breathing among middle-aged adults. *New England Journal of Medicine, 328*(17), 1230–1235.

Young, T., Skatrud, J., & Peppard, P. E. (2004). Risk factors for obstructive sleep apnea in adults. *Journal of the American Medical Association, 291*(16), 2013–2016.

Youngstedt, S. D., Kripke, D. F., Klauber, M. R., Sepulveda, R. S., & Mason, W. J. (1998). Periodic leg movements during sleep and sleep disturbances in elders. *Journals of Gerontology. Series A: Biological Sciences and Medical Sciences, 53*(5), M391–M394.

Zeitzer, J. M., Daniels, J. E., Duffy, J. F., Klerman, E. B., Shanahan, T. L., Dijk, D. J., & Czeisler, C. A. (1999). Do plasma melatonin concentrations decline with age? *American Journal of Medicine, 107*, 432–436.

Zhou, J.-N., Hofman, M. A., & Swaab, D. F. (1995). VIP neurons in the human SCN in relation to sex, age, and Alzheimer's disease. *Neurobiology of Aging, 16*(4), 571–576.

Zhou, J.-N., & Swaab, D. F. (1999). Activation and degeneration during aging: A morphometric study of the human hypothalamus. *Microscopy Research and Technique, 44*, 36–48.

Zitting, K. M., Munch, M. Y., Cain, S. W., Wang, W., Wong, A., Ronda, J. M., Aeschbach, D., Czeisler, C. A., & Duffy, J. F. (2018). Young adults are more vulnerable to chronic sleep deficiency and recurrent circadian disruption than older adults. *Scientific Reports, 8*(1), Article 11052.

CHAPTER

5 The Genetics of Sleep

James B. Jaggard, Keri J. Ngo, *and* Philippe Mourrain

Abstract

In comparison to many other medical and biological fields, sleep science and medicine have only more recently begun using genetic approaches to uncover questions regarding the nature, regulation, and function of sleep. This is due in part to the challenge of phenotyping sleep, a phenomenon that can only be fully defined with multiple behavioral and electrophysiological characteristics. Sleep research has yet to uncover a gene(s) that is the core, master, or critical regulator of sleep, instead finding that many genes with diverse functions impact sleep. Thus, the question of whether a core sleep gene(s) exists remains unanswered. In this chapter, the authors review what constitutes successful genetic screening and how multiple model organisms from nematodes, flies, fish, mice, and human genetics have helped uncover the evolutionarily conserved mechanisms behind sleep. They categorize conserved genes and molecular systems that are necessary for normal sleep or that contribute to pathological sleep into four main categories: circadian, neurotransmission, brain development, and sleep need genes. Finally, they discuss the direction of the sleep field and the current and impending challenges for uncovering the genetics and molecular mechanisms of sleep and its functions.

Key Words: sleep, circadian, genetics, development, neurotransmission, evolution

Introduction

As we progress through the 21st century, significant gaps remain in our understanding regarding the nature, regulation, and function of sleep. In comparison to other biological and medical phenomena, genetic approaches have only recently been applied to the field of sleep research. In contrast, investigations into the genetics of human disorders, such as brachydactyly (Mathew, 1908), congenital cataracts (Chance, 1907), and Huntington's chorea (for review Lanska, 2000) began early in the 19th century, revealing the underlying genetic mechanisms. Similarly, since the 1970s, the field of circadian biology identified the genes underlying the core transcriptional loop of 24-hour endogenous oscillators by harnessing genetic approaches in numerous model systems. Relative to these foundational discoveries, genetic approaches to sleep are still in a contemporary phase. Despite many concerted efforts since 2000, sleep research has not revealed a single core sleep gene but rather has found that sleep is influenced by numerous genes—many of which impact diverse aspects of behavior and physiology other than sleep. This leads to the question of whether core sleep genes even exist or if we are currently ill-equipped to identify them. To better understand the specificity and current limitations associated with the genetics of sleep, it is necessary to take a step back and comprehend what constitutes successful genetic screening.

In 1900, the rediscovery of Mendelian genetics by three plant biologists—Hugo DeVries, Carl Correns, and Erich von Tschermak—ushered in a new era of biology, revolutionizing our understanding of trait transmission and molecular mechanisms of eukaryotic organisms (Simunek et al., 2011). Thomas Hunt Morgan, in 1910, pioneered what would be the very first genetic screen using the fruit fly, *Drosophila melanogaster*, and identified a white-eyed mutant among red-eyed wild types. After crossing the flies, Morgan demonstrated that the "white" gene was not inherited according to the Mendelian laws and resided at a specific location on a sex chromosome where only males displayed the white-eyed phenotype, thereby establishing sex-dependent genetic linkage. Subsequent work from his team analyzing thousands of flies and inheritance of their traits led to the concept of gene linkage and the establishment of the first genetic map using the Morgan as a unit (Sturtevant et al., 1919). Genetic mapping using the centimorgan as the modern unit continued across all plant and animal species for over eight decades until the development of whole-genome sequencing and physical DNA maps in the 1990s (Vassarotti & Goffeau, 1992; Watson, 1990).

The discovery of the role played by chromosomes in heredity would see Professor Hunt awarded the Nobel Prize in 1933, the first of six Nobel Prizes in Biology relying on *Drosophila* genetics to unravel broader biological processes (Rieder & Larschan, 2014). Dr. Hermann Joseph Muller was awarded the Nobel Prize in 1946 for the use of X-ray irradiation to increase mutation rates. In 1995, Dr. Edward B. Lewis, Dr. Christiane Nüsslein-Volhard, and Dr. Eric F. Wieschaus received the prize for their work on the genetic control of embryonic development shared from invertebrates to humans. Dr. Linda Buck and Dr. Richard Axel's 2004 prize celebrated their research on odor receptors and the organization of the olfactory system. In 2011, Dr. Jules A. Hoffmann received the award for his research on the activation of innate immunity. Finally, in 2017, Dr. Jeffrey C. Hall, Dr. Michael Rosbash, and Dr. Michael W. Young won the prize for uncovering the molecular mechanisms that control circadian rhythms.

Following the early steps of *Drosophila*, the 20th century saw the development of many more genetic screening methods using eukaryotic model organisms such as the yeast *Saccharomyces cerevisiae*, the plant *Arabidopsis thaliana*, the worm *Caenorhabditis elegans*, the zebrafish *Danio rerio*, and the mouse *Mus musculus*. Genetic comparison across species gave a new life to evolutionary developmental biology. With the discovery of the homeotic genes, antennapedia and bithorax, in *Drosophila* and the identification of their homologs (Homeobox genes, Hox) in mammals, a major breakthrough was the realization that developmental processes from insects to humans are evolutionarily conserved (Akam, 1989). Despite looking so different in size and morphology, the embryology, body plan, and organ development of flies and vertebrates rely on highly conserved pathways. Foundational genes of famous signaling pathways such as transforming growth factor beta (TGFβ), Wnt, Notch, Sonic hedgehog (Shh), fibroblast growth factor (FGF), and vascular endothelial growth factor were often first discovered in flies and other animal models (fish, *Xenopus*, chick, mouse) before their human counterparts were identified (Mitashov & Vassetzky, 2000). A comparative approach has revealed central features of rostrocaudal (head–tail) and dorsoventral axis formation and patterning in bilaterally symmetric animals regulated by such conserved pathways (Mitashov & Vassetzky, 2000). Overall, from yeast to mammals, the genetic investigations that these invertebrate and vertebrate eukaryotic model systems provide have uncovered a plethora of genes involved in biological processes ranging from cell division and metabolism to body development and physiology. A century of such genetic studies leveraging evolution has revolutionized modern medicine and established many of the standard approaches used in fields such as gastroenterology, cardiology, oncology, immunology, and more.

From the outset, biologists and physicians recognized the value of the similarities between eukaryotes. To this end, yeast has been used as a major model for studying basic metabolic and cell biology processes. Similarly, researchers have long leveraged the similarities between invertebrate and vertebrate animals to investigate body and organ development, maintenance, and pathologies. Even more specific features relevant to human health have been widely elucidated by studying diverse genetic model systems. In fact, by the end of the 20th century, most medical fields had fully taken advantage of forward and reverse genetic approaches and successfully leveraged comparative biology and evolutionary conservation. In stark contrast, the first sleep genetic screen was only published in 2000.

Thus, while significant strides were made across the medical field due to this genetic revolution, psychiatry, including sleep medicine, has lagged behind by at least 50 years. It is crucial to reflect on more than a century of genetic screens and studies to grasp the contrast between the progress made in these other fields and the delay in sleep medicine. Through this reflection, we can extract valuable lessons on the key factors that contribute to the success of genetic approaches and identify the limitations we must overcome in sleep science.

For an unbiased genetic screen to be successful, one usually needs a conserved trait (e.g., cell division or neuron formation), a high-throughput model organism (e.g., *Caenorhabditis elegans*, fly, zebrafish, and, to some extent, mouse), and, critically, a very precise and easy phenotype to screen (e.g., pigmentation). Below we will discuss how difficulties in both phenotyping and the late development of genetically amenable models have been a hindrance in the quest for sleep genes. We will review the categories of genes that have been involved in normal and pathological sleep (Figure 5.1). Finally,

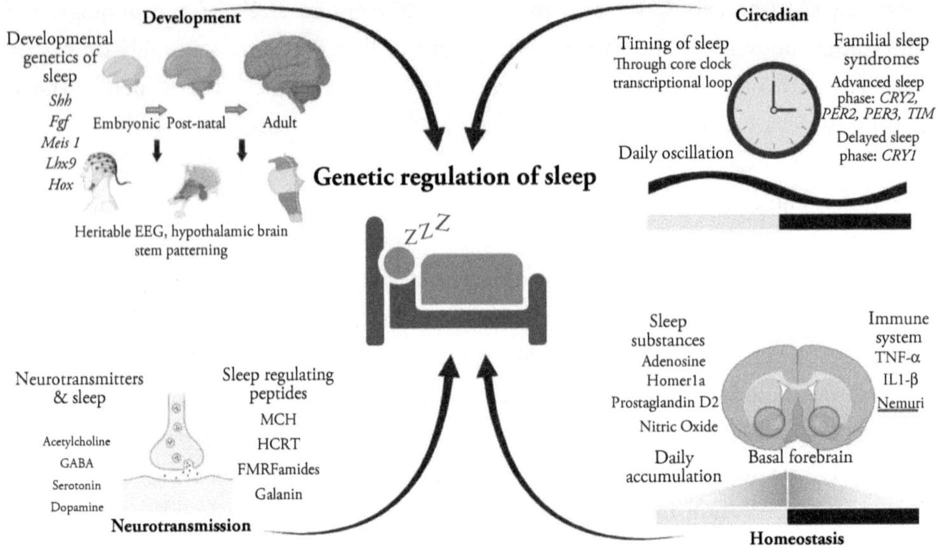

Figure 5.1 The genetic regulation of sleep occurs through multiple biological pathways, including through development, neurotransmission, circadian rhythms, and homeostatic function

Note. Some examples are given for genes that are known to regulate aspects of sleep within each category. Developmental patterning of the brain through transcription factors can alter the size and makeup of nuclei and circuits within the hypothalamus and brainstem to alter sleep. Electroencephalographic signals are known to be genetically determined from studies using monozygotic twins. Sleep is tightly controlled through the actions of neuropeptides and fast neurotransmitters. The circadian clock controls the timing of sleep with day–night cycles through the oscillation of clock transcription factors. Homeostatic factors accumulate as a function of time spent awake, dissipate as a function of time spent in sleep, and include classical somnogens and substances that regulate both sleep and immune function. EEG = electroencephalography; *Fgf* = fibroblast growth factor; GABA = gamma-aminobutyric acid; HCRT = hypocretin/orexin neuropeptide; Hox = homeobox; IL1-β = interleukin 1 beta; MCH = melanin concentrating hormone; *Shh* = Sonic hedgehog; TNF-α = tumor necrosis factor alpha.

we will reflect on where the field is going and what are the next challenges and directions for sleep genetics to deliver the promises of a molecular understanding of sleep functions.

What Is Sleep? The Limits of Sleep Phenotyping

To efficiently discover genes underpinning a biological phenomenon, it is essential to have a precise and reliable trait, known as a *phenotype*, that can be observed across generations and used as a screening tool after mutagenesis. Phenotypes can either be qualitative, such as eye, skin, or petal pigmentation, or quantitative, such as the number or length of fingers. In yeast, genetic screens based on small colony size (also known as *petite*) have uncovered the mitochondrial genome and key genes involved in cellular respiration (for review Slonimski et al., 2016). Mutations in key genes for the aerobic respiratory pathway prevent the normal growth of yeast colonies (Slonimski et al., 1968). Similarly, easily identifiable developmental defects in fly, *Xenopus*, zebrafish, chick, mouse, and human have led to the discovery of well-established gene pathways like those mentioned in the introduction (including TGFβ, Wnt, and FGF) that are necessary for body and organ specification, differentiation, and growth. Even if the phenotype is not as obvious as a limb defect or change in pigmentation, a genetic approach is still possible so long as a reliable trait can be followed and is consistent enough to be recognized across different labs throughout time. This approach has been used by circadian biologists, taking advantage of the stable periodicity of Tau, the circadian period, within many species ranging from bacteria, fungi, plants, insects, and mammals to unravel the conserved genes and transcriptional mechanisms responsible for the stable circadian clock (Allada et al., 2001; Doolittle et al., 1996; Dunlap, 1996; Dvornyk et al., 2003; Feldman & Hoyle, 1973; Kondo et al., 1993; Pentikäinen et al., 1976; Sehgal, 1995).

In 2017, Dr. Jeffrey C. Hall, Dr. Michael Rosbash, and Dr. Michael W. Young won the Nobel Prize for uncovering the molecular mechanisms that control circadian rhythms. In contrast to this success, the genetics of sleep has been more challenging; and as of yet, there has not been any specific gene identified like *Bmal1* or *Per2* in circadian biology that can serve as a master or critical regulator of sleep. Understanding the challenges associated with sleep genetics requires acknowledging that sleep does not yet have a single defining parameter to screen with. Unlike a "small" yeast colony or "red" *Drosophila* eyes or the duration of a circadian period (Tau) in hours and minutes, sleep lacks a simple unifying trait that defines it. Although intuitively one may think that sleep is easy to recognize, sleep definitions have evolved over the past century, and the concept of what constitutes sleep is still debated. Therefore, identifying genes associated with sleep has proven to be a more complex process.

Although modern sleep research is still in a contemporary phase, sleep research began to emerge at the same time Dr. Hunt and others were founding the field of genetics in the early 20th century. Dr. Henri Piéron established the first scientific definition of sleep in 1913, in his famous thesis entitled "Le problème physiologique du sommeil" ("The Physiological Problem of Sleep"; Howell, 1913). In his comparative studies on sleep physiology, Piéron reports the existence of sleep periods in crustaceans, in larval and adult insects, in fresh- and saltwater fishes, in frogs, in aquatic and terrestrial reptiles, as well as in birds and mammals. From his comparative studies on sleep physiology, he established a list of the most obvious and less debatable sleep characteristics encountered across species, including (1) reduced mobility, (2) a loss of muscle tone and a sleeping position compatible with this change, (3) rapid reversibility, and (4) absence of reactivity to stimulus, known as an *increased arousal threshold.* With these behavioral criteria, Piéron established the first scientific definition of sleep. Interestingly, his foundational work already raised the issue that to define sleep one must use a combinatorial examination, rather than relying on a single defining trait.

More than four decades later, in the 1950s–1960s, Nathaniel Kleitman and Michel Jouvet defined sleep states in humans (Fisch, 2012; Jouvet & Michel, 1958; Jouvet et al., 1959a, 1959b). They characterized deep sleep/slow-wave sleep (SWS) and rapid-eye-movement (REM) sleep/paradoxical sleep (PS) based on electrophysiological hallmarks captured by polysomnography (PSG)—a combination of measures including electroencephalogram (EEG), electromyogram (EMG), electrocardiogram, and electro-oculogram (EOG). SWS, the deepest stage of non-REM (NREM) sleep, is characterized by slow, synchronized cortical waves recorded by EEG, accompanied by low muscle tone, regular cardiorespiratory activity, and no eye movement. In contrast, PS has a core characteristic of muscle atonia with a wake-like desynchronized EEG. Furthermore, cardiorespiratory irregularities and episodic bursts of rapid eye movements define the more widely known PS/REM stage of sleep.

Thus, similar to the behavioral definition first established by Piéron, the electrophysiological definition of sleep requires the combination of up to five measures, making sleep state phenotyping cumbersome and not amenable for high-throughput screening. Additionally, while PSG is an elegant way to quantify sleep states, it relies on neocortical activity signatures. The neocortex—as indicated in its name, "neo" for new—is a relatively novel evolution of the vertebrate telencephalon and mostly represents the outer layer of the human and mammalian brain, thus making the transposition of such measures to non-mammalian species difficult for comparative biological studies such as those started by Piéron.

It is interesting to note that in his first paper on sleep in 1925, Kleitman praised Piéron's thesis as one of the best books on the subject ever published (Morrison, 2014). However, the research of Kleitman and Jouvet has unfortunately biased subsequent generations of sleep researchers toward a human/mammalian-centric vision of sleep focusing on PSG/EEG, with many rejecting the idea that sleep can be found throughout the animal kingdom. Fortunately, Dr. Irene Tobler's seminal work on cockroaches in the late 1970s challenged this perspective and re-established Piéron's definition of sleep across phylogeny. Dr. Tobler added a fifth characteristic, homeostasis, to the four criteria established by Piéron. She observed that even in insects, sleep deprivation led to a sleep rebound, suggesting conservation of homeostatic processes in sleep regulation across invertebrate and vertebrate animals (Tobler, 1983; Tobler & Neuner-Jehle, 1992).

Thus, the sleep field has faced challenges in adopting simple, straightforward genetic models and approaches to perform high-throughput screens due to the existence of both behavioral and neurological definitions of sleep, both of which rely upon numerous criteria to fully define them. Alarmingly, this multi-criteria complexity makes the sleep field ill-equipped for standard genetic approaches and high-throughput screens leveraging amenable models. Nevertheless, researchers have demonstrated tenacity and resourcefulness in identifying many genes involved in sleep timing, regulation, and homeostasis. Although no core, master regulator "sleep gene" has been identified yet, these studies have greatly contributed to the progression of the field from behavioral and electrophysiological perspectives to a cellular and molecular exploration of sleep regulation and of its nature and functions. The purpose of this chapter is not to review all the genes and mutants that impact sleep or that have a sleep-related phenotype published so far but instead to reflect on the main classes of genes involved in the genetics of sleep. In the next sections, we will hence discuss four main categories of genes necessary for the normal expression of sleep: (1) circadian genes, (2) neurotransmission genes, (3) brain development genes, and (4) sleep need genes (Figure 5.1).

Circadian Clock Genes Regulate Sleep Timing

Circadian Rhythm and Gene Discovery

The 4.6 billion years of our solar system's existence and the ~24 hours it takes the Earth to complete a rotation have imposed irradiation, light, and physical constraints on the development and natural rhythm of life on our planet. Repetition of night and day cycles has set the pace of biological processes across all organisms. This tremendous astronomical and evolutionary pressure has led to the development of ingrained rhythm independently of environmental cues such as light. Animals, plants, fungi, and even bacteria display behavioral patterns that follow a near-24-hour cycle, known as *circadian rhythm* (from Latin *circa*, "approximately," and *diem*, "day"). The first scientific observation of circadian rhythm was made in 1729 by the French astronomer Jean Jacques d'Ortous de Mairan when he placed a mimosa plant in a dark cabinet and observed that the leaves continued to unfold in the morning and close in the evening, suggesting an endogenous origin of the daily rhythm independent of sunlight cycle. This endogenous rhythm, also later coined as an *internal clock*, was then reported across prokaryotes and eukaryotes; and it has long been evident that circadian regulation has a critical impact on all aspects of life, including sleep in animals. An incredible feature of the circadian cycle is the stability of its period (also known as *Tau/τ*) within each species. It is measured in context free from strong time cues (*zeitgebers*, "time givers") such as sunlight or regular environmental cues (e.g., feeding time). For example, in the absence of time cues, the average human circadian rhythm cycles about once every 24.2 hours, while in fly, Tau is 24.4 hours (Czeisler et al., 1999; Konopka & Benzer, 1971). This near-24-hour rhythm was also previously reported in plants and filamentous fungi such as *Neurospora crassa* (Bianchi, 1964; Neurath & Berliner, 1964). Even cyanobacteria which were present 3.4 billion years ago are highly circadian (Kondo et al., 1993, 1994). Not only is the circadian period very stable within an organism, but the range of period lengths across species is extremely narrow, between 23 and 25 hours despite billions of years of evolution (Allada et al., 2001; Doolittle et al., 1996; Dunlap, 1996; Dvornyk et al., 2003; Kondo et al., 1993, Pentikäinen et al., 1976; Sehgal, 1995).

Thus, in contrast to the complex multifactorial sleep definition and phenotyping described above, circadian biologists were able to leverage a single, stable, easily quantifiable trait that is highly conserved across species, allowing for comparative studies and the ability to investigate circadian genetics in model organisms such as the fruit fly. In 1971, the first fly circadian mutants with arrhythmic, short (19-hour) and long

(28-hour) periods based on inactivity–activity patterns were identified (Konopka & Benzer, 1971), thus pioneering a field that would be rewarded with the Nobel Prize in Medicine 46 years later (Rosbash, Young, and Hall) for the discoveries of the genes and mechanisms at the core of the circadian rhythm. Investigations in cyanobacteria, *Neurospora*, *Arabidopsis*, fly, and mouse models also uncovered many of the genetic elements of circadian rhythms. While each species employs a different set of clock genes that are not all phylogenetically conserved across animals, plants, fungi, and bacteria, they all generate a genuine clock using a common mechanism in which a molecular negative feedback loop based on transcription and translation runs its course over about a day. The core components of the mammalian circadian clock are the genes encoding the transcription factors BMAL1 and CLOCK and the genes *Per1*, *Per2*, *Cry1*, and *Cry2* (Koike et al., 2012; Lowrey & Takahashi, 2004, 2011; Padmanabhan et al., 2012). They encode the proteins PER and CRY that dimerize and translocate to the nucleus after binding with casein kinase 1δ (CSNK1D/CK1δ) or CK1ϵ, where they repress their own transcription (Eng et al., 2017). The stability of PER and CRY is regulated both in the cytoplasm and within the nucleus by several proteins, including FBXL21 and FBXL3 (Hirano et al., 2013; Yoo et al., 2013), leading to a near 24-hour molecular oscillation. This core transcription-translation negative feedback loop mechanism as well as numerous secondary inputs, feedback loops, and interacting modulators are responsible for the tight control of the 24-hour circadian cycle.

Sleep Timing Is Under Circadian Genetic Control

We owe to forward genetics the identification of most, if not all, of the genes involved in the circadian clock. Interestingly, when such genetic screens were first performed in flies or in mice (see previous section), to identify mutants with abnormal period length, motor activity was used as a readout for a 24-hour cycle of active versus rest behaviors, even though the focus was on circadian rhythm but not sleep *per se*. In contrast, the involvement of circadian genes in the regulation of sleep mostly originated from human studies, followed by reverse genetic studies (from gene to phenotype) in animal models (fly and mouse). It will come as no surprise to the reader that humans are diurnal and mostly sleep at night. Even though our development, aging, and sociocultural and environmental surroundings will impact our sleep quantity and timing, we consolidate sleep at night, usually within a fairly well-defined time window. In modern societies, based on population average, the conventional sleep period is often considered to be from 10:00 p.m. to 7:00 a.m. (Gentry et al., 2021). While such a period is voluntarily disrupted in the case of shift workers, it would not be the workers' preferred and natural sleep–wake timing. In stark contrast, some individuals will present an extreme shift in their sleep phase by preferring to go to bed very early in the afternoon/early evening or extremely late in the wee hours of the night (after 3:00 a.m.; Gentry et al., 2021). Considering that such traits run in specific families, it suggests a genetic component. These hereditary phase shifts are known as familial advanced sleep phase syndrome (FASP; Curtis et al., 2019) and familial delayed sleep phase syndrome (FDSP; Patke et al., 2017).

Using the classic family pedigree chart approach, researchers have revealed that both FASP and FDSP can be transmitted as autosomal dominant traits. FASP human genome sequencing revealed mutations in several genes of the circadian clock, including *CK1δ/CSNK1D*, *CRY2*, *PER2*, *PER3*, and *TIMELESS* (Kurien et al., 2019; Toh et al., 2001; Xu et al., 2005; Zhang et al., 2016). Implementation of these rare genetic variations in animal models has allowed mechanistic and functional investigation. They showed that these mutations overall lead to a faster oscillation of the clock, shortening the circadian period. Conversely, for FDSP, only one gene has been identified so far; but it is also due to another core element of the clock, the transcriptional repressor *CRY1* (Patke et al., 2017), where a splicing site mutation in the human *CRY1* gene leads to an internal deletion of the protein. Reverse genetic modeling of this *CRY1* deletion in cell cultures showed that it lengthens the circadian molecular oscillation, providing a mechanistic explanation for FDSP disorder symptoms (Patke et al., 2017).

Thus, the genetics of our circadian rhythms predict the pace of many of our daily activities and behaviors, of which sleep is no exception. In this regard, the genetics of sleep has benefited from the breakthroughs of circadian molecular biology. The circadian clock is genetically encoded and is susceptible to modification by spontaneous mutations affecting human biological rhythms including sleep timing. By using reverse targeted mutations of the respective factors in animal models, researchers have shone light on the underpinning mechanisms including how short and long Tau/circadian periods are responsible for FASP and FDSP, respectively. The success of forward and reverse genetic screens in animal models combined with classic human genetics has been instrumental in the deciphering of the clock genetic elements and how they can be affected in humans. This has been and continues to be inspirational for sleep science and medicine.

Genetics of Neurotransmission and Conservation of Sleep–Wake Regulation Across Invertebrates and Vertebrates

These elegant circadian studies showed that the normal timing of sleep and wakefulness phases was (in the absence of sleep deprivation and other factors) genetically encoded by the clock. By demonstrating at the molecular level that sleep was under tight circadian regulation in both invertebrates and vertebrates, researchers confirmed that the "Process C" or circadian process often mentioned in the sleep regulation literature was under the same genetic control as all other chronobiological traits. However, this did not shine much light on the nature and function of sleep.

Despite the first findings of fly circadian mutants in 1971, it was not until 2000 that a sleep state was formally demonstrated in *Drosophila* and the first mutants and genes directly affecting sleep in this species were described (Hendricks et al., 2000; Shaw et al., 2000). Five years later, the first fly "sleep" mutant screen was published (Cirelli et al.,

2005). In addition to fruit fly work, the late 1990s and early 2000s was a turning point for sleep genetics with the discovery of the hypocretin/orexin system in mice and its implication in canine and human narcolepsy. It was also during this time that the development of additional genetic models of sleep regulation was underway, including zebrafish and *Caenorhabditis elegans*. In this section, we discuss how these studies uncovered a second category of genes, all involved in neurotransmission, critical for sleep-wake regulation and instrumental to our understanding of sleep's neural nature.

The Hypocretin/Orexin and Melanin Concentrating Hormone Neurotransmission Genes

The first evidence that sleep disorders had a genetic component came from quite an unusual species to biomedical research, *Canis familiaris*, known as the common dog. As he was pioneering sleep medicine on several fronts, Dr. Bill Dement recognized the importance of animal research and established the first colony of narcoleptic Dobermans at Stanford (Foutz et al., 1979). These dogs display the striking symptom of cataplexy, losing their muscle tone and collapsing into a sleep state during the normal wake period. This phenotype was easy to observe across progeny as it was transmitted and segregated according to the Mendelian laws as a fully penetrant single autosomal recessive locus, one of the simplest case scenarios for genetic pedigree. However, due to dogs not being amenable for molecular genetics studies, it took over a decade of positional cloning to reveal that the locus was in the region where the gene encoding the orexin/hypocretin receptor 2 was located. Of which, the hypocretin/orexin systems had been previously discovered in mice (Chemelli et al., 1999; de Lecea et al., 1998). It is composed of three genes, one gene encoding the preproprotein that is cleaved into the two hypocretin/orexin ligands and two genes encoding receptors 1 and 2 (Chemelli et al., 1999). Knockout disruption of the hypocretin/orexin ligand gene in mouse and spontaneous mutations in the canine hypocretin receptor 2 gene both led to a narcoleptic-like phenotype, thus linking this neuropeptidergic system to human narcolepsy (Chemelli et al., 1999; Takahashi, 1999). Like in humans, both narcoleptic mice and dogs have severe fragmentation of both wake and sleep phases, especially NREM sleep. These studies provided the first genetic evidence that sleep is not the default form of quiescence but instead is an actively regulated state. It also showed the conservation of this peptidergic system and its function across mammals. Interestingly, genomic studies have since shown that the HCRT/ORX and HCRTR2 genes are conserved across vertebrates but that HCRTR1 is only found in mammals (Yokogawa et al., 2007). Based on the Ensembl genome database, it is present neither in the 27 sequenced genomes of birds and reptiles nor in the 65 fishes available so far, suggesting a reinforcement of this signaling pathway in mammals following the mammalian radiation 160–190 million years ago. Still, HCRT and HCRTR2 have been shown to have conserved functions down to fish. HCRTR2$^{-/-}$ zebrafish mutants isolated with TILLING following ENU mutagenesis display a similar narcoleptic-like sleep phenotype including sleep fragmentation and early sleep onset (Yokogawa et al., 2007). Furthermore, as observed in mammals, in zebrafish, and in cavefish (see later section, "Genetics of Sleep and Arousal States or Genetics of Brain Development"), HCRT overexpression increases wakefulness quantity (Jaggard et al., 2018). Altogether, these findings showed that the hypocretin/orexin ligand and receptor genes are critical for wake promotion as well as sleep–wake state consolidation across vertebrates.

While the most famous, the HCRT/ORX neuropeptidergic system is not the only one to be involved in sleep regulation in mammals and vertebrates at large. Another striking example of the genetic conservation of sleep regulation is the melanin concentrating hormone (MCH) system. The MCH peptide was originally isolated in salmon in 1983 (Kawauchi et al., 1983). Composed of 17 amino acids, its injection/overexpression in fish leads to shrinkage of the melanin-containing granules around the nuclei of the melanophores. As they concentrate around these pigment cell nuclei, they reveal the lighter color of the tissue underneath the skin, therefore making the fish look paler and allowing for background camouflage adaptation. Three years later, in 1986, a 19–amino acid (AA) coding sequence that is 68% identical to the salmon MCH was discovered in rats (Zamir et al., 1986). Surprisingly, subsequent MCH and MCH receptor gene knockouts in mice did not show skin or fur pigmentation defects, instead these mutations were shown to regulate sleep, especially PS/REM sleep (Jego et al., 2013; Peyron et al., 2009; Verret et al., 2003). For the next 33 years, this strong discrepancy led to a biased perception that fishes do not sleep and could not have REM sleep or that fishes and mammals are so different that they cannot share sleep regulation. However, in 2009, it was first demonstrated that fish genomes contain two *MCH* genes: a single-exon gene, which we named *mch1*, as it encodes the preproprotein encoding the 17-AA peptide first discovered in salmon, and *mch2*, a three-exon gene that shares genomic structure, splicing sites, and the 19-AA coding sequence with the mammalian MCH gene first discovered in rats (Berman et al., 2009). This discovery of two *MCH* genes in the fish genome explained the discrepancy in previous findings involving the function of MCH in fish compared to its function in mammals. Thus, like the *HCRTR2* ancestral gene duplication in mammalian genomes leading to *HCRTR1*, *mch2* was likely duplicated with intron loss during the teleost genome duplication event 300–350 million years ago, generating the fish-specific *mch1* gene (Berman et al., 2009).

Thus, only more recently have the *mch2* and *mch receptor* genes been demonstrated to be involved in sleep regulation even in fish (Leung et al., 2019), more precisely during propagating wave sleep (PWS), a sleep state sharing many commonalities with REM/PS, including pontine activation, ponto-midbrain-telencephalic (PMT) wave propagation, rostrocaudal voluntary muscle atonia propagation, heart arrhythmia, and wake-like activity of the dorsal pallium (analogous region to neocortex). Like in mammals, disruption of MCHR signaling in zebrafish impairs REM-like sleep cellular dynamics. MCH2 neuron–ablated fish produced far fewer pontine activations or PMT waves and had a marked decrease in the amount of sleep during the night. Consistently, double mutants against both subtypes of MCHR1 (MCHR1a and MCHR1b) using CRISPR-Cas9 and TILLING also displayed greatly reduced sleep quantity and impaired PWS cellular dynamics. This genetic study showed that disruption of the MCH signal perturbs PWS/REM and greatly reduces sleep quantity, which suggests that it has a sleep-promoting function in fishes that is similar to its role in mammals.

Overall, genetic studies in humans, dogs, rodents, and fishes have demonstrated the conservation of the main sleep–wake regulatory functions of the HCRT and MCH systems, ending the debate of mammalian-specific regulation. Many other peptides have been subsequently shown to have conserved influence on sleep across vertebrate species. In fact, most of the neuropeptide-encoding genes are highly conserved across vertebrate genomes, as are their regulatory impacts on a wide range of physiological functions such as stress, reproduction, metabolism, homeostasis, and more.

(FM)RFamides Neuropeptide VF and Neuropeptide Y

While there is a very strong difference between pools of genes encoding neuropeptides in vertebrates and invertebrates, a few like the FMRFamides/RFamides are found across the entire animal kingdom with conserved influence on sleep.

FMRFamides are a family of very diverse peptides, sharing the tetrapeptide Phe–Met–Arg–Phe–NH2 (hence the name *FMRFamide*), originally discovered in mollusks such as *Aplysia*, a sea snail with a wide range of behaviors including sleep (Belkin & Abrams, 1993; Gerstner et al., 2009; Vorster et al., 2014). However, the involvement of RFamides in 24-hour rhythm and sleep–wake regulation was first discovered in mice and *Caenorhabditis elegans* (Nelson et al., 2014). In these worms, periods of sleep can be observed at the transition between developmental stages (molting; Raizen et al., 2008), or sleep can be induced by stress (stress-induced sleep; Iannacone et al., 2017). When stressed, the worms release the neuropeptide Flp-13 (FMRFamide-like peptide-13), which promotes the transition to sleep (Nelson et al., 2014). To find effectors of this sleep-promoting effect, Flp-13-overexpressing worms were mutagenized, and by leveraging worm self-fertilization, mutants from a single parent were isolated for their suppressed Flp-13 somnogenic effect. The affected gene was found to encode the G protein–coupled receptor Dmsr1 (Iannacone et al., 2017). This receptor for Flp-13 is coupled to the $G_{i/o}$ alpha subunit Goa-1, which was identified in another mutagenesis screen for genes regulating normal worm sleep phase/molting, along with Gpb-2, encoding another G-protein subunit (Iannacone et al., 2017). Subsequently, studies of the pro-FMRFamide-related neuropeptide VF in zebrafish also demonstrated a sleep-regulating role in vertebrates for this family of peptides via projections to the serotonergic raphe (Lee et al., 2020; Madelaine et al., 2017), known for its sleep–wake regulating functions previously demonstrated in rodents and cats (Dresse & Scuvée-Moreau, 1986; Jouvet et al., 1966).

Another interesting case of the genetic conservation of sleep peptides from mammals to invertebrates is the neuropeptide Y (NPY), a peptide that was first isolated from pig brains in 1982 (Tatemoto et al., 1982). Besides mammals, this peptide-encoding gene was also found in a wide variety of species including amphibians, fishes, insects, worms, and octopuses. The impact of NPY on sleep was first observed in rats during overexpression experiments (Zini et al., 1984). However, depending on the site of injection in the basal forebrain, NPY could also promote wakefulness. NPY also exerts a strong influence on sedation—in anesthetized mammals, it increases synchronized activity and decreases desynchronized EEG components. In humans, NPY was also found to have hypnotic properties and can shorten sleep onset latency if administered at the beginning of the night. Following genetic studies, NPY and its receptors were implicated in the regulation of sleep in humans, rats, fruit flies, and nematodes (Antonijevic et al., 2000; Dyzma et al., 2010; He et al., 2013; H. Huang et al., 2017; Tóth et al., 2007; van den Pol, 2012). A similar sleep-promoting effect was later described in a zebrafish genetic screen (Singh et al., 2017), further confirming the conservation of neuropeptidergic regulation in sleep across both vertebrates and invertebrates.

Genetics of Sleep Regulation by Monoamines and Fast Neurotransmitters

For decades, neuropharmacology in mammals has demonstrated the importance of the monoaminergic systems including histamine, serotonin, dopamine, and noradrenaline as well as faster neurotransmitters such as acetylcholine and gamma-aminobutyric acid (GABA) in the control of sleep and wakefulness. Genetic studies have shown that the roles of these monoamines and fast neurotransmitters are conserved down to invertebrates.

As previously mentioned, a major hindrance to the field of sleep biology and the development of genetic models was, and still is, the belief that sleep was a state only found in mammalian and avian species. Recent decades have seen a shift away from this bias thanks to *Drosophila* genetics and the discovery of fly mutants with sleep phenotypes. In 2000, Dr. Paul Shaw and colleagues described that mutations in arylalkylamine *N*-acetyltransferase, an enzyme involved in the catabolism of monoamines, can cause dysregulated sleep homeostasis. Involvement of other monoaminergic transmissions such as histamine and octopamine, the insect homolog of norepinephrine, was also later shown to be critical in sleep–wake regulation (Crocker & Sehgal, 2008; Oh et al., 2013).

In 2005, the first fly "sleep" mutant screen identified *shaker*, a mutant affected in a gene encoding a voltage-gated potassium channel that promotes sleep via GABA transmission (Cirelli et al., 2005). Another short sleeper fly mutant, *Wide awake*, was also later described to be affected in a GABA receptor regulator, confirming the importance of inhibitory GABA transmission during sleep in flies like in mammals. Similarly, a role for acetylcholine regulation in sleep was genetically demonstrated in *Drosophila*, and another unbiased genetic screen identified the short-sleeping mutant *redeye* (Shi et al., 2014). Cloning of *redeye* revealed that it encodes a nicotinic acetylcholine receptor α subunit required for *Drosophila* sleep. Likewise, CRISPR-Cas9 gene editing of homologous acetyl receptor family genes showed that mice lacking the muscarinic acetylcholine receptor genes *Chrm1* and *Chrm3* lacked REM sleep (Niwa et al., 2018).

Overall, in contrast to studies uncovering circadian genes and neuropeptide-encoding genes, these genetic approaches did not reveal new genes and mechanisms *per se* as pharmacology had previously pointed toward the roles of these neurotransmitters in sleep regulation. For example, cholinergic agonists such as carbachol and eserine have been used since the 1960s in rats and cats and were even more recently shown to induce PS-like pontine and REM sleep neural dynamics in fish. These genetic findings were impactful as they demonstrated that sleep regulation most likely shares evolutionarily conserved core mechanisms involving neurotransmitter molecules such as RFamides, monoamines, acetylcholine, and GABA found in nematodes, insects, annelids, mollusks, and vertebrates.

Genetics of Sleep and Arousal States or Genetics of Brain Development

Genetics of EEG Spectral Bands

Some of the first quantifiable evidence of the heritability of sleep and arousal states in humans came from twin studies, focusing not on sleep neurotransmission specifically but instead on the resulting neocortical activity. In classic genetics, identical/monozygotic (MZ) and fraternal/dizygotic (DZ) twins are frequently used to divide quantitative traits into environmental and genetic components and to estimate heritability. Developmental biology and genetics have demonstrated long ago that the identical morphological features of MZ twins are due to their shared genetic programs. Notably, as genetic clones, the development and positions of the internal organs in MZ twins are strictly identical. Even in the extremely rare cases of *situ inversus*, the organs' precise morphology is not affected, but they have a left–right mirror organization between twins. However, when it comes to the human mind, behaviors, and brain activity, fields like psychiatry and psychology often have a vision biased toward the "uniqueness" of each individual's brain features and animation. Nevertheless, it is unsurprising that neocortical arousal state signatures recorded by EEG were found to also be genetically determined.

In the 1980s, Webb and Campbell (1983) as well as Linkowski and colleagues (1989) were among the first to apply PSG composed of EEG, EMG, and EOG to MZ and DZ pairs to investigate the genetic regulation of sleep. The first group studied 14 identical and 14 fraternal young adult twin pairs (mean age was 19 years, both genders were represented) during 1 night. The second group studied 14 MZ and 12 DZ twins (mean age was 24 years, all males) during 3 consecutive nights. In both studies, EEG measures of sleep structure of the fraternal/DZ twins showed no evidence of significant correlations. In contrast, in MZ/identical twins, many characteristics of sleep architecture seemed to have a genetic component. Webb and Campbell reported that onset latencies, awakening measures, stage changes, and amounts of rapid eye movement were significantly correlated in the identical twins. The second team found that NREM Stages 2, 4, and delta sleep (Stages 3 and 4) unequivocally showed a strong genetic component. To a lesser extent, REM density was also correlated in DZ pairs. However, the total amount of REM, NREM Stage 1, and total sleep in identical twins had a marked environmental confound. These pioneering studies provided the first data supporting the existence of genetic determinants of structural aspects of human sleeping EEG. It was consistent with previous reports that had shown the importance of genetic factors in the spontaneous human waking EEG (Stassen et al., 1988; Whitton et al., 1985).

Building on these early studies, in 1996, van Beijsterveldt and colleagues similarly wanted to study the genetic and environmental contributions to individual differences in brain functioning. They measured EEG activity at rest in 91 MZ and 122 DZ twins at age 16 from both genders. EEG was recorded on 14 scalp positions during quiet resting with eyes closed during 3.5-hour sessions. They leveraged the fact that although the EEG is a complex trait that varies in many dimensions, such as distribution of frequencies, amplitudes over the different brain areas, and morphology of waveforms, it tends to be a stable individual characteristic. As a proxy of brain activity, spectral powers were extracted for delta, theta, alpha, and beta frequency bands. Strikingly, they found that the averaged heritability for the delta, theta, alpha, and beta frequencies was 76%, 89%, 89%, and 86%, respectively. In addition, the genetic correlations among all scalp locations and left–right hemispheres were also very high, indicating that the same genetic contributions are underpinning the different brain areas and hemispheres. Finally, genetic factors determining EEG were similarly high in male and female DZ twin pairs, dismissing sex influence. The authors concluded rightly that "This study shows that brain functioning, as indexed by rhythmic brain-electrical activity, is one of the most heritable characteristics in humans" (van Beijsterveldt et al., 1996, p. 562).

Moreover, the same group had previously published a similar study on 209 5-year old twin pairs (Van Baal et al., 1996). In contrast to their more recent study, while the heritability for theta and alpha was still relatively high (averaged over electrode positions, it was 81% and 79%, respectively, for theta and alpha), the heritability for beta and delta was ~50%, substantially lower than that in 16-year-old twin pairs. These observations suggest (1) that the organization of the whole-brain EEG is mainly of a genetic nature and (2) that this genetic program is involved in the development of the brain/neocortex prior to 5 years old but continues to be engaged between 5- and 16-year-old stages of development.

Even though the mechanism that generates EEG rhythms is largely unknown, we do know that the synchronous activity of pyramidal neurons in the cortex is involved in (Nunez, 1981) and generated by corticocortical, thalamocortical interactions and regulated by subcortical nuclei down to the brainstem. We know from the famous experiment on *cerveau isolé*, or decerebration, from Dr. Frédéric Bremer in 1937 on cats (Gottesmann, 1988) that the neocortex can display slow, synchronized activity similar to delta EEG/SWS in the absence of ascending connections.

Developmental Genetics of Sleep-Regulating Brain Regions

The strong genetic determination of EEG patterns/brain activity observed by all these groups is consistent with the high conservation of developmental genetic programs that establish brain morphology and circuitry starting from early gastrulation and neurulation, when formation of the forebrain, midbrain, and hindbrain occurs via nuclear differentiation, axon guidance, and synaptic wiring. In contrast to the very slow start of genetic studies in the sleep field and psychiatry at large, developmental biologists have deciphered and demonstrated for decades the genetic programming of animal development. Following the early pioneering studies of Browne in 1909, Spemann and Mangold in 1924, and Nieuwkoop in 1947 in sea urchin and *Xenopus* that demonstrated the existence of cellular determinants and signals able to induce and organize the embryo body and central nervous system (CNS; see Lenhoff, 1991; Nieuwkoop, 1947), scores of scientists have uncovered the genetic programs and signaling pathways responsible for brain and body development. Transcription factors such as beta-catenin, vegT, and veg1, for example, were some of the first genetic factors identified. Many more were cloned and organized in famous genetic signaling pathways such as WNT, TGF-β, FGF, Notch, and SHH, as previously mentioned. Again, *Drosophila* genetics has been instrumental in discovering the fly genes and subsequently the mammalian homologs responsible for animal development conserved from invertebrates to vertebrates. Thus, these findings became the field of evolutionary developmental biology, where scientists compared developmental processes across species and demonstrated the strong conservation of the genetic and molecular mechanisms across phylogeny (see example of common patterning for the thalamus in Scholpp & Lumsden, 2010).

The cloning of the homeotic genes in the fly and the identification of their homologs, the homeo(tic)box genes in mammals, also similarly responsible for body segmentation, are among the most striking examples of evolutionary conservation. Since the 1970s, their roles in the hindbrain/brainstem patterning and organization have been carefully investigated using a variety of vertebrate species including mice, *Xenopus*, fish, chicken, and quails (Krumlauf & Wilkinson, 2021; Scholpp & Lumsden, 2010). It is one of the most classic and famous examples of the very strong conservation of the genetic determination of the vertebrate CNS. Whether a fish, a chick, or a mouse, the rhombomere segmentation of the hindbrain is under the same genetic program (Krumlauf & Wilkinson, 2021; Moens & Prince, 2002). This conserved genetic programming does not stop in early development but also guides most vertebrate CNS differentiation. Thus, for example, whether in mouse, chicken, or fish, the noradrenergic locus coeruleus in the rostral pons of the brainstem originates from rhombomere 1, differentiates the same way (Aroca et al., 2006), and has the same functions including arousal and wake/sleep regulation (Aston-Jones & Bloom, 1981; Bourgin et al., 2000; Hobson et al., 1975; Singh et al., 2015).

The brainstem is not a unique case; the development of other brain structures critical for sleep regulation, such as the hypothalamus, is also under the same genetic control across vertebrate species. Experiments in mice, chicks, and fish have revealed the genes involved in the specification, regionalization, and differentiation of the hypothalamus and preoptic region of the forebrain (Alvarez-Bolado, 2019; Pearson & Placzek, 2013). Many of the secreted signaling factors that confer regional identity elsewhere in the CNS, in particular Shh, bone morphogenetic protein (BMP), FGF, and Wnt, operate similarly within the hypothalamus independent of species differences (Briscoe & Novitch, 2008; Edlund & Jessell, 1999; Shirasaki & Pfaff, 2002). Numerous studies have substantially advanced our appreciation of hypothalamic development, demonstrating that hypothalamic transcription factors and neuropeptides have been highly conserved during evolution (Burbridge et al., 2016; Löhr & Hammerschmidt, 2011; Machluf et al., 2011; Pearson & Placzek, 2013), leading to a good understanding of the embryonic origins of defined hypothalamic nuclei and neurons (Jo & Chua, 2009; Szarek et al., 2010). Most, if not all, hypothalamic peptides/nuclei found in the mammalian brain are found down to the fish brain. A few relevant to this chapter include key sleep regulators such as hypocretin/orexin, MCH, thyrotropin releasing hormone (TRH), NPY, adrenocorticotropic hormone, corticotropin releasing factor (CRF), arginine vasopressin, oxytocin, pro-opiomelanocortin (POMC)/melanocyte stimulating hormone and somatostatin. Because these neurohormones are encoded by genes, the genetic programming of the regionalization and differentiation of the neuropeptidergic hypothalamus has received much attention. Downstream the major Wnt, FGF, Shh, and BMP patterning signals, the transcriptional pathways controlling the precise specification and differentiation of progenitors into neurons in organized nuclei expressing neuropeptides, have been studied for decades (for review, Burbridge et al., 2016). It is not the purpose of this chapter to review the entirety of these pathways as many reviews and textbooks are available. However, one may mention a few transcription factors such as Pax6, Nkx2.1, Nkx2.2, Aristaless, Distal-less 5, Six3, Vax1, and Orthopedia; LIM domain Lhx family members; basic helix–loop–helix (bHLH) factors such as Sim1; the Forkhead domain protein Foxb1; and T-box family members, involved in the dorsoventral regionalization of the hypothalamus into alar, basal, and floor plate longitudinal subdivisions, which are conserved in all species examined. Similarly, the genes involved in neurogenesis, commitment, and differentiation such as Achaete–scute-like 1 (Mash1), a bHLH proneural transcription factor, or atonal-like genes Neurogenin1 (Ngn1) and Neurogenin3 (Ngn3) have similar functions in the differentiation of the vertebrate hypothalamus (Anthwal et al., 2013). These factors are responsible for the transcriptional control and identity fating of neuropeptidergic neurons. For example, Mash1 function is required for expression of the homeodomain transcription factor genomic screen homeobox 1, which in turn is necessary for growth hormone releasing hormone expression (McNay et al., 2006; Mutsuga et al., 2001). The homeodomain protein Nkx2.1 is expressed in progenitor cells that occupy the hypothalamic basal plate and differentiate into GABA, NPY, POMC, and dopaminergic neurons (Yee et al., 2009). SIM1 and its dimerization partner aryl hydrocarbon receptor nuclear translocator 2 are required for expression of TRH, CRF, oxytocin, and arginine vasopressin (Hosoya et al., 2001; Keith et al., 2001). In conclusion, the vertebrate hypothalamus development is under the control of a very precise and conserved genetic program. Any deregulation of this program may underlie complex human pathological conditions and dysfunctional behaviors, including stress, eating disorders, and, most importantly for this chapter, sleep/wake changes.

Developmental Genetics of Sleep Loss

A striking example in the wild of how a genetic change in brain and hypothalamus development can lead to a major change in sleep-wake quantity has been reported in the freshwater fish *Astyanax mexicanus*. This fish exists as two distinct morphotypes of the same species: surface populations that inhabit rivers and multiple cave populations that have evolutionarily converged on sleep loss. Cavefish are derived from surface ancestors, which arose from colonization events that are estimated to have taken place within the past 2–5 million years (Gross, 2012; Jeffery, 2009; Yoshizawa et al., 2015). While *Astyanax mexicanus* surface fish sleep from 6 to 8 hours a day, independently evolved cave populations share converging morphological and behavioral traits including eye loss and a marked reduction in sleep, only sleeping 1 to 3 hours over 24 hours. Additionally, evolutionary convergence of brain morphology has been found in multiple populations of cavefish, suggesting that major neuroanatomical variation is driven by genetically determined factors (Jaggard et al., 2020). Pharmacological or genetic inhibition of the wake-promoting hypocretin/HCRT system increased sleep in cavefish, suggesting that enhanced HCRT signaling underlies the evolution of sleep loss. Precise neuroanatomical analysis and *Hcrt* gene expression quantification showed not only that the number of HCRT-positive hypothalamic neurons is increased significantly in cavefish but also that *Hcrt* gene expression is upregulated at both the transcript and protein levels (Jaggard et al., 2018). This study showed that HCRT overexpression was the main cause of sleep loss in cavefish.

Moreover, careful examination of the basal forebrain in surface fish and cavefish showed marked differences in neurodevelopmental evolution. Quantitative differences in terms of numbers of cells in specific clusters of neuropeptidergic cell types include more HCRT and agouti-related protein neurons and fewer POMC and arginine vasotocin neurons in cavefish compared to the surface variant. These hypothalamic changes are consistent with some of the cavefish behaviors compared to surface fish such as sleep loss and hyperphagia. Developmental genetic investigation of these changes in cavefish showed that enlarged ventral midline Shh expression during gastrulation and neurulation (Yamamoto et al., 2004) results in a larger hypothalamic region, presumably via extension of Nkx2.1a, Lhx6, and Lhx7 transcription factor expression domains and increased cell proliferation (Menuet et al., 2007; Rétaux et al., 2008). Fgf8 maintains Shh expansion in the cavefish developing forebrain basal plate, with consequences on neural plate patterning at the onset of neurulation: the expression domains of transcription factors such as Lhx2, Lhx7, Lhx9, Pax6, or Zic1 are different in surface fish and cavefish at the neural plate stage (Hinaux et al., 2016; Pottin et al., 2011; Strickler et al., 2001). Critically, Lhx9 is expressed in HCRT progenitors, where it precisely delineates *Hcrt*-expressing neuron territories. Functional analyses showed that, in cavefish, the wider domain of expression of Lhx9 is responsible for an enlargement of the *Hcrt*-expressing neuron cluster and, in turn, likely responsible for a stronger wake-promoting impact. Conversely, in the absence of Lhx9, HCRT+ cell number in cavefish is reduced to a level close to that of surface fish.

Overall, this elegant work showed how genetic changes in the Shh and Fgf signaling pathway at the end of gastrulation and during neurulation via Lhx9 can change the number of wake-promoting HCRT neurons and, in turn, be responsible for ~60% sleep loss in cavefish (Jaggard et al., 2018). It illustrates a category of potential "sleep genes" that are often overlooked: the entire genetic program required for the development of the brain. It not only includes the sleep–wake regulating nuclei but also the telencephalic/neocortex circuit organization necessary for the expression of the EEG spectral bands discussed above. Another critical reflection arising from this cavefish example is how early in development such a genetic impact can take place; here, the change happens during late gastrulation and neurulation when the broad subdivisions of the CNS, such as the forebrain, midbrain, and hindbrain, are established, likely much earlier than the behavioral and physiological consequences that these changes have on the genetic regulation of sleep. In conclusion, one can see how the genetics of sleep and of brain development share significant overlap and could act in concert with a large fraction of the 22,000+ protein-encoding genes of the human genome involved in CNS development, integrity/maintenance, and functions.

Sleep Need—Genetic Factors Driving Sleep Homeostasis

Beyond the genes involved in the timing and development of sleep and arousal states already described are the less understood genetic and molecular components underpinning sleep need and functions. We have all experienced the feeling of lethargy that stems from insufficient sleep, causing us to yearn for our beds. Sleep is seemingly vital for maintaining both short- and long-term health and homeostasis. Critical and yet unanswered questions in the sleep sciences surround what causes this daily tiredness, what purpose(s) it serves, and how it is regulated. As far back as the early 1900s, both Henri Piéron and Kuniomi Ishimori proposed that endogenous chemicals that drive sleep need built up during waking periods, a theory known as the *hypnogenic* or *endotoxic* regulation of sleep (Howell, 1913; Kubota, 1989). Despite the long-standing curiosity surrounding these questions, we still lack a comprehensive understanding of the physiological and molecular balance between waking and sleeping. In this section, we will discuss the history and genetics of sleep homeostasis research and contemplate how the next generation of sleep research can build on our current knowledge base.

Broadly, sleep homeostasis is the process regulating the need for sleep that accumulates during wakefulness and dissipates during sleep (Borbély & Achermann, 1999). Behaviorally, this is characterized by a decrease in the amount of time it takes to fall asleep and a total increase in sleep time upon the first opportunity to sleep. The homeostatic regulation of sleep is widely conserved across species from humans down to hydra, demonstrating that this drive to sleep is intrinsic to animals (Kanaya et al., 2020; Porkka-Heiskanen, 2013). In the 1980s, Dr. Irene Tobler added sleep homeostasis to Piéron's four original behavioral characterizations of sleep after defining a rebound phase of sleep in cockroaches after a day of sleep deprivation, thus creating the five criteria of behavioral sleep now widely accepted as the defining parameters for behavioral sleep research (Borbély & Tobler, 2011; Tobler, 1983).

The duration or intensity of waking activity significantly impacts the architecture of neural sleep patterns. Sleep deprivation and/or intense experiences during wakefulness are compensated by deeper sleep. In vertebrates, this is referred to as *slow-wave activity* (SWA; 0.5–4.0 Hz in EEG) during NREM sleep and is a widely accepted biomarker for increased sleep depth in response to sleep pressure (Deboer, 2015; Jaggard et al., 2021). It is likely that the overall role of this deeper sleep is restorative and that it eliminates damages accumulated during wake. Several of these functions have been observed in fly, fish, and mammals; they include toxic waste and cellular stress clearing, synaptic normalization, and neuronal genomic DNA repair (Coulson et al., 2022; Eide et al., 2021; Mourrain & Wang, 2019; Tononi & Cirelli, 2014; van Alphen et al., 2021; Xie et al., 2013). The genetics that underlie sleep homeostasis involve multiple neural and nonneural systems including both defined circuits and global levels of circulating signaling molecules, making dissection of the cellular and molecular mechanisms challenging. During wakefulness, global sleep-promoting factors are thought to accumulate, thereby increasing the pressure for sleep. Here, we will review some of the known literature on this class of somnogens.

Global Sleep Need Substances: Adenosine

Adenosine (ADO) is an important molecule found in all cells throughout the body that serves many biological functions, including nucleotide synthesis, cellular metabolism, and immunological function (Novotný, 2015). ADO is thought to accumulate throughout the waking period, as cells deplete their energy stores (Lazarus et al., 2019). ADO is mainly produced through metabolism of adenosine 5′-triphosphate (ATP); dephosphorylation of ATP occurs through two nucleotidase genes—*CD39/ENTPD*, which hydrolyzes ATP to adenosine monophosphate (AMP), and *CD73/NT5e*, which converts AMP to ADO (Le Hir & Kaissling, 1993; Robson et al., 2006). Additionally, ADO is directly produced through equilibrative nucleoside transport actions—both of these processes are thought to be directly coupled to the level of activity a cell is experiencing (Novotný, 2015).

Both neurons and nonneuronal cells produce extracellular ADO. Interestingly, astrocytes have been shown to be an important source of ADO related to sleep–wake balance, suggesting that both neuronal and glial activity drives sleep pressure (Nadjar et al., 2013; Petit & Magistretti, 2016). Glial regulation of ADO in sleep homeostasis has been carried out by expressing a dominant-negative form of SNARE protein under a glial fibrillary acidic protein promoter which prevents vesicular gliotransmission of ADO (Nadjar et al., 2013). Animals expressing this construct have impaired responses to sleep deprivation and reduced SWA and do not respond to ADO A1R receptor signaling, directly implicating gliotransmission in sleep homeostasis (Halassa et al., 2009). However, very recent findings suggest that astrocytic signaling regulating sleep occurs independently of ADO (Peng et al., 2023). Using an elegant set of chemogenetic, optogenetic, and imaging experiments, researchers were able to partially disentangle Ca^{2+} activity from ADO release and found that Ca^{2+} from astrocytes, and not ADO, may be the main mechanism through which astrocytes regulate sleep. While this study was able to eliminate the production of ADO through CD73, there remain several other ways for cells to produce ADO; and future studies will need to systematically test other potential sources of ADO in astrocytes as the source of gliotransmission in sleep homeostasis.

ADO influences the activity of both wake- and sleep-promoting circuits, indicating that this global signal has specific functions on defined cell types (for detailed review, see Donlea et al., 2017). Based on microdialysis measurements of ADO throughout the brain, the basal forebrain and cortex have been identified as the main locations of ADO elevation related to sleep regulation (Porkka-Heiskanen et al., 2000). ADO A1R receptors are G_i-coupled and thought to function to inhibit wake-promoting systems including cholinergic, histamine, and hypocretin neurons in the basal forebrain and ventrolateral hypothalamus (Alam et al., 1999; Liu & Gao, 2007; Rainnie et al., 1994; Thakkar et al., 2003). A2 receptors are G-coupled and seemingly activate sleep-promoting systems, including cholinergic neurons lining the ventricular space below the basal forebrain, as well as GABA and galanin neurons in the ventrolateral preoptic area (Coleman et al., 2006; Gallopin et al., 2005; Hong et al., 2005). In humans, interindividual variations in EEG signals have been linked to mutations in both A2 receptor genes and adenosine deaminase genetic polymorphisms that induce enhanced SWA during sleep, as well as alter EEG during both sleep and wake, suggesting that ADO regulation may serve as a hub for calculating sleep depth and amount by genotype (Rétey et al., 2005).

Until recently, how ADO is dynamically regulated during wake and sleep was unknown. Peng and colleagues (2020) developed a novel genetically encoded G protein–coupled receptor activation-based sensor bound to A2 receptors that allows for the quantification of ADO signals with high spatial and temporal dynamics that were previously lacking from past microdialysis studies. As expected, the authors found that ADO sensor activity was tightly coupled to EEG and Ca^{2+} activity, where during wake and REM sleep—in periods of high-frequency neural activity—ADO levels were also high. During NREM sleep, however, ADO levels were significantly lower, showing that specific phases of sleep, particularly SWA of NREM, are critical for dissipating ADO accumulation.

This study focused specifically on A2 receptors in the basal forebrain to profile specific cell type–ADO dynamics and identified the importance of a previously unknown group of VGLUT+ neurons required for ADO baseline sleep regulation. Harnessing this novel approach, future studies could be carried out using agnostic whole-brain recordings to further identify other nuclei, circuits, and cells that are likely involved in ADO sleep homeostasis.

A foundational conundrum of ADO sleep regulation is that while pharmacological manipulation of A1R and A2R has been shown to strongly modulate sleep, genetic knockout models for these receptors have much more subtle/conflicting sleep changes compared to controls (Fredholm et al., 2005). Pharmacologically, the role of ADO in sleep regulation is clear from the wake-promoting effects of its receptor antagonism by caffeine and the sleep-promoting effect that both ADO and its analogues have on sleep (Lazarus et al., 2019). The first report of a full knockout of *A1R* observed no changes to either baseline sleep or sleep after deprivation (Stenberg et al., 2003). Others, using the Cre-loxP system to conditionally knock out *A1R* in mice, have found that this induces significant reductions in SWA and sleep time after both acute and chronic sleep deprivation (Bjorness & Greene, 2009). Using both *A1R* and *A2R* receptor knockout mice, it was shown that the wake-promoting effect of caffeine relies solely on intact A2R receptors, while A1Rs are dispensable (Z. L. Huang et al., 2005). Using an inducible Cre system, the waking effect of caffeine was localized to the nucleus accumbens where A2Rs modulate dopaminergic signaling to regulate both sleep and wake. Recently, using a conditional inducible system, researchers found that chemogenic activation of A2 receptors in the olfactory bulb of mice significantly increased NREM sleep, and optogenetic activation of these cells induces GABA release in both the hypothalamus and preoptic areas to modulate sleep (Li et al., 2020). While there is still much to decipher concerning the nature of ADO and sleep, these findings largely demonstrate a simple testable model for the role of ADO in sleep: As energy stores are depleted through ATP metabolism, ADO accumulates, providing a counterbalance for cells to promote their need to rest and restore during sleep phases.

Global Sleep Need Substances: Prostaglandin D2

Prostaglandin (PG) D2 (PGD2) is part of a large family of polyunsaturated fatty acids with 20 carbons with a five-carbon ring, which until the 1980s was considered a minor and biologically unimportant molecule as no function or expression pattern was yet known. However, PGD2 was subsequently discovered to be the most enriched PG in the brain, suggesting that it may play an important role in the nervous system (Narumiya et al., 1982; Ogorochi et al., 1984). The role of PGD2 as a sleep-inducing agent was first shown in 1982 by exogenous injection of nanomolar levels into the rodent brain, which caused significant increases in both NREM and REM sleep (Ueno et al., 1982).

Subsequently, it was found that PGD2 levels are coupled to the circadian timing of the sleep–wake cycle (Pandey et al., 1995). Additionally, sleep deprivation drastically increases the amount of PGD2 in the brain as a function of increased sleep pressure (Ram et al., 1997). PGD2 is produced in oligodendrocytes, leptomeninges, and the choroid plexus, where it is secreted into the cerebrospinal fluid (CSF) and acts as a sleep-inducing agent (Urade et al., 1993). The effect of PGD2 on both basal sleep and its role in sleep homeostasis requires intact PGD2 receptor type 1 (DP1); these receptors are nearly exclusively expressed along the ventricle lining of the brain near the basal forebrain, suggesting that these cells may integrate signals from the CSF and signal to downstream sleep circuitry in the hypothalamus and forebrain (Mizoguchi et al., 2001).

Recently, conditional knockout models for tissue-specific deletion of the *PGD2 synthase* gene revealed that only expression in the leptomeninges is necessary for sleep regulation; this pathway allows for direct secretion into the CSF along the same pathway where ADO signaling integrates global CSF signals into the basal forebrain (Cherasse et al., 2018). Indeed, PGD2 signaling through DP1 receptors increases extracellular ADO, and this effect is completely abrogated in *DP1*-knockout animals. There appears to be reciprocal feedback within this system as well: ADO A2A receptor deficiency significantly attenuates the sleep-promoting effects of PGD2. Further studies harnessing modern genetic approaches and diverse model organisms are needed to better understand how PGD2 and ADO interact functionally.

Nitric Oxide: A Link Between Somnogens and Immune Functions

Nitric oxide (NO) is a short-lived (half-life <1 second) gas that can be generated in cells through a family of NO synthase (NOS)–encoding genes (Amitai, 2010). In 1996, researchers reported that NO levels were tightly correlated to circadian timing, where during waking time NO increased and then dissipated during the sleep phase (Cespuglio et al., 2004; Kalinchuk et al., 2010). This led to the idea that NO may act as a classic somnogen similar to ADO and PGD2. The first forays into testing the effect of NO on sleep found that injecting NO donors into pontine hindbrain areas strongly induced sleep, while NOS inhibitors drastically reduced sleep (Clément et al., 2005; Kalinchuk, Lu, et al., 2006). Prior to the elevation of ADO due to sleep deprivation, NO is significantly increased in both the basal forebrain and cortex (Kalinchuk et al., 2011). Whether there is a direct relationship between ADO and NO is still unclear, but they may have functional connections through glutamatergic signals (Sims et al., 2013).

Further support of NO's role in sleep homeostasis has come from genetic models examining the effect that specific NOSs play on sleep. Both neural NOS (nNOS), which produces small amounts of NO, and inducible NOS (iNOS), which can produce large amounts of NO up to cytotoxic levels, are known to be involved in sleep regulation and have specific functions relating to sleep homeostasis (Brown, 2010; Chen et al., 2003). Of particular interest, while nNOS is expressed widely throughout the brain in adult animals, iNOS is only expressed in response to sleep deprivation or inflammation. However, iNOS is also expressed early in development, as well as much later during aging (Gautier-Sauvigné et al., 2005). The context-dependent nature of iNOS expression is of significant interest when considering the relationship between stress and sleep deprivation.

Sleep deprivation triggers a complex sequence of events involving a steep increase in iNOS and NO, which happens prior to the elevation of ADO (Kalinchuk et al., 2011). Whether there is functional connectivity between ADO and NO signals remains poorly understood. However, adding an iNOS inhibitor during sleep deprivation prevents the increase in extracellular ADO that is expected (Kalinchuk et al., 2010). Infection is the other main driver of iNOS expression. It is known that pathological conditions provide a permissive environment that enhances sleep, especially NREM SWA (Besedovsky et al., 2019). Rodents whose iNOS has been genetically deleted do have a homeostatic sleep response to virus challenge like that found in wild-type animals (Chen et al., 2004). Additionally, iNOS inhibitors that prevent SWA are associated with lipopolysaccharide challenge, which promotes NREM sleep. There may be unique contributions from neurons and glial cells that distinguish iNOS regulation of sleep after deprivation compared to during sickness—an intriguing idea that warrants further exploration in future studies (Freyer et al., 1996; Kalinchuk, Stenberg, et al., 2006).

Sleep Homeostasis and Immune Function: Tumor Necrosis Factor-Alpha, Interleukin-1-Beta, and Nemuri

While the majority of sleep research over time has focused on the brain, there is a growing appreciation for the role of sleep in somatic tissues throughout the body because of the wide range of functions they perform (Anafi et al., 2019). Sleep affects nearly all physiological functions: body temperature, hormones, cardiorespiratory system, kidney function, and the immune system (Besedovsky et al., 2019). But why when we have a simple chest infection do we feel so tired? What signals underlie this sensation, and how are they computed by the brain? The need for sleep is especially sensitive to sickness and follows the logic of sleep homeostasis, where sleep is increased at the first opportunity with enhanced SWA (Zielinski et al., 2013). Several factors have been identified that regulate both immune function and sleep homeostasis; we will discuss some of the genetics involved in regulating both sleep and immune function.

Tumor necrosis factor-alpha (TNF-α) is an adipokine and a cytokine which has many functions related to immune response. Similar to all somnogens, the expression levels of the *TNF-α* gene are activity-dependent and coupled to increased time spent awake (Arias-Carrión et al., 2011). TNF-α was first identified as a sleep substance in 1987 in rabbits, where it strongly induced SWA at the expense of REM, enhanced SWA EEG amplitude, and increased total sleep time (Shoham et al., 1987). Since this initial study, TNF-α has been shown to regulate sleep in many organisms, ranging from *Drosophila* to humans (Dickstein et al., 1999; Fang et al., 1997; Vanderheyden et al., 2018).

For instance, fruit flies with deletions in the *EGR1* and *EGR3* genes (homologs to human TNF-α) sleep significantly less, and through tissue-specific RNA interference knockdown, it was found that astrocytes are the main source of EGR that regulates sleep and sleep homeostasis (Vanderheyden et al., 2018). Similarly, mice lacking the 55-kD TNF-α receptor sleep less than controls, through reduction of both NREM and REM sleep (Fang et al., 1997). And mice with deletions in both the 55-kD and 75-kD TNF-α receptors exhibit significantly less NREM, with fragmentation (Rockstrom et al., 2018). Interestingly, when these mice are challenged with sickness, they still sleep a similar amount as controls but have a compressed NREM EEG power, suggesting that the quality of their sleep is reduced compared to wild-type animals in an immune-dependent manner (Kapás et al., 2008).

Interleukin-1-beta (IL1β) was first discovered in 1955 for its role in inducing a strong fever response in rabbits (Atkins & Wood, 1955). Its role in sleep was first characterized in the 1980s, again in rabbits, after observing that injecting IL1β strongly promotes sleep and NREM activity (Krueger et al., 1983, 1984). The exogenous application of IL1β produces large increases in NREM, which have been shown in rats, mice, cats, monkeys, and humans. Additionally, IL1β expression varies by day and night, and levels are significantly increased through sleep deprivation.

Genetic studies have shown that IL1β signaling through IL1-receptor 1 is required for the sleep-promoting effects of IL1β (Fang et al., 1998). Mice with genetic deletion of *IL-R1* neither increase time asleep nor have any changes in NREM activity when exogenous IL1β is applied to them. Mice lacking both IL-R1 and TNF receptor 1 were more active and experienced less NREM sleep during the night (Krueger et al., 1998). After sleep deprivation, *IL-R1/TNF-R1* KO mice have a deeply attenuated NREM sleep rebound and do not produce any REM rebound. In humans, *IL-R1* genetic polymorphisms have significantly shortened time spent asleep, reduced SWA activity, and increased risk of developing Alzheimer's disease (Yin et al., 2016). While these studies have provided meaningful insights into the relationship between immune function and sleep by IL1β, there have been very few studies of this in recent years. Modern genetic tools, such as optogenetic and chemogenic systems, and tissue-specific knockouts through CRISPR/Cas9 have not yet been applied to better understand the deeper genetic underpinnings of immune function and sleep through genetic regulators such as *IL1β*.

The idea that molecules associated with being awake build up as we get tired goes back over 100 years. Yet the genetic deciphering of this process is still very much in its beginning phase. Several recent studies have identified novel genes and proteins involved in both sleep homeostasis and immune regulation. A forward gain-of-function screen in *Drosophila* discovered the novel protein Nemuri, which increases with time awake, induces increased sleep, and has potent antimicrobial properties (Toda et al., 2019). Another recent study that used quantitative proteomics to profile synapses as they undergo wake–sleep cycles found that glutamatergic alpha-amino-3-hydroxy-5-methyl-4-isoxazolepropionic acid receptors are responsible for synaptic restoration during sleep and that this is controlled by Homer1a, which interacts with ADO signaling to modulate the strength of sleep need (Diering et al., 2017). Here, our discussion of the genetics of sleep homeostasis is by no means exhaustive (see other extensive reviews: Allada et al., 2017; Mang & Franken, 2015) but rather focused on the systems that have been studied in the most detail, such as ADO and TNF-α. Despite the concerted efforts to understand these sleep-promoting substances, the genetic control of these systems remains largely elusive. This is likely partially due to the global nature in which these substances build up throughout the brain and body. This presents an intriguing opportunity to apply cellular-level whole-brain or even whole-body imaging studies in conjunction with modern genetics to better capture how sleep homeostasis is regulated by the body and how its actions are genetically determined at the cellular level.

Conclusion

The study of genetics has played a critical role in revolutionizing our understanding of biology and its applications to medicine, enabling us to uncover the underlying genetic workings of numerous human disorders. In comparison to other fields of research, such as cell metabolism or circadian biology, sleep research is still in a more contemporary phase in our understanding of the genetics that regulate sleep. Throughout this chapter we have discussed many genetic mechanisms that have been implicated in sleep regulation, yet despite two decades filled with elegant and robust studies, no single gene is known to be both necessary and sufficient to encompass the complexities of sleep regulation. There remains a major challenge in effective genetic screening to find such sleep genes as there are so many complex physiological components that define sleep. Here, we have argued for the need to reflect on what constitutes an effective genetic screen: a strong and heritable phenotype or trait. But what does this mean for sleep? The future generation of researchers in sleep genetics should advocate for genetic techniques that have proven to be so successful in other fields of biology, such as (1) honing the precision of the phenotype that is screened, (2) continuing to expand the horizons of sleep genetics to tissues and cellular pathways across the whole body, and (3) promoting the development of diverse model systems to better understand the genetic basis of sleep across phylogeny.

However, sleep definitions currently lack a simple unifying trait that could be used for more effective genetic screening. Rather, sleep can be defined behaviorally or through PSG but only by combining a total of five components or multimodal measures that may use cumbersome techniques that are not amenable to high-throughput screens. It is therefore clear that there is a need to define sleep differently to move past the more ambiguous behavioral/neurological sleep definitions we are currently burdened with. Ideally, this would be best addressed by forming a defined cellular-level explanation of what sleep is and does. With advances in genetic and imaging techniques, the sleep field is now beginning to tackle these problems by performing whole-brain and whole-body cellular imaging. In zebrafish and fly, this has already uncovered novel cell types involved in the regulation of sleep, and extending these techniques into other species will likely uncover more novel regulators and functions of sleep at the cellular level. Yet experiments such as these pose a non-trivial hurdle for the field of sleep sciences. In order to establish a novel cellular signature associated with sleep, this defining sleep signature will need to be validated as a *bona fide* sleep state by using the current behavioral/neurological definitions, and performing such detailed analyses in current model organisms in a state-dependent manner will be extremely difficult. To date, the observed cellular signatures of sleep from humans to *Drosophila* fall into two categories: neurological dynamic signatures, including oscillations, silencing, and paradoxical wake-like activity, and metabolic changes, such as energy balance and cellular respiration. This makes for a complex system to disentangle. However, using comparative studies across evolutionarily distinct species could provide the precision needed to better understand the state of sleep as a cellular process. Hopefully, to complement the mammalian systems, "simpler" high-throughput genetic models, such as zebrafish, fly, *Caenorhabditis elegans*, or one of the earliest diverging lineages, cniderians (jellyfish and hydra) and placozoans (e.g., *Trichoplax adhaerens*), could be key in uncovering sleep-dependent cellular features. Such cellular processes will be under precise genetic control—an exciting prospect for the current and future generation of sleep scientists to tackle. Integrative studies that combine developmental patterning, circadian regulation, cellular transmission, and sleep homeostasis are the new frontier of sleep genetics. Harnessing a comprehensive view of sleep as a whole-body physiological state that is critical for the continued development and health of all animal species, along with the application of modern genetic techniques, will be essential in uncovering the mystery of what sleep is.

References

Akam, M. (1989). *Hox* and HOM: Homologous gene clusters in insects and vertebrates. *Cell, 57*(3), 347–349. https://doi.org/10.1016/0092-8674(89)90909-4

Alam, M. N., Szymusiak, R., Gong, H., King, J., & McGinty, D. (1999). Adenosinergic modulation of rat basal forebrain neurons during sleep and waking: Neuronal recording with microdialysis. *The Journal of Physiology, 521*(Pt. 3), 679–690. https://doi.org/10.1111/j.1469-7793.1999.00679.x

Allada, R., Cirelli, C., & Sehgal, A. (2017). Molecular mechanisms of sleep homeostasis in flies and mammals. *Cold Spring Harbor Perspectives in Biology, 9*(8), Article a027730. https://doi.org/10.1101/cshperspect.a027730

Allada, R., Emery, P., Takahashi, J. S., & Rosbash, M. (2001). Stopping time: The genetics of fly and mouse circadian clocks. *Annual Review of Neuroscience, 24*, 1091–1119. https://doi.org/10.1146/annurev.neuro.24.1.1091

Alvarez-Bolado, G. (2019). Development of neuroendocrine neurons in the mammalian hypothalamus. *Cell and Tissue Research, 375*(1), 23–39. https://doi.org/10.1007/s00441-018-2859-1

Amitai, Y. (2010). Physiologic role for "inducible" nitric oxide synthase: A new form of astrocytic–neuronal interface. *Glia, 58*(15), 1775–1781. https://doi.org/10.1002/glia.21057

Anafi, R. C., Kayser, M. S., & Raizen, D. M. (2019). Exploring phylogeny to find the function of sleep. *Nature Reviews Neuroscience, 20*(2), 109–116. https://doi.org/10.1038/s41583-018-0098-9

Anthwal, N., Pelling, M., Claxton, S., Mellitzer, G., Collin, C., Kessaris, N., Richardson, W. D., Gradwohl, G., & Ang, S. L. (2013). Conditional deletion of neurogenin-3 using Nkx2.1iCre results in a mouse model for the central control of feeding, activity and obesity. *Disease Models & Mechanisms, 6*(5), 1133–1145. https://doi.org/10.1242/dmm.011916

Antonijevic, I. A., Murck, H., Bohlhalter, S., Frieboes, R. M., Holsboer, F., & Steiger, A. (2000). Neuropeptide Y promotes sleep and inhibits ACTH and cortisol release in young men. *Neuropharmacology*, *39*(8), 1474–1481. https://doi.org/10.1016/s0028-3908(00)00057-5

Arias-Carrión, O., Huitron-Resendiz, S., Arankowsky-Sandoval, G., & Murillo-Rodriguez, E. (2011). Biochemical modulation of the sleep–wake cycle: Endogenous sleep-inducing factors. *Journal of Neuroscience Research*, *89*(8), 1143–1149. https://doi.org/10.1002/jnr.22666

Aroca, P., Lorente-Canovas, B., Mateos, F. R., & Puelles, L. (2006). Locus coeruleus neurons originate in alar rhombomere 1 and migrate into the basal plate: Studies in chick and mouse embryos. *The Journal of Comparative Neurology*, *496*(6), 802–818. https://doi.org/10.1002/cne.20957

Aston-Jones, G., & Bloom, F. E. (1981). Activity of norepinephrine-containing locus coeruleus neurons in behaving rats anticipates fluctuations in the sleep–waking cycle. *The Journal of Neuroscience*, *1*(8), 876–886. https://doi.org/10.1523/JNEUROSCI.01-08-00876.1981

Atkins, E., & Wood, W. B. (1955). Studies on the pathogenesis of fever. II. Identification of an endogenous pyrogen in the blood stream following the injection of typhoid vaccine. *The Journal of Experimental Medicine*, *102*(5), 499–516. https://doi.org/10.1084/jem.102.5.499

Belkin, K. J., & Abrams, T. W. (1993). FMRFamide produces biphasic modulation of the LFS motor neurons in the neural circuit of the siphon withdrawal reflex of *Aplysia* by activating Na^+ and K^+ currents. *The Journal of Neuroscience*, *13*(12), 5139–5152. https://doi.org/10.1523/JNEUROSCI.13-12-05139.1993

Berman, J. R., Skariah, G., Maro, G. S., Mignot, E., & Mourrain, P. (2009). Characterization of two melanin-concentrating hormone genes in zebrafish reveals evolutionary and physiological links with the mammalian MCH system. *The Journal of Comparative Neurology*, *517*(5), 695–710. https://doi.org/10.1002/cne.22171

Besedovsky, L., Lange, T., & Haack, M. (2019). The sleep–immune crosstalk in health and disease. *Physiological Reviews*, *99*(3), 1325–1380. https://doi.org/10.1152/physrev.00010.2018

Bianchi, D. E. (1964). An endogenous circadian rhythm in *Neurospora crassa*. *Journal of General Microbiology*, *35*, 437–445. https://doi.org/10.1099/00221287-35-3-437

Bjorness, T. E., & Greene, R. W. (2009). Adenosine and sleep. *Current Neuropharmacology*, *7*(3), 238–245. https://doi.org/10.2174/157015909789152182

Borbély, A. A., & Achermann, P. (1999). Sleep homeostasis and models of sleep regulation. *Journal of Biological Rhythms*, *14*(6), 557–568. https://doi.org/10.1177/074873099129000894

Borbély, A. A., & Tobler, I. (2011). Manifestations and functional implications of sleep homeostasis. In P. Montagna & S. Chokorverty (Eds.), *Sleep disorders part I. Handbook of clinical neurology* (Vol. 98, pp. 205–213). Elsevier. https://doi.org/10.1016/B978-0-444-52006-7.00013-7

Bourgin, P., Huitron-Resendiz, S., Spier, A. D., Fabre, D., Morte, B., Criado, J. R., Sutcliffe, J. G., Henriksen, S. J., & de Lecea, L. (2000). Hypocretin-1 modulates rapid eye movement sleep through activation of locus coeruleus neurons. *The Journal of Neuroscience*, *20*(20), 7760–7765. https://doi.org/10.1523/JNEUROSCI.20-20-07760.2000

Briscoe, J., & Novitch, B. G. (2008). Regulatory pathways linking progenitor patterning, cell fates and neurogenesis in the ventral neural tube. *Philosophical Transactions of the Royal Society of London. Series B, Biological Sciences*, *363*(1489), 57–70. https://doi.org/10.1098/rstb.2006.2012

Brown, G. C. (2010). Nitric oxide and neuronal death. *Nitric Oxide*, *23*(3), 153–165. https://doi.org/10.1016/j.niox.2010.06.001

Burbridge, S., Stewart, I., & Placzek, M. (2016). Development of the neuroendocrine hypothalamus. *Comprehensive Physiology*, *6*(2), 623–643. https://doi.org/10.1002/cphy.c150023

Cespuglio, R., Debilly, G., & Burlet, S. (2004). Cortical and pontine variations occurring in the voltammetric no signal throughout the sleep–wake cycle in the rat. *Archives Italiennes de Biologie*, *142*(4), 551–556.

Chance, B. (1907). Unusual form of hereditary congenital cataract in several members of a family. *Transactions of the American Ophthalmological Society*, *11*(Pt. 2), 334–337.

Chemelli, R. M., Willie, J. T., Sinton, C. M., Elmquist, J. K., Scammell, T., Lee, C., Richardson, J. A., Williams, S. C., Xiong, Y., Kisanuki, Y., Fitch, T. E., Nakazato, M., Hammer, R. E., Saper, C. B., & Yanagisawa, M. (1999). Narcolepsy in *orexin* knockout mice: Molecular genetics of sleep regulation. *Cell*, *98*(4), 437–451. https://doi.org/10.1016/s0092-8674(00)81973-x

Chen, L., Duricka, D., Nelson, S., Mukherjee, S., Bohnet, S. G., Taishi, P., Majde, J. A., & Krueger, J. M. (2004). Influenza virus-induced sleep responses in mice with targeted disruptions in neuronal or inducible nitric oxide synthases. *Journal of Applied Physiology*, *97*(1), 17–28. https://doi.org/10.1152/japplphysiol.01355.2003

Chen, L., Majde, J. A., & Krueger, J. M. (2003). Spontaneous sleep in mice with targeted disruptions of neuronal or inducible nitric oxide synthase genes. *Brain Research*, *973*(2), 214–222. https://doi.org/10.1016/s0006-8993(03)02484-3

Cherasse, Y., Aritake, K., Oishi, Y., Kaushik, M. K., Korkutata, M., & Urade, Y. (2018). The leptomeninges produce prostaglandin D2 involved in sleep regulation in mice. *Frontiers in Cellular Neuroscience*, *12*, Article 357. https://doi.org/10.3389/fncel.2018.00357

Cirelli, C., Bushey, D., Hill, S., Huber, R., Kreber, R., Ganetzky, B., & Tononi, G. (2005). Reduced sleep in Drosophila Shaker mutants. *Nature*, *434*(7037), 1087–1092. https://doi.org/10.1038/nature03486

Clément, P., Sarda, N., Cespuglio, R., & Gharib, A. (2005). Potential role of inducible nitric oxide synthase in the sleep–wake states occurrence in old rats. *Neuroscience*, *135*(2), 347–355. https://doi.org/10.1016/j.neuroscience.2005.05.064

Coleman, C. G., Baghdoyan, H. A., & Lydic, R. (2006). Dialysis delivery of an adenosine A2A agonist into the pontine reticular formation of C57BL/6J mouse increases pontine acetylcholine release and sleep. *Journal of Neurochemistry*, *96*(6), 1750–1759. https://doi.org/10.1111/j.1471-4159.2006.03700.x

Coulson, R. L., Mourrain, P., & Wang, G. X. (2022). Sleep deficiency as a driver of cellular stress and damage in neurological disorders. *Sleep Medicine Reviews*, *63*, Article 101616. https://doi.org/10.1016/j.smrv.2022.101616

Crocker, A., & Sehgal, A. (2008). Octopamine regulates sleep in *Drosophila* through protein kinase A–dependent mechanisms. *The Journal of Neuroscience*, *28*(38), 9377–9385. https://doi.org/10.1523/JNEUROSCI.3072-08a.2008

Curtis, B. J., Ashbrook, L. H., Young, T., Finn, L. A., Fu, Y.-H., Ptacek, L. J., & Jones, C. R. (2019). Extreme morning chronotypes are often familial and not exceedingly rare: The estimated prevalence of advanced sleep phase, familial advanced sleep phase, and advanced sleep–wake phase disorder in a sleep clinic population. *Sleep*, *42*(10), Article zsz148. https://doi.org/10.1093/sleep/zsz148

Czeisler, C. A., Duffy, J. F., Shanahan, T. L., Brown, E. N., Mitchell, J. F., Rimmer, D. W., Ronda, J. M., Silva, E. J., Allan, J. S., Emens, J. S., Dijk, D.-J., & Kronauer, R. E. (1999). Stability, precision, and near-24-hour period of the human circadian pacemaker. *Science*, *284*(5423), 2177–2181. https://doi.org/10.1126/science.284.5423.2177

Deboer, T. (2015). Behavioral and electrophysiological correlates of sleep and sleep homeostasis. *Current Topics in Behavioral Neurosciences*, *25*, 1–24. https://doi.org/10.1007/7854_2013_248

de Lecea, L., Kilduff, T. S., Peyron, C., Gao, X.-B., Foye, P. E., Danielson, P. E., Fukuhara, C., Battenberg, E. L. F., Gautvik, V. T., Bartlett, F. S., II, Frankel, W. N., van den Pol, A. N., Bloom, F. E., Gautvik, K. M., & Sutcliffe, J. G. (1998). The hypocretins: Hypothalamus-specific peptides with neuroexcitatory activity. *Proceedings of the National Academy of Sciences of the United States of America*, *95*(1), 322–327. https://doi.org/10.1073/pnas.95.1.322

Dickstein, J. B., Moldofsky, H., Lue, F. A., & Hay, J. B. (1999). Intracerebroventricular injection of TNF-alpha promotes sleep and is recovered in cervical lymph. *The American Journal of Physiology*, *276*(4), R1018–R1022. https://doi.org/10.1152/ajpregu.1999.276.4.R1018

Diering, G. H., Nirujogi, R. S., Roth, R. H., Worley, P. F., Pandey, A., & Huganir, R. L. (2017). Homer1a drives homeostatic scaling-down of excitatory synapses during sleep. *Science*, *355*(6324), 511–515. https://doi.org/10.1126/science.aai8355

Donlea, J. M., Alam, M. N., & Szymusiak, R. (2017). Neuronal substrates of sleep homeostasis; Lessons from flies, rats and mice. *Current Opinion in Neurobiology*, *44*, 228–235. https://doi.org/10.1016/j.conb.2017.05.003

Doolittle, R. F., Feng, D.-F., Tsang, S., Cho, G., & Little, E. (1996). Determining divergence times of the major kingdoms of living organisms with a protein clock. *Science*, *271*(5248), 470–477. https://doi.org/10.1126/science.271.5248.470

Dresse, A., & Scuvée-Moreau, J. (1986). Influence of the alpha-2 agonist oxaminozoline (S3341) on firing rate of central noradrenergic and serotonergic neurons in the rat. Comparison with clonidine. *Archives Internationales de Physiologie et de Biochimie*, *94*(2), 99–106.

Dunlap, J. C. (1996). Genetics and molecular analysis of circadian rhythms. *Annual Review of Genetics*, *30*, 579–601. https://doi.org/10.1146/annurev.genet.30.1.579

Dvornyk, V., Vinogradova, O., & Nevo, E. (2003). Origin and evolution of circadian clock genes in prokaryotes. *Proceedings of the National Academy of Sciences of the United States of America*, *100*(5), 2495–2500. https://doi.org/10.1073/pnas.0130099100

Dyzma, M., Boudjeltia, K. Z., Faraut, B., & Kerkhofs, M. (2010). Neuropeptide Y and sleep. *Sleep Medicine Reviews, 14*(3), 161–165. https://doi.org/10.1016/j.smrv.2009.09.001

Edlund, T., & Jessell, T. M. (1999). Progression from extrinsic to intrinsic signaling in cell fate specification: A view from the nervous system. *Cell, 96*(2), 211–224. https://doi.org/10.1016/s0092-8674(00)80561-9

Eide, P. K., Vinje, V., Pripp, A. H., Mardal, K.-A., & Ringstad, G. (2021). Sleep deprivation impairs molecular clearance from the human brain. *Brain, 144*(3), 863–874. https://doi.org/10.1093/brain/awaa443

Eng, G. W. L., Edison, & Virshup, D. M. (2017). Site-specific phosphorylation of casein kinase 1 δ (CK1δ) regulates its activity towards the circadian regulator PER2. *PLOS ONE, 12*(5), Article e0177834. https://doi.org/10.1371/journal.pone.0177834

Fang, J., Wang, Y., & Krueger, J. M. (1997). Mice lacking the TNF 55 kDa receptor fail to sleep more after TNFα treatment. *The Journal of Neuroscience, 17*(15), 5949–5955. https://doi.org/10.1523/JNEUROSCI.17-15-05949.1997

Fang, J., Wang, Y., & Krueger, J. M. (1998). Effects of interleukin-1 beta on sleep are mediated by the type I receptor. *The American Journal of Physiology: Regulatory, Integrative and Comparative Physiology, 274*(3), R655–R660. https://doi.org/10.1152/ajpregu.1998.274.3.R655

Feldman, J. F., & Hoyle, M. N. (1973). Isolation of circadian clock mutants of *Neurospora crassa. Genetics, 75*(4), 605–613.

Fisch, A. (2012). *Neuroanatomy: Draw it to know it.* Oxford University Press. https://doi.org/10.1093/med/9780199845712.003.0321

Foutz, A. S., Mitler, M. M., Cavalli-Sforza, L. L., & Dement, W. C. (1979). Genetic factors in canine narcolepsy. *Sleep, 1*(4), 413–421. https://doi.org/10.1093/sleep/1.4.413

Fredholm, B. B., Chen, J. F., Masino, S. A., & Vaugeois, J.-M. (2005). Actions of adenosine at its receptors in the CNS: Insights from knockouts and drugs. *Annual Review of Pharmacology and Toxicology, 45*, 385–412. https://doi.org/10.1146/annurev.pharmtox.45.120403.095731

Freyer, D., Weih, M., Weber, J. R., Burger, W., Scholz, P., Manz, R., Ziegenhorn, A., Angestwurm, K., & Dirnagl, U. (1996). Pneumococcal cell wall components induce nitric oxide synthase and TNF-alpha in astroglial-enriched cultures. *Glia, 16*(1), 1–6. https://doi.org/10.1002/(SICI)1098-1136(199601)16:1<1::AID-GLIA1>3.0.CO;2-8

Gallopin, T., Luppi, P.-H., Cauli, B., Urade, Y., Rossier, J., Hayaishi, O., Lambolez, B., & Fort, P. (2005). The endogenous somnogen adenosine excites a subset of sleep-promoting neurons via A2A receptors in the ventrolateral preoptic nucleus. *Neuroscience, 134*(4), 1377–1390. https://doi.org/10.1016/j.neuroscience.2005.05.045

Gautier-Sauvigné, S., Colas, D., Parmantier, P., Clement, P., Gharib, A., Sarda, N., & Cespuglio, R. (2005). Nitric oxide and sleep. *Sleep Medicine Reviews, 9*(2), 101–113. https://doi.org/10.1016/j.smrv.2004.07.004

Gentry, N. W., Ashbrook, L. H., Fu, Y.-H., & Ptacek, L. J. (2021). Human circadian variations. *The Journal of Clinical Investigation, 131*(16), Article e148282. https://doi.org/10.1172/JCI148282

Gerstner, J. R., Lyons, L. C., Wright, K. P., Jr., Loh, D. H., Rawashdeh, O., Eckel-Mahan, K. L., & Roman, G. W. (2009). Cycling behavior and memory formation. *The Journal of Neuroscience, 29*(41), 12824–12830. https://doi.org/10.1523/JNEUROSCI.3353-09.2009

Gottesmann, C. (1988). What the cerveau isolé preparation tells us nowadays about sleep–wake mechanisms? *Neuroscience & Biobehavioral Reviews, 12*(1), 39–48. https://doi.org/10.1016/s0149-7634(88)80072-1

Gross, J. B. (2012). The complex origin of *Astyanax* cavefish. *BMC Evolutionary Biology, 12*, Article 105. https://doi.org/10.1186/1471-2148-12-105

Halassa, M. M., Florian, C., Fellin, T., Munoz, J. R., Lee, S.-Y., Abel, T., Haydon, P. G., & Frank, M. G. (2009). Astrocytic modulation of sleep homeostasis and cognitive consequences of sleep loss. *Neuron, 61*(2), 213–219. https://doi.org/10.1016/j.neuron.2008.11.024

Hendricks, J. C., Finn, S. M., Panckeri, K. A., Chavkin, J., Williams, J. A., Sehgal, A., & Pack, A. I. (2000). Rest in *Drosophila* is a sleep-like state. *Neuron, 25*(1), 129–138. https://doi.org/10.1016/s0896-6273(00)80877-6

He, C., Yang, Y., Zhang, M., Price, J. L., & Zhao, Z. (2013). Regulation of sleep by neuropeptide Y-like system in *Drosophila melanogaster. PLOS ONE, 8*(9), Article e74237. https://doi.org/10.1371/journal.pone.0074237

Hinaux, H., Devos, L., Blin, M., Elipot, Y., Bibliowicz, J., Alie, A., & Retaux, S. (2016). Sensory evolution in blind cavefish is driven by early embryonic events during gastrulation and neurulation. *Development, 143*(23), 4521–4532. https://doi.org/10.1242/dev.141291

Hirano, A., Yumimoto, K., Tsunematsu, R., Matsumoto, M., Oyama, M., Kozuka-Hata, H., Nakagawa, T., Lanjakornsiripan, D., Nakayama, K. I., & Fukada, Y. (2013). FBXL21 regulates oscillation of the circadian clock through ubiquitination and stabilization of cryptochromes. *Cell, 152*(5), 1106–1118. https://doi.org/10.1016/j.cell.2013.01.054

Hobson, J. A., McCarley, R. W., & Wyzinski, P. W. (1975). Sleep cycle oscillation: Reciprocal discharge by two brainstem neuronal groups. *Science, 189*(4196), 55–58. https://doi.org/10.1126/science.1094539

Hong, Z.-Y., Huang, Z.-L., Qu, W.-M., Eguchi, N., Urade, Y., & Hayaishi, O. (2005). An adenosine A receptor agonist induces sleep by increasing GABA release in the tuberomammillary nucleus to inhibit histaminergic systems in rats. *Journal of Neurochemistry, 92*(6), 1542–1549. https://doi.org/10.1111/j.1471-4159.2004.02991.x

Hosoya, T., Oda, Y., Takahashi, S., Morita, M., Kawauchi, S., Ema, M., Yamamoto, Y., & Fujii-Kuriyama, Y. (2001). Defective development of secretory neurones in the hypothalamus of Arnt2-knockout mice. *Genes to Cells, 6*(4), 361–374. https://doi.org/10.1046/j.1365-2443.2001.00421.x

Howell, W. H. (1913). *Le problème physiologique du sommeil.* By Henri Piéron. Paris, Masson et Cie. 1913. Pp. xv + 520, six figures in text. *Science, 37*(953), 525–526. https://doi.org/10.1126/science.37.953.525

Huang, H., Zhu, Y., Eliot, M. N., Knopik, V. S., McGeary, J. S., Carskadon, M. A., & Hart, A. C. (2017). Combining human epigenetics and sleep studies in *Caenorhabditis elegans*: A cross-species approach for finding conserved genes regulating sleep. *Sleep, 40*(6), Article zsx063. https://doi.org/10.1093/sleep/zsx063

Huang, Z.-L., Qu, W.-M., Eguchi, N., Chen, J.-F., Schwarzschild, M. A., Fredholm, B. B., Urade, Y., & Hayaishi, O. (2005). Adenosine A2A, but not A1, receptors mediate the arousal effect of caffeine. *Nature Neuroscience, 8*(7), 858–859. https://doi.org/10.1038/nn1491

Iannacone, M. J., Beets, I., Lopes, L. E., Churgin, M. A., Fang-Yen, C., Nelson, M. D., Schoofs, L., & Raizen, D. M. (2017). The RFamide receptor DMSR-1 regulates stress-induced sleep in C. elegans. *eLife, 6*, Article e19837. https://doi.org/10.7554/eLife.19837

Jaggard, J. B., Lloyd, E., Yuiska, A., Patch, A., Fily, Y., Kowalko, J. E., Appelbaum, L., Duboue, E. R., & Keene, A. C. (2020). Cavefish brain atlases reveal functional and anatomical convergence across independently evolved populations. *Science Advances, 6*(38), Article eaba3126. https://doi.org/10.1126/sciadv.aba3126

Jaggard, J. B., Stahl, B. A., Lloyd, E., Prober, D. A., Duboue, E. R., & Keene, A. C. (2018). Hypocretin underlies the evolution of sleep loss in the Mexican cavefish. *eLife, 7*, Article e32637. https://doi.org/10.7554/eLife.32637

Jaggard, J. B., Wang, G. X., & Mourrain, P. (2021). Non-REM and REM/paradoxical sleep dynamics across phylogeny. *Current Opinion in Neurobiology, 71*, 44–51. https://doi.org/10.1016/j.conb.2021.08.004

Jeffery, W. R. (2009). Regressive evolution in *Astyanax* cavefish. *Annual Review of Genetics, 43*, 25–47. https://doi.org/10.1146/annurev-genet-102108-134216

Jego, S., Glasgow, S. D., Herrera, C. G., Ekstrand, M., Reed, S. J., Boyce, R., Friedman, J., Burdakov, D., & Adamantidis, A. R. (2013). Optogenetic identification of a rapid eye movement sleep modulatory circuit in the hypothalamus. *Nature Neuroscience, 16*(11), 1637–1643. https://doi.org/10.1038/nn.3522

Jo, Y.-H., & Chua, S. (2009). Transcription factors in the development of medial hypothalamic structures. *American Journal of Physiology: Endocrinology and Metabolism, 297*(3), E563–E567. https://doi.org/10.1152/ajpendo.00064.2009

Jouvet, M., & Michel, F. (1958). Recherches sur l'activité électrique cérébrale au cours du sommeil [Study of the cerebral electrical activity during sleep]. *Comptes rendus des seances de la societe de biologie et de ses filiales, 152*(7), 1167–1170.

Jouvet, M., Michel, F., & Courjon, J. (1959a). Sur la mise en jeu de deux mécaismes à expression électro-encéphalographique différente au cours du sommeil physiologique chez le Chat [Bringing into play of two mechanisms with different electroencephalographic expression during physiological sleep in the cat]. *Comptes rendus hebdomadaires des séances de l'Académie des sciences, 248*(1), 3043–3045.

Jouvet, M., Michel, F., & Courjon, J. (1959b). Sur un stade d'activité électrique rapide au cours du sommeil physiologique [On a stage of rapid cerebral electrical activity in the course of physiological sleep]. *Comptes rendus des séances de la Société de biologie et de ses filiales, 151*(3), 1024–1028.

Jouvet, M., Bobillier, P., Pujol, J. F., & Renault, J. (1966). Effets des lésions du système du raphé sur le sommeil et la sérotonine cérébrale [Effects of lesions of the raphe system on sleep and cerebral serotonin]. *Comptes rendus des seances de la societe de biologie et de ses filiales, 160*(12), 2343–2346.

Kalinchuk, A. V., Lu, Y., Stenberg, D., Rosenberg, P. A., & Porkka-Heiskanen, T. (2006). Nitric oxide production in the basal forebrain is required for recovery sleep. *Journal of Neurochemistry, 99*(2), 483–498. https://doi.org/10.1111/j.1471-4159.2006.04077.x

Kalinchuk, A. V., Stenberg, D., Rosenberg, P. A., & Porkka-Heiskanen, T. (2006). Inducible and neuronal nitric oxide synthases (NOS) have complementary roles in recovery sleep induction. *The European Journal of Neuroscience, 24*(5), 1443–1456. https://doi.org/10.1111/j.1460-9568.2006.05019.x

Kalinchuk, A. V., McCarley, R. W., Porkka-Heiskanen, T., & Basheer, R. (2010). Sleep deprivation triggers inducible nitric oxide-dependent nitric oxide production in wake-active basal forebrain neurons. *The Journal of Neuroscience, 30*(40), 13254–13264. https://doi.org/10.1523/JNEUROSCI.0014-10.2010

Kalinchuk, A. V., McCarley, R. W., Porkka-Heiskanen, T., & Basheer, R. (2011). The time course of adenosine, nitric oxide (NO) and inducible NO synthase changes in the brain with sleep loss and their role in the non-rapid eye movement sleep homeostatic cascade. *Journal of Neurochemistry, 116*(2), 260–272. https://doi.org/10.1111/j.1471-4159.2010.07100.x

Kanaya, H. J., Park, S., Kim, J.-H., Kusumi, J., Krenenou, S., Sawatari, E., Sato, A., Lee, J., Bang, H., Kobayakawa, Y., Lim, C., & Itoh, T. Q. (2020). A sleep-like state in *Hydra* unravels conserved sleep mechanisms during the evolutionary development of the central nervous system. *Science Advances, 6*(41), Article eabb9415. https://doi.org/10.1126/sciadv.abb9415

Kapás, L., Bohnet, S. G., Traynor, T. R., Majde, J. A., Szentirmai, E., Magrath, P., Taishi, P., & Krueger, J. M. (2008). Spontaneous and influenza virus-induced sleep are altered in TNF-alpha double-receptor deficient mice. *Journal of Applied Physiology, 105*(4), 1187–1198. https://doi.org/10.1152/japplphysiol.90388.2008

Kawauchi, H., Kawazoe, I., Tsubokawa, M., Kishida, M., & Baker, B. I. (1983). Characterization of melanin-concentrating hormone in chum salmon pituitaries. *Nature, 305*(5932), 321–323. https://doi.org/10.1038/305321a0

Keith, B., Adelman, D. M., & Simon, M. C. (2001). Targeted mutation of the murine arylhydrocarbon receptor nuclear translocator 2 (Arnt2) gene reveals partial redundancy with Arnt. *Proceedings of the National Academy of Sciences of the United States of America, 98*(12), 6692–6697. https://doi.org/10.1073/pnas.121494298

Koike, N., Yoo, S.-H., Huang, H.-C., Kumar, V., Lee, C., Kim, T.-K., & Takahashi, J. S. (2012). Transcriptional architecture and chromatin landscape of the core circadian clock in mammals. *Science, 338*(6105), 349–354. https://doi.org/10.1126/science.1226339

Kondo, T., Strayer, C. A., Kulkarni, R. D., Taylor, W., Ishiura, M., Golden, S. S., & Johnson, C. H. (1993). Circadian rhythms in prokaryotes: Luciferase as a reporter of circadian gene expression in cyanobacteria. *Proceedings of the National Academy of Sciences of the United States of America, 90*(12), 5672–5676. https://doi.org/10.1073/pnas.90.12.5672

Kondo, T., Tsinoremas, N. F., Golden, S. S., Johnson, C. H., Kutsuna, S., & Ishiura, M. (1994). Circadian clock mutants of cyanobacteria. *Science, 266*(5188), 1233–1236. https://doi.org/10.1126/science.7973706

Konopka, R. J., & Benzer, S. (1971). Clock mutants of *Drosophila melanogaster*. *Proceedings of the National Academy of Sciences of the United States of America, 68*(9), 2112–2116. https://doi.org/10.1073/pnas.68.9.2112

Krueger, J., Dinarello, C., & Chedd, L. (1983). Promotion of slow-wave sleep (SWS) by a purified interleukin-1 (IL-1) preparation. *Federation Proceedings, 42*(3), Article 356.

Krueger, J. M., Fang, J., Taishi, P., Chen, Z., Kushikata, T., & Gardi, J. (1998). Sleep. A physiologic role for IL-1 beta and TNF-alpha. *Annals of the New York Academy of Sciences, 856*, 148–159. https://doi.org/10.1111/j.1749-6632.1998.tb08323.x

Krueger, J. M., Walter, J., Dinarello, C. A., Wolff, S. M., & Chedid, L. (1984). Sleep-promoting effects of endogenous pyrogen (interleukin-1). *American Journal of Physiology, 246*(6 Pt. 2), R994–R999. https://doi.org/10.1152/ajpregu.1984.246.6.R994

Krumlauf, R., & Wilkinson, D. G. (2021). Segmentation and patterning of the vertebrate hindbrain. *Development, 148*(15), Article dev.186460. https://doi.org/10.1242/dev.186460

Kubota, K. (1989). Kuniomi Ishimori and the first discovery of sleep-inducing substances in the brain. *Neuroscience Research, 6*(6), 497–518. https://doi.org/10.1016/0168-0102(89)90041-2

Kurien, P., Hsu, P. K., Leon, J., Wu, D., McMahon, T., Shi, G., Xu, Y., Lipzen, A., Pennacchio, L. A., Jones, C. R., Fu, Y.-H., & Ptacek, L. J. (2019). TIMELESS mutation alters phase responsiveness and causes advanced sleep phase. *Proceedings of the National Academy of Sciences of the United States of America, 116*(24), 12045–12053. https://doi.org/10.1073/pnas.1819110116

Lanska, D. J. (2000). George Huntington (1850–1916) and hereditary chorea. *Journal of the History of the Neurosciences, 9*(1), 76–89. https://doi.org/10.1076/0964-704X(200004)9:1;1-2;FT076

Lazarus, M., Chen, J.-F., Huang, Z.-L., Urade, Y., & Fredholm, B. B. (2019). Adenosine and sleep. In H.-P. Landolt & D.-J. Dijk (Eds.), *Sleep–wake neurobiology and pharmacology. Handbook of experimental pharmacology* (Vol. 253, pp. 359–381). Springer. https://doi.org/10.1007/164_2017_36

Lee, D. A., Oikonomou, G., Cammidge, T., Andreev, A., Hong, Y., Hurley, H., & Prober, D. A. (2020). Neuropeptide VF neurons promote sleep via the serotonergic raphe. *eLife*, 9, Article e54491. https://doi.org/10.7554/eLife.54491

Le Hir, M., & Kaissling, B. (1993). Distribution and regulation of renal ecto-5′-nucleotidase: Implications for physiological functions of adenosine. *American Journal of Physiology: Renal Physiology*, 264(3 Pt. 2), F377–F387. https://doi.org/10.1152/ajprenal.1993.264.3.F377

Lenhoff, H. M. (1991). Ethel Browne, Hans Spemann, and the discovery of the organizer phenomenon. *The Biological Bulletin, 181*(1), 72–80. https://doi.org/10.2307/1542490

Leung, L. C., Wang, G. X., Madelaine, R., Skariah, G., Kawakami, K., Deisseroth, K., Urban, A. E., & Mourrain, P. (2019). Neural signatures of sleep in zebrafish. *Nature, 571*(7764), 198–204. https://doi.org/10.1038/s41586-019-1336-7

Li, R., Wang, Y.-Q., Liu, W.-Y., Zhang, M.-Q., Li, L., Cherasse, Y., Schiffmann, S. N., de Kerchove d'Exaerde, A., Lazarus, M., Qu, W.-M., & Huang, Z.-L. (2020). Activation of adenosine A2A receptors in the olfactory tubercle promotes sleep in rodents. *Neuropharmacology, 168*, Article 107923. https://doi.org/10.1016/j.neuropharm.2019.107923

Linkowski, P., Kerkhofs, M., Hauspie, R., Susanne, C., & Mendlewicz, J. (1989). EEG sleep patterns in man: A twin study. *Electroencephalography and Clinical Neurophysiology, 73*(4), 279–284. https://doi.org/10.1016/0013-4694(89)90106-5

Liu, Z.-W., & Gao, X.-B. (2007). Adenosine inhibits activity of hypocretin/orexin neurons by the A1 receptor in the lateral hypothalamus: A possible sleep-promoting effect. *Journal of Neurophysiology, 97*(1), 837–848. https://doi.org/10.1152/jn.00873.2006

Löhr, H., & Hammerschmidt, M. (2011). Zebrafish in endocrine systems: Recent advances and implications for human disease. *Annual Review of Physiology, 73*, 183–211. https://doi.org/10.1146/annurev-physiol-012110-142320

Lowrey, P. L., & Takahashi, J. S. (2004). Mammalian circadian biology: Elucidating genome-wide levels of temporal organization. *Annual Review of Genomics and Human Genetics, 5*, 407–441. https://doi.org/10.1146/annurev.genom.5.061903.175925

Lowrey, P. L., & Takahashi, J. S. (2011). Genetics of circadian rhythms in mammalian model organisms. In S. Brody (Ed.), *The genetics of circadian rhythms. Advances in genetics* (Vol. 74, pp. 175–230). Academic Press. https://doi.org/10.1016/B978-0-12-387690-4.00006-4

Machluf, Y., Gutnick, A., & Levkowitz, G. (2011). Development of the zebrafish hypothalamus. *Annals of the New York Academy of Sciences, 1220*, 93–105. https://doi.org/10.1111/j.1749-6632.2010.05945.x

Madelaine, R., Lovett-Barron, M., Halluin, C., Andalman, A. S., Liang, J., Skariah, G. M., Leung, L. C., Burns, V. M., & Mourrain, P. (2017). The hypothalamic NPVF circuit modulates ventral raphe activity during nociception. *Scientific Reports, 7*, Article 41528. https://doi.org/10.1038/srep41528

Mang, G. M., & Franken, P. (2015). Genetic dissection of sleep homeostasis. *Current Topics in Behavioral Neurosciences, 25*, 25–63. https://doi.org/10.1007/7854_2013_270

Mathew, P. W. (1908). A case of hereditary brachydactyly. *British Medical Journal, 2*(2492), Article 969. https://doi.org/10.1136/bmj.2.2492.969

McNay, D. E. G., Pelling, M., Claxton, S., Guillemot, F., & Ang, S.-L. (2006). *Mash1* is required for generic and subtype differentiation of hypothalamic neuroendocrine cells. *Molecular Endocrinology, 20*(7), 1623–1632. https://doi.org/10.1210/me.2005-0518

Menuet, A., Alunni, A., Joly, J.-S., Jeffery, W. R., & Retaux, S. (2007). Expanded expression of Sonic Hedgehog in *Astyanax* cavefish: Multiple consequences on forebrain development and evolution. *Development, 134*(5), 845–855. https://doi.org/10.1242/dev.02780

Mitashov, V. I., & Vassetzky, S. G. (2000). L. Wolpert "Principles of development," Oxford University Press, 1998. *Russian Journal of Developmental Biology, 31*(3), 193–196. https://doi.org/10.1007/BF02758827

Mizoguchi, A., Eguchi, N., Kimura, K., Kiyohara, Y., Qu, W.-M., Huang, Z.-L., Mochizuki, T., Lazarus, M., Kobayashi, T., Kaneko, T., Narumiya, S., Urade, Y., & Hayaishi, O. (2001). Dominant localization of prostaglandin D receptors on arachnoid trabecular cells in mouse basal forebrain and their involvement in the regulation of non-rapid eye movement sleep. *Proceedings of the National Academy of Sciences of the United States of America, 98*(20), 11674–11679. https://doi.org/10.1073/pnas.201398898

Moens, C. B., & Prince, V. E. (2002). Constructing the hindbrain: Insights from the zebrafish. *Developmental Dynamics, 224*(1), 1–17. https://doi.org/10.1002/dvdy.10086

Morgan, T. H. (1910). Sex limited inheritance in *Drosophila*. *Science, 32*(812), 120–122. https://doi.org/10.1126/science.32.812.120

Morrison, A. R. (2014). Henri Piéron and Nathaniel Kleitman: Two major figures of 20th century sleep research. *Sleep, 37*(3), 621. https://doi.org/10.5665/sleep.3512

Mourrain, P., & Wang, G. X. (2019). Sleep: DNA repair function for better neuronal aging? *Current Biology, 29*(12), R585–R588. https://doi.org/10.1016/j.cub.2019.05.018

Mutsuga, N., Iwasaki, Y., Morishita, M., Nomura, A., Yamamori, E., Yoshida, M., Asai, M., Ozaki, N., Kambe, F., Seo, H., Oiso, Y., & Saito, H. (2001). Homeobox protein Gsh-1-dependent regulation of the rat GHRH gene promoter. *Molecular Endocrinology, 15*(12), 2149–2156. https://doi.org/10.1210/mend.15.12.0747

Nadjar, A., Blutstein, T., Aubert, A., Laye, S., & Haydon, P. G. (2013). Astrocyte-derived adenosine modulates increased sleep pressure during inflammatory response. *Glia, 61*(5), 724–731. https://doi.org/10.1002/glia.22465

Narumiya, S., Ogorochi, T., Nakao, K., & Hayaishi, O. (1982). Prostaglandin D2 in rat brain, spinal cord and pituitary: Basal level and regional distribution. *Life Sciences, 31*(19), 2093–2103.

Nelson, M. D., Lee, K. H., Churgin, M. A., Hill, A. J., Van Buskirk, C., Fang-Yen, C., & . (2014). FMRFamide-like FLP-13 neuropeptides promote quiescence following heat stress in *Caenorhabditis elegans*. *Current Biology, 24*(20), 2406–2410. https://doi.org/10.1016/j.cub.2014.08.037

Neurath, P. W., & Berliner, M. D. (1964). Biological rhythms: A new type in strains of a mutant of *Neurospora crassa*. *Science, 146*(3644), 646–647. https://doi.org/10.1126/science.146.3644.646

Nieuwkoop, P. D. (1947). Investigations on the regional determination of the central nervous system. *Journal of Experimental Biology, 24*(1–2), 145–183.

Niwa, Y., Kanda, G. N., Yamada, R. G., Shi, S., Sunagawa, G. A., Ukai-Tadenuma, M., Fujishima, H., Matsumoto, N., Masumoto, K.-h., Nagano, M., Kasukawa, T., Galloway, J., Perrin, D., Shigeyoshi, Y., Ukai, H., Kiyonari, H., Sumiyama, K., & Ueda, H. R. (2018). Muscarinic acetylcholine receptors chrm1 and chrm3 are essential for REM sleep. *Cell Reports, 24*(9), 2231–2247.e7. https://doi.org/10.1016/j.celrep.2018.07.082

Novotný, J. (2015). Adenosin a jeho role ve fyziologii [Adenosine and its role in physiology]. *Ceskoslovenska fysiologie/Ustredni ustav biologicky, 64*(1), 35–44.

Nunez, P. L. (1981). A study of origins of the time dependencies of scalp EEG: I—Theoretical basis. *IEEE Transactions on Bio-Medical Engineering, 28*(3), 271–280. https://doi.org/10.1109/tbme.1981.324700

Ogorochi, T., Narumiya, S., Mizuno, N., Yamashita, K., Miyazaki, H., & Hayaishi, O. (1984). Regional distribution of prostaglandins D2, E2, and F2 alpha and related enzymes in postmortem human brain. *Journal of Neurochemistry, 43*(1), 71–82. https://doi.org/10.1111/j.1471-4159.1984.tb06680.x

Oh, Y., Jang, D., Sonn, J. Y., & Choe, J. (2013). Histamine–HisCl1 receptor axis regulates wake-promoting signals in *Drosophila melanogaster*. *PLOS ONE, 8*(7), Article e68269. https://doi.org/10.1371/journal.pone.0068269

Padmanabhan, K., Robles, M. S., Westerling, T., & Weitz, C. J. (2012). Feedback regulation of transcriptional termination by the mammalian circadian clock PERIOD complex. *Science, 337*(6094), 599–602. https://doi.org/10.1126/science.1221592

Pandey, H. P., Ram, A., Matsumura, H., & Hayaishi, O. (1995). Concentration of prostaglandin D2 in cerebrospinal fluid exhibits a circadian alteration in conscious rats. *Biochemistry and Molecular Biology International, 37*(3), 431–437.

Patke, A., Murphy, P. J., Onat, O. E., Krieger, A. C., Ozcelik, T., Campbell, S. S., & Young, M. W. (2017). Mutation of the human circadian clock gene CRY1 in familial delayed sleep phase disorder. *Cell, 169*(2), 203–215.e13. https://doi.org/10.1016/j.cell.2017.03.027

Pearson, C. A., & Placzek, M. (2013). Development of the medial hypothalamus: Forming a functional hypothalamic–neurohypophyseal interface. In P. Thomas (Ed.), *Endocrine gland development and disease. Current Topics in Developmental Biology* (Vol. 106, pp. 49–88). Academic Press. https://doi.org/10.1016/B978-0-12-416021-7.00002-X

Peng, W., Liu, X., Ma, G., Wu, Z., Wang, Z., Fei, X., Qin, M., Wang, L., Li, Y., Zhang, S., & Xu, M. (2023). Adenosine-independent regulation of the sleep–wake cycle by astrocyte activity. *Cell Discovery*, *9*(1), Article 16. https://doi.org/10.1038/s41421-022-00498-9

Peng, W., Wu, Z., Song, K., Zhang, S., Li, Y., & Xu, M. (2020). Regulation of sleep homeostasis mediator adenosine by basal forebrain glutamatergic neurons. *Science*, *369*(6508), Article eabb0556. https://doi.org/10.1126/science.abb0556

Pentikäinen, P. J., Valtonen, V. V., & Miettinen, T. A. (1976). Deaths in connection with chlormethiazole (heminevrin) therapy. *International Journal of Clinical Pharmacology and Biopharmacy*, *14*(3), 225–230.

Petit, J. M., & Magistretti, P. J. (2016). Regulation of neuron–astrocyte metabolic coupling across the sleep–wake cycle. *Neuroscience*, *323*, 135–156. https://doi.org/10.1016/j.neuroscience.2015.12.007

Peyron, C., Sapin, E., Leger, L., Luppi, P.-H., & Fort, P. (2009). Role of the melanin-concentrating hormone neuropeptide in sleep regulation. *Peptides*, *30*(11), 2052–2059. https://doi.org/10.1016/j.peptides.2009.07.022

Porkka-Heiskanen, T. (2013). Sleep homeostasis. *Current Opinion in Neurobiology*, *23*(5), 799–805. https://doi.org/10.1016/j.conb.2013.02.010

Porkka-Heiskanen, T., Strecker, R. E., & McCarley, R. W. (2000). Brain site-specificity of extracellular adenosine concentration changes during sleep deprivation and spontaneous sleep: An in vivo microdialysis study. *Neuroscience*, *99*(3), 507–517. https://doi.org/10.1016/s0306-4522(00)00220-7

Pottin, K., Hinaux, H., & Rétaux, S. (2011). Restoring eye size in *Astyanax mexicanus* blind cavefish embryos through modulation of the Shh and Fgf8 forebrain organising centres. *Development*, *138*(12), 2467–2476. https://doi.org/10.1242/dev.054106

Rainnie, D. G., Grunze, H. C. R., McCarley, R. W., & Greene, R. W. (1994). Adenosine inhibition of mesopontine cholinergic neurons: Implications for EEG arousal. *Science*, *263*(5147), 689–692. https://doi.org/10.1126/science.8303279

Raizen, D. M., Zimmerman, J. E., Maycock, M. H., Ta, U. D., You, Y.-J., Sundaram, M. V., & Pack, A. I. (2008). Lethargus is a *Caenorhabditis elegans* sleep-like state. *Nature*, *451*(7178), 569–572. https://doi.org/10.1038/nature06535

Ram, A., Pandey, H. P., Matsumura, H., Kasahara-Orita, K., Nakajima, T., Takahata, R., Satoh, S., Terao, A., & Hayaishi, O. (1997). CSF levels of prostaglandins, especially the level of prostaglandin D2, are correlated with increasing propensity towards sleep in rats. *Brain Research*, *751*(1), 81–89. https://doi.org/10.1016/s0006-8993(96)01401-1

Rétaux, S., Pottin, K., & Alunni, A. (2008). Shh and forebrain evolution in the blind cavefish *Astyanax mexicanus*. *Biology of the Cell*, *100*(3), 139–147. https://doi.org/10.1042/BC20070084

Rétey, J. V., Adam, M., Honegger, E., Khatami, R., Luhmann, U. F. O., Jung, H. H., Berger, W., & Landolt, H.-P. (2005). A functional genetic variation of adenosine deaminase affects the duration and intensity of deep sleep in humans. *Proceedings of the National Academy of Sciences of the United States of America*, *102*(43), 15676–15681. https://doi.org/10.1073/pnas.0505414102

Rieder, L. E., & Larschan, E. N. (2014). Wisdom from the fly. *Trends in Genetics*, *30*(11), 479–481. https://doi.org/10.1016/j.tig.2014.08.003

Robson, S. C., Sévigny, J., & Zimmermann, H. (2006). The E-NTPDase family of ectonucleotidases: Structure function relationships and pathophysiological significance. *Purinergic Signalling*, *2*(2), 409–430. https://doi.org/10.1007/s11302-006-9003-5

Rockstrom, M. D., Chen, L., Taishi, P., Nguyen, J. T., Gibbons, C. M., Veasey, S. C., & Krueger, J. M. (2018). Tumor necrosis factor alpha in sleep regulation. *Sleep Medicine Reviews*, *40*, 69–78. https://doi.org/10.1016/j.smrv.2017.10.005

Scholpp, S., & Lumsden, A. (2010). Building a bridal chamber: Development of the thalamus. *Trends in Neurosciences*, *33*(8), 373–380. https://doi.org/10.1016/j.tins.2010.05.003

Sehgal, A. (1995). Molecular genetic analysis of circadian rhythms in vertebrates and invertebrates. *Current Opinion in Neurobiology*, *5*(6), 824–831. https://doi.org/10.1016/0959-4388(95)80112-x

Shaw, P. J., Cirelli, C., Greenspan, R. J., & Tononi, G. (2000). Correlates of sleep and waking in *Drosophila melanogaster*. *Science*, *287*(5459), 1834–1837. https://doi.org/10.1126/science.287.5459.1834

Shi, M., Yue, Z., Kuryatov, A., Lindstrom, J. M., & Sehgal, A. (2014). Identification of Redeye, a new sleep-regulating protein whose expression is modulated by sleep amount. *eLife*, *3*, Article e01473. https://doi.org/10.7554/eLife.01473

Shirasaki, R., & Pfaff, S. L. (2002). Transcriptional codes and the control of neuronal identity. *Annual Review of Neuroscience, 25*, 251–281. https://doi.org/10.1146/annurev.neuro.25.112701.142916

Shoham, S., Davenne, D., Cady, A. B., Dinarello, C. A., & Krueger, J. M. (1987). Recombinant tumor necrosis factor and interleukin 1 enhance slow-wave sleep. *American Journal of Physiology: Regulatory, Integrative and Comparative Physiology, 253*(1 Pt. 2), R142–R149. https://doi.org/10.1152/ajpregu.1987.253.1.R142

Sims, R. E., Wu, H. H. T., & Dale, N. (2013). Sleep–wake sensitive mechanisms of adenosine release in the basal forebrain of rodents: An in vitro study. *PLOS ONE, 8*(1), Article e53814. https://doi.org/10.1371/journal.pone.0053814

Simunek, M., Hossfeld, U., & Wissemann, V. (2011). "Rediscovery" revised—The cooperation of Erich and Armin von Tschermak-Seysenegg in the context of the "rediscovery" of Mendel's laws in 1899–1901. *Plant Biology, 13*(6), 835–841. https://doi.org/10.1111/j.1438-8677.2011.00491.x

Singh, C., Oikonomou, G., & Prober, D. A. (2015). Norepinephrine is required to promote wakefulness and for hypocretin-induced arousal in zebrafish. *eLife, 4*, Article e07000. https://doi.org/10.7554/eLife.07000

Singh, C., Rihel, J., & Prober, D. A. (2017). Neuropeptide Y regulates sleep by modulating noradrenergic signaling. *Current Biology, 27*(24), 3796–3811.e5. https://doi.org/10.1016/j.cub.2017.11.018

Slonimski, P. P., Cooper, T. G., & von Borstel, R. C. J. (2016). Piotr P. Slonimski—The Warrior Pope: The discovery of mitochondrial (petite) mutants and split genes. *FEMS Yeast Research, 16*(2), Article fow004. https://doi.org/10.1093/femsyr/fow004

Slonimski, P. P., Perrodin, G., & Croft, J. H. (1968). Ethidium bromide induced mutation of yeast mitochondria: Complete transformation of cells into respiratory deficient non-chromosomal "petites." *Biochemical and Biophysical Research Communications, 30*(3), 232–239. https://doi.org/10.1016/0006-291X(68)90440-3

Stassen, H. H., Lykken, D. T., Propping, P., & Bomben, G. (1988). Genetic determination of the human EEG. Survey of recent results on twins reared together and apart. *Human Genetics, 80*(2), 165–176. https://doi.org/10.1007/BF00702862

Stenberg, D., Litonius, E., Halldner, L., Johansson, B., Fredholm, B. B., & Porkka-Heiskanen, T. (2003). Sleep and its homeostatic regulation in mice lacking the adenosine A1 receptor. *Journal of Sleep Research, 12*(4), 283–290. https://doi.org/10.1046/j.0962-1105.2003.00367.x

Strickler, A. G., Yamamoto, Y., & Jeffery, W. R. (2001). Early and late changes in *Pax6* expression accompany eye degeneration during cavefish development. *Development Genes and Evolution, 211*(3), 138–144. https://doi.org/10.1007/s004270000123

Sturtevant, A. H., Bridges, C. B., & Morgan, T. H. (1919). The spatial relations of genes. *Proceedings of the National Academy of Sciences of the United States of America, 5*(5), 168–173. https://doi.org/10.1073/pnas.5.5.168

Szarek, E., Cheah, P.-S., Schwartz, J., & Thomas, P. (2010). Molecular genetics of the developing neuroendocrine hypothalamus. *Molecular and Cellular Endocrinology, 323*(1), 115–123. https://doi.org/10.1016/j.mce.2010.04.002

Takahashi, J. S. (1999). Narcolepsy genes wake up the sleep field. *Science, 285*(5436), 2076–2077. https://doi.org/10.1126/science.285.5436.2076

Tatemoto, K., Carlquist, M., & Mutt, V. (1982). Neuropeptide Y—A novel brain peptide with structural similarities to peptide YY and pancreatic polypeptide. *Nature, 296*(5858), 659–660. https://doi.org/10.1038/296659a0

Thakkar, M. M., Delgiacco, R. A., Strecker, R. E., & McCarley, R. W. (2003). Adenosinergic inhibition of basal forebrain wakefulness-active neurons: A simultaneous unit recording and microdialysis study in freely behaving cats. *Neuroscience, 122*(4), 1107–1113. https://doi.org/10.1016/j.neuroscience.2003.08.006

Tobler, I. (1983). Effect of forced locomotion on the rest–activity cycle of the cockroach. *Behavioural Brain Research, 8*(3), 351–360. https://doi.org/10.1016/0166-4328(83)90180-8

Tobler, I., & Neuner-Jehle, M. (1992). 24-h variation of vigilance in the cockroach *Blaberus giganteus*. *Journal of Sleep Research, 1*(4), 231–239. https://doi.org/10.1111/j.1365-2869.1992.tb00044.x

Toda, H., Williams, J. A., Gulledge, M., & Sehgal, A. (2019). A sleep-inducing gene, *nemuri*, links sleep and immune function in *Drosophila*. *Science, 363*(6426), 509–515. https://doi.org/10.1126/science.aat1650

Toh, K. L., Jones, C. R., He, Y., Eide, E. J., Hinz, W. A., Virshup, D. M., Ptacek, L. J., & Fu. Y.-H. (2001). An h*Per2* phosphorylation site mutation in familial advanced sleep phase syndrome. *Science, 291*(5506), 1040–1043. https://doi.org/10.1126/science.1057499

Tononi, G., & Cirelli, C. (2014). Sleep and the price of plasticity: From synaptic and cellular homeostasis to memory consolidation and integration. *Neuron*, *81*(1), 12–34. https://doi.org/10.1016/j.neuron.2013.12.025

Tóth, A., Hajnik, T., Zaborszky, L., & Detari, L. (2007). Effect of basal forebrain neuropeptide Y administration on sleep and spontaneous behavior in freely moving rats. *Brain Research Bulletin*, *72*(4–6), 293–301. https://doi.org/10.1016/j.brainresbull.2007.01.006

Ueno, R., Ishikawa, Y., Nakayama, T., & Hayaishi, O. (1982). Prostaglandin D2 induces sleep when microinjected into the preoptic area of conscious rats. *Biochemical and Biophysical Research Communications*, *109*(2), 576–582. https://doi.org/10.1016/0006-291x(82)91760-0

Urade, Y., Kitahama, K., Ohishi, H., Kaneko, T., Mizuno, N., & Hayaishi, O. (1993). Dominant expression of mRNA for prostaglandin D synthase in leptomeninges, choroid plexus, and oligodendrocytes of the adult rat brain. *Proceedings of the National Academy of Sciences of the United States of America*, *90*(19), 9070–9074. https://doi.org/10.1073/pnas.90.19.9070

van Alphen, B., Semenza, E. R., Yap, M., van Swinderen, B., & Allada, R. (2021). A deep sleep stage in *Drosophila* with a functional role in waste clearance. *Science Advances*, *7*(4), Article eabc2999. https://doi.org/10.1126/sciadv.abc2999

Van Baal, G. C., De Geus, E. J., & Boomsma, D. I. (1996). Genetic architecture of EEG power spectra in early life. *Electroencephalography and Clinical Neurophysiology*, *98*(6), 502–514. https://doi.org/10.1016/0013-4694(96)95601-1

van Beijsterveldt, C. E., Molenaar, P. C., de Geus, E. J., & Boomsma, D. I. (1996). Heritability of human brain functioning as assessed by electroencephalography. *American Journal of Human Genetics*, *58*(3), 562–573.

van den Pol, A. N. (2012). Neuropeptide transmission in brain circuits. *Neuron*, *76*(1), 98–115. https://doi.org/10.1016/j.neuron.2012.09.014

Vanderheyden, W. M., Goodman, A. G., Taylor, R. H., Frank, M. G., Van Dongen, H. P. A., & Gerstner, J. R. (2018). Astrocyte expression of the *Drosophila* TNF-alpha homologue, Eiger, regulates sleep in flies. *PLOS Genetics*, *14*(10), Article e1007724. https://doi.org/10.1371/journal.pgen.1007724

Vassarotti, A., & Goffeau, A. (1992). Sequencing the yeast genome: The European effort. *Trends in Biotechnology*, *10*(1–2), 15–18. https://doi.org/10.1016/0167-7799(92)90160-w

Verret, L., Goutagny, R., Fort, P., Cagnon, L., Salvert, D., Leger, L., Boissard, R., Salin, P., Peyron, C., & Luppi, P.-H. (2003). A role of melanin-concentrating hormone producing neurons in the central regulation of paradoxical sleep. *BMC Neuroscience*, *4*, Article 19. https://doi.org/10.1186/1471-2202-4-19

Vorster, A. P. A., Biol, D., Krishnan, H. C., Cirelli, C., & Lyons, L. C. (2014). Characterization of sleep in *Aplysia californica*. *Sleep*, *37*(9), 1453–1463. https://doi.org/10.5665/sleep.3992

Watson, J. D. (1990). The Human Genome Project: Past, present, and future. *Science*, *248*(4951), 44–49. https://doi.org/10.1126/science.2181665

Webb, W. B., & Campbell, S. S. (1983). Relationships in sleep characteristics of identical and fraternal twins. *Archives of General Psychiatry*, *40*(10), 1093–1095. https://doi.org/10.1001/archpsyc.1983.01790090055008

Whitton, J. L., Elgie, S. M., Kugel, H., & Moldofsky, H. (1985). Genetic dependence of the electroencephalogram bispectrum. *Electroencephalography and Clinical Neurophysiology*, *60*(4), 293–298. https://doi.org/10.1016/0013-4694(85)90002-1

Xie, L., Kang, H., Xu, Q., Chen, M. J., Liao, Y., Thiyagarajan, M., O'Donnell, J., Christensen, D. J., Nicholson, C., Iliff, J. J., Takano, T., Deane, R., & Nedergaard, M. (2013). Sleep drives metabolite clearance from the adult brain. *Science*, *342*(6156), 373–377. https://doi.org/10.1126/science.1241224

Xu, Y., Padiath, Q. S., Shapiro, R. E., Jones, C. R., Wu, S. C., Saigoh, N., Saigoh, K., Ptacek, L. J., & Fu, Y.-H. (2005). Functional consequences of a CKIdelta mutation causing familial advanced sleep phase syndrome. *Nature*, *434*(7033), 640–644. https://doi.org/10.1038/nature03453

Yamamoto, Y., Stock, D. W., & Jeffery, W. R. (2004). Hedgehog signalling controls eye degeneration in blind cavefish. *Nature*, *431*(7010), 844–847. https://doi.org/10.1038/nature02864

Yee, C. L., Wang, Y., Anderson, S., Ekker, M., & Rubenstein, J. L. R. (2009). Arcuate nucleus expression of NKX2.1 and DLX and lineages expressing these transcription factors in neuropeptide Y(+), proopiomelanocortin(+), and tyrosine hydroxylase(+) neurons in neonatal and adult mice. *The Journal of Comparative Neurology*, *517*(1), 37–50. https://doi.org/10.1002/cne.22132

Yin, Y., Liu, Y., Pan, X., Chen, R., Li, P., Wu, H.-J., Zhao, Z.-Q., Li, Y.-P., Huang, L.-Q., Zhuang, J.-H., & Zhao, Z.-X. (2016). Interleukin-1β promoter polymorphism enhances the risk of sleep disturbance in Alzheimer's disease. *PLOS ONE, 11*(3), Article e0149945. https://doi.org/10.1371/journal.pone.0149945

Yokogawa, T., Marin, W., Faraco, J., Pezeron, G., Appelbaum, L., Zhang, J., Rosa, F., Mourrain, P., & Mignot, E. (2007). Characterization of sleep in zebrafish and insomnia in hypocretin receptor mutants. *PLOS Biology, 5*(10), Article e277. https://doi.org/10.1371/journal.pbio.0050277

Yoo, S.-H., Mohawk, J. A., Siepka, S. M., Shan, Y., Huh, S. K., Hong, H.-K., Kornblum, I., Kumar, V., Koike, N., Xu, M., Nussbaum, J., Liu, X., Chen, Z., Chen, Z. J., Green, C. B., & Takahashi, J. S. (2013). Competing E3 ubiquitin ligases govern circadian periodicity by degradation of CRY in nucleus and cytoplasm. *Cell, 152*(5), 1091–1105. https://doi.org/10.1016/j.cell.2013.01.055

Yoshizawa, M., Robinson, B. G., Duboue, E. R., Masek, P., Jaggard, J. B., O'Quin, K. E., Borowsky, R. L., Jeffery, W. R., & Keene, A. C. (2015). Distinct genetic architecture underlies the emergence of sleep loss and prey-seeking behavior in the Mexican cavefish. *BMC Biology, 13*, Article 15. https://doi.org/10.1186/s12915-015-0119-3

Zamir, N., Skofitsch, G., Bannon, M. J., & Jacobowitz, D. M. (1986). Melanin-concentrating hormone: Unique peptide neuronal system in the rat brain and pituitary gland. *Proceedings of the National Academy of Sciences of the United States of America, 83*(5), 1528–1531. https://doi.org/10.1073/pnas.83.5.1528

Zhang, L., Hirano, A., Hsu, P.-K., Jones, C. R., Sakai, N., Okuro, M., McMahon, T., Yamazaki, M., Xu, Y., Saigoh, N., Saigoh, K., Lin, S.-T., Kaasik, K., Nishino, S., Ptacek, L. J., & Fu, Y.-H. (2016). A PERIOD3 variant causes a circadian phenotype and is associated with a seasonal mood trait. *Proceedings of the National Academy of Sciences of the United States of America, 113*(11), E1536–E1544. https://doi.org/10.1073/pnas.1600039113

Zielinski, M. R., Dunbrasky, D. L., Taishi, P., Souza, G., & Krueger, J. M. (2013). Vagotomy attenuates brain cytokines and sleep induced by peripherally administered tumor necrosis factor-α and lipopolysaccharide in mice. *Sleep, 36*(8), 1227–1238. https://doi.org/10.5665/sleep.2892

Zini, I., Pich, E. M., Fuxe, K., Lenzl, P. L., Agnati, L. F., Harfstrand, A., Mutt, V., Tatemoto, K., & Moscara, M. (1984). Actions of centrally administered neuropeptide Y on EEG activity in different rat strains and in different phases of their circadian cycle. *Acta Physiologica Scandinavica, 122*(1), 71–77. https://doi.org/10.1111/j.1748-1716.1984.tb07483.x

CHAPTER

6 Local Sleep

Vladyslav V. Vyazovskiy *and* Thomas Andrillon

Abstract

Sleep–wake states arise from a dynamic interplay across local and brain-wide brain circuitries, which allow the coordination of intrinsic homeostatic needs with environmental contingencies. Historically, sleep was viewed as a global phenomenon imposed on the organism from a limited set of subcortical neural centers, yet the role of local, activity-dependent processes in sleep control is becoming increasingly appreciated. Likewise, while the suprachiasmatic nucleus has been established as a central master clock of the brain, local clocks distributed throughout the brain and the body are now recognized as an essential component in the circadian regulation of a range of essential functions from metabolism to synaptic plasticity. Recent studies demonstrate that intrusion of local sleep-like patterns of neural activity into wakefulness reflect use-dependent processes, related to metabolism and synaptic plasticity. In turn, local sleep affects the responsiveness of neurons to incoming inputs and the processing of external information and may underlie a range of subjective experiences—from sleep inertia to mind-wandering. The function of local sleep remains not sufficiently understood, and the authors only begin to unravel how coordinated activity within the hierarchy of local and global brain networks involved in sleep regulation render stability and homeostasis.

Key Words: sleep–wake state, brain, suprachiasmatic nucleus, neural activity, local sleep, brain network, sleep regulation

Multilayered Regulation of Sleep

Behaviorally, sleep is defined as a reversible state of inactivity, whereby sensory responsiveness is reduced (Campbell & Tobler, 1984). Electrophysiologically, the predominant stage of sleep—non-rapid-eye-movement (NREM) sleep—is defined by the presence of so-called slow-wave activity (SWA; electroencephalographic [EEG] or local field potential oscillations occurring at around 1–4 Hz) recorded from the neocortex and other brain areas (Adamantidis et al., 2019; Vyazovskiy & Harris, 2013). It is now widely accepted that sleep is not an all-or-none phenomenon. Instead, sleep is characterized by pronounced fluctuations or systematic trends at several distinct temporal scales—from a moment-to-moment fast modulation of the activity in cortical and subcortical networks to slow changes in sleep propensity and sleep intensity across hours or days.

Two fundamental processes are responsible for the amount, intensity, and temporal dynamics of sleep and wakefulness at the level of an individual organism. The first process arises from a 24-hour rhythmicity, imposed by the circadian clock, which is controlled by the central pacemaker in the suprachiasmatic nucleus (SCN; Hastings et al., 2018; Mendoza & Challet, 2009). The existence of a circadian control is thought to ensure that a broad range of bodily functions, behavior, and physiology are precisely timed with respect to periodic changes in the environment (Bass & Takahashi, 2010; Fisher et al., 2013). The second process refers to the maintenance of a species-specific amount of sleep across 24 hours, whereby an initial sleep loss is compensated by a later increase in its amount and intensity (Borbely et al., 2016). This latter process, traditionally called *sleep homeostasis*, accounts for daily deviations in the amount of sleep from a species-specific set point, while ensuring that it is maintained within a stable range (Thomas et al., 2020).

The circadian system has a complex organization, which is thought to be essential for generation and maintenance of stable 24-hour rhythms (Pilorz et al., 2020). Circadian rhythms can be measured at two distinct levels: from isolated cells taken from different tissues and organs (Saini et al., 2011) to the whole-animal behavior (L. A. Brown et al., 2019; Siepka & Takahashi, 2005). Circadian gene expression was found in most, if not all, cells of the brain and the body (Brancaccio et al., 2019; Castillo et al., 2011; Saini et al., 2011), but only in the SCN were the molecular rhythms shown to be tightly coupled with electrical activity of neurons (Colwell, 2011). Since each cell in the SCN represents an autonomous oscillator with a period different from the majority of other cells, intra-SCN coupling mechanisms are essential to allow averaging of diverse phases, which results in a stable circadian period of the whole SCN and the whole animal (C. Liu et al., 1997; Pilorz et al., 2020). Furthermore, environmental factors also appear to play a critical role. The endogenous circadian rhythm in the SCN is entrained through photic and non-photic cues (Hastings et al., 2018; S. Hughes et al., 2015). While the molecular mechanisms involved in the effects of light on the molecular clockwork in the SCN have been well elucidated (Golombek & Rosenstein, 2010; Jagannath et al., 2013), the role of non-photic cues in circadian entrainment has received less attention (Hastings et al., 1997; Maywood et al., 1999).

There is a bidirectional relationship between brain state, reflected in the patterns of neural network activity, and behavior, which are both modulated by preceding sleep–wake history. For example, wheel-running decreases cortical neural activity, especially during high-speed stereotypic locomotion (Fisher et al., 2016), and was shown to influence the amount and timing of sleep (Vyazovskiy & Tobler, 2012). Sleep homeostasis is a ubiquitous phenomenon found in all animal species studied so far, suggesting that it concerns some fundamental function (Tobler, 2005; Vyazovskiy & Harris, 2013). Sleep pressure increases as a function of time spent awake and decreases in the course of sleep. The best-characterized physiological indicator of sleep–wake history is the level of cortical EEG SWA during NREM sleep (Borbely, 1982; Borbely & Achermann, 2000; Daan et al.,

1984; Vyazovskiy, Achermann, & Tobler, 2007). In mammals, sleep SWA is high in early sleep and after sleep deprivation, when sleep pressure is increased physiologically, and decreases progressively to reach low levels in late sleep (Franken et al., 2001; Tobler & Borbely, 1986; Vyazovskiy, Achermann, & Tobler, 2007). Typically, SWA during wakefulness is low, when the high tone of arousal-promoting neuromodulators prevents large-scale synchronization among the cortical neurons (Steriade, Amzica, & Nunez, 1993). Although it has been long suggested that SWA is linked to restorative processes occurring during sleep, this possibility, albeit intuitive and attractive, has not been conclusively proven or disproven (Frank & Heller, 2019).

The common view is that the molecular and cerebral networks responsible for the occurrence and temporal organization of sleep and its numerous characteristics represent a distributed system. Indeed, sleep is thought to be regulated through a dynamic interplay across a widely distributed network of subcortical nuclei, including the hypothalamus, the basal forebrain, the brainstem, the basal ganglia, and the neocortex (D. Liu & Dan, 2019; Saper et al., 2010). Numerous studies have been performed to dissect the contribution of specific subcortical structures into sleep behavior and regulation, yet these result in the ever-growing complexity of the network of putative sleep- or wake-promoting structures, whose function as a whole is still not understood (Yamagata et al., 2021). Likewise, while the SCN represents a major node in the neuroanatomical circadian network, there is evidence for a widely distributed network of tightly coupled local circadian oscillators across the brain (Pilorz et al., 2020). It remains to be understood how the balance between local and global control of sleep is achieved and what the contribution of specific levels of organization is in the overall sleep-wake organization.

Regulation of Local Sleep

First and foremost, sleep is defined as a global behavioral state, characterized by immobility and elevated arousal threshold. In recent decades considerable progress has been made with respect to delineating the role of specific brain structures and neurophysiological correlates of these fundamental characteristics of sleep. However, the question remains how fine is the spatial and temporal resolution that can be achieved to provide meaningful insights into brain mechanisms of sleep and wakefulness without losing the big picture?

The now prevailing idea that global wakefulness and sleep are imposed on the brain and the body by a limited set of subcortical structures was motivated by pioneering observations made by Constantin von Economo in patients with encephalitis lethargica (Economo, 1930). Importantly, polysomnography did not exist when the consequences of encephalitis lethargica were first described, and therefore caution is warranted when interpreting these early observations (Ward, 2011). The first sleep recordings were performed in the 1930s by Alfred Loomis et al. (1935a, 1935b), and it was not until several decades later that full-night EEG was first obtained and became a gold-standard approach for sleep studies (Dement & Kleitman, 1957). Although sleep is typically viewed as a global behavioral state, observations that sleep patterns occur locally were first made more than 50 years ago.

> We are now faced with a much more complex mechanism of sleep than was previously thought. . . . Clinicians have long suspected that partial sleep must be possible, i.e., that parts of the brain may rest while others are involved in waking activity, although they thought that these were exceptions. It now seems that this is rather the rule. And when we come to think of it, it may not be surprising that neuronal networks with such different structures, different functions and different loads of work need also different modes of rest and recovery. (Hess, 1964, pp. 45–55)

Electrophysiologically, sleep is distinguished from wakefulness by characteristic patterns of cortical neuronal activity, such as sleep spindles (bursts of neural activity of 10–15 Hz) and slow waves (0.5–4 Hz), occurring in isolation or in trains (Adamantidis et al., 2019). At the neuronal level, slow waves are characterized by an alternation between off (inactive) and on (active) periods in large neuronal assemblies (Vyazovskiy & Harris, 2013). However, these two types of brain oscillations reflect not only and not simply whether the subject is awake or asleep. Sleep is not a stable, homogenous process but shows substantial variations in activity across the brain and across time. These regional modulations of sleep are especially prominent in marine mammals, who display a phenomenon of unihemispheric sleep in which the two brain hemispheres show brain activity characteristic of either sleep or wakefulness (Mukhametov et al., 1977). Unihemispheric sleep has been thought of as an adaptation to the environmental niche of marine mammals, which cannot remain immobile during their sleep (Rattenborg et al., 2000). In humans, parasomnias, such as sleepwalking, are dissociated states in which some brain regions (e.g., frontal cortices) display sleep activity while other brain regions (e.g., motor cortices) show signs of arousal, demonstrating that sleep and wake patterns of activity can coexist in distinct neural networks (Baldini et al., 2019; Castelnovo et al., 2018; Nobili et al., 2012).

Recent research has demonstrated how the concept of "local sleep" can extend beyond these specific animal species or sleep disorders. Sleep is not an all-or-none phenomenon but a dynamic process characterized by specific spatiotemporal dynamics of cortical activity. It is especially apparent within individual single sleep episodes, when sleep progresses from the thalamus to the cortex (Magnin et al., 2010) and invariably starts with shallow stages, as characterized by low values of SWA and sparse occurrence of local slow waves but becomes progressively more intense, as tracked by an increase in SWA across time (Aeschbach et al., 1996; Vyazovskiy et al., 2004b). The mechanisms governing this dynamic are not known, and at least two factors can play a role. First, as is well known, falling asleep is precipitated by a withdrawal of ascending activating influence arising from neuromodulatory subcortical areas (Steriade, 1993; Steriade & Amzica,

1998; Steriade, Amzica, & Nunez, 1993). The change in neuromodulatory milieu alters voltage-dependent properties of fast-acting ionic channels, thereby producing global shifts in neuronal membrane potential (McCormick, 1992). In addition, withdrawal of global generalized activation can tilt the balance toward increased local neuromodulation that could involve slow-acting metabotropic receptors, such as gamma-aminobutyric acid (GABA) B, which are responsible for producing slow hyperpolarization potentials (Kohl & Paulsen, 2010; Mann et al., 2009). It is yet unclear whether arousal-promoting neuromodulators change gradually across the sleep episode or decrease all at once at sleep onset.

It was shown that upon falling sleep there are consistent delays in the range of minutes in the measures of deactivation between the thalamus and the neocortex, and "falling asleep" time was also heterogeneous between cortical regions (Magnin et al., 2010). Consistently, another human study showed pronounced frequency-specific regional differences in the EEG during the first 30 minutes of the first sleep episode (Ferrara et al., 2002). Conversely, in the first minutes of wakefulness, brain activity is characterized by sleep-like patterns, which likely underlies the subjective experience of sleep inertia (Vyazovskiy et al., 2014).

Since the size of slow waves is directly related to synchronization in local and global cortical networks (Nir et al., 2011; Vyazovskiy, Olcese, et al., 2009), a progressive increase in the number of high-amplitude slow waves should, at least indirectly, reflect a progressive increase in global cortical synchrony. Indeed, it has been shown in both humans (Massimini et al., 2004) and rats (Vyazovskiy, Faraguna, et al., 2009) that incidence of high-amplitude slow waves increases across individual sleep episodes. It remains to be determined, however, whether such an increase is accounted by intracortical networks or involves the thalamocortical loop or other subcortical areas. Efficient mechanisms of intracortical synchronization are known to be crucially important for shaping cortical network oscillations on a faster timescale of hundreds of milliseconds. For example, it has been shown that cortical propagation of sleep slow waves is facilitated by long-range recruitment of distributed cortical networks in the global slow oscillation (Esser et al., 2007; Massimini et al., 2004; Nir et al., 2011; Riedner et al., 2007; Vyazovskiy, Faraguna, et al., 2009; Vyazovskiy, Olcese, et al., 2011; Vyazovskiy, Riedner, et al., 2007). The progression of local events into global slow waves can be facilitated by their propagation along specific pathways with strongest synaptic connectivity (Murphy et al., 2009). Direct corticocortical connections are likely to play an important role in such propagation as the latencies were invariably shortest to the contralateral homotopic areas connected to the origins by the direct callosal excitatory fibers (Cisse et al., 2004).

As sleep progresses, moment-to-moment variations in SWA within a local recording site remain substantial (Tobler & Borbely, 1986; Trachsel et al., 1989; Vyazovskiy, Faraguna, et al., 2009) and show pronounced systematic changes on a slow timescale. Generally, sleep SWA is high at the beginning of the period of sleep, especially after sleep deprivation or extended periods of spontaneous wakefulness, and decreases during subsequent sleep (Achermann et al., 1993; Vyazovskiy & Tobler, 2012). But even at the very same moment of time different parts of the brain may manifest vastly different levels of SWA, and even individual cortical slow waves may occur in isolation (McKillop & Vyazovskiy, 2019; Nir et al., 2011). For example, in both humans and animals, SWA appears to be more "intense" in the frontal derivations, especially in early sleep or after sleep deprivation (Cajochen et al., 1999; Finelli et al., 2001; Huber et al., 2000; Vyazovskiy et al., 2002; Werth et al., 1996; Zavada et al., 2009), and shows sleep state–dependent interhemispheric asymmetries (Achermann et al., 2001; Vyazovskiy et al., 2002).

What is the neurophysiological basis for the regional differences in SWA during sleep? Several studies suggested that different cortical areas have a different capacity for generating sleep slow waves. Early studies noted that neuronal activity linked to EEG slow waves originates in a certain location and propagates to the neighboring areas in a three-dimensional pattern (Calvet et al., 1973; Verzeano & Negishi, 1960), and more recent studies confirmed these findings. One can argue that substantial regional differences in the total EEG power or the frequency content of EEG signals could be expected given that cortical areas exhibit differences in their anatomy, patterns of connectivity, or proximity to powerful generators of specific oscillations (e.g., the hippocampus). However, the topographic gradients in SWA do not merely reflect the absolute values of the EEG amplitude. Instead, different cortical regions differ in the relative dynamics of SWA across sleep, quantified as, for example, percentage increase or decrease compared to baseline. Therefore, such topographic differences have been attributed to different levels of "sleep need" among different cortical areas, in exactly the same way as SWA in general is considered a marker of sleep need referring to the whole brain. This notion is further supported by observations that regional enhancement of slow waves is related to preceding local neural activity during wakefulness. For example, peripheral sensory stimulation leads to more intense local EEG slow waves in humans (Huber et al., 2004; Kattler et al., 1994) and rodents (Vyazovskiy et al., 2000; Vyazovskiy & Tobler, 2008; Vyazovskiy, Welker, et al., 2004). Conversely, the immobilization of an arm (Huber et al., 2006) leads to reduced SWA during the night in the contralateral motor cortex. It was suggested that the sleep process emerges at the level of local neuronal populations in an activity-dependent fashion, as a direct consequence of fine synaptic modifications and local changes in neuronal connectivity arising from specific preceding waking activities (Krueger & Tononi, 2011; Roy et al., 2008). Important evidence suggesting the link between wake- or experience-dependent changes in SWA and neural plastic process is the observation that preceding sleep/wake history affects the degree of neuronal synchrony at both the local and global scales (Vyazovskiy, Cirelli, & Tononi, 2011; Vyazovskiy, Faraguna, et al., 2009; Vyazovskiy, Olcese, et al., 2011).

The most intriguing aspect of local sleep regulation is that it effectively blurs the distinction between global behavioral states (Figure 6.1). EEG SWA was noted in awake animals after sleep deprivation as early as 1984 (Borbely et al., 1984). Since then several

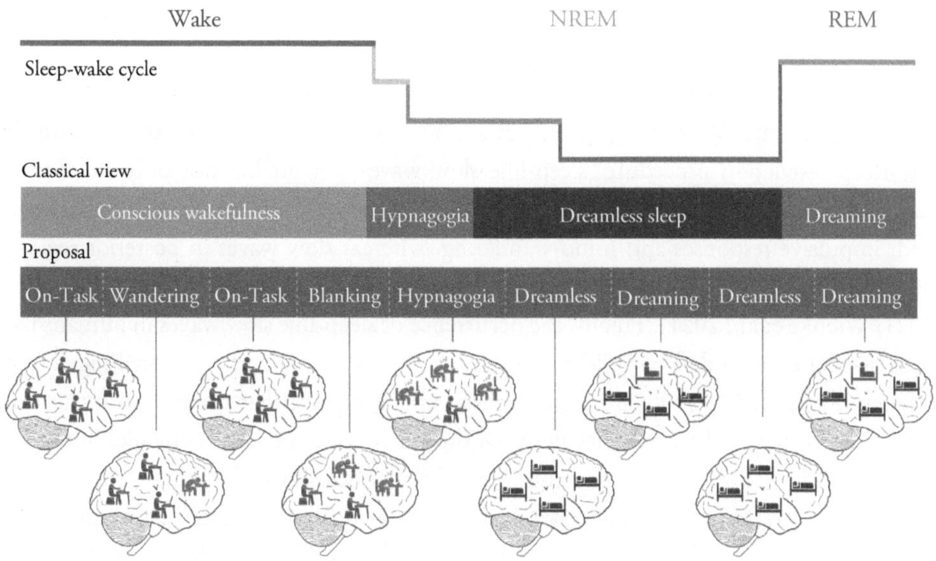

Figure 6.1 Schematic depiction of the relationship between classically defined global states of vigilance and a wide spectrum of substates defined based on local patterns of brain activity
Note. NREM = non-rapid eye movement; REM = rapid eye movement.

studies have demonstrated that NREM-like patterns of cortical activity can manifest during "activated" brain states, such as wakefulness and REM sleep (Funk et al., 2016; Soltani et al., 2019; Vyazovskiy, Olcese, et al., 2011). In humans, isolated slow waves similar to K-complexes can be induced by electrical stimulations of the anterior cingulate gyrus (Voysey et al., 2015), suggesting that the generation of slow waves does not depend on a global cortical state of sleep. In rodents, spontaneous episodes of local sleep are neurophysiologically characterized by the presence of delta/theta waves, accompanied by a reduction of single-unit firing rate ("off" period). In humans, sleep-like delta/theta waves have also been observed and represent a reliable index of vigilance: They increase with the time spent on task, even more so in brain regions recruited by a recurring task (Hung et al., 2013), and negatively correlate with subjective ratings of vigilance and pupil size (Andrillon et al., 2021). However, the link between the individual waves detected at the scalp level and off periods at the single-unit level has yet to be established in humans.

Functions of Local Sleep

The observation that sleep has local aspects of regulation provided a unifying framework for understanding the role of sleep in metabolic/energy homeostasis and synaptic plasticity and may account for sleep deprivation–induced changes in cognitive functions and performance (Vyazovskiy & Harris, 2013). Sleep intrusions during wakefulness, including the context of sleep deprivation, have been linked to the deterioration of various cognitive functions in a region-specific fashion (Andrillon et al., 2019). For example, in humans, the increase of theta waves over motor regions with time spent awake has been associated with visuomotor impairments, while the increase of similar theta waves over frontal cortices has been associated with executive failures (Bernardi et al., 2015; similarly as in rats [Vyazovskiy, Olcese, et al., 2011]). Within the same task and outside any sleep restriction procedure, sleep-like slow waves can predict not only the occurrence but also the type of attentional lapses: Slow waves in frontal regions are associated with impulsive responses and mind-wandering, whereas slow waves in posterior regions were more predictive of sluggish or missed responses and mind-blanking (Andrillon et al., 2021; Wienke et al., 2021). Finally, the occurrence of sleep-like slow waves in humans has been associated with deficits in learning (Quercia et al., 2018) and emotional regulation (Avvenuti et al., 2021). Taken together, these results suggest that these sleep intrusions represent a functional switch that perturbs the functioning of local networks impacted by these sleep intrusions and prevents them from processing information correctly or efficiently. Conversely, local reduction of slow waves during sleep could allow enhanced processing of external information (Andrillon & Kouider, 2020; Andrillon et al., 2016) or the occurrence of dreams (Siclari et al., 2017).

If increase in EEG SWA reflects both the duration of preceding waking and some aspects of wake "intensity" (Vyazovskiy & Tobler, 2012), the mechanisms triggering an increase in sleep intrusions during wakefulness remain unclear. Evidence suggests that activity-dependent release of cytokines or products of neuronal metabolism may have an important contribution (Krueger et al., 2008, 2013; Obal & Krueger, 2003; Roy et al., 2008). For example, it was shown that the levels of expression of tumor necrosis factor in the brain are dependent on peripheral activity, such as unilateral whisker stimulation (Churchill et al., 2008; Rockstrom et al., 2018), consistent with a local increase of SWA after the same manipulation (Vyazovskiy et al., 2000; Vyazovskiy, Welker, et al., 2004). Arguably, local activity is metabolically costly (Harris et al., 2012), and therefore a local decrease in spiking and synaptic activity may provide a necessary break (Vyazovskiy & Harris, 2013). Adenosine has been proposed as an important mediator of this effect (Benington & Heller, 1995; R. E. Brown et al., 2012; Krueger et al., 2008), and, given its important modulatory influence on inhibitory and excitatory synaptic neurotransmission in the neocortex (Zhang et al., 2015), the link between local energy metabolism and changes in sleep oscillations can be expected (Scharf et al., 2008). In rodents, intracellular levels of chloride could encode tiredness within cortical regions and underlie local increases in SWA (Alfonsa et al., 2022). In humans and along the same line, exerting self-control for long periods of time has been associated with behavioral impulsivity (Blain et al., 2016) and the accumulation of metabolites in the nucleus accumbens (Strasser et al., 2020) or the lateral prefrontal cortex (Wiehler et al., 2022), which are key regions for motivation and decision-making. Consistent with this notion, "intense" wake state was shown to be consistently associated with a greater buildup of SWA during subsequent sleep (Leemburg et al., 2010; Milinski et al., 2021; Yamagata et al., 2021). Thus, changes in the metabolism of neurons and the depletion of metabolic resources or the accumulation of metabolic waste could be mechanistically linked to local sleep intrusions within wakefulness. An alternative, but not mutually exclusive, mechanism for local sleep could be linked to synaptic plasticity. Indeed, an increase in connections or increased synaptic strength within a cortical network (as obtained through synaptic plasticity) could lead to more within-network synchrony (Olcese et al., 2010) and sleep-like slow waves (Vyazovskiy & Faraguna, 2015). Thus, both metabolic and plastic changes could represent major determinants of local sleep. It is worth noting that the homeostatic regulation of energetic resources, metabolic waste, and synaptic plasticity has been proposed as a key function of sleep in general (Frank & Heller, 2019).

Neural Responsiveness and Local Sleep

How is the occurrence of local sleep related to the key defining characteristic of sleep—sensory unresponsiveness? An essential function of the brain is to perceive complex external and internal stimuli and translate them into adequate behavioral responses. There is continuous fluctuation in the brain state, which impacts the responsiveness of neural networks to incoming stimuli, even in an awake state. It is widely agreed that the brain state accounts to a large extent for the trial-to-trial variability in the responses to stimuli (Churchland et al., 2010; Crochet et al., 2005; Fontanini & Katz, 2008; Foster et al., 1989; Haider et al., 2007; Kahn et al., 2022; Krueger et al., 2008; Rector et al., 2005; Scheeringa et al., 2011; Vyazovskiy, Faraguna, et al., 2009). Neuronal sensitivity to synaptic input is dictated by several mechanisms including membrane potential, ionic conductances, plasticity, neuromodulators, and a balance of excitation/inhibition (Bezdudnaya et al., 2006; Cano et al., 2006; Haider & McCormick, 2009; Okun & Lampl, 2008; Priebe & Ferster, 2008; Swadlow, 2002). Importantly, neuronal responsiveness depends on previous activity (Abbott & Nelson, 2000) and on the levels of neuromodulators that vary with the activity state of the brain (McCormick, 1992; McCormick et al., 1991) and impose both a global (extrinsic) and a local, synapse-specific (intrinsic) control (Gil et al., 1997; Laplante et al., 2005; Lawrence, 2008; Marrocco et al., 1987). An intriguing possibility is that the interaction between internal activity and afferent activity, on the one hand, and the balance between local and global neuromodulation, on the other hand, determine both spontaneous brain states and neuronal responsiveness.

Whether the capacity to respond to stimuli during sleep is reduced and whether it is related to the occurrence of slow waves have not been entirely understood, and the function of global behavioral unresponsiveness during sleep has not yet been determined (Rattenborg et al., 2012). One hypothesis is that this has metabolic implications as fast and adequate responding to incoming stimuli is, on the one hand, vital for survival but, on the other hand, highly energy-demanding (Attwell & Laughlin, 2001). Thus, a reduction of responsivity during sleep could result from the balance between energy-saving and the maintenance of neuronal responsiveness to enable survival. Indeed, the responsiveness to stimuli is drastically different between wake and sleep (Hall & Borbely, 1970; Massimini et al., 2005) as well as between periods of neuronal depolarization (up) and hyperpolarization (down) states that are typical for NREM sleep (Kahn et al., 2022; Steriade, Nunez, & Amzica, 1993; Steriade et al., 2001; Vyazovskiy et al., 2013). This bi-stable dynamics is brought about by neuromodulatory changes affecting voltage dependency of ionic conductances (Bazhenov et al., 2002; Compte et al., 2003; Hill & Tononi, 2005; Massimini & Amzica, 2001; McCormick, 1992). Specifically, excitatory postsynaptic potentials (EPSPs) elicited during the down states are less variable and have higher amplitude and duration as compared to those induced during up states (Crochet et al., 2005; Leger et al., 2005). However, studies suggest that generally the auditory cortex retains responsiveness to incoming stimuli regardless of the state of vigilance, although some aspects of neural processing may be selectively altered during sleep (Hayat et al., 2022; Nir et al., 2015; Sela et al., 2016). It has been proposed that reactive patterns of brain activity such as K-complexes (Halasz, 2005, 2016) could help achieve this balance by inhibiting sensory stimuli while subsequently opening a period of activation that can help sleepers track sensory inputs (Andrillon et al., 2016; Destexhe et al., 2007; Legendre et al., 2019).

In addition to the suppression of sensory inputs, it has been proposed that the occurrence of slow waves and off periods contributes to the reduction of awareness or consciousness (Nir et al., 2017; Pigorini et al., 2015). While the underlying mechanisms remain unclear, it is possibly related to the breakdown of functional connectivity between cortical areas, which interrupts the spread and processing of information (Massimini et al., 2005). Furthermore, when neurons are deprived of an input, they undergo continuous hyperpolarization and do not produce spikes (Timofeev et al., 2000). Conversely, a local reduction of SWA in parietal regions is a reliable correlate not only of dream occurrence in both NREM and REM sleep but also of dream contents (Siclari et al., 2017), which suggests that conscious experiences come and go according to the presence or absence of SWA in key brain regions. In conclusion, a growing body of work shows that the fine spatiotemporal dynamics of brain activity shapes the processing of external inputs as well as the generation of endogenous conscious experiences such as dreaming.

The question remains whether the mechanisms underlying the variability of spontaneous activity in awake brain (Bezdudnaya et al., 2006; Vyazovskiy, Olcese, et al., 2009) are similar to those present during sleep. One of the important factors that affect spontaneous activity during waking is preceding history of sleep, waking, and behavior (Borbely et al., 1984; Cirelli & Tononi, 2008; Leemburg et al., 2010; Vyazovskiy, Olcese, et al., 2009, 2011). During acute and chronic sleep deprivation, slower EEG activity, including SWA (0.5–4 Hz) or low theta (5–7 Hz) activity, leaks into periods of waking, and it does so in a region-specific manner (Franken et al., 1991; Leemburg et al., 2010; Vyazovskiy & Tobler, 2005). Moreover, when wake is prolonged beyond its physiological duration, brain metabolism tends to decrease (Everson et al., 1994; Wu et al., 2006), suggesting that the brain may partially switch into a sleep-like mode (Vyazovskiy, Olcese, et al., 2011).

While the continual changes and variability in spontaneous brain states and the responsiveness of individual cortical neurons are well established, their origin remains unknown. It is possible that the occurrence of different cortical states is regulated by preceding wake duration and experience.

Mechanisms of Local Sleep

The question of what triggers individual episodes of local sleep remains largely open. While intrinsic mechanisms are undoubtedly important for shaping the activity of individual neurons (S. W. Hughes et al., 2002), state-dependent network mechanisms perhaps play a crucial role (Compte et al., 2003; Haider & McCormick, 2009; Sanchez-Vives & McCormick, 2000; Timofeev et al., 2001). It was suggested (Haider et al., 2006) that neocortical pyramidal cells form a significant number of long-range excitatory connections, while inhibitory interneurons mostly communicate with principal cells within a local circuit (McGuire et al., 1991). Thus, at least three spatial scales can be identified, which might be responsible for the initiation and maintenance of network synchrony at the local level. One scale can be defined by the radius of an individual inhibitory GABA-ergic interneuron, such as a basket cell, that projects simultaneously to several hundreds of principal pyramidal neurons and could contribute to an off-period initiation. The second spatial scale refers to the extent of intracortical horizontal connectivity. It is usually postulated that the number of intracortical monosynaptic connections decays rapidly with distance and fades within a few hundred milliseconds. However, it is now widely accepted that intracortical excitatory horizontal connections are abundant—most neurons in supragranular layers are interconnected by short-range and long-range connections and are believed to play an important functional role in intracortical processing (Boucsein et al., 2011; Gonzalez-Burgos et al., 2000). Excitatory connections arriving from distant neurons are crucial not only for conveying specific sensory information but also for providing a necessary level of cortical excitability (Stepanyants et al., 2009). It is possible that long-range effective connectivity is fully developed at the beginning of an up-state, when the supragranular neurons reach a sufficient level of depolarization as a result of EPSP summation (Haider et al., 2006). On the other hand, it was suggested that an increase in excitation toward the end of the up-state, accounted for by depolarizing inputs from long-distant neurons, can drive a critical population of excitatory neurons simultaneously into refractoriness, precipitating the occurrence of a synchronous down-state (Gutkin et al., 2001). Third, long-range major commissures, such as the corpus callosum, are likely important to enable truly global cortical synchronization, encompassing not only local neuronal populations within a hemisphere but also an entire brain (Achermann & Borbely, 1998; Avvenuti et al., 2020; Vyazovskiy et al., 2004a).

The view of sleep as a local, activity-dependent process stimulated efforts toward the development of ex vivo, "sleep in a dish" preparations (Bandarabadi et al., 2020; Hinard et al., 2012; Jewett et al., 2015). These studies revealed important commonalities in both circuit and molecular mechanisms and consequences of sleep at the local and global levels. Intriguingly, studies in neuronal cultures revealed that sleep-like patterns of activity spontaneously emerge and can be maintained for days in neuronal cultures, leading to the hypothesis that the slow oscillation represents a default mode of cortical network function (Bandarabadi et al., 2020; Jewett et al., 2015; Sanchez-Vives et al., 2017).

The fundamental gap, however, remains, with respect to how local changes within neocortical circuits relate to global manifestation of sleep. In other words, if local sleep can occur, why is global behavioral shutdown necessary? One scenario that was proposed recently is that, due to extensive interconnectivity among individual neurons and neuronal populations, it is, at least, inefficient if individual neurons obtain "rest" independently; and this can compromise the function of the large distributed networks they are part of (Rattenborg et al., 2012; Vyazovskiy & Harris, 2013). Yet, on the other hand, the emergence of sleep need at the local level in the cortex may represent an important signal to subcortical sleep–wake-promoting neurons, which are ultimately responsible for the occurrence of global sleep (Krone et al., 2021; D. Liu & Dan, 2019). Several sleep–wake-controlling areas have been identified based on their functional properties and patterns of connectivity. Crucially, none of these is exclusively sleep- or wake-related, but they typically contain a mixture of neurons, selectively active during a specific state of vigilance, or fire in a manner which is state-unspecific. This raises an important question of how to establish the causal, active role of a specific brain structure or a local neuronal circuit in sleep state control.

The proponents of the idea of sleep as a local, activity-dependent process argue that if subcortical sleep–wake switching were to occur in a top-down fashion at the level of specific hypothalamic or brainstem circuitry, then how does it "know" when this should be happening? This view implies an existence of other, higher-order, pathways, which are more important in this context. One scenario is that specific dedicated cortical or subcortical circuits are responsible for "sensing" the levels of specific variables that need to be renormalized and thus signal global sleep need or play a role in translating the levels of sleep need accumulated elsewhere into the global sleep signal (Krone et al., 2021; Thomas et al., 2020). If this were the case, the neurons responsible for these functions must possess unique properties, for example, with respect to the patterns of their anatomical connectivity, which yet remains to be established. It is worthwhile remembering, however, that neurons are "flexible" entities, to the extent that they can fire at different rates and patterns depending on the level of depolarization (Steriade, 2004). In any case, quasi-independent frequent occurrence of local neuronal bi-stability across the neocortex might be an important factor precipitating the global synchronization of cortical slow waves and the initiation of global sleep. Evidence suggests that fast spread of slow waves might be facilitated by long-range recruitment of distributed cortical networks in the global slow oscillation (Esser et al., 2007; Massimini et al., 2004; Nir et al., 2011; Riedner et al.,

2007; Vyazovskiy, Faraguna, et al., 2009; Vyazovskiy, Olcese, et al., 2011; Vyazovskiy, Riedner, et al., 2007).

When dealing with complex brain networks, it is often difficult to establish whether the local state of a specific neuronal population is a cause or a consequence of the global activity across the rest of the network (Okun et al., 2015). As the amount and strength of synaptic connections are not equally distributed across the network, simple tuning up or down of the excitability across the entire network (Bridi et al., 2019) can, at least in theory, lead to dramatic changes in the behavioral state, which will be determined by which areas or connections prevail or "rule" the rest of the brain (Banks et al., 2020). To this end, the key open question remains how, in such a scenario, the signals are transferred and coordinated across widely distributed brain networks to allow physiological sleep and wake to occur when they are ecologically relevant.

Conclusions

In summary, sleep timing and intensity, as well as the spatiotemporal dynamics of brain activity during sleep, are regulated at both the local and global levels; and there is a continual bidirectional interaction between the respective levels. Local regulation of sleep manifests both in the role of specific subcortical structures in sleep control as well as in activity-dependent emergence of sleep-like patterns of activity in the neocortical structures. We argue that sleep regulation is conceptually similar to the functioning of the circadian system, where global temporal coordination of physiology and behavior requires not only the central clock in the SCN but also numerous local clocks in the brain in the periphery. While the underlying neurophysiological mechanisms of local sleep remain not entirely understood, evidence suggests its role in metabolic regulation, cellular maintenance, synaptic plasticity, and sensory processing. Evidence suggests that it is not merely an exotic phenomenon, found in a few animal species or sleep disorders, but a fundamental property of normal sleep. It is even possible that local sleep is in fact the expression of a general tendency of cortical networks to default to certain patterns of activity (such as the bi-stable on and off alternation), which can be achieved through pharmacological interventions (Vyazovskiy, Tobler, & Winsky-Sommerer, 2007), electric stimulations (Voysey et al., 2015), or following brain lesions (Sarasso et al., 2020) and not only in association with wake–sleep transitions.

An important challenge remains how to tackle the complexity of sleep control, given the increasing realization of its multilayered network organization. There is little doubt that multiple brain areas and many cell types are necessary for coordination of behavioral and brain-state changes with external changes in the environment and homeostatic needs. Furthermore, the phylogeny of sleep and circadian rhythmicity needs to be considered as they coevolved together, in parallel with the development of increasingly complex brains and elaborate behaviors and as new spatial and temporal niches were conquered. Undoubtedly, this favored the emergence of a distributed hierarchical system for the control of sleep, where each level played a defined role in a specific subtask. To this end, useful lessons can be learned from other systems, such as the hierarchical organization of the image-forming visual system, which has components arranged in both a serial and a parallel fashion and consisting of numerous sequential stages of information processing (Van Essen et al., 1992). Within such a framework, new rules could be established with respect to how information about the time of day or preceding sleep–wake history is represented by individual neurons or specific neuronal populations and how it is transformed and processed across successive levels to allow adaptive behavioral patterns to emerge.

Future Directions

We identify the following key questions that need to be answered:

1. How can we bridge the gap between slow waves observed in scalp EEG and bi-stable dynamics at the level of individual neurons?
2. What triggers the transition from locally occurring sleep to global behavioral shutdown, and is this a gradual or an abrupt process?
3 Is local sleep fundamentally adaptive or dysfunctional?
4. How does local sleep and its underlying neurophysiological substrates evolve throughout the life span—from early ontogeny to aging?
5. Do bi-stable dynamics in wake and sleep always share the same mechanisms?
6. What is the best definition of *local sleep*, and is this an adequate term?

References

Abbott, L. F., & Nelson, S. B. (2000). Synaptic plasticity: Taming the beast. *Nature Neuroscience, 3*, 1178–1183.

Achermann, P., & Borbely, A. A. (1998). Temporal evolution of coherence and power in the human sleep electroencephalogram. *Journal of Sleep Research, 7*(S1), 36–41.

Achermann, P., Dijk, D. J., Brunner, D. P., & Borbely, A. A. (1993). A model of human sleep homeostasis based on EEG slow-wave activity: Quantitative comparison of data and simulations. *Brain Research Bulletin, 31*, 97–113.

Achermann, P., Finelli, L. A., & Borbely, A. A. (2001). Unihemispheric enhancement of delta power in human frontal sleep EEG by prolonged wakefulness. *Brain Research, 913*, 220–223.

Adamantidis, A. R., Gutierrez Herrera, C., & Gent, T. C. (2019). Oscillating circuitries in the sleeping brain. *Nature Reviews Neuroscience, 20*, 746–762.

Aeschbach, D., Cajochen, C., Landolt, H., & Borbely, A. A. (1996). Homeostatic sleep regulation in habitual short sleepers and long sleepers. *American Journal of Physiology, 270*, R41–R53.

Alfonsa, H., Burman, R. J., Brodersen, P. J. N., Newey, S. E., Mahfooz, K., Yamagata, T., Panayi, M. C., Bannerman, D. M., Vyazovskiy, V. V., & Akerman, C. J. (2022). Intracellular chloride regulation mediates local sleep pressure in the cortex. *Nature Neuroscience, 26*, 64–78.

Andrillon, T., Burns, A., Mackay, T., Windt, J., & Tsuchiya, N. (2021). Predicting lapses of attention with sleep-like slow waves. *Nature Communications, 12*, Article 3657.

Andrillon, T., & Kouider, S. (2020). The vigilant sleeper: Neural mechanisms of sensory (de)coupling during sleep. *Current Opinion in Physiology, 15*, 47–59.

Andrillon, T., Poulsen, A. T., Hansen, L. K., Leger, D., & Kouider, S. (2016). Neural markers of responsiveness to the environment in human sleep. *Journal of Neuroscience, 36*, 6583–6596.

Andrillon, T., Windt, J., Silk, T., Drummond, S. P. A., Bellgrove, M. A., & Tsuchiya, N. (2019). Does the mind wander when the brain takes a break? Local sleep in wakefulness, attentional lapses and mind-wandering. *Frontiers in Neuroscience, 13*, Article 949.

Attwell, D., & Laughlin, S. B. (2001). An energy budget for signaling in the grey matter of the brain. *Journal of Cerebral Blood Flow & Metabolism, 21*, 1133–1145.

Avvenuti, G., Bertelloni, D., Lettieri, G., Ricciardi, E., Cecchetti, L., Pietrini, P., & Bernardi, G. (2021). Emotion regulation failures are preceded by local increases in sleep-like activity. *Journal of Cognitive Neuroscience, 33*, 2342–2356.

Avvenuti, G., Handjaras, G., Betta, M., Cataldi, J., Imperatori, L. S., Lattanzi, S., Riedner, B. A., Pietrini, P., Ricciardi, E., Tononi, G., Siclari, F., Polonara, G., Fabri, M., Silvestrini, M., Bellesi, M., & Bernardi, G. (2020). Integrity of corpus callosum is essential for the cross-hemispheric propagation of sleep slow waves: A high-density EEG study in split-brain patients. *Journal of Neuroscience, 40*, 5589–5603.

Baldini, T., Loddo, G., Sessagesimi, E., Mignani, F., Cirignotta, F., Mondini, S., Licchetta, L., Bisulli, F., Tinuper, P., & Provini, F. (2019). Clinical features and pathophysiology of disorders of arousal in adults: A window into the sleeping brain. *Frontiers in Neurology, 10*, Article 526.

Bandarabadi, M., Vassalli, A., & Tafti, M. (2020). Sleep as a default state of cortical and subcortical networks. *Current Opinion in Physiology, 15*, 60–67.

Banks, G. T., Guillaumin, M. C. C., Heise, I., Lau, P., Yin, M., Bourbia, N., Aguilar, C., Bowl, M. R., Esapa, C., Brown, L. A., Hasan, S., Tagliatti, E., Nicholson, E., Bains, R. S., Wells, S., Vyazovskiy, V. V., Volynski, K., Peirson, S. N., & Nolan, P. M. (2020). Forward genetics identifies a novel sleep mutant with sleep state inertia and REM sleep deficits. *Science Advances, 6*, Article eabb3567.

Bass, J., & Takahashi, J. S. (2010). Circadian integration of metabolism and energetics. *Science, 330*, 1349–1354.

Bazhenov, M., Timofeev, I., Steriade, M., & Sejnowski, T. J. (2002). Model of thalamocortical slow-wave sleep oscillations and transitions to activated states. *Journal of Neuroscience, 22*, 8691–704.

Benington, J. H., & Heller, H. C. (1995). Restoration of brain energy metabolism as the function of sleep. *Progress in Neurobiology, 45*, 347–360.

Bernardi, G., Siclari, F., Yu, X., Zennig, C., Bellesi, M., Ricciardi, E., Cirelli, C., Ghilardi, M. F., Pietrini, P., & Tononi, G. (2015). Neural and behavioral correlates of extended training during sleep deprivation in humans: Evidence for local, task-specific effects. *Journal of Neuroscience, 35*, 4487–500.

Bezdudnaya, T., Cano, M., Bereshpolova, Y., Stoelzel, C. R., Alonso, J. M., & Swadlow, H. A. (2006). Thalamic burst mode and inattention in the awake LGNd. *Neuron, 49*, 421–432.

Blain, B., Hollard, G., & Pessiglione, M. (2016). Neural mechanisms underlying the impact of daylong cognitive work on economic decisions. *Proceedings of the National Academy of Sciences of the United States of America, 113*, 6967–6972.

Borbely, A. A. (1982). A two process model of sleep regulation. *Human Neurobiology, 1*, 195–204.

Borbely, A. A., & Achermann, P. (2000). *Homeostasis of human sleep and models of sleep regulation*. W. B. Saunders.

Borbely, A. A., Daan, S., Wirz-Justice, A., & Deboer, T. (2016). The two-process model of sleep regulation: A reappraisal. *Journal of Sleep Research, 25*, 131–143.

Borbely, A. A., Tobler, I., & Hanagasioglu, M. (1984). Effect of sleep deprivation on sleep and EEG power spectra in the rat. *Behavioural Brain Research, 14*, 171–182.

Boucsein, C., Nawrot, M. P., Schnepel, P., & Aertsen, A. (2011). Beyond the cortical column: Abundance and physiology of horizontal connections imply a strong role for inputs from the surround. *Frontiers in Neuroscience, 5*, Article 32.

Brancaccio, M., Edwards, M. D., Patton, A. P., Smyllie, N. J., Chesham, J. E., Maywood, E. S., & Hastings, M. H. (2019). Cell-autonomous clock of astrocytes drives circadian behavior in mammals. *Science, 363*, 187–192.

Bridi, M. C. D., Zong, F. J., Min, X., Luo, N., Tran, T., Qiu, J., Severin, D., Zhang, X. T., Wang, G., Zhu, Z. J., He, K. W., & Kirkwood, A. (2019). Daily oscillation of the excitation-inhibition balance in visual cortical circuits. *Neuron, 105*, 621–629.e4.

Brown, L. A., Fisk, A. S., Pothecary, C. A., & Peirson, S. N. (2019). Telling the time with a broken clock: Quantifying circadian disruption in animal models. *Biology (Basel), 8*, Article 18.

Brown, R. E., Basheer, R., McKenna, J. T., Strecker, R. E., & McCarley, R. W. (2012). Control of sleep and wakefulness. *Physiological Review, 92*, 1087–1187.

Cajochen, C., Foy, R., & Dijk, D. J. (1999). Frontal predominance of a relative increase in sleep delta and theta EEG activity after sleep loss in humans. *Sleep Research Online, 2*, 65–69.
Calvet, J., Fourment, A., & Thiefry, M. (1973). Electrical activity in neocortical projection and association areas during slow wave sleep. *Brain Research, 52*, 173–187.
Campbell, S. S., & Tobler, I. (1984). Animal sleep: A review of sleep duration across phylogeny. *Neuroscience and Biobehavioral Reviews, 8*, 269–300.
Cano, M., Bezdudnaya, T., Swadlow, H. A., & Alonso, J. M. (2006). Brain state and contrast sensitivity in the awake visual thalamus. *Nature Neuroscience, 9*, 1240–1242.
Castelnovo, A., Lopez, R., Proserpio, P., Nobili, L., & Dauvilliers, Y. (2018). NREM sleep parasomnias as disorders of sleep-state dissociation. *Nature Reviews Neurology, 14*, 470–481.
Castillo, C., Molyneux, P., Carlson, R., & Harrington, M. E. (2011). Restricted wheel access following a light cycle inversion slows re-entrainment without internal desynchrony as measured in Per2Luc mice. *Neuroscience, 182*, 169–176.
Churchill, L., Rector, D. M., Yasuda, K., Fix, C., Rojas, M. J., Yasuda, T., & Krueger, J. M. (2008). Tumor necrosis factor alpha: Activity dependent expression and promotion of cortical column sleep in rats. *Neuroscience, 156*, 71–80.
Churchland, M. M., Yu, B. M., Cunningham, J. P., Sugrue, L. P., Cohen, M. R., Corrado, G. S., Newsome, W. T., Clark, A. M., Hosseini, P., Scott, B. B., Bradley, D. C., Smith, M. A., Kohn, A., Movshon, J. A., Armstrong, K. M., Moore, T., Chang, S. W., Snyder, L. H., Lisberger, S. G., . . . Shenoy, K. V. (2010). Stimulus onset quenches neural variability: A widespread cortical phenomenon. *Nature Neuroscience, 13*, 369–378.
Cirelli, C., & Tononi, G. (2008). Is sleep essential? *PLOS Biology, 6*, Article e216.
Cisse, Y., Crochet, S., Timofeev, I., & Steriade, M. (2004). Synaptic responsiveness of neocortical neurons to callosal volleys during paroxysmal depolarizing shifts. *Neuroscience, 124*, 231–239.
Colwell, C. S. (2011). Linking neural activity and molecular oscillations in the SCN. *Nature Reviews Neuroscience, 12*, 553–569.
Compte, A., Sanchez-Vives, M. V., McCormick, D. A., & Wang, X. J. (2003). Cellular and network mechanisms of slow oscillatory activity (<1 Hz) and wave propagations in a cortical network model. *Journal of Neurophysiology, 89*, 2707–2725.
Crochet, S., Chauvette, S., Boucetta, S., & Timofeev, I. (2005). Modulation of synaptic transmission in neocortex by network activities. *European Journal of Neuroscience, 21*, 1030–1044.
Daan, S., Beersma, D. G., & Borbely, A. A. (1984). Timing of human sleep: Recovery process gated by a circadian pacemaker. *American Journal of Physiology, 246*, R161–R183.
Dement, W., & Kleitman, N. (1957). Cyclic variations in EEG during sleep and their relation to eye movements, body motility, and dreaming. *Electroencephalography and Clinical Neurophysiology, 9*, 673–690.
Destexhe, A., Hughes, S. W., Rudolph, M., & Crunelli, V. (2007). Are corticothalamic "up" states fragments of wakefulness? *Trends in Neuroscience, 30*, 334–342.
Economo, C. V. (1930). Sleep as a problem of localization. *The Journal of Nervous and Mental Disease, 71*, 249–259.
Esser, S. K., Hill, S. L., & Tononi, G. (2007). Sleep homeostasis and cortical synchronization: I. Modeling the effects of synaptic strength on sleep slow waves. *Sleep, 30*, 1617–1630.
Everson, C. A., Smith, C. B., & Sokoloff, L. (1994). Effects of prolonged sleep deprivation on local rates of cerebral energy metabolism in freely moving rats. *Journal of Neuroscience, 14*, 6769–6778.
Ferrara, M., De Gennaro, L., Curcio, G., Cristiani, R., & Bertini, M. (2002). Regional differences of the temporal EEG dynamics during the first 30 min of human sleep. *Neuroscience Research, 44*, 83–89.
Finelli, L. A., Borbely, A. A., & Achermann, P. (2001). Functional topography of the human nonREM sleep electroencephalogram. *European Journal of Neuroscience, 13*, 2282–2290.
Fisher, S. P., Cui, N., McKillop, L. E., Gemignani, J., Bannerman, D. M., Oliver, P. L., Peirson, S. N., & Vyazovskiy, V. V. (2016). Stereotypic wheel running decreases cortical activity in mice. *Nature Communications, 7*, Article 13138.
Fisher, S. P., Foster, R. G., & Peirson, S. N. (2013). The circadian control of sleep. In A. Kramer, & M. Merrow (Eds.), *Circadian clocks. Handbook of experimental pharmacology* (Vol. 217, pp. 157–183). Springer.
Fontanini, A., & Katz, D. B. (2008). Behavioral states, network states, and sensory response variability. *Journal of Neurophysiology, 100*, 1160–1168.

Foster, T. C., Castro, C. A., & McNaughton, B. L. (1989). Spatial selectivity of rat hippocampal neurons: Dependence on preparedness for movement. *Science, 244,* 1580–1582.

Frank, M. G., & Heller, H. C. (2019). The function(s) of sleep. In H. P. Landolt & D. J. Dijk (Eds.), *Sleep–wake neurobiology and pharmacology. Handbook of experimental pharmacology* (Vol. 253, pp. 3–34). Springer.

Franken, P., Chollet, D., & Tafti, M. (2001). The homeostatic regulation of sleep need is under genetic control. *Journal of Neuroscience, 21,* 2610–2621.

Franken, P., Dijk, D. J., Tobler, I., & Borbely, A. A. (1991). Sleep deprivation in rats: Effects on EEG power spectra, vigilance states, and cortical temperature. *American Journal of Physiology, 261,* R198–R208.

Funk, C. M., Honjoh, S., Rodriguez, A. V., Cirelli, C., & Tononi, G. (2016). Local slow waves in superficial layers of primary cortical areas during REM sleep. *Current Biology, 26,* 396–403.

Gil, Z., Connors, B. W., & Amitai, Y. (1997). Differential regulation of neocortical synapses by neuromodulators and activity. *Neuron, 19,* 679–686.

Golombek, D. A., & Rosenstein, R. E. (2010). Physiology of circadian entrainment. *Physiological Reviews, 90,* 1063–1102.

Gonzalez-Burgos, G., Barrionuevo, G., & Lewis, D. A. (2000). Horizontal synaptic connections in monkey prefrontal cortex: An in vitro electrophysiological study. *Cerebral Cortex, 10,* 82–92.

Gutkin, B. S., Laing, C. R., Colby, C. L., Chow, C. C., & Ermentrout, G. B. (2001). Turning on and off with excitation: The role of spike-timing asynchrony and synchrony in sustained neural activity. *Journal of Computational Neuroscience, 11,* 121–134.

Haider, B., Duque, A., Hasenstaub, A. R., & McCormick, D. A. (2006). Neocortical network activity in vivo is generated through a dynamic balance of excitation and inhibition. *Journal of Neuroscience, 26,* 4535–4545.

Haider, B., Duque, A., Hasenstaub, A. R., Yu, Y., & McCormick, D. A. (2007). Enhancement of visual responsiveness by spontaneous local network activity in vivo. *Journal of Neurophysiology, 97,* 4186–4202.

Haider, B., & McCormick, D. A. (2009). Rapid neocortical dynamics: Cellular and network mechanisms. *Neuron, 62,* 171–189.

Halasz, P. (2005). K-complex, a reactive EEG graphoelement of NREM sleep: An old chap in a new garment. *Sleep Medicine Reviews, 9,* 391–412.

Halasz, P. (2016). The K-complex as a special reactive sleep slow wave—A theoretical update. *Sleep Medicine Reviews, 29,* 34–40.

Hall, R. D., & Borbely, A. A. (1970). Acoustically evoked potentials in the rat during sleep and waking. *Experimental Brain Research, 11,* 93–110.

Harris, J. J., Jolivet, R., & Attwell, D. (2012). Synaptic energy use and supply. *Neuron, 75,* 762–777.

Hastings, M. H., Duffield, G. E., Ebling, F. J., Kidd, A., Maywood, E. S., & Schurov, I. (1997). Non-photic signalling in the suprachiasmatic nucleus. *Biology of the Cell, 89,* 495–503.

Hastings, M. H., Maywood, E. S., & Brancaccio, M. (2018). Generation of circadian rhythms in the suprachiasmatic nucleus. *Nature Reviews Neuroscience, 19,* 453–469.

Hayat, H., Marmelshtein, A., Krom, A. J., Sela, Y., Tankus, A., Strauss, I., Fahoum, F., Fried, I., & Nir, Y. (2022). Reduced neural feedback signaling despite robust neuron and gamma auditory responses during human sleep. *Nature Neuroscience, 25,* 935–943.

Hess, R. (1964). The electroencephalogram in sleep. *Electroencephalography and Clinical Neurophysiology, 16,* 44–55.

Hill, S., & Tononi, G. (2005). Modeling sleep and wakefulness in the thalamocortical system. *Journal of Neurophysiology, 93,* 1671–1698.

Hinard, V., Mikhail, C., Pradervand, S., Curie, T., Houtkooper, R. H., Auwerx, J., Franken, P., & Tafti, M. (2012). Key electrophysiological, molecular, and metabolic signatures of sleep and wakefulness revealed in primary cortical cultures. *Journal of Neuroscience, 32,* 12506–12517.

Huber, R., Deboer, T., & Tobler, I. (2000). Topography of EEG dynamics after sleep deprivation in mice. *Journal of Neurophysiology, 84,* 1888–1893.

Huber, R., Ghilardi, M. F., Massimini, M., Ferrarelli, F., Riedner, B. A., Peterson, M. J., & Tononi, G. (2006). Arm immobilization causes cortical plastic changes and locally decreases sleep slow wave activity. *Nature Neuroscience, 9,* 1169–1176.

Huber, R., Ghilardi, M. F., Massimini, M., & Tononi, G. (2004). Local sleep and learning. *Nature, 430,* 78–81.

Hughes, S., Jagannath, A., Hankins, M. W., Foster, R. G., & Peirson, S. N. (2015). Photic regulation of clock systems. *Methods in Enzymology, 552,* 125–143.

Hughes, S. W., Cope, D. W., Blethyn, K. L., & Crunelli, V. (2002). Cellular mechanisms of the slow (<1 Hz) oscillation in thalamocortical neurons in vitro. *Neuron, 33*, 947–958.

Hung, C. S., Sarasso, S., Ferrarelli, F., Riedner, B., Ghilardi, M. F., Cirelli, C., & Tononi, G. (2013). Local experience-dependent changes in the wake EEG after prolonged wakefulness. *Sleep, 36*, 59–72.

Jagannath, A., Butler, R., Godinho, S. I., Couch, Y., Brown, L. A., Vasudevan, S. R., Flanagan, K. C., Anthony, D., Churchill, G. C., Wood, M. J., Steiner, G., Ebeling, M., Hossbach, M., Wettstein, J. G., Duffield, G. E., Gatti, S., Hankins, M. W., Foster, R. G., & Peirson, S. N. (2013). The CRTC1–SIK1 pathway regulates entrainment of the circadian clock. *Cell, 154*, 1100–1111.

Jewett, K. A., Taishi, P., Sengupta, P., Roy, S., Davis, C. J., & Krueger, J. M. (2015). Tumor necrosis factor enhances the sleep-like state and electrical stimulation induces a wake-like state in co-cultures of neurons and glia. *European Journal of Neuroscience, 42*, 2078–2090.

Kahn, M., Krone, L. B., Blanco-Duque, C., Guillaumin, M. C. C., Mann, E. O., & Vyazovskiy, V. V. (2022). Neuronal-spiking-based closed-loop stimulation during cortical ON- and OFF-states in freely moving mice. *Journal of Sleep Research, 31*, Article e13603.

Kattler, H., Dijk, D. J., & Borbely, A. A. (1994). Effect of unilateral somatosensory stimulation prior to sleep on the sleep EEG in humans. *Journal of Sleep Research, 3*, 159–164.

Kohl, M. M., & Paulsen, O. (2010). The roles of GABAB receptors in cortical network activity. *Advances in Pharmacology, 58*, 205–229.

Krone, L. B., Yamagata, T., Blanco-Duque, C., Guillaumin, M. C. C., Kahn, M. C., Van Der Vinne, V., McKillop, L. E., Tam, S. K. E., Peirson, S. N., Akerman, C. J., Hoerder-Suabedissen, A., Molnar, Z., & Vyazovskiy, V. V. (2021). A role for the cortex in sleep–wake regulation. *Nature Neuroscience, 24*, 1210–1215.

Krueger, J. M., Huang, Y. H., Rector, D. M., & Buysse, D. J. (2013). Sleep: A synchrony of cell activity–driven small network states. *European Journal of Neuroscience, 38*, 2199–2209.

Krueger, J. M., Rector, D. M., Roy, S., Van Dongen, H. P., Belenky, G., & Panksepp, J. (2008). Sleep as a fundamental property of neuronal assemblies. *Nature Reviews Neuroscience, 9*, 910–919.

Krueger, J. M., & Tononi, G. (2011). Local use-dependent sleep; synthesis of the new paradigm. *Current Topics in Medicinal Chemistry, 11*, 2490–2492.

Laplante, F., Morin, Y., Quirion, R., & Vaucher, E. (2005). Acetylcholine release is elicited in the visual cortex, but not in the prefrontal cortex, by patterned visual stimulation: A dual in vivo microdialysis study with functional correlates in the rat brain. *Neuroscience, 132*, 501–510.

Lawrence, J. J. (2008). Cholinergic control of GABA release: Emerging parallels between neocortex and hippocampus. *Trends in Neuroscience, 31*, 317–327.

Leemburg, S., Vyazovskiy, V. V., Olcese, U., Bassetti, C. L., Tononi, G., & Cirelli, C. (2010). Sleep homeostasis in the rat is preserved during chronic sleep restriction. *Proceedings of the National Academy of Sciences of the United States of America, 107*, 15939–15944.

Legendre, G., Andrillon, T., Koroma, M., & Kouider, S. (2019). Sleepers track informative speech in a multitalker environment. *Nature Human Behavior, 3*, 274–283.

Leger, J. F., Stern, E. A., Aertsen, A., & Heck, D. (2005). Synaptic integration in rat frontal cortex shaped by network activity. *Journal of Neurophysiology, 93*, 281–293.

Liu, C., Weaver, D. R., Strogatz, S. H., & Reppert, S. M. (1997). Cellular construction of a circadian clock: Period determination in the suprachiasmatic nuclei. *Cell, 91*, 855–860.

Liu, D., & Dan, Y. (2019). A motor theory of sleep–wake control: Arousal–action circuit. *Annual Review of Neuroscience, 42*, 27–46.

Loomis, A. L., Harvey, E. N., & Hobart, G. (1935a). Further observations on the potential rhythms of the cerebral cortex during sleep. *Science, 82*, 198–200.

Loomis, A. L., Harvey, E. N., & Hobart, G. (1935b). Potential rhythms of the cerebral cortex during sleep. *Science, 81*, 597–598.

Magnin, M., Rey, M., Bastuji, H., Guillemant, P., Mauguiere, F., & Garcia-Larrea, L. (2010). Thalamic deactivation at sleep onset precedes that of the cerebral cortex in humans. *Proceedings of the National Academy of Sciences of the United States of America, 107*, 3829–3833.

Mann, E. O., Kohl, M. M., & Paulsen, O. (2009). Distinct roles of GABA(A) and GABA(B) receptors in balancing and terminating persistent cortical activity. *Journal of Neuroscience, 29*, 7513–7518.

Marrocco, R. T., Lane, R. F., McClurkin, J. W., Blaha, C. D., & Alkire, M. F. (1987). Release of cortical catecholamines by visual stimulation requires activity in thalamocortical afferents of monkey and cat. *Journal of Neuroscience, 7*, 2756–2767.

Massimini, M., & Amzica, F. (2001). Extracellular calcium fluctuations and intracellular potentials in the cortex during the slow sleep oscillation. *Journal of Neurophysiology, 85*, 1346–1350.

Massimini, M., Ferrarelli, F., Huber, R., Esser, S. K., Singh, H., & Tononi, G. (2005). Breakdown of cortical effective connectivity during sleep. *Science, 309*, 2228–2232.

Massimini, M., Huber, R., Ferrarelli, F., Hill, S., & Tononi, G. (2004). The sleep slow oscillation as a traveling wave. *Journal of Neuroscience, 24*, 6862–6870.

Maywood, E. S., Mrosovsky, N., Field, M. D., & Hastings, M. H. (1999). Rapid down-regulation of mammalian period genes during behavioral resetting of the circadian clock. *Proceedings of the National Academy of Sciences of the United States of America, 96*, 15211–15216.

McCormick, D. A. (1992). Neurotransmitter actions in the thalamus and cerebral cortex. *Journal of Clinical Neurophysiology, 9*, 212–223.

McCormick, D. A., Pape, H. C., & Williamson, A. (1991). Actions of norepinephrine in the cerebral cortex and thalamus: Implications for function of the central noradrenergic system. *Progress in Brain Research, 88*, 293–305.

McGuire, B. A., Gilbert, C. D., Rivlin, P. K., & Wiesel, T. N. (1991). Targets of horizontal connections in macaque primary visual cortex. *Journal of Comparative Neurology, 305*, 370–392.

McKillop, L. E., & Vyazovskiy, V. V. (2019). Sleep- and wake-like states in small networks in vivo and in vitro. In H. P. Landolt & D. J. Dijk (Eds.), *Sleep–wake neurobiology and pharmacology. Handbook of experimental pharmacology* (Vol. 253, pp. 97–121). Springer.

Mendoza, J., & Challet, E. (2009). Brain clocks: From the suprachiasmatic nuclei to a cerebral network. *Neuroscientist, 15*, 477–488.

Milinski, L., Fisher, S. P., Cui, N., McKillop, L. E., Blanco-Duque, C., Ang, G., Yamagata, T., Bannerman, D. M., & Vyazovskiy, V. V. (2021). Waking experience modulates sleep need in mice. *BMC Biology, 19*, Article 65.

Mukhametov, L. M., Supin, A. Y., & Polyakova, I. G. (1977). Interhemispheric asymmetry of the electroencephalographic sleep patterns in dolphins. *Brain Research, 134*, 581–584.

Murphy, M., Riedner, B. A., Huber, R., Massimini, M., Ferrarelli, F., & Tononi, G. (2009). Source modeling sleep slow waves. *Proceedings of the National Academy of Sciences of the United States of America, 106*, 1608–1613.

Nir, Y., Andrillon, T., Marmelshtein, A., Suthana, N., Cirelli, C., Tononi, G., & Fried, I. (2017). Selective neuronal lapses precede human cognitive lapses following sleep deprivation. *Nature Medicine, 23*, 1474–1480.

Nir, Y., Staba, R. J., Andrillon, T., Vyazovskiy, V. V., Cirelli, C., Fried, I., & Tononi, G. (2011). Regional slow waves and spindles in human sleep. *Neuron, 70*, 153–169.

Nir, Y., Vyazovskiy, V. V., Cirelli, C., Banks, M. I., & Tononi, G. (2015). Auditory responses and stimulus-specific adaptation in rat auditory cortex are preserved across NREM and REM sleep. *Cerebral Cortex, 25*, 1362–1378.

Nobili, L., De Gennaro, L., Proserpio, P., Moroni, F., Sarasso, S., Pigorini, A., De Carli, F., & Ferrara, M. (2012). Local aspects of sleep: Observations from intracerebral recordings in humans. *Progress in Brain Research, 199*, 219–232.

Obal, F., Jr., & Krueger, J. M. (2003). Biochemical regulation of non-rapid-eye-movement sleep. *Frontiers in Bioscience, 8*, d520–d550.

Okun, M., & Lampl, I. (2008). Instantaneous correlation of excitation and inhibition during ongoing and sensory-evoked activities. *Nature Neuroscience, 11*, 535–537.

Okun, M., Steinmetz, N. A., Cossell, L., Iacaruso, M. F., Ko, H., Bartho, P., Moore, T., Hofer, S. B., Mrsic-Flogel, T. D., Carandini, M., & Harris, K. D. (2015). Diverse coupling of neurons to populations in sensory cortex. *Nature, 521*, 511–515.

Olcese, U., Esser, S. K., & Tononi, G. (2010). Sleep and synaptic renormalization: A computational study. *Journal of Neurophysiology, 104*, 3476–3493.

Pigorini, A., Sarasso, S., Proserpio, P., Szymanski, C., Arnulfo, G., Casarotto, S., Fecchio, M., Rosanova, M., Mariotti, M., Lo Russo, G., Palva, J. M., Nobili, L., & Massimini, M. (2015). Bistability breaks-off deterministic responses to intracortical stimulation during non-REM sleep. *Neuroimage, 112*, 105–113.

Pilorz, V., Astiz, M., Heinen, K. O., Rawashdeh, O., & Oster, H. (2020). The concept of coupling in the mammalian circadian clock network. *Journal of Molecular Biology, 432*, 3618–3638.

Priebe, N. J., & Ferster, D. (2008). Inhibition, spike threshold, and stimulus selectivity in primary visual cortex. *Neuron, 57*, 482–497.

Quercia, A., Zappasodi, F., Committeri, G., & Ferrara, M. (2018). Local use-dependent sleep in wakefulness links performance errors to learning. *Frontiers in Human Neuroscience, 12*, Article 122.
Rattenborg, N. C., Amlaner, C. J., & Lima, S. L. (2000). Behavioral, neurophysiological and evolutionary perspectives on unihemispheric sleep. *Neuroscience and Biobehavioral Reviews, 24*, 817–842.
Rattenborg, N. C., Lima, S. L., & Lesku, J. A. (2012). Sleep locally, act globally. *Neuroscientist, 18*, 533–546.
Rector, D. M., Topchiy, I. A., Carter, K. M., & Rojas, M. J. (2005). Local functional state differences between rat cortical columns. *Brain Research, 1047*, 45–55.
Riedner, B. A., Vyazovskiy, V. V., Huber, R., Massimini, M., Esser, S., Murphy, M., & Tononi, G. (2007). Sleep homeostasis and cortical synchronization: III. A high-density EEG study of sleep slow waves in humans. *Sleep, 30*, 1643–1657.
Rockstrom, M. D., Chen, L., Taishi, P., Nguyen, J. T., Gibbons, C. M., Veasey, S. C., & Krueger, J. M. (2018). Tumor necrosis factor alpha in sleep regulation. *Sleep Medicine Reviews, 40*, 69–78.
Roy, S., Krueger, J. M., Rector, D. M., & Wan, Y. (2008). A network model for activity-dependent sleep regulation. *Journal of Theoretical Biology, 253*, 462–468.
Saini, C., Suter, D. M., Liani, A., Gos, P., & Schibler, U. (2011). The mammalian circadian timing system: Synchronization of peripheral clocks. *Cold Spring Harbor Symposia on Quantitative Biology, 76*, 39–47.
Sanchez-Vives, M. V., Massimini, M., & Mattia, M. (2017). Shaping the default activity pattern of the cortical network. *Neuron, 95*, 993–1001.
Sanchez-Vives, M. V., & McCormick, D. A. (2000). Cellular and network mechanisms of rhythmic recurrent activity in neocortex. *Nature Neuroscience, 3*, 1027–1034.
Saper, C. B., Fuller, P. M., Pedersen, N. P., Lu, J., & Scammell, T. E. (2010). Sleep state switching. *Neuron, 68*, 1023–1042.
Sarasso, S., D'Ambrosio, S., Fecchio, M., Casarotto, S., Vigano, A., Landi, C., Mattavelli, G., Gosseries, O., Quarenghi, M., Laureys, S., Devalle, G., Rosanova, M., & Massimini, M. (2020). Local sleep-like cortical reactivity in the awake brain after focal injury. *Brain, 143*, 3672–3684.
Scharf, M. T., Naidoo, N., Zimmerman, J. E., & Pack, A. I. (2008). The energy hypothesis of sleep revisited. *Progress in Neurobiology, 86*, 264–280.
Scheeringa, R., Mazaheri, A., Bojak, I., Norris, D. G., & Kleinschmidt, A. (2011). Modulation of visually evoked cortical FMRI responses by phase of ongoing occipital alpha oscillations. *Journal of Neuroscience, 31*, 3813–3820.
Sela, Y., Vyazovskiy, V. V., Cirelli, C., Tononi, G., & Nir, Y. (2016). Responses in rat core auditory cortex are preserved during sleep spindle oscillations. *Sleep, 39*, 1069–1082.
Siclari, F., Baird, B., Perogamvros, L., Bernardi, G., Larocque, J. J., Riedner, B., Boly, M., Postle, B. R., & Tononi, G. (2017). The neural correlates of dreaming. *Nature Neuroscience, 20*, 872–878.
Siepka, S. M., & Takahashi, J. S. (2005). Methods to record circadian rhythm wheel running activity in mice. *Methods in Enzymology, 393*, 230–239.
Soltani, S., Chauvette, S., Bukhtiyarova, O., Lina, J. M., Dube, J., Seigneur, J., Carrier, J., & Timofeev, I. (2019). Sleep–wake cycle in young and older mice. *Frontiers in Systems Neuroscience, 13*, Article 51.
Stepanyants, A., Martinez, L. M., Ferecsko, A. S., & Kisvarday, Z. F. (2009). The fractions of short- and long-range connections in the visual cortex. *Proceedings of the National Academy of Sciences of the United States of America, 106*, 3555–3560.
Steriade, M. (1993). Cholinergic blockage of network- and intrinsically generated slow oscillations promotes waking and REM sleep activity patterns in thalamic and cortical neurons. *Progress in Brain Research, 98*, 345–355.
Steriade, M. (2004). Neocortical cell classes are flexible entities. *Nature Reviews Neuroscience, 5*, 121–134.
Steriade, M., & Amzica, F. (1998). Coalescence of sleep rhythms and their chronology in corticothalamic networks. *Sleep Research Online, 1*, 1–10.
Steriade, M., Amzica, F., & Nunez, A. (1993a). Cholinergic and noradrenergic modulation of the slow (approximately 0.3 Hz) oscillation in neocortical cells. *Journal of Neurophysiology, 70*, 1385–1400.
Steriade, M., Nunez, A., & Amzica, F. (1993b). A novel slow (<1 Hz) oscillation of neocortical neurons in vivo: Depolarizing and hyperpolarizing components. *Journal of Neuroscience, 13*, 3252–3265.
Steriade, M., Timofeev, I., & Grenier, F. (2001). Natural waking and sleep states: A view from inside neocortical neurons. *Journal of Neurophysiology, 85*, 1969–1985.
Strasser, A., Luksys, G., Xin, L., Pessiglione, M., Gruetter, R., & Sandi, C. (2020). Glutamine-to-glutamate ratio in the nucleus accumbens predicts effort-based motivated performance in humans. *Neuropsychopharmacology, 45*, 2048–2057.

Swadlow, H. A. (2002). Thalamocortical control of feed-forward inhibition in awake somatosensory "barrel" cortex. *Philosophical Transactions of the Royal Society of London. Series B, Biological Sciences, 357*, 1717–1727.

Thomas, C. W., Guillaumin, M. C., McKillop, L. E., Achermann, P., & Vyazovskiy, V. V. (2020). Global sleep homeostasis reflects temporally and spatially integrated local cortical neuronal activity. *Elife*, 9, Article e54148.

Timofeev, I., Grenier, F., Bazhenov, M., Sejnowski, T. J., & Steriade, M. (2000). Origin of slow cortical oscillations in deafferented cortical slabs. *Cerebral Cortex, 10*, 1185–1199.

Timofeev, I., Grenier, F., & Steriade, M. (2001). Disfacilitation and active inhibition in the neocortex during the natural sleep–wake cycle: An intracellular study. *Proceedings of the National Academy of Sciences of the United States of America, 98*, 1924–1929.

Tobler, I. (2005). Phylogeny of sleep regulation. In M. H. Kryger, T. Roth, & W. C. Dement (Eds.), *Principles and practice of sleep medicine* (4th ed., pp. 77–90). W. B. Saunders.

Tobler, I., & Borbely, A. A. (1986). Sleep EEG in the rat as a function of prior waking. *Electroencephalography and Clinical Neurophysiology, 64*, 74–76.

Trachsel, L., Tobler, I., & Borbely, A. A. (1989). Effect of sleep deprivation on EEG slow wave activity within non-REM sleep episodes in the rat. *Electroencephalography and Clinical Neurophysiology, 73*, 167–171.

Van Essen, D. C., Anderson, C. H., & Felleman, D. J. (1992). Information processing in the primate visual system: An integrated systems perspective. *Science, 255*, 419–423.

Verzeano, M., & Negishi, K. (1960). Neuronal activity in cortical and thalamic networks. *Journal of General Physiology, 43*(S6), 177–195.

Voysey, Z., Martin-Lopez, D., Jimenez-Jimenez, D., Selway, R. P., Alarcon, G., & Valentin, A. (2015). Electrical stimulation of the anterior cingulate gyrus induces responses similar to K-complexes in awake humans. *Brain Stimulation, 8*, 881–890.

Vyazovskiy, V., Achermann, P., Borbely, A. A., & Tobler, I. (2004). Interhemispheric coherence of the sleep electroencephalogram in mice with congenital callosal dysgenesis. *Neuroscience, 124*, 481–488.

Vyazovskiy, V., Borbely, A. A., & Tobler, I. (2000). Unilateral vibrissae stimulation during waking induces interhemispheric EEG asymmetry during subsequent sleep in the rat. *Journal of Sleep Research, 9*, 367–371.

Vyazovskiy, V. V., Achermann, P., Borbely, A. A. & Tobler, I. (2004). The dynamics of spindles and EEG slow-wave activity in NREM sleep in mice. *Archives Italienne de Biologie, 142*, 511–523.

Vyazovskiy, V. V., Achermann, P., & Tobler, I. (2007). Sleep homeostasis in the rat in the light and dark period. *Brain Research Bulletin, 74*, 37–44.

Vyazovskiy, V. V., Borbely, A. A., & Tobler, I. (2002). Interhemispheric sleep EEG asymmetry in the rat is enhanced by sleep deprivation. *Journal of Neurophysiology, 88*, 2280–2286.

Vyazovskiy, V. V., Cirelli, C., & Tononi, G. (2011). Electrophysiological correlates of sleep homeostasis in freely behaving rats. *Progress in Brain Research, 193*, 17–38.

Vyazovskiy, V. V., Cui, N., Rodriguez, A. V., Funk, C., Cirelli, C., & Tononi, G. (2014). The dynamics of cortical neuronal activity in the first minutes after spontaneous awakening in rats and mice. *Sleep, 37*, 1337–1347.

Vyazovskiy, V. V., & Faraguna, U. (2015). Sleep and synaptic homeostasis. *Current Topics in Behavioral Neurosciences, 25*, 91–121.

Vyazovskiy, V. V., Faraguna, U., Cirelli, C., & Tononi, G. (2009). Triggering slow waves during NREM sleep in the rat by intracortical electrical stimulation: Effects of sleep/wake history and background activity. *Journal of Neurophysiology, 101*, 1921–1931.

Vyazovskiy, V. V., & Harris, K. D. (2013). Sleep and the single neuron: The role of global slow oscillations in individual cell rest. *Nature Reviews Neuroscience, 14*, 443–451.

Vyazovskiy, V. V., Olcese, U., Cirelli, C., & Tononi, G. (2013). Prolonged wakefulness alters neuronal responsiveness to local electrical stimulation of the neocortex in awake rats. *Journal of Sleep Research, 22*, 239–250.

Vyazovskiy, V. V., Olcese, U., Hanlon, E. C., Nir, Y., Cirelli, C., & Tononi, G. (2011). Local sleep in awake rats. *Nature, 472*, 443–447.

Vyazovskiy, V. V., Olcese, U., Lazimy, Y. M., Faraguna, U., Esser, S. K., Williams, J. C., Cirelli, C., & Tononi, G. (2009). Cortical firing and sleep homeostasis. *Neuron, 63*, 865–878.

Vyazovskiy, V. V., Riedner, B. A., Cirelli, C., & Tononi, G. (2007). Sleep homeostasis and cortical synchronization: II. A local field potential study of sleep slow waves in the rat. *Sleep, 30*, 1631–1642.

Vyazovskiy, V. V., & Tobler, I. (2005). Theta activity in the waking EEG is a marker of sleep propensity in the rat. *Brain Research, 1050*, 64–71.

Vyazovskiy, V. V., & Tobler, I. (2008). Handedness leads to interhemispheric EEG asymmetry during sleep in the rat. *Journal of Neurophysiology, 99*, 969–975.

Vyazovskiy, V. V., & Tobler, I. (2012). The temporal structure of behaviour and sleep homeostasis. *PLOS ONE, 7*, Article e50677.

Vyazovskiy, V. V., Tobler, I., & Winsky-Sommerer, R. (2007). Alteration of behavior in mice by muscimol is associated with regional electroencephalogram synchronization. *Neuroscience, 147*, 833–841.

Vyazovskiy, V. V., Welker, E., Fritschy, J. M., & Tobler, I. (2004). Regional pattern of metabolic activation is reflected in the sleep EEG after sleep deprivation combined with unilateral whisker stimulation in mice. *European Journal of Neuroscience, 20*, 1363–1370.

Ward, C. D. (2011). On doing nothing: Descriptions of sleep, fatigue, and motivation in encephalitis lethargica. *Movement Disorders, 26*, 599–604.

Werth, E., Achermann, P., & Borbely, A. A. (1996). Brain topography of the human sleep EEG: Antero-posterior shifts of spectral power. *Neuroreport, 8*, 123–127.

Wiehler, A., Branzoli, F., Adanyeguh, I., Mochel, F., & Pessiglione, M. (2022). A neuro-metabolic account of why daylong cognitive work alters the control of economic decisions. *Current Biology, 32*, 3564–3575.e5.

Wienke, C., Bartsch, M. V., Vogelgesang, L., Reichert, C., Hinrichs, H., Heinze, H. J., & Durschmid, S. (2021). Mind-wandering is accompanied by both local sleep and enhanced processes of spatial attention allocation. *Cerebral Cortex Communications, 2*, Article tgab001.

Wu, J. C., Gillin, J. C., Buchsbaum, M. S., Chen, P., Keator, D. B., Khosla Wu, N., Darnall, L. A., Fallon, J. H., & Bunney, W. E. (2006). Frontal lobe metabolic decreases with sleep deprivation not totally reversed by recovery sleep. *Neuropsychopharmacology, 31*, 2783–2792.

Yamagata, T., Kahn, M. C., Prius-Mengual, J., Meijer, E., Sabanovic, M., Guillaumin, M. C. C., Van Der Vinne, V., Huang, Y. G., McKillop, L. E., Jagannath, A., Peirson, S. N., Mann, E. O., Foster, R. G., & Vyazovskiy, V. V. (2021). The hypothalamic link between arousal and sleep homeostasis in mice. *Proceedings of the National Academy of Sciences of the United States of America, 118*, Article e2101580118.

Zavada, A., Strijkstra, A. M., Boerema, A. S., Daan, S., & Beersma, D. G. (2009). Evidence for differential human slow-wave activity regulation across the brain. *Journal of Sleep Research, 18*, 3–10.

Zhang, P., Bannon, N. M., Ilin, V., Volgushev, M., & Chistiakova, M. (2015). Adenosine effects on inhibitory synaptic transmission and excitation–inhibition balance in the rat neocortex. *Journal of Physiology, 593*, 825–841.

SECTION 2

The Roles and Functions of Sleep

CHAPTER

7 Why We Sleep

H. Craig Heller

Abstract

The function of sleep is an enduring question in biomedical sciences. Many hypotheses are discussed in the chapters in this section. However, the question has become more complex in recent decades with the expansion of defining characteristics of sleep beyond its electrophysiological manifestations in mammals and birds. Acceptance of possible homologies between traditionally defined sleep and behavioral rest states widely observed in the animal kingdom has led to the view that sleep has very deep phylogenetic roots. That view requires an evolutionary approach to understand functions of sleep and distinguish between basal or primal functions and more complex derived functions. A primal function could have been simple rest/activity phases in response to environmental geophysical cycles. Energetic consequences of such cycling could have been preadaptations for maximizing efficiency of energy acquisition, utilization, and conservation through processes that became basal sleep. That energetic function of sleep may have been retained through phylogeny as selection added functions such as those associated with more complex nervous systems and more complex physiology. An unavoidable conclusion from this line of evolutionary thinking is that sleep, broadly speaking, serves many functions. The challenge is to discover those diverse functions and seek homologies between species.

Key Words: adenosine, glycogen, glymphatics, learning/memory, REM–NREM homeostasis, neural plasticity

Introduction

"Why do we sleep?" is a common question received by sleep researchers. Yet, there is no easy answer. Why we sleep is one of the largest unanswered questions in the life sciences. There are many leading hypotheses, and most are covered extensively in the chapters in this section. The substance of these hypotheses, however, is broader now than it was 20+ years ago. Prior to that time, sleep sensu stricto was considered to be what was observed in mammals and birds. The reason for this distinction was that the electrical signals recorded from the cerebral cortex in mammals and the pallium in birds showed distinctive patterns in behavioral wake and sleep. These electroencephalographic (EEG) signatures became the standard metric for studying sleep. Since nonavian and nonmammalian vertebrates do not have similar elaborations of the telencephalon and therefore do not show these characteristic EEG features, they were assumed not to have neurophysiological states homologous to mammalian and avian non–rapid-eye-movement (NREM) and rapid-eye-movement (REM) sleep. Even though a broad diversity of species had been shown to have clear changes in activity, in sensory receptivity, and in behavior, usually on a daily basis, the terminology used for these daily cycles was simply *rest/activity*. An example is the pioneering work on cockroaches and fish by Tobler (1983) and Tobler and Borbely (1985). There were no assumptions or implications of homology with the electrophysiologically characterized sleep/wake states in mammals and birds. However, clear behavioral state changes with characteristic changes in posture, arousal thresholds, and responses to prolonged activity were observed and characterized. One conclusion of a massive review of "animal sleep" was, "In summary, the presence of sleep among insects remains highly debatable" (Campbell & Tobler, 1984, p. 273).

A sea change in the possible relationships between avian/mammalian sleep and what had been carefully distinguished as rest in other species occurred in the early 2000s. At the Associated Professional Sleep Societies' SLEEP meeting in Philadelphia in 2004, I was struck by the almost universal shift from the year before in the use of *sleep* instead of *rest phase* in talks and posters about research in fruit flies (*Drosophila*). This transition in the scope of what is considered sleep was heralded by two influential papers (Hendricks et al., 2000; Shaw et al., 2000). Since that time, *Drosophila* has become a model system in sleep research, and there has been enormous growth in the number of studies claiming to characterize sleep in species other than birds and mammals: for example, fish (Yokogawa et al., 2007; Zhdanova, 2006), amphibians and reptiles (review by Libourel & Herrel, 2016), cephalopods (Frank et al., 2012; Iglesias et al., 2019; Meisel et al., 2011), coelenterates (Nath et al., 2017), nematodes (Raizen et al., 2008), and more.

Broadening Our Perspective

The significance of this enormous expansion of sleep research in model and non-model organisms is that it changes the questions we might ask about the function or functions of sleep. When the scope of our perspective was limited to mammals and birds, many questions about why we sleep focused on complex higher vertebrate functions such as cognition, memory, and emotion regulation. Those may be sleep functions in species with more complex nervous systems, but now we must consider the possibility that the phylogeny of sleep stretches deep into the distant origins of life, or at least multicellular life. Thus, if there is a unitary or primal function of sleep, it must pertain to very basic properties of organisms. That function could have remained throughout phylogeny while serving as a preadaptation for adding more specialized functions found in more complex organisms. It is time to abandon the concept of a single function of sleep. An important reason for searching for functions of sleep in diverse organisms and different physiological systems is that discovering a sleep function in one group of organisms would lead to questions as to whether that same function exists in other lineages. Finding such commonalities across phylogenetic groups could lead to discovering which sleep functions are basal and primal and which sleep functions have evolved along with increased complexity of living systems.

Rest–Activity Cycles Are Primal

An obvious feature of early life forms that could have served as a preadaptation for additional sleep functions is daily rest/activity cycles that evolved as adaptations to geophysical cycles and perhaps to avoidance of ultraviolet radiation. The existence of light/dark activity phases was surely a major selective factor in the evolution of early life forms. That selection would have been important in the evolution of specializations for energy acquisition and the sensory systems involved. Those specializations along with the rise of predation would have resulted naturally in physiological and behavioral cycles with phases dominated by anabolism or catabolism. A selective advantage in this scenario would have been conservation of energy during the inactive phase. Thus, an important early function of the rest phase of the daily rest/activity cycle could have been energy conservation, as proposed by Walker and Berger (1980). Inactivity limits acquisition of energy; but it has lower energetic costs than activity, and it could be of value in avoiding predation during the daily phase in which a potential prey species is at a sensory disadvantage. The phylogenetic continuity of energy conservation as a function of rest/sleep is supported by the fact that body temperature is regulated at lower levels during the sleep phase in mammals and birds, resulting in significant energy savings (Glotzbach & Heller, 1976; Heller et al., 1983). The idea of a rest phase as a preadaptation for the evolution of a sleep function involving energetics is supported by the evolutionary extensions of sleep as torpor and hibernation in endotherms—clear adaptations for energy conservation (Heller, 1979; Walker et al., 1977, 1979, 1981).

Energetics and Sleep

A connection between energetics and a sleep function was supported by the finding that adenosine—a breakdown product of adenosine triphosphate—is a somnogen. Radulovacki et al. (1984) showed that adenosine analogues increased sleep duration. Furthermore, that effect was blocked by wake-promoting caffeine, which was known to block adenosine receptors. Around this same time quantitative EEG studies of the effects of sleep deprivation on subsequent sleep in rats and in humans established the homeostatic relationship between prior wake duration and the spectral power of slow waves (delta waves, 0.5–4.4 Hz; Borbely, 1982, 2022). The association between NREM delta power and adenosine was subsequently shown (Figure 7.1; Benington, Kodali, & Heller, 1995; Porkka-Heisskanen et al., 1997). This connection between a breakdown product of energy metabolism and the regulation of sleep homeostasis supported the concept that sleep serves a function supporting energetics. More recent support for the link between

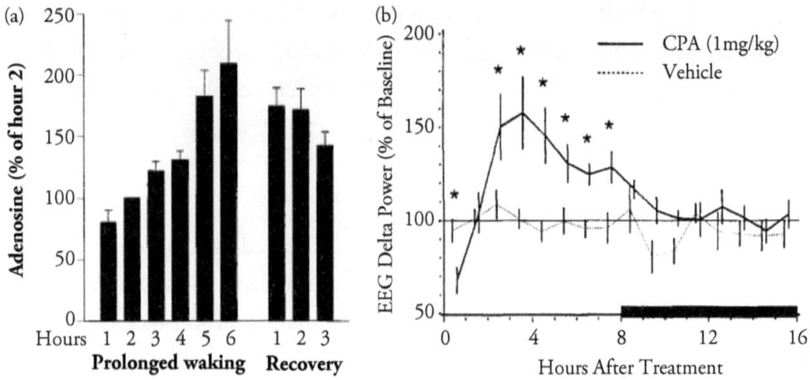

Figure 7.1 Relationships between cerebral extracellular adenosine, sleep/wake, and electroencephalographic (EEG) slow-wave activity

Note. Panel A: Microdialysis reveals that extracellular adenosine in the cat brain increases with prolonged wake and declines during recovery sleep. From Porkka-Heisskanen T, Strecker RE, Thakkar M, Bjorkum AA, Greene RW, and McCarley RW (1997) Adenosine: A mediator of the sleep-inducing effects of prolonged wakefulness. *Science 276*: 1265–1268. Reprinted with permission from AAAS. Panel B. Intracerebroventricular injection of the adenosine A1 receptor agonist cyclopentyladenosine increases EEG slow-wave activity in a sleep-satiated rat (Benington, Woudenberg, & Heller, 1995). AAAS = American Association for the Advancement of Science; CPA = cyclopentyladenosine.

sleep and energy conservation came from the demonstration that adenosine and the adenosine A1 receptor are a major controlling mechanism for the entrance into torpor by hibernators (Jinka et al., 2011).

Linking energetics with sleep, arguably a brain function, led to a consideration of the major energy reserve of the brain, glycogen (Greutter, 2003). We proposed that a function of sleep was the restoration of brain glycogen reserves that were depleted regionally during waking activities (Benington & Heller, 1995b). Experiments on rats by Kong et al. (2002) showed that prolonged wakefulness depletes brain glycogen and that restorative sleep replenishes it. Subsequent studies on mice and rats showed a more complicated relationship between wake, sleep, and cerebral glycogen that was influenced by brain region, genotype, and glucocorticoid levels (Allaman et al., 2004; Franken et al., 2003, 2006; Gip et al., 2002, 2004). The reasons for these discrepant results may have been that glycogen synthesis and degradation are not discretely separated by wake and sleep and that the dynamics of glycogen synthesis and glycogenolysis have different time frames. Sorg and Magistretti (1992) showed biphasic effects of neurotransmitters and adenosine on glycogen homeostasis in astrocytes. Immediate responses (minutes) elevate cyclic adenosine monophosphate (cAMP), leading to phosphorylations and glycogenolysis; but the longer-term (hours) effects of the elevated cAMP are transcription events leading to new protein synthesis that elevates glycogenesis. Whereas the initial investigations of brain glycogen amounts were snapshots of glycogen levels at specific time points, the relationship between rates of glycogen synthesis and catabolism is a continuous but variable function.

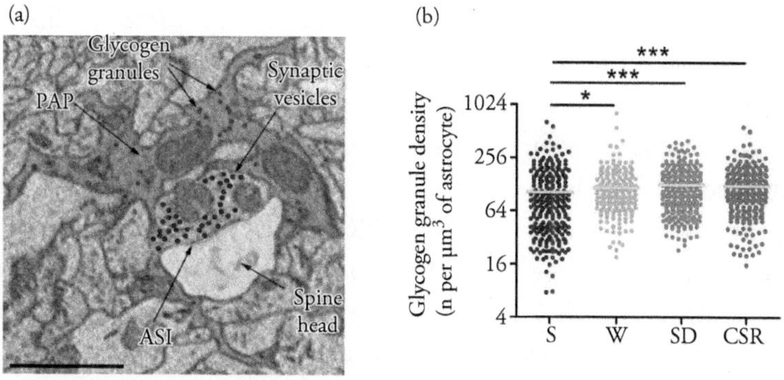

Figure 7.2 Glycogen distribution and dynamics in the tripartite synapse

Note. Panel A: In this tridimensional electron micrograph, the dendritic spine head is colored yellow. Blue circles in the presynaptic terminal are neurotransmitter vesicles. Peripheral astrocytic process is colored blue, and glycogen granules are red circles. Panel B: During all wake conditions, the number of glycogen granules around the synapses was greater; but the granules were smaller, suggesting greater turnover, and the estimated glucose content of the granules was smaller (Bellesi et al., 2018). Figure reproduced under a CC BY 4.0 license. ASI = axon-spine interface; CSR = chronic sleep restriction; PAP = peripheral astrocytic process; S = sleep; SD = sleep deprivation; W = wake.

Thus, the limited technology in the early 2000s did not allow a definitive examination of the relationship between glycogen dynamics and sleep/wake.

New technology has enabled a closer look at glycogen dynamics in the synapses between astrocytes and neurons as a function of sleep and wake (Bellesi et al., 2018). Glycogen granules are highly branched polymers of glucose. The branches of those chains lose glucose units during glycogenolysis and gain glucose units during glycogen synthesis. Tridimensional electron microscopy enabled quantification of glycogen granules at the synapses of astrocytic processes and the neurons they support (Figure 7.2). The findings were that there are more glycogen granules in the astrocyte terminals during wake, but with longer duration of wake the granules get smaller and closer to the synaptic membrane. During sleep the granules get bigger. The estimated glucose content of the granules is greater during sleep. The conclusion of the authors was that wake leads to increased glycogen turnover around synapses and sleep promotes glycogen accumulation. Thus, from the perspectives of energy utilization, temperature regulation, and management of brain energy reserves, the hypothesis that sleep serves a fundamental energy conservation and restoration function remains plausible.

Homeostasis of the Intercellular Environment

Just as the efficient utilization of energy resources can be a primal benefit of rest/activity cycles and a preadaptation in the evolution of sleep, so can the need to deal with the consequences of energy metabolism and other nervous system functions—the need to eliminate waste products. That problem is the focus of a recently proposed function of sleep—the glymphatic hypothesis (Hablitz & Nedergaard, 2021; Hablitz et al., 2020;

Iliff et al., 2012; Xie et al., 2013). The mammalian brain is protected from intrusion of circulating substances by the blood–brain barrier (BBB) consisting of astrocytic processes. But that BBB could also be expected to impede the extrusion of waste products such as protein complexes, referred to as *amyloids*. The discovery of the glymphatic system suggests a solution to this problem. The glymphatic system consists of perivascular spaces that allow cerebrospinal fluid (CSF) to flow from the surface of the brain through the brain and have access to the intercellular spaces through aquaporin channels in the astrocytic membranes (Figure 7.3). Circulatory pulsations move the CSF through the perivascular spaces and move the intercellular fluid through the parenchyma and into venous perivascular spaces, and thereby out of the brain into the lymphatic system (Fultz et al., 2019; Iliff et al., 2013). How is this elegant clearance system through CSF flow related to sleep? The researchers infused fluorescent dyes iontophoretically into the subarachnoid CSF and then imaged their spread in the cortex with two-photon microscopy (Hablitz et al., 2019; Xie et al., 2013). The spread of tracer was greater in sleep than in wake. In fact, the spread was almost nil in wake in comparison to sleep. Subsequent experiments infused the dyes into the cisterna magna, and the spread of the dye throughout the brain was subsequently measured 30 minutes postinfusion. These experiments were also done on mice anesthetized with six different anesthetic agents that were known to produce different levels of slow-wave activity (SWA). The spread of the dye throughout the brain parenchyma was proportional to the SWA (Hablitz et al., 2019). The functioning of the glymphatic system has also been demonstrated in humans awake and asleep (Fultz et al., 2019). That study showed that the slow waves are

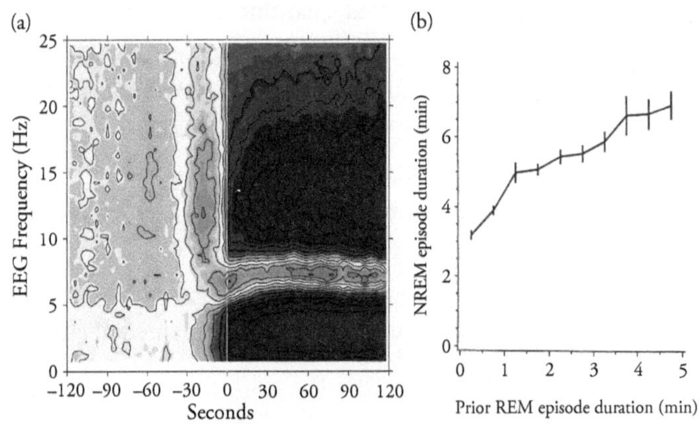

Figure 7.3 A model of the process of encoding and consolidating spatial and declarative information into short- and long-term memories

Note. During spatial and declarative experiences, information registers in the neocortex but is predominantly stored in the hippocampus. During non-rapid-eye-movement sleep the information stored in the hippocampus is reactivated/replayed within the structure of sharp-wave ripples—highly synchronous 150–250 hz oscillations. The sharp-wave ripple events are synchronized with thalamocortical spindles and, as such, are registered in the neocortex in windows of activity framed by the cortical slow waves (Born & Wilhelm, 2012). Reproduced with permission from Springer Nature. EEG = electroencephalography; NREM = non–rapid eye movement; REM = rapid eye movement.

followed by hemodynamic oscillations that are coupled to CSF flow (Figure 7.3). We can conclude that in mammals with closed skulls there is a tight functional relationship between sleep, hemodynamics, CSF flow, and waste clearance—certainly an important function of sleep in mammals.

Is waste clearance a derived function of sleep found only in vertebrates, which have closed circulatory systems and BBBs? Work on *Drosophila* indicates that the answer is "no." Insects like *Drosophila*, and indeed all arthropods, have open circulatory systems, yet they do have the equivalent of the BBB of vertebrates consisting of barrier glial cells that separate the hemolymph from the interstitial fluids of the brain—a hemolymph–brain barrier (HBB). Experiments have shown that endocytotic activity in the HBB is more active during sleep than wake (Artiushin et al., 2018). Also, inhibition of the endocytotic activity of the barrier glial cells increases sleep pressure. Apparently, clearance of waste from the nervous system is a function of sleep that goes further back in sleep phylogeny than the origin of the vertebrates.

Repair and Reorganization

Waste removal is not the only activity necessary for maintenance of any complex machine or living organism; there are also repair and reorganization. Neural tissue is composed of long-lived cells with extensive membranous structures that require maintenance and repair. By analogy with complex machinery, maintenance and repair in the nervous system are more likely to be done offline (i.e., during inactivity) to avoid interfering with ongoing functions. In addition to maintenance and repair, there are changes in neuronal structures and synaptic processes involved in development, seasonal adaptations, behavioral adaptations, physiological alterations, and learning/memory. Many of these changes, generally referred to as *synaptic plasticity*, have been shown to be associated with sleep (Wang et al., 2011).

Acquisition and processing of information during wake involve the growth of new and/or modification of existing synapses. As pointed out by Tononi and Cirelli (2003), synapses cannot continue to be added over time due to spatial and perhaps energetic considerations. Also, modifications of learned information and the behavioral manifestations of that information require weakening or losing synapses as well as gaining new ones. Forgetting is an important component of learning. There is considerable evidence that sleep plays essential roles in synaptic plasticity (Born & Wilhelm, 2012; Rasch & Born, 2012; Stickgold, 2005; Stickgold et al., 2001). Whereas Tononi and Cirelli (2014) make a strong case for synaptic downscaling during sleep resulting in the loss of weaker synapses, there is also evidence for synaptic strengthening during sleep (Frank et al., 2001; Yang et al., 2014). It is reasonable to expect that synaptic remodeling during sleep should involve both weakening and strengthening of synapses depending on wakeful experience and its integration with stored information (Heller, 2014).

Beyond synaptic plasticity, neuronal circuit processes of learning and memory in mammals have been the subjects of extensive study, as reviewed by Rasch and Born (2013); and such research has only expanded since that review. Learning and memory involve acquisition, storage, and integration of information through changes in the structures and functions of neurons in circuits. Current views based on experiments with spatial memories are that wakeful experience is registered short-term in patterned activity in hippocampal circuits, as has been shown in elegant studies by Wilson and colleagues (Lee & Wilson, 2002; Louie & Wilson, 2001; Siapas & Wilson, 1998). These patterns of activity are then organized and transferred to the cortex during sleep (e.g., Ji & Wilson, 2007; Sanda et al., 2021; Siapas et al., 2005). The neuronal events demonstrated in these studies involve several brain structures and broader electrical activity reflected in local field potentials, and they have been modeled by Born and Wilhelm (2012; Figure 7.4). It is unlikely that homologies with these complex mechanisms of information processing and integration considered to be functions of sleep exist in simpler organisms that are now described as sleeping. This is not to say that sleep is not involved in learning and memory in older lineages of animals. Long-term potentiation, considered to be a basic element of learning and memory, was discovered in a mollusk, *Aplysia* (Kandel & Schwartz, 1982), and has been shown to be affected by sleep deprivation (Krishnan et al., 2016); but the higher-order memory phenomena ascribed to specific sleep events in mammals are likely to be without homologies in older lineages of animals. Therefore, types and mechanisms of synaptic remodeling

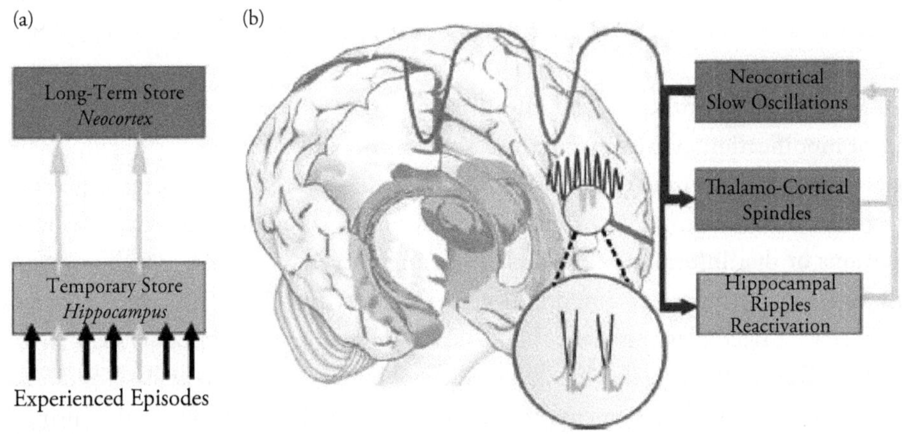

Figure 7.4 The transition from non-rapid-eye-movement (NREM) to rapid-eye-movement (REM) sleep has a distinctive electroencephalographic spectral profile that can be used to quantify sleep cycles

Note. Panel A: The transition from NREM to REM in the rat takes about 30 seconds and is a distinctive feature of sleep even if no scorable REM sleep follows (i.e. an aborted REM bout; figure courtesy of Paul Franken). Panel B: If the length of NREM bouts is plotted as a function of the length of the prior REM bouts, the results indicate a homeostatic relationship between NREM and REM sleep. Long REM bouts are followed by long NREM bouts and vice versa (Benington & Heller, 1994).

and reorganization that are described as functions of NREM and REM sleep and sleep events in mammals are most likely to be derived, rather than primal, functions of rest phases.

Accepting the possibility that sleep-related functions in mammals are derived rather than primal adaptations can influence how we approach the question of the evolution of sleep. A frequently expressed rationale supporting cellular/molecular sleep research is that discovery of cellular/molecular homologies to mammalian sleep (rather than EEG features) would be valuable criteria for establishing evolutionary relationships across widely different phylogenetic groups. However, if the selective pressures on different lineages produced different derived functions of a primal rest state, the search for cellular/molecular homologies might not produce definitive results. In other words, the absence of such homologies would not be evidence that putative sleep in different lineages does not share common evolutionary origins.

Assumptions About Sleep Can Bias Research for Functions

Searches for answers to why we sleep have been shaped by the broad assumption that sleep—including both NREM and REM sleep—serves needs generated by wake. The accepted view is that processes of wake create non-homeostatic conditions that must be corrected by the two sleep states that oscillate with each other. But why are there two sleep states, and why do they oscillate, with NREM always coming first except in some pathological conditions? These questions led to studies probing an alternative to the idea that both NREM and REM serve needs generated by wake. The alternative view is that only NREM is in a homeostatic relationship with wake, and the expression of NREM generates a homeostatic need for REM. Only when REM need gets reduced can the animal have another robust bout of NREM (Benington & Heller, 1995a).

The evidence supporting the hypothesis that the need for REM builds during NREM came from the discovery of an EEG signature of the NREM to REM transition (NRT; Benington, Woudenberg, & Heller, 1994; Figure 7.5). That signature event was frequently not followed by any sustained REM as scored by standard methods and was therefore ignored in sleep cycle analysis. However, when sleep cycles were scored by these NRTs, the homeostatic relationship between NREM and REM was revealed. Short or interrupted REM episodes were always followed by short NREM episodes. Long NREM episodes depended on prior sustained REM episodes (Benington & Heller, 1994). Similar relationships between NREM and REM sleep were subsequently found in human EEG recordings (Barbato & Wehr, 1998). Experiments on rats probed the homeostatic relationship between NREM and REM by interrupting NRTs with minor electrical stimulation of the dorsal raphe nucleus. The response of the animals was to attempt another transition to REM sooner. With only 2 hours of REM being disturbed by this method, the NRTs were occurring at 40 to 50 per hour. After another 2 hours, the

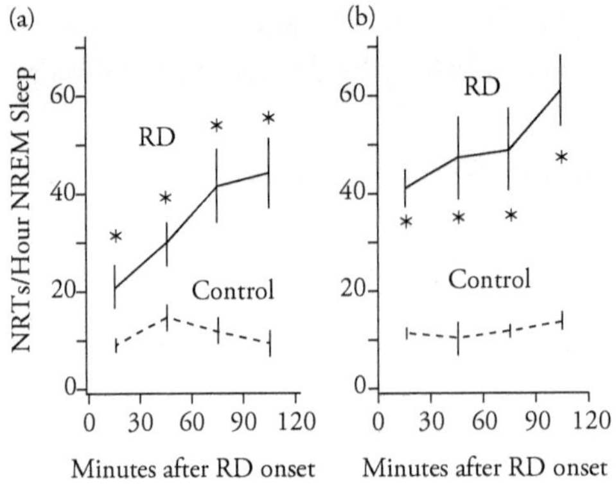

Figure 7.5 A homeostatic relationship between non-rapid-eye-movement (NREM) and rapid-eye-movement (REM) sleep is tested by selective REM interruption by brief, mild electrical stimulation of the dorsal raphe whenever a transition to REM is detected by its spectral profile

Note. Panel A: Early in the rest phase, selective REM deprivation for 2 hours results in a steady increase in the frequency of attempts to enter REM. Panel B: Similar effects of selective REM deprivation are seen in the later half of the rest phase, but they begin with a higher level of NREM to REM transitions. In both experiments, the controls are rats that receive the same number of dorsal raphe stimulations but delivered randomly and not linked to NREM to REM transitions (Benington, Woudenberg, & Heller 1994). NRTs = NREM to REM transitions.

NRTs were occurring at 60 per hour (Figure 7.6; Benington, Kodali, & Heller, 1994). Since the transition to full-blown NREM sleep is not instantaneous but takes many seconds to reach full SWA, this short-term blockage of REM sleep severely compromised the quality of NREM sleep. An important conclusion drawn from these results is that there can be no valid experimental approach that seeks to understand the function of REM sleep by imposing REM deprivation. That manipulation impairs NREM sleep as well.

What could be a homeostatic function of REM sleep with respect to NREM sleep? This question has not been asked previously because of the assumption that REM is serving a function related to wake, even if that function is in concert with an NREM function such as memory consolidation or synaptic pruning. One possibility was suggested by considering what is required to maintain NREM sleep. That is high potassium (K^+) conductance to achieve sufficient hyperpolarization to sustain the synchronous bursting discharges of thalamocortical neurons generating the EEG slow waves (McCormick & Pape, 1990). Maybe it is necessary to periodically reduce that hyperpolarization to re-establish the K^+ concentration gradient across the neuronal membranes. When the K^+ conductance was reduced slightly by low-dose application of apamin, an SK^+ channel blocker (small-conductance calcium-activated potassium channel blocker), rats sustained long bouts of NREM sleep with no REM sleep; and when the drug wore off, there was no REM rebound, suggesting that the need for REM sleep had been reduced or eliminated (Benington, Woudenberg, & Heller, 1995).

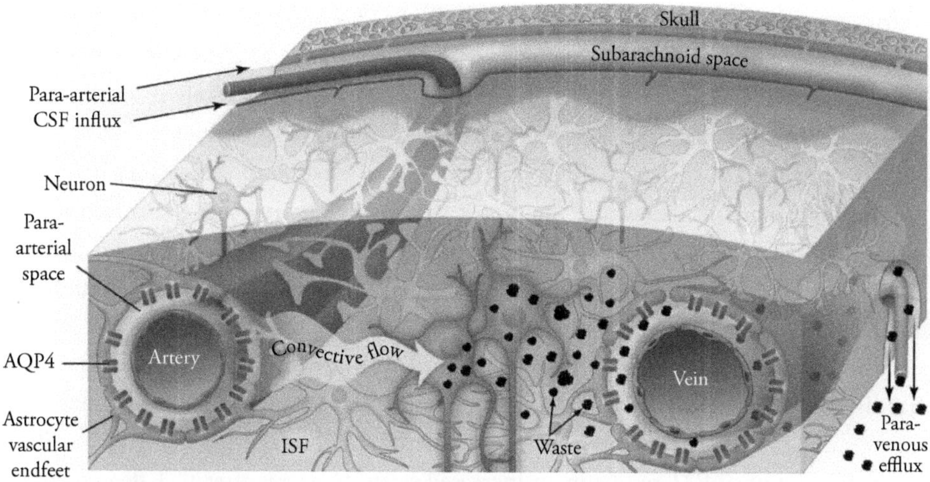

Figure 7.6 A model of the glymphatic hypothesis

Note. Superficial arteries serving the brain course through the subarachnoid space from which they penetrate the parenchyma. Cerebrospinal fluid (CSF) from the subarachnoid space also flows into the brain through the para-arterial space between the blood vessel wall and the astrocyte vascular endfeet that encapsulate the blood vessels. Aquaporins in the astrocytic membranes allow CSF to flow into the astrocytes and then into the intercellular spaces. Flow of this intercellular fluid is driven by hemodynamic pulsations and eventually recollects in the para venous spaces, from which it flows out of the brain parenchyma carrying with it waste products shed into the intercellular fluids. This flow of CSF through the brain is much higher during sleep than during wake. From Nedergaard, M. (2013). Garbage truck of the brain. *Science, 340*(6140), 1529–1530. Reprinted with permission from AAAS. AAAS = American Association for the Advancement of Science; AQP4 = aquaporin 4; ISF = interstitial fluid.

If REM sleep serves a need created by NREM sleep, then why is it generally assumed that REM sleep arises first in mammalian development and predominates in early life? That quandary is based in part on another possibly flawed assumption—that neonatal active sleep is REM sleep. All neonatal sleep is characterized by a low-amplitude, desynchronous EEG that cannot be used to differentiate sleep states. The difference between neonatal active and neonatal quiet sleep is the presence of frequent muscle twitches in active sleep. The combination of those phasic events along with the desynchronous EEG results in active sleep resembling REM sleep, but is it? In one study of EEG development in neonatal rats, slow waves first appeared about postnatal day (P) 11.5, and they were equally likely in quiet or active sleep (Frank & Heller, 1997). Slow waves were gradually consolidated into quiet sleep by P16. A marker of REM sleep is intermittent theta activity in the EEG, and that feature was seen to emerge around P12–14. Thus, this EEG study supports the possibility that both NREM sleep and REM sleep emerge from behavioral active sleep, with NREM sleep preceding REM sleep in sleep development. What about the muscle twitches? These phasic events in the neonate clearly play a role in the development of sensory motor circuits, as shown by Del Rio-Bermudez and Blumberg (2018). However, this developmental function does not define active sleep as

REM sleep. It can be a totally separate process that becomes aligned with REM sleep as REM sleep emerges. In fact, Dooley and Blumberg (2018) have shown that in active sleep in P8–10 rats, motor neurons behave as sensory neurons receiving information from twitching muscles. But they do not respond to muscle movements during wake. By P12, after the emergence of NREM sleep, during active sleep the sensory neuron in a sensorimotor circuit fires before the motor neuron, suggesting that the twitches are a developmental process in the wiring of sensorimotor circuits. In conclusion, it is possible and reasonable that the EEG in both neonatal active and quiet sleep reflects an undifferentiated brain state from which NREM and REM sleep gradually emerge, with NREM preceding REM. A further developmental feature of the sleep EEG in the neonatal rat is that after slow waves first appear, they gradually increase in amplitude until about P20; but over this time, they do not show a homeostatic response to sleep deprivation. Sleep deprivation up until P21 results in an increased sleep time, but after P21 sleep deprivation results in an increase in SWA as occurs in the adult homeostatic response to sleep deprivation (Frank et al., 1998).

I raise this issue of the timing of the developmental appearance of NREM versus REM sleep because it influences how we might think of the previous question of whether REM sleep supports wake or NREM sleep. Solid evidence that REM emerges first in development would tend to support the view that REM is in a homeostatic relationship with wake, but evidence that NREM emerges first in development would tend to support the view that REM could be serving a function related to wake. This is another example of how assumptions or conclusions based on incomplete evidence can influence the course of subsequent hypothesis generation, experimental design, and interpretation.

Sleep Has Many Functions, Both Primal and Advanced

The title of this chapter—"Why We Sleep"—seems at first to be a simple enough statement. But the words in this title require deeper consideration. *Why* is straightforward, it seeks a link between causes and effects. The causes may be proximate (physiological) or ultimate (evolutionary selective pressure), and the effect is the phenomena we want to understand—sleep, NREM sleep, REM sleep. As I have indicated, however, *we* and *sleep* complicate the focus of the quest for answers to the why questions and in opposite directions. *We* usually refers to humans, or at most to other mammalian species. *We* therefore narrows the scope of possibilities for causes and effects. *Sleep*, on the other hand, broadens the scope of possibilities. As pointed out at the beginning of this chapter, there is a rapidly growing perspective that the phenomenon considered *sleep* has much deeper phylogenetic roots than is subsumed by the use of *we*. *We* justifies the focus of much of this chapter on research focusing on properties of advanced, complex nervous systems; but our reference to *sleep* suggests that we should consider functions that are more basal and primal in animal life. This is not to say that functions such as synaptic plasticity, memory consolidation, and glymphatic waste removal are not primary functions of sleep in us and other complex life forms, but these functions could be evolutionary add-ons to a preadaptation that was, and perhaps still is, a more basal and primal function.

As discussed above, selective pressures due to the daily geophysical cycles surely shaped adaptations of even early life forms to optimize their organization of biochemical, physiological, and behavioral processes to maximize survival and/or reproductive success. Candidates for these processes are obviously energetics, growth, repair, and temporal organization. Temporal organization is key because it enables optimization of the other candidate processes. Time and place influence the success of energy acquisition and energy usage. Temporal organization enables reduction in conflict between processes and therefore improves efficiency of metabolism. Temporal organization also enables anticipation of future conditions or events. Temporal organization enables coordination of physiology and behavior with other organisms. Thus, I propose that rest/activity cycles and circadian rhythms are basal, primal functions that were preadaptations for sleep in various and divergent lineages of animals.

In the *we* mode of discussing sleep functions, we frequently encounter the absolute statement that sleep is for the brain. There are good reasons for this statement. Comparing sleep and quiet rest, there are few differences between physiological processes in the body but major differences in neural system functions. When animals sleep, they are maximally vulnerable to predators, so sleep must be really important for some brain functions to require taking the brain offline to accomplish those functions. However, abundant evidence shows that many non-brain physiological systems are severely affected by sleep deprivation. The classical studies of complete sleep deprivation by Rechtschaffen and colleagues (summarized in Rechtschaffen et al., 1989) showed that rats die of sleep deprivation sooner than they would die from total food deprivation. Yet, the investigators of these many studies could not come up with a single cause of death in these experiments. Virtually all physiological systems in these animals deteriorated. Septicemia was usually the end state in these animals, but the extensive damage to other systems was serious enough to have proven lethal even without the loss of integrity of the gut. Granted, the condition of total sleep deprivation to death was an extreme method for revealing the role of sleep in normal cell, tissue, and organ system functions just as total food deprivation would not be a good way of investigating nutrition. Nevertheless, the Rechtschaffen team's experiments certainly pointed to the fact that sleep had to play important roles in non-brain physiological systems.

Subsequent to the Rechtschaffen et al.'s experiments with total sleep deprivation, investigators have taken more nuanced approaches, examining shorter sleep deprivations or restrictions on specific cellular functions. A notable example is the work of Everson and Szabo (2011) on the chronic effects of repeated episodes of sleep restriction. Rather than extreme and continuous sleep deprivation, these experiments used the disk over water method (Bergmann et al., 1989) to expose rats to six 10-day periods of sleep fragmentation and partial deprivation separated by 2 days of ad-lib sleep. NREM sleep across these

10-day periods was reduced by 30%, and REM sleep was reduced about 60%. Animals were then followed for 16 weeks of undisturbed sleep/wake cycles. Forced ambulation of the control rats was the same but limited to a consolidated period of time during the day allowing substantial time for ad-lib sleep. The effects of the sleep restriction on whole-body metabolism were substantial. The sleep-restricted rats lost body mass in spite of being hyperphagic. The main tissue loss was adipose tissue. For 3 months following the sleep restriction episodes the experimental rats continued to have less body mass than controls in spite of remaining hyperphagic.

A following experiment by the Everson group (2012) used the same experimental protocol to investigate in depth one physiological system—bone maintenance. The sleep restriction protocol resulted in a 45-fold reduction in osteoid covered bone, and the remaining osteoid was dramatically reduced in thickness. A blood marker of osteoclast activity was elevated, bone mineral density was reduced, and the composition of the bone marrow was altered. Sleep restriction clearly has a major impact on the physiology of bone health.

Another example of research revealing negative effects of sleep deprivation at the cellular level in a non-neural system is that of Rolls et al. (2015). The focus of that work was the ability of hematopoietic stem cells (HSCs) to migrate into and populate the bone marrow. Mice received lethal exposures to radiation and then received HSC infusions from donor mice. The remarkable result was that these HSC transplantations were 50% less likely to succeed if the donor mice had been sleep-deprived for 4 or 6 hours prior to the transplantation. The ability of the HSCs to migrate into the bone marrow was restored if the donor animal had the opportunity of recovery sleep prior to the bone marrow extraction. The researchers identified the molecular mechanism responsible for this determinant of the ability of the HSCs to migrate into and populate the bone marrow of the recipients. For our discussion here, the significance of this work is that it shows effects of sleep deprivation and recovery sleep at the cellular level, not involving the nervous system and not even in the individual where the deficit is observed.

I do not mean to imply that the nervous system is not involved in functions of the peripheral physiological systems, but rather I am saying that in looking for functions of sleep, we have to consider that major functions of sleep may be found in peripheral, non-neuronal systems and that these sleep functions would be more likely to represent basal, primal functions of sleep than phenomena we study in the mammalian or even the vertebrate nervous system.

Conclusions

In this introductory chapter to the Roles and Functions of Sleep section of this handbook, I have emphasized three main messages: (1) Sleep has deep phylogenetic origins and therefore a complex evolutionary history. Therefore, it is unlikely that studies of sleep function in mammals and birds, or even studies limited to "model systems," will yield a single answer to the question "what is the function of sleep?" (2) We can think of a diversity of potential sleep functions as being on a basal-derived spectrum. Energy management and conservation is likely a basal function, whereas memory consolidation is likely a derived function. (3) There must be a multitude of sleep functions that extend from cells, tissues, and physiological systems to complex activities of the mammalian nervous system. A conclusion from these considerations is that the way we will learn about the evolution and the functions of sleep will be to study different organisms, different systems, and different levels of organization to seek out homologies. Sleep phenomena that are homologous across a diversity of species and levels of biological organization are likely to be basal/primal functions of sleep and those found only in certain species are likely to be more specialized and more recent adaptations.

Future Directions

Several lines of enquiry appear to be particularly important for further research. I have framed these in the following questions.

1. Does REM sleep serve a need created by wake or by NREM sleep, and what is that need?
2. What cellular functions are associated with sleep, and do those functions extend over different cell types and in different species?
3. What is the role of cortical slow waves in mammalian (and, more generally, vertebrate) brain functions?
4. What differences occur in glycogen dynamics in different brain regions and in cortical regions working at different levels during wake?
5. What is a memory transcript in the brain, how is it formed, and how is it transferred and consolidated during sleep?

References

Allaman, I., Pellerin, L., & Magistretti, P. J. (2004). Glucocorticoids modulate neurotransmitter-induced glycogen metabolism in cultured cortical astrocytes. *Journal of Neurochemistry*, *88*(4), 900–908. https://doi.org/10.1046/j.1471-4159.2003.02235.x

Artiushin, G., Shang, S., Tricore, H., & Sehgal, A. (2018). Endocytosis at the *Drosophila* blood–brain barrier as a function for sleep. *eLife*, *7*, Article 43326. https://doi.org/10.7554/eLife.43326

Barbato, G., & Wehr, T. A. (1998). Homeostatic regulation of REM sleep in humans during extended sleep. *Sleep*, *21*, 267–276.

Bellesi, M., de Vivo, L., Koeb, S., Tononi, G., & Cirelli, C. (2018). Sleep and wake affect glycogen content and turnover at perisynaptic astrocytic processes. *Frontiers in Cellular Neuroscience*, *12*, Article 308. https://doi.org/10.3389/fncel.2018.00308

Benington, J. H., & Heller, H. C. (1994). REM-sleep timing is controlled homeostatically by accumulation of REM-sleep propensity in non-REM sleep. *American Journal of Physiology: Regulatory, Integrative and Comparative Physiology*, *266*, R1992–R2000.

Benington, J. H., & Heller, H. C. (1995a). Does the function of REM sleep concern nonREM sleep or waking? *Progress in Neurobiology*, *44*, 433–449.

Benington, J. H., & Heller, H.C. (1995b). Restoration of brain energy metabolism as the function of sleep. *Progress in Neurobiology*, *45*, 347–360.

Benington, J. H., Kodali, S. K., & Heller, H. C. (1994). Scoring transitions to REM-sleep in rats based on the EEG phenomena of pre-REM-sleep: An improved analysis of sleep structure. *Sleep, 17*, 28–36.
Benington, J. H., Kodali, S. K., & Heller, H. C. (1995). Stimulation of A1 adenosine receptors mimics the electroencephalographic effects of sleep deprivation. *Brain Research, 692*, 79–85.
Benington, J. H., Woudenberg, M. C., & Heller, H. C. (1994). REM-sleep propensity accumulates during 2-h REM-sleep deprivation in the rest period in rats. *Neuroscience Letters, 180*, 76–80.
Benington, J. H., Woudenberg, M. C., & Heller, H. C. (1995). Apamin, a selective SK potassium channel blocker, suppresses REM sleep without a compensatory rebound. *Brain Research, 692*, 86–92.
Bergmann, B. M., Kushida, C. A., Everson, C. A., Gilliland, M. A., Obermeyer, W., & Rechtschaffen, A. (1989). Sleep deprivation in the rat: II. Methodology. *Sleep, 12*(1), 5–12. https://doi.org/10.1093/sleep/12.1.5
Borbely, A. (1982). A two process model of sleep regulation. *Human Neurobiology, 1*, 195–204.
Borbely, A. (2022). The two-process model of sleep regulation: Beginnings and outlook. *Journal of Sleep Research, 31*(4), Article e13598. https://doi.org/10.1111/jsr.13598
Born, J., & Wilhelm, I. (2012). System consolidation of memory during sleep. *Psychological Research, 76*(2), 192–203. https://doi.org/10.1007/s00426-011-0335-6
Campbell, S. S., & Tobler, I. (1984). Animal sleep: A review of sleep duration across phylogeny. *Neuroscience and Biobehavioral Reviews, 8*, 269–300.
Del Rio-Bermudez, C., & Blumberg, M. S. (2018). Active sleep promotes functional connectivity in developing sensorimotor networks. *Bioessays, 40*(4), Article e1700234. https://doi.org/10.1002/bies.201700234
Dooley, J. C., & Blumberg, M. S. (2018). Developmental "awakening" of primary motor cortex to the sensory consequences of movement. *eLife, 7*, Article e41841. https://doi.org/10.7554/eLife.41841
Everson, C. A., Folley, A. E., & Toth, J. M. (2012). Chronically inadequate sleep results in abnormal bone formation and abnormal bone marrow in rats. *Experimental Biology and Medicine, 237*(9), 1101–1109. https://doi.org/10.1258/ebm.2012.012043
Everson, C. A., & Szabo, A. (2011). Repeated exposure to severely limited sleep results indistinctive and persistent physiological imbalances in rats. *PLOS ONE, 6*, Article e22987.
Frank, M. G., & Heller, H. C. (1997). The development of REM and slow wave sleep in the rat. *American Journal of Physiology: Regulatory, Integrative and Comparative Physiology, 272*(41), R1792–R1799.
Frank, M. G., Issa, N. P., & Stryker, M. P. (2001). Sleep enhances plasticity in the developing visual cortex. *Neuron, 30*(1), 275–287. https://doi.org/10.1016/S0896-6273(01)00279-3
Frank, M. G., Morrissette, R. N., & Heller, H. C. (1998). Effects of sleep deprivation in neonatal rats. *American Journal of Physiology: Regulatory, Integrative and Comparative Physiology, 275*, R145–R157.
Frank, M. G. Waldrop, R. H., Dumoulin, M., Aton, S., & Boal, J. G. (2012). A preliminary analysis of sleep-like states in the cuttlefish *Sepia officinalis*. *PLOS ONE, 7*(6), Article e38125. https://doi.org/10.1371/journal.pone.0038125
Franken, P., Gip, P., Hagiwara, G., Ruby, N. F., & Heller, H. C. (2003). Changes in brain glycogen after sleep deprivation vary with genotype. *American Journal of Physiology: Regulatory, Integrative and Comparative Physiology, 285*, R413–R419.
Franken, P., Gip, P., Hagiwara, G., Ruby, N. F., & Heller, H. C. (2006). Glycogen content in the cerebral cortex increases with sleep loss in C57BL/6J mice. *Neuroscience Letters, 402*, 176–179.
Fultz, N. E., Bonmassar, G., Setsompop, K., Stickgold, R. A., Rosen, B. R. Polimeni, J. R., & Lewis, L. D. (2019). Coupled electrophysiological, hemodynamic, and cerebrospinal fluid oscillations in human sleep. *Science, 366*, 628–631.
Gip, P., Hagiwara, G., Ruby, N. F., & Heller, H. C. (2002). Sleep deprivation decreases glycogen in the cerebellum but not in the cortex of young rats. *American Journal of Physiology: Regulatory, Integrative and Comparative Physiology, 283*, R54–R59.
Gip, P., Hagiwara, G., Sapolsky, R. M., Cao, V. H., Heller, H. C., & Ruby, N. F. (2004). Glucocorticoids influence brain glycogen levels during sleep deprivation. *American Journal of Physiology: Regulatory, Integrative and Comparative Physiology, 286*, R1057–R1062.
Glotzbach, S. F., & Heller, H. C. (1976). Central nervous regulation of body temperature during sleep. *Science, 194*, 537–539.
Greutter, R. (2003). Glycogen: The forgotten cerebral energy store. *Journal of Neuroscience Research, 74*(2), 179–183. https://doi.org/10.1002/jnr.10785
Hablitz, L. M., & Nedergaard, M. (2021). The glymphatic system. *Current Biology, 31*(20), R1371–R1375. https://doi.org/10.1016/j.cub.2021.08.026

Hablitz, L. M., Plá, V., Giannetto, M., Vinitsky, H. D., Staeger, F. F., Metcalfe, T., Nguyen, R. B., Benrais, A., & Nedergaard, M. (2020). Circadian control of brain glymphatic and lymphatic fluid flow. *Nature Communications, 11*(1), Article 4411. https://doi.org/10.1038/s41467-020-18115-2

Hablitz, L. M., Vinitsky H. S., Sun, Q., Stæger, F. F., Sigurdsson. B., Mortensen, K. N., Lilius, T. O., & Nedergaard, M. (2019). Increased glymphatic influx is correlated with high EEG delta power and low heart rate in mice under anesthesia. *Science Advances, 5*(2), Article aav5447.

Heller, H. C. (1979). Hibernation: Neural aspects. *Annual Review of Physiology, 41*, 305–321.

Heller, H. C. (2014). The ups and downs of synapses during sleep and learning. *Sleep, 37*(7), 1157–1158. https://doi.org/10.5665/sleep.3824

Heller, H. C., Graf, R., & Rautenberg, W. (1983). Circadian and arousal state influences on thermoregulation in the pigeon. *American Journal of Physiology, 245*, R321–R328.

Hendricks, J. C., Finn, S. M., Panckeri, K. A., Chavkin, J., Williams, J. A., Sehgal, A., & Pack, A. I. (2000). Rest in *Drosophila* is a sleep-like state. *Neuron, 25*(1), 129–138. https://doi.org/10.1016/s0896-6273(00)80877-6

Iglesias, T. L., Boal, J. G., Frank, M. G., Zeil, J., & Hanlon, R. T. (2019). Cyclic nature of the REM-like state in the cuttlefish *Sepia officinalis*. *Journal of Experimental Biology, 222*, Article 174862.

Iliff, J. J., Wang, M., Liao, Y., Plogg, B. A., Peng, P., Gundersen, G. A., Benveniste, H., Vates, G. E., Deane, R., Goldman, S. A., Nagelhus, E. A., & Nedergaard, M. (2012). A paravascular pathway facilitates CSF flow through the brain parenchyma and the clearance of interstitial solutes, including amyloid beta. *Science Translational Medicine, 4*, Article 147ra111.

Iliff, J. J., Wang, M., Zeppenfeld, D. M., Venkataraman, A., Plogg, B. A. M., Liao, Y., Deane, R., Goldman, S. A., Nagelhus, E. A., & Nedergaard, M. (2013). Cerebral arterial pulsation drives paravascular CSF–interstitial fluid exchange in the murine brain. *Journal of Neuroscience, 33*, 18190–18199.

Ji, D., & Wilson, M. A. (2007). Coordinated memory replay in the visual cortex and hippocampus during sleep. *Nature Neuroscience, 10*, 100–107. https://doi.org/10.1038/nn1825

Jinka, T. R., Toien, O., & Drew, K. L. (2011). Season primes the brain in an arctic hibernator to facilitate entrance into torpor mediated by adenosine A_1 receptors. *Journal of Neuroscience*, 31(30), 10752–10758. https://doi.org/10.1523/JNEUROSCI.1240-11.2011

Kandel, E. R., & Schwartz, J. H. (1982). Molecular biology of learning: Modulation of transmitter release, *Science, 218*, 433–443.

Kong, J., Shepel, P. N., Holden, C. P., Mackiewicz, M., Pack, A. I., & Geiger, J. D. (2002). Brain glycogen decreases with increased periods of wakefulness: Implications for homeostatic drive to sleep. *Journal of Neuroscience, 22*, 5581–5587. https://doi.org/10.1523/JNEUROSCI.22-13-05581.2002

Krishnan, H. C., Gandour, C. E., Ramos, J. L., Wrinkle, M. C., Sanchez-Pacheco, J. J., & Lyons, L. C. (2016). Acute sleep deprivation blocks short- and long-term operant memory in *Aplysia*. *Sleep, 39*(12), 2161–2171. https://doi.org/10.5665/sleep.6320

Lee, A. K., & Wilson, M. A. (2002). Memory of sequential experience in the hippocampus during slow wave sleep. *Neuron, 36*, 1183–1194.

Libourel, P.-A., & Herrel, A. (2016). Sleep in amphibians and reptiles: A review and a preliminary analysis of evolutionary patterns. *Biological Reviews of the Cambridge Philosophical Society, 91*(3), 833–866. https://doi.org/10.1111/brv.12197

Louie, K., & Wilson, M. A. (2001). Temporally structured replay of awake hippocampal ensemble activity during rapid eye movement sleep. *Neuron, 29*(1), 145–156. https://doi.org/10.1016/s0896-6273(01)00186-6

McCormick, D. A., & Pape, H. C. (1990). Properties of a hyperpolarization activated cation current and its role in rhythmic oscillation in thalamic relay neurons. *Journal of Physiology, 431*, 291–318.

Meisel, D. V., Byrne, R. A., Mather, J. A., & Kuba, M. (2011). Behavioral sleep in *Octopus vulgaris*. *Vie et Milieu, 61*(4), 185–190.

Nath, R. D., Bedbrook, C. N., Abrams, M. J., Basinger, T., Bois, J. S., Prober, D. A., Sternberg, P. W., Gradinaru, V., & Geontoro, L. (2017). The jellyfish *Cassiopea* exhibits a sleep-like state. *Current Biology, 27*(19), 2984–2990. https://doi.org/10.1016/j.cub.2017.08.014

Nedergaard, M. (2013). Garbage truck of the brain. *Science, 340*(6140), 1529–1530.

Porkka-Heisskanen, T., Strecker, R. E., Thakkar, M., Bjorkum, A. A., Greene, R. W., & McCarley, R. W. (1997). Adenosine: A mediator of the sleep-inducing effects of prolonged wakefulness. *Science, 276*, 1265–1268.

Radulovacki, M., Virus, R. M., Djuricic-Nedelson, M., & Green, R. D. (1984). Adenosine analogs and sleep in rats. *The Journal of Pharmacology and Experimental Therapeutics, 228*, 268–274.

Raizen, D. M., Zimmerman, J. E., Maycock, M. H., Ta, U. D., You, Y.-J., Sundaram, M. V., & Pack, A. I. (2008). Lethargus is a *Caenorhabditis elegans* sleep-like state. *Nature, 451*, 569–572.

Rasch, B., & Born, J. (2013). About sleep's role in memory. *Physiological Reviews, 93*(2), 681–766. https://doi.org/10.1152/physrev.00032.2012

Rechtschaffen, A., Bergmann, B. M., Everson, C. A., Kushida, C. A., & Gilliland, M. A. (1989). Sleep deprivation in the rat: X. Integration and discussion of the findings. *Sleep, 12*(1), 68–87.

Rolls, A., Pang, W. W., Ibarrra, I., Colas, D., Bonnavion, P., Korin, B., Heller, H. C., Weissman, I. L., & deLecea, L. (2015). Sleep disruption impairs haematopoietic stem cell transplantation in mice. *Nature Communication, 6*, Article 8516.

Sanda, P., Malerba, P., Jiang, X., Krishnan, G. P., Gonzalez-Martinez, J., Halgren, E., & Bazhenov, M. (2021). Bidirectional interaction of hippocampal ripples and cortical slow waves leads to coordinated spiking activity during NREM sleep. *Cerebral Cortex, 31*, 324–340. https://doi.org/10.1093/cercor/bhaa228

Shaw, P. J., Cirelli, C., Greenspan, R. J., & Tononi, G. (2000). Correlates of sleep and waking in *Drosophila melanogaster*. *Science, 287*, 1834–1837.

Siapas, A. G., Lubenov, E. V., & Wilson, M. (2005). Prefrontal phase locking to hippocampal theta oscillations. *Neuron, 46*(1), 141–151. https://doi.org/10.1016/j.neuron.2005.02.028

Siapas, A. G., & Wilson, M. A. (1998). Coordinated interactions between hippocampal ripples and cortical spindles during slow-wave sleep. *Neuron, 21*, 1123–1128.

Sorg, O., & Magistretti, P. (1992). Vasoactive intestinal peptide and noradrenaline exert long-term control on glycogen levels in astrocytes: Blockade by protein synthesis inhibition. *Journal of Neuroscience, 12*(12), 4923–4931.

Stickgold, R. (2005). Sleep-dependent memory consolidation. *Nature, 437*, 1272–1278.

Stickgold, R., Hobson, J. A., Fosse, R., & Fosse, M. (2001). Sleep, learning, and dreams: Off-line memory reprocessing. *Science, 294*, 1052–1057. https://doi.org/10.1126/science.1063530

Tobler, I. (1983). Effect of forced locomotion on the rest–activity cycle of the cockroach. *Behavioural Brain Research, 8*, 351–360.

Tobler, I., & Borbely, A. A. (1985). Effect of rest deprivation on motor activity in fish. *Journal of Comparative Physiology, 157*, 817–822.

Tononi, G., & Cirelli, C. (2003). Sleep and synaptic homeostasis: A hypothesis. *Brain Research Bulletin, 62*, 143–150. https://doi.org/10.1016/j.brainresbull.2003.09.004

Tononi, G. C., & Cirelli, C. (2014). Sleep and the price of plasticity: From synaptic and cellular homeostasis to memory consolidation and integration. *Neuron, 8*(1), 12–34.

Walker, J. M., & Berger, R. J. (1980). Sleep as an adaptation for energy conservation functionally related to hibernation and shallow torpor. *Progress in Brain Research, 53*, 255–278.

Walker, J. M., Garber, A., Berger, R. J., & Heller, H. C. (1979). Sleep and estivation (shallow torpor): Continuous processes of energy conservation. *Science, 204*, 1098–1100.

Walker, J. M., Glotzbach, S. F., Berger, R. J., & Heller, H. C. (1977). Sleep and hibernation in ground squirrels (*Citellus* spp.): Electrophysiological observations. *American Journal of Physiology, 223*, R213–R221.

Walker, J. M., Haskell, E. H., Berger, R. J., & Heller, H. C. (1981). Hibernation at moderate temperatures: A continuation of slow wave sleep. *Experientia, 37*, 726–728.

Wang, G., Grone, B., Colas, D., Appelbaum, L., & Mourrain, P. (2011). Synaptic plasticity in sleep: Learning, homeostasis, and disease. *Trends in Neurosciences, 34*(9), 452–463. https://doi.org/10.1016/j.tins.2011.07.005

Xie, L., Kang, H., Xu, Q., Chen, M. J., Liao, Y., Thiyagarajan, M., O'Donnell, J., Christensen, D. J., Nicholson, C., Iliff, J. J., Takano, T., Deane, R., & Nedergaard, M. (2013). Sleep drives metabolite clearance from the adult brain. *Science, 342*, 373–377. https://doi.org/10.1126/science.1241224

Yang, G., Lai, C. S. W., Cichon, J., Ma, L., Li, W., & Gan, W.-B. (2014). Sleep promotes branch-specific formation of dendritic spines after learning. *Science, 344*(6188), 1173–1178.

Yokogawa, T., Marin, W., Faraco, J., Pézeron, G., Appelbaum, L., Zhang, J., Rosa, F., Mourrain, P., & Mignot, E. (2007). Characterization of sleep in zebrafish and insomnia in hypocretin receptor mutants. *PLOS Biology, 5*, 2379–2397.

Zhdanova, I. V. (2006). Sleep in zebrafish. *Zebrafish, 3*, 215–226.

CHAPTER

8 Brain Clearance, Sleep, and Circadian Rhythms: Implications for Brain Health

Eva M. van Heese, Erik N. T. P. Bakker, *and* Ysbrand D. van der Werf

Abstract

This chapter provides an overview on the implications of brain clearance, sleep, and circadian rhythms for the brain. It highlights brain clearance as a significant function of sleep, referencing how brain clearance becomes less efficient with aging, hypertension, and several pathological conditions. The chapter then discusses the anatomy of the brain clearance system, particularly cerebrospinal fluid, aquaporin-4 perivascular spaces, and the glymphatic system. It then elaborates on the enhanced brain clearance during sleep in relation to proposed drivers of brain clearance, such as synchronized vasomotion and norepinephrine. It lastly explains the relevance of brain clearance for brain disorders, such as neurodegeneration and Alzheimer's disease.

Key Words: brain clearance, circadian rhythm, cerebrospinal fluid, perivascular space, glymphatic system, vasomotion, norepinephrine, aquaporin-4, neurodegeneration, Alzheimer's disease

General Introduction

Sleep is an important brain and bodily state that supports physiological, hormonal, immune-related, and cognitive processes. Recent studies add another important function to sleep: brain clearance. This groundbreaking idea comes from work in mice, showing efficient clearance of metabolic waste during sleep (Xie et al., 2013). Brain clearance becomes less efficient with aging, hypertension, and several pathological conditions, which has led to the hypothesis that clearance failure may be a final common pathway in diseases of protein aggregation such as dementia (Nedergaard & Goldman, 2020). Thus far, the exact mechanism through which sleep contributes to brain clearance is unclear, and translation from animal studies to humans has only just begun; but it is becoming evident that the field of brain clearance in relation to sleep will be a vast and productive area of research in the upcoming years, with ramifications for the understanding and management of brain disorders and for interventions aimed at improving sleep, brain clearance, and brain health.

This chapter will review the purpose and anatomical routes of brain clearance, discuss different views on the mechanism, describe the role of sleep and circadian factors in relation to driving forces, discuss the relevance of brain clearance for brain disorders, and review ways of harnessing the potential of brain clearance for brain health through medicated and unmedicated approaches.

Anatomy of the Brain Clearance System

Clearance takes place through degradation, transport across the blood–brain barrier into the bloodstream, and uptake in the choroid plexus and via perivascular spaces that surround the cerebral vasculature (Hladky & Barrand, 2018). In these spaces, cerebrospinal fluid (CSF) interacts with interstitial fluid (ISF), facilitating removal of waste products from the brain parenchyma. It is important to note that this interaction is bidirectional: Waste products are removed, while hormones, neurotransmitters, and nutrients are delivered to the brain via the CSF at the same time.

Fluid Compartments in the Brain

The brain consists of four aqueous compartments: CSF, ISF, intracellular fluid, and blood. The blood compartment is separated from the brain by two barriers (Hladky & Barrand, 2016; Plog & Nedergaard, 2018). The blood–brain barrier is located throughout the brain, following the outline of the vasculature. Tight junctions between endothelial cells block the entry of macromolecules and most solutes, but the barrier allows diffusion of certain small molecules (e.g., oxygen and carbon dioxide). Astrocytes and pericytes contribute to the blood–brain barrier but permit solute exchange with brain tissue through small gaps between the astrocytic endfeet. Aquaporin-4 (AQP4) channels within the astrocytic endfeet provide water transportation and function to maintain homeostatic balance and decrease resistance to CSF–ISF exchange (Plog & Nedergaard, 2018). Active transport is necessary for most other substances (Hladky & Barrand, 2016). The blood–CSF barrier is located within the choroid plexus of the two lateral, third and fourth ventricles. It has fenestrated endothelial cells, allowing larger molecules to enter into the stroma of the choroid plexus; but its epithelial cells have an abundance of tight junctions in order to control CSF composition (Jessen et al., 2015). Transport of macromolecules and ions including Na, K, Cl, and HCO_3 occurs through active transport, in which Na/K adenosine triphosphatase is the principal component (Hladky & Barrand, 2016; Plog & Nedergaard, 2018). The choroid plexus epithelium resembles secretory epithelia with a high density of mitochondria, a high transcription rate of genes encoding membrane transport mechanisms, and the presence of microvilli. Taken together, the choroid plexus is fully equipped for secreting the majority of CSF, perhaps with a minor contribution from the cerebral vasculature (MacAulay et al., 2022). The production of CSF adds up to around 500 ml each day in humans, flowing from the lateral ventricles to the third and then fourth, entering the subarachnoid space and cisterna. Exit of CSF from the brain, once thought to occur via arachnoid granulations into the cerebral veins, is now believed to occur primarily via perineural spaces of the cranial nerves along the internal carotid artery, the olfactory–nasal submucosa pathway, both draining into deep cervical lymph nodes. Additional outflow may occur via dural lymphatics and via the spinal cord (Jessen et al., 2015; Plog & Nedergaard, 2018; Proulx, 2021; Spera et al., 2023).

Perivascular Spaces

CSF flows along the brain surface following the perivascular spaces lining meningeal vessels, which appear as expansions of the subarachnoid space (Bedussi et al., 2017, 2018). These spaces thereby form low-resistance pathways from which CSF may either directly drain into the exit routes from the brain (bypassing the brain parenchyma) or contribute to brain clearance via perivascular spaces along penetrating vessels. The interaction of CSF with brain tissue depends on the experimental conditions, such as type of anesthesia, and brain state (sleep vs. awake; Ma et al., 2019). Perivascular spaces have been imaged and described in many studies but in vivo almost exclusively identified along arteries using optical imaging in rodents (Iliff et al., 2012). In humans, magnetic resonance imaging (MRI) has located perivascular spaces adjacent to arteries but rarely along veins (Jochems et al., 2020). Perivascular spaces continue along penetrating arteries and arterioles into the brain tissue and appear to merge with basement membranes along smaller vessels. Thus, while perivascular spaces along the arterial bed are prominent, perivenous spaces remain enigmatic and await further studies.

Competing Theories

How perivascular spaces facilitate waste removal is subject to ongoing research. The field of brain clearance is dominated by the glymphatic theory on waste removal (Jessen et al., 2015). This model proposes CSF flow from the arterial perivascular space, through the brain parenchyma, leaving through the venous perivascular space. It should be noted, however, that alternative views exist, and the model has been criticized (Hladky & Barrand, 2022). The intramural periarterial drainage (IPAD) pathway theory shares the view on perivascular entry of CSF along arteries but proposes a removal path along basement membranes of smooth muscle cells within the arterial wall in the opposite direction of blood flow (Carare et al., 2008). This is a fundamental difference with the glymphatic concept, which proposes exit along perivenous spaces. According to a third theory, bulk flow is present along meningeal vessels within the subarachnoid space, but flow is hypothesized not to continue along perivascular spaces upon entering the brain tissue. In this view, mixing of CSF and ISF occurs within perivascular spaces around the penetrating arteries (Asgari et al., 2016; Bakker et al., 2019; Martinac et al., 2021). This would allow both influx of CSF-derived nutrients and efflux of waste from the ISF, based upon concentration gradients. In this view, mixing in the perivascular spaces would accelerate the exchange of solutes between the CSF and ISF by means of facilitated diffusion, enhanced by pulsations of CSF. The sources of these pulsations could be the heartbeat, respiration, and vasomotion. Within the parenchyma itself, there are also contrasting views on whether bulk flow is present or diffusion is the dominant mode of solute dispersion within the ISF (Smith & Verkman, 2018). A schematic overview of the three competing models of perivascular space waste drainage is provided in Figure 8.1.

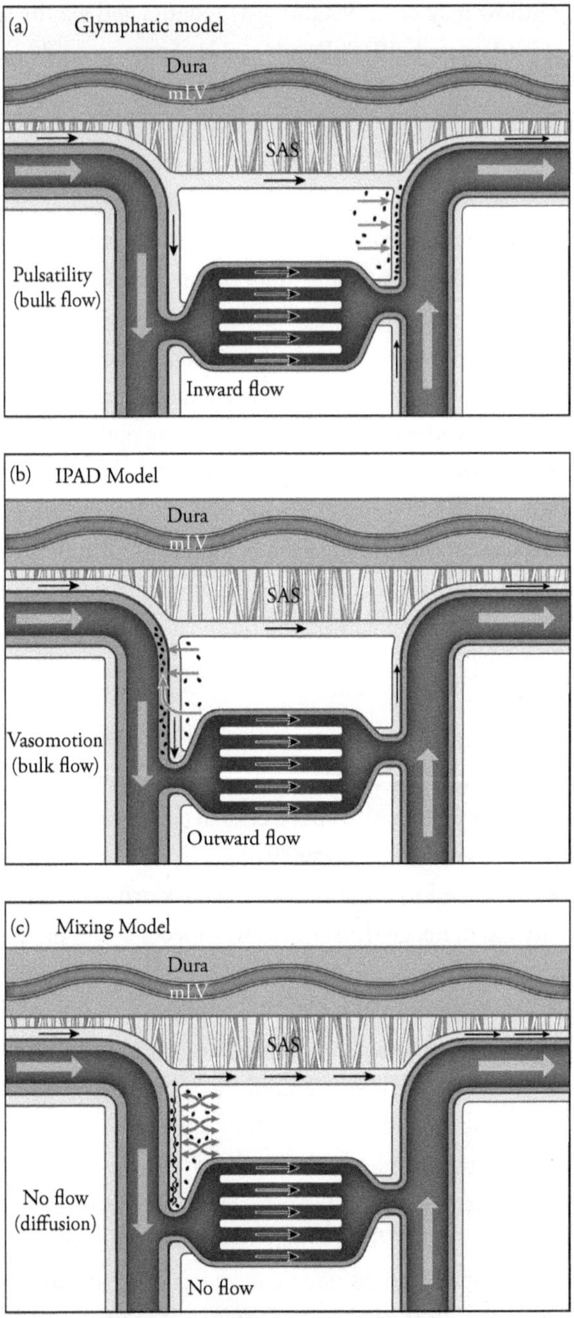

Figure 8.1 Three models describing perivascular space waste drainage in the brain clearance system
Note. Panel A: Glymphatic model. Panel B: Intramural periarterial drainage (IPAD) model. Panel C: Mixing model. The glymphatic model proposes perivascular inflow along arteries, flow through the interstitium, and drainage of waste via perivenous spaces. The IPAD model proposes inflow along arteries and removal of waste along basement membranes of arteries, flowing retrograde to the blood flow. The mixing model proposes flow in the subarachnoid space, but exchange of solutes between cerebrospinal fluid and interstitial fluid in perivascular spaces along penetrating arteries that is enhanced through mixing. mLV = meningeal lymphatic vasculature; SAS = subarachnoid space. Reproduced from Zhao et al. (2022).

Brain Clearance During Sleep

A major breakthrough in the field of brain clearance research was the work of Xie and colleagues (2013). This paper showed that in mice the vast majority of brain clearance occurs during sleep. Both influx and efflux of tracers were found to be considerably enhanced by sleep or anesthesia, with twofold faster amyloid-β clearance during sleep compared to wake. Sleep is, therefore, a primary driver of waste removal and may be crucial in its modulation. Mechanistically, the work of Xie and colleagues (2013) in mice suggested that during sleep the interstitial space of the brain parenchyma enlarges, which facilitates influx of CSF and subsequent exchange with ISF. In the study, iontophoresis was used to measure extracellular volume, a technique that is not readily transferable to humans. Changes in interstitial volume are expected to alter diffusivity of tissue, which is detectable with MRI using diffusion-weighted imaging. Indeed, in a study by Demiral and colleagues (2019), some brain regions showed increases in diffusivity, while other regions showed a decrease during human sleep. Altogether, changes in brain diffusivity during sleep seem limited, and other factors may contribute.

Recent work by Eide and colleagues (2022) more directly addressed the role of sleep in waste clearance. These authors showed that poor sleep in humans is associated with higher brain tissue levels of intrathecally infused tracer, indicating reduced clearance. This suggests that the removal pathways from the brain are negatively affected by sleep deprivation. In another study, the amyloid-β burden was increased in certain brain areas already after 1 night of sleep deprivation (Shokri-Kojori et al., 2018). Of course, it should be acknowledged that the level of waste products in CSF is determined not only by clearance rates but also by the production rate, which may also be dependent on the sleep–wake cycle.

In the next paragraphs, we will discuss evidence for enhanced brain clearance during sleep in relation to proposed drivers of brain clearance: synchronized vasomotion, cardiac pulsations, respiration, CSF production, and norepinephrine. The drivers discussed in this section are visualized in Figure 8.2.

Slow-Wave Sleep

Slow-wave sleep, synonymous with the N3 sleep stage, is characterized by slow oscillations: high-voltage synchronized waveforms as measured with the electroencephalogram at the scalp level (Benveniste et al., 2019). Slow-wave sleep has numerous functions including learning, memory, and metabolite clearance (Léger et al., 2018). In young adults, slow-wave sleep makes up 10%–25% of total sleep time, but slow-wave sleep is not evenly distributed throughout the night, with the majority occurring in the first half and then ceding to rapid-eye-movement (REM) sleep occurring predominantly in the second half (Léger et al., 2018). Slow waves usually lie between 0.5 and 4.5 Hz and have been linked to sleep pressure. The phenomenon of large bundles of neurons coordinating their electrical activity, rhythmically and repetitively depolarizing, termed *slow oscillatory neuronal activity*, is

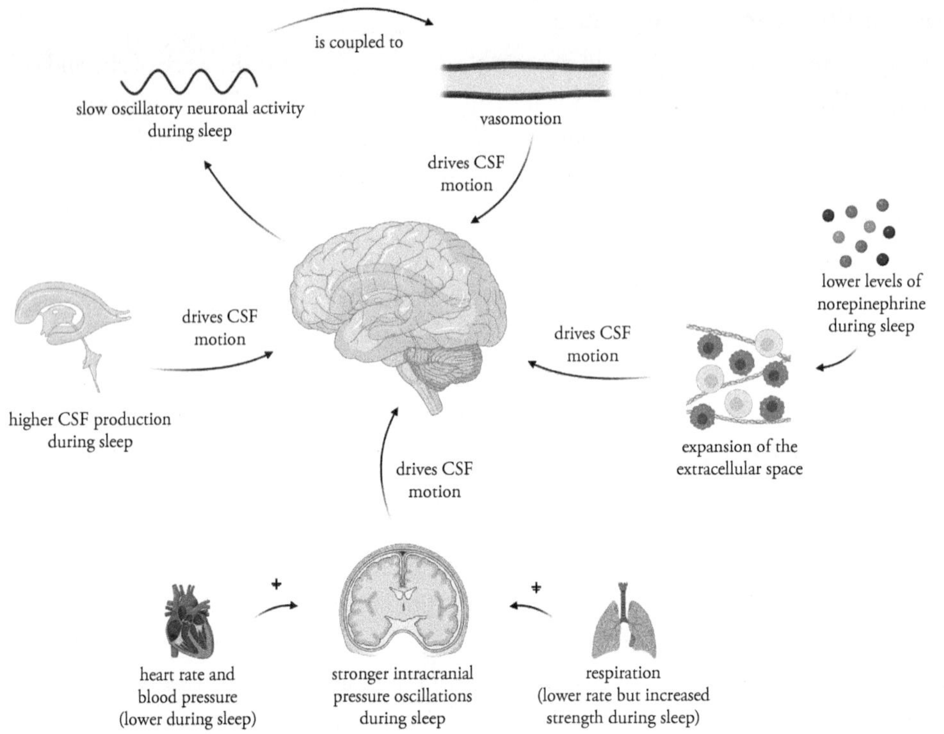

Figure 8.2 Proposed driving forces of brain clearance in wake and sleep
Note. This visual overview summarizes the proposed drivers of brain clearance that are amplified during sleep: vasomotion, cardiovascular and respiratory factors, cerebrospinal fluid production, and norepinephrine. CSF = cerebrospinal fluid. Created with BioRender.com.

embedded in pulsations ranging from 20 to 30 seconds that reflect important physiological restoration of the brain and blood oxygenation (Léger et al., 2018). The reoxygenation and the pulsatory movement of tracers from the brain through CSF-mediated clearance precisely match the time, rhythm, and electrical activity of the N3 stage, confirming that this waste clearance system is primarily active during slow-wave sleep.

Synchronized Vasomotion During Sleep

The presence of large, synchronized oscillations in neuronal activity during slow-wave sleep drives oscillations in blood flow and CSF motility; the report by Fultz and colleagues (2019) showed a pattern of coupled, oscillating electrophysiological, hemodynamic, and CSF dynamics that emerges during sleep. These large waves in CSF movement that appear during sleep may promote brain clearance. The waves of CSF motion arise from expansions of cerebral blood volume (caused by vascular changes), allowing for CSF inflow into the brain or pushing CSF out. A recent paper from van Veluw and colleagues (2020) demonstrated that vasomotion, the spontaneous oscillation in blood vessel walls, is indeed an important driver of brain clearance. In that paper, the authors promoted vasomotion via visual stimulation. It should be noted, however, that vasomotion is an intrinsic property of arteries (not veins). It is a rhythmic oscillation in diameter, with a frequency around 0.1 Hz. Apparently, this property of arteries is uncovered, or synchronized, during sleep. Given the magnitude of the effects, we speculate that it may be one of the most important drivers for brain clearance as it produces relatively large changes in diameter and, consequently, a large displacement of CSF volume (Bojarskaite et al., 2023).

Cardiovascular Aspects of Sleep

Sleep may also impact brain clearance via its effect on cardiovascular parameters. Sleep is associated with a lowering of the heart rate and blood pressure. There is indirect evidence that heart rate is important for brain clearance. Thus, heart rate is negatively correlated with brain clearance when comparing the effects of different types of anesthesia (Hablitz et al., 2019). A concomitant lowering of heart rate and blood pressure has strong effects on the pulsatility of blood vessels. Hypertensive rats that were treated with atenolol, a selective β-adrenergic inhibitor, showed lower heart rate and blood pressure with treatment. This drug also prevented impaired pulsatility of the larger carotid artery by increasing its diameter (Naessens et al., 2023). As pulsations of arteries have been suggested to be an important driving force for brain clearance (Iliff et al., 2013), one may speculate that lowering of heart rate and blood pressure during sleep may promote brain clearance through an increase in vascular pulsatility. Additionally, as opposed to systemic arterial pulsations dissipating at an arteriolar and venous level, in the brain, the rigid skull promotes propagation of arterial pulsations in the form of intracranial pressure oscillations, which are still measurable in the microvasculature and venous outflow. Even acute decreases in arterial pulsations impair brain clearance. Paradoxically, the N3 sleep stage which has the highest levels of CSF influx and amyloid-β removal, also has the lowest rates of arterial pulsations (Benveniste et al., 2019), suggesting other factors are at play.

Respiratory Aspects of Sleep

Similar to heart rate and blood pressure, respiratory rate decreases during sleep. Spontaneous ventilation, as compared to mechanical ventilation, was found to be more effective for tracer dispersion in the subarachnoid space of rats (Liu et al., 2022). These authors also suggested that pressure oscillations resulting from respiration are more important for brain clearance than oscillations that result from cardiac pulsations. In rats, pulsations in intracranial pressure that result from respiration are much larger than those from cardiac pulsation (Bedussi et al., 2017). In humans, non-REM (NREM) sleep is associated with increased strength of respiratory pulsations (Helakari et al., 2022). Finally, recent work has shown that lower-frequency intracranial pressure oscillations produced by respiration complement cardiac pulsations, which could alternatively drive clearance. Ultrafast MRI demonstrated that forced inspiration was a main driver of CSF flow in both the lateral ventricles and the subarachnoid space (Benveniste et al., 2019). So although there is no final answer to the question of whether cardiac or respiratory rate drives intracranial pressure pulsations, the likely answer is a combination of the two.

CSF Production During Sleep

Independent of the exact route and mechanisms of perivascular waste removal, the CSF is an important sink for waste that is not removed across the blood–brain barrier. CSF production and removal are therefore of utmost importance. It not only directly sweeps away waste but also provides a concentration gradient for diffusion from the brain tissue toward the CSF compartment. The production of CSF is attributed largely to the choroid plexus. As reviewed by Christensen and colleagues (2022), the choroid plexus is also strongly under the control of circadian rhythms, with CSF production being highest during sleep. The time course of CSF production negatively correlates with CSF levels of amyloid-β. Sleep, particularly NREM sleep, may therefore prove important for waste clearance as it constitutes an important stimulus for CSF production. Sleep and circadian rhythmicity are closely related but not identical. The production of CSF in humans shows a circadian rhythm, with the highest production, as measured in the cerebral aqueduct, in the beginning of the night (Nilsson et al., 1992). It should be noted though that participants in this study were woken up for the measurements to be performed and did not experience a full night of sleep. The production of CSF is also highest during the night in rats, which are nocturnal animals (Steffensen et al., 2023). Thus, while rats have evolved as nocturnal animals to avoid predation, their circadian rhythm with respect to CSF formation has been maintained. In these animals, therefore, sleep and CSF production seem "out of phase."

Norepinephrine

As stated above, natural sleep is associated with improved tracer penetration along the periarterial spaces and increased interstitial solute clearance, such as amyloid-β (Plog & Nedergaard, 2018). As we sleep, the central levels of norepinephrine decline due to a lower locus coeruleus–derived noradrenergic tone. Experimental evidence suggests that this decrease in adrenergic tone has an important contribution to the beneficial effect of sleep. Thus, awake mice show limited tracer influx into the brain, while both sleeping mice and mice anaesthetized with ketamine/xylazine show much larger tracer influx (Miyakoshi et al., 2023). Xylazine and (dex)medetomidine are anesthetics or sedative drugs that are α2-adrenergic antagonists. These types of drugs are quite effective at promoting brain clearance as compared to other types of anesthesia (Hablitz et al., 2019). This is attributed to their effect on slow-wave brain activity, astrocyte volume, and lymphatic outflow routes (Benveniste et al., 2019; Persson et al., 2022). In addition, norepinephrine suppresses choroid plexus CSF production (Jessen et al., 2015). Taken together, these data have led to the suggestion that dexmedetomine could be used therapeutically to enhance brain clearance (Persson et al., 2022).

Brain Clearance and Brain Health

The Aging Brain: Sleep and Brain Clearance

Sleep changes greatly with the aging brain. Changes in sleep duration and quality are widely reported, most prominently in the stages of slow-wave sleep (Li et al., 2022). Slow-wave sleep duration peaks in adolescence and declines with age. As aging is often accompanied by a significant loss of cortical gray matter in regions essential for the origination of slow oscillations, this neuronal loss is proposed to underlie the decrease in slow-wave sleep duration (Léger et al., 2018). Poor sleep (as a result of aging) is an important risk factor for the development of many somatic, neurological, and psychiatric disorders and can accelerate physical and mental deterioration. It remains unclear to what extent this can be attributed to a declining brain clearance system. Mice studies show that waste solute clearance is efficient for a large part of the life span and starts to deteriorate at a fast pace toward the end of the reproductive period (Jessen et al., 2015). Impairment of the brain clearance system could be the result of declining driving forces (weaker and fewer arterial pulsations, higher breathing rates of shallower breaths) or changes in AQP4 expression and localization. A proposed pathway by Rasmussen and colleagues (2022) describes how poor sleep in the elderly contributes to the inhibition of brain clearance pathways, resulting in cognitive impairment and progression of neurodegeneration. In brief, poor sleep would lead to an accumulation of waste products, such as protein aggregates (e.g., amyloid and tau proteins). The buildup of these protein deposits would then make the tissue less permeable, causing reduced subsequent clearance; this could result in a downward spiral of decremental efficient brain clearance and incremental protein aggregation, resulting in tissue damage consistent with Alzheimer's disease and other neurodegenerative disorders.

Brain Clearance in Neurodegenerative Disorders

Many of the neurodegenerative disorders are characterized by protein aggregation: These include Alzheimer's disease, Parkinson's disease, prion diseases, tauopathies, Huntington's disease, and others. The presence of these accumulations proposes a central role for the brain clearance system in neurodegenerative disorders and has been studied in both health and disease to better understand brain clearance impairments (Rasmussen et al., 2022). Studies in mice have highlighted the effect of healthy sleep and, thus, brain clearance on protein accumulation levels in ISF and CSF. Results showed that higher levels of amyloid-β (two times) and tau (a third increase) exist during wake, a state with limited clearance activity. Additionally, clearance of injected amyloid-β in mice doubled during sleep. In healthy humans, similar effects were found, showing large increases in amyloid-β (30%) and tau (50%) CSF levels after a night of sleep deprivation (Eide et al., 2021). In neurodegenerative disorders, the brain clearance system fails to efficiently clear depositions of amyloid-β, tau, oxidative stress, microglial proliferation, and reactive gliosis from the extracellular space. Mouse models of Alzheimer's disease have shown strong increases

(25%–50%) in amyloid-β brain levels after prolonged brain clearance attenuation (by AQP4 knockout) compared to normal clearance (Xu et al., 2015). Interestingly, natural failure of the brain clearance system (associated with astrogliosis) in Alzheimer's mouse models appeared before the onset of amyloid-β deposition, suggesting it to be an important risk factor for developing Alzheimer's disease. In contrast to a more uniform, gradual appearance of brain clearance deficits in animal models, human clearance impairments show large interindividual variability on a continuous spectrum, possibly related to single-nucleotide polymorphisms in the gene for the AQP4 channels (Chandra et al., 2021). In human Alzheimer's disease, a strong reduction (33%) of CSF clearance rates (de Leon et al., 2017) and altered latency and propagation speed of clearance drivers are observed in patients compared to healthy controls (Rajna et al., 2021; Tuovinen et al., 2020). After the onset of neurodegeneration, other factors (e.g., weakened cardiovascular pumping of CSF) may worsen brain clearance function even further. The link between brain clearance deficits and Alzheimer's disease hints at the idea that poor sleep predisposes or at least enhances the development of the disease. This notion would be corroborated by a recent long-term study showing that chronic sleep deficit (<6 h) for 25 years can lead to the development of dementia (Sabia et al., 2021) and, conversely, findings that sleep improvement via bright-light treatment in people with early dementia slows cognitive decline (Riemersma-van der Lek et al., 2008). Admittedly, the relationship with brain clearance remains circumstantial for now as other sleep-related health benefits may play a role in these findings as well.

Brain Clearance in Sleep Disorders

Sleep disorders, unlike neurodegenerative disorders, are not directly linked to protein aggregates and thus altered brain clearance. Because of sleep–wake rhythm disruptions in people with sleep disorders, however, brain clearance mechanisms are likely to be involved. In sleep apnea, the study of perivascular space morphology (MRI) and fluid dynamics showed alterations in brain clearance (J. Wang et al., 2023). In elderly with chronic insomnia, an increase of MRI-visible, enlarged perivascular spaces is observed and found to be associated with higher levels of CSF amyloid-β and tau (X.-X. Wang et al., 2022). These enlarged perivascular spaces naturally occur in the aging brain and are emerging as an MRI marker to reflect brain clearance. The effects of sleep deprivation on CSF protein aggregates, as discussed above, confirm the notion that insomnia, much like a single night of sleep deprivation, is characterized by impaired brain clearance. With respect to sleep medication, its influence on brain clearance through improved sleep remains unclear and understudied. A recent study showed that administration of suvorexant, an orexin antagonist approved to treat people with insomnia, resulted in acutely decreased tau phosphorylation and amyloid-β concentrations in CSF measurements without significant changes in sleep architecture (Lucey et al., 2023). Other than that, we can only speculate about possible enhancement of brain clearance by, for example, sodium oxybate to increase slow-wave sleep. The potential of sleep medication to modulate brain clearance warrants attention and further exploration within the scientific community.

Improving Brain Clearance

It would appear that certain behavioral factors impact the efficacy of brain clearance, meaning that lifestyle choices can potentially be used for optimal or improved clearance that could be of aid in the management or even prevention of brain disorders characterized by waste product accumulation in the brain, such as protein aggregate disorders (Reddy & van der Werf, 2020). The most obvious and general lifestyle choice to improve brain clearance would be to sleep; while this may sound trivial, in this context we take it to mean that improvement of sleep could play a role in the optimization of brain clearance processes. Sleep improvement falls along the lines of the recommendations for sleep hygiene as part of the cognitive behavioral treatment for insomnia, encompassing recommendations for regular bedtimes, exercise, stimulus control, food and fluid intake etc. A better understanding of the role of sleep in brain clearance will allow us in the upcoming years to firmly place sleep health, sleep treatment, and sleep recommendations at the heart of preventative medicine (Figure 8.3).

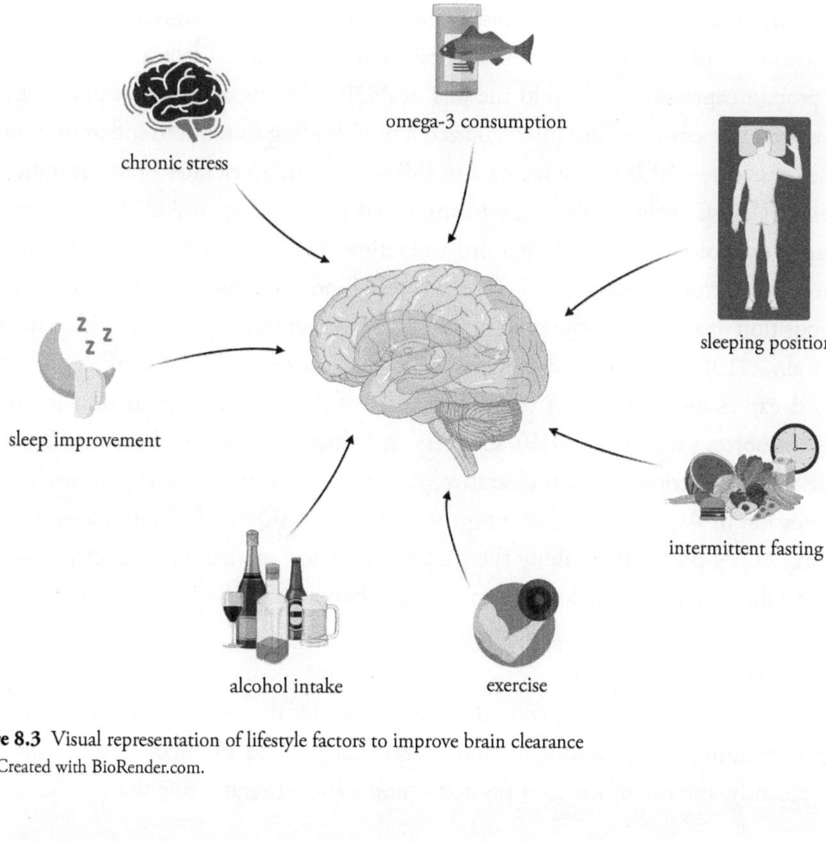

Figure 8.3 Visual representation of lifestyle factors to improve brain clearance
Note. Created with BioRender.com.

Specific recommendations for optimizing brain clearance may include sleep position, alcohol intake, exercise, omega-3 consumption, intermittent fasting, and chronic stress that all appear to modulate brain clearance. Gravity affects the movement of blood and CSF throughout the brain, and therefore sleep position will play a role in the clearance of waste products from the brain: Neurodegenerative patients were found to spend a much larger percentage of time in the supine position compared to controls, establishing an association between time in supine position and dementia (Levendowski et al., 2019). Fluid transport was most efficient in the right lateral sleeping position, with more CSF clearance occurring compared to the supine and prone positions, showing that clearance is more efficient in the lateral position (Lee et al., 2015). High levels of both endogenous and exogenous marine-based fish oils known as omega-3 polyunsaturated fatty acids (n3-PUFAs) are associated with lower incidence of neurodegenerative disease, and n3-PUFA supplementation has been suggested to delay or prevent the onset of Alzheimer's disease. N3-PUFAs promote, among other functions, amyloid-β clearance and reduce aggregate formation by inhibiting the activation of astrocytes, protecting against the loss of AQP4 polarization, exhibiting anti-amyloidogenic activity, decreasing amyloid-β production, modulating aggregation, and decreasing downstream toxicity (Ren et al., 2017). Alcohol consumption can either boost or hinder brain clearance, depending on dosage and chronic or acute consumption. Acute and chronic exposure of high doses of alcohol (1 g/kg) dramatically reduces transport in awake mice. On the other hand, both acute and chronic exposure of low doses of alcohol (0.5 g/kg) may increase brain clearance due to decreased glial fibrillary acidic protein expression and avoid the loss of AQP4 (Lundgaard et al., 2018). Physical exercise decreases astrocyte and microglia activation, leading to reduced inflammation and increased movement of ISF. The increase in ISF movement accelerates brain clearance and reduces amyloid-β accumulation due to improved polarization of AQP4, resulting in a decrease in amyloid plaques and neuroinflammation (He et al., 2017). Chronic stress is a common risk factor for Alzheimer's disease through an acceleration of the accumulation and deposition of amyloid-β, the protein thought to reflect the ongoing neurodegeneration (Wei et al., 2019). Mice exposed to stress exhibit decreased glymphatic influx and efflux, decreased expression and loss of the polarization of AQP4, and a reduction in AQP4-bearing astrocytes (Wei et al., 2019). Conversely, reducing stress would conceivably aid in optimizing the function of brain clearance pathways. Intermittent fasting downregulates the expression of AQP4-M1, decreasing the AQP4-M1/AQP4-M23 ratio, and therefore increasing AQP4 polarization along the paravenous space, increasing brain clearance, and decreasing the amount of amyloid-β deposition (Zhang et al., 2017).

Conclusions

As this field is burgeoning and will continue to rapidly develop, novel approaches and attempts to optimize the action of brain clearance will no doubt appear in the near future; recently, the use of infrared photobiomodulation therapy to enhance the activity of brain clearance has been reviewed (Semyachkina-Glushkovskaya et al., 2023), while breathing exercises have been put forward as a possible intervention technique (Chavez & Zappaterra, 2023). Pharmaceutical approaches to changing AQP4 channel activity appear to be a logical point of focus, although the aquaporins have been notoriously hard to target (Salman et al., 2022). Well-powered and scientifically executed drug discovery, clinical trials, and replication studies will need to inform the field of brain clearance in the next exciting years about the efficacy of such novel approaches.

Future Directions

To increase understanding of brain clearance, the following questions should be addressed:

- As it currently stands, there are several competing theories to explain CSF motion in and around perivascular spaces. Which of the models is an accurate representation?
- What is the relative contribution of the different proposed drivers on clearance?
- Is there a relationship between clearance and the various sleep stages? Is there clearance during REM sleep?
- Is there a causal relationship between sleep, waste clearance, and neurodegeneration?

To improve or manipulate brain clearance, it is necessary to identify the following:

- Which drivers or factors to target. Does altering sleep architecture affect brain clearance?
- Which manipulations are most effective? To what degree do lifestyle factors and medication modulate brain clearance?

References

Asgari, M., de Zélicourt, D., & Kurtcuoglu, V. (2016). Glymphatic solute transport does not require bulk flow. *Scientific Reports, 6*, Article 38635.

Bakker, E. N. T. P., Naessens, D. M. P., & VanBavel, E. (2019). Paravascular spaces: Entry to or exit from the brain? *Experimental Physiology, 104*(7), 1013–1017.

Bedussi, B., Almasian, M., de Vos, J., VanBavel, E., & Bakker, E. N. (2018). Paravascular spaces at the brain surface: Low resistance pathways for cerebrospinal fluid flow. *Journal of Cerebral Blood Flow and Metabolism, 38*(4), 719–726.

Bedussi, B., van der Wel, N. N., de Vos, J., van Veen, H., Siebes, M., VanBavel, E., & Bakker, E. N. (2017). Paravascular channels, cisterns, and the subarachnoid space in the rat brain: A single compartment with preferential pathways. *Journal of Cerebral Blood Flow and Metabolism, 37*(4), 1374–1385.

Benveniste, H., Heerdt, P. M., Fontes, M., Rothman, D. L., & Volkow, N. D. (2019). Glymphatic system function in relation to anesthesia and sleep states. *Anesthesia and Analgesia, 128*(4), 747–758.

Bojarskaite, L., Vallet, A., Bjørnstad, D. M., Gullestad Binder, K. M., Cunen, C., Heuser, K., Kuchta, M., Mardal, K.-A., & Enger, R. (2023). Sleep cycle–dependent vascular dynamics in male mice and the predicted effects on perivascular cerebrospinal fluid flow and solute transport. *Nature Communications, 14*(1), Article 953.

Carare, R. O., Bernardes-Silva, M., Newman, T. A., Page, A. M., Nicoll, J. A. R., Perry, V. H., & Weller, R. O. (2008). Solutes, but not cells, drain from the brain parenchyma along basement membranes of capillaries and arteries: Significance for cerebral amyloid angiopathy and neuroimmunology. *Neuropathology and Applied Neurobiology, 34*(2), 131–144.

Chandra, A., Farrell, C., Wilson, H., Dervenoulas, G., De Natale, E. R., Politis, M., & Alzheimer's Disease Neuroimaging Initiative. (2021). Aquaporin-4 polymorphisms predict amyloid burden and clinical outcome in the Alzheimer's disease spectrum. *Neurobiology of Aging, 97*, 1–9.

Chavez, J. A., & Zappaterra, M. (2023). Can Wim Hof method breathing induce conscious metabolic waste clearance of the brain? *Medical Hypotheses, 177*, Article 111118.

Christensen, J., Li, C., & Mychasiuk, R. (2022). Choroid plexus function in neurological homeostasis and disorders: The awakening of the circadian clocks and orexins. *Journal of Cerebral Blood Flow and Metabolism, 42*(7), 1163–1175.

de Leon, M. J., Li, Y., Okamura, N., Tsui, W. H., Saint-Louis, L. A., Glodzik, L., Osorio, R. S., Fortea, J., Butler, T., Pirraglia, E., Fossati, S., Kim, H.-J., Carare, R. O., Nedergaard, M., Benveniste, H., & Rusinek, H. (2017). Cerebrospinal fluid clearance in Alzheimer disease measured with dynamic PET. *Journal of Nuclear Medicine, 58*(9), 1471–1476.

Demiral, Ş. B., Tomasi, D., Sarlls, J., Lee, H., Wiers, C. E., Zehra, A., Srivastava, T., Ke, K., Shokri-Kojori, E., Freeman, C. R., Lindgren, E., Ramirez, V., Miller, G., Bandettini, P., Horovitz, S., Wang, G.-J., Benveniste, H., & Volkow, N. D. (2019). Apparent diffusion coefficient changes in human brain during sleep—Does it inform on the existence of a glymphatic system? *NeuroImage, 185*, 263–273.

Eide, P. K., Pripp, A. H., Berge, B., Hrubos-Strøm, H., Ringstad, G., & Valnes, L. M. (2022). Altered glymphatic enhancement of cerebrospinal fluid tracer in individuals with chronic poor sleep quality. *Journal of Cerebral Blood Flow and Metabolism, 42*(9), 1676–1692.

Eide, P. K., Vinje, V., Pripp, A. H., Mardal, K.-A., & Ringstad, G. (2021). Sleep deprivation impairs molecular clearance from the human brain. *Brain, 144*(3), 863–874.

Fultz, N. E., Bonmassar, G., Setsompop, K., Stickgold, R. A., Rosen, B. R., Polimeni, J. R., & Lewis, L. D. (2019). Coupled electrophysiological, hemodynamic, and cerebrospinal fluid oscillations in human sleep. *Science, 366*(6465), 628–631.

Hablitz, L. M., Vinitsky, H. S., Sun, Q., Stæger, F. F., Sigurdsson, B., Mortensen, K. N., Lilius, T. O., & Nedergaard, M. (2019). Increased glymphatic influx is correlated with high EEG delta power and low heart rate in mice under anesthesia. *Science Advances, 5*(2), Article eaav5447.

He, X.-F., Liu, D.-X., Zhang, Q., Liang, F.-Y., Dai, G.-Y., Zeng, J.-S., Pei, Z., Xu, G.-Q., & Lan, Y. (2017). Voluntary exercise promotes glymphatic clearance of amyloid beta and reduces the activation of astrocytes and microglia in aged mice. *Frontiers in Molecular Neuroscience, 10*, Article 144.

Helakari, H., Korhonen, V., Holst, S. C., Piispala, J., Kallio, M., Väyrynen, T., Huotari, N., Raitamaa, L., Tuunanen, J., Kananen, J., Järvelä, M., Tuovinen, T., Raatikainen, V., Borchardt, V., Kinnunen, H., Nedergaard, M., & Kiviniemi, V. (2022). Human NREM sleep promotes brain-wide vasomotor and respiratory pulsations. *The Journal of Neuroscience, 42*(12), 2503–2515.

Hladky, S. B., & Barrand, M. A. (2016). Fluid and ion transfer across the blood–brain and blood–cerebrospinal fluid barriers; a comparative account of mechanisms and roles. *Fluids and Barriers of the CNS, 13*(1), Article 19.

Hladky, S. B., & Barrand, M. A. (2018). Elimination of substances from the brain parenchyma: Efflux via perivascular pathways and via the blood–brain barrier. *Fluids and Barriers of the CNS, 15*(1), Article 30.

Hladky, S. B., & Barrand, M. A. (2022). The glymphatic hypothesis: The theory and the evidence. *Fluids and Barriers of the CNS, 19*(1), Article 9.

Iliff, J. J., Wang, M., Liao, Y., Plogg, B. A., Peng, W., Gundersen, G. A., Benveniste, H., Vates, G. E., Deane, R., Goldman, S. A., Nagelhus, E. A., & Nedergaard, M. (2012). A paravascular pathway facilitates CSF flow through the brain parenchyma and the clearance of interstitial solutes, including amyloid β. *Science Translational Medicine, 4*(147), Article 147ra111.

Iliff, J. J., Wang, M., Zeppenfeld, D. M., Venkataraman, A., Plog, B. A., Liao, Y., Deane, R., & Nedergaard, M. (2013). Cerebral arterial pulsation drives paravascular CSF–interstitial fluid exchange in the murine brain. *The Journal of Neuroscience, 33*(46), 18190–18199.

Jessen, N. A., Munk, A. S. F., Lundgaard, I., & Nedergaard, M. (2015). The glymphatic system: A beginner's guide. *Neurochemical Research*, *40*(12), 2583–2599.

Jochems, A. C. C., Blair, G. W., Stringer, M. S., Thrippleton, M. J., Clancy, U., Chappell, F. M., Brown, R., Jaime Garcia, D., Hamilton, O. K. L., Morgan, A. G., Marshall, I., Hetherington, K., Wiseman, S., MacGillivray, T., Valdés-Hernández, M. C., Doubal, F. N., & Wardlaw, J. M. (2020). Relationship between venules and perivascular spaces in sporadic small vessel diseases. *Stroke*, *51*(5), 1503–1506.

Lee, H., Xie, L., Yu, M., Kang, H., Feng, T., Deane, R., Logan, J., Nedergaard, M., & Benveniste, H. (2015). The effect of body posture on brain glymphatic transport. *The Journal of Neuroscience*, *35*(31), 11034–11044.

Léger, D., Debellemaniere, E., Rabat, A., Bayon, V., Benchenane, K., & Chennaoui, M. (2018). Slow-wave sleep: From the cell to the clinic. *Sleep Medicine Reviews*, *41*, 113–132.

Levendowski, D. J., Gamaldo, C., St Louis, E. K., Ferini-Strambi, L., Hamilton, J. M., Salat, D., Westbrook, P. R., & Berka, C. (2019). Head position during sleep: Potential implications for patients with neurodegenerative disease. *Journal of Alzheimer's Disease*, *67*(2), 631–638.

Li, J., Vitiello, M. V., & Gooneratne, N. S. (2022). Sleep in normal aging. *Sleep Medicine Clinics*, *17*(2), 161–171.

Liu, S., Bilston, L. E., Flores Rodriguez, N., Wright, C., McMullan, S., Lloyd, R., Stoodley, M. A., & Hemley, S. J. (2022). Changes in intrathoracic pressure, not arterial pulsations, exert the greatest effect on tracer influx in the spinal cord. *Fluids and Barriers of the CNS*, *19*(1), Article 14.

Lucey, B. P., Liu, H., Toedebusch, C. D., Freund, D., Redrick, T., Chahin, S. L., Mawuenyega, K. G., Bollinger, J. G., Ovod, V., Barthélemy, N. R., & Bateman, R. J. (2023). Suvorexant acutely decreases tau phosphorylation and Aβ in the human CNS. *Annals of Neurology*, *94*(1), 27–40.

Lundgaard, I., Wang, W., Eberhardt, A., Vinitsky, H. S., Reeves, B. C., Peng, S., Lou, N., Hussain, R., & Nedergaard, M. (2018). Beneficial effects of low alcohol exposure, but adverse effects of high alcohol intake on glymphatic function. *Scientific Reports*, *8*(1), Article 2246.

Ma, Q., Ries, M., Decker, Y., Müller, A., Riner, C., Bücker, A., Fassbender, K., Detmar, M., & Proulx, S. T. (2019). Rapid lymphatic efflux limits cerebrospinal fluid flow to the brain. *Acta Neuropathologica*, *137*(1), 151–165.

MacAulay, N., Keep, R. F., & Zeuthen, T. (2022). Cerebrospinal fluid production by the choroid plexus: A century of barrier research revisited. *Fluids and Barriers of the CNS*, *19*(1), Article 26.

Martinac, A. D., Fletcher, D. F., & Bilston, L. E. (2021). Phase offset between arterial pulsations and subarachnoid space pressure fluctuations are unlikely to drive periarterial cerebrospinal fluid flow. *Biomechanics and Modeling in Mechanobiology*, *20*(5), 1751–1766.

Miyakoshi, L. M., Stæger, F. F., Li, Q., Pan, C., Xie, L., Kang, H., Pavan, C., Dang, J., Sun, Q., Ertürk, A., & Nedergaard, M. (2023). The state of brain activity modulates cerebrospinal fluid transport. *Progress in Neurobiology*, *229*, Article 102512.

Naessens, D. M. P., de Vos, J., Richard, E., Wilhelmus, M. M. M., Jongenelen, C. A. M., Scholl, E. R., van der Wel, N. N., Heijst, J. A., Teunissen, C. E., Strijkers, G. J., Coolen, B. F., VanBavel, E., & Bakker, E. N. T. P. (2023). Effect of long-term antihypertensive treatment on cerebrovascular structure and function in hypertensive rats. *Scientific Reports*, *13*(1), Article 3481.

Nedergaard, M., & Goldman, S. A. (2020). Glymphatic failure as a final common pathway to dementia. *Science*, *370*(6512), 50–56.

Nilsson, C., Ståhlberg, F., Thomsen, C., Henriksen, O., Herning, M., & Owman, C. (1992). Circadian variation in human cerebrospinal fluid production measured by magnetic resonance imaging. *The American Journal of Physiology*, *262*(1 Pt. 2), R20–R24.

Persson, N. D. Å., Uusalo, P., Nedergaard, M., Lohela, T. J., & Lilius, T. O. (2022). Could dexmedetomidine be repurposed as a glymphatic enhancer? *Trends in Pharmacological Sciences*, *43*(12), 1030–1040.

Plog, B. A., & Nedergaard, M. (2018). The glymphatic system in central nervous system health and disease: Past, present, and future. *Annual Review of Pathology*, *13*, 379–394.

Proulx, S. T. (2021). Cerebrospinal fluid outflow: A review of the historical and contemporary evidence for arachnoid villi, perineural routes, and dural lymphatics. *Cellular and Molecular Life Sciences*, *78*(6), 2429–2457.

Rajna, Z., Mattila, H., Huotari, N., Tuovinen, T., Krüger, J., Holst, S. C., Korhonen, V., Remes, A. M., Seppänen, T., Hennig, J., Nedergaard, M., & Kiviniemi, V. (2021). Cardiovascular brain impulses in Alzheimer's disease. *Brain*, *144*(7), 2214–2226.

Rasmussen, M. K., Mestre, H., & Nedergaard, M. (2022). Fluid transport in the brain. *Physiological Reviews, 102*(2), 1025–1151.

Reddy, O. C., & van der Werf, Y. D. (2020). The sleeping brain: Harnessing the power of the glymphatic system through lifestyle choices. *Brain Sciences, 10*(11), Article 868. https://doi.org/10.3390/brainsci10110868

Ren, H., Luo, C., Feng, Y., Yao, X., Shi, Z., Liang, F., Kang, J. X., Wan, J.-B., Pei, Z., & Su, H. (2017). Omega-3 polyunsaturated fatty acids promote amyloid-β clearance from the brain through mediating the function of the glymphatic system. *FASEB Journal, 31*(1), 282–293.

Riemersma-van der Lek, R. F., Swaab, D. F., Twisk, J., Hol, E. M., Hoogendijk, W. J. G., & Van Someren, E. J. W. (2008). Effect of bright light and melatonin on cognitive and noncognitive function in elderly residents of group care facilities: A randomized controlled trial. *JAMA, 299*(22), 2642–2655.

Sabia, S., Fayosse, A., Dumurgier, J., van Hees, V. T., Paquet, C., Sommerlad, A., Kivimäki, M., Dugravot, A., & Singh-Manoux, A. (2021). Association of sleep duration in middle and old age with incidence of dementia. *Nature Communications, 12*(1), Article 2289.

Salman, M. M., Kitchen, P., Yool, A. J., & Bill, R. M. (2022). Recent breakthroughs and future directions in drugging aquaporins. *Trends in Pharmacological Sciences, 43*(1), 30–42.

Semyachkina-Glushkovskaya, O., Penzel, T., Poluektov, M., Fedosov, I., Tzoy, M., Terskov, A., Blokhina, I., Sidorov, V., & Kurths, J. (2023). Phototherapy of Alzheimer's disease: Photostimulation of brain lymphatics during sleep: A systematic review. *International Journal of Molecular Sciences, 24*(13), Article 10946. https://doi.org/10.3390/ijms241310946

Shokri-Kojori, E., Wang, G.-J., Wiers, C. E., Demiral, S. B., Guo, M., Kim, S. W., Lindgren, E., Ramirez, V., Zehra, A., Freeman, C., Miller, G., Manza, P., Srivastava, T., De Santi, S., Tomasi, D., Benveniste, H., & Volkow, N. D. (2018). β-Amyloid accumulation in the human brain after one night of sleep deprivation. *Proceedings of the National Academy of Sciences of the United States of America, 115*(17), 4483–4488.

Smith, A. J., & Verkman, A. S. (2018). The "glymphatic" mechanism for solute clearance in Alzheimer's disease: Game changer or unproven speculation? *FASEB Journal, 32*(2), 543–551.

Spera, I., Cousin, N., Ries, M., Kedracka, A., Castillo, A., Aleandri, S., Vladymyrov, M., Mapunda, J. A., Engelhardt, B., Luciani, P., Detmar, M., & Proulx, S. T. (2023). Open pathways for cerebrospinal fluid outflow at the cribriform plate along the olfactory nerves. *EBioMedicine, 91*, Article 104558.

Steffensen, A. B., Edelbo, B. L., Barbuskaite, D., Andreassen, S. N., Olsen, M. H., Møller, K., & MacAulay, N. (2023). Nocturnal increase in cerebrospinal fluid secretion as a circadian regulator of intracranial pressure. *Fluids and Barriers of the CNS, 20*(1), Article 49.

Tuovinen, T., Kananen, J., Rajna, Z., Lieslehto, J., Korhonen, V., Rytty, R., Mattila, H., Huotari, N., Raitamaa, L., Helakari, H., Elseoud, A. A., Krüger, J., LeVan, P., Tervonen, O., Hennig, J., Remes, A. M., Nedergaard, M., & Kiviniemi, V. (2020). The variability of functional MRI brain signal increases in Alzheimer's disease at cardiorespiratory frequencies. *Scientific Reports, 10*(1), Article 21559.

van Veluw, S. J., Hou, S. S., Calvo-Rodriguez, M., Arbel-Ornath, M., Snyder, A. C., Frosch, M. P., Greenberg, S. M., & Bacskai, B. J. (2020). Vasomotion as a driving force for paravascular clearance in the awake mouse brain. *Neuron, 105*(3), 549–561.e5.

Wang, J., Tian, Y., Qin, C., Meng, L., Feng, R., Xu, S., Zhai, Y., Liang, D., Zhang, R., Tian, H., Liu, H., Chen, Y., Fu, Y., Chen, P., Zhu, Q., Teng, J., & Wang, X. (2023). Impaired glymphatic drainage underlying obstructive sleep apnea is associated with cognitive dysfunction. *Journal of Neurology, 270*(4), 2204–2216.

Wang, X.-X., Cao, Q.-C., Teng, J.-F., Wang, R.-F., Yang, Z.-T., Wang, M.-G., & Cao, Z.-H. (2022). MRI-visible enlarged perivascular spaces: Imaging marker to predict cognitive impairment in older chronic insomnia patients. *European Radiology, 32*(8), 5446–5457.

Wei, F., Song, J., Zhang, C., Lin, J., Xue, R., Shan, L.-D., Gong, S., Zhang, G.-X., Qin, Z.-H., Xu, G.-Y., & Wang, L.-H. (2019). Chronic stress impairs the aquaporin-4-mediated glymphatic transport through glucocorticoid signaling. *Psychopharmacology, 236*(4), 1367–1384.

Xie, L., Kang, H., Xu, Q., Chen, M. J., Liao, Y., Thiyagarajan, M., O'Donnell, J., Christensen, D. J., Nicholson, C., Iliff, J. J., Takano, T., Deane, R., & Nedergaard, M. (2013). Sleep drives metabolite clearance from the adult brain. *Science, 342*(6156), 373–377.

Xu, Z., Xiao, N., Chen, Y., Huang, H., Marshall, C., Gao, J., Cai, Z., Wu, T., Hu, G., & Xiao, M. (2015). Deletion of aquaporin-4 in APP/PS1 mice exacerbates brain Aβ accumulation and memory deficits. *Molecular Neurodegeneration, 10*, Article 58.

Zhang, J., Zhan, Z., Li, X., Xing, A., Jiang, C., Chen, Y., Shi, W., & An, L. (2017). Intermittent fasting protects against Alzheimer's disease possible through restoring aquaporin-4 polarity. *Frontiers in Molecular Neuroscience, 10,* Article 395.

Zhao, L., Tannenbaum, A., Bakker, E. N. T. P., & Benveniste, H. (2022). Physiology of glymphatic solute transport and waste clearance from the brain. *Physiology, 37*(6), 349–362.

CHAPTER

9 Sleep and Circadian Rhythms and Metabolism

Anne-Marie Chang, Praneet C. Kaki, Robin K. Yuan, Christopher M. Depner, and Orfeu M. Buxton

Abstract

Diabetes and obesity remain two of the most prominent diseases and causes of morbidity and mortality in the United States and across the world. Approaches to curbing these epidemics primarily revolve around lifestyle adjustments to diet and exercise. However, recent research continues to further inform the important role that sleep deficiency and sleep health behaviors play in diabetes, obesity, and health. Both sleep restriction and circadian disruption represent risk factors for weight gain and diabetes, via physiological mechanisms including adverse impacts on glucose and lipid metabolism, and energy expenditure. This chapter summarizes evidence from epidemiological and experimental laboratory studies regarding a role for sleep health in metabolism, obesity, and diabetes.

Key Words: glucose metabolism, lipid metabolism, sleep restriction, sleep deficiency, circadian misalignment, circadian disruption, artificial light, obesity risk, diabetes risk

Introduction

"Sleep restriction" refers to curtailing the sleep opportunity over days to weeks in experimental studies or as a habitual practice in population studies. "Circadian disruption" refers to the misalignment of daily physical activity, dietary intake, and light–dark cycles with endogenous circadian rhythms. Both sleep restriction and circadian disruption increase risks for obesity and diabetes. Most aspects of metabolism exhibit diurnal variation. Acute circadian misalignment and circadian disruption are associated with impaired glucose metabolism in ways that differ from sleep restriction yet still increase obesity and diabetes risk. The timing of many behavioral, physiological, and environmental factors is simultaneously altered during circadian disruption. Circadian disruption often results from exposure to artificial light at night (ALAN), common in modern society, and is associated with health risks including overweight and obesity. Laboratory studies have begun to tease apart the mechanistic contributions of sleep restriction, circadian disruption, and ALAN in causing adverse metabolic consequences.

Although this field of research linking sleep deficiency and circadian disruption to diabetes, obesity, and lipid metabolism continues to evolve, findings to date can inform future interventions. The following sections review the epidemiological and laboratory evidence for circadian disruption and adverse consequences for metabolism and obesity and diabetes risk.

Epidemiology of Obesity and Diabetes Risk

Obesity, defined as a body mass index (BMI) >30 kg/m^2, is a pervasive problem worldwide in children and adults. Per the Centers for Disease Control and Prevention (CDCP, 2023), "Obesity is a serious chronic disease, and the prevalence of obesity continues to increase in the United States. Obesity is common, serious, and costly. This epidemic is putting a strain on American families, affecting overall health, health care costs, productivity, and military readiness." According to the CDCP (2022a), obesity rates across adults in the United States have increased from 30.5% in 1999–2000 to 41.9% in 2017–2020. Childhood obesity rates (people aged 2–19 years) in the United States were at 19.7% in 2017–2020 (CDCP, 2022a), compared to 18.5% in 2015–2016 (Hales et al., 2017). Outside the United States, worldwide obesity rates nearly tripled from 1975 to 2016. World Health Organization (WHO) data from 2016 indicate that over 1.9 billion adults were overweight (BMI >25) and 650 million were obese (BMI >30). Similarly, there were 39 million obese or overweight children under the age of 5, and this trend continues to worsen in both high-income and low-income countries, especially in urban areas (WHO, 2021).

Fundamentally, obesity is caused by an energy imbalance that results in the prolonged intake of more calories than expended. This can be due to a combination of factors such as eating energy-dense foods, low physical activity, and high levels of sedentary behavior that can adversely impact energy expenditure. Obesity is associated with a myriad of health complications including heart disease, stroke, musculoskeletal conditions, cancer, and diabetes. In the setting of experimental studies, obesity and overweight are largely preventable and treatable by reducing energy intake (less fat- and sugar-rich foods), eating a healthier diet including fruits and vegetables, and regular physical activity (WHO, 2021). However, as evidenced by the increasing rates of obesity over recent decades, such treatment and prevention strategies from experimental studies have not translated into effective prevention and treatment strategies in the real world.

Diabetes, a chronic disease of glucose and lipid metabolism, is diagnosed by high levels of glucose in the blood, primarily due to a lack of insulin production (Type 1 diabetes) or an impaired sensitivity to insulin (Type 2 diabetes). Glucose is a vital source of energy for the body's tissues, and elevated levels in the bloodstream could interfere with other bodily functions. Diabetes is also frequently accompanied by dyslipidemia and increased risk of heart disease, stroke, kidney disease, and vision impairment. The leading cause of death in people with diabetes is cardiovascular disease (CVD; Dal Canto et al., 2019).

In 2019, 11.3% of the US adult population (37.3 million) had diabetes, of which ~8.5 million were undiagnosed (American Diabetes Association [ADA], 2022). Diabetes continues to remain rampant in the United States, with 1.4 million new diagnoses every year, and ranks as the seventh leading cause of death (87,647 deaths) (ADA, 2022). From 1980 to 2014, the number of cases of diabetes more than tripled worldwide. Moreover, in 2019, diabetes caused 1.5 million deaths worldwide, of which about half occurred in people under the age of 70 (WHO, 2022). Diabetes became the ninth leading cause of death worldwide, making it a major cause of morbidity and mortality.

Type 2 diabetes is often linked to obesity but has other contributing causes including low physical activity, age over 45 years, previous diagnosis of gestational diabetes, and a family member with Type 2 diabetes (CDCP, 2022b). The ADA recognizes factors such as age, gender, a "first-degree relative with diabetes," hypertension, low high-density lipoprotein (HDL) and high triglyceride levels, history of CVD, physical inactivity, and obesity as risk factors for diabetes (Davies et al., 2022). As of September 2022, the ADA acknowledged sleep as an important determinant in the management of diabetes. Specifically, it highlighted sleep disorders (such as obstructive sleep apnea), short and long sleep, and the quality of sleep as being associated with impairments in glucose metabolism (Davies et al., 2022). Sleep restriction is associated with increased risk for weight gain in children (Ruan et al., 2015), obesity in adults (Guimaraes et al., 2022), and diabetes (Lu et al., 2021); circadian disruption, such as light at night, is associated with increased risk for obesity (Lai et al., 2020); and occupational circadian disruption by shift work increases risk for diabetes (Gao et al., 2020).

In 2022, the American Heart Association (AHA) defined sleep as one of the key pillars of cardiovascular health (Lloyd-Jones et al., 2022). With this addition, what was previously "Life's Simple 7" is now "Life's Essential 8," consisting of diet, physical activity, nicotine exposure, BMI, blood lipids, blood glucose, blood pressure, and sleep health. Sleep duration ties into the original seven factors of cardiovascular health (CVH) but also exerts its own independent influence on CVH. Although the focus is on sleep duration, the AHA also mentions that there are various aspects of sleep—such as timing, regularity, efficiency, and satisfaction—that contribute to CVH.

Epidemiologic Evidence for the Role of Sleep Deficiency and Circadian Disruption on Weight Gain and Obesity Risk

A meta-analysis identified a dose–response relationship between sleep and weight change, such that, for each additional hour of daily sleep duration, children exhibited a 0.05 kg/m^2 (95% confidence interval [CI] [–0.09, –0.01]) lower annual BMI gain over a 3.4-year average follow-up, corresponding to a 21% reduction in obesity risk (Ruan et al., 2015). However, there was relatively high heterogeneity across the relevant studies. A systematic review and meta-analysis involving 32 cohorts of preschool-aged children observed that each additional hour of daily sleep duration was associated with a 0.3 kg/m^2 lower BMI

(Miller et al., 2021). Another systematic review of cohort studies in adult populations found an association between short sleep (<7 hours) and obesity that remained even after removing potentially biased studies (Guimaraes et al., 2022). A 2021 systematic review and meta-analysis of short sleep and obesity in preschool children identified an association between short sleep duration and increased obesity risk in preschool children (risk ratio [RR] = 1.54, 95% CI [1.33, 1.77]; $p < .001$) from 13 prospective studies (Miller et al., 2021). The same meta-analysis, using 11 prospective studies, also found a 0.02-unit reduction in BMI *z*-score per hour of additional sleep (mean difference –0.02 unit per hour sleep; [–0.03, –0.01]; $p < .001$). However, in contrast, a 2022 study examining the relationship between longitudinal sleep and BMI change in a low-income, predominantly Black sample based in two Pittsburgh neighborhoods found no significant association (Brooks Holliday et al., 2022). Further longitudinal work is needed.

Epidemiologic Evidence for the Role of Sleep Deficiency and Circadian Disruption on Diabetes Risk

A meta-analysis assessed 17 cohort studies comprised of over 700,000 participants to study the relationship between short sleep duration and Type 2 diabetes mellitus (T2DM; Lu et al., 2021). In this meta-analysis, they found a higher incidence of T2DM in people with short sleep duration (≤6 hours) compared to normal sleep duration (6–9 hours). There was an RR of 1.22 (95% CI [1.15, 1.29], $p < .001$) for T2DM incidence for short sleep duration conditions compared to normal sleep duration. Another meta-analysis of 10 prospective studies describes a U-shaped curve relating sleep duration and T2DM risk, which was observed to be at a minimum at 7–8 hours of sleep/day (Shan et al., 2015). Short sleep durations of 6 hours/day and ≤5 hours/day were associated with increasing risk of T2DM compared to a 7 hours/day reference, with RR values of 1.06 and 1.37, respectively. On the other hand, long sleep durations of 8 hours/day and ≥9 hours/day were associated with increasing risk of T2DM (compared to 7 hours/day), with RR values of 1.11 and 1.40, respectively. Moreover, sleep has also been shown to be relevant in pre-diabetic patients in a meta-analysis (of only three studies) that found a significant association (hazard ratio = 1.59, $p < .0001$) between short sleep duration (<5 hours and 5–6 hours) and progression from pre-diabetes to Type 2 diabetes (Mostafa et al., 2022). The authors do, however, discuss the need for further research and data on specific sleep disorders to aid in the development of targeted interventions to prevent progression to T2DM. In a meta-analysis of 12 cohort studies and nine cross-sectional studies, a significant relationship was observed between shift work, an occupational driver of circadian disruption, and increased type 2 diabetes risk, RR = 1.10 (Gao et al., 2020).

Epidemiological Evidence Linking Sleep Duration and Lipids

A 2017 meta-analysis of 13 prospective studies did not find a significant relationship between sleep duration and dyslipidemia, a categorical variable that was assessed in different ways by the individual studies (Kruisbrink et al., 2017). Variables that were measured to assess this outcome included high total cholesterol (TC), low HDL, high low-density lipoprotein (LDL), high non-HDL, TC/HDL ratio ≥5, and high triglycerides (TG). When considering the rate ratios between short sleep duration and these individual variables on their own, one study included in the meta-analysis found a negative association between short sleep (<6 hours/night) and low HDL cholesterol (serum HDL <40 mg/dl for men or <50 mg/dl for women) levels (RR = 0.75, 95% CI [0.57, 0.99]; J.-Y. Kim et al., 2015). Another study found a positive association between short sleep (5–7 hours/night) and high TG (≥200 mg/dl) levels in men (RR = 1.23, 95% CI [1.03, 1.48]; Kinuhata et al., 2014). However, the pooled results of the meta-analysis combining the studies did not show a significant result for any of these variables. These findings on limited clinical measures of lipid metabolism may not tell the full story. Experimental evidence presented below from inpatient studies using perturbation analyses in controlled conditions describes multiple pathways by which sleep restriction impacts lipid metabolism (Kruisbrink et al., 2017).

Experimental Evidence of the Effects of Sleep Restriction on Glucose Metabolism

A laboratory study published in 1999 used intravenous glucose tolerance tests (IVGTTs) and carbohydrate-rich test meals to assess the impact of experimental sleep restriction on glucose metabolism in healthy young men (Spiegel et al., 1999). The sleep restriction condition (termed "sleep debt") consisted of 6 nights with sleep opportunities restricted to 4 hours of time in bed (TIB), from 1:00 a.m. to 5:00 a.m. Following sleep restriction, participants completed a "sleep-recovery" condition with 7 nights of sleep opportunities extended to 12 hours TIB, from 9:00 p.m. to 9:00 a.m. In the sleep restriction versus recovery condition there was a 15 mg/dl higher peak glucose response to the carbohydrate-rich meal and a 30% decrease in glucose effectiveness and the acute insulin response to glucose on the IVGTT, with no change in insulin sensitivity between conditions. In subsequent analyses, however, the homeostasis model assessment of insulin resistance was elevated in the sleep restriction versus recovery condition (Spiegel et al., 2005). In aggregate, these findings demonstrate that glucose metabolism was impaired during the sleep restriction condition. Notably, in both conditions TIB was centered around 3:00 a.m., and participants were required to live in the laboratory on Days 5 and 6 of data collection. However, on Days 1–4 of each condition participants were free to leave the laboratory and continue their normal daily activities, including obtaining exposure to natural and electrical lighting throughout the day. During Days 1–4 participants returned to the laboratory by 7:00 p.m. and remained in the laboratory until 9:00 the following morning. Although light exposure was not reported, participants were allowed to watch television and use laptop computers during scheduled wakefulness in the laboratory. Accordingly, it is highly probable that participants were exposed to light levels in the laboratory that could have impacted the timing of their central circadian clock differently in the sleep restriction versus sleep-recovery conditions. Because the timing of the central circadian clock was not assessed in this study, it is not known if the potentially altered timing of light exposure between conditions impacted the clock and therefore potentially contributed to the impaired glucose metabolism during sleep restriction.

In another randomized crossover sleep restriction study, 2 nights of 4 hours/night sleep restriction compared to 2 nights of 8 hours/night (regular) sleep resulted in a significant increase in both glucose (p = .022) and insulin (p = .007) peaks following an ad libitum standardized breakfast buffet (Schmid et al., 2011). An increase in the postprandial glucose peak despite a concurrent increased insulin peak points to reduced glucose tolerance and insulin sensitivity following 2 nights of sleep restriction. There were no changes in pre-breakfast glucose and insulin levels, however, between the two conditions. Moreover, there were no significant differences in any of the markers of glucose metabolism throughout the afternoon and evening. Although caloric intake from the ad libitum buffet was not statistically different between conditions, this was not a controlled test meal, and it is possible that differences in food intake patterns between conditions may have contributed to the differences observed in the glucose and insulin responses.

Findings from a double-blind, randomized clinical study by Buxton and colleagues (2010), where healthy young men spent 7 days with 5 hours/night TIB (sleep-restricted condition), demonstrate the negative consequences of short sleep on insulin sensitivity, which was measured by using both IVGTTs and the gold-standard euglycemic-hyperinsulinemic clamps. Subjects spent 10 hours/night TIB in a sleep-replete condition before sleep restriction. They were restricted to the laboratory with isocaloric diets and minimal activity. The results of both IVGTT and euglycemic-hyperinsulinemic clamp showed that insulin sensitivity was significantly reduced, and the IVGTT data indicated that insulin secretion was not increased to compensate for the impaired insulin sensitivity in the sleep-restricted condition compared to resting state. Although the IVGTT results did not show a significant change in the acute insulin response, the disposition index and glucose tolerance were both significantly reduced in the sleep-restricted condition. A reduced disposition index—which is calculated as the product of insulin sensitivity and insulin secretion—is a sign of increased risk for diabetes (Lorenzo et al., 2010). Notably, light levels were <90 lux during scheduled wakefulness, and circadian phase was not measured (Buxton et al., 2010). As data indicates that light levels as low as 6 lux can shift the central circadian clock (Phillips et al., 2019), it is possible that altered light exposure during sleep restriction induced a shift of the central circadian clock, which could potentially contribute to impaired insulin sensitivity.

In another randomized crossover study by Nedeltcheva and colleagues (2009), middle-aged adult participants spent either 5.5 or 8.5 hours/night in bed for 2 weeks with an ad libitum diet and sedentary activity. Such sleep restriction (5 hours/night) resulted in elevated glucose levels and insulin resistance without a compensatory increase in insulin secretion. The controlled diet and activity in the laboratory combined with chronic partial sleep restriction are all common aspects of Western lifestyles and make the results of this study more relevant to real life. Importantly, light exposure and circadian phase were not reported in this study, and therefore it is not known if potential shifts in circadian phase may have also contributed to the observed impairments in glucose metabolism.

In a brief sleep restriction study by Schmid and colleagues (2011) using a randomized-order crossover design including 2 consecutive nights of either 8-hour (regular) sleep or 4-hour (sleep-restricted condition) sleep, blood concentrations of glucose, insulin, C-peptide, glucagon, adrenocorticotropic hormone, cortisol, and interleukin-6 were measured. Following the 2 nights of controlled sleep, an ad libitum standardized breakfast buffet and a subsequent snack buffet and other main dishes were used to evaluate metabolic responses throughout the day. Under the 2 nights of the sleep-restricted condition following a standardized breakfast buffet, glucagon area under the curve (AUC) levels exhibited a decrease as the normal spike in glucagon following breakfast intake showed a diminished increase.

In a more recent study published by Ness, Strayer, Nahmod, Chang, et al. (2019), following 5 days of sleep restriction (5 hours TIB/night), glucagon levels during a morning IVGTT were reduced relative to the baseline fully rested condition (see Figure 9.1). These differences were no longer present after a recovery condition of 2 days (10 hours TIB/night). Another paper based on this study (Ness, Strayer, Nahmod, Schade, et al., 2019) evaluated postprandial responses to an evening high-fat dinner (HFD) after 4 nights of sleep restriction. Although pre-meal glucagon levels were not different from the fully rested condition, postprandial glucagon levels varied across time, exhibiting a significant and sustained decrease in the sleep restriction condition from the pre-meal baseline, compared to a characteristic dip and subsequent postprandial increase observed in the rested condition. Moreover, there were no significant differences in glucagon levels—both pre-meal and time-dependent—between the baseline and recovery conditions.

Glucagon levels normally increase after a meal and peak a few hours later. These two sleep restriction studies using three different meal/caloric intake challenges yielded altered responses following sleep restriction, pointing to a potential role for sleep restriction to influence pancreatic α-cell function (Schmid et al., 2011). As noted by the authors, circadian timing was not assessed in this study, and it is possible that altered light exposure during sleep restriction altered the timing of the central circadian clock. Like the prior studies mentioned, it is thus possible that circadian phase differences between conditions are contributing to these findings.

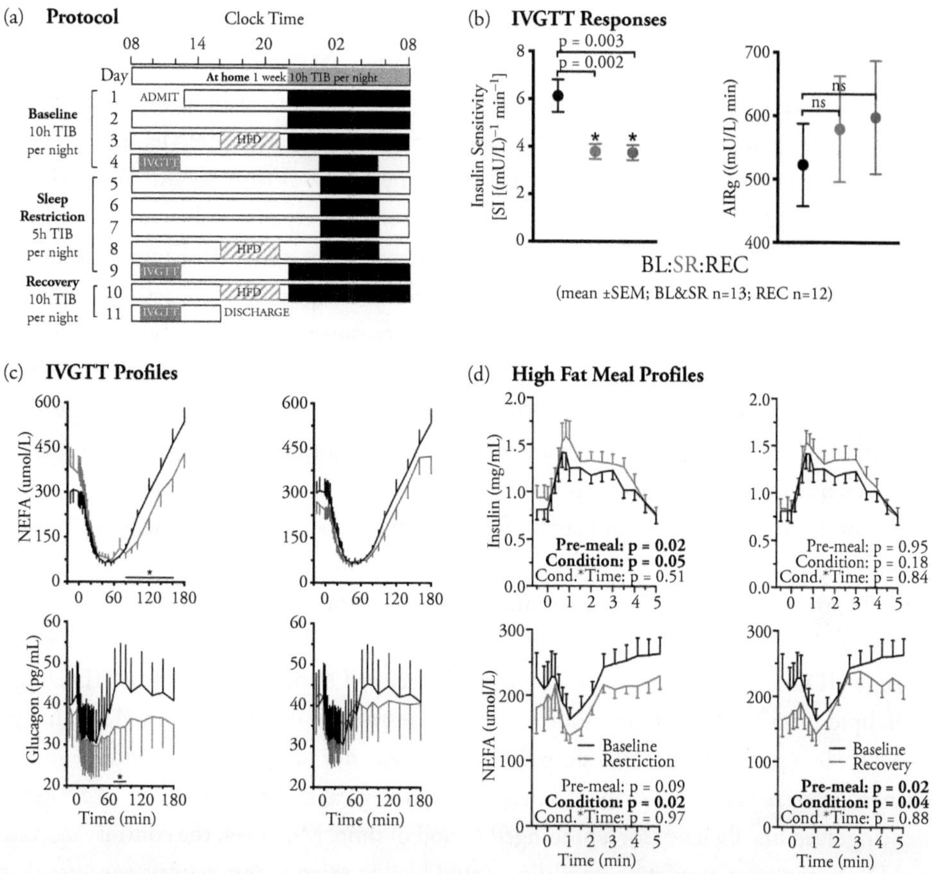

Figure 9.1 Sleep restriction effects on glucose and lipid metabolism during a standardized morning intravenous glucose tolerance test (IVGTT) and on lipid metabolism during evening meal response

Note. Panel A: Protocol. Participants completed an 11-day protocol involving sleep restriction followed by recovery sleep. Pre-study at home time in bed (TIB) was 10 hours for 1 week. Sleep restriction study protocol with three conditions: 3-night baseline of 10-hour TIB per night, 5-night restriction of 5-hour TIB per night, and 2-night recovery of 10-hour TIB per night. High-fat dinner (HFD) response (striped bars on Days 3, 8, and 10) and morning IVGTT (gray bars on Days 4, 9, and 11) were conducted during each condition. Panel B: IVGTT responses. Sleep restriction effects on glucose and lipid metabolism during a morning IVGTT. Insulin sensitivity was significantly reduced after sleep restriction (red) compared to baseline (black) and remained decreased even after 2 nights of recovery sleep (gray). The acute insulin response (insulin secretion in response to glucose) was not significantly changed after sleep restriction or recovery sleep compared to baseline. Panel C: Morning IVGTT profiles. An IVGTT condition × time interaction showed that the non-esterified fatty acid (NEFA) rebound was reduced in the sleep restriction condition (red) compared to baseline (p = .01). IVGTT showed no significant change in NEFA levels in the recovery condition compared to baseline. The response following 5 days of sleep restriction showed a significant reduction in glucagon levels compared to baseline (p = .01). IVGTT glucagon after recovery sleep no longer showed a reduction compared to baseline, although there was a significant condition × time interaction (p = .03). Panel D: Evening HFD profiles. Sleep restriction effects on lipid metabolism during an evening HFD. Pre-meal insulin was elevated following 4 nights of sleep restriction compared to baseline (p = .02) and remained elevated over the course of the HFD (p = .05). Insulin levels pre-meal and during the HFD returned to baseline in the recovery condition compared to baseline and showed no condition × time interaction. NEFA levels were significantly decreased over the course of the HFD after sleep restriction compared to baseline (p = .02). NEFA levels were reduced before the HFD (p = .02) and remained suppressed during the HFD even after recovery sleep compared to baseline (p = .04). AIRg = acute insulin response (insulin secretion in response to glucose); BL = baseline; REC = recovery; SEM = standard error of the mean; SR = sleep restriction. Adapted from Ness, Strayer, Nahmod, Chang, et al. (2019); Ness, Strayer, Nahmod, Schade, et al. (2019).

Experimental Studies of the Effects of Sleep Restriction on Lipid Metabolism

A partial sleep restriction study that subjected participants to 4 hours sleep/night for 5 nights, along with two epidemiological studies (The Dietary, Lifestyle, and Genetic Determinants of Obesity and Metabolic Syndrome Study, $N = 518$, and Young Finns Study, $N = 2221$) that used questionnaires to assess participants' subjective feelings of insufficient sleep, analyzed the effect of sleep restriction on cholesterol metabolism and inflammatory responses (Aho et al., 2016). At the transcriptional level, results showed a down-regulation in cholesterol transport and lipid transport pathways in both the experimental sleep restriction condition and the epidemiological study subjects who reported subjective sleep insufficiency. Reverse cholesterol transport pathways were downregulated in both the sleep restriction study and the epidemiological studies in subjects with subjective sleep insufficiency. The experimental condition in the sleep restriction study showed a reduction in small, medium, and large LDL ($p < .01$) and small very low-density lipoprotein ($p < .05$) concentrations compared to baseline. The sleep restriction condition did not result in any change in HDL concentrations after correction, however. In both epidemiological studies, individuals reporting subjective sleep insufficiency exhibited a reduction in large HDL levels. Risk for CVD is typically increased in people with a low HDL/high LDL lipid profile. Although the short-term sleep restriction condition showed no change in HDL, it is plausible that this sleep deprivation was not long enough to induce such a change, whereas HDL was reduced in the epidemiological subjects who were likely experiencing sleep insufficiency for a prolonged period of time. Moreover, the contrary *decrease* in LDL in the sleep restriction condition could be due to an inflammatory response that was also observed in this condition.

Recent findings from a laboratory-based sleep restriction study evaluated lipid metabolism in perturbation analyses evaluating responses to morning glucose infusions (IVGTT) and evening standardized meals. The study design included 3 baseline nights (10 hours TIB/night) of sleep, followed by 5 sleep-restricted nights (5 hours TIB/night), and finally 2 days of sleep recovery (10 hours TIB/night) in 15 healthy males. Specifically, one paper based on this study found that 5 nights of such sleep restriction led to a significant reduction in the non-esterified fatty acid (NEFA) rebound response following an IVGTT, which was restored following the 2 nights of recovery sleep (Ness, Strayer, Nahmod, Chang, et al., 2019). There was also a significant reduction in insulin sensitivity, which was not restored by the recovery sleep. NEFAs are a particularly important class of lipids that are a major source of energy for skeletal muscle and are normally suppressed by the action of insulin on adipose tissues. However, whereas NEFA levels normally rebound after glucose is cleared, 5 days of sleep restriction led to a significantly delayed rebound. Another paper based on this study found that 4 nights of 5 hours TIB led to a significant reduction in both the standard postprandial lipemic response and the feeling of satiety following an HFD (Ness, Strayer, Nahmod, Schade, et al., 2019). More specifically, sleep restriction led to reduced NEFA levels during the entirety of the HFD, an effect that persisted even during the days of recovery sleep. It also led to a reduced postprandial TG AUC, which, however, returned to baseline after 1 night of recovery sleep. Participant-reported satiety was also decreased following sleep restriction despite no change in the satiety hormones.

Recovery From Sleep Restriction (Hint: A Weekend Is Not Enough)

Regarding glucose metabolism, some laboratory studies have investigated the influence of recovery sleep following experimental sleep restriction. In three studies, insulin sensitivity was assessed after 4–5 nights of experimental sleep restriction followed by 2 nights of recovery sleep (designed to simulate a weekend of recovery sleep). Findings from two of these three studies suggest that weekend recovery sleep does not restore insulin sensitivity to baseline levels observed prior to the experimental sleep restriction. Specifically, in the study from Depner et al. (2019), participants had ad libitum access to food and were exposed to recurrent sleep restriction following the weekend of recovery sleep. Insulin sensitivity was measured by the euglycemic-hyperinsulinemic clamp on the second morning following weekend recovery sleep, when participants had 1 night of recurrent sleep restriction of 5 hours TIB. Thus, the findings show that weekend recovery sleep did not prevent impaired insulin sensitivity when participants had recurrent sleep restriction following the weekend. In the studies by Ness, Strayer, Nahmod, Chang, et al. (2019) and Broussard et al. (2016), energy intake was controlled and insulin sensitivity was measured by the IVGTT immediately following weekend recovery sleep, without recurrent sleep restriction. Findings from Ness, Strayer, Nahmod, Chang, et al. (2019) show that insulin sensitivity did not improve during weekend recovery sleep, whereas findings from Broussard et al. (2016) did show that insulin sensitivity improved to baseline levels during weekend recovery sleep. Intriguingly, findings from another study (Eckel et al., 2015) that analyzed insulin sensitivity by the IVGTT after 5 days of experimental sleep restriction followed by 5 days of recovery sleep with 9 hours TIB also showed no improvements in insulin sensitivity, consistent with data from Ness, Strayer, Nahmod, Chang, et al. (2019) In aggregate, this data suggests that a weekend of recovery sleep is not adequate to fully counteract the impairments in insulin sensitivity that occur in response to a workweek of insufficient sleep. Because the timing and intensity of light exposure differed between the weekend recovery protocols, future studies are needed to better characterize the impact of weekend recovery sleep on circadian timing and to determine if altered circadian timing following weekend recovery sleep is linked with changes in insulin sensitivity. Furthermore, longer-term studies that investigate the impact of weekend recovery sleep on insulin sensitivity, over many cycles of insufficient sleep and weekend recovery sleep, are needed to better understand the long-term consequences of weekend recovery sleep on cardiometabolic risk.

Under Conditions of Sleep Restriction Symmetrically Around the Midpoint of Habitual Sleep, the Extent of Observed Circadian Misalignment Is Associated With the Degree of Impaired Insulin Sensitivity

In a study published in 2015 by Eckel et al., insulin sensitivity measured by the IVGTT was similarly reduced during a sleep restriction condition versus baseline and a control condition (Figure 9.2). Here, the sleep restriction condition consisted of 5 nights with sleep opportunities restricted to 5 hours TIB, the control condition consisted of 5 nights with sleep opportunities of 9 hours TIB, and baseline consisted of 3 nights with 9 hours TIB. Prior to completing baseline, all participants maintained an ~9-hour sleep schedule for 1 week in their home environment, based on individual participants' habitual sleep and wake times. In the laboratory, the 9-hour sleep schedules matched the participants' habitual sleep schedules, and during sleep restriction participants went to bed 2 hours later and woke up 2 hours earlier relative to their habitual 9-hour TIB schedules, keeping the midpoint of sleep centered throughout the study. During scheduled wakefulness light exposure in the laboratory was room lighting and sunlight through a window. Circadian melatonin phase was measured in dim light (<8 lux maximum) during the final 24 hours of each condition. Although the midpoint of sleep remained centered during sleep restriction and participants were exposed to 2 hours of additional light in the evening and morning, dim-light melatonin onset was delayed ~1.5 hours and the phase angle between wake time and dim-light melatonin offset (DLMOff) was wider during sleep restriction relative to baseline and control conditions. These findings provide support that sleep restriction, even when the midpoint of sleep is centered, can alter the timing of the central circadian clock and result in circadian misalignment, especially in the morning. Furthermore, the magnitude of circadian misalignment in these participants, quantified as the phase angle between wake time and DLMOff, was associated (Figure 9.2C; $p < .05$, beta estimate -0.29 ± 0.14 [standard error of the mean]) with the magnitude of impaired insulin sensitivity. These findings suggest that circadian misalignment resulting from sleep restriction in laboratory studies may contribute to impaired insulin sensitivity. Similar findings were also published from a study in adolescents with polycystic ovary syndrome (Simon et al., 2019). Specifically, data showed that worse circadian misalignment was associated with worse insulin sensitivity in adolescents with polycystic ovary syndrome who were getting insufficient sleep duration. In aggregate, these findings help raise the intriguing hypothesis that circadian misalignment induced by short sleep duration may be a key factor contributing to impaired insulin sensitivity and therefore risk of Type 2 diabetes associated with habitual short sleep duration. However, because the insulin sensitivity testing occurred at different circadian phases between conditions in these studies, the influence of prior circadian misalignment (during the 5 days of sleep restriction) versus testing at a different circadian phase cannot be disentangled in this dataset.

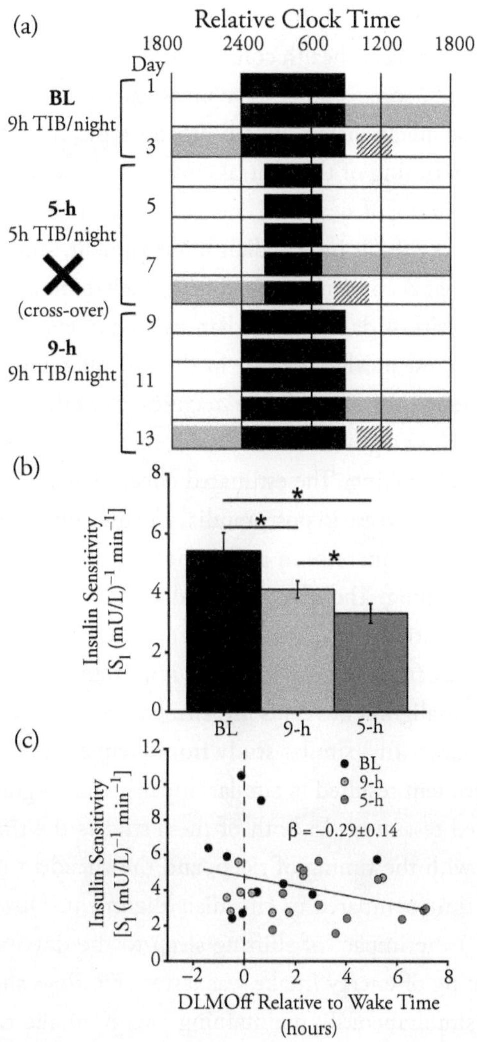

Figure 9.2 Morning circadian misalignment during experimental sleep restriction is associated with impaired insulin sensitivity

Note. Panel A: Protocol. Participants completed a 13–14-day laboratory protocol consisting of a 3-day baseline (BL) condition, followed by control (9-hour) and short sleep (5-hour) conditions lasting 5 days each, in a randomized crossover counterbalanced order. For 1 week prior to the in-laboratory study, participants time in bed was set to 9 hours per night based on habitual bed and waketimes (±30 minutes). Black boxes represent scheduled sleep opportunities, with sleep timing based on individual habitual sleep schedules. Gray shading represents dim light (<8 lux) to permit assessment of 24-hour plasma melatonin profiles. Intravenous glucose tolerance tests were administered after the final sleep opportunity of each condition (diagonal cross-hatched lines) to assess insulin sensitivity. Panel B: Insulin sensitivity was significantly reduced in the 5-hour versus 9-hour and BL conditions and in the 9-hour versus BL condition. Food intake was ad libitum during the 9-hour and 5-hour conditions, and participants tended to overeat during these conditions relative to BL. This higher food intake over 9 hours is likely contributing to the reduced insulin sensitivity during 9-hour versus BL condition (*$p < .05$). Panel C: Association between morning circadian misalignment and insulin sensitivity. Scheduled wake time is represented by the vertical dashed line. A negative value on the *x*-axis indicates that dim-light melatonin offset occurred before scheduled wake time, whereas a positive value on the *x*-axis indicates that dim-light melatonin offset occurred after scheduled waketime. The beta estimate (±standard error) is derived from a linear mixed model regression of the association between dim-light melatonin offset and insulin sensitivity when controlled for condition order, body weight, and energy balance, with participant entered as a random factor. S_I = insulin sensitivity; DLMOff = dim-light melatonin offset; TIB = time in bed. Adapted from Eckel et al. (2015).

Acute Circadian Misalignment and Metabolism

In addition to probing the adverse health consequences of altered circadian timing during insufficient sleep schedules, some studies have investigated the impact of acute circadian misalignment on glucose metabolism. These protocols typically use dim-light conditions to minimize shifts in the timing of the central circadian clock and then abruptly impose 8–12-hour shifts in the timing of sleep and energy intake. Such abrupt shifts in behaviors like sleep and energy intake result in circadian misalignment, similar to night-shift work where people are awake and consume food during their biological night. Morris et al. (2015) used a protocol with 4 days of circadian misalignment and assessed the glucose and insulin responses to test meals provided in the morning and evening. This allowed the investigators to somewhat disentangle the magnitude of effects of acute circadian misalignment compared to the magnitude of effects in meal responses during the biological morning versus biological evening. The estimated effect of acute circadian misalignment versus alignment was a 6% increase in postprandial glucose, whereas the effect of circadian timing was larger with a 17% increase in postprandial glucose during the biological evening versus biological morning. The effect of circadian misalignment was presumed to be from impaired insulin sensitivity, whereas the effect of the biological evening appeared to be from impaired beta-cell function, showing it is important to understand impairments due to acute circadian misalignment versus impairments due to measurements conducted at different circadian phases. In a similar study from Depner et al. (2018), just 2 days of acute circadian misalignment resulted in similar impairments in glucose metabolism, also analyzed by a controlled test meal. In both of these studies the timing of energy intake was shifted in parallel with the timing of sleep, and the circadian misalignment resulted in reduced total sleep time compared to circadian alignment. However, in a study from Chellappa et al. (2021) the impact of shifting sleep to the daytime, with or without a parallel shift in the timing of energy intake was tested. Findings show that shifting sleep to the daytime while simultaneously maintaining energy intake to the typical daytime hours prevented the impairments in glucose tolerance compared to the condition where sleep was shifted to the daytime and energy intake was shifted to the nighttime hours. These findings suggest the altered timing of energy intake during acute circadian misalignment is a large contributor to the adverse impacts of acute circadian misalignment on glucose metabolism. Additionally, in the study from Chellappa et al. (2021), total sleep time was similarly reduced in both conditions, suggesting that these findings are independent of shorter sleep duration that typically accompanies acute circadian misalignment. All of these studies used controlled test meals to assess changes in glucose metabolism, and therefore studies using more sensitive techniques such as the IVGTT or euglycemic-hyperinsulinemic clamp are needed to more rigorously characterize the impairments in glucose metabolism during acute circadian misalignment. Additionally, further studies focused on tissue-specific changes and the role of peripheral circadian clock timing in these findings are needed to help advance the field.

The Effect of Semi-Chronic Sleep Restriction Combined With or Without Abrupt and Repeated Circadian Misalignment on Glucose Metabolism

A study published in 2014 was designed to test the adverse cardiometabolic consequences of 8 days of experimentally imposed sleep restriction to 5 hours TIB per night, with continued circadian alignment of sleep versus abrupt circadian misalignment (Leproult et al., 2014), as commonly experienced in night/shift work. The study had two conditions, circadian alignment and abrupt circadian misalignment, with insulin sensitivity measured by the IVGTT at baseline and the end of each condition. For the circadian alignment condition the timing of sleep remained centered throughout the protocol. For the abrupt circadian misalignment condition the timing of sleep was delayed by 8.5 hours on Days 2–3 and 5–6 of the 8 days of sleep restriction to repeat the abrupt circadian misalignment twice. Sleep opportunities were equally restricted to 5 hours TIB in both conditions, and there were no significant differences in total sleep time between conditions. Light levels were <50 lux during scheduled wakefulness and complete darkness during scheduled sleep. Insulin sensitivity was decreased in both study conditions, but the percent decrease in the circadian misalignment group was nearly twice as large as the decrease in the circadian alignment group. Because of the small number of female participants, these between-group analyses were limited to the male participants. Similar to other studies of experimental sleep restriction, these findings also show that sleep restriction in healthy adults results in significant decreases in insulin sensitivity and that abrupt circadian misalignment in addition to sleep restriction causes further impairments in insulin sensitivity. Notably, at the end of sleep restriction relative to baseline, the timing of dim-light melatonin onset (DLMO) was delayed ~3 hours in the abrupt circadian misalignment group, whereas DLMO was not significantly different from baseline in the circadian alignment group. Thus, the IVGTT occurred at different circadian phases between groups, and it is not possible to disentangle the effects of prior circadian misalignment (during the sleep restriction phase of the study) versus testing at a different circadian phase. This finding supports the idea that minimizing circadian misalignment during sleep restriction may help minimize the magnitude of adverse cardiometabolic effects of sleep restriction.

The Combination of Sleep Restriction Plus Recurrent Circadian Disruption (3 Weeks Forced Desynchrony, Young and Old Men and Women) Increases Postprandial Glucose Levels Due to a Reduction in Postprandial Insulin Secretion

A study in 2012 by Buxton et al. tested the effects of the combination of prolonged sleep restriction and circadian disruption on glucose regulation and metabolism. A prestudy baseline included at-home sleep extension (10 hours TIB/night). After admission, 3 weeks of sleep restriction (5.6 hours TIB/night) in a forced desynchrony protocol (T = 28 hours), followed by 9 days of recovery sleep with TIB realigned to the baseline circadian phase (Figure 9.3). Resting metabolic rate (RMR) was measured via indirect calorimetry in all three conditions. Prior exposure to sleep restriction with circadian disruption resulted in a significant decrease in RMR of 8% (mean 120 kcal/day) in both younger and older adults, which recovered—although incompletely—in the 9-day recovery phase. In the absence of changes to diet, activity, and energy balance, this would lead to a weight gain of ~12 lb per year, thus dramatically increasing obesity risk.

A standardized high-carbohydrate breakfast meal was used to evaluate postprandial glucose metabolism. Importantly, this meal challenge was timed to occur at the same circadian phase in each condition (±2 hours), thus eliminating the potential confounding by testing at different circadian phases. This exposure to prior circadian disruption combined with sleep restriction resulted in significantly elevated fasting glucose levels in older adults. Postprandial glucose levels (both peak and AUC) were significantly elevated relative to the baseline sleep condition in both younger and older and male and female participants.

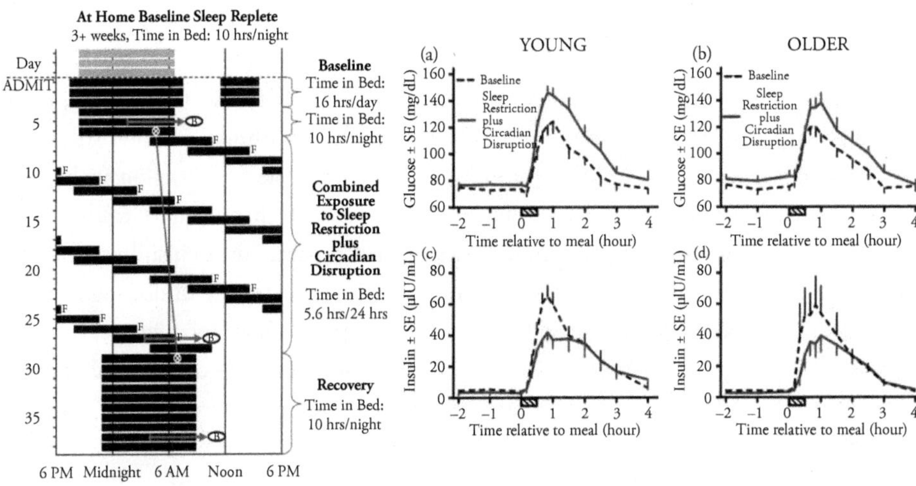

Figure 9.3 Prior exposure to circadian disruption and sleep restriction impairs glucose metabolism in young and older adults

Note. Participants completed a 39-day protocol (left panel) involving prior exposure to chronic circadian disruption and sleep restriction. Pre-study time in bed (TIB) was centered around habitual sleep duration and set to 10 hours TIB for 3+ weeks. After admission to the laboratory, baseline "sleep replete" condition (3 weeks of 10 hours TIB/day at home followed by 6 days with ≥10 hours TIB/day). Sleep opportunities were then systematically spread across the circadian cycle on a 28-hour "forced desynchrony" (FD) protocol, with 6.5 hours TIB, equivalent to 5.6 hours per 24 hours, and 21.5 hours of monitored wakefulness for 3 weeks. A subsequent period of 10 days of circadian re-entrainment with sleep recovery (10 hours TIB/24 hours) with the sleep period adjusted to the same circadian phase as the baseline sleep condition by modification of the duration of the wake period after the last FD day. Dark bars represent scheduled sleep intervals. Standardized breakfast meal responses (B); daily fasted blood samples for assessment of glucose, insulin, cortisol (F); core body temperature minimum (white X, depicted on days 6 and 29 in this example). Time from midpoint of sleep to start of breakfast (gray horizontal arrow) was maintained by choosing a day in the last week of sleep restriction plus circadian disruption such that the standardized meal occurred during this exposure at the same circadian phase as baseline within 4 hours (0.7 ± 1.8 hours), resulting in an average exposure duration of 19.2 ± 2.8 24-hour days (range 15–22 days). Postprandial peak and area under the curve (AUC) glucose levels were significantly elevated in both younger and older adults due to reduced peak and AUC insulin levels. SE = standard error. Adapted from Buxton et al. (2012).

Postprandial glucose levels in the prediabetic ranges were observed in 3 of the 21 participants following exposure to circadian disruption and sleep restriction. Postprandial hyperglycemia resulted from a significant reduction of postprandial insulin secretion, both peak and AUC (Figure 9.3). Fortunately, postprandial glucose and insulin returned to baseline patterns after a week of sleep recovery. The inability of beta cells to produce adequate insulin in response to elevated blood glucose levels points to pancreatic dysfunction as a consequence of chronic exposure to the combination of sleep restriction and circadian disruption, increasing diabetes risk (Buxton et al., 2012).

Circadian Disruption (While Minimizing Sleep Loss) Impairs Glucose Tolerance, but Only When Combined With a High-Fat Diet

Following up on the previous finding that a history of chronic circadian disruption with concurrent sleep restriction impaired glucose metabolism, a 2022 study investigated whether prior exposure to chronic circadian disruption alone (without sleep restriction) would also impair glucose metabolism evaluated by standardized meal responses (Zitting et al., 2022). After completing 3 weeks of at-home sleep extension (10 hours TIB/night), participants (mean age, #F of total n) were admitted to the 37-day inpatient study, which included 3 weeks of a 28-hour forced desynchrony protocol. Importantly, scheduled TIB during forced desynchrony was maintained at 10 hours TIB/night (11.67 hours/28 hours) in order to minimize inadvertent sleep loss due to reduced sleep efficiency when participants slept at adverse circadian phases. Thus, the authors were able to examine the influence of chronic circadian disruption without sleep loss on glucose metabolism. Because data from rodent studies suggested that circadian disruption may interact with a high-fat diet to impact metabolism (Arble et al., 2009; Espitia-Bautista et al., 2017; S. M. Kim et al., 2018; Kohsaka et al., 2007), both high- and lower-fat diets were used in conjunction with the exposure to circadian disruption (Figure 9.4).

Postprandial glucose metabolism was assessed using a standardized breakfast meal at baseline, following 3 weeks of circadian disruption, and after 1 week of recovery. As in the 2012 study (Buxton et al., 2012), all three of these meal challenges occurred at the same circadian phase, verified by core body temperature, ensuring that there was no acute circadian misalignment. Surprisingly, adverse metabolic outcomes were observed only in participants who consumed a high-fat diet (45%–50% fat) during the study. In participants who consumed a lower-fat diet (25%–27% fat), postprandial glucose levels were not significantly different from baseline, suggesting that a lower-fat diet may be somewhat protective against the adverse glycemic effects of chronic circadian disruption. However, participants who were exposed to chronic circadian disruption and consumed the high-fat diet exhibited elevated postprandial glucose levels and increased dual-energy X-ray absorptiometry–assessed body fat (+1%), suggesting that chronic circadian disruption, when it occurs in conjunction with additional insults such as high-fat diet, may lead to adverse metabolic outcomes (Zitting et al., 2022).

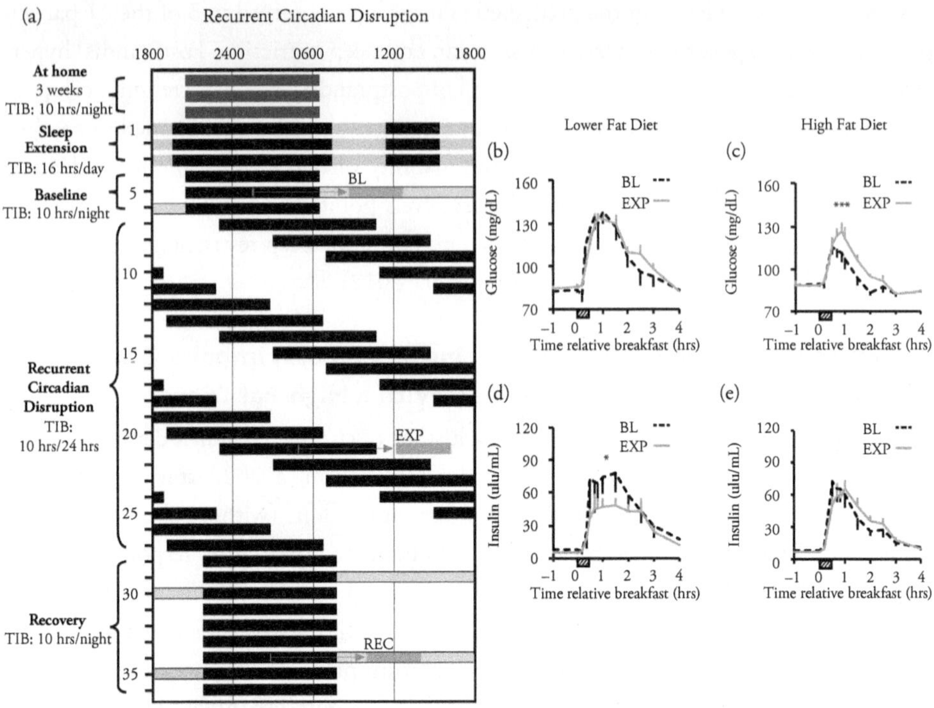

Figure 9.4 Effects of recurrent circadian disruption vary with diet (lower-fat diet versus high-fat diet)
Note. Panel A: Study day is indicated along the left side and representative clock hour along the top axis. Prior to admission, participants maintained a consistent, at-home sleep schedule of 10 hours time in bed for 3 weeks, centered on the same midpoint of sleep as inpatient baseline sleep opportunities. Solid black bars represent scheduled sleep episodes in darkness, while gray and white indicate parts of the study conducted under 4-lux and 90-lux lighting levels, respectively. The timing of standardized breakfast meal responses (blue bars), conducted at a consistent circadian phase from midpoint of sleep, is also indicated. Panels B–E: Postprandial glucose and insulin profiles are depicted following a standardized breakfast meal at baseline and after exposure to recurrent circadian disruption while on a lower-fat diet (B, D) or a high-fat diet (C, E). BL = baseline; EXP = exposure; REC = recovery; TIB = time in bed. Adapted from Zitting et al. (2022).

Sleep Restriction (While Minimizing Concurrent Circadian Disruption) Does Not Increase Postprandial Glucose Levels

Sleep restriction commonly occurs with circadian disruption through extended exposure to ALAN. Therefore, a 2021 study in older adults sought to compare the metabolic effects of chronic sleep restriction with and without concurrent circadian disruption (Yuan et al., 2021). In the chronic sleep restriction with circadian disruption condition, participants were exposed to 3 weeks of a 28-hour forced desynchrony protocol with 5.6 hours/24 hours of scheduled TIB. Meanwhile, in the chronic sleep restriction without circadian disruption group, participants were also sleep-restricted to 5.6 hours scheduled TIB; however, participants maintained a semi-recumbent posture in bed under very dim (1 lux) lighting during periods of extended and monitored wakefulness. Thus, the duration of light exposure during sleep restriction was the same on all days throughout the study, minimizing circadian disruption and enabling the authors to examine the metabolic impact of sleep restriction alone. Glucose metabolism was evaluated by postprandial responses to a standardized high-carbohydrate breakfast meal at similar circadian phase in all conditions and thus in the absence of any acute circadian misalignment. Consistent with earlier findings in younger and older adults on a standardized high-carbohydrate breakfast meal response (Buxton et al., 2012), exposure to sleep restriction combined with prior history of circadian disruption elevated postprandial glucose levels and reduced insulin levels. In contrast, when extended exposure to artificial light at night was minimized, no significant effects on postprandial glucose and insulin were observed following 3 weeks of exposure to sleep restriction alone. Indeed, more recent findings suggest that light at night may be a risk factor for cardiometabolic disease independent of sleep loss (Mason et al., 2022), further highlighting the importance of accounting for inadvertent circadian disruption by ALAN when assessing the metabolic effects of sleep restriction (Figure 9.5).

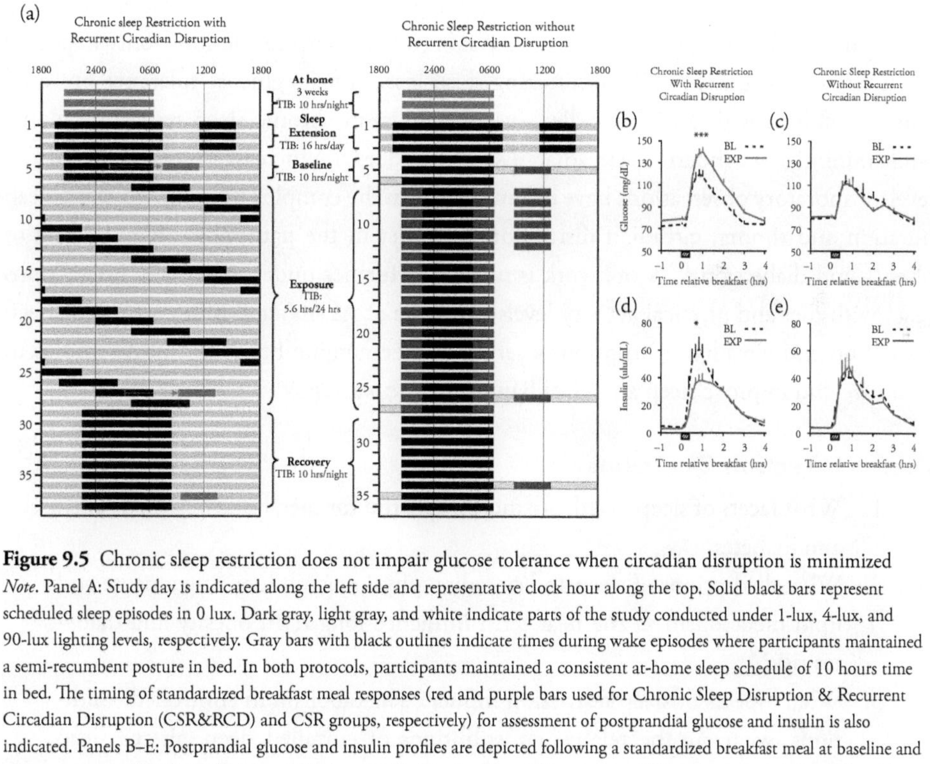

Figure 9.5 Chronic sleep restriction does not impair glucose tolerance when circadian disruption is minimized
Note. Panel A: Study day is indicated along the left side and representative clock hour along the top. Solid black bars represent scheduled sleep episodes in 0 lux. Dark gray, light gray, and white indicate parts of the study conducted under 1-lux, 4-lux, and 90-lux lighting levels, respectively. Gray bars with black outlines indicate times during wake episodes where participants maintained a semi-recumbent posture in bed. In both protocols, participants maintained a consistent at-home sleep schedule of 10 hours time in bed. The timing of standardized breakfast meal responses (red and purple bars used for Chronic Sleep Disruption & Recurrent Circadian Disruption (CSR&RCD) and CSR groups, respectively) for assessment of postprandial glucose and insulin is also indicated. Panels B–E: Postprandial glucose and insulin profiles are depicted following a standardized breakfast meal at baseline and after exposure to CSR&RCD (B, D) or CSR alone (C, E). BL = baseline; EXP = exposure; TIB = time in bed. Adapted from Yuan et al. (2021).

Conclusion

In this chapter we reviewed the epidemiology of sleep deficiency and circadian disruption as risk factors for obesity and diabetes. Epidemiologic evidence supports the association of sleep deficiency and circadian disruption with weight gain, obesity, and diabetes risk. Additional evidence links sleep deficiency and circadian disruption with dyslipidemia. Varied experimental, laboratory-based evidence from controlled studies examining the effects of sleep deficiency and circadian disruption on metabolism informs our understanding of the physiological mechanisms of these population-level findings. Sleep restriction, from several days to a week in duration, impairs glucose metabolism. More than 2 days of recovery sleep is necessary to restore baseline (well-rested) levels of function. Under conditions of sleep restriction symmetrically around the midpoint of habitual sleep (attempting to minimize changes in circadian phase), the extent of observed circadian misalignment is associated with the degree of impaired insulin sensitivity. Acute circadian misalignment influences metabolism including postprandial glucose and insulin responses that exhibit diurnal variation. Semi-chronic sleep restriction combined with abrupt and repeated circadian misalignment (e.g., a forced-desynchrony protocol) negatively impacts glucose metabolism by increasing postprandial glucose levels due to a reduction in insulin secretion, not changes in insulin sensitivity as seen with sleep restriction alone. Exposure to circadian disruption, while minimizing sleep loss, impairs glucose tolerance but only when combined with a high-fat diet. In contrast, semi-chronic sleep restriction alone, while minimizing concurrent circadian disruption, does not increase postprandial glucose levels. Laboratory observations have begun to inform the complex interplay between sleep duration and timing, circadian disruption, and diet in the pathophysiology leading to obesity and diabetes risk. More work is needed to further understand these interactions (e.g., with diet and physical activity levels), the role of ALAN, and other aspects of sleep restriction and circadian disruption observed in free-ranging humans. Future studies to prioritize and improve sleep and circadian health are warranted.

Future Direction Questions

1. What facets of sleep health are most impactful for metabolic health, obesity, and diabetes?
2. What disruptions of sleep and circadian physiology influencing glucose and lipid metabolism in the near term influence long-term obesity and diabetes risk?
3. What aspects of sleep restriction influence metabolism in controlled conditions; what are the relative contributions of curtailed sleep, altered sleep architecture, ALAN, and/or circadian disruption?
4. What aspects of sleep restriction influence metabolism in real-world conditions; what are the relative contributions of curtailed sleep, altered sleep

architecture, ALAN, and/or circadian disruption, as well as changes in other health behaviors such as diet or physical activity and sedentary behavior?

5. Moving beyond "just do it" or "go to sleep," what are the crucial elements of behavioral change interventions to optimize sleep health and thereby improve metabolic health?

References

Aho, V., Ollila, H. M., Kronholm, E., Bondia-Pons, I., Soininen, P., Kangas, A. J., Hilvo, M., Seppälä, I., Kettunen, J., Oikonen, M., Raitoharju, E., Hyötyläinen, T., Kähönen, M., Viikari, J. S. A., Härmä, M., Sallinen, M., Olkkonen, V. M., Alenius, H., Jauhiainen, M., . . . Porkka-Heiskanen, T. (2016). Prolonged sleep restriction induces changes in pathways involved in cholesterol metabolism and inflammatory responses. *Scientific Reports, 6*, Article 24828. https://doi.org/10.1038/srep24828

American Diabetes Association. (2022). *Statistics about diabetes*. Retrieved September 28, 2022, from https://diabetes.org/about-us/statistics/about-diabetes

Arble, D. M., Bass, J., Laposky, A. D., Vitaterna, M. H., & Turek, F. W. (2009). Circadian timing of food intake contributes to weight gain. *Obesity, 17*(11), 2100–2102. http://www.ncbi.nlm.nih.gov/pubmed/19730426?dopt=Citation

Brooks Holliday, S., Dong, L., Haas, A., Ghosh-Dastidar, M. B., Dubowitz, T., Buysse, D. J., Hale, L., & Troxel, W. M. (2022). Longitudinal associations between sleep and BMI in a low-income, predominantly Black American sample. *Sleep Health, 9*(1), 11–17. https://doi.org/10.1016/j.sleh.2022.10.012

Broussard, J. L., Wroblewski, K., Kilkus, J. M., & Tasali, E. (2016). Two nights of recovery sleep reverses the effects of short-term sleep restriction on diabetes risk. *Diabetes Care, 39*(3), e40–e41. https://doi.org/10.2337/dc15-2214

Buxton, O. M., Cain, S. W., O'Connor, S. P., Porter, J. H., Duffy, J. F., Wang, W., Czeisler, C. A., & Shea, S. A. (2012). Adverse metabolic consequences in humans of prolonged sleep restriction combined with circadian disruption. *Science Translational Medicine, 4*(129), Article 129ra143. https://doi.org/10.1126/scitranslmed.3003200

Buxton, O. M., Pavlova, M., Reid, E. W., Wang, W., Simonson, D. C., & Adler, G. K. (2010). Sleep restriction for 1 week reduces insulin sensitivity in healthy men. *Diabetes, 59*(9), 2126–2133. https://doi.org/10.2337/db09-0699

Centers for Disease Control and Prevention. (2022a). *Adult obesity facts*. Retrieved September 28, 2022, from https://www.cdc.gov/obesity/data/adult.html

Centers for Disease Control and Prevention. (2022b). *Diabetes risk factors*. Retrieved September 28, 2022, from https://www.cdc.gov/diabetes/basics/risk-factors.html

Centers for Disease Control and Prevention. (2023). *About overweight & obesity*. Retrieved March 24, 2023, from https://www.cdc.gov/obesity/about-obesity/index.html

Chellappa, S. L., Qian, J., Vujovic, N., Morris, C. J., Nedeltcheva, A., Nguyen, H., Rahman, N., Heng, S. W., Kelly, L., Kerlin-Monteiro, K., Srivastav, S., Wang, W., Aeschbach, D., Czeisler, C. A., Shea, S. A., Adler, G. K., Garaulet, M., & Scheer, F. (2021). Daytime eating prevents internal circadian misalignment and glucose intolerance in night work. *Science Advances, 7*(49), Article eabg9910. https://doi.org/10.1126/sciadv.abg9910

Dal Canto, E., Ceriello, A., Ryden, L., Ferrini, M., Hansen, T. B., Schnell, O., Standl, E., & Beulens, J. W. (2019). Diabetes as a cardiovascular risk factor: An overview of global trends of macro and micro vascular complications. *European Journal of Preventive Cardiology, 26*(S2), 25–32. https://doi.org/10.1177/2047487319878371

Davies, M. J., Aroda, V. R., Collins, B. S., Gabbay, R. A., Green, J., Maruthur, N. M., Rosas, S. E., Del Prato, S., Mathieu, C., Mingrone, G., Rossing, P., Tankova, T., Tsapas, A., & Buse, J. B. (2022). Management of hyperglycemia in Type 2 diabetes, 2022. A consensus report by the American Diabetes Association (ADA) and the European Association for the Study of Diabetes (EASD). *Diabetes Care, 45*(11), 2753–2786. https://doi.org/10.2337/dci22-0034

Depner, C. M., Melanson, E. L., Eckel, R. H., Snell-Bergeon, J. K., Perreault, L., Bergman, B. C., Higgins, J., Guerin, M. K., Stothard, E. R., Morton, S. J., & Wright, K. P., Jr. (2019). Ad libitum weekend recovery sleep fails to prevent metabolic dysregulation during a repeating pattern of insufficient sleep and weekend recovery sleep. *Current Biology, 29*(6), 957–967.e4. https://doi.org/10.1016/j.cub.2019.01.069

Depner, C. M., Melanson, E. L., McHill, A. W., & Wright, K. P., Jr. (2018). Mistimed food intake and sleep alters 24-hour time-of-day patterns of the human plasma proteome. *Proceedings of the National Academy of Sciences of the United States of America, 115*(23), E5390–E5399. https://doi.org/10.1073/pnas.1714813115

Eckel, R. H., Depner, C. M., Perreault, L., Markwald, R. R., Smith, M. R., McHill, A. W., Higgins, J., Melanson, E. L., & Wright, K. P., Jr. (2015). Morning circadian misalignment during short sleep duration impacts insulin sensitivity. *Current Biology, 25*(22), 3004–3010. https://doi.org/10.1016/j.cub.2015.10.011

Espitia-Bautista, E., Velasco-Ramos, M., Osnaya-Ramirez, I., Angeles-Castellanos, M., Buijs, R. M., & Escobar, C. (2017). Social jet-lag potentiates obesity and metabolic syndrome when combined with cafeteria diet in rats. *Metabolism, 72*, 83–93. https://doi.org/10.1016/j.metabol.2017.04.006

Gao, Y., Gan, T., Jiang, L., Yu, L., Tang, D., Wang, Y., Li, X., & Ding, G. (2020). Association between shift work and risk of Type 2 diabetes mellitus: A systematic review and dose–response meta-analysis of observational studies. *Chronobiology International, 37*(1), 29–46. https://doi.org/10.1080/07420528.2019.1683570

Guimaraes, K. C., Silva, C. M., Latorraca, C. O. C., Oliveira, R. A., & Crispim, C. A. (2022). Is self-reported short sleep duration associated with obesity? A systematic review and meta-analysis of cohort studies. *Nutrition Reviews, 80*(5), 983–1000. https://doi.org/10.1093/nutrit/nuab064

Hales, C. M., Carroll, M. D., Fryar, C. D., & Ogden, C. L. (2017). *Prevalence of obesity among adults and youth: United States, 2015–2016* (NCHS Data Brief No. 288). National Center for Health Statistics. https://www.ncbi.nlm.nih.gov/pubmed/29155689

Kim, J.-Y., Yadav, D., Ahn, S. V., Koh, S.-B., Park, J. T., Yoon, J., Yoo, B.-S., & Lee, S. H. (2015). A prospective study of total sleep duration and incident metabolic syndrome: The ARIRANG study. *Sleep Medicine, 16*(12), 1511–1515. https://doi.org/10.1016/j.sleep.2015.06.024

Kim, S. M., Neuendorff, N., Alaniz, R. C., Sun, Y., Chapkin, R. S., & Earnest, D. J. (2018). Shift work cycle-induced alterations of circadian rhythms potentiate the effects of high-fat diet on inflammation and metabolism. *FASEB Journal, 32*(6), 3085–3095. https://doi.org/10.1096/fj.201700784R

Kinuhata, S., Hayashi, T., Sato, K. K., Uehara, S., Oue, K., Endo, G., Kambe, H., & Fukuda, K. (2014). Sleep duration and the risk of future lipid profile abnormalities in middle-aged men: The Kansai Healthcare Study. *Sleep Medicine, 15*(11), 1379–1385. https://doi.org/10.1016/j.sleep.2014.06.011

Kohsaka, A., Laposky, A. D., Ramsey, K. M., Estrada, C., Joshu, C., Kobayashi, Y., Turek, F. W., & Bass, J. (2007). High-fat diet disrupts behavioral and molecular circadian rhythms in mice. *Cell Metabolism, 6*(5), 414–421. https://doi.org/10.1016/j.cmet.2007.09.006

Kruisbrink, M., Robertson, W., Ji, C., Miller, M. A., Geleijnse, J. M., & Cappuccio, F. P. (2017). Association of sleep duration and quality with blood lipids: A systematic review and meta-analysis of prospective studies. *BMJ Open, 7*(12), Article e018585. https://doi.org/10.1136/bmjopen-2017-018585

Lai, K. Y., Sarkar, C., Ni, M. Y., Gallacher, J., & Webster, C. (2020). Exposure to light at night (LAN) and risk of obesity: A systematic review and meta-analysis of observational studies. *Environmental Research, 187*, Article 109637. https://doi.org/10.1016/j.envres.2020.109637

Leproult, R., Holmback, U., & Van Cauter, E. (2014). Circadian misalignment augments markers of insulin resistance and inflammation, independently of sleep loss. *Diabetes, 63*(6), 1860–1869. https://doi.org/10.2337/db13-1546

Lloyd-Jones, D. M., Allen, N. B., Anderson, C. A. M., Black, T., Brewer, L. C., Foraker, R. E., Grandner, M. A., Lavretsky, H., Perak, A. M., Sharma, G., & Rosamond, W.; American Heart Association. (2022). Life's essential 8: Updating and enhancing the American Heart Association's construct of cardiovascular health: A presidential advisory from the American Heart Association. *Circulation, 146*(5), Article 101161CIR0000000000001078. https://doi.org/10.1161/CIR.0000000000001078

Lorenzo, C., Wagenknecht, L. E., Rewers, M. J., Karter, A. J., Bergman, R. N., Hanley, A. J., & Haffner, S. M. (2010). Disposition index, glucose effectiveness, and conversion to Type 2 diabetes: The Insulin Resistance Atherosclerosis Study (IRAS). *Diabetes Care, 33*(9), 2098–2103. https://doi.org/10.2337/dc10-0165

Lu, H., Yang, Q., Tian, F., Lyu, Y., He, H., Xin, X., & Zheng, X. (2021). A meta-analysis of a cohort study on the association between sleep duration and Type 2 diabetes mellitus. *Journal of Diabetes Research, 2021*, Article 8861038. https://doi.org/10.1155/2021/8861038

Mason, I. C., Grimaldi, D., Reid, K. J., Warlick, C. D., Malkani, R. G., Abbott, S. M., & Zee, P. C. (2022). Light exposure during sleep impairs cardiometabolic function. *Proceedings of the National Academy of Sciences of the United States of America, 119*(12), Article e2113290119. https://doi.org/10.1073/pnas.2113290119

Miller, M. A., Bates, S., Ji, C., & Cappuccio, F. P. (2021). Systematic review and meta-analyses of the relationship between short sleep and incidence of obesity and effectiveness of sleep interventions on weight gain in preschool children. *Obesity Reviews, 22*(2), Article e13113. https://doi.org/10.1111/obr.13113

Morris, C. J., Yang, J. N., Garcia, J. I., Myers, S., Bozzi, I., Wang, W., Buxton, O. M., Shea, S. A., & Scheer, F. A. (2015). Endogenous circadian system and circadian misalignment impact glucose tolerance via separate mechanisms in humans. *Proceedings of the National Academy of Sciences of the United States of America, 112*(17), E2225–E2234. https://doi.org/10.1073/pnas.1418955112

Mostafa, S. A., Mena, S. C., Antza, C., Balanos, G., Nirantharakumar, K., & Tahrani, A. A. (2022). Sleep behaviours and associated habits and the progression of pre-diabetes to Type 2 diabetes mellitus in adults: A systematic review and meta-analysis. *Diabetes & Vascular Disease Research, 19*(3), Article 14791641221088824. https://doi.org/10.1177/14791641221088824

Nedeltcheva, A. V., Kessler, L., Imperial, J., & Penev, P. D. (2009). Exposure to recurrent sleep restriction in the setting of high caloric intake and physical inactivity results in increased insulin resistance and reduced glucose tolerance. *The Journal of Clinical Endocrinology and Metabolism, 94*(9), 3242–3250. http://www.ncbi.nlm.nih.gov/pubmed/19567526?dopt=Citation

Ness, K. M., Strayer, S. M., Nahmod, N. G., Chang, A.-M., Buxton, O. M., & Shearer, G. C. (2019). Two nights of recovery sleep restores the dynamic lipemic response, but not the reduction of insulin sensitivity, induced by five nights of sleep restriction. *American Journal of Physiology: Regulatory, Integrative and Comparative Physiology, 316*(6), R697–R703. https://doi.org/10.1152/ajpregu.00336.2018

Ness, K. M., Strayer, S. M., Nahmod, N. G., Schade, M. M., Chang, A.-M., Shearer, G. C., & Buxton, O. M. (2019). Four nights of sleep restriction suppress the postprandial lipemic response and decrease satiety. *Journal of Lipid Research, 60*(11), 1935–1945. https://doi.org/10.1194/jlr.P094375

Phillips, A. J. K., Vidafar, P., Burns, A. C., McGlashan, E. M., Anderson, C., Rajaratnam, S. M. W., Lockley, S. W., & Cain, S. W. (2019). High sensitivity and interindividual variability in the response of the human circadian system to evening light. *Proceedings of the National Academy of Sciences of the United States of America, 116*(24), 12019–12024. https://doi.org/10.1073/pnas.1901824116

Ruan, H., Xun, P., Cai, W., He, K., & Tang, Q. (2015). Habitual sleep duration and risk of childhood obesity: Systematic review and dose–response meta-analysis of prospective cohort studies. *Scientific Reports, 5*, Article 16160. https://doi.org/10.1038/srep16160

Schmid, S. M., Hallschmid, M., Jauch-Chara, K., Wilms, B., Lehnert, H., Born, J., & Schultes, B. (2011). Disturbed glucoregulatory response to food intake after moderate sleep restriction. *Sleep, 34*(3), 371–377. http://www.ncbi.nlm.nih.gov/pubmed/21358855?dopt=Citation

Shan, Z., Ma, H., Xie, M., Yan, P., Guo, Y., Bao, W., Rong, Y., Jackson, C. L., Hu, F. B., & Liu, L. (2015). Sleep duration and risk of Type 2 diabetes: A meta-analysis of prospective studies. *Diabetes Care, 38*(3), 529–537. https://doi.org/10.2337/dc14-2073

Simon, S. L., McWhirter, L., Diniz Behn, C., Bubar, K. M., Kaar, J. L., Pyle, L., Rahat, H., Garcia-Reyes, Y., Carreau, A.-M., Wright, K. P., Jr., Nadeau, K. J., & Cree-Green, M. (2019). Morning circadian misalignment is associated with insulin resistance in girls with obesity and polycystic ovarian syndrome. *The Journal of Clinical Endocrinology and Metabolism, 104*(8), 3525–3534. https://doi.org/10.1210/jc.2018-02385

Spiegel, K., Knutson, K., Leproult, R., Tasali, E., & Van Cauter, E. (2005). Sleep loss: A novel risk factor for insulin resistance and Type 2 diabetes. *Journal of Applied Physiology, 99*(5), 2008–2019. https://doi.org/10.1152/japplphysiol.00660.2005

Spiegel, K., Leproult, R., & Van Cauter, E. (1999). Impact of sleep debt on metabolic and endocrine function. *Lancet, 354*, 1435–1439.

World Health Organization. (2021). *Obesity and overweight.* Retrieved September 28, 2022, from https://www.who.int/news-room/fact-sheets/detail/obesity-and-overweight

World Health Organization. (2022). *Diabetes.* Retrieved September 28, 2022, from https://www.who.int/news-room/fact-sheets/detail/diabetes

Yuan, R. K., Zitting, K. M., Duffy, J. F., Vujovic, N., Wang, W., Quan, S. F., Klerman, E. B., Scheer, F. A. J. L., Buxton, O. M., Williams, J. S., & Czeisler, C. A. (2021). Chronic sleep restriction while minimizing circadian disruption does not adversely affect glucose tolerance. *Frontiers in Physiology, 12,* Article 764737. https://doi.org/10.3389/fphys.2021.764737

Zitting, K. M., Vetrivelan, R., Yuan, R. K., Vujovic, N., Wang, W., Bandaru, S. S., Quan, S. F., Klerman, E. B., Scheer, F. A. J. L., Buxton, O. M., Williams, J. S., Duffy, J. F., Saper, C. B., & Czeisler, C. A. (2022). Chronic circadian disruption on a high-fat diet impairs glucose tolerance. *Metabolism: Clinical and Experimental, 130,* Article 155158. https://doi.org/10.1016/j.metabol.2022.155158

CHAPTER

10 Sleep, Neurocognitive Function, Learning, and Memory

Daniel Baena, Alyssa Pozzobon, Joel Hordijk, Laura B. Ray, *and* Stuart M. Fogel

Abstract

Sleep has been shown to play a central role in the optimal consolidation of memory and maintenance of neurocognitive function. This chapter first provides a comprehensive review of the various sleep-specific electrophysiological markers related to learning and memory consolidation. Second, accumulating evidence for the role of sleep in declarative memory consolidation will be discussed, differentiating between the contribution of slow wave–spindle–ripple coupling during non-rapid-eye-movement (NREM) sleep and the specific contribution of rapid-eye-movement (REM) sleep in memory consolidation. Third, the authors explore the contribution of sleep in cognitively simple motor procedural memories, suggesting that NREM sleep and, critically, sleep spindles play a central role in this process. Finally, the specific case of cognitively complex procedural memory consolidation will be considered, suggesting that, as compared to the case of simple procedural memories, REM sleep may be involved when the task demands are more challenging and cognitively complex (e.g., new rules, novel strategies, problem-solving skills), whereas spindles are involved when the task requires well-established skills (e.g., cognitively simple motor skills).

Key Words: sleep, memory, consolidation, EEG, fMRI, slow-wave sleep, spindle, slow wave, ripple

Introduction

What is the relationship between sleep and cognition? Do our brains continue to process newly acquired information while we are asleep? Do we need sleep to remember and, perhaps, to forget? While it is obvious that sleep is good for our bodies and minds, the precise nature, variety, extent, and mechanisms of memory processing during sleep continues to be the subject of rigorous scientific investigation. This chapter will highlight evidence supporting a role for sleep in learning and memory and summarizing evidence which shows that sleep is an essential component in maintaining good cognitive health.

Origins of Sleep and Memory Research

The earliest laboratory demonstration of the involvement of sleep in remembering was shown by Ebbinghaus (1885/2013). In his now famous "forgetting curve" study,

Ebbinghaus performed a series of memory experiments on himself and showed that the rate of forgetting information over time is slowed over a period of sleep. However, Ebbinghaus himself rejected this notion and attributed his findings to anomalies in his experiments. In 1924, Jenkins and Dallenbach directly tested the hypothesis that memory decays at a slower rate over a period of sleep compared to a period of wakefulness and attributed these findings to a lack of sensory interference during the unconscious state. As research techniques became more sophisticated, in particular with the advent of polysomnography to measure and define the different stages of sleep (Aserinsky & Kleitman, 1953) as well as the identification of encephalographic (EEG) patterns representing brain processes unique to sleep (Loomis et al., 1937), modern studies began to focus on differences between rapid-eye-movement (REM) sleep and non-rapid-eye-movement (NREM) sleep, including the different types of memory supported by each sleep state as well as the brain mechanisms underlying these processes. The following section briefly describes the most common EEG markers associated with sleep, which are theorized to support learning and memory.

Electrophysiological Markers of Neurocognitive Function

There are a number of sleep-specific electrophysiological markers of learning, memory, and cognitive abilities, including spindles, slow waves (SWs), hippocampal ripples, and rapid eye movements (REMs).

Sleep Spindles

Sleep spindles are characteristic features of NREM sleep. They are short-duration (~0.5–3 seconds), waxing and waning oscillations in the sigma (σ) range (~11–16 Hz), whose maximal amplitude is typically found over central regions (De Gennaro et al., 2000; McCormick et al., 1997). Behavioral, electrophysiological (Gennaro & Ferrara, 2003), and neuroimaging (Schabus et al., 2007) data further suggest a functional differentiation and distinct neuroanatomical substrates for slow (~11–13.5 Hz) and fast (~13.5–16 Hz) spindles. Slow spindles are typically distributed over frontal sites, and fast spindles typically have a posterior distribution (De Gennaro et al., 2000). Sleep spindles are thought to be generated by communication between the thalamus and the neocortex and are a result of the synaptic interactions between thalamocortical neurons and rhythmic depolarization (Steriade, 1995), modulated by gamma-aminobutyric acid–ergic pathways (Bazhenov et al., 1999, 2000), although Bonjean and colleagues (2011) provide compelling evidence suggesting that spindles are actually initiated in the neocortex.

Spindles are considered to serve three main (known) functions: (1) memory consolidation (for reviews, see Fogel & Smith, 2011; Rasch & Born, 2013), (2) sleep maintenance and protection (Dang-Vu et al., 2010; Elton et al., 1997; A. Kim et al., 2012; Lecci et al., 2017), and (3) support of cognitive abilities (Fang et al., 2017, 2019; Fogel & Smith, 2011; Gais et al., 2002; Ujma et al., 2014).

SWs

SWs are characteristic features of NREM Stage 3 (NREM3) sleep (i.e., "deep sleep" or SW sleep [SWS]). SWs have frequencies of ~0.5–2.0 Hz with large peak-to-peak amplitudes of >75 μV (Amzica & Steriade, 1998). SWs are thought to reflect the large-scale synchronous firing of cortical neurons, originating from the thalamus (Steriade, 2006). More specifically, the oscillations appear between the "up"-state (depolarizing and generating action potentials) and "down"-state (hyperpolarizing and terminating action potentials; for a review, see Contreras & Steriade, 1995). Another sleep parameter related to SWs is slow-wave activity (SWA), defined as the EEG spectral power at ~0.5–4.0 Hz. SWA is used as a quantitative measure of NREM sleep dynamics and an indicator of sleep depth (Borb & Achermann, 1999).

SWA has been implicated in a great variety of functions that sleep supports (covered throughout the other chapters in this section). In terms of neurocognitive function, SWs and SWA are important for memory consolidation (for a review, see Rasch & Born, 2013), daytime cognitive performance (Aeschbach et al., 2008; Landsness et al., 2009), and sleep-dependent synaptic homeostasis (Tononi & Cirelli, 2006, 2014). In addition, SWs predominate as the sleep stage most resilient to environmental interference (Buxton et al., 2012; Dijk, 2009; Ferrara et al., 1999), thus providing a state where processes can transpire uninterrupted and be internally focused.

Ripples

Hippocampal sharp-wave ripple, or "ripples," 100–200 Hz oscillations, lasting 40–100 ms, are generated in the hippocampus (Buzsaki, 2015) and typically occur during "offline" brain states. Ripples are believed to reflect hippocampal–neocortical communication and occur in-phase together with sleep spindles and SW up-states (Siapas & Wilson, 1998) in humans (Bragin et al., 1999; Le Van Quyen et al., 2010) and animals (Buzaki et al., 1996; Sirota et al., 2003).

Hippocampal ripples have been shown to play a role in memory consolidation during sleep via the process of neuronal replay (Ego-Stengel & Wilson, 2010; Girardeau et al., 2009) and spatial navigation during wakefulness (Jadhav et al., 2012). To date, the relationship between ripples occurring during sleep and those appearing during the awake state remains unclear. Suppression of awake ripples and associated replay has been shown to leave sleep replay unaffected (Jadhav et al., 2012), suggesting a complementary mechanism to bridge the gap between sequences established during behavior and those consolidated during sleep.

REMs

REMs are characteristic features of REM sleep. REMs appear on the electro-oculogram as conjugate, high-amplitude, sharply peaked, horizontal eye movements. The ponto-geniculate-occipital (PGO) circuitry is involved in the generation of REMs (Morrison &

Bowker, 1975). Until only recently, human PGO activity was only presumed to underlie REM activity as PGO activity is predominantly subcortical and not detectable with superficial EEG recordings. However, recent evidence from deep brain recordings in epileptic patients and neuroimaging studies has confirmed REM-PGO activity in humans (Fernández-Mendoza et al., 2009; Peigneux et al., 2001).

REMs are important markers of memory consolidation (for reviews, see Rasch & Born, 2013; Siegel, 2001; Vertes et al., 2000), and there is some evidence suggesting REMs may also support certain intellectual abilities (Fogel, Nader, et al., 2007; Fogel & Smith, 2011; Lafortune et al., 2014); more recently, REMs have been found to be associated with increased theta activity over the course of natural language learning (Thompson et al., 2021), suggesting that REMs may be a marker of underlying neural oscillations involved in REM-related memory processing.

Sleep and Memory Consolidation

Modern studies of sleep and memory have largely sought to delineate specific types of memory and their relationship to the different sleep stages and related brain activity. While there is evidence to suggest that memory is processed in some sort of sequential manner, involving several distinct stages of sleep (Giuditta, 2014; Redondo & Morris, 2011), the distinct brain states and processes unique to each stage of sleep support cognition in dissociable ways. For example, it has been traditionally thought that memory for places and objects is supported primarily by NREM sleep, whereas REM sleep primarily supports consolidation of motor memory for procedures, as well as emotional processing. However, recent studies challenge this differentiation between NREM and REM sleep, proposing a complementary function between the two stages to optimize memory consolidation, especially in complex problem-solving skills (Fogel et al., 2015; Lewis et al., 2018; T. A. Nielsen et al., 2015). The following sections describe current knowledge relating different types of memory with sleep and sleep-related brain activity.

Declarative Memory

Declarative memory is the "what" of long-term memory, as opposed to knowing "how." Declarative memory is comprised of events and facts that are usually explicitly known (i.e., freely accessible to conscious knowledge; Cohen et al., 1985; Moscovitch et al., 2006; Nadel & Moscovitch, 1997; Squire, 1992; Squire & Zola-Morgan, 1996). Declarative memory is normally acquired through rehearsal and rote memorization (Graf et al., 1984; Moscovitch et al., 1986). Traditionally, declarative memory has been subdivided into episodic memory (e.g., autobiographical events associated with a specific spatiotemporal context) and semantic memory (e.g., precise details and information about objects, facts, and figures, independent of context; Squire & Zola-Morgan, 1996; Tulving, 1985). Declarative learning is dependent on the hippocampus and is impaired in patients with medial temporal lobe damage (Scoville & Milner, 1957; Warrington, 1996), especially when those memories are in the recent past (Winocur & Moscovitch, 2011).

New memory traces initially exist in a labile state, and following long periods of post-acquisition time (ranging anywhere from hours to years), that memory changes via consolidation into a state that is stable, lasting, integrated, and more easily retrieved (Haist et al., 2001; J. J. Kim & Fanselow, 1992; Scoville & Milner, 1957; Zola-Morgan et al., 1992). The hippocampus and thalamus are the brain structures thought to be primarily involved in the declarative memory consolidation process. During declarative memory consolidation, the involvement of the hippocampus and/or thalamus is gradually reduced until the memory is stored in the neocortex (Dudai & Eisenberg, 2004; Frankland et al., 2004). The hippocampus is generally thought to be less involved in recalling/recollecting the memory as time passes (Frankland & Bontempi, 2005; Winocur & Moscovitch, 2011).

Although declarative memory consolidation has traditionally been thought to be dependent on NREM sleep (Fowler et al., 1973; Gais et al., 2000; Maquet, 2001; Plihal & Born, 1997; Smith, 1995; Yaroush et al., 1971), evidence also suggests REM sleep may be involved, especially when the memories are acquired in an emotional context (Gais & Born, 2004; Nishida & Walker, 2007; U. Wagner et al., 2002, 2011). Sleep thus acts differently on newly formed memories, depending on the form and context of the memory, the nature of the memory trace, and the related neurobiological substrates recruited at the time of encoding.

NREM SLEEP AND DECLARATIVE MEMORY CONSOLIDATION

NREM (i.e., NREM Stage 2 [NREM2] and SWS) sleep enhances declarative memory consolidation. This conclusion is supported by a variety of sources, including studies on sleep deprivation (Castaldo et al., 1974; Chernik, 1972; Ekstrand et al., 1971; Empson & Clarke, 1970; Lewin & Glaubman, 1975; Smith, 1993; Tilley & Empson, 1978), sleep-dependent behavioral improvements (Clemens et al., 2005; Fogel & Smith, 2006; Gais et al., 2002; Schabus et al., 2004; Tucker & Fishbein, 2008; Tucker et al., 2006), sleep recording techniques (Gais et al., 2002, 2007; Jegou et al., 2019; Ruch et al., 2012; Schabus et al., 2004), and targeted memory reactivation (TMR) studies (Cairney et al., 2014; Fuentemilla et al., 2013; Lehmann, Schreiner, et al., 2016; Rasch et al., 2007; van Dongen et al., 2012; Wang et al., 2018).

For example, after semantically associating and memorizing new word pairs (i.e., paired associates learning), early studies demonstrated that depriving participants of REM sleep did not impair recall performance at retest (Castaldo et al., 1974; Chernik, 1972; Ekstrand et al., 1971; Empson & Clarke, 1970; Lewin & Glaubman, 1975; Smith, 1993; Tilley & Empson, 1978), suggesting that other types of sleep (e.g., NREM) may be required for optimal declarative memory consolidation. Additional support for the notion that declarative memory is enhanced following naps containing mainly NREM sleep was provided by behavioral studies using a variety of declarative learning tasks (e.g., paired associates and face-scene pairs) (Ruch et al., 2012; Schmidt et al., 2006; Tucker & Fishbein, 2008; Tucker et al., 2006). Although, these studies do not reveal what features of NREM sleep are involved in the consolidation process.

Certain EEG features of NREM sleep have since been linked to declarative memory consolidation including increases in spindle density, amplitude, and frequency (Clemens et al., 2005; Fogel, Smith, & Cote, 2007; Gais et al., 2002; Ruch et al., 2012; Schabus et al., 2004, 2006; Schmidt et al., 2006; Wolansky et al., 2006), as well as sigma power (Berner et al., 2006; Schabus et al., 2006). These changes in spindles are observed following extensive repetition of declarative memory tasks and normally as compared with a non-learning condition in both overnight and daytime (e.g., nap) sleep paradigms. The results of these studies suggest that declarative learning impacts post-learning sleep and that spindles are likely involved in consolidation processes or, at a minimum, are markers of the intensity of declarative memory consolidation that is occurring. Recently, EEG–functional magnetic resonance imaging (fMRI) studies (Bergmann et al., 2012; Jegou et al., 2019) have shown that during subsequent sleep, reactivation of the memory trace of brain regions recruited during declarative learning (e.g., the hippocampus) occurs. Importantly, these memory trace reactivations were time-locked to spindle events, providing additional support and possibly causal involvement of spindles in declarative memory consolidation, via repeated reactivation of the newly formed memory trace.

A few studies (Lau et al., 2010; Marshall et al., 2006) have suggested that SWS may also play a role in declarative memory consolidation, possibly via the action of SWs. It is known that SWs group with faster-frequency events which originate from thalamocortical circuitry (e.g., spindles; for a review, see Steriade, 2006). The functional significance of the phase–amplitude interactions for memory consolidation have recently been revealed (Bergmann & Born, 2018; Helfrich et al., 2018). Following declarative learning, SWs are coupled to spindles, suggesting that these two temporally related events may work together, whereby spindles reflect synaptic strengthening (Rosanova & Ulrich, 2005; Werk & Chapman, 2003; Werk et al., 2005) which act in coordination with SWs for synaptic downscaling (Massimini et al., 2009; Tononi, 2009; Tononi & Cirelli, 2006) to optimize declarative memory consolidation.

Hippocampal ripples have also been shown to be temporally coupled to spindle events and SWs (forming SW–spindle–ripple complexes) in rats (Siapas & Wilson, 1998; Sirota et al., 2003) and, more recently, in humans (Clemens et al., 2007, 2011; Latchoumane et al., 2017; Staresina et al., 2015). This SW–spindle–ripple coupling has been suggested as a possible mechanism for transfer of newly encoded learning from the hippocampus to the neocortex (Figure 10.1; Axmacher et al., 2006; Siapas & Wilson, 1998; Sirota et al., 2003). By using auditory or olfactory mnemonic cues during sleep, TMR studies have recently provided convincing causal evidence that sleep-dependent consolidation of declarative memories can be enhanced by externally triggering reactivation (for a review,

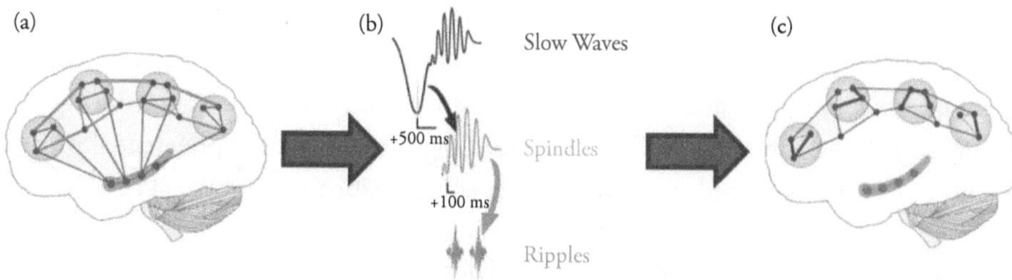

Figure 10.1 Sleep and memory consolidation
Note. Panel A: Neocortical (larger nodes) and hippocampal (smaller nodes) distribution of a newly acquired memory. Panel B: Slow-wave (SW)–spindle–ripple complexes. SWs (first waveform) set the temporal frame for memory processing during the up-state transition. The SW up-state acts on thalamic networks (indicated by the first arrow) driving spindle activity (second waveform) in thalamocortical networks (with! a peak ~500 ms after the SW down-state peak). Spindles that reach the hippocampus act on these networks (second arrow), increasing ripples (third waveform) and associated memory replay starting ~100 ms after spindle onset. Panel C: Changes in the memory trace of newly acquired memory after a period of sleep. These changes include the strengthening of corticocortical connections as well as the reduction/disappearance of hippocampal–cortical connections. Adapted from Jens G. Klinzing et al. (2019), Mechanisms of systems memory consolidation during sleep, *Nature Neuroscience*, *22*, 1598–1610, Springer Nature.

see Tambini et al., 2017). This evidence suggests that NREM sleep enhances declarative memory consolidation, resulting from communication between the hippocampal, thalamocortical, and neocortical NREM oscillations (Diekelmann & Born, 2010; Eschenko et al., 2006; Marshall & Born, 2007; Mölle et al., 2002, 2004; Nadasdy et al., 1999; Schmidt et al., 2006; Wilson & McNaughton, 1994). These coupled oscillations (ripples, spindles, and SWs) coordinate with one another in the reactivation and replay of memory traces. Animal studies suggest that this reactivation may serve to strengthen newly acquired memory traces by means of changes at the synaptic level (e.g., long-term potentiation [LTP]) and at the systems level.

Studies have also shown that artificially increasing coupling either between SWs and spindles (Ladenbauer et al., 2017; Niknazar et al., 2015; Zhang et al., 2020) or between SWs, spindles, and ripples (Latchoumane et al., 2017; Maingret et al., 2016) improves declarative memory, whereas its disruption, whether artificial (Garside et al., 2015; Novitskaya et al., 2016) or promoted by aging (Helfrich et al., 2018), the presence of any psychiatric disorder (Bartsch et al., 2019; Demanuele et al., 2017), or neurological damage (Mendes et al., 2021), has negative consequences for memory. Moreover, Helfrich and colleagues (2019) demonstrated that only SW-coupled spindles, but not isolated spindles, induce hippocampal–neocortical information transfer, implying that SW–spindle coupling may support subcortical–cortical network dialog.

Finally, recent studies have shown that TMR can trigger SW–spindle coupling, allowing successful decoding of memories (Antony et al., 2018; Cairney et al., 2018; Schönauer et al., 2017; Schönauer & Pöhlchen, 2018), supporting the notion that coupling constitutes a key mechanism for memory consolidation. In addition, the role of SW–spindle coupling in memory consolidation can change depending on initial memory encoding quality. Some studies have shown that the degree of coupling of spindles in the up-state of SW depends not only on the extent of the activation of the regions involved in the acquisition of new memories but also on the quality of the representations encoded during that learning session. In particular, SW–spindle coupling seems to have a preferential protective effect on weakly encoded memories (Baena et al., 2020; Yordanova et al., 2017).

REM SLEEP AND DECLARATIVE MEMORY CONSOLIDATION

A limited number of studies suggest there is a relationship between REM sleep and declarative memory consolidation (De Koninck et al., 1989; Fogel, Smith, & Cote, 2007; Grosmark et al., 2012). The first evidence for such a relationship was provided by De Koninck and colleagues (1989) via a series of studies investigating the sleep architecture of native English speakers during an intensive French immersion second language–learning course. Immediately preceding performance improvements, increased REM sleep was observed. This increase in REM sleep was also associated with the first occurrence of dreaming in French during REM sleep (De Koninck, 1995; De Koninck et al., 1989, 1990), suggesting that the reprocessing of newly acquired declarative learning occurs during REM sleep and that learning is also reflected in dream content. However, a recent revisitation of these data using more modern EEG techniques has taken into account the different stages of natural language acquisition and suggests that sleep spindles during NREM sleep support the early, declarative aspect of natural language acquisition, whereas REM sleep, and specifically theta activity time-locked to REMs, might be primarily involved in the consolidation of the later, procedural aspects of language acquisition (Thompson et al., 2021).

In addition, declarative information encoded by the hippocampus is reactivated via the synchronization of hippocampal theta oscillations (4–8 Hz) during REM sleep (Boyce et al., 2016; Jones & Wilson, 2005; Remondes et al., 2014; Vijayan et al., 2017). This is demonstrated by an increase in REM sleep theta power following learning in an emotional picture recognition task (Nishida et al., 2009), providing evidence that REM neural oscillations are electrophysiological markers of sleep-related declarative memory consolidation. Additionally, these oscillations may reflect a means of strengthening the memory traces during sleep (U. Wagner et al., 2011).

REM sleep also appears to play a critical role in the processing of emotionally charged declarative memories by further processing the emotional content of the memories (Marshall & Born, 2007; Moroni et al., 2008; G. Wagner et al., 2006; U. Wagner et al., 2002). Specifically, better recall of emotionally charged episodic memories is observed after a period of REM sleep but not following NREM sleep (Hu et al., 2006; Nishida et al., 2009). This may be particularly important under abnormal psychiatric conditions (e.g., post-traumatic stress disorder [PTSD]) where memory strengthening can be maladaptive or problematic. In individuals with depression, an increase in REM density and a prolonged initial REM period (Tsuno et al., 2005) have been suggested (Germain et al.,

2013; Murkar & De Koninck, 2018; Pace-Schott et al., 2015) as a mechanism resulting in dysfunction of consolidation processes, resulting in continued processing/reactivation of past negative emotional memories (Nishida et al., 2009; Tsuno et al., 2005). This could further exacerbate the clinical features of PTSD, considering that PTSD is often comorbid with depression.

SUMMARY

The benefits of sleep for declarative memory consolidation are primarily dependent on the unique EEG features which characterize different stages of sleep. Sleep spindles, which characterize NREM2 sleep, facilitate the transfer of declarative memories into long-term memories, suggesting that they support the stabilization of declarative memory (Clemens et al., 2005; Fogel, Smith, & Cote, 2007; Gais et al., 2002; Tucker & Fishbein, 2008; Tucker et al., 2006). Hippocampal ripples, thalamocortical spindles, and SWA during SWS mediate communication between subcortical structures and the neocortex, suggesting that they also play a critical role in the consolidation of declarative memory via hippocampal–neocortical transfer (Diekelmann & Born, 2010; Eschenko et al., 2006; Schmidt et al., 2006). Lastly, REM sleep appears to enhance the consolidation of emotionally charged declarative memories (Marshall & Born, 2007; G. Wagner et al., 2006; U. Wagner et al., 2002, 2011).

PROCEDURAL MEMORY

By contrast, procedural memory, or non-declarative memory, is memory for learning and knowing "how" as opposed to knowing "what." Traditionally, procedural memory has been subdivided into procedural skills and habits, classical conditioning, priming, and non-associative learning (Gabrieli, 1998; B. Milner et al., 1998; Squire & Zola-Morgan, 1998), which are usually independent of conscious retrieval. A large volume of evidence supports the notion that sleep enhances procedural memory consolidation (Albouy et al., 2015; Barakat et al., 2012; Doyon et al., 2009; Fischer et al., 2002; Fogel et al., 2015, 2017; King et al., 2013; Kuriyama et al., 2004; Laventure et al., 2016; Peters et al., 2007; Schönauer et al., 2014; Sio et al., 2013; Smith, 2001a; Smith & MacNeill, 1994; Stickgold, 2005; Vahdat et al., 2017; Vien et al., 2016; Walker et al., 2003), although various aspects of procedural memory appear to be influenced and differentiated by the various stages of sleep. Accordingly, and depending on the cognitive complexity or novelty of the task, procedural skills can be further subdivided into motor procedural skills and complex cognitive procedural skills. For example, motor skills involve the use and refinement of preexisting skills. Classic examples of such tasks include the pursuit rotor (Adams, 1952; Ammons, 1955) and the finger-tapping task (Karni et al., 1995). In contrast, procedural skills can also comprise cognitively complex procedural skills (Fogel, Smith, & Cote, 2007; Smith, 1995, 2001b) that typically (and sometimes in addition to simple motor skills) involve the acquisition of entirely new rules or strategies necessary in order to improve performance (Smith, 1995, 2001b; Smith, Aubrey, & Peters, 2004). Classic examples of such tasks include the artificial grammar task (Cleeremans & McClelland, 1991; Fischer et al., 2006), the Tower of Hanoi, and the mirror tracing task (Fogel, Smith, & Cote, 2007; Smith, 1995, 2001a; Starch, 1910). However, other terminology is also commonly used to describe the same types of tasks (Gabrieli, 1998).

In amnesia resulting from damage to the medial temporal lobe, procedural memory is largely spared. Procedural learning is dependent on a variety of structures including the striatum, cerebellum, pons, globus pallidus, and cortical regions (independent of the hippocampus; Doyon et al., 2003; Schacter, 1997). The categorization of different types of procedural memory to different brain structures suggests that there may be separate mechanisms for consolidating the various subtypes of memory.

More specifically, memory for procedural skills and habits is associated with the striatum, simple classical conditioning involves the cerebellum, priming involves the neocortex, and non-associative learning is dependent on reflex pathways (Squire & Zola-Morgan, 1998). The thalamus may play a role in earlier stages of declarative memory consolidation and has been suggested as one possible structure that may be an analog to the hippocampus (Winocur, 1985). The thalamus may also be of importance for procedural learning (Asanuma & Pavlides, 1997). Repeated trials or practiced learning is required for long-term storage of procedural memory, which mainly occurs in the neocortex. For cortical LTP to occur, this type of memory encoding requires spaced and repeated stimulation (Chapman et al., 1998; Trepel & Racine, 1998). Oscillatory firing of thalamocortical projections is involved in such spaced and repeated neocortical stimulation, which is characteristic of sleep spindles and SWs during NREM sleep (Steriade, 1999). This oscillatory activation has been implicated as one of the mechanisms for LTP (Destexhe & Sejnowski, 2001).

First proposed by Smith, Aubrey, and Peters (2004), the differentiation of procedural memory into subtypes helps to clarify some of the uncertainty in the literature concerning sleep's role in the consolidation of procedural memory. Although procedural memory consolidation has traditionally been thought to be dependent on REM sleep (Smith, Aubrey, & Peters, 2004), some evidence suggests a role for NREM sleep, whereby NREM sleep appears to benefit simple procedural memory and serves to fine-tune explicitly learned skills, especially for motor sequence learning (Fogel et al., 2015; T. A. Nielsen et al., 2015). Thus, sleep acts differently on memory consolidation, depending on the type of learning and the related neurobiological substrates recruited at the time of encoding.

Sleep and Cognitively Simple Procedural Memory Consolidation

The majority of studies demonstrating a link between sleep and procedural memory consolidation have mostly focused on learning through repetition of a cognitively simple sequence of motor skills (Maier et al., 2017; Nettersheim et al., 2015; Walker et al., 2003; Witt et al., 2010). Following motor sequence learning, early studies demonstrated that offline gains in performance were identified after an intervening period of sleep but not wake (Karni et al., 1995; Walker et al., 2002, 2003), suggesting that memory consolidation for procedural learning (i.e., newly acquired motor sequences) is sleep-dependent. However, more recent evidence suggests that when the sequence is learned without conscious awareness (i.e., implicitly), performance does not differ following a night of sleep or an equivalent period of wake (Nemeth et al., 2010; Robertson, 2009; Robertson et al., 2004; Viczko et al., 2018), suggesting that the benefit that sleep affords to motor skills occurs only if the task is learned with conscious awareness (i.e., explicitly). Evidence for this conclusion comes from sleep deprivation (Conway & Smith, 1994; Sandys-Wunsch & Smith, 1991; Smith & Fazekas, 1997; Smith & MacNeill, 1994; Tweed et al., 1999), EEG/behavioral (Karni et al., 1995; Walker, 2005; Walker et al., 2002), and TMR studies (Antony et al., 2012; Antony & Paller, 2017; Cousins et al., 2014; Diekelmann et al., 2016; Laventure et al., 2016; Schönauer et al., 2015).

NREM Sleep and Cognitively Simple Procedural Memory Consolidation

To investigate whether sleep played a role in memory consolidation and, if so, what type of sleep might be important, early studies utilized sleep deprivation paradigms. These studies found that NREM2 sleep is primarily involved in motor skill memory consolidation (Conway & Smith, 1994; Sandys-Wunsch & Smith, 1991; Smith & MacNeill, 1994; Tweed et al., 1999). For example, task performance on the pursuit rotor and finger-tapping task was unaffected following REM sleep deprivation; however, disrupting NREM2 sleep resulted in impaired performance equivalent to total sleep deprivation (Smith & Fazekas, 1997; Smith & MacNeill, 1994; Tweed et al., 1999). While these studies provided evidence that simple motor procedural memory is NREM sleep–dependent, they cannot inform what features of NREM sleep are involved in the consolidation process. EEG studies have since demonstrated that increased amount of NREM2 sleep occurs (Fogel et al., 2001; Fogel, Smith, & Cote, et al., 2007; Fogel & Smith, 2006; Mantua et al., 2016; Nader & Smith, 2001; Walker et al., 2002), suggesting an active role for NREM sleep in the consolidation of procedural memory, with sleep spindles of particular importance for motor procedural memory consolidation (Barakat et al., 2012; Fogel & Smith, 2006; Fogel, Smith, & Cote, 2007; Laventure et al., 2016; Morin et al., 2008; Nader & Smith, 2001; Nishida et al., 2016; Nishida & Walker, 2007; Schabus et al., 2006; van Schalkwijk et al., 2020). For example, compared with an equivalent period of wake, daytime naps have been shown to improve motor memory consolidation (Korman et al., 2007; C. E. Milner et al., 2006). For habitual nappers, this improvement is associated with an increase in sleep spindles (C. E. Milner et al., 2006). Additionally, the characteristics of spindles (e.g., duration, amplitude, and density) are modulated by new motor procedural learning (Fogel & Smith, 2006; Nishida & Walker, 2007; Peters et al., 2007, 2008). More recently, TMR studies have provided evidence of a causal link between sleep and memory consolidation. TMR paradigms often involve introducing auditory or odor cues during training and subsequently reintroducing the cues time-locked to specific sleep oscillations. These studies have shown that motor sequence memory consolidation is enhanced following cuing during NREM2 (Antony et al., 2012; Laventure et al., 2016; Schönauer et al., 2014) and SWS (Cousins et al., 2014; Schönauer et al., 2014) but not REM sleep (Laventure et al., 2016). For example, better task performance and more spindles were found in participants who learned a finger-tapping task in the presence of an odor and were subsequently re-exposed to the odor during NREM2 sleep, compared to participants who were not previously exposed to the odor during the task (Laventure et al., 2016). Further insights into the neural substrates supporting the sleep-dependent consolidation of motor skill memory are provided by recent fMRI studies. Specifically, during motor sequence learning the striatum and motor cortical regions are recruited (Doyon & Benali, 2005; Doyon & Ungerleider, 2002; Friederici & Ungerleider, 2005; Karni et al., 1995; Ungerleider et al., 2002), and when the motor skill memory consolidation period contains sleep (vs. wake) striatal activity is enhanced at retest (Debas et al., 2010). This increased activation has been shown to be linked to increases in spindle amplitude (Barakat et al., 2012), suggesting that sleep spindles might be actively involved in the strengthening of the memory trace. In addition, simultaneous EEG–fMRI recordings have allowed brain activations during motor sequence training and post-training sleep to be observed (Boutin et al., 2018; Fogel et al., 2017; Vahdat et al., 2017). Collectively, these studies have identified that functional connectivity, a measure of communication within neural networks recruited during training, is restored during sleep (Vahdat et al., 2017). And after a consolidation period of NREM sleep (but not wake), functional connectivity within the network of brain regions recruited at retest (i.e., the consolidated memory trace) is strengthened. Furthermore, brain regions recruited during motor skill learning, including the putamen and motor cortical regions, are reactivated during NREM sleep, time-locked to sleep spindle events (Fogel et al., 2017). Importantly, the extent of this spindle-related reactivation was correlated to the magnitude of the offline performance gains. Taken together, these studies suggest that sleep is required for optimal motor skill memory consolidation. At the behavioral and neural levels, NREM sleep and sleep spindles specifically are markers of the extent of the consolidation in terms of enhancement and transformation, with sleep spindles actively involved in this process. Evidence suggests a role for NREM2 in motor skill memory consolidation; however, a specific/distinct role for SWS remains less clear. On a perceptual, texture discrimination task, post-sleep performance improvements were hindered following SWA suppression via acoustic stimulation (Aeschbach et al., 2008), although it is not clear what aspect of the task (e.g., motor or discrimination) was impaired. Following motor skill learning, an increase in the duration of SWS has been shown (Moroni et al., 2008), although this study also included a declarative task, for which SWS has been implicated, making it difficult to discriminate between the two types of learning and/or establish a specific link between SWS and motor skill memory. Cousins and colleagues (2014) found that following auditory cuing during SWS motor sequence memory is consolidated; however, several other studies were unable to identify a role for SWS in motor learning (Diekelmann et al., 2016; Huber et al., 2004; Marshall et al., 2006). While SWS does not appear to play a critical role in the consolidation of motor skill memory, spindles during SWS have been linked to improvements in simple procedural tasks (Fogel, Smith, & Cote, 2007), suggesting that spindles are an important factor regardless of the stage of sleep during which they occur. The underlying mechanism mediating the reorganizing and strengthening of memory traces has been proposed to be related to the reactivation of recently learned memories during sleep (Born et al., 2006). Spindles appear to play a central role in this process, possibly through the transient synchronization and coordination of specialized cortical/subcortical networks (Boutin et al., 2018), via memory trace reactivation (Fogel et al., 2017) and transformation/strengthening (Debas et al., 2010; Vahdat et al., 2017). Therefore, NREM sleep and sleep spindles are a possible mechanism for the strengthening of new memory traces during sleep.

REM Sleep and Cognitively Simple Procedural Memory Consolidation

Ample evidence suggests that NREM2 sleep and spindles are actively involved in memory transformation and enhancement via the process of memory trace reactivation. By comparison, little to no evidence supports a role for REM sleep in motor memory consolidation. Specifically, performance improvements were observed on a simple procedural task only when an odor cue conditioned during training was re-presented during NREM2, but not REM, sleep (Laventure et al., 2016). In addition, suppressing REM sleep by zolpidem administration did not affect the consolidation of motor memory, despite improvements on a word-pair memory task (Mednick et al., 2013). However, several studies (Maquet et al., 2000; G. Nielsen et al., 2014; Peigneux et al., 2003; Smith, Aubrey, & Peters, 2004) have reported increases in REM sleep following learning on tasks with a motor procedural component (e.g., a probabilistic sequential finger-tapping task and the Corsi block-tapping task). However, these studies employed cognitively complex tasks which may be dependent on REM sleep as the tasks require the acquisition of a new strategy in order to improve on the task, thus suggesting that the cognitive complexity of the procedural task is a critical factor to consider. This also may be the case when the individual's initial skill level is low, and thus the task is introducing a novel (more complex) quality to the training experience (Fogel et al., 2015; Peters et al., 2007; Smith, Aubrey, & Peters, 2004).

SLEEP AND COGNITIVELY COMPLEX PROCEDURAL MEMORY

A large volume of evidence suggests that for optimal procedural memory consolidation, especially when an underlying cognitive strategy is to be learned, sleep is required (Mantua et al., 2016; Plihal & Born, 1997; Smith, 1993, 1996; Smith, Aubrey, & Peters, 2004; Smith & Smith, 2003; Smith & Wong, 1991). And the benefit that sleep affords to this cognitively complex procedural learning is specific to sleep and does not take place as a factor of the passage of time (Doyon et al., 2009; Fogel, Smith, & Cote, 2007; Kuriyama et al., 2004; G. Nielsen et al., 2014; Plihal & Born, 1997). Evidence supporting this comes from sleep deprivation (Conway & Smith, 1994; Sandys-Wunsch & Smith, 1991; Smith, 1993; Smith & MacNeill, 1994; Smith & Smith, 2003), behavioral (Buchegger et al., 1991; De Koninck & Prévost, 1991; Mantua et al., 2016; Morita et al., 2012; Peters et al., 2007; Smith, Aubrey, & Peters, 2004; Sugawara et al., 2017; van Schalkwijk et al., 2017; Verschoor & Holdstock, 1984), and a small handful of TMR studies, investigating complex grammatical rule learning (Guerrien et al., 1989; Smith & Weeden, 1990). Taken together, these studies suggest that REM sleep contributes to improvements on cognitively complex procedural tasks. There is also evidence suggesting that existing skills previously enhanced by REM sleep may be "fine-tuned" by NREM sleep (Fogel et al., 2015; G. Nielsen et al., 2014; Peters et al., 2007; Smith, Aubrey, & Peters, 2004). Therefore, REM and NREM sleep both appear to play distinctive roles in procedural memory consolidation, even though the precise behavioral and cognitive aspects as well as the neural mechanisms remain to be fully understood.

REM Sleep and Cognitively Complex Procedural Memory

Evidence supporting the role of REM sleep in the consolidation of cognitively complex procedural memory comes from REM sleep–suppression studies that either administered alcohol (Sandys-Wunsch & Smith, 1991; Smith & Smith, 2003) or selectively REM-deprived participants (Conway & Smith, 1994; Smith, 1993; Smith & MacNeill, 1994). Both methods of REM-sleep suppression led to impaired sleep-dependent consolidation of cognitively complex procedural skills. Specifically, participants performed worse on the Tower of Hanoi post-sleep when they had consumed alcohol immediately before sleep versus those who consumed alcohol early in the afternoon (which allowed enough time for the dissipation of the diminishing effects of alcohol on REM sleep to occur; Smith & Smith, 2003). These participants also had a significantly reduced number of REMs, suggesting that neural activity associated with eye movements may be involved in offline memory processing. Post-learning increases in REM sleep were observed in behavioral and physiological studies utilizing whole-night EEG monitoring following cognitively complex procedural learning (Smith, Aubrey, & Peters, 2004) and following training on a trampoline, which requires the acquisition of highly novel and complex motor skills (e.g., backflips and other complex aerial maneuvers), but not simpler, preexisting motor skills (Buchegger et al., 1991; Buchegger & Meier-Koll, 1988). By contrast, studies comparing little or no REM sleep (i.e., during daytime naps) versus an equivalent period of quiet wakefulness have shown that little or no REM sleep might stabilize, but not enhance, procedural task performance while still enhancing declarative word-pair memory (Antonenko et al., 2013; Tucker et al., 2006; van Schalkwijk et al., 2017). In addition, on the post-training night immediately prior to the acquisition of the cognitive strategy required to solve the Tower of Hanoi task, a single study found increases in frontal delta activity during REM sleep, reflecting an increase in the intensity of the REMs (Fogel et al., 2015). Increases in post-sleep memory performance for cognitive procedural tasks have repeatedly been shown following the presentation of auditory or odor cues during task training and again specifically during post-learning REM sleep (Guerrien et al., 1989; Smith & Weeden, 1990). Such an effect might result from reactivating the contextual cues involved during the consolidation process (Parker et al., 2001; Smith & Weeden, 1990) as they only occurred when auditory stimuli were time-locked to bursts of REMs during REM sleep (Mandai et al., 1989; Smith & Weeden, 1990). In humans, REMs, generated by phasic PGO activity, are difficult to non-invasively measure. However, animal studies have established that PGO wave density is associated with improved avoidance learning in rats (Datta, 2000; Datta & Maclean, 2007). Avoidance training in rodents has similarities to procedural learning in humans; thus, this has implications for non-declarative memory in humans (Datta, 2000; Datta & Maclean, 2007). In humans, REMs during REM sleep are associated with activation of the pontine tegmentum, thalamus, and putamen, thereby providing converging fMRI evidence for PGO generation of REMs (Miyauchi et al., 2009; Wehrle et al., 2007). Future simultaneous EEG–fMRI studies could provide insight into the underlying neural substrates and patterns of brain communication that occur during procedural memory consolidation for cognitively complex skills and problem-solving.

NREM Sleep and Cognitively Complex Procedural Memory

While REM sleep is required for optimal memory consolidation of cognitively complex procedural skills, a limited number of studies have recently suggested that NREM sleep may play a role as well. For example, Peters and colleagues (2007) found that an increase in REM density and post-training performance improvements were correlated in a low-skill group but not in a high-skill group. On the other hand, the increase in spindle density and post-training performance improvements were correlated in a high-skill group but not in a low-skill group (Peters et al., 2007), suggesting that spindles are involved in memory consolidation when the task requires well-established skills, whereas REM sleep may be involved when the task demands are more challenging/complex. Recently, Fogel and colleagues (2015) found that an increase in REM sleep occurred immediately prior to the acquisition of a cognitive strategy, whereas increases in NREM2 sleep and sleep spindles were found following mastery of the task (once they were well learned). Thus, REM sleep may be involved in the consolidation of cognitively complex and novel rule learning, whereas NREM sleep may be involved in the refinement of preexisting/well-learned skills. While evidence from TMR studies exists supporting the role of REM sleep in cognitively complex motor procedural skills, no changes in post-sleep procedural memory performance were observed following reactivation targeting SWS (Rasch et al., 2007). Following reactivation targeting NREM2 using a similar odor-cuing paradigm, enhancement of motor skills was observed (Laventure et al., 2016), and this enhancement was associated with sleep spindles.

SUMMARY

The benefits of sleep for procedural memory consolidation depend on both the cognitive complexity or novelty of the task and the unique EEG features which characterize the different stages of sleep. NREM sleep and sleep spindles appear to play a central role in the consolidation of preexisting cognitively simple procedural skills, possibly through the transient synchronization and coordination of specialized cortical/subcortical networks (Boutin et al., 2018), memory trace reactivation (Fogel et al., 2017), and transformation/strengthening of the memory trace (Debas et al., 2010; Vahdat et al., 2017). However, little to no consistent evidence supports a role for REM sleep in this type of memory. However, REM is necessary for the consolidation of newly acquired, cognitively complex procedural skills and strategies, whereas NREM2 sleep and sleep spindles are necessary for the refinement of existing skills (Fogel et al., 2015; G. Nielsen et al., 2014; Peters et al., 2007; Smith, Aubrey, & Peters, 2004; van den Berg et al., 2019). The relationship between various sleep stages and their respective sleep EEG features with different types of memory consolidation are summarized in Table 10.1.

Conclusions and Future Directions

It has been a century since modern scientific research formally pursued the hypothesis that sleep benefits cognition. Great strides have been made with the use of refined experimental paradigms, the identification of sleep-dependent neurophysiological events such as spindles, the development of technologies such as simultaneous EEG and fMRI recording, causal evidence in humans from TMR paradigms, longitudinal and/or large-sample studies, and significant technological advancements (e.g., brain imaging, sophisticated EEG techniques, brain stimulation techniques, computerized behavioral and cognitive testing, etc.). Thanks to these advancements, and an accompanying development in the nature of human memory systems, instead of the initial conception of a protective/passive role, it is now widely accepted that sleep is actively involved in memory consolidation. This view is supported by studies showing that sleep in some cases is not only sufficient for memory consolidation to take place but actually necessary/critical. Studies showing reactivation of newly encoded memories and enhancement via TMR show the extent to which sleep is involved in the transformation and enhancement of newly formed memory traces, as well as actively involved in memory improvements. The pursuit of understanding the relationships between sleep-related neural events, such as SW–spindle coupling, and their relationship to different types of cognitive processes will likely continue to be a promising direction in understanding the underlying mechanisms involved in sleep-specific memory consolidation. Indeed, save for sleep-altering pharmaceuticals, there are few ways to alter the architecture, microarchitecture, and brain activity during sleep other than an intense period of learning. While sleep supports a myriad of biological, psychological, cognitive, and restorative functions, current evidence suggests that one of the primary functions of sleep is optimizing memory consolidation.

Table 10.1 Overview of the relationship between sleep electroencephalographic features and different types of memory consolidation

Memory type	Sleep stage	Sleep EEG feature	Description	References
Declarative memory	NREM		Consolidation enhanced[1] by, and thought to be dependent on, NREM,[2] later suggested that REM may be involved,[3] demonstrated by declarative learning tasks.[1,4]	[1](Cairney et al., 2014; Castaldo et al., 1974; Chernik, 1972; Ekstrand et al., 1971; Empson & Clarke, 1970; Fuentemilla et al., 2013; Gais et al., 2002, 2007; Jegou et al., 2019; Lehmann, Seifritz, & Rasch, 2016; Lewin & Glaubman, 1975; Ruch et al., 2012; Schabus et al., 2004; Smith, 1993; Tilley & Empson, 1978; van Dongen et al., 2012; Wang et al., 2018) [2](Fowler et al., 1973; Gais et al., 2000; Maquet, 2001; Plihal & Born, 1997; Smith, 1995; Yaroush et al., 1971) [3](Gais & Born, 2004; Nishida & Walker, 2007; U. Wagner et al., 2002, 2011) [4](Schmidt et al., 2006; Tucker & Fishbein, 2008; Tucker et al., 2006)
Declarative memory	NREM	Spindles, sigma power	Increased density, amplitude, and frequency,[5] as well as sigma power,[6] following declarative learning tasks.	[5](Clemens et al., 2005; Fogel, Nader, et al., 2007; Gais et al., 2002; Ruch et al., 2012; Schabus et al., 2004, 2006; Schmidt et al., 2006; Wolansky et al., 2006) [6](Berner et al., 2006; Schabus et al., 2006)
Declarative memory	NREM	SWs, spindles, SW–spindle coupling	Following declarative learning tasks, SWs are coupled to spindles, suggesting[7] SWS plays a role in optimizing consolidation through synaptic strengthening by spindles[8] and synaptic downscaling by SWs[9]	[7](Lau et al., 2010; Marshall et al., 2006) [8](Rosanova & Ulrich, 2005; Werk & Chapman, 2003; Werk et al., 2005) [9](Massimini et al., 2009; Tononi, 2009; Tononi & Cirelli, 2006)

Continued

Table 10.1 *Continued*

Memory type	Sleep stage	Sleep EEG feature	Description	References
Declarative memory	NREM	SWs, spindles, ripples, SW–spindle–ripple coupling	SW–spindle–ripple complexes have been shown in rats[10a] and humans,[10b] suggesting a possible transfer mechanism from the hippocampus to neocortex enhancing consolidation for newly encoded learning[10a,11] presented as NREM oscillations.[12]	[10a](Siapas & Wilson, 1998; Sirota et al., 2003) [10b](Clemens et al., 2007, 2011; Latchoumane et al., 2017; Staresina et al., 2015) [11](Axmacher et al., 2006) [12](Diekelmann & Born, 2010; Eschenko et al., 2006; Marshall & Born, 2007; Mölle et al., 2004; Nadasdy et al., 1999; Schmidt et al., 2006; Wilson & McNaughton, 1994)
Declarative memory	NREM	SWs, spindles, ripples SW–spindle–ripple coupling	Artificially increasing SWs, spindles,[13] and ripples[14] improves declarative memory. TMR studies[15] provide further support.	[13](Ladenbauer et al., 2017; Niknazar et al., 2015; Zhang et al., 2020) [14](Latchoumane et al., 2017; Maingret et al., 2016) [15](Antony et al., 2018; Cairney et al., 2018; Schönauer et al., 2017; Schönauer & Pöhlchen, 2018)
Declarative memory	REM and NREM	Spindles	Limited studies suggest a relationship between REM and declarative memory consolidation.[16] Increased REM was seen after performance improvements,[17] dreaming,[17] and recently declarative aspects of language acquisition.[18]	[16](De Koninck et al., 1989; Fogel, Nader, et al., 2007; Grosmark et al., 2012) [17](De Koninck, 1995; De Koninck et al., 1989, 1990) [18](Thompson et al., 2021)

Simple/motor procedural memory	NREM	Spindles	Sleep enhances procedural memory consolidation.[19] Studies through motor procedural skill (pursuit rotor and finger tapping)[20] or cognitive procedural skills[21] (artificial grammar task, tower of Hanoi, mirror tracing task).[22]	[19](Albouy et al., 2015; Barakat et al., 2012; Doyon et al., 2009; Fischer et al., 2002; Fogel et al., 2015, 2017; King et al., 2013; Kuriyama et al., 2004; Laventure et al., 2016; Peters et al., 2007; Schönauer et al., 2014; Sio et al., 2013; Smith, 2001a; Smith & MacNeill, 1994; Stickgold, 2005; Vahdat et al., 2017; Vien et al., 2016; Walker et al., 2003) [20](Adams, 1952; Ammons, 1955) [21](Fogel, Smith, & Cote, 2007; Smith, 1995, 2001b) [22](Cleeremans & McClelland, 1991; Fischer et al., 2006; Fogel, Smith, & Cote, 2007; Smith, 1995, 2001a; Starch, 1910)
Simple/motor procedural memory	NREM	Spindles	Sleep deprivation paradigms found NREM 2 is primarily involved in motor skill memory consolidation,[23] with sleep spindles showing particular importance for consolidation.[24]	[23](Conway & Smith, 1994; Sandys-Wunsch & Smith, 1991; Smith & MacNeill, 1994; Tweed et al., 1999) [24](Barakat et al., 2012; Fogel & Smith, 2006; Fogel, Smith, & Cote, 2007; Laventure et al., 2016; Morin et al., 2008; Nader & Smith, 2001; Nishida et al., 2016; Nishida & Walker, 2007; Peters et al., 2007; Plihal & Born, 1997; Schabus et al., 2006; van Schalkwijk et al., 2020; Walker et al., 2002)
Simple/motor procedural memory	SWS	Spindles	Distinct role is unclear. Few studies found a possible relationship[25] with consolidation, but several studies found no role for SWS in motor learning.[26] However, spindles during SWS were linked to improved procedural tasks.[27]	[25](Aeschbach et al., 2008; Cousins et al., 2014; Moroni et al., 2008) [26](Diekelmann et al., 2016; Huber et al., 2004; Marshall et al., 2006) [27](Fogel, Smith, & Cote, 2007)

Continued

Table 10.1 *Continued*

Memory type	Sleep stage	Sleep EEG feature	Description	References
Simple/motor procedural memory	REM		Increased REM has been reported following learning on tasks with a motor procedural component.[28] However, these studies employed cognitively complex tasks.	[28](Maquet et al., 2000; G. Nielsen et al., 2014; Peigneux et al., 2003; Smith et al., 2004)
Complex/cognitive procedural memory	REM and NREM	Rapid eye movements, theta power	Existing skills, previously enhanced by REM sleep, are "fine-tuned" by NREM sleep.[29] Recently procedural aspects of language acquisition were linked to theta power time-locked to rapid eye movements.[30]	[29](Fogel et al., 2015; G. Nielsen et al., 2014; Peters et al., 2007; Smith, Aubrey, & Peters, 2004) [30](Thompson et al., 2021)
Complex/cognitive procedural memory	REM	Rapid eye movements	REM sleep suppression studies[31] show evidence of impaired sleep-dependent consolidation of complex procedural skills.	[31](Conway & Smith, 1994; Sandys-Wunsch & Smith, 1991; Smith, 1993; Smith & MacNeill, 1994; Smith & Smith, 2003)

Note. EEG = electroencephalography; NREM = non-rapid eye movement; REM = rapid eye movement; SWs = slow waves; SWS = slow-wave sleep; TMR = targeted memory reactivation.

References

Adams, J. A. (1952). Warm-up decrement in performance on the pursuit-rotor. *The American Journal of Psychology, 65*(3), 404–414.

Aeschbach, D., Cutler, A. J., & Ronda, J. M. (2008). A role for non-rapid-eye-movement sleep homeostasis in perceptual learning. *Journal of Neuroscience, 28*(11), 2766–2772. https://doi.org/10.1523/JNEUROSCI.5548-07.2008

Albouy, G., Fogel, S., King, B. R., Laventure, S., Benali, H., Karni, A., Carrier, J., Robertson, E. M., & Doyon, J. (2015). Maintaining vs. enhancing motor sequence memories: Respective roles of striatal and hippocampal systems. *NeuroImage, 108*, 423–434. https://doi.org/10.1016/j.neuroimage.2014.12.049

Ammons, R. B. (1955). Rotary pursuit apparatus: I. Survey of variables. *Psychological Bulletin, 52*(1), 69–76. https://doi.org/10.1037/h0040849

Amzica, F., & Steriade, M. (1998). Electrophysiological correlates of sleep delta waves. *Electroencephalography and Clinical Neurophysiology, 107*(2), 69–83. https://doi.org/10.1016/s0013-4694(98)00051-0

Antonenko, D., Diekelmann, S., Olsen, C., Born, J., & Mölle, M. (2013). Napping to renew learning capacity: Enhanced encoding after stimulation of sleep slow oscillations. *European Journal of Neuroscience, 37*(7), 1142–1151. https://doi.org/10.1111/ejn.12118

Antony, J. W., Gobel, E. W., O'Hare, J. K., Reber, P. J., & Paller, K. A. (2012). Cued memory reactivation during sleep influences skill learning. *Nature Neuroscience, 15*(8), 1114–1116. https://doi.org/10.1038/nn.3152

Antony, J. W., & Paller, K. A. (2017). Using oscillating sounds to manipulate sleep spindles. *Sleep, 40*(3), Article zsw068. https://doi.org/10.1093/sleep/zsw068

Antony, J. W., Piloto, L., Wang, M., Pacheco, P., Norman, K. A., & Paller, K. A. (2018). Sleep spindle refractoriness segregates periods of memory reactivation. *Current Biology, 28*(11), 1736–1743.e4. https://doi.org/10.1016/j.cub.2018.04.020

Asanuma, H., & Pavlides, C. (1997). Neurobiological basis of motor learning in mammals. *Neuroreport, 8*(4), i–vi.

Aserinsky, E., & Kleitman, N. (1953). Regularly occurring periods of eye motility, and concomitant phenomena, during sleep. *Science, 118*(3062), 273–274. https://doi.org/10.1176/appi.neuropsych.15.4.454

Axmacher, N., Mormann, F., Fernandez, G., Elger, C. E., & Fell, J. (2006). Memory formation by neuronal synchronization. *Brain Research Reviews, 52*(1), 170–182. https://doi.org/10.1016/j.brainresrev.2006.01.007

Baena, D., Cantero, J. L., Fuentemilla, L., & Atienza, M. (2020). Weakly encoded memories due to acute sleep restriction can be rescued after one night of recovery sleep. *Scientific Reports, 10*(1), Article 1449. https://doi.org/10.1038/s41598-020-58496-4

Barakat, M., Doyon, J., Debas, K., Vandewalle, G., Morin, A., Poirier, G., Martin, N., Lafortune, M., Karni, A., Ungerleider, L. G., Benali, H., & Carrier, J. (2012). Fast and slow spindle involvement in the consolidation of a new motor sequence. *Behavioural Brain Research, 217*(1), 117–121. https://doi.org/10.1016/j.bbr.2010.10.019

Bartsch, U., Simpkin, A. J., Demanuele, C., Wamsley, E., Marston, H. M., & Jones, M. W. (2019). Distributed slow-wave dynamics during sleep predict memory consolidation and its impairment in schizophrenia. *NPJ Schizophrenia, 5*(1), Article 18. https://doi.org/10.1038/s41537-019-0086-8

Bazhenov, M., Timofeev, I., Steriade, M., & Sejnowski, T. (1999). Self-sustained rhythmic activity in the thalamic reticular nucleus mediated by depolarizing GABAA receptor potentials. *Nature Neuroscience, 2*(2), 168–174. https://doi.org/10.1038/5729

Bazhenov, M., Timofeev, I., Steriade, M., & Sejnowski, T. (2000). Spiking-bursting activity in the thalamic reticular nucleus initiates sequences of spindle oscillations in thalamic networks. *Journal of Neurophysiology, 84*(2), 1076–1087.

Bergmann, T. O., & Born, J. (2018). Phase-amplitude coupling: A general mechanism for memory processing and synaptic plasticity? *Neuron, 97*(1), 10–13. https://doi.org/10.1016/J.NEURON.2017.12.023

Bergmann, T. O., Mölle, M., Schmidt, M. A., Lindner, C., Marshall, L., Born, J., & Siebner, H. R. (2012). EEG-guided transcranial magnetic stimulation reveals rapid shifts in motor cortical excitability during the human sleep slow oscillation. *Journal of Neuroscience, 32*(1), 243–253. https://doi.org/10.1523/JNEUROSCI.4792-11.2012

Berner, I., Schabus, M., Wienerroither, T., & Klimesch, W. (2006). The significance of sigma neurofeedback training on sleep spindles and aspects of declarative memory. *Applied Psychophysiology and Biofeedback, 31*(2), 97–114. https://doi.org/10.1007/s10484-006-9013-7

Bonjean, M., Baker, T., Lemieux, M., Timofeev, I., Sejnowski, T., & Bazhenov, M. (2011). Corticothalamic feedback controls sleep spindle duration in vivo. *Journal of Neuroscience, 31*(25), 9124–9134. https://doi.org/10.1523/JNEUROSCI.0077-11.2011

Borb, A. A., & Achermann, P. (1999). Sleep homeostasis and models of sleep regulation. *Journal of Biological Rhythms, 14*(6), 559–570. https://doi.org/10.1177/074873099129000894

Born, J., Rasch, B., & Gais, S. (2006). Sleep to remember. *The Neuroscientist, 12*(5), 410–424.

Boutin, A., Pinsard, B., Boré, A., Carrier, J., Fogel, S., & Doyon, J. (2018). Transient synchronization of hippocampo-striato-thalamo-cortical networks during sleep spindle oscillations induces motor memory consolidation. *NeuroImage, 169*, 419–430. https://doi.org/10.1016/j.neuroimage.2017.12.066

Boyce, R., Glasgow, S. D., Williams, S., & Adamantidis, A. (2016). Causal evidence for the role of REM sleep theta rhythm in contextual memory consolidation. *Science, 352*(6287), 812–816.

Bragin, A., Engel, J., Wilson, C. L., Fried, I., & Buzsáki, G. (1999). High-frequency oscillations in human brain. *Hippocampus, 9*(2), 137–142. https://doi.org/10.1002/(SICI)1098-1063(1999)9:2<137::AID-HIPO5>3.0.CO;2-0

Buchegger, J., Fritsch, R., Meier-Koll, A., & Riehle, H. (1991). Does trampolining and anaerobic physical fitness affect sleep? *Perceptual and Motor Skills, 73*(1), 243–252. https://doi.org/10.2466/pms.1991.73.1.243

Buchegger, J., & Meier-Koll, A. (1988). Motor learning and ultradian sleep cycle: An electroencephalographic study of trampoliners. *Perceptual and Motor Skills, 67*(2), 635–645. https://doi.org/10.2466/pms.1988.67.2.635

Buxton, O. M., Ellenbogen, J. M., Wang, W., Carballeira, A., O'Connor, S., Cooper, D., Gordhandas, A. J., McKinney, S. M., & Solet, J. M. (2012). Sleep disruption due to hospital noises: A prospective evaluation. *Annals of Internal Medicine, 157*(3), 170–179. https://doi.org/10.7326/0003-4819-156-12-201208070-00472

Buzsáki, G. (2015). Hippocampal sharp wave-ripple: A cognitive biomarker for episodic memory and planning. *Hippocampus, 25*(10), 1073–1188. https://doi.org/10.1002/hipo.22488

Buzsáki, G., Pentfonen, M., Nadasdy, Z., & Bragin, A. (1996). Pattern and inhibition-dependent invasion of pyramidal cell dendrites by fast spikes in the hippocampus in vivo. *Proceedings of the National Academy of Sciences of the United States of America, 93*(18), 9921–9925. https://doi.org/10.1073/pnas.93.18.9921

Cairney, S. A., Durrant, S. J., Hulleman, J., & Lewis, P. A. (2014). Targeted memory reactivation during slow wave sleep facilitates emotional memory consolidation. *Sleep, 37*(4), 701–707. https://doi.org/10.5665/sleep.3572

Cairney, S. A., Guttesen, A. V., El Marj, N., & Staresina, B. P. (2018). Memory consolidation is linked to spindle-mediated information processing during sleep. *Current Biology, 28*(6), 948–954. https://doi.org/10.1016/j.cub.2018.01.087

Castaldo, V., Krynicki, V., & Goldstein, J. (1974). Sleep stages and verbal memory. *Perceptual and Motor Skills, 39*(3), 1023–1030. https://doi.org/10.2466/pms.1974.39.3.1023

Chapman, C. A., Trepel, C., Ivanco, T. L., Froc, D. J., Wilson, K., & Racine, R. J. (1998). Changes in field potentials and membrane currents in rat sensorimotor cortex following repeated tetanization of the corpus callosum in vivo. *Cerebral Cortex, 8*(8), 730–742.

Chernik, D. A. (1972). Effect of REM sleep deprivation on learning and recall by humans. *Perceptual and Motor Skills, 34*(1), 283–294. https://doi.org/10.2466/pms.1972.34.1.283

Cleeremans, A., & McClelland, J. L. (1991). Learning the structure of event sequences. *Journal of Experimental Psychology: General, 120*(3), 235–253.

Clemens, Z., Fabó, D., & Halász, P. (2005). Overnight verbal memory retention correlates with the number of sleep spindles. *Neuroscience, 132*(2), 529–535. https://doi.org/10.1016/j.neuroscience.2005.01.011

Clemens, Z., Mölle, M., Eross, L., Barsi, P., Halász, P., & Born, J. (2007). Temporal coupling of parahippocampal ripples, sleep spindles and slow oscillations in humans. *Brain, 130*(Pt. 11), 2868–2878. https://doi.org/10.1093/brain/awm146

Clemens, Z., Mölle, M., Eross, L., Jakus, R., Rásonyi, G., Halász, P., & Born, J. (2011). Fine-tuned coupling between human parahippocampal ripples and sleep spindles. *European Journal of Neuroscience, 33*(3), 511–520. https://doi.org/10.1111/j.1460-9568.2010.07505.x

Cohen, N., Eichenbaum, H., Deacedo, B., & Corkin, S. (1985). Different memory systems underlying acquisition of procedural and declarative knowledge. *Annals of the New York Academy of Sciences*, *444*(1), 54–71. https://doi.org/10.1111/J.1749-6632.1985.Tb37579.X

Contreras, D., & Steriade, M. (1995). Cellular basis of EEG slow rhythms: A study of dynamic corticothalamic relationships. *Journal of Neuroscience*, *15*(1), 604–622.

Conway, J. M., & Smith, C. T. (1994). REM sleep and learning in humans: A sensitivity to specific types of learning tasks. *Journal of Sleep Research*, *3*(1), 48. [Paper presentation], 12th Congress of the European Sleep Research Society in Florence, Italy, May 22–27, 1994.

Cousins, J. N., El-Deredy, W., Parkes, L. M., Hennies, N., & Lewis, P. A. (2014). Cued memory reactivation during slow-wave sleep promotes explicit knowledge of a motor sequence. *Journal of Neuroscience*, *34*(48), 15870–15876. https://doi.org/10.1523/JNEUROSCI.1011-14.2014

Dang-Vu, T. T., McKinney, S. M., Buxton, O. M., Solet, J. M., & Ellenbogen, J. M. (2010). Spontaneous brain rhythms predict sleep stability in the face of noise. *Current Biology*, *20*(15), R626–R627. https://doi.org/10.1016/j.cub.2010.06.032

Datta, S. (2000). Avoidance task training potentiates phasic pontine-wave density in the rat: A mechanism for sleep-dependent plasticity. *Journal of Neuroscience*, *20*(22), 8607–8613.

Datta, S., & Maclean, R. R. (2007). Neurobiological mechanisms for the regulation of mammalian sleep–wake behavior: Reinterpretation of historical evidence and inclusion of contemporary cellular and molecular evidence. *Neuroscience and Biobehavioral Reviews*, *31*(5), 775–824. https://doi.org/10.1016/j.neubiorev.2007.02.004

Debas, K., Carrier, J., Orban, P., Barakat, M., Lungu, O., Vandewalle, G., Hadj Tahar, A., Bellec, P., Karni, A., Ungerleider, L. G., Benali, H., & Doyon, J. (2010). Brain plasticity related to the consolidation of motor sequence learning and motor adaptation. *Proceedings of the National Academy of Sciences of the United States of America*, *107*(41), 17839–17844. https://doi.org/10.1073/pnas.1013176107

De Gennaro, L., Ferrara, M., & Bertini, M. (2000). Topographical distribution of spindles: Variations between and within NREM sleep cycles. *Sleep Research Online*, *3*(4), 155–160.

De Koninck, J. (1995). Intensive learning, REM sleep and REM sleep mentation. *Sleep Research Bulletin*, *1*(2), 39–40.

De Koninck, J., Christ, G., Hébert, G., & Rinfret, N. (1990). Language learning efficiency, dreams and REM sleep. *Psychiatric Journal of the University of Ottawa: Revue de Psychiatrie de L'Université d'Ottawa*, *15*(2), 91–92.

De Koninck, J., Lorrain, D., Christ, G., Proulx, G., & Coulombe, D. (1989). Intensive language learning and increases in rapid eye movement sleep: Evidence of a performance factor. *International Journal of Psychophysiology*, *8*(1), 43–47. https://doi.org/10.1016/0167-8760(89)90018-4

De Koninck, J., & Prévost, F. (1991). Paradoxical sleep and information processing: Exploration by inversion of the visual field. *Canadian Journal of Psychology*, *45*(2), 125–139.

Demanuele, C., Bartsch, U., Baran, B., Khan, S., Vangel, M. G., Cox, R., Hämäläinen, M., Jones, M. W., Stickgold, R., & Manoach, D. S. (2017). Coordination of slow waves with sleep spindles predicts sleep-dependent memory consolidation in schizophrenia. *Sleep*, *40*(1), Article zsw013. https://doi.org/10.1093/sleep/zsw013

Destexhe, A., & Sejnowski, T. (2001). *Thalamocortical assemblies: How ion channels, single neurons and large-scale networks organize sleep oscillations*. Oxford University Press.

Diekelmann, S., & Born, J. (2010). The memory function of sleep. *Nature Reviews Neuroscience*, *11*(2), 114–126. https://doi.org/10.1038/nrn2762

Diekelmann, S., Born, J., & Rasch, B. (2016). Increasing explicit sequence knowledge by odor cueing during sleep in men but not women. *Frontiers in Behavioral Neuroscience*, *10*, Article 74. https://doi.org/10.3389/fnbeh.2016.00074

Dijk, D. J. (2009). Regulation and functional correlates of slow wave sleep. *Journal of Clinical Sleep Medicine*, *5*(2), S6–S15.

Doyon, J., Bellec, P., Amsel, R., Penhune, V. B., Monchi, O., Carrier, J., Lehéricy, S., & Benali, H. (2009). Contributions of the basal ganglia and functionally related brain structures to motor learning. *Behavioural Brain Research*, *199*(1), 61–75. https://doi.org/10.1016/j.bbr.2008.11.012

Doyon, J., & Benali, H. (2005). Reorganization and plasticity in the adult brain during learning of motor skills. *Current Opinion in Neurobiology*, *15*(2), 161–167. https://doi.org/10.1016/J.CONB.2005.03.004

Doyon, J., Penhune, V. B., & Ungerleider, L. G. (2003). Distinct contribution of the cortico-striatal and cortico-cerebellar systems to motor skill learning. *Neuropsychologia, 41*(3), 252–262. https://doi.org/10.1016/s0028-3932(02)00158-6

Doyon, J., & Ungerleider, L. G. (2002). Functional anatomy of motor skill learning. *Neuropsychology of Memory, 3*, 225–238.

Dudai, Y., & Eisenberg, M. (2004). Rites of passage of the engram: Reconsolidation and the lingering consolidation hypothesis. *Neuron, 44*(1), 93–100. https://doi.org/10.1016/j.neuron.2004.09.003

Ebbinghaus, H. (2013). Memory: A contribution to experimental psychology. *Annals of Neurosciences, 20*(4), 155–156. https://doi.org/10.5214/ans.0972.7531.200408 (Original work published 1885).

Ego-Stengel, V., & Wilson, M. A. (2010). Disruption of ripple-associated hippocampal activity during rest impairs spatial learning in the rat. *Hippocampus, 20*(1), 1–10. https://doi.org/10.1002/hipo.20707

Ekstrand, B. R., Sullivan, M. J., Parker, D. F., & West, J. N. (1971). Spontaneous recovery and sleep. *Journal of Experimental Psychology, 88*(1), 142–144.

Elton, M., Winter, O., Heslenfeld, D., Loewy, D., Campbell, K., & Kok, A. (1997). Event-related potentials to tones in the absence and presence of sleep spindles. *Journal of Sleep Research, 6*(2), 78–83.

Empson, J. A. C., & Clarke, P. R. F. (1970). Rapid eye movements and remembering. *Nature, 227*(5255), 287–288.

Eschenko, O., Molle, M., Born, J., &Sara, S. J. (2006). Elevated sleep spindle density after learning or after retrieval in rats. *Journal of Neuroscience, 26*(50), 12914–12920. https://doi.org/10.1523/JNEUROSCI.3175-06.2006

Fang, Z., Ray, L. B. B., Owen, A. M. M., & Fogel, S. (2019). Brain activation time-locked to sleep spindles associated with human cognitive abilities. *Frontiers in Neuroscience, 13*, Article 46. https://doi.org/10.3389/fnins.2019.00046

Fang, Z., Sergeeva, V., Ray, L. B., Viczko, J., Owen, A. M., & Fogel, S. (2017). Sleep spindles and intellectual ability: Epiphenomenon or directly related? *Journal of Cognitive Neuroscience, 29*(1), 167–182. https://doi.org/10.1162/jocn_a_01034

Fernández-Mendoza, J., Lozano, B., Seijo, F., Santamarta-Liébana, E., Ramos-Platón, M. J., Vela-Bueno, A., & Fernández-González, F. (2009). Evidence of subthalamic PGO-like waves during REM sleep in humans: A deep brain polysomnographic study. *Sleep, 32*(9), 1117–1126.

Ferrara, M., De Gennaro, L., Casagrande, M., & Bertini, M. (1999). Auditory arousal thresholds after selective slow-wave sleep deprivation. *Clinical Neurophysiology, 110*(12), 2148–2152. https://doi.org/10.1016/S1388-2457(99)00171-6

Fischer, S., Drosopoulos, S., Tseng, I. J., & Born, J. (2006). Implicit learning—Explicit knowing: A role for sleep in memory system interaction. *Journal of Cognitive Neuroscience, 18*(3), 311–319.

Fischer, S., Hallschmid, M., Elsner, A. L., & Born, J. (2002). Sleep forms memory for finger skills. *Proceedings of the National Academy of Sciences of the United States of America, 99*(18), 11987–11991. https://doi.org/10.1073/pnas.182178199

Fogel, S. M., Jacob, J., & Smith, C. T. (2001). Increased sleep spindle activity following simple motor procedural learning in humans. *Proceedings of the Congress Physiological Basis for Sleep Medicine, 7*, 123. [Paper presentation], Congress Physiological Basis for Sleep Medicine. Uruguay, October 21–26, 2001.

Fogel, S. M., Nader, R., Cote, K., & Smith, C. (2007). Sleep spindles and learning potential. *Behavioral Neuroscience, 121*(1), 1–10. https://doi.org/10.1037/0735-7044.121.1.1

Fogel, S. M., Ray, L. B., Binnie, L., & Owen, A. M. (2015). How to become an expert: A new perspective on the role of sleep in the mastery of procedural skills. *Neurobiology of Learning and Memory, 125*(1), 236–248. https://doi.org/10.1016/j.nlm.2015.10.004

Fogel, S. M., & Smith, C. T. (2006). Learning-dependent changes in sleep spindles and Stage 2 sleep. *Journal of Sleep Research, 15*(3), 250–255. https://doi.org/10.1111/j.1365-2869.2006.00522.x

Fogel, S. M., & Smith, C. (2011). The function of the sleep spindle: A physiological index of intelligence and a mechanism for sleep-dependent memory consolidation. *Neuroscience and Biobehavioral Reviews, 35*(5), 1154–1165. https://doi.org/10.1016/j.neubiorev.2010.12.003

Fogel, S. M., Smith, C., & Cote, K. (2007). Dissociable learning-dependent changes in REM and non-REM sleep in declarative and procedural memory systems. *Behavioural Brain Research, 180*(1), 48–61. https://doi.org/10.1016/j.bbr.2007.02.037

Fogel, S. M., Vien, C., Karni, A., Benali, H., Carrier, J., Doyon, J., & Albouy, G. (2017). Sleep spindles: A physiological marker of age-related changes in grey matter in brain regions supporting motor skill memory consolidation. *Neurobiology of Aging, 49*, 154–164. https://doi.org/10.1016/j.neurobiolaging.2016.10.009

Fowler, M. J., Sullivan, M. J., & Ekstrand, B. R. (1973). Sleep and memory. *Science, 179*, 302–304.

Frankland, P. W., & Bontempi, B. (2005). The organization of recent and remote memories. *Nature Reviews Neuroscience, 6*(2), 119–130. https://doi.org/10.1038/nrn1607

Frankland, P. W., Bontempi, B., Talton, L. E., Kaczmarek, L., & Silva, A. J. (2004). The involvement of the anterior cingulate cortex in remote contextual fear memory. *Science, 304*(5672), 881–883. https://doi.org/10.1126/science.1094804

Friederici, A. D., & Ungerleider, L. G. (2005). Cognitive neuroscience. *Current Opinion in Neurobiology, 15*(2), 131–134. https://doi.org/10.1016/j.conb.2005.03.019

Fuentemilla, L., Miró, J., Ripollés, P., Vilà-Balló, A., Juncadella, M., Castañer, S., Salord, N., Monasterio, C., Falip, M., Rodríguez-Fornells, A. (2013). Hippocampus-dependent strengthening of targeted memories via reactivation during sleep in humans. *Current Biology, 23*(18), 1769–1775. https://doi.org/10.1016/j.cub.2013.07.006

Gabrieli, J. D. E. (1998). Cognitive neuroscience of human memory. *Annual Review of Psychology, 49*, 87–115.

Gais, S., Albouy, G., Boly, M., Dang-Vu, T. T., Darsaud, A., Desseilles, M., Rauchs, G., Schabus, M., Sterpenich, V., Vandewalle, G., Maquet, P., & Peigneux, P. (2007). Sleep transforms the cerebral trace of declarative memories. *Proceedings of the National Academy of Sciences of the United States of America, 104*(47), 18778–18783. https://doi.org/10.1073/pnas.0705454104

Gais, S., & Born, J. (2004). Declarative memory consolidation: Mechanisms acting during human sleep. *Learning & Memory, 11*(6), 679–685. https://doi.org/10.1101/lm.80504

Gais, S., Mölle, M., Helms, K., & Born, J. (2002). Learning-dependent increases in sleep spindle density. *Journal of Neuroscience, 22*(15), 6830–6834. https://doi.org/10.1523/JNEUROSCI.22-15-06830-2002

Gais, S., Plihal, W., Wagner, U., & Born, J. (2000). Early sleep triggers memory for early visual discrimination skills. *Nature Neuroscience, 3*(12), 1335–1339. https://doi.org/10.1038/81881

Garside, P., Arizpe, J., Lau, C.-I., Goh, C., & Walsh, V. (2015). Cross-hemispheric alternating current stimulation during a nap disrupts slow wave activity and associated memory consolidation. *Brain Stimulation, 8*(3), 520–527. https://doi.org/10.1016/j.brs.2014.12.010

Gennaro, L. D., & Ferrara, M. (2003). Sleep spindles: An overview. *Sleep Medicine Reviews, 7*(5), 423–440. https://doi.org/10.1053/smrv.2002.0252

Germain, A., James, J., Insana, S., Herringa, R. J., Mammen, O., Price, J., & Nofzinger, E. A. (2013). A window into the invisible wound of war: Functional neuroimaging of REM sleep in returning combat veterans with PTSD. *Psychiatry Research: Neuroimaging, 211*(2), 176–179. https://doi.org/10.1016/j.pscychresns.2012.05.007

Girardeau, G., Benchenane, K., Wiener, S. I., Buzsaki, G., & Zugaro, M. (2009). Selective suppression of hippocampal ripples impairs spatial memory. *Nature Neuroscience, 12*(10), 1222–1223. https://doi.org/10.1038/nn.2384

Giuditta, A. (2014). Sleep memory processing: The sequential hypothesis. *Frontiers in Systems Neuroscience, 8*, Article 219. https://doi.org/10.3389/fnsys.2014.00219

Graf, P., Squire, L. R., & Mandler, G. (1984). The information that amnesic patients do not forget. *Journal of Experimental Psychology, 10*(1), 164–178. https://doi.org/10.1037//0278-7393.10.1.164

Grosmark, A. D., Mizuseki, K., Pastalkova, E., Diba, K., Buzsaki, G., & Buzsáki, G. (2012). REM sleep reorganizes hippocampal excitability. *Neuron, 75*(6), 1001–1007. https://doi.org/10.1016/j.neuron.2012.08.015

Guerrien, A., Dujardin, K., Mandai, O., Sockeel, P., Leconte, P., Mandal, O., Sockeel, P., & Leconte, P. (1989). Enhancement of memory by auditory stimulation during postlearning REM sleep in humans. *Physiology & Behavior, 45*(5), 947–950. https://doi.org/10.1016/0031-9384(89)90219-9

Haist, F., Bowden Gore, J., & Mao, H. (2001). Consolidation of human memory over decades revealed by functional magnetic resonance imaging. *Nature Neuroscience, 4*(11), 1139–1145. https://doi.org/10.1038/nn739

Helfrich, R. F., Lendner, J. D., Mander, B. A., Guillen, H., Paff, M., Mnatsakanyan, L., Vadera, S., Walker, M. P., Lin, J. J., & Knight, R. T. (2019). Bidirectional prefrontal-hippocampal dynamics organize information transfer during sleep in humans. *Nature Communications, 10*(1), Article 3572. https://doi.org/10.1038/s41467-019-11444-x

Helfrich, R. F., Mander, B. A., Jagust, W. J., Knight, R. T., & Walker, M. (2018). Old brains come uncoupled in sleep: Slow wave-spindle synchrony, brain atrophy, and forgetting. *Neuron, 97*(1), 221–230. https://doi.org/10.1016/J.NEURON.2017.11.020

Hu, P. T., Stylos-Allan, M., & Walker, M. P. (2006). Sleep facilitates consolidation of emotionally arousing declarative memory. *Psychological Science*, *17*(10), 891–898.

Huber, R., Ghilardi, M. F., Massimini, M., & Tononi, G. (2004). Local sleep and learning. *Nature*, *430*(6995), 78–81. https://doi.org/10.1038/nature02663

Jadhav, S. P., Kemere, C., German, P. W., & Frank, L. M. (2012). Awake hippocampal sharp-wave ripples support spatial memory. *Science*, *336*(6087), 1454–1458. https://doi.org/10.1126/science.1217230

Jegou, A., Schabus, M., Gosseries, O., Dahmen, B., Albouy, G., Desseilles, M., Sterpenich, V., Phillips, C., Maquet, P., Grova, C., & Dang-Vu, T. T. (2019). Cortical reactivations during sleep spindles following declarative learning. *NeuroImage*, *195*, 104–112. https://doi.org/10.1016/j.neuroimage.2019.03.051

Jenkins, J., & Dallenbach, K. M. (1924). Obliviscence during sleep and waking. *American Journal of Psychology*, *35*(4), 605–612.

Jones, M. W., & Wilson, M. A. (2005). Phase precession of medial prefrontal cortical activity relative to the hippocampal theta rhythm. *Hippocampus*, *15*(7), 867–873. https://doi.org/10.1002/hipo.20119

Karni, A., Meyer, G., Jezzard, P., Adams, M. M., Turner, R., & Ungerleider, L. G. (1995). Functional MRI evidence for adult motor cortex plasticity during motor skill learning. *Nature*, *377*(6545), 155–158. https://doi.org/10.1038/377155a0

Kim, A., Latchoumane, C. V., Lee, S., Kim, G. B., Cheong, E., Augustine, G. J., & Shin, H.-S. (2012). Optogenetically induced sleep spindle rhythms alter sleep architectures in mice. *Proceedings of the National Academy of Sciences of the United States of America*, *109*(50), 20673–20678. https://doi.org/10.1073/pnas.1217897109

Kim, J. J., & Fanselow, M. S. (1992). Modality-specific retrograde amnesia of fear. *Science*, *256*(5057), 675–677.

King, B. R., Fogel, S., Albouy, G., & Doyon, J. (2013). Neural correlates of the age-related changes in motor sequence learning and motor adaptation in older adults. *Frontiers in Human Neuroscience*, *7*, Article 142. https://doi.org/10.3389/fnhum.2013.00142

Korman, M., Doyon, J., Doljansky, J., Carrier, J., Dagan, Y., & Karni, A. (2007). Daytime sleep condenses the time course of motor memory consolidation. *Nature Neuroscience*, *10*(9), 1206–1213. https://doi.org/10.1038/nn1959

Kuriyama, K., Stickgold, R., & Walker, M. P. (2004). Sleep-dependent learning and motor-skill complexity. *Learning & Memory*, *11*(6), 705–713. https://doi.org/10.1101/lm.76304

Ladenbauer, J., Ladenbauer, J., Külzow, N., de Boor, R., Avramova, E., Grittner, U., & Flöel, A. (2017). Promoting sleep oscillations and their functional coupling by transcranial stimulation enhances memory consolidation in mild cognitive impairment. *Journal of Neuroscience*, *37*(30), 7111–7124. https://doi.org/10.1523/JNEUROSCI.0260-17.2017

Lafortune, M., Gagnon, J. F., Martin, N., Latreille, V., Dubé, J., Bouchard, M., Bastien, C. H., & Carrier, J. (2014). Sleep spindles and rapid eye movement sleep as predictors of next morning cognitive performance in healthy middle-aged and older participants. *Journal of Sleep Research*, *23*(2), 159–167. https://doi.org/10.1111/jsr.12108

Landsness, E. C., Crupi, D., Hulse, B. K., Peterson, M. J., Huber, R., Ansari, H., Coen, M., Cirelli, C., Benca, R. M., Ghilardi, M. F., & Tononi, G. (2009). Sleep-dependent improvement in visuomotor learning: A causal role for slow waves. *Sleep*, *32*(10), 1273–1284.

Latchoumane, C.-F. V., Ngo, H.-V. V., Born, J., & Shin, H.-S. (2017). Thalamic spindles promote memory formation during sleep through triple phase-locking of cortical, thalamic, and hippocampal rhythms. *Neuron*, *95*(2), 424–435. https://doi.org/10.1016/j.neuron.2017.06.025

Lau, H., Tucker, M. A., & Fishbein, W. (2010). Daytime napping: Effects on human direct associative and relational memory. *Neurobiology of Learning and Memory*, *93*(4), 554–560. https://doi.org/10.1016/j.nlm.2010.02.003

Laventure, S., Fogel, S., Lungu, O., Albouy, G., Sévigny-Dupont, P., Vien, C., Sayour, C., Carrier, J., Benali, H., & Doyon, J. (2016). NREM2 and sleep spindles are instrumental to the consolidation of motor sequence memories. *PLOS Biology*, *14*(3), Article e1002429. https://doi.org/10.1371/journal.pbio.1002429

Lecci, S., Fernandez, L. M. J., Weber, F. D., Cardis, R., Chatton, J.-Y., Born, J., & Lüthi, A. (2017). Coordinated infraslow neural and cardiac oscillations mark fragility and offline periods in mammalian sleep. *Science Advances*, *3*(2), Article e1602026. https://doi.org/10.1126/SCIADV.1602026

Lehmann, M., Schreiner, T., Seifritz, E., & Rasch, B. (2016). Emotional arousal modulates oscillatory correlates of targeted memory reactivation during NREM, but not REM sleep. *Scientific Reports, 6*(1), Article 39229. https://doi.org/10.1038/srep39229
Lehmann, M., Seifritz, E., & Rasch, B. (2016). Sleep benefits emotional and neutral associative memories equally. *Somnologie, 20*(1), 47–53. https://doi.org/10.1007/s11818-015-0034-4
Le Van Quyen, M., Staba, R., Bragin, A., Dickson, C., Valderrama, M., Fried, I., & Engel, J. (2010). Large-scale microelectrode recordings of high-frequency gamma oscillations in human cortex during sleep. *Journal of Neuroscience, 30*(23), 7770–7782. https://doi.org/10.1523/JNEUROSCI.5049-09.2010
Lewin, I., & Glaubman, H. (1975). The effect of REM deprivation: Is it detrimental, beneficial, or neutral? *Psychophysiology, 12*(3), 349–353.
Lewis, P. A., Knoblich, G., & Poe, G. (2018). How memory replay in sleep boosts creative problem-solving. *Trends in Cognitive Sciences, 22*(6), 491–503. https://doi.org/10.1016/j.tics.2018.03.009
Loomis, A. L., Harvey, E. N., & Hobart, G. A. (1937). Cerebral states during sleep, as studied by human brain potentials. *Journal of Experimental Psychology, 21*(2), 127–144.
Maier, J. G., Piosczyk, H., Holz, J., Landmann, N., Deschler, C., Frase, L., Kuhn, M., Klöppel, S., Spiegelhalder, K., Sterr, A., Riemann, D., Feige, B., Voderholzer, U., & Nissen, C. (2017). Brief periods of NREM sleep do not promote early offline gains but subsequent on-task performance in motor skill learning. *Neurobiology of Learning and Memory, 145*, 18–27. https://doi.org/10.1016/j.nlm.2017.08.006
Maingret, N., Girardeau, G., Todorova, R., Goutierre, M., & Zugaro, M. (2016). Hippocampo-cortical coupling mediates memory consolidation during sleep. *Nature Neuroscience, 19*(7), 959–966. https://doi.org/10.1038/nn.4304
Mandai, O., Guerrien, A., Sockeel, P., Dujardin, K., & Leconte, P. (1989). REM sleep modifications following a Morse code learning session in humans. *Physiology & Behavior, 46*(4), 639–642. https://doi.org/10.1016/0031-9384(89)90344-2
Mantua, J., Baran, B., & Spencer, R. M. C. (2016). Sleep benefits consolidation of visuo-motor adaptation learning in older adults. *Experimental Brain Research, 234*(2), 587–595. https://doi.org/10.1007/s00221-015-4490-7
Maquet, P. (2001). The role of sleep in learning and memory. *Science, 294*(5544), 1048–1052. https://doi.org/10.1126/science.1062856
Maquet, P., Laureys, S., Peigneux, P., Fuchs, S., Petiau, C., Phillips, C., Aerts, J., Del Fiore, G., Degueldre, C., Meulemans, T., Luxen, A., Franck, G., Van Der Linden, M., Smith, C. T., & Cleeremans, A. (2000). Experience-dependent changes in cerebral activation during human REM sleep. *Nature Neuroscience, 3*(8), 831–836. https://doi.org/10.1038/77744
Marshall, L., & Born, J. (2007). The contribution of sleep to hippocampus-dependent memory consolidation. *Trends in Cognitive Sciences, 11*(10), 442–450. https://doi.org/10.1016/j.tics.2007.09.001
Marshall, L., Helgadóttir, H., Mölle, M., & Born, J. (2006). Boosting slow oscillations during sleep potentiates memory. *Nature, 444*(7119), 610–613. https://doi.org/10.1038/nature05278
Massimini, M., Tononi, G., & Huber, R. (2009). Slow waves, synaptic plasticity and information processing: Insights from transcranial magnetic stimulation and high-density EEG experiments. *European Journal of Neuroscience, 29*(9), 1761–1770. https://doi.org/10.1111/j.1460-9568.2009.06720.x
McCormick, L., Nielsen, T., Nicolas, A., Ptito, M., & Montplaisir, J. (1997). Topographical distribution of spindles and K-complexes in normal subjects. *Sleep, 20*(11), 939–941. https://doi.org/10.1093/sleep/20.11.939
Mednick, S. C., McDevitt, E. A., Walsh, J. K., Wamsley, E. J., Paulus, M., Kanady, J. C., & Drummond, S. P. A. (2013). The critical role of sleep spindles in hippocampal-dependent memory: A pharmacology study. *Journal of Neuroscience, 33*(10), 4494–4504. https://doi.org/10.1523/JNEUROSCI.3127-12.2013
Mendes, R. A. V., Zacharias, L. R., Ruggiero, R. N., Leite, J. P., Moraes, M. F. D., & Lopes-Aguiar, C. (2021). Hijacking of hippocampal–cortical oscillatory coupling during sleep in temporal lobe epilepsy. *Epilepsy & Behavior, 121*, Article 106608. https://doi.org/10.1016/j.yebeh.2019.106608
Milner, B., Squire, L. R., & Kandel, E. R. (1998). Cognitive neuroscience and the study of memory. *Neuron, 20*(3), 445–468. https://doi.org/10.1016/s0896-6273(00)80987-3
Milner, C. E., Fogel, S., & Cote, K. A. (2006). Habitual napping moderates motor performance improvements following a short daytime nap. *Biological Psychiatry, 73*(2), 141–156. https://doi.org/10.1016/j.biopsycho.2006.01.015

Miyauchi, S., Misaki, M., Kan, S., Fukunaga, T., & Koike, T. (2009). Human brain activity time-locked to rapid eye movements during REM sleep. *Experimental Brain Research, 192*(4), 657–667. https://doi.org/10.1007/s00221-008-1579-2

Mölle, M., Marshall, L., Gais, S., & Born, J. (2002). Grouping of spindle activity during slow oscillations in human non-rapid eye movement sleep. *Journal of Neuroscience, 22*(24), 10941–10947. https://doi.org/10.1523/JNEUROSCI.22-24-10941.2002

Mölle, M., Marshall, L., Gais, S., & Born, J. (2004). Learning increases human electroencephalographic coherence during subsequent slow sleep oscillations. *Proceedings of the National Academy of Sciences of the United States of America, 101*(38), 13963–13968. https://doi.org/10.1073/pnas.0402820101

Morin, A., Doyon, J., Dostie, V., Barakat, M., Hadj Tahar, A., Korman, M., Benali, H., Karni, A., Ungerleider, L. G., & Carrier, J. (2008). Motor sequence learning increases sleep spindles and fast frequencies in post-training sleep. *Sleep, 31*(8), 1149–1156.

Morita, Y., Ogawa, K., & Uchida, S. (2012). The effect of a daytime 2-hour nap on complex motor skill learning. *Sleep and Biological Rhythms, 10*(4), 302–309. https://doi.org/10.1111/j.1479-8425.2012.00576.x

Moroni, F., Nobili, L., Curcio, G., De Carli, F., Tempesta, D., Marzano, C., De Gennaro, L., Mai, R., Francione, S., Lo Russo, G., & Ferrara, M. (2008). Procedural learning and sleep hippocampal low frequencies in humans. *Neuroimage, 42*(2), 911–918. https://doi.org/10.1016/j.neuroimage.2008.05.027

Morrison, A. R., & Bowker, R. M. (1975). The biological significance of PGO spikes in the sleeping cat. *Acta Neurobiologiae Experimentalis, 35*, 821–840.

Moscovitch, M., Nadel, L., Winocur, G., Gilboa, A., & Rosenbaum, R. S. (2006). The cognitive neuroscience of remote episodic, semantic and spatial memory. *Current Opinion in Neurobiology, 16*(2), 179–190. https://doi.org/10.1016/j.conb.2006.03.013

Moscovitch, M., Winocur, G., & McLachlan, D. (1986). Memory as assessed by recognition and reading time in normal and memory-impaired people with Alzheimer's disease and other neurological disorders. *Journal of Experimental Psychology: General, 115*(4), 331–347. https://doi.org/10.1037/0096-3445.115.4.331

Murkar, A. L. A., & De Koninck, J. (2018). Consolidative mechanisms of emotional processing in REM sleep and PTSD. *Sleep Medicine Reviews, 41*, 173–184. https://doi.org/10.1016/j.smrv.2018.03.001

Nadasdy, Z., Hirase, H., Czurko, A., Csicsvari, J., & Buzsaki, G. (1999). Replay and time compression of recurring spike sequences in the hippocampus. *Journal of Neuroscience, 19*(21), 9497–9507.

Nadel, L., & Moscovitch, M. (1997). Memory consolidation, retrograde amnesia and the hippocampal complex. *Current Opinion in Neurobiology, 7*(2), 217–227.

Nader, R., & Smith, C. T. (2001). The relationship between Stage 2 sleep spindles and intelligence. *Sleep, 24*, Article A160.

Nemeth, D., Janacsek, K., Londe, Z., Ullman, M. T., Howard, D. V., & Howard, J. H. (2010). Sleep has no critical role in implicit motor sequence learning in young and old adults. *Experimental Brain Research, 201*(2), 351–358. https://doi.org/10.1007/s00221-009-2024-x

Nettersheim, A., Hallschmid, M., Born, J., & Diekelmann, S. (2015). The role of sleep in motor sequence consolidation: Stabilization rather than enhancement. *Journal of Neuroscience, 35*(17), 6696–6702. https://doi.org/10.1523/JNEUROSCI.1236-14.2015

Nielsen, G., Wikman, J. M., Jensen, C. J., Schmidt, J. F., Gliemann, L., & Andersen, T. R. (2014). Health promotion: The impact of beliefs of health benefits, social relations and enjoyment on exercise continuation. *Scandinavian Journal of Medicine and Science in Sports, 24*(S1), 66–75. https://doi.org/10.1111/sms.12275

Nielsen, T. A., O'Reilly, C., Carr, M., Dumel, G., Godin, I., Solomonova, E., Lara-Carrasco, J., Blanchette-Carrière, C., & Paquette, T. (2015). Overnight improvements in two REM sleep-sensitive tasks are associated with both REM and NREM sleep changes, sleep spindle features, and awakenings for dream recall. *Neurobiology of Learning and Memory, 122*, 88–97. https://doi.org/10.1016/j.nlm.2014.09.007

Niknazar, M., Krishnan, G. P., Bazhenov, M., & Mednick, S. C. (2015). Coupling of thalamocortical sleep oscillations are important for memory consolidation in humans. *PLOS ONE, 10*(12), Article e0144720. https://doi.org/10.1371/journal.pone.0144720

Nishida, M., Nakashima, Y., & Nishikawa, T. (2016). Slow sleep spindle and procedural memory consolidation in patients with major depressive disorder. *Nature and Science of Sleep, 8*, 63–72. https://doi.org/10.2147/NSS.S100337

Nishida, M., Pearsall, J., Buckner, R. L., & Walker, M. (2009). REM sleep, prefrontal theta, and the consolidation of human emotional memory. *Cerebral Cortex, 19*(5), 1158–1166. https://doi.org/10.1093/cercor/bhn155

Nishida, M., & Walker, M. P. (2007). Daytime naps, motor memory consolidation and regionally specific sleep spindles. *PLOS ONE, 2*(4), Article e341. https://doi.org/10.1371/journal.pone.0000341

Novitskaya, Y., Sara, S. J., Logothetis, N. K., & Eschenko, O. (2016). Ripple-triggered stimulation of the locus coeruleus during post-learning sleep disrupts ripple/spindle coupling and impairs memory consolidation. *Learning & Memory, 23*(5), 238–248. https://doi.org/10.1101/LM.040923.115

Pace-Schott, E. F., Germain, A., & Milad, M. R. (2015). Sleep and REM sleep disturbance in the pathophysiology of PTSD: The role of extinction memory. *Biology of Mood & Anxiety Disorders, 5*(1), Article 3. https://doi.org/10.1186/s13587-015-0018-9

Parker, A., Ngu, H., & Cassaday, H. J. (2001). Odour and Proustian memory: Reduction of context-dependent forgetting and multiple forms of memory. *Applied Cognitive Psychology, 15*(2), 159–171. https://doi.org/10.1002/1099-0720(200103/04)15:2<159::AID-ACP694>3.0.CO;2-D

Peigneux, P., Laureys, S., Fuchs, S., Delbeuck, X., Degueldre, C., Aerts, J., Delfiore, G., Luxen, A., & Maquet, P. (2001). Generation of rapid eye movements during paradoxical sleep in humans. *Neuroimage, 14*(3), 701–708. https://doi.org/10.1006/nimg.2001.0874

Peigneux, P., Laureys, S., Fuchs, S., Destrebecqz, A., Collette, F., Delbeuck, X., Phillips, C., Aerts, J., Del Fiore, G., Degueldre, C., Luxen, A., Cleeremans, A., & Maquet, P. (2003). Learned material content and acquisition level modulate cerebral reactivation during posttraining rapid-eye-movements sleep. *Neuroimage, 20*(1), 125–134.

Peters, K. R., Ray, L. B., Smith, V., & Smith, C. T. (2008). Changes in the density of Stage 2 sleep spindles following motor learning in young and older adults. *Journal of Sleep Research, 17*(1), 23–33. https://doi.org/10.1111/j.1365-2869.2008.00634.x

Peters, K. R., Smith, V., & Smith, C. T. (2007). Changes in sleep architecture following motor learning depend on initial skill level. *Journal of Cognitive Neuroscience, 19*(5), 817–829. https://doi.org/10.1162/jocn.2007.19.5.817

Plihal, W., & Born, J. (1997). Effects of early and late nocturnal sleep on declarative and procedural memory. *Journal of Cognitive Neuroscience, 9*(4), 534–547. https://doi.org/10.1162/jocn.1997.9.4.534

Rasch, B., & Born, J. (2013). About sleep's role in memory. *Physiological Reviews, 93*(2), 681–766. https://doi.org/10.1152/physrev.00032.2012

Rasch, B., Büchel, C., Gais, S., & Born, J. (2007). Odor cues during slow-wave sleep prompt declarative memory consolidation. *Science, 315*(5817), 1426–1429. https://doi.org/10.1126/science.1138581

Redondo, R. L., & Morris, R. G. M. (2011). Making memories last: The synaptic tagging and capture hypothesis. *Nature Reviews Neuroscience, 12*(1), Article 1. https://doi.org/10.1038/nrn2963

Remondes, M., Wilson, M. A., Flint, J., & Kendler, K. S. (2014). Cingulate-hippocampus coherence and trajectory coding in a sequential choice task [Erratum]. *Neuron, 81*(5), 484–503. https://doi.org/10.1016/j.neuron.2014.02.035

Robertson, E. M. (2009). From creation to consolidation: A novel framework for memory processing. *PLOS Biology, 7*(1), Article e1000019. https://doi.org/10.1371/journal.pbio.1000019

Robertson, E. M., Pascual-Leone, A., & Press, D. Z. (2004). Awareness modifies the skill-learning benefits of sleep. *Current Biology, 14*(3), 208–212. https://doi.org/10.1016/j.cub.2004.01.027

Rosanova, M., & Ulrich, D. (2005). Pattern-specific associative long-term potentiation induced by a sleep spindle-related spike train. *Journal of Neuroscience, 25*(41), 9398–9405. https://doi.org/10.1523/JNEUROSCI.2149-05.2005

Ruch, S., Markes, O., Duss, S. B., Oppliger, D., Reber, T. P., Koenig, T., Mathis, J., Roth, C., & Henke, K. (2012). Sleep Stage II contributes to the consolidation of declarative memories. *Neuropsychologia, 50*(10), 2389–2396. https://doi.org/10.1016/j.neuropsychologia.2012.06.008

Sandys-Wunsch, H., & Smith, C. T. (1991). The effect of alcohol consumption on sleep and memory [Abstract]. *Sleep Research, 20*, 419.

Schabus, M., Dang-Vu, T. T., Albouy, G., Balteau, E., Boly, M., Carrier, J., Darsaud, A., Degueldre, C., Desseilles, M., Gais, S., Phillips, C., Rauchs, G., Schnakers, C., Sterpenich, V., Vandewalle, G., Luxen, A., & Maquet, P. (2007). Hemodynamic cerebral correlates of sleep spindles during human non-rapid eye movement sleep. *Proceedings of the National Academy of Sciences of the United States of America, 104*(32), 13164–13169. https://doi.org/10.1073/PNAS.0703084104

Schabus, M., Gruber, G., Parapatics, S., Sauter, C., Klösch, G., Anderer, P., Klimesch, W., Saletu, B., & Zeitlhofer, J. (2004). Sleep spindles and their significance for declarative memory consolidation. *Sleep, 27*(8), 1479–1485. https://doi.org/10.1093/sleep/27.7.1479

Schabus, M., Hödlmoser, K., Gruber, G., Sauter, C., Anderer, P., Klösch, G., Parapatics, S., Saletu, B., Klimesch, W., & Zeitlhofer, J. (2006). Sleep spindle-related activity in the human EEG and its relation to general cognitive and learning abilities. *European Journal of Neuroscience, 23*(7), 1738–1746. https://doi.org/10.1111/j.1460-9568.2006.04694.x

Schacter, D. L. (1997). The cognitive neuroscience of memory: Perspectives from neuroimaging research. *Philosophical Transactions of the Royal Society of London B: Biological Sciences, 352*(1362), 1689–1695. https://doi.org/10.1098/rstb.1997.0150

Schmidt, C., Peigneux, P., Muto, V., Schenkel, M., Knoblauch, V., Münch, M., de Quervain, D. J.-F., Wirz-Justice, A., & Cajochen, C. (2006). Encoding difficulty promotes postlearning changes in sleep spindle activity during napping. *Journal of Neuroscience, 26*(35), 8976–8982. https://doi.org/10.1523/JNEUROSCI.2464-06.2006

Schönauer, M., Alizadeh, S., Jamalabadi, H., Abraham, A., Pawlizki, A., & Gais, S. (2017). Decoding material-specific memory reprocessing during sleep in humans. *Nature Communications, 8*, Article 15404. https://doi.org/10.1038/ncomms15404

Schönauer, M., Geisler, T., & Gais, S. (2014). Strengthening procedural memories by reactivation in sleep. *Journal of Cognitive Neuroscience, 26*(1), 143–153. https://doi.org/10.1162/jocn_a_00471

Schönauer, M., Grätsch, M., & Gais, S. (2015). Evidence for two distinct sleep-related long-term memory consolidation processes. *Cortex, 63*, 68–78. https://doi.org/10.1016/j.cortex.2014.08.005

Schönauer, M., & Pöhlchen, D. (2018). Sleep spindles. *Current Biology, 28*(19), R1129–R1130. https://doi.org/10.1016/j.cub.2018.07.035

Scoville, W. B., & Milner, B. (1957). Loss of recent memory after bilateral hippocampal lesions. *Journal of Neurology, Neurosurgery and Psychiatry, 20*(1), 11–21.

Siapas, A. G., & Wilson, M. A. (1998). Coordinated interactions between hippocampal ripples and cortical spindles during slow-wave sleep. *Neuron, 21*(5), 1123–1128. https://doi.org/10.1016/S0896-6273(00)80629-7

Siegel, J. M. (2001). The REM sleep–memory consolidation hypothesis. *Science, 294*(5544), 1058–1063. https://doi.org/10.1126/science.1063049

Sio, U. N., Monaghan, P., & Ormerod, T. (2013). Sleep on it, but only if it is difficult: Effects of sleep on problem solving. *Memory & Cognition, 41*(2), 159–166. https://doi.org/10.3758/s13421-012-0256-7

Sirota, A., Csicsvari, J., Buhl, D., & Buzsaki, G. (2003). Communication between neocortex and hippocampus during sleep in rodents. *Proceedings of the National Academy of Sciences of the United States of America, 100*(4), 2065–2069. https://doi.org/10.1073/pnas.0437938100

Smith, C. T. (1993). REM sleep and learning: Some recent findings. In A. Moffitt, M. Kramer, & R. Hoffmann (Eds.), *The functions of dreaming* (pp. 341–361). State University of New York Press.

Smith, C. T. (1995). Sleep states and memory processes. *Behavioural Brain Research, 69*(1–2), 137–145. https://doi.org/10.1016/0166-4328(95)00024-n

Smith, C. T. (1996). Sleep states, memory processes and synaptic plasticity. *Behavioural Brain Research, 78*(1), 49–56. https://doi.org/10.1016/0166-4328(95)00218-9

Smith, C. T. (2001a). Changes in density of REM sleep following acquisition of cognitive procedural tasks in humans [Abstract]. *Actas de Fisiologia, 7*, 27.

Smith, C. T. (2001b). Sleep states and memory processes in humans: Procedural versus declarative memory systems. *Sleep Medicine Reviews, 5*(6), 491–506. https://doi.org/10.1053/smrv.2001.0164

Smith, C. T., Aubrey, J. B., & Peters, K. R. (2004). Different roles for REM and Stage 2 sleep in motor learning: A proposed model. *Psychologica Belgica, 44*(1–2), 81–104. https://doi.org/10.5334/pb.1018

Smith, C. T., & Fazekas, A. (1997). Amounts of REM sleep and Stage 2 required for efficient learning [Abstract]. *Sleep Research, 26*, 690.

Smith, C. T., & MacNeill, C. (1994). Impaired motor memory for a pursuit rotor task following Stage 2 sleep loss in college students. *Journal of Sleep Research, 3*(4), 206–213. https://doi.org/10.1111/j.1365-2869.1994.tb00133.x

Smith, C. T., Nixon, M., & Nader, R. S. (2004). Posttraining increases in REM sleep intensity implicate REM sleep in memory processing and provide a biological marker of learning potential. *Learning & Memory, 11*(6), 714–719. https://doi.org/10.1101/lm.74904

Smith, C. T., & Smith, D. (2003). Ingestion of ethanol just prior to sleep onset impairs memory for procedural but not declarative tasks. *Sleep, 26*(2), 185–191. https://doi.org/10.1093/sleep/26.2.185

Smith, C. T., & Weeden, K. (1990). Post training REMs coincident auditory stimulation enhances memory in humans. *Psychiatric Journal of the University of Ottawa, 15*(2), 85–90.

Smith, C. T., & Wong, P. T. P. (1991). Paradoxical sleep increases predict successful learning in a complex operant task. *Behavioral Neuroscience, 105*(2), 282–288. https://doi.org/10.1037/0735-7044.105.2.282

Squire, L. R. (1992). Declarative and nondeclarative memory: Multiple brain systems supporting learning and memory. *Journal of Cognitive Neuroscience, 4*(3), 232–243. https://doi.org/10.1162/jocn.1992.4.3.232

Squire, L. R., & Zola-Morgan, S. (1996). Structure and function of declarative and nondeclarative memory systems. *Proceedings of the National Academy of Sciences of the United States of America, 93*(24), 13515–13522. https://doi.org/10.1073/pnas.93.24.13515

Squire, L. R., & Zola-Morgan, S. (1998). Episodic memory, semantic memory, and amnesia. *Hippocampus, 8*(3), 205–211. https://doi.org/10.1002/(SICI)1098-1063(1998)8:3<205::AID-HIPO3>3.0.CO;2-I

Starch, D. A. (1910). A demonstration of the trial and error method of learning. *Psychological Bulletin, 7*(1), 20–23. https://doi.org/10.1037/h0063796

Staresina, B. P., Ole Bergmann, T., Bonnefond, M., Van Der Meij, R., Jensen, O., Deuker, L., Elger, C. E., Axmacher, N., & Fell, J. (2015). Hierarchical nesting of slow oscillations, spindles and ripples in the human hippocampus during sleep. *Nature Neuroscience, 18*(11), 1679–1686. https://doi.org/10.1038/nn.4119

Steriade, M. (1995). Thalamic origin of sleep spindles: Morison and Bassett (1945). *Journal of Neurophysiology, 73*(3), 921–922.

Steriade, M. (1999). Brainstem activation of thalamocortical systems. *Brain Research Bulletin, 50*(5–6), 391–392. https://doi.org/10.1016/s0361-9230(99)00119-7

Steriade, M. (2006). Grouping of brain rhythms in corticothalamic systems. *Neuroscience, 137*(4), 1087–1106. https://doi.org/10.1016/j.neuroscience.2005.10.029

Stickgold, R. (2005). Sleep-dependent memory consolidation. *Nature, 437*(7063), 1272–1278. https://doi.org/10.1038/nature04286

Sugawara, S. K., Koike, T., Kawamichi, H., Makita, K., Hamano, Y. H., Takahashi, H. K., Nakagawa, E., & Sadato, N. (2017). Qualitative differences in offline improvement of procedural memory by daytime napping and overnight sleep: An fMRI study. *Neuroscience Research, 132*, 37–45. https://doi.org/10.1016/j.neures.2017.09.006

Tambini, A., Berners-Lee, A., & Davachi, L. (2017). Brief targeted memory reactivation during the awake state enhances memory stability and benefits the weakest memories. *Scientific Reports, 7*(1), Article 15325. https://doi.org/10.1038/s41598-017-15608-x

Thompson, K., Gibbings, A., Shaw, J., Ray, L., Hébert, G., De Koninck, J., & Fogel, S. (2021). Sleep and second-language acquisition revisited: The role of sleep spindles and rapid eye movements. *Nature and Science of Sleep, 13*, 1887–1902. https://doi.org/10.2147/NSS.S326151

Tilley, A. J., & Empson, J. A. C. (1978). REM sleep and memory consolidation. *Biological Psychology, 6*(4), 293–300.

Tononi, G. (2009). Slow wave homeostasis and synaptic plasticity. *Journal of Clinical Sleep Medicine, 5*(2), 16–19.

Tononi, G., & Cirelli, C. (2006). Sleep function and synaptic homeostasis. *Sleep Medicine Reviews, 10*(1), 49–62. https://doi.org/10.1016/j.smrv.2005.05.002

Tononi, G., & Cirelli, C. (2014). Sleep and the price of plasticity: From synaptic and cellular homeostasis to memory consolidation and integration. *Neuron, 81*(1), 12–34. https://doi.org/10.1016/j.neuron.2013.12.025

Trepel, C., & Racine, R. J. (1998). Long-term potentiation in the neocortex of the adult, freely moving rat. *Cerebral Cortex, 8*(8), 719–729.

Tsuno, N., Besset, A., & Ritchie, K. (2005). Sleep and depression. *Journal of Clinical Psychiatry, 66*(10), 1254–1269.

Tucker, M. A., & Fishbein, W. (2008). Enhancement of declarative memory performance following a daytime nap is contingent on strength of initial task acquisition. *Sleep, 31*(2), 197–203.

Tucker, M. A., Hirota, Y., Wamsley, E. J., Lau, H., Chaklader, A., & Fishbein, W. (2006). A daytime nap containing solely non-REM sleep enhances declarative but not procedural memory. *Neurobiology of Learning and Memory, 86*(2), 241–247. https://doi.org/10.1016/j.nlm.2006.03.005

Tulving, E. (1985). How many memory systems are there? *American Psychologist, 40*(4), 385–398. https://doi.org/10.1037/0003-066X.40.4.385

Tweed, S., Aubrey, J. B., Nader, R., & Smith, C. T. (1999). Deprivation of REM sleep or stage 2 sleep differentially affects cognitive procedural and motor procedural memory. *Sleep, 22*(1), Article S241.

Ujma, P. P., Konrad, B. N., Genzel, L., Bleifuss, A., Simor, P., Pótári, A., Körmendi, J., Gombos, F., Steiger, A., Bódizs, R., & Dresler, M. (2014). Sleep spindles and intelligence: Evidence for a sexual dimorphism. *Journal of Neuroscience, 34*(49), 16358–16368. https://doi.org/10.1523/JNEUROSCI.1857-14.2014

Ungerleider, L. G., Doyon, J., & Karni, A. (2002). Imaging brain plasticity during motor skill learning. *Neurobiology of Learning and Memory, 78*(3), 553–564.

Vahdat, S., Fogel, S., Benali, H., & Doyon, J. (2017). Network-wide reorganization of procedural memory during NREM sleep revealed by fMRI. *eLife, 6*, Article 24987. https://doi.org/10.7554/ELIFE.24987

van den Berg, N. H., Al-Kuwatli, J., Paulin, J., Ray, L. B., Owen, A. M., & Fogel, S. M. (2019). Sleep preferentially enhances memory for a cognitive strategy but not the implicit motor skills used to acquire it. *Neurobiology of Learning and Memory, 161*, 135–142. https://doi.org/10.1016/j.nlm.2019.04.005

van Dongen, E. V., Takashima, A., Barth, M., Zapp, J., Schad, L. R., Paller, K. A., & Fernandez, G. (2012). Memory stabilization with targeted reactivation during human slow-wave sleep. *Proceedings of the National Academy of Sciences of the United States of America, 109*(26), 10575–10580. https://doi.org/10.1073/pnas.1201072109

van Schalkwijk, F. J., Hauser, T., Hoedlmoser, K., Ameen, M. S., Wilhelm, F. H., Sauter, C., Klösch, G., Moser, D., Gruber, G., Anderer, P., Saletu, B., Parapatics, S., Zeitlhofer, J., & Schabus, M. (2020). Procedural memory consolidation is associated with heart rate variability and sleep spindles. *Journal of Sleep Research, 29*(3), Article e12910. https://doi.org/10.1111/jsr.12910

van Schalkwijk, F. J., Sauter, C., Hoedlmoser, K., Heib, D. P. J. J., Klösch, G., Moser, D., Gruber, G., Anderer, P., Zeitlhofer, J., & Schabus, M. (2017). The effect of daytime napping and full-night sleep on the consolidation of declarative and procedural information. *Journal of Sleep Research, 28*(1), Article e12649. https://doi.org/10.1111/jsr.12649

Verschoor, G. J., & Holdstock, T. L. (1984). REM bursts and REM sleep following visual and auditory learning. *South African Journal of Psychology, 14*(3), 69–74. https://doi.org/10.1177/008124638401400301

Vertes, R. P., Eastman, K. E., El-shanti, H., Lidral, A. C., Mar-, M. L., Cooper, M. E., & Jarrah, N. (2000). The case against memory consolidation in REM sleep. *Behavioural and Brain Sciences, 23*(6), 867–876.

Viczko, J., Sergeeva, V., Ray, L. B., Owen, A. M. M., & Fogel, S. (2018). Does sleep facilitate the consolidation of allocentric or egocentric representations of implicitly learned visual-motor sequence learning? *Learning & Memory, 25*(2), 67–77. https://doi.org/10.1101/lm.044719.116

Vien, C., Boré, A., Lungu, O., Benali, H., Carrier, J., Fogel, S., & Doyon, J. (2016). Age-related white-matter correlates of motor sequence learning and consolidation. *Neurobiology of Aging, 48*, 13–22. https://doi.org/10.1016/j.neurobiolaging.2016.08.006

Vijayan, S., Lepage, K. Q., Kopell, N. J., & Cash, S. S. (2017). Frontal beta-theta network during REM sleep. *eLife, 6*, Article e18894. https://doi.org/10.7554/eLife.18894

Wagner, G., Koch, K., Reichenbach, J. R., Sauer, H., & Schlösser, R. G. M. (2006). The special involvement of the rostrolateral prefrontal cortex in planning abilities: An event-related fMRI study with the Tower of London paradigm. *Neuropsychologia, 44*(12), 2337–2347. https://doi.org/10.1016/j.neuropsychologia.2006.05.014

Wagner, U., Fischer, S., & Born, J. (2002). Changes in emotional responses to aversive pictures across periods rich in slow-wave sleep versus rapid eye movement sleep. *Psychosomatic Medicine, 64*(4), 627–634. https://doi.org/10.1097/01.psy.0000021940.35402.51

Wagner, U., Gais, S., & Born, J. (2011). Emotional memory formation is enhanced across sleep intervals with high amounts of rapid eye movement sleep. *Learning & Memory, 8*(2), 112–119. https://doi.org/10.1101/lm.36801

Walker, M. P. (2005). A refined model of sleep and the time course of memory formation. *Behavioral Brain Sciences, 28*(1), 51–64.

Walker, M. P., Brakefield, T., Morgan, A., Hobson, J. A., & Stickgold, R. (2002). Practice with sleep makes perfect: Sleep-dependent motor skill learning. *Neuron, 35*(1), 205–211. https://doi.org/10.1016/S0896-6273(02)00746-8

Walker, M. P., Brakefield, T., Seidman, J., Morgan, A., Hobson, J. A., & Stickgold, R. (2003). Sleep and the time course of motor skill learning. *Learning & Memory, 10*(4), 275–284. https://doi.org/10.1101/lm.58503

Wang, B., Antony, J. W., Lurie, S., Brooks, P. P., Paller, K. A., & Norman, K. A. (2018). Targeted memory reactivation during sleep elicits neural signals related to learning content. *BioRxiv*. https://doi.org/10.1101/449389

Warrington, E. K. (1996). Studies of retrograde memory: A long-term view. *Proceedings of the National Academy of Sciences of the United States of America, 93*(24), 13523–13526.

Wehrle, R., Kaufmann, C., Wetter, T. C., Holsboer, F., Auer, D. P., Pollmächer, T., & Czisch, M. (2007). Functional microstates within human REM sleep: First evidence from fMRI of a thalamocortical network specific for phasic REM periods. *European Journal of Neuroscience, 25*(3), 863–871. https://doi.org/10.1111/j.1460-9568.2007.05314.x

Werk, C. M., & Chapman, C. A. (2003). Long-term potentiation of polysynaptic responses in Layer V of the sensorimotor cortex induced by theta-patterned tetanization in the awake rat. *Cerebral Cortex, 13*(5), 500–507. https://doi.org/10.1093/cercor/13.5.500

Werk, C. M., Harbour, V. L., & Chapman, C. A. (2005). Induction of long-term potentiation leads to increased reliability of evoked neocortical spindles in vivo. *Neuroscience, 131*(4), 793–800. https://doi.org/10.1016/j.neuroscience.2004.12.020

Wilson, M. A., & McNaughton, B. L. (1994). Reactivation of hippocampal ensemble memories during sleep. *Science, 265*(5172), 676–679. https://doi.org/10.1126/science.8036517

Winocur, G. (1985). The hippocampus and thalamus: Their roles in short- and long-term memory and the effects of interference. *Behavioural Brain Research, 16*(2–3), 135–152.

Winocur, G., & Moscovitch, M. (2011). Memory transformation and systems consolidation. *Journal of the International Neuropsychological Society, 17*(5), 766–780. https://doi.org/10.1017/S1355617711000683

Witt, K., Margraf, N., Bieber, C., Born, J., & Deuschl, G. (2010). Sleep consolidates the effector-independent representation of a motor skill. *Neuroscience, 171*(1), 227–234. https://doi.org/10.1016/j.neuroscience.2010.07.062

Wolansky, T., Clement, E. A., Peters, S. R., Palczak, M. A., & Dickson, C. T. (2006). Hippocampal slow oscillation: A novel EEG state and its coordination with ongoing neocortical activity. *Journal of Neuroscience, 26*(23), 6213–6229. https://doi.org/10.1523/JNEUROSCI.5594-05.2006

Yaroush, R., Sullivan, M. J., & Ekstrand, B. R. (1971). Effect of sleep on memory. II. Differential effect of the first and second half of the night. *Journal of Experimental Psychology, 88*(3), 361–366.

Yordanova, J., Kirov, R., Verleger, R., & Kolev, V. (2017). Dynamic coupling between slow waves and sleep spindles during slow wave sleep in humans is modulated by functional pre-sleep activation. *Scientific Reports, 7*(1), Article 14496. https://doi.org/10.1038/S41598-017-15195-X

Zhang, J., Yetton, B., Whitehurst, L. N., Naji, M., & Mednick, S. C. (2020). The effect of zolpidem on memory consolidation over a night of sleep. *Sleep, 43*(11), Article zsaa084. https://doi.org/10.1093/sleep/zsaa084

Zola-Morgan, S., Squire, L. R., Rempel, N. L., Clower, R. P., & Amaral, D. G. (1992). Enduring memory impairment in monkeys after ischemic damage to the hippocampus. *Journal of Neuroscience, 12*(7), 2582–2596.

CHAPTER

11 Sleep and Human Performance

Courtney A. Kurinec, Jonah A. Scott, *and* Hans P. A. Van Dongen

Abstract

The criticality of sleep to human performance is well documented; however, the performance impairments that result when people are deprived of sleep are multifaceted and only partially understood. This chapter provides an overview of cognitive performance changes due to sleep loss, which are driven by homeostatic, circadian, and allostatic processes of sleep regulation. A pervasive consequence of sleep loss is degradation of bottom-up information processing, but sleep loss also diminishes the ability to effectively use top-down attentional control and the ability to bind information together in memory. These deficits are distinct but interrelated and may be connected and integrated in complex ways to produce a variety of cognitive performance outcomes, including real-world performance failures leading to errors and accidents. This chapter reviews the current understanding of the relationship between sleep and human performance.

Key Words: sleep, sleep loss, cognitive performance, bottom-up processing, top-down attentional control, binding, memory, accident

Introduction

Most of what is known about the link between human performance and sleep comes from studies in which people were deprived of sleep, or their sleep was otherwise altered in terms of duration, timing, or structure. When sleep is curtailed or displaced in time, sleepiness ensues, and impairments are observed on tasks involving cognitive performance. These impairments are undone by subsequent sleep. As such, it appears that there is something about wakefulness that exacts a price on cognition, which leads to reduced performance capability, whereas sleep evidently supports cognition, presumably by restoring and/or protecting performance capability for the next waking period. However, what it is exactly in wakefulness and sleep that makes this happen is not well understood, although theories have been formulated that provide some insight. In this chapter, the enigmatic link between sleep and cognitive performance is discussed from multiple angles, with an emphasis on principles and concepts, and illustrated with examples drawn from laboratory studies in healthy adult populations.

Temporal Dynamics of Sleep and Waking Cognitive Performance

In humans, as a diurnal species, the optimal timing of wakefulness is during the daytime hours. The temporal regulation of wakefulness and sleep is such that when sufficient nighttime sleep is obtained on a routine basis—where *sufficient* in this context is estimated to be approximately 8 hours per night for the average individual (Van Dongen et al., 2003; Wehr et al., 1993)—cognitive performance is near optimal and relatively stable through most of the day. This is achieved by the interplay of two physiological processes. The first is a circadian process, which originates from the biological clock in the suprachiasmatic nuclei of the hypothalamus (Moore, 1992); it provides a day/night rhythm in pressure for wakefulness, with the highest pressure during the "wake-maintenance zone" in the late afternoon or early evening (Strogatz et al., 1987). The second is a homeostatic process, for which understanding of the neurobiological basis is far from complete (Benington & Heller, 1995; Porkka-Heiskanen et al., 1997; Tononi & Cirelli, 2020); it provides a pressure for sleep that accumulates in a saturating exponential manner with time awake and dissipates exponentially with time asleep (Borbély, 1982). The two processes balance each other out: During the day, rising circadian pressure for wakefulness offsets the accumulating homeostatic pressure for sleep across time awake, providing a stable level of arousal to support wakefulness and cognitive functioning until well into the evening. During the night, on the other hand, the dissipating pressure for sleep across the sleep period goes hand in hand with falling circadian pressure for wakefulness, providing a stable level of low arousal to facilitate consolidated sleep (Dijk & Czeisler, 1994).

When sleep is curtailed or displaced, the balance between the two processes is lost, and waking cognitive performance suffers. During sleep periods, the dissipation of homeostatic pressure for sleep is left incomplete, leaving residual sleep pressure upon awakening. Moreover, during wake periods, the circadian pressure for wakefulness no longer offsets the homeostatic pressure for sleep consistently, leading to periods of increased sleepiness. The resulting temporal dynamics depend on the specific sleep/wake schedule and require a biomathematical model to describe in detail (Riedy et al., 2022) but typically involve a progressive degradation of performance through nighttime wakefulness and into the early morning, while performance tends to be less impaired during the wake-maintenance zone (Daan et al., 1984). There is also a brief period of impairment immediately after awakening when the brain transitions from sleep to wakefulness (Balkin et al., 2002). This is referred to as *sleep inertia* and usually passes in 30 minutes or less, but it is more prominent under conditions of sleep curtailment.

While sleep/wake regulation through the circadian and homeostatic processes is directly related to cognitive performance over periods of hours to a few days, there are longer-term dynamics where that relationship breaks down. This is particularly evident when nighttime sleep is restricted to between approximately 4 and 7 hours per day across multiple consecutive days. The homeostatic process rapidly reaches equilibrium, such that the buildup of homeostatic sleep pressure across each of the extended wake periods equals the dissipation of homeostatic sleep pressure across each of the restricted sleep periods (Van Dongen et al., 2003). As a consequence, the intensity of slow-wave sleep—presumed to be the most restorative component of sleep and a putative marker of sleep homeostasis (Frank, 2021)—stabilizes after just a few days of sleep restriction, as if there were no further need for sleep to restore performance capability for the next waking period (Skorucak et al., 2018). This occurs even though the brain's capacity to generate intense slow-wave sleep is much higher (Van Dongen et al., 2003). However, laboratory studies have shown that average daily performance deteriorates steadily across days of sleep restriction in a dose–response manner—that is, the greater the amount of sleep restriction and the greater the number of consecutive days, the greater the level of performance impairment (Belenky et al., 2003; Van Dongen et al., 2003). This profound breakdown in the link between sleep regulation, through the homeostatic and circadian processes, and the temporal dynamics of waking cognitive performance constitutes a significant challenge for theories of sleep function (Grant & Van Dongen, 2013).

Brain Mechanisms Underlying the Regulation of Sleep, Wakefulness, and Performance

The mechanisms underlying the regulation of sleep and wakefulness are multilayered and complex (Krueger et al., 2008; Saper, Scammell, & Lu, 2005; Tononi & Cirelli, 2014). Multiple schemes have been proposed for the mechanisms underlying the temporal dynamics, and they have different implications for the role of sleep and sleep loss in cognitive performance. We discuss four that have particular relevance for how the link between sleep and performance may be understood.

In one perspective, wakefulness is essentially the product of the activity of the ascending arousal system (Munn et al., 2021), modulated by circadian rhythmicity (Saper, Lu, et al., 2005), and sleep is triggered by a neuronal switch in the ventrolateral preoptic area of the hypothalamus, which blocks the ascending arousal system from activating the thalamus and cerebral cortex (Saper et al., 2001). Recent evidence suggests that the neuronal circuitry involved is more complex (Eban-Rothschild et al., 2018) and more widely distributed across the brain (e.g., Ma et al., 2019). Even so, this perspective leaves unspecified what it is exactly that produces sleep homeostasis and determines when the hypothalamic sleep/wake switch is thrown. Nonetheless, this view gave rise to the idea that sleep loss produces cognitive impairment due to the global influence of sleep-initiating mechanisms on the endogenous capacity to maintain alertness and attention. According to this *state instability hypothesis*, interaction of growing homeostatic pressure for sleep with circadian pressure for wakefulness and activation from compensatory effort or external stimulation produces an increasingly unstable brain state that cannot be characterized as either fully awake or asleep, fluctuates within seconds, and can rapidly progress to physiological sleep if not resisted (Doran et al., 2001). The unstable brain state would have downstream consequences for cognitive performance across the board but would be most readily observable on sustained attention performance tasks that probe brain function frequently and thereby expose the instability, such as simple reaction time tasks (Lim & Dinges, 2008).

An alternative view is based on the notion that sleep is not principally a global brain phenomenon but rather occurs locally at the level of neuronal/glial cell assemblies in a use-dependent manner (Krueger et al., 2008). According to this *local sleep theory*, neural circuitry that is repeatedly stimulated by task performance builds up a homeostatic pressure for sleep locally, thereby providing a neurobiological basis for global sleep homeostasis (Krueger et al., 2013). Moreover, it has been posited that expression of a local, sleep-like state in response to repeated circuit stimulation causes information processing in the neural circuit at hand to be degraded (Van Dongen et al., 2011b). This would occur stochastically and with increasing likelihood the longer the circuit has been kept "awake," leading to instability in cognitive performance equivalent to what is predicted by the state instability hypothesis (Hudson et al., 2020). However, local sleep theory expressly predicts that the effects of sleep deprivation on cognitive performance would be task-dependent (Van Dongen et al., 2011a).

An early and more regionally focused variant on local sleep theory posits that the prefrontal cortex is particularly vulnerable to degradation of the effectiveness of neural circuitry (Harrison et al., 2000) because of its high cerebral metabolic rate during wakefulness (Drummond et al., 2000; Maquet et al., 1990; Thomas et al., 2000). In this view, sleep deprivation would be most impactful for executive functioning, which would be exposed by tasks involving complex cognitive performance such as decision-making and particularly tasks that require adjusting to novel information (Harrison & Horne, 1998; Harrison & Horne, 1999). Supporting evidence for this assertion has been found in the intensification of slow-wave sleep in (pre)frontal areas during recovery sleep after sleep deprivation (Cajochen et al., 1999; Horne, 1986), although the lack of responsiveness of slow-wave sleep across days of sleep restriction (Skorucak et al., 2018; Van Dongen et al., 2003) puts the interpretation of that evidence into question.

Finally, the *synaptic homeostasis hypothesis* (or SHY) posits that synaptic plasticity is the driving force underlying sleep regulation (Tononi & Cirelli, 2020). The main premise of the SHY is that continual strengthening of neuronal connections as a result of ongoing learning during wakefulness would increase metabolic needs in the circuitry, degrade information processing, and saturate learning. During sleep, the net synaptic strength would be renormalized and cellular homeostasis restored (Tononi & Cirelli, 2014). Experiments have revealed associations between the use of brain circuits for learning during wakefulness and regional intensification of subsequent sleep (e.g., Huber et al., 2004), providing indirect evidence for the SHY and connecting its presumed phenomenology with local sleep theory (Krueger & Obál, 1993). Although the SHY makes no specific predictions about the nature of performance impairment due to loss of sleep, other than (in the extreme case) a failure to learn new information, the hypothesis underscores the importance of sleep for memory consolidation (Walker & Stickgold, 2004) and gist extraction, integration, and insight (e.g., Wagner et al., 2004).

Sleep Loss and Degradation of Bottom-Up Information Processing

Arguably the best-known and most extensively used tool to study the impact of sleep deprivation on performance is the psychomotor vigilance test (PVT; see Figure 11.1A). In its most common implementation, it is a 10-minute one-choice reaction time task with a random inter-trial interval of 2–10 seconds (Dinges & Powell, 1985). On each trial, subjects taking the test are required to respond to a visual stimulus as quickly as possible, which creates a significant demand for sustained attention. This is evident in the presence of a vigilance decrement or "time-on-task effect" over the course of the test duration. The time-on-task effect is amplified under conditions of sleep deprivation (Lim & Dinges, 2008). There is no appreciable practice effect on the PVT (Van Dongen et al., 2003).

Much of what is known about the temporal dynamics of performance impairment due to sleep loss is based at least in part on research using the PVT. An important finding is that sleep deprivation is associated with a rightward skewing of the response time (RT) distribution (see Figure 11.1B). This is in fact a hallmark characteristic of sleep loss–induced performance impairment on the PVT (Dinges & Kribbs, 1991). Well-rested, healthy young adults produce stable, fast responses on the PVT, with the vast majority of RTs in the 200–300 ms range. In sleep-deprived individuals, however, these fast responses are interspersed with notably slower responses, which occur stochastically (Doran et al., 2001). For a given time of day (i.e., at fixed circadian pressure for wakefulness), the greater the amount of sleep loss, the stronger the skewing of the RT distribution. The longer tail of the skewed RT distribution means more RTs fall beyond the threshold for "lapses of attention," which is conventionally set at 500 ms (Dorrian et al., 2005). Counting the number of lapses of attention defined that way (i.e., the number of RTs >500 ms) thus provides an easy way to quantify how much the RT distribution is skewed, and thereby the degree to which performance on the PVT is impaired (Van Dongen et al., 2003).

The phenomenon of lapses of attention (or "blocking") as a consequence of sleep deprivation has been observed extensively and originally gave rise to the *lapse hypothesis* (Williams et al., 1959), which regarded the slower RTs as evidence of actual interruptions in attention or brief periods when information presented to the brain would literally be missed. However, the continuity of the RT distribution, even when skewed, makes such a dichotomous interpretation (i.e., the attentive brain vs. the lapsing brain) untenable, and the lapse hypothesis has been replaced by the state instability hypothesis (Doran et al., 2001).

Neuroimaging studies have shown reduced activation in widely distributed areas of the brain during PVT performance while sleep deprived (Ma et al., 2015), although

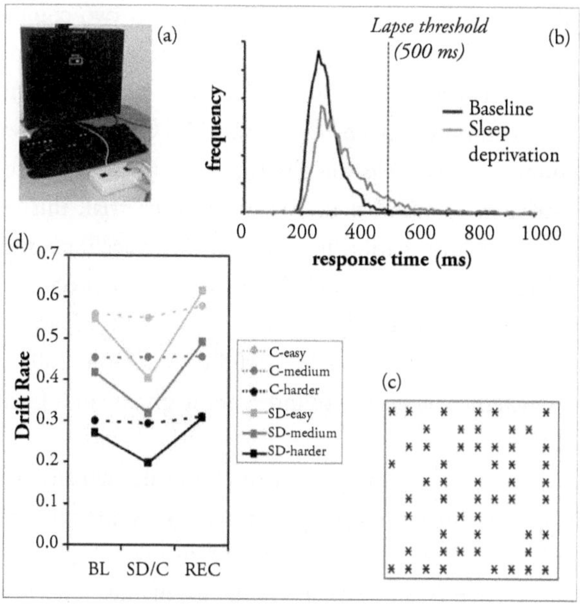

Figure 11.1 Sleep deprivation and bottom-up information processing

Note. Panel a: Picture of the psychomotor vigilance test (PVT) as implemented on a desktop computer. In a little red box, a stimulus (a rolling millisecond counter) appears at random intervals of 2–10 seconds for 10 consecutive minutes, and subjects are asked to respond to the appearance of the stimulus as quickly as possible by pressing a button. The task generates a significant demand for sustained attention. Panel b: Sleep deprivation causes a rightward skewing of the response time (RT) distribution. Data of 16 healthy young adults are aggregated over daytime test administrations (at 08:45, 11:45, 14:45, and 17:45) at well-rested baseline (black) and 24 hours later after a night of total sleep deprivation (grey). Conventionally, RTs beyond a 500-ms threshold are counted as lapses of attention, a measure of the skewing of the distribution and therefore the degree of performance impairment on the PVT. Figure adapted from Grant et al. (2017) with permission. Panel c: Example trial on the two-choice numerosity discrimination task, during which a variable number of asterisks are placed in random locations on a 10 by 10 array. Subjects are asked to respond quickly and accurately, without actually counting the asterisks, whether the number of asterisks is greater or less than 50. The closer to 50 the actual number of asterisks, the lesser the quality of the information provided as the basis for the response and the harder the trial. This particular trial is considered extremely hard. Panel d: Sleep deprivation reduces the quality of information processing. Means are shown of 25 healthy young adults who performed the numerosity discrimination task three times, at 2-day intervals, during an in-laboratory study. Of the 25 subjects, 12 had been sleep-deprived for 57 hours during the second task administration; the other 13 served as controls. In the controls (circles), drift rate—a computational model measure of the quality of information processing—varied predictably as a function of trial difficulty. In the sleep deprivation group (square), the same was observed, but during the second task administration the quality of information processing was further reduced by the loss of sleep. As such, easy trials became moderately hard, moderately hard trials became harder, etc. (Ratcliff & Van Dongen, 2009). BL = baseline; REC = recovery; SD/C = sleep deprivation or control.

increased activation has been seen in the thalamus except during lapses (Chee et al., 2008). Lapses have also been related to greater activation of the "default mode network" (Drummond et al., 2005), a set of brain regions often found to be more active during passive wakefulness (Raichle et al., 2001). Although the available evidence is largely limited to studies with a night of total sleep deprivation, these brain changes may be interpreted as broadly consistent with the state instability hypothesis.

Yet, there is reason to believe the state instability hypothesis does not fully capture the essence of the effects of sleep deprivation on sustained attention task performance

(Hudson et al., 2020). Consider, for example, data from a two-choice numerosity discrimination task (Ratcliff & Van Dongen, 2009). Subjects completed 30 blocks of 40 trials, and in each trial between 31 and 70 asterisks were placed in random positions in a 10 by 10 array on a computer screen (see Figure 11.1C). Subjects were instructed to judge whether the number of asterisks was greater or less than 50 and to respond quickly and accurately. By varying the number of asterisks in each trial, this task systematically manipulates the quality of information provided, making accurate and fast responding easy (31–35 or 66–70 asterisks), moderately hard (36–40 or 61–65 asterisks), harder yet (41–45 or 56–60 asterisks), or extremely hard (46–55 asterisks). Data from the task were analyzed with the diffusion decision model (Ratcliff & McKoon, 2008), yielding an estimate of "drift rate" which may be seen as an index of the quality of information processing (cf. Chavali et al., 2017).

During a multiday laboratory study, the two-choice numerosity discrimination task was administered a total of three times, at 2-day intervals. While subjects were well rested for the first and third administrations, for the second they were either well rested or sleep-deprived. Predictably, drift rate reflected the difficulty of the trials—that is, the harder (i.e., closer to 50 asterisks) the trials, the lower the drift rate—such that the quality of information processing matched the quality of the information provided. When subjects were sleep-deprived, however, they responded more slowly and less accurately, such that drift rate characterized the trials as progressively more difficult (see Figure 11.1D). In other words, sleep deprivation degraded the quality of information processing, further diminishing the quality of the information provided as the basis for responding (Ratcliff & Van Dongen, 2009).

The state instability hypothesis does not really offer an explanation for this result. Rather, the finding points to a more general degradation of neuronal processing, brought about by external information in a *bottom-up* fashion, as an overarching mechanism by which sleep deprivation impairs sustained attention task performance (Hudson et al., 2020). This interpretation is consistent with the implications of local sleep theory (Van Dongen et al., 2011a). Further supporting this latter point of view, a study involving single-neuron recordings from intracranial electrodes in the medial temporal lobe of neurosurgical patients found evidence of degraded neuronal functioning that could be associated with a use-dependent, local sleep-like state. That is, while the patients performed a PVT-like task after sleep deprivation, the selective spiking responses of individual neurons in the medial temporal lobe preceding the slowest responses on the task were attenuated and delayed, suggesting that local sleep in neurons subserving task performance led to the observed lapses of attention (Nir et al., 2017).

Seemingly a universal consequence of sleep deprivation, evidence of the degradation of bottom-up information processing, whether or not due to local sleep, has been found in all kinds of performance tasks, including those that are not sustained attention tasks per se (Honn et al., 2018, 2020). However, as we shall see, degradation of bottom-up information processing does not, by itself, explain all effects of sleep deprivation on cognitive performance.

Interindividual Differences and Dissociable Components of Cognition

While the characteristic effects of sleep deprivation on cognitive performance are qualitatively similar from one person to another, there are substantial differences between individuals in the magnitude of performance impairment while sleep-deprived (Wilkinson, 1961). These interindividual differences have been shown to be stable and robust, constituting a human phenotype (Van Dongen et al., 2004), which is observed in both acute total sleep deprivation and sustained sleep restriction (Rupp et al., 2012). The phenotype is determined in part by genetic makeup (Satterfield et al., 2019), developmental state and aging (Campbell et al., 2018; Philip et al., 2004), and probably long-term sleep history (Grant & Van Dongen, 2013; Rupp et al., 2009) but for the larger part has remained unexplained.

Paradoxically, the phenotypic interindividual differences in performance impairment while sleep-deprived appear to be fundamentally task-dependent (Van Dongen et al., 2004), such that one person compared to another may be more vulnerable to impairment from sleep loss on one task and more resilient on another task. This divergence in the link between sleep and waking cognitive performance cannot be understood solely on the idea that sleep (and sleep intensity) and wakefulness (and sleepiness level) form a (quasi-) continuum of vigilance states (Ulrich & Frick, 1986) regulated centrally and modulated by physiological arousal (Saper & Fuller, 2017). Rather, consistent with local sleep theory (Van Dongen et al., 2011a), it implies that there are multiple, distinct aspects of cognition that may be affected by sleep deprivation independently (Jackson et al., 2013). In line with efforts to differentiate the effects of sleep deprivation on attentional networks (e.g., Riontino & Cavallero, 2022; Whitney et al., 2017) and other conceptual dissections of cognitive functioning (e.g., Habeck et al., 2005; Kurinec et al., 2021; Tucker et al., 2010), dissociation of separable components of cognition is critical for a more complete understanding of the impact of sleep loss on performance (Whitney & Hinson, 2010).

Sleep Loss and Impairment of Top-Down Attentional Control

Sleep deprivation has been found to impair a wide range of ostensibly unrelated, complex cognitive abilities, such as decision-making, problem-solving, and creativity (Harrison & Horne, 2000b; Killgore, 2010; Pilcher & Huffcut, 1996). However, the effects of sleep loss on tasks involving these abilities are generally much less pronounced than those on relatively "simple" tasks like the PVT (Lim & Dinges, 2010; Wickens et al., 2015). Functional neuroimaging evidence has revealed increasing activation of brain regions that appear to provide compensatory processing with increasing task difficulty and may thereby lessen the impact of sleep deprivation on more difficult tasks (Drummond et al., 2004). Although degraded bottom-up information processing may explain a range of performance impairments due to sleep deprivation (e.g., Mao et al., 2021), the diversity of cognitive functions involved in complex tasks and the variety of performance effects observed on such tasks in sleep-deprived people defy a universal explanation in terms of bottom-up information processing alone.

In addition to decreased brain activation in areas associated with bottom-up processing, neuroimaging studies investigating changes in selective attention during sleep deprivation (Chee et al., 2008, 2011; Chee & Tan, 2010) have observed decreased activation in frontoparietal brain areas linked to top-down attentional control (Corbetta & Shulman, 2002). Top-down attentional control refers to the ability for contextual or previously learned information to influence the allocation of attention, directly or indirectly, in a goal-directed manner (Braver, 2012; Draheim et al., 2022; Egner, 2017; Katsuki & Constantinidis, 2014). To examine top-down control, the aforementioned neuroimaging studies used selective attention tasks that manipulated the need for top-down attentional control during functional brain imaging and investigated brain activation during portions of tasks that specifically required top-down control.

For instance, Chee and Tan (2010) had subjects complete a visual selective attention task in the scanner after a night of normal sleep and after a night of sleep deprivation. Subjects were shown a large, global letter (H or S) composed of smaller, local letters (H or S) and had to identify the local letters, which were either congruent (same letter) or incongruent (different letter) with the global letter. The difficulty of the task varied by level of contrast (5%, 25%, or 50%); less contrast made the task more difficult. Compared to their rested performance, subjects were worse at identifying the local letters during sleep deprivation and, regardless of the level of task difficulty, showed reduced activation in the frontoparietal regions where top-down signals that guide attention are believed to originate (see Figure 11.2A). The diminished frontoparietal activation during sleep deprivation is thought to reflect a disruption of the signals critical for capturing top-down attentional control (Chee & Tan, 2010; Chee et al., 2011), which makes it more difficult to direct attention in a top-down, goal-directed manner when sleep-deprived.

Separate neuroimaging studies have found that in sleep-deprived individuals, frontoparietal regions related to top-down attentional control have altered functional connectivity with brain networks pivotal for bottom-up processing (Chuah et al., 2010; Ning et al., 2022; Yoo et al., 2007). Collectively, these neuroimaging findings suggest that sleep deprivation disrupts the generation or processing of signals that should focus attention on information that is relevant with regard to goals or expectations, and thereby makes top-down attentional control less efficient. This conclusion is supported by behavioral studies showing that sleep deprivation impairs performance on a variety of tasks that require top-down attentional control (e.g., Gevers et al., 2015; Kusztor et al., 2019).

However, while top-down attentional control may be impaired during sleep deprivation, it may not be entirely absent or ineffective. This was well illustrated by Stenson et

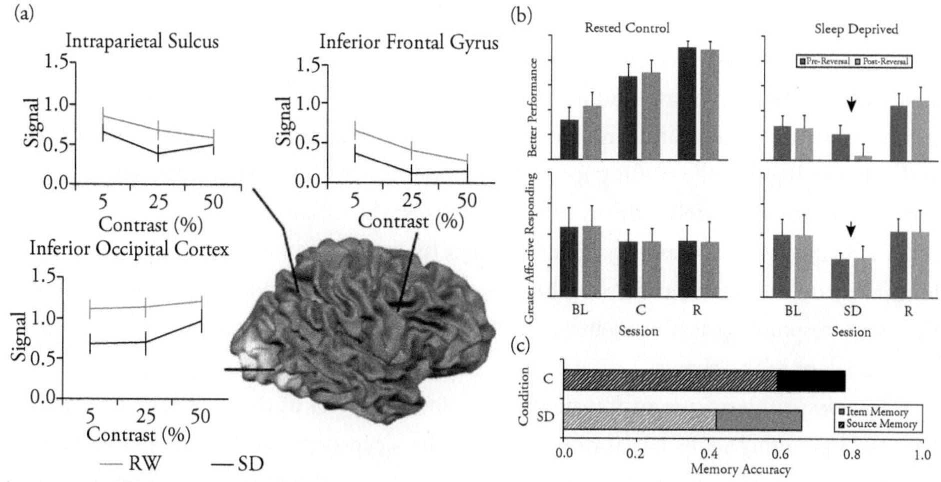

Figure 11.2 Sleep deprivation and top-down attentional control

Note. Panel a: Sleep deprivation reduces activation in frontoparietal areas where top-down control signals are thought to originate. Subjects' patterns of brain activation were measured with functional magnetic resonance imaging while they performed a visual selective attention task with varying degrees of stimulus contrast, under both rested wakefulness (grey) and sleep deprivation (black) conditions. Means (± standard error) of 20 healthy young adults are shown. Regardless of the degree of stimulus contrast level, the sleep deprivation condition was associated with lower activation in the intraparietal sulcus, inferior frontal gyrus, and inferior occipital cortex. Activated areas during rested wakefulness are shown in as brighter areas on the image of the brain. Figure taken from Chee and Tan (2010) with permission. Panel b: Sleep deprivation impairs the ability to flexibly adapt top-down attentional control to adjust to a change in contingencies (top) and blunts physiological responses to feedback (bottom). Subjects completed a modified go/no-go reversal learning task three times (once every 2 days) during a 7-day in-laboratory study. This task involved learning stimulus–response pairings based on feedback (pre-reversal phase) and adapting to a reversal of contingencies about midway through the task, also based on feedback (post-reversal phase). Data of 26 healthy young adults were analyzed; half the sample was randomly assigned to 62 hours of sleep deprivation during the second session; the other half served as rested controls. Means (bars) and standard errors (whiskers) are shown. Rested controls showed a steady improvement in their ability to identify the stimulus–response pairings and correctly discriminate between go and no-go stimuli across the three task administrations, both pre-reversal (dark grey bars) and post-reversal (light grey bars). By contrast, sleep-deprived subjects showed poorer performance during the second session, when they were sleep-deprived (top graphs, downward arrow), especially in the post-reversal phase. This poorer performance was accompanied by decreased affective reactions to feedback, giving rise to the concept of "feedback blunting" (bottom graphs, downward arrow). The sleep-deprived subjects' performance also did not improve as much as that of their well-rested counterparts during the third session, after recovery sleep (top right graph). This reduced learning suggests that binding of information together in memory was impaired during sleep deprivation (cf. panel c), such that sleep-deprived subjects benefited less from practice. Figure adapted from Whitney et al. (2015) with permission. Panel c: Sleep deprivation impairs the ability to bind, or associate, information in memory. Subjects completed an item and source memory task twice during a 4-day in-laboratory study. This task required them to remember individual items (words) and the source or context of those items (male or female speaker). Data of 68 healthy young adults were analyzed; approximately half the sample was assigned to 38 hours of sleep deprivation, and the remaining half served as rested controls. During the second session, unlike rested subjects, sleep-deprived subjects showed poorer recognition memory accuracy for individual words (item memory, solid bars) and, for those items they did correctly recognize, poorer memory for the associated speakers (source memory, hashed bars). Figure adapted from Kurinec et al. (2021) with permission. BL = baseline; R = recovery; RW = rested wakefulness; SD/C = sleep deprivation or control.

al. (2023) using the Flexible Attentional Control Task (FACT). On this task, subjects are shown cues followed by target stimuli consisting of either a smiling icon or an angry icon. The cues can be valid (e.g., the word *friend* before a smiling icon), invalid (e.g., the word *friend* before an angry icon), or uninformative (i.e., the phrase *no hint*). Subjects must indicate, as quickly as possible before an individualized deadline, whether the displayed icon is a smiling "friend" or an angry "foe"; they are given feedback to inform them whether their response was correct. In the first half of the task, the majority of trials have valid cues (pre-switch phase). Subjects can thus use cues to anticipate the appearance of the corresponding icons and prepare to respond accordingly (e.g., seeing the cue *friend* and anticipating that the smiling icon will be shown), which yields accurate responses on most trails. Approximately halfway through the task, the validity of the cues changes, such that the majority of trials now have invalid cues (post-switch phase). Subjects can thus no longer rely on the cues to anticipate the appearance of the corresponding icons; as a result, they start responding less accurately, and based on the feedback they receive they must learn to adapt to the change.

To assess subjects' use of top-down attentional control during the FACT to anticipate the upcoming icons based on the cues while sleep-deprived, Stenson et al. (2023) investigated the facilitation effect—the extent to which valid cues increase performance accuracy compared to uninformative cues—and the interference effect—the extent to which invalid cues decrease performance accuracy compared to uninformative cues. Of note, the higher frequency of valid cue trials in the pre-switch phase and invalid cues in the post-switch phase could result in automatic priming through repetition, which would improve performance on these respective trials. However, when the facilitation effect and the interference effect are observed in conjunction, automatic priming cannot be the sole explanation, and it can be inferred that top-down attentional control was being used.

Stenson et al. (2023) had subjects complete the FACT under both rested and sleep-deprived conditions. When the subjects were rested, they showed evidence of both facilitation and interference effects (i.e., use of top-down attentional control) in the pre-switch phase of the task. Whereas they continued to show the facilitation effect in the post-switch phase, the interference effect was smaller, indicating subjects partially abandoned the use of top-down control after being confronted with the change in cue validity. The same thing happened in the post-switch phase when subjects were sleep-deprived. In the pre-switch phase, however, the facilitation effect increased while the interference effect decreased, indicating that automatic priming contributed to sleep-deprived subjects' performance while the effectiveness of top-down control was diminished. Collectively, these results suggest that although sleep-deprived subjects primarily benefited from implicit priming, they were also able to use top-down attentional control; but sleep deprivation reduced the use or effectiveness of top-down control to overcome degraded bottom-up processing.

The finding that sleep deprivation disrupts processes involved in top-down attentional control, but not more automatic processes like implicit priming, helps to explain deficits on tasks that are unlikely to be related to problems with bottom-up processing, such as tasks involving emotion regulation. *Emotion regulation* is the ability to influence one's emotional state or expression, usually in a goal-directed manner (McRae &

Gross, 2020). To regulate their emotions successfully, subjects must deliberately use top-down control mechanisms to implement specific strategies (e.g., distracting their attention from a displeasing stimulus or suppressing an emotional response). Various strategies for emotion regulation have been linked to interindividual differences in attentional control (Hendricks & Buchanan, 2016; Ochsner & Gross, 2005; Pruessner et al., 2020).

Sleep deprivation has been shown to impair the ability to regulate emotions (Harrington et al., 2021; Stenson et al., 2021; Tomaso et al., 2021; J. Zhang et al., 2019). For instance, in a study with a sleep deprivation condition and a rested control condition (Stenson et al., 2021), subjects were shown images from a standardized image database (Lang et al., 2008). When shown images known to elicit a negative emotional response (e.g., spiders, snakes), the sleep-deprived subjects reported similar ratings of how negative they felt as the rested subjects. However, when instructed to engage in emotion regulation strategies to reduce their emotional reaction while viewing the negative images, the sleep-deprived individuals reported higher negative ratings than their rested counterparts, indicating less effective emotion regulation. In a similar study with sleep deprivation and rested control conditions (J. Zhang et al., 2019), individuals viewed four trial blocks of negative images drawn from the same image database. During each block, subjects either viewed the images normally or applied one of three emotion regulation strategies, while event-related potentials were measured in the electroencephalogram. The rested controls showed reductions in experienced emotion when using the emotion regulation strategies compared to viewing them normally, as reflected by a reduced amplitude of the late positive component of the event-related potentials, which indexes emotional processing. By contrast, the sleep-deprived subjects did not show any differences in late positive potential amplitude when using the emotion regulation strategies, suggesting less effective strategy use. Together, these findings suggest that while bottom-up processing of affective stimuli (e.g., the ability for negative stimuli to elicit an emotional response) is preserved, sleep deprivation renders people less able to redirect their attention from the negative stimuli, which is in line with the proposition that sleep deprivation produces deficits in top-down attentional control. Issues with top-down control could potentially contribute to other self-regulation problems reported to be associated with sleep loss as well, such as deviations from socially acceptable behavior (Dorrian et al., 2019).

Impairments in Cognitive Flexibility Due to Sleep Deprivation

Deficits in top-down attentional control during sleep deprivation may extend to problems with cognitive control more broadly. In laboratory tasks, the use of top-down control is often manipulated by making the task environments predictable so that subjects can develop expectations about the stimuli and their subsequent responses. But not all environments are consistently predictable, and people may have to adapt when information in the environment indicates that conditions have changed. Research has shown that sleep deprivation impairs cognitive flexibility, or the ability to reallocate one's attention when task contingencies change (Bratzke et al., 2009; Couyoumdjian et al., 2010; Heuer et al., 2004; Slama et al., 2018; Whitney et al., 2015, 2017). This impairment is particularly evident on reversal learning tasks, which require subjects to first learn to discriminate between two or more choices based on feedback regarding choice outcomes, then recognize when the choice–outcome relationships change or reverse at some point during the task and modify their behavior accordingly (Izquierdo et al., 2017; Yaple & Yu, 2019).

In a study with a sleep deprivation condition and a rested control condition (Whitney et al., 2015), subjects performed a modified go/no-go reversal learning task where they had to learn, from feedback, which stimuli required a response (button press) and which required withholding a response (no button press). Halfway through the task the contingencies reversed unannounced, such that unexpectedly the original go stimuli were now no-go stimuli and vice versa, and subjects had to use feedback to detect and adapt to the reversal. Subjects completed the task three times: after 2 nights of baseline sleep, after either 2 nights of extended wakefulness (sleep deprivation condition) or sleep (rested control condition), and after 2 nights of recovery sleep. Those who had been deprived of sleep performed worse than their rested counterparts and worse than their own baseline (non-sleep-deprived) performance (see Figure 11.2B, top panels). Notably, while sleep-deprived performance was poorer both before and after the reversal, the impairment was especially profound after the reversal, suggesting a near-complete inability to flexibly reallocate attention.

The poorer cognitive flexibility exhibited by sleep-deprived subjects on reversal learning tasks has been demonstrated to be distinct from the effects of sleep deprivation on bottom-up processing. In rested subjects, simulating the possible effects of lapsing on information processing in up to 40% of trials of the modified go/no-go reversal learning task by withholding outcome feedback failed to reproduce the pattern of effects seen during sleep deprivation (Whitney et al., 2015). Separately, upon embedding a probe recognition procedure in the task, sleep-deprived subjects showed no difficulty identifying which stimuli they had been shown during trials, with similarly high rates of accuracy as their rested counterparts (Honn et al., 2019). Thus, the problems with cognitive flexibility did not appear to be related to issues with attending to or processing of stimuli. Evidence from skin conductance responses to feedback, which were blunted in sleep-deprived individuals, pointed to a reduction in the salience of the feedback—a phenomenon termed *feedback blunting* (Whitney et al., 2015; see Figure 11.2B, bottom panels).

Although it is as yet unclear whether feedback blunting is a direct or indirect consequence of sleep deprivation, the reduced salience of feedback makes it less likely for the feedback to spontaneously capture and guide attention. This contributes to poorer performance when cognitive flexibility is required and may underlie perseverative behavior and other performance impairments when sleep-deprived individuals are in uncertain, dynamic environments and must use feedback in order to determine the appropriate course of action (Whitney et al., 2015).

The Effects of Extended Wakefulness on Learning and Memory

It is well established that sleep plays a role in the consolidation of memories (Jenkins & Dallenback, 1924; MacDonald & Cote, 2021; Rasch & Born, 2013; Walker & Stickgold, 2004) and that forgoing sleep therefore has significant impact on learning and memory retention (see Chapter 10 of this volume). However, learning and memory are affected not only by whether or not individuals are sleep deprived *after* learning new information but also by whether or not they are sleep-deprived during learning itself. How lack of sleep affects memory processes depends on the type of memory in question. Researchers generally differentiate between short-term memory or working memory, a memory store with limited capacity where information in the focus of attention can be manipulated in pursuit of a given goal, and long-term memory, a memory store with effectively unlimited capacity where memories from across the life span can be stored and retrieved (Cowan, 2008; Engle, 2002; Jeneson & Squire, 2012). Working memory and long-term memory are connected, and information can be transferred from working memory to long-term memory and vice versa (Bartsch & Shepherdson, 2022; McCabe, 2008). Moreover, how well information is maintained in working memory has been linked to how well information is later stored in long-term memory, suggesting a critical relationship between the two with regard to learning (Forsberg et al., 2021; Hartshorne & Makovski, 2019). Although exactly how working and long-term memory are connected remains a topic of investigation, these two types of memory are dissociable and can be studied separately (Baddeley & Warrington, 1970; Unsworth, 2010).

Working memory is essential for retaining and manipulating information within a short period of time. Aspects of working memory that are of particular interest in the context of sleep deprivation include working memory maintenance and the updating of working memory. Tasks that measure working memory maintenance, such as digit span and working memory scanning tasks, focus on how much information can be maintained in the focus of attention at a given time and how well information maintained in working memory can be searched and retrieved. Updating tasks, on the other hand, assess the ability to replace information in working memory that is no longer relevant. Although research on the effect of sleep deprivation on working memory has generally been mixed, the findings suggest that information in the focus of attention can be maintained during sleep loss (Drummond et al., 2012; Giacobbo et al., 2016; Tucker et al., 2010; Whitney et al., 2015). For example, Whitney and colleagues (2015) found that although sleep-deprived subjects had difficulties encoding or learning new information, their ability to maintain and scan information that did get into working memory was preserved. Thus, once information is contained in working memory, it appears it can be maintained, searched, and retrieved during sleep deprivation.

By contrast, sleep deprivation has been found to impair the ability to update information in working memory (Song et al., 2022; L. Zhang et al., 2019). Song and colleagues (2022) assigned subjects to complete two versions of a two-back task during baseline and during 36 hours of sleep deprivation. On a location version of the two-back task, subjects viewed black squares located in one of the four corners of a screen. They indicated on each trial whether the location of the black square matched that of the one shown two trials back. On an object version of the two-back task, subjects viewed a series of shapes. They indicated on each trial whether the shape shown matched that shown two trials back. On both versions of the task, it was found that subjects had lower accuracy when sleep-deprived than when rested, indicating that the ability to update information in working memory is impaired by sleep loss. These problems with working memory updating imply that sleep-deprived individuals are less able to replace outdated information when contingencies change (Whitney et al., 2019) and, as such, may be linked to performance impairments on cognitive flexibility tasks during sleep deprivation.

Long-term memory is critical for remembering information over the long run. Most studies of long-term memory in the context of sleep deprivation have focused on the ability to learn and later remember stimuli that are not intrinsically associated, such as random pictures or words. There is a well-documented, negative impact of sleep deprivation on memory retention subsequent to learning, which has revealed the active role of sleep in memory consolidation processes; this is covered elsewhere (see Chapter 10 of this volume). Sleep deprivation during encoding, or initial learning, also results in poorer memory (Drummond et al., 2000; Kaida et al., 2015; Kurinec et al., 2021; Poh & Chee, 2017; Ratcliff & Van Dongen, 2018; Saletin et al., 2016)—even if sleep-deprived subjects are allowed to sleep before memory testing occurs (Tempesta et al., 2016; Yoo et al., 2007). Given that the ability to retrieve already-consolidated information out of long-term memory does not appear to be impaired by sleep deprivation (Idzikowski, 1984; Schönauer et al., 2015), it follows that individuals are less able to encode new information into long-term memory if they are sleep-deprived. Moreover, whereas memory consolidation processes interrupted by sleep loss can sometimes be resumed at the next sleep opportunity (Schönauer et al., 2015), disruptions to initial learning are unlikely to be ameliorated by later sleep. As such, impairments to encoding may help explain why sleep-deprived individuals continue to show poorer performance than rested counterparts even after recovery sleep (Chai et al., 2020; Sallinen et al., 2008; Whitney et al., 2015).

Extended Wakefulness Disrupts Binding in Memory

Sleep deprivation also appears to disrupt the ability to associate pieces of information together in memory, which is sometimes referred to as *associative* or *relational memory*. Studies investigating associative memory for pairs of words or images have found that sleep deprivation impairs performance in this respect (Falleti et al., 2003; Ratcliff & Van Dongen, 2018). While remembering pairs of words or images may have limited utility in the real world, the ability to make associations among similar or different items in memory is critical for daily life. Crucially, being able to associate or "bind" an item with the context it was presented in is necessary for forming memories of events (Zimmer et al., 2006). Such memories could be as simple as remembering that one left one's key (item) in the kitchen (context), but they could also be more complex, with an item being bound to additional spatial, temporal, and other contextual elements of the scene. For example, a memory for a colleague's visit could be associated with contextual information on who was present for the visit, when it occurred, why the colleague was in town, and how the visit was perceived.

The ability to bind items with their context and form memories of events depends on the hippocampus (Olsen et al., 2012; Yonelinas, 2013). During sleep deprivation, the hippocampus shows compromised functioning (Van Der Werf et al., 2009; Yoo et al., 2007) and reduced functional connectivity with other brain regions critical for memory, such as the prefrontal cortex (Chai et al., 2020; Yoo et al., 2007). As a result, people exhibit poorer memory for context during sleep deprivation (Harrison & Horne, 2000a; Kaida et al., 2015; Kurinec et al., 2021; Tempesta et al., 2016). They may also be less likely to benefit from practice in tasks that rely on subjects' actions to be associated with feedback in order to learn from one's successes and mistakes, like in reversal learning tasks (Whitney et al., 2015; see Figure 11.2B). Notably, problems with binding during sleep deprivation are not caused merely by failure to learn the individual pieces of information, as sleep-deprived subjects show poorer memory for the bound contextual information even when memory for the individual items is intact (Kurinec et al., 2021).

In a study with a sleep deprivation and rested control condition, Kurinec and colleagues (2021) tested subjects for words (items) that had originally been heard as spoken by either a male or a female speaker (context). The researchers found that sleep-deprived subjects were less likely to remember that a given word had been heard at study than their rested counterparts. Importantly, for words they did correctly recognize as having been studied, they were less likely to correctly remember the speaker (male or female; see Figure 11.2C). Because subjects had to listen to the words during study, they processed the words and the associated speaker identities at the same time. Intact memory of a word was therefore evidence that the speaker information was also encoded. As such, failures to remember speakers did not reflect a problem learning the speaker information per se but rather indicated a problem associating speakers with words (i.e., a binding problem).

Sleep deprivation–induced binding problems have significant consequences for people's ability to correctly remember the spatial, temporal, and other contextual information of events and experiences (who, what, when, where, and how). Difficulty forming intact memories of events and experiences due to binding failures induced by sleep loss is arguably a threat to one's ability to function well in daily life, in particular in operational settings where accurate situational awareness is crucial. In many high-stakes occupations, such as emergency services, transportation, search-and-rescue, law enforcement, and the military, people must bind spatial, temporal, and other contextual information in order to navigate their environment. If individuals working in these fields have trouble binding contextual information during sleep deprivation, either because they are unable to bind the information at all or because their bindings are less precise and thus harder to retrieve (Ekstrom & Yonelinas, 2020), they will be less able to maintain situational awareness and remember the information they need to successfully carry out their mission (e.g., the location an enemy last fired from or where a missing hiker's wallet was found). Research on this issue is scarce, but the implications for those types of occupations, as well as other activities that depend on accurate memory—like eyewitness testimony (Frenda et al., 2014)—are significant.

Distinct but Interrelated and Integrated Mechanisms

As discussed throughout this chapter, sleep deprivation has distinct effects on different aspects of cognition, which also exhibit differential interindividual differences. As performance tasks involve multiple, interrelated cognitive abilities, deficits in any one of these abilities may lead to diminished performance. This makes it difficult to predict how sleep loss will impair performance on any given task. Careful task analysis is required to determine which cognitive abilities, such as facets of attention or memory, are directly impaired by sleep deprivation and which, if any, are downstream consequences (Whitney & Hinson, 2010).

The effects of sleep deprivation on bottom-up information processing are well established, such that individuals are more likely to miss the presentation of stimuli in the environment and the quality of the information they do receive is poorer, making it more difficult to respond in a timely and accurate manner. Current knowledge about the temporal dynamics of performance and the involvement of the circadian, homeostatic, and allostatic processes, as described earlier in this chapter, has been established primarily on the basis of observed deficits in bottom-up information processing (Hudson et al., 2020). However, these deficits in bottom-up processing are unlikely to explain all the disparate impairments from sleep loss that have been documented in the literature.

Rather, many of the other sleep deprivation–related deficits involve failures in the engagement of top-down attentional control, resulting in a reduced or even extinguished ability to use contextual or learned information to facilitate performance and/or overcome bottom-up processing-related impairments. Because many tasks require individuals to engage attention in a goal-directed manner, failures of top-down control during sleep deprivation may unite a range of performance deficits on seemingly unrelated tasks, from emotion regulation to cognitive flexibility to divided attention (Gevers et al., 2015; Jackson et al., 2011; Stenson et al., 2021). It has been suggested that even the deficits observed on the archetypal task for assessing bottom-up impairment in information processing, the PVT, may be in part due to a disrupted ability to engage top-down attentional control to anticipate and prepare responses and/or to overcome the challenge posed by degraded bottom-up information processing (Honn & Van Dongen, 2023; Kong et al., 2015; Sarter et al., 2001).

How sleep deprivation disrupts top-down attentional control remains unclear. Top-down attentional control signals originate primarily in the prefrontal cortex (Katsuki & Constantinidis, 2014), which is thought to be especially vulnerable to sleep loss (Harrison et al., 2000). Sleep deprivation may disrupt the dissemination of those signals, leaving individuals unable to focus attention in a goal-directed manner. Another possibility is that sleep deprivation has an indirect effect on top-down control because it impairs underlying cognitive components that are necessary for engaging attention. Problems employing top-down attentional control may thus be the manifestation of upstream impairments in other cognitive abilities. Indeed, there are multiple ways for sleep deprivation–induced impairments in other cognitive abilities to contribute to deficits in top-down attentional control.

For example, degradation of bottom-up processing may lead to less effective binding of information together in long-term memory. In turn, this binding problem may explain some of the deficits in adjusting top-down attentional control in decision-making tasks that require learning correct or advantageous responses from feedback, including the previously described "feedback blunting" phenomenon observed by Whitney and colleagues (2015). On the modified go/no-go reversal learning task used in their study, subjects had to use information from feedback to learn the stimulus–response pairings of the task and adapt to the reversal of contingencies occurring about midway through the task (Figure 11.2B). If sleep-deprived individuals were less able to bind the stimulus–response pairings or the response–feedback associations, they would be impaired in learning the correct stimulus–response pairings and would thus be less able to form clear expectations about what the outcomes of their response choices should be. Without clear expectations about these choice outcomes, the feedback they received would be less salient, and signals from the prefrontal cortex indicating that a change in contingencies had occurred would be less likely to change the focus of attention. This would reduce cognitive flexibility following the reversal of contingencies in the task and would manifest as perseveration on a response strategy that no longer produces optimal performance. Thus, a sleep loss–induced binding problem may be the root cause of the reduction in the salience of feedback, resulting in diminished affective reactions as measured by skin conductance responses, as well as the concomitant top-down attentional control deficit resulting in poorer decision-making on the reversal learning task. While there is some reasoned speculation included in this example, it illustrates how the mechanisms underlying performance impairment due to sleep deprivation on a given task may involve multiple, interrelated cognitive abilities.

Their integrated impact may not be readily apparent from the observed performance outcomes and necessitates careful experimentation and in-depth analysis to uncover (Jackson et al., 2013; Whitney & Hinson, 2010).

Conclusion and Future Directions

In addition to performance impairment on relatively well-defined tasks used to study the effects of sleep and sleep loss on human performance in laboratory settings, it has long been recognized that sleep deprivation contributes to performance errors and accidents in the real world (Dinges, 1995; Van Dongen et al., 2022). Future research is needed to determine the extent to which sleep deprivation–related impairments in performance inside and outside of the laboratory can be ascribed to deficits in bottom-up processing and/or top-down attentional control. In many contexts, problems with bottom-up processing during sleep loss are well recognized, and countermeasures of varying efficacy have been developed and evaluated (Rosekind et al., 1997; Wesensten, 2012). However, problems associated with top-down attentional control are often more difficult to discern and address; for instance, perseverative behavior may only become apparent when people fail to adapt to changing circumstances, at which point it may be too late to intervene. Research on what deficits may presage loss of top-down control during sleep deprivation, such as problems with working memory updating or long-term memory binding, could provide valuable information for the development of novel countermeasures.

Sleep loss has been cited as a factor in numerous incidents and accidents, particularly in settings where sleep loss is common, such as healthcare, transportation, and the military (Åkerstedt et al., 2011; Caldwell, 2012; Gurubhagavatula et al., 2021; Landrigan et al., 2005; LoPresti et al., 2016). Individuals with sleep disorders may also be more predisposed to cognitive impairments commonly associated with sleep loss, which may contribute to poorer work performance (Swanson et al., 2011) and a higher rate of driving accidents (Catarino et al., 2014; Philip et al., 2010). Exploring how the effects of sleep deprivation on cognitive performance manifest outside of the laboratory and contribute to real-world outcomes is an important future direction for understanding the relationship between sleep and human performance (Monk, 2007; Raslear et al., 2011; Van Dongen et al., 2022).

Lastly, most research in this context has focused on understanding the consequences of sleep loss in individuals, but in fields like medicine or the military individuals rarely work alone. More work is needed to determine how individual deficits in performance and the underlying cognitive components contribute to failures in team situational awareness and decision-making (Banks et al., 2019; Miller & Shattuck, 2005). Such work would help explain how sleep deprivation contributes to disasters such as aviation or nuclear accidents, where multiple people fail to either detect an error or intervene upon doing so. As long as sleep loss continues to be widespread (Basner et al., 2014), the importance of further research in these areas cannot be overstated.

References

Åkerstedt, T., Philip, P., Capelli, A., & Kecklund, G. (2011). Sleep loss and accidents—Work hours, life style, and sleep pathology. In H. P. A. Van Dongen & G. A. Kerkhof (Eds.), *Human sleep and cognition Part II: Clinical and applied research. Progress in Brain Research* (Vol. 190, pp. 169–188). Elsevier.

Baddeley, A. D., & Warrington, E. K. (1970). Amnesia and the distinction between long- and short-term memory. *Journal of Verbal Learning and Verbal Behavior, 9*(2), 176–189.

Balkin, T. J., Braun, A. R., Wesensten, N. J., Jeffries, K., Varga, M., Baldwin, P., Belenky, G., & Herscovitch, P. (2002). The process of awakening: A PET study of regional brain activity patterns mediating the re-establishment of alertness and consciousness. *Brain, 125*(10), 2308–2319.

Banks, S., Landon, L. B., Dorrian, J., Waggoner, L. B., Centofanti, S. A., Roma, P. G., & Van Dongen, H. P. A. (2019). Effects of fatigue on teams and their role in 24/7 operations. *Sleep Medicine Reviews, 48*, Article 101216.

Bartsch, L. M., & Shepherdson, P. (2022). Freeing capacity in working memory (WM) through the use of long-term memory (LTM) representations. *Journal of Experimental Psychology: Learning, Memory, and Cognition, 48*(4), 465–482.

Basner, M., Spaeth, A. M., & Dinges, D. F. (2014). Sociodemographic characteristics and waking activities and their role in the timing and duration of sleep. *Sleep, 37*(12), 1889–1906.

Belenky, G., Wesensten, N.J., Thorne, D. R., Thomas, M. L., Sing, H. C., Redmond, D. P., Russo, M. B., & Balkin, T. J. (2003). Patterns of performance degradation and restoration during sleep restriction and subsequent recovery: A sleep dose–response study. *Journal of Sleep Research, 12*(1), 1–12.

Benington, J. H., & Heller, H. C. (1995). Restoration of brain energy metabolism as the function of sleep. *Progress in Neurobiology, 45*, 347–360.

Borbély, A. A. (1982). A two process model of sleep regulation. *Human Neurobiology, 1*, 195–204.

Bratzke, D., Rolke, B., Steinborn, M. B., & Ulrich, R. (2009). The effect of 40 h constant wakefulness on task-switching efficiency. *Journal of Sleep Research, 18*(2), 167–172.

Braver, T. S. (2012). The variable nature of cognitive control: A dual mechanisms framework. *Trends in Cognitive Sciences, 16*(2), 106–113.

Cajochen, C. A., Foy, R., & Dijk, D.-J. (1999). Frontal predominance of a relative increase in sleep delta and theta EEG activity after sleep loss in humans. *Journal of Sleep Research, 2*(3), 65–69.

Caldwell, J. A. (2012). Crew schedules, sleep deprivation, and aviation performance. *Current Directions in Psychological Science, 21*(2), 85–89.

Campbell, I. G., Van Dongen, H. P. A., Gainer, M., Karmouta, E., & Feinberg, I. (2018). Differential and interacting effects of age and sleep restriction on daytime sleepiness and vigilance in adolescence: A longitudinal study. *Sleep, 41*(12), Article zsy177.

Catarino, R., Spratley, J., Catarino, I., Lunet, N., & Pais-Clemente, M. (2014). Sleepiness and sleep-disordered breathing in truck drivers. *Sleep and Breathing, 18*(1), 59–68.

Chai, Y., Fang, Z., Yang, F. N., Xu, S., Deng, Y., Raine, A., Wang, J., Yu, M., Basner, M., Goel, N., Kim, J. J., Wolk, D. A., Detre, J. A., Dinges, D. F., & Rao, H. (2020). Two nights of recovery sleep restores hippocampal connectivity but not episodic memory after total sleep deprivation. *Scientific Reports, 10*(1), Article 8774.

Chavali, V. P., Riedy, S. M., & Van Dongen, H. P. A. (2017). Signal-to-noise ratio in PVT performance as a cognitive measure of the effect of sleep deprivation on the fidelity of information processing. *Sleep, 40*(3), Article zsx016.

Chee, M. W. L., Goh, C. S. F., Namburi, P., Parimal, S., Seidl, K. N., & Kastner, S. (2011). Effects of sleep deprivation on cortical activation during directed attention in the absence and presence of visual stimuli. *NeuroImage, 58*(2), 595–604.

Chee, M. W. L., & Tan, J. C. (2010). Lapsing when sleep deprived: Neural activation characteristics of resistant and vulnerable individuals. *NeuroImage, 51*(2), 835–843.

Chee, M. W. L., Tan, J. C., Zheng, H., Parimal, S., Weissman, D. H., Zagorodnov, V., & Dinges, D. F. (2008). Lapsing during sleep deprivation is associated with distributed changes in brain activation. *Journal of Neuroscience, 28*(21), 5519–5528.

Chuah, L. Y. M., Dolcos, F., Chen, A. K., Zheng, H., Parimal, S., & Chee, M. W. L. (2010). Sleep deprivation and interference by emotional distracters. *Sleep, 33*(10), 1305–1313.

Corbetta, M., & Shulman, G. L. (2002). Control of goal-directed and stimulus-driven attention in the brain. *Nature Reviews Neuroscience, 3*(3), 201–215.

Couyoumdjian, A., Sdoia, S., Tempesta, D., Curcio, G., Rastellini, E., Gennaro, L. D., & Ferrara, M. (2010). The effects of sleep and sleep deprivation on task-switching performance. *Journal of Sleep Research, 19*(1 Pt. 1), 64–70.

Cowan, N. (2008). What are the differences between long-term, short-term, and working memory? In W. S. Sossin, J.-C. Lacaille, V. F. Castellucci, & S. Belleville (Eds.), *Essence of memory. Progress in Brain Research* (Vol. 169, pp. 323–338). Elsevier.

Daan, S., Beersma, D. G. M., & Borbély, A. A. (1984). Timing of human sleep: Recovery process gated by a circadian pacemaker. *American Journal of Physiology, 246*(18), R161–R178.

Dijk, D.-J., & Czeisler, C. A. (1994). Paradoxical timing of the circadian rhythm of sleep propensity serves to consolidate sleep and wakefulness in humans. *Neuroscience Letters, 166*(1), 63–68.

Dinges, D. F. (1995). An overview of sleepiness and accidents. *Journal of Sleep Research, 4*(S2), 4–14.

Dinges, D. F., & Kribbs, N. B. (1991). Performing while sleepy: Effects of experimentally-induced sleepiness. In T. H. Monk (Ed.), *Sleep, sleepiness and performance* (pp. 97–128). John Wiley & Sons.

Dinges, D. F., & Powell, J. W. (1985). Microcomputer analyses of performance on a portable, simple visual RT task during sustained operations. *Behavior Research Methods, Instruments, & Computers, 17*, 652–655.

Doran, S. M., Van Dongen, H. P. A., & Dinges, D.F. (2001). Sustained attention performance during sleep deprivation: Evidence of state instability. *Archives Italiennes de Biologie, 139*(3), 253–267.

Dorrian, J., Centofanti, S., Smith, A., & McDermott, K. D. (2019). Self-regulation and social behavior during sleep deprivation. In H. P. A. Van Dongen, P. Whitney, J. M. Hinson, K. A. Honn, & M. W. L. Chee (Eds.), *Sleep deprivation and cognition. Progress in Brain Research* (Vol. 246, pp. 73–110). Elsevier.

Dorrian, J., Rogers, N. L., & Dinges, D. F. (2005). Psychomotor vigilance performance: Neurocognitive assay sensitive to sleep loss. In C. A. Kushida (Ed.), *Sleep deprivation: Clinical issues, pharmacology, and sleep loss effects* (pp. 39–70). Marcel Dekker.

Draheim, C., Pak, R., Draheim, A. A., & Engle, R. W. (2022). The role of attention control in complex real-world tasks. *Psychonomic Bulletin & Review, 29*, 1143–1197.

Drummond, S. P. A., Anderson, D. E., Straus, L. D., Vogel, E. K., & Perez, V. B. (2012). The effects of two types of sleep deprivation on visual working memory capacity and filtering efficiency. *PLOS ONE, 7*(4), Article e35653.

Drummond, S. P. A., Bischoff-Grethe, A., Dinges, D. F., Ayalon, L., Mednick, S. C., & Meloy, M. J. (2005). The neural basis of the psychomotor vigilance task. *Sleep, 28*(9), 1059–1068.

Drummond, S. P. A., Brown, G. G., Gillin, J. C., Stricker, J. L., Wong, E. C., & Buxton, R. B. (2000). Altered brain response to verbal learning following sleep deprivation. *Nature, 403*(6770), 655–657.

Drummond, S. P. A., Brown, G. G., Salamat, J. S., & Gillin, J. C. (2004). Increasing task difficulty facilitates the cerebral compensatory response to total sleep deprivation. *Sleep, 27*(3), 445–451.

Eban-Rothschild, A., Appelbaum, L., & de Lecea, L. (2018). Neuronal mechanisms for sleep/wake regulation and modulatory drive. *Neuropsychopharmacology, 43*, 937–952.

Egner, T. (Ed.). (2017). *The Wiley handbook of cognitive control.* John Wiley & Sons.

Ekstrom, A. D., & Yonelinas, A. P. (2020). Precision, binding, and the hippocampus: Precisely what are we talking about? *Neuropsychologia, 138*, Article 107341.

Engle, R. W. (2002). Working memory capacity as executive attention. *Current Directions in Psychological Science, 11*(1), 19–23.

Falleti, M. G., Maruff, P., Collie, A., Darby, D. G., & McStephen, M. (2003). Qualitative similarities in cognitive impairment associated with 24 h of sustained wakefulness and a blood alcohol concentration of 0.05%. *Journal of Sleep Research, 12*(4), 265–274.

Forsberg, A., Guitard, D., & Cowan, N. (2021). Working memory limits severely constrain long-term retention. *Psychonomic Bulletin & Review, 28*(2), 537–547.

Frank, M. G. (2021). Challenging sleep homeostasis. *Neurobiology of Sleep and Circadian Rhythms, 10*, Article 100060.

Frenda, S. J., Patihis, L., Loftus, E. F., Lewis, H. C., & Fenn, K. M. (2014). Sleep deprivation and false memories. *Psychological Science, 25*(9), 1674–1681.

Gevers, W., Deliens, G., Hoffmann, S., Notebaert, W., & Peigneux, P. (2015). Sleep deprivation selectively disrupts top-down adaptation to cognitive conflict in the Stroop test. *Journal of Sleep Research, 24*(6), 666–672.

Giacobbo, B. L., Corrêa, M. S., Vedovelli, K., de Souza, C. E. B., Spitza, L. M., Gonçalves, L., Paludo, N., Molina, R. D., da Rosa, E. D., de Lima Argimon, I. I., & Bromberg, E. (2016). Could BDNF be involved in compensatory mechanisms to maintain cognitive performance despite acute sleep deprivation? An exploratory study. *International Journal of Psychophysiology, 99*, 96–102.

Grant, D. A., Honn, K. A., Layton, M. E., Riedy, S. M., & Van Dongen, H. P. A. (2017). 3-Minute smartphone-based and tablet-based psychomotor vigilance tests for the assessment of reduced alertness due to sleep deprivation. *Behavior Research Methods, 49*, 1020–1029.

Grant, D. A., & Van Dongen, H. P. A. (2013). Individual differences in sleep duration and responses to sleep loss. In P. J. Shaw, M. Tafti, & M. J. Thorpy (Eds.), *The genetic basis of sleep and sleep disorders* (pp. 189–196). Cambridge University Press.

Gurubhagavatula, I., Barger, L. K., Barnes, C. M., Basner, M., Boivin, D. B., Dawson, D., Drake, C. L., Flynn-Evans, E. E., Mysliwiec, V., Patterson, P. D., Reid, K. J., Samuels, C., Shattuck, N. L., Kazmi, U., Carandang, G., Heald, J. L., & Van Dongen, H. P. A. (2021). Guiding principles for determining work shift duration and addressing the effects of work shift duration on performance, safety, and health: Guidance from the American Academy of Sleep Medicine and the Sleep Research Society. *Sleep, 44*(11), Article zsab161.

Habeck, C., Rakitin, B. C., Moeller, J., Scarmeas, N., Zarahn, E., Brown, T., & Stern, Y. (2005). An event-related fMRI study of the neural networks underlying the encoding, maintenance, and retrieval phase in a delayed-match-to-sample task. *Cognitive Brain Research, 23*, 207–220.

Harrington, M. O., Ashton, J. E., Sankarasubramanian, S., Anderson, M. C., & Cairney, S. A. (2021). Losing control: Sleep deprivation impairs the suppression of unwanted thoughts. *Clinical Psychological Science, 9*(1), 97–113.

Harrison, Y., & Horne, J. A. (1998). Sleep loss impairs short and novel language tasks having a prefrontal focus. *Journal of Sleep Research, 7*(2), 95–100.

Harrison, Y., & Horne, J. A. (1999). One night of sleep loss impairs innovative thinking and flexible decision making. *Organizational Behavior and Human Decision Processes, 78*(2), 128–145.

Harrison, Y., & Horne, J. A. (2000a). Sleep loss and temporal memory. *The Quarterly Journal of Experimental Psychology Section A, 53*(1), 271–279.

Harrison, Y., & Horne, J. A. (2000b). The impact of sleep deprivation on decision making: A review. *Journal of Experimental Psychology: Applied, 6*(3), 236–249.

Harrison, Y., Horne, J. A., & Rothwell, A. (2000). Prefrontal neuropsychological effects of sleep deprivation in young adults—A model for healthy aging? *Sleep, 23*(8), 1067–1073.

Hartshorne, J. K., & Makovski, T. (2019). The effect of working memory maintenance on long-term memory. *Memory & Cognition, 47*(4), 749–763.

Hendricks, M. A., & Buchanan, T. W. (2016). Individual differences in cognitive control processes and their relationship to emotion regulation. *Cognition and Emotion, 30*(5), 912–924.

Heuer, H., Kleinsorge, T., Klein, W., & Kohlisch, O. (2004). Total sleep deprivation increases the costs of shifting between simple cognitive tasks. *Acta Psychologica, 117*(1), 29–64.

Honn, K. A., Grant, D. A., Hinson, J. M., Whitney, P., & Van Dongen, H. P. A. (2018). Total sleep deprivation does not significantly degrade semantic encoding. *Chronobiology International, 35*(6), 746–749.

Honn, K. A., Halverson, T., Jackson, M. L., Krusmark, M., Chavali, V. P., Gunzelmann, G., & Van Dongen, H. P. A. (2020). New insights into the cognitive effects of sleep deprivation by decomposition of a cognitive throughput task. *Sleep, 43*(7), Article zsz319.

Honn, K. A., Hinson, J. M., Whitney, P., & Van Dongen, H. P. A. (2019). Cognitive flexibility: A distinct element of performance impairment due to sleep deprivation. *Accident Analysis & Prevention, 126*, 191–197.

Honn, K. A., & Van Dongen, H. P. A. (2023). Paradoxical effects from stimulus density manipulation provide new insight into the impact of sleep deprivation on PVT performance. *Sleep Advances, 4*, Article zpac045.

Horne, J. A. (1986). Human slow wave sleep. *European Neurology, 25*(S2), 18–21.

Huber, R., Ghilardi, M. F., Massimini, M., & Tononi, G. (2004). Local sleep and learning. *Nature, 430*, 78–81.

Hudson, A. N., Van Dongen, H. P. A., & Honn, K. A. (2020). Sleep deprivation, vigilant attention, and brain function: A review. *Neuropsychopharmacology, 45*(1), 21–30.

Idzikowski, C. (1984). Sleep and memory. *British Journal of Psychology, 75*(4), 439–449.

Izquierdo, A., Brigman, J. L., Radke, A. K., Rudebeck, P. H., & Holmes, A. (2017). The neural basis of reversal learning: An updated perspective. *Neuroscience, 345*, 12–26.

Jackson, M. L., Gunzelmann, G., Whitney, P., Hinson, J. M., Belenky, G., Rabat, A., & Van Dongen, H. P. A. (2013). Deconstructing and reconstructing cognitive performance in sleep deprivation. *Sleep Medicine Reviews, 17*(3), 215–225.

Jackson, M. L., Hughes, M. E., Croft, R. J., Howard, M. E., Crewther, D., Kennedy, G. A., Owens, K., Pierce, R. J., O'Donoghue, F. J., & Johnston, P. (2011). The effect of sleep deprivation on BOLD activity elicited by a divided attention task. *Brain Imaging and Behavior, 5*(2), 97–108.

Jeneson, A., & Squire, L. R. (2012). Working memory, long-term memory, and medial temporal lobe function. *Learning & Memory, 19*(1), 15–25.

Jenkins, J. G., & Dellenbach, K. M. (1924). Obliviscence during sleep and waking. *American Journal of Psychology, 35*(4), 605–612.

Kaida, K., Niki, K., & Born, J. (2015). Role of sleep for encoding of emotional memory. *Neurobiology of Learning and Memory, 121*, 72–79.

Katsuki, F., & Constantinidis, C. (2014). Bottom-up and top-down attention: Different processes and overlapping neural systems. *The Neuroscientist, 20*(5), 509–521.

Killgore, W. D. S. (2010). Effects of sleep deprivation on cognition. In G. A. Kerkhof & H. P. A. Van Dongen (Eds.), *Human sleep and cognition. Part 1: Basic research. Progress in Brain Research* (Vol. 185, pp. 105–129). Elsevier.

Kong, D., Asplund, C. L., Ling, A., & Chee, M. W. L. (2015). Increased automaticity and altered temporal preparation following sleep deprivation. *Sleep, 38*(8), 1219–1227.

Krueger, J. M., Huang, Y. H., Rector, D. M., & Buysse, D. J. (2013). Sleep: A synchrony of cell activity–driven small network states. *European Journal of Neuroscience, 38*(2), 2199–2209.

Krueger, J. M., & Obál, F., Jr. (1993). A neuronal group theory of sleep function. *Journal of Sleep Research, 2*(2), 63–69.

Krueger, J. M., Rector, D. M., Roy, S., Van Dongen, H. P. A., Belenky, G., & Panksepp, J. (2008). Sleep as a fundamental property of neuronal assemblies. *Nature Reviews Neuroscience, 9*(12), 910–919.

Kurinec, C. A., Whitney, P., Hinson, J. M., Hansen, D. A., & Van Dongen, H. P. A. (2021). Sleep deprivation impairs binding of information with its context. *Sleep, 44*(8), Article zsab113.

Kusztor, A., Raud, L., Juel, B. E., Nilsen, A. S., Storm, J. F., & Huster, R. J. (2019). Sleep deprivation differentially affects subcomponents of cognitive control. *Sleep, 42*(4), Article zsz016.

Landrigan, C. P., Lockley, S. W., & Czeisler, C. A. (2005). Effect of intern's consecutive work hours on safety, medical education and professionalism. *Critical Care, 9*(5), 528–530.

Lang, P. J., Bradley, M. M., & Cuthbert, B. N. (2008). *International Affective Picture System (IAPS): Affective ratings of pictures and instruction manual* (Technical Report A-8). University of Florida.

Lim, J., & Dinges, D. F. (2008). Sleep deprivation and vigilant attention. *Annals of the New York Academy of Sciences, 1129*, 305–322.

Lim, J., & Dinges, D. F. (2010). A meta-analysis of the impact of short-term sleep deprivation on cognitive variables. *Psychological Bulletin, 136*(3), 375–389.

LoPresti, M. L., Anderson, J. A., Saboe, K. N., McGurk, D. L., Balkin, T. J., & Sipos, M. L. (2016). The impact of insufficient sleep on combat mission performance. *Military Behavioral Health, 4*(4), 356–363.

Ma, C., Zhong, P., Liu, D., Barger, Z. K., Zhou, L., Chang, W., Kim, B., & Dan, Y. (2019). Sleep regulation by neurotensinergic neurons in a thalamo-amygdala circuit. *Neuron, 103*(2), 323–334.

Ma, N., Dinges, D. F., Basner, M., & Rao, H. (2015). How acute total sleep loss affects the attending brain: A meta-analysis of neuroimaging studies. *Sleep, 38*(2), 233–240.

MacDonald, K. J., & Cote, K. A. (2021). Contributions of post-learning REM and NREM sleep to memory retrieval. *Sleep Medicine Reviews, 59*, Article 101453.

Mao, T., Dinges, D., Deng, Y., Zhao, K., Yang, Z., Lei, H., Fang, Z., Yang, F. N., Galli, O., Goel, N., Basner, M., & Rao, H. (2021). Impaired vigilant attention partly accounts for inhibition control deficits after total sleep deprivation and partial sleep restriction. *Nature and Science of Sleep, 13*, 1545–1560.

Maquet, P., Dive, D., Salmon, E., Sadzot, B., Franco, G., Poirrier, R., von Frenckell, R., & Franck, G. (1990). Cerebral glucose utilization during sleep–wake cycle in man determined by positron emission tomography and [^{18}F]2-fluoro-2-deoxy-D-glucose method. *Brain Research, 513*(1), 136–143.

McCabe, D. P. (2008). The role of covert retrieval in working memory span tasks: Evidence from delayed recall tests. *Journal of Memory and Language, 58*(2), 480–494.

McRae, K., & Gross, J. J. (2020). Emotion regulation. *Emotion, 20*(1), 1–9.

Miller, N. L., & Shattuck, L. G. (2005). Applying a dynamic model of situated cognition to the investigation of mishaps. *Proceedings of the Human Factors and Ergonomics Society Annual Meeting, 49*(3), 219–223.

Monk, T. H. (2007). Practical consequences of fatigue-related performance failures. *Sleep, 30*(11), 1402–1403.

Moore, R. Y. (1992). Symposium: Adjusting the clock. *Journal of Interdisciplinary Research, 23*(3), 101–117.

Munn, B. R., Müller, E. J., Wainstein, G., & Shine, J. M. (2021). The ascending arousal system shapes neural dynamics to mediate awareness of cognitive states. *Nature Communications, 12*(1), Article 6016.

Ning, Y., Zheng, S., Feng, S., Li, K., & Jia, H. (2022). Altered functional connectivity and topological organization of brain networks correlate to cognitive impairments after sleep deprivation. *Nature and Science of Sleep, 14*, 1285–1297.

Nir, Y., Andrillon, T., Marmelshtein, A., Suthana, N., Cirelli, C., Tononi, G., & Fried, I. (2017). Selective neuronal lapses precede human cognitive lapses following sleep deprivation. *Nature Medicine, 23*(12), 1474–1480.

Ochsner, K. N., & Gross, J. J. (2005). The cognitive control of emotion. *Trends in Cognitive Sciences, 9*(5), 242–249.

Olsen, R., Moses, S., Riggs, L., & Ryan, J. (2012). The hippocampus supports multiple cognitive processes through relational binding and comparison. *Frontiers in Human Neuroscience, 6*, Article 146.

Philip, P., Sagaspe, P., Lagarde, E., Leger, D., Ohayon, M. M., Bioulac, B., Boussuge, J., & Taillard, J. (2010). Sleep disorders and accidental risk in a large group of regular registered highway drivers. *Sleep Medicine, 11*(10), 973–979.

Philip, P., Taillard, J., Sagaspe, P., Valtat, C., Sanchez-Ortuno, M., Moore, N., Charles, A., & Bioulac, B. (2004). Age, performance and sleep deprivation. *Journal of Sleep Research, 13*(2), 105–110.

Pilcher, J. J., & Huffcutt, A. I. (1996). Effects of sleep deprivation on performance: A meta-analysis. *Sleep, 19*(4), 318–326.

Poh, J.-H., & Chee, M. W. L. (2017). Degradation of cortical representations during encoding following sleep deprivation. *NeuroImage, 153*, 131–138.

Porkka-Heiskanen, T., Strecker, R. E., Thakkar, M., Bjorkum, A. A., Greene, R. W., & McCarley, R. W. (1997). Adenosine: A mediator of the sleep-inducing effects of prolonged wakefulness. *Science, 276*(5316), 1265–1268.

Pruessner, L., Barnow, S., Holt, D. V., & Schulze, K. (2020). A cognitive control framework for understanding emotion regulation flexibility. *Emotion, 20*(1), 21–29.

Raichle, M. E., MacLeod, A. M., Snyder, A. Z., Powers, W. J., Gusnard, D. A., & Shulman, G. L. (2001). A default mode of brain function. *Proceedings of the National Academy of Sciences of the United States of America, 98*(2), 676–682.

Rasch, B., & Born, J. (2013). About sleep's role in memory. *Physiological Reviews, 93*(2), 681–766.

Raslear, T. G., Hursh, S. R., & Van Dongen, H. P. A. (2011). Predicting cognitive impairment and accident risk. In H. P. A. Van Dongen & G. A. Kerkhof (Eds.), *Human sleep and cognition. Part 2: Clinical and applied research. Progress in Brain Research* (Vol. 190, pp. 155–167). Elsevier.

Ratcliff, R., & McKoon, G. (2008). The diffusion decision model: Theory and data for two-choice decision tasks. *Neural Computation, 20*(4), 873–922.

Ratcliff, R., & Van Dongen, H. P. A. (2009). Sleep deprivation affects multiple distinct cognitive processes. *Psychonomic Bulletin & Review, 16*, 742–751.

Ratcliff, R., & Van Dongen, H. P. A. (2018). The effects of sleep deprivation on item and associative recognition memory. *Journal of Experimental Psychology: Learning, Memory, and Cognition, 44*(2), 193–208.

Riedy, S., Hursh, S. R., Dawson, D., Balkin, T. J., & Van Dongen, H. P. A. (2022). Sleep, sleepiness, and performance prediction modeling. In M. Kryger, T. Roth, C. A. Goldstein, & W. C. Dement (Eds.), *Principles and practice of sleep medicine* (7th ed., pp. 780–787). Elsevier.

Riontino, L., & Cavallero, C. (2022). Impact of sleep deprivation on attentional networks: Disentangling orienting components. *Brain and Cognition, 159*, Article 105863.

Rosekind, M. R., Gander, P. H., Gregory, K. B., Smith, R. M., Miller, D. L., Oyung, R., Webbon, L. L., & Johnson, J. M. (1997). Managing fatigue in operational settings 1: Physiological considerations and countermeasures. *Hospital Topics, 75*(3), 23–30.

Rupp, T. L., Wesensten, N. J., & Balkin, T. J. (2012). Trait-like vulnerability to total and partial sleep loss. *Sleep, 35*(8), 1163–1172.

Rupp, T. L., Wesensten, N. J., Bliese, P. D., & Balkin, T. J. (2009). Banking sleep: Realization of benefits during subsequent sleep restriction and recovery. *Sleep, 32*(3), 311–321.

Saletin, J. M., Goldstein-Piekarski, A. N., Greer, S. M., Stark, S., Stark, C. E., & Walker, M. P. (2016). Human hippocampal structure: A novel biomarker predicting mnemonic vulnerability to, and recovery from, sleep deprivation. *Journal of Neuroscience, 36*(8), 2355–2363.

Sallinen, M., Holm, A., Hiltunen, J., Hirvonen, K., Härmä, M., Koskelo, J., Letonsaari, M., Luukkonen, R., Virkkala, J., & Müller, K. (2008). Recovery of cognitive performance from sleep debt: Do a short rest pause and a single recovery night help? *Chronobiology International, 25*(2–3), 279–296.

Saper, C. B., Chou, T. C., & Scammell, T. E. (2001). The sleep switch: Hypothalamic control of sleep and wakefulness. *Trends in Neurosciences, 24*(12), 726–731.

Saper, C. B., & Fuller, P. M. (2017). Wake–sleep circuitry: An overview. *Current Opinion in Neurobiology, 44*, 186–192.

Saper, C. B., Lu, J., Chou, T. C., & Gooley, J. (2005). The hypothalamic integrator for circadian rhythms. *Trends in Neurosciences, 28*(3), 152–157.

Saper, C. B., Scammell, T. E., & Lu, J. (2005). Hypothalamic regulation of sleep and circadian rhythms. *Nature, 437*, 1257–1263.

Sarter, M., Givens, B., & Bruno, J. P. (2001). The cognitive neuroscience of sustained attention: Where top-down meets bottom-up. *Brain Research Reviews, 35*(2), 146–160.

Satterfield, B. C., Stucky, B., Landolt, H.-P., & Van Dongen, H. P. A. (2019). Unraveling the genetic underpinnings of sleep deprivation-induced impairments in human cognition. In H. P. A. Van Dongen, P. Whitney, J. M. Hinson, K. A. Honn, & M. W. L. Chee (Eds.), *Sleep deprivation and cognition. Progress in Brain Research* (Vol. 246, pp. 127–158). Elsevier.

Schönauer, M., Grätsch, M., & Gais, S. (2015). Evidence for two distinct sleep-related long-term memory consolidation processes. *Cortex, 63*, 68–78.

Skorucak, J., Arbon, E. L., Dijk, D.-J., & Achermann, P. (2018). Response to chronic sleep restriction, extension, and subsequent total sleep deprivation in humans: Adaptation or preserved sleep homeostasis? *Sleep, 41*(7), Article zsy078.

Slama, H., Chylinski, D. O., Deliens, G., Leproult, R., Schmitz, R., & Peigneux, P. (2018). Sleep deprivation triggers cognitive control impairments in task-goal switching. *Sleep, 41*(2), Article zsx200.

Song, T., Yu, K., Wang, L., Xu, L., Xu, M., Peng, Z., Dai, C., Wang, H., Yang, T., Shao, Y., Wang, X., & Lv, J. (2022). Total sleep deprivation triggers greater activation in the parietal brain in the visual working memory updating processes: An event-related potentials study. *Frontiers in Neuroscience, 16*, Article 736437.

Stenson, A. R., Kurinec, C. A., Hinson, J. M., Whitney, P., & Van Dongen, H. P. A. (2021). Total sleep deprivation reduces top-down regulation of emotion without altering bottom-up affective processing. *PLOS ONE, 16*(9), Article e0256983.

Stenson, A. R., Whitney, P., Hinson, J. M., Hansen, D. A., Lawrence-Sidebottom, D., Skeiky, L., Riedy, S. M., Kurinec, C. A., & Van Dongen, H. P.A. (2023). Effects of total sleep deprivation on components of top-down attentional control using a flexible attentional control task. *Journal of Sleep Research, 32*(2), Article e13744.

Strogatz, S. H., Kronauer, R. E., & Czeisler, C. A. (1987). Circadian pacemaker interferes with sleep onset at specific times each day: Role in insomnia. *American Journal of Physiology, 253*(1, Pt. 2), R172–R178.

Swanson, L. M., Arnedt, J. T., Rosekind, M. R., Belenky, G., Balkin, T. J., & Drake, C. (2011). Sleep disorders and work performance: Findings from the 2008 National Sleep Foundation Sleep in America poll. *Journal of Sleep Research, 20*(3), 487–494.

Tempesta, D., Socci, V., Coppo, M., Dello Ioio, G., Nepa, V., De Gennaro, L., & Ferrara, M. (2016). The effect of sleep deprivation on the encoding of contextual and non-contextual aspects of emotional memory. *Neurobiology of Learning and Memory, 131*, 9–17.

Thomas, M., Sing, H., Belenky, G., Holcomb, H., Mayberg, H., Dannals, R., Wagner, H., Thorne, D., Popp, K., Rowland, L., Welsh, A., Balwinski, S., & Redmond, D. (2000). Neural basis of alertness and cognitive performance impairments during sleepiness. I. Effects of 24 h of sleep deprivation on waking human regional brain activity. *Journal of Sleep Research, 9*(4), 335–352.

Tomaso, C. C., Johnson, A. B., & Nelson, T. D. (2021). The effect of sleep deprivation and restriction on mood, emotion, and emotion regulation: Three meta-analyses in one. *Sleep, 44*(6), Article zsaa289.

Tononi, G., & Cirelli, C. (2014). Sleep and the price of plasticity: From synaptic and cellular homeostasis to memory consolidation and integration. *Neuron, 81*(1), 12–34.

Tononi, G., & Cirelli, C. (2020). Sleep and synaptic down-selection. *The European Journal of Neuroscience, 51*(1), 413–421.

Tucker, A. M., Whitney, P., Belenky, G., Hinson, J. M., & Van Dongen, H. P. A. (2010). Effects of sleep deprivation on dissociated components of executive functioning. *Sleep, 33*(1), 47–57.

Ulrich, G., & Frick, K. (1986). A new quantitative approach to the assessment of stages of vigilance as defined by spatiotemporal EEG patterning. *Perceptual Motor Skills, 62*(2), 567–576.

Unsworth, N. (2010). On the division of working memory and long-term memory and their relation to intelligence: A latent variable approach. *Acta Psychologica, 134*(1), 16–28.

Van Der Werf, Y. D., Altena, E., Schoonheim, M. M., Sanz-Arigita, E. J., Vis, J. C., De Rijke, W., & Van Someren, E. J. W. (2009). Sleep benefits subsequent hippocampal functioning. *Nature Neuroscience, 12*(2), 122–123.

Van Dongen, H. P.A., Balkin, J. T., Hursh, S. R., & Dorrian, J. (2022). Performance deficits during sleep loss and their operational consequences. In M. H. Kryger, T. Roth, & C. A. Goldstein (Eds.), *Principles and practice of sleep medicine* (7th ed., pp. 742–749). Elsevier.

Van Dongen, H. P. A., Belenky, G., & Krueger, J. M. (2011a). A local, bottom-up perspective on sleep deprivation and neurobehavioral performance. *Current Topics in Medicinal Chemistry, 11*(19), 2414–2422.

Van Dongen, H. P. A., Belenky, G., & Krueger, J. M. (2011b). Investigating the temporal dynamics and underlying mechanisms of cognitive fatigue. In P. L. Ackerman (Ed.), *Cognitive fatigue: Multidisciplinary perspectives on current research and future applications* (pp. 127–147). American Psychological Association.

Van Dongen, H. P. A., Maislin, G., Mullington, J. M., & Dinges, D. F. (2003). The cumulative cost of additional wakefulness: Dose–response effects on neurobehavioral functions and sleep physiology from chronic sleep restriction and total sleep deprivation. *Sleep, 26*(2), 117–126.

Van Dongen, H. P. A., Maurice, D. B., Maislin, G., & Dinges, D. F. (2004). Systematic interindividual differences in neurobehavioral impairment from sleep loss: Evidence of trait-like differential vulnerability. *Sleep, 27*(3), 423–433.

Wagner, U., Gais, S., Haider, H., Verleger, R., & Born, J. (2004). Sleep inspires insight. *Nature, 427*(6972), 352–355.

Walker, M. P., & Stickgold, R. (2004). Sleep-dependent learning and memory consolidation. *Neuron, 44*(1), 121–133.

Wehr, T. A., Moul, D. E., Barbato, G., Giesen, H. A., Seidal, J. A., Barker, C., & Bender, C. (1993). Conservation of photoperiod-responsive mechanisms in humans. *American Journal of Physiology, 265*(4), R846–R857.

Wesensten, N. J. (2012). *Sleep deprivation, stimulant medications, and cognition*. Cambridge University Press.

Whitney, P., & Hinson, J. M. (2010). Measurement of cognition in studies of sleep deprivation. In G. A. Kerkhof & H. P. A. Van Dongen (Eds.), *Human sleep and cognition. Part 1: Basic research. Progress in Brain Research* (Vol. 185, pp. 37–48). Elsevier.

Whitney, P., Hinson, J. M., Jackson, M. L., & Van Dongen, H. P. A. (2015). Feedback blunting: Total sleep deprivation impairs decision making that requires updating based on feedback. *Sleep, 38*(5), 745–754.

Whitney, P., Hinson, J. M., & Nusbaum, A. T. (2019). A dynamic attentional control framework for understanding sleep deprivation effects on cognition. In H. P. A. Van Dongen, P. Whitney, J. M. Hinson, K. A. Honn, & M. W. L. Chee (Eds.), *Sleep deprivation and cognition. Progress in Brain Research* (Vol. 246, pp. 111–126). Elsevier.

Whitney, P., Hinson, J. M., Satterfield, B. C., Grant, D. A., Honn, K. A., & Van Dongen, H. P. A. (2017). Sleep deprivation diminishes attentional control effectiveness and impairs flexible adaptation to changing conditions. *Scientific Reports, 7*(1), 1–9.

Wickens, C. D., Hutchins, S. D., Laux, L., & Sebok, A. (2015). The impact of sleep disruption on complex cognitive tasks: A meta-analysis. *Human Factors, 57*(6), 930–946.

Wilkinson, R. T. (1961). Interaction of lack of sleep with knowledge of results, repeated testing, and individual differences. *Journal of Experimental Psychology, 62*, 263–271.

Williams, H. L., Lubin, A., & Goodnow, J. J. (1959). Impaired performance with acute sleep loss. *Psychological Monographs, 73*(14), 1–26.

Yaple, Z. A., & Yu, R. (2019). Fractionating adaptive learning: A meta-analysis of the reversal learning paradigm. *Neuroscience & Biobehavioral Reviews, 102*, 85–94.

Yonelinas, A. P. (2013). The hippocampus supports high-resolution binding in the service of perception, working memory and long-term memory. *Behavioural Brain Research, 254*, 34–44.

Yoo, S. S., Gujar, N., Hu, P., Jolesz, F. A., & Walker, M. P. (2007). The human emotional brain without sleep—A prefrontal amygdala disconnect. *Current Biology, 17*(20), R877–R878.

Zhang, J., Lau, E. Y. Y., & Hsiao, J. H. (2019). Using emotion regulation strategies after sleep deprivation: ERP and behavioral findings. *Cognitive, Affective, & Behavioral Neuroscience, 19*(2), 283–295.

Zhang, L., Shao, Y., Liu, Z., Li, C., Chen, Y., & Zhou, Q. (2019). Decreased information replacement of working memory after sleep deprivation: Evidence from an event-related potential study. *Frontiers in Neuroscience, 13*, Article 408.

Zimmer, H. D., Mecklinger, A., & Lindenberger, U. (2006). Levels of binding: Types, mechanisms, and functions of binding in remembering. In H. D. Zimmer, A. Mecklinger, & U. Lindenberger (Eds.), *Handbook of binding and memory: Perspectives from cognitive neuroscience* (pp. 3–22). Oxford University Press.

CHAPTER

12 Sleep and Emotion Regulation

Debora Meneo, Monica Martoni, *and* Chiara Baglioni

Abstract

Sleep and emotional processes are closely linked, yet there are still difficulties in grasping the relationship. Emotion regulation is believed to be a transdiagnostic mechanism explaining how disrupted sleep may lead to psychopathology. The dynamics of affect is an aspect of emotional experience that might contribute to the understanding of the path from sleep disturbance to mood disorders. In this chapter, two models of emotional processes are considered: the process model of emotion regulation and the DynAffect model. Selected literature is discussed to shed light on the relationship between emotional and sleep processes, considering the effect of disruption in sleep duration (sleep deprivation), efficiency (insomnia disorder), and timing (circadian misalignment) on emotion regulation and affective dynamics. Future directions for research practice will be discussed from the perspective of an integrated framework.

Key Words: sleep disruption, insomnia disorder, sleep deprivation, circadian misalignment, emotion regulation, affect, process model, DynAffect model

Introduction

The transdiagnostic nature of sleep disruption for mental health has been more and more recognized in research and clinical practice, with sleep problems being a contributing and risk factor to psychiatric disorders (Baglioni et al., 2011, 2016; Freeman et al., 2020; Harvey et al., 2011; Hertenstein et al., 2019). When sleep is disrupted, it may be of insufficient duration (quantity), characterized by difficulties in sleep initiation and/or maintenance (efficiency), or placed at an inappropriate time in the 24-hour day (timing). Other aspects are also relevant, such as satisfaction for sleep and the level of alertness during the day, as well as sleep variability across days. The quantity, efficiency, and timing of sleep are among the dimensions that constitute good sleep health (Buysse, 2014); their alteration may span from acute momentary disturbance to chronic sleep–wake disorders and is associated with negative health outcomes. Emotional processes have been regarded as one mechanism that may explain how disrupted sleep leads to or maintains psychopathological symptoms (Kahn et al., 2013; Palmer & Alfano, 2017). This line of research is rooted in the bidirectional relationship observed between altered sleep regulation and disturbed emotional processes (Gruber & Cassoff, 2014), which is a transdiagnostic factor for internalizing and externalizing mental disorders (Aldao et al., 2016). Intense emotional states that are not appropriately managed affect sleep duration, continuity, and timing. On the other hand, sleep disruption impairs the processing and regulation of emotions (Gruber & Cassoff, 2014).

Emotions and Affects

While *emotion* is often used as an umbrella term for different processes and states, James Gross (1998) proposed a useful distinction between emotions, affects, and mood for research purposes. Emotions are multicomponent responses to stimuli: When the person attends to and appraises a situation as relevant to current goals, a response is generated that involves changes in subjective experience, behavior, and physiology. These characteristics make emotion a whole-body process, which makes us both feel and incline to act (Frijda, 1986). Mood, on the other hand, lasts longer than emotions, is more diffused, and therefore is not always contingent to a specific object or situation. Superordinate to emotion and mood is affect, which encompasses various emotions, something closer to a dye. Affect does not differentiate between discrete states; instead, it has two features: valence, which may be negative or positive, and arousal, which is either high or low. In this context, *affective regulation* is also used as an umbrella term that embraces efforts to influence the valence and arousal of affective experience, including efforts to shape the timing, expression, experience, and content of emotions to adapt to the context, which is called *emotion regulation* (Gross, 1998). Emotion regulation refers not just to the suppression or dampening of intense emotional states but also to their modulation to meet environmental demands or hedonic needs (Gratz & Roemer, 2004; Gross, 2015). Failure to manage emotional responses to everyday events leads to more intense and prolonged distress, which may predispose the individual to develop a major psychiatric disorder (Aldao et al., 2010). For instance, sustained negative affect is a core feature of clinical depression according to the *Diagnostic and Statistical Manual of Mental Disorder*—fifth edition (DSM-5; American Psychiatric Association, 2013).

The link between mood disturbance and emotion regulation is a cardinal argument in many models of emotional processes; nonetheless, the field is vast, and theoretical stances vary, with consequently different research and clinical practices. A widely used model is the *process model of emotion regulation*, developed by Gross (1998), which focuses on the different actions that we employ to influence what emotions we have, when we have them, and how we have them. The model identifies five stages of emotional processes in which regulation may occur: situation selection, situation modification, attentional deployment, cognitive change, and response modulation (Gross, 1998). The point at which the regulation happens distinguishes between types of strategies, which may be centered on the antecedent, such as the re-evaluation of an emotional stimulus (*cognitive reappraisal*), or response-focused, such as the suppression of emotional expression (*suppression*; Gross,

1998; Gross & John, 2003). Furthermore, some strategies are considered adaptive on their own; for example, cognitive reappraisal is adaptive in the way that it guides the emotional response back to baseline values. Other strategies are considered maladaptive, such as suppression, given that it tends to maintain elevated emotional arousal levels for longer periods (Aldao et al., 2010). The distinction between adaptive and maladaptive emotion regulation strategies has guided many research efforts to try and draw a dividing line between good and bad outcomes in terms of psychopathology and to understand the road that leads from normal emotional experiences to psychopathological ones. The tendency to adopt maladaptive emotion regulation strategies is considered transdiagnostic to psychopathology, while adaptive strategies may be protective against mood disturbance (see Aldao et al., 2010, 2016; Gross & Jazaieri, 2014; Sloan et al., 2017; Webb et al., 2012).

In recent years, the field has been rapidly expanding with new models of emotional processes to address aspects beyond regulation strategies, such as the dynamic nature of affect. Gross's model may be not suitable to capture individual differences in the variability of affective experiences across time. This point is at the center of a recent model developed by Kuppens and colleagues (2010), called the *DynAffect model.* The model focuses on the individual differences in core affect dynamics, which entails the valence and arousal of core affect (*home base*), the affective fluctuations in response to salient events (*affective variability*), and the regulatory processes that redirect affect back toward the home base (*attractor strength*; Kuppens et al., 2010). The dynamics of affects are postulated to be in some way related to emotion regulation processes. For instance, the attractor strength, or *emotional recovery*, is partly a function of emotion regulation; and a slower recovery may be responsible for the experience of prolonged affective states with high arousal (Kuppens et al., 2010). These three main mechanisms have been investigated in relation to psychopathology. For instance, the model has been applied to emotional experiences of borderline personality disorder, which is characterized by more negative intense affect, more variability in response to events, and slower emotional recovery (Ebner-Priemer et al., 2015).

Evidence is accumulating on the role of both affective states and the ability to regulate emotions in the development of internalizing and externalizing psychopathology (Aldao et al., 2016; Heininga & Kuppens, 2021; Lynch et al., 2021). The two models attend to different aspects of what we call emotional processes, and terminology differs because of individual theoretical grounds. Nonetheless, emotion regulation as conceptualized by Gross and affect dynamics as detailed by Kuppens and colleagues are not contradictory; on the contrary, each model is suitable to capture a different aspect of the vast, complex phenomenon that is emotional experience.

Firstly, the use and effectiveness of an emotion regulation strategy may be rooted in the valence and arousal of the core affect: The stronger a negative affective state, the higher is the effort to regulate emotions. In terms of the DynAffect model, the ability to emotionally recover from an event is dependent on both the home-base values and the amplitude of the fluctuation around it. Secondly, the kind of emotion regulation strategy frequently adopted may shape the course of affect over time. Failure to regulate emotional experiences might lead to a vicious circle with more and stronger negative emotions being generated, while the attractor strength is more and more weak. This interplay between affective and emotion regulation processes might perpetuate negative emotional experiences, leading to higher vulnerability to psychopathology.

An Integrated View of the Relationship Between Sleep and Emotions

Recent empirical evidence assessed the role of emotions and emotion regulatory processes in the relationship between sleep and psychopathology (e.g., O'Leary et al., 2017; Semplonius & Willoughby, 2018). At the neurobiological level, sleep and emotional processes share substrates and mechanisms that influence one another (Gruber & Cassoff, 2014; Harvey et al., 2011). On the psychological level, emotional states that are intense and have a negative valence disrupt sleep, mainly due to heightened psychophysiological arousal (Baglioni et al., 2010; Harvey, 2002). On the other hand, disruption in sleep regulation alters the way in which emotions are appraised, recognized, regulated, and, ultimately, experienced (Kahn et al., 2013; Palmer & Alfano, 2017).

The vast literature on emotions and sleep needs integration to better address open questions on how the relationship between sleep and emotions is formed and what aspects of emotional processes are involved. Palmer and Alfano (2017) reviewed the association between sleep and emotions through the lens of Gross's framework. Inadequate sleep is linked with the generation of negative emotions and the dampening of positive emotions, as well as impairment in emotion regulation at each proposed step in Gross's model (Palmer & Alfano, 2017). Firstly, the experience of sleep loss and dissatisfaction may lead to cognitive and motivational changes that reduce the likelihood of experiencing positive emotions (*situation selection* and *modification*). Secondly, sleep loss alters the way in which emotional stimuli are appraised, heightening the salience of negative and threatening stimuli with low implementation of distraction strategies (*attentional deployment*). Furthermore, it may reduce the use of cognitive reappraisal (*cognitive change*) and make the use of suppression more frequent (*response modulation*).

Gross's model is an important framework to explain sleep–emotion processes. Nonetheless, the model focuses on the way a person responds to emotional stimuli and the affective experience that is elicited. The model do no directly address questions pertaining to the dynamics of affects, such as how it shapes and is shaped by the experience of sleep disruption. In our view, a more complete understanding of emotional experience in the context of sleep disruption might come from the integration of Gross's conceptualization of emotion regulation and the dynamics of affect as captured by the DynAffect model. In the field of sleep research, this integration might be useful to synthetize the available literature and to address questions concerning individual vulnerability and emotional response to sleep disruption, considering the quantity, efficiency, and timing of sleep.

In the following sections, we will discuss the relationship between sleep and emotions in the context of emotion regulation strategies and the dynamics of core affect, also considering the possible repercussions in terms of vulnerability to psychopathology. We will consider alterations in the duration, efficiency, and timing of sleep, applying an integrated view to evaluate emotional processes in three main areas of sleep research: sleep deprivation, insomnia disorder, and circadian misalignment. Figure 12.1 summarizes the associations between sleep disruption and both affective dynamics and emotion regulation strategies that will guide our discussion. While recognizing the bidirectional link between sleep and emotions, here we focalize on the effect of sleep disruption on emotional processes.

THE DURATION OF SLEEP: SLEEP DEPRIVATION

Sleep deprivation indicates the state in which a person does not get enough sleep hours. Meeting the age-appropriate recommended amount of sleep is not sufficient to obtain enough sleep; other factors, such as sleep quality and continuity, influence what can be defined as good sleep. Here we focused on the reduction of sleeping hours to review the literature on the function of sleep for emotion regulation and affect dynamics, approaching the matter from the perspective of sleep deprivation.

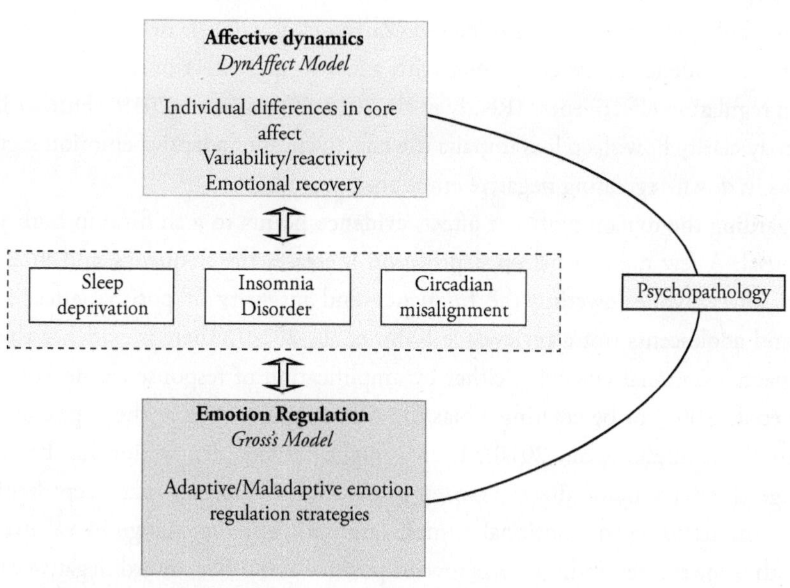

Figure 12.1 Interplay between sleep disruption and emotional processes

Note. A framework for the interplay between sleep disruption and emotional processes, integrating the process model of emotion regulation and the DynAffect model. The three main alterations in sleep are sleep deprivation (duration), insomnia disorder (efficiency), and circadian misalignment (timing). The arced line indicates the interplay between emotion regulation strategies in Gross's model and affective dynamics in the DynAffect model. The bidirectional relationship between emotions and sleep disruption might lead to the development of psychopathology.

Periods of sleep reduction have been shown to alter the processing, appraisal, and response to emotional stimuli (Watling et al., 2017). How continued sleep deprivation alters emotion regulation has been relatively less investigated. Neurobiological findings suggest that the functional connectivity between the prefrontal and limbic areas, which is fundamental for the monitoring and regulation of emotional processes, is altered by sleep deprivation (Simon et al., 2015; Yoo et al., 2007). This and other evidence (e.g., Mauss et al., 2013) may suggest that sleep loss interferes with the ability to cope with the cognitive load of emotion regulation (Watling et al., 2017). Adaptive emotion regulation strategies may be less adopted and less effective at modulating affective states. This is particularly of concern in adolescents, as we are witnessing an epidemic of sleep deprivation during this developmental stage, which is also vulnerable to emotion dysregulation due to the neurobiological substrates being still not fully mature (Giedd, 2004; Talbot et al., 2010). Under conditions of sleep deprivation, the ability of the adolescent to regulate intense negative emotions is in fact impaired (Baum et al., 2014).

The *effectiveness* of a strategy in regulating emotions is another important aspect of emotional functioning under sleep loss (Watling et al., 2017). A recent study by Zhang and colleagues (2019) recorded the centroparietal late positive potential, a neural index of emotion regulation, while participants applied a given emotion regulation strategy in viewing negative pictures. After 24 hours of sleep deprivation, the effectiveness of adaptive emotion regulation strategies was impaired (Zhang et al., 2019). At the behavioral level, it seems that evidence is less consistent, with a low to null effect of sleep deprivation on emotion regulation effectiveness (Reddy et al., 2017; Zhang et al., 2019). Further investigation may clarify how sleep loss impairs the effectiveness of adaptive emotion regulation strategies in down-regulating negative emotions.

Regarding the dynamic of core affect, evidence points to a shifting in both valence and arousal: A few nights of sleep deprivation increases the frequency and intensity of negative affect, while lowering the frequency and intensity of positive affect in both adults and adolescents (for a review, see Kahn et al., 2013). There is evidence that sleep loss impacts emotional reactivity, either by amplification of responses to negative events (Zohar et al., 2005) or by creating a bias toward a negative tone in the appraisal of neutral stimuli (Tempesta et al., 2010). Even 1 night of sleep deprivation has been found to change the dynamic of affect (Franzen et al., 2008). It seems that sleep deprivation increases the response to emotional stimuli (arousal), but the change in valence is less clear, with some studies finding a bias toward positive and other toward negative categorization of emotional stimuli (Watling et al., 2017). Possible explanations for contradictory findings are differences in the procedure by which emotional responses are measured or in sleep restriction periods and protocols (Watling et al., 2017). Another possibility is the existence of baseline differences in core affect that influence the emotional response to sleep loss (Zhang et al., 2019). For instance, individual differences in anxiety, coupled with emotion dysregulation, amplify the effect of sleep loss on emotional functioning and mood (Palmer & Alfano, 2020). This is in line with evidence suggesting that individual differences in neurobehavioral response to sleep are trait-like characteristics that demonstrate consistency (Tkachenko & Dinges, 2018).

Taking together the evidence from research on core affect and on emotion regulation strategies, the experience of sleep deprivation may have a profound impact on adjustment to daily life. If a person does not achieve enough sleep hours, they may become more reactive to emotional stimuli and experience more frequent and intense negative emotions. Furthermore, their ability to regulate these emotional states may be compromised, creating a vicious circle in which affective fluctuations are wider and regulation efforts fail to restore a home-base value. With time, it is reasonable to expect that the rise of negative emotions further impairs sleep, leading to its reduction. Repeated experiences of sleep loss over a longer period may have profound effects on emotional processes and lead to long-lasting emotional difficulties. In fact, emotional experience may be limited in time as emotions are short-lived; nonetheless, the sum of emotional responses may contribute to the insurgence of mood disturbance (Watling et al., 2017). The field needs further investigation on how individual differences in affective dynamics shape the emotional response to sleep loss and how sleep loss changes the dynamics of affect over time.

THE EFFICIENCY OF SLEEP: INSOMNIA DISORDER

Insomnia disorder is primarily a clinical impairment in sleep continuity: The person has a persistent difficulty in initiating or maintaining sleep, which is nonrestorative, and suffers daytime consequences, such as reduced attention, mood alterations, and fatigue (*International Classification of Sleep Disorders*, third edition [ICSD-3]; American Academy of Sleep Medicine, 2014; DSM-5; American Psychiatric Association, 2013). The field of emotional processes in insomnia disorder has gained considerable attention in recent years, given the role of insomnia as a risk factor for depression (Baglioni et al., 2011; Hertenstein et al., 2019).

Etiological models of insomnia have integrated the emotional components as one predisposing and perpetuating factor (Espie, 2002; Harvey, 2002; Perlis et al., 1997; Riemann et al., 2010). Sleep deprivation, as discussed above, is linked to the processing of emotional stimuli and to the regulative efforts to adjust emotional experiences and responses. While acute sleep deprivation may be an occurrence in everyone's life, and chronic sleep loss may also present, insomnia disorder is not only sleep deprivation. In some predisposed individuals, the experience of a few nights of sleep loss may trigger an array of negative responses and cognitive hyperarousal. The nights of poor sleep are then associated with negative emotions and stress that also permeate daytime experience. The negatively toned cognitive activity that characterizes insomnia disorder (Harvey, 2002) may then lead to a sequence of effects that span from withdrawal from social activities to excessive preoccupation with sleep. At the emotion generation level, negative emotions become more and more frequent, and social interactions are also restricted, causing the person with insomnia disorder to have fewer occasions to experience positive emotional states (Palmer & Alfano, 2017). There is a need to both characterize emotional processes linked to sleep disturbance and trace a possible pattern from insomnia disorder to psychopathology. In response to this, an emerging field of research is investigating how insomnia patients regulate their emotional states, assumed to have a negative valence and high intensity. The ability to employ adaptive emotion regulation strategies appears impaired by the presence of poor sleep quality and insomnia symptoms; on the other hand, the use of maladaptive strategies, with consequent sustained intense negative emotions, predicts the quality of nocturnal sleep (for an overview, see Vanek et al., 2020). Tavernier and Willoughby (2015) performed a longitudinal study in college students, finding that sleep problems predicted problems in emotion regulation and that difficulties in emotion regulation predicted sleep problems. While researchers have focused on the relationship between sleep quality or insomnia symptoms and emotion regulation, investigations in insomnia patients are scarce. Pioneering studies comparing insomnia patients to good sleepers found that the former use more suppression and worry as thought control strategies (Harvey, 2001; Ree et al., 2005).

Different lines of research have investigated how the properties of core affect, namely valence and arousal, are impacted by the experience of poor sleep. Studies on healthy adults showed that the experience of poor sleep quality reduces positive states and induces negative states (e.g., McCrae et al., 2008; Simor et al., 2015; Takano et al., 2014). Insomnia patients have been found to have a more negative attitude in the evaluation of their surroundings (Buysse et al., 2007) and intensified and more lasting processing of negative emotional stimuli (Schiel et al., 2020).

Reactivity to emotional stimuli and insomnia disorders seems to be bidirectionally connected (Altena et al., 2016). Having an insomnia disorder leads to higher variability in affective experience and more reactivity to emotional stimuli (for an overview, see Baglioni et al., 2010; Hertenstein et al., 2019). An interesting result observed by Buysse and colleagues (2007) using ecological momentary assessment was that the time course of affect during the day was different in insomnia disorder patients and good sleepers: Negative emotions increased in insomnia disorder patients and decreased in good sleepers from morning to evening, while positive affect was variable only in good sleepers. More vulnerability to negative emotions and more fluctuations in them, without positive emotions balancing them, may implicate more regulatory efforts to regain a home-base value in core affect. Given an already depleted cognitive system due to sleep loss, it is reasonable that efforts to regulate emotions often fail and, therefore, negative emotions intensify. A recent study found that sleep efficiency predicted the affective recovery following a laboratory-induced stressor (Leger & Charles, 2020). Poor sleepers were less able to recover from a stressful experience: Their negative affect remained high at post-recovery, and their positive affect was lower. This might in fact indicate that emotional recovery is impaired by poor sleep, but investigations in insomnia disorder patients are lacking.

An ecological momentary assessment study investigated the emotional experience of insomnia patients within a theoretical framework grounded in both the process model and the DynAffect model (Baglioni et al., 2023). Over five consecutive days, patients with insomnia disorder experienced more frequent negative emotions and decreased positive emotions compared to good sleepers, either in a control condition or under sleep deprivation. This may indicate a difference in the dynamics of core affect between those with insomnia disorder, who were also sleep deprived, and good sleepers, who were momentarily under sleep restriction. Furthermore, insomnia patients showed higher use of maladaptive emotion regulation strategies, compared to both groups of good sleepers. Regarding adaptive strategies, both insomnia and sleep-deprived groups used such strategies less frequently than controls. This may suggest that insomnia disorder might be characterized by individual difference in core affect and in the use of emotion regulation strategies.

While it is clear, from a theoretical point of view and from neurobiological findings, how emotional processes are impacted by sleep and may lead insomnia patients to higher vulnerability to psychopathology, what shapes this intersection at the individual level is less clear (Hertenstein et al., 2019). New insight may come by considering the dynamic nature of affect. Those who develop insomnia may be the same individuals with a predisposition for hyperarousal. This may entail a core affect which is already higher in arousal and more negative in valence, coupled with less ability to adaptively regulate emotions, even before sleep disturbance occurs. After a precipitating factor (a life stressor, for instance), sleep is perturbed. The fluctuations of affect that follow may be different from individual to individual, as may the ability to emotionally recover from the original stressor (partly due to ineffective emotion regulation strategies). The intersection of these differences with known perpetuating factors (e.g., beliefs, attitudes, cognitive processes; Harvey, 2002) may maintain insomnia symptoms to the point of a chronic disorder. Further evidence is needed to sustain this framework and shed light on the effect of emotional processes as consequence and part of the etiology of insomnia disorder.

THE TIMING OF SLEEP: CIRCADIAN MISALIGNMENT

The timing of sleep is an important, even if relatively overlooked, aspect of sleep health. It refers to the time for which one allocates sleep or, in other words, when one goes to bed and rises in respect to an external clock. The circadian clock is synchronized by environmental signals (*zeitgeber*), among which the light–dark cycle is the principal (solar clock), along with social schedules (social clock). The synchronization between the solar day and the circadian clock is important for the appropriate timing of psychophysiological functions, including, but not limited to, the sleep–wake cycle. Being synchronized with the social clock is also essential in our society, in which most activities are allocated at specific time windows. An ideal situation of synchronization happens when the three clocks are in phase, while an excessive difference between the phase angles of two or more rhythms is defined as *circadian misalignment*. It is a widespread phenomenon in our society, in which biological and societal times are often not synchronized (Vetter, 2020). In fact, "Societal determination of work times, and sometimes also of free times, interferes with individual sleep preferences" (Wittman et al., 2006, p. 504). Circadian misalignment seems to play an important role in mood disorders, but the mechanism of association is unclear; genetic vulnerabilities are being investigated (McClung, 2011).

Extreme cases of desynchronization can take the form of an actual circadian disorder, which has endogenous causes or environmental determinants. The DSM-5 and the ICSD-3 recognize six circadian disorders: advanced sleep phase disorder, delayed sleep phase disorder, irregular sleep–wake type, non-entrained type (or non-24 hours disorder), shiftwork disorder, and jetlag disorder (American Academy of Sleep Medicine, 2014; American Psychiatric Association, 2013). Even with different manifestations and phenomenology, circadian disorders are characterized by a misalignment between two or more rhythms, which has been associated with emotional difficulties, depressive symptoms, and negative health outcomes, including cardiovascular disease and mood disorders (Baron & Reid, 2014).

While circadian disorders are relatively uncommon, circadian misalignment is almost a modern-day disease. In modern society, electronic illumination has extended the daytime well into nighttime; moreover, the exposure to clock-delaying lights in the evening is more and more common, from childhood to old age. Given that social schedules still impose an early rhythm on most people, sleep hours are shortened during the week and, to compensate, extended during the weekend or free days. In chronobiological terms, the biological clock appears to be unable to fully synchronize with the social clock, resuming a spontaneous rhythm as soon as societal demands are lifted (Roenneberg et al., 2019). The effect of the desynchronization between circadian and social clocks is similar to the effect of traveling across zones, from which it took the name of *social jetlag* (Wittmann et al., 2006). The differences between sleep timing on work (or school) and free days is considered a proxy of circadian misalignment (Roenneberg et al., 2019; Vetter et al., 2020), and it has been linked to negative health outcomes, psychiatric symptoms, and conduct problems (Beauvalet et al., 2017). In particular, social jetlag is associated with depression (Henderson et al., 2019; Islam et al., 2020). While circadian misalignment may shorten sleep hours and disrupt sleep continuity, the effect on mood also may be due to other factors, such as alteration in the biological rhythm of hormone secretion and blood pressure and reduced exposure to sunlight (Dumont & Beaulieu, 2007). Overall, circadian rhythm and mood disturbance appear closely linked, but explaining mechanisms are still debated (for an overview, see McClung, 2013). Circadian misalignment may impair emotional processes, and this, in turn, may be a factor of vulnerability to mood disturbance. Emotions, like other cognitive, behavioral, and physiological events, are rhythmic and thus under the influence of the circadian clock (Wright et al., 2012). The desynchronization between internal clock and environmental demand may alter the reactivity to emotional stimuli because the "time is not right." In fact, negative emotional reactivity tends to be higher when there is a demand to perform an emotional task at the circadian off-peak time of day for cognitive performance (Tucker et al., 2012).

While social jetlag to some degree affects most people, there is an individual difference in sleep–wake rhythm that might influence the likelihood of the desynchronization: circadian typology (or chronotype). The term *chronotype* describes not a disorder or a pathological condition but a continuum created by differences in the phase of entrainment to the solar clock, which are expressed as the preferred time for sleep onset and offset. At the behavioral level, circadian typology may express as an effect of acquired habits and/or of biological characteristics: Early chronotypes tend to wake up early in the morning and have difficulty staying up late in the evening, while late chronotypes stay up until late in the night and find it difficult to wake up at an early hour. While not pathological per se, extreme circadian preference has been investigated in association with emotional processes and mood disturbance more than most circadian disorders. Morningness has been regarded as a protective factor for psychopathology, while eveningness is considered a risk factor for behavioral and mood problems (Lotti et al., 2022; Taylor & Hasler, 2018). Emotional processes appear influenced by chronotype: Evening types recur more often to maladaptive emotion regulation strategies, such as suppression (Antúnez, 2020; Van den Berg et al., 2018; Watts & Norbury, 2017); show more unstable daily variations in valence and arousal of core affect (Ottoni et al., 2012); are more reactive to negative emotional stimuli (Antypa et al., 2017); and experience low positive emotions (Carciofo, 2020; Dagys et al., 2012). An interesting result is that chronotype may be one individual difference that shapes the affective response to sleep loss: While positive affect is consistently decreased after sleep loss, late chronotypes seem more vulnerable to experiencing negative affect following sleep deprivation (e.g., Cox & Olatunji, 2021).

What makes late chronotypes vulnerable to emotional difficulties is still to be explored (Au & Reece, 2017). A higher vulnerability to circadian misalignment, in the form of social jetlag, might play an important role in the observed associations. The social clock, which demands an early rise time and a higher morning vigilance, is most suited for morning types, while evening types might struggle to keep up with social rhythms. Due to social jetlag, evening types have difficulties initiating sleep at a time that would allow enough rest, considering early rise time. This may suggest that emotional processes are impaired in late chronotypes just because they do not sleep well. Nonetheless, sleep quality seems to play only a partial role in explaining the association between evening chronotype and emotional impairments (Horne et al., 2017; Watts et al., 2017). There is more in social jetlag than sleep: Desynchronization also affects other rhythmic functions, such as attention and inhibitory control, which in turn are implicated in the monitoring and adjustment of emotional experiences. When different chronotypes are asked to perform a cognitive task at their optimal time of day (evening for late chronotypes, morning for early chronotypes), they perform much better. Late chronotypes may perform worse in cognitive, emotional, and social tasks because they are asked to attend to them at an off-peak time of the day. Fatigue may explain why emotion regulation strategies which implicate less cognitive burden are preferred over strategies such as reappraisal that need more effort. Moreover, evening types are constantly off-time, forced to go to bed and rise at a rhythm that is not their own (Wittman et al., 2006); and this may become a strain that gives rise to emotional problems.

Overall, the field of circadian–emotion interactions is a promising one to shed light on the effect of appropriate timing of sleep on mood disturbance. Emotional perturbations seem difficult to regulate in conditions of chronic desynchronization such as those often experienced by late chronotypes, due to social jetlag. This, in turn, might lead to a vicious circle of intense negative emotions and failed regulative efforts. The focus on the emotional experience of chronotypes raises several questions that need to be answered. While genetic influences may mediate the association between chronotypes and emotional processes, the role of the desynchronization often experienced by late chronotypes merits consideration. Social jetlag in late chronotypes may offer new insight on how circadian misalignment influences emotions.

While evening types seem to suffer more strongly from social jetlag, the phenomenon is a common experience among most people. The tendency to change sleep–wake hours during the weekend to compensate for sleep debt is a known perpetuating factor of sleep disturbance. Social jetlag is a common problem in our society and a good indicator of how much strain is imposed on the biological clock by societal demands (Roenneberg et al., 2019). Understanding the impact of social jetlag on the sleep–emotion relationship may benefit not only evening types, and new insights on its role in emotional experiences are needed.

Conclusions

As it is an emerging and growing field, the literature on sleep and emotions is scattered across different models and theoretical frameworks, and an integration is needed. Here we attempted to integrate research on affective dynamics and emotion regulation using two models: the process model of emotion regulation (Gross, 1998) and the DynAffect model (Kuppens et al., 2010).

The framework we adopted appears suitable to investigate sleep–emotion processes in sleep deprivation, insomnia disorder, and circadian misalignment. As shown in Figure 12.2, there is evidence supporting the interplay between emotion regulation and the dynamic of affect in sleep disturbance, but some mechanisms need further investigation and empirical evidence to confirm the associations.

Sleep deprivation has been extensively connected to lowered positive affect, while the association with negative affect is less consistent. The variability of affect following sleep loss is also less clear, but it appears that without enough sleep hours the reactivity

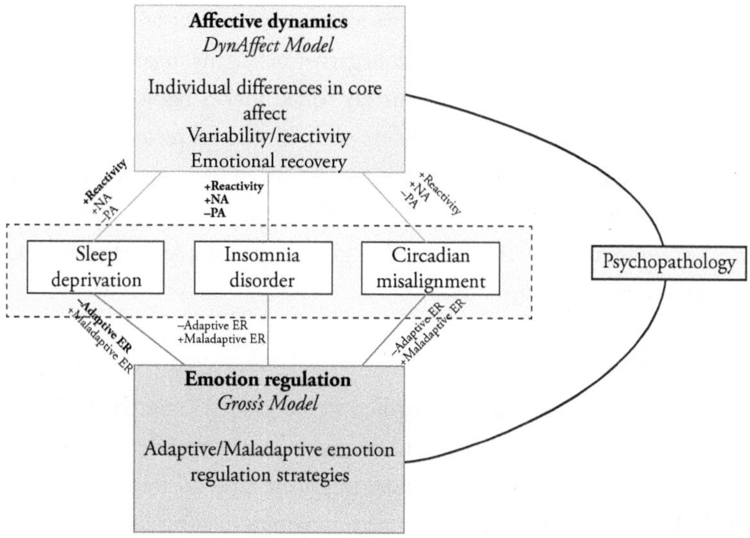

Figure 12.2 Associations between sleep disruption and both emotion regulation and affective dynamics
Note. Graphical depiction of the research status on the association between sleep disruption and the dimensions postulated by the process model of emotion regulation and the DynAffect model. Bold text indicates more consistent and coherent evidence. It should be noted that emotional recovery is not included in the associations as there is not enough literature that examines emotional recovery and sleep deprivation, insomnia disorder, or circadian misalignment. ER = emotion regulation; NA = negative affect, PA = positive affect.

to negative stimuli is altered. Emotion regulation is impaired after sleep reduction, probably due to depleted cognitive resources. How much individual differences in home-base valence and arousal shape the emotional response to sleep loss is yet to be fully explored.

Etiological models of insomnia disorder posit emotional processes as vulnerability factors. Insomnia disorder is also linked to a more intense negative emotional state and difficulties in emotion regulation, but more investigations are needed, especially on the latter matter.

The study of the circadian misalignment–emotion relationship has received less attention. Much research has focused on late chronotypes as a risk factor for mood disorders and behavioral problems. While it appears that late chronotypes experience more negative and less positive affective states, are more reactive to negative emotional stimuli, and have difficulties in regulating emotions, the literature is not enough to understand how circadian typology and emotional processes are connected and how the association may lead to psychopathological outcomes. Understanding the impact of social jetlag may shed light on how sleep alterations under the societal schedule affect emotional processes and may lead to mood disturbance.

Overall, sleep regulation appears closely linked to emotional processes, to the point that how and when we sleep shape the way emotions are experienced and regulated.

Individual differences in the dynamic of core affect may interact with our ability to regulate emotional states that are intense and negative or highly reactive and variable. An emotional experience that is strongly negatively toned makes regulative efforts more difficult and less effective, and this may interfere with emotional recovery, perpetuate negative affect, and reduce positive affect. In this context, sleep loss, insomnia symptoms, and circadian misalignment fuel a negative emotional experience, which further deteriorates sleep. This may represent the perfect ground to give rise to long-lasting emotional difficulties and, ultimately, mood disturbance.

Future Directions

1. The process model of emotion regulation has guided research in the context of sleep disruption, while the dynamics of affective experiences has received less attention. The DynAffect model might be a useful framework to study the individual difference in core affect dynamics in sleep disturbance.
2. Both emotion regulation and affective dynamics are impacted by sleep alterations. Taking both into account when investigating emotional processes in sleep disruption is important as the two processes influence each other. A moment-by-moment assessment that takes together emotion regulation and affective dynamics may help to better address the consequences of sleep disruption.
3. For some areas of research, the relationship between emotions and sleep is less clear: alterations in the dynamics of affect following sleep deprivation, particularly the valence of core affect; emotion regulation in insomnia disorder; how circadian misalignment affects emotional experience.

References

Aldao, A., Gee, D. G., De Los Reyes, A., & Seager, I. (2016). Emotion regulation as a transdiagnostic factor in the development of internalizing and externalizing psychopathology: Current and future directions. *Development and Psychopathology, 28*(4, Pt. 1), 927–946. https://doi.org/10.1017/S0954579416000638

Aldao, A., Nolen-Hoeksema, S., & Schweizer, S. (2010). Emotion-regulation strategies across psychopathology: A meta-analytic review. *Clinical Psychology Review, 30*(2), 217–237. https://doi.org/10.1016/j.cpr.2009.11.004

Altena, E., Micoulaud-Franchi, J.-A., Geoffroy, P.-A., Sanz-Arigita, E., Bioulac, S., & Philip, P. (2016). The bidirectional relation between emotional reactivity and sleep: From disruption to recovery. *Behavioral Neuroscience, 130*(3), 336–350. https://doi.org/10.1037/bne0000128

American Academy of Sleep Medicine. (2014). *International classification of sleep disorders* (3rd ed.).

American Psychiatric Association. (2013). *Diagnostic and statistical manual of mental disorders* (5th ed.). https://doi.org/10.1176/appi.books.9780890425596

Antúnez, J. M. (2020). Circadian typology is related to emotion regulation, metacognitive beliefs and assertiveness in healthy adults. *PLOS ONE, 15*(3), Article e0230169. https://doi.org/10.1371/journal.pone.0230169

Antypa, N., Verkuil, B., Molendijk, M., Schoevers, R., Penninx, B., & Van Der Does, W. (2017). Associations between chronotypes and psychological vulnerability factors of depression. *Chronobiology International, 34*(8), 1125–1135. https://doi.org/10.1080/07420528.2017.1345932

Au, J., & Reece, J. (2017). The relationship between chronotype and depressive symptoms: A meta-analysis. *Journal of Affective Disorders*, *218*, 93–104. https://doi.org/10.1016/j.jad.2017.04.021

Baglioni, C., Battagliese, G., Feige, B., Spiegelhalder, K., Nissen, C., Voderholzer, U., Lombardo, C., & Riemann, D. (2011). Insomnia as a predictor of depression: A meta-analytic evaluation of longitudinal epidemiological studies. *Journal of Affective Disorders*, *135*(1–3), 10–19. https://doi.org/10.1016/j.jad.2011.01.011

Baglioni, C., Johann, A. F., Benz, F., Steinmetz, L., Meneo, D., Frase, L., Kuhn, M., Ohler, M., Huart, S., Speiser, N., Tuschen-Caffier, B., Riemann, D., & Feige, B. (2023). Interactions between insomnia, sleep duration and emotional processes: An ecological momentary assessment of longitudinal influences combining self-report and physiological measures. *Journal of Sleep Research*, e14001. https://doi.org/10.1111/jsr.14001

Baglioni, C., Nanovska, S., Regen, W., Spiegelhalder, K., Feige, B., Nissen, C., Reynolds, C. F., & Riemann, D. (2016). Sleep and mental disorders: A meta-analysis of polysomnographic research. *Psychological Bulletin*, *142*(9), 969–990. https://doi.org/10.1037/bul0000053

Baglioni, C., Spiegelhalder, K., Lombardo, C., & Riemann, D. (2010). Sleep and emotions: A focus on insomnia. *Sleep Medicine Reviews*, *14*(4), 227–238. https://doi.org/10.1016/j.smrv.2009.10.007

Baron, K. G., & Reid, K. J. (2014). Circadian misalignment and health. *International Review of Psychiatry*, *26*(2), 139–154. https://doi.org/10.3109/09540261.2014.911149

Baum, K. T., Desai, A., Field, J., Miller, L. E., Rausch, J., & Beebe, D. W. (2014). Sleep restriction worsens mood and emotion regulation in adolescents. *Journal of Child Psychology and Psychiatry, and Allied Disciplines*, *55*(2), 180–190. https://doi.org/10.1111/jcpp.12125

Beauvalet, J. C., Quiles, C. L., Oliveira, M. A. B. D., Ilgenfritz, C. A. V., Hidalgo, M. P. L., & Tonon, A. C. (2017). Social jetlag in health and behavioral research: A systematic review. *ChronoPhysiology and Therapy*, *7*, 19–31. https://doi.org/10.2147/CPT.S108750

Buysse, D. J. (2014). Sleep health: Can we define it? Does it matter? *Sleep*, *37*(1), 9–17. https://doi.org/10.5665/sleep.3298

Buysse, D. J., Thompson, W., Scott, J., Franzen, P. L., Germain, A., Hall, M., Moul, D. E., Nofzinger, E. A., & Kupfer, D. J. (2007). Daytime symptoms in primary insomnia: A prospective analysis using ecological momentary assessment. *Sleep Medicine*, *8*(3), 198–208. https://doi.org/10.1016/j.sleep.2006.10.006

Carciofo, R. (2020). Morningness–eveningness and affect: The mediating roles of sleep quality and metacognitive beliefs. *Sleep and Biological Rhythms*, *18*(1), 17–26. https://doi.org/10.1007/s41105-019-00238-9

Cox, R. C., & Olatunji, B. O. (2021). Eveningness predicts negative affect following sleep restriction. *Behavior Therapy*, *52*(4), 797–805. https://doi.org/10.1016/j.beth.2020.10.004

Dagys, N., McGlinchey, E. L., Talbot, L. S., Kaplan, K. A., Dahl, R. E., & Harvey, A. G. (2012). Double trouble? The effects of sleep deprivation and chronotype on adolescent affect. *Journal of Child Psychology and Psychiatry, and Allied Disciplines*, *53*(6), 660–667. https://doi.org/10.1111/j.1469-7610.2011.02502.x

Dumont, M., & Beaulieu, C. (2007). Light exposure in the natural environment: Relevance to mood and sleep disorders. *Sleep Medicine*, *8*(6), 557–565. https://doi.org/10.1016/j.sleep.2006.11.008

Ebner-Priemer, U. W., Houben, M., Santangelo, P., Kleindienst, N., Tuerlinckx, F., Oravecz, Z., Verleysen, G., Van Deun, K., Bohus, M., & Kuppens, P. (2015). Unraveling affective dysregulation in borderline personality disorder: A theoretical model and empirical evidence. *Journal of Abnormal Psychology*, *124*(1), 186–198. https://doi.org/10.1037/abn0000021

Espie, C. A. (2002). Insomnia: Conceptual issues in the development, persistence, and treatment of sleep disorder in adults. *Annual Review of Psychology*, *53*, 215–243. https://doi.org/10.1146/annurev.psych.53.100901.135243

Franzen, P. L., Siegle, G. J., & Buysse, D. J. (2008). Relationships between affect, vigilance, and sleepiness following sleep deprivation. *Journal of Sleep Research*, *17*(1), 34–41. https://doi.org/10.1111/j.1365-2869.2008.00635.x

Freeman, D., Sheaves, B., Waite, F., Harvey, A. G., & Harrison, P. J. (2020). Sleep disturbance and psychiatric disorders. *The Lancet: Psychiatry*, *7*(7), 628–637. https://doi.org/10.1016/S2215-0366(20)30136-X

Frijda, N. H. (1986). *The emotions*. Cambridge University Press.

Giedd, J. N. (2004). Structural magnetic resonance imaging of the adolescent brain. *Annals of the New York Academy of Sciences*, *1021*, 77–85. https://doi.org/10.1196/annals.1308.009

Gratz, K. L., & Roemer, L. (2004). Multidimensional assessment of emotion regulation and dysregulation: Development, factor structure, and initial validation of the difficulties in emotion regulation scale. *Journal of Psychopathology and Behavioral Assessment*, *26*(1), 41–54. https://doi.org/10.1023/B:JOBA.0000007455.08539.94

Gross, J. J. (1998). Antecedent- and response-focused emotion regulation: Divergent consequences for experience, expression, and physiology. *Journal of Personality and Social Psychology*, *74*(1), 224–237. https://doi.org/10.1037/0022-3514.74.1.224

Gross, J. J. (2015). Emotion regulation: Current status and future prospects. *Psychological Inquiry*, *26*(1), 1–26. https://doi.org/10.1080/1047840X.2014.940781

Gross, J. J., & Jazaieri, H. (2014). Emotion, emotion regulation, and psychopathology: An affective science perspective. *Clinical Psychological Science*, *2*(4), 387–401. https://doi.org/10.1177/2167702614536164

Gross, J. J., & John, O. P. (2003). Individual differences in two emotion regulation processes: Implications for affect, relationships, and well-being. *Journal of Personality and Social Psychology*, *85*, 348–362. https://doi.org/10.1037/0022-3514.85.2.348

Gruber, R., & Cassoff, J. (2014). The interplay between sleep and emotion regulation: Conceptual framework empirical evidence and future directions. *Current Psychiatry Reports*, *16*(11), Article 500. https://doi.org/10.1007/s11920-014-0500-x

Harvey, A. G. (2001). I can't sleep, my mind is racing! An investigation of strategies of thought control in insomnia. *Behavioural and Cognitive Psychotherapy*, *29*(1), 3–11. https://doi.org/10.1017/S1352465801001023

Harvey, A. G. (2002). A cognitive model of insomnia. *Behaviour Research and Therapy*, *40*(8), 869–893. https://doi.org/10.1016/s0005-7967(01)00061-4

Harvey, A. G., Murray, G., Chandler, R. A., & Soehner, A. (2011). Sleep disturbance as transdiagnostic: Consideration of neurobiological mechanisms. *Clinical Psychology Review*, *31*(2), 225–235. https://doi.org/10.1016/j.cpr.2010.04.003

Heininga, V. E., & Kuppens, P. (2021). Psychopathology and positive emotions in daily life. *Current Opinion in Behavioral Sciences*, *39*, 10–18. https://doi.org/10.1016/j.cobeha.2020.11.005

Henderson, S., Brady, E. M., & Robertson, N. (2019). Associations between social jetlag and mental health in young people: A systematic review. *Chronobiology International*, *36*(10), 1316–1333. https://doi.org/10.1080/07420528.2019.1636813

Hertenstein, E., Feige, B., Gmeiner, T., Kienzler, C., Spiegelhalder, K., Johann, A., Jansson-Fröjmark, M., Palagini, L., Rücker, G., Riemann, D., & Baglioni, C. (2019). Insomnia as a predictor of mental disorders: A systematic review and meta-analysis. *Sleep Medicine Reviews*, *43*, 96–105. https://doi.org/10.1016/j.smrv.2018.10.006

Horne, C. M., Marr-Phillips, S. D. M., Jawaid, R., Gibson, E. L., & Norbury, R. (2017). Negative emotional biases in late chronotypes. *Biological Rhythm Research*, *48*(1), 151–155. https://doi.org/10.1080/09291016.2016.1236461

Islam, Z., Hu, H., Akter, S., Kuwahara, K., Kochi, T., Eguchi, M., Kurotani, K., Nanri, A., Kabe, I., & Mizoue, T. (2020). Social jetlag is associated with an increased likelihood of having depressive symptoms among the Japanese working population: The Furukawa Nutrition and Health Study. *Sleep*, *43*(1), Article zsz204. https://doi.org/10.1093/sleep/zsz204

Kahn, M., Sheppes, G., & Sadeh, A. (2013). Sleep and emotions: Bidirectional links and underlying mechanisms. *International Journal of Psychophysiology*, *89*(2), 218–228. https://doi.org/10.1016/j.ijpsycho.2013.05.010

Kuppens, P., Oravecz, Z., & Tuerlinckx, F. (2010). Feelings change: Accounting for individual differences in the temporal dynamics of affect. *Journal of Personality and Social Psychology*, *99*(6), 1042–1060. https://doi.org/10.1037/a0020962

Leger, K. A., & Charles, S. T. (2020). Affective recovery from stress and its associations with sleep. *Stress and Health*, *36*(5), 693–699. https://doi.org/10.1002/smi.2966

Lotti, S., Pagliai, G., Colombini, B., Sofi, F., & Dinu, M. (2022). Chronotype differences in energy intake, cardiometabolic risk parameters, cancer, and depression: A systematic review with meta-analysis of observational studies. *Advances in Nutrition*, *13*(1), 269–281. https://doi.org/10.1093/advances/nmab115

Lynch, S. J., Sunderland, M., Newton, N. C., & Chapman, C. (2021). A systematic review of transdiagnostic risk and protective factors for general and specific psychopathology in young people. *Clinical Psychology Review*, *87*, Article 102036. https://doi.org/10.1016/j.cpr.2021.102036

Mauss, I. B., Troy, A. S., & LeBourgeois, M. K. (2013). Poorer sleep quality is associated with lower emotion-regulation ability in a laboratory paradigm. *Cognition & Emotion*, *27*(3), 567–576. https://doi.org/10.1080/02699931.2012.727783

McClung, C. A. (2011). Circadian rhythms and mood regulation: Insights from pre-clinical models. *European Neuropsychopharmacology, 21*(S4), S683–S693. https://doi.org/10.1016/j.euroneuro.2011.07.008
McClung, C. A. (2013). How might circadian rhythms control mood? Let me count the ways . . . *Biological Psychiatry, 74*(4), 242–249. https://doi.org/10.1016/j.biopsych.2013.02.019
McCrae, C. S., McNamara, J. P., Rowe, M. A., Dzierzewski, J. M., Dirk, J., Marsiske, M., & Craggs, J. G. (2008). Sleep and affect in older adults: Using multilevel modeling to examine daily associations. *Journal of Sleep Research, 17*(1), 42–53. https://doi.org/10.1111/j.1365-2869.2008.00621.x
O'Leary, K., Bylsma, L. M., & Rottenberg, J. (2017). Why might poor sleep quality lead to depression? A role for emotion regulation. *Cognition & Emotion, 31*(8), 1698–1706. https://doi.org/10.1080/02699931.2016.1247035
Ottoni, G. L., Antoniolli, E., & Lara, D. R. (2012). Circadian preference is associated with emotional and affective temperaments. *Chronobiology International, 29*(6), 786–793. https://doi.org/10.3109/07420528.2012.679329
Palmer, C. A., & Alfano, C. A. (2017). Sleep and emotion regulation: An organizing, integrative review. *Sleep Medicine Reviews, 31*, 6–16. https://doi.org/10.1016/j.smrv.2015.12.006
Palmer, C. A., & Alfano, C. A. (2020). Anxiety modifies the emotional effects of sleep loss. *Current Opinion in Psychology, 34*, 100–104. https://doi.org/10.1016/j.copsyc.2019.12.001
Perlis, M. L., Giles, D. E., Mendelson, W. B., Bootzin, R. R., & Wyatt, J. K. (1997). Psychophysiological insomnia: The behavioural model and a neurocognitive perspective. *Journal of Sleep Research, 6*(3), 179–188. https://doi.org/10.1046/j.1365-2869.1997.00045.x
Reddy, R., Palmer, C. A., Jackson, C., Farris, S. G., & Alfano, C. A. (2017). Impact of sleep restriction versus idealized sleep on emotional experience, reactivity and regulation in healthy adolescents. *Journal of Sleep Research, 26*(4), 516–525. https://doi.org/10.1111/jsr.12484
Ree, M. J., Harvey, A. G., Blake, R., Tang, N. K., & Shawe-Taylor, M. (2005). Attempts to control unwanted thoughts in the night: Development of the Thought Control Questionnaire-Insomnia Revised (TCQI-R). *Behaviour Research and Therapy, 43*(8), 985–998. https://doi.org/10.1016/j.brat.2004.07.003
Riemann, D., Spiegelhalder, K., Feige, B., Voderholzer, U., Berger, M., Perlis, M., & Nissen, C. (2010). The hyperarousal model of insomnia: A review of the concept and its evidence. *Sleep Medicine Reviews, 14*(1), 19–31. https://doi.org/10.1016/j.smrv.2009.04.002
Roenneberg, T., Pilz, L. K., Zerbini, G., & Winnebeck, E. C. (2019). Chronotype and social jetlag: A (self-) critical review. *Biology, 8*(3), Article 54. https://doi.org/10.3390/biology8030054
Schiel, J. E., Holub, F., Petri, R., Leerssen, J., Tamm, S., Tahmasian, M., Riemann, D., & Spiegelhalder, K. (2020). Affect and arousal in insomnia: Through a lens of neuroimaging studies. *Current Psychiatry Reports, 22*(9), Article 44. https://doi.org/10.1007/s11920-020-01173-0
Semplonius, T., & Willoughby, T. (2018). Psychosocial adjustment throughout university: A longitudinal investigation of the roles of sleep quality and emotion dysregulation. *Journal of Youth and Adolescence, 47*(6), 1267–1278. https://doi.org/10.1007/s10964-018-0826-5
Simon, E. B., Oren, N., Sharon, H., Kirschner, A., Goldway, N., Okon-Singer, H., Tauman, R., Deweese, M. M., Keil, A., & Hendler, T. (2015). Losing neutrality: The neural basis of impaired emotional control without sleep. *Journal of Neuroscience, 35*(38), 13194–13205. https://doi.org/10.1523/JNEUROSCI.1314-15.2015
Simor, P., Krietsch, K. N., Köteles, F., & McCrae, C. S. (2015). Day-to-day variation of subjective sleep quality and emotional states among healthy university students—A 1-week prospective study. *International Journal of Behavioral Medicine, 22*(5), 625–634. https://doi.org/10.1007/s12529-015-9464-4
Sloan, E., Hall, K., Moulding, R., Bryce, S., Mildred, H., & Staiger, P. K. (2017). Emotion regulation as a transdiagnostic treatment construct across anxiety, depression, substance, eating and borderline personality disorders: A systematic review. *Clinical Psychology Review, 57*, 141–163. https://doi.org/10.1016/j.cpr.2017.09.002
Takano, K., Sakamoto, S., & Tanno, Y. (2014). Repetitive thought impairs sleep quality: An experience sampling study. *Behavior Therapy, 45*(1), 67–82. https://doi.org/10.1016/j.beth.2013.09.004
Talbot, L. S., McGlinchey, E. L., Kaplan, K. A., Dahl, R. E., & Harvey, A. G. (2010). Sleep deprivation in adolescents and adults: Changes in affect. *Emotion, 10*(6), 831–841. https://doi.org/10.1037/a0020138
Tavernier, R., & Willoughby, T. (2015). A longitudinal examination of the bidirectional association between sleep problems and social ties at university: The mediating role of emotion regulation. *Journal of Youth and Adolescence, 44*(2), 317–330. https://doi.org/10.1007/s10964-014-0107-x

Taylor, B. J., & Hasler, B. P. (2018). Chronotype and mental health: Recent advances. *Current Psychiatry Reports, 20*(8), Article 59. https://doi.org/10.1007/s11920-018-0925-8

Tempesta, D., Couyoumdjian, A., Curcio, G., Moroni, F., Marzano, C., De Gennaro, L., & Ferrara, M. (2010). Lack of sleep affects the evaluation of emotional stimuli. *Brain Research Bulletin, 82*(1–2), 104–108. https://doi.org/10.1016/j.brainresbull.2010.01.014

Tkachenko, O., & Dinges, D. F. (2018). Interindividual variability in neurobehavioral response to sleep loss: A comprehensive review. *Neuroscience and Biobehavioral Reviews, 89*, 29–48. https://doi.org/10.1016/j.neubiorev.2018.03.017

Tucker, A. M., Feuerstein, R., Mende-Siedlecki, P., Ochsner, K. N., & Stern, Y. (2012). Double dissociation: Circadian off-peak times increase emotional reactivity; aging impairs emotion regulation via reappraisal. *Emotion, 12*(5), 869–874. https://doi.org/10.1037/a0028207

Van den Berg, J. F., Kivelä, L., & Antypa, N. (2018). Chronotype and depressive symptoms in students: An investigation of possible mechanisms. *Chronobiology International, 35*(9), 1248–1261. https://doi.org/10.1080/07420528.2018.1470531

Vanek, J., Prasko, J., Genzor, S., Ociskova, M., Holubova, M., Sova, M., Kantor, K., Slepecky, M., & Nesnidal, V. (2020). Insomnia and emotion regulation. *Neuro Endocrinology Letters, 41*(5), 255–269.

Vetter, C. (2020). Circadian disruption: What do we actually mean? *European Journal of Neuroscience, 51*(1), 531–550. https://doi.org/10.1111/ejn.14255

Watling, J., Pawlik, B., Scott, K., Booth, S., & Short, M. A. (2017). Sleep loss and affective functioning: More than just mood. *Behavioral Sleep Medicine, 15*(5), 394–409. https://doi.org/10.1080/15402002.2016.1141770

Watts, A. L., & Norbury, R. (2017). Reduced effective emotion regulation in night owls. *Journal of Biological Rhythms, 32*(4), 369–375. https://doi.org/10.1177/0748730417709111

Webb, T. L., Miles, E., & Sheeran, P. (2012). Dealing with feeling: A meta-analysis of the effectiveness of strategies derived from the process model of emotion regulation. *Psychological Bulletin, 138*(4), 775–808. https://doi.org/10.1037/a0027600

Wittmann, M., Dinich, J., Merrow, M., & Roenneberg, T. (2006). Social jetlag: Misalignment of biological and social time. *Chronobiology International, 23*(1–2), 497–509. https://doi.org/10.1080/07420520500545979

Wright, K. P., Lowry, C. A., & Lebourgeois, M. K. (2012). Circadian and wakefulness–sleep modulation of cognition in humans. *Frontiers in Molecular Neuroscience, 5*, Article 50. https://doi.org/10.3389/fnmol.2012.00050

Yoo, S. S., Gujar, N., Hu, P., Jolesz, F. A., & Walker, M. P. (2007). The human emotional brain without sleep—A prefrontal amygdala disconnect. *Current Biology, 17*(20), R877–R878. https://doi.org/10.1016/j.cub.2007.08.007

Zhang, J., Lau, E., & Hsiao, J. H. (2019). Using emotion regulation strategies after sleep deprivation: ERP and behavioral findings. *Cognitive, Affective & Behavioral Neuroscience, 19*(2), 283–295. https://doi.org/10.3758/s13415-018-00667-y

Zohar, D., Tzischinsky, O., Epstein, R., & Lavie, P. (2005). The effects of sleep loss on medical residents' emotional reactions to work events: A cognitive-energy model. *Sleep, 28*(1), 47–54. https://doi.org/10.1093/sleep/28.1.47

CHAPTER

13 Sleep, Dreams, and Dreaming

Joseph De Koninck

Abstract

Dreams have fascinated humans from the earliest of times. Yet modern research is still struggling to understand the nature and functions of dreaming. It has been observed that sleep mentation tends to be in continuity with waking mentation but that the memory sources of dreams are significantly transformed into new expressions of experience and current concerns. Some dreams are creative and useful. Dreams can also be used to increase self-knowledge or as a complement in psychotherapy. Negative emotions and outcomes prevail in dreams and can culminate in nightmares. Fortunately, dreams can be controlled by suggestion, imagery rehearsal, and lucid dreaming. Electrophysiological and neuroimaging studies suggest that the unique features of dreaming are due to the key brain structures that are activated and interact differently in sleep, particularly rapid-eye-movement sleep, than in waking. While many new and original dream function theories have been proposed very recently, more rigorous scientific research is needed to determine whether dreaming by itself serves an adaptive function.

Key Words: dream, dreaming, dream formation, dream function, dream control

Introduction

From the earliest times, humans have been intrigued by their dreams and have sought to understand their meaning and function. This chapter attempts to cover a large spectrum of our current knowledge of the phenomenon of dreaming. First, an overview of the history of conceptions and uses of dreams reveals interesting roots to modern dream research and to the use of dreams in psychological practice. Then a review of factors influencing dream recall is followed by an overview of modern scientific methods of studying dreams. A description of characteristics of dream content as a function of age, gender, and personality and psychopathology provides a broad picture of dream features. Recent developments in the identification of the sources of dreams and the mechanisms of dream formation will serve as a basis for an examination of current hypotheses regarding the impact of dreams on waking life and of dream function theories. The practical uses of dreams, notably in problem-solving and psychotherapy, will culminate on methods of controlling dreams not only to reduce nightmares but to enhance the dream experience.

Historical Roots and Definitions

In the most primitive groups, dreams were not distinguished from waking reality and could lead to erroneous behaviors (Van de Castle, 1971). For example, a dream that a neighbor had stolen a good could trigger an undeserved retaliation. It is interesting to note here that this primitive attitude from a phylogenetic perspective mimics the ontogeny of modern humans. Indeed, the young child does not distinguish dreams from reality and will wake up fearing an imminent danger and will try to convince their parents of its reality (Foulkes, 1982; Strauch & Lederbogen, 1999). In more evolved cultures dreams have played a major role not only by influencing day-to-day behaviors but at a collective level by influencing major political decisions (Callois & Von Grunebaum, 1967; Van de Castle, 1994). There are many accounts of leaders using their dreams to decide on invasions and wars. It has been the same for major religions, for which dreams could be used by gods to guide humans (Van de Castle, 1994). *The Iliad*, *The Odyssey*, the Bible, and the Koran provide good examples of such interventions. The value of dreams in early societies is also exemplified by the establishment of temples to allow individuals to sleep and upon awakening narrate their dreams to priests who would interpret them. Egyptians, Greeks, and Romans have all adhered to these practices. It is, however, with the Greek philosophers that the bases of modern scientific study of dreams were established. They viewed dreams as natural phenomena, explored many of their facets, and formulated propositions that are still relevant to modern dream formation and dream function theories. Hippocrates's proposition that dreams could provide signs of illness and their origin is consistent with modern studies of incorporation of endogenous stimulation in dreams. Plato's views that dreams expressed hidden desires and were dominated by negative emotions are well in tune with Freud's wish fulfillment theory (Freud, 1900/1991) and the recent surge of interest in dream emotions as the central element of dream construction (Hartmann, 2008). Aristotle's essay on dreams ("De Insomnii") went further in investigating the relationship of dreams with waking life (Gallop, 1991). Anticipating the notion of continuity between waking and dreaming, he reflected on how dreams incorporate past experience and external and internal bodily sensations, and he noted that it was done in a distorted fashion. This notion is at the core of modern dream formation theories. His proposition that dreams are acts of imagination is congruent with Foulkes's (1985) cognitive theory of dreams and leads the way to the creative potential of dreams that is recognized today. Aristotle also noted that dreams can impact subsequent waking experience, which is central to modern dream function theories (e.g., Kuiken & Smith, 1991). Finally, Aristotle pointed out that dreamers can realize that they are dreaming, which is the first condition for lucid dreaming (Laberge, 1985), that is, when dreamers take control of the dream experience. It is the subject of modern research for its intense electrophysiological and neuronal activation correlates.

Another important Greek contribution came in the second century AD from Artemidorus de Daldis, who wrote a most impressive dream encyclopedia (*Oneirocritica*).

He produced a comprehensive taxonomy of dreams and established principles of dream interpretation. The methods proposed were precursors of modern dream content analyses and dream interpretation techniques (Van de Castle, 1994; White, 1975).

In early Christianity, dreams still played a significant role and were often referred to in accounts of the lives of saints and martyrs (Davis, 2005). Tertullian, an important Christian theologian and dream theoretician, proposed explanations on the formation of dreams (Salisbury, 2004). He notably remarked that dreams were more elaborated in the latter part of the night, an observation corroborated today by modern research (Antrobus et al., 1995). However, the propositions that dreams are influenced by seasons, the position of the dreamer, and food and wine intake are more marginally supported today. In his analyses of the sources of dreams, he noted that dreams can reflect day-to-day life events but could also contain messages from God. His view that most dreams are sent by demons and "can deceive humans, flatter them, and lure them into misbehavior" (Salisbury, 2004, p. 81) is one that has prevailed for many centuries and perhaps may explain why dreams were demoted during the Middle Ages, with little progress in their study realized (Van de Castle, 1994).

The systematic study of dreams resumed with the renewed interest in science in the 17th and 18th centuries, but the appearance of experimental approaches to the study of dreams came about only in the second half of the 19th century (Delboeuf, 1885). Notable contributions came from Maury (1865), who conducted experiments where he exposed himself to stimulations during his sleep and noted their influence on his dreams. Similar experiments were conducted by Léon D'Hervey de St-Denys (1867/1995). He went further to develop an elaborated method to control dreams in a manner that has become known in modern research as *lucid dreaming*.

Lavie and Hobson (1986) have pointed out that other important contributions in the 18th and 19th centuries by philosophers such as Leibnitz and psychophysiologists like Müller and Wundt, who recognized the endogenous and neurological basis of dream formation, have been mostly ignored, notably by Freud. Their contributions were clear precursors of modern theories of dream physiology.

There is no doubt that dreams came back to the attention of both the public and mental health professionals with Freud's *Interpretation of Dreams*, which appeared at the turn of the 20th century (1900/1991). He proposed that dreams were the guardians of sleep by preventing disruption by external and internal stimuli, the most important disruptions being repressed childhood conflicts trying to seek expression during sleep. This function was achieved by the transformation (dream work) of this latent content into acceptable manifest dream content, notably using sexual symbols. So dreams were not relevant to contemporary life but instead were the "royal road to the unconscious," thus a tool relevant in psychoanalytic therapy. There have been many reviews of the legacy and scientific values of Freud's hypotheses (e.g., Domhoff, 2003; Lavie & Hobson, 1986), and there have been vigorous debates about their survival to modern scientific evidence

(Domhoff, 2003; Hobson, 2004; Hobson et al., 2000; Solms, 2000, 2004). While there is now research evidence that dreams do incorporate external and internal stimulations during sleep and that these can prevent and delay awakenings, there is no evidence that dreams are essential for sleep maintenance and consolidation (Domhoff, 2003). Similarly, there is little support for the childhood sexual substrate of dreams (Foulkes, 1999). Freud's immediate followers saw a more direct relationship between dreams and contemporary life and concerns, and their influence prevails today. Adler (1929) viewed dreams as reflecting current coping attempts to solve contemporary problems. For Jung (1933), waking experience was represented in a compensatory and complementary fashion in dreams. Dreams were viewed as creative representations of the "subjective state" of the dreamer. The influence of these latter approaches has received support from modern research and has been integrated into research-based psychotherapeutic techniques (Hill, 2004; Rossner et al., 2004; Schredl & Hoffman, 2003). It is also interesting to point out that Jung's (1933) proposition that archetypes arising from the collective unconscious were expressed in dreams gave a phylogenetic component to dream formation that was echoed by Jouvet's (1974) hypothesis of a genetic expression role of rapid-eye-movement (REM) sleep towards acquired sensorimotor and adaptive behaviors echoed recently by Casaglia and Luppi (2022) and Revonsuo's (2000) more recent model of an evolutionary heritance of a threat simulation function of REM dreaming.

Modern studies of dreaming emerged from the discovery of REM sleep and its association with vivid dreaming (Aserinsky & Kleitman, 1953; Dement & Kleitman, 1957). Equating dreaming with REM sleep seemed to provide a definite tool for the scientific study of dreams. Waking up subjects during REM sleep would provide a detailed account of dream content, and REM sleep deprivation would cause dream deprivation (Dement, 1960). But as it became clear that dreaming was not limited to REM sleep and that indeed dreaming occurs during all stages of sleep (Foulkes, 1962), the scientific study of dreams was facing new challenges. Modern electroencephalography (EEG) and brain imaging are now offering very promising tools for the understanding of dreaming.

Definitions of Dreaming

Mental activity can vary in quality and quantity during sleep, and there is still a debate on the definition of what constitutes a dream. Even the International Association for the Study of Dreams has not come to a clear consensus on a definition (Pagel et al., 2001). One approach is to distinguish between different levels of dreaming. For example, Orlinsky (Dement, 1976, p. 41) has proposed an eight-point scale on the quality of dream content. It ranges from *no dream* (0) to *several disconnected thoughts, scenes, or actions* (3) to *a detailed dream sequence* (5) to *an extremely long and detailed sequence of five or more stages* (7). Although all levels of dream quality can be obtained from all stages of sleep, Levels 0 to 3 are more likely to emerge from non-REM (NREM) sleep and Levels 4 to 7 from REM sleep. More recent scales have been proposed (e.g., Nielsen, 2000) that essentially distinguish between levels of quality and complexity of the dream experience (dream-like) in an attempt to separate dreams arising from REM sleep and dreams arising from NREM sleep. A more recent arising consensus is that the underlying state of neuronal activity is the best determinant of the quality of the dream experience rather than the classification of dream stages that continue to be based on visual polygraphy parameters (Scarpelli, Alfonsi, et al., 2022).

Despite the above, it is still of interest to distinguish between different types of mental activities that occur during sleep with a typical place along the sleep cycle. Box 13.1 defines them, and Figure 13.1 situates them on a hypnogram of a young healthy adult. Expressed broadly, dreaming can be equated with *sleep mentation*, which Stickgold defines as "all perceptions, thoughts, and emotions experienced during sleep, or the process of perceiving, thinking, emoting during sleep" (2005a, p. 519). However, since most of the research has been carried out with either REM sleep–collected dreams or detailed home diaries, it will become evident that this chapter will focus on dreams that are more elaborated and dream-like and that would fall into categories 3–7 of the Orlinsky (Dement, 1976) scale.

Dream Recall

Until it is possible to directly record dreaming activity from brain activity, the study of mental activity in sleep must rely on the introspective recall of the dreamer. This limitation has always constituted and continues to be a challenge for dream research. The identification of factors influencing dream recall in both frequency and quality has been studied extensively in both the laboratory and the home environment, and several models

Box 13.1 A Brief Description of Types of Mental Activities in Sleep in Their Typical Order of Placement During the Sleep Cycle

1. ***Hypnagogic reverie:*** This sleep onset mentation (N1 and N2) is typically characterized by simple images, but it can also be elaborated. Recall frequency can reach 80%.
2. ***Reflections:*** Thoughts mainly observed in stages N2, 3, the dreamer reports thoughts with no hallucinatory content. Recall frequency in NREM sleep is approximately 40%–50%.
3. ***Night terrors:*** These very brief episodes of panic sometimes accompanied by mental activity occur in deep NREM sleep (N3: stages 3 and 4) at the beginning of the night.
4. ***Vivid dreams:*** These are classic dreams characterized by vivid imagery and sequences and involve characters, interactions, and emotions. This type of dream occurs mainly in REM sleep but can be observed in NREM. Recall frequency is up to 80% in REM sleep.
5. ***Lucid dreams:*** The dreamer is conscious of dreaming but remains asleep. In its purest form, the dreamer controls the scenario. They have been observed mainly in REM sleep but also in stage N2.
6. ***Nightmares and bad dreams:*** These dreams of highly anxiogenic content are observed in REM sleep, especially toward the end of the night. The content of nightmares actually awakens the dreamer.
7. ***Hypnopompic reverie:*** Obtained at the time of spontaneous arousal, typically in the morning. It can also be characterized by elaborate imagery.

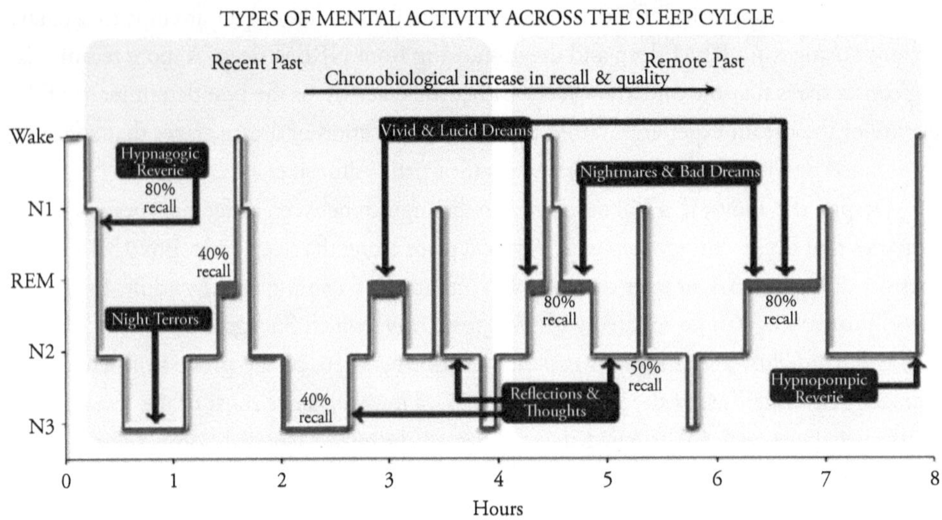

Figure 13.1 Hypnogram of a normal young adult and illustration of the situation of types of mental activity
Note. REM = rapid eye movement.

integrating them have been formulated (e.g., Cohen, 1974; Koulack & Goodenough, 1976; Schredl, Wittman, et al., 2003; Schredl, 2019a).

The main factors are as follows:

The sleep cycle, electrophysiological activity, and neuronal structures: Dream recall frequency from awakenings during a typical night of sleep is significantly higher after waking up from a state with activated EEG, such as at sleep onset (80%) and during REM sleep (80%), compared to slow EEG activity like in NREM sleep (40%–50%; Nielsen, 1995, 2000, 2004; Vogel, 1991). During REM sleep, recall is favored by sudden arousals, particularly during bursts of eye movements on the electro-oculogram. Kramer et al. (1974) have shown that the successive periods of REM sleep during the course of the night lead to the recall of increasingly rich content (for a review, see Nielsen, 2004). Within long periods of REM sleep, recall appears better and the content more elaborated in the window between 10 and 20 minutes (Kramer et al., 1979). Recent work suggests that, regardless of sleep stage, it is the electrophysiological activity that seems associated with dream recall. The levels of arousal including appearance of sleep spindles can predict the quality of the dream experience even during REM sleep when they are not present (Nielsen et al., 2017). In addition, in both REM and NREM sleep, reports of dream experience were found to be associated with local decreases in low-frequency activity in posterior cortical regions (Siclari et al., 2017). There is also evidence that stable individual features of the brain structure and activation patterns can explain interindividual differences in dream experience in the same way that similarities of dream quality are associated with the implications of similar underlying neuronal structures (Scarpelli, Alfonsi, et al., 2022). Finally a Topographic-dynamic Re-organization model of Dreams (TRoD) according to which the Default Mode

Network, that is characteristically present during REM sleep, is responsible for fluctuations in dream content characteristics in terms of activity and for example bizarreness (Northoff et al., 2023).

Memory processes: The basic principles of waking memory apply to dream recall. On arousal from sleep, distractions and interference will reduce recall quality and frequency (Cohen, 1974). The dreamer must pay attention immediately to the dream. The primacy and recency effect applies as well: Elements at the beginning and end of the same dream experience are more accessible to the dreamer upon awakening. Similarly, the first and last dreams of the night are easier to recall the following morning (Pivik, 1991). Dreams that are vivid and have a salient content are better remembered (Cohen, 1974), and individuals with good visual memory are advantaged in their recall of dreams (Buisink & Kuiken, 1996). Recently, it has been documented that during NREM sleep, dream recall is positively correlated with fast sleep spindles, which are also associated with memory consolidation during sleep (Nielsen et al., 2017). It is not surprising therefore that, as mentioned earlier, fast sleep spindles were also correlated with REM dream recall frequency even though they are not actually present in REM sleep.

Psychological factors: Individuals with interest and motivation in dreams will recall dreams more frequently (Halliday, 1992). For example, women are typically more interested in dreams and accordingly have higher dream recall frequency (Schredl, 2007). In periods of real-life stress, dream recall is enhanced (Lavie & Kaminer, 1991; Schredl, Ciric, Gottz, & Witmann, 2003; Valli et al., 2006), perhaps because of their enhanced emotionality and vividness (Malinowski & Horton, 2014a). The recent pandemic has fostered a host of studies that unsurprisingly observed an increase of dream recall and of nightmares in the general population (e.g., Scarpelli, Alfonsi, et al., 2021; Scarpelli, Nadoorff, et al., 2022).

Age and gender: According to a large-scale survey study by Nielsen (2012), dream recall frequency increases from adolescence to early adulthood and then decreases starting in middle adulthood. There are various proposed explanations of this decrease in dream recall in late adulthood including the well-documented decrease in REM sleep percentage with age. As for gender, consistent with a number of earlier studies, there is overall a higher recall for females, but that seems concentrated in those between 14 and 44 years old (Nielsen, 2012).

Personality factors: There have been many studies exploring the relationship between dream recall frequency and many personality dimensions, notably introversion/extroversion, field dependence, anxiety trait, locus of control, and, more recently, thick versus thin boundaries and openness to experience (see early reviews by Blagrove, 2007; Cohen, 1979; recently Schredl, 2019a; Schredl & Ruthman, 2022). While in most cases, the correlations have been low, the latter two dimensions remain the most significant; that is, there is better recall with thinner boundaries (Hartmann, 1991) and higher openness to experience (Watson, 2003).

Dream Research Methodologies

Dream Collection

It transpires from above that for research purposes it is important to obtain dream reports as close as possible to their occurrence. Traditionally, research work employed two approaches: collecting dreams either in the laboratory by waking up subjects during polysomnographic recording or at home in the subject's natural surroundings through dream diaries, optimally by dream writing upon morning awakening (Antrobus et al., 1991). While laboratory awakenings during polysomnography can provide detailed accounts of mental activity in sleep, the dreams obtained are often affected by the laboratory situations and have been found to be less salient and to contain less aggression (Foulkes, 1962). Indeed, Picard-Deland et al. (2021) reported that 36% of dreams collected from the lab, largely from REM sleep, include lab incorporations 40% of the time. The dream diary recorded at home is more likely to contain elaborations extending beyond the original content (for a discussion, see Domhoff, 2003, Ch. 2). Direct recordings by telephone protocols seem to facilitate spontaneity in reporting and avoiding writing artifacts. While portable polysomnography with close to full montage has been used for home monitoring of sleep, more recent approaches use simplified ambulatory monitoring in the home environment that should allow REM sleep detection and dream reporting during the night (e.g., Arnal et al., 2020). That is not the case for recent smartphone applications to monitor sleep quality and even measure deep sleep and REM sleep. So far, they have not yet been validated to serve as REM detectors for the purpose of dream collection (Ananth, 2021).

It should be mentioned that the use of naps instead of full-night laboratory recordings is gaining popularity because of the increased interest in sleep onset mentation and that more than 90-minute naps can give opportunities to collect dreams from all stages.

Finally, in order to probe information on dreams from large samples, some researchers use questionnaires that ask subjects to retroactively indicate the frequency of appearances of particular dream content features or themes (e.g., Nielsen et al., 2003; Schredl et al., 2004).

Dream Content Analyses

Dream reports are typically analyzed by judges with scales on various dream dimensions (Winget & Kramer, 1979). The most comprehensive system still used today is that of Hall and Van de Castle (1966), which deciphers dreams notably on objects, characters, interactions, emotions, activities, and outcomes. Its use has been adapted to computation on spreadsheets by Domhoff (1996, 2003). There are now attempts to develop automatic dream content analyses (e.g., Barcaro et al., 2005; Wong et al., 2016; Fogli et al., 2020), particularly using text mining software such as the Linguistic Inquiry and Word Count program (Bulkeley & Graves, 2018; Mota et al., 2020). It has also been possible using artificial intelligence and machine learning to match human judges in the evaluation of the emotional tone of dreams at over 60% accuracy and to trace the evolution of emotional tone across dream reports (Amini et al., 2011; Pesonen et al., 2020). Even the gender of the dreamer can be detected, with machine learning reaching comparable accuracy to human judges (Amini et al., 2011).

Dream Norms

The Hall and Van de Castle studies from the 1950s and 1960s (combined in Hall & Van de Castle, 1966) have provided a global profile of dream content dimensions in the young adult as obtained from home diary methods. It was based on five dreams from 100 female and 100 male college students. It remains today the major reference since it has proven stable over at least one generation (Hall et al., 1982). Table 13.1 provides a brief résumé of

Table 13.1 Normative data on the dreams of young American adults[a] compared to those of young Canadian adults[b]

	Men 1966	Men 2016	Women 1966	Women 2016
Environment (per dream)	1.29	1.49	1.31	1.64
Interior (%)	44	50	55	67
Exterior (%)	47	43	35	34
Familiar (%)	31	29	37	33
Unfamiliar (%)	19	10	10	14
Characters (per dream)	2.4	3.13	2.8	3.89
Male (%)	53	59	37	36
Female (%)	26	48	40	35
Animal (%)	6	13	4	9
Social interaction		1.36		1.48
Aggressive (%)	47	46	44	47
Friendly (%)	38	33	42	40
Sexual (%)	12	4	3	7
Emotions		0.85		1.10
Positive (%)	20	18	20	19
Negative (%)	80	40	80	81
Outcome		0.33		0.23
Success (%)	15	11	8	9
Failure (%)	15	16	10	11
Fortune		0.72		0.65
Good fortune (%)	6	10	6	5
Misfortune (%)	36	40	33	39

[a]Data obtained in the early 1950s, based on five dreams of 100 men and 100 women aged 18–25. Summarized from Hall and Van de Castle (1966).

[b]Data obtained between 2005 and 2016 at the University of Ottawa, based on the dreams of 300 men and 300 women aged 18–24, who each contributed two dreams.

the incidences and proportions on several dream dimensions derived from the initial Hall and Van de Castle sample and recent data obtained from a comparable but smaller sample at the University of Ottawa (Dale et al., 2016). While norms have been well established for young adults, there are only a few studies that have looked at developmental trends in dream content (Dale et al., 2015, 2017; Lortie-Lussier et al., 2019). From recent results, it transpires that aggression decreases from adolescence to old age, which includes aggression initiated by the dreamer and targeted at the dreamer. Also, a gender difference that permeates across age is that verbal aggression is the dominant form of aggressive interactions in women's dreams and physical aggression in men's dreams (Lortie-Lussier et al., 2019).

The main observation emerging from all these normative studies is that dreams tend to be more negative than positive on many dimensions. Indeed, the most common emotion is apprehension; aggressions are more frequent than friendly interactions, and misfortunes outnumber good fortunes. This is also observed in laboratory-collected dreams during REM sleep (Roussy et al., 2000) and in studies of typical dream themes. For example, in a sample of more than 1,000 Canadian university students, the most frequent dream theme remembered was that of being chased (Nielsen et al., 2003). It has been observed since then by other studies and seems universal (Mathes et al., 2014). However, the issue of unpleasantness and emotional tone of dreams has recently been the subject of debate since it has been observed that when dreamers rate the emotions of their dreams their evaluation can be more positive than the traditional evaluation by external judges (e.g., Röver & Schredl, 2017). While this may be due to methodologic artifacts, it can also be interpreted as indicative of some adaptive function since it is present even in dreams that contain threats, misfortunes, and failures (Barbeau, Turpin, et al., 2022; Sikka et al., 2017).

Dream Formation

With the discovery of REM sleep's association with vivid dreaming, it was hoped that by obtaining a large and systematic sample of the dreaming activity from a single night, it would be possible to determine which waking experiences find their way into dreams, how they are transformed, and when this occurs. However, more than 60 years of laboratory research have revealed that REM dream construction is overly complex and multifactorial (see discussion in Domhoff, 2018; Barbeau, Lafrenière, et al., 2022). There is a substantial proportion of dream elements whose source is unidentified by independent judges and even by the dreamer. Even when elements appear, they are so transformed that in most cases only the dreamer can recognize the link. Independent judges can identify pre-sleep concerns in REM dreams of subjects in less than 20% of instances (Saredi et al., 1997). They can match descriptions of daily events or pre-sleep concerns with dreams from different days and nights at a rate not above chance (Roussy et al., 1996). It is evident that several factors contribute to this transformation and lead to an original expression that is typically far from episodic sources of waking experience.

Figure 13.2 illustrates an updated proposed layer approach for conceptualizing the contributions of the sources and factors in a hierarchical manner. It proposes that the lower-level factors are predominant and that higher ones still shape the content of dreams but with decreasing influence. The lower layers are also more difficult to influence or manipulate. Of course, in special situations, such as following traumatic events, certain factors can gain more influence.

Sleep Stage and Electrophysiology, Neurophysiological Organization, Chronobiological Position

SLEEP STAGE AND ELECTROPHYSIOLOGY

The electrophysiological correlates of dreaming have been studied extensively by waking subjects during polysomnographic recordings. For example, sleep onset mentation, which can be very vivid and dream-like, typically refers to the recent past such as the preceding hours and days (Nielsen, 1995; Vogel, 1991; Wamsley et al., 2010). REM dreams are also vivid and story-like. In most cases, reports from subjects awakened from REM sleep are longer than those obtained from NREM sleep, and this contributes to their higher quality. REM dreams from the first half of the night tend to refer to pre-sleep experiences, while later REM periods are typically associated with more remote temporal references (Roussy et al., 1998; Verdone, 1965). Dreams arising from NREM sleep contain more day residues and episodic memory than dreams from REM sleep (Foulkes, 1962). Using high-density EEG, Siclari et al. (2017) recorded dreams from both REM and NREM sleep and observed that reports of dream experience were associated with local decreases in low-frequency activity in posterior cortical regions. In addition, they reported that high-frequency activity correlated with the thinking dream dimension in frontal brain

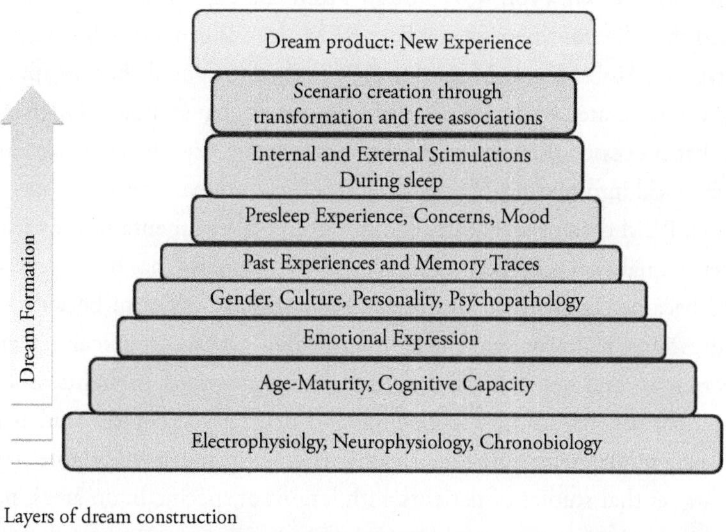

Figure 13.2 Layers of dream construction

Note. The various factors in the elaboration of dreaming are illustrated as a pyramid, suggesting their order and importance (see text).

regions and with the perceiving dream dimension in parietal, occipital, and temporal areas. As pointed out earlier, there is thus emerging evidence that intense dreaming can appear outside of REM sleep, notably when the underlying activation is present (Scarpelli, Alfonsi, et al., 2022).

At the time of discovery of the association between REM sleep and dreaming, it was reported that eye movements during REM sleep were related to the actual visual activity in dreams (Aserinsky & Kleitman, 1953; Dement & Kleitman, 1957). Other phasic events in REM sleep were also thought to be directly related to the dream experience. For example, penile erections during REMs were hypothesized to reflect the underlying sexual drive of dreams as proposed by Freud (1900/1991). These isomorphism hypotheses have not been corroborated. For example, for eye movements, the presence of vivid dreams outside of REM sleep and the fact that the eye movements come in bursts, are often in diagonal directions, and are present in the congenitally blind does not support this contention (see Arnulf, 2011). There are special situations, however, where eye movements seem to correspond to the dreaming activity, as reported recently in cases of REM sleep behavior disorder (Leclair-Visonneau et al., 2010; Oudiette et al., 2010). One consistent finding is that the density of eye movements in REM sleep as well as other phasic events in REM sleep are positively related to the level of activity and affect of dreams (see Maranci et al., 2022; Pivik, 1991).

NEUROPHYSIOLOGICAL SUBSTRATE

The close association of vivid dreaming with REM sleep and the undeniable fact that mental activity occurs throughout all sleep stages are still the sources of considerable debate concerning the brain generators of dreaming. It has been notably expressed in debates that appeared in *Behavioral and Brain Sciences* (Vol. 23, 2000), *Scientific American* (May 2004), and *Nature* (Vol. 437, 2005). From the early work of Jouvet (1962), it was assumed that the pontine region where REM sleep is generated was responsible for dream activation. Hobson and McCarley (1977) then proposed that dream imagery in REM sleep was generated by giant cells of the brainstem that stimulated higher centers of the cortex that processed them to create the actual dream experience while normal waking neurochemical information-processing filters (i.e., monoamines) are shut. According to this model, REM dreams are clearly distinct from NREM mentation, which is significantly lower in quality. Their "activation-synthesis hypothesis" has had a very significant impact and became the mainstream model, while raising criticism because it gave the origin of dreaming to lower brain centers, provided a neurochemical explanation for dream bizarreness, and negated the contribution of processed thoughts. Solms (2000, 2019) used pharmacological, neuroimaging, and neuropsychological studies to formulate an alternate model proposing that dreams are actively generated by forebrain mechanisms. He argues that studies of patients with lesions of specific brain areas, notably the temporoparietooccipital junction and the ventromedian quadrant of the frontal lobes, suggest that dreaming can be generated only through these higher centers and that they have no relation with the frequency, duration, and density of REM sleep (Solms, 1997). According to this model, not only can dreaming occur outside of REM sleep, but it is not dependent on brain generators of REM sleep. Foulkes (1985) has proposed that a dream is essentially a cognitive product that depends on the cognitive capacity of the dreamer and the level of memory activation during sleep. It accounts for differences between REM and NREM mentation on the basis of the difference in cognitive capacity associated with these sleep stages.

Nielsen (2000) has offered a distinction between one-generator and two-generator models of dream formation. The former stipulates that a "single set of imagery processes produce sleep mentation regardless of sleep stage in which it occurs" (p. 852). Solms's (2000) and Foulkes's (1985) propositions fall into the one-generator category of models. On the other hand, the two-generator model asserts that "REM and NREM mentation reports stem from qualitatively different imagery generation systems" (Nielsen, 2000, p. 852). Hobson and McCarley's (1977) activation synthesis hypothesis is the prototype of two-generator models. To reconcile these two opposing models, Nielsen (2000) points out that there are components of REM sleep, such as reductions in muscle tone and high-frequency EEG, that spill over into NREM sleep. They are notably better observed in case of REM sleep deprivation. These components would be responsible for the mental activity produced in NREM sleep, and their relative weakness would account for the lower quality of NREM dreaming. This model thus explains the presence of mental activity through all the sleep stages yet still attributes the mentation generator to that of REM sleep mechanisms.

The important issue that has been very rarely mentioned in this debate is the sleep onset mentation (Foulkes & Vogel, 1965; Vogel, 1991). More recent studies with advanced EEG recording techniques and imaging have offered new perspectives of mental activity during sleep that include sleep onset mentation. Domhoff, in several contributions along the development of his neurocognitive theory of dream formation, points out the importance of the default mode network (DMN) that prevails during REM sleep as well as at sleep onset (Domhoff, 2019, 2023; Hong et al., 2021). The cognitive constraints associated with the DMN explain why dreams contain little or no instances of reading, writing, and counting (Domhoff, 2023; Hartmann, 1996; Hartmann, 2000). On the other hand, this feature leads the way to the expression of emotions and of associative thinking. Indeed, it is well documented that, during REM sleep, there is significant activation of the limbic/paralimbic areas including the amygdala (Dang-Vu et al., 2007). This observation is consistent with the prevalence of emotions, particularly on the negative side, in REM dreams. Scarpelli et al. (2019) offer a more global picture by pointing out that the several neural substrates that regulate emotions in REM sleep are like those involved in waking emotions. The associative feature of the DMN is congruent with the creative potential of both REM dreams and sleep onset mentation. Lacaux et al. (2021) have indeed undertaken an interesting series of studies focusing on the sleep onset period and reported promising observations explaining its use by artists and scientists for its creative value.

Despite all this progress, the neural correlates of dreaming have not been identified satisfactorily yet (Ruby, 2020). Continued improvements in imaging techniques and high-density EEG will provide more and more precise localization of dreaming activity. An innovative line of research uses imagery to uncover subjective contents of dreaming using objective neural measurement. More precisely, functional magnetic resonance imaging–recorded activity and image decoders with machine learning have been used to reconstruct visual images from the human brain, particularly the occipital regions, that are replayed in REM sleep. Findings show that specific visual experience during sleep is represented by brain activity patterns, providing a window to subjective contents of dreaming and to dream formation (Horikawa & Katamini, 2017).

CHRONOBIOLOGICAL POSITION

Nielsen (2004) has reviewed studies suggesting that dream formation is also modulated by chronobiological factors. For example, the ultradian 90-minute basic rest–activity cycle proposed by Kleitman (1962), which is expressed notably in waking by an alternation of states of vigilance and fantasy, corresponds in sleep to the 90-minute NREM/REM rhythm expressed by alternation between thought-like mentation and dream-like mentation. This phenomenon was proposed to be associated with an alternation between left (NREM) and right (REM) hemispheric dominance (Broughton, 1975). Subsequent studies suggested, however, that both hemispheres were active in dreaming and that hemispheric dominance corresponds to actual dream activity in the same fashion as in waking mental activity (Pivik, 1991). This ultradian 90-minute variation in type of sleep mentation seems to correspond to alternations in brain activation levels (Llinas & Pare, 1991) and is present in narcoleptic daytime sleep episodes (De Koninck et al., 1986; Lacaux, 2021). Within a night's sleep in the young adult, it has just been documented that recent memory sources are more frequent at sleep onset and from REM sleep episodes (Picard-Deland et al., 2022) and confirmed as well that late-night dreams from all stages contain more remote sources than early-night temporal memories. A second level of rhythm is the 12-hour circasemidian oscillation in slow-wave sleep expression and sleep propensity (Broughton & Mullington, 1992). It corresponds to the increased sleep pressure in the early part of the night and in mid-afternoon (napping zone). These two periods are associated with decreased sleep mentation and dream recall (Chellappa et al., 2009). The infradian rhythm of the menstrual cycle has an impact on dream emotions and social interactions, with increases in anxiety and aggressive interactions during the premenstrual phase of the cycle (e.g., Sirois-Berliss & De Koninck, 1982; Wiebe et al., 2007).

Age-Maturity, Cognitive Capacity

According to the cognitive approach to dream formation, dreams are dependent not on perception but on "how the brain thinks" during sleep (Foulkes, 1985). A most obvious determinant of capacity is age and maturation. There is clearly an ontogenetic evolution in both the organization and the content of dreams (Zepelin, 1981). Foulkes and his collaborators have characterized extensively dreams in children in both longitudinal and cross-sectional studies (e.g., Foulkes, 1982; Foulkes et al., 1990; Foulkes 2017). They have demonstrated that the cognitive organization of dreams follows the cognitive development of the child as described by Piaget (1962). Before the age of 5, dreams are poor in narrative structure and not elaborated. Later they become more organized with themes, characters, and scenarios. In the 5- to 8-year-old range, the authors observed high correlations between dream-report rates and the Wechsler Bloc Design (Foulkes et al., 1990). In adult life and in aging, the quality of the dreams parallels the waking cognitive ability of the dreamer (see Cavallero & Foulkes, 1993; Fogel et al., 2018). As mentioned above in the dream norms section, the actual content of dreams follows developmental patterns of waking social and emotional experience (Lortie-Lussier et al., 2019).

Emotional Expression

Hartmann (2007) has proposed that emotions are not only important components of dreams but that they are the primary source of dream formation. According to his theory, each dream starts with a central image that expresses the dominant emotion of the dreamer and guides the creation of connections to existing memory systems that in turn lead to new associations that have an adaptive value (Hartmann, 2008).

Consistent with the neuronal basis of REM sleep outlined above, there is a rising consensus that indeed waking emotionality and current concerns are important contributors to dream formation and are most predominant in dreams (Malinowski & Horton 2014b; Nielsen, 2005). Even the perception of the emotions and feelings of others appears to be preserved in dreams (Kahn & Hobson, 2005). As mentioned earlier, in normative studies where dreams are rated by judges, negative emotions tend to prevail (e.g., Dale et al., 2016; Hall & Van de Castle, 1966). However, some studies of REM dreams where emotions were rated by the dreamer instead of a judge showed that positive emotions were more frequent than negative ones (e.g., Barbeau, Turpin, et al., 2022; Fosse et al., 2001; Sikka et al., 2017). Several studies referred to below support the notion that this predominance of emotions is part of a mood regulation function of REM sleep itself that transpires into the expressed dream emotions that accompany it (Scarpelli et al., 2019).

Gender, Social Role, Culture, Personality, and Psychopathology

Gender differences in dream content have been documented in adolescents (Winegar & Levin, 1997) and in adults (Hall & Van de Castle, 1966) and integrated into young adult norms that have been replicated over three generations (Dale et al., 2016; Hall et al., 1982). It has been postulated that the observation that dreams of women are more pleasant and contain less aggression, more friendliness, and pleasant emotions reflects a long-lasting impact of biological differences and/or early socialization. However, it has been reported that social roles enacted in adulthood attenuate some of the gender differences (Lortie-Lussier et al., 1992). Table 13.1 reveals that some of the dream content gender differences observed several decades ago by Hall and Van de Castle (1966), such as aggression and positive emotions, seem to disappear.

Anthropologists have studied dreams in a large number of ancient cultures (see special issue of *Dreaming*, Vol. 14, 2004), and cross-cultural comparisons have been made between modern societies such as American, Mexican, Japanese, Canadian, German, and Chinese (Dale et al., 2016; Griffith et al., 1960; Roll & Brenneis, 1975; Roll et al., 1974; Schredl, Ciric, Bishop, et al., 2003; Yu, 2008). The main normative observations made by Hall and Van de Castle (1966) appear to be present across cultures (see Table 13.1 and Domhoff, 1996, 2019). Thematic preferences also appear universal, such as the prevalent theme of being chased but not physically abused (Nielsen et al., 2003). Other studies suggest that some features correspond to cultural identity. For example, death themes are more frequent in dreams of Mexicans than Americans (Roll & Brenneis, 1975). It seems also that cultural values transpire in dreams, notably in incidences of aggression (Tartz & Krippner, 2008).

Many studies have attempted to link personality characteristics to the construction of dreams (Blagrove, 2007; Domhoff, 1996; Samson-Daoust et al., 2019; Schrell, 2019b). However, research has not revealed much relationship between personality traits and dream characteristics. Instead, it seems that dreams express more current concerns and conceptions of the dreamer than personality dimensions. Yet, the personality dimension that has received much attention in connection with dreams and nightmares is that of thin/thick boundary (Hartmann et al., 1991). Individuals with thin boundaries are open, trusting, vulnerable, and sensitive and have a rich fantasy life. Those with thick boundaries are very focused and rigid and differentiate clearly between thoughts and feelings. Thin-boundary persons have been found to have dreams that are more vivid, are more emotional, and have more interactions than those of thick-boundary persons. According to Hartmann (1991), they are also more susceptible to frequent nightmares. However, Samson-Daoust et al. (2019) observed that the best predictor of emotional valence in everyday dreams is trait anxiety. The latest study revealed that openness to experience was significantly related to nightmare frequency, whereas neuroticism was related to nightmare distress (Brekke et al., 2023).

Psychopathological conditions can also affect dreams (for a first review, see Kramer & Nuhic, 2007 and Khazaie, 2012). For example, the dreams of schizophrenia sufferers are brief and have very little hallucinatory content, apparently in a compensatory fashion to waking fantasy predominance (Kramer & Roth, 1979; Lusignan et al., 2009). In addition, their dreams exhibit surprisingly few depressive themes (Kramer & Roth, 1979).

However, they contain more aggression, particularly directed toward the dreamer (e.g., Strompe et al., 2003). Most interestingly, it has been observed that dreams containing vivid expressions of violence can precede severe psychotic episodes in waking and that, as the patient deteriorates, dreams can become less distinguishable from waking state mentation (Herz & Melville, 1980; Khazaie et al., 2012; Levin & Daly, 1998; Wolman, 1979).

The relationship between dream content and depression also seems to depend on the severity of the condition. Some studies show that depressed individuals report short and bland dreams (e.g., Barrett & Loeffler, 1992; Beauchemin & Hays, 1996). However, it has also been observed that dreams during depression were more negative and contained more masochistic elements (e.g., Beck & Ward, 1961; Trenholme et al., 1984). With improvements in depression, "hostility is decreased while intimacy, heterosexuality, and motility are increased" in dreams (Kramer & Roth, 1979, p. 379). One possible explanation for these divergent results is the different severity of depressive symptoms from one study to another. Thus, negative dreams were observed mainly in cases of mild, moderate, or remitted depression, while neutral dreams have generally been obtained from samples of people with severe depression or with psychotic features.

More recently, Glucksman and Kramer (2017) in a psychodynamic study reported that dream themes of death and/or dying, violence, injury, or murder were more frequent in the dream reports of depressed patients with suicidal ideation and/or attempts than in those of depressed patients without suicidal ideation or behavior.

A study of subjects suffering from autism spectrum disorder revealed that they had a lower dream recall, shorter dreams with fewer features including fewer emotions, and lower negative tone than in controls (Daoust et al., 2008). These results reflect the neurocognitive dimension of this condition.

As for studies of dreams in psychopathologies such as post-traumatic stress disorder (PTSD) and in parasomnias such as nightmares, night terrors, and REM sleep behavior disorder, they are the subject of other chapters, so we will simply provide here an overview. Foremost are night terrors and nightmares. As mentioned earlier and illustrated in Figure 13.1, night terrors occur in NREM sleep in the first part of the night. Typically they are characterized by a sudden arousal with little or no mental content recall. When there is recall, it is usually concentrated on one theme, often a suffocation sensation, which is why night terrors are also called "incubus attack." In some instances, night terrors may lead to somnambulism accompanied by more elaborated mental content of a negative tone (Oudiette et al., 2009).

Nightmares are twice as frequent in individuals with mood or psychotic disorders than in healthy controls (Akkaoui et al., 2020). They are mainly produced in the latter part of the night, mostly in REM sleep, but can also occur in Stage 2 (Kellerman, 1987). They are dreams with elaborate and highly anxious and stressful content (Zadra, Pilon, & Donderi, 2006). Some authors distinguish those whose stressful content provokes awakening from those where it does not. The latter are labeled as *bad dreams* instead of nightmares (Nielsen & Levin, 2007). There is, however, the unanswered question of whether it is possible to remember dreams without awakening during or at the end of their course. It may be that if the nightmare is salient enough, it leads to a spontaneous observation by dreamers that its very negative content was responsible for the awakening (Blagrove & Haywood, 2006). In cases of less stressful content, the dreamers do not mention that its negative content awakened them.

Nightmares and night terrors are prevalent in 5- to 9-year-olds and normally disappear by early adolescence. They persist in adulthood in 2% to 10% of the population. When present in adulthood, they tend to be associated with sensitive personalities and individuals who are artists or creative persons, and nightmares are more prevalent in periods of stress. Persistent nightmares are also reported after traumatic events, are a key feature of PTSD, and can occur across the night (Lamarche & De Koninck, 2007). The most systematically studied were those of war survivors, notably after the Holocaust (Lavie & Kaminer, 1991), the wars in the Middle East (Valli et al., 2006), and Afghanistan. Currently, out of dozens of studies of the impact of the 2019 pandemic on sleep, a host of them have included dreaming and consistently confirm an increased dream recall and nightmares (e.g., Scarpelli, Alfonsi, et al., 2022). We just recently observed that adolescents who were hospitalized for suicide attempt reported having frequent nightmares. They also incorporated higher prevalence of destructive themes and failures, as well as self-directed and death-resulting aggressions. Their morning mood seemed negatively influenced by their dreams (Desjardins et al., 2024).

Studies of dreaming in parasomnias have been reviewed recently by Arnulf (2019). Both those present in NREM (night terrors, sleepwalking, sexsomnia) and in REM (REM sleep behavior disorder) as well as sleep paralysis include dream content that can mirror the accompanied movements, behaviors, and emotions. For example, in REM sleep behavior disorder, the person exhibits vigorous motor activity and speech usually associated with dreaming activity and sleep talking (Arnulf et al., 2017). However, the apparent aggressive movements are not associated with elevated aggression in waking (Fantini et al., 2005).

Pre-Sleep Experience, Concerns, Mood

There is ample evidence that waking experience finds its way into dreams. For example, throughout adulthood both men's and women's dreams refer to family life and work, and in the elderly themes of death surface (Lortie-Lussier et al., 1992; Winget et al., 1972). The time course for the integration of waking experience into dreams is, however, more complex.

A host of REM dream studies have been carried out in which subjects have been exposed to unusual pre-sleep events. Typically, they have been conducted in the laboratory involving polysomnographic recording and REM period awakening with the caveats of the effect of the lab setting itself, as mentioned earlier. Manipulations of pre-sleep experiences have included social isolation (Wood, 1962), water deprivation (Bokert, 1968), stressful or unusual films (De Koninck & Koulack, 1975), stressful intellectual activity (Koulack et al., 1985), and even subliminal stimulation (Shevrin, 1986). Other studies have focused on the effects of real-life experiences and/or stress on dream content, such as divorce (Cartwright et al., 1998), pregnancy (Sabourin et al., 2018), postpartum depression (Forest et al., 2023), premenstrual symptoms (Wiebe et al., 2007), trauma (Valli et al., 2006), and recently the 2019 pandemic (Scarpelli, Nadorff, et al., 2022). Overall, these conditions have had more potent impacts on dreams than experimentally induced stress. The bulk of the literature supports the notion that the mode of representation of waking activity in dreams is that of continuity (e.g., that waking stress induces anxiety in dreams, and relaxation induces pleasant dreams; Lafrenière et al., 2018). However, there are instances of compensation for waking needs or drives. For example, social isolation can trigger dreams of social interactions (Wood, 1962), thirst may induce dreams of drinking (Bokert, 1968), and regular exposure to video games involving threats is accompanied by reduced threat severity variables in dreams (Gackenbach & Kuruvilla, 2008). It can be argued, however, that these latter instances are in continuity with waking experience but in a complementary fashion.

Direct incorporations of pre-sleep experiences tend to be few. And that applies to salient ones. For example, we have observed, in subjects who wore goggles inverting vertically their visual field for 4 days, very few incorporations of inverted vision in REM dreams and that in only four of eight subjects (De Koninck et al., 1996). The incorporations were mostly indirect and referred to frustrations related to the inverted vision experience. Direct incorporations have tended to be more prominent in the cases of real-life emotionally stressful experiences, for example, during war traumas (e.g., Valli et al., 2006).

Certain types of activities have more difficulty finding their way into dreams. Hartmann (1996) noted that reading, writing, and counting, which are common everyday activities, are seldom reported in dreams. It has also been observed that episodic memory is essentially absent from the manifest content of REM dreams (Fosse et al., 2003). Indeed, a 6-week intensive language learning program led to incorporations of the new language in most cases after several weeks of constant daytime learning exposure (De Koninck et al., 1990).

Marquandt et al. (1996) reported that almost half of incorporations of waking experiences come from the preceding day, close to 20% from the preceding week, and the remaining third from earlier experiences. Although a large proportion of dream elements therefore refer to preceding-day activities, thoughts, and concerns, there is good evidence that incorporation of some experiences and memories can be significantly delayed (see Nielsen, 2005). Jouvet (1979), from his own multiyear dream diary, noted first a lag of 6 to 9 days before a new environment or situation would be incorporated into his dreams. This 1-week *dream lag effect* has since been clearly demonstrated in laboratory studies (Grenier et al., 2005; Nielsen & Powel, 1992). More recently, Eichenlaub et al.

(2018) reported that the dream lag effect is particularly present in the case of personally significant events. Beyond 1 week, there is a sharp decline in references to remote waking experiences in dreams. However, Grenier et al. (2005), in a study of temporal references in REM dreams of elderly persons, dream elements that refer to waking events during adolescence and early adulthood were more prominent than those referring to adulthood. This observation is consistent with the predominance of autobiographical memories of adolescence and early childhood over the life span (Rubin et al., 1986). It is therefore well documented that dreams can readily use memory traces that go back to childhood (for further discussion, see Nielsen, 2005; Picard-Deland et al., 2022).

External and Internal Stimulation During Sleep

Early studies by Maury (1865) and Léon D'Hervey de St-Denys (1867/1995) already demonstrated that various sensory stimulations such as exposition to perfumes, tactile sensations, and sounds can be incorporated into dreams but that they were markedly distorted. The transformations can take different forms. For example, Berger (1963) noted that pronouncing nouns during REM sleep could lead to a variety of incorporations by *assonance* ("Gillian" transformed into "Chile" [Chilian]), *association* ("Richard": dreams of a shop by the same name), and represen*tation* ("Paul" appears in the dream but it is a different person). Not surprisingly, meaningful stimulations such as the dreamer's name are more likely to be incorporated into REM dreams, illustrating the capacity of the brain to process stimuli from the outside world during REM sleep (Perrin et al., 1999).

Of all external stimulations, the one that seems the most likely to influence dream content and emotional valence is olfactory (Schredl et al., 2009). It seems also efficient for inducing lucid dreaming (Erlacher et al., 2020).

The Product of Dream Formation: New Content in Dreams

A prevailing observation of dream production that is reflected in most dream formation theories is the capacity of dreams to produce new material that is far from directly mirroring waking experience except in abnormal conditions (Stickgold & Walker, 2004). Indeed, in his cognitive model of dreaming, Foulkes proposed that dreams constitute "a creative recombination of memory and knowledge" (1985, p. 123). Perhaps the best demonstration of this phenomenon comes from a study by Uga et al. (2006), who studied dreams in 35 professional musicians and a control group. As expected, musicians did hear more music in their dreams than controls; but, most interestingly, in 28% of instances it had never been heard before and was new music. It seems that dreaming activity is "open season" for the mind to explore new associations. It is not surprising that many novels were written from a scenario laid out in dreams. Painters such as Dali reported systematically using dream imagery as a starting canvas (Van de Castle, 1994) Interestingly, Dali used to nap with a key in his hand that would fall into a plate next to his bed and wake him up. He would then use the images of his dreams for his paintings (Dali, 1992). It can be speculated that he was experiencing hypnagogic reverie at sleep onset. A similar approach was used by Thomas Edison, the famous inventor. Lacaux (2021), in a doctoral thesis, has explored this phenomenon and confirmed that the sleep onset period does facilitate creativity. Numerous other scientific discoveries were reportedly made because of dreams containing new associations. The best known are the molecular formula of benzine, the light bulb, and the sewing machine needle (for examples, see Mazarello, 2000). In all instances, however, credit must be given to the dreamers who have recognized the innovative associations in their dreaming material.

As pointed out earlier, this creative potential of dreaming arises because its cognitive activity is essentially associative and not limited by the operational constraints of waking (Klinger, 1978) arising with the neural substrate of the DMN (Domhoff, 2023). It therefore facilitates unrestricted sequences of associations between memory traces and cognitive operations. Such new associations seem effective for problem-solving at a personal level. Klinger notes that "Dreams, like play and fantasy, are fractionated, unsystematic approaches that work over the dreamer's real concerns, and in the process sometimes yield solutions by generating new combinations of pre-established schemata" (1978, p. 83). Other models of dream function also describe this enhanced connectivity found in the dreaming process (Domhoff, 2003, 2023; Hartmann, 1996; Maquet & Ruby, 2004; Stickgold, 2005b; Wagner et al., 2004). Renewed interest in exploring the creative process of sleep and dreaming phenomena more systematically is emerging (e.g., Lacaux, 2021).

In brief, as Figure 13.2 illustrates, the evidence suggests that REM dreams are constructed from external and internal stimulations during sleep, previous waking experiences, memory traces that can go back to early childhood, personality characteristics, gender, social roles, and culture. Most importantly, these elements appear to be orchestrated with the cognitive capacity present, rely on underlying current emotions, and are transformed by the unique brain processes that prevail during REM sleep. This process generates a new and unique expression and associations, the adaptive value of which is discussed below.

Consequences of Dreams, Dream Function Theories, and Dreams in Psychotherapy

The fact that dreams are not simply a replay of waking experience, tend to carry a negative tone, and contain new images and associations suggests that they should have an impact on subsequent waking states. Despite more than 60 years of research on the potential effects of dreams on waking life, there is no consistent empirical evidence that dreams serve a biological function. There was an interesting debate published in a special issue of *Behavioral and Brain Sciences* (2000, Vol. 23) in which a large number of sleep and dream researchers exchanged opinions on the state of our knowledge on sleep and dreaming that is still of interest today. Notable authors, such as Blagrove (2000) and Flanagan (2000) echoed Foulkes (1985), that dream content *by itself* does not have a function, a view that we share along with Domhoff (2018). There is significant support for dream formation theories that consider remembered dreams as reflecting the state of our cognitive activity and capacity as well as our emotional status and concerns and can provide insight and new associations that can be harnessed and useful for waking life. However, most dreams are not remembered; and, according to a recent CBS poll (Backus, 2021), one-third of the population either rarely (24%) or never (10%) remembers dreams. It becomes an important challenge to demonstrate that unremembered dreams serve a necessary function without reaching consciousness other than reflecting undergoing neural sleep function activity.

One of the additional challenges for the theories of dream function has been methodological, particularly when it comes to clarifying the variables that can intervene between dreaming per se and its potential effects on subsequent waking state and adaptation (for elaboration, see Blagrove, 1993; De Koninck, 1991). Figure 13.3 illustrates the links between chronologically implicated events and states: *pre-sleep psychological state*, *sleep and dreaming activity*, *dream recall*, *post-sleep psychological state*, *dream work or interpretation*, and *long-term adaptation*. It also illustrates on the *y*-axis that each level of dream function is associated with higher levels of consciousness or more involvement of waking mental activity, and therefore further away from the endogenous dreaming experience. Depending on which links are examined, different questions arise:

- F1: Do dreams serve a function in maintaining or protecting sleep even if they are not remembered and no consciousness is involved? A good example is Freud's (1900/1991) hypotheses that dreams that were not remembered were those that fulfilled their function of *guardians of sleep* by preventing the dreamer from waking up and discovering their disguised meaning.
- F2: Do dreams serve an adaptive function toward the following post-sleep state and long-term psychological adaptation even if they do not reach consciousness and are not remembered? For example, following pleasant dreams, will the dreamer feel better in the morning even if the dreams are not remembered, and conversely if dreams are unpleasant? This is also the view of some formulations of the mood regulation theory of dreaming that describe desensitization of negative components.
- F3: Do remembered dreams affect post-sleep state (F3.1) and/or serve a long-term adaptation function (F3.2)? Once dreams become part of consciousness, they have a life of their own. What impact do they have on morning state and adaptation?
- F4: Is it only once remembered dreams are worked on or interpreted that they serve an adaptive function? Here, Freud's use of dreams in psychoanalysis as the "royal road to the unconscious" to uncover unresolved conflicts was conceived as an essential component for them to serve a long-term adaptive function. This type of dream function is at the center of modern psychotherapies that use dreams.

Since the beginning of the scientific studies of dreaming, there have been many theories and hypotheses of both the construction and the usefulness of dreams. Originally, two main notions prevailed. The mastery hypothesis proposed that dreams "may serve a unique function in the assimilation and mastery of aroused material into the solutions embodied in existing memory systems" (Breger 1967, p.1). It was expanded to problem-solving, information-processing, and ego consolidation. The compensation hypothesis originally formulated by Jung stated that "dreams function to balance and complete waking consciousness" (Dallet 1973, p. 408). Then emerged the continuity hypothesis (Hall & Nordby, 1972) that served as an umbrella for most recent theories of dream formation and dream function since it postulated a continuity between waking and dreaming experience in a reciprocal fashion, encompassing both mastery and compensation. In a recent textbook, Valli and Hoss (2019) offer a collection of more than a dozen current hypotheses synthesized by a host of contributing researchers. In recent years, several new theories and updates of older formulations have been published (e.g., Domhoff, 2023; Hoel, 2021; Lemyre et al., 2022; Wamsley, 2022). Surprisingly, a number them do not specify where their propositions fall in the continuum of variables identified in Figure 13.3.

We briefly present some dream function theories in each of the types and attempt an outline of some of the current research evidence supporting them. Interestingly, Zadra and Stickgold (2021), in a book-length synthesis, propose an original multifaceted integration of research and theories in a multifunction model called NEXTUP. Since it covers the whole spectrum of types of dream functions, the following examination of theories may help in understanding this latter complex contribution.

Types of Dream Function Theories Including Dreams in Psychotherapy

Unremembered Dream Theories (Types F1 and F2)

One of the more recent theories that have received much interest is the threat simulation theory formulated by Revonsuo (2000). It proposes that dreams serve a function that

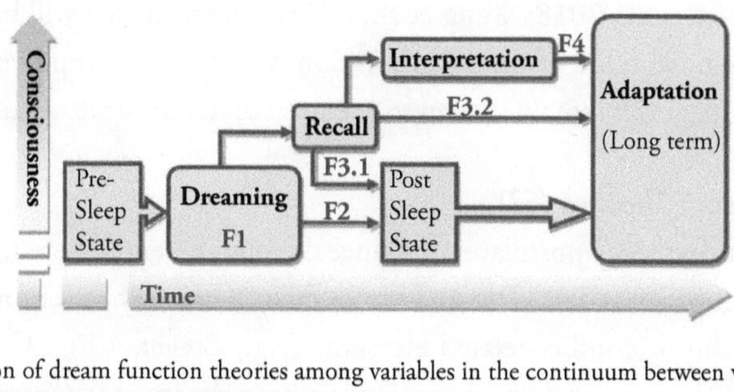

Figure 13.3 Situation of dream function theories among variables in the continuum between waking, dreaming, and post-sleep psychological state and adaptation

Note. F1 to F4 represent increasing involvement of consciousness: F1 = dreams preserve sleep; F2 = dreams impact waking even if they are not remembered; F3.1 = remembered dreams impact waking; F3.2 = remembered dreams impact long-term adaptation; F4 = dreams that are interpreted or worked with impact psychological adaptation.

emerged in the evolution of our ancestors to prepare them, in a form of virtual reality or imagery rehearsal, to face upcoming dangers in waking life. More specifically, it is proposed that "dreaming is to stimulate threatening events, and to rehearse threat perception and threat avoidance" (Revonsuo, 2000, p. 877). The model postulates that the threat rehearsal episodes in dreaming do not need to be explicitly remembered to have their adaptive value. This evolutionary model has been expanded to give a more global function of this imagery rehearsal process (Barrett, 2007; Franklin & Zyphur, 2005). Recently, a social simulation version has been added (Revonsuo et al., 2016). In brief, it suggests that dreams provide a virtual simulation not only of threats but also of other contemporary problems faced by the dreamer and allow the testing of solutions.

Ideally, experimentally testing the function of dreams that are not remembered (F1 and F2) would require having access to the dream experience and influencing it without awakening subjects, as future developments in imaging techniques may permit (Horikawa & Katamini, 2017). It seems, however, that an interesting avenue has emerged with the demonstration that olfactory stimulation can impact dream emotional tone (Schredl et al., 2009). The smell of rotten eggs induced a negative tone in dreams and that of roses a positive tone. It will be interesting to test the effects of such manipulation when subjects are not awakened for dream collection, and hopefully do not remember their dreams, on morning mood. It would be the first experimental study of the effects of dreams that do not reach consciousness on morning mood and adaptation.

In the meantime, given the paucity of methods for significantly manipulating dream content without confounding the manipulation with arousals, very little is being achieved except in demonstrating the value of concepts involved in the formation of dreams and examining their predictive correlational value on subsequent morning psychological status and beyond. In the case of the threat simulation theory, attempts are being made using observations of threats in, for example, recurrent dreams to draw conclusions on their adaptive value (e.g., Zadra, Desjardins, & Marcotte, 2006). Recent studies have, among other things, documented the relation between waking stress including the type arising from the 2019 pandemic and the emergence of threats in dreams (Barbeau, Lafrenière, et al., 2022; Lafrenière et al., 2018; Wang et al., 2021). The next step will be to evaluate the correlational predictive value of the incorporation of threats for improved morning psychological state. There will remain, however, the need to demonstrate a causal relationship.

Remembered Dream Theories (F3)

This type of function theory postulates that once dreams are remembered, they can impact waking life (F3 in Figure 13.3). The main ones favor a mastery function through incorporation of stressful or conflict-related elements (e.g., Breger, 1967; Cartwright, 2005; Wamsley, 2022). The mastery hypotheses focuses on a dream mechanism that integrates current concerns with past experiences. On the other hand, compensation hypotheses focuses on complementary mechanisms through dreams. Wright and Koulack (1987) have proposed that compensation and integration alternate as adaptive mechanisms of dreams to the previous day's events.

The impact of remembered dreams on waking state has been studied in experimental laboratory situations and more extensively in natural situations. Early studies showed that incorporations of elements of pre-sleep stress into dreams seem to impact negatively on morning adaptation to the stressful situation (e.g., De Koninck & Koulack, 1975; Koulack et al., 1985). However, when dreams compensate for a negative pre-sleep condition, the impact on morning state can be positive. For example, subjects who had been water-deprived before sleep and who drank during their dreams were less thirsty in the morning (Bokert, 1968). It seemed then that dreams would need not simply to mirror the stressful situation but to reduce its memory trace in some fashion.

The same seemed to apply to the impact of dreams on mood. Laboratory studies show that forcing the recall of REM dreams has a negative impact on morning mood. The more dysphoric the dreams are, the more negative the impact is on morning mood (Koulack et al., 1985). However, Cartwright et al. (1998) reported that in cases of elevated depressed mood at night, negative feelings in REM sleep dreams decrease across the night and interpreted this finding as supporting the mood regulation hypothesis of dreaming. In a study of dreams during premenstrual stress, dream mood was more negative than pre-sleep mood and post-sleep mood, the latter being the most positive (Sirois-Berliss & De Koninck, 1982). This was corroborated by Yu (2007). It seems that in natural settings and in normal circumstances, only dreams that are particularly salient appear to affect the following day. Kuiken and Sikora define these impactful dreams as those that directly and noticeably "influence thoughts and feelings during wakefulness" (1993, p. 422). They contain strong images that draw the attention of the dreamer and influence them in one form or another and recently replicated (Nixon et al., 2017).

There is an emerging consensus that mood regulation, which has been demonstrated to be achieved with REM sleep (Murkar & De Koninck, 2018), may be reflected in dream content. These models take into account recent findings on factors involved in dream formation that emphasize the expression of emotions in dreams (Malinowski & Horton, 2014b). Their roots come mainly from a series of contributions from Milton Kramer and collaborators in the early 1970s (Kramer et al., 1974) that are still present in the literature (Kramer, 2007). They proposed that dreams serve a mood regulation function by integrating past emotional experience with new connections that have an adaptive value. Other formulations followed (Cartwright 2005; Stickgold, 2005b), suggesting that a form of desensitization of negative dream components is achieved by combining them with positive components or by the muscle relaxation that takes place with the atonia of REM sleep (Perlis & Nielsen, 1993). This view is currently updated by several interesting contributions that integrate improvement in the understanding of the role of REM sleep in consolidating processes of emotions and the dream's preferential expression of emotions stemming from the neuronal basis of REM sleep (Scarpelli et al.,

2019). Another example is Lemyre et al. (2022), who emphasized the importance of the expression of feelings in dreams beyond emotions and their adaptive value to the following waking emotions.

More recent research does support some of the predictions of the mood regulation theories (Barbeau, Turpin, et al., 2022; Scarpelli et al., 2019; Sterpenich et al., 2019). Indeed, it has been observed that dreams do include negative emotions, but they can be combined with positive emotions (Barbeau, Lafrenière, et al., 2022; Vallat et al., 2017) This at least partially explains the positive bias that dreamers exhibit when they evaluate their dream mood compared to when an independent judge does so (Sikka et al., 2017). Moreover, this positive bias has been found to be a good predictor of morning mood, particularly when the bias appears in more negative dreams (Barbeau, Turpin, et al., 2022). A similar point is made by Kramer (2007), who originally suggested that mood regulation is best achieved during undisrupted sleep with the normal REM sleep components. Despite this notion, the desensitizing mechanism that is thought to be attributed to muscle relaxation during REM (Perlis & Nielsen, 1993) and/or its neuronal basis (Scarpelli et al., 2019) therefore still primarily applies to non-remembered REM dreams. In other words, it may be that this desensitization apparent within dreams may simply reflect the underlying REM sleep mood regulation.

A second prominent approach that regained interest in the early 2000s is the role of sleep in learning and memory (see special issues of *Science*, 2001; *Nature*, 2005). It has also brought back to the limelight the potential role of dreams in memory consolidation including REM dreams with most recent updated versions (Wamsley, 2022; Wamsley et al., 2010).

The testing of the role of dreaming on memory consolidation is progressing. Studies suggest that transformed dream elements that are related to pre-sleep learning tasks are accompanied by improved declarative memory (Cipolli et al., 2005). There is, however, very little support for the notion that actual learning takes place in dream imagery and scenarios. For example, while it has been observed that during intensive language learning there is a significant increase in REM sleep percentage that is correlated with learning efficiency (De Koninck et al., 1989), the concurrent dreaming activity contains very few instances of the new language (De Koninck et al., 1990). More specifically, the few incorporations of the new language are not indicative of a learning process but simply express the frustration accompanying the learning efforts ("I was trying to understand what he was saying"). This observation reinforces the notion just expressed above that emotions rather than complex cognitive operation prevail in dreams. Recent analyses of our second language learning (SLL) immersion studies do show that in the early weeks of learning, NREM sleep spindles increased and in later weeks of SLL, REM sleep theta rapid eye movement increased in parallel to learning performance (Thompson et al., 2021). It suggests that in early SLL, when grammar depends on declarative memory, sleep spindles prevail, whereas cortical theta activity is time-locked to rapid eye movements in late SLL, when grammar depends on procedural memory. This is congruent with the recent consensus that NREM sleep is involved in the early phases of memory consolidation, notably expressed in sleep spindles, while REM sleep is involved in the more stabilizing phase of the consolidation process (Picard-Deland et al., 2022). It would explain why, in our language learning studies, incorporations of language related in dream only appeared after several weeks and in conjunction with learning progress. Dream content from both NREM and REM sleep would reflect the status rather than be involved in it. This would also explain why NREM dreams are closer to episodic memories, while REM dreams would utilize the consolidated memories to simulate potential challenges (Wamsley, 2022). This latter hypothesis thus fits with the next type of function (F3.2) as it is linked to long-term adaptation.

Looking at the potential long-term impact of remembered dreams on psychological adaptation (F3.2), there are some indications that incorporation of preoccupations or conflicts may have a positive value. Cartwright (1992) observed in a group of women who had experienced a divorce that those who were frequently incorporating their ex-partner in their dreams were those better adapting to the divorce. The design of the study could not determine, however, if the incorporations were adaptive or simply a reflection of an adaptation already in progress. In other words, no causal role can yet be attributed to the dreams.

Nightmares present a special case, and theories of their formation are covered in Chapter 29. Briefly, as mentioned earlier, they are dreams that are so negative that they wake up the dreamer and evoke morning distress (see Nielsen & Levin, 2007). Bad dreams, which can be equally stressful but do not appear to wake up the dreamer and are remembered in the morning, also have a negative impact. Both nightmares and bad dreams are associated with poor well-being (Zadra & Donderi, 2000). Nightmares are also provoked by stress and are part of the aggravating conditions in PTSD.

Dreams in Psychotherapy (F4)

In contrast with Freud's use of dreams in psychoanalysis to access so-called repressed conflicts and wishes from early childhood, most modern psychotherapy approaches use dreams to work on the contemporary problems of their patients (F4 type of dream function in Figure 13.3). They rely on the assumptions that (1) dreams are in continuity with the waking experience without input from the external world (Hill, 2004), (2) central to their formation is the expression of emotions and concerns, and (3) they can create new connections (Domhoff, 2023; Hartmann, 2007). In approaches labeled *dreamwork*, therapists seek in dreams new expressions of current preoccupations of patients and work with them to derive associations with past experiences (e.g., Mahrer, 1989; Ullman & Zimmerman, 1979). These become tools in therapeutic attempts to increase self-knowledge and plan behavior change. For example, Maher's approach of using dreams in psychotherapy follows these steps:

1. Selecting and recounting a dream.
2. Identifying recent situations connected with the dream.
3. Identifying and clarifying the "peak moment" in the dream—in other words, one that is central to the scenario.
4. Identifying an earlier life experience connected with the peak moment and re-experiencing in the therapy the dream blended with this earlier life situation as well as more recent life situations.
5. As a result, rehearsing behavior change and establishing behavioral commitments for the future.

These models also integrate dreams in cognitive therapies, including cognitive behavior therapy (CBT; Rossner et al., 2004). For example, Montangero (2009) has proposed a technique that uses dream analysis as a complementary technique in CBT. It is interestingly close to Maher's (1989) approach and that of Hill (2004) in its use of a dream that is interpreted in the context of a link with past experience and is used to plan for the future. More specifically, the dream interpretation is more systematic in that it takes three steps: description, memory sources, and reformulation. Given their research tradition, these cognitive approaches have been subjected to studies on their efficacy, which offer positive future perspectives (e.g., Hill & Goates, 2004; Pesant & Zadra, 2004). A more recent analysis of the different facets of the use of dreams in CBT is found in Skrzypińska et al. (2018).

There is quite a bit of interest in using dreams for self-knowledge and well-being that, although not yet strongly supported by experimental research, is gaining strength in the research community. Applying principles as outlined above but outside a formal psychotherapeutic relationship may be very useful for the layperson to gain insight and develop coping capabilities for daily stress and life challenges (e.g., Delaney, 1988). Such systems as that of Ullman and Zimmerman (1979) receive favorable results in empirical studies (e.g., DeCicco, 2007).

Dream Control

Since dreams tend to have a negative tone that can impact waking mood, it is of interest to examine whether they can be influenced or controlled. The most efficient pre-sleep technique of influencing dream content is suggestion, be it in the form of hypnotic or non-hypnotic suggestion or pre-sleep incubation (Barrett, 1993; Walker & Johnson, 1974). For example, De Koninck and Brunette (1991) successfully trained subjects with pre-sleep suggestion to incorporate phobic objects or a pleasant counterpart (snakes, squirrels) into their dreams. More importantly, they were able, also with pre-sleep suggestion, to induce more positive emotions in dreams and improve dream pleasantness. Others have developed techniques of incubation to induce subjects to dream of topics or induce problem-solving dreams (Barrett, 1993; Saredi et al., 1997). There is empirical evidence that CBT that uses dream imagery rehearsal for the treatment of nightmares is effective (Krakow et al., 1995), and its practice has been integrated into behavioral sleep medicine. More specifically, in imagery rehearsal therapy subjects suffering from frequent nightmares, such as in PTSD, can learn to eliminate them by rehearsing a positively modified scenario of their nightmares during the day (Krakow et al., 1995). This technique has proven successful with adults (Krakow et al., 1995), adolescents (Krakow et al., 2001; Long et al., 2011), and children who rehearsed their dream scenario at bedtime (St-Onge et al., 2009).

The most spectacular situation of comprehensive dream control is that of lucid dreaming. Already well elaborated by Léon D'Hervey de Saint Denys (1867/1995), it consists first of becoming aware that one is dreaming but, instead of waking up, taking control of the dream elaboration (Laberge, 1985). Frightening or strange images or unusual activities in dreams such as flying can facilitate the onset of lucidity. Research on characteristics of lucid dreams collected in the laboratory reveals that they have salient and vivid contents closely related to reality with more emotions and more pleasantness than typical REM dreams (Laberge, 1988). While lucid dreaming occurs spontaneously in some individuals, most need to train extensively to achieve it (see, e.g., the technique of Laberge, 1985). Recently, we have reported that lucid dreaming could be a useful addition in CBT for insomnia by reducing the negative emotional dream experiences that typically affect insomniacs (Ellis et al., 2020). Lemyre et al. (2020) have documented the various techniques that lucid dreamers use to attain lucidity to help future research determine their respective efficiency.

Even if lucid dreams appear to be produced essentially in REM sleep, they have also been observed in hypnagogic dreaming at the onset of sleep and during Stage 2 (Laberge, 1988). Intrusion of alpha waves in the EEG, which could be instances of "micro-arousals," have been found to accompany dream lucidity in laboratory studies (Ogilvie et al., 1982). This has been challenged by Laberge (1988), who was able to have lucid dreamers who slept in the laboratory signal to the experimenter when a lucid dream started and ended using voluntary codified eye movements. He did not observe any unusual activation level during lucidity but noted that the interhemispheric activation levels corresponded with the dominant activity in the lucid dream. For example, the right hemisphere was dominant when the dreamer sang. It has also been observed that cardiovascular activity levels correspond to physical exercise during REM lucid dreaming (Erlacher & Schredl, 2008). Voss et al. (2009) have observed that during lucid dreaming there is increased EEG activation in the frontal and frontolateral regions of the brain, which suggests that it is a state that is distinguishable from both waking and REM sleep. Brain imaging has been used to link neural correlates of lucid dreaming with levels of arousal and neurocognitive mechanisms inducing lucid dreaming (Simor et al., 2022).

Lucid dreaming has notably been claimed to enhance creativity (Garfield, 1974), but there have not been systematic studies of their adaptive potential except for their capacity to increase dream pleasantness and treat nightmares (Halliday, 1987). Mallet et al. (2022) have explored the potential benefits and risks of the practice of lucid dreaming and point out that it can be used for therapeutic benefits such as the treatment of nightmares but can have negative outcomes when pre-sleep induction attempts fail. It may also be that extensive use of lucid dreaming may alter the natural course of REM sleep and inhibit its potential functions, notably in mood regulation.

Conclusion and Future Research

In recent decades there has been significant progress in our understanding of the mechanisms of dream formation. The dreaming brain works differently than in waking and opens the way for memory traces, emotions, and waking experiences to be expressed in original fashions. The typical content is very mundane and has little effect on waking life, but some dreams can also be very vivid and original and offer new associations and impact on waking life. Their tone tends to be negative in terms of emotions, interactions, and outcome and can culminate in nightmares. Fortunately, dreams can be controlled. Finally, there is progress in the scientific validation of the use of dreams in psychotherapy and for improvements in self-knowledge. In the future, it will be interesting to further explore by imaging techniques the brain generators of dreaming. As pointed out earlier, most dream research has focused on REM dreaming, but considerable progress has been made to better understand dreaming that occurs at sleep onset and in NREM sleep. The study of mental activity in parasomnias also provides valuable information on dream formation. Further exploration of the sources of dreams will help us to better understand their potential usefulness in enhancing self-knowledge and their use in psychotherapy, as well as shedding light on psychopathological conditions such as schizophrenia and depression. The potential use of dreaming for creative purposes is most promising but will require more stringent methodology. Lucid dreaming constitutes a fruitful avenue to explore the physiological correlates of REM dreaming and its potential value for adaptation and psychological well-being.

In the scientific study of dreams, the main remaining challenge is the experimental demonstration of a causal adaptive function of dreaming that applies to non-remembered dreams because of the still limited access to the actual dream experience that does not reach consciousness. Again, further advances in methodology, notably neural imaging, offer the best opportunity to understand this fascinating dimension of the human mind.

Acknowledgments

This is an updated version of the chapter from the 2012 version of the handbook. The author wishes to thank those who have helped in different stages of the preparation of both versions: Reza Amini, Daniel Ouellet, Roger Godbout, and Allyson Dale. Sections on norms, gender differences, culture, and psychotherapy benefited from previous collaborative work with Monique Lortie-Lussier.

References

Adler, A. (1929). *Individual psychology*. Routledge & Kegal Paul.

Akkaoui, M. A., Lejoyeux, M., d'Ortho, M. P., & Geoffroy, P. A. (2020). Nightmares in patients with major depressive disorder, bipolar disorder, and psychotic disorders: A systematic review. *Journal of Clinical Medicine, 9*(12), Article 3990. https://doi.org/10.3390/jcm9123990

Amini, R., Sabourin, C., & De Koninck, J. (2011). Word associations improve automatic analysis of dream emotional tone. *Consciousness and Cognition, 20*, 1570–1576. https://doi.org/10.1016/j.concog.2011.08.003

Ananth, S. (2021). Sleep apps: Current limitations and challenges. *Sleep Science, 14*(1), 83–86. https://doi.org/10.5935/1984-0063.20200036

Antrobus, J. S., Fein, G., Jordan, L., Ellman, S. J., & Arkin, A. M. (1991). Measurement and design in research on sleep reports. In S. J. Ellman & J. S. Antrobus (Eds.), *The mind in sleep* (pp. 83–123). John Wiley & Sons.

Antrobus, J., Kondo, T., Reinsel, R., & Fein, R. (1995). Dreaming in the late morning: Summation of REM and diurnal cortical activation. *Consciousness and Cognition, 4*(3), 275–299. https://doi.org/10.1006/ccog.1995.1039

Arnal, P. J., Thorey, V., Debellemaniere, E., Ballard, M. E., Bou Hernandez, A., Guillot, A., Jourde, H., Harris, M., Guillard, M., Van Beers, P., Chennaoui, M., & Sauvet, F. (2020). The Dreem Headband compared to polysomnography for electroencephalographic signal acquisition and sleep staging. *Sleep, 43*(11), Article zsaa097. https://doi.org/10.1093/sleep/zsaa097

Arnulf, I. (2011). The "scanning hypothesis" of rapid eye movements during REM sleep: A review of the evidence. *Archives Italienne de Biologie, 149*, 367–382. https://doi.org/10.4449/aib.v149i4.1246

Arnulf, I. (2019). Dreaming in parasomnias. In K. Valli & R. Hoss (Eds.), *Dreams: Understanding biology, psychology, and culture* (Vol. 1, pp. 238–248). ABC-CLIO.

Arnulf, I., Uguccioni, G., Gay, F., Baldeyrou, E., Golmard, J. L., Gayraud, F., & Devevey, A. (2017). What does the sleeping brain say? Syntax and semantics of sleep talking in healthy subjects and in parasomnia patients. *Sleep, 40*(11), Article zsx159. https://doi.org/10.1093/sleep/zsx159

Aserinsky, E., & Kleitman, N. (1953). Regularly occurring periods of eye motility and concomitant phenomena during sleep. *Science, 118*, 273–274. https://doi.org/10.1126/science.118.3062.273

Backus, F. (2021). *CBS News poll: How often do you remember your dreams?* https://www.cbsnews.com/news/remember-dreams-opinion-poll/

Barbeau, K., Lafrenière, A., Ben Massaoud, H., Campbell, E., & De Koninck, J. (2022). Dissociated effects of age and recent troubling experiences on nightmares, threats and negative emotions in dreams. *Frontiers in Psychiatry*, 13, Article 770380. https://doi.org/10.3389/fpsyt.2022.770380

Barbeau, K., Turpin, C., Lafrenière, A., Campbell, E., & De Koninck, J. (2022). Dreamers' evaluation of the emotional valence of their day-to-day dreams is indicative of some mood regulation function. *Frontiers in Behavioral Neuroscience*, 16, Article 947396. https://doi.org/10.3389/fnbeh.2022.947396

Barcaro, U., Cavallero, C., & Navona, C. (2005). A method for recognizing and describing the links among dream sources. *Dreaming, 15*, 271–287. https://doi.org/10.1037/1053-0797.15.4.271

Barrett, D. (1993). The "committee of sleep": A study of dream incubation for problem solving. *Dreaming, 3*, 115–122. https://doi.org/10.1037/h0094375

Barrett, D. (2007). An evolutionary theory of dreams and problem-solving. In D. Barrett & P. McNamara (Eds.), *The new science of dreaming* (Vol. 3, pp. 133–153). Praeger.

Barrett, D., & Loeffler, M. (1992). Comparison of dream content of depressed vs nondepressed dreamers. *Psychological Reports, 70*, 403–406. https://doi.org/10.2466/pr0.1992.70.2.403

Beauchemin, K. M., & Hays, P. (1996). Dreaming away depression: The role of REM sleep and dreaming in affective disorders. *Journal of Affective Disorders, 41*, 125–133. https://doi.org/10.1016/S0165-0327(96)00080-8

Beck, A. T., & Ward, C. H. (1961). Dreams of depressed patients: Characteristic themes in manifest content. *Archives of General Psychiatry, 5*, 462–467. https://doi.org/10.1001/archpsyc.1961.01710170040004

Berger, R. J. (1963). Experimental modification of dream content by meaningful verbal stimuli. *British Journal of Psychiatry, 109*, 722–740. https://doi.org/10.1192/bjp.109.463.722

Blagrove, M. (1993). Dreams as the reflection of our waking concerns and abilities: A critique of the problem-solving paradigm in dream research. *Dreaming, 2*, 205–220. https://doi.org/10.1037/h0094361

Blagrove, M. (2000). Dreams have meaning but no function. *Behavioral and Brain Sciences, 23*(6), 910–911. https://doi.org/10.1017/S0140525X00244026

Blagrove, M. (2007). Dreams and personality. In D. Barrett & P. McNamara (Eds.), *The new science of dreaming* (Vol. 2, pp. 115–158). Praeger.

Blagrove, M., & Haywood, S. (2006). Evaluating the awakening criterion in the definition of nightmares: How certain are people in judging whether a nightmare woke them up? *Journal of Sleep Research, 15*, 117–124. https://doi.org/10.1111/j.1365-2869.2006.00507.x

Bokert, E. (1968). The effects of thirst and related verbal stimulus on dream reports. *Dissertation Abstracts, 28*, Article 4753B.

Breger, L. (1967). The functions of dreams. *Journal of Abnormal Psychology Monograph, 72*, 1–28. https://doi.org/10.1037/h0025040

Brekke, F., Hodges Dale, T., & Pallesen, S. (2023). Who has nightmares? An investigation into the relationship between personality and nightmares. *Dreaming, 33*(1), 32–44. https://doi.org/10.1037/drm0000235

Broughton, R. (1975). Biorhythmic variations, in consciousness and psychological functions. *Canadian Psychological Review, 16*(4), 217–240.

Broughton, R., & Mullington, J. (1992). Circasemidian sleep propensity and the phase amplitude maintenance model of human sleep/wake regulation. *Journal of Sleep Research, 1*, 93–98. https://doi.org/10.1111/j.1365-2869.1992.tb00017.x

Buisink, R., & Kuiken, D. (1996). Identifying types of impactful dreams: A replication. *Dreaming, 6*, 97–119.

Bulkeley, K., & Graves, M. (2018). Using the LIWC program to study dreams. *Dreaming, 28*(1), 43–58. https://doi.org/10.1037/drm0000071

Callois, R., & Von Grunebaum, G. E. (1967). *Le rêve et les sociétés humaines*. Gallimard.

Cartwright, R. D. (1992). Dreams that work: The relation of dream incorporation to adaptation to stressful events. *Dreaming, 1*, 3–9. https://doi.org/10.1037/h0094312

Cartwright, R. D. (2005). Dreaming as a mood regulatory system. In M. Kryger, T. Roth, & W. C. Dement (Eds.), *Principles and practice of sleep medicine* (pp. 565–572). Saunders.

Cartwright, R., Young, M., Mercer, J., & Bears, M. (1998). Role of REM sleep and dream variables in the prediction of remission from depression. *Psychiatry Research, 80*, 249–255. https://doi.org/10.1016/s0165-1781(98)00071-7

Casaglia, E., & Luppi, P. H. (2022). Is paradoxical sleep setting up innate and acquired complex sensorimotor and adaptive behaviours? A proposed function based on literature review. *Journal of Sleep Research, 31*(4), Article e13633. https://doi.org/10.1111/jsr.13633

Cavallero, C., & Foulkes, D. (Eds.). (1993). *Dreaming as cognition*. Harvester Wheatsheaf.

Chellappa, S. L., Munch, M., Blatter, K., Knoblauch, V., & Cajochen, C. (2009). Does the circadian modulation of dream recall modify with age? *Sleep, 32*(9), 1201–1209. https://doi.org/10.1093/sleep/32.9.1201

Cipolli, C., Fagioli, I., Mazzetti, M., & Tuozzi, G. (2005). Consolidation effect of the processing of declarative knowledge during human sleep: Evidence from long-term retention of interrelated contents of mental sleep experiences. *Brain Research Bulletin, 65*(2), 97–104. https://doi.org/10.1016/j.brainresbull.2004.10.014

Cohen, D. B. (1974). Toward a theory of dream recall. *Psychological Bulletin, 81*, 138–154. https://doi.org/10.1037/h0037616

Cohen, D. B. (1979). *Sleeping and dreaming*. Pergamon Press.

Dale, A., Lafrenière, A., & De Koninck, J. (2017). Dream content of Canadian males from adolescence to old age: An exploration of ontogenetic patterns. *Consciousness and Cognition, 49*, 145–156. http://dx.doi.org/10.1016/j.concog.2017.01.008

Dale, A., Lortie-Lussier, M., & De Koninck, J. (2015). Ontogenetic patterns in the dreams of women across the lifespan. *Consciousness and Cognition, 37*, 214–224. https://doi.org/10.1016/j.concog.2015.09.008

Dale, A., Lortie-Lussier, M., Wong, C., & De Koninck, J. (2016). Dreams of Canadian students: Norms, gender differences, and comparison with Americans. *Journal of Cross Cultural Psychology, 47*(7), 941–955. https://doi.org/10.1177/0022022116655788

Dali, S. (1992). *50 Secrets of magic craftsmanship*. H. M. Chevalier (Trans., illustrated ed.). Dover Publications.

Dallet, J. (1973). Theories of dream function. *Psychological Bulletin, 79*(6), 408–416. https://doi.org/10.1037/h0034485

Dang-Vu, T. T., Schabus, M., Desseilles, M., Schwarts, S., & Maquet, P. (2007). Neuroimaging of REM sleep dreaming. In D. Barrett & P. McNamara (Eds.), *The new science of dreaming* (Vol. 1, pp. 95–114). Praeger.

Daoust, A. M., Lusignan, F. A., Braun, C., Mottron, L., & Godbout, R. (2008). Dream content analysis in persons with an autism spectrum disorder. *Journal of Autism and Developmental Disorders, 38*, 634–643. https://doi.org/10.1007/s10803-007-0431-z

Davis, P. M. (2005). The weaning of perpetua: Female embodiment and spiritual growth metaphor in the dream of an early Christian martyr. *Dreaming, 15*(4), 261–270. https://doi.org/10.1037/1053-0797.15.4.261

DeCicco, T. L. (2007). Dreams of female university students: Content analysis and the relationship to discovery via the Ullman method. *Dreaming, 17*, 98–112. https://doi.org/10.1037/1053-0797.17.2.98

Desjardings, E., Gaber, L., Larking, E., Benoit, A., Boafo, A., & De Koninck, J. (2024). The dream experience and its relationship with morning mood in adolescents hospitalized after a suicide attempt. *Brain Sciences, 14*(8), 804. https://doi.org/10.3390/brainsci14080804

De Koninck, J., Salva, M. Q., Besset, A., & Billiard, M. (1986). Are REM cycles in narcoleptic patients governed by an ultradian rhythm? *Sleep, 9*(1 Pt 2), 162–166. https://doi.org/10.1093/sleep/9.1.162

De Koninck, J. (1991). Sources and consequences of dreams: Experimental manipulations and their effects. In J. Gachenbac & A. Sheikh (Eds.), *Dream images: A call to mental arms* (pp. 17–30). Baywood Publishing.

De Koninck, J., & Brunette, R. (1991). Presleep suggestion related to a phobic object: Successful manipulation of reported dream affect. *Journal of General Psychology, 118*(3), 185–200. https://doi.org/10.1080/00221309.1991.9917780

De Koninck, J., Christ, G., Hébert, G., & Rinfret, N. (1990). Language learning efficiency, dreams, and REM sleep. *Psychiatric Journal of the University of Ottawa, 15*, 91–92.

De Koninck, J.-M., & Koulack, D. (1975). Dream content and adaptation to a stressful situation. *Journal of Abnormal Psychology, 84*(3), 250–260. https://doi.org/10.1037/h0076648

De Koninck, J., Lorrain, D., Christ, G., Proulx, G., & Coulombe, D. (1989). Intensive language learning and increases in REM sleep: Evidence of a performance factor. *International Journal of Psychophysiology, 8*, 43–47. https://doi.org/10.1016/0167-8760(89)90018-4

De Koninck, J., Prévost, F., & Lortie-Lussier, M. (1996). Vertical inversion of the visual field on REM sleep mentation. *Journal of Sleep Research, 5*, 16–20. https://doi.org/10.1046/j.1365-2869.1996.00001.x

Delaney, G. (1988). *Living your dreams: Using sleep to solve problems and enrich your life*. Harper and Row.

Delboeuf, J.-R. L. (1885). *Le sommeil et les rêves* (*Sleep and dreams*). Alcan.

Dement, W. C. (1960). The effect of dream deprivation. *Science, 131*, 1705–1707. https://doi.org/10.1126/science.131.3415.1705

Dement, W. C. (1976). *Some must watch while some must sleep*. W. W. Norton.

Dement, W. C., & Kleitman, N. (1957). The relation of eye movements during sleep to dream activity: An objective method for the study of dreaming. *Journal of Experimental Psychology, 53*, 339–346. https://doi.org/10.1037/h0048189

D'Hervey de Saint-Denys, L. (1995). *Les rêves et les moyens de les diriger* (*Dreams and how to guide them*). Oniros. (Original work published 1867).

Domhoff, G. W. (2003). *The scientific study of dreams*. American Psychological Association.

Domhoff, G. W. (1996). *Finding meaning in dreams*. Plenum Press.

Domhoff, G. W. (2019). *The emergence of dreaming: Mind-wandering, embodied simulation, and the default network*. Oxford University Press.

Domhoff, G. W. (2023). The relationship between dreaming and autonoetic consciousness: The neurocognitive theory of dreaming gains in explanatory power by drawing upon the multistate hierarchical model of consciousness. *Dreaming, 33*(1), 1–18.

Eichenlaub, J. B., van Rijn, E., Gaskell, M. G., Lewis, A. L., Maby, E., Malinowski, J. E., Walker, M. P., Boy, F., & Blagrove, M. S. (2018). Incorporation of recent waking-life experiences in dreams correlates with frontal theta activity in REM sleep. *Social Cognitive and Affective Neuroscience, 13*(6), 637–647. https://doi.org/10.1093/scan/nsy041

Ellis, J. S., De Koninck, J., & Bastien, C. H. (2020). Managing insomnia using lucid dreaming training: A pilot study. *Behavioral Sleep Medicine, 19*(2), 273–283. https://doi.org/10.1080/15402002.2020.1739688

Erlacher, D., Schmid, D., Schuler, S., & Rasch, B. (2020). Inducing lucid dreams by olfactory-cued reactivation of reality testing during early-morning sleep: A proof of concept. *Consciousness and Cognition, 83*, Article 10297. https://doi.org/10.1016/j.concog.2020.102975

Erlacher, D., & Schredl, M. (2008). Cardiovascular responses to dreamed physical exercise during REM lucid dreaming. *Dreaming, 18*, 112–121. https://doi.org/10.1037/1053-0797.18.2.112

Fantini, M. L., Corona, A., Clerici, S., & Ferini-Strambi, L. (2005). Aggressive dream content without day-time aggressiveness in REM sleep behavior disorder. *Neurology, 65*, 1010–1015. https://doi.org/10.1212/01.wnl.0000179346.39655.e0

Flanagan, O. (2000). Dreaming is not an adaptation. *Behavioral and Brain Sciences, 23*, 936–939.

Fogel, S., Ray, L., Sergeeva, V., De Koninck, J., & Owen, A. M. (2018). A novel approach to dream content analysis reveals links between learning-related dream incorporation and cognitive abilities. *Frontiers in Psychology, 9*, Article 1398. https://doi.org/10.3389/fpsyg.2018.01398

Fogli, A., Aiello, L. M., & Quercia, D. (2020). Our dreams, our selves: Automatic analysis of dream reports. *Royal Society Open Science, 7*, Article 192080. http://dx.doi.org/10.1098/rsos.192080

Forest, G., Sabourin, C., Pétrin, R., Robidoux, R., & De Koninck, J. (2023). Dream content and depressive symptoms during pregnancy and postpartum. *Journal of Affective Disorders Reports*, 11, Article 100480. https://doi.org/10.1016/j.jadr.2023.100480

Fosse, M. J., Fosse, R., Hobson, J. A., & Stickgold, R. J. (2003). Dreaming and episodic memory: A functional dissociation? *Journal of Cognitive Neuroscience, 15*, 1–9. https://doi.org/10.1162/089892903321107774

Fosse, M. J., Stickgold, R. J., & Hobson, J. A. (2001). The mind in REM sleep: Reports of emotional experience. *Sleep, 24*, 947–955.

Foulkes, D. (1962). Dream reports from different stages of sleep. *Journal of Abnormal and Social Psychology, 65*, 14–25. https://doi.org/10.1037/h0040431

Foulkes, D., & Vogel, G. (1965). Mental activity at sleep onset. *Journal of Abnormal Psychology, 70*(4), 231–243. https://doi.org/10.1037/h0022217

Foulkes, D. (1982). *Children's dreams*. Wiley.

Foulkes, D. (1985). *Dreaming: A cognitive psychological analysis*. Lawrence Erlbaum Associates.

Foulkes, D. (1999). *Children's dreams and the development of consciousness*. Harvard University Press.

Foulkes, D. (2017). Dreaming, reflective consciousness, and feelings in the preschool child. *Dreaming, 27*(1), 1–13. https://doi.org/10.1037/drm0000040

Foulkes, D., Hollifield, M., Sullivan, B., Bradley, L., & Terry, R. (1990). REM dreaming and cognitive skills at ages 5–8: A cross sectional study. *International Journal of Behavioral Development, 13*, 447–465. https://doi.org/10.1177/016502549001300404

Franklin, M. S., & Zyphur, M. J. (2005). The role of dreams in the evolution of human mind. *Evolutionary Psychology, 3*, 59–78. https://doi.org/10.1177/147470490500300106

Freud, S. (1991). *The interpretation of dreams*. Penguin Books. (Original work published 1900)

Gackenbach, J., & Kuruvilla, B. (2008). The relationship between video game play and threat simulation dreams. *Dreaming, 18*, 236–256. https://doi.org/10.1037/a0013782

Gallop, D. (1991). *Aristotle on sleep and dreams*. Broadview Press.

Garfield, P. (1974). *Creative dreaming*. Simon and Schuster.

Glucksman, M. L., & Kramer, M. (2017). Manifest dream content as a predictor of suicidality. *Psychodynamic Psychiatry, 45*(2), 175–185. https://doi.org/10.1521/pdps.2017.45.2.175

Grenier, J., Cappeliez, P., St-Onge, M., Vachon, J., Vinette, S., Roussy, F., & De Koninck, J. (2005). Temporal references in dreams and autobiographical memory. *Memory and Cognition, 33*, 280–288. https://doi.org/10.3758/BF03195317

Griffith, R. M., Miyagi, O., & Tako, A. (1960). Universality of typical dreams: Japanese versus Americans. *American Anthropologist, 58*, 1174–1179.

Hall, C. S., Domhoff, G. W., Blick, K. A., & Weesner, K. E. (1982). The dreams of college men and women in 1950 and 1980: A comparison of dream content and sex differences. *Sleep, 5*, 188–194. https://doi.org/10.1093/sleep/5.2.188

Hall, C. S., & Nordby, V. J. (1972). *The individual and his dreams*. New American Library.

Hall, C. S., & Van de Castle, R. L. (1966). *The content analysis of dreams*. Appleton Century Croft.

Halliday, G. (1987). Direct psychological therapies for nightmares: A review. *Clinical Psychology Review, 7*, 501–523. https://doi.org/10.1016/0272-7358(87)90041-9

Halliday, G. (1992). Effects of encouragement on dream recall. *Dreaming, 9*, 32–44.

Hartmann, E. (1991). *Boundaries in the mind*. Basic Books.

Hartmann, E. (1996). Outline for a theory on the nature and functions of dreaming. *Dreaming, 6*(2), 147–170. https://doi.org/10.1037/h0094452

Hartmann, E. (2000). We do not dream of the 3 R's: Implications for the nature of dream mentation. *Dreaming, 10*, 103–110. https://doi.org/10.1023/A:1009400805830

Hartmann, E. (2007). The nature and function of dreaming. In D. Barrett & P. McNamara (Eds.), *The new science of dreaming* (Vol. 3, pp. 171–172). Praeger.
Hartmann, E. (2008). The central image makes "big" dreams big: The central image as the emotional heart of the dreams. *Dreaming, 18*, 44–57. https://doi.org/10.1037/1053-0797.18.1.44
Hartmann, E., Elkin, R., & Garg, M. (1991). Personality and dreaming: The dreams of people with very thick or very thin boundaries. *Dreaming, 1*, 311–324. https://doi.org/10.1037/h0094342
Herz, M. I., & Melville, C. (1980). Relapse in schizophrenia. *American Journal of Psychiatry, 137*, 801–805. https://doi.org/10.1176/ajp.137.7.801
Hill, C. E. (2004). *Dream work in therapy*. American Psychological Association.
Hill, C. E., & Goates, M. I. (2004). Research on the cognitive-experiential dream model. In C. E. Hill (Ed.), *Dream work in therapy: Exploration, insight and action* (pp. 245–288). American Psychological Association.
Hobson, J. A. (2004). Freud returns? Like a bad dream. *Scientific American, 290*, 89–89. https://doi.org/10.1038/scientificamerican0504-89
Hobson, J. A., & McCarley, R W. (1977). The brain as a dream state generator: An activation-synthesis hypothesis of the dream process. *American Journal of Psychiatry, 134*, 1335–1348. https://doi.org/10.1176/ajp.134.12.1335
Hobson, J. A., Pace-Schott, E. F., & Stickgold, R. (2000). Dreaming and the brain: Toward a cognitive neuroscience of conscious states. *Behavioral and Brain Sciences, 23*, 793–842.
Hoel, E. (2021). The overfitted brain: Dreams evolved to assist generalization. *Patterns, 2*(5), Article 100244. https://doi.org/10.1016/j.patter.2021.100244
Hong, C. C.-H., Fallon, J. H., & Friston, K. J. (2021). fMRI evidence for default mode network deactivation associated with rapid eye movements in sleep. *Brain Sciences, 11*, Article 1528. https://doi.org/10.3390/brainsci11111528
Horikawa, T., & Katamini, Y. (2017). Hierarchical neural representation of dreamed objects revealed by brain decoding with deep neural network features. *Frontiers in Computational Neuroscience, 31*, Article 4. https://doi.org/10.3389/fncom.2017.00004
Jouvet, M. (1962). Recherches sur les structures nerveuses et les mécanismes responsables des différentes phases du sommeil physiologique(Reflection on brain physilogical mechanisms responsible for sleep stage). *Archives Italiennes de Biologie, 100*, 125–206.
Jouvet, M. (1974). Essai sur le rêve (Essay on dreams). *Archives Italiennes de Biologie, 3*, 564–576.
Jouvet, M. (1979). Mémoire et "cerveau dédoublé" au cours du rêve à propos de 130 souvenirs de rêve (Memory and "split brain" during dreams about 130 dream memories). *L'année du Praticien, 29*, 27–32.
Jung, C. G. (1933). *Modern man in search of a soul*. Harcourt, Brace and World.
Kahn, D., & Hobson, A. (2005). The theory of mind in sleep: Awareness of feelings and thoughts of others in dreams. *Dreaming, 15*, 48–57. https://doi.org/10.1037/1053-0797.15.1.48
Kellerman, H. (1987). *The nightmare*. Columbia University Press.
Khazaie, H., Tahmasian, M., Younesi, G. C., Schwebel, D., Rezaei, M., Rezaie, L., Mohamadi, M., & Ghanbari, A. (2012). Evaluation of dream content among patients with schizophrenia, their siblings, patients with psychiatric diagnoses other than schizophrenia, and healthy control. *Iranian Journal of Psychiatry, 7*(1), 26–30.
Kleitman, N. (1962). *Sleep and wakefulness*. University of Chicago Press.
Klinger, E. (1978). *The structure and function of fantasy*. John Wiley & Sons.
Koulack, D., & Goodenough, D. R. (1976). Dream recall and dream recall failure: An arousal-retrieval model. *Psychological Bulletin, 83*, 975–984. https://doi.org/10.1037/0033-2909.83.5.975
Koulack, D., Prévost, F., & De Koninck, J. (1985). Sleep, dreaming, and adaptation to a stressful intellectual activity. *Sleep, 8*, 244–254. https://doi.org/10.1093/sleep/8.3.244
Krakow, B., Kellner, R., Pathak, D., & Lambert, L. (1995). Imagery rehearsal treatment for chronic nightmares. *Behavior, Research & Therapy, 33*, 837–843. https://doi.org/10.1016/0005-7967(95)00009-m
Krakow, B., Sandoval, D., Schrader, R., Kuehne, B., McBride, L., Yau, C. L., & Chen, D.T. (2001). Treatment of chronic nightmares in adjudicated adolescent girls in a residential facility. *Journal of Adolescent Health, 29*, 94–100. https://doi.org/10.1016/s1054-139x(00)00195-6
Kramer, M. (2007). *The dream experience*. Routledge.
Kramer, M., Czaya, J., Arand, D., & Roth, T. (1974). The development of psychological content across the REMP [Abstract]. *Sleep Research, 3*, 121.

Kramer, M., McQuarreie, E., & Bonnet, M. (1979). Dream differences as a function of REM period progression [Abstract]. *Sleep Research, 9,* 155.

Kramer, M., & Nuhic, Z. (2007). A review of dreaming by psychiatric patients: An update. In S. R. Padi-Perumal, R. R. Ruoti, & M. Kramer (Eds.), *Sleep and psychosomatic medicine* (pp. 137–156). Informa.

Kramer, M., & Roth, T. (1979). Dreams in psychopathology. In B. B. Wolman (Ed.), *Handbook of dreams* (pp. 361–387). Van Nostrand.

Kuiken, D., & Sikora, S. (1993). The impact of dreams on waking thoughts and feelings. In A. Moffitt, M. Kramer, & R. Hoffman (Eds.), *The functions of dreaming* (pp. 419–476). State University of New York Press.

Kuiken, D., & Smith, L. (1991). Impactful dreams and metaphor generation. *Dreaming, 1,* 135–145. https://doi.org/10.1037/h0094326

Laberge, S. (1985). *Lucid dreaming.* Ballantine.

Laberge, S. (1988). The psychophysiology of lucid dreaming. In J. Gackenbach & S. Laberge (Eds.), *Conscious mind, sleeping brain* (pp. 135–153). Plenum.

Lacaux, C. (2021). *The borderland between wakefulness and sleep, a doorway into creativity* [Doctoral dissertation, Sorbonne Université]. HAL Theses. https://theses.hal.science/tel-03541702

Lacaux, C., Andrillon, T., Bastoul, C., Idir, Y., Fonteix-Galet, A., Arnulf, I., & Oudiette, D. (2021). Sleep onset is a creative sweet spot. *Sciences Advances, 7*(50), Article eabj5866. https://doi.org/10.1126/sciadv.abj5866

Lafrenière, A., Lortie-Lussier, M., Dale, A., Robidoux, R., & De Koninck, J. (2018). Autobiographical memory sources of threats in dreams. *Consciousness and Cognition, 58,* 124–135. https://doi.org/10.1016/j.concog.2017.10.017

Lamarche, L., & De Koninck, J. (2007). Sleep disturbance in adults with post traumatic stress disorder: Clinical integration and future research. *Journal of Clinical Psychiatry, 68,* 1257–1270. https://doi.org/10.4088/jcp.v68n0813

Lavie, P., & Hobson, J. A. (1986). Origin of dreams: Anticipation of modern theories in the philosophy and physiology of the eighteenth and nineteenth centuries. *Psychological Bulletin, 100,* 229–240. https://doi.org/10.1037/0033-2909.100.2.229

Lavie, P., & Kaminer, H. (1991). Dreams that poison sleep: Dreaming in Holocaust survivors. *Dreaming, 1,* 11–23. https://doi.org/10.1037/h0094313

Leclair-Visonneau, L., Oudiette, D., Gaymard, B., Leu-Seimenescu, S., & Arnulf, I. (2010). Do the eyes scan dream images during rapid eye movement sleep? Evidence from the rapid eye movement sleep behaviour disorder model. *Brain, 133*(6), 1737–1746. https://doi.org/10.1093/brain/awq110

Lemyre, A., Bastien, C., & Vallieres, A. (2022). The feeling priming theory (FPT) of dreaming. *Dreaming, 33*(3), 316–367. https://doi.org/10.1037/drm0000202

Lemyre, A., Légaré-Bergeron, L., Landry, R. B., Garon, D., & Vallières, A. (2020). High-level control in lucid dreams. *Imagination, Cognition and Personality, 40*(1), 20–42. https://doi.org/10.1177/0276236620909544

Levin, R., & Daly, R. S. (1998). Nightmares and psychotic decompensation: A case study. *Psychiatry, 61*(3), 217–222. https://doi.org/10.1080/00332747.1998.11024833

Llinas, R. R., & Pare, D. (1991). Of dreaming and wakefulness. *Neuroscience, 44,* 521–535. https://doi.org/10.1016/0306-4522(91)90075-y

Long, M. E., Hammonsa, M. E., Frueh, C., Khana, M. M., Elhaif, J. D., & Tenga, E. J. (2011). Imagery rescripting and exposure group treatment of posttraumatic nightmares in veterans with PTSD. *Journal of Anxiety Disorders, 25,* 531–535. https://doi.org/10.1016/j.janxdis.2010.12.007

Lortie-Lussier, M., Dale, A., & De Koninck, J. (2019). Ontogenetic development of dreaming. In K. Valli & R. Hoss (Eds.), *Dreams: Understanding biology, psychology, and culture* (Vol. 1, pp. 201–208). ABC-CLIO.

Lortie-Lussier, M., Simond, S., Rinfret, N., & De Koninck, J. (1992). Beyond sex differences: Family and occupational roles' impact on women's and men's dreams. *Sex Roles, 26,* 79–96. https://doi.org/10.1007/BF00289751

Lusignan, F. A., Zadra, A., Dubuc, M. J., Daoust, A. M., Mottard, J. P., & Godbout, R. (2009). Dream content in chronically-treated persons with schizophrenia. *Schizophrenia Research, 112,* 164–173. https://doi.org/10.1016/j.schres.2009.03.032

Mahrer, A. (1989). *Dream work.* W. W. Norton.

Malinowski, J., & Horton, C. (2014a). Memory sources of dreams: The incorporation of autobiographical rather than episodic experiences. *Journal of Sleep Research, 23,* 441–447. https://doi.org/10.1111/jsr.12134

Malinowski, J., & Horton, C. L. (2014a). Evidence for the preferential incorporation of emotional waking-life experiences into dreams. *Dreaming, 24*, 18–31. https://doi.org/10.1037/a0036017

Mallet, R., Sowin, L., Raider, R., Konkoly, K. R., & Paller, K. A. (2022). Benefits and concerns of seeking and experiencing lucid dreams: Benefits are tied to successful induction and dream control. *Sleep Advances, 3*(1), Article zpac027. https://doi.org/10.1093/sleepadvances/zpac027

Maquet, P., & Ruby, P. (2004). Psychology: Insight and the sleep committee. *Nature, 427*, 304–305. https://doi.org/10.1038/427304a

Maranci, J. B., Nigam, M., Masset, L., Msika, E., Vionnet, M. C., Chaumereil, C., Vidailhet, M., Leu-Semenescu, S., & Arnulf, I. (2022). Eye movement patterns correlate with overt emotional behaviours in rapid eye movement sleep. *Scientific Reports, 12*, Article 1770. https://doi.org/10.1038/s41598-022-05905-5

Marquandt, C. J. G., Bonato, R. A., & Hoffman R. F. (1996). An empirical investigation into the day-residue and dream lag effects. *Dreaming, 6*, 57–65. https://doi.org/10.1037/h0094446

Mathes, J., Schredl, M., & Göritz, A. S. (2014). Frequency of typical dream themes in most recent dreams: An online study. *Dreaming, 24*(1), 57–66. https://doi.org/10.1037/a0035857

Maury, A. (1865). *Le sommeil et les rêves* (*Sleep and dreams*). Didier.

Mazzarello, P. (2000). What dreams may come? *Nature, 408*, 523. https://doi.org/10.1038/35046170

Montangero, J. (2009). Using dreams in cognitive behavioral psychotherapy: Theory, method, and examples. *Dreaming, 19*(4), 239–254. https://doi.org/10.1037/a0017613

Mota, N. B., Weissheimer, J., Ribeiro, M., de Paiva, M., Avilla-Souza, J., Simabucuru, G., Chaves, M. F., Cecchi, L., Cirne, J., Cecchi, G., Rodrigues, C., Copelli, M., & Ribeiro, S. (2020). Dreaming during the Covid-19 pandemic: Computational assessment of dream reports reveals mental suffering related to fear of contagion. *PLoS One, 15*(11), e0242903. https://doi.org/10.1371/journal.pone.0242903

Murkar, A. L. A., & De Koninck, J. (2018). Consolidative mechanisms of emotional processing in REM sleep and PTSD. *Sleep Medicine Reviews, 41*, 173–184. https://doi.org/10.1016/j.smrv.2018.03.001

Nielsen, T. A. (1995). Describing and modeling hypnagogic imagery using a systematic self-observation procedure. *Dreaming, 5*, 75–94.

Nielsen, T. A. (2000). A review of mentation in REM and NREM sleep: "Covert" REM sleep as a possible reconciliation of two opposing models. *Behavioral and Brain Sciences, 23*, 851–866. https://doi.org/10.1017/S0140525X0000399X

Nielsen, T. A. (2004). Chronobiological features of dream production. *Sleep Medicine Reviews, 8*, 403–424. https://doi.org/10.1016/j.smrv.2004.06.005

Nielsen, T. A. (2005). What are the memory sources of dreams? *Nature, 437*, 1286–1289. https://doi.org/10.1038/nature04288

Nielsen, T. (2012). Variations in dream recall frequency and dream theme diversity by age and sex. *Frontiers in Neurology, 3*, Article 106. https://doi.org/10.3389/fneur.2012.00106

Nielsen, T. A., Carr, M., Blanchette-Carrière, C., Marquis, L.-P., Dumel, G., Solomonova, E., Julien, S. H., Picard-Deland, C., & Paquette, T. (2017). NREM sleep spindles are associated with dream recall. *Sleep Spindles and Cortical Up States, 1*, 27–41. https://doi.org/10.1556/2053.1.2016.003

Nielsen, T., & Levin, R. (2007). Nightmares: A new neurocognitive model. *Sleep Medicine Reviews, 11*(4), 295–310. https://doi.org/10.1016/j.smrv.2007.03.004

Nielsen, T. A., & Powell, R. A. (1992). The day-residue and dream-lag effects: A literature review and limited replication of two temporal effects in dream formation. *Dreaming, 2*, 67–78.

Nielsen, T. A., Zadra, A. L., Simard, V., Saucier, S., Stenstrom, P., Smith, C., & Kuiken, D. (2003). The typical dreams of Canadian university students. *Dreaming, 13*, 211–236. https://doi.org/10.1023/B:DREM.0000003144.40929.0b

Nixon, A., Robidoux, R., Dale, A., & De Koninck, J. (2017). Pre-sleep and post-sleep mood as a complementary evaluation of emotionally impactful dreams. *International Journal of Dream Research 10*, 141–150. https://doi.org/10.11588/ijodr.2017.2.35411

Northoff, G., Scalabrini, A., & Fogel, S. (2023). Topographic-dynamic reorganisation model of dreams (TRoD) – A spatiotemporal approach. *Neuroscience and Biobehavioral Reviews, 148*, 105117. https://doi.org/10.1016/j.neubiorev.2023.105117

Ogilvie, R. D., Hunt, H. T., Tyson, P. D., Lucescu, M. L., & Jeakins, D. B. (1982). Lucid dreaming and alpha activity: A preliminary report. *Perceptual and Motor Skills, 55*(3, Pt. 1), 795–808. https://doi.org/10.2466/pms.1982.55.3.795

Oudiette, D., Dealberto, M.-J., Uguccioni, G., Golmard, J.-L., Merino-Andreu, M., Tafti, M., Garma, L, Schwartz, S., & Arnulf, I. (2012). Dreaming without REM sleep. *Consciousness and Cognition*, *21*(3), 1129–1140. https://doi.org/10.1016/j.concog.2012.04.010
Oudiette, D., Leclair-Visonneau, L., Gaymard, B., Leu, S., & Arnulf, I. (2010) Do the eyes scan dream images during REM sleep? Evidence from the REM sleep behaviour disorder model. *Brain*, 133(Pt6), 1737–1746.
Oudiette, D., Leu, S., Pottier, M., Buzare, M. A., Brion, A., & Arnulf, I. (2009). Dreamlike mentations during sleepwalking and sleep terrors in adults. *Sleep*, *32*(12), 1621–1627. https://doi.org/10.1093/sleep/32.12.1621
Pagel, J. F., Blagrove, M., Levin, R., States, B., Stickgold, B., & White, S. (2001). Definitions of dream: A paradigm for comparing field descriptive specific studies of dream. *Dreaming*, *11*(4), 195–202. https://doi.org/10.1023/A:1012240307661
Perlis, M. L., & Nielsen, T. A. (1993). Mood regulation, dreaming and nightmares: Evaluation of a desensitization function for REM sleep. *Dreaming*, *3*, 243–257.
Perrin, F., García-Larrea, L., Mauguière, F., & Bastuji, H. A. (1999). Differential brain response to the subject's own name persists during sleep. *Clinical Neurophysiology*, *110*, 2153–2164. https://doi.org/10.1016/s1388-2457(99)00177-7
Pesant, N., & Zadra, A. (2004). Working with dreams in therapy: What do we know and what should we do? *Clinical Psychology Review*, *24*, 489–512. https://doi.org/10.1016/j.cpr.2004.05.002
Pesonen, A.-K., Lipsanen, J., Halonen, R., Elovainio, M., Sandman, N., Mäkelä, J.-M., Antila, M., Béchard, D., Ollila, H. M., & Kuula, L. (2020). Pandemic dreams: Network analysis of dream content during the COVID-19 lockdown. *Frontiers in Psychology*, *11*, Article 573961. https://doi.org/10.3389/fpsyg.2020.573961
Piaget, J. (1962). *Play, dreams and imitation in childhood.* W. W. Norton.
Picard-Deland, C., Konkoly, K., Raider, K., Paller, K., Nielsen, T., Pigeon, R., & Carr, M. (2022). The memory sources of dreams: Serial awakenings across sleep stages and time of night. *Sleep*, *46*(4), Article zsac292. https://doi.org/10.1093/sleep/zsac292
Picard-Deland, C., Nielsen, T., & Carr, M. (2021). Dreaming of the sleep lab. *PLOS ONE*, *16*(10), Article e0257738. https://doi.org/10.1371/journal.pone.0257738
Pivik, R. T. (1991). Tonic states and phasic events in relation to sleep mentation. In S. J. Euman & J. Antrobus (Eds.), *The mind in sleep* (pp. 214–248). Wiley.
Revonsuo, A. (2000). The reinterpretation of dreams: An evolutionary hypothesis of the function of dreaming. *Behavioral and Brain Sciences*, *23*, 877–901.
Revonsuo, A., Jarno, T., & Katja, V. (2016). The avatars in the machine-dreaming as a simulation of social reality. In T. Metzinger & J. Windt (Eds.), *Open MIND: Philosophy and the mind sciences in the 21st century* (pp. 1295–1322). MIT Press.
Roll, S. R., & Brenneis, C. B. (1975). Chicano and Anglo dreams of death: A replication. *Journal of Cross-Cultural Psychology*, *6*, 377–383.
Roll, S. R., Hinton, J. A., & Glazer, M. (1974). Dreams of death: Mexican-American versus Anglo-American dreams. *Interamerican Journal of Psychology*, *8*, 111–115.
Rossner, R. I., Lyddon, W. J., & Freeman, A. (2004). *Cognitive therapy and dreams.* Springer.
Roussy, F., Camirand, C., Foulkes, D., De Koninck, J., Loftis, M., & Kerr, N. H. (1996). Does early-night REM dream content reliably reflect presleep state of mind? *Dreaming*, *6*, 121–130. https://doi.org/10.1037/h0094450
Roussy, F., Raymond, I., & De Koninck, J. (2000). Affect in REM dreams: Exploration of a time-of-night effect. *Sleep*, *23*, A174–A175.
Roussy, F., Raymond, I., Gonthier, I., Grenier, J., & De Koninck, J. (1998). Temporal references in manifest dream content: Confirmation of increased remoteness as the night progresses [Abstract]. *Sleep*, *21*, 285.
Röver, S. A., & Schredl, M. (2017). Measuring emotions in dreams: Effects of dream length and personality. *International Journal of Dream Research*, *10*, 65–68. https://doi.org/10.11588/ijodr.2017.1.34565
Rubin, D. C., Wetzler, S. E., & Nebes, R. D. (1986). Autobiographical memory across the life-span. In D. C. Rubin (Ed.), *Autobiographical memory* (pp. 202–221). Cambridge University Press.
Ruby, P. M. (2020). The neural correlates of dreaming have not been identified yet. Commentary on "The NeuralCorrelates of Dreaming. Nat Neurosci.2017". *Frontiers in Neuroscience*, *14*, 585470. https://doi.org/10.3389/fnins.2020.585470

Sabourin, C., Robidoux, R., Pérusse, A., & De Koninck, J. (2018). Dream content in pregnancy and postpartum: Refined exploration of continuity between waking and dreaming. *Dreaming, 28*(2), 122–139. https://doi.org/10.1037/drm0000070

Salisbury, J. E. (2004). *The blood of martyrs: Unintended consequences of ancient violence.* Routledge.

Samson-Daoust, E., Julien, S. H., Beaulieu-Prévost, D., & Zadra, A. (2019). Predicting the affective tone of everyday dreams: A prospective study of state and trait variables. *Scientific Reports*, 9, Article 14780. https://doi.org/10.1038/s41598-019-50859-w

Saredi, R., Baylor, G., Meier, B., & Strauch, I. (1997). Current concerns and REM-dreams: A laboratory study of dream incubation. *Dreaming, 7*, 195–208. https://doi.org/10.1037/h0094474

Scarpelli, S., Alfonsi, V., Gorgoni, M., & De Gennaro, L. (2022). What about dreams? State of the art and open question. *Journal of Sleep Research, 31*, Article e13609. https://doi.org/10.1111/jsr.13609

Scarpelli, S., Bartolacci, C., D'Atri, A., Gorgoni, M., & De Gennaro, L. (2019). The functional role of dreaming in emotional processes. *Frontiers in Psychology, 10*, Article 459. https://doi.org/10.3389/fpsyg.2019.00459

Scarpelli, S., Nadorff, M. R., Bjorvatn, B., Chung, F., Dauvilliers, Y., Espie, C. A., Inoue, Y., Matsui, K., Merikanto, I., Morin, C. M., Penzel, T., Sieminski, M., Fang, H., Macêdo, T., Mota-Rolim, S. A., Leger, D., Plazzi, G., Chan, N. Y., Partinen, M., . . . De Gennaro L (2022). Nightmares in people with COVID-19: Did coronavirus infect our dreams? *Nature and Science of Sleep, 14*, 93–108. https://doi.org/10.2147/NSS.S344299

Schredl, M. (2019a). Dream recall and individual differences. In K. Valli & R. J. Hoss (Eds.), *Dreams: Understanding biology, psychology, and culture* (Vol. 1, pp. 201–208). ABC-CLIO.

Schredl, M. (2019b). Continuity hypothesis of dreaming. In K. Valli & R. Hoss (Eds.), *Dreams: Understanding biology, psychology and culture* (Vol. 1, pp. 88–94). ABC-CLIO.

Schredl, M., Ciric, P., GÖtz, S., & Wittmann, L. (2004). Typical dreams: Stability and gender differences. *The Journal of Psychology, 138*(6), 485–494. https://doi.org/10.3200/JRLP.138.6.485-494

Schredl, M., Atanasova, D., Horman, K., Maurer, J. T., Hummel, T., & Stuck, B. A. (2009). Information processing during sleep: The effect of olfactory stimuli on dream content and dream emotions. *Journal of Sleep Research, 18*(3), 285–290. https://doi.org/10.1111/j.1365-2869.2009.00737.x

Schredl, M., Ciric, P., Bishop, A., Gölitz, E., & Buschtöns, D. (2003). Content analysis of German students' dreams: Comparison to American findings. *Dreaming, 13*, 237–243. https://doi.org/10.1023/B:DREM.0000003145.26849.37

Schredl, M., Ciric, P., Gottz, S., & Witmann, L. (2003). Dream recall frequency, attitude towards dreams and openness to experience. *Dreaming, 13*, 145–154. https://doi.org/10.1023/A:1025369311813

Schredl, M., & Hoffman, F. (2003). Continuity between waking activities and dream activities. *Consciousness and Cognition, 12*, 298–308. https://doi.org/10.1016/s1053-8100(02)00072-7

Schredl, M., & Rauthmann, J. (2022). Dream recall, nightmares, dream sharing, and personality: A replication study. *Dreaming, 32*(2), 163–172. https://doi.org/10.1037/drm0000200

Schredl, M., Wittman, L., Ciric, P., & Götz, S. (2003). Factors of home dream recall: A structural equation model. *Journal of Sleep Research, 12*, 133–141. https://doi.org/10.1046/j.1365-2869.2003.00344.x

Shevrin, H. (1986). Subliminal perception and dreaming. *Journal of Mind and Behavior, 7*, 379–395.

Siclari, F., Baird, B., Perogamvros, L., Bernardi, G., LaRocque, J. J., Riedner, B., Boly, M., Postle, B. & Tononi, G. (2017). The neural correlates of dreaming. *Nature Neuroscience, 20*(6), 872–878. https://doi.org/10.1038/nn.4545

Sikka, P., Feilhauer, D., Valli, K., & Revonsuo, A. (2017). How you measure is what you get: Differences in self- and external ratings of emotional experiences in home dreams. *American Journal of Psychology, 130*(3), 367–384. https://doi.org/10.5406/amerjpsyc.130.3.0367

Sikka, P., Pesonen, H. & Revonsuo, A. (2018). Peace of mind and anxiety in the waking state are related to the affective content of dreams. *Scientific Reports, 8*, 12762. https://doi.org/10.1038/s41598-018-30721-1

Simor, P., Bogdanya, T., & Peigneux, P. (2022). Predictive coding, multisensory integration, and attentional control: A multicomponent framework for lucid dreaming. *Proceedings of the National Academy of Sciences of the United States of America, 119*(44), Article e2123418119. https://doi.org/10.1073/pnas.2123418119

Sirois-Berliss, M., & De Koninck, J. (1982). Menstrual stress and dreams: Adaptation or interference. *The Psychiatric Journal of the University of Ottawa, 7*, 77–86.

Skancke, J. F., Holsen, I., & Schredl, M. (2014). Continuity between waking life and dreams of psychiatric patients: A review and discussion of the implications for dream research. *International Journal of Dream Research, 7*(1), 39–53. https://doi.org/10.11588/ijodr.2014.1.12184

Skrzypińska, D., Szmigielska, B., Skrzypińńska, D., & Szmigielska, B. (2018). Dreams in cognitive-behavioral therapy. In O. Şenormancı & G. Şenormancı (Eds.), *Cognitive behavioral therapy and clinical applications*. IntechOpen. https://doi.org/10.5772/INTECHOPEN.70893
Solms, M. (1997). *The neuropsychology of dreams*. Lawrence Erlbaum Associates.
Solms, M. (2000). Dreaming and REM sleep are controlled by different brain mechanisms. *Behavioral and Brain Sciences, 23*, 843–850.
Solms, M. (2004). Freud returns. *Scientific American, 290*, 82–88.
Solms, M. (2019). Effects of brain legions on dreaming. In K. Valli & R. J. Hoss (Eds.), *Dreams: Understanding biology, psychology, and culture* (Vol. 1, pp. 78–87). ABC-CLIO.
Sterpenich, V., Perogamvros, L., Tononi, G., & Schwartz, S. (2019). Fear in dreams and in wakefulness: Evidence for day/night affective homeostasis. *bioRxiv*. https://doi.org/10.1101/534099
Stickgold, R. (2005a). Introduction to dreams and their pathology. In M. Kryger, T. Roth, & W. C. Dement (Eds.), *Principles and practice of sleep medicine* (pp. 519–521). Saunders.
Stickgold, R. (2005b). Why we dream. In M. Kryger, T. Roth, & W. C. Dement (Eds.), *Principles and practice of sleep medicine* (pp. 579–587). Saunders.
Stickgold, R., & Walker, M. (2004). To sleep, perchance to gain creative insight? *Trends in Cognitive Science, 8*(5), 191–192. https://doi.org/10.1016/j.tics.2004.03.003
St-Onge, M., Mercier, P., & De Koninck, J. (2009). Imagery rehearsal therapy for frequent nightmares in children. *Behavioral Sleep Medicine, 7*, 81–98. https://doi.org/10.1080/15402000902762360
Strauch, I., & Lederbogen, S. (1999). The home dreams and waking fantasies of boys and girls between ages 9 and 15: A longitudinal study. *Dreaming, 9*, 153–161. https://doi.org/10.1023/A:1021341732185
Strompe, T., Ritter, K., Ortwein-Swoboda, G., Schmid-Siegel, B., Zitterl, W., Strobl, R., & Schanda, H. (2003). Anxiety and hostility in the manifest dreams of schizophrenic patients. *Journal of Nervous and Mental Diseases, 191*(12), 806–812.
Tartz, R. S., & Krippner, S. (2008). Cognitive differences in dream content between Argentine males and females using quantitative content analysis. *Dreaming, 18*, 217–235. https://doi.org/10.1037/a0013780
Thompson, K., Gibbings, A., Shaw, J., Ray, L., Hébert, G., De Koninck, J., & Fogel, S. (2021). Sleep and second language acquisition revisited: The role of sleep spindles and rapid eye movements, *Nature and Science of Sleep, 13*, 1887–1902. https://doi.org/10.2147/NSS.S326151
Trenholme, I., Cartwright, R. D., & Greenberg, G. (1984). Dream dimension differences during a life change. *Psychiatry Research, 12*, 35–45. https://doi.org/10.1016/0165-1781(84)90136-7
Uga, V., Lemut, M. C., Zampi, C., Zilli, I., & Salzarulo, P. (2006). Music in dreams. Con*sciousness and Cognition, 15*, 351–357. https://doi.org/10.1016/j.concog.2005.09.003
Ullman, M., & Zimmerman, N. (1979). *Working with dreams*. Delacorte Press.
Vallat, R., Chatard, B., Blagrove, M., & Ruby, P. (2017). Characteristics of the memory sources of dreams: A new version of the content-matching paradigm to take mundane and remote memories into account. *PLOS ONE, 12*(10), Article e0185262. https://doi.org/10.1371/journal.pone.0185262
Valli, K., & Hoss, R. J. (2019). *Dreams: Understanding biology, psychology, and culture*. ABC-CLIO.
Valli, K., Revonsuo, A., Pälkäs, O., & Punamäki, R. L. (2006). The effect of trauma on dream content: A field study of Palestinian children. *Dreaming, 16*, 63–87. https://doi.org/10.1037/1053-0797.16.2.63
Van de Castle, R. (1971). *The psychology of dreaming*. General Learning Corp.
Van de Castle, R. L. (1994). *Our dreaming mind*. Ballantine Books.
Verdone, P. (1965). Temporal reference of manifest dream content. *Perceptual and Motor Skills, 20*, 262–271.
Vogel, G. (1991). Sleep onset mentation. In S. J. Ellman & J. Antrobus (Eds.), *The mind in sleep* (pp. 125–136). Wiley.
Voss, U., Holzmann, R., Tuin, I., & Hobson, J. A. (2009). Lucid dreaming: A state of consciousness with features of both waking and non-lucid dreaming. *Sleep, 32*(9), 1191–1200. https://doi.org/10.1093/sleep/32.9.1191
Wagner, U., Gais, S., Haider, H., Verleger, R., & Born J. (2004). Sleep inspires insight. *Nature, 427*, 352–355. https://doi.org/10.1038/nature02223
Walker, P. C., & Johnson, R. F. (1974). The influence of presleep suggestions on dream content: Evidence and methodological problems. *Psychological Bulletin, 81*, 362–370. https://doi.org/10.1037/h0036335
Wamsley, E. J. (2022). Constructive episodic simulation in dreams. *PLOS ONE, 17*, Article e0264574. https://doi.org/10.1371/journal.pone.0264574

Wamsley, E. J., Tucker, M., Payne, J., Benavides, J. A., & Stickgold, R. (2010). Dreaming of a learning task is associated with enhanced sleep-dependent memory consolidation. *Current Biology*, *20*, 850–855. https://doi.org/10.1016/j.cub.2010.03.027

Wang, J., & Feng, X. (2024). Dreaming of being chased reflects waking-life experiences related to negative relationships with others metaphorically. *Frontiers in Psychology*, *15*, 1413011. https://doi.org/10.3389/fpsyg.2024.1413011

Wang, J., Zemmelman, S. E., Hong, D., Feng, X., & Shen, H. (2021). Does COVID-19 impact the frequency of threatening events in dreams? An exploration of pandemic dreaming in light of contemporary dream theories. *Consciousness and Cognition*, *87*, Article 103051. https://doi.org/10.1016/j.concog.2020.103051

Watson, D. (2003). To dream, perchance to remember: Individual differences in dream recall. *Personality and Individual Differences*, *34*, 1271–1286. https://doi.org/10.1016/S0191-8869(02)00114-9

White, R. J. (1975). *The interpretation of dreams.* Park Ridge.

Wiebe, S., Lamarche, L., Sabourin, C., Lortie-Lussier, M., & De Koninck, J. (2007). The dreams of women with severe emotional/behavioral premenstrual symptoms. *Dreaming*, *17*, 199–207. https://doi.org/10.1037/1053-0797.17.4.199

Winegar, R., & Levin, R. (1997). Sex differences in the object representations in the dreams of adolescents. *Sex Roles*, *36*, 503–516. https://doi.org/10.1007/BF02766687

Winget, C., & Kramer, M. (1979). *Dimensions of dreams.* University of Florida Press.

Winget, C., Kramer, M., & Whitman, R. (1972). Dreams and demography. *Canadian Psychiatric Association Journal*, *17*, 203–208. https://doi.org/10.1177/07067437720176s232

Wolman, B. B. (1979). Dreams and schizophrenia. In B. B. Wolman (Ed.), *Handbook of dreams* (pp. 388–405). Van Nostrand.

Wong, C., Amini, R., & De Koninck, J. (2016). Automatic gender detection of dream reports: A promising approach. *Consciousness and Cognition*, *44*, 20–28. https://doi.org/10.1016/j.concog.2016.06.004

Wood, P. (1962). *Dreaming and social isolation* [Unpublished doctoral dissertation]. University of North Carolina, Chapel Hill.

Wright, J., & Koulack, D. (1987). Dreams and contemporary stress: A disruption–avoidance–adaptation model. *Sleep*, *10*, 172–179. https://doi.org/10.1093/sleep/10.2.172

Yu, C. K.-C. (2007). Emotions before, during, and after dreaming sleep. *Dreaming*, *17*(2), 73–86. https://doi.org/10.1037/1053-0797.17.2.73

Yu, C. K.-C. (2008). Typical dreams experienced by Chinese people. *Dreaming*, *18*, 1–10. https://doi.org/10.1037/1053-0797.18.1.1

Zadra, A., Desjardins, S., & Marcotte, E. (2006). Evolutionary function of dreams: A test of the threat simulation theory in recurrent dreams. *Consciousness and Cognition*, *15*, 450–463. https://doi.org/10.1016/j.concog.2005.02.002

Zadra, A., & Donderi, D. C. (2000). Nightmares and bad dreams: Their prevalence and relationship to well-being. *Journal of Abnormal Psychology*, *109*, 273–281. https://doi.org/10.1037/0021-843X.109.2.273

Zadra, A., Pilon, M., & Donderi, D. C. (2006). Variety and intensity of emotions in nightmares and bad dreams. *Journal of Nervous and Mental Diseases*, *194*, 249–254. https://doi.org/10.1097/01.nmd.0000207359.46223.dc

Zadra, A., & Stickgold, R. (2021). *When brains dream.* W. W. Norton.

Zepelin, H. (1981). Age differences in dreams. I: Men's dreams and thematic apperceptive fantasy. *International Journal of Aging and Human Development*, *12*, 171–186. https://doi.org/10.2190/L7HQ-1U3K-46Q5-HD82

SECTION 3

Societal Factors Influencing Sleep

CHAPTER

14 Multidimensional Sleep Health: An Emerging Framework for Understanding Sleep in Relation to Multiple Health Outcomes

Caitlan A. Tighe, Meredith L. Wallace, Rachel P. K. Conlon, Marquis S. Hawkins, Christopher C. Imes, *and* Daniel J. Buysse

Abstract

Sleep is inextricably linked to health. Sleep disorders and the adverse consequences of suboptimal sleep have been a primary focus of empirical sleep research and clinical sleep medicine. However, suboptimal sleep and sleep disorders do not reflect the full spectrum of sleep and sleep-related experiences. Recently, there has been growing interest in better understanding not only suboptimal sleep and sleep disorders but also sleep health. This chapter defines multidimensional sleep health, discusses methods for measuring and analyzing sleep health in relation to health outcomes, discusses sleep health in relation to some specific health outcomes, and considers behavioral interventions from a sleep health framework.

Key Words: multidimensional sleep health, sleep, physical health, mental health, intervention

Introduction

Sleep is inextricably linked to health. Poor sleep in adults is related to prevalent obesity and weight gain (Cappuccio et al., 2008; Ogilvie & Patel, 2017), metabolic syndrome and cardiovascular disease (CVD; Cappuccio et al., 2011; Krittanawong et al., 2019; Xie et al., 2021; Yin et al., 2017), depression and other mental disorders (Baglioni et al., 2010; Bao et al., 2017; Hertenstein et al., 2019), substance use (Roehrs et al., 2021), and early mortality (Cappuccio et al., 2010; Wallace, Buysse, et al., 2019; Yin et al., 2017). Poor sleep in adolescents is related to poor school performance, motor vehicle accidents, substance use, and suicidal thoughts and behavior (Kearns et al., 2020; Kwon et al., 2019; J.-W. Liu et al., 2019; R. T. Liu et al., 2020; Shochat et al., 2014). Yet, while we now know a great deal about the adverse consequences of poor sleep, we have focused less on defining what constitutes good sleep. At first glance, it may seem obvious that good sleep is simply the opposite of poor. However, this is not necessarily the case. Just as overall health is not simply the absence of disease, so too good sleep health is not the absence of sleep disorders. In this chapter, we will focus on the emerging definition of multidimensional sleep health (MDSH), examine methods for measuring and analyzing sleep health in relation to health outcomes, examine sleep health in relation to some specific health outcomes, and consider behavioral interventions from a sleep health framework.

Definition and Rationale for MDSH

In order to define sleep health, we might first consider the larger question of the function of sleep. Sleep has been considered from perspectives of ecological adaptation, energy metabolism and conservation, and effects on immune and neuronal function. However, in a larger sense, sleep may also be thought of as the price we pay for synaptic plasticity and, ultimately, consciousness (Tononi & Cirelli, 2014). In other words, sleep appears to be a necessary restorative state that permits high levels of functioning during waking or active hours. While it is not a mechanistic explanation, it is empirically true that sleep optimizes adaptation and function during wakefulness at every level of biological function: from molecular energy regulation to function at the cellular, tissue, circuit, and organ system levels to systemic physiology to cognition, affect, and learning and to behavior. Disrupting sleep interferes with function at each of these levels, and optimizing sleep optimizes waking function.

Defining sleep health also requires the recognition that sleep can be defined and measured from several different perspectives. First, sleep can be viewed as a complex neurobehavioral state distinguished from that of wakefulness. Within sleep, the states of non-rapid-eye-movement (NREM) and rapid-eye-movement (REM) sleep are also distinct from each other. Second, sleep can be viewed as a neurobiological process that unfolds in a temporally ordered fashion over a period of time. For instance, in adult humans, wakefulness transitions to light and then deep stages of NREM sleep, followed by a transition to REM sleep, and proceeds through alternating NREM–REM cycles across the entire sleep period. Of course, the temporal structure of sleep is distinct for each species, with polyphasic sleep bouts and a less clear day–night distinction being common in many. Third, sleep can be defined as a set of behaviors. For instance, in humans, sleep is behaviorally defined by recumbent posture, closed eyelids, and seeking of a safe, dark, quiet environment. Whether we define sleep as a state, a process, or a behavior, we strive to describe and measure it in quantitative terms, which allow us to indicate when one person's sleep, or one bout of sleep, is "better" than another.

Recognizing that sleep in all of its complexities is related to health outcomes of various sorts, we then need to ask how it is that sleep affects health. At a broad level, three different frameworks have been considered. First is the medical or sleep disorders perspective. The establishment and development of sleep medicine as a medical specialty has brought with it an emphasis on sleep disorders. Currently, the *International Classification of Sleep Disorders*, third edition (American Academy of Sleep Medicine, 2014), recognizes six broad categories of sleep disorders: insomnia, sleep-related breathing disorders, central disorders of hypersomnolence, circadian rhythm sleep disorders, parasomnias, and sleep-related movement disorders. The presence of each of these disorders has been associated with adverse health outcomes. While describing the full range of such relationships is beyond the scope of this chapter, a few brief examples will suffice. Insomnia is associated both cross-sectionally and longitudinally with the development of depression and other mental disorders (Baglioni et al., 2010; Hertenstein et al., 2019) and has been associated less consistently with the development of hypertension and early mortality (Ge et al., 2019; Jarrin et al., 2018; Lovato & Lack, 2019). Specific phenotypes of insomnia, such as insomnia with short objective sleep duration, may carry particular risk (Jarrin et al., 2018; K. A. Johnson et al., 2021). Sleep-related breathing disorders include obstructive sleep apnea syndrome (OSAS) and central sleep apnea disorders. OSAS is associated with prevalent and incident obesity, hypertension, CVD, atrial fibrillation and other arrhythmias, and early mortality in a dose-dependent fashion (Khokhrina et al., 2022; Yeghiazarians et al., 2021). Central disorders of hypersomnolence such as narcolepsy are associated with tremendous functional impairment, but narcolepsy itself may also be associated with obesity (Mohammadi et al., 2021; Tadrous et al., 2021). Circadian rhythm sleep–wake disorders such as delayed sleep phase disorder and shift-work sleep–wake disorder are also associated with substantial functional impairment. Moreover, they too may be associated with obesity and metabolic dysfunction (Shah et al., 2022). Among the parasomnias, REM behavior disorder is strongly associated with the onset of Parkinson's disease and other alpha-synucleinopathies and, in fact, may be an early indicator of the presence of these diseases (Galbiati et al., 2019). Finally, restless legs syndrome, the prototype sleep-related movement disorder, may be associated with increased risk for cardiovascular events (Kendzerska et al., 2017). In summary, poor sleep may lead to poor health through the presence of specific sleep disorders. This sleep disorders perspective is a useful one because it focuses on case identification and because specific treatments are available for all or most sleep disorders.

However, the absence of sleep disorders is not equivalent to having good sleep. As an analogy, consider that myocardial infarction indicates the presence of CVD, but the absence of a myocardial infarction does not necessarily indicate the presence of good heart health. An individual who has never had a myocardial infarction may still have hypertension, atherosclerosis, and increased arterial stiffness. In the same way, a person who does not have significant sleep apnea does not necessarily have good sleep, nor does the treatment of sleep apnea guarantee good sleep.

An alternative perspective, widely used in epidemiologic studies, has been to focus on specific sleep characteristics, the most common of which is sleep duration. Although specific studies have varied in whether they measure 24-hour sleep duration or sleep duration at night or whether they measure sleep duration by self-report versus behaviorally, with actigraphy, they largely converge on the conclusion that very short and very long sleep duration are associated with adverse health consequences both cross-sectionally and longitudinally (Cappuccio et al., 2008, 2010, 2011; Itani et al., 2017; Jike et al., 2018). Measuring specific sleep characteristics is useful because such characteristics can be measured in every individual, rather than the more dichotomous method of diagnosing individuals with or without a particular condition.

However, the complexities of defining sleep as a state, a process, and a behavior led to the recognition that sleep cannot be adequately measured with any single characteristic. Rather, sleep can be characterized along multiple dimensions simultaneously. For instance, in addition to duration, sleep can be characterized by efficiency or continuity (i.e., the degree to which it is consolidated or interrupted by frequent or prolonged awakenings); the time of day at which it occurs and whether this timing is aligned with other circadian rhythms; its subjective quality, satisfaction, or the "degree of goodness" an individual perceives in their sleep; the amount of sleepiness (i.e., the propensity to fall asleep during usual waking hours or, conversely, the degree of alertness an individual feels); and the regularity of sleep timing and duration across successive nights. Other dimensions may also be considered and vary depending on the means of measurement. However, each of the dimensions noted above has the advantage of being measurable by self-report, behavioral (i.e., actigraphy), and physiological (i.e., polysomnography [PSG]) methods. The one exception is sleep satisfaction, which is inherently self-reported. Moreover, each of these dimensions has been individually associated with a range of adverse health outcomes. An exhaustive review of this literature is beyond the scope of this chapter, but Table 14.1 indicates a few references substantiating the relationship between each dimension and health outcomes.

Moreover, each of these dimensions can be characterized for every individual at every point in time, leading to several important implications. First, individuals may vary in how "good" or "poor" they are along each individual dimension. Second, different individuals will vary in the particular *pattern* of sleep dimensions they possess. Third, different sleep dimensions may have cumulative or interacting effects on good or poor health outcomes. An example of this final point is suggested by the phenotype of insomnia with short objective sleep duration. Insomnia is characterized by poor quality sleep (i.e., poor sleep satisfaction, combined with symptoms of poor sleep efficiency or continuity). However, a subset of individuals with insomnia also have short sleep duration when measured by objective means such as PSG. Cross-sectional and longitudinal studies have suggested that this particular collection of characteristics, or phenotype, is distinct from the phenotype of insomnia symptoms in the presence of normal objective sleep duration. Specifically, individuals who have insomnia with short sleep have increased risk for depression, hypertension, Type 2 diabetes, neurocognitive impairment, and poor response to cognitive behavioral treatment for insomnia compared to individuals with insomnia

Table 14.1 Example papers reporting on sleep health characteristics and outcomes

Outcomes	Regularity	Satisfaction	Alertness/sleepiness/napping	Timing	Efficiency	Duration
Mortality	(Omichi et al., 2022; Wallace et al., 2022)	(Ge et al., 2019[a])	(Sun et al., 2022[a]; Wallace, Lee, et al., 2019)	(Knutson & von Schantz, 2018; Wallace et al., 2022)	(Wallace, Lee, et al., 2019)	(da Silva et al., 2016[a]; Itani et al., 2017[a]; Jike et al., 2018[a]; Kabat et al., 2018; Tao et al., 2021; Wallace, Lee, et al., 2019)
Metabolic	(Chaput et al., 2020[a]; Lunsford-Avery et al., 2018; Zhu et al., 2022[a])	(Anothaisintawee et al., 2016[a]; Brouwer et al., 2020)	(Léger et al., 2019; Sun et al., 2022[a]; van der Pal et al., 2018)	(Anothaisintawee et al., 2016[a]; Chaput et al., 2020[a])	(Brouwer et al., 2020; Lian et al., 2019[a]; Tsereteli et al., 2022)	(Dejenie et al., 2022[a]; Hua et al., 2021[a]; Itani et al., 2017[a]; Jike et al., 2018[a]; Mostafa et al., 2022[a]; Xie et al., 2021[a])
Cardiovascular	(Lunsford-Avery et al., 2018)	(Bertisch et al., 2018; C. Li & Shang, 2021; Yuan et al., 2021)	(Cheungpasitporn et al., 2016[a]; Léger et al., 2019; Salari et al., 2022[a])	(Lee et al., 2022)	(Didikoglu et al., 2020; Lee et al., 2022; Yan et al., 2021; Yuan et al., 2021)	(Dejenie et al., 2022[a]; Itani et al., 2017[a]; Jike et al., 2018[a]; Krittanawong et al., 2019 [a]; C. Li & Shang, 2021)
Depression	(Lunsford-Avery et al., 2018)	(Hertenstein et al., 2019[a]; Hill Almeida et al., 2022[a]; Pigeon et al., 2017[a]; Smagula et al., 2016[a])	(Devine & Wolf, 2016; Léger et al., 2019)	(Furihata et al., 2017; Morita et al., 2015)	(Didikoglu et al., 2020)	(X. Li et al., 2023 [a])
Neurobehavioral and cognitive	(Chaput et al., 2020[a])	(Fortier-Brochu et al., 2012[a]; Shi et al., 2018[a])	(Owusu et al., 2019; Ru et al., 2019)	(Chaput et al., 2020[a]; Suh et al., 2018)	(Philbrook et al., 2017)	(Fan et al., 2019[a]; Lo et al., 2016 [a])

Note. References listed here are intended to be representative examples that highlight reviews or larger, more recent studies. In some cases associations among sleep health characteristics and outcomes were only significant in a subset of patients or under certain circumstances (e.g., varied based on study design, methods, etc.).

[a]Review paper.

with normal sleep duration (Fernandez-Mendoza et al., 2010, 2015; He et al., 2023; K. A. Johnson et al., 2021).

To illustrate the importance of considering sleep health from a multidimensional perspective, consider three individuals, each of whom has a sleep duration of 5 hours. Individual A works night shifts, most often sleeps during daylight hours but moves to nocturnal sleep on days off, and overall reports moderate sleep quality and efficiency. Individual B sleeps for 5 hours at night but reports low quality/satisfaction and poor sleep efficiency and meets the characteristics for insomnia. Individual C, who also sleeps 5 hours, is busy working two jobs and raising a family and reports limited available time for sleep and that, when they sleep, they sleep deeply and with high efficiency. In most epidemiologic studies, individuals A, B, and C would all be characterized as having the same sleep duration, which fails to account for the very different causes of short sleep duration and other sleep characteristics they possess.

Thus, sleep disorders are distinct from sleep characteristics; each individual can be characterized by multiple sleep characteristics; each of these characteristics is individually associated with health outcomes; and these characteristics may combine and interact with each other. In recognition of these observations, we offered the following definition for *sleep health* in 2014: "Sleep health is a multidimensional pattern of sleep wakefulness, adapted to individual, social, and environmental demands, that promotes physical and mental well-being" (Buysse, 2014, p. 12). We have subsequently adopted the term *MDSH* to highlight the importance of the multiple factors that can characterize sleep health. In adults, we have typically focused on six sleep health dimensions: satisfaction/quality, alertness, timing, efficiency, duration, and regularity (Figure 14.1). However, different sleep dimensions may be more appropriate for categorizing the sleep health of other groups. For instance, sleep behavior has been emphasized as a critical component of pediatric sleep health (Meltzer, 2021).

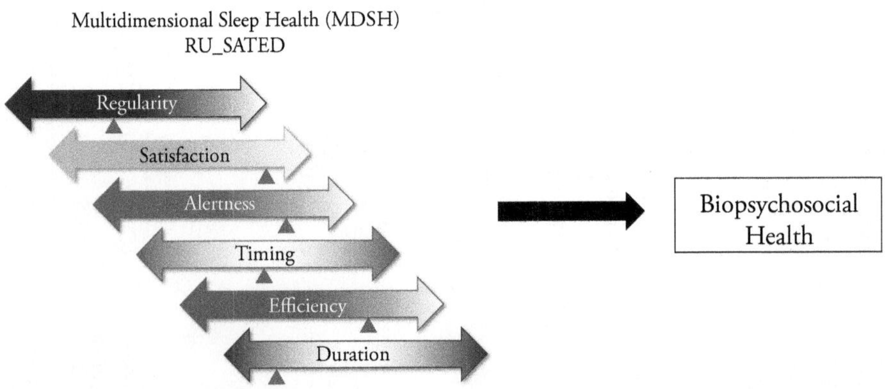

Figure 14.1 Multidimensional sleep health (MDSH) conceptual framework

Measurement of MDSH

The different components of MDSH can be measured with a variety of tools, including retrospective self-report questionnaires, sleep diaries, wrist actigraphy, PSG, and even functional neuroimaging. These different measurement tools assess different levels of analysis, ranging from experience to behavior, physiology, and brain circuits. The specific components of MDSH that are assessed with each method may vary. For instance, self-reports can evaluate all six dimensions of regularity, satisfaction, alertness, timing, efficiency, and duration. Behavioral measures such as actigraphy cannot assess the satisfaction component, and PSG, when conducted for 1 or 2 nights, cannot assess regularity. Thus, the specific choice of measurement tool depends on the goals and resources available to a study or clinic and affects the specific dimensions that can be evaluated.

Examples of retrospective self-report tools to assess MDSH are the SATED and RU_SATED v2.0 questionnaires (Buysse, 2014; Ravyts et al., 2021); the SATED questionnaire assesses sleep **s**atisfaction/quality, **a**lertness, **t**iming, **e**fficiency, and **d**uration and the RU_SATED v2.0 questionnaire assesses the aforementioned sleep dimensions plus **regu**larity. Although these were initially proposed as examples of how MDSH might be measured efficiently as a self-report, they have subsequently been evaluated in a number of empirical studies (e.g., Benítez et al., 2020; Brandolim Becker et al., 2018; Dalmases et al., 2018; Ravyts et al., 2021). These studies have generally found adequate internal consistency and item total correlation, with low interitem correlation, indicating that each item assesses a distinct dimension, all of which load on a larger construct of sleep health. However, some studies have found that a two-factor solution fits RU_SATED v2.0 better than a one-factor solution (Ravyts et al., 2021). Ongoing studies are using more robust psychometric techniques to refine RU_SATED v2.0, based on cognitive interviews, classic test theory validation, item response theory validation, and external validation against other self-report, behavioral, and physiologic measures such as wrist actigraphy.

Other studies have used a combination of self-report and actigraphy data to empirically derive cutoff values for "good" and "poor" sleep health on different MDSH dimensions (e.g., Brindle et al., 2019; Wallace, Lee, et al., 2019). Resulting MDSH scores, whether representing specific sleep dimensions, total number of "poor" dimensions, or latent multidimensional clusters, have been related to health outcomes such as cardiac arrhythmias (Li, Zhou, et al., 2021), cardiometabolic morbidity (Brindle et al., 2019), and mortality (Wallace, Lee, et al., 2019).

Analysis of MDSH: Methods and Examples

Challenges in Analyzing MDSH Data

There are abundant statistical challenges related to the inherent multidimensionality of sleep health. Multiple interconnected sleep characteristics (e.g., mean and variability of sleep/wake timing, daytime sleepiness, total sleep time, sleep latency and efficiency) can be measured through one or more data modalities (e.g., retrospective self-report, daily sleep diary, actigraphy, PSG). These sleep characteristics can be organized into broader conceptual domains (e.g., timing, continuity, regularity, depth)—although there are often discrepancies between homologous features measured through different sources—and associations among characteristics can differ depending on the population. Sleep health characteristics may be differentially associated with multiple outcomes, and these associations can further fluctuate across different populations. Finally, multiple plausible statistical models can provide complementary information about sleep health and its associations with outcomes of interest.

Unfortunately, the multidimensionality and multimodality of sleep health can lead to disorganization in data analytic strategies, which ultimately reduces rigor and reproducibility in model building and selection and increases false-positive rates. Consider, for example, the process of testing and reporting each possible feature separately. Such univariate approaches increase multiple comparison problems, may suggest relatively small associations given that each feature is examined in isolation, and fail to identify which features are most important when considered in the context of others. These problems may be mitigated by using organized and rigorous approaches for analysis of MDSH data—specifically, multivariable modeling strategies. When used correctly and thoughtfully, such approaches have the potential to enhance predictive power, reproducibility, and interpretation.

The first step in developing an organized data analytic approach is to carefully consider the question being addressed. Here, we focus on four questions that are often of interest in sleep health research (Table 14.2): (1) How are sleep health characteristics associated with each other (or, put another way, how do *sleep health characteristics* group together)? (2) Does a composite score indicating overall sleep health relate to the outcome (or exposure) of interest? (3) Which combinations of sleep health characteristics relate to the outcome (or exposure) of interest (or, put another way, how do *people* group together based on their sleep profiles)? (4) Which features have the strongest associations with the outcome of interest?

How Are Sleep Health Characteristics Associated with Each Other?

We can use exploratory and confirmatory factor analysis to understand how sleep health characteristics relate to each other. Factor analysis assumes that there exist multiple latent (unobserved) underlying factors (i.e., sleep health domains) and that each latent factor is actualized through the measurement of multiple observed sleep health characteristics. Through exploratory factor analysis, we can determine the number of latent factors that exist in a sample, often through plotting and examining the eigenvalues of the correlation matrix, which essentially summarize the extent to which a particular latent factor explains the variability in the data. One can also use factor loadings to identify which specific characteristics best represent a particular latent factor. Confirmatory factor analysis on an

Table 14.2 Multidimensional sleep health approaches

Question	Method	Benefit	Limitation
How are sleep health characteristics associated with each other?	• Exploratory or confirmatory factor analysis	• Defines which specific sleep–wake measures are related to each other and distinct from each other • Empirically derived solution • Guides variable selection	• Factors not always clinically interpretable • Does not clarify how characteristics may co-occur within an individual
Does a composite score relate to the outcome of interest?	• Sum the number of potentially adverse MDSH characteristics (can be equal weights or empirically weighted) • Relate to outcome of interest	• Easy to administer and score • Generalizable across outcomes (equally weighted) • Optimizes prediction and clarify which MDSH features have largest effects in multivariable context (empirically weighted) • Interpretable and clinically practical • Composite measure reduces dimensionality	• Cannot compare relative effects of each MDSH characteristic • Non-predictive MDSH characteristics dampen the overall effect (if equally weighted) • More complex scoring (if empirically weighted)
Which combinations of sleep health characteristics relate to the outcome of interest?	• Use clustering to reveal common combinations of MDSH characteristics (i.e., profiles or phenotypes)	• Composite measure reduces dimensionality • Generalizable across outcomes • Compares effects of each phenotype • Can suggest novel intervention strategies	• Does not optimize prediction (i.e., common phenotypes not necessarily related to outcome of interest) • Cannot compare relative effects of each individual MDSH characteristic
Which features have the strongest associations with the outcome of interest?	• Include set of MDSH characteristics within a single statistical model (e.g., regression or more complex ML)	• Examines value of overall MDSH construct (regression and ML) • Evaluates/interprets the effect of each MDSH characteristic in context of the other characteristics (regression and ML) • Few a priori assumptions (ML) • Can optimize prediction (ML)	• Requires larger sample size for power • Findings not necessarily easy to interpret • Logic for ML decisions not transparent • Less clinically practical

Note. MDSH = multidimensional sleep health; ML = machine learning.

independent sample can be used to further establish the existence of the latent factors via goodness-of-fit statistics and evaluation of the correlations among the latent factors themselves. For established factor solutions, a factor score for each domain can be computed for each individual; the score on each particular domain summarizes the extent to which a person's observed data on that domain is higher or lower than others' observed data.

An example of this approach is a factor analysis of 28 actigraphy features from the Osteoporotic Fractures in Men Study (MrOS) and the Study of Osteoporotic Fractures (SOF; Wallace, Yu, et al., 2021). Using exploratory and confirmatory factor analyses of actigraphy summary features (e.g., means and standard deviations of nightly features) as well as rest–activity-rhythm parameters extracted from an extended cosine model, we identified five actigraphy sleep health factors: timing, efficiency, duration, sleepiness/wakefulness, and regularity. In follow-up work in a separate sample of older adults with a longer period of actigraphy observation, Ji et al. (2023) replicated these findings and extended them to include a rhythmicity domain.

Does a Composite Score Indicating Overall Sleep Health Relate to the Outcome (or Exposure) of Interest?

A composite sleep health score describes the extent to which a person has better or worse sleep health across several sleep health characteristics of interest, typically with each characteristic representing an underlying domain. Self-report tools for quantifying composite sleep health, including RU_SATED v2.0, are one example. However, several ad hoc composite approaches can also be used across any measurement type, and such approaches have been gaining popularity in recent years. Here, we focus on methods for ad hoc approaches.

The first step in computing a composite sleep health score is to select which variables should be included. Ideally, we might want to select one variable to represent each sleep health dimension, or domain, of interest. Such domains can be identified conceptually (e.g., based on the RU_SATED framework) or empirically (e.g., using factor analysis). If a factor analysis is used, it is also possible to compute the factor scores instead of selecting individual items. Ideally, the selected features should be relatively independent (if two highly correlated features are selected, the score could be biased toward that construct) and clinically meaningful. The second step is to determine whether one prefers to prioritize a composite score that is more generalizable across outcomes and samples versus a score that is more predictive of the particular outcome in the sample of interest. We describe each of these approaches below.

GENERALIZABLE COMPOSITE SCORES

When the selected features are categorical—or can be easily categorized into meaningful categories representing "good" or "poor" sleep health—the simplest approach to compute a composite score is to count the number of "good" or "poor" sleep health characteristics within each individual. However, if the features are not easily categorized (or if a more continuous approach is preferred), one may also standardize the items and then sum the standardized variables.

Composite scores are deemed generalizable because each characteristic contributes an equal weight to the score, making the score nonspecific to any particular outcome or sample. However, if the standardization or selection of cut-points is specific to the sample, this will reduce generalizability. For this reason, we recommend using clinically meaningful and established cutoffs (e.g., see Brindle et al., 2019) or standardization based on established population means and standard deviations whenever possible. In the absence of such established values, empirically determined values specific to the sample can be used. Several recent sources have published associations between composite scores and health outcomes (see Tables 14.3–14.5 for examples).

OPTIMALLY PREDICTIVE COMPOSITE SCORES

A limitation of generalizable composite scores is that they weight each feature equally, even if it is not associated with the outcome of interest. In this case, the noise added to the composite score can reduce its overall predictive abilities. As an alternative, one can fit a regression model of the health outcome on each selected feature to extract the weights, which can then be used to compute the overall sleep health score. An added advantage is that they also indicate which features are driving the associations. However, such weights should be developed on a "training" sample and then subsequently applied to an independent "testing" sample to determine predictive abilities; otherwise, the model will be overly optimistic regarding actual associations.

Which Combinations of Sleep Health Characteristics Relate to the Outcome (or Exposure) of Interest?

The composite sleep health score indicates whether the number of potentially adverse sleep characteristics relates to health outcomes. However, we may also be interested in understanding whether there are important *combinations* of sleep health characteristics (i.e., sleep health profiles) within a sample and whether these combinations relate to health outcomes. To accomplish this, we can use clustering. The specific clustering approach depends on whether features are categorical/ordinal, continuous, or both.

CATEGORICAL

When features can be categorized into meaningful "good" or "poor" sleep health groups, one may be interested in making a large contingency table to examine which features tend to group together. Latent class analysis (LCA) is a modeling technique that can identify the patterns in such contingency tables to suggest subgroups of people with similar combinations of sleep health characteristics. Because not everyone's categorical characteristics perfectly match within a given latent class, LCA estimates the probability that

Table 14.3 Cross-sectional studies of multidimensional sleep health and health outcomes

Reference	Sample	MDSH method	Outcome(s)	Main findings
(Dalmases et al., 2019)	*N* = 4,385 adults	SATED questionnaire	Overall health	MDSH stronger risk factor than physical activity, diet, tobacco, alcohol
(Dalmases et al., 2018)	*N* = 4,385 adults	SATED questionnaire and self-reported sleep duration	Number of chronic conditions	SATED has higher AUC than sleep duration for association with number of chronic conditions
(Lee & Lawson, 2021)	*N* = 441 adults	RU_SATED dimensions from self-report and actigraphy	Chronic conditions, stress	Worse MDSH associated with more chronic conditions, stress
(Brindle et al., 2019)	*N* = 432 and 268 from MIDUS	RU_SATED dimensions from diaries and actigraphy	Cardiometabolic outcomes	Better MDSH associated with lower cardiometabolic morbidity
(Makarem et al., 2022)	*N* = 4,555 adults aged ≥20 years old from NHANES	Five dimensions from self-report	Cardiovascular and cardiometabolic risk factors and outcomes	Better MDSH associated with lower odds of hypertension, obesity, central adiposity, prevalent CVD and Type 2 diabetes, and lower blood pressure, BMI, waist circumference, & fasting glucose
(Lee et al., 2022)	*N* = 6,820 adults from MIDUS for self-report *N* = 663 adults from MIDUS for actigraphy	RU_SATED from self-report and actigraphy	Cardiac disease	Worse MDSH associated with cardiac disease
(Hawkins et al., 2021)	*N* = 4,837 adults from NHANES	Five dimensions from self-report	Intention to lose weight, self-report prior year weight change, BMI	For those who attempted weight loss, good sleep health inversely associated with current BMI and weight change
(Kubala et al., 2020)	*N* = 114 adults	RU_SATED questionnaire	Self-reported physical activity, pedometer steps	MDSH associated with reported moderate/vigorous physical activity, not pedometer
(Chen et al., 2022)	*N* = 2,015 adults ≥65 years from Taiwan Longitudinal Study on Aging	SATED dimensions from self-report	Frailty	Better MDSH associated with lower likelihood of frailty in women, not men

(Tighe et al., 2021)	*N* = 158 adults ≥65 years old from MIDUS studies	RU_SATED from diaries and actigraphy	Physical functioning	Better MDSH associated with faster gait speed, not grip or lower extremity strength
(Desantis et al., 2019)	*N* = 738 low-income Black adults	Five dimensions from self-report and actigraphy	Physical functioning, psychological distress, BMI	Better MDSH associated with better physical functioning, lower psychological distress, not with BMI
(Dong et al., 2019)	*N* = 176 adolescents at risk for poor health	RU_SATED dimensions from diaries and self-report	Functioning in emotional, cognitive, behavioral, social, and physical domains	Better MDSH associated with lower risk in emotional, cognitive, and social domains
(Furihata et al., 2020)	*N* = 2,482 hospital nurses	SATED dimensions from self-report questions	Depressed mood, loss of interest	MDSH associated with greater odds of depression symptoms
(Furihata et al., 2017)	*N* = 3,806–6,485 older women, SOF study	Five dimensions from self-report	Depression symptoms	MDSH associated with cross-sectional depression in graded fashion
(Barham et al., 2022)	*N* = 1,576 adults	RU_SATED questionnaire	Depression symptoms	Better MDSH associated with lower levels of depression symptoms
(Appleton et al., 2022)	*N* = 2,044 community-dwelling adults aged 18–90 years	SATED and RU_SATED from self-report	Depression and anxiety symptoms	Better MDSH associated with absence of depression and anxiety symptoms, fewer chronic depression symptoms

Note. AUC = area under the curve; BMI = body mass index; CVD = cardiovascular disease; MDSH = multidimensional sleep health; MIDUS = Midlife in the United States; NHANES = National Health and Nutrition Examination Survey; SATED/RU_SATED = **s**atisfaction/quality, **a**lertness, **t**iming, **e**fficiency, **d**uration and **regu**larity sleep dimensions; SOF = Study of Osteoporotic Fractures.

Table 14.4 Longitudinal studies of multidimensional sleep health and health outcomes

Reference	Sample	MDSH method	Outcome(s)	Main findings
(Wallace, Stone, et al., 2018)	*N* = 2,887 older men from MrOS	Seven dimensions from self-report and actigraphy	Mortality risk	MDSH related to mortality risk in graded fashion
(Wallace, Buysse, et al., 2019)	*N* = 8,668 adults 65–99 years old from SOF, MrOS, SHHS	Nine self-report items	Mortality	MDSH significant predictor of all-cause and cardiovascular mortality; stronger than self-rated health, heart failure
(Wallace, Lee, et al., 2019)	*N* = 1,722 adults ≥65 years old from SOF, MrOS	Five dimensions from self-report	Time to mortality	Time to mortality shorter in "high sleep propensity" versus "good sleep" or "insomnia short sleep duration"
(Bowman et al., 2020)	*N* = 221 midlife women from SWAN study	RU_SATED dimensions from self-report and actigraphy	BMI, waist–hip ratio	MDSH not associated with adiposity cross-sectionally or longitudinally in adjusted models
(Kline et al., 2021)	*N* = 125 adults with overweight or obesity in weight loss program	RU_SATED questionnaires and actigraphy	Change in percentage weight, fat mass, fat-free mass	Better MDSH associated with greater subsequent weight loss, fat loss; attenuated after accounting for apnea
(Lee & Lawson, 2021)	*N* = 441 adults	RU_SATED dimensions from self-report and actigraphy	Chronic conditions	Worse MDSH associated with more chronic conditions
(Lunyera et al., 2021)	*N* = 33,497 adult women	Five dimensions from self-report	Hypertension risk	Each unit increase in poor MDSH score was associated with increase in incident hypertension risk
(Makarem et al., 2022)	*N* = 1,920 from MESA	Four to five dimensions from actigraphy and self-report	CVD	Cardiovascular health scores including MDSH associated with lower odds of CVD prevalence and incidence
(Li, Zhou, et al., 2021)	*N* = 403,187 adults	Five sleep dimensions from self-report	Arrhythmias	Better sleep health associated with lower risk of atrial fibrillation, bradyarrhythmias
(Furihata et al., 2017)	*N* = 3,806-6,485 older women, SOF study	Five dimensions from self-report	Depression symptoms	MDSH associated with longitudinal depression in graded fashion
(Bowman et al., 2021)	*N* = 302 midlife women from SWAN study	RU_SATED dimensions from self-report and actigraphy	Depression symptoms	Higher depressive symptoms longitudinally associated with poorer MDSH

Note. BMI = body mass index; CVD = cardiovascular disease; MDSH = multidimensional sleep health; MESA = Multi-Ethnic Study of Atherosclerosis; MrOS = Osteoporotic Fractures in Men Study; RU_SATED = **s**atisfaction/quality, **a**lertness, **t**iming, **e**fficiency, **d**uration, and **regu**larity sleep dimensions; SHHS = Sleep Heart Health Study; SOF = Study of Osteoporotic Fractures; SWAN = Study of Women's Health Across the Nation.

Table 14.5 Studies of multidimensional sleep health and healthcare utilization and costs				
Reference	Sample	MDSH method	Outcome(s)	Main findings
(Ensrud et al., 2020)	*N* = 1,459 women from SOF	Five dimensions from self-report	Total healthcare costs and utilization (36 months)	Costs increase in graded fashion with MDSH scores; accounted for by medical conditions, functional limitations, depressive symptoms
(Schousboe et al., 2020)	*N* = 1,413 older men in MrOS study	Five dimensions from self-report	Healthcare costs and utilization over 3 years	MDSH associated with higher total healthcare costs

Note. MDSH = multidimensional sleep health; MrOS = Osteoporotic Fractures in Men Study; SOF = Study of Osteoporotic Fractures.

an individual is a member of each latent class based on their characteristics; and they are assigned to the latent class for which they have the highest probability of being a member (Collins & Lanza, 2010).

LCA has been used to identify latent sleep health classes in older men and women from the MrOS and SOF studies, considering self-report satisfaction, daytime sleepiness, timing, efficiency, and duration (Wallace, Lee, et al., 2019). This study identified three subgroups (latent classes) of people with similar combinations of these features: heightened sleep propensity, insomnia with short sleep, and average sleep. These latent class profiles were more strongly associated with the outcome of interest (time to mortality) than individual features that they comprised.

Finally, a more recent interest is in modeling mixed data types, such as both continuous and categorical data that one might obtain through multimodal data (e.g., self-report, actigraphy, PSG). Recent approaches that allow for these mixed data types are becoming available and may allow for novel insights regarding multimodal sleep health profiles (McParland & Gormley, 2016).

CONTINUOUS

Many sleep characteristics are measured continuously and may not be easily categorized into meaningful groupings. By clustering these measures as continuous features, we can leverage the natural heterogeneity of the data to identify subgroups with similar multivariable profiles on these continuous features. Traditional clustering models (e.g., k-means clustering or latent profile analysis) assume clusters are elliptically shaped. However, given the naturally skewed nature of many sleep characteristics, it is also worth considering whether the clusters themselves may be skewed (Wallace, Buysse, et al., 2018). New model-based clustering approaches including multiple coalesced generalized hyperbolic distribution (MCGHD) mixture modeling (Tortora et al., 2019) can be used to model clusters with more flexible shapes that may better conform to the natural heterogeneity of the data.

For example, we applied MCGHD mixture modeling to actigraphy data on five characteristics selected based on the prior factor analysis in the same sample (Wallace et al., 2022). Three factors were identified in older men and women from MrOS and SOF: high sleep propensity, inadequate sleep, and average sleep. These clusters had stronger associations with the outcome (time to all-cause mortality) than any of the individual features they comprised.

Which Features Have the Strongest Associations with the Outcome of Interest?

When it is of interest to understand which features have the strongest associations with the outcome, one may use a relatively independent set of selected features (e.g., selected a priori or based on a factor analysis) in a multivariable regression model. For instance, the multivariable regression approach was used to predict all-cause mortality in older men from MrOS (Wallace, Stone, et al., 2018).

It may also be of interest to leverage "big data" to enhance predictive power. In such situations, one can use machine learning (ML). ML requires a trade-off between predictive power and interpretability. Thus, ML should be used when the focus is more on predictive power rather than developing a highly interpretable model that can "explain" an association or test a hypothesis. Through use of ML models, we may allow higher dimensional data and features that are more highly correlated, thus limiting the amount of preselection that is needed. However, it is still essential to be thoughtful about the features that are being included in the model as this has implications if any level of interpretability is desired. Examples of ML models include regularized regression (which essentially tests additive associations without overfitting) and random forest (which allows for complex empirically driven combinations of features). In all ML modeling, training/testing sets should always be used to avoid overfitting.

As an example of this approach, we aimed to clarify whether PSG data could predict mortality and stroke above and beyond traditional risk factors and enhance risk screening (Wallace, Coleman, et al., 2021; Wallace et al., 2023). Using the Sleep Heart Health Study and the Wisconsin Sleep Cohort, we fit random forest ML models and extracted novel feature importance measures that quantify the extent to which the model improves relative to a model where the feature is altered (e.g., using permutation or knockoff variable importance metrics that address limitations in default "out of bag" importance metrics). PSG-assessed features were important predictors of time to all-cause mortality and incident stroke, on par with other traditional predictors such as demographic characteristics and health behaviors.

Application of MDSH to Health Outcomes

Having described the conceptualization of MDSH and analytic approaches to MDSH data, we next provide some examples of how this concept might deepen our understanding of the relationships between sleep and health. A rapidly growing body of research has linked MDSH to health outcomes and suggested how an MDSH framework might be useful in developing interventions (see Tables 14.3–14.5). In this section, we provide examples from four specific domains to highlight the range of such studies: pregnancy/postpartum, cardiovascular and cardiometabolic, depression, and physical functioning. Other domains of health outcomes have also been investigated; for instance, the previous section on analysis of MDSH data provided multiple examples using MDSH in relation to mortality outcomes. Although many studies have examined one or more individual sleep characteristics to health outcomes, we focus here on studies that have considered multiple sleep characteristics in aggregate.

MDSH During Pregnancy and Postpartum

The application of MDSH has particular salience during pregnancy and postpartum. Sleep patterns are significantly impacted during pregnancy and after delivery, with most studies focusing on challenges with and changes in sleep duration and/or sleep quality that prenatal individuals experience (Conlon et al., 2021; Ladyman & Signal, 2018). Multiple biopsychosocial influences contribute to the effect of pregnancy on patterns, including gradual increases in sex hormones (estradiol and progesterone) over pregnancy which impact sleep architecture. Gradual increases in cortisol and changes in nutrient metabolism (e.g., iron and folate) are also associated with emerging sleep disorders including insomnia, sleep apnea, and restless legs syndrome. Nocturia is common, leading to frequent sleep disruptions. In addition, comfort with sleeping and body positioning change during pregnancy as body size, shape, and weight change, which may also affect breathing and snoring during sleep, as well as factors such as depressive symptoms or anxiety related to pregnancy and the developing fetus, delivery, and parenting (Hall et al., 2009). During the postpartum period, numerous changes to individuals' bodies and lives can reduce sleep duration and quality, including caring for the baby around-the-clock and overnight feeding, hormonal shifts, discomfort while recovering from delivery and associated procedures, and psychological distress related to depressive symptoms or anxiety about factors related to the baby's health and development, returning to work, and navigating childcare challenges. Short sleep duration and poor sleep quality during pregnancy predict higher gestational weight gain and greater risk for cardiometabolic disease (Gay et al., 2017; Pauley et al., 2022). Sleep duration and sleep quality also interact with other health behaviors during pregnancy to predict gestational weight gain, such as physical activity and eating behaviors (Hawkins, Conlon, et al., 2023; Pauley et al., 2022).

However, sleep duration and sleep quality do not account for the many ways in which sleep is affected during pregnancy and postpartum or how such shifts in sleep affect birthing individuals, their support people, and caregivers of infants. For example, recent data from a large cohort study of pregnant individuals suggests that excessive gestational weight gain, a critical predictor of weight and cardiometabolic health during pregnancy, postpartum, and in the long term, was more strongly associated with MDSH than individual sleep domains during pregnancy (Hawkins, Pokutnaya, et al., 2023). Thus, the MDSH framework provides a more comprehensive understanding of ways in which pregnant and postpartum people experience sleep problems or are able to acclimate and maintain or achieve sufficient levels of sleep health (Buysse, 2014; Ladyman & Signal, 2018).

Adaptations may be needed to characterize sleep health dimensions in the context of pregnancy and the postpartum period. For instance, rather than focusing on obtaining a certain number of hours of continuous sleep at night during the first month postpartum, it might be more realistic and more helpful for birthing individuals and caregivers of newborns to consider sleep duration concurrently with timing and regularity. Given that newborns have a developing circadian timing system (CTS) and thus do not display regular, well-established 24-hour patterns of sleep and wakefulness during the first several weeks, birthing individuals and caregivers of newborns often also experience disruptions in diurnal sleep patterns, meaning that sleep may not be consolidated at night or occur regularly from day to day. Thus, encouraging the evaluation and targeting of multiple sleep dimensions might yield a better indicator of impairment and specific factors to address to support sleep health during pregnancy and postpartum.

MDSH and Cardiovascular and Cardiometabolic Health

Data from large, observational studies conducted in the United States has provided initial insights into associations of MDSH and cardiometabolic outcomes. Two complementary studies from the Midlife in the United States (MIDUS) studies examined cross-sectional associations of MDSH with cardiometabolic outcomes. In the first study, Brindle et al. (2019) found that better MDSH scores were associated with lower odds of total cardiometabolic morbidity and hypertension. In a subsequent study, Lee et al. (2022) examined associations of MDSH with heart disease by calculating a MDSH scores wherein sleep health dimensions were weighted based on their differential associations with risk of heart disease. Findings generally converged with those of Brindle et al. (2019). Each unit increase in the self-report composite measure of poor MDSH was associated with a 54% higher risk of heart disease; for the self-report/actigraphy MDSH composite, each unit increase was associated with a 141% higher risk of heart disease (Lee et al., 2022).

Analyses of data from the National Health and Nutrition Examination Survey (NHANES) corroborate cross-sectional links to cardiometabolic outcomes identified in the MIDUS studies. For instance, Makarem et al. (2022) found that ideal versus poor MDSH scores were associated with lower body mass index (BMI), waist circumference, fasting glucose, systolic blood pressure, and diastolic blood pressure. Further, ideal versus poor MDSH scores were associated with lower odds of obesity, central obesity, and hypertension. In a separate sample of NHANES participants, Xiao et al. (2016) found that sleep quality (defined as two or more poor sleep health dimensions) was cross-sectionally associated with higher BMI, percent body fat, waist circumference, and android/gynoid fat ratio.

In contrast to the MIDUS and NHANES studies, DeSantis et al. (2019) found that MDSH was not associated with BMI in a cross-sectional study of community-dwelling adults recruited from low-income, predominantly African American neighborhoods. Similarly, Bowman and colleagues (2020) examined cross-sectional and longitudinal associations of MDSH with BMI and waist-to-hip ratio among women participants in the Study of Women's Health Across the Nation (SWAN). Although MDSH was cross-sectionally and longitudinally associated with BMI and waist-to-hip ratio in unadjusted models, the significant associations did not persist in models that adjusted for covariates (age, race, study site, menopausal status, vasomotor symptoms, apnea–hypopnea index, negative affect). These equivocal findings may be due to study sample and design differences but also suggest that associations of MDSH with cardiometabolic outcomes may vary based on factors such as race, socioeconomic status, gender, and age.

Although longitudinal associations of MDSH and select metabolic outcomes were not supported in the study by Bowman and colleagues (2020), other longitudinal analyses have identified significant associations. For example, Lunyera et al. (2021) evaluated MDSH and incident hypertension and found that each unit increase in poor MDSH score was associated with a 6% increase in incident hypertension risk. More recently, analyzing data from the Multi-Ethnic Study of Atherosclerosis (MESA) Sleep Study, Makarem et al. (2022) found that, when added to the American Heart Association's Life's Simple 7, MDSH scores were associated with CVD prevalence and incidence; individuals in the highest (better sleep health) versus lowest tertile had lower odds of CVD prevalence and CVD incidence. Finally, work by Kline et al. (2021) identified that, in the context of a weight loss intervention, better MDSH at the beginning of a given interval (baseline to 6 months, 6 to 12 months) was associated with greater weight loss over the subsequent 6-month interval; additionally, better MDSH was associated with greater fat loss. However, after adjusting for apnea–hypopnea index, the association between MDSH and weight loss was no longer statistically significant.

The majority of studies discussed in this subsection support the importance of MDSH in relation to cardiovascular and cardiometabolic health. Additional prospective and longitudinal studies explicitly examining MDSH and cardiovascular/cardiometabolic health are needed to further elucidate the underlying mechanisms. Studies of diverse samples, in terms of age, race/ethnicity, gender, and menopausal, socioeconomic, employment, caregiver, and health status, are needed to further advance our understanding of MDSH and health among various populations and across the life span.

MDSH and Depression

Existing literature points to a bidirectional relationship between different dimensions of sleep and depression, and emerging studies examining associations of MDSH with depression are suggesting a similar association. Two studies have examined longitudinal associations of MDSH and depression, both in samples of women. In the first study of older women in SOF, Furihata and colleagues (2017) found that MDSH from self-report was associated in a graded fashion with prevalent and incident depression symptoms approximately 6 years later. In a sample of midlife women from the SWAN study, Bowman et al. (2021) examined the reverse association—symptoms of depression predicting MDSH—and found that higher levels of depression symptoms assessed annually for 6–9 years significantly predicted MDSH (defined by actigraphy and self-report). Decreases in depressive symptoms over time were associated with better MDSH but only among African American women.

Cross-sectional investigations of MDSH–depression links have been more common and conducted in broader samples. Two studies that included community-dwelling adults found that better MDSH was associated with lower likelihood of having depression symptoms; another study including a sample of nurses found the same (Appleton et al., 2022; Barham et al., 2022; Furihata et al., 2020). Other cross-sectional studies suggest that better MDSH is also associated with lower levels of psychological distress in adults and better emotional functioning in adolescents (DeSantis et al., 2019; Dong et al., 2019).

Additional research is needed in diverse samples to further characterize the associations between MDSH and depression symptoms on multiple timescales. Aligned with the sleep health approach, it will be of particular interest to better understand the potential protective role MDSH plays with regard to depression and whether interventions to promote sleep health have value in preventing depression. It will also be important to understand whether and how MDSH is associated with other psychological health outcomes, including those that are positively oriented (e.g., flourishing, psychological flexibility) and, again, whether MDSH interventions can support psychological well-being.

MDSH and Physical Functioning

Physical functioning is a broad term that generally refers to one's ability to engage in physical activities common in daily life (e.g., mobility, lifting/carrying materials, activities of daily living, etc.). Compared to other health outcomes, fewer studies have examined MDSH as it relates to physical functioning. Most have tested associations of MDSH with self-report measures of physical functioning and have used similar approaches to calculating composite MDSH scores.

In a cross-sectional study of community-dwelling adults, DeSantis et al. (2019) examined associations of MDSH with self-reported physical functioning as well as psychological distress. Sleep health was significantly associated with physical functioning and psychological distress, such that higher levels of sleep health were associated with better self-reported physical functioning and lower levels of psychological distress. Cross-sectional associations of MDSH with frailty among older adults were examined in the Taiwan Longitudinal Study on Aging (Chen et al., 2022). In this sample, better MDSH was significantly associated with lower likelihood of frailty in women but not men. In one of the few studies involving adolescents, Dong et al. (2019) examined associations of MDSH with functioning in five health domains, including physical functioning. Results demonstrated significant associations of MDSH with functioning in cognitive, emotional, and social domains; MDSH was not significantly associated with physical functioning. Cross-sectional associations of MDSH with gait speed, grip strength, and lower extremity strength have been examined in community-dwelling adults ≥65 years old from the MIDUS-2 study (Tighe et al., 2021). Better MDSH was significantly associated with faster gait speed. Importantly, statistical models that treated sleep health as a multidimensional construct accounted for greater variance in gait speed relative to those that examined sleep dimensions separately.

Together, these studies provide preliminary evidence of associations of MDSH with gait speed (considered an indicator of functional status) and self-reported functional limitations, with some indications that these associations may vary by sex. The small number of studies paired with the shared limitations in study design point to several directions for future research. Each of the reviewed studies used cross-sectional and observational methods, precluding conclusions regarding causality. Microlongitudinal, longitudinal, and experimental study designs will help clarify the directionality and causal links between these constructs. Exploration among samples diverse in age, race/ethnicity, health status, and gender will also be important for understanding the extent to which associations generalize across sociodemographic and clinical characteristics.

Interventions in an MDSH Framework

The dimensions of sleep included in the MDSH framework are all amenable, at least in theory, to manipulation with behavioral and pharmacologic measures. Three of the dimensions—duration, regularity, and timing—are likely to be more primary, and the main focus of such interventions. In other words, sleep duration can be more directly affected by behavioral choices regarding the amount of time in bed, as well as by medications. Likewise, regularity and timing of sleep are amenable to voluntary choices regarding sleep behavior and may likewise be affected by medications or substances such as melatonin. The other three dimensions—satisfaction, alertness, and efficiency—may be secondarily affected by interventions targeting duration, regularity, and timing. For instance, sleep efficiency is affected primarily by behavioral choices regarding the amount of time in bed. The MDSH framework is not an alternative to our understanding of homeostatic and circadian sleep regulatory processes but, rather, builds on those processes for effective interventions.

Transdiagnostic Sleep and Circadian Intervention

The Transdiagnostic Sleep and Circadian Intervention (TranS-C) is a behavioral intervention developed to promote MDSH across a range of sleep problems (Harvey & Buysse,

2017). TranS-C was developed based on the premise that sleep and circadian disturbance is a transdiagnostic feature of multiple mental health disorders (e.g., depressive disorders, bipolar disorders) and may contribute to their development and exacerbation. The goal of TranS-C is to improve sleep health across key sleep health dimensions (RU_SATED). As a result, anyone with suboptimal experiences on any one dimension of sleep health (e.g., someone with short sleep, someone with poor sleep quality, someone with irregular sleep timing) could be a candidate for, and potentially benefit from, the TranS-C intervention. Thus, TranS-C is also transdiagnostic in that it can be used to promote sleep health across different types of sleep disorders (e.g., insomnia disorder, advanced/delayed sleep phase disorder) and sleep problems of varying severity, including subsyndromal or complex sleep problems.

The TranS-C intervention is informed by the two-process model of sleep regulation (Borbély, 1982) and incorporates components of treatments such as cognitive behavioral therapy for insomnia (CBT-I), interpersonal and social rhythm therapy, imagery rehearsal therapy, systematic desensitization, and motivational interviewing. Personalized and modular in nature, TranS-C includes four core modules, seven optional modules, and four cross-cutting modules (Table 14.6). The cross-cutting modules of TranS-C are those that are incorporated throughout the intervention, core modules are those that are delivered

Table 14.6 Transdiagnostic Sleep and Circadian Intervention (TranS-C) modules
Cross-cutting modules
Case formulation
Sleep and circadian education
Behavior change and motivation
Goal setting
Core modules
Establishing regular sleep–wake times
Improving daytime functioning
Correcting unhelpful sleep-related beliefs
Maintenance of behavior change
Optional modules
Improving sleep efficiency
Reducing time in bed
Dealing with delayed or advanced circadian rhythms
Reducing sleep-related worry and vigilance
Promoting compliance with continuous positive airway pressure
Negotiating sleep in a complicated environment
Reducing nightmares

to the majority of patients, and optional modules are those that are delivered as needed/appropriate based on case conceptualization. TranS-C was originally designed to be delivered over 4–10 sessions lasting approximately 50 minutes each. Since its development, however, it has undergone adaptation to be delivered in fewer sessions that are shorter in duration to increase implementation potential.

A growing literature supports the efficacy of TranS-C for individuals across the life span. In a randomized controlled trial involving adults living with serious mental illness and sleep and circadian dysfunction, TranS-C plus usual care yielded greater post-treatment improvements in functional impairment, psychiatric symptoms, sleep disturbance, and sleep-related impairment compared to usual care followed by delayed treatment with TranS-C (Harvey et al., 2021). With the exception of functional impairment, improvements were maintained at 6-month follow-up. Subsequent analysis of treatment mediators and moderators indicated that changes in sleep-related impairment and sleep health mediated effects on post-treatment functional impairment and psychiatric symptoms (Armstrong et al., 2022). Symptom severity, race, and age emerged as moderators of treatment effects. Treatment benefits were greater for those with worse symptom severity at baseline and those who identified as Black/African American; treatment benefits were mitigated for older participants (Armstrong et al., 2022). Among adolescents with evening chronotypes who were considered at risk in at least one health domain, TranS-C yielded treatment effects on eveningness circadian preference, global sleep quality, and weeknight–weekend wake-up time discrepancies compared to psychoeducation (Dong et al., 2020; Harvey et al., 2018); treatment effects on eveningness circadian preference were maintained at 12-month follow-up (Dolsen et al., 2023).

Integrating Sleep Health into Other Behavioral Health Interventions

By definition, MDSH focuses on multiple dimensions of sleep and recognizes the CTS as a major determinant of those dimensions. However, other health behaviors, including physical activity and eating, also show feedback regulation by the CTS. This recognition leads to the possibility of linking MDSH interventions with interventions for other such health behaviors. Below we present two examples of how MDSH may be integrated with other health behavior interventions.

EXAMPLE 1: PREGNANCY AND POSTPARTUM HEALTH BEHAVIORS/WEIGHT MANAGEMENT

Pregnancy and the postpartum period are critical windows for intervention and may be well suited to interventions that address MDSH. Studies suggest that addressing sleep and incorporating sleep targets into behavioral interventions for gestational weight gain are feasible and acceptable and have demonstrated initial efficacy in helping individuals to improve their sleep patterns and achieve recommended amounts of gestational weight gain (Hawkins, Pokutnaya, et al., 2023; Sheynblyum et al., 2022). Of note, most of the extant literature on interventions for pregnancy and postpartum people has used sleep hygiene education (e.g., creating a comfortable sleep environment, adopting a consistent sleep schedule), exercise (e.g., walking, swimming, yoga), relaxation techniques (e.g., music therapy, massage, mindful techniques, guided imagery), and CBT-I (Bacaro et al., 2020; Felder et al., 2020; Kalmbach et al., 2023; Mancinelli et al., 2022; Owais et al., 2018; Paulino et al., 2022; Yang et al., 2020).

Novel interventions that address the multiple dimensions of health, rather than sleep disorders per se, offer promise for sleep and related health behaviors during pregnancy and the postpartum period. Our team has been developing the *ClockWork* intervention, which uses the CTS as an underlying framework for addressing multiple health behaviors that affect many health outcomes, and has been designing and testing the intervention among postpartum individuals (Conlon et al., 2023). Specifically, ClockWork targets eating, sleep, light/dark exposure, and physical activity because they are key health behaviors related to weight management and cardiometabolic health. These four key health behaviors also serve to regulate and are regulated by the CTS (Vitaterna et al., 2001). The CTS and misalignment of health behaviors are emerging as critical factors that impact weight and cardiometabolic health (Page et al., 2020; Rana et al., 2020). However, most extant interventions do not harness the CTS and the role of time in multiple key health behaviors (Siega-Riz et al., 2010; Yuhas et al., 2022). We posit that targeting the amount, regularity, and timing of multiple key health behaviors using a CTS framework will innovate and enhance intervention to promote eating, sleep, light/dark exposure, activity, as well as weight management.

In particular, the postpartum period is a time in individuals' lives when eating, sleep, light/dark exposure, and activity fall rapidly out of sync with the 24-hour light–dark cycle (Ehlers, 1988; Ross et al., 2005). Implementing health behavior programs postpartum is challenging due to stress, hormonal fluctuations, healing from delivery, and caring for a newborn. Such challenges are exacerbated by the "chrono-chaos" of infants, given that their CTS and related biobehavioral patterns are still developing (Herring et al., 2019; Yuhas et al., 2022). Notably, observational studies show that postpartum weight retention and health behaviors predict poorer cardiometabolic health outcomes in the year postpartum and later in life (Linné et al., 2004; Siega-Riz et al., 2010; Yuhas et al., 2022), with greater cardiometabolic disease risk among individuals who begin pregnancy with a BMI $\geq 25 kg/m^2$ (Rong et al., 2015; Smith et al., 2019; Yuhas et al., 2022). Thus, postpartum promotion of health behavior change and weight management is important for birthing individuals' short- and long-term cardiometabolic health (Phelan, 2010).

The ClockWork intervention addresses health behavior change by harnessing our knowledge of the CTS to jointly optimize key behaviors related to weight and cardiometabolic health. Digital monitoring tools help to monitor and reinforce these changes. Specifically, the ClockWork intervention targets the **a**mount of eating, sleep, light/dark exposure, and physical activity and on their **r**egularity and **t**iming—the ART of ClockWork (Conlon et al., 2023). In addition to using the CTS as a unifying framework, the ClockWork intervention is unique in that it addresses multiple dimensions (i.e., the amount, regularity, and timing) not only of sleep but of three other key health behaviors (eating, physical activity, light–dark exposure) as well. Initial data from postpartum individuals with BMI ≥25kg/m^2 suggests that the MDSH goals, along with the goals for the other behavioral domains, are feasible and acceptable during the postpartum period (Conlon et al., 2023). Future work will optimize the intervention and evaluate the impact of addressing multidimensional sleep and circadian health on postpartum cardiometabolic health.

Another intervention being developed by our team is called *Sleep GOALS* (Goal-focused Online Access to Lifestyle Support). Sleep GOALS is an internet-assisted weight loss intervention that integrates key concepts from TranS-C and the Diabetes Prevention Program's (DPP's) lifestyle core material to address circadian-related behaviors, sleep, diet, and physical activity among postpartum individuals. Sleep GOALS utilizes an online platform that coordinates with clinical care to deliver interactive lessons, self-monitoring tools, personalized e-coaching, and resources to support healthy behavior change (McTigue et al., 2009; Simkin-Silverman et al., 2011). The development of Sleep GOALS included qualitative interviews with over 40 postpartum individuals, who shared their experiences with sleep, physical activity, and diet after childbirth and provided insights into what they would like to see in an intervention for postpartum individuals. Interviews confirmed the complex relationship between sleep, diet, and physical activity. Some participants noted the impact of sleep on their physical activity and diet choices, while others felt energized by adopting a physical activity routine. Based on these interviews, we selected key concepts from TranS-C that address concerns specific to postpartum individuals. TranS-C interactive lessons cover adopting a regular sleep schedule, healthy wake-up and wind-down routines, and tips to improve sleep efficiency. TranS-C modules regarding daytime functioning were integrated with DPP's physical activity lessons. As part of Sleep GOALS, we also address sleep beliefs to help postpartum individuals connect their thoughts, feelings, and behaviors to their sleep health; set realistic expectations about sleep; and develop action plans to reduce sleep-related worry. Additionally, we link sleep and eating behaviors, providing tips on how changes to each behavior can support better health in the other. We are currently pilot-testing Sleep GOALS to assess the intervention's feasibility, acceptability, and preliminary efficacy. Future research will compare the effects of Sleep GOALS with the original DPP's lifestyle intervention to determine the additive benefits of integrating MDSH concepts.

EXAMPLE 2: EXCESS WEIGHT AND OBESITY

Poor sleep health can contribute to excess weight and obesity through various pathways. Poor sleep timing can result in eating out of phase with our biological clock. When this happens, food intake occurs when leptin levels are lower than when eating in-phase. Leptin plays a role in energy balance by signaling satiety. Thus, eating out-of-phase results in excess consumption of high-fat, calorie-dense foods (Cain et al., 2015; Dennis et al., 2016). Misaligned eating not only affects energy balance but also impairs glucose tolerance and insulin sensitivity (Depner et al., 2014). Several studies examining individual sleep dimensions have demonstrated the association between poor sleep timing and body fat percentage (Kline et al., 2021; Wirth et al., 2015), weight outcomes (Hawkins et al., 2021), and cardiometabolic markers (Matricciani et al., 2022). Furthermore, short sleep duration and mistimed sleep result in altered metabolic and inflammatory pathways that contribute to obesity and poor cardiometabolic health (Archer & Oster, 2015; Möller-Levet et al., 2013). Short sleep duration is associated with anthropometric measures (body fat mass, waist circumference, and BMI; Chaput & Tremblay, 2012; Ogilvie et al., 2016; Wirth et al., 2015; Xiao et al., 2016) and weight loss success (Thomson et al., 2012).

Meeting calorie and fat intake recommendations is an essential component of weight loss. Greater wake after sleep onset (WASO) has been associated with reduced odds of meeting energy intake recommendations in the context of a weight loss intervention (Creasy et al., 2022). In a cross-sectional study of sleep and weight, Wirth et al. (2015) found that less WASO was associated with lower BMI and body fat percentage. Increased adherence to daily calorie and fat recommendations could be the underlying mechanism responsible for this finding. Poor sleep may also impair cognitive control and individuals' ability to make healthy choices. Lower sleep quality and increased morning tiredness predicted lower self-efficacy for adherence to a healthy lifestyle plan when engaged in weight loss (Burke et al., 2022). Similarly, Dehghan et al. (2022) found significant correlations between worse sleep quality and efficiency and reduced self-efficacy and lower healthy eating behaviors.

Lastly, poor sleep predicts reduced levels of physical activity (Kline, 2014). Sleep health, specifically later wake times, greater time in bed, higher WASO, more awakenings, and greater sleep latency, was associated with reduced odds of meeting the moderate-to-vigorous physical activity guidelines in a weight loss intervention (Creasy et al., 2022).

Interventions to improve sleep health represent a potential multifaceted approach to addressing the various biological and behavioral pathways contributing to excess weight and obesity. Integrating components of behavioral sleep and circadian interventions, such as sleep and circadian education and establishing regular sleep–wake times, into standardized behavioral treatment for weight loss (Butryn et al., 2011) may improve MDSH. Given that sleep timing, duration, and quality are individually associated with anthropometric measures, improvements in these areas may help optimize weight loss through multiple pathways. Future studies should examine if, and when, adding these components to standardized behavioral treatment for weight loss optimizes weight outcomes.

MULTILEVEL MDSH INTERVENTIONS

We have largely discussed sleep health interventions that focus on changing individual behavioral factors. However, determinants of sleep health extend beyond individual

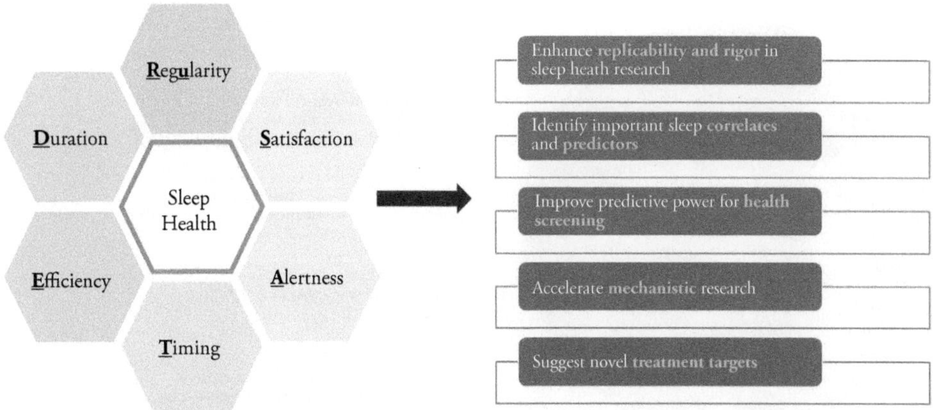

Figure 14.2 Sleep and circadian health interventions in a socioecological context
Note. Figure modified from Hale, Troxel, Buysse, 2020, *Ann Rev Public Health.* 41:81–99; Creative Commons Attribution 4.0 International License.

behaviors to also include sociodemographic and identity, interpersonal, community, and societal factors (Hale et al., 2020). Interventions that consider and address multiple levels of sleep health determinants may have added value compared to those that address individual-level behavioral factors alone, but they have been comparatively understudied (Billings et al., 2021; Hale et al., 2020; Meltzer et al., 2021; Figure 14.2).

A growing number of intervention development and adaptation studies are being conducted in an effort to increase the accessibility of sleep health interventions. For example, Williamson and colleagues (2022) used an iterative, community-engaged approach to adapt an intervention to address insomnia and insufficient sleep among children presenting to primary care in urban settings whose families have lower socioeconomic status. Feedback from advisory boards and study participants led to adaptations to intervention delivery strategies and intervention content, and in preliminary pilot testing, participating family members rated the adapted intervention high in acceptability and cultural humility. Other research groups are similarly taking iterative and community-engaged approaches, adapting and developing multilevel interventions across the life span (L. C. M. Johnson et al., 2023; Levenson et al., 2021; Rottapel et al., 2020; Spadola et al., 2020). Continued work in this area is pivotal to improving sleep health at the individual, group, and population health levels.

Conclusions

We have discussed the conceptual and empirical basis for MDSH, as well as the challenges and methods for measuring and analyzing MDSH data, and provided examples of how this construct relates to important health outcomes. We assert that MDSH is a useful construct theoretically and clinically, that it can be measured empirically and reliably, and that it relates

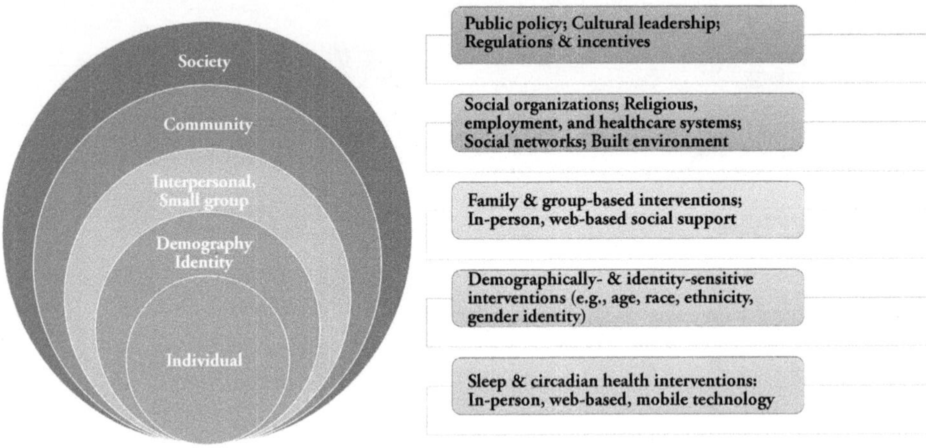

Figure 14.3 Potential benefits of a multidimensional sleep health framework

to health outcomes in ways that provide more information than single indices of sleep (Figure 14.3). At the same time, we recognize that a great deal of additional work is needed to evaluate the validity and utility of MDSH in observational, experimental, and intervention studies.

Future Directions

We suggest that the following research priorities will address these needs:

- Conduct further psychometric analyses of self-report MDSH scales.
- Define metrics for "good" and "poor" sleep on each dimension for self-report, behavioral, and physiologic measures. These metrics will likely vary according to age.
- Adopt consistent measurement tools for MDSH in future clinical, cohort, intervention, and population studies. Such tools must be sensitive to differences and disparities among different populations.
- Examine physiological and neural correlates of MDSH, contrasting these with correlates of individual sleep dimensions.
- Develop and evaluate interventions for poor MDSH. Such interventions would likely be behaviorally based and would need to be flexible enough to accommodate different profiles of poor MDSH. As such, these interventions could potentially apply to a larger number of individuals than disorder-based treatments such as CBT-I. The TranS-C intervention is one example of such a treatment and has already shown preliminary efficacy for improving sleep and non-sleep outcomes (Harvey & Buysse, 2017; Harvey et al., 2021).
- Develop and evaluate community- and policy-based interventions for improving MDSH.

References

American Academy of Sleep Medicine. (2014). *International classification of sleep disorders* (3rd ed.).

Anothaisintawee, T., Reutrakul, S., Van Cauter, E., & Thakkinstian, A. (2016). Sleep disturbances compared to traditional risk factors for diabetes development: Systematic review and meta-analysis. *Sleep Medicine Reviews, 30*, 11–24. https://doi.org/10.1016/j.smrv.2015.10.002

Appleton, S. L., Melaku, Y. A., Reynolds, A. C., Gill, T. K., de Batlle, J., & Adams, R. J. (2022). Multidimensional sleep health is associated with mental well-being in Australian adults. *Journal of Sleep Research, 31*(2), Article e13477. https://doi.org/10.1111/jsr.13477

Archer, S. N., & Oster, H. (2015). How sleep and wakefulness influence circadian rhythmicity: Effects of insufficient and mistimed sleep on the animal and human transcriptome. *Journal of Sleep Research, 24*(5), 476–493. https://doi.org/10.1111/jsr.12307

Armstrong, C. C., Dong, L., & Harvey, A. G. (2022). Mediators and moderators of outcome from the Transdiagnostic Sleep and Circadian Intervention for adults with severe mental illness in a community setting. *Behaviour Research and Therapy, 151*, Article 104053. https://doi.org/10.1016/j.brat.2022.104053

Bacaro, V., Benz, F., Pappaccogli, A., De Bartolo, P., Johann, A. F., Palagini, L., Lombardo, C., Feige, B., Riemann, D., & Baglioni, C. (2020). Interventions for sleep problems during pregnancy: A systematic review. *Sleep Medicine Reviews, 50*, Article 101234. https://doi.org/10.1016/j.smrv.2019.101234

Baglioni, C., Spiegelhalder, K., Lombardo, C., & Riemann, D. (2010). Sleep and emotions: A focus on insomnia. *Sleep Medicine Reviews, 14*(4), 227–238.

Bao, Y.-P., Han, Y., Ma, J., Wang, R.-J., Shi, L., Wang, T.-Y., He, J., Yue, J.-L., Shi, J., Tang, X.-D., & Lu, L. (2017). Cooccurrence and bidirectional prediction of sleep disturbances and depression in older adults: Meta-analysis and systematic review. *Neuroscience and Biobehavioral Reviews, 75*, 257–273. https://doi.org/10.1016/j.neubiorev.2017.01.032

Barham, W. T., Buysse, D. J., Kline, C. E., Kubala, A. G., & Brindle, R. C. (2022). Sleep health mediates the relationship between physical activity and depression symptoms. *Sleep & Breathing, 26*(3), 1341–1349. https://doi.org/10.1007/s11325-021-02496-9

Benítez, I., Roure, N., Pinilla, L., Sapiña-Beltran, E., Buysse, D. J., Barbé, F., & de Batlle, J. (2020). Validation of the Satisfaction, Alertness, Timing, Efficiency and Duration (SATED) Questionnaire for sleep health measurement. *Annals of the American Thoracic Society, 17*(3), 338–343. https://doi.org/10.1513/AnnalsATS.201908-628OC

Bertisch, S. M., Pollock, B. D., Mittleman, M. A., Buysse, D. J., Bazzano, L. A., Gottlieb, D. J., & Redline, S. (2018). Insomnia with objective short sleep duration and risk of incident cardiovascular disease and all-cause mortality: Sleep Heart Health Study. *Sleep, 41*(6), Article zsy047. https://doi.org/10.1093/sleep/zsy047

Billings, M. E., Cohen, R. T., Baldwin, C. M., Johnson, D. A., Palen, B. N., Parthasarathy, S., Patel, S. R., Russell, M., Tapia, I. E., Williamson, A. A., & Sharma, S. (2021). Disparities in sleep health and potential intervention models. *Chest, 159*(3), 1232–1240. https://doi.org/10.1016/j.chest.2020.09.249

Borbély, A. A. (1982). A two process model of sleep regulation. *Human Neurobiology, 1*(3), 195–204.

Brandolim Becker, N., Martins, R. I. S., de Neves Jesus, S., Chiodelli, R., & Stephen Rieber, M. (2018). Sleep health assessment: A scale validation. *Psychiatry Research, 259*, 51–55. https://doi.org/10.1016/j.psychres.2017.10.014

Brindle, R. C., Yu, L., Buysse, D. J., & Hall, M. H. (2019). Empirical derivation of cutoff values for the sleep health metric and its relationship to cardiometabolic morbidity: Results from the Midlife in the United States (MIDUS) study. *Sleep, 42*(9), Article zsz116. https://doi.org/10.1093/sleep/zsz116

Brouwer, A., van Raalte, D. H., Rutters, F., Elders, P. J. M., Snoek, F. J., Beekman, A. T. F., & Bremmer, M. A. (2020). Sleep and HbA_{1c} in patients with Type 2 diabetes: Which sleep characteristics matter most? *Diabetes Care, 43*(1), 235–243. https://doi.org/10.2337/dc19-0550

Burke, L. E., Kline, C. E., Mendez, D. D., Shiffman, S., Chasens, E. R., Zheng, Y., Imes, C. C., Cajita, M. I., Ewing, L., Goode, R., Mattos, M., Kariuki, J. K., Kriska, A., & Rathbun, S. L. (2022). Nightly variation in sleep influences self-efficacy for adhering to a healthy lifestyle: A prospective study. *International Journal of Behavioral Medicine, 29*(3), 377–386. https://doi.org/10.1007/s12529-021-10022-0

Butryn, M. L., Webb, V., & Wadden, T. A. (2011). Behavioral treatment of obesity. *Psychiatric Clinics of North America, 34*(4), 841–859. https://doi.org/10.1016/j.psc.2011.08.006

Buysse, D. J. (2014). Sleep health: Can we define it? Does it matter? *Sleep, 37*(1), 9–17.

Cain, S. W., Filtness, A. J., Phillips, C. L., & Anderson, C. (2015). Enhanced preference for high-fat foods following a simulated night shift. *Scandinavian Journal of Work, Environment & Health*, *41*(3), 288–293. https://doi.org/10.5271/sjweh.3486

Cappuccio, F. P., Cooper, D., D'Elia, L., Strazzullo, P., & Miller, M. A. (2011). Sleep duration predicts cardiovascular outcomes: A systematic review and meta-analysis of prospective studies. *European Heart Journal*, *32*(12), 1484–1492. https://doi.org/10.1093/eurheartj/ehr007

Cappuccio, F. P., D'Elia, L., Strazzullo, P., & Miller, M. A. (2010). Sleep duration and all-cause mortality: A systematic review and meta-analysis of prospective studies. *Sleep*, *33*(5), 585–592. https://doi.org/10.1093/sleep/33.5.585

Cappuccio, F. P., Taggart, F. M., Kandala, N.-B., Currie, A., Peile, E., Stranges, S., & Miller, M. A. (2008). Meta-analysis of short sleep duration and obesity in children and adults. *Sleep*, *31*(5), 619–626. https://doi.org/10.1093/sleep/31.5.619

Chaput, J.-P., Dutil, C., Featherstone, R., Ross, R., Giangregorio, L., Saunders, T. J., Janssen, I., Poitras, V. J., Kho, M. E., Ross-White, A., Zankar, S., & Carrier, J. (2020). Sleep timing, sleep consistency, and health in adults: A systematic review. *Applied Physiology, Nutrition, and Metabolism*, *45*(10, S2), S232–S247. https://doi.org/10.1139/apnm-2020-0032

Chaput, J.-P., & Tremblay, A. (2012). Sleeping habits predict the magnitude of fat loss in adults exposed to moderate caloric restriction. *Obesity Facts*, *5*(4), 561–566. https://doi.org/10.1159/000342054

Chen, T.-Y., Lee, S., & Buxton, O. M. (2022). Multidimensional sleep health is associated with physical frailty in a national sample of Taiwanese community-dwelling older adults: Sex matters. *Sleep Health*, *8*(5), 528–535. https://doi.org/10.1016/j.sleh.2022.05.003

Cheungpasitporn, W., Thongprayoon, C., Srivali, N., Vijayvargiya, P., Andersen, C. A., Kittanamongkolchai, W., Sathick, I. J. J., Caples, S. M., & Erickson, S. B. (2016). The effects of napping on the risk of hypertension: A systematic review and meta-analysis. *Journal of Evidence-Based Medicine*, *9*(4), 205–212. https://doi.org/10.1111/jebm.12211

Collins, L. M., & Lanza, S. T. (2010). *Latent class and latent transition analysis: With applications in the social behavioral, and health sciences*. Wiley.

Conlon, R. P. K., Hu, H., Saptono, A., Hawkins, M. S., Parmanto, B., Levine, M. D., & Buysse, D. J. (2023). Formative development of ClockWork for the postpartum period: A theory-based intervention to harness the circadian timing system to address cardiometabolic health-related behaviors. *International Journal of Environmental Research and Public Health*, *20*(4), Article 3669. https://doi.org/10.3390/ijerph20043669

Conlon, R. P. K., Wang, B., Germeroth, L. J., Cheng, Y., Buysse, D. J., & Levine, M. D. (2021). Demographic, pregnancy-related, and health-related factors in association with changes in sleep among pregnant women with overweight or obesity. *International Journal of Behavioral Medicine*, *28*(2), 200–206. https://doi.org/10.1007/s12529-020-09887-4

Creasy, S. A., Ostendorf, D. M., Blankenship, J. M., Grau, L., Arbet, J., Bessesen, D. H., Melanson, E. L., & Catenacci, V. A. (2022). Effect of sleep on weight loss and adherence to diet and physical activity recommendations during an 18-month behavioral weight loss intervention. *International Journal of Obesity*, *46*(8), 1510–1517. https://doi.org/10.1038/s41366-022-01141-z

Dalmases, M., Benítez, I. D., Mas, A., Garcia-Codina, O., Medina-Bustos, A., Escarrabill, J., Saltó, E., Buysse, D. J., Roure, N., Sánchez-de-la-Torre, M., Rué, M., Barbé, F., & de Batlle, J. (2018). Assessing sleep health in a European population: Results of the Catalan Health Survey 2015. *PLOS ONE*, *13*(4), Article e0194495. https://doi.org/10.1371/journal.pone.0194495

Dalmases, M., Benítez, I., Sapiña-Beltran, E., Garcia-Codina, O., Medina-Bustos, A., Escarrabill, J., Saltó, E., Buysse, D. J., Plana, R. E., Sánchez-de-la-Torre, M., Barbé, F., & de Batlle, J. (2019). Impact of sleep health on self-perceived health status. *Scientific Reports*, *9*(1), Article 7284. https://doi.org/10.1038/s41598-019-43873-5

da Silva, A. A., Mello, R. G. B. de, Schaan, C. W., Fuchs, F. D., Redline, S., & Fuchs, S. C. (2016). Sleep duration and mortality in the elderly: A systematic review with meta-analysis. *BMJ Open*, *6*(2), Article e008119. https://doi.org/10.1136/bmjopen-2015-008119

Dehghan, P., Aynehchi, A., Saleh-Ghadimi, S., Asghari Jafarabadi, M., & Moslemi, E. (2022). Association of self-efficacy and coping with sleep quality and disturbances with an emphasis on mediating role of eating behaviors and body mass index: A structural equation modeling approach. *Current Psychology*, *41*(11), 7471–7481. https://doi.org/10.1007/s12144-021-01774-9

Dejenie, T. A., G/Medhin, M. T., Admasu, F. T., Adella, G. A., Enyew, E. F., Kifle, Z. D., Seid, M. A., Mengstie, M. A., & Abebe, E. C. (2022). Impact of objectively-measured sleep duration on cardiometabolic health: A systematic review of recent evidence. *Frontiers in Endocrinology, 13*, Article 1064969. https://www.frontiersin.org/articles/10.3389/fendo.2022.1064969

Dennis, L., Spaeth, A., & Goel, N. (2016). Phenotypic stability of energy balance responses to experimental total sleep deprivation and sleep restriction in healthy adults. *Nutrients, 8*(12), Article 823. https://doi.org/10.3390/nu8120823

Depner, C. M., Stothard, E. R., & Wright, K. P. (2014). Metabolic consequences of sleep and circadian disorders. *Current Diabetes Reports, 14*(7), Article 507. https://doi.org/10.1007/s11892-014-0507-z

DeSantis, A. S., Dubowitz, T., Ghosh-Dastidar, B., Hunter, G. P., Buman, M., Buysse, D. J., Hale, L., & Troxel, W. M. (2019). A preliminary study of a composite sleep health score: Associations with psychological distress, body mass index, and physical functioning in a low-income African American community. *Sleep Health, 5*(5), 514–520. https://doi.org/10.1016/j.sleh.2019.05.001

Devine, J. K., & Wolf, J. M. (2016). Integrating nap and night-time sleep into sleep patterns reveals differential links to health-relevant outcomes. *Journal of Sleep Research, 25*(2), 225–233. https://doi.org/10.1111/jsr.12369

Didikoglu, A., Maharani, A., Tampubolon, G., Canal, M. M., Payton, A., & Pendleton, N. (2020). Longitudinal sleep efficiency in the elderly and its association with health. *Journal of Sleep Research, 29*(3), Article e12898. https://doi.org/10.1111/jsr.12898

Dolsen, E. A., Dong, L., & Harvey, A. G. (2023). Transdiagnostic Sleep and Circadian Intervention for adolescents plus text messaging: Randomized controlled trial 12-month follow-up. *Journal of Clinical Child and Adolescent Psychology, 52*(6), 750–762. https://doi.org/10.1080/15374416.2021.1978295

Dong, L., Dolsen, E. A., Martinez, A. J., Notsu, H., & Harvey, A. G. (2020). A transdiagnostic sleep and circadian intervention for adolescents: Six-month follow-up of a randomized controlled trial. *Journal of Child Psychology and Psychiatry, 61*(6), 653–661. https://doi.org/10.1111/jcpp.13154

Dong, L., Martinez, A. J., Buysse, D. J., & Harvey, A. G. (2019). A composite measure of sleep health predicts concurrent mental and physical health outcomes in adolescents prone to eveningness. *Sleep Health, 5*(2), 166–174. https://doi.org/10.1016/j.sleh.2018.11.009

Ehlers, C. L. (1988). Social zeitgebers and biological rhythms: A unified approach to understanding the etiology of depression. *Archives of General Psychiatry, 45*(10), 948–952. https://doi.org/10.1001/archpsyc.1988.01800340076012

Ensrud, K. E., Kats, A. M., Schousboe, J. T., Langsetmo, L., Vo, T. N., Blackwell, T. L., Buysse, D. J., Ancoli-Israel, S., & Stone, K. L. (2020). Multidimensional sleep health and subsequent health-care costs and utilization in older women. *Sleep, 43*(2), zsz230. https://doi.org/10.1093/sleep/zsz230

Fan, L., Xu, W., Cai, Y., Hu, Y., & Wu, C. (2019). Sleep duration and the risk of dementia: A systematic review and meta-analysis of prospective cohort studies. *Journal of the American Medical Directors Association, 20*(12), 1480–1487.e5. https://doi.org/10.1016/j.jamda.2019.06.009

Felder, J. N., Epel, E. S., Neuhaus, J., Krystal, A. D., & Prather, A. A. (2020). Efficacy of digital cognitive behavioral therapy for the treatment of insomnia symptoms among pregnant women. *JAMA Psychiatry, 77*(5), 484–492. https://doi.org/10.1001/jamapsychiatry.2019.4491

Fernandez-Mendoza, J., Calhoun, S., Bixler, E. O., Pejovic, S., Karataraki, M., Liao, D., Vela-Bueno, A., Ramos-Platon, M. J., Sauder, K. A., & Vgontzas, A. N. (2010). Insomnia with objective short sleep duration is associated with deficits in neuropsychological performance: A general population study. *Sleep, 33*(4), 459–465. https://doi.org/10.1093/sleep/33.4.459

Fernandez-Mendoza, J., Shea, S., Vgontzas, A. N., Calhoun, S. L., Liao, D., & Bixler, E. O. (2015). Insomnia and incident depression: Role of objective sleep duration and natural history. *Journal of Sleep Research, 24*(4), 390–398. https://doi.org/10.1111/jsr.12285

Fortier-Brochu, E., Beaulieu-Bonneau, S., Ivers, H., & Morin, C. M. (2012). Insomnia and daytime cognitive performance: A meta-analysis. *Sleep Medicine Reviews, 16*(1), 83–94. https://doi.org/10.1016/j.smrv.2011.03.008

Furihata, R., Hall, M. H., Stone, K. L., Ancoli-Israel, S., Smagula, S. F., Cauley, J. A., Kaneita, Y., Uchiyama, M., & Buysse, D. J.; Study of Osteoporotic Fractures (SOF) Research Group. (2017). An aggregate measure of sleep health is associated with prevalent and incident clinically significant depression symptoms among community-dwelling older women. *Sleep, 40*(3), Article zsw075. https://doi.org/10.1093/sleep/zsw075

Furihata, R., Saitoh, K., Suzuki, M., Jike, M., Kaneita, Y., Ohida, T., Buysse, D. J., & Uchiyama, M. (2020). A composite measure of sleep health is associated with symptoms of depression among Japanese female hospital nurses. *Comprehensive Psychiatry, 97*, Article 152151. https://doi.org/10.1016/j.comppsych.2019.152151

Galbiati, A., Verga, L., Giora, E., Zucconi, M., & Ferini-Strambi, L. (2019). The risk of neurodegeneration in REM sleep behavior disorder: A systematic review and meta-analysis of longitudinal studies. *Sleep Medicine Reviews, 43*, 37–46. https://doi.org/10.1016/j.smrv.2018.09.008

Gay, C. L., Richoux, S. E., Beebe, K. R., & Lee, K. A. (2017). Sleep disruption and duration in late pregnancy is associated with excess gestational weight gain among overweight and obese women. *Birth, 44*(2), 173–180. https://doi.org/10.1111/birt.12277

Ge, L., Guyatt, G., Tian, J., Pan, B., Chang, Y., Chen, Y., Li, H., Zhang, J., Li, Y., Ling, J., & Yang, K. (2019). Insomnia and risk of mortality from all-cause, cardiovascular disease, and cancer: Systematic review and meta-analysis of prospective cohort studies. *Sleep Medicine Reviews, 48*, Article 101215. https://doi.org/10.1016/j.smrv.2019.101215

Hale, L., Troxel, W., & Buysse, D. J. (2020). Sleep health: An opportunity for public health to address health equity. *Annual Review of Public Health, 41*(1), 81–99. https://doi.org/10.1146/annurev-publhealth-040119-094412

Hall, W. A., Hauck, Y. L., Carty, E. M., Hutton, E. K., Fenwick, J., & Stoll, K. (2009). Childbirth fear, anxiety, fatigue, and sleep deprivation in pregnant women. *Journal of Obstetric, Gynecologic & Neonatal Nursing, 38*(5), 567–576. https://doi.org/10.1111/j.1552-6909.2009.01054.x

Harvey, A. G., & Buysse, D. J. (2017). *Treating sleep problems: A transdiagnostic approach*. Guilford Press.

Harvey, A. G., Dong, L., Hein, K., Yu, S. H., Martinez, A. J., Gumport, N. B., Smith, F. L., Chapman, A., Lisman, M., Mirzadegan, I. A., Mullin, A. C., Fine, E., Dolsen, E. A., Gasperetti, C. E., Bukosky, J., Alvarado-Martinez, C. G., Kilbourne, A. M., Rabe-Hesketh, S., & Buysse, D. J. (2021). A randomized controlled trial of the Transdiagnostic Intervention for Sleep and Circadian Dysfunction (TranS-C) to improve serious mental illness outcomes in a community setting. *Journal of Consulting and Clinical Psychology, 89*(6), 537–550. https://doi.org/10.1037/ccp0000650

Harvey, A. G., Hein, K., Dolsen, E. A., Dong, L., Rabe-Hesketh, S., Gumport, N. B., Kanady, J., Wyatt, J. K., Hinshaw, S. P., Silk, J. S., Smith, R. L., Thompson, M. A., Zannone, N., & Blum, D. J. (2018). Modifying the impact of eveningness chronotype ("Night-Owls") in youth: A randomized controlled trial. *Journal of the American Academy of Child and Adolescent Psychiatry, 57*(10), 742–754. https://doi.org/10.1016/j.jaac.2018.04.020

Hawkins, M. S., Conlon, R. K., Donofry, S., Buysse, D. J., Venditti, E. M., Cheng, Y., & Levine, M. D. (2023). Sleep characteristics modify the associations of physical activity during pregnancy and gestational weight gain. *Archives of Gynecology and Obstetrics, 308*, 101–109. https://doi.org/10.1007/s00404-022-06677-z

Hawkins, M. S., Levine, M. D., Buysse, D. J., Abebe, K. Z., Hsiao, W.-H., McTigue, K. M., & Davis, E. M. (2021). Sleep health characteristics among adults who attempted weight loss in the past year: NHANES 2017–2018. *International Journal of Environmental Research and Public Health, 18*(19), Article 10170. https://doi.org/10.3390/ijerph181910170

Hawkins, M. S., Pokutnaya, D. Y., Bodnar, L. M., Levine, M. D., Buysse, D. J., Davis, E. M., Wallace, M. L., Zee, P. C., Grobman, W. A., Reid, K. J., & Facco, F. L. (2023). The association between multidimensional sleep health and gestational weight gain: nuMoM2b Sleep Duration and Continuity Study. *medRxiv*. https://doi.org/10.1101/2023.02.21.23285931

He, D., Guo, Z., McClure, M. A., Mu, Q., & Jiang, B. (2023). Cognitive-behavioral therapy for insomnia with objective short sleep duration phenotype: A systematic review with meta-analysis. *Sleep Medicine Reviews, 67*, Article 101736. https://doi.org/10.1016/j.smrv.2022.101736

Herring, S. J., Yu, D., Spaeth, A., Pien, G., Darden, N., Riis, V., Bersani, V., Wallen, J., Davey, A., & Foster, G. D. (2019). Influence of sleep duration on postpartum weight change in Black and Hispanic women. *Obesity, 27*(2), 295–303. https://doi.org/10.1002/oby.22364

Hertenstein, E., Feige, B., Gmeiner, T., Kienzler, C., Spiegelhalder, K., Johann, A., Jansson-Fröjmark, M., Palagini, L., Rücker, G., Riemann, D., & Baglioni, C. (2019). Insomnia as a predictor of mental disorders: A systematic review and meta-analysis. *Sleep Medicine Reviews, 43*, 96–105. https://doi.org/10.1016/j.smrv.2018.10.006

Hill Almeida, L. M., Flicker, L., Hankey, G. J., Golledge, J., Yeap, B. B., & Almeida, O. P. (2022). Disrupted sleep and risk of depression in later life: A prospective cohort study with extended follow up and a systematic review and meta-analysis. *Journal of Affective Disorders, 309*, 314–323. https://doi.org/10.1016/j.jad.2022.04.133

Hua, J., Jiang, H., Wang, H., & Fang, Q. (2021). Sleep duration and the risk of metabolic syndrome in adults: A systematic review and meta-analysis. *Frontiers in Neurology, 12*, Article 635564. https://www.frontiersin.org/articles/10.3389/fneur.2021.635564

Itani, O., Jike, M., Watanabe, N., & Kaneita, Y. (2017). Short sleep duration and health outcomes: A systematic review, meta-analysis, and meta-regression. *Sleep Medicine, 32*, 246–256. https://doi.org/10.1016/j.sleep.2016.08.006

Jarrin, D. C., Alvaro, P. K., Bouchard, M.-A., Jarrin, S. D., Drake, C. L., & Morin, C. M. (2018). Insomnia and hypertension: A systematic review. *Sleep Medicine Reviews, 41*, 3–38. https://doi.org/10.1016/j.smrv.2018.02.003

Ji, L., Wallace, M. L., Master, L., Schade, M. M., Shen, Y., Derby, C. A., & Buxton, O. M. (2023). Six multidimensional sleep health facets in older adults identified with factor analysis of actigraphy: Results from the Einstein Aging Study. *Sleep Health, 9*(5), 758–766. https://doi.org/10.1016/j.sleh.2023.03.002

Jike, M., Itani, O., Watanabe, N., Buysse, D. J., & Kaneita, Y. (2018). Long sleep duration and health outcomes: A systematic review, meta-analysis and meta-regression. *Sleep Medicine Reviews, 39*, 25–36. https://doi.org/10.1016/j.smrv.2017.06.011

Johnson, K. A., Gordon, C. J., Chapman, J. L., Hoyos, C. M., Marshall, N. S., Miller, C. B., & Grunstein, R. R. (2021). The association of insomnia disorder characterised by objective short sleep duration with hypertension, diabetes and body mass index: A systematic review and meta-analysis. *Sleep Medicine Reviews, 59*, Article 101456. https://doi.org/10.1016/j.smrv.2021.101456

Johnson, L. C. M., Aiello, J. J., Jagtiani, A., Moore, K. N., Barber, L., Gujral, U. P., & Johnson, D. A. (2023). Feasibility, appropriateness, and acceptability of a mobile mindfulness meditation intervention to improve sleep quality among a racially/ethnically diverse population. *Sleep Health, 9*(2), 196–202. https://doi.org/10.1016/j.sleh.2022.09.014

Kabat, G. C., Xue, X., Kamensky, V., Zaslavsky, O., Stone, K. L., Johnson, K. C., Wassertheil-Smoller, S., Shadyab, A. H., Luo, J., Hale, L., Qi, L., Cauley, J. A., Brunner, R. L., Manson, J. E., & Rohan, T. E. (2018). The association of sleep duration and quality with all-cause and cause-specific mortality in the Women's Health Initiative. *Sleep Medicine, 50*, 48–54. https://doi.org/10.1016/j.sleep.2018.05.015

Kalmbach, D. A., Cheng, P., Reffi, A. N., Seymour, G. M., Ruprich, M. K., Bazan, L. F., Pitts, D. S., Walch, O., & Drake, C. L. (2023). Racial disparities in treatment engagement and outcomes in digital cognitive behavioral therapy for insomnia among pregnant women. *Sleep Health, 9*(1), 18–25. https://doi.org/10.1016/j.sleh.2022.10.010

Kearns, J. C., Coppersmith, D. D. L., Santee, A. C., Insel, C., Pigeon, W. R., & Glenn, C. R. (2020). Sleep problems and suicide risk in youth: A systematic review, developmental framework, and implications for hospital treatment. *General Hospital Psychiatry, 63*, 141–151. https://doi.org/10.1016/j.genhosppsych.2018.09.011

Kendzerska, T., Kamra, M., Murray, B. J., & Boulos, M. I. (2017). Incident cardiovascular events and death in individuals with restless legs syndrome or periodic limb movements in sleep: A systematic review. *Sleep, 40*(3), Article zsx013. https://doi.org/10.1093/sleep/zsx013

Khokhrina, A., Andreeva, E., & Degryse, J.-M. (2022). A systematic review on the association of sleep-disordered breathing with cardiovascular pathology in adults. *NPJ Primary Care Respiratory Medicine, 32*(1), Article 41. https://doi.org/10.1038/s41533-022-00307-6

Kline, C. E. (2014). The bidirectional relationship between exercise and sleep: Implications for exercise adherence and sleep improvement. *American Journal of Lifestyle Medicine, 8*(6), 375–379. https://doi.org/10.1177/1559827614544437

Kline, C. E., Chasens, E. R., Bizhanova, Z., Sereika, S. M., Buysse, D. J., Imes, C. C., Kariuki, J. K., Mendez, D. D., Cajita, M. I., Rathbun, S. L., & Burke, L. E. (2021). The association between sleep health and weight change during a 12-month behavioral weight loss intervention. *International Journal of Obesity, 45*(3), 639–649. https://doi.org/10.1038/s41366-020-00728-8

Knutson, K. L., & von Schantz, M. (2018). Associations between chronotype, morbidity and mortality in the UK Biobank cohort. *Chronobiology International, 35*(8), 1045–1053. https://doi.org/10.1080/07420528.2018.1454458

Krittanawong, C., Tunhasiriwet, A., Wang, Z., Zhang, H., Farrell, A. M., Chirapongsathorn, S., Sun, T., Kitai, T., & Argulian, E. (2019). Association between short and long sleep durations and cardiovascular

outcomes: A systematic review and meta-analysis. *European Heart Journal: Acute Cardiovascular Care, 8*(8), 762–770. https://doi.org/10.1177/2048872617741733
Kubala, A. G., Buysse, D. J., Brindle, R. C., Krafty, R. T., Thayer, J. F., Hall, M. H., & Kline, C. E. (2020). The association between physical activity and a composite measure of sleep health. *Sleep & Breathing, 24*(3), 1207–1214. https://doi.org/10.1007/s11325-019-02007-x
Kwon, M., Park, E., & Dickerson, S. S. (2019). Adolescent substance use and its association to sleep disturbances: A systematic review. *Sleep Health, 5*(4), 382–394. https://doi.org/10.1016/j.sleh.2019.06.001
Ladyman, C., & Signal, T. L. (2018). Sleep health in pregnancy: A scoping review. *Sleep Medicine Clinics, 13*(3), 307–333. https://doi.org/10.1016/j.jsmc.2018.04.004
Lee, S., & Lawson, K. M. (2021). Beyond single sleep measures: A composite measure of sleep health and its associations with psychological and physical well-being in adulthood. *Social Science & Medicine, 274*, 113800. https://doi.org/10.1016/j.socscimed.2021.113800
Lee, S., Mu, C. X., Wallace, M. L., Andel, R., Almeida, D. M., Buxton, O. M., & Patel, S. R. (2022). Sleep health composites are associated with the risk of heart disease across sex and race. *Scientific Reports, 12*(1), Article 2023. https://doi.org/10.1038/s41598-022-05203-0
Léger, D., Torres, M. J., Bayon, V., Hercberg, S., Galan, P., Chennaoui, M., & Andreeva, V. A. (2019). The association between physical and mental chronic conditions and napping. *Scientific Reports, 9*(1), Article 1795. https://doi.org/10.1038/s41598-018-37355-3
Levenson, J. C., Ford, H. A., Reyes, Z. M. D., Mukundan, A., Patel, G., Bahary, S., & Miller, E. (2021). Designing adolescent sleep interventions with stakeholder input. *Sleep Health, 7*(5), 581–587. https://doi.org/10.1016/j.sleh.2021.07.007
Li, X., Zhou, T., Ma, H., Huang, T., Gao, X., Manson, J. E., & Qi, L. (2021). Healthy sleep patterns and risk of incident arrhythmias. *Journal of the American College of Cardiology, 78*(12), 1197–1207. https://doi.org/10.1016/j.jacc.2021.07.023
Li, C., & Shang, S. (2021). Relationship between sleep and hypertension: Findings from the NHANES (2007–2014). *International Journal of Environmental Research and Public Health, 18*(15), Article 7867. https://doi.org/10.3390/ijerph18157867
Li, X., Wei, J., Zhang, X., Meng, Z., & Zhu, W. (2023). Relationship between night-sleep duration and risk for depression among middle-aged and older people: A dose–response meta-analysis. *Frontiers in Physiology, 14*, Article 1085091. https://www.frontiersin.org/articles/10.3389/fphys.2023.1085091
Lian, Y., Yuan, Q., Wang, G., & Tang, F. (2019). Association between sleep quality and metabolic syndrome: A systematic review and meta-analysis. *Psychiatry Research, 274*, 66–74. https://doi.org/10.1016/j.psychres.2019.01.096
Linné, Y., Dye, L., Barkeling, B., & Rössner, S. (2004). Long-term weight development in women: A 15-year follow-up of the effects of pregnancy. *Obesity Research, 12*(7), 1166–1178. https://doi.org/10.1038/oby.2004.146
Liu, J.-W., Tu, Y.-K., Lai, Y.-F., Lee, H.-C., Tsai, P.-S., Chen, T.-J., Huang, H.-C., Chen, Y.-T., & Chiu, H.-Y. (2019). Associations between sleep disturbances and suicidal ideation, plans, and attempts in adolescents: A systematic review and meta-analysis. *Sleep, 42*(6), Article zsz054. https://doi.org/10.1093/sleep/zsz054
Liu, R. T., Steele, S. J., Hamilton, J. L., Do, Q. B. P., Furbish, K., Burke, T. A., Martinez, A. P., & Gerlus, N. (2020). Sleep and suicide: A systematic review and meta-analysis of longitudinal studies. *Clinical Psychology Review, 81*, Article 101895. https://doi.org/10.1016/j.cpr.2020.101895
Lo, J. C., Groeger, J. A., Cheng, G. H., Dijk, D. J., & Chee, M. W. (2016). Self-reported sleep duration and cognitive performance in older adults: A systematic review and meta-analysis. *Sleep Medicine, 17*, 87–98. https://doi.org/10.1016/j.sleep.2015.08.021
Lovato, N., & Lack, L. (2019). Insomnia and mortality: A meta-analysis. *Sleep Medicine Reviews, 43*, 71–83. https://doi.org/10.1016/j.smrv.2018.10.004
Lunsford-Avery, J. R., Engelhard, M. M., Navar, A. M., & Kollins, S. H. (2018). Validation of the Sleep Regularity Index in older adults and associations with cardiometabolic risk. *Scientific Reports, 8*(1), Article 14158. https://doi.org/10.1038/s41598-018-32402-5
Lunyera, J., Park, Y.-M. M., Ward, J. B., Gaston, S. A., Bhavsar, N. A., Muntner, P., Sandler, D. P., & Jackson, C. L. (2021). A prospective study of multiple sleep dimensions and hypertension risk among White, Black and Hispanic/Latina women: Findings from the Sister Study. *Journal of Hypertension, 39*(11), 2210–2219. https://doi.org/10.1097/HJH.0000000000002929

Makarem, N., Castro-Diehl, C., St-Onge, M., Redline, S., Shea, S., Lloyd-Jones, D., Ning, H., & Aggarwal, B. (2022). Redefining cardiovascular health to include sleep: Prospective associations with cardiovascular disease in the MESA Sleep Study. *Journal of the American Heart Association, 11*(21), Article e025252. https://doi.org/10.1161/JAHA.122.025252

Mancinelli, E., Bassi, G., Gabrielli, S., & Salcuni, S. (2022). The efficacy of digital cognitive–behavioral interventions in supporting the psychological adjustment and sleep quality of pregnant women with sub-clinical symptoms: A systematic review and meta-analysis. *International Journal of Environmental Research and Public Health, 19*(15), Article 9549. https://doi.org/10.3390/ijerph19159549

Matricciani, L., Paquet, C., Dumuid, D., Lushington, K., & Olds, T. (2022). Multidimensional sleep and cardiometabolic risk factors for Type 2 diabetes: Examining self-report and objective dimensions of sleep. *The Science of Diabetes Self-Management and Care, 48*(6), 533–545. https://doi.org/10.1177/26350106221137896

McParland, D., & Gormley, I. C. (2016). Model based clustering for mixed data: clustMD. *Advances in Data Analysis and Classification, 10*(2), 155–169. https://doi.org/10.1007/s11634-016-0238-x

McTigue, K. M., Conroy, M. B., Hess, R., Bryce, C. L., Fiorillo, A. B., Fischer, G. S., Milas, N. C., & Simkin-Silverman, L. R. (2009). Using the internet to translate an evidence-based lifestyle intervention into practice. *Telemedicine Journal and E-Health, 15*(9), 851–858. https://doi.org/10.1089/tmj.2009.0036

Meltzer, L. J., Williamson, A. A., & Mindell, J. A. (2021). Pediatric sleep health: It matters, and so does how we define it. *Sleep Medicine Reviews, 57*, Article 101425. https://doi.org/10.1016/j.smrv.2021.101425

Mohammadi, S., Moosaie, F., Saghazadeh, A., Mahmoudi, M., & Rezaei, N. (2021). Metabolic profile in patients with narcolepsy: A systematic review and meta-analysis. *Sleep Medicine, 81*, 268–284. https://doi.org/10.1016/j.sleep.2021.02.040

Möller-Levet, C. S., Archer, S. N., Bucca, G., Laing, E. E., Slak, A., Kabiljo, R., Lo, J. C. Y., Santhi, N., von Schantz, M., Smith, C. P., & Dijk, D.-J. (2013). Effects of insufficient sleep on circadian rhythmicity and expression amplitude of the human blood transcriptome. *Proceedings of the National Academy of Sciences of the United States of America, 110*(12), E1132–E1141. https://doi.org/10.1073/pnas.1217154110

Morita, Y., Sasai-Sakuma, T., Asaoka, S., & Inoue, Y. (2015). The impact of a delayed sleep–wake schedule on depression is greater in women—A web-based cross-sectional study in Japanese young adults. *Chronobiology International, 32*(7), 952–958. https://doi.org/10.3109/07420528.2015.1055756

Mostafa, S. A., Mena, S. C., Antza, C., Balanos, G., Nirantharakumar, K., & Tahrani, A. A. (2022). Sleep behaviours and associated habits and the progression of pre-diabetes to type 2 diabetes mellitus in adults: A systematic review and meta-analysis. *Diabetes and Vascular Disease Research, 19*(3), Article 14791641221088824. https://doi.org/10.1177/14791641221088824

Ogilvie, R. P., & Patel, S. R. (2017). The epidemiology of sleep and obesity. *Sleep Health, 3*(5), 383–388. https://doi.org/10.1016/j.sleh.2017.07.013

Ogilvie, R. P., Redline, S., Bertoni, A. G., Chen, X., Ouyang, P., Szklo, M., & Lutsey, P. L. (2016). Actigraphy measured sleep indices and adiposity: The Multi-Ethnic Study of Atherosclerosis (MESA). *Sleep, 39*(9), 1701–1708. https://doi.org/10.5665/sleep.6096

Omichi, C., Koyama, T., Kadotani, H., Ozaki, E., Tomida, S., Yoshida, T., Otonari, J., Ikezaki, H., Hara, M., Tanaka, K., Tamura, T., Nagayoshi, M., Okada, R., Kubo, Y., Oze, I., Matsuo, K., Nakamura, Y., Kusakabe, M., Ibusuki, R., . . . Wakai, K. (2022). Irregular sleep and all-cause mortality: A large prospective cohort study. *Sleep Health, 8*(6), 678–683. https://doi.org/10.1016/j.sleh.2022.08.010

Owais, S., Chow, C. H. T., Furtado, M., Frey, B. N., & Van Lieshout, R. J. (2018). Non-pharmacological interventions for improving postpartum maternal sleep: A systematic review and meta-analysis. *Sleep Medicine Reviews, 41*, 87–100. https://doi.org/10.1016/j.smrv.2018.01.005

Owusu, J. T., Wennberg, A. M. V., Holingue, C. B., Tzuang, M., Abeson, K. D., & Spira, A. P. (2019). Napping characteristics and cognitive performance in older adults. *International Journal of Geriatric Psychiatry, 34*(1), 87–96. https://doi.org/10.1002/gps.4991

Page, A. J., Christie, S., Symonds, E., & Li, H. (2020). Circadian regulation of appetite and time restricted feeding. *Physiology & Behavior, 220*, Article 112873. https://doi.org/10.1016/j.physbeh.2020.112873

Pauley, A. M., Moore, G. A., Mama, S. K., Molenaar, P., & Downs, D. S. (2022). Systematic review of the associations between prenatal sleep behaviours and components of energy balance for regulating weight gain. *Journal of Sleep Research*, 32(2), Article e13619. https://doi.org/10.1111/jsr.13619

Paulino, D. S. M., Borrelli, C. B., Faria-Schützer, D. B., Brito, L. G. O., & Surita, F. G. (2022). Non-pharmacological interventions for improving sleep quality during pregnancy: A systematic review and

meta-analysis. *Revista Brasileira de Ginecologia e Obstetrícia, 44*(8), 776–784. https://doi.org/10.1055/s-0042-1746200
Phelan, S. (2010). Pregnancy: A "teachable moment" for weight control and obesity prevention. *American Journal of Obstetrics and Gynecology, 202*(2), 135.e1–135.e8. https://doi.org/10.1016/j.ajog.2009.06.008
Philbrook, L. E., Hinnant, J. B., Elmore-Staton, L., Buckhalt, J. A., & El-Sheikh, M. (2017). Sleep and cognitive functioning in childhood: Ethnicity, socioeconomic status, and sex as moderators. *Developmental Psychology, 53*, 1276–1285. https://doi.org/10.1037/dev0000319
Pigeon, W. R., Bishop, T. M., & Krueger, K. M. (2017). Insomnia as a precipitating factor in new onset mental illness: A systematic review of recent findings. *Current Psychiatry Reports, 19*(8), Article 44. https://doi.org/10.1007/s11920-017-0802-x
Rana, S., Prabhu, S. D., & Young, M. E. (2020). Chronobiological influence over cardiovascular function: The good, the bad, and the ugly. *Circulation Research, 126*(2), 258–279. https://doi.org/10.1161/CIRCRESAHA.119.313349
Ravyts, S. G., Dizerzewski, J. M., Perez, E., Donovan, E. K., & Dautovich, N. (2021). Sleep health as measured by RU SATED: A psychometric evaluation. *Behavioral Sleep Medicine, 19*(1), 48–56. https://doi.org/10.1080/15402002.2019.1701474
Roehrs, T., Sibai, M., & Roth, T. (2021). Sleep and alertness disturbance and substance use disorders: A bi-directional relation. *Pharmacology, Biochemistry, and Behavior, 203*, Article 173153. https://doi.org/10.1016/j.pbb.2021.173153
Rong, K., Yu, K., Han, X., Szeto, I. M., Qin, X., Wang, J., Ning, Y., Wang, P., & Ma, D. (2015). Pre-pregnancy BMI, gestational weight gain and postpartum weight retention: A meta-analysis of observational studies. *Public Health Nutrition, 18*(12), 2172–2182. https://doi.org/10.1017/S1368980014002523
Ross, L. E., Murray, B. J., & Steiner, M. (2005). Sleep and perinatal mood disorders: A critical review. *Journal of Psychiatry and Neuroscience, 30*(4), 247–256.
Rottapel, R. E., Zhou, E. S., Spadola, C. E., Clark, C. R., Kontos, E. Z., Laver, K., Chen, J. T., Redline, S., & Bertisch, S. M. (2020). Adapting sleep hygiene for community interventions: A qualitative investigation of sleep hygiene behaviors among racially/ethnically diverse, low-income adults. *Sleep Health, 6*(2), 205–213. https://doi.org/10.1016/j.sleh.2019.12.009
Ru, T., Chen, Q., You, J., & Zhou, G. (2019). Effects of a short midday nap on habitual nappers' alertness, mood and mental performance across cognitive domains. *Journal of Sleep Research, 28*(3), Article e12638. https://doi.org/10.1111/jsr.12638
Salari, N., Moradi, S., Bagheri, R., Talebi, S., Wong, A., Babavaisi, B., Kermani, M. a. H., & Hemati, N. (2022). Daytime napping and coronary heart disease risk in adults: A systematic review and dose–response meta-analysis. *Sleep and Breathing, 27*, 1255–1267. https://doi.org/10.1007/s11325-022-02759-z
Schousboe, J. T., Kats, A. M., Stone, K. L., Langsetmo, L., Vo, T. N., Blackwell, T. L., Buysse, D. J., Ancoli-Israel, S., & Ensrud, K. E. (2020). Self-reported poor sleep on multiple dimensions is associated with higher total health care costs in older men. *Sleep, 43*(10), zsaa073. https://doi.org/10.1093/sleep/zsaa073
Shah, A., Turkistani, A., Luenam, K., Yaqub, S., Ananias, P., Jose, A. M., Melo, J. P., & Mohammed, L. (2022). Is shift work sleep disorder a risk factor for metabolic syndrome and its components? A systematic review of cross-sectional studies. *Metabolic Syndrome and Related Disorders, 20*(1), 1–10. https://doi.org/10.1089/met.2021.0070
Sheynblyum, M., Conlon, R. P. K., Donofry, S. D., & Levine, M. D. (2022). Incorporating skills for managing mood, stress, and sleep into a gestational weight gain intervention. *Journal of Contemporary Psychotherapy, 53*, 157–163. https://doi.org/10.1007/s10879-022-09577-0
Shi, L., Chen, S.-J., Ma, M.-Y., Bao, Y.-P., Han, Y., Wang, Y.-M., Shi, J., Vitiello, M. V., & Lu, L. (2018). Sleep disturbances increase the risk of dementia: A systematic review and meta-analysis. *Sleep Medicine Reviews, 40*, 4–16. https://doi.org/10.1016/j.smrv.2017.06.010
Shochat, T., Cohen-Zion, M., & Tzischinsky, O. (2014). Functional consequences of inadequate sleep in adolescents: A systematic review. *Sleep Medicine Reviews, 18*(1), 75–87. https://doi.org/10.1016/j.smrv.2013.03.005
Siega-Riz, A. M., Herring, A. H., Carrier, K., Evenson, K. R., Dole, N., & Deierlein, A. (2010). Sociodemographic, perinatal, behavioral, and psychosocial predictors of weight retention at 3 and 12 months postpartum. *Obesity, 18*(10), 1996–2003. https://doi.org/10.1038/oby.2009.458
Simkin-Silverman, L. R., Conroy, M. B., Bhargava, T., & McTigue, K. M. (2011). Development of an online diabetes prevention lifestyle intervention coaching protocol for use in primary care practice. *The Diabetes Educator, 37*(2), 263–268. https://doi.org/10.1177/0145721710396587

Smagula, S. F., Stone, K. L., Fabio, A., & Cauley, J. A. (2016). Risk factors for sleep disturbances in older adults: Evidence from prospective studies. *Sleep Medicine Reviews, 25*, 21–30. https://doi.org/10.1016/j.smrv.2015.01.003

Smith, G. N., Louis, J. M., & Saade, G. R. (2019). Pregnancy and the postpartum period as an opportunity for cardiovascular risk identification and management. *Obstetrics & Gynecology, 134*(4), 851–862. https://doi.org/10.1097/AOG.0000000000003363

Spadola, C. E., Rottapel, R. E., Zhou, E. S., Chen, J. T., Guo, N., Khalsa, S. B. S., Redline, S., & Bertisch, S. M. (2020). A sleep hygiene and yoga intervention conducted in affordable housing communities: Pilot study results and lessons for a future trial. *Complementary Therapies in Clinical Practice, 39*, Article 101121. https://doi.org/10.1016/j.ctcp.2020.101121

Suh, S. W., Han, J. W., Lee, J. R., Byun, S., Kwon, S. J., Oh, S. H., Lee, K. H., Han, G., Hong, J. W., Kwak, K. P., Kim, B.-J., Kim, S. G., Kim, J. L., Kim, T. H., Ryu, S.-H., Moon, S. W., Park, J. H., Seo, J., Youn, J. C., . . . Kim, K. W. (2018). Sleep and cognitive decline: A prospective nondemented elderly cohort study. *Annals of Neurology, 83*(3), 472–482. https://doi.org/10.1002/ana.25166

Sun, J., Ma, C., Zhao, M., Magnussen, C. G., & Xi, B. (2022). Daytime napping and cardiovascular risk factors, cardiovascular disease, and mortality: A systematic review. *Sleep Medicine Reviews, 65*, Article 101682. https://doi.org/10.1016/j.smrv.2022.101682

Tadrous, R., O'Rourke, D., Mockler, D., & Broderick, J. (2021). Health-related quality of life in narcolepsy: A systematic review and meta-analysis. *Journal of Sleep Research, 30*(6), Article e13383. https://doi.org/10.1111/jsr.13383

Tao, F., Cao, Z., Jiang, Y., Fan, N., Xu, F., Yang, H., Li, S., Zhang, Y., Zhang, X., Sun, L., & Wang, Y. (2021). Associations of sleep duration and quality with incident cardiovascular disease, cancer, and mortality: A prospective cohort study of 407,500 UK biobank participants. *Sleep Medicine, 81*, 401–409. https://doi.org/10.1016/j.sleep.2021.03.015

Thomson, C. A., Morrow, K. L., Flatt, S. W., Wertheim, B. C., Perfect, M. M., Ravia, J. J., Sherwood, N. E., Karanja, N., & Rock, C. L. (2012). Relationship between sleep quality and quantity and weight loss in women participating in a weight-loss intervention trial. *Obesity, 20*(7), 1419–1425. https://doi.org/10.1038/oby.2012.62

Tighe, C. A., Brindle, R. C., Stahl, S. T., Wallace, M. L., Bramoweth, A. D., Forman, D. E., & Buysse, D. J. (2021). Multidimensional sleep health and physical functioning in older adults. *Gerontology & Geriatric Medicine, 7*, Article 23337214211016224. https://doi.org/10.1177/23337214211016222

Tononi, G., & Cirelli, C. (2014). Sleep and the price of plasticity: From synaptic and cellular homeostasis to memory consolidation and integration. *Neuron, 81*(1), 12–34. https://doi.org/10.1016/j.neuron.2013.12.025

Tortora, C., Franczak, B. C., Browne, R. P., & McNicholas, P. D. (2019). A mixture of coalesced generalized hyperbolic distributions. *Journal of Classification, 36*(1), 26–57. https://doi.org/10.1007/s00357-019-09319-3

Tsereteli, N., Vallat, R., Fernandez-Tajes, J., Delahanty, L. M., Ordovas, J. M., Drew, D. A., Valdes, A. M., Segata, N., Chan, A. T., Wolf, J., Berry, S. E., Walker, M. P., Spector, T. D., & Franks, P. W. (2022). Impact of insufficient sleep on dysregulated blood glucose control under standardised meal conditions. *Diabetologia, 65*(2), 356–365. https://doi.org/10.1007/s00125-021-05608-y

van der Pal, K. C., Koopman, A. D. M., Lakerveld, J., van der Heijden, A. A., Elders, P. J., Beulens, J. W., & Rutters, F. (2018). The association between multiple sleep-related characteristics and the metabolic syndrome in the general population: The New Hoorn study. *Sleep Medicine, 52*, 51–57. https://doi.org/10.1016/j.sleep.2018.07.022

Vitaterna, M. H., Takahashi, J. S., & Turek, F. W. (2001). Overview of circadian rhythms. *Alcohol Research & Health, 25*(2), 85–93.

Wallace, M. L., Buysse, D. J., Germain, A., Hall, M. H., & Iyengar, S. (2018). Variable selection for skewed model-based clustering: Application to the identification of novel sleep phenotypes. *Journal of the American Statistical Association, 113*(521), 95–110. https://doi.org/10.1080/01621459.2017.1330202

Wallace, M. L., Buysse, D. J., Redline, S., Stone, K. L., Ensrud, K., Leng, Y., Ancoli-Israel, S., & Hall, M. H. (2019). Multidimensional sleep and mortality in older adults: A machine-learning comparison with other risk factors. *The Journals of Gerontology. Series A, Biological Sciences and Medical Sciences, 74*(12), 1903–1909. https://doi.org/10.1093/gerona/glz044

Wallace, M. L., Coleman, T. S., Mentch, L. K., Buysse, D. J., Graves, J. L., Hagen, E. W., Hall, M. H., Stone, K. L., Redline, S., & Peppard, P. E. (2021). Physiological sleep measures predict time to 15-year mortality in community adults: Application of a novel machine learning framework. *Journal of Sleep Research, 30*(6), Article e13386. https://doi.org/10.1111/jsr.13386

Wallace, M. L., Lee, S., Hall, M. H., Stone, K. L., Langsetmo, L., Redline, S., Schousboe, J. T., Ensrud, K., LeBlanc, E. S., & Buysse, D. J.; MrOS and SOF Research Groups. (2019). Heightened sleep propensity: A novel and high-risk sleep health phenotype in older adults. *Sleep Health, 5*(6), 630–638. https://doi.org/10.1016/j.sleh.2019.08.001

Wallace, M. L., Lee, S., Stone, K. L., Hall, M. H., Smagula, S. F., Redline, S., Ensrud, K., Ancoli-Israel, S., & Buysse, D. J. (2022). Actigraphy-derived sleep health profiles and mortality in older men and women. *Sleep, 45*(4), Article zsac015. https://doi.org/10.1093/sleep/zsac015

Wallace, M. L., Mentch, L., Wheeler, B. J., Tapia, A. L., Richards, M., Zhou, S., Yi, L., Redline, S., & Buysse, D. J. (2023). Use and misuse of random forest variable importance metrics in medicine: Demonstrations through incident stroke prediction. *BMC Medical Research Methodology, 23*(1), Article 144. https://doi.org/10.1186/s12874-023-01965-x

Wallace, M. L., Stone, K., Smagula, S. F., Hall, M. H., Simsek, B., Kado, D. M., Redline, S., Vo, T. N., & Buysse, D. J.; Osteoporotic Fractures in Men (MrOS) Study Research Group. (2018). Which sleep health characteristics predict all-cause mortality in older men? An application of flexible multivariable approaches. *Sleep, 41*(1), Article zsx189. https://doi.org/10.1093/sleep/zsx189

Wallace, M. L., Yu, L., Buysse, D. J., Stone, K. L., Redline, S., Smagula, S. F., Stefanick, M. L., Kritz-Silverstein, D., & Hall, M. H. (2021). Multidimensional sleep health domains in older men and women: An actigraphy factor analysis. *Sleep, 44*(2), Article zsaa181. https://doi.org/10.1093/sleep/zsaa181

Williamson, A. A., Okoroji, C., Cicalese, O., Evans, B. C., Ayala, A., Harvey, B., Honore, R., Kratchman, A., Beidas, R. S., Fiks, A. G., Power, T. J., & Mindell, J. A. (2022). *Sleep Well!* An adapted behavioral sleep intervention implemented in urban primary care. *Journal of Clinical Sleep Medicine, 18*(4), 1153–1166. https://doi.org/10.5664/jcsm.9822

Wirth, M. D., Hébert, J. R., Hand, G. A., Youngstedt, S. D., Hurley, T. G., Shook, R. P., Paluch, A. E., Sui, X., James, S. L., & Blair, S. N. (2015). Association between actigraphic sleep metrics and body composition. *Annals of Epidemiology, 25*(10), 773–778. https://doi.org/10.1016/j.annepidem.2015.05.001

Xiao, Q., Gu, F., Caporaso, N., & Matthews, C. E. (2016). Relationship between sleep characteristics and measures of body size and composition in a nationally-representative sample. *BMC Obesity, 3*(1), Article 48. https://doi.org/10.1186/s40608-016-0128-y

Xie, J., Li, Y., Zhang, Y., Vgontzas, A. N., Basta, M., Chen, B., Xu, C., & Tang, X. (2021). Sleep duration and metabolic syndrome: An updated systematic review and meta-analysis. *Sleep Medicine Reviews, 59*, Article 101451. https://doi.org/10.1016/j.smrv.2021.101451

Yan, B., Yang, J., Zhao, B., Fan, Y., Wang, W., & Ma, X. (2021). Objective sleep efficiency predicts cardiovascular disease in a community population: The Sleep Heart Health Study. *Journal of the American Heart Association, 10*(7), Article e016201. https://doi.org/10.1161/JAHA.120.016201

Yang, S.-Y., Lan, S.-J., Yen, Y.-Y., Hsieh, Y.-P., Kung, P.-T., & Lan, S.-H. (2020). Effects of exercise on sleep quality in pregnant women: A systematic review and meta-analysis of randomized controlled trials. *Asian Nursing Research, 14*(1), 1–10. https://doi.org/10.1016/j.anr.2020.01.003

Yeghiazarians, Y., Jneid, H., Tietjens, J. R., Redline, S., Brown, D. L., El-Sherif, N., Mehra, R., Bozkurt, B., Ndumele, C. E., & Somers, V. K.; on behalf of the American Heart Association Council on Clinical Cardiology; Council on Peripheral Vascular Disease; Council on Arteriosclerosis, Thrombosis and Vascular Biology; Council on Cardiopulmonary, Critical Care, Perioperative and Resuscitation; Stroke Council; and Council on Cardiovascular Surgery and Anesthesia. (2021). Obstructive sleep apnea and cardiovascular disease: A scientific statement from the American Heart Association. *Circulation, 144*(3), e56–e67. https://doi.org/10.1161/CIR.0000000000000988

Yin, J., Jin, X., Shan, Z., Li, S., Huang, H., Li, P., Peng, X., Peng, Z., Yu, K., Bao, W., Yang, W., Chen, X., & Liu, L. (2017). Relationship of sleep duration with all-cause mortality and cardiovascular events: A systematic review and dose-response meta-analysis of prospective cohort studies. *Journal of the American Heart Association, 6*(9), Article e005947. https://doi.org/10.1161/JAHA.117.005947

Yuan, Y., Heizhati, M., Wang, L., Li, M., Lin, M., Gan, L., Cai, X., Yang, W., Yao, L., Wang, Z., Abudereyimu, R., & Li, N. (2021). Poor sleep quality is associated with new-onset hypertension in a diverse young and middle-aged population. *Sleep Medicine, 88*, 189–196. https://doi.org/10.1016/j.sleep.2021.10.021

Yuhas, M., Moore, C. F., Garay, J., & Brown, S. D. (2022). Improving maternal cardiovascular health in underserved populations: A narrative review of behavioral intervention trials targeting postpartum weight retention. *Current Atherosclerosis Reports, 24*(9), 689–699. https://doi.org/10.1007/s11883-022-01045-3
Zhu, B., Wang, Y., Yuan, J., Mu, Y., Chen, P., Srimoragot, M., Li, Y., Park, C. G., & Reutrakul, S. (2022). Associations between sleep variability and cardiometabolic health: A systematic review. *Sleep Medicine Reviews, 66*, Article 101688. https://doi.org/10.1016/j.smrv.2022.101688

CHAPTER

15 Sleep, Social Inequalities, and Societal Costs

Mari Hysing, Tormod Bøe, *and* Børge Sivertsen

Abstract

This chapter describes how socioeconomic status (SES) is associated with sleep characteristics and sleep problems. Core markers of SES, such as income, occupation, and educational level, are associated with both the quality and quantity of sleep throughout different life stages. The chapter also describes different mechanisms that may be important in explaining the social gradient in sleep from early childhood to adulthood. Furthermore, the chapter illustrates how the social inequalities in sleep exist across the globe, including low- to middle-income countries. It also describes how sleep not only may be a consequence of social disadvantage but also may drive future socioeconomic disparities, for both individuals and the society.

Key Words: social gradient, social inequality, sleep disparity, societal cost, socioeconomic status

Introduction

Systematic health inequalities are present across a range of health indicators during the life span and exist both between social strata and between countries or regions. In the current chapter, we will review core markers of socioeconomic status (SES), such as income, occupation, and education level, and how these are linked to the quality and quantity of sleep. Taking a life-span perspective, we will begin by investigating social inequalities in sleep in childhood, adolescence, and adulthood and describe mechanisms that are important in the different life stages. We will then take a more global perspective on the social gradient in sleep, examining sleep in low- to middle-income countries (LMICs) and which mechanisms may drive the association in these settings. Finally, we will discuss how impaired sleep not only may be a consequence of social disadvantage but also may drive future socioeconomic disparities, for both individuals and the society.

Sleep and Social Inequalities in Children

The literature demonstrating how different markers of family or parental SES may be associated with sleep problems in children and adolescents has increased. Figure 15.1 illustrates

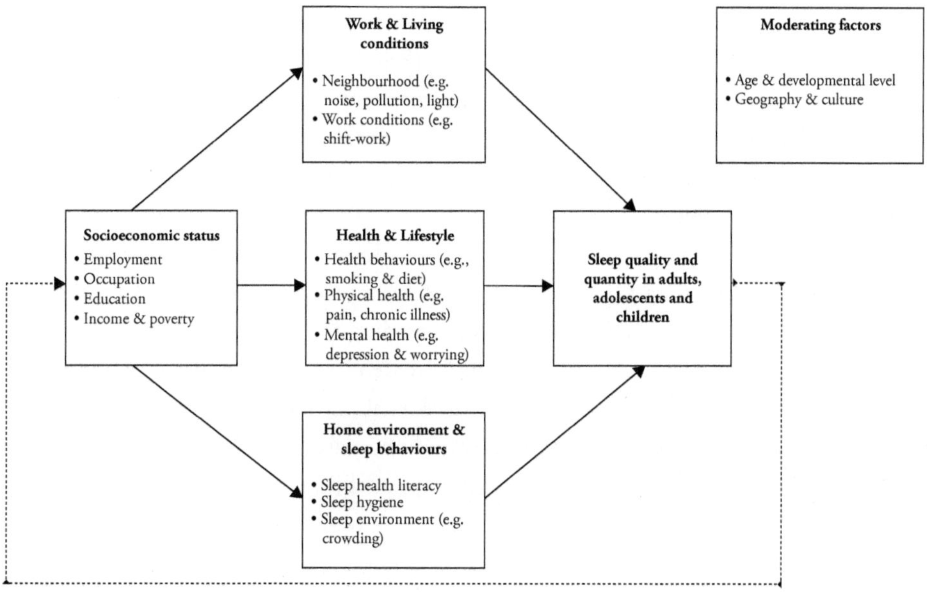

Figure 15.1 A model of the relationship between markers of socioeconomic status and sleep and possible mechanisms and moderators

the complex relationship between SES and sleep, as well as potential mechanisms and moderators this chapter will focus on. For infants and children, SES is determined based on their parents' educational level or occupation or according to their parents' income or the level of income in their family household. These can be aggregated into composite measures. In a systematic review of several risk factors for sleep problems among preschool and early school-aged children, six studies using such composite measure of SES were identified (Newton et al., 2020). Low SES was significantly associated with shorter sleep duration, sleep onset problems, as well as parent-reported sleep problems, thereby supporting low SES as a general risk factor across sleep indicators.

There are also indications that it may be fruitful to examine different markers of social inequity separately, rather than employing a composite SES measure, when studying the SES–sleep link in young childhood. This is exactly what Cameron et al. (2022) did in the so far only meta-analysis of different SES markers and subjectively measured sleep in children, identifying a total of 46 studies. The overall conclusion from this meta-analysis was that the associations differed substantially according to which marker of SES and outcome of sleep was examined. For example, higher parental education was significantly associated with longer child sleep duration but not sleep problems. Conversely, family income was only related to sleep problems and not sleep duration, suggesting that there may be specific associations for different sleep outcomes. Most of the studies investigating sleep have used questionnaire-based assessments with parents as informants. This may give rise to biases, and a meta-analysis of objective actigraphic measurement of sleep confirmed a consistent association between the different SES markers and sleep parameters, supporting the robustness of the social gradient in sleep (Etindele Sosso et al., 2021).

Improved knowledge of the pathways and mechanisms through which SES impacts sleep may give us a deeper understanding of the complex associations, as well as point to possible targets for preventive interventions. For infants and children, parental sleep health literacy and parental behavior recommended to promote child sleep may be such driving factors. For example, bedsharing has been found to be more prevalent among lower educated mothers, and bedsharing has also been prospectively linked to more sleep problems (Nulty et al., 2022). Regular bedtime, reading for the child before going to bed, and having the child fall asleep in their own bed were more common among high-SES families in a study of British preschoolers (Patrick et al., 2016). Similarly, low sleep health literacy has been shown to be more prevalent among parents with low SES, and poorer sleep health literacy was also associated with a range of child sleep problems (Bonuck et al., 2016). Sleep-promoting behavior and routines that were less frequent among families with low education in a large-scale study of preschoolers included regular bedtime and bedtime routines, especially interactive bedtime routines such as storytelling and reading.

A higher level of sleep problems, including later bedtimes, longer sleep onset latency, and shorter nocturnal sleep duration, was more prevalent among children living in communities with socioeconomic disadvantage, as demonstrated in a large US study based on data from a sleep app (Williamson et al., 2021). That study also showed that these families were less likely to have consistent bedtime routines. However, the parents from socioeconomically disadvantaged areas were also less likely to perceive sleep problems and more likely to be confident in managing sleep. Given the importance of parental perception of child sleep problems in help-seeking behavior, this distinction is important but also requires further exploration. For instance, whether these differences indicate underreporting in the disadvantaged areas or overreporting in the more prosperous areas remains uncertain. Further, implementing behavior may be difficult in an insecure and unpredictable everyday life. Families with housing insecurity and food insecurity were, for example, less likely to implement bedtime routines among toddlers (Covington et al., 2019). Using an observer-based method of family chaos, it was found that both the physical organization of the house and parents' ability to manage intrusions mediated the association between family SES and actigraphy-measured sleep among children entering kindergarten (Fronberg et al., 2022).

Other mechanisms may not be as easily modifiable through interventions, such as some unfavorable sleep environments. The quality of the physical home environment was identified as a significant pathway between socioeconomic disparity and actigraphy-measured sleep in a socioeconomically diverse sample of children (Doane et al., 2019). A similar association was found in a study of toddlers, confirming the importance of some sleep environment factors, including comfort, cleanliness, and noise and light levels of the child's sleep space, as pathways between SES and sleep problems in young children, in addition to bedtime routines (Hoyniak et al., 2021). While the strongest associations between SES and sleep are found at the parental and family levels, more distant indicators of social deprivation may also influence sleep. In a systematic review and meta-analysis of eight studies including nearly 70,000 participants, Tomfohr-Madsen et al. (2020) found poorer neighborhood SES to be associated with shorter sleep duration in children. Families in disadvantaged neighborhoods with high crime rates could influence infant sleep through maternal perceptions of safety, as shown in a study of families with 12-month-old children (MacKinnon et al., 2021). This also indicates how the mothers' mental health may influence sleep in these settings. Knowing, for instance, that the rate of postpartum depression is higher among mothers with low SES (Goyal et al., 2010) and that postpartum depression is associated with sleep problems in infants (Gress-Smith et al., 2012), this may be an overlooked but important pathway between SES and sleep in infants.

Thus, preventive interventions need to target multiple levels, spanning from the family to the broader society. The observed social inequity in sleep hygiene behavior may be one such modifiable risk factor that may be easily targeted. In an intervention study aimed at increasing sleep health literacy, the observed effects were similar across educational backgrounds (Jones et al., 2013).

Sleep and Social Inequalities in Adolescents

Adolescent sleep and its link to SES has received less focus, at least compared to the above literature on younger children. The lack of well-conducted studies focusing on adolescents was also evident in the systematic review of how SES was related to actigraphy-measured sleep (Etindele Sosso et al., 2021), with only one or two studies providing data on adolescents, precluding subgroup meta-analyses for adolescents. There are some studies that have examined the social gradient of self-reported sleep in adolescents, including a large-scale study of Norwegian adolescents which found a consistent association across multiple SES indicators and sleep parameters (Hysing et al., 2016). Insomnia was more frequent among adolescents who had less educated parents or parents who were outside the workforce and in adolescents who perceived their economic well-being to be poorer than that of others. Adolescents from lower socioeconomic backgrounds also had shorter sleep duration, later bedtimes, and larger weekday–weekend differences compared to peers with higher SES. However, such clear associations are not always consistent across studies. For instance, inadequate sleep was found to be more prevalent among adolescents from high-SES families in a nationally representative survey in the United States, and this social pattern of sleep became even more pronounced with age (Hawkins & Takeuchi, 2016).

Mirroring the complex patterns described above for studies on children, a study encompassing both children and adolescents (from age 8 to 16 years; Jarrin et al., 2014) showed that while all three SES markers (parental income and education and subjective SES) influenced most sleep parameters among the children in the sample, with income and education showing the strongest associations; subgroup analyses of the adolescents showed that poorer subjective SES was strongly associated with poorer sleep quality and parent-reported sleep quality, also after adjusting for parental income and education.

A possible differential impact of the various markers of SES was suggested in a study using actigraphy-measured sleep of middle adolescents in the United States (Marco et al., 2011). While the timing and consistency of school-night sleep were associated with parental SES and sleep hygiene practices, weekend sleep was additionally associated with the neighborhood-level SES, including a busier street environment. The importance of the adolescents' own perceived economic well-being was also confirmed in a study of young adolescents, including almost 6,000 11–13-year-old participants from the Bergen Child Study. In that study, it was found that children who perceived their family to have poorer economic well-being had significantly higher odds of reporting difficulties initiating and/or maintaining sleep and short time-in-bed, compared to peers with better perceived economic well-being (Bøe et al., 2012). The importance of the adolescents' own perception of SES may be an indication of both the development of a personal SES, independent of the family, as well as the factors that contribute to sleep during adolescence.

The importance of pre-sleep arousal, worry, and mood in understanding social disparities in sleep also points to the central role of mental health when addressing the SES–sleep link. Mental health shows a consistent social gradient (Quon & McGrath, 2014), and sleep can be viewed as a transdiagnostic factor for mental health problems (Harvey et al., 2011). The understanding of how the bidirectional association between mental health and sleep is influenced by SES is still in its infancy. Some mental health pathways have been explored. For example, pre-sleep worry is a strong driver of common sleep problems, including the long sleep onset latency and insomnia that characterize adolescence (Bagley et al., 2015). Pre-sleep worry, along with somatic and cognitive arousal, is a well-established risk factors for low sleep efficiency and prolonged sleep onset latency. These factors may be particularly significant for adolescents, especially those from low socioeconomic backgrounds. This was demonstrated in a study of adolescents which included measures of both pre-sleep worries and arousal. In that study, the authors concluded that in the context of better pre-sleep conditions and fewer environmental disturbances, sleep health disparities would be reduced or eliminated (McWood et al., 2022). And importantly, family concerns were a risk factor specifically for low-SES youth. Similarly, low-SES youth may be more prone to the negative effect of poor sleep on poor mood the next day (Kouros et al., 2022). Thus, low-SES youth may both have a higher rate of cognitive and emotional risk factors for poor sleep and be more sensitive to their impact on sleep.

In addition to cognitive arousal, physiological arousal before bedtime may be of importance. Stressors related to low SES could increase physiological activation; the functioning of the hypothalamic–pituitary–adrenal axis has been hypothesized to be a mediator between SES and adolescent sleep, but the evidence to date is scarce and inconclusive (Rocha et al., 2022).

While adolescents are in the process of establishing their own SES and have increased independence, family-level factors are still influential during adolescence. For instance, family chaos, noise, unpredictability, and interruptions in the family environment were more prevalent among low-SES youth in a longitudinal study of adolescence; and this mediated the association between family SES and adolescents' sleep (Philbrook et al., 2020). That study also examined sleep problems that are especially frequent at that age, such as insomnia and delayed sleep phase, and how family environment exacerbated these sleep problems. Sleep hygiene practices may also be affected by living conditions, related to both crowdedness and household rules. For instance, adolescents in low-SES families have been shown to be more likely to have TVs in their bedroom, which again is related to poor sleep (Barr-Anderson et al., 2008). Further, having rules regarding sleep-related practices, such as bedtimes and caffeine intake, has also been shown to be less common among parents with lower education and would expectedly be related to poorer sleep habits among the adolescents (Buxton et al., 2015).

Sleep and Social Inequalities in Adults

A social gradient in sleep in adults is robustly present across most markers of SES, including educational level, work affiliation, and household income, and has been demonstrated in studies employing both subjective and objective measures of sleep (Etindele Sosso et al., 2022; Lallukka et al., 2012). For example, income, lower educational level, living in rented housing, and unemployment were consistently associated with reporting sleep problems more than four times a week among more than 8,500 adult participants in the British Psychiatric Morbidity Survey 2000 (Arber et al., 2009). This pattern was also observed in a longitudinal study that investigated sleep duration trajectories over 10 years, which found higher odds of more suboptimal sleep trajectories across individual SES indicators and neighborhood-level SES (Nyarko et al., 2023). Whereas most studies find poorer sleep among those with lower SES, the mechanisms through which sleep may be impaired may be differently associated across different SES markers.

Lower educational level has been linked to poorer self-reported sleep quality and symptoms of insomnia in multiple studies (Moore et al., 2002; Stewart et al., 2006). The educational gradient in sleep problems has been associated with sleep health literacy, as mentioned in relation to children, but may also be related to awareness of strategies of how to improve sleep in adults. Other SES-related barriers may be of a more structural nature, effectively hindering the implementation of sound sleep hygiene principles. Crowding, where families share bedrooms, may cause family members to disturb each other's sleep, while disturbances from noisy neighbors may be a larger problem in poor-quality housing and in apartment buildings where noise may travel more easily. A noisy sleep environment may cause sleep to become more fragmented, delay the onset of sleep, and contribute to early awakenings. In a study of more than 2,000 US Hispanic/Latino adults, those who lived in a noisy neighborhood had higher risk of insomnia compared to those who lived in non-noisy neighborhoods (Simonelli et al., 2016). Excessive light exposure has been associated with shorter sleep duration (Xiao et al., 2020), which is likely influenced by depressed melatonin secretion delaying initiation of sleep and prolonging sleep onset latency. In addition to poor urban neighborhoods having more artificial light at night, the association has been shown to be stronger in this setting (Xiao et al., 2020). Residents in disadvantaged neighborhoods are also more often exposed to air pollution, and in a study of almost 2,000 US adults, higher exposure to air pollution was associated with a 60% increased odds of sleep apnea (Billings et al., 2019). These environmental risk factors are often investigated in isolation, while they often will appear in concert. For instance, in urban and poor neighborhoods, these risk factors may often be interlinked, and thus increase the negative impact on sleep. In addition to these environmental factors that may be pathways from neighborhood-level disadvantaged communities, psychological factors may be an important mechanism. For example, neighborhood-level crime rates and social cohesion were associated with sleep characteristics, and part of these associations could be explained by psychological distress (Kim et al., 2022).

Living conditions were also found to be the most important moderators in a review of studies investigating SES and polysomnography-measured sleep in adults (Etindele Sosso, 2022). The central role of living conditions in sleep health disparities was also confirmed in a study of short sleep duration in relation to SES (Stamatakis et al., 2007), where also more proximal health risk factors accounted for some of these associations, suggesting the importance of other health conditions. A social gradient in health is evident across multiple health parameters, as well as lifestyle behaviors that increase the risk of poor health (Petrovic et al., 2018). Lifestyle behaviors may thus be likely candidates for factors that can account for some of the social gradients in sleep. While a large-scale study did find that lifestyle behaviors, such as smoking, did mediate part of the association, poor somatic health accounted for more of the co-occurrence of low SES and sleep problems (Arber et al., 2009). Similarly, with poor health being more frequent among low-SES adults in a large-scale German study, these other health problems also partly mediated the observed social gradient found in sleep (Lallukka et al., 2012). Pain is also more prevalent in disadvantaged communities, closely related to sleep problems. Using neighborhood-level SES indicators, one study suggested that pain was more closely related to sleep problems for those in disadvantaged communities (Rumble et al., 2021).

Other sleep disorders, such as sleep apnea, also show a consistent social gradient (Etindele Sosso & Matos, 2021), and body mass index partly mediated the SES–sleep apnea link in a population-based study (Petrovic et al., 2019). Thus, sleep apnea may be one of the sleep disorders where behavior may be important for sleep health disparities. However, while consistent associations between low SES and both short sleep duration and insomnia were found in the same population as described above, the authors did not find that these associations were mediated by any lifestyle or behavioral factors (Stringhini et al., 2015). Furthermore, given the strong association between the type of occupation and various sleep problems, it is likely that work-related variables may be even more important to investigate further. For example, an unstable work schedule, which is more common in low-SES groups, is one important risk factor for sleep problems (Stringhini et al., 2015); and shift work and psychosocial stress at work have been found to account for some of the difference in sleep patterns across SES in a Japanese study (Sekine et al., 2006), further highlighting the importance of occupational work factors in such studies. However, some work-related SES indicators may not show the standard social gradient. In a recent review, employment showed a differential association to sleep duration compared to the other investigated indicators, such as education and subjective SES, with shorter sleep duration among those employed (Papadopoulos & Etindele Sosso, 2022). This is not unexpected, given that work life often includes early-morning start times and routines that may impede sleep duration.

Changes in SES

We have focused on concurrent associations between sleep and SES. However, a static perspective may be insufficient to cover how SES may shape future health, as well as the fluctuating and complex aspects of SES. In a systematic review of 80 articles on the association between impact of changes in SES and children and adolescent health, the authors found a consistent pattern of improved health and functioning with increased income and deteriorating health with reductions in income (Levesque et al., 2021). However, only one of the included studies had investigated sleep as an outcome. This was a study that investigated childhood poverty and adolescent sleep, using registry data on family income linked to a population-based study (Sivertsen, Bøe, et al., 2017). Downward social mobility was associated with more adolescent sleep problems, including short sleep duration, lower sleep efficiency, and more nocturnal awakenings, even more so than for those who were in a chronically poor group. Potential mechanisms for these findings were not certain, and depressive symptoms could only account for some of the observed associations.

Sleep and Social Inequalities Across the Globe

Taking a bird's-eye view on the social gradient of sleep problems and patterns across the globe, sleep health epidemiology for LMICs is a starting point. In a meta-analysis of sleep duration and sleep quality for adults in LMICs, the large variability across the 50 included studies and substantial bias impeded any firm conclusion, mainly caused by a notable lack of high-quality studies and nearly half of the included studies being based on middle-income countries, such as China and Brazil (Simonelli et al., 2018). The lack of firm conclusions may also be related to the fact that the term *LMIC* covers such diverse countries culturally, geographically, and sociodemographically that one common estimate is not realistic; and we need to address sleep health in more defined populations. Indeed, some studies in more narrowly defined populations have shown support for more impaired sleep health in LMICs. For example, a population-based study among adults in Sri Lanka found a short mean sleep duration of 6 hours as measured by actigraphy (Schokman et al., 2018). And in a meta-analysis of sleep health epidemiology in Ethiopia including nine studies, the pooled estimate of poor sleep quality was 53%, suggesting a high rate of sleep problems (Manzar et al., 2020). The sleep pattern may also be qualitatively different and not directly comparable to that in high-income countries (HICs). Using data from a large-scale Brazilian population, this was exemplified by a shift in rhythms for infants and preschoolers, with later bedtimes and later wake-up times, and even more so for families with higher SES (Patrick et al., 2016).

There are also large differences across regions, populations, and demographic characteristics, with substantial changes over time. For instance, the urban poor in LMICs may be one high-risk group that is on the rise due to urbanization (Bessone et al., 2021). Furthermore, LMICs are particularly vulnerable to climate change–related disasters and the consequences of climate change when they occur, with poor sleep health being one of many negative health outcomes (Rifkin et al., 2018). Climate-related disasters may have both direct consequences, such as poor sleeping conditions due to forced displacement, and indirect consequences through a likely increase of post-traumatic stress disorder and depression, two mental disorders with sleep problems as core symptoms (Sharpe & Davison, 2021).

To further understand such sleep disparities, investigating factors that drive this pattern may be a fruitful approach. The populations in the least developed countries are likely to have both a higher rate of established risk factors for sleep problems relative to HICs as well as more unique risk factors that arise from poverty in these settings, including biological, psychological, cultural, and environmental risks. With regard to environmental risk factors, living in impoverished conditions and the sleep environment itself may lead to both sleep deprivation and lower sleep quality. Among an urban poor population in India, sleep efficiency was low, and the participants reported a range of barriers to sleep, such as heat, noise, and light that interrupted their sleep (Bessone et al., 2021). Some of these risk factors may also be on the rise. For example, heat impedes sleep, and climate change will give rise to increasing nighttime temperatures, which again may lead to sleep loss (Obradovich et al., 2017). This will disproportionately affect poor populations since many do not have the resources for proper housing and air conditioning or other measures for temperature regulation. Further, the basic needs of being in an environment which is safe and without disturbances may be violated in certain impoverished areas (Simonelli et al., 2015). In a study of perceived neighborhood safety and sleep quality in six LMICs, it was found that a lack of feeling safe from violence and crime was strongly associated with insomnia symptoms, moderately with sleepiness, and inconsistently with shorter sleep duration (Hill et al., 2016). For farmers, the use of pesticides may be a specific risk factor for sleep problems, as indicated in a study of Ugandan farmers in a low-income context with an exposure-dependent risk of sleep problems in relation to pesticide use (Fuhrimann et al., 2022). There may also be unique sleep environments for some groups, such as in a study of rural and Indigenous families in Ghana, where children who lived in houses without electricity had longer actigraphy-measured sleep duration compared to children in houses with electricity (Kundel et al., 2022).

Crowded sleep environments, including room sharing and bedsharing with other family members, may also be a result of poverty, as well as cultural practices which may impact sleep. This was investigated using actigraphy-measured sleep in Congo. Both the quantity and quality of sleep were poorer on nights with more crowded sleeping conditions (Gettler et al., 2022). For many families, crowded sleeping areas, which often include combined kitchen and sleeping accommodation due to limited space, are also related to another associated risk factor for sleep: indoor air pollution due to solid fuels used for cooking (Yu, 2020). The association between solid fuels and sleep disturbances has been shown across multiple populations, including China, and becomes even stronger the longer the participants are exposed to the air pollution (Yu, 2020). Indeed, intervention studies have shown that reducing solid fuel use has significant sleep benefits, as demonstrated in a study of Peruvian children where symptoms of sleep apnea were reduced when changing the stove, leading to a reduction in biomass pollution (Castañeda et al., 2013).

Malnutrition in LMICs is a well-established biological risk factor for development in general and is also related to poor sleep (Cheruku et al., 2002). Stunted children, a hallmark sign of malnutrition, have been shown to have shorter parent-reported nighttime sleep and total sleep compared to their better-nourished peers (Kordas et al., 2008). A randomized controlled trial (RCT) in Nepal and Zanzibar showed improved sleep in children at high risk for iron deficiency after receiving micronutrient supplementation (Kordas et al., 2009). However, other nutritional interventions in this setting have not led to improved sleep, such as an RCT on vitamin B_{12} in stunted children in Nepal (Hysing et al., 2022). While malnutrition is an important risk factor for poor health in LMICs, obesity is another growing public health problem in these settings. One example is Nepal, showing an increase in obesity with related increases in sleep apnea and sleep problems (Singh et al., 2021). Other lifestyle factors that are related to sleep may also be important in these settings, which was highlighted in a study from Indonesia showing that the high rate of smoking was associated with sleep disturbances and concluding that this could be a target for preventive interventions (Sujarwoto, 2020).

Mental health and sleep problems have a strong bidirectional association, and this is also the case in LMICs (Khadka et al., 2020). The high rate of mental health problems and related burden of disease of mental disorders in LMICs may give rise to sleep problems, which in turn may further exacerbate mental health problems. The consequences of these co-occurring problems on daily functioning may be especially concerning, given that the co-occurrence between sleep and depression has been shown to be related to risk of decrements in health among community-dwelling adults in 46 LMICs (Stickley et al., 2019).

To adequately identify and address sleep problems, sleep health literacy among the population needs to be taken into consideration. For instance, large-scale interventions focusing on safe sleeping environments have been effective at reducing sudden infant death syndrome. In some areas, knowledge about safe sleeping environments, including sleeping positions, is low in the population, as shown in studies from both Brazil (Cesar et al., 2019) and Ecuador (Feld et al., 2021). However, this may be improved through sleep education, as demonstrated by an educational intervention for mothers which increased the rate of infants sleeping in the supine position in Brazil (Issler et al., 2009). How interventions need to be adapted to the specific needs, knowledge gaps, and sleep health status of the population was also exemplified in randomized study on adults' sleep in Chennai, India, where increasing nocturnal sleep did not show detectable improvements in productivity and daytime functioning, while short afternoon naps did improve productivity in cognition and psychological well-being (Bessone et al., 2021).

Interventions may also need to address the barriers to sleep health that are present in that population and may differ from HICs, for example, by assuring that basic requirements for sleep-friendly environments are available. An intervention aimed at improving housing in a slum was associated with improved sleep quality, which was facilitated by a feeling of safety after the house upgrade (Simonelli et al., 2013). Thus, sleep interventions to reduce sleep disparity on both a population-based level and an individual level need to consider the context.

Societal Costs of Sleep Problems

While sleep problems, as demonstrated, may represent an important consequence of different socioeconomic markers, the opposite directionality has also been explored, that is, to what extent sleep problems may serve as a risk factor for socioeconomic or societal outcomes.

From a health-related outlook, the many adverse consequences of sleep problems are well documented. If left untreated, insomnia strongly increases the risk of developing a wide range of common conditions and diseases and is also linked to reduced quality of life. Also, beyond studies demonstrating cross-sectional and prospective links to a variety of health outcomes, there is now a growing body of evidence showing how sleep problems represent an independent risk factor for several adverse occupational outcomes. The combination of high prevalence of sleep problems with the potential severity of consequences suggests that sleep problems indeed do have a societal cost. Although the overarching term *sleep problems* encompasses a variety of disorders and complaints related to sleep, most of the literature on societal costs has been limited to insomnia and, to some extent, obstructive sleep apnea. As such, the following text will mainly focus on the costs related to insomnia or symptoms of insomnia.

In terms of the monetary aspect of societal costs, providing accurate estimates of the economic burden of insomnia is not an easy task; and most approaches suffer from some methodological restrictions, potentially limiting the generalizability of the findings (Bolge et al., 2009; Ozminkowski et al., 2007; Swanson et al., 2011). One common approach is to divide the costs into direct and indirect costs (Drummond & McGuire, 2001). While direct costs include the consumption of resources (assessment and treatments), indirect costs mainly relate to the loss of resources. It has also been suggested that a third group of costs should be distinguished, so-called intangible costs. These costs may be of a non-financial nature, and thereby more difficult to quantify or estimate.

The direct costs of insomnia typically include prescription medications, healthcare consultations aimed at the sleep problem (live or virtual), and various over-the-counter products (including alcohol) as a sleep aid. Indirect costs mainly encompass reduced workplace productivity (presenteeism), short- and long-term absenteeism (missing scheduled work time), and permanent work disability. While some studies have specifically focused on either treatment costs or risk or work disability, a few studies have also provided detailed monetary estimates of the direct, indirect, and total costs of insomnia.

In terms of the latter, a Canadian study by Daley and colleagues (2009) estimated the total costs of insomnia per year in the province of Quebec to be CA$6.6 billion, which equates to 1.3% of the gross domestic product in Quebec. In that study, specifically designed to assess several detailed aspects of direct and indirect costs, the authors demonstrated that the indirect costs far superseded the direct costs, with lost productivity comprising by far the largest proportion (76%) of all costs. Relatedly, Kessler and colleagues (2011) provided a detailed analysis of the work-related costs of insomnia, showing that presenteeism (i.e., attending work while ill) accounted for about two-thirds of the lost work performance, whereas absenteeism (i.e., missed work due to illness) accounted for the remainder. In all, that study concluded that the annual loss of work performance caused by insomnia in the United States amounted to US$63.2 billion per year, after accounting for comorbid conditions.

Not focusing specifically on the monetary loss of untreated insomnia, some earlier studies, mainly from the Nordic countries, demonstrated how insomnia has important occupational consequences. Employing large data sets from the general adult population, these studies showed how insomnia may be associated with subsequent absenteeism, including both sick leave and permanent work disability. Using strong methodological designs, which include linkages between large epidemiological health surveys and official employment registries, insomnia has been established as a strong risk factor for work disability as indicated by sickness absence (Rahkonen et al., 2012; Sivertsen, Overland, Bjorvatn, et al., 2009) and disability retirement (Lallukka et al., 2011; Salo et al., 2010; Sivertsen et al., 2006; Sivertsen, Overland, Pallesen, et al., 2009). In fact, in a study comparing the predictive effect of insomnia and depression in relation to subsequent work disability, Sivertsen, Overland, Pallesen, et al. (2009) found that insomnia had an equally important and independent role, further suggesting that insomnia may be an underappreciated problem in terms of the ability to remain in the workforce.

However, such findings are not limited to the adult population, and recent studies have now turned their focus on the equivalence of work affiliation in adolescence, namely school attendance. Sleep problems in adolescence represent a public health concern in their own right, both because the prevalence increases sharply following puberty (Sivertsen, Harvey, et al., 2017) and because they are associated with several health-related problems and increased use of healthcare services (Cousins et al., 2011; Roberts et al., 2008). As for adults, the link between sleep problems and school/work attendance is likely bidirectional. On the one hand, a Danish community study found high rates of sleep problems in children and adolescents with school absence behavior (Egger et al., 2003), which may be explained by school obligations possibly disrupting the sleep–wake cycle. On the other hand, a large population-based study linked with objective register data on school attendance showed a clear dose–response association between several sleep parameters (insomnia, sleep duration, sleep deficit, etc.) and subsequent register-based days of school absence, even after controlling for mental health (Hysing et al., 2015). Relatedly, adolescents with delayed sleep phase have also been shown to have increased risk of school non-attendance (Sivertsen et al., 2013). As such, these studies on adolescents mirror the functional importance of sleep in adults, where sick leave and work absence represent the occupational consequences.

The literature covered in this chapter shows the consistent social gradient in sleep health across the life span. The associations are complex and nuanced, differing both across SES indicators and with different types of sleep characteristics and sleep problems. Further, the nature of the associations changes through developmental periods, as demonstrated in both the various aspects of SES as well as the developmentally pertinent sleep indicators at that time. Similarly, the mechanisms that drive the association, although wide-ranging from micro to macro levels, show developmental changes. It is important to understand these associations globally, taking into consideration the unique risk factors in LMICs and being mindful of cultural differences in sleep behavior. Further, we are just starting to unravel these complex associations and their drivers, and we still need more and more high-quality studies before we can fully understand how social inequities impact sleep across development. The importance of enhancing our understanding of the social gradient in health is underpinned by the gross negative outcomes on the individual and societal levels.

Conclusion

In the current chapter we have demonstrated how core markers of SES, including income, occupation, and education level, are linked to quality and quantity of sleep. We have shown that social inequalities in sleep exist in childhood, adolescence, and adulthood and that different mechanisms may be more important across different life stages. We have also shown how social inequality in sleep is present across the globe, focusing on risk factors in LMICs. Finally, we have briefly outlined the social costs that are linked to untreated sleep problems.

Future Directions

Future studies should further investigate the mechanisms that drive social inequality in sleep, and there is also a need for more knowledge on the effect of preventive intervention to combat sleep inequalities. Most of the studies are conducted in Western HICs, and more knowledge on sleep disparities and related risks and consequences in LMICs is called for.

References

Arber, S., Bote, M., & Meadows, R. (2009). Gender and socio-economic patterning of self-reported sleep problems in Britain. *Social Science & Medicine, 68*(2), 281–289. https://doi.org/10.1016/j.socscimed.2008.10.016

Bagley, E. J., Kelly, R. J., Buckhalt, J. A., & El-Sheikh, M. (2015). What keeps low-SES children from sleeping well: The role of presleep worries and sleep environment. *Sleep Medicine, 16*(4), 496–502. https://doi.org/10.1016/j.sleep.2014.10.008

Barr-Anderson, D. J., van den Berg, P., Neumark-Sztainer, D., & Story, M. (2008). Characteristics associated with older adolescents who have a television in their bedrooms. *Pediatrics, 121*(4), 718–724. https://doi.org/10.1542/peds.2007-1546

Bessone, P., Rao, G., Schilbach, F., Schofield, H., & Toma, M. (2021). The economic consequences of increasing sleep among the urban poor. *Quarterly Journal of Economics, 136*(3), 1887–1941.

Billings, M. E., Gold, D., Szpiro, A., Aaron, C. P., Jorgensen, N., Gassett, A., Leary, P. J., Kaufman, J. D., & Redline, S. R. (2019). The association of ambient air pollution with sleep apnea: The Multi-Ethnic Study of Atherosclerosis. *Annals of the American Thorac Society, 16*(3), 363–370. https://doi.org/10.1513/AnnalsATS.201804-248OC

Bøe, T., Hysing, M., Stormark, K. M., Lundervold, A. J., & Sivertsen, B. (2012). Sleep problems as a mediator of the association between parental education levels, perceived family economy and poor mental health in children. *Journal of Psychosomatic Research, 73*(6), 430–436. https://doi.org/10.1016/j.jpsychores.2012.09.008

Bolge, S. C., Doan, J. F., Kannan, H., & Baran, R. W. (2009). Association of insomnia with quality of life, work productivity, and activity impairment. *Quality of Life Research, 18*(4), 415–422. https://doi.org/10.1007/s11136-009-9462-6

Bonuck, K. A., Schwartz, B., & Schechter, C. (2016). Sleep health literacy in Head Start families and staff: Exploratory study of knowledge, motivation, and competencies to promote healthy sleep. *Sleep Health, 2*(1), 19–24. https://doi.org/10.1016/j.sleh.2015.12.002

Buxton, O. M., Chang, A. M., Spilsbury, J. C., Bos, T., Emsellem, H., & Knutson, K. L. (2015). Sleep in the modern family: Protective family routines for child and adolescent sleep. *Sleep Health, 1*(1), 15–27. https://doi.org/10.1016/j.sleh.2014.12.002

Cameron, E. E., Watts, D., Silang, K., Dhillon, A., Sohal, P. R., MacKinnon, A. L., Roos, L. E., & Tomfohr-Madsen, L. M. (2022). Parental socioeconomic status and childhood sleep: A systematic review and meta-analysis. *Sleep Epidemiology, 2*, 100047.

Castañeda, J. L., Kheirandish-Gozal, L., Gozal, D., & Accinelli, R. A.; & Pampa Cangallo Instituto de Investigaciones de la Altura Research Group. (2013). Effect of reductions in biomass fuel exposure on symptoms of sleep apnea in children living in the peruvian andes: A preliminary field study. *Pediatric Pulmonology, 48*(10), 996–999.

Cesar, J. A., Marmitt, L. P., Carpena, M. X., Pereira, F. G., Neto, J. D. M., Neumann, N. A., & Acevedo, J. D. (2019). Maternal knowledge and unsafe baby sleep position: A cross-sectional survey in Southern Brazil. *Maternal and Child Health Journal, 23*(2), 183–190.

Cheruku, S. R., Montgomery-Downs, H. E., Farkas, S. L., Thoman, E. B., & Lammi-Keefe, C. J. (2002). Higher maternal plasma docosahexaenoic acid during pregnancy is associated with more mature neonatal sleep-state patterning. *American Journal of Clinical Nutrition, 76*(3), 608–613. http://www.ncbi.nlm.nih.gov/pubmed/12198007

Cousins, J. C., Whalen, D. J., Dahl, R. E., Forbes, E. E., Olino, T. M., Ryan, N. D., & Silk, J. S. (2011). The bidirectional association between daytime affect and nighttime sleep in youth with anxiety and depression. *Journal of Pediatric Psychology, 36*(9), 969–979. https://doi.org/10.1093/jpepsy/jsr036

Covington, L. B., Rogers, V. E., Armstrong, B., Storr, C. L., & Black, M. M. (2019). Toddler bedtime routines and associations with nighttime sleep duration and maternal and household factors. *Journal of Clinical Sleep Medicine, 15*(6), 865–871. https://doi.org/10.5664/jcsm.7838

Daley, M., Morin, C. M., LeBlanc, M., Gregoire, J. P., & Savard, J. (2009). The economic burden of insomnia: Direct and indirect costs for individuals with insomnia syndrome, insomnia symptoms, and good sleepers. *Sleep, 32*(1), 55–64. https://www.ncbi.nlm.nih.gov/pubmed/19189779

Doane, L. D., Breitenstein, R. S., Beekman, C., Clifford, S., Smith, T. J., & Lemery-Chalfant, K. (2019). Early life socioeconomic disparities in children's sleep: The mediating role of the current home environment. *Journal of Youth and Adolescence, 48*(1), 56–70. https://doi.org/10.1007/s10964-018-0917-3

Drummond, M., & McGuire, A. (2001). *Economic evaluation in health care*. Oxford University Press.

Egger, H. L., Costello, E. J., & Angold, A. (2003). School refusal and psychiatric disorders: A community study. *Journal of the American Academy of Child & Adolescent Psychiatry, 42*(7), 797–807. https://doi.org/10.1097/01.CHI.0000046865.56865.79

Etindele Sosso, F. A. (2022). Measuring sleep health disparities with polysomnography: A systematic review of preliminary findings. *Clocks Sleep, 4*(1), 80–87. https://doi.org/10.3390/clockssleep4010009

Etindele Sosso, F. A., Holmes, S. D., & Weinstein, A. A. (2021). Influence of socioeconomic status on objective sleep measurement: A systematic review and meta-analysis of actigraphy studies. *Sleep Health, 7*(4), 417–428. https://doi.org/10.1016/j.sleh.2021.05.005

Etindele Sosso, F. A., Kreidlmayer, M., Pearson, D., & Bendaoud, I. (2022). Towards a socioeconomic model of sleep health among the Canadian population: A systematic review of the relationship between age, income, employment, education, social class, socioeconomic status and sleep disparities. *European Journal of Investigation in Health, Psychology and Education, 12*(8), 1143–1167. https://www.mdpi.com/2254-9625/12/8/80

Etindele Sosso, F. A., & Matos, E. (2021). Socioeconomic disparities in obstructive sleep apnea: A systematic review of empirical research. *Sleep and Breathing, 25*(4), 1729–1739.

Feld, H., Ceballos Osorio, J., Bahamonde, M., Young, T., Boada, P., & Rayens, M. K. (2021). Poverty and paternal education associated with infant safe sleep intentions in a peri-urban community in Ecuador. *Global Pediatric Health, 8*, Article 2333794X211044112.

Fronberg, K. M., Bai, S., & Teti, D. M. (2022). Household chaos mediates the link between family resources and child sleep. *Sleep Health, 8*(1), 121–129. https://doi.org/10.1016/j.sleh.2021.10.005

Fuhrimann, S., van den Brenk, I., Atuhaire, A., Mubeezi, R., Staudacher, P., Huss, A., & Kromhout, H. (2022). Recent pesticide exposure affects sleep: A cross-sectional study among smallholder farmers in Uganda. *Environment International, 158*, Article 106878. https://doi.org/10.1016/j.envint.2021.106878

Gettler, L. T., Samson, D. R., Kilius, E., Sarma, M. S., Ouamba, Y. R., Miegakanda, V., Boyette, A. H., & Lew-Levy, S. (2022). Links between household and family social dynamics with sleep profiles among BaYaka foragers of the Congo Basin. *Social Science & Medicine, 311*, Article 115345.

Goyal, D., Gay, C., & Lee, K. A. (2010). How much does low socioeconomic status increase the risk of prenatal and postpartum depressive symptoms in first-time mothers? *Women's Health Issues, 20*(2), 96–104. https://doi.org/10.1016/j.whi.2009.11.003

Gress-Smith, J. L., Luecken, L. J., Lemery-Chalfant, K., & Howe, R. (2012). Postpartum depression prevalence and impact on infant health, weight, and sleep in low-income and ethnic minority women and infants. *Maternal and Child Health Journal, 16*(4), 887–893. https://doi.org/10.1007/s10995-011-0812-y

Harvey, A. G., Murray, G., Chandler, R. A., & Soehner, A. (2011). Sleep disturbance as transdiagnostic: Consideration of neurobiological mechanisms. *Clinical Psychology Review, 31*(2), 225–235. https://doi.org/10.1016/j.cpr.2010.04.003

Hawkins, S. S., & Takeuchi, D. T. (2016). Social determinants of inadequate sleep in US children and adolescents. *Public Health, 138*, 119–126. https://doi.org/10.1016/j.puhe.2016.03.036

Hill, T. D., Trinh, H. N., Wen, M., & Hale, L. (2016). Perceived neighborhood safety and sleep quality: A global analysis of six countries. *Sleep Medicine, 18*, 56–60.

Hoyniak, C. P., Bates, J. E., McQuillan, M. E., Albert, L. E., Staples, A. D., Molfese, V. J., Rudasill, K. M., & Deater-Deckard, K. (2021). The family context of toddler sleep: Routines, sleep environment, and emotional security induction in the hour before bedtime. *Behavioral Sleep Medicine, 19*(6), 795–813. https://doi.org/10.1080/15402002.2020.1865356

Hysing, M., Haugland, S., Stormark, K. M., Bøe, T., & Sivertsen, B. (2015). Sleep and school attendance in adolescence: Results from a large population-based study. *Scandinavian Journal of Public Health, 43*(1), 2–9. https://doi.org/10.1177/1403494814556647

Hysing, M., Petrie, K. J., Bøe, T., Lallukka, T., & Sivertsen, B. (2016). The social gradient of sleep in adolescence: Results from the youth@hordaland survey. *European Journal of Public Health, 27*(1), 65–71. https://doi.org/10.1093/eurpub/ckw200

Hysing, M., Strand, T. A., Chandyo, R. K., Ulak, M., Ranjitkar, S., Schwinger, C., Shrestha, M., & Kvestad, I. (2022). The effect of vitamin B12-supplementation on actigraphy measured sleep pattern; a randomized control trial. *Clinical Nutrition, 41*(2), 307–312.

Issler, R. M., Marostica, P. J., & Giugliani, E. R. (2009). Infant sleep position: A randomized clinical trial of an educational intervention in the maternity ward in Porto Alegre, Brazil. *Birth, 36*(2), 115–121. https://doi.org/10.1111/j.1523-536X.2009.00308.x

Jarrin, D. C., McGrath, J. J., & Quon, E. C. (2014). Objective and subjective socioeconomic gradients exist for sleep in children and adolescents. *Health Psychology, 33*(3), 301–305. https://doi.org/10.1037/a0032924

Jones, C. H., Owens, J. A., & Pham, B. (2013). Can a brief educational intervention improve parents' knowledge of healthy children's sleep? A pilot-test. *Health Education Journal, 72*(5), 601–610. https://doi.org/10.1177/0017896912464606

Kessler, R. C., Berglund, P. A., Coulouvrat, C., Hajak, G., Roth, T., Shahly, V., Shillington, A. C., Stephenson, J. J., & Walsh, J. K. (2011). Insomnia and the performance of US workers: Results from the America Insomnia Survey. *Sleep, 34*(9), 1161–1171. https://doi.org/10.5665/SLEEP.1230

Khadka, R., Hong, S. A., & Chang, Y.-S. (2020). Prevalence and determinants of poor sleep quality and depression among postpartum women: A community-based study in Ramechhap district, Nepal. *International Health, 12*(2), 125–131.

Kim, B., Troxel, W. M., Dubowitz, T., Hunter, G. P., Ghosh-Dastidar, B., Chaix, B., Rudolph, K. E., Morrison, C. N., Branas, C. C., & Duncan, D. T. (2022). Mediating role of psychological distress in the associations between neighborhood social environments and sleep health. *Sleep, 45*(8), Article zsac087. https://doi.org/10.1093/sleep/zsac087

Kordas, K., Siegel, E. H., Olney, D. K., Katz, J., Tielsch, J. M., Chwaya, H. M., Kariger, P. K., Leclerq, S. C., Khatry, S. K., & Stoltzfus, R. J. (2008). Maternal reports of sleep in 6–18 month-old infants from Nepal and Zanzibar: Association with iron deficiency anemia and stunting. *Early Human Development, 84*(6), 389–398. https://doi.org/10.1016/j.earlhumdev.2007.10.007

Kordas, K., Siegel, E. H., Olney, D. K., Katz, J., Tielsch, J. M., Kariger, P. K., Khalfan, S. S., LeClerq, S. C., Khatry, S. K., & Stoltzfus, R. J. (2009). The effects of iron and/or zinc supplementation on maternal reports of sleep in infants from Nepal and Zanzibar. *Journal of Developmental & Behavioral Pediatrics, 30*(2), 131–139. https://doi.org/10.1097/DBP.0b013e31819e6a48

Kouros, C. D., Keller, P. S., Martin-Pinon, O., & El-Sheikh, M. (2022). Bidirectional associations between nightly sleep and daily happiness and negative mood in adolescents. *Child Development, 93*(5), e547–e562. https://doi.org/10.1111/cdev.13798

Kundel, V., Agyapong, P. D., Parekh, A., Kaali, S., Prah, R. K. D., Taweesedt, P., Tawiah, T., Ayappa, I., Mujtaba, M. N., Agyei, O., Jack, D., Osei, M., Kwarteng, A. A., Lee, A., & Asante, K. P. (2022). Characterizing sleep–wake patterns in mothers and children in an agrarian community: Results from the Ghana Randomized Air Pollution and Health Study. *Sleep, 45*(8), Article zsac033. https://doi.org/10.1093/sleep/zsac033

Lallukka, T., Haaramo, P., Lahelma, E., & Rahkonen, O. (2011). Sleep problems and disability retirement: A register-based follow-up study. *American Journal of Epidemiology, 173*(8), 871–881. https://doi.org/10.1093/aje/kwq462

Lallukka, T., Sares-Jäske, L., Kronholm, E., Sääksjärvi, K., Lundqvist, A., Partonen, T., Rahkonen, O., & Knekt, P. (2012). Sociodemographic and socioeconomic differences in sleep duration and insomnia-related symptoms in Finnish adults. *BMC Public Health, 12*(1), Article 565.

Levesque, A. R., MacDonald, S., Berg, S. A., & Reka, R. (2021). Assessing the impact of changes in household socioeconomic status on the health of children and adolescents: A systematic review. *Adolescent Research Review, 6*(2), 91–123.

MacKinnon, A. L., Tomfohr-Madsen, L., & Tough, S. (2021). Neighborhood socio-economic factors and associations with infant sleep health. *Behavioral Sleep Medicine, 19*(4), 458–470. https://doi.org/10.1080/15402002.2020.1778478

Manzar, M. D., Bekele, B. B., Noohu, M. M., Salahuddin, M., Albougami, A., Spence, D. W., Pandi-Perumal, S. R., & Bahammam, A. S. (2020). Prevalence of poor sleep quality in the Ethiopian population: A systematic review and meta-analysis. *Sleep and Breathing, 24*(2), 709–716.

Marco, C. A., Wolfson, A. R., Sparling, M., & Azuaje, A. (2011). Family socioeconomic status and sleep patterns of young adolescents. *Behavioral Sleep Medicine, 10*(1), 70–80. https://doi.org/10.1080/15402002.2012.636298

McWood, L. M., Zeringue, M. M., Piñón, O. M., Buckhalt, J. A., & El-Sheikh, M. (2022). Linear and nonlinear associations between the sleep environment, presleep conditions, and sleep in adolescence: Moderation by race and socioeconomic status. *Sleep Medicine, 93*, 90–99. https://doi.org/10.1016/j.sleep.2021.11.004

Moore, P. J., Adler, N. E., Williams, D. R., & Jackson, J. S. (2002). Socioeconomic status and health: The role of sleep. *Psychosomatic Medicine, 64*(2), 337–344. https://journals.lww.com/psychosomaticmedicine/Fulltext/2002/03000/Socioeconomic_Status_and_Health__The_Role_of_Sleep.18.aspx

Newton, A. T., Honaker, S. M., & Reid, G. J. (2020). Risk and protective factors and processes for behavioral sleep problems among preschool and early school-aged children: A systematic review. *Sleep Medicine Reviews, 52*, Article 101303. https://doi.org/10.1016/j.smrv.2020.101303

Nulty, A. K., Thompson, A. L., Wasser, H. M., & Bentley, M. E. (2022). Directionality of the associations between bedsharing, maternal depressive symptoms, and infant sleep during the first 15 months of life. *Sleep Health, 8*(1), 39–46. https://doi.org/10.1016/j.sleh.2021.11.001

Nyarko, S. H., Luo, L., Schlundt, D. G., & Xiao, Q. (2023). Individual and neighborhood socioeconomic status and long-term individual trajectories of sleep duration among Black and White adults: The Southern Community Cohort Study. *Sleep, 46*(1), Article zsac225.

Obradovich, N., Migliorini, R., Mednick, S. C., & Fowler, J. H. (2017). Nighttime temperature and human sleep loss in a changing climate. *Science Advances, 3*(5), Article e1601555.

Ozminkowski, R. J., Wang, S., & Walsh, J. K. (2007). The direct and indirect costs of untreated insomnia in adults in the United States. *Sleep, 30*(3), 263–273. https://doi.org/10.1093/sleep/30.3.263

Papadopoulos, D., & Etindele Sosso, F. A. (2022). Socioeconomic status and sleep health: A narrative synthesis of three decades of empirical research. *Journal of Clinical Sleep Medicine, 19*(3), 605–620. https://doi.org/10.5664/jcsm.10336

Patrick, K. E., Millet, G., & Mindell, J. A. (2016). Sleep differences by race in preschool children: The roles of parenting behaviors and socioeconomic status. *Behavioral Sleep Medicine, 14*(5), 467–479. https://doi.org/10.1080/15402002.2015.1017101

Petrovic, D., de Mestral, C., Bochud, M., Bartley, M., Kivimäki, M., Vineis, P., Mackenbach, J., & Stringhini, S. (2018). The contribution of health behaviors to socioeconomic inequalities in health: A systematic review. *Preventive Medicine, 113*, 15–31. https://doi.org/10.1016/j.ypmed.2018.05.003

Petrovic, D., Haba-Rubio, J., Carmeli, C., Vollenweider, P., Heinzer, R., & Stringhini, S. (2019). Social inequalities in sleep-disordered breathing: Evidence from the CoLaus|HypnoLaus study. *Journal of Sleep Research, 28*(5), Article e12799. https://doi.org/10.1111/jsr.12799

Philbrook, L. E., Saini, E. K., Fuller-Rowell, T. E., Buckhalt, J. A., & El-Sheikh, M. (2020). Socioeconomic status and sleep in adolescence: The role of family chaos. *Journal of Family Psychology, 34*(5), 577–586. https://doi.org/10.1037/fam0000636

Quon, E. C., & McGrath, J. J. (2014). Subjective socioeconomic status and adolescent health: A meta-analysis. *Health Psychology, 33*(5), 433–447.

Rahkonen, O., Lallukka, T., Kronholm, E., Vahtera, J., Lahelma, E., & Laaksonen, M. (2012). Sleep problems and sickness absence among middle-aged employees. *Scandinavian Journal of Work, Environment & Health, 38*(1), 47–55. https://doi.org/10.5271/sjweh.3186

Rifkin, D. I., Long, M. W., & Perry, M. J. (2018). Climate change and sleep: A systematic review of the literature and conceptual framework. *Sleep Medicine Reviews, 42*, 3–9.

Roberts, R. E., Roberts, C. R., & Duong, H. T. (2008). Chronic insomnia and its negative consequences for health and functioning of adolescents: A 12-month prospective study. *Journal of Adolescent Health, 42*(3), 294–302. https://doi.org/10.1016/j.jadohealth.2007.09.016

Rocha, S., Almeida, D. M., Chiang, J. J., Cole, S. W., Irwin, M. R., Seeman, T., & Fuligni, A. J. (2022). The relationship between family socioeconomic status and adolescent sleep and diurnal cortisol. *Psychosomatic Medicine, 84*(7), 848–855. https://journals.lww.com/psychosomaticmedicine/Fulltext/2022/09000/The_Relationship_Between_Family_Socioeconomic.14.aspx

Rumble, D. D., O'Neal, K., Overstreet, D. S., Penn, T. M., Jackson, P., Aroke, E. N., Sims, A. M., King, A. L., Hasan, F. N., Quinn, T. L., Long, D. L., Sorge, R. E., & Goodin, B. R. (2021). Sleep and neighborhood socioeconomic status: A micro longitudinal study of chronic low-back pain and pain-free individuals. *Journal of Behavioral Medicine, 44*(6), 811–821. https://doi.org/10.1007/s10865-021-00234-w

Salo, P., Oksanen, T., Sivertsen, B., Hall, M., Pentti, J., Virtanen, M., Vahtera, J., & Kivimaki, M. (2010). Sleep disturbances as a predictor of cause-specific work disability and delayed return to work. *Sleep, 33*(10), 1323–1331. https://doi.org/10.1093/sleep/33.10.1323

Schokman, A., Bin, Y. S., Simonelli, G., Pye, J., Morris, R., Sumathipala, A., Siribaddana, S. H., Hotopf, M., Rijsdijk, F., & Jayaweera, K. (2018). Agreement between subjective and objective measures of sleep duration in a low-middle income country setting. *Sleep Health, 4*(6), 543–550.

Sekine, M., Chandola, T., Martikainen, P., Marmot, M., & Kagamimori, S. (2006). Work and family characteristics as determinants of socioeconomic and sex inequalities in sleep: The Japanese Civil Servants Study. *Sleep, 29*(2), 206–216. https://doi.org/10.1093/sleep/29.2.206

Sharpe, I., & Davison, C. M. (2021). Climate change, climate-related disasters and mental disorder in low-and middle-income countries: a scoping review. *BMJ Open, 11*(10), Article e051908.

Simonelli, G., Dudley, K. A., Weng, J., Gallo, L. C., Perreira, K., Shah, N. A., Alcantara, C., Zee, P. C., Ramos, A. R., Llabre, M. M., Sotres-Alvarez, D., Wang, R., & Patel, S. R. (2016). Neighborhood factors as predictors of poor sleep in the Sueño ancillary study of the Hispanic Community Health Study/Study of Latinos. *Sleep, 40*(1), Article zsw025. https://doi.org/10.1093/sleep/zsw025

Simonelli, G., Leanza, Y., Boilard, A., Hyland, M., Augustinavicius, J. L., Cardinali, D. P., Vallières, A., Pérez-Chada, D., & Vigo, D. E. (2013). Sleep and quality of life in urban poverty: The effect of a slum housing upgrading program. *Sleep, 36*(11), 1669–1676.

Simonelli, G., Marshall, N. S., Grillakis, A., Miller, C. B., Hoyos, C. M., & Glozier, N. (2018). Sleep health epidemiology in low and middle-income countries: A systematic review and meta-analysis of the prevalence of poor sleep quality and sleep duration. *Sleep Health, 4*(3), 239–250.

Simonelli, G., Patel, S. R., Rodríguez-Espínola, S., Pérez-Chada, D., Salvia, A., Cardinali, D. P., & Vigo, D. E. (2015). The impact of home safety on sleep in a Latin American country. *Sleep Health, 1*(2), 98–103.

Singh, D. R., Sunuwar, D. R., Dahal, B., & Sah, R. K. (2021). The association of sleep problem, dietary habits and physical activity with weight status of adolescents in Nepal. *BMC Public Health, 21*(1), Article 938.

Sivertsen, B., Bøe, T., Skogen, J. C., Petrie, K. J., & Hysing, M. (2017). Moving into poverty during childhood is associated with later sleep problems. *Sleep Medicine, 37*, 54–59. https://doi.org/10.1016/j.sleep.2017.06.005

Sivertsen, B., Harvey, A. G., Pallesen, S., & Hysing, M. (2017). Trajectories of sleep problems from childhood to adolescence: A population-based longitudinal study from Norway. *Journal of Sleep Research, 26*(1), 55–63. https://doi.org/10.1111/jsr.12443

Sivertsen, B., Overland, S., Bjorvatn, B., Maeland, J. G., & Mykletun, A. (2009). Does insomnia predict sick leave? The Hordaland Health Study. *Journal of Psychosomatic Research, 66*(1), 67–74. https://doi.org/10.1016/j.jpsychores.2008.06.011

Sivertsen, B., Overland, S., Neckelmann, D., Glozier, N., Krokstad, S., Pallesen, S., Nordhus, I. H., Bjorvatn, B., & Mykletun, A. (2006). The long-term effect of insomnia on work disability: The HUNT-2 historical cohort study. *American Journal of Epidemiology, 163*(11), 1018–1024. https://doi.org/10.1093/aje/kwj145

Sivertsen, B., Overland, S., Pallesen, S., Bjorvatn, B., Nordhus, I. H., Maeland, J. G., & Mykletun, A. (2009). Insomnia and long sleep duration are risk factors for later work disability. The Hordaland Health Study. *Journal of Sleep Research, 18*(1), 122–128. https://doi.org/10.1111/j.1365-2869.2008.00697.x

Sivertsen, B., Pallesen, S., Stormark, K. M., Bøe, T., Lundervold, A. J., & Hysing, M. (2013). Delayed sleep phase syndrome in adolescents: Prevalence and correlates in a large population based study. *BMC Public Health, 13*, Article 1163. https://doi.org/10.1186/1471-2458-13-1163

Stamatakis, K. A., Kaplan, G. A., & Roberts, R. E. (2007). Short sleep duration across income, education, and race/ethnic groups: Population prevalence and growing disparities during 34 years of follow-up. *Annals of Epidemiology, 17*(12), 948–955.

Stewart, R., Besset, A., Bebbington, P., Brugha, T., Lindesay, J., Jenkins, R., Singleton, N., & Meltzer, H. (2006). Insomnia comorbidity and impact and hypnotic use by age group in a national survey population aged 16 to 74 years. *Sleep, 29*(11), 1391–1397. https://doi.org/10.1093/sleep/29.11.1391

Stickley, A., Leinsalu, M., DeVylder, J. E., Inoue, Y., & Koyanagi, A. (2019). Sleep problems and depression among 237 023 community-dwelling adults in 46 low-and middle-income countries. *Scientific Reports, 9*(1), Article 12011.

Stringhini, S., Haba-Rubio, J., Marques-Vidal, P., Waeber, G., Preisig, M., Guessous, I., Bovet, P., Vollenweider, P., Tafti, M., & Heinzer, R. (2015). Association of socioeconomic status with sleep disturbances in the Swiss population-based CoLaus study. *Sleep Medicine, 16*(4), 469–476. https://doi.org/10.1016/j.sleep.2014.12.014

Sujarwoto, S. (2020). Sleep disturbance in Indonesia: How much does smoking contribute? *Behavioral Sleep Medicine, 18*(6), 760–773.

Swanson, L. M., Arnedt, J. T., Rosekind, M. R., Belenky, G., Balkin, T. J., & Drake, C. (2011). Sleep disorders and work performance: Findings from the 2008 National Sleep Foundation Sleep in America poll. *Journal of Sleep Research, 20*(3), 487–494. https://doi.org/10.1111/j.1365-2869.2010.00890.x

Tomfohr-Madsen, L., Cameron, E. E., Dhillon, A., MacKinnon, A., Hernandez, L., Madigan, S., & Tough, S. (2020). Neighborhood socioeconomic status and child sleep duration: A systematic review and meta-analysis. *Sleep Health, 6*(5), 550–562. https://doi.org/10.1016/j.sleh.2020.02.012

Williamson, A. A., Gould, R., Leichman, E. S., Walters, R. M., & Mindell, J. A. (2021). Socioeconomic disadvantage and sleep in early childhood: Real-world data from a mobile health application. *Sleep Health, 7*(2), 143–152. https://doi.org/10.1016/j.sleh.2021.01.002

Xiao, Q., Gee, G., Jones, R. R., Jia, P., James, P., & Hale, L. (2020). Cross-sectional association between outdoor artificial light at night and sleep duration in middle-to-older aged adults: The NIH-AARP Diet and Health Study. *Environmental Research, 180*, Article 108823. https://doi.org/10.1016/j.envres.2019.108823

Yu, H. (2020). *Solid fuel-related indoor air pollution and poor sleep quality in adults aged 45 years and older; a national longitudinal study in China* [Unpublished master's thesis, Yale University]. Yale University EliScholar. https://elischolar.library.yale.edu/ysphtdl/2007/

CHAPTER

16 Sleep, Health, and Shift Work

Siri Waage *and* Bjørn Bjorvatn

Abstract

Shift work is common in our modern society, and the number of shift workers is increasing. There is strong evidence linking shift work to a variety of adverse biological, psychological, and social consequences. The potential health consequences are most likely related to sleep loss and the circadian misalignment between the light–dark cycle and the human activity–rest cycle. However, there are large interindividual differences in tolerance to shift work, and many workers cope well with such work hours. It is important to understand both why some people experience negative health effects and how countermeasures can be used to limit the negative consequences both for the individual and for the society. In this chapter, these issues are highlighted.

Key Words: shift work, night work, sleep, sleepiness, health, circadian rhythm

Introduction

The society has changed toward a 24/7 society where shift work is implemented due to financial causes, social structure, and the need for 24-hour services. This applies to many sectors, for instance, in healthcare, security, transportation, and recreation. In some sectors around-the-clock work is needed due to critical societal requirements such as emergency services, while other societal benefits of shift work include increased production and number of jobs. Consequently, the number of shift workers has increased during the last decades. More and more people are not working during standard hours, defined as 8-hour workdays Monday to Friday. For instance, in the United States, about 16% of wage and salaried employees follow shift work schedules according to the US Bureau of Labor Statistics (2019), and about 29% have work arrangements outside the normal workday from 6:00 a.m. to 6:00 p.m. In Europe more than one in three workers are engaged in nonstandard work schedules (Gracia et al., 2021). From a societal perspective it is therefore useful to summarize the knowledge about shift work and sleep and to use this knowledge to best facilitate health-promoting working schedules. In this chapter we will give an overview of shift work as a concept and how shift work affects the society in terms of sleep, sleepiness, and other health problems related to different types of shift work.

The Concept of Shift Work

Nonstandard working schedules include shift work, extended working hours and extended working weeks, on-call duties, weekend work, and combinations of these work schedules. Shift work is described as a form of work scheduling in which a group of workers succeeds one another temporally at the workplace in order to maintain operation (International Labour Organization, 1995). It is often defined as work which takes place between 7:00 p.m. and 6:00 a.m. Several different shift work schedules are described, and they differ widely in respect to their structure and organization. Such dimensions include, among others, type of shift according to their start and end times, inclusion of night work, combination of shifts, duration of shifts, regularity, and time for rest and recovery (Stevens et al., 2011). Shift work may be permanent or fixed, meaning that workers stay on a given shift (i.e., early morning, evening, or night work). Another commonly used shift schedule is rotating shifts (more or less regular), that is, to alternate or rotate between morning, evening, and/or night shifts. To maintain a 24/7 service, rotating shift work often also includes what is described as quick returns, defined as a rest period between two following shifts of less than 11 hours. This is most common between an evening shift and a day shift but is also seen in night shifts followed by evening shifts or in morning shifts followed by night shifts. This specific work schedule therefore deviates from the rule of having a minimum of 11 hours off duty time, defined in some national working time directives or working time acts. Rotating shift work involving quick returns is a common shift system in the healthcare sector in many Scandinavian countries, including Norway. Shift work is also often defined by the presence or absence of night work, where night work refers to shifts where most of the work hours take place during the night, between 10:00 p.m. and 6:00 a.m. Night work is regarded as one of the most demanding dimensions of shift work as night work entails work that coincides with workers' habitual sleep periods. Approximately 19% of the workforce in Europe are reported to be engaged in night work at least once a month (Eurofound 2016). Evening work typically takes place somewhere between 2:00 p.m. and midnight. About 27% of the European workforce work five or more evening shifts per month (Eurofound 2007). Usually, such a schedule is not associated with the same amount of sleep-related complaints compared to night work. For instance, sleep (total sleep time, Stage 2 sleep, rapid-eye-movement [REM] sleep, and slow-wave sleep) was reduced in connection with night work and mornings shifts compared to evening shifts among Swedish three-shift workers (Akerstedt et al., 1991). However, evening work may have more negative social consequences compared to other shifts since people working evening shifts have to work when family and friends have their leisure time. Also evening workers may find it difficult to unwind before going to bed after a shift and tend to have later bedtimes compared to what they usually have (Akerstedt et al., 1991; Pilcher et al., 2000). The use of the described work schedules differs between countries. While permanent or fixed shift work is more common in the United States, rotating shifts dominate in Europe (Akerstedt & Wright, 2009). However, both on a societal and on an individual level, nonstandard working hours and different shift work schedules come with a cost. Precise economic costs have not been quantified, although the economic impact of individual elements provides some idea. In general, shift work disrupts biological rhythms and is associated with a variety of adverse health outcomes for the individual. Possible negative health effects that are reported include sleep problems, increased risk of cardiovascular disease, metabolic disorders, certain types of cancer, gastrointestinal problems, and psychological distress (Kecklund & Axelsson, 2016). For an overview of short- term and long-term consequences, see Table 16.1. However, research has shown that the negative effects of shift work are likely to arise from several schedule specific characteristics.

Sleep is known to be important for health and functional capacity, and poor sleep leads to sleepiness and fatigue. Humans typically sleep better at night and perform better during the daytime. Night workers are exposed to light and dark at the wrong time according to their endogenous circadian rhythm and are forced to be active when their circadian rhythms are prepared to rest and the opposite, to sleep when their bodily rhythms are set to be active. Sleep problems are the most frequent consequence of disrupted circadian

Table 16.1 Complaints, diseases, and other consequences related to shift work

	Acute effects of shift work	Long-term risk effects of shift work
Sleepiness and fatigue	Yes	Yes
Sleep problems	Yes	Yes
Difficulty concentrating, irritability, and bad mood	Yes	Yes
Decreased work ability and productivity	Yes	Yes
Social and family conflict	Yes	Yes
Traffic accidents	Yes	Yes
Other accidents/near accidents	Yes	Yes
Gastrointestinal problems	Yes	Yes
Infections and other common health complaints	Yes	Yes
Cardiovascular disease	No	Yes
Overweight	No	Yes
Diabetes	No	Yes
Infertility and reproduction problems	No	Yes
Mental problems	No	Yes
Dementia	No	Yes
Cancer	No	Yes
Shift work disorder	No	Yes
Worsening of health problems	Yes	Yes

Note. Based on table 2.1 in Shift work and Sleep (Bjorvatn, 2019).

rhythms. Therefore, sleep disturbances and associated excessive sleepiness are among the most common and persistent health complaints of shift work. Most commonly reported are complaints of insomnia (i.e., sleep onset and maintenance difficulties), reduced sleep duration, and excessive sleepiness during work. Prevalences of insomnia among shift workers range between 47% and 55%, and between 26% and 30% of shift workers experience excessive sleepiness (Oyane et al., 2013). Shift workers are found to sleep approximately 10 hours less than daytime workers during a week (Akerstedt, 2003). Excessive sleepiness is in turn associated with impaired safety and increased accident risk; consequently, there is an established link between shift work and increased risk of accidents and workplace injuries (Folkard & Tucker, 2003). The reduced safety is linked to the negative effects of sleep deprivation and disrupted circadian rhythm. The reported sleep problems in shift work vary widely between different work schedules (Flo et al., 2012). Most important, the direction and speed of shift rotation, the length of recovery period between shifts, the distribution of rest days during the shift system, and the number of consecutive work shifts play important roles (Knauth & Hornberger, 2003).

Shift Work, Sleep, and Sleepiness

Night Work

The effects of night work on sleep involve both quality and quantity. Night-shift work is particularly associated with disturbances in the sleep–wake patterns both during and outside the shifts. Night workers have an irregular sleep schedule, which is often abruptly displaced at unconventional circadian phases. For night-shift workers, sleep is usually initiated 1 hour after the night shift has ended, which is close to the core body temperature nadir. Sleep initiated around the nadir most often results in shortened sleep duration and increased amount of wakefulness in the latter part of the sleep period. Typically, the sleep period after night work is reduced by 2 to 4 hours compared to normal night sleep (Akerstedt, 2003). This is mainly explained by the fact that it is difficult for night workers to sleep when the circadian rhythm is rising and setting the body for wakefulness.

Most of the sleep loss related to night work involves Stage N2 sleep and REM sleep, whereas N3 (deep sleep) is relatively unaffected. Since the curtailed sleep duration is related to the endogenous circadian rhythm, several consecutive night shifts most likely will gradually adapt the circadian rhythm to night work, resulting in better and longer daytime sleep. Typically, the human circadian rhythm adjusts 1 to 2 hours daily (Bjorvatn & Pallesen, 2009). When working consecutive night shifts, a complete adaptation to night work is beneficial. However, such complete adaptation to night work is rare, and studies have shown that even after seven consecutive shifts a night worker is not yet fully adapted. Still, in some occupations, like in the offshore oil industry, full adaptation to night work is easier and more common compared with adaptation to night work onshore. Suggested explanations for this faster entrainment are related to the fact that the offshore environment is better adapted to 24-hour operations with similar routines for day- and night-shift workers, in addition to the fact that night workers offshore normally are not exposed to morning bright light between work and bedtime after night work (Bjorvatn et al., 1998).

Night work is also characterized by increased sleepiness, measured both subjectively and objectively; and this increased sleepiness is associated with an increased risk of accidents. At night, the human body is typically prepared for rest and sleep, with a dropping core body temperature and rising levels of melatonin. Night work is associated with severe sleepiness and unintended sleep episodes during shifts, where levels of alertness are especially reduced during the second half of the night (Tucker et al., 1998). The human circadian rhythm is set to be active during the day, and sleepiness is often the first negative consequence related to night work. Sleepiness is especially problematic if the work tasks are monotonous. In addition, night workers often experience work in dimmed light. Studies on permanent night shift often compare permanent night workers with rotating shift workers; however, there are small differences between permanent night workers and rotating night workers regarding sleep duration during daytime and sleepiness during night work, where permanent night workers sleep slightly longer than rotating shift workers after the night shift (Akerstedt & Wright, 2009).

Rotating Shift Work

The effects of rotating shift work will vary with direction and speed of the rotation. The main assumption is that the sleep–wake pattern of workers on a regular three-shift system is influenced by early morning shifts and night shifts with reduced sleep duration prior to early morning shifts and after night shifts and that the organization of the shift system plays a role. Studies on irregular two- or three-shift rotations often highlight the start and finish times of the shifts in addition to shift lengths and rest periods. Slowly rotating shifts are considered better for the workers' sleep because the workers get better circadian adaptation to night work when they work several consecutive night shifts. In contrast, circadian adaptation to a new shift schedule may not be warranted for rotating shift workers since they must readapt their circadian rhythm to a daytime schedule when not working nights. Regarding the rotation of the shifts, forward or clockwise rotation of shifts is considered better for adaptation to shifts compared to backward rotation. This is based on the knowledge about circadian rhythms and that it is easier to extend the length of a day compared to shorten it (Bjorvatn & Pallesen, 2009).

Quick Returns

Quick returns are defined as short rest periods between two shifts (less than 11 hours) and are demanding for sleep. This shift characteristic in general limits the time available for rest since the workers also need to commute and to take care of domestic tasks and personal needs in between the two work shifts. Quick returns are reported to be associated with sleep problems, primarily shortened sleep duration but also disturbed sleep and excessive daytime sleepiness (Vedaa et al., 2016). Typically sleep durations between 5 and 6.5 hours are reported in relation to quick returns compared to 7 to 8 hours when not having quick returns. Quick returns are also shown to be associated with more fatigue, higher levels of sleepiness, insomnia, and shift work disorder (SWD; Eldevik et al., 2013). Some studies have also reported that quick returns are associated with poorer sleep quality. In addition to the limited hours available for sleep between the shifts, one could speculate that the limited time to unwind after the shift before going to bed makes it difficult to fall asleep. It is also suggested that the limited hours available for rest when working quick returns may cause activation, which in turn may disturb sleep with higher frequency of awakenings during the night.

Other Shift Schedules

Also, other work hours influence sleep, for instance, long working hours or extended working weeks. Long working hours are described as working for a length of time which exceeds standard working hours. What is defined as standard working hours varies from country to country. However, long working hours are often specified as working more than 40 hours per week or more than 8 hours per day. The findings from a review suggested that long work hours are associated with both sleep disturbances and reduced sleep duration (Caruso, 2014). Shifts lasting 12 hours or longer are found to reduce the opportunity to obtain enough sleep between the shifts (Sallinen & Kecklund, 2010). In addition, results have suggested that extended work weeks (>55 hours) are associated with increased risk of incidents (Matre et al., 2021). Long work shifts lasting more than 12 hours are associated with twice the risk of having an incident compared to 8-hour shifts (Matre et al., 2021).

Shift Work Disorder

Shift and especially night-shift workers may experience sleep and sleepiness problems associated with the work schedule that could be defined as SWD. SWD is a circadian rhythm sleep disorder that includes symptoms of insomnia during the sleep period and/or excessive sleepiness during the wake period. The symptoms are related to reduced sleep duration due to work hours overlapping with the worker's habitual sleep period. This definition confirms that not only night workers can experience these symptoms but also early morning shifts can lead to problems, especially for people who are extreme evening types (night owls). The prevalence rates vary between different types of work schedules, but approximately 30% of shift workers experience symptoms that may be consistent with SWD (Pallesen et al., 2021). SWD is associated with substantial adverse consequences to the individual, employers, and the society and is associated with impaired health. Shift workers having this circadian rhythm sleep disorder have reported, among other things, more health complaints and sleepiness-related accidents compared to workers without SWD (Waage et al., 2021).

Shift Work and Other Health Issues

Cardiovascular Disease

Night work is related to an increased risk of cardiovascular disease. This risk is reported to be approximately 40%, including both men and women (Boggild & Knutsson, 1999), but this risk has been modified in more recent research (Torquati et al., 2018). The possible mechanisms of this relationship have been linked to poor sleep, changes in the circadian rhythm, increase in psychosocial stress, and unfavorable changes in lifestyle such as smoking and eating habits. Several major risk factors for cardiovascular disorders, such as smoking, obesity, and dyslipidemia, are in many cases reportedly more prevalent among shift workers compared to day workers.

Metabolic Disorders

Shift work is associated with increased weight and obesity. A recent review concluded with a pooled odds ratio of 1.23 (95% confidence interval [CI; 1.17, 1.29]) for the association between night-shift work and obesity/overweight (Sun et al., 2018). Suggested mechanisms are related to changes in the hormones ghrelin and leptin associated with sleep loss and that shift workers report exercising less than day workers. As weight and diabetes are related, shift work is also associated with diabetes Type 2 (Canuto et al., 2013). A systematic review from 2015 concluded that there was moderate evidence for an association between shift work and Type 2 diabetes, supported by a meta-analysis showing a pooled adjusted odds ratio of 1.09 (95% confidence interval [CI; 1.05, 1.12]) for the association between ever compared to never being exposed to shift work and diabetes (Gan et al., 2015).

Cancer

Shift work is described as a risk factor for certain types of cancer, particularly breast and prostate cancers. A review of 13 studies on night work and breast cancer risk shows an increased breast cancer risk among women (Megdal et al., 2005). More recent studies show that the increased risk of breast cancer among shift-working women is related to having worked many years on schedules involving many consecutive night shifts, with a dose–response relationship (Lin et al., 2015). The International Agency for Research on Cancer (IARC) has classified night work with circadian disruption as one probable human carcinogen (Ward et al., 2019). Night work is described by the IARC as shifts where ≥3 hours of work is situated between midnight and 5:00 a.m. (Stevens et al., 2011). Causal links between shift work and cancer are not yet established (Ward et al., 2019). However, exposure to light at night (LAN) leading to circadian disruption has long been considered as a possible cause of breast cancer related to shift work (Costa et al., 2010; Stevens et al., 2014; Straif et al., 2007). Other possible mechanisms for the probable carcinogenesis of LAN are related to melatonin suppression, sleep deprivation affecting the immune system, adverse changes to lifestyle factors, and irregularity in cell proliferation (Fritschi et al., 2011; Truong et al., 2014).

Gastrointestinal Problems

Working at different hours of the day may be problematic for our gastrointestinal system. Shift workers experience greater prevalence of gastrointestinal problems such as abdominal pain, constipation, and diarrhea. Such symptoms are reported by 20%–75% of shift workers with night work compared to 10%–25% of day workers and shift workers without night work (Knutsson, 2003). One review on gastrointestinal disorders among shift workers including 20 studies also concluded with an increased risk of gastrointestinal symptoms and peptic ulcers in shift workers (Knutsson & Boggild, 2010). Gastrointestinal symptoms are usually explained as an effect of disruption of food and eating habits, particularly due to night shifts (Costa, 1996).

Mental Health

Poor sleep is associated with poor mental health. Shift work has been linked to mental health beyond problems related to sleep. Several psychosomatic complaints like anxiety and depression are more common among shift workers compared to day workers (Torquati et al., 2019). Shift workers often complain about irritability, nervousness, and anxiety in relation to more stressful working conditions and higher difficulties balancing family and social life. Furthermore, psychological symptoms such as fatigue (Yuan et al., 2011) and burnout (Jamal, 2004) are reported to be more common among night than day workers. However, the evidence of the impact of shift work on mental health is mixed. A review published in 2012 concluded that the causal relationship between shift work and mental health is not sufficiently established (Vogel et al., 2012).

Reproductive Health

Shift work is considered to be a risk factor for miscarriage, preterm labor, and low birth weight; but the results from scientific studies are divergent. However, employers do have a responsibility to facilitate the work for pregnant employees, including the work hours; and a recent Scandinavian discussion paper recommended, for instance, no more than one night shift in a week for pregnant women in order to reduce risk of miscarriage (Garde et al., 2020).

Shift Work and Safety

Sleep loss will, among other factors, contribute to reduced performance, impaired physical and mental reaction time, increased errors, impaired memory, and fatigue. Many of the most serious accidents in the world have taken place during the night, like the nuclear accident in *Chernobyl* in 1986, the *Exxon Valdez* oil spill in 1989, and the sinking of the cruise ferry *Estonia* in 1994. In retrospect, accident commissions have focused on fatigue, night work, and unfavorable work hours as contributing factors to these fatal accidents. The reduced performance is partly illustrated by the fact that after 17–19 hours of sustained wakefulness, curtailments in task performance are equivalent to or worse than those seen with a blood alcohol concentration of 0.05%. Further, after about 24 hours of sustained wakefulness, performance on some tasks is equivalent to a blood alcohol concentration of 0.1% (Rajaratnam & Arendt, 2001). Shift work is thus considered a significant contributor to excessive sleepiness and impaired alertness, with severe consequences such as road and workplace accidents. Several reviews have demonstrated a relationship between shift work and accidents. The risk of incidents covering both accidents and injuries was found to be dependent on type of shift, number of successive shifts, and hours on duty in one review (Folkard & Tucker, 2003). Night-shift workers do not usually adapt their circadian rhythm, and during night work they work at a time when the activation is at its lowest. This can lead to an increased accident rate and discounted or reduced performance and productivity. Since sleep and performance are closely related, shift work could be considered a safety risk mainly due to the reduced sleep duration associated with night work. Research has demonstrated that both safety and productivity are reduced by night work. This reduction probably reflects several underlying factors, which include impaired health, a disturbed social life, shortened and disturbed sleep, and disrupted circadian rhythms. The risk of accidents and near-miss events is reported to be significantly elevated in shift workers. The relative risk of accidents increases in line with the number of consecutive night shifts, as well as at the end of long night shifts. Regarding number of successive night shifts, the risk gradually increases for each successive shift, accumulating to a 36% higher risk on the fourth compared to the first night shift (Folkard & Tucker, 2003). It is estimated that the risk of accidents is increased by 18% in the afternoon shift and by 30% in night shifts compared to morning shifts in the same review including five studies and a total of eight data sets from different shift work populations (Folkard & Tucker, 2003).

Mechanisms/Models

Several models and theories describing the mechanisms between shift work and negative health exist. Most of them focus on the disrupted sleep and circadian rhythm, and insufficient sleep is suggested as a probable mechanism of the impaired health outcomes experienced by shift workers. Yet, the underlying mechanisms for the negative health consequences are not fully understood but involve most likely circadian disruption, curtailed and disturbed sleep, and risk behaviors and psychosocial stress with cognitive impairment as a consequence. Models have also included limited possibilities for recovery between shifts to better explain the association between shift work and nonstandard working hours and health.

Shift Work Tolerance

Most people working shifts are healthy individuals who do not report sleep problems, excessive sleepiness, or diseases like cancer, cardiovascular disease, or diabetes. The ability to adapt to shift work without adverse health consequences is described as *shift work tolerance*. Both individual and situational factors could affect the tolerance for shift work and may explain why some individuals cope better compared to others. Factors that are found to affect shift work tolerance are, among other things, age and sex, where sleep problems related to shift work increase with increasing age and men seem to tolerate shift work better than women. The critical age for reduced tolerance to shift and night work is reported to be between 40 and 50 years (Harma et al., 1994). The increased vulnerability of aging workers to the negative effects of shift and night work may be related to circadian factors, reduced sleep duration with following sleepiness, as well as social factors and the working conditions (Costa & Sartori, 2007). Aging is associated with a decreased ability for circadian adjustment and with increased sleep disturbances (Harma et al., 1994). Furthermore, some personality traits seem also to play a significant role in shift work tolerance. Such traits include circadian preference (being a morning or an evening type), languidity (tendency to become tired/sleepy upon losing sleep), and flexibility (ability to sleep and work at odd times). Morning types are, for instance, suggested to be less tolerant to night work, and aging is normally associated with morningness (e.g., becoming a morning type; Costa & Sartori, 2007). Situational factors such as the interaction between work and private life may also play an important role. Both night work and rotating shift work are reported to have a negative effect on family life. However, which work schedule best suits in combination with family life or a general social life will vary from individual to individual, and for some, night work may be the most beneficial work schedule, at least during some periods of life.

The "healthy worker effect" implies that shift workers in general are more fit for such work hours compared to others. Workers who do not cope with such work hours quit shift work, leaving a group of workers who cope better with shift work than the average person. In addition, individuals who assume they may not cope with shift work and nonstandard work hours may not apply for work where shift work is implemented. This means that the risk of reporting health problems related to shift work might be higher than what is found in research studies since the shift workers participating in the studies in general cope better with these work hours.

There exist many interventions and recommendations to reduce the consequences related to shift work (Pallesen et al., 2010). The interventions are often divided into three categories, depending on the different types of shifts. First, there are recommendations to help the shift worker to adapt the circadian rhythm to the working hours, for instance, for workers working several consecutive night shifts. Those measures include bright light and melatonin for adjusting the circadian rhythm. Second, in order to reduce sleepiness at work, which many night workers experience, the recommendations include several behavioral measures such as social interaction with others, light, activity, meals, napping, and caffeine that will help night workers to stay alert and awake. Third, to improve sleep both

Table 16.2 Summary of key interventions to minimize sleep/circadian problems among shift workers		
Interventions for adapting the circadian rhythm to the work schedule	Interventions to reduce sleepiness at work	Interventions to sleep better before/after work
Bright light	Social interaction	Sleep hygiene
Melatonin	Increased lighting	Sleep restriction
	Activity/exercise	Stimulus control
	Meals	Cognitive therapy
	Naps	Mindfulness
	Caffeine	Sleep medications
	Other stimulants	

Note. Based on table 3.1 in Shift work and Sleep (Bjorvatn, 2019).

before and after work, which is relevant for workers on both permanent shifts and rotating shifts, measures like sleep hygiene advice, sleep restriction, stimulus control, cognitive therapy, sleep medication, and mindfulness are useful (Table 16.2).

Considering the high numbers of workers involved in night and shift work, the increased risk of negative health for the individuals, and the associated reduced productivity, accident risks, and economic costs, society has a responsibility for and would benefit from both preventing and acting on the consequences of shift work. The effort may include designing interventions and policies that keep both the shift workers and the public as safe as possible. Governments should be responsible for making rules on night work and shift scheduling. Optimizing the shift schedule by including adequate time for recovery between shifts, minimizing extended work hours, facilitating napping during shifts, minimizing night work, and arranging shifts in a forward direction can reduce the risks of negative health and maximize productivity. From a societal perspective it may also be useful if one could prescreen individuals for tolerance to shift work before starting work. A prescreen may ensure safety for society and the workers' health, with possibilities of both identifying risk factors and advising and making recommendations.

Conclusion

More and more people are working shifts as society has moved toward a 24/7 society. Shift work may lead to negative consequences, both for the individual and for society. However, many workers also tolerate shift work well. Knowledge about the associations between shift work, sleep, and circadian rhythm is important as well as information about how to use this knowledge both for the shift workers themselves and to best facilitate health-promoting working schedules.

Future Directions for Research

There is a large selection both in and out of shift work. It is likely that people who remain in demanding shift work schedules are more robust against the potential consequences compared to those who quit shift work. To be able to address both preselection effects as well as survival effects, future studies should include participants from before they are exposed to shift work to investigate causal relationships. More longitudinal studies are therefore needed, where in addition to those who remain in shift work, workers leaving shift work should be followed.

References

Akerstedt, T. (2003). Shift work and disturbed sleep/wakefulness. *Occupational Medicine, 53*(2), 89–94. http://occmed.oxfordjournals.org/cgi/content/abstract/53/2/89

Akerstedt, T., Kecklund, G., & Knutsson, A. (1991). Spectral analysis of sleep electroencephalography in rotating three-shift work. *Scandinavian Journal of Work, Environment & Health, 17*(5), 330–336. https://doi.org/10.5271/sjweh.1694

Akerstedt, T., & Wright, K. P. (2009). Sleep loss and fatigue in shift work and shift work disorder. *Sleep Medicine Clinics, 4*(2), 257–271.

Bjorvatn, B. (2019). *Skiftarbeid og søvn.* Fagbokforlaget.

Bjorvatn, B., Kecklund, G., & Akerstedt, T. (1998). Rapid adaptation to night work at an oil platform, but slow readaptation after returning home. *Journal of Occupational and Environmental Medicine, 40*(7), 601–608.

Bjorvatn, B., & Pallesen, S. (2009). A practical approach to circadian rhythm sleep disorders. *Sleep Medicine Reviews, 13*(1), 47–60.

Boggild, H., & Knutsson, A. (1999). Shift work, risk factors and cardiovascular disease. *Scandinavian Journal of Work, Environment & Health, 25*(2), 85–99.

Canuto, R., Garcez, A. S., & Olinto, M. T. A. (2013). Metabolic syndrome and shift work: A systematic review. *Sleep Medicine Reviews, 17*(6), 425–431. https://doi.org/10.1016/j.smrv.2012.10.004

Caruso, C. C. (2014). Negative impacts of shiftwork and long work hours. *Rehabilitation Nursing Journal, 39*(1), 16–25. https://doi.org/10.1002/rnj.107

Costa, G. (1996). The impact of shift and night work on health. *Applied Ergonomics, 27*(1), 9–16.

Costa, G., Haus, E., & Stevens, R. (2010). Shift work and cancer—Considerations on rationale, mechanisms, and epidemiology. *Scandinavian Journal of Work, Environment & Health, 36*(2), 163–179.

Costa, G., & Sartori, S. (2007). Ageing, working hours and work ability. *Ergonomics, 50*(11), 1914–1930.

Eldevik, M. F., Flo, E., Moen, B. E., Pallesen, S., & Bjorvatn, B. (2013). Insomnia, excessive sleepiness, excessive fatigue, anxiety, depression and shift work disorder in nurses having less than 11 hours in-between shifts. *PLOS ONE, 8*(8), Article e70882. https://doi.org/10.1371/journal.pone.0070882

Eurofound. (2007). *Fourth European working conditions survey.* https://www.eurofound.europa.eu/en/publications/2007/fourth-european-working-conditions-survey

Eurofound. (2016). *Working time developments in the 21st century: Work duration and its regulation in the EU.* https://www.eurofound.europa.eu/en/publications/2016/working-time-developments-21st-century-work-duration-and-its-regulation-eu

Flo, E., Bjorvatn, B., Folkard, S., Moen, B. E., Gronli, J., Nordhus, I. H., & Pallesen, S. (2012). A reliability and validity study of the Bergen Shift Work Sleep Questionnaire in nurses working three-shift rotations. *Chronobiology International, 29*(7), 937–946. https://doi.org/10.3109/07420528.2012.699120

Folkard, S., & Tucker, P. (2003). Shift work, safety and productivity. *Occupational Medicine, 53*(2), 95–101. http://occmed.oxfordjournals.org/cgi/content/abstract/53/2/95

Fritschi, L., Glass, D. C., Heyworth, J. S., Aronson, K., Girschik, J., Boyle, T., Grundy, A., & Erren, T. C. (2011). Hypotheses for mechanisms linking shiftwork and cancer. *Medical Hypotheses, 77*(3), 430–436. https://doi.org/10.1016/j.mehy.2011.06.002

Gan, Y., Yang, C., Tong, X., Sun, H., Cong, Y., Yin, X., Li, L., Cao, S., Dong, X., Gong, Y., Shi, O., Dong, J., Bi, H., & Lu, Z. (2015). Shift work and diabetes mellitus: A meta-analysis of observational studies. *Occupational & Environmental Medicine, 72*(1), 72–78. https://doi.org/10.1136/oemed-2014-102150

Garde, A. H., Begtrup, L., Bjorvatn, B., Bonde, J. P., Hansen, J., Hansen, A. M., Härmä, M., Jensen, M. A., Kecklund, J., Kolstand, H. A., Larsen, A. D., Lie, J. A., Moreno, C. R. C., Nabe-Nielsen, K., & Sallinen, M. (2020). How to schedule night shift work in order to reduce health and safety risks. *Scandinavian Journal of Work, Environment & Health, 46*(6), 557–569. https://doi.org/10.5271/sjweh.3920

Gracia, P., Han, W., & Li, J. (2021). Nonstandard work schedules in cross-national perspective: A study of 29 European countries, 2005–2015. SocArXiv Papers. https://doi.org/10.31235/osf.io/mz53c

Harma, M. I., Hakola, T., Akerstedt, T., & Laitinen, J. T. (1994). Age and adjustment to night work. *Occupational & Environmental Medicine, 51*(8), 568–573.

International Labour Organization. (1995). *World employment 1995. An ILO report.*

Jamal, M. (2004). Burnout, stress and health of employees on non-standard work schedules: A study of Canadian workers. *Stress and Health, 20*(3), 113–119. https://doi.org/10.1002/smi.1012

Kecklund, G., & Axelsson, J. (2016). Health consequences of shift work and insufficient sleep. *BMJ, 355*, Article i5210. https://doi.org/10.1136/bmj.i5210

Knauth, P., & Hornberger, S. (2003). Preventive and compensatory measures for shift workers. *Occupational Medicine, 53*(2), 109–116. http://occmed.oxfordjournals.org/cgi/content/abstract/53/2/109

Knutsson, A. (2003). Health disorders of shift workers. *Occupational Medicine, 53*(2), 103–108. http://occmed.oxfordjournals.org/cgi/content/abstract/53/2/103

Knutsson, A., & Boggild, H. (2010). Gastrointestinal disorders among shift workers. *Scandinavian Journal of Work, Environment & Health, 36*(2), 85–95.

Lin, X., Chen, W., Wei, F., Ying, M., Wei, W., & Xie, X. (2015). Night-shift work increases morbidity of breast cancer and all-cause mortality: A meta-analysis of 16 prospective cohort studies. *Sleep Medicine, 16*(11), 1381–1387. https://doi.org/10.1016/j.sleep.2015.02.543

Matre, D., Skogstad, M., Sterud, T., Nordby, K. C., Knardahl, S., Christensen, J. O., & Lie, J. S. (2021). Safety incidents associated with extended working hours. A systematic review and meta-analysis. *Scandinavian Journal of Work, Environment & Health, 47*(6), 415–424. https://doi.org/10.5271/sjweh.3958

Megdal, S. P., Kroenke, C. H., Laden, F., Pukkala, E., & Schernhammer, E. S. (2005). Night work and breast cancer risk: A systematic review and meta-analysis. *European Journal of Cancer, 41*(13), 2023–2032.

Oyane, N. M., Pallesen, S., Moen, B. E., Akerstedt, T., & Bjorvatn, B. (2013). Associations between night work and anxiety, depression, insomnia, sleepiness and fatigue in a sample of Norwegian nurses. *PLOS ONE, 8*(8), Article e70228. https://doi.org/10.1371/journal.pone.0070228

Pallesen, S., Bjorvatn, B., Mageroy, N., Saksvik, I. B., Waage, S., & Moen, B. E. (2010). Measures to counteract the negative effects of night work. *Scandinavian Journal of Work, Environment & Health, 36*(2), 109–120. https://doi.org/10.5271/sjweh.2886

Pallesen, S., Bjorvatn, B., Waage, S., Harris, A., & Sagoe, D. (2021). Prevalence of shift work disorder: A systematic review and meta-analysis. *Frontiers in Psychology, 12*, Article 638252. https://doi.org/10.3389/fpsyg.2021.638252

Pilcher, J. J., Lambert, B. J., & Huffcutt, A. I. (2000). Differential effects of permanent and rotating shifts on self-report sleep length: A meta-analytic review. *Sleep, 23*(2), 155–163. https://www.ncbi.nlm.nih.gov/pubmed/10737332

Rajaratnam, S. M., & Arendt, J. (2001). Health in a 24-h society. *Lancet, 358*(9286), 999–1005.

Sallinen, M., & Kecklund, G. (2010). Shift work, sleep, and sleepiness—Differences between shift schedules and systems. *Scandinavian Journal of Work, Environment & Health, 36*(2), 121–133.

Stevens, R. G., Brainard, G. C., Blask, D. E., Lockley, S. W., & Motta, M. E. (2014). Breast cancer and circadian disruption from electric lighting in the modern world. *CA: A Cancer Journal for Clinicians, 64*(3), 207–218. https://doi.org/10.3322/caac.21218

Stevens, R. G., Hansen, J., Costa, G., Haus, E., Kauppinen, T., Aronson, K. J., Castaño-Vinyals, G., Davis, S., Frings-Dresen, M. H. W., Fritschi, L., Kogevinas, M., Kogi, K., Lie, J.-A., Lowden, A., Peplonska, B., Pesch, B., Pukkala, E., Schernhammer, E., Travis, R. C., . . . Straif, K. (2011). Considerations of circadian impact for defining "shift work" in cancer studies: IARC Working Group Report. *Occupational & Environmental Medicine, 68*(2), 154–162. https://doi.org/10.1136/oem.2009.053512

Straif, K., Baan, R., Grosse, Y., Secretan, B., El, G. F., Bouvard, V., Altieri, A., Benbrahim-Tallaa, L., & Cogliano, V.; WHO International Agency for Research on Cancer Monograph Working Group. (2007). Carcinogenicity of shift-work, painting, and fire-fighting. *Lancet Oncology, 8*(12), 1065–1066.

Sun, M., Feng, W., Wang, F., Li, P., Li, Z., Li, M., Tse, G., Vlaanderen, J., Vermeulen, R., & Tse, L. A. (2018). Meta-analysis on shift work and risks of specific obesity types. *Obesity Reviews, 19*(1), 28–40. https://doi.org/10.1111/obr.12621

Torquati, L., Mielke, G. I., Brown, W. J., Burton, N. W., & Kolbe-Alexander, T. L. (2019). Shift work and poor mental health: A meta-analysis of longitudinal studies. *American Journal of Public Health, 109*(11), E13–E20. https://doi.org/10.2105/Ajph.2019.305278

Torquati, L., Mielke, G. I., Brown, W. J., & Kolbe-Alexander, T. (2018). Shift work and the risk of cardiovascular disease. A systematic review and meta-analysis including dose–response relationship. *Scandinavian Journal of Work, Environment & Health, 44*(3), 229–238. https://doi.org/10.5271/sjweh.3700

Truong, T., Liquet, B., Menegaux, F., Plancoulaine, S., Laurent-Puig, P., Mulot, C., Cordina-Duverger, E., Sanchez, M., Arveux, P., Kerbrat, P., Richardson, S., & Guénel, P. (2014). Breast cancer risk, nightwork, and circadian clock gene polymorphisms. *Endocrine-Related Cancer, 21*(4), 629–638. https://doi.org/10.1530/erc-14-0121

Tucker, P., Smith, L., Macdonald, I., & Folkard, S. (1998). Shift length as a determinant of retrospective on-shift alertness. *Scandinavian Journal of Work, Environment & Health, 24*(S3), 49–54. https://www.ncbi.nlm.nih.gov/pubmed/9916817

US Bureau of Labor Statistics. (2019). *Job flexibilities and work schedules summary.* https://www.bls.gov/news.release/flex2.nr0.htm

Vedaa, O., Harris, A., Bjorvatn, B., Waage, S., Sivertsen, B., Tucker, P., & Pallesen, S. (2016). Systematic review of the relationship between quick returns in rotating shift work and health-related outcomes. *Ergonomics, 59*(1), 1–14. https://doi.org/10.1080/00140139.2015.1052020

Vogel, M., Braungardt, T., Meyer, W., & Schneider, W. (2012). The effects of shift work on physical and mental health. *Journal of Neural Transmission, 119*(10), 1121–1132. https://doi.org/10.1007/s00702-012-0800-4

Waage, S., Pallesen, S., Moen, B. E., Vedaa, O., Thun, E., Buchvold, H. V., Blytt, K. M., Harris, A., & Bjorvatn, B. (2021). Changes in work schedule affect the prevalence of shift work disorder among Norwegian nurses—A two year follow-up study. *Chronobiology International, 38*(6), 924–932. https://doi.org/10.1080/07420528.2021.1896535

Ward, E. M., Germolec, D., Kogevinas, M., McCormick, D., Vermeulen, R., Anisimov, V. N., Aronson, K. J., Bhatti, P., Cocco, P., Costa, G., Dorman, D. C., Fu, L., Garde, A. H., Guénel, P., Hansen, J., Härmä, M. I., Kawai, K., Khizkhin, E. A., Knutsson, A., . . . Schubauer-Berigan, M. K. (2019). Carcinogenicity of night shift work. *The Lancet Oncology, 20*(8), 1058–1059. https://doi.org/10.1016/S1470-2045(19)30455-3

Yuan, S. C., Chou, M. C., Chen, C. J., Lin, Y. J., Chen, M. C., Liu, H. H., & Kuo, H. W. (2011). Influences of shift work on fatigue among nurses. *Journal of Nursing Management, 19*(3), 339–345. https://doi.org/10.1111/j.1365-2834.2010.01173.x

CHAPTER

17 Sex Differences in Sleep

Fiona C. Baker, Rena Wang, *and* Helen S. Driver

Abstract

In this chapter the authors discuss sex differences in sleep behavior, sleep structure, and aspects of three sleep disorders. Women report a greater need for sleep and sleep longer than men, as determined from self-report as well as actigraphy and wearable sleep trackers, although this difference is heavily influenced by family and work responsibilities. Women are also more likely to have earlier bedtimes and a morning chronotype, which may in part be a consequence of their phase-advanced circadian rhythms and shorter circadian period compared with men. Women are more likely than men to report poorer sleep quality and greater difficulty sleeping; however, polysomnographic recordings reveal other sex differences, including better sleep efficiency and more slow-wave sleep that is better preserved with aging in women than in men. Sex differences are evident in the prevalence, presentation, and etiology of some sleep disorders. Women are more likely than men to have insomnia disorder, a difference that becomes evident in adolescence and continues across the life span. Restless legs syndrome is more prevalent in women than men, and they also experience worse symptoms, particularly during pregnancy and postmenopause. Men are at greater risk for obstructive sleep apnea, at least until women reach menopause, when the sex difference lessens.

Key Words: sex, sleep behavior, sleep structure, sleep disorder, women, men, restless legs syndrome, obstructive sleep apnea

Introduction

Sex Differences and Dimorphisms

Sexual dimorphism and the resulting battle between the sexes began with a single mutation some 300 million years ago in ordinary autosomal chromosomes (Lahn & Page, 1999). This resulted in the SRY gene that determines the sexual fate of the embryo (Lahn & Page, 1999; Waters et al., 2007). After the creation of the SRY gene, the Y chromosome became genetically isolated owing to its lack of recombination with a "sister chromosome," and it has been forced down a distinct evolutionary path from that of its natural companion, the X chromosome. Indeed, there are only 19 genes shared on both the X and Y chromosomes, and the genetic differences in these two chromosomes give rise to the many physical, emotional, mental, and physiological differences between the sexes (Bachtrog, 2006). It is often hard to comprehend that although men and women share more than 99% of their genetic makeup, such vast gender differences can arise through the modifications of just a single chromosome pair.

While differences in sexual traits and morphology are to be expected between males and females, it is not inherently intuitive to expect differences with respect to sleep need, quality, and architecture. Yet, given that the X and Y chromosomes determine physical and emotional characteristics and that these in turn influence the behavioral state of sleep, one would expect to find sex differences in sleep. Indeed, there are sex-specific differences in sleep across several mammalian species (Mong & Cusmano, 2016). In humans, there are differences according to sex in objective sleep parameters as recorded electrographically, subjective ratings of sleep, sleep-endocrine regulation, and the prevalence of sleep disorders (for reviews, see Carrier et al., 2017; Collop et al., 2004; Dzaja et al., 2005; Kumar et al., 2021; Mong & Cusmano, 2016). Subtle sex differences in sleep may be evident in childhood; however, they become most evident after puberty when differences in cycling sex steroid levels influence many aspects of mammalian physiology and give rise to pronounced sexual dimorphism in phenotype. After puberty, as women enter their reproductive phase, sleep may be impacted in association with cyclical changes in hormones and physiology that characterize the menstrual cycle and pregnancy. As women approach menopause, with dramatic declines and increased variability in reproductive hormones, also in the context of midlife psychosocial changes and aging, they are more vulnerable to sleep disturbances. Here, we highlight key differences in sleep quality, duration, timing, and architecture between men and women across the life span. We also summarize sex differences in prevalence, presentation, and pathophysiology of major sleep disorders, insomnia, restless legs syndrome, and sleep disordered breathing.

Definitions of Sex Versus Gender

It is important to acknowledge the limitations of our definitions of men and women. The discussion of sex in this chapter refers to biological sex differences, as defined by the X and Y chromosomes and the various associated genetic and hormonal influences. The majority of health surveys and research quantify sex and gender as a self-defined dualistic variable: male or female (Eliason, 2014). However, it is important to recognize that gender identity is complex, exists on a continuum, and has significant cultural influences (Eliason, 2014). Many health questionnaires do not identify participants on a gender continuum, limiting the understanding to biological sexual-identity influences. For example, there is negligible data on the sleep physiology and prevalence of certain sleep disorders in the transgender population. The first sex-dependent analysis of quality of life in transgender populations in 2017 found that sleep quality was an independent and strong determinant of quality of life and that around 80% reported poor sleep quality (Auer et al., 2017). This suggests that transgender people experience different societal stressors that transcend the genetic foundation underpinning sleep-quality differences as traditionally discussed. Research limited to understanding only the two "opposite" genders fails to recognize a population who are influenced not just by genetics but by the expectations of society. Given the paucity of data in the transgender population, having highlighted that there is much work to be done to gather more inclusive research that categorizes gender on a spectrum, this chapter will address sex differences rather than gender differences in sleep physiology and pathology.

Self-Reported and Physiological Sleep and Circadian Rhythms

Sex Differences in Self-Reported Sleep

Common findings from general population studies are that women report a greater need for sleep, spend more time in bed, and sleep longer than men (Ferrara & De Gennaro, 2001; Lindberg et al., 1997). Women are also more likely than men to report poorer sleep quality, insufficient sleep, and more sleep disruption (difficulty falling asleep, frequent and prolonged nighttime awakenings) across the life span (Chaput et al., 2017; Collop et al., 2004; Groeger et al., 2004), which corresponds with their increased risk for insomnia disorder. One contributing factor to the increased prevalence of poor sleep quality in women is the response to changes in female reproductive hormones across the life span. Insomnia symptoms can emerge in some women premenstrually and during the menopausal transition, as discussed in Chapter 41. An important issue when considering self-reports of sleep quality that has received limited attention is the potential for differences in how men and women interpret sleep quality. For example, an analysis of the components of the Pittsburgh Sleep Quality Index found that "daytime dysfunction" and "sleep disturbances" were important for women's ratings of sleep quality, whereas "sleep efficiency" and "sleep duration" were important for men's ratings (Morris et al., 2018), although others did not replicate this finding (Li et al., 2019).

Several studies from around the world support a sex difference in self-reported sleep duration and potentially subjective sleep need, both being higher in women (Burgard & Ailshire, 2013; Groeger et al., 2004; Lindberg et al., 1997; Reyner et al., 1995; Ursin et al., 2005). In an analysis of minutes of time allocated for sleep in a nationally representative sample of working-age adults (N = 56,149, 18–64 years old) in the American Time Use Surveys (2003–2007), women reported about 23 minutes more time for sleep than men (Burgard & Ailshire, 2013) in models adjusting for sociodemographic factors, although the difference was reduced when also adjusting for paid and unpaid work. The influence of work and family responsibilities on time for sleep varied for men and women—partnered men with young children sleep significantly less than men who are young, single, and childless, an effect going in the opposite direction for women. These data highlight the importance of considering work–family responsibilities and gendered social expectations for their fulfillment when examining gender differences in sleep (Burgard & Ailshire, 2013). Similarly, an interview-based study of a nationally representative sample of almost

2,000 Britons (16–93 years) found an influence of family and work conditions on sleep duration in men and women, and there was only a difference in sleep duration—longer for women in the age group of 40–49 years (Groeger et al., 2004). Women consistently reported more sleep problems than men. Ursin and colleagues (2005) found in a sample of almost 9,000 Norwegian men and women (40–45 years) that women reported a longer mean sleep duration during the weekdays (7 hours, 11 minutes) than did men (6 hours, 52 minutes) and that mean subjective sleep need was also higher in women (7 hours, 45 minutes) than in men (7 hours, 16 minutes). A study of Swedish adults also reported an association between female sex and longer sleep duration and greater need for sleep (Lindberg et al., 1997). A higher subjective sleep need in women may be one factor contributing to the higher frequency of insomnia, though the reason for the higher sleep need in women is not clear and could be influenced by life-stage conditions, including work and family responsibilities.

Limited studies using activity monitoring at home in large groups have reported similar sex differences in sleep duration: In a sample of almost 300 adults aged 40 to 64 years, women slept more than men (Jean-Louis et al., 2000), a finding supported by subsequent community-based actigraphy studies of middle-aged (Lauderdale et al., 2006) and elderly (van den Berg et al., 2009) adults. A longer sleep duration in adolescent girls and adult women compared with men has also been found based on "big data" from thousands of participants' wearable sleep trackers (Jonasdottir et al., 2021). Analysis of this large data set showed sex differences in sleep timing that differed according to age, with an earlier bedtime in women than men until midlife, after which bedtimes converged but women had later wake-up times such that sleep duration was still longer in older women than older men (Jonasdottir et al., 2021). Taken together, with different methodologies, women tend to have a longer sleep duration than men, which likely reflects the influence of a combination of biological, environmental, lifestyle, and socioeconomic factors.

Sex Differences in Sleep Architecture and Sleep Electroencephalography

Paradoxically, self-reports from women describing poorer sleep quality than men are not borne out in polysomnographic (PSG) measures of sleep quality and continuity. Several studies have reported sex differences in PSG measures, with women having better sleep efficiency, fewer arousals, and more slow-wave sleep (SWS; the deepest stage of sleep, now called non-rapid-eye-movement [NREM] N3 sleep; Della Monica et al., 2018; Ehlers & Kupfer, 1997; Hume et al., 1998; Redline et al., 2004; Yetton et al., 2018). A large study controlling for respiratory disturbance index (RDI), age, ethnicity, body mass index (BMI), and medical comorbidities found that women had more N3, less Stage 1 (N1) sleep, and fewer arousals at night than men (Redline et al., 2004). Further, there was a significant age-related decline in N3 (SWS) sleep and an increase in N1 and N2 sleep in men but not in women. These findings were replicated in another large study of adult men and women across a wide age range, showing that women had more N3 (SWS), less

Stage 1 sleep, and a better sleep efficiency than men and that these PSG sleep measures were better preserved with aging in women (Della Monica et al., 2018). Also, there were stronger associations between objective and subjective measures of sleep quality in women than in men, suggesting that women more accurately perceived their sleep. An analysis of 3,202 records of sleep from 14 databases of nonclinical samples also found that men had less N3 sleep than women and that there was a steeper age-related increase in N1 sleep and decrease in N3 sleep in men than in women (Yetton et al., 2018). Examination of the dynamics of sleep patterns across the night informs the age–sex interaction, showing that differences extend beyond duration, with men being more likely than women to have fewer transitions to deeper NREM stages (N2 and N3) and greater propensity to transition to wakefulness and N1 sleep starting in midlife. In contrast, a meta-analysis of 5,273 adult healthy controls in PSG studies found no sex difference or sex–age interaction in N3 sleep or sleep efficiency. However, male sex was associated with a higher mean arousal index as well as differences in clinical measures, such as lower oxygen saturation and higher apnea hypopnea index (AHI; Boulos et al., 2019).

Analysis of the sleep electroencephalography (EEG) has revealed additional sex differences beyond those found in measures of sleep stages and continuity across the night. The sleep EEG provides continuous and detailed information beyond time spent in a particular sleep stage. Typically, a fast Fourier transform is applied to the signal, after which power spectral density can be calculated for EEG bands, of which delta (slow-wave activity [SWA], 1–4 Hz) has received the most attention. Consistently, studies have found that women have greater EEG absolute power than men across a broad frequency range, including the slow frequency ranges (delta, theta) and sigma frequency (12.25–15.0 Hz reflecting spindle frequency activity) in NREM sleep (Carrier et al., 2017). Consistent with their findings for sleep macrostructure, Della Monica and colleagues (2018) found that men had lower SWA (0.75–4.5 Hz) and a steeper age-related reduction in SWA than women. Others found greater spindle density, higher peak frequency and amplitude, and maintenance of spindle density with age in women more than in men (Carrier et al., 2017; Purcell et al., 2017). With this focus on the sleep EEG, questions have persisted as to whether sex differences in sleep stages and sleep EEG reflect differences in sleep regulatory mechanisms or differences in anatomical features that influence EEG amplitude, and thus absolute SWA and N3. In a data-driven approach, Rosinvil and colleagues (2021) addressed this question directly by adapting slow-wave amplitude criteria to age and sex. They showed that sex-related differences in slow-wave density were no longer evident, suggesting that differences between men and women in SWA are strongly dependent on anatomical features affecting amplitude. Further work is needed to determine the contributions of brain anatomy to the measurement of sleep EEG as well as the use of interventions to challenge sleep to determine whether there are functional differences in aspects of sleep as well as next-day consequences (e.g., alertness, cognitive performance) between men and women. For example, one study showed that young women have a greater increase in SWA in the first sleep cycle during a recovery night following sleep deprivation than do men (Armitage et al., 2001).

Sex Differences in Sleep Across Infancy, Childhood, and Adolescence

Infant boys may have less total sleep and more frequent awakenings than girls (Bach et al., 2000). In a Thai study of 3,172 infants aged 3 months, where a large proportion of infants shared a bed (68%) or room (32%) with the parents, the mean number of night awakenings was 2.7, with infant boys having a higher odds ratio (OR = 1.5) of being frequent wakers (more than 14 night awakenings per week; Anuntaseree et al., 2008). Compared to girls, boys are at higher risk for sudden infant death syndrome (SIDS), which occurs in infants under 1 year of age, peaking between 2 and 5 months of age (Byard & Krous, 2004). Bedsharing, although not routine as it is in Asian and African cultures, still commonly occurs in Western culture and has been associated with an increased SIDS risk in infants younger than 11 weeks of age, especially if their position in bed was between their parents (Tappin et al., 2005). Two preventable risk factors for SIDS are household smoking and infant sleeping position, where supine sleep is advocated (e.g., "Back to Sleep" campaigns).

In prepubertal children there are few sex differences in sleep. However, changes are noted from puberty, starting earlier in girls than boys. During the teenage years, there is a strong tendency toward later bedtimes and even later rise times. This delay in bedtime is due to a circadian phase delay in adolescents (Carskadon et al., 2004). This "eveningness" tendency starts at around 13 years of age and peaks at around 20 years old, the peak occurring earlier in girls (19.5 years) than in boys (20.9 years; Roenneberg et al., 2004). Along with a shift toward later bedtimes across adolescence, sleep duration declines during school and non-school days at a slightly faster pace in girls, although sleep duration on both school days and non-school days remains longer overall for girls than for boys (Olds et al., 2010), matching findings in adults.

Activity monitors worn for 7 consecutive days in 91 schoolchildren aged 13–14 years (47 girls, 44 boys) showed that girls had longer sleep times and that during the weekdays an earlier wake time than boys (Gaina et al., 2005). Along with later bedtimes on the weekends, boys had a tendency to spend more time watching television and playing games, with concomitant lower sleep efficiency, higher activity, and more movement time than girls. Similarly, others found a greater amount of nighttime wake after sleep onset and sleep fragmentation in adolescent boys compared to girls (Short et al., 2012).

PSG studies in adolescents have extended knowledge about sex differences in the initiation of changes in the sleep EEG that characterize this critical developmental phase and reflect underlying changes in brain structure and function, with extensive synaptic pruning (Campbell et al., 2012; Goldstone et al., 2018). There are sex differences in the timing of the typical adolescent decline in N3 and SWA, with the decline starting approximately 1.2 years earlier in girls than in boys (Campbell et al., 2012). Other differences in sleep architecture in adolescents include more awakenings per hour of sleep and more wakefulness after sleep onset in boys compared to girls, although this effect was small (Baker et al., 2016). These findings suggest that several sex differences in PSG measures emerge during adolescence.

SEX DIFFERENCES IN CIRCADIAN TYPE AND RHYTHMS

Sex differences in circadian rhythms have been identified, which may in turn impact sleep (Kervezee et al., 2018). Morning or evening preference is a reflection of circadian type, or *chronotype.* Women tend more toward being morning types, with a preference for going to bed earlier and waking up early, a greater propensity for sleep in the evening, and earlier peak time for optimal mental performance (Adan & Natale, 2002; Fischer et al., 2017). This greater tendency for "morningness" may reflect, at least in part, phase-advanced circadian rhythms in women compared to men (Adan & Natale, 2002; Mongrain et al., 2004). Constant routine or forced desynchrony studies, which control photic and non-photic influences on the circadian system, have shown that women have phase-advanced melatonin and temperature rhythms, as well as a higher melatonin amplitude and lower temperature amplitude, compared with men (Cain et al., 2010). A mechanism contributing to this sex difference in circadian alignment and morningness tendency is a shorter circadian period in women, with a period of the temperature rhythm of 24.09 (0.2 hours) in women versus 24.19 (0.19 hours) in men and a significantly greater proportion of women than men having intrinsic circadian periods shorter than 24.0 hours (Duffy et al., 2011).

Impact of Sex on Shift Work

Sex differences in circadian rhythms may impact adaptability to shift work. Morning types, who have phase-advanced rhythms, are less tolerant of shift work than are evening types (Saksvik et al., 2011). Indeed, findings overall suggest that women are less tolerant of shift work and are more likely to report sleep difficulties and more fatigue than men (Saksvik et al., 2011). Women also show greater deterioration than do men in accuracy on cognitive tasks in the early morning hours when body temperature is at its nadir (Santhi et al., 2016). Other factors are also important for shift-work tolerance and may differentially impact women, including family and domestic responsibilities, which reduce time available for sleep and add stress.

Sex Steroids and Sleep

Sleep exerts modulatory influences on endocrine regulation, metabolism, immune functions, and cardiovascular activities. A probable factor contributing to sex differences in sleep is the difference in levels and cyclical changes of reproductive hormones in men and women. Endocrine regulation of reproductive function is complex and involves the hypothalamic–pituitary–adrenal (HPA) axis, gonads, and reproductive tract. Their effects are not specific to reproduction and have widespread actions throughout the body; not surprisingly, sex steroid receptors have been identified in the brain, including the suprachiasmatic nucleus, and somatic tissues. Although both men and women produce the same suite of reproductive hormones, the pronounced differences in levels and sensitivity are significant contributors to the sexually dimorphic phenotype. The effects of reproductive hormones on sleep specifically in women are discussed in Chapter 41.

Sleep Disorders

Insomnia Disorder

Insomnia disorder is currently defined in the *Diagnostic and Statistical Manual of Mental Disorders*, fifth edition (DSM-5; American Psychiatric Association, 2013) as a complaint of dissatisfaction with sleep quantity or quality (difficulty initiating sleep, maintaining sleep, or early morning awakenings) for at least 3 months, causing clinically significant distress or impairment. The disturbance must occur at least 3 nights a week despite adequate opportunity for sleep and cannot be explained by a concurrent sleep–wake disorder, breathing disorder, circadian rhythm disorder, substance use, mental disorder, or medical condition. Data from community-dwelling samples shows that the prevalence of insomnia disorder as formally and conservatively diagnosed is 6% (based on DSM-4 classification), whereas insomnia symptoms have a prevalence of 33% and insomnia symptoms with daytime consequences, a prevalence of 9%–15% (Ohayon, 2002). Consistently, the prevalence rate of insomnia symptoms and insomnia disorder is higher in women than in men (Ohayon, 1997, 2002; Figure 17.1).

A meta-analysis of 29 epidemiologic studies with more than 1.25 million participants identified that women had a risk ratio of 1.41 (95% confidence interval [CI] [1.28, 1.55]) to develop insomnia compared to men (Zhang & Wing, 2006). The trend of female predisposition for insomnia was persistent through various iterations of insomnia criteria and across all ages, with increased significance in the elderly population (Zhang & Wing,

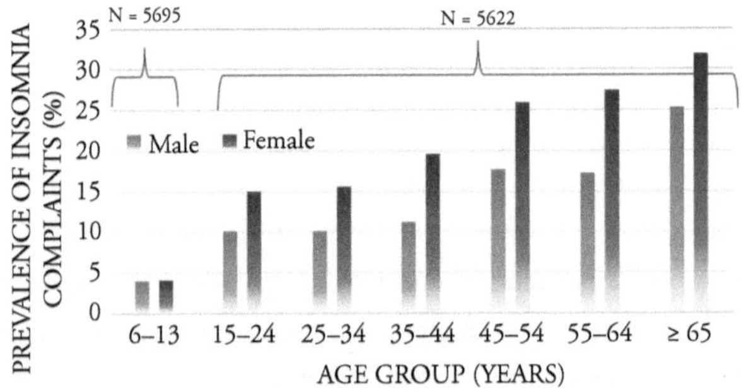

Figure 17.1 Prevalence of insomnia complaints in community samples of male and female children in Hong Kong (N = 5,695, 6–13 years) and male and female adults in France (N = 5,622, 15 years or older)

Note. Insomnia complaints are more common in women across the life span, with this difference emerging in late puberty. Data are taken from Zhang et al. (2009) and Ohayon (1997).

2006). Given that untreated insomnia can lead to significant comorbidities, it is important to recognize how women are disproportionately affected throughout several stages of life, from puberty to postmenopause.

The rate of insomnia in adolescents ranges between 4% and 39%, with a strong female preponderance emerging after puberty (de Zambotti et al., 2018, Zhang et al., 2009). Insomnia in adolescents emerges in the context of normal physiological changes in sleep timing and architecture that reflect reorganization of the adolescent brain (de Zambotti et al., 2018). A study of 7,507 children and adolescents (49% female) ages 6–17 recruited from 31 schools in Hong Kong found that the prevalence of insomnia increased 3.6-fold in girls and 2.1-fold in boys from Tanner Stages 1 to 5 (Zhang et al., 2016). The female preponderance for insomnia arose at Tanner Stage 4 and was associated with poor mental health, behavioral problems, and general poor health in both sexes (Zhang et al., 2016). Interestingly, boys with insomnia had more maladaptive lifestyles (smoking, alcohol use, energy drink use), while girls with insomnia experienced more emotional and relationship stress (Zhang et al., 2016). Crucially, insomnia experienced by adolescents is often chronic, with 88% of those with a history of insomnia reporting ongoing symptoms (de Zambotti et al., 2018). Insomnia is also an independent risk factor for suicidality in adolescents, making it particularly important to diagnose early with the aim to reduce the risk of adverse outcomes (de Zambotti et al., 2018). Given the higher prevalence of insomnia in teenage girls, it is important to examine potential sex-specific causal factors and determine whether treatment strategies should be differentially targeted to boys and girls.

While women are at greater risk for insomnia throughout their lives, insomnia symptoms can also emerge, or worsen, during certain reproductive phases, in particular the perimenopause period (Baker et al., 2018). A longitudinal analysis of insomnia symptoms among perimenopausal women in the Study of Women Across the Nation, which included multiethnic pre- and perimenopausal midlife women ($N = 3{,}302$) with an average age of 46 years (Ciano et al., 2017; Kravitz & Joffe, 2011), identified insomnia symptoms in 31%–42% of perimenopausal women at any 1-year study interval, especially in the late stage of perimenopause (Ciano et al., 2017). The odds of having insomnia symptoms in the late stage of perimenopause were 1.3 times greater than for women at the early stage of perimenopause (95% CI [1.2, 1.5]), suggesting that the stage of perimenopause heightens the risk of developing insomnia disorder (Ciano et al., 2017). A study aiming to quantify sleep disturbances and the contribution of hot flashes in 72 perimenopausal women with clinical insomnia versus without clinical insomnia found that women with insomnia in the approach to menopause had a significant sleep deficit, with 50% having less than 6 hours of sleep (Baker et al., 2015). Women with insomnia were more likely to have physiological hot flashes, had 44 minutes less PSG-measured sleep time, and had more wakefulness after sleep onset, as measured in the lab, and more night-to-night variability in wakefulness after sleep onset, as tracked using diaries at home (Baker et al., 2015). A myriad of factors can contribute to either the exacerbation or emergence of insomnia in the context of the menopausal transition, ranging from the sleep disruptive effects of hot flashes, changes in the hormonal milieu, and life stress.

In the elderly population insomnia has been associated with age-related sleep changes as well as an increase in medical conditions linked to insomnia, yet women continue to be disproportionately impacted. Furthermore, older adults are more vulnerable to the psychiatric and clinical effects of insomnia than are younger adults (Patel et al., 2018). In individuals older than 65 years with any type of insomnia diagnosis, a cross-sectional study found there was a significant association with female gender (OR = 2.21), consumption of psychotropic drugs (OR = 1.83), presence of four or more health problems (OR = 1.88), and being single, widowed, or divorced (OR = 1.43; Lopez-Torres Hidalgo et al., 2012). A review of late-life insomnia found that women who are caregivers have an increased prevalence of sleep complaints, specifically those who are primary caregivers for family members in addition to working outside the home (Patel et al., 2018). Indeed, while age itself is a contributor to increased sleep disturbances, additional obstacles that women face in older age include social obligations and comorbid health problems that could contribute to their impaired sleep.

It is likely that the predilection to insomnia in women is multifactorial. Beyond sex and female-specific changes in reproductive life stages together with age, the prevalence of insomnia could also be influenced by factors including mental health disorders, organic disease, marital status, socioeconomic class, drug use, and more (Hsu et al., 2013; Lopez-Torres Hidalgo et al., 2012; Ohayon, 2002; Patel et al., 2018). Anxiety and hyperarousal and biologic factors involving the HPA axis may enhance female vulnerability to insomnia (Beaulieu-Bonneau et al., 2007; Mai & Buysse, 2008; Voderholzer et al., 2003; Zhang & Wing, 2006), although sex differences in insomnia are not solely explained by the higher prevalence of anxiety and depression in women (Zhang & Wing, 2006).

Insomnia, when left undiagnosed and untreated, is associated with significant comorbidities in individuals at all ages. Older individuals with insomnia have a 23% increased risk of depression (Patel et al., 2018). Insomnia can precipitate or maintain mental disorders including major depressive illness and increase the risk of substance use disorders (Krystal et al., 2019; Ohayon, 2002). Overall, insomnia and mental disorders have a bidirectional relationship and can increase the risk of suicidal tendencies (Patel et al., 2018). Chronic insomnia is also a risk factor for cardiovascular disease, obesity, hypertension, and diabetes, with poor long-term outcomes (Kaur et al., 2022). Addressing the increased prevalence of insomnia specifically at critical time points could prevent or alleviate associated negative health consequences.

Restless Legs Syndrome

The International Restless Legs Syndrome Study Group (IRLSSG) defines restless legs syndrome (RLS) as a chronic movement disorder with an irresistible urge to move the legs with relief from movement, particularly in the evenings (IRLSSG 2021). Chronic RLS must occur at least twice a week for over a year, often causing significant sleep disturbance and decreased quality of life (IRLSSG 2021).

In America, RLS impacts approximately 5%–15% of the population (Mansur et al., 2022). RLS affects individuals at all ages starting from childhood, with an established predominance in women (Mallampalli & Carter, 2014; Mansur et al., 2022). A cross-sectional study of 4,310 randomly selected participants in Germany who were evaluated based on the IRLSSG criteria (Berger et al., 2004) found that women were affected twice as often as men, with an increased prevalence with age. The etiology behind this female predominance is unclear, but RLS has been associated with iron and dopamine homeostasis, chronic kidney disease, diabetes mellitus, rheumatic disease, and genetic factors.

Not only do more women develop RLS but they also experience worse symptoms, particularly during pregnancy and postmenopause. A retrospective study including 42 men and 42 women with RLS found that women self-reported worse RLS symptoms, while men had increased periodic leg movements during sleep (Holzknecht et al., 2020). Several of the participants, including 22 women and 8 men, also had lower serum ferritin levels, below 75 μg/L (Holzknecht et al., 2020). This finding demonstrates that there might be a sex difference in the phenotypical presentation of RLS, with women having more severe sensory symptoms, while men have more motor symptoms (Holzknecht et al., 2020).

The predominance and severity of RLS also change for women during hormonal milestones, including pregnancy, menses, and menopause. A study of 536 women who fulfilled IRLSSG criteria was evaluated for RLS symptoms at various life stages (Ghorayeb et al., 2008). A significant percentage perceived worsening of symptoms during pregnancy (23%), menses (23%), and postmenopause (23%; Ghorayeb et al., 2008). The study also identified that earlier age of RLS onset and increased parity were correlated to increased severity of RLS symptoms (Ghorayeb et al., 2008). Around 23%–26% of pregnant women develop symptoms of RLS by the third trimester, possibly due to lower iron levels, relative folate deficiency, or hormonal changes (Khan et al., 2017; Mansur et al., 2022). Increased estrogen is also hypothesized to precipitate RLS—estrogen is increased in the third trimester, and women using estrogen-based therapies are prone to develop RLS (Didato et al., 2020). Pregnancy-related RLS is often transient and resolves after delivery but is a risk factor for future chronic RLS and recurrent RLS in future pregnancies (Cesnik et al., 2010). Interestingly, nulliparous women had a similar prevalence to men up to age 64, confirming that pregnancy does have a significant role in the pathophysiology of RLS (Berger et al., 2004).

People with RLS have increased risk of several comorbidities and experience significantly lower quality-of-life outcomes (Berger et al., 2004; Didato et al., 2020; Mallampalli & Carter, 2014). Women are a vulnerable population for developing RLS, and understanding the pathophysiology and sequelae of RLS would contribute to improving long-term health outcomes.

Obstructive Sleep Apnea

Obstructive sleep apnea (OSA) is classically diagnosed via PSG identification of apneas (cessation of airflow) and hypopneas (reduced airflow) lasting at least 10 seconds during sleep. The American Academy of Sleep Medicine classifies OSA as mild, moderate, or severe based on an AHI of 5–15, 15–30, or >30 apneic events per hour of sleep, respectively (American Academy of Sleep Medicine Task Force, 1999).

OSA has classically been shown to disproportionately impact men more than women (Senaratna et al., 2017), in up to a 3:1 ratio in the general population and up to an 8:1 ratio in the clinical population (Ye et al., 2009). The etiology behind the discrepancy is attributed to a multitude of reasons, including foundational anatomical differences, the potential protective effect of female hormones, and missed or misdiagnoses in women due to different symptom presentations (Ye et al., 2009).

Anatomical differences in the upper airway between men and women could account for some of the increased prevalence of OSA diagnosed in men. A study of 71 patients with OSA compared the upper airway dimensions between men and women and the change in pharyngeal cross section with retrusive movement of the mandible during sleep (Mohsenin, 2003). The study concluded that men tend to have a larger but more collapsible airway in sleep, especially dependent on positioning (Mohsenin, 2003). OSA was more severe in men in the supine position, and the difference in supine versus side apnea–hypopnea was significantly increased in men (43.7 ± 5.2 events/hour) compared to that in women (10.7 ± 7.6 events/hour; Mohsenin, 2003).

Obesity is also a well-established risk factor for OSA, yet apnea severity in women is found to be less weight-dependent. A cross-sectional analysis of 686 patients with OSA in the preoperative period was made in relation to BMI and RDI (Walker et al., 2001). The correlation between OSA and BMI was stronger in male patients ($r = 0.40$) compared to female patients ($r = 0.21$; Walker et al., 2001). Male patients were generally younger and had a lower BMI associated with a higher RDI, suggesting the BMI threshold might be higher in women before symptoms appear (Walker et al., 2001).

While physical differences could influence OSA, women experience a change in the prevalence of OSA after menopause, which cannot be explained by anatomy alone. A sample of 589 midlife women in the Wisconsin Sleep Cohort Study compared the risk of OSA in perimenopausal versus postmenopausal women (Young et al., 2003). After adjusting for age, body habitus, and smoking status, postmenopausal women had increased odds of developing OSA (OR = 2.6, 95% CI [1.4, 4.8]) compared to perimenopausal women (OR = 1.2, 95% CI [0.7, 2.2]; Young et al., 2003). Postmenopausal women had a threefold increased risk of severe OSA, defined as over 15 apnea/hypopnea events per hour (Young et al., 2003). In fact, the sex differences in OSA prevalence diminish between older men and older women. When comparing individuals with OSA among three age groups (18–39, 40–59, 60–88), the sex difference between men and women was nonsignificant as the frequency of OSA doubled from middle-aged to older women (Ware et al., 2000). In the longitudinal analyses of the Wisconsin Sleep Cohort, AHI increased from premenopause to peri- and postmenopause, independent of age and changes in body habitus, although these factors were also associated with AHI (Mirer et al., 2017). The increased likelihood of sleep disordered breathing after menopause could be partially attributed to the hormonal shift during this pivotal life stage (Young et al., 2003): The hormonal milieu of women in the reproductive stages protects them from developing sleep apnea before the menopause. Indeed, there is a menstrual phase effect on upper airway resistance, possibly related to a benefit from progesterone, with less airway resistance during the luteal phase than in the follicular phase (Driver et al., 2005). Changes in fat distribution after menopause can also contribute to increased risk for OSA (Polesel et al., 2015). In postmenopausal women, hormone therapy has been associated with a lower prevalence of sleep apnea (Lindberg et al., 2020). While there may be potential for hormone therapy in the management of OSA in older women, the health risks associated with using hormone therapy need to be carefully considered, and continuous positive airway pressure remains the treatment of choice. Healthy lifestyle changes (e.g., weight loss and exercise) should also be implemented.

As referred to above, it is important to consider that women might be underrepresented in the diagnosis of OSA due to variable symptom presentations. Large cohort studies in the general population coupled with changes in technology (e.g., more accurate airflow measurement via nasal cannula pressure transducers than with thermal sensors), the increase in obesity with higher prevalence in women than men (in most countries), and the referral bias in favor of men indicate that OSA is more common in women than previously recognized (Banno & Kryger, 2008). A sample of 1,166 patients (male:female ratio of 4.9:1) with OSA contrasted the frequency of common OSA complaints between the male and female participants (Quintana-Gallego et al., 2004). Snoring and daytime hypersomnolence were similar between the sexes, while morning headache, insomnia, depression, fatigue, and use of sedatives were more frequent in women (Quintana-Gallego et al., 2004). The symptoms of OSA that are more common in women—particularly insomnia, depression, and fatigue—can easily be labeled as a mood disorder rather than a sleep disorder (Banno & Kryger, 2008). Notably, more men came to clinical interviews accompanied by their partners, and witnessed apneas were more frequent in men (Quintana-Gallego et al., 2004). Another study of OSA participants (N = 36) including family members and neighbors found that women consistently underreported classic symptoms of OSA, including snoring, snorting, gasping, and apnea in sleep (Redline et al., 1994). Furthermore, there are also differences in PSG findings of OSA between men and women, further complicating the diagnosis. A retrospective study of 830 patients with OSA found that women had milder OSA during NREM sleep and more respiratory events clustered during REM sleep (O'Connor et al., 2000). The disruption of REM sleep with OSA could contribute to the symptom differences experienced by women compared to men.

The etiology of OSA is not well understood, and its sex disparity likely has contributions from a combination of the factors discussed above. While it appears that men are disadvantaged based on physical and hormonal differences to develop OSA, there is a chance that women are being underdiagnosed due to their symptom presentation and PSG findings. Chronic OSA can cause significant sequelae including hypertension, coronary vascular disease, insulin resistance, stroke, and diminished quality of life (Lin et al., 2008); and it is unclear whether women are at a higher risk for developing cardiovascular problems and metabolic disorders as a consequence (Hegner et al., 2021). More work needs to be done to understand OSA for improved diagnosis and potential for novel management options.

Conclusion and Future Directions

There are sex differences in sleep behavior, architecture, and the prevalence, presentation, and severity of some sleep disorders. These differences are summarized in Table 17.1. Women have a greater sleep need, longer sleep duration, and earlier bedtimes yet a poorer sleep quality and more sleep difficulties than men. These differences should be explored further and contextualized within a psychosocial framework while considering caregiving and work responsibilities, underlying mood or physical health issues, as well as stage of the reproductive life cycle. PSG and quantitative sleep EEG measures reveal more SWS and delta (slow wave) power and better preservation of SWS with

Table 17.1 Summary of sex differences in sleep

Parameter	Women compared to men
Sleep duration—self-report, actigraphy, big data	Longer
Sleep quality—subjective	Worse
Sleep quality—objective polysomnography	Better
N3%	Higher
Age-related decrease N3	Later
Absolute delta power (slow-wave activity) and sleep spindle activity	Greater
Circadian type	Morning-type
Circadian period	Shorter
Shift work	Less tolerant
Insomnia	More likely
Restless legs syndrome	Higher incidence, including pregnancy
Obstructive sleep apnea	Lower incidence premenopause

aging in women than men as consistent findings. However, some studies have questioned whether these sex differences are true physiological differences or rather reflect sex differences in brain anatomy influencing measurement of the sleep EEG. Future studies that use interventions to challenge sleep, for example, sleep restriction or sleep interruption, and examining possible sex differences in cognitive and other performance measures are needed to determine whether there are functional sex differences in sleep. Women are at greater risk for both insomnia disorder and RLS, and the prevalence and severity of both these disorders can fluctuate according to reproductive hormonal milestones. The higher risk for insomnia in women emerges in adolescence, making this period an important focus for future studies to understand underlying mechanisms to prevent the chronicity of insomnia from persisting into adulthood. Men are at higher risk for OSA, with women being relatively protected at least until midlife due to several factors including anatomical differences of the upper airway and the potential protective effect of female hormones. However, the potential for underdiagnosis of OSA in women due to a different symptom profile cannot be discounted and may affect the true prevalence in women. Furthermore, it is unclear whether comorbidity differs according to sex and how this might impact symptom presentation or outcomes. Given the significant long-term health effects of all three of these sleep disorders, further studies are needed to improve our understanding of the underlying etiology, clinical presentation, and diagnosis, as well as the potential for novel management options that may be customized for women and men.

References

Adan, A., & Natale, V. (2002). Gender differences in morningness-eveningness preference. *Chronobiology International, 19*, 709–720.

American Academy of Sleep Medicine Task Force. (1999). Sleep-related breathing disorders in adults: Recommendations for syndrome definition and measurement techniques in clinical research. The Report of an American Academy of Sleep Medicine Task Force. *Sleep, 22*(5), 667–689.

American Psychiatric Association. (2013). *Diagnostic and statistical manual of mental disorders* (5th ed.). https://doi.org/10.1176/appi.books.9780890425596

Anuntaseree, W., Mo-Suwan, L., Vasiknanonte, P., Kuasirikul, S., Ma-A-Lee, A., & Choprapawan, C. (2008). Night waking in Thai infants at 3 months of age: Association between parental practices and infant sleep. *Sleep Medicine, 9*, 564–571.

Armitage, R., Smith, C., Thompson, S., & Hoffmann, R. (2001). Sex differences in slow-wave activity in response to sleep deprivation. *Sleep Research Online, 4*, 33–41.

Auer, M. K., Liedl, A., Fuss, J., Nieder, T., Briken, P., Stalla, G. K., Hildebrandt, T., Biedermann, S. V., & Sievers, C. (2017). High impact of sleeping problems on quality of life in transgender individuals: A cross-sectional multicenter study. *PLOS ONE, 12*, Article e0171640.

Bach, V., Telliez, F., Leke, A., & Libert, J. P. (2000). Gender-related sleep differences in neonates in thermoneutral and cool environments. *Journal of Sleep Research, 9*, 249–254.

Bachtrog, D. (2006). A dynamic view of sex chromosome evolution. *Current Opinion in Genetics & Development, 16*, 578–585.

Baker, F. C., De Zambotti, M., Colrain, I. M., & Bei, B. (2018). Sleep problems during the menopausal transition: Prevalence, impact, and management challenges. *Nature and Science of Sleep, 10*, 73–95.

Baker, F. C., Willoughby, A. R., De Zambotti, M., Franzen, P. L., Prouty, D., Javitz, H., Hasler, B., Clark, D. B., & Colrain, I. M. (2016). Age-related differences in sleep architecture and electroencephalogram in

adolescents in the National Consortium on Alcohol and Neurodevelopment in Adolescence sample. *Sleep, 39*, 1429–1439.
Baker, F. C., Willoughby, A. R., Sassoon, S. A., Colrain, I. M., & De Zambotti, M. (2015). Insomnia in women approaching menopause: Beyond perception. *Psychoneuroendocrinology, 60*, 96–104.
Banno, K., & Kryger, M. H. (2008). The circuitous route to diagnosing sleep disorders in women: Healthcare utilization and benefits of improved awareness for sleep disorders. *Sleep Medicine Clinics, 3*, 133–140.
Beaulieu-Bonneau, S., Leblanc, M., Merette, C., Dauvilliers, Y., & Morin, C. M. (2007). Family history of insomnia in a population-based sample. *Sleep, 30*, 1739–1745.
Berger, K., Luedemann, J., Trenkwalder, C., John, U., & Kessler, C. (2004). Sex and the risk of restless legs syndrome in the general population. *Archives of Internal Medicine, 164*, 196–202.
Boulos, M. I., Jairam, T., Kendzerska, T., Im, J., Mekhael, A., & Murray, B. J. (2019). Normal polysomnography parameters in healthy adults: A systematic review and meta-analysis. *Lancet: Respiratory Medicine, 7*, 533–543.
Burgard, S. A., & Ailshire, J. A. (2013). Gender and time for sleep among U.S. adults. *American Sociological Review, 78*, 51–69.
Byard, R. W., & Krous, H. F. (2004). Research and sudden infant death syndrome: Definitions, diagnostic difficulties and discrepancies. *Journal of Paediatric and Child Health, 40*, 419–421.
Cain, S. W., Dennison, C. F., Zeitzer, J. M., Guzik, A. M., Khalsa, S. B., Santhi, N., Schoen, M. W., Czeisler, C. A., & Duffy, J. F. (2010). Sex differences in phase angle of entrainment and melatonin amplitude in humans. *Journal of Biologica Rhythms, 25*, 288–296.
Campbell, I. G., Grimm, K. J., De Bie, E., & Feinberg, I. (2012). Sex, puberty, and the timing of sleep EEG measured adolescent brain maturation. *Proceedings of the National Academy of Sciences of the United States of America, 109*, 5740–5743.
Carrier, J., Semba, K., Deurveilher, S., Drogos, L., Cyr-Cronier, J., Lord, C., & Sekerovick, Z. (2017). Sex differences in age-related changes in the sleep–wake cycle. *Frontiers in Neuroendocrinology, 47*, 66–85.
Carskadon, M. A., Acebo, C., & Jenni, O. G. (2004). Regulation of adolescent sleep: Implications for behavior. *Annals of the New York Academy of Sciences, 1021*, 276–291.
Cesnik, E., Casetta, I., Turri, M., Govoni, V., Granieri, E., Strambi, L. F., & Manconi, M. (2010). Transient RLS during pregnancy is a risk factor for the chronic idiopathic form. *Neurology, 75*, 2117–2120.
Chaput, J. P., Wong, S. L., & Michaud, I. (2017). Duration and quality of sleep among Canadians aged 18 to 79. *Health Reports, 28*, 28–33.
Ciano, C., King, T. S., Wright, R. R., Perlis, M., & Sawyer, A. M. (2017). Longitudinal study of insomnia symptoms among women during perimenopause. *Journal of Obstetric, Gynecologic, and Neonatal Nursing, 46*, 804–813.
Collop, N. A., Adkins, D., & Phillips, B. A. (2004). Gender differences in sleep and sleep-disordered breathing. *Clinics in Chest Medicine, 25*, 257–268.
Della Monica, C., Johnsen, S., Atzori, G., Groeger, J. A., & Dijk, D.-J. (2018). Rapid eye movement sleep, sleep continuity and slow wave sleep as predictors of cognition, mood, and subjective sleep quality in healthy men and women, aged 20–84 years. *Frontiers in Psychiatry, 9*, Article 255.
De Zambotti, M., Goldstone, A., Colrain, I. M., & Baker, F. C. (2018). Insomnia disorder in adolescence: Diagnosis, impact, and treatment. *Sleep Medicine Reviews, 39*, 12–24.
Didato, G., Di Giacomo, R., Rosa, G. J., Dominese, A., De Curtis, M., & Lanteri, P. (2020). Restless legs syndrome across the lifespan: Symptoms, pathophysiology, management and daily life impact of the different patterns of disease presentation. *International Journal of Environmental Research and Public Health*, 17, Article 3658.
Driver, H. S., Mclean, H., Kumar, D. V., Farr, N., Day, A. G., & Fitzpatrick, M. F. (2005). The influence of the menstrual cycle on upper airway resistance and breathing during sleep. *Sleep, 28*, 449–456.
Duffy, J. F., Cain, S. W., Chang, A. M., Phillips, A. J., Munch, M. Y., Gronfier, C., Wyatt, J. K., Dijk, D. J., Wright, K. P., Jr., & Czeisler, C. A. (2011). Sex difference in the near-24-hour intrinsic period of the human circadian timing system. *Proceedings of the National Academy of Sciences of the United States of America, 108*(S3), 15602–15608.
Dzaja, A., Arber, S., Hislop, J., Kerkhofs, M., Kopp, C., Pollmacher, T., Polo-Kantola, P., Skene, D. J., Stenuit, P., Tobler, I., & Porkka-Heiskanen, T. (2005). Women's sleep in health and disease. *Journal of Psychiatric Research, 39*, 55–76.

Ehlers, C. L., & Kupfer, D. J. (1997). Slow-wave sleep: Do young adult men and women age differently? *Journal of Sleep Research, 6*, 211–215.

Eliason, M. J. (2014). An exploration of terminology related to sexuality and gender: Arguments for standardizing the language. *Social Work in Public Health, 29*, 162–75.

Ferrara, M., & De Gennaro, L. (2001). How much sleep do we need? *Sleep Medicine Reviews, 5*, 155–179.

Ferri, R., DelRosso, L. M., Provini, F., Stefani, A., Walters, A. S., & Picchietti, D. L., on behalf of the International Restless Legs Syndrome Study Group (IRLSSG). (2021). Scoring of large muscle group movements during sleep: An International Restless Legs Syndrome Study Group position statement. *Sleep, 44*(9), zsab092. https://doi.org/10.1093/sleep/zsab092

Fischer, D., Lombardi, D. A., Marucci-Wellman, H., & Roenneberg, T. (2017). Chronotypes in the US—Influence of age and sex. *PLOS ONE, 12*, Article e0178782.

Gaina, A., Sekine, M., Hamanishi, S., Chen, X., & Kagamimori, S. (2005). Gender and temporal differences in sleep–wake patterns in Japanese schoolchildren. *Sleep, 28*, 337–342.

Ghorayeb, I., Bioulac, B., Scribans, C., & Tison, F. (2008). Perceived severity of restless legs syndrome across the female life cycle. *Sleep Medicine, 9*, 799–802.

Goldstone, A., Willoughby, A. R., De Zambotti, M., Franzen, P. L., Kwon, D., Pohl, K. M., Pfefferbaum, A., Sullivan, E. V., Muller-Oehring, E. M., Prouty, D. E., Hasler, B. P., Clark, D. B., Colrain, I. M., & Baker, F. C. (2018). The mediating role of cortical thickness and gray matter volume on sleep slow-wave activity during adolescence. *Brain Structure & Function, 223*, 669–685.

Groeger, J. A., Zijlstra, F. R., & Dijk, D. J. (2004). Sleep quantity, sleep difficulties and their perceived consequences in a representative sample of some 2000 British adults. *Journal of Sleep Research, 13*, 359–371.

Hegner, P., Lebek, S., Maier, L. S., Arzt, M., & Wagner, S. (2021). The effect of gender and sex hormones on cardiovascular disease, heart failure, diabetes, and atrial fibrillation in sleep apnea. *Frontiers in Physiology, 12*, Article 741896.

Holzknecht, E., Hochleitner, M., Wenning, G. K., Hogl, B., & Stefani, A. (2020). Gender differences in clinical, laboratory and polysomnographic features of restless legs syndrome. *Journal of Sleep Research, 29*, Article e12875.

Hsu, Y. W., Ho, C. H., Wang, J. J., Hsieh, K. Y., Weng, S. F., & Wu, M. P. (2013). Longitudinal trends of the healthcare-seeking prevalence and incidence of insomnia in Taiwan: An 8-year nationally representative study. *Sleep Medicine, 14*, 843–849.

Hume, K. I., Van, F., & Watson, A. (1998). A field study of age and gender differences in habitual adult sleep. *Journal of Sleep Research, 7*, 85–94.

Jean-Louis, G., Kripke, D. F., & Ancoli-Israel, S. (2000). Sleep and quality of well-being. *Sleep, 23*, 1115–1121.

Jonasdottir, S. S., Minor, K., & Lehmann, S. (2021). Gender differences in nighttime sleep patterns and variability across the adult lifespan: A global-scale wearables study. *Sleep, 44*, Article zsaa169.

Kaur, H., Spurling, B. C., & Bollu, P. C. (2022). *Chronic insomnia.* StatPearls.

Kervezee, L., Shechter, A., & Boivin, D. B. (2018). Impact of shift work on the circadian timing system and health in women. *Sleep Medicine Clinics, 13*, 295–306.

Khan, F. H., Ahlberg, C. D., Chow, C. A., Shah, D. R., & Koo, B. B. (2017). Iron, dopamine, genetics, and hormones in the pathophysiology of restless legs syndrome. *Journal of Neurology, 264*, 1634–1641.

Kravitz, H. M., & Joffe, H. (2011). Sleep during the perimenopause: A SWAN story. *Obstetrics and Gynecology Clinics of North America, 38*, 567–586.

Krystal, A. D., Prather, A. A., & Ashbrook, L. H. (2019). The assessment and management of insomnia: An update. *World Psychiatry, 18*, 337–352.

Kumar, S., Anton, A., & D'Ambrosio, C. M. (2021). Sex differences in obstructive sleep apnea. *Clinics in Chest Medicine, 42*, 417–425.

Lahn, B. T., & Page, D. C. (1999). Four evolutionary strata on the human X chromosome. *Science, 286*, 964–967.

Lauderdale, D. S., Knutson, K. L., Yan, L. L., Rathouz, P. J., Hulley, S. B., Sidney, S., & Liu, K. (2006). Objectively measured sleep characteristics among early-middle-aged adults: The CARDIA study. *American Journal of Epidemiology, 164*, 5–16.

Li, L., Sheehan, C. M., & Thompson, M. S. (2019). Measurement invariance and sleep quality differences between men and women in the Pittsburgh Sleep Quality Index. *Journal of Clinical Sleep Medicine, 15*, 1769–1776.

Lin, C. M., Davidson, T. M., & Ancoli-Israel, S. (2008). Gender differences in obstructive sleep apnea and treatment implications. *Sleep Medicine Reviews, 12*, 481–496.
Lindberg, E., Bonsignore, M. R., & Polo-Kantola, P. (2020). Role of menopause and hormone replacement therapy in sleep-disordered breathing. *Sleep Medicine Reviews, 49*, Article 101225.
Lindberg, E., Janson, C., Gislason, T., Bjornsson, E., Hetta, J., & Boman, G. (1997). Sleep disturbances in a young adult population: Can gender differences be explained by differences in psychological status? *Sleep, 20*, 381–387.
Lopez-Torres Hidalgo, J., Navarro Bravo, B., Parraga Martinez, I., Andres Pretel, F., Tellez Lapeira, J., & Boix Gras, C. (2012). Understanding insomnia in older adults. *International Journal of Geriatric Psychiatry, 27*, 1086–1093.
Mai, E., & Buysse, D. J. (2008). Insomnia: Prevalence, impact, pathogenesis, differential diagnosis, and evaluation. *Sleep Medicine Clinics, 3*, 167–174.
Mallampalli, M. P., & Carter, C. L. (2014). Exploring sex and gender differences in sleep health: A Society for Women's Health Research report. *Journal of Women's Health, 23*, 553–562.
Mansur, A., Castillo, P. R., Rocha Cabrero, F., & Bokhari, S. R. A. (2022). *Restless legs syndrome*. StatPearls.
Mirer, A. G., Young, T., Palta, M., Benca, R. M., Rasmuson, A., & Peppard, P. E. (2017). Sleep-disordered breathing and the menopausal transition among participants in the Sleep in Midlife Women Study. *Menopause, 24*, 157–162.
Mohsenin, V. (2003). Effects of gender on upper airway collapsibility and severity of obstructive sleep apnea. *Sleep Medicine, 4*, 523–529.
Mong, J. A., & Cusmano, D. M. (2016). Sex differences in sleep: Impact of biological sex and sex steroids. *Philosophical Transactions of the Royal Society of London B: Biological Sciences, 371*, Article 20150110.
Mongrain, V., Lavoie, S., Selmaoui, B., Paquet, J., & Dumont, M. (2004). Phase relationships between sleep–wake cycle and underlying circadian rhythms in morningness-eveningness. *Journal of Biological Rhythms, 19*, 248–257.
Morris, J. L., Rohay, J., & Chasens, E. R. (2018). Sex differences in the psychometric properties of the Pittsburgh Sleep Quality Index. *Journal of Women's Health, 27*, 278–282.
O'Connor, C., Thornley, K. S., & Hanly, P. J. (2000). Gender differences in the polysomnographic features of obstructive sleep apnea. *American Journal of Respiratory and Critical Care Medicine, 161*, 1465–1472.
Ohayon, M. M. (1997). Prevalence of DSM-IV diagnostic criteria of insomnia: Distinguishing insomnia related to mental disorders from sleep disorders. *Journal of Psychiatric Research, 31*, 333–346.
Ohayon, M. M. (2002). Epidemiology of insomnia: What we know and what we still need to learn. *Sleep Medicine Reviews, 6*, 97–111.
Olds, T., Blunden, S., Petkov, J., & Forchino, F. (2010). The relationships between sex, age, geography and time in bed in adolescents: A meta-analysis of data from 23 countries. *Sleep Medicine Reviews, 14*, 371–378.
Patel, D., Steinberg, J., & Patel, P. (2018). Insomnia in the elderly: A review. *Journal of Clinical Sleep Medicine, 14*, 1017–1024.
Polesel, D. N., Hirotsu, C., Nozoe, K. T., Boin, A. C., Bittencourt, L., Tufik, S., Andersen, M. L., & Hachul, H. (2015). Waist circumference and postmenopause stages as the main associated factors for sleep apnea in women: A cross-sectional population-based study. *Menopause, 22*, 835–844.
Purcell, S. M., Manoach, D. S., Demanuele, C., Cade, B. E., Mariani, S., Cox, R., Panagiotaropoulou, G., Saxena, R., Pan, J. Q., Smoller, J. W., Redline, S., & Stickgold, R. (2017). Characterizing sleep spindles in 11,630 individuals from the National Sleep Research Resource. *Nature Communications, 8*, Article 15930.
Quintana-Gallego, E., Carmona-Bernal, C., Capote, F., Sanchez-Armengol, A., Botebol-Benhamou, G., Polo-Padillo, J., & Castillo-Gomez, J. (2004). Gender differences in obstructive sleep apnea syndrome: A clinical study of 1166 patients. *Respiratory Medicine, 98*, 984–989.
Redline, S., Kirchner, H. L., Quan, S. F., Gottlieb, D. J., Kapur, V., & Newman, A. (2004). The effects of age, sex, ethnicity, and sleep-disordered breathing on sleep architecture. *Archives of Internal Medicine, 164*, 406–418.
Redline, S., Kump, K., Tishler, P. V., Browner, I., & Ferrette, V. (1994). Gender differences in sleep disordered breathing in a community-based sample. *American Journal of Respiratory and Critical Care Medicine, 149*, 722–726.
Reyner, L. A., Horne, J. A., & Reyner, A. (1995). Gender- and age-related differences in sleep determined by home-recorded sleep logs and actimetry from 400 adults. *Sleep, 18*, 127–134.

Roenneberg, T., Kuehnle, T., Pramstaller, P. P., Ricken, J., Havel, M., Guth, A., & Merrow, M. (2004). A marker for the end of adolescence. *Current Biology, 14*, R1038–R1039.

Rosinvil, T., Bouvier, J., Dube, J., Lafreniere, A., Bouchard, M., Cyr-Cronier, J., Gosselin, N., Carrier, J., & Lina, J. M. (2021). Are age and sex effects on sleep slow waves only a matter of electroencephalogram amplitude? *Sleep, 44*, Article zsaa186.

Saksvik, I. B., Bjorvatn, B., Hetland, H., Sandal, G. M., & Pallesen, S. (2011). Individual differences in tolerance to shift work—A systematic review. *Sleep Medicine Reviews, 15*, 221–235.

Santhi, N., Lazar, A. S., McCabe, P. J., Lo, J. C., Groeger, J. A., & Dijk, D. J. (2016). Sex differences in the circadian regulation of sleep and waking cognition in humans. *Proceedings of the National Academy of Sciences of the United States of America, 113*, E2730–E2739.

Senaratna, C.V., Perret, J. L. Lodge, C. J., Lowe, A. J., Campbell, B. E., Matheson, M. C., Hamilton, G. S., & Dharmage, S. C. (2017). Prevalence of obstructive sleep apnea in the general population: A systematic review. *Sleep Medicine Reviews, 34*, 70–81.

Short, M. A., Gradisar, M., Lack, L. C., Wright, H., & Carskadon, M. A. (2012). The discrepancy between actigraphic and sleep diary measures of sleep in adolescents. *Sleep Medicine, 13*, 378–384.

Tappin, D., Ecob, R., & Brooke, H. (2005). Bedsharing, roomsharing, and sudden infant death syndrome in Scotland: A case–control study. *Journal of Pediatrics, 147*, 32–37.

Ursin, R., Bjorvatn, B., & Holsten, F. (2005). Sleep duration, subjective sleep need, and sleep habits of 40- to 45-year-olds in the Hordaland Health Study. *Sleep, 28*, 1260–1269.

van den Berg, J. F., Miedema, H. M., Tulen, J. H., Hofman, A., Neven, A. K., & Tiemeier, H. (2009). Sex differences in subjective and actigraphic sleep measures: A population-based study of elderly persons. *Sleep, 32*, 1367–1375.

Voderholzer, U., Al-Shajlawi, A., Weske, G., Feige, B., & Riemann, D. (2003). Are there gender differences in objective and subjective sleep measures? A study of insomniacs and healthy controls. *Depression and Anxiety, 17*, 162–172.

Walker, R. P., Durazo-Arvizu, R., Wachter, B., & Gopalsami, C. (2001). Preoperative differences between male and female patients with sleep apnea. *Laryngoscope, 111*, 1501–1505.

Ware, J. C., McBrayer, R. H., & Scott, J. A. (2000). Influence of sex and age on duration and frequency of sleep apnea events. *Sleep, 23*, 165–170.

Waters, P. D., Wallis, M. C., & Marshall Graves, J. A. (2007). Mammalian sex—Origin and evolution of the Y chromosome and SRY. *Seminars in Cell & Developmental Biology, 18*, 389–400.

Ye, L., Pien, G. W., & Weaver, T. E. (2009). Gender differences in the clinical manifestation of obstructive sleep apnea. *Sleep Medicine, 10*, 1075–1084.

Yetton, B. D., Mcdevitt, E. A., Cellini, N., Shelton, C., & Mednick, S. C. (2018). Quantifying sleep architecture dynamics and individual differences using big data and Bayesian networks. *PLOS ONE, 13*, Article e0194604.

Young, T., Finn, L., Austin, D., & Peterson, A. (2003). Menopausal status and sleep-disordered breathing in the Wisconsin Sleep Cohort Study. *American Journal of Respiratory and Critical Care Medicine, 167*, 1181–1185.

Zhang, B., & Wing, Y. K. (2006). Sex differences in insomnia: A meta-analysis. *Sleep, 29*, 85–93.

Zhang, J., Chan, N. Y., Lam, S. P., Li, S. X., Liu, Y., Chan, J. W., Kong, A. P., Ma, R. C., Chan, K. C., Li, A. M., & Wing, Y. K. (2016). Emergence of sex differences in insomnia symptoms in adolescents: A large-scale school-based study. *Sleep, 39*, 1563–1570.

Zhang, J., Li, A. M., Kong, A. P., Lai, K. Y., Tang, N. L., & Wing, Y. K. (2009). A community-based study of insomnia in Hong Kong Chinese children: Prevalence, risk factors and familial aggregation. *Sleep Medicine, 10*, 1040–1046.

CHAPTER

18 The Impact of Prescription and Recreational Drugs on Sleep

Kai Spiegelhalder, Christoph Nissen, *and* Dieter Riemann

Abstract

This chapter provides an overview of the effects of psychotropic substances on sleep including over-the-counter sleep medications, synthetic drugs for insomnia, and recreational drugs. For each class of substances, a short description of the pharmacological properties is given. This is followed by a review of its effects on polysomnographic sleep and insomnia as well as of potential risks and side effects. In an evidence-based approach, meta-analyses are referred to where available. Although significant progress has been made over recent decades in understanding the fundamentals of sleep–wake regulation and in treating sleep disturbances, future research is needed to develop better pharmacological treatment options and to better meet the individual needs of patients with disordered sleep.

Key Words: sleep, insomnia, medication, over-the-counter medication, benzodiazepine, benzodiazepine receptor agonist, sedating antidepressant, orexin receptor antagonist, antipsychotic, recreational drug

The Problematic History of Sleep Medication

The search for and the use of substances to alleviate sleep complaints and to induce restful sleep have a very long history. In ancient times, opium and alcohol-containing beverages were not only used for recreational or religious purposes but also for the treatment of insomnia (Shiyi & Inoué, 1995). Also, scopolamine and herbal substances were frequently used prior to the 20th century to induce or improve sleep. The bromides became fashionable in the early 20th century. Yet this class of drugs turned out to be very problematic due to the risk of bromide poisoning and associated health risks, including nausea, an acne-like rash, ataxia, and psychotic symptoms. The barbiturates that act at the γ-aminobutyric acid A (GABA-A) receptor were introduced in 1903 and dominated the treatment of insomnia until the early 1960s (Mendelson, 2005). Though initially praised as effective and harmless, it became known in the 1930s that barbiturates are associated with a high risk of abuse, dependence, and accidental overdosing (Oswald, 1984). Due to their strong inhibition of the respiratory drive and the small range between therapeutic and lethal doses, barbiturates are now considered obsolete for insomnia treatment.

Another reason for the widespread negative image of sleep medication was the thalidomide scandal. Thalidomide was introduced in 1957 for the treatment of insomnia; however, it turned out that the substance is highly teratogenic, and, in consequence, more than 10,000 children were born with malformations of their extremities. In the 1960s, benzodiazepines (BZs) were introduced into clinical practice. BZs act as agonists at the GABA-A receptor and were frequently prescribed for the treatment of anxiety and insomnia. Initially, it was claimed that these substances were effective and bore no risk of abuse. However, the risk for the development of tolerance and dependence as well as the risk for nocturnal falls have led experts to question their widespread use (Mendelson et al., 2004). In the following sections, the effects of over-the-counter sleep medication, synthetic drugs for insomnia, and recreational drugs are summarized.

Over-the-Counter Sleep Medications

Valerian

EFFECTS ON POLYSOMNOGRAPHIC SLEEP

The phytotherapeutic agent that has probably most often been used for improving sleep is valerian. However, only few studies have investigated the effects of valerian on polysomnographically recorded sleep. The majority of the few randomized placebo-controlled studies that were conducted showed no significant effect on polysomnographic sleep (Leach & Page, 2015).

EFFECTS ON INSOMNIA

A systematic review and meta-analysis on the effects of valerian on insomnia included 14 randomized controlled trials involving 1,602 participants with insomnia (Leach & Page, 2015). The quantitative synthesis did not show any superiority of valerian in comparison to placebo. Consequently, the authors concluded that there is insufficient evidence to support the use of valerian for insomnia.

SIDE EFFECTS

There is preliminary evidence that valerian results in an increased number of adverse events compared to placebo (Leach & Page, 2015). Serious adverse events have, however, not been reported after the intake of valerian. In addition, clinical experience in Europe indicates a low incidence of interactions with alcohol or other drugs and that residual morning sleepiness is uncommon. Use near conception and during pregnancy and lactation is not recommended due to potential mutagenic effects of valepotriates.

Antihistamines

EFFECTS ON POLYSOMNOGRAPHIC SLEEP

Despite their widespread use, the effects of antihistamines on polysomnographic sleep have rarely been investigated. Early studies have shown a reduction of sleep onset latency after diphenhydramine and doxylamine (Rickels et al., 1983, 1984). However, it seems that effects beyond 1 week of drug intake have not been studied.

EFFECTS ON INSOMNIA

The evidence concerning the efficacy of antihistamines in the treatment of insomnia is insufficient. A systematic review has concluded that there are no high-quality randomized controlled trials, the efficacy appears to be weak at best, and tolerance against antihistamines develops rapidly (VanDe Griend & Anderson, 2012). Thus, antihistamines can currently not be recommended for the treatment of insomnia.

SIDE EFFECTS

Most prominently, central nervous system (CNS) side effects of antihistamines include sedation, dizziness, muscle relaxation (potentially leading to falls), fatigue, and headache.

Melatonin and Melatonin Receptor Agonists

EFFECTS ON POLYSOMNOGRAPHIC SLEEP

The literature concerning the effects of melatonin and melatonin receptor agonists on polysomnographic sleep suggests a small to moderate improvement of both sleep onset latency and total sleep time (Marupuru et al., 2022; Salanitro et al., 2022). Clinically meaningful effects on slow-wave sleep or rapid-eye-movement (REM) sleep have not been reported so far.

EFFECTS ON INSOMNIA

The latest meta-analysis on the efficacy of melatonin and melatonin receptor agonists in insomnia has summarized data from 17 studies (Marupuru et al., 2022). The quantitative analysis demonstrated significant small to moderate improvements in objective total sleep time and objective and subjective sleep onset latency after the intake of these substances. However, in line with previous meta-analyses, the positive effects were primarily reported for patients with an age of at least 55 years. This has affected the approval of melatonin by the European Medicines Agency, which is limited to patients with an age of 55 years or above.

SIDE EFFECTS

The published literature on melatonin and melatonin receptor agonists does not suggest any serious side effects of these substances (see, e.g., Salanitro et al., 2022). The primary side effects that were observed in clinical trials were nasopharyngitis, somnolence, sore throat, and headache. There seems to be no risk for abuse, dependence, or rebound effects upon withdrawal.

Synthetic Drugs for Insomnia

BZs/BZ Receptor Agonists

BZs and BZ receptor agonists (BZRAs) are probably still the most widely prescribed drugs for insomnia. The mechanism of action is characterized by the effects of BZs/BZRAs on the BZ receptor (also referred to as the *GABA-A–BZ receptor complex*). This receptor belongs to a group of ligand-gated ion channel complexes. BZs bind to a hyperjunction of the alpha- and gamma-subunits of this receptor complex, comprising a Type 1 and a Type 2 configuration. The Type 1 configuration represents roughly 40% of GABA-A receptors and is found in most areas of the brain, including hippocampal and cortical interneurons. The Type 2 configuration is predominantly located in spinal cord motor nerves and hippocampal parental neurons. BZ hypnotics bind to both receptor types. In contrast, zolpidem binds with greater specificity to the Type 1 receptor. Whether this more selective binding relates to differential pharmacological profiles remains a matter of controversy.

EFFECTS ON POLYSOMNOGRAPHIC SLEEP

In general, the administration of BZs/BZRAs shortens polysomnographic sleep onset latency and prolongs polysomnographic total sleep time (Winkler et al., 2014). The duration of the effect depends on the half-life of the substance. Substances with shorter half-lives exert their effects mainly in the first half of the night and are usually not well suited for sleep maintenance problems, whereas substances with longer half-lives act throughout the night. Mild to moderate REM sleep suppression is observed with many BZs and BZRAs. The development of tolerance (i.e., the relative loss of effect after repeated intake of a constant dose) has been observed with BZs/BZRAs. Interestingly, studies using spectral analysis of sleep electroencephalography have discovered a typical BZ/BZRA signature. All of these substances decrease spectral power in the delta range (1–4 Hz) and enhance spectral power in the spindle range from 12 to 14 Hz (see, e.g., Feige et al., 1999). The physiological significance of this finding is unclear.

EFFECTS ON INSOMNIA

A number of meta-analyses have evaluated the efficacy of BZs and BZRAs in the short-term treatment of insomnia (Glass et al., 2005; Holbrook et al., 2000; Huedo-Medina et al., 2012; Nowell et al., 1997; Rösner et al., 2018; Winkler et al., 2014). For example, the meta-analysis by Winkler et al. (2014) included 24 study groups receiving BZs or BZRAs with N = 1,003 patients and demonstrated the short-term efficacy of these substances on subjective sleep outcomes. However, the meta-analysis by Huedo-Medina et al. (2012), which focused on the data that was submitted to the US Food and Drug Administration, found rather small effects for BZs and BZRAs. In addition, the vast majority of the randomized trials restricted the treatment duration to 7–14 days without investigating long-term effects.

There are a few notable exceptions. For example, Krystal et al. (2003) reported continued efficacy of eszopiclone over a period of 6 months in a randomized placebo-controlled trial that included almost 800 patients with primary insomnia. Uchimura et al. (2012) supported these findings in another randomized trial of eszopiclone given over a period of 6 months. Moreover, Ancoli-Israel et al. (2005) reported continued efficacy of zaleplone for treatment durations of up to 12 months in an open-label trial including 260 patients with primary insomnia. Nevertheless, since there is rather little data on the long-term efficacy and safety of BZs and BZRAs, current guidelines do not recommend the long-term use of these substances in insomnia (Riemann et al., 2017).

SIDE EFFECTS

Initially praised as ideal hypnotics, many reports have shown that BZs and BZRAs have problematic side effects. These include morning hangover effects, next-day performance deficits, amnestic effects, unwanted muscle relaxation during the night leading to falls, sleepwalking, nocturnal eating, development of tolerance, abuse, and dependence (Glass et al., 2005; Holbrook et al., 2000). In addition, Kripke (2006) and Kripke et al. (2002) have emphasized the risk of an increased morbidity/mortality with BZ/BZRA usage, arguing against general long-term use of these substances. Since tolerance and dependence are important side effects, prescription guidelines restrict the intake of BZs and BZRAs to 3–4 weeks. This creates an unsatisfactory situation as insomnia is a chronic disorder in most individuals (Morin et al., 2009), and there is no effect of pharmacological treatment beyond the actual treatment period.

Sedating Antidepressants

Off-label treatment of insomnia with sedating antidepressants is very common. For example, in Germany, mirtazapine and trimipramine are among the four pharmacological agents most frequently prescribed for patients with insomnia. Of note, dosages for antidepressants to treat insomnia are usually substantially lower than the recommended doses for the treatment of depression. It is assumed that the most important sleep-related mechanism of action of sedating antidepressants is an antagonism at histamine receptors.

EFFECTS ON POLYSOMNOGRAPHIC SLEEP

Few studies have investigated the effects of sedating antidepressants on polysomnographic sleep. However, tentative evidence suggests positive effects of tricyclic antidepressants and trazodone on sleep continuity and total sleep time, whereas an increase of slow-wave sleep was only suggested for trazodone (Everitt et al., 2018; Zheng et al., 2022). Tricyclic antidepressants have been shown to substantially suppress REM sleep, whereas such effects are mild or nonexistent with mirtazapine or trazodone (Everitt et al., 2018). After administration of doxepin and mirtazapine, increases in periodic limb movements during sleep and the experience of restless legs syndrome symptoms have been observed.

EFFECTS ON INSOMNIA

The prescription of sedating antidepressants for insomnia has become a "mainstream" clinical practice today (e.g., Bertisch et al., 2014). However, there is surprisingly little evidence on the efficacy and safety of sedating antidepressants as hypnotic drugs (Everitt et al., 2018; Liu et al., 2017). A meta-analysis by Everitt et al. (2018) showed significant small effects for the short-term use of doxepin and trazodone; however, no long-term studies have been carried out so far, raising doubts about the long-term efficacy and long-term safety of these substances in individuals with insomnia. In addition, the evidence supporting short-term use is mainly based on a few small-scaled studies with design limitations (Everitt et al., 2018).

SIDE EFFECTS

A variety of adverse events can be encountered when treating insomnia with sedating antidepressants. These include sedation (especially on the day after intake), dry mouth and other anticholinergic effects, weight gain, and sometimes cardiovascular complications. So far it is clear that sedating antidepressants are not a harmless alternative to BZs/BZRAs devoid of side effects. Specific caution must be taken, including electrocardiography and routine blood monitoring, in order to exclude patients with relevant medical diseases.

Orexin Receptor Antagonists

In recent years, the orexin receptor antagonists suvorexant, lemborexant, and daridorexant have been approved for the treatment of insomnia in various countries.

EFFECTS ON POLYSOMNOGRAPHIC SLEEP

A network meta-analysis by De Crescenzo et al. (2022) has investigated the effects of orexin receptor antagonists on polysomographic outcomes. The results suggest significant effects of lemborexant and daridorexant on total sleep time; of suvorexant, lemborexant, and daridorexant on wake time after sleep onset; and of lemborexant on sleep onset latency.

EFFECTS ON INSOMNIA

Two recent network meta-analyses have analyzed the evidence of orexin receptor antagonists for the treatment of insomnia (De Crescenzo et al., 2022; Xue et al., 2022). Both meta-analyses suggest that orexin receptor antagonists are effective treatments and improve subjective sleep outcomes. According to De Crescenzo et al. (2022), lemborexant has the most favorable profile of the orexin receptor antagonists; however, safety data for lemborexant was regarded as inconclusive. With respect to daridorexant, surprisingly, subjectively reported difficulties in initiating/maintaining sleep, the core nighttime symptoms of insomnia, were not among the primary and secondary outcomes of the Phase 3 trials (Mignot et al., 2022).

SIDE EFFECTS

The meta-analysis published by Xue et al. (2022) showed that the administration of orexin receptor antagonists is associated with an increased risk of somnolence, abnormal dreams, fatigue, and dry mouth. In contrast with this data, the newest approved substance, daridorexant, does not appear to be associated with enhanced daytime somnolence relative to placebo (Mignot et al., 2022).

Antipsychotics

Due to their strong sedating effects, some antipsychotics tend to be used in clinical practice to treat patients with insomnia, either with or without comorbid psychiatric conditions. However, antipsychotics like levomepromazine, olanzapine, and quetiapine are not recommended for this indication since there is insufficient evidence supporting their usage (Riemann et al., 2017).

EFFECTS ON POLYSOMNOGRAPHIC SLEEP AND INSOMNIA

Antipsychotics and their effects on sleep have been mainly studied in patients with schizophrenia (Cohrs, 2008; Monti & Monti, 2004; Monti et al., 2017; Thompson et al., 2016). The corresponding evidence from small-sample studies suggests that antipsychotics may increase total sleep time and the amount of slow-wave sleep in this patient group. Stronger effects on sleep in good sleepers were reported with the newer atypical antipsychotics like clozapine, olanzapine, quetiapine, risperidone, and ziprasidone. However, there are no randomized controlled trials on the efficacy of antipsychotics for the treatment of insomnia without schizophrenia.

SIDE EFFECTS

Adverse events of first- and second-generation antipsychotics are summarized in handbooks on clinical psychopharmacology (e.g., Benkert & Hippius, 2021). In short, substances of the first generation may produce strong extrapyramidal side effects, frequently leading to noncompliance. These side effects include early and tardive dyskinesias, akathisia, and, in severe cases, the malignant neuroleptic syndrome with life-threatening consequences. Furthermore, epileptic seizures, deliriant syndromes, and an increased incidence of cardiovascular and cerebrovascular events have been noted. Sedation, fatigue, and impairments in attention also frequently occur. Second-generation antipsychotics show a lower incidence of extrapyramidal side effects. However, some of the compounds have other side effects, including significant increases in weight coupled with a number of long-term sequelae, including an increased risk for cardiovascular disease or new-onset diabetes.

Recreational Drugs and Sleep

Caffeine

Caffeine is one of the most frequently consumed psychoactive substances in the world and is, besides in coffee, contained in a variety of dietary sources as teas, cola, soft drinks, and candy bars. Orally taken caffeine is absorbed rapidly, with peak plasma concentrations reached after 30–75 minutes. The half-life of a single dose of caffeine is 3–7 hours, and with higher levels of consumption the duration of action is extended, due to a delayed clearance of caffeine from the body. The primary mode of action of caffeine is the blockade of A1 and A2 adenosine receptors. A1 receptors can be found throughout the brain including the hippocampus, cerebral and cerebellar cortex, and thalamus, while A2 receptors are primarily distributed in the striatum, nucleus accumbens, and olfactory tubercle. Adenosine promotes sleep, and caffeine blocks these sleep-promoting effects (Reichert et al., 2022).

EFFECTS ON POLYSOMNOGRAPHIC SLEEP

Gardiner et al. (2023) have summarized data on the effects of caffeine on sleep. According to this meta-analysis, caffeine delays sleep onset, reduces total sleep time and sleep efficiency, increases the amount of N1 sleep, decreases the amount of slow-wave sleep, and has no substantial effect on REM sleep. The sleep-disturbing effects of caffeine have also been used as a model for insomnia (Bonnet & Arand, 1992). Thus, caffeine mimics many of the polysomnographic characteristics of psychophysiological insomnia with hyperarousal (Baglioni et al., 2014; Riemann et al., 2010).

EFFECTS ON INSOMNIA

Epidemiological studies suggest an association between daily caffeine intake and sleep problems (e.g., Chaudhary et al., 2016). Sleep hygiene usually includes the recommendation to avoid caffeine, especially in the afternoon and evening (Irish et al., 2015). Yet, up to now, the impact of avoiding caffeine has never been systematically tested in patients with insomnia.

SIDE EFFECTS

The occurrence of adverse events of caffeine depends on the dosage and probably on genetic factors and previous exposure to the substance. Typically, after high doses of caffeine, anxiety, insomnia, and changes of mood occur. Peripheral effects include an increase of blood pressure, a racing heart, cardiac arrhythmias, and gastrointestinal symptoms. In vulnerable subjects, even panic attacks may be induced.

Nicotine

Cigarette smoking is a major public health problem. Half of all long-term smokers die prematurely as a consequence of tobacco consumption (Doll et al., 2004). In industrialized countries smoking is recognized as the most significant avoidable single cause for a multiplicity of chronic diseases. Nicotine stimulates cholinergic neurotransmission via the widespread $\alpha7$ and $\alpha4\beta2$ nicotinergic acetylcholine receptors and indirectly alters the glutaminergic, dopaminergic, and serotonergic systems in the brain (Benowitz, 2010). The half-life of inhaled nicotine is approximately 2 hours in chronic smokers, thereby stimulating the smoking person to apply the substance frequently in order to avoid symptoms of withdrawal. Cigarettes usually contain 0.1–1.4 mg of nicotine. In the CNS, nicotine stimulates attention and memory functions, psychomotor activity, and cognitive functions. Peripherally, heart rate and blood pressure are increased, whereas healthy blood vessels are dilated and atherosclerotic blood vessels contracted.

EFFECTS ON POLYSOMNOGRAPHIC SLEEP AND INSOMNIA

Jaehne et al. (2009) have summarized the literature on the effects of nicotine on polysomnographic sleep. According to this review, direct administration of nicotine impairs sleep in healthy nonsmokers by prolonging sleep onset latency, increasing wakefulness after sleep onset, and reducing slow-wave sleep. Findings on the effects of nicotine on REM sleep are inconsistent, with some studies reporting increases after nicotine administration and some documenting decreases. Chronic smokers display impaired sleep continuity and reduced slow-wave sleep compared to nonsmokers. In addition, in smokers, nicotine withdrawal further disturbs sleep, both in the objective and in the subjective domains.

SIDE EFFECTS

Chronic nicotine consumption is usually coupled with physical and psychological dependence. Withdrawal symptoms include sleep disturbances, craving, dysphoria, fear, anhedonia, irritability or restlessness, and increased appetite. In addition, the tobacco consumption is one of the most important risk factors for a large number of diseases which could be prevented by giving up smoking.

Alcohol

Alcohol use is a major risk factor for death and global disease burden, and alcohol use disorders are very prevalent (Carvalho et al., 2019; GBD 2016 Alcohol Collaborators, 2018). Acute alcohol consumption leads to a reinforcement of neuronal inhibition mediated by GABA-A receptors. However, chronic exposure to alcohol leads to diminished GABAergic neuronal inhibition via biochemical adaptation and to alterations of the subunit structure of the GABA-A receptors (Cagetti et al., 2003). Another well-documented effect of alcohol is the inhibition of the *N*-methyl-D-aspartate subtype of glutamate receptors (Kumari & Ticku, 2000). Glutamate acts as the neurotransmitter of a population of neurons in the reticular activating system in the brainstem, which also controls the cholinergic neurons in the basal forebrain.

EFFECTS ON POLYSOMNOGRAPHIC SLEEP

Alcohol consumed by healthy individuals shortens sleep onset latency, reduces the amount of wake time after sleep onset and REM sleep, and increases the amount non-REM (NREM) sleep (Ebrahim et al., 2013; Feige et al., 2006). Since alcohol is metabolized relatively quickly, changes in sleep architecture are often limited to the first half of the night, while during the second half, the effects of alcohol withdrawal disturb sleep

(Ebrahim et al., 2013; Feige et al., 2006). In particular, late sleep following alcohol ingestion prior to going to bed can be "shallow" and interrupted by frequent periods of wakefulness, and dreams and nightmares frequently occur (Rundell et al., 1972). It should also be noted that alcohol use disorders are associated with severe (and often non-reversible) disturbances of sleep continuity and sleep architecture (Koob & Colrain, 2020). In addition to these effects, alcohol is a muscle relaxant and consequently can lead to or worsen sleep-related breathing disorders (Kolla et al., 2018).

EFFECTS ON INSOMNIA

Alcohol consumption and insomnia are epidemiologically associated (Hipson & Fischer, 2016; Husberg et al., 2022). Alcohol use is a risk factor for the development of insomnia (Koob & Colrain, 2020), and, vice versa, insomnia is a risk factor for the development of alcohol use disorders (Hertenstein et al., 2019), maybe because alcohol is used as self-medication by many patients suffering from insomnia. Consequently, sleep hygiene education includes the recommendation to avoid alcohol before bedtime (Irish et al., 2015). However, there have been very few attempts to investigate the effects of this recommendation on nighttime sleep in well-designed randomized controlled trials (Irish et al., 2015).

SIDE EFFECTS

The consumption of alcohol at high doses or its abuse has a negative impact on practically every organ system including the CNS. According to the World Health Organization (WHO), the harmful use of alcohol is a causal factor in more than 200 diseases, injuries, and other health conditions (WHO, 2024b).

Illicit Drugs: Cannabis, 3,4-Methylenedioxymethamphetamine, Cocaine

Estimating the prevalence of illicit drug usage is difficult (Degenhardt & Hall, 2012), but the WHO (2024a) states that about 2.5% of the world population consumes cannabis, and 0.2% consumes cocaine. The cannabis plant contains over 60 cannabinoids, with Δ-9-tetrahydrocannabinol being the constituent that is mainly responsible for the psychotropic effects. These psychotropic effects are mainly mediated by cannabinoid CB_1 receptors, which can be found in high concentrations in the frontal cortex, cerebellum, and basal ganglia (Iversen, 2003). CB_1 receptors activate a variety of signal transduction pathways and interact with numerous neurotransmitters and neuromodulators. The half-life of cannabis when inhaled through smoking is estimated to be around 2–3 hours. 3,4-Methylenedioxymethamphetamine (MDMA) is an amphetamine analog that induces rapid release of serotonin via inverse interaction with presynaptic serotonin reuptake carriers. MDMA also induces rapid dopamine release and binds to serotonin $5\text{-}HT_2$ receptors (Green et al., 2003). The half-life of MDMA is 6–10 hours. Cocaine is a stimulant that inhibits presynaptic dopamine transporters in the nucleus accumbens and prefrontal cortex, leading to an increase in dopamine availability (Nestler et al., 2004). The half-life of cocaine is 1–1.5 hours.

EFFECTS ON POLYSOMNOGRAPHIC SLEEP AND INSOMNIA

So far, it is difficult to interpret studies on the effects of cannabis on polysomnographic sleep and insomnia due to a number of methodological limitations, for example, small sample sizes and heterogeneity of participants and outcomes (Bhagavan et al., 2020; Gates et al., 2014; Schierenbeck et al., 2008). According to these systematic reviews, several studies have suggested that the acute administration of cannabis decreases sleep onset latency; however, there are also opposing findings in the literature. Furthermore, it has been reported rather consistently that cannabis decreases the amount of REM sleep and REM density. Studies in chronic cannabis users have suggested that many individuals develop tolerance against the effects of cannabis on sleep. Cannabis withdrawal appears to lead to disturbances in subjective sleep continuity and an increase in dreaming. These phenomena may persist for 6–8 weeks. Correspondingly, polysomnographic studies have demonstrated that cannabis withdrawal leads to an increased sleep onset latency, increased wakefulness after sleep onset, and an increased amount of REM sleep.

Many MDMA users report restless, disturbed sleep following MDMA intake (Schierenbeck et al., 2008); and there may be long-term effects of MDMA consumption on sleep, at least in the subjective domain (Taurah et al., 2014). In addition, epidemiologically, MDMA users are likely to use sleep medications than nonusers (Tait et al., 2013). In line with this, one experimental polysomnographic study reported disrupted NREM and REM sleep after MDMA administration (Randall et al., 2009).

Sleep continuity disturbances are often experienced by cocaine users. Polysomnography studies have supported the stimulant properties of cocaine, demonstrating a prolonged sleep onset latency, reduced total sleep time, and suppression of REM sleep after acute cocaine administration (Schierenbeck et al., 2008). During withdrawal, cocaine-dependent individuals experience even more severe sleep disturbances and unpleasant dreams. During this phase, studies have demonstrated a significant reduction of total sleep time, a prolonged sleep onset latency, decreased sleep efficiency, and an increase in the amount of REM sleep (Schierenbeck et al., 2008).

SIDE EFFECTS

Cannabis, MDMA, and cocaine have a variety of unwanted side effects and can lead to substance abuse. The interested reader is referred to reviews by Connor et al. (2021), Parrott (2013), and Havakuk et al. (2017).

Other CNS-Active Drugs

In this section, the effects of stimulants, antiepileptics, antihypertensive agents, pain medications, glucocorticoids, and thyroid hormones on sleep will be reviewed as these substances are clinically relevant and at least some evidence exists regarding their effects on sleep.

Stimulants

Stimulants like methylphenidate, modafinil, and solriamfetol are used to treat excessive daytime sleepiness, for example, in patients with narcolepsy. Furthermore, methylphenidate, an amphetaminergic substance, is frequently prescribed to treat children and adolescents with attention deficit hyperactivity disorder. Methylphenidate inhibits the reuptake of dopamine and norepinephrine and, thus, increases their neurotransmission. The plasma half-life is about 2 hours. Modafinil acts as a dopamine reuptake inhibitor and activates the histaminergic and orexinergic system. However, the mechanism of action of modafinil remains to be fully elucidated. The plasma half-life of the substance is 10–12 hours. Solriamfetol is a norepinephrine–dopamine reuptake inhibitor with a plasma half-life of around 7 hours.

EFFECTS ON POLYSOMNOGRAPHIC SLEEP AND INSOMNIA

Stimulants have been shown to enhance wakefulness and to reduce sleepiness, which are primary aims in the treatment of narcolepsy (Bassetti et al., 2021). There are no or almost no negative effects on nocturnal sleep in patients suffering from narcolepsy when the last dose is taken around noon. However, stimulants disturb sleep when administered in close proximity to the sleep period and are generally believed to be problematic in patients with insomnia. In two small-scaled clinical studies, modafinil and armodafinil were investigated as adjunct treatment to cognitive behavioral therapy for insomnia (CBT-I) with the aim of reducing side effects of sleep restriction therapy (Judge et al., 2023; Perlis et al., 2004). While Perlis et al. (2004) showed a beneficial adjunctive effect of modafinil on daytime symptoms of insomnia compared to a placebo treatment, the results of Judge et al. (2023) did not support these earlier findings for armodafinil.

SIDE EFFECTS

Stimulants carry a risk for abuse and dependence if not properly controlled. Therefore, the prescription of stimulants is highly regulated in most countries. Common side effects of stimulants include headache, irritability, tachycardia, decreased appetite, and insomnia.

Antiepileptics

EFFECTS ON POLYSOMNOGRAPHIC SLEEP AND INSOMNIA

The effects of antiepileptics on sleep have been systematically reviewed by Carvalho et al. (2022). According to this review, negative effects on sleep were found for carbamazepine, while gabapentin, lamotrigine, pregabalin, and tiagabine increase slow-wave sleep. Moreover, gabapentin and pregabalin are recommended for the treatment of restless legs syndrome by clinical guidelines (Winkelman et al., 2016). Overall, however, the evidence about the effects of antiepileptics on sleep is rather limited and deserves further attention.

SIDE EFFECTS

Antiepileptics usage is associated with diverse side effects. Please refer to the textbook *Basic & Clinical Pharmacology* for more detailed information (Katzung & Vanderah, 2020). Sleep-related negative effects have primarily reported for older antiepileptics like carbamazepine.

Antihypertensive Agents

Antihypertensive drugs are widely prescribed to decrease the risk of cardiovascular morbidity and mortality associated with hypertension. Major classes of antihypertensives include beta blockers, calcium channel blockers, angiotensin-converting enzyme inhibitors, angiotensin II receptor antagonists, and diuretics.

EFFECTS ON POLYSOMNOGRAPHIC SLEEP AND INSOMNIA

The use of beta blockers has been demonstrated to be associated with sleep disturbances in a significant number of patients (Dahlöf & Dimenäs, 1990). Because of this, there is a need to assess medical history including current and previous pharmacotherapeutic treatment in those with insomnia. In contrast to the findings for beta blockers, the few available studies indicate that calcium channel blockers, angiotensin-converting enzyme inhibitors, and diuretics have few to no marked effects on polysomnographic or subjective sleep (e.g., Monti, 1987).

SIDE EFFECTS

For an overview of the broad spectrum of side effects of antihypertensive drugs, the interested reader is referred to the textbook *Basic & Clinical Pharmacology* (Katzung & Vanderah, 2020). With regard to sleep, it is of additional interest that nightmares have been frequently reported after drug-induced attenuation of REM sleep (e.g., after the intake of beta blockers), presumably related to REM rebounds (Thompson & Pierce, 1999).

Pain Medication

Pain is a common symptom of many medical conditions and often leads to severe disturbances of sleep, especially when pain occurs at nighttime. Many different substances are used to treat pain and pain-related sleep disorders. In this section, only substances that are specifically indicated for the treatment of pain are reviewed, including acetylsalicylic acid, acetaminophen, ibuprofen, and opioids.

EFFECTS ON POLYSOMNOGRAPHIC SLEEP AND INSOMNIA

Overall, the impact of pain medication on sleep and insomnia has not been well studied for either non-opioid or opioid drugs. In a small study, acetylsalicylic acid had negative effects on slow-wave sleep but increased Stage 2 sleep (Horne et al., 1980). Acetaminophen is presumably not associated with changes in sleep parameters (see Beaulieu & Walczak,

2007). Ibuprofen seems to cause an increase in nocturnal awakenings and a decrease in slow-wave sleep (Cairns, 2007). Animal and human studies have provided evidence that the acute administration of opioids results in a significant suppression of REM sleep and slow-wave sleep (Cairns, 2007). These effects have been linked to complex alterations of endogenous cholinergic, adenosinergic, and GABAergic neurotransmission in brain areas relevant to sleep regulation (Lydic & Baghdoyan, 2007). With chronic administration, the amount of slow-wave sleep appears to return to baseline levels, while REM sleep suppression seems to persist. Clear-cut effects on sleep continuity have not been reported.

SIDE EFFECTS

Pain medication is associated with diverse side effects. Please refer to the textbook *Basic & Clinical Pharmacology* for more detailed information (Katzung & Vanderah, 2020).

Glucocorticoids

Glucocorticoids are steroid hormones that bind to intracellular glucocorticoid receptors and are involved in the response to stress. Their main effects comprise an attenuation of inflammatory processes and an enhancement of catabolic processes such as gluconeogenesis and lipolysis. Endogenous cortisol is released under control of the hypothalamic–pituitary–adrenal (HPA) axis. A number of glucocorticoids that differ in their affinity to glucocorticoid and mineralocorticoid receptors and in their half-lives are used in the treatment of acute pain, severe allergic reactions, asthma, rheumatic diseases, and other chronic inflammatory diseases.

EFFECTS ON POLYSOMNOGRAPHIC SLEEP AND INSOMNIA

The close relationship between HPA activity, stress, and sleep has been investigated for decades (Elder et al., 2014; van Dalfsen & Markus, 2018). In experimental and clinical studies, the administration of cortisol and synthetic glucocorticoids in animals and humans consistently results in sleep fragmentation and a suppression of REM sleep (Chrousos et al., 1993; Steiger, 2002). Dressle et al. (2022) recently reviewed studies on the activity of the HPA axis in insomnia. According to this meta-analysis, patients with insomnia, on average, present with moderately increased cortisol levels both during the day and before bedtime. However, the cross-sectional nature of this literature does not allow conclusions about causality yet.

SIDE EFFECTS

Acute glucocorticoid administration may cause a number of side effects including increased blood glucose levels, alterations of mood, and disrupted sleep. Long-term administration in higher doses can lead to Cushing syndrome, including abdominal obesity, hypertension, diabetes mellitus, as well as tiredness, depression, and anxiety. Please refer to a textbook of pharmacology for further information (e.g., Katzung & Vanderah, 2020).

Thyroid Hormones

The thyroid hormones thyroxine (T4) and triiodothyronine (T3) are synthesized and released by the thyroid gland, a process that is controlled by the thyroid-stimulating hormone (TSH). T4 and T3 regulate the metabolism of the body, and both hormones are also used medically to treat hypothyroidism.

EFFECTS ON POLYSOMNOGRAPHIC SLEEP AND INSOMNIA

Brief periods of acute sleep deprivation are associated with significant increases in TSH, T4, and T3 in animals and humans (Gary et al., 1996). In contrast, longer periods of partial sleep deprivation rather lead to a reduction of TSH and T4 (Kessler et al., 2010). Clinically, hypothyroidism has been demonstrated to be associated with fatigue, increased total sleep time, and sleep-related breathing disorders, whereas hyperthyroidism is associated with insomnia (Xia et al., 2013). Although causality has not been definitely established for all of these associations, these findings suggest that it is clinically important to screen for thyroid dysfunction when diagnosing patients with sleep-related symptoms or disorders (see also Riemann et al., 2017).

Conclusion

Over recent decades, significant progress has been made in understanding the neural basis of sleep regulation and the impact of disrupted sleep on individual functioning and public health. Compared to older compounds, such as bromides or barbiturates, substances currently used for the induction of sleep provide significant steps forward in terms of risks and safety. Yet some compounds, such as melatonin, herbal substances, and other over-the-counter medications, are relatively safe but not effective enough for severe sleep disturbances. Other substances have been demonstrated to induce sleep (e.g., BXs, BZRAs, and sedative antidepressants); however, there is insufficient data on the long-term efficacy. Moreover, BZs and BZRAs are associated with the significant risk of developing tolerance, dependency, and withdrawal symptoms; and antidepressants show a variety of potential side effects spanning from mild vegetative complaints to severe dysfunction. Thus, even after significant progress has been made, persistently high prevalence rates of patients suffering from insomnia and associated health risks indicate the need for the development of novel, more effective, and safer pharmacological treatments. These may be used in those who do not or only partially respond to the first-line treatment, CBT-I (Riemann et al., 2017), or when CBT-I is refused or not available.

Future Directions

Based on the literature review outlined in this chapter, one may postulate that the characteristics of an ideal hypnotic include a specified mechanism of action; a broad therapeutic range and high safety in the case of overdosing; a fast induction of sleep; a defined and limited duration of action; induction of a physiological sleep pattern; no impairing of cognitive or emotional effects; no psychomotor, vegetative, or other side effects; no interaction with other medication; and, importantly, no development of tolerance, dependency, and withdrawal symptoms or rebound insomnia. Since none of the hypnotics described in this chapter meet all of these requirements, there is a lot of potential for future research in this area. Moreover, patients should be individually informed about potential benefits and risks associated with sleep medications and about other evidence-based treatment options.

References

Ancoli-Israel, S., Richardson, G. S., Mangano, R. M., Jenkins, L., Hall, P., & Jones, W. S. (2005). Long-term use of sedative hypnotics in older patients with insomnia. *Sleep Medicine, 6*, 107–113.

Baglioni, C., Regen, W., Teghen, A., Spiegelhalder, K., Feige, B., Nissen, C., & Riemann, D. (2014). Sleep changes in the disorder of insomnia: A meta-analysis of polysomnographic studies. *Sleep Medicine Reviews, 18*, 195–213.

Bassetti, C. L. A., Kallweit, U., Vignatelli, L., Plazzi, G., Lecendreux, M., Baldin, E., Dolenc-Groselj, L., Jennum, P., Khatami, R., Manconi, M., Mayer, G., Partinen, M., Pollmächer, T., Reading, P., Santamaria, J., Sonka, K., Dauvilliers, Y., & Lammers, G. J. (2021). European guideline and expert statements on the management of narcolepsy in adults and children. *Journal of Sleep Research, 30*, Article e13387.

Beaulieu, P., & Walczak, J. S. (2007). Drugs for sleep pain/interactions. In G. Lavigne, B. J. Sessle, M. Choiniere, & P. J. Soja (Eds.), *Sleep and pain* (pp. 391–415). IASP Press.

Benkert, O., & Hippius, H. (2021). *Kompendium der psychiatrischen pharmakotherapie* (13th ed.). Springer.

Benowitz, N. L. (2010). Nicotine addiction. *New England Journal of Medicine, 362*, 2295–2303.

Bertisch, S. M., Herzig, S. J., Winkelman, J. W., & Buettner, C. (2014). National use of prescription medications for insomnia: NHANES 1999–2010. *Sleep, 37*, 343–349.

Bhagavan, C., Kung, S., Doppen, M., John, M., Vakalalabure, I., Oldfield, K., Braithwaite, I., & Newton-Howes, G. (2020). Cannabinoids in the treatment of insomnia disorder: A systematic review and meta-analysis. *CNS Drugs, 34*, 1217–1228.

Bonnet, M. H., & Arand, D. L. (1992). Caffeine use as a model of acute and chronic insomnia. *Sleep, 15*, 526–536.

Cagetti, E., Liang, J., Spigelman, I., & Olsen, R. W. (2003). Withdrawal from chronic intermittent ethanol treatment changes subunit composition, reduces synaptic function, and decreases behavioral responses to positive allosteric modulators of GABA (A) receptors. *Molecular Pharmacology, 63*, 53–64.

Cairns, B. E. (2007). Pain medication and sleep quality. In G. Lavigne, B. J. Sessle, M. Choiniere, & P. J. Soja (Eds.), *Sleep and pain* (pp. 371–390). IASP Press.

Carvalho, A. F., Heilig, M., Perez, A., Probst, C., & Rehm, J. (2019). Alcohol use disorders. *Lancet, 394*, 781–792.

Carvalho, B. M. S., Chaves, J., & da Silva, A. M. (2022). Effects of antiepileptic drugs on sleep architecture parameters in adults. *Sleep Science, 15*, 224–244.

Chaudhary, N. S., Grandner, M. A., Jackson, N. J., & Chakravorty, S. (2016). Caffeine consumption, insomnia, and sleep duration: Results from a nationally representative sample. *Nutrition, 32*, 1193–1199.

Chrousos, G. A., Kattah, J. C., Beck, R. W., & Cleary, P. A. (1993). Side effects of glucocorticoid treatment. Experience of the Optic Neuritis Treatment Trial. *JAMA, 269*, 2110–2112.

Cohrs, S. (2008). Sleep disturbances in patients with schizophrenia. *CNS Drugs, 22*, 939–962.

Connor, J. P., Stjepanovic, D., Le Foll, B., Hoch, E., Budney, A. J., & Hall, W. D. (2021). Cannabis use and cannabis use disorder. *Nature Reviews Disease Primers, 7*, Article 16.

Dahlöf, C., & Dimenäs, E. (1990). Side effects of beta-blocker treatments as related to the central nervous system. *American Journal of the Medical Sciences, 299*, 236–244.

De Crescenzo, F., D'Alò, G. L., Ostinelli, E. G., Ciabattini, M., Di Franco, V., Watanabe, N., Kurtulmus, A., Tomlinson, A., Mitrova, Z., Foti, F., Del Giovane, C., Quested, D. J., Cowen, P. J., Barbui, C., Amato, L., Efthimiou, O., & Cipriani, A. (2022). Comparative effects of pharmacological interventions for the acute and long-term management of insomnia disorder in adults: A systematic review and network meta-analysis. *Lancet, 400*, 170–184.

Degenhardt, L., & Hall, W. (2012). Extent of illicit drug use and dependence, and their contribution to the global burden of disease. *Lancet, 379*, 55–70.

Doll, R., Peto, R., Boreham, J., & Sutherland, I. (2004). Mortality in relation to smoking: 50 years observation on male British doctors. *British Medical Journal, 328*, Article 1519.

Dressle, R. J., Feige, B., Spiegelhalder, K., Schmucker, C., Benz, F., Mey, N. C., & Riemann, D. (2022). HPA axis activity in patients with chronic insomnia: A systematic review and meta-analysis of case-control studies. *Sleep Medicine Reviews, 62*, Article 101588.

Ebrahim, I. O., Shapiro, C. M., Williams, A. J., & Fenwick, P. B. (2013). Alcohol and sleep I: Effects on normal sleep. *Alcohol: Clinical and Experimental Research, 37*, 539–549.

Elder, G. J., Wetherell, M. A., Barclay, N. L., & Ellis, J. G. (2014). The cortisol awakening response—Applications and implications for sleep medicine. *Sleep Medicine Reviews, 18*, 215–224.

Everitt, H., Baldwin, D. S., Stuart, B., Lipinska, G., Mayers, A., Malizia, A. L., Manson, C. C., & Wilson, S. (2018). Antidepressants for insomnia in adults. *Cochrane Database of Systematic Reviews, 5*, CD010753.

Feige, B., Gann, H., Brueck, R., Hornyak, M., Litsch, S., Hohagen, F., & Riemann, D. (2006). Effects of alcohol on polysomnographically recorded sleep in healthy subjects. *Alcoholism: Clinical and Experimental Research, 30*, 1527–1537.

Feige, B., Voderholzer, U., Riemann, D., Hohagen, F., & Berger, M. (1999). Independent sleep EEG slow-wave and spindle band dynamics associated with 4 weeks of continuous application of short-half-life hypnotics in healthy subjects. *Clinical Neurophysiology, 110*, 1965–1974.

Gardiner, C., Weakley, J., Burke, L. M., Roach, G. D., Sargent, C., Maniar, N., Townshend, A., & Halson, S. L. (2023). The effect of caffeine on subsequent sleep: A systematic review and meta-analysis. *Sleep Medicine Reviews, 69*, Article 101764.

Gary, K. A., Winokur, A., Douglas, S. D., Kapoor, S., Zaugg, L., & Dinges, D. F. (1996). Total sleep deprivation and the thyroid axis: Effects of sleep and waking activity. *Aviation, Space, and Environmental Medicine, 67*, 513–519.

Gates, P. J., Albertella, L., & Copeland, J. (2014). The effects of cannabinoid administration on sleep: A systematic review of human studies. *Sleep Medicine Reviews, 18*, 477–487.

GBD 2016 Alcohol Collaborators. (2018). Alcohol use and burden for 195 countries and territories, 1990–2016: A systematic analysis for the Global Burden of Disease Study 2016. *Lancet, 392*, 1015–1035.

Glass, J., Lanctot, K. L., Herrmann, N., Sproule, B. A., & Busto, U. E. (2005). Sedative hypnotics in older people with insomnia: Meta-analysis of risks and benefits. *BMJ, 331*, Article 1169.

Green, A. R., Mechan, A. O., Elliott, J. M., O'Shea, E., & Colado, M. I. (2003). The pharmacology and clinical pharmacology of 3,4-methylenedioxymethamphetamine (MDMA, "ecstasy"). *Pharmacology Reviews, 55*, 463–508.

Havakuk, O., Rezkalla, S. H., & Kloner, R. A. (2017). The cardiovascular effects of cocaine. *Journal of the American College of Cardiology, 70*, 101–113.

Hertenstein, E., Feige, B., Gmeiner, T., Kienzler, C., Spiegelhalder, K., Johann, A., Jansson-Fröjmark, M., Palagini, L., Rücker, G., Riemann, D., & Baglioni, C. (2019). Insomnia as a predictor of mental disorders: A systematic review and meta-analysis. *Sleep Medicine Reviews, 43*, 96–105.

Hipson, W. E., & Fisher, D. J. (2016). The association between acute stress-related insomnia and alcohol use. *Sleep Health, 2*, 246–252.

Holbrook, A. M., Crowther, R., Lotter, A., Cheng, C., & King, D. (2000). Meta-analysis of benzodiazepine use in the treatment of insomnia. *Canadian Medical Association Journal, 162*, 225–233.

Horne, J. A., Percival, J. E., & Traynor J. R. (1980). Aspirin and human sleep. *Electroencephalography and Clinical Neurophysiology, 49*, 409–413.

Huedo-Medina, T. B., Kirsch, I., Middlemass, J., Klonizakis, M., & Siriwardena, A. N. (2012). Effectiveness of non-benzodiazepine hypnotics in treatment of adult insomnia: Meta-analysis of data submitted to the Food and Drug Administration. *BMJ, 345*, Article e8343.

Husberg, V. H., Hopstock, L. A., Friborg, O., Rosenvinge, J. H., Bergvik, S., & Rognmo, K. (2022). Epidemiology of comorbid hazardous alcohol use and insomnia in 19 185 women and men attending the population-based Tromsø Study 2015–2016. *BMC Public Health, 22*, Article 844.

Irish, L. A., Kline, C. E., Gunn, H. E., Buyse, D. J., & Hall, M. H. (2015). The role of sleep hygiene in promoting public health: A review of empirical evidence. *Sleep Medicine Reviews, 22*, 23–36.

Iversen, L. (2003). Cannabis and the brain. *Brain, 126*, 1252–1270.

Jaehne, A., Loessl, B., Bárkai, Z., Riemann, D., & Hornyak, M. (2009). Effects of nicotine on sleep during consumption, withdrawal and replacement therapy. *Sleep Medicine Reviews, 13*, 363–377.

Judge, D. J., Miller, C. B., Bartlett, D. J., Jomaa, I., Wong, K. K. W., Saini, B., Semsarian, C. R., Espie, C. A., Kyle, S. D., Grunstein, R. R., Yee, B. J., & Marshall, N. S. (2023). Armodafinil to reduce the sleepiness related side-effects of sleep restriction therapy being used to treat insomnia disorder: An open label clinical trial pilot study compared with historical controls. *Journal of Sleep Research, 32*, Article e13699.

Katzung, B. G., & Vanderah, T. W. (2020). *Basic & clinical pharmacology* (15th ed.). McGraw Hill Lange.

Kessler, L., Nedeltcheva, A., Imperial, J., & Penev, P. D. (2010). Changes in serum TSH and free T4 during human sleep restriction. *Sleep, 33*, 1115–1118.

Kolla, B. P., Foroughi, M., Saeidifard, F., Chakravorty, S., Wang, Z., & Mansukhani, M. P. (2018). The impact of alcohol on breathing parameters during sleep: A systematic review and meta-analysis. *Sleep Medicine Reviews, 42*, 59–67.

Koob, G. F., & Colrain, I. A. (2020). Alcohol use disorders and sleep disturbances: A feed-forward allostatic framework. *Neuropsychopharmacology, 45*, 141–165.

Kripke, D. F. (2006). Risks of chronic hypnotic use. In M. Lader, D. P. Cardinali, & S. R. Pandi-Perumal (Eds.), *Sleep and sleep disorders—A neuropsychopharmacological approach* (pp. 141–145). Springer.

Kripke, D. F., Garfinkel, I., & Wingard, D. L. (2002). Mortality associated with sleep duration and insomnia. *Archives of General Psychiatry, 59*, 131–136.

Krystal, A. D., Walsh, J. K., Laska, E., Caron, J., Amto, D. A., Wessel, T. C., & Roth, T. (2003). Sustained efficacy of eszopiclone over 6 months of nightly treatment: Results of a randomized, double-blind, placebo-controlled study in adults with chronic insomnia. *Sleep, 26*, 793–799.

Kumari, M., & Ticku, M. K. (2000). Regulation of NMDA receptors by ethanol. *Progress in Drug Research, 54*, 152–189.

Leach, M. J., & Page, A. T. (2015). Herbal medicine for insomnia: A systematic review and meta-analysis. *Sleep Medicine Reviews, 24*, 1–12.

Liu, Y., Xu, X., Dong, M., Jia, S., & Wie, Y. (2017) Treatment of insomnia with tricyclic antidepressants: A meta-analysis of polysomnographic randomized controlled trials. *Sleep Medicine, 34*, 126–133.

Lydic, R., & Baghodoyan, H. (2007). Neuronal mechanisms mediating opioid-induced REM sleep disruption. In G. Lavigne, B. J. Sessle, M. Choiniere, & P. J. Soja (Eds.), *Sleep and pain* (pp. 99–122). IASP Press.

Marupuru, S., Arku, D., Campbell, A. M., Slack, M. K., & Lee, J. K. (2022). Use of melatonin and/or ramelteon for the treatment of insomnia in older adults: A systematic review and meta-analysis. *Journal of Clinical Medicine, 11*, Article 5138.

Mendelson, W. B. (2005). Hypnotic medications: Mechanisms of action and pharmacological effects. In M. H. Kryger, T. Roth, & W. C. Dement (Eds.), *Principles and practice of sleep medicine* (4th ed., pp. 444–451). Elsevier Saunders.

Mendelson, W. B., Roth, T., Cassella, J., Roehrs, T., Walsh, J. K., Woods, J. H., Buysse, D. J., & Meyer, R. E. (2004). The treatment of chronic insomnia: Drug indications, chronic use and abuse liability. Summary of a 2001 new clinical drug evaluation unit meeting symposium. *Sleep Medicine Reviews, 8*, 7–17.

Mignot, E., Mayleben, D., Fietze, I., Leger, D., Zammit, G., Bassetti, C. L. A., Pain, S., Kinter, D. S., & Roth, T. (2022). Safety and efficacy of daridorexant in patients with insomnia disorder: Results from two multicenter, randomised, double-blind, placebo-controlled, Phase 3 trials. *Lancet Neurology, 21*, 125–139.

Monti, J. M. (1987). Disturbances of sleep and wakefulness associated with the use of antihypertensive agents. *Life Sciences, 41*, 1979–1988.

Monti, J. M., & Monti, D. (2004). Sleep in schizophrenia patients and the effects of antipsychotic drugs. *Sleep Medicine Reviews, 8*, 133–148.

Monti, J. M., Torterolo, P., & Pandi Perumal, S. R. (2017). The effects of second generation antipsychotics in healthy subjects and patients with schizophrenia. *Sleep Medicine Reviews, 33*, 51–57.

Morin, C. M., Bélanger, L., LeBlanc, M., Ivers, H., Savard, J., Espie, C. A., Mérette, C., Baillargeon, L., & Grégoire, J.-P. (2009). The natural history of insomnia: A population-based 3-year longitudinal study. *Archives of Internal Medicine, 169*, 447–453.

Nestler, E. J. (2004). Historical review: Molecular and cellular mechanisms of opiate and cocaine addiction. *Trends in Pharmacological Sciences, 25*, 210–218.

Nowell, P. D., Mazumdar, S., Buysse, D. J., Dew, M. A., Reynolds, C. F., & Kupfer, D. J. (1997). Benzodiazepines and zolpidem for chronic insomnia: A meta-analysis of treatment efficacy. *JAMA, 278*, 2170–2177.

Oswald, I. (1984). Hypnotic drugs for 1984. In I. Hindmarch, H. Ott, & T. Roth (Eds.), *Sleep, benzodiazepines and performance* (pp. 84–90). Springer-Verlag.
Parrott, A. C. (2013). Human psychobiology of MDMA or "ecstasy": An overview of 25 years of empirical research. *Human Psychopharmacology, 28*, 289–307.
Perlis, M. L., Smith, M. T., Orff, H., Enright, T., Nowakowski, S., Jungquist, C., & Plotkin, K. (2004). The effects of modafinil and cognitive behavior therapy on sleep continuity in patients with primary insomnia. *Sleep, 27*, 715–725.
Randall, S., Johanson, C. E., Tancer, M., & Roehrs, T. (2009). Effects of acute 3,4-methylenedioxymethamphetamine on sleep and daytime sleepiness in MDMA users: A preliminary study. *Sleep, 32*, 1513–1519.
Reichert, C. F., Deboer, T., & Landolt, H. P. (2022). Adenosine, caffeine, and sleep–wake regulation: State of the science and perspectives. *Journal of Sleep Research, 31*, Article e13597.
Rickels, K., Ginsberg, J., Morris, R., Newman, H., Schiller, H., Weinstock, A., & Schilling, A. (1984). Doxylamine succinate in insomniac family practice patients: A double-blind study. *Current Therapeutic Research, 35*, 532–540.
Rickels, K., Morris, R. J., Newman, H., Rosenfeld, H., Schiller, H., & Weinstock, R. (1983). Diphenhydramine in insomniac family practice patients: A double-blind study. *Journal of Clinical Pharmacology, 23*, 234–242.
Riemann, D., Baglioni, C., Bassetti, C., Bjorvatn, B., Dolenc Groselj, L., Ellis, J., Espie, C., Garcia-Borreguero, D., Gjerstad, M., Gonçalves, M., Hertenstein, E., Jansson-Fröjmark, M., Jennum, P., Léger, D., Nissen, C., Parrino, L., Paunio, T., Pevernagie, D., Verbraecken, J., . . . Spiegelhalder, K. (2017). European guideline for the diagnosis and treatment of insomnia. *Journal of Sleep Research, 26*, 675–700.
Riemann, D., Spiegelhalder, K., Feige, B., Voderholzer, U., Berger, M., Perlis, M., & Nissen, C. (2010). The hyperarousal model of insomnia: A review of the concept and its evidence. *Sleep Medicine Reviews, 14*, 19–31.
Rösner, S., Englbrecht, C., Wehrle, R., Hajak, G., & Soyka, M. (2018). Eszopiclone for insomnia. *Cochrane Database of Systematic Reviews, 10*, Article CD010703.
Rundell, O. H., Lester, B. K., Griffiths, W. J., & Williams, H. L. (1972). Alcohol and sleep in young adults. *Psychopharmacologia, 26*, 201–218.
Salanitro, M., Wrigley, T., Ghabra, H., de Haan, E., Hill, C. M., Solmi, M., & Cortese, S. (2022). Efficacy on sleep parameters and tolerability of melatonin in individuals with sleep or mental disorders: A systematic review and meta-analysis. *Neuroscience and Biobehavioral Reviews, 139*, Article 104723.
Schierenbeck, T., Riemann, D., Berger, M., & Hornyak, M. (2008). Effect of illicit recreational drugs upon sleep: Cocaine, ecstasy and marijuana. *Sleep Medicine Reviews, 12*, 381–389.
Shiyi, L., & Inoué, S. (1995). *Sleep—Ancient and modern*. Shanghai Scientific and Technological Literature Publishing House, Asian Sleep Research Society.
Steiger, A. (2002). Sleep and the hypothalamo–pituitary–adrenocortical system. *Sleep Medicine Reviews, 6*, 125–138.
Tait, R. J., George, A., & Olesen, S. (2013). "Ecstasy" and the use of sleep medications in a general community sample: A 4-year follow-up. *Addiction, 108*, 1640–1648.
Taurah, L., Chandler, C., & Sanders, G. (2014). Depression, impulsiveness, sleep, and memory in past and present polydrug users of 3,4-methylenedioxymethamphetamine (MDMA, ecstasy). *Psychopharmacology, 231*, 737–751.
Thompson, D. F., & Pierce, D. R. (1999). Drug-induced nightmares. *Annals of Pharmacotherapy, 33*, 93–98.
Thompson, W., Quay, T. A. W., Rojas-Fernandez, C., & Farrell, B. (2016). Atypical antipsychotics for insomnia: A systematic review. *Sleep Medicine, 22*, 13–17.
Uchimura, N., Kamijo, A., & Takase, T. (2012). Effects of eszopiclone on safety, subjective measures of efficacy, and quality of life in elderly and nonelderly Japanese patients with chronic insomnia, both with and without comorbid psychiatric disorders: A 24-week, randomized, double-blind study. *Annals of General Psychiatry, 11*, Article 15.
Van Dalfsen, J. H., & Markus, C. R. (2018). The influence of sleep on human hypothalamic–pituitary–adrenal (HPA) axis reactivity: A systematic review. *Sleep Medicine Reviews, 39*, 187–194.
Vande Griend, J. P., & Anderson, S. L. (2012). Histamine-1 receptor antagonism for treatment of insomnia. *Journal of the American Pharmaceutical Association, 52*, e210–e219.
Winkelman, J. W., Armstrong, M. J., Allen, R. P., Chaudhuri, K. R., Ondo, W., Trenkwalder, C., Zee, P. C., Gronseth, G. S., Gloss, D., & Zesiewicz, T. (2016). Practice guideline summary: Treatment of restless

legs syndrome in adults: Report of the Guideline Development, Dissemination, and Implementation Subcommittee of the American Academy of Neurology. *Neurology, 87*, 2585–2593.
Winkler, A., Auer, C., Doering, B. K., & Rief, W. (2014). Drug treatment of primary insomnia: A meta-analysis of polysomnographic randomized controlled trials. *CNS Drugs, 28*, 799–816.
World Health Organization. (2024a). *Alcohol, Drugs and Addictive Behaviours Unit.* https://www.who.int/teams/mental-health-and-substance-use/alcohol-drugs-and-addictive-behaviours/drugs-psychoactive/cannabis
World Health Organization. (2024b). *Alcohol.* https://www.who.int/news-room/fact-sheets/detail/alcohol
Xia, L., Chen, G. H., Li, Z. H., Jiang, S., & Shen, J. (2013). Alterations in hypothalamus-pituitary-adrenal/thyroid axes and gonadotropin-releasing hormone in the patients with primary insomnia: A clinical research. PLoS One, 8, e71065.
Xue, T., Wu, X., Chen, S., Yang, Y., Yan, Z., Song, Z., Zhang, W., Zhang, J., Chen, Z., & Wang, Z. (2022). The efficacy and safety of dual orexin receptor antagonists in primary insomnia: A systematic review and network meta-analysis. *Sleep Medicine Reviews, 61*, Article 101573.
Zheng, Y., Lv, T., Wu, J., & Lyu, Y. (2022). Trazodone changed the polysomnographic sleep architecture in insomnia disorder: A systematic review and meta-analysis. *Scientific Reports, 12*, Article 14453.

CHAPTER

19 Bedtime Social Media Use and Sleep: A New Understanding of Social, Emotional, and Cognitive Processes

Holly Scott *and* Heather Cleland Woods

Abstract

It has become established that there are important links between the use of technology and sleep. Consequently, contemporary frameworks for understanding, researching, and managing sleep need to address the media-rich sleep environment in which young people typically continue with online social interactions after bedtime. This chapter summarizes and discusses such matters and provides recommendations on how to support healthy sleep in young people, cognizant of contemporary challenges associated with their use of social media. The chapter outlines the importance of considering models within educational programs as a potential vehicle for sleep improvement in young people. It highlights how the historical focus on "screen time," "addiction," or specific (but now outdated) platforms has limited the scope and the impact of available evidence and discusses how novel measurement tools open a promising avenue for future work in this field.

Key Words: sleep, technology, adolescence, social media, bedtime, social interaction

Introduction

This chapter provides an overview of recent advances in understanding the social, cognitive, and emotional processes involved in bedtime social media interactions and discusses how new evidence may be integrated into the major models that refer to technology use and sleep. It then outlines the importance of considering these adapted models within educational programs as a potential vehicle for sleep improvement in young people. Finally, the chapter highlights how the historical focus on "screen time," "addiction," or specific (but now outdated) platforms has limited the scope and the impact of available evidence and discusses how novel measurement tools open a promising avenue for future work in this field.

Underpinning the chapter is the Sleepyteens project, which was motivated by our interest in supporting young people to recognize the value of sleep to their health and well-being, while simultaneously acknowledging the priority they place on social interactions with peers. This has taken us on a journey, alongside our colleagues, of discovering the nuances of bedtime social interactions through the adolescent voice and places us in the privileged position of having insight into the importance of these interactions being balanced with good quality and quantity of sleep.

Mechanisms Linking Social Media Use and Sleep: Recent Insights

In this section, we provide examples of how our understanding of the links between social media use and sleep have evolved in recent years. We highlight where these new contributions could be incorporated into the widely influential model of technology and sleep pioneered by Cain and Gradisar (2010) and updated by Bartel and Gradisar (2017). Specifically, we focus on fresh understanding of the social processes that drive bedtime social media use and increase pre-sleep cognitive arousal and describe how online interactions can fragment the sleep onset process. To illustrate this fragmentation, we extend Exelmans and Van den Bulck's (2017) two-step process of sleep displacement by technology use to propose a third step. We then briefly explain other relevant mechanisms, contextualizing the modest effect of screen light, and offer new suggestions of possible bidirectional links, such as social media as a coping mechanism among poor sleepers.

Social Drivers for Bedtime Social Media Use

MacKenzie et al.'s (2022) systematic review suggested that sleep researchers and clinicians would benefit from an updated framework for conceptualizing bedtime social media use, one which recognizes the developing social context of the sleep environment, whereby increased availability and immediacy of online interactions with peers can fuel concerns about disengaging due to the fear of missing out (FoMO) or violating perceived norms. Research with young people has identified powerful social drivers that lead some individuals to prioritize social media over sleep (Jakobsson et al., 2020; Paterson et al., 2019), even struggling to disengage in the context of acknowledging sleepiness and impaired daytime functioning (Scott et al., 2019a). It may be difficult for young people to disengage due to concerns about "staying connected," to avoid feeling left out of either live online peer group interactions or subsequent in-person interactions that comprise shared references to online content (MacKenzie et al., 2022). Additional concerns can arise in relation to following etiquette, with some individuals continuing late-night online interactions to avoid causing offense to peers by ending an interaction or by not responding promptly (Scott et al., 2019a). As new generations experience social media less as a form of technology separate from "real life" and more as an extension of face-to-face interactions, we must recognize that online experiences can be underpinned by the same drivers as any other form of social interaction, such as a desire to feel included and to follow group norms (Assunção & Matos, 2014; Hogg & Reid, 2006). Figure 19.1 illustrates (see sections in bold) where this insight into social drivers of bedtime social media use can be incorporated into established models relating technology and sleep (Bartel & Gradisar, 2017; Cain & Gradisar, 2010). More specifically, the model outlines the social drivers for bedtime social media use

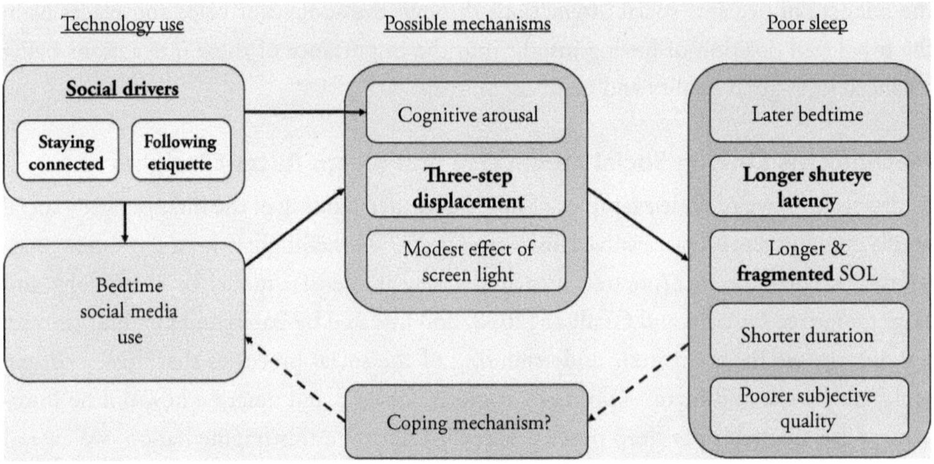

Figure 19.1 Integrating new understanding of bedtime social media drivers and mechanisms
Note. Figure 19.1 draws on aspects of the field's prominent model of technology use and sleep (Bartel & Gradisar, 2017; Cain & Gradisar, 2010) and highlights (in bold) where recent work on the experiences of bedtime social media could be incorporated into this model. SOL = sleep onset latency.

and elaborates on the sleep displacement mechanism that fragments sleep onset. It also adds the potential for effects in the opposite direction, where social media may be used as a coping mechanism by poor sleepers. In simple terms, the longitudinal evidence suggests bidirectional associations.

As can be seen, these social drivers not only impact bedtime social media *behaviour*, but they may also increase pre-sleep *cognitive arousal* (Scott & Woods, 2018), for example, rumination about potentially missing out on peer group interactions while offline at night (MacKenzie et al., 2022; Scott et al., 2019a). An understanding of the social processes that can result in continued social media engagement late at night can also help to explain the process of sleep displacement, by elucidating *why* individuals may choose to "trade" an hour of sleep for an extra hour online (Blakemore, 2018; Blakemore & Mills, 2014). Such influences may apply to individuals of all ages, but among young people there may be heightened sensitivity to social cues because the adolescent "social brain" might prioritize the opportunity for peer acceptance over the opportunity for longer sleep. This process of sleep displacement by technology use has long been hypothesized (Van den Bulck, 2004), but recent research is leading to a reconceptualization of the steps involved.

Redefining Sleep Displacement as a Three-Step Process

We, like others, have hypothesized that links between social media use and sleep quality may be explained by disruptions to nighttime sleep from "notifications." Early models certainly suggested this as a potential mechanism that merited further investigation (Cain & Gradisar, 2010). However, we were surprised to find that this was rarely reported by our participants, either quantitatively or qualitatively (e.g., Scott et al., 2019a; Woods & Scott, 2016). Rather, and more commonly, the potential sleep disruption from social media use has arisen as a factor in fragmenting the bedtime and sleep onset process. Exelmans and Van den Bulck (2017) conceptualized this fragmentation by introducing the notion of sleep displacement as a *two-step* process, where individuals' media use can delay not only bedtime (the time at which they get into bed) but also what Exelmans and Van Den Bulck referred to as "shuteye time" (the time at which they close their eyes and try to go to sleep). Indeed, these authors found that 88% of participants reported a non-zero shuteye latency (SEL), whereby they got into bed and did not immediately try to go to sleep, instead spending time on other activities including media use. The emergence of SEL as a construct suggests that sleep measurement scales require updating to clearly distinguish bedtime and shuteye time and to avoid miscategorizing some individuals as having sleep-onset insomnia when the delay between bedtime and sleep onset is in fact spent engaging in other activities with no intention of sleeping.

Accordingly, we have recently updated sleep displacement as a *three-step* process, taking account of the evidence that many individuals report using social media in bed for longer than their initial SEL (Scott et al., 2021). This is consistent also with self-reports of re-engaging with social media after initially closing one's eyes to try to sleep (Jakobsson et al., 2020; Scott et al., 2019a). This can result in an even more fragmented process involving social media displacing sleep. Figure 19.2 therefore extends Exelmans and Van den Bulck's (2017) two-step process by adding a third stage of displacement whereby

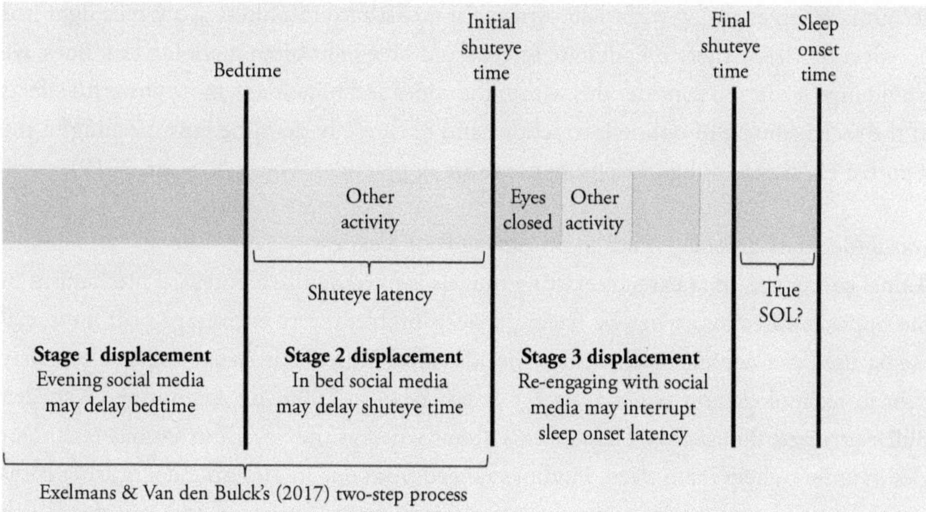

Figure 19.2 The three stages of sleep displacement by social media use
Note. SOL = sleep onset latency.

individuals may re-engage with social media after their initial shuteye time, interrupting sleep onset latency and delaying their final shuteye time.

By introducing the question "after going to bed, how long are you awake (doing other things than sleeping) before trying to go to sleep?" it becomes possible to distinguish *initial* shuteye time (when respondents first close their eyes to go to sleep) and *final* shuteye time (when they stop other activities, such as rechecking their phone or responding to messages, for the final time and try to sleep). There is a parallel here in the insomnia field where sleep diaries commonly incorporate the notion of "lying down intending to sleep" or "light out time" to mark the effective start of the sleep onset period, rather than the literal time of getting into bed (e.g., Carney et al., 2012).

Modest Effect of Screen Light

Beyond displacement and increased cognitive arousal, a third proposed mechanism that Figure 19.1 has retained from prominent models (Bartel & Gradisar, 2017; Cain & Gradisar, 2010) is the effect of screen light on alertness and circadian rhythm. While this chapter focuses primarily on a new understanding of the social, emotional, and cognitive processes of online interactions relevant to sleep, we should note that the parallel effect of screen light is modest when it comes to sleep. For example, Chang et al. (2015) found that although 5 hours of evening screen light from an e-book (vs. a printed book) repeated for 5 consecutive evenings did produce a meaningful delay in young adults' circadian timing, the impact on sleep measures was not very meaningful, with just a 10-minute increase in sleep onset latency and no difference in total sleep time. In another experimental design, Bowler and Bourke (2019) found that filtering out blue light from iPads before bed only had a positive impact on sleep quality when participants were viewing a mock social media account. When engaging with their own social media account, filtering out blue light had no effect on sleep. Therefore, despite screens and blue light often grabbing headlines, we would urge readers to consider this within the wider and potentially more powerful effects of the social context of online interactions and to carefully examine how meaningful the reported effect sizes of light exposure per se are in practice (Woods & Scott, 2019).

Social Media as a Coping Mechanism Among Poor Sleepers

A final component that extends existing models is to recognize a potential mechanism in the opposite direction, whereby having a sleep problem may encourage bedtime social media use, as a coping mechanism. The idea that individuals struggling to sleep may turn to technology as a coping strategy is not new. In 2006, Eggermont and Van den Bulck surveyed thousands of adolescents about whether they ever use various technologies in order to help them sleep. Findings ranged from one in 10 respondents using computer games to one in two using music for this purpose. Exelmans and Van den Bulck (2016) replicated reports of using media as a sleep aid a decade later in a sample of adults. Of course, this prevalence may only increase with the growth of smartphone ownership facilitating entertainment and social interactions via handheld devices. Recent qualitative work has added further insight into the potential use of social media as part of some individuals' bedtime relaxation routine, as a tool to combat rumination (Griggs et al., 2020). Despite the link from sleep problems to technology use having been identified as an important alternative perspective (Bartel & Gradisar, 2017), this mechanism has continued to receive comparatively little attention, in contrast to the wealth of studies arguing (or assuming) that technology use is responsible for poor sleep (see Alonzo et al., 2021, for a recent systematic review). The coping mechanism perspective merits further investigation, particularly in light of longitudinal work which indicated as early as 2014 that sleep problems predicted future media habits (Tavernier & Willoughby, 2014) and which has continued to confirm that there are bidirectional effects between sleep and technology use (Mazzer et al., 2018; Richardson et al., 2021).

Balancing Sleep and Social Media Use Through Educational Interventions

The adolescent voice has provided understanding of the nuances and drivers for using social media around bedtime (Scott et al., 2019a). With this perspective comes the insight that devices provide peer interaction opportunities that are very important to young people (Casey et al., 2008). Whereas the instinct may be to remove the device to prevent use in order to promote earlier sleep onset, there is evidence to suggest that understanding the rationale for, and complying with, disengaging from social media needs to be part of the discussion.

Pillon et al. (2022) took the novel approach of investigating the impact of rules set by parents around technology use and adolescent sleep. Parental rules improved sleep parameters, such as earlier lights-out times and increased sleep duration. Bedtime procrastination and FoMO were associated with later bedtimes, later lights-out times, longer sleep onset latency, shorter sleep duration, and more daytime sleepiness. Within this study, there was a significant interaction between rule-setting and age, with older adolescents either not having parental rules or not complying with them and younger adolescents having them and complying. Following Crowley et al.'s (2018) perfect storm model, we would expect to see an increase in bedtime autonomy in older adolescents. It could be that the compliance is a function of age rather than of understanding the need for good sleep. However, the Pillon et al. study offers evidence that when rules are in place, and when they are adhered to, sleep parameters do improve. This may be particularly relevant to younger adolescents and children but less so for older adolescents who are becoming more autonomous. Consequently, discussion about social media use and sleep should be undertaken within the context of developmental considerations, such as age. Device removal is not necessarily the most effective approach.

There will likely be advantages to moving away from a compliance model where parents set the rules and the boundaries and toward a model of good sleep as a positive health behavior choice, in which young people may invest. Undoubtedly, devices and the social interaction they facilitate are now part of life. Arguments concerning potential negative impacts, of course, remain valid (e.g., Twenge et al., 2020), and we will discuss "pathologizing" these social behaviors later in this chapter; but there are voices that provide a more balanced view (Orben & Przybylski, 2019) rather than a zero-tolerance approach. Indeed, Mahalingham et al. (2023) found no reduction of insomnia (on the Insomnia Severity Index) or anxiety symptoms following a 7-day removal of social media apps from their phones. Although this study did not take other devices into consideration and was not focused specifically on the pre-sleep period, the findings nevertheless suggest that limitation of access to social media use has less positive impact than might be expected on sleep.

Clearly it is important that young people are provided with more information. In the United Kingdom, for example, recommendations have been made to develop and signpost high-quality curriculum resources to help young people navigate the issues around social media (UK House of Commons Science and Technology Committee, 2019). The school curriculum also offers an accessible way to reach adolescents with initiatives in health promotion, defined as "the process of enabling people to increase control over, and to improve, their health" (World Health Organization, 1986). School-based health promotion appears to positively influence a range of health behaviors, such as smoking (Thomas et al., 2015), physical activity (Kriemler et al., 2011), and mental health (Weare & Nind, 2011). Curricula produce long-term positive effects, particularly when they move beyond simply providing information to also supporting young people to develop awareness, skills, strategies, and self-control (Thomas et al., 2015). School-based programs also provide a population-level focus on prevention and early intervention (Whitley et al., 2013). Of course, there are delivery challenges such as restrictions within school timetables, available teaching and support resources, and workload (Humphrey et al., 2016); and it is prudent to first explore barriers and facilitators to implementation, prior to investing in producing and rolling out such programs, if we want to maximize effectiveness (Durlak et al., 2011; Weare & Nind, 2011).

There are reasons to be encouraged that helpful learning can be achieved (Blunden & Rigney, 2015; Gruber, 2017). However, improving sleep knowledge may be more attainable than sustained improvements in sleep practices (Cain et al., 2011; de Sousa et al., 2007; Illingworth et al., 2020; Moseley & Gradisar, 2009). It has been argued that a key factor preventing this knowledge from translating into behavior is motivation (Cassoff et al., 2013). Even if adolescents know about the importance of adequate sleep, motivational barriers—such as social influence—can prevent them from implementing and maintaining sleep behavior changes (Owens et al., 2006). Several health behavior change models have been applied to sleep promotion, and these consistently highlight the importance of identifying and overcoming this type of motivational barrier (Grandner, 2019; Knowlden, 2019). For example, the attitude-social influence-self-efficacy model (De Vries & Mudde, 1998) draws together common aspects from the theory of planned behavior (Ajzen &

Madden, 1986), social learning theory (Bandura, 1986), and the transtheoretical model (Prochaska & Velicer, 1997). This has been used as a conceptual framework for school-based sleep promotion (Cassoff et al., 2013), with social influence being highlighted as an especially salient motivational element for adolescent populations (Blakemore, 2018; Blakemore & Mills, 2014). Therefore, a greater emphasis upon social influence and self-efficacy (helping adolescents feel more able to implement pro-sleep behaviors) is important. Identifying and directly addressing social media interactions is a major barrier to healthy sleep habits (Godsell & White, 2019; Quante et al., 2019) because some adolescents feel helplessly "stuck" in social media interactions at night (Scott et al., 2019a). The sense of obligation and/or fear of exclusion must not be underestimated as a powerful motivational barrier that stands in the way of implementing appropriate bedtimes, even when the young person "knows" what optimal sleep should look like.

In our own work with Sleepyteens we have adopted a stakeholder consultation approach, comprising phone interviews, focus groups, and workshop events with recent school leavers, teachers, teaching support staff, and management team members at both local school levels and across district education authorities (Scott, 2019). We are interested in both facilitators and barriers, and it has become clear that there is a need to bridge the teacher–pupil generational gap in social media experiences, to balance teacher-led and pupil-led input, to ensure pupils view content as personally relevant, and to engage parents. Such insights informed our approach to designing curriculum materials for three lessons that were then piloted by teachers in a partner school. Half of participating pupils reported feeling more aware of how social media affects their sleep, and one-quarter reported making changes to their habits as a result of the lessons. Participating pupils greatly appreciated the opportunity to learn new information about social media and sleep and to engage in peer group discussions on the subject of sleep. They also benefited from "discovering" the survey results on typical habits for *their* school as an integral part of the lesson content.

Our experience has been that more can be achieved by adopting a pragmatic approach, utilizing the only three 50-minute lessons that were available, and by devoting a modest proportion of time to teaching the benefits of sleep, relative to prioritizing pupil-led discussions about their sleep profiles and to potential changes to their online social interactions at night. Students perhaps need greater opportunity to become more convinced of sleep's benefits (Blunden & Rigney, 2015), and this may be better achieved by helping young people reflect on how to address and overcome the challenges associated with their nighttime social world. As well as accommodating student needs, it is important to do likewise with the educational environment. Busy school timetables are a common barrier to implementing comprehensive school-based sleep promotion programs (Humphrey et al., 2016). This makes it all the more important to ensure that the content delivered within inevitably restricted opportunity is as balanced as it can be, to optimize for engagement and best outcomes.

In summary of this section, knowledge is important, but it is just one contributory component to behavior change. Having the confidence and readiness to change are also essential (Cain et al., 2011). The evidence on such matters highlights the importance of properly understanding social aspects of teenagers' nighttime media use. While young people may understand why good sleep is good for them, having the confidence to disengage from their peers in order to sleep requires specific attention. Their readiness to leave social interactions in favor of sleep needs to be understood in the context of developmental challenges where peer approval and social interaction are likely rated higher than sleep. Consequently, any intervention intending to do more than simply educate needs to embrace such motivational factors.

Limitations of Existing Literature

In this section, we discuss three ways in which sleep research has historically, and in our view unhelpfully, framed technology such as social media use, thus limiting the scope of the available evidence and limiting our current understanding. We will take each of these three, the focus on social media "addiction," the focus on "screen time," and the focus on outdated social media platforms, in turn. We will go on to propose that developing more meaningful measurement tools in this space is an important priority and one that might help to integrate and unify research efforts. In this regard we highlight one contemporary development in questionnaire measurement that may support the field going forward.

A Focus on Social Media "Addiction"

Even in recent years, many studies have continued to explore associations between sleep and so-called addiction to smartphones, the internet, or social media (e.g., Chen et al., 2017; Gupta et al., 2021; Mamun & Griffiths, 2019). However, despite many researchers taking the existence of such "addictions" for granted, closer examination has provided insufficient evidence for applying an addiction-based framework to these behaviors (Davidson & Ellis, 2019; Panova & Carbonell, 2018). Importantly, while many popular questionnaire measures are based on clinical symptoms of addiction (e.g., "How often have you become irritable if you have been prohibited from using Facebook?"; Bergen Facebook Addiction Scale; Andreassen et al., 2012), social media, smartphone, or internet "addictions" were not added to the *Diagnostic and Statistical Manual of Mental Disorders*, fifth edition, or the *International Classification of Diseases*, 11th revision, due to lack of evidence (Grant & Chamberlain, 2016). In fact, simply replacing "social media" or "Facebook" in these popular scales with the words "spending time with friends" leads to a classification of 69% of participants as being "addicted" to interacting with their offline friends (Satchell et al., 2021). Moving away from applying addiction models and measurements, a more accurate and constructive approach would afford greater scope to acknowledge that some people do identify technology and online interactions as impacting on their sleep (Godsell

& White, 2019; Scott et al., 2021), without unnecessarily pathologizing behavior that is a normal part of modern life.

This tendency to pathologize social media habits is partly fueled by the lack of availability of appropriate measurement tools. As exemplified above with the satirical validation of the Offline-Friend Addiction Questionnaire (Satchell et al., 2021), many widely used, validated social media use measures tend to pathologize social media use (Andreassen et al., 2012; Holmgren & Coyne, 2017; van den Eijnden et al., 2016). It is crucial to remember that the measurement tools available to researchers and clinicians limit the questions we can ask participants and patients, the conclusions we can draw, and the recommendations we can make. Therefore, if we only ask about participants' or patients' experience of supposed "addictive" symptoms, then we are limiting our understanding and discussions—as well as wider public dialogue—by missing insights into other relevant aspects of social media interactions.

A Focus on "Screen Time"

Even in cases where social media is not actively pathologized, existing literature on its implications for sleep has not always distinguished social media from other forms of technology use. Social media has often been grouped together with markedly different technology-based activities—such as all types of internet use, smartphone use, and even TV viewing—under generic umbrella terms such as *screen time*. However, social media's unique social affordances offer a different (inherently social and interactive) experience compared to other activities that also happen to be facilitated by devices (Carr & Hayes, 2015). Therefore, this "screen time"–focused technocentric approach fails to capture the unique social, emotional, and cognitive aspects of adolescent social media use that are specifically relevant to an improved understanding of sleep and well-being in today's connected world (Scott & Woods, 2019). It is important that future research acknowledges social media use in its own right, recognizing its different properties. The richly varied opportunities for social interactions offered by today's platforms have contributed not only to increased time devoted to social media use (Auxier & Anderson, 2021) but importantly to evolving social norms around expected availability and the urgency of online interactions, which have become increasingly relevant for sleep as platforms have become more accessible with the move from computers to smartphones (Fox & Moreland, 2015; Thomee et al., 2010).

A core underlying issue that feeds into this continued focus on the screens and devices, rather than the experiences of online interactions, is measurement. With existing evidence frequently reliant upon single-item measures of "screen time" or of daily social media use (in hours and minutes), it is important to interpret the literature within the marked limitations of what it can and cannot tell us. Crucially, to meaningfully inform sleep education and clinical practice, we must remember that conceptualizing social media use solely in minutes and hours only gives one part of the picture. As we have seen, it is also important to consider the motivations for—and experiences of—this time spent using social media, to avoid oversimplification that reduces "social media use" from a complex range of experiences and social interactions to a singular construct, and most typically a single number, such as hours per day.

A Focus on Specific Social Media Platforms

A further challenge facing sleep researchers interested in social media use has been the rapidly changing media landscape. Available multi-item questionnaires that do focus on social media separate from other technologies are often specific to one platform and its features, meaning that they can quickly become outmoded ("Social Media, Screen Time, and Young People's Mental Health," 2019). For example, given its prevalence in the 2010s, several available measures are specific to Facebook (Andreassen et al., 2012; Ellison et al., 2007; Ross et al., 2009). However, particularly among adolescents, the popularity of Facebook was overtaken several years ago by image-based platforms Snapchat and Instagram (Anderson & Jiang, 2018), which have now in turn lost their top spot to TikTok among this age group (Vogels et al., 2022). Shifting platforms with changing features, often by design, inevitably facilitate qualitatively different social interactions and user experiences (Pittman & Reich, 2016). Researchers are left scrambling to rigorously develop and validate new versions of established questionnaire measures for the current most popular platforms, taking an "insert platform name here" approach; meanwhile, trends continue to move on, for example, with TikTok's prime position no doubt in time giving way to future platforms. Maintaining pace with current platforms and features is an inevitable and unrelenting challenge in this field, particularly for researchers responding to calls for longitudinal analysis (Bhat et al., 2018; Li et al., 2019), because platform- or feature-specific measures often become outmoded during the course of the study (Scott & Woods, 2019). This highlights the pressing need to establish validated measures that offer greater longevity, to support the valuable contribution of longitudinal studies, which have so far yielded important findings, for example, on the bidirectional links between sleep and technology use (Mazzer et al., 2018; Richardson et al., 2021).

Moving Forward: A New Focus on Meaningful Measurement

The prevalent measurement approaches in the sleep literature of pathologizing technology or social media use as a supposed "addiction," measuring generic "screen time" in hours per day, and focusing upon specific platforms whose popularity declines over time need to be reconsidered. We are heartened to see that the field has been making advances toward a more nuanced understanding of the social and emotional processes involved in balancing social media and sleep habits. Indeed, we are actively supporting this movement through our own work by developing and validating a questionnaire which captures the sleep-specific implications of bedtime social media experiences. The Index of Nighttime Offline Distress (iNOD; Scott et al., 2021; Figure 19.3) enables researchers to move beyond

Thinking about how you use social media at night, please rate each of the following statements from 'not at all true of me' to 'extremely true of me'.

Not at all true of me	Slightly true of me	Moderately true of me	Very true of me	Extremely true of me
0	1	2	3	4

1. I feel like I am missing out on something if I am not on social media around bedtime
2. I would feel left out from my friends if I could not use social media at night
3. I feel like my friends expect me to be on social media around my bedtime
4. I feel like my friends expect me to be on social media throughout the night
5. I need to be up to date with things on social media before I can relax at bedtime
6. If I am not on social media around bedtime, I wonder if my friends are
7. I feel like a bad friend if I do not answer a message quickly
8. I worry that I will offend someone if I leave a conversation
9. If I end a conversation, I feel like a bad friend
10. I feel rude if I end a conversation

Scoring instructions:
Sum scores for items 1–6 for *Staying Connected* subscale total (0–24).
Sum scores for items 7–10 for *Following Etiquette* subscale total (0–16).

Figure 19.3 The Index of Nighttime Offline Distress
Note. From Scott et al. (2021).

unvalidated and often single-item measures of frequency and duration of social media use toward a validated multi-item measure that does not pathologize social media interactions but instead captures related concerns about staying connected, which young people themselves identify as highly relevant to their sleep behaviors. We hope that the iNOD will facilitate efficient research which ensures that measurement keeps pace with the rapidly evolving social media landscape. By tapping into underlying social processes, around peer approval and belonging, that drive sleep-relevant social media habits, the iNOD offers better longevity than the existing platform- or feature-specific measures, which can quickly become outdated ("Social Media, Screen Time, and Young People's Mental Health," 2019). This is especially relevant given calls for longitudinal work on adolescent sleep and social media use (Bhat et al., 2018; Li et al., 2019), where sustained relevance across the course of the study is crucial to maximize meaningful and useful conclusions from the considerable investment of research resources.

Conclusions

Scientific understanding of how technology shapes sleep is evolving as devices and platforms—and the associated social norms and etiquette around their use—continue to develop. It is now clear that one aspect of technology that deserves focused consideration in relation to sleep onset processes is the opportunity to continue online social interactions after bedtime. This inherently social and interactive experience is driven by important social drivers, such as the universal human desire to find belonging and acceptance. Crucially, this has also highlighted the fragmented process of sleep onset for many individuals, whereby bedtime, initial shuteye time, and final shuteye time now need to be differentiated. This has important implications for anyone working in sleep research, education, or clinical practice. However, our understanding of these issues has been limited in scope by the measurement tools available to researchers and practitioners, which have focused on "screen time," on supposed social media "addiction," and on specific platforms that quickly become outmoded. As our understanding of the social nature of nighttime social media use has developed, we are now at the juncture of being able to provide more relevant and informed measurement and rhetoric.

Future Directions

Our recent work has added new validated questionnaire measures to the available toolkit, which focus on the experience of balancing online social interactions with sleep in today's connected world. Crucially, sleep research and practice must reframe social media use as an inherently social and interactive experience, rather than simply another hour of generic "screen time" or as a pathological phenomenon. This shift in emphasis can enhance existing models of sleep, support more efficient future research, inform more effective intervention and education strategies, and help shape a more constructive narrative in wider dialogue moving forward.

References

Ajzen, I., & Madden, T. J. (1986). Prediction of goal-directed behavior: Attitudes, intentions, and perceived behavioral control. Journal of Experimental Social Psychology, 22(5), 453–474.

Alonzo, R., Hussain, J., Stranges, S., & Anderson, K. K. (2021). Interplay between social media use, sleep quality, and mental health in youth: A systematic review. *Sleep Medicine Reviews, 56*, Article 101414. https://doi.org/10.1016/j.smrv.2020.101414

Anderson, M., & Jiang, J. (2018, May 31). *Teens, social media & technology 2018*. Pew Research Center. https://www.pewinternet.org/2018/05/31/teens-social-media-technology-2018/

Andreassen, C. S., Torsheim, T., Brunborg, G. S., & Pallesen, S. (2012). Development of a Facebook addiction scale. *Psychological Reports, 110*(2), 501–517. https://doi.org/10.2466/02.09.18.pr0.110.2.501-517

Assunção, R. S., & Matos, P. M. (2014). Perspectives of adolescents about Facebook use: A qualitative study. *Psicologia em Estudo, 19*, 539–547. https://doi.org/10.1590/1413-73722133716

Auxier, B., & Anderson, M. (2021, April 7). *Social media use in 2021*. Pew Research Center. https://www.pewresearch.org/internet/2021/04/07/social-media-use-in-2021/

Bandura, A., & National Inst of Mental Health. (1986). Social foundations of thought and action: A social cognitive theory. Prentice-Hall, Inc.

Bartel, K., & Gradisar, M. (2017). New directions in the link between technology use and sleep in young people. In S. Nevšímalová & O. Bruni (Eds.), *Sleep disorders in children* (pp. 69–80). Springer.

Bhat, S., Pinto-Zipp, G., Upadhyay, H., & Polos, P. G. (2018). "To sleep, perchance to tweet": In-bed electronic social media use and its associations with insomnia, daytime sleepiness, mood, and sleep duration in adults. *Sleep Health, 4*(2), 166–173. https://doi.org/10.1016/j.sleh.2017.12.004

Blakemore, S. J., & Mills, K. L. (2014). Is adolescence a sensitive period for sociocultural processing? Annual Review of Psychology, 65, 187–207. https://doi.org/10.1146/annurev-psych-010213-115202

Blakemore, S.-J. (2018). Avoiding social risk in adolescence. Current Directions in Psychological Science, 27(2), 116–122. https://doi.org/10.1177/0963721417738144

Blunden, S., & Rigney, G. (2015). Lessons learned from sleep education in schools: A review of dos and don'ts. Journal of Clinical Sleep Medicine, 11(6), 671–680. https://doi.org/10.5664/jcsm.4782

Bowler, J., & Bourke, P. (2019). Facebook use and sleep quality: Light interacts with socially induced alertness. *British Journal of Psychology, 110*(3), 519–529.

Cain, N., & Gradisar, M. (2010). Electronic media use and sleep in school-aged children and adolescents: A review. *Sleep Medicine*, 11(8), 735–742. https://doi.org/10.1016/j.sleep.2010.02.006

Cain, N., Gradisar, M., & Moseley, L. (2011). A motivational school-based intervention for adolescent sleep problems. *Sleep Medicine*, *12*(3), 246–251. https://doi.org/10.1016/j.sleep.2010.06.008

Carney, C. E., Buysse, D. J., Ancoli-Israel, S., Edinger, J. D., Krystal, A. D., Lichstein, K. L., & Morin, C. M. (2012). The consensus sleep diary: Standardizing prospective sleep self-monitoring. *Sleep*, *35*(2), 287–302.

Carr, C. T., & Hayes, R. A. (2015). Social media: Defining, developing, and divining. *Atlantic Journal of Communication*, *23*(1), 46–65. https://doi.org/10.1080/15456870.2015.972282

Casey, B. J., Getz, S., & Galvan, A. (2008). The adolescent brain. *Developmental Review*, *28*(1), 62–77. https://doi.org/10.1016/j.dr.2007.08.003

Cassoff, J., Knäuper, B., Michaelsen, S., Gruber, R. (2013). School-based sleep promotion programs: Effectiveness, feasibility and insights for future research. *Sleep Medicine Reviews*, *17*(3), 207–214. https://doi.org/10.1016/j.smrv.2012.07.001

Chang, A. M., Aeschbach, D., Duffy, J. F., & Czeisler, C. A. (2015). Evening use of light-emitting eReaders negatively affects sleep, circadian timing, and next-morning alertness. *Proceedings of the National Academy of Sciences of the United States of America*, *112*(4), 1232–1237.

Chen, B., Liu, F., Ding, S., Ying, X., Wang, L., & Wen, Y. (2017). Gender differences in factors associated with smartphone addiction: A cross-sectional study among medical college students. *BMC Psychiatry*, *17*(1), Article 341. https://doi.org/10.1186/s12888-017-1503-z

Crowley, S. J., Wolfson, A. R., Tarokh, L., & Carskadon, M. A. (2018). An update on adolescent sleep: New evidence informing the perfect storm model. *Journal of Adolescence*, *67*, 55–65. https://doi.org/10.1016/j.adolescence.2018.06.001

Davidson, B. I., & Ellis, D. A. (2019). Social media addiction: Technological déjà vu. *BMJ*, *365*, Article l4277.

De Sousa, I. C., Araújo, J. F., & De Azevedo, C. V. M. (2007). The effect of a sleep hygiene education program on the sleep-wake cycle of Brazilian adolescent students. *Sleep and Biological Rhythms*, *5*(4): 251–258.

Durlak, J. A., Weissberg, R. P., Dymnicki, A. B., Taylor, R. D., & Schellinger, K. B. (2011). The impact of enhancing student's social and emotional learning: A meta-analysis of school-based universal interventions: Social and emotional learning. *Child Development*, *82*(1), 405 432. https://doi.org/10.1111/j.1467-8624.2010.01564.x

Eggermont, S., & Van den Bulck, J. (2006). Nodding off or switching off? The use of popular media as a sleep aid in secondary-school children. *Journal of Paediatrics and Child Health*, *42*(7–8), 428–433. https://doi.org/10.1111/j.1440-1754.2006.00892.x

Ellison, N. B., Steinfield, C., & Lampe, C. (2007). The benefits of Facebook "friends": Social capital and college students' use of online social network sites. *Journal of Computer-Mediated Communication*, *12*(4), 1143–1168. https://doi.org/10.1111/j.1083-6101.2007.00367.x

Exelmans, L., & Van den Bulck, J. (2016). The use of media as a sleep aid in adults. *Behavioral Sleep Medicine*, *14*(2), 121–133. https://doi.org/10.1080/15402002.2014.963582

Exelmans, L., & Van den Bulck, J. (2017). Bedtime, shuteye time and electronic media: Sleep displacement is a two-step process. *Journal of Sleep Research*, *26*(3), 364–370. https://doi.org/10.1111/jsr.12510

Fox, J., & Moreland, J. J. (2015). The dark side of social networking sites: An exploration of the relational and psychological stressors associated with Facebook use and affordances. *Computers in Human Behavior*, *45*, 168–176. https://doi.org/10.1016/j.chb.2014.11.083

Godsell, S., & White, J. (2019). Adolescent perceptions of sleep and influences on sleep behaviour: A qualitative study. *Journal of Adolescence*, *73*, 18–25. https://doi.org/10.1016/j.adolescence.2019.03.010

Grandner, M. A. (2019). Social-ecological model of sleep health. In M. A. Grandner (Ed.), *Sleep and health* (pp. 45–53). Elsevier Academic Press. https://doi.org/10.1016/B978-0-12-815373-4.00005-8

Grant, J. E., & Chamberlain, S. R. (2016). Expanding the definition of addiction: DSM-5 vs. ICD-11. *CNS Spectrums*, *21*(4), 300–303.

Griggs, S., Whittemore, R., Redeker, N. S., & Grey, M. (2020). Facilitators and barriers of sleep in young adults with Type 1 diabetes. *The Diabetes Educator*, *46*(3), 242–251.

Gruber, R. (2017). School-based sleep education programs: A knowledge-to-action perspective regarding barriers, proposed solutions, and future directions. *Sleep Medicine Reviews*, *36*, 13–28.

Gupta, R., Taneja, N., Anand, T., Gupta, A., Gupta, R., Jha, D., & Singh, S. (2021). Internet addiction, sleep quality and depressive symptoms amongst medical students in Delhi, India. *Community Mental Health Journal*, *57*(4), 771–776. https://doi.org/10.1007/s10597-020-00697-2

Hogg, M. A., & Reid, S. A. (2006). Social identity, self-categorization, and the communication of group norms. *Communication Theory, 16*(1), 7–30. https://doi.org/10.1111/j.1468-2885.2006.00003.x

Holmgren, H. G., & Coyne, S. M. (2017). Can't stop scrolling!: Pathological use of social networking sites in emerging adulthood. *Addiction Research & Theory, 25*(5), 375–382. https://doi.org/10.1080/16066359.2017.1294164

House of Commons Science and Technology Committee. (2019). *Impact of social media and screen-use on young people's health [HC 22]: Government Response to the Committee's Fourteenth Report.* UK Parliament.

Humphrey, N., Barlow, A., Wigelsworth, M., Lendrum, A., Pert, K., Joyce, C., Stephens, E., Wo, L., Squires, G., Woods, K., Calam, R., & Turner, A. (2016). A cluster randomized controlled trial of the Promoting Alternative Thinking Strategies (PATHS) curriculum. *Journal of School Psychology, 58*, 73–89. https://doi.org/10.1016/j.jsp.2016.07.002

Illingworth, G., Sharman, R., Harvey, C. J., Foster, R. G., & Espie, C. A. (2020). The Teensleep study: The effectiveness of a school-based sleep education programme at improving early adolescent sleep. *Sleep Medicine: X, 2*, Article 100011. https://doi.org/10.1016/j.sleepx.2019.100011

Jakobsson, M., Josefsson, K., & Högberg, K. (2020). Reasons for sleeping difficulties as perceived by adolescents: A content analysis. *Scandinavian Journal of Caring Sciences, 34*(2), 464–473.

Kriemler, S., Meyer, U., Martin, E., van Sluijs, E. M., Andersen, L. B., & Martin, B. W. (2011). Effect of school-based interventions on physical activity and fitness in children and adolescents: a review of reviews and systematic update. *British Journal of Sports Medicine, 45*(11), 923–930. https://doi.org/10.1136/bjsports-2011-090186

Knowlden, A. P. (2019). Models and theories of behavior change relevant to sleep health. In M. A. Grandner (Ed.), *Sleep and health* (pp. 171–186). Elsevier Academic Press. https://doi.org/10.1016/B978-0-12-815373-4.00014-9

Li, X., Buxton, O. M., Lee, S., Chang, A. M., Berger, L. M., & Hale, L. (2019). Sleep mediates the association between adolescent screen time and depressive symptoms. *Sleep Medicine, 57*, 51–60. https://doi.org/10.1016/j.sleep.2019.01.029

MacKenzie, M. D., Scott, H., Reid, K., & Gardani, M. (2022). Adolescent perspectives of bedtime social media use: A qualitative systematic review and thematic synthesis. *Sleep Medicine Reviews, 63*, Article 101626. https://doi.org/10.1016/j.smrv.2022.101626

Mahalingham, T., Howell, J., & Clarke, P. J. F. (2023) Assessing the effects of acute reductions in mobile device social media use on anxiety and sleep. *Journal of Behavior Therapy and Experimental Psychiatry, 78*, Article 101791. https://doi.org/10.1016/j.jbtep.2022.101791

Mamun, M. A. A., & Griffiths, M. D. (2019). The association between Facebook addiction and depression: A pilot survey study among Bangladeshi students. *Psychiatry Research, 271*, 628–633. https://doi.org/10.1016/j.psychres.2018.12.039

Mazzer, K., Bauducco, S., Linton, S. J., & Boersma, K. (2018). Longitudinal associations between time spent using technology and sleep duration among adolescents. *Journal of Adolescence, 66*, 112–119. https://doi.org/10.1016/j.adolescence.2018.05.004

Moseley, L., & Gradisar, M. (2009). Evaluation of a school-based intervention for adolescent sleep problems. *Sleep, 32*(3), 334–341. https://doi.org/10.1093/sleep/32.3.334

Orben, A., & Przybylski, A. K. (2019). The association between adolescent well-being and digital technology use. *Nature Human Behavior, 3*, 173–182.

Owens, J. A., Stahl, J., Patton, A., Reddy, U., & Crouch, M. (2006). Sleep practices, attitudes, and beliefs in inner city middle school children: A mixed-methods study. *Behavioral Sleep Medicine, 4*(2), 114–134. https://doi.org/10.1207/s15402010bsm0402_4

Panova, T., & Carbonell, X. (2018). Is smartphone addiction really an addiction? *Journal of Behavioral Addictions, 7*(2), 252–259.

Paterson, J. L., Reynolds, A. C., Duncan, M., Vandelanotte, C., & Ferguson, S. A. (2019). Barriers and enablers to modifying sleep behavior in adolescents and young adults: A qualitative investigation. *Behavioral Sleep Medicine, 17*(1), 1–11.

Pillion, M., Gradisar, M., Bartel, K., Whittall, H., Mikulcic, J., Daniels, A., Rullo, B., & Kahn, M. (2022). Wi-Fi off, devices out: do parent-set technology rules play a role in adolescent sleep? *Sleep Medicine*, 4. https://doi.org/10.1016/j.sleepx.2022.100046

Pittman, M., & Reich, B. (2016). Social media and loneliness: Why an Instagram picture may be worth more than a thousand Twitter words. *Computers in Human Behavior, 62*, 155–167. https://doi.org/10.1016/j.chb.2016.03.084

Prochaska, J. O., & Velicer, W. F. (1997). The transtheoretical model of health behavior change. *American Journal of Health Promotion: AJHP, 12*(1), 38–48. https://doi.org/10.4278/0890-1171-12.1.38

Quante, M., Khandpur, N., Kontos, E. Z., Bakker, J. P., Owens, J. A., & Redline, S. (2019). "Let's talk about sleep": A qualitative examination of levers for promoting healthy sleep among sleep-deprived vulnerable adolescents. *Sleep Medicine, 60*, 81–88. https://doi.org/10.1016/j.sleep.2018.10.044

Richardson, C., Magson, N., Fardouly, J., Oar, E., Johnco, C., & Rapee, R. (2021). A longitudinal investigation of sleep and technology use in early adolescence: Does parental control of technology use protect adolescent sleep? *Sleep Medicine*, 84, 368–379. https://doi.org/10.1016/j.sleep.2021.06.003

Ross, C., Orr, E. S., Sisic, M., Arseneault, J. M., Simmering, M. G., & Orr, R. R. (2009). Personality and motivations associated with Facebook use. *Computers in Human Behavior, 25*(2), 578–586. https://doi.org/10.1016/j.chb.2008.12.024

Satchell, L. P., Fido, D., Harper, C. A., Shaw, H., Davidson, B., Ellis, D. A., Hart, C. M., Jalil, R., Bartoli, A. J., Kaye, L. K., Lancaster, G. L. J., & Pavetich, M. (2021). Development of an Offline-Friend Addiction Questionnaire (O-FAQ): Are most people really social addicts? *Behavior Research Methods, 53*(3), 1097–1106.

Scott, H. (2019). *Beyond "screentime": Reframing bedtime social media use as a social interaction with unique implications for adolescent sleep* [Unpublished doctoral dissertation]. University of Glasgow.

Scott, H., Biello, S. M., & Woods, H. C. (2019a). Identifying drivers for bedtime social media use despite sleep costs: The adolescent perspective. *Sleep Health, 5*(6), 539–545. https://doi.org/10.1016/j.sleh.2019.07.006

Scott, H., Biello, S. M., & Woods, H. C. (2019b). Social media use and adolescent sleep patterns: Cross-sectional findings from the UK millennium cohort study. *BMJ Open, 9*(9), Article e031161. https://doi.org/10.1136/bmjopen-2019-031161

Scott, H., Biello, S. M., & Woods, H. C. (2021). Nodding off but can't disconnect: Development and validation of the iNOD index of nighttime offline distress. *Sleep Medicine, 81*, 430–438. https://doi.org/10.1016/j.sleep.2021.02.045

Scott, H., & Woods, H. C. (2018). Fear of missing out and sleep: Cognitive behavioural factors in adolescents' nighttime social media use. *Journal of Adolescence, 68*, 61–65. https://doi.org/10.1016/j.adolescence.2018.07.009

Scott, H., & Woods, H. C. (2019). Understanding links between social media use, sleep and mental health: Recent progress and current challenges. *Current Sleep Medicine Reports, 5*(3), 141–149.

Social media, screen time, and young people's mental health [Editorial]. (2019). *The Lancet, 393*(10172), 611. https://doi.org/10.1016/S0140-6736(19)30358-7

Tavernier, R., & Willoughby, T. (2014). Sleep problems: Predictor or outcome of media use among emerging adults at university? *Journal of Sleep Research, 23*(4), 389–396. https://doi.org/10.1111/jsr.12132

Thomas, R. E., McLellan, J., & Perera, R. (2015). Effectiveness of school-based smoking prevention curricula: Systematic review and meta-analysis. *BMJ Open, 5*(3), e006976. https://doi.org/10.1136/bmjopen-2014-006976

Thomee, S., Dellve, L., Harenstam, A., & Hagberg, M. (2010). Perceived connections between information and communication technology use and mental symptoms among young adults—A qualitative study. *BMC Public Health, 10*, Article 66. https://doi.org/10.1186/1471-2458-10-66

Twenge, J. M., Haidt, J., Joiner, T. E., & Campbell, W. K. (2020). Underestimating digital media harm. *Nature Human Behavior, 4*, 346–348. https://doi.org/10.1038/s41562-020-0839-4

Van den Bulck, J. (2004). Television viewing, computer game playing, and internet use and self-reported time to bed and time out of bed in secondary-school children. *Sleep, 27*(1), 101–104.

van den Eijnden, R. J. J. M., Lemmens, J. S., & Valkenburg, P. M. (2016). The Social Media Disorder Scale. *Computers in Human Behavior, 61*, 478–487. https://doi.org/10.1016/j.chb.2016.03.038

Vogels, E. A., Gelles-Watnick, R., & Massarat, N. (2022, August 10). *Teens, social media & technology*. Pew Research Center. https://www.pewresearch.org/internet/2022/08/10/teens-social-media-and-technology-2022/

Vries, H. D., & Mudde, A. N. (1998). Predicting stage transitions for smoking cessation applying the attitude-social influence-efficacy model. *Psychology & Health, 13*(2), 369–385. https://doi.org/10.1080/08870449808406757

Weare, K., & Nind, M. (2011). Mental health promotion and problem prevention in schools: What does the evidence say? *Health Promotion International*, 26(Suppl 1), i29-69. https://doi.org/10.1093/heapro/dar075
Whitley, J., Smith, J. D., & Vaillancourt, T. (2013). Promoting mental health literacy among educators: Critical in school-based prevention and intervention. *Canadian Journal of School Psychology*, *28*(1), 56–70. https://doi.org/10.1177/0829573512468852
Woods, H. C., & Scott, H. (2016). #Sleepyteens: Social media use in adolescence is associated with poor sleep quality, anxiety, depression and low self-esteem. *Journal of Adolescence*, *51*, 41–49. https://doi.org/10.1016/j.adolescence.2016.05.008
Woods, H. C., & Scott, H. (2019). Merging the biological and cognitive processes of sleep and screens. *Current Sleep Medicine Reports*, *5*(3), 150–155.
World Health Organization. (1986). *The 1st international conference on health promotion*, Ottawa, November 21st, 1986. https://www.who.int/teams/health-promotion/enhanced-wellbeing/first-global-conference

SECTION 4

Disorders of Sleep and Circadian Function: Epidemiology, Classification, and Assessment

CHAPTER

20 Epidemiology of Sleep and Circadian Health

Qian Xiao *and* Katie Stone

Abstract

A growing body of basic, clinical, and epidemiological research has convincingly established sleep as one of the core biological and behavioral determinants of human health and a prime target for interventions for disease prevention and health promotion. In this chapter, the authors review epidemiological evidence concerning four important aspects of sleep and circadian research. They begin by discussing the epidemiology of sleep disorders, 24-hour rest–activity rhythms, and multidimensional sleep health, with specific emphasis on sleep across the life span and gender and sex differences in sleep. They then discuss the individual-level and contextual determinants of sleep. Following this, they review the health consequences of sleep deficiency and circadian impairment. Finally, they discuss methodological considerations in epidemiological research of sleep and circadian health.

Key Words: sleep, circadian rhythm, life span, cardiometabolic health, cognition, cancer, epidemiology

Introduction

Sleep is a fundamental phenomenon and essential requirement of human life. Defined as "a recurring, reversible neuro-behavioral state of relative perceptual disengagement from and unresponsiveness to the environment" (Kryger et al., 2010), sleep encompasses a multitude of physiological processes that are regulated by neuroendocrine systems and constrained or facilitated by environmental factors (Borbely et al., 2016; Grandner, 2017). A growing body of basic, clinical, and epidemiological research has convincingly established sleep as one of the core biological and behavioral determinants of human health and a prime target for interventions for disease prevention and treatment. In this chapter, we will review epidemiological evidence concerning sleep health, focusing on both determinants and health consequences of sleep deficiencies and circadian disruptions, and discuss methodological considerations in epidemiological studies in the area of sleep and circadian rhythms. Key considerations in conducting epidemiologic research on sleep as a risk factor for health outcomes require insight and careful attention to detail in defining the sleep characteristics of interest; key age- and sex-specific difference in sleep characteristics; as well as the many health, behavioral, and environmental factors that contribute to poor sleep across the life span.

Epidemiology of Sleep and Circadian Rhythms

Emergence of "Sleep Epidemiology"

The field of epidemiology originally emerged as a methodological approach to study and control epidemics, but modern epidemiology has expanded to encompass "the study of health and illness in human populations" (Kleinbaum et al., 1982, p. 2), covering both acute and chronic physical and mental health conditions and a myriad of risk factors including biological, environmental, sociocultural, and behavioral factors linked to human health. Epidemiologic research employs a variety of types of study designs, including experimental designs, clinical trials, and observational study designs (e.g., cohort studies, cross-sectional studies, and case–control studies). Whereas clinical trials and experiments are essential to establish causality, observational studies may often be more feasible and have other advantages including allowing for more flexibility to explore a broader set of hypotheses.

Much of the observational epidemiologic research on poor sleep as a risk factor for health outcomes has been cross-sectional (i.e., sleep and presence of health outcomes were ascertained at the same time). For example, numerous studies have explored the association of short and long self-reported sleep duration and cognitive function, assessed concurrently (Blackwell et al., 2006; Ding et al., 2020; Miller et al., 2014), While such findings are important and can be hypothesis-generating, it is impossible to determine whether poor sleep may be contributing to impaired cognition or vice versa; it is also possible that both conditions may be impacted by some unmeasured factor and that no direct relationship exists.

The prospective cohort study, in which exposures are assessed in study subjects at an initial time point and outcomes are ascertained through prospective population surveillance or repeat examinations, is generally considered to be among the most rigorous observational study designs (Kleinbaum et al., 1982). A key advantage of cohort study is its ability to establish temporality between exposures and outcomes (e.g., that the presence of an exposure preceded the outcome of interest) which helps strengthen causal inference. However, it is worth emphasizing that as a type of observational study, evidence from prospective cohorts often cannot be used to directly establish a causal link. Additional strengths include the ability to explore multiple risk factors for a given outcome in a single study, and minimizing selection bias related to outcome status. Increased cost given the need for repeat visits or longer follow-up is a limitation.

Over the past few decades, there has been considerable expansion in the number of prospective cohort studies focused on objective and subjective sleep as a risk factor for health and disease outcomes. Among the first such studies with objectively characterized sleep were the Wisconsin Sleep Cohort (Young, 2009), the Sleep Heart Health Study (SHHS; Quan et al., 1997), and the Osteoporotic Fractures in Men (MrOS) Sleep Study (Mehra et al., 2007). These early studies characterized sleep comprehensively using in-home polysomnography (PSG) and, in some cases, actigraphy and paved the way for incorporation of subjective and objective sleep measures into many other ongoing cohort studies, yielding new findings establishing sleep health and sleep disorders as key determinants for a variety of health outcomes across the life span. The availability of richly characterized sleep data in large cohort studies has also provided new opportunities to explore a broader array of sleep exposures beyond self-reported sleep duration, including specific-sleep disorders (e.g., sleep apnea and insomnia), 24-hour rest–activity rhythms, and multidimensional sleep health, which are discussed in the following sections. In addition, the epidemiology of sleep across the life span and sex and gender differences in sleep are discussed as cross-cutting factors that are essential to consider in all epidemiologic studies concerning sleep and health.

Common Sleep Disorders

INSOMNIA

Insomnia is defined as persistent difficulty with sleep initiation, duration, or consolidation that is associated with impaired function or distress (American Academy of Sleep Medicine, 2014). While insomnia is common in most demographic groups, it tends to be more common in women and increasingly more prevalent with advancing age, particularly in older adults with comorbid mental or physical health problems (National Institutes of Health, 2005). Estimates for the prevalence of insomnia vary widely, depending on the specific population and definition of insomnia (e.g., insomnia symptoms or insomnia disorder which is accompanied by daytime distress or functional impairment). In a large study of over 9,000 older adults (aged 65 and above), more than 50% of participants reported at least one sleep complaint as frequently occurring, and up to a third of the population reported symptoms of insomnia (Foley et al., 1995). High prevalence of insomnia symptoms (ranging 15%–25%) has also been reported based on data from the SHHS (Unruh et al., 2008). Estimates for insomnia disorder in older adults tend to be somewhat lower (12%–20%) as many older adults may report symptoms of insomnia but do not meet all of the formal criteria for insomnia disorder including daytime consequences (Patel et al., 2018). It is also important to note that insomnia symptoms in older adults are frequently comorbid with other physical and mental health conditions which may exacerbate sleep problems, including depression and anxiety, dementia, chronic pain, and chronic illnesses such as pulmonary and cardiovascular diseases (CVDs). One study reported that, among older adults without other comorbid conditions, the prevalence of insomnia is reported to be only 1%–2% (Vitiello et al., 2002). It is essential to consider underlying health conditions, and use of concomitant medications, in epidemiologic studies investigating the health outcomes associated with insomnia.

SLEEP DISORDERED BREATHING

Sleep disordered breathing (SDB), a broad spectrum of sleep-related breathing disorders of which obstructive sleep apnea (OSA) is the most common (Foldvary-Schaefer & Waters, 2017), is estimated to affect 30%–60% of older adults, depending on the definition used and specific population (Ancoli-Israel & Kripke, 1991; Ancoli-Israel et al., 1991, 1993; Mehra et al., 2007). This contrasts with much lower prevalence, ranging 5%–15% in younger adults (Young et al., 1993). Despite higher prevalence of SDB and other common sleep disorders in older adults, in many cases these conditions are undiagnosed and untreated. Further, SDB is linked to adverse health outcomes, as described in more detail in the sections that follow.

24-Hour Rest–Activity Cycle

Many human behaviors exhibit a diurnal pattern, and one of the most prominent examples is the rest–activity cycle, which encompasses physical activity, sedentary behaviors, and sleep. The rest–activity cycle is orchestrated by the internal circadian timing system, consisting of a master clock in the suprachiasmatic nucleus and numerous peripheral clocks located in various organs, such as muscle, heart, liver, and adipose tissue (Dibner et al., 2010). Master and peripheral clocks maintain autonomous circadian cycles but are also influenced by external stimuli including physical cues (e.g., light, temperature) as well as lifestyle and social factors (e.g., work and school schedule, nutrient intakes, exercise), forming an intricate relationship between circadian clocks and diurnal behaviors. More recently, there has been growing interest in investigating the health consequences of impaired rest–activity patterns.

The growing popularity of multi-day, 24-hour actigraphy in large epidemiological studies has provided rich and complex data for characterizing rest–activity rhythms by various methods, the most popular of which included cosine-based parametric models (Marler et al., 2006) and nonparametric algorithms (Van Someren et al., 1999; Table 20.1). The former assumes a cosine or cosine-like shape of daily activity patterns. A widely used parametric approach is the extended cosine model that applies anti-logistic transformation and fits activity data to derive multiple rest–activity parameters, including amplitude, mean estimating statistic of rhythm (MESOR), acrophase, and overall rhythmicity (Marler et al., 2006). In contrast, the nonparametric methods have no underlying assumption about activity patterns and derive metrics that measure specific aspects of the rest–activity cycle, such as stability, variability/fragmentation, and activity levels and timing during the most and least active periods. Recent studies have also applied functional principal component analysis (fPCA; R. Fan et al., 2015; Shou et al., 2015; S. Y. Xu et al., 2019; Zeitzer et al., 2018), which fits activity data to Fourier-based functions with no a

Table 20.1 Commonly used measures of rest–activity rhythms

Parametric (cosine or modified cosine models)	
Amplitude	Peak-to-nadir difference
Acrophase	Time of peak activity
MESOR	Minimum + one-half amplitude
Pseudo-F	Goodness-of-fit statistics, a measure of overall rhythmicity
Nonparametric	
L5	Activity in the least active 5 hours
M10	Activity in the most active 10 hours
Relative amplitude	(L5 – M10)/(L5 + M10)
Interdaily stability	The ratio between the variance of activity around the mean at each hour and the overall variance, a measure of stability
Intradaily variability	The ratio between the mean squares (MS) of the difference between all successive hours and the MS around the overall mean, a measure of rhythm fragmentation
Dichotomy index I < O	Percentage of rest period when activity is lower than the median activity during wakefulness
fPCA and FDA	Fourier-based functions or smoothing algorithms

Note. FDA = functional data analysis; fPCA = functional principal component analysis; MESOR = mean estimating statistic of rhythm.

priori assumptions about activity patterns to identify components that explain the greatest amount of variance of all the individual functions. In addition, functional data analysis such as function regression and bivariate smoothing have been applied to examine rest–activity rhythms (Goldsmith et al., 2015; Schrack et al., 2019; L. Xiao et al., 2015), which allows for incorporating important covariates such as sex and age in the model fitting process. These methods all have their unique features, assumptions, strengths, and limitations; and it requires careful consideration to select the right method for different study objectives and populations. Some studies showed that using multiple methods may be beneficial as they provide more comprehensive profiling of rest–activity rhythms (Q. Xiao, Shadyab, et al., 2022).

Growing research suggests that rest–activity rhythm profiles are unique predictors for mortality and various disease risks, including obesity, Type 2 diabetes, CVD, and dementia (McHill et al., 2017; Paudel et al., 2010; Posner et al., 2021; Rogers-Soeder et al., 2018; Tranah et al., 2010, 2011; Q. Xiao, Garaulet, & Scheer, 2019; Q. Xiao et al., 2020, 2021; Q. Xiao, Sampson, et al., 2022; Q. Xiao, Shadyab, et al., 2022). For example, in the MrOS study, Paudel et al. (2010) reported that men in the lowest quintile of overall rhythmicity as measured by pseudo-F value derived by an extended cosine model had a 57% higher mortality rate when compared with those in the highest quintile. This relationship was mainly driven by an increased risk of CVD mortality in this population. In the same cohort, we also found that multiple rest–activity characteristics, such as lower amplitude, lower MESOR, weakened overall rhythmicity, increased rhythm fragmentation, and decreased stability, were predictive of higher risk of Type 2 diabetes (Q. Xiao et al., 2020) and dementia (Rogers-Soeder et al., 2018; Q. Xiao, Sampson, et al., 2022); and similar findings were also observed in cohorts of older women such as the Women's Health Initiative and Study of Osteoporotic Fractures study (Posner et al., 2021; Tranah et al., 2011; Q. Xiao, Shadyab, et al., 2022). More recently, an analysis in the nationally representative sample of National Health and Nutrition Examination Survey (NHANES) reported that the link between weakened rest–activity rhythms and higher odds of diabetes and impaired glycemic control was consistently observed across all age, gender, racial/ethnic, and body mass index (BMI) groups and robust to various metabolic biomarkers including fasting glucose, insulin, homeostatic model assessment of insulin resistance, and oral glucose tolerance test results (Q. Xiao, Matthews, et al., 2022). Finally, in another study in NHANES, we applied fPCA to characterize rest–activity patterns in American adults and identified four distinct profiles (i.e., high amplitude, early rise, prolonged activity window, biphasic pattern) that together accounted for 86.8% of total variation. Moreover, we observed considerable variation in rest–activity profiles across subgroups by age, gender, race/ethnicity, education, income, and employment status, suggesting that biological, demographic, socioeconomic, and work-related factors play a role in shaping rest–activity patterns in human populations (Q. Xiao, Lu, et al., 2022). Taken together, recent evidence in this growing research area suggests that 24-hour rest–activity characteristics are important indicators and predictors of health status and that variations in rest–activity patterns may play a role in the uneven distribution of health outcomes in the population.

Multidimensional Sleep Health

Like many areas in medicine, clinical research on sleep and health conventionally focused on various forms of sleep disorders, such as insomnia and sleep apnea, or tended to focus on single self-reported sleep characteristics, such as sleep duration. In recent decades, there has been a growing trend in medicine and public health to take a holistic and multifaceted approach to evaluate health (Larson, 1999), following the example of the World Health Organization, which defined health as "a state of complete physical, mental and social well-being and not merely the absence of disease or infirmity" (World Health Organization, 1995). Similarly, a multidimensional framework has been developed to define sleep health (Buysse, 2014). This model is based on the notion that multiple measurable aspects of sleep–wake function are critically involved in health and well-being and shaped by complex biological, behavioral, social, and environmental demands, and thus should be incorporated in sleep health research. Specifically, the framework proposed the following dimensions of sleep health: duration, continuity or efficiency, timing and regularity, alertness/sleepiness, and subjective satisfaction/quality (Table 20.2).

Table 20.2 Sleep dimensions, definitions, and associated health outcomes

Sleep dimension	Definition	Common measures	Associated health outcomes
Duration	The total amount of sleep obtained per 24 hours	Questionnaire-based sleep duration; objectively measured total sleep time	Mortality, obesity, metabolic syndrome, diabetes, cardiovascular diseases, impaired neurobehavioral performance, cognitive impairment, mental disorders
Continuity/efficiency	The ease of falling asleep, maintaining sleep, and returning to sleep	Self-reported and objectively measured sleep efficiency, sleep latency, wake after sleep onset	Mortality, metabolic syndrome, diabetes, cardiovascular diseases, depression, cognitive impairment
Timing and timing regularity	The placement of sleep within the 24-hour day (timing) and the consistency of sleep timing	Self-reported and objectively measured bedtime, wake-up time, midpoint of sleep; self-reported chronotype or morningness–eveningness propensities; standard deviation of sleep timing measures; sleep regularity index	Obesity, cardiovascular diseases, mental disorders, diabetes, impaired neurobehavioral performance
Alertness/sleepiness	The ability to maintain attentive wakefulness	Self-reported daytime sleepiness, objectively measured sleep propensity, objectively measured alertness, self-reported and objectively measured napping	Mortality, diabetes, cardiovascular diseases, dementia, depression, impaired neurobehavioral performance
Satisfaction/quality	The subjective assessment of "good" or "poor" sleep	Self-reported sleep quality and satisfaction	Mortality, obesity, diabetes, cardiovascular diseases, depression

Note. Adapted from Buysse (2014).

Since its publication, the multidimensional framework of sleep has been increasingly adopted in sleep epidemiology research. Several studies have applied statistical algorithms to self-reported and objectively measured sleep data to characterize sleep profiles and reported associations of different sleep dimensions and/or overall sleep profiles with multiple health outcomes, including mortality, depression, CVD, and general physical function (Chung et al., 2021; Furihata et al., 2017; Tighe et al., 2021; Wallace et al., 2019, 2021, 2022). Findings from some of these studies also suggested that the predictive value of sleep on specific health outcomes may vary across different dimensions of sleep and/or between sexes (Tighe et al., 2021; Wallace et al., 2022). Together, these studies not only demonstrated the utility of the multidimensional approach in assessing sleep characteristics as determinants of health and disease risk in human populations but also pinpointed specific sleep aspects as modifiable risk factors for health promotion and disease prevention strategies.

Sleep Over the Life Course—Age Effects

Human sleep patterns are highly dynamic and undergo considerable changes across the life span. Human development and aging processes are associated with changes in almost all sleep dimensions, including duration, timing, efficiency, and quality, and in the sleep architecture. At different life stages, individuals present different sleep patterns and face unique challenges in sleep health. Age-related changes in sleep patterns are driven by biological changes with age, are influenced by changes in environment with which individuals interact, and may be unique predictors of health and disease risks. Guidelines for sleep health typically vary according to age groups (Ohayon et al., 2017).

SLEEP IN YOUNG CHILDREN

Healthy sleep is essential to physical growth and mental and psychological development in children. The amount of sleep needed in early childhood is high, and it is recommended that infants 4–12 months get 12–16 hours of sleep and young children 1–2 and 3–5 years of age get 11–14 hours and 10–13 hours of sleep per 24 hours, respectively (Paruthi et al., 2016). Sleep patterns undergo dramatic changes during the course of child development. During the first ~4 months of life, infants do not possess a fully developed circadian system and tend to sleep around the clock, with intervals often coordinated with feeding schedules (Davis et al., 2004). Newborns also have less organized sleep stages and lower sleep efficiency when compared to older children and exhibit shorter and less efficient sleep periods. Throughout the first year of life, circadian rhythms and other sleep-related brain functions mature, leading to sleep consolidation to primarily nighttime hours and longer sleep periods with less interruption (Anders et al., 1995). As children grow, nocturnal sleep duration continues to decrease, sleep periods lengthen, and the number of nighttime wakenings decreases. At the same time, daytime naps, although still common among preschool children, become gradually shorter (Galland et al., 2012). In addition, as children mature, their sleep architecture evolves to become more similar to that in adults, including extension of sleep cycles to ~90 min and reorganization of sleep stages (Anders et al., 1995). It has been postulated that sleep and child development, especially brain development, may have a bidirectional relationship. On the one hand, changes in sleep patterns may be important markers reflecting brain maturation; on the other hand, a large body of evidence supports the benefit of healthy sleep in cognitive development in children (Mason et al., 2021).

SLEEP IN ADOLESCENTS

Adolescence is a period during which children undergo drastic physical, psychological, cognitive, and social changes to transition into adulthood. The rapid development in body and brain in adolescence is often accompanied by unique changes in sleep. A well-recognized pattern in adolescent populations throughout the world and particularly in Western countries is a delay in sleep timing (Fischer et al., 2017; Roenneberg et al., 2007). This trend typically starts to manifest around puberty, with the average sleep timing in the population continuing to delay until around age 20 and starting to gradually advance afterward. Several studies also suggested that males show a higher peak in delayed sleep timing than females (Fischer et al., 2017; Roenneberg et al., 2007). It has been suggested that such a delaying trend in adolescent sleep timing is driven by neuroendocrine changes that lead to alterations in circadian clocks and influenced by social and environmental factors (Hagenauer & Lee, 2012; Touitou, 2013). For example, it has been shown that the endogenous circadian timing system among adolescents, including in adolescent animal models, exhibits a shorter period and higher sensitivity to environmental cues such as light exposure at night. These changes can be partially explained by alterations in gonadal hormone levels and result in delayed timing in sleep propensity (Hagenauer & Lee, 2012). On the other hand, in human adolescent populations, the growing need for social autonomy and use of modern electronic devices such as computers and smart phones may also cause and/or exacerbate the delay in bedtime. When delayed bedtime is combined with an early school start time and/or a morning schedule of extracurricular activities, this typically leads to shortened sleep duration and substantial social jet lag, a phenomenon describing weekday–weekend differences in sleep schedule in individuals (Roenneberg et al., 2007). Indeed, numerous epidemiological studies have reported alarmingly high prevalence of short sleep in adolescents. For example, a recent study using data from the nationally representative sample of the Youth Behavior Risk Surveillance System reported that only 31.1% of high school students met the recommended 8–10 hours of sleep (Wheaton et al., 2016). Given the importance of sleep in both physical and mental health, misaligned sleep timing and insufficient sleep quantity represent a great public health challenge in this population.

SLEEP IN OLDER ADULTS

Sleep changes with age and sleep problems are common in the elderly (Mander et al., 2017), as documented in a growing body of research. For example, in the Established Populations for Epidemiologic Studies of the Elderly Study, Foley et al. (1995) assessed the frequencies of reporting common insomnia symptoms, including trouble falling asleep, waking up, waking too early, and nonrestorative sleep in more than 9,000 people aged 65 and above. The study found that more than half of the participants reported at least one complaint as frequently occurring, and as high as a third of the population showed symptoms of insomnia. Similarly, in the SHHS, self-reported prevalence of difficulty falling asleep was significantly higher among men and women aged 80 and above when compared to younger groups, and women were more likely to report frequent nighttime waking and waking up too early (Unruh et al., 2008). Moreover, although studies have shown that healthy elderly subjects reported a lower level of daytime sleepiness than younger adults (Dijk et al., 2010), in the general aging population, sleepiness during daytime is a common complaint; and in the National Sleep Foundation's "2003 Sleep in America Poll," 15% of respondents 55–84 years of age reported regular napping (Foley et al., 2007). SDB, a common sleep disorder, has also been found to increase with age. In the SHHS, it has been estimated that ~20% of participants who were 60 or older have an Apnea/Hypopnea Index of 15 or higher (Young et al., 2002).

A growing body of literature has documented changes in various sleep characteristics based on objective measurements as people enter older adulthood. A meta-analysis synthesized findings from 65 studies with PSG- or actigraphy-based measurement of sleep in adults (Ohayon et al., 2004) and reported that older age is associated with decreases in total sleep time, sleep efficiency, and percentage of slow-wave sleep and rapid-eye-movement (REM) sleep; on the other hand, sleep latency, percentage of light sleep, and wake after sleep onset significantly increased with age. Interestingly, the authors found that most age-related changes in sleep tended to become smaller, sleep trajectories became more stable in the elderly, and only sleep efficiency continued to decrease after people reached age 60. Such changes in sleep structure are consistent with an increase in sleep complains in the older population. Numerous factors may account for age-related change in sleep, including alterations in both homeostatic and circadian regulation of sleep (Dijk et al., 1999; Hood & Amir, 2017), changes in working schedule and living environment, as well as chronic diseases and side effects of medications. As discussed in detail below, sleep deficiencies and impaired circadian function are important predictors of a wide range of health outcomes in the older population, and several promising interventions have been developed to enhance sleep hygiene and circadian rhythmicity to improve health and reduce disease risk in the older population.

Gender and Sex and Sleep Health

There are notable sex differences in sleep health across the life span. While there are generally no well-established sex differences in sleep that manifest during childhood, the onset of puberty and beginning of the menstrual cycle in females corresponds with changes in sex hormones which may impact sleep differentially in females as compared to males (Pengo et al., 2018). Mood disorders are also more common during puberty in females and may adversely impact sleep quality (Kessler & Walters, 1998). While females tend to report more sleep problems during adolescence, objective assessments of sleep during adolescence have shown conflicting findings (Elkhatib Smidt et al., 2021). For example, some studies that used actigraphy to assess sleep in adolescent boys and girls have found that sleep duration is shorter on average in boys (Matthews et al., 2014; Mitchell et al., 2020; Short et al., 2012).

Throughout adulthood, women are more likely to experience sleep complaints and are at increased risk of insomnia. In contrast, they have considerably lower risk for SDB compared to men. Somewhat paradoxically, objectively women tend to have longer sleep duration than men, and younger women may have more resistance to external stressors impacting sleep (Bixler et al., 2009). However, in a large multinational study of non-shift workers providing data from wearable devices to assess sleep, nighttime awakenings were found to be more common in women, particularly during child-rearing ages. Furthermore, sleep onset in younger and middle-aged women tended to be earlier as compared to similar-aged men until converging in late life (Jonasdottir et al., 2021). Sleep in women may also be negatively impacted during pregnancy, caused by anatomical, metabolic, and hormonal changes that occur during this time (Pengo et al., 2018). Risk of SDB is also higher during pregnancy (Pengo et al., 2018).

Sleep in women is also differentially impacted during the menopausal transition, with a decline in levels of female sex hormones and onset of sleep-disrupting symptoms such as hot flashes. Insomnia symptoms are common in women during menopause and continue to be elevated in older women compared to similar-aged men (Guidozzi, 2015).

Given the growing evidence of key sex differences impacting sleep during various stages throughout life, it is critical to consider sex as a covariate or effect modifier when conducting epidemiologic research on sleep and health outcomes. In some cases, the sleep disruption may relate differently to risk of health outcomes in males and females. In such situations, simple adjustment for sex as a covariate is not sufficient. Effect modification should be explored through sex-stratified analyses and formal tests of interaction. For example, in a study of 5,422 middle- to older-aged adults participating in the SHHS, OSA was examined as a risk factor for incident stroke over 8.7 years of follow-up. A strong dose–response association was observed across quartiles of the OSA–hypopnea index and stroke risk in men, but in women no significant trend was observed (Redline et al., 2010).

Factors Impacting Sleep Health

Physical and Mental Health

Sleep problems are frequently comorbid with other physical and mental health conditions that may exacerbate sleep problems, including depression and anxiety, dementia, chronic pain, and chronic illnesses such as pulmonary disease and CVD (Stone & Xiao, 2018). However, much of the epidemiologic research on sleep and physical or mental health is focused on sleep as a risk factor for such outcomes; virtually all of these comorbidities which may negatively impact sleep quality are also outcomes that have been linked to poor sleep. Sleep as a risk factor for physical and mental health outcomes is discussed in more detail in the next section ("Sleep and Health Outcomes"). In most cases, epidemiologic studies have not been designed to fully investigate the bidirectional associations between sleep and physical and mental health outcomes. Methodological issues related to the bidirectionality of sleep and health outcomes are discussed later in the chapter ("Methodological Considerations in Sleep Epidemiology Research").

Lifestyle Behaviors

A variety of lifestyle factors and health behaviors may have detrimental effects on sleep, including smoking (Amiri & Behnezhad, 2020), use of alcohol (Otsuka et al., 2022; Park et al., 2015), caffeine intake (Clark & Landolt, 2017), and other factors including sedentary behavior, diet, and use of the internet and social media (Dzierzewski et al., 2021).

SMOKING

A number of studies have examined the association between smoking and sleep-related issues. Studies with prospective designs (i.e., smoking behaviors or nicotine dependence and risk of developing sleeping problems over time) were examined in a systematic review including articles published through 2018 (Amiri & Behnezhad, 2020). Overall, those with smoking and nicotine exposures had about a 50% increase in risk of developing sleep-related issues (risk ratio [RR] = 1.47, 95% confidence interval [CI; 1.20, 1.79]) compared to nonsmokers. It was hypothesized that this association may be explained by increased risks of other health-related issues related to smoking and comorbid with sleep such as CVD and depression. Smoking has also been associated with sleep-related breathing problems (Jaehne et al., 2009).

ALCOHOL USE

Although there is well-documented evidence that alcohol use impacts sleep physiology (Ebrahim et al., 2013; Roehrs & Roth, 2001; Roehrs & Roth, 2001), there is relatively little epidemiologic evidence to document this association (Ebrahim et al., 2013). In a cross-sectional study of 393 Korean adults, alcohol use was associated with poorer subjective sleep quality, short sleep duration, and snoring, but only among men (Park et al., 2015). In women, but not in men, alcohol use was associated with increased sleep-related daytime dysfunction. In contrast, in a large nationwide cross-sectional survey of 35,717 men and 39,911 women conducted in Japan, heavy alcohol consumption was found to significantly predict subjective nonrestorative sleep in both men and women (adjusted odds ratios [ORs] = 1.3 and 1.4, respectively; Otsuka et al., 2022). More research is warranted to determine patterns of alcohol use and temporal patterns linking alcohol to sleep health.

CAFFEINE

Results of a systematic review concluded that evidence form epidemiological studies and clinical trials support an overall detrimental effect of coffee and caffeine on sleep (Clark &

Landolt, 2017). However, individual effects vary based on age and a variety of other factors, possibly including genetics, impacting sensitivity levels. There was some consistency of findings indicating effects on prolonged sleep latency, reduction in slow-wave sleep, and increased arousals and wakefulness. Most studies were conducted in Western countries, primarily in male subjects, limiting the generalizability. In addition, there is very little longitudinal data; thus, future studies are warranted (Clark & Landolt, 2017).

PHYSICAL ACTIVITY AND SEDENTARY BEHAVIOR

The epidemiologic literature has been fairly consistent in supporting a positive impact of physical activity on sleep health. A systematic review published in 2021 incorporated information from previously published meta-analyses including both observational and experimental studies about physical activity and sleep (Kline et al., 2021). Overall, there was strong evidence linking physical activity to more positive sleep outcomes, including more acute bouts of activity as well as regular activity levels. These relationships were generally observed across the life span and were fairly consistent for both men and women. Further, there was moderate evidence of beneficial effects of exercise on sleep among individuals with insomnia and sleep apnea.

In a more recent study of middle-aged and older adults using accelerometry data derived from the population-based Rotterdam Study cohort, compositional isotemporal substitution analysis was employed to determine the potential impact of reallocating time spent in sleep to sedentary behavior or light physical activity (Hofman et al., 2022). The results suggested a significant decrease in sleep quality resulting from shifting 30 minutes of sleep time to either sedentary or light physical activity. Overall results from prior epidemiological studies suggest that physical activity could be a potential intervention target for improving sleep health, potentially across the life span. This work also underscores the importance of future clinical trials to establish the benefits of physical activity on sleep.

Social and Environmental Determinants of Sleep

Social factors at both the individual and neighborhood levels have been widely recognized as important determinants of health behaviors and outcomes and critical contributors to health disparities in human societies. Decades of research has revealed substantial sleep disparities with disadvantaged groups disproportionately exhibiting high prevalence of various forms of sleep deficiencies including short and long sleep durations, poor sleep quality, misaligned and irregular sleep timing, sleep disorders, and excessive daytime sleepiness (Duncan et al., 2019). It has been proposed that a social–ecological framework may be applied to understand myriad social and environmental factors and complex pathways that influence sleep patterns in human populations. Previous research has identified multiple social determinants that are associated with sleep characteristics and can potentially shape sleep health. Below we briefly discuss several such factors with consistent research evidence supporting their role in sleep.

RACE AND ETHNICITY

Mounting evidence suggests that certain racial and ethnic minority groups are more likely to experience suboptimal sleep. For example, an analysis in the nationally representative sample NHANES (2007–2008) reported that Black Americans were 2.34 and 1.85 times more likely to report very short (<5 hours) and short (5–6 hours) sleep when compared to non-Hispanic White Americans, and similarly high prevalence of very short and short sleep was also observed among Asians (Whinnery et al., 2014). However, findings for Hispanic groups in this analysis were mixed, with Mexican-born adults showing a lower likelihood of reporting short sleep and other Hispanics/Latinos showing a higher likelihood of very short sleep. Another analysis in the 2014 Behavioral Risk Factor Surveillance System showed that age-adjusted percentages of adults reporting adequate sleep duration (7 hours or more) over the 24-hour period were substantially and significantly lower in Black (54.2%), Native Hawaiian/Pacific Islander (53.7%), and multiracial (53.6%) groups when compared to non-Hispanic White adults (66.8%). Notably, a recent study in the National Health Interview Survey (NHIS; 2004–2018) reported that not only did Black adults show persistently higher prevalence of self-reported short sleep than White adults did throughout this period but the Black–White gap appeared to increase from a 7.51 percentage point difference in 2004 to a 10.68 point difference in 2018, suggesting worsening racial disparity in sleep duration. The study also found that the racial difference in sleep duration was more pronounced among women and individuals with middle to high household income levels (Caraballo et al., 2022). A more limited number of studies also investigated objectively measured sleep characteristics and reported disparities in various sleep parameters between racial/ethnic minority groups and Whites. For instance, an earlier investigation in the Multi-Ethnic Study of Atherosclerosis (MESA) showed that Black adults had higher PSG-measured sleep apnea and higher actigraphy-measured short sleep and poor sleep quality. The study also showed that both Hispanics and Chinese had higher odds of SDB and short sleep than Whites (X. Chen et al., 2015). Moreover, several studies reported racial/ethnic differences in characteristics of 24-hour rest–activity rhythms. For example, in NHANES, one study reported that Hispanics had the least fragmented (low intradaily variability [IV]) and most stable (high interdaily stability [IS]) rhythms among all racial/ethnic groups, while non-Hispanic Black adults had the least stable rhythmic patterns and lowest amplitude derived from cosine-based algorithms (J. Li et al., 2021). Another study applied fPCA to characterize rest–activity patterns in the same NHANES data set and reported that when compared to those of non-Hispanic White adults, the rhythmic profiles of non-Hispanic Black adults were characterized by a lower amplitude, later rise time, a prolonged activity window, and a more monophasic pattern (Q. Xiao, Lu, et al., 2022). Finally, it is worth noting that persistent and structural racism is an important contributor to racial and ethnic disparities in sleep health in the United States. For example, multiple studies found that greater exposure to identity-based discrimination among racial/ethnic minority groups was a consistent predictor of poor sleep health (Slopen et al., 2016). Moreover, it has been reported that exposure to discrimination is an important mediator of the relationship between racial/ethnic identity and differences in sleep architecture as measured by PSG (Thomas et al., 2006).

EDUCATION AND INCOME

Education attainment and income are commonly used measures of individual-level socioeconomic status (SES). Previous studies investigating individual-level SES in relation to sleep patterns generally reported an association between lower SES and less healthy sleep patterns in multiple dimensions (Grandner et al., 2016). For example, in the NHANES data set, both lower education levels and lower household income were linked to self-reported very short sleep (Whinnery et al., 2014). In the Southern Community Cohort Study (SCCS), a large prospective study of middle- to older-aged Black and White Americans enrolled from predominantly low-SES communities, a recent study found that lower education and income levels were significantly associated with suboptimal long-term sleep trajectories, such as consistent short or long sleep, deteriorating sleep, and unstable sleep patterns (Nyarko et al., 2023). Interestingly, the association between SES and sleep may vary across different race and sex groups. For example, in the SCCS, the relationship between lower income and suboptimal sleep trajectories was stronger among White than Black adults (Nyarko et al., 2023). In the NHIS, one study reported opposite educational gradients in sleep duration in Black and White populations: higher education levels were associated with lower odds of short sleep among White adults but higher odds among Black adults (Luo et al., 2021). Such findings highlight the importance of considering the interaction of multiple social factors in the context of sleep health.

WORK-RELATED FACTORS

Employment status, occupation, and other work-related factors play important roles in shaping health behaviors including sleep patterns. Previous studies based on national surveys in the United States found that unemployment is associated with a lower prevalence of healthy sleep duration (Y. Liu et al., 2016) and higher likelihood to report both short (<7 hours) and long (10+ hours) sleep duration (Blanchflower & Bryson, 2021). In a large cross-sectional study of workers in 31 European countries, Mai et al. (2019) found that employment insecurity was associated with higher odds of reporting "insomnia or general sleep difficulties" in the past year, and the results were consistent across different countries and persisted after controlling for other sociodemographic, socioeconomic, and family-related factors. Among workers, the prevalence of short sleep duration varies by industry and occupation: A higher prevalence was found in management (40.5%), transportation/warehousing (37.1%), and manufacturing (34.8%) sectors (Luckhaupt et al., 2010) and among occupation groups of production (42.9%), healthcare support (40.1%), healthcare practitioners and technical (40.0%), food preparation and service-related (39.8%), and protective service (39.2%; Shockey & Wheaton, 2017). The disparate patterns of sleep duration across different industry and occupation groups may be partially attributable to different work schedules for different types: One study reported that night-shift work is more common among workers in transportation and warehousing, healthcare, and social assistance than in other industry and occupation types; and short sleep prevalence appeared to be much higher among night-shift workers (44.0%) than day-shift workers (28.8%; Centers for Disease Control and Prevention, 2012). Finally, an earlier study suggested that not only the prevalence of short sleep but also racial disparities in short sleep vary across different occupations and industries, with the largest Black–White gap in short sleep observed in finance/information/real estate (prevalence ratio, Black vs. White, = 1.44, 95% CI [1.30, 1.59]), professional/administrative/management (1.30 [1.18, 1.44]), educational services (1.39 [1.25, 1.54]), public administration/arts/other services (1.30 [1.21, 1.41]), healthcare/social assistance (1.23 [1.14, 1.32]), and manufacturing/construction (1.14 [1.07, 1.20]). These findings also suggested a complex relationship at the intersection of employment, occupation, work schedule, and race/ethnicity in determining sleep duration.

NEIGHBORHOOD AND HOUSING CONDITIONS

Like many other health behaviors such as diet and physical activity, sleep is shaped not only by biological and individual factors but also by characteristics of the larger macroenvironment (Grandner, 2017). Recent studies have found that physical and social aspects of the neighborhood environment are associated with sleep deficiency. For example, exposure to ambient light and noise have an adverse effect on sleep (Chepesiuk, 2009; Muzet, 2007). In addition, neighborhood disadvantage, including low social cohesion, poor safety, and high poverty, is associated with sleep deficiency (Desantis et al., 2013; Fuller-Rowell et al., 2016; Hale et al., 2010, 2013; T. D. Hill et al., 2009, 2016; Johnson et al., 2016, 2017; Simonelli et al., 2017; Troxel et al., 2017). A cross-sectional study in US Hispanic adults linked unsafe neighborhoods to short sleep, low sleep efficiency, and late sleep timing (Simonelli et al., 2017). Similarly, among African Americans in the Jackson Heart Study, high neighborhood violence was also associated with shorter sleep duration and poorer sleep quality (Johnson et al., 2016). An international study using data from Mexico, Ghana, South Africa, India, China, and Russia found that respondents who felt safe in their neighborhoods reported better sleep outcomes (Hale et al., 2013). Two cross-sectional studies in the MESA study examined multiple aspects of the neighborhood social environment and found that neighborhood disorder, poor safety, and low social cohesion were associated with both self-reported and objectively measured short sleep duration (Desantis et al., 2013; Johnson et al., 2017). Using the 2004 Survey of Texas Adults, a statewide probability sample of Texas adults, two studies reported that a higher perception of neighborhood disorder was associated with poor sleep quality (Hale et al., 2010; T. D. Hill et al., 2009). Moreover, an earlier investigation of predominantly White adults in Wisconsin reported that a poorer perception of neighborhood quality was correlated with worse sleep quality (Hale et al., 2013). In addition, three studies used composite measures of neighborhood SES and examined their relationships with sleep (Desantis et al., 2013; Fuller-Rowell et al., 2016; Johnson et al., 2016; Q. Xiao & Hale, 2018). However, only the largest two of the four studies (Jackson Heart Study and NIH-AARP Diet and Health Study) found a significant association between low neighborhood SES and shorter sleep duration (Johnson et al., 2016; Q. Xiao & Hale, 2018); and the other two smaller studies (MESA and Midlife in the United States Study) reported a similar trend, but the results were not statistically significant (Desantis et al., 2013; Fuller-Rowell et al., 2016). A recent analysis in the SCCS found that lower neighborhood SES was associated with multiple suboptimal long-term sleep patterns in both Black and White adults, although the specific sleep trajectories associated with neighborhood SES differed by race (Nyarko et al., 2023). Finally, one earlier study also reported that change in neighborhood SES over 10 years was a unique predictor of sleep duration, and the effect was independent of that of average neighborhood SES during the same period. Specifically, women who lived in neighborhoods with deteriorating SES were more likely to report very short sleep (<5 hours) when compared to women living in more stable neighborhoods. On the other hand, an upward trajectory in neighborhood SES were associated with a higher likelihood of reporting long sleep (9+ hours) in men (Q. Xiao & Hale, 2018). Besides neighborhood characteristics, several earlier studies also reported a relationship between housing conditions and sleep duration. For example, a study in the NHIS (2004–2015) reported that people living in mobile homes and trailers were more likely to report short sleep than those living in apartments and houses. Moreover, the study also reported an interaction between housing conditions and race such that a Black–White difference in short sleep was only observed among those living in apartments and houses but not among those living in mobile homes and trailers (Johnson et al., 2018). Taken together, findings from these studies support an important role of neighborhood environment and housing conditions in sleep health and suggested that effects of environmental factors on sleep may differ by individual sociodemographic characteristics such as gender and race/ethnicity.

Genetics

Human sleep genetic studies showed that multiple sleep traits are heritable. Earlier twin studies showed modest heritability (30%–70%) for various sleep characteristics, including self-reported sleep length, quality, timing, sleep onset delay, and diurnal preference, as well as FitBit-based measures of various sleep and rest–activity characteristics (e.g., duration of total, light, and deep sleep; sleep efficiency; IS; IV; relative amplitude; M10; L5; and rhythmic index; Barclay et al., 2011; Gehrman et al., 2019; Heath et al., 1990; Partinen et al., 1983). However, the specific degree of estimated heritability varied by studies, likely influenced by study sample characteristics and sleep measures; and not all studies found significant heredity in sleep traits (Boomsma et al., 2008). More recently, advances in genome sequencing techniques and statistical methods have led to increasing popularity of genome-wide association studies (GWASs) in genetic epidemiology. Over the years, multiple GWAS investigations have been conducted to identify several genetic variants associated with various sleep phenotypes. A recent review summarized findings from 13 GWASs on genetic loci and sleep duration (nine focusing on self-reported sleep duration and four on objective measurements) and identified several genetic variants of interest (Garfield, 2021). For example, several genetic variants near and within the paired box thyroid-specific transcription factor (PAX8) gene were shown to be associated with both self-reported and objectively measured sleep duration in several study samples including the Cohorts for Heart and Aging Research and Genomic Epidemiology and UK Biobank studies (Dashti et al., 2019; Gottlieb et al., 2015). Another gene of which the signal was replicated in multiple studies was vaccinia related kinase 2 (VRK2; Dashti et al., 2019; Jones et al., 2016), a gene that has been previously linked to psychiatric disorders such as schizophrenia and epilepsy (International League Against Epilepsy Consortium on Complex Epilepsies, 2014; Steinberg et al., 2011). However, the overall conclusion from the review was that the heritability of sleep duration was lower than previously assumed. A number of other GWAS investigations also examined other sleep characteristics, including daytime sleepiness, sleep disturbances and insomnia symptoms, sleep apnea, and diurnal preferences of sleep timing or chronotype (Jones et al., 2016, 2019; Lane et al., 2017; Strausz et al., 2021; H. Wang et al., 2019). These studies provided valuable information for identifying biological mechanisms in determining sleep patterns and paved the way for investigating causal relationships between sleep and rest–activity rhythms and various health outcomes using genotypes as instrumental variables (i.e., Mendelian randomization studies).

Sleep and Health Outcomes

Safety and Injury

Sleep deficiency has been widely recognized as an important risk factor for workplace and non-work injuries and accidents and a threat to public safety. It has been shown that not only severe sleep deprivation but even relatively moderate sleep restriction, especially when accumulated over an extended period of time, can lead to serious neurobehavioral impairment including attention lapse and poor decision-making (Czeisler et al., 2016). A widely cited study by Dawson and Reid (1997) reported that after 17 hours of continuous wakefulness, the reduction in cognitive psychomotor performance among subjects was equivalent to that at 0.05% blood alcohol concentration, the legal threshold for drunk driving adopted by many industrialized countries. This finding was later confirmed by multiple studies (Lowrie & Brownlow, 2020; Roehrs et al., 2003; Van Dongen et al., 2003; Williamson & Feyer, 2000). In 2015, the National Highway Traffic Safety Administration and the National Sleep Foundation convened a panel of researchers and stakeholders to address drowsy driving. The panel concluded that drivers with a sleep duration of less than 3 hours in the past 24 hours are "too impaired to safely operate a motor vehicle" (Czeisler et al., 2016). However, the panels also found a high prevalence of drowsy driving in the United States and called for a national plan of concerted efforts to eliminate the problem (Higgins et al., 2017).

Another area where sleep deficiency represents an important threat to safety and performance is healthcare. Long work hours, unpredictable and irregular work schedule including rotating and night shifts, and high job demand and stress make health workers particularly susceptible to sleep deficiency and related adverse effects on work performance and their own health. Mounting evidence has linked sleep deficiency with a wide range of deficits in cognitive and motor functions critical to clinical performance among physicians, surgeons, and nurses (Howard et al., 2002; Robbins & Gottlieb, 1990; Rollinson et al., 2003; Taffinder et al., 1998; Wesnes et al., 1997). Working extended shifts (24 hours or longer) has been found to increase attention failures, medical errors, and adverse events in patient care in residents (Barger et al., 2006). Conversely, a randomized trial in medical interns showed that eliminating extended work shifts and reducing work hours significantly reduced serious medical errors. Among surgeons, sleep deprivation can lead to impaired technical proficiency and negatively impact nontechnical kills including decision-making, situational awareness, and communication (Quan et al., 2023; Whelehan et al., 2020). Moreover, sleep deficiencies are also linked to increased burnout and decreased wellness among physicians, with a higher level of sleep-related impairment and potential burnout found among trainee physicians and in surgery programs (Trockel et al., 2020). The authors also postulated that work-related sleep deficiency among healthcare workers may contribute to a vicious cycle where excessive and highly demanding work reduces efficiency, which further increases the need and tendency for overworking, which in turn exacerbates sleep problems.

Among athletes, there is increasing recognition of the link between sleep and sports injury, recovery, and performance. Emerging evidence from recent research suggested that insufficient sleep is highly prevalent among athletes. For example, in a recent survey of over 8,000 collegiate athletes, 57% of the participants reported insufficient sleep on 4 nights per week or more, and 61% reported daytime tiredness (Turner et al., 2021). Sleep restriction among athletes can lead to higher risk for injury, poorer physical performance, suboptimal recovery, and impaired mental health (Charest & Grandner, 2020). For example, a recent study including 190 National Collegiate Athletic Association Division-1 athletes reported that moderate to severe insomnia and excessive daytime sleepiness were associated with a threefold increase in concussion risk (Raikes et al., 2019). A meta-analysis found that adolescent athletes with chronic sleep deficiencies were 58% more likely to sustain sports injuries when compared to peers who reported sufficient sleep (Gao et al., 2019). There has been a call for promoting sleep health among athletes through better education, training schedule, and screening for and treatment of sleep disorders (Charest & Grandner, 2020).

Finally, among older adults, disturbed sleep has been linked to increased risk of falls and fractures (Cauley et al., 2014; Rogers et al., 2017; Stone, Ancoli-Israel, et al., 2008; Stone et al., 2014). Importantly, treatments for insomnia (e.g., benzodiazepines) have also been linked to increased fall risk (Stone, Ensrud, & Ancoli-Israel, 2008). While effective non-pharmacological treatments for insomnia are available and may prove to be safer in older adults, there remain issues with access to such therapy and inadequate comparative effectiveness data.

Cardiometabolic Disease

Multiple aspects of sleep have been linked to cardiometabolic health outcomes, such as obesity, metabolic syndrome, diabetes, and CVD. In general, suboptimal sleep patterns including short and long sleep durations, poor sleep quality, misaligned sleep timing and irregular sleep schedules, various sleep disorders, and impaired 24-hour rest–activity patterns have been linked to higher risk of cardiometabolic diseases.

SLEEP DURATION

Two meta-analyses summarized evidence from prospective cohort studies on the relationship between short and long sleep duration (mostly self-reported) and a wide range of cardiometabolic diseases (Itani et al., 2017; Jike et al., 2018). The authors reported that short sleep was associated with significantly higher risks for obesity (RR = 1.38, 95% CI [1.25, 1.53]), diabetes (1.37 [1.22, 1.53]), hypertension (1.17 [1.09, 1.26]), coronary heart disease (1.26 [1.15, 1.38]), and CVD in general (1.16 [1.10, 1.23]), while long sleep was associated with increased risks for obesity (1.08 [1.02, 1.15]), diabetes (1.26 [1.11, 1.43]), coronary heart disease (1.24 [1.13, 1.37]), stroke (1.46 [1.26, 1.69]), and total CVD (1.25 [1.14, 1.37]). Meta-regression analysis also found a linear relationship between the duration of long sleep and incident CVD. Previous studies also suggested that the relationship between sleep and cardiometabolic health may vary in different age, sex, and racial and ethnic groups. For example, while the relationship with short sleep appeared stronger among younger (<65) individuals, the relationship with long sleep appeared stronger among older individuals (Itani et al., 2017; Jike et al., 2018). Moreover, several studies also reported a weaker association between sleep and cardiometabolic health outcomes among Black than White individuals (S. Lee et al., 2022; Q. Xiao, Blot, & Matthews, 2019).

SLEEP QUALITY

Numerous studies examined self-reported overall quality of sleep in relation to various cardiometabolic conditions and generally reported a relationship between poorer sleep quality and higher disease risks. For example, a meta-analysis found that poor sleep quality was associated with metabolic syndrome, and the strengths of association varied across different measures of sleep quality, with sleep inefficiency showing the strongest effect

(Lian et al., 2019). In another systematic review and meta-analysis, poor sleep quality, along with a few other sleep measures, was found to be a significant predictor of diabetes risk; and the effect sizes appeared to be comparable to traditional risk factors such as overweight, family history, and lack of physical activity (Anothaisintawee et al., 2016). Observational studies found that among patients with Type 2 diabetes, poor sleep quality was associated with worse glycemic control as indicated by a higher level of hemoglobin A1c (S. W. H. Lee et al., 2017). However, a meta-analysis of intervention studies found that although sleep interventions, such as sleep extension, sleep education, or cognitive behavioral therapy, and pharmacological treatments led to significantly improved sleep quality, their effects on glycemic control were not statistically significant (Kothari et al., 2021). Self-reported poor sleep quality was also found to be a predictor of higher risk of coronary heart disease in a meta-analysis, but the results were not statistically significant for other cardiovascular outcomes including stroke, cardiovascular mortality, and overall CVD incidence (Kwok et al., 2018). Another more recent study found that poor sleep quality was associated with increased arterial stiffness (Saz-Lara et al., 2022). Finally, there has been evidence showing that the association of sleep quality with cardiometabolic conditions such as obesity was independent of that of sleep duration (Fatima et al., 2016), suggesting that sleep quality is a unique predictor and highlighting the importance of using multidimensional measures of sleep.

SLEEP TIMING AND REGULARITY

It has been well established that night-shift workers, who frequently experience severe circadian misalignment and sleep deficiencies, are at a higher risk of developing many cardiometabolic conditions. For example, a meta-analysis synthesized evidence from 12 cohorts and found a 14% increase in the risk of developing diabetes among shift workers when compared to non-shift workers, and the study also found a highly significant linear dose–response curve, with each 5-year increase in the duration of shift work associated with a 7% increase in risk (W. Li et al., 2019). Similar findings were also reported for CVD: The pooled RR for ischemic heart disease comparing shift work with non-shift work was 1.13 (95% CI [1.08, 1.20]), and each year increase in shift-work was associated with a 0.9% increase (Cheng et al., 2019). Another two studies found similar associations with total CVD and CVD mortality (Torquati et al., 2018; D. Wang et al., 2018).

Beside night-shift work, more subtle differences in sleep timing and the degree of its alignment with the internal biological clock may also contribute to cardiometabolic risk. For example, mounting evidence suggests that chronotype (i.e., a person's propensity to sleep at a certain time) may be a predictor of cardiometabolic disease risk. In particular, a later chronotype has been linked to diabetes (Knutson & von Schantz, 2018; Tan et al., 2020; Vetter et al., 2015; Yu et al., 2015), metabolic syndrome (Yu et al., 2015), CVD (Kobayashi Frisk et al., 2022; Yu et al., 2015), and obesity (Teixeira et al., 2022). Interestingly, several studies shed light on the mechanisms by which chronotype may be associated with cardiometabolic risk: For example, in the Nurses' Health Study 2, the relationship between late chronotype and higher diabetes risk was only observed among day workers (RR = 1.51, 95% CI [1.13, 2.02]), while among night-shift workers, late chronotype was associated with a nonsignificant decrease in diabetes risk, suggesting that it was not chronotype itself but a more severe misalignment between sleep/work schedule with the internal circadian clock that contributed to a higher risk of diabetes. Moreover, mediation analysis in several studies suggested that the relationship between eveningness and cardiometabolic diseases was at least partially explained by lifestyle factors such as a sedentary lifestyle and poor diet (Kobayashi Frisk et al., 2022; Teixeira et al., 2022). Finally, findings from a limited but growing number of Mendelian randomization studies generally reported a lack of causal relationship between chronotype and cardiometabolic conditions, suggesting that the observed relationships may be explained by confounding factors (Cai et al., 2020; M. Fan et al., 2020; J. Liu et al., 2022).

Recent evidence suggested that not only sleep timing, but the consistency or regularity in sleep schedules is also an important predictor of cardiometabolic risk. For example, in a Hispanic population in the United States, a recent analysis found a cross-sectional relationship between lower regularity in sleep schedules and higher odds of diabetes; also, the prospective analysis in the same sample produced null findings (Fritz et al., 2021). Moreover, greater bedtime variability was also associated with poorer dietary quality (Rusu et al., 2022). Finally, several studies have reported associations between variability in sleep duration and various cardiometabolic outcomes, including obesity, diabetes, and CVD (Rosique-Esteban et al., 2018; Slavish et al., 2019); and the relationships persisted even after adjusting for average sleep duration. However, a role of inconsistent sleep timing in these conditions can only be inferred from these studies as they did not specifically examine variability in sleep timing. More studies are needed to clarify the role of inconsistent sleep schedules in cardiometabolic health.

24-HOUR REST–ACTIVITY PATTERNS

Emerging evidence suggests that not only nighttime sleep patterns but characteristics of the overall rest–activity rhythms are important predictors of cardiometabolic outcomes. For example, an analysis in older men in the MrOS study reported that characteristics of the rest–activity rhythms consistent with weakened diurnal rhythmicity were associated with both higher prevalence and incidence of diabetes. For example, older men in the lowest quartile of overall rhythmicity as measured by the pseudo-F statistic were 3.5 times more likely to develop diabetes than those in the highest quartile (Q. Xiao et al., 2020). Similar results were also reported in the NHANES, showing that weakened rest–activity rhythms were associated with higher odds of diabetes and impaired glycemic control measures (Q. Xiao, Matthews, et al., 2022). A recent publication including over 3,000 patients with Type 2 diabetes in the UK Biobank cohort found that the lowest quartile of interdaily stability and relative amplitude was associated with elevated risk of CVD (Yang et al., 2023). Finally, an analysis in the MrOS using a novel harmonic hidden Markov model to characterize the overall strength of rest–activity rhythms reported both cross-sectional and prospective relationships between impaired rhythmic strength and obesity (Heckler et al., 2023). It is worth mentioning that these findings typically persisted after controlling for sleep, physical activity, and sedentary variables, suggesting that rhythmic profiles of the 24-hour rest and activity are independent predictors of cardiometabolic health.

Dementia and Cognitive Outcomes

Sleep plays a key role in the consolidation of memory, maintenance of daytime alertness, and optimal cognitive functioning (Diekelmann & Born, 2010; Durmer & Dinges, 2005; Stickgold, 2005). Older adults have impaired overnight memory consolidation, which may be caused by specific age-related changes in sleep (A. Lam et al., 2021; Mander et al., 2015). While it has long been established that older adults with dementia are more likely to experience sleep disturbances, more recent evidence from epidemiologic studies suggests a bidirectional relationship, such that sleep disturbance may also play a causal role in the progression of Alzheimer's disease and related dementias (ADRD).

There is considerable emerging evidence from both epidemiological and experimental studies that sleep disorders could contribute to cognitive decline and risk of ADRD. In addition, there is supporting evidence from experimental studies indicating that sleep plays a key role in clearing key proteins involved in dementia pathogenesis, including β-amyloid and tau, via the glymphatic system (Xie et al., 2013). Furthermore, short sleep duration and poor sleep quality have been associated with greater cerebral β-amyloid burden among community-dwelling older adults (Spira et al., 2013).

Systematic reviews and meta-analyses revealed that older adults with sleep disturbances had higher risks of incident all-cause dementia (L. Shi et al., 2018), vascular dementia (L. Shi et al., 2018), cognitive impairment (Bubu et al., 2017), Alzheimer's disease (AD; Bubu et al., 2017; L. Shi et al., 2018), and preclinical AD (Bubu et al., 2017) compared to individuals without sleep problems. Specific findings suggest that insomnia, sleep fragmentation, daytime dysfunction, prolonged sleep latency, REM sleep behavior disorder, and excessive time in bed were linked to risks of all-cause cognitive disorders with moderate to high levels of evidence (W. Xu et al., 2020). Insomnia has been linked to a 53% increased risk for dementia in older adults (de Almondes et al., 2016). These results, together with emerging experimental evidence of a potential role of sleep in dementia risk and AD pathogenesis, indicate that future research is needed to assess whether sleep interventions may result in a reduced risk of cognitive decline and ADRD. A growing body of epidemiologic evidence has also linked disrupted circadian rest–activity rhythms to increased risk of cognitive impairment and decline and risk for dementia (Posner et al., 2021; Rogers-Soeder et al., 2018; Tranah et al., 2010; Walsh et al., 2014; Q. Xiao, Qian, et al., 2022; Q. Xiao, Sampson, et al., 2022; Q. Xiao, Shadyab, et al., 2022).

Growing evidence also suggests a strong link between SDB (including OSA; Bubu et al., 2022) and increased risk of all-cause dementia, AD, and vascular dementia (L. Shi et al., 2018). Data from the Study of Osteoporotic Fractures showed that cognitively normal older women with SDB had a nearly twofold increase in risk of developing mild cognitive impairment (MCI) or dementia over 5 years of follow-up; the effects appeared to be largely driven by nocturnal hypoxia (Yaffe et al., 2011). OSA may induce neurodegenerative changes through the effects on intermittent hypoxia, sleep fragmentation, and excessive daytime sleepiness (Bubu et al., 2020). The accumulation of AD biomarkers (β-amyloid and tau protein) increases MCI and AD progression risk and predicts shorter progression time to MCI and AD (Bubu et al., 2021). Treatment of OSA, for example, using continuous positive airway pressure, may help to delay age at MCI onset, reduce MCI or AD incidence, and slow cognitive decline, although large randomized controlled trials are still exploring these relationships (Kuo et al., 2020; Shieu et al., 2022), and future trials are needed to determine if treating presymptomatic (i.e. cognitively normal) individuals can prevent MCI and ultimately AD.

While much of the research on the effects of sleep and cognition has been focused on older adults, the role of sleep in maintaining cognitive health is essential across the life span. For example, a meta-analysis of studies investigating sleep disturbance and cognition in school-aged children found significant effects of shorter sleep duration with overall cognitive performance, executive function, and school performance but not with intelligence, attention, or memory (Astill et al., 2012). Neurocognitive deficits are also more common in children with SDB (Bourke et al., 2011).

Depression and Anxiety

The epidemiologic literature suggests that sleep is a likely contributor to mental health problems such as depression and anxiety across the life span. In children and adolescents, not only are mental health problems such as depression and anxiety frequently comorbid with insomnia and other sleep problems (Simonds & Parraga, 1984), but results from longitudinal and prospective cohort studies have established that early childhood sleep disorders predict later development of mental health problems during adolescence, suggesting a possible causal relationship (L. T. Lam & Lam, 2021). Similarly, in a meta-analysis of longitudinal epidemiologic studies it was shown that nondepressed adults with insomnia have a twofold risk of incident depression as compared to adults without insomnia (Baglioni et al., 2011). In prospective studies of nondepressed older adults, insomnia (Jaussent et al., 2011) as well as subjective and actigraphic measures of sleep (Maglione et al., 2014) and circadian rest–activity rhythms (Smagula et al., 2015) have been linked to increased risk of developing depressive symptoms over time. These findings together suggest a potential role for sleep therapies to relieve symptoms of depression and anxiety. Overall, the compendium of evidence from randomized trials has suggested that treatment of insomnia symptoms in patients with depression has a positive effect on mood

(Gebara et al., 2018). More research in this area is needed, for example, clinical trials designed to determine if treatment of insomnia and circadian disruption can prevent new onset of depression across the life span.

Cancer

It has long been suggested that sleep deficiencies and circadian disruptions may play a role in cancer development and survival due to the myriad effects of sleep and circadian rhythms on biological pathways involved in cancer (Mogavero et al., 2021). Although the relationship between sleep and cancer has been investigated by numerous epidemiological studies, there is considerable heterogeneity in study findings according to sleep characteristics and types of cancer examined. A meta-analysis that included 65 studies on sleep duration and risk of cancer found no relationship between either short or long sleep and total cancer risk (OR = 1.01, 95% CI [0.97, 1.05], and 1.02 [0.97, 1.07] for short and long sleep, respectively; Y. Chen et al., 2018). Further subgroup analysis showed a significant relationship between short sleep and cancer risk among Asian populations and between long sleep and colorectal cancer. Similarly, another meta-analysis that focused on breast cancer, the most studied cancer type in studies that investigated the sleep–cancer relationship, also found no association between short or long sleep duration and breast cancer risk (Wong et al., 2021). However, a meta-analysis of cohort studies that examined the relationship between sleep duration and all-cancer mortality found that both very short sleep (≤5 hours) and long sleep (≥8 hours) were associated with a small but statistically significant increase in cancer mortality (RR = 1.08, 95% CI [1.02, 1.13], and 1.05 [1.02, 1.08], respectively; Y. Li et al., 2019).

Studies that examined sleep disorders, such as sleep apnea and insomnia, generally reported stronger associations with cancer risk. For example, a meta-analysis including seven studies on sleep apnea and lung cancer reported a 30% increase in lung cancer among patients with OSA (Cheong et al., 2022). Another study reported a 36% increase in breast cancer risk among women with SDB (Wei et al., 2021). An earlier systematic review and meta-analysis also concluded that OSA/SDB was associated with a significant increase in cancer incidence (RR = 1.53, 95% CI [1.31, 1.79]; Shantha et al., 2015). Multiple studies also examined the relationship between insomnia and cancer risk. For example, in a cohort study in Norway that included over 30,000 women, those who reported symptoms in all three aspects of insomnia (nonrestorative sleep, difficulty initiating sleep, and difficulty maintaining sleep) were 2.38 times (95% CI [1.11, 5.09]) more likely to develop breast cancer than women who reported no symptom in any of the aspects (Sen et al., 2017). Frequent insomnia symptoms were found to be associated with lung cancer in the UK Biobank (Peeri et al., 2022), and a Mendelian randomization analysis in the same cohort suggested that there may be a causal relationship between insomnia and lung cancer risk (J. Wang et al., 2021). Finally, a systematic review and meta-analysis that included eight studies reported that insomnia was associated with a 24% and 28%

increase in total cancer risk in women and men, respectively; but the association in men was not statistically significant due to smaller sample size (T. Shi et al., 2020).

It has long been postulated that circadian disruption may play a role in breast cancer carcinogenesis (Blakeman et al., 2016). Epidemiological studies in long-time night-shift workers, who often experience severe and frequent circadian misalignment, have shown higher breast cancer incidence compared to the general population (Hansen, 2017). Notably, the effect was only observed among long-term night-shift workers (≥10 years), a finding that was further confirmed by a meta-analysis that included 26 studies (Manouchehri et al., 2021). It has been postulated that one of the mechanisms that may drive the link between night-shift work and breast cancer may be the suppression of melatonin, a hormone critical to circadian regulation. Melatonin is involved in a wide range of biological pathways involved in breast cancer carcinogenesis, such as estrogen production and signaling, cell proliferation, DNA repair, and inflammation pathways (Ball et al., 2016; S. M. Hill et al., 2015). In 2007, the International Agency for Cancer Research (IARC) listed shift work that involves circadian disruption as a Class 2a or probable carcinogen, and the designation was reaffirmed by IARC in 2019 (Zhang & Papantoniou, 2019). More recently, an increasing body of literature has examined the relationship between chronotype and the risk of various cancer types. For example, in the UK Biobank study, a morning preference was shown to be associated with a lower risk of breast cancer, and subsequent two-sample Mendelian randomization analysis suggested a causal effect (Richmond et al., 2019). Another studying using both the UK Biobank and the FinnGen studies also showed a modest protective effect of morningness on overall digestive tract cancer, stomach cancer, and colorectal cancer (Yuan et al., 2023). Moreover, a large case–control study showed that a genetic profile related to morningness was associated with reduced risk of prostate cancer (Sun et al., 2021). Collectively, these findings suggested that circadian disruptions may increase cancer risk, particularly breast cancer risk, while an earlier chronotype may have a protective effect.

Inflammation

Sleep is critical to immune function and inflammation regulation (Irwin, 2019). There is compelling evidence suggesting that sleep deficiencies and circadian disruptions are linked to chronic inflammation and immune dysfunction, which are important risk factors for morbidity and mortality. In experimental studies, both partial and total sleep deprivation have been shown to increase levels of multiple inflammatory markers, including C-reactive protein (CRP), interleukin 6 (IL-6), and tumor necrosis factor (TNF; Chennaoui et al., 2011; Sauvet et al., 2010; Sauvet et al., 2010Schmid et al., 2011; Vgontzas et al., 2004). In observational studies, both short and long sleep duration and sleep disturbances have also been linked to elevated inflammation. For example, in the Whitehall II study, both short sleep and a decrease in sleep duration over time were found to be associated with higher levels of inflammatory markers, including CRP and IL-6 (Ferrie et al., 2013). Another study in the same cohort found that the relationship between sleep duration and inflammatory markers was only observed among women (Miller et al., 2009). A systematic review and meta-analysis of 72 studies on this topic concluded that sleep disturbances and long sleep, but not short sleep, were associated with chronic inflammation (Irwin et al., 2016).

The circadian system plays an important role in immune function and inflammatory responses, and prior research has linked circadian disruption with elevated inflammation (Scheiermann et al., 2013, 2018). For example, an inverted sleep–wake cycle that mimicked night work led to higher levels of multiple inflammatory markers under laboratory conditions (Leproult et al., 2014; Morris et al., 2016, 2017; Wright et al., 2015). Similar findings were also reported by observational studies. For example, among healthy adults, Morris et al. (2016) showed that a multi-day lab protocol to induce circadian misalignment similar to night-shift work led to significant increases in IL-6, CRP, and TNF alpha by 15%, 7%, and 3%, respectively. In a large cross-sectional study of almost 2,000 middle-aged adults in Finland, working the night shift was associated with significantly higher levels of CRP in men after adjusting for infection and multiple lifestyle factors (Puttonen et al., 2011). In a recent analysis in a large cohort of older men, we also found that multiple rest–activity characteristics, such as lower amplitude and relative amplitude and decreased overall rhythmicity, were associated with higher levels of CRP, IL-6, TNF alpha, and TNF alpha soluble receptor II. Moreover, these rest–activity parameters were also associated with changes in these inflammatory markers such that weakened rest–activity rhythms predicted a greater increase in these inflammatory markers over 3.5 years of follow-up (Q. Xiao, Qian, et al., 2022).

Methodological Considerations in Sleep Epidemiology Research

Sleep Measurement in Epidemiologic Studies

Assessing sleep in large epidemiologic studies presents challenges because the cost and burden of comprehensive objective sleep assessments may not always be feasible, yet multidimensional data on sleep may be essential to identify and interpret key relationships of sleep health and disorders with health and disease. Described below are some of the primary methods that have been used to measure sleep in epidemiologic studies, including PSG, actigraphy and other wearable devices, and questionnaires. This is by no means an exhaustive summary of devices available, and new technologies are rapidly emerging. Key advantages and disadvantages of each approach are discussed.

PSG

PSG is considered the "gold standard" for evaluating sleep but is the most difficult to implement in epidemiologic studies given the increased burden and cost of multichannel overnight recording of information that is required. Sleep–wake and sleep staging information can be derived from the PSG signals, and inclusion of respirations and oximetry is utilized to identify individuals with SDB including sleep apnea. Most epidemiologic studies that have utilized PSG to assess sleep have used in-home monitoring rather than bringing participants in to a sleep laboratory for overnight assessments.

PSG provides a very rich source of information about sleep which has yielded numerous important findings linking sleep to health outcomes. For example, findings have underscored the associations between sleep apnea and risk of incident CVD (Gottlieb et al., 2010), stroke (Redline et al., 2010; Stone et al., 2016), and onset of MCI or dementia (Yaffe et al., 2011). In addition, a recent multicohort analysis linked decreased percent time in REM sleep to increased risk of mortality. Increasingly, researchers are utilizing machine learning methods and deep neural networks applied to raw PSG signal data to predict outcomes such as biological age and life expectancy (Brink-Kjaer et al., 2022), highlighting the potential for powerful and novel uses of this data in epidemiologic research.

Despite the very rich data afforded by use of PSG in epidemiologic studies, there are some clear disadvantages. In addition to substantially increased burden and cost, typically only one single night of recording is feasible, and the recording period is restricted to a nighttime interval lasting 6–10 hours. As a result, there is no information on daytime sleep; and the recording process itself may disrupt the participant's sleep, resulting in data that is less representative of the participant's usual sleep patterns.

It is worth noting that there are less cumbersome devices designed and validated to capture some of the specific exposures typically derived from PSG, such as sleep apnea (Tauman et al., 2020) or electroencephalogram (Lunsford-Avery et al., 2020).

ACTIGRAPHY AND WEARABLE DEVICES

In comparison with PSG, actigraphy is much less expensive and provides 24-hour recordings of activity (movement) from which wake and sleep can be scored. When used to measure sleep, the actigraph is typically worn on the wrist. A variety of research-grade actigraphs are available and are designed to provide access to raw acceleration data, epoch-by-epoch activity counts, and estimated average nightly sleep–wake variables (e.g., sleep duration, sleep efficiency, and minutes of wake after sleep onset). Many such devices have been validated against PSG and are reasonably reliable (Stone & Li, 2022). A distinct advantage of actigraphic devices is the ability to estimate daytime activity variables in addition to nighttime sleep variables, although it is widely believed that waist or hip placement of the device is preferred for assessment of physical activity to more accurately pick up center of mass acceleration (Kerr et al., 2018).

In recent years, there has been a wealth of consumer-grade wearable devices developed that estimate sleep, typically using proprietary algorithms. While initially these devices were underutilized in research settings due to lack of transparency about the validity of the algorithms for estimation of sleep, increasingly there have been partnerships between

directionality of associations between sleep and health outcomes, multiple measurements of both exposures and outcomes with relevant time intervals (usually several years apart for chronic diseases) are required. When such data is available, appropriate methods may be employed to explore bidirectional associations of sleep and related health outcomes. For example, in one multi-wave study with measures of sleep and cognitive function conducted in China, latent growth and cross-lagged models were used to explore the bidirectional associations of short and long sleep duration and cognition (Hua et al., 2021). This particular study with subjective measures of sleep found stronger associations of cognition with subsequent sleep problems than the reverse association. However, another study which explored longitudinal associations between disturbed sleep and depressive symptoms in children and adolescents using cross-lagged models confirmed a bidirectional association of these conditions (Marino et al., 2022). Further epidemiologic research is needed with multiple time points of objective and subjective sleep assessments and other potential health outcomes linked to poor sleep in order to better establish the directionality of such associations.

Approaches to Studying Multidimensional Sleep Characteristics

The emphasis on multidimensionality of sleep and rest–activity behaviors presents a unique challenge and opportunity for researchers to identify the best sleep and rest–activity profiles as behavioral predictors of disease risk. A large number of distinct yet interrelated parameters of sleep and rest–activity rhythms can be derived using various survey instruments and wearable devices in epidemiological studies. It is informative to simultaneously evaluate the comparative importance of these parameters in predicting health outcomes, but this is challenging when using traditional regression models. Recently, several statistical methods have been applied for this purpose and have generated intriguing findings. In particular, several machine learning methods have been applied to model complex, nonlinear relationships and quantify the relative importance of sleep and rest–activity variables in relation to health outcomes. For example, Wallace et al. (2018) used random survival forest, a flexible machine-learning method, to rank multiple sociodemographic, medical, and lifestyle factors based on their predictive values for total mortality among MrOS participants. In this analysis, overall rhythmicity, as measured by the pseudo-F statistic (indicating how strongly the extended cosine model curve fits the data), emerged among the strongest predictors for mortality (ranked eighth among 43 predictors), ranking higher than many nonmodifiable factors such as education, race, and histories of hypertension and diabetes. This finding suggests that the regularity of sleep-wake patterns from day to day may be more important to overall health than sleep duration and other demographic and health-related factors. In two other studies in older men and women, cluster analysis and factor analysis were used to extract sleep health profiles from actigraphy data (Wallace et al., 2021, 2022). One of these studies reported relationships between several sleep profiles and mortality risk (Wallace et al., 2022). Findings from these and other similar studies may help in the development of algorithms for better risk prediction and disease management.

Elucidating Biological Pathways by Omics Studies

High-throughput technologies offer powerful agnostic tools for elucidating the biological pathways underlying the wide range of health effects of sleep deficiencies and circadian disruptions. Multiple omics studies have examined the biological effects of sleep deficiencies in human subjects. For example, by using a forced-desynchrony protocol, Archer et al. (2014) showed that delaying sleep by 4 hours for 3 consecutive days led to a significant reduction in circadian amplitude and a loss of rhythmicity in the expression patterns of many genes involved in circadian regulation, chromatin modification, ribosome biogenesis, and gene transcription and translation regulators. Another study using a sleep deprivation protocol and proteomics approach showed significant alterations in multiple proteins involved in metabolic pathways, the immune system, and blood coagulation following a 6-hour sleep deprivation (Bjørkum et al., 2021). In a metabolomics study, 12 healthy men underwent total sleep deprivation for 24 hours, and the study showed that the majority of metabolites exhibited circadian fluctuation in blood levels. Moreover, sleep deprivation significantly altered the levels of many metabolites, including amino acids, carbohydrates, and lipids (Davies et al., 2014). Multiple studies also have examined the associations between metabolomic profiles and sleep characteristics in free-living populations. For example, in one of the first population studies on sleep and metabolomics, we used an untargeted approach to identify metabolomic markers in relation to habitual sleep timing (midpoint of sleep) and sleep duration in a group of Chinese men and women. Our study found over 60 metabolites in many biochemical pathways that were associated with sleep timing but not duration. Notably, these metabolites included amino acids, particularly branched chain amino acids and their gamma-glutamyl dipeptides, and lipids including bile acids, carnitines, and fatty acids; and many of the observed associations were consistent with a link between a later sleep time and higher disease risks as suggested by metabolomic profiles (e.g., higher branched chain amino acids and bile acids; Q. Xiao et al., 2017). In a recent investigation that included over 9,000 women, Fritz et al. (2023) reported that short sleep was associated with 20 metabolites, including several lysophospholipids, amino acids, and triacylglycerols, as well as the acylcarnitine pathway. The study did not find a relationship between long sleep and any individual metabolites but did report suggestive evidence linking long sleep with lipid pathways. Finally, in a study of postmenopausal women, Huang et al. (2019) found that a sleep quality score derived from self-reported sleep problems was associated with multiple metabolites. Importantly, using a least absolute shrinkage and selection operator algorithm, the authors derived a nine-metabolite score. This sleep-associated plasma metabolite score was associated with conventional coronary heart disease (CHD) biomarkers, such as cholesterol, CRP, and fasting glucose, and predicted CHD risk after controlling for multiple CHD risk factors including conventional biomarkers (Huang et al., 2019). Future studies should focus on identifying metabolomic and other omics profiles that may mediate the adverse health effects of sleep deficiency and circadian disruption and investigate if and how these biomarker profiles can be incorporated into risk prediction algorithms for various chronic diseases.

The Future of Sleep Epidemiology

The epidemiology of sleep has seen tremendous growth over recent decades, with multiple epidemiologic cohort studies specifically designed to assess associations of subjective and objective sleep with health and disease outcomes. These studies have led to key findings linking various characteristics of sleep to risks to mortality (Tranah et al., 2010; Wallace et al., 2018, 2019; Zeitzer et al., 2018), CVD (Kwok et al., 2018), obesity and diabetes (Fatima et al., 2016; Fritz et al., 2023), cognitive decline and dementia (Blackwell et al., 2006; Bubu et al., 2017; Posner et al., 2021; Yaffe et al., 2011), and other mental (Baglioni et al., 2011; Furihata et al., 2017; Maglione et al., 2014) and physical (Stone & Xiao, 2018) health outcomes. However, future research is needed with more comprehensive assessments of sleep and novel statistical approaches (e.g., machine learning) to elucidate which aspects of sleep health are driving the observed associations; this is essential to inform which sleep interventions may be most effective at preventing or alleviating poor health outcomes.

New technological advances including wearable devices and novel and more feasible sleep monitoring approaches will continue to offer possibilities for larger epidemiologic studies, with longitudinal assessments needed to establish the directionality of associations. Given the decreasing costs and more feasible approaches to monitoring sleep, larger-scale studies with longitudinal designs should be considered to explore new associations and key interactions such as whether associations fundamentally differ with age, race and ethnicity, or sex or gender.

While observational epidemiology has revolutionized the study of the potential role of sleep in a wide range of health outcomes, the time is ripe to translate these findings into randomized trials to test whether improving sleep can slow the onset of health problems and/or alleviate symptoms of physical and mental health conditions. For example, can we reduce the risk of AD by treating sleep apnea? Does treating insomnia alleviate chronic pain or improve mood? To inform the design of such trials, it is essential to incorporate a more comprehensive set of sleep exposures into epidemiologic studies to inform which aspects of sleep are the optimal targets for intervention studies.

References

Ali, R. M., Zolezzi, M., & Awaisu, A. (2020). A systematic review of instruments for the assessment of insomnia in adults. *Nature and Science of Sleep*, *12*, 377–409. https://doi.org/10.2147/NSS.S250918

American Academy of Sleep Medicine. (2014). *International classification of sleep disorders* (3rd ed.).

Amiri, S., & Behnezhad, S. (2020). Smoking and risk of sleep-related issues: A systematic review and meta-analysis of prospective studies. *Canadian Journal of Public Health, 111*(5), 775–786. https://doi.org/10.17269/s41997-020-00308-3

Ancoli-Israel, S., & Kripke, D. F. (1991). Prevalent sleep problems in the aged. *Biofeedback and Self-regulation, 16*(4), 349–359. https://doi.org/10.1007/BF00999989

Ancoli-Israel, S., Kripke, D. F., Klauber, M. R., Mason, W. J., Fell, R., & Kaplan, O. (1991). Sleep-disordered breathing in community-dwelling elderly. *Sleep, 14*(6), 486–495. https://doi.org/10.1093/sleep/14.6.486

Ancoli-Israel, S., Kripke, D. F., Klauber, M. R., Parker, L., Stepnowsky, C., Kullen, A., & Fell, R. (1993). Natural history of sleep disordered breathing in community dwelling elderly. *Sleep, 16*(S8), S25–S29. https://doi.org/10.1093/sleep/16.suppl_8.s25

Anders, T., Sadeh, A., & Appareddy, V. J. P. (1995). Normal sleep in neonates and children. In R. Ferber & M. H. Kryger (Eds.), Principles and practice of sleep medicine in the child (pp. 7–18). Saunders.

Anothaisintawee, T., Reutrakul, S., Van Cauter, E., & Thakkinstian, A. (2016). Sleep disturbances compared to traditional risk factors for diabetes development: Systematic review and meta-analysis. *Sleep Medicine Reviews, 30,* 11–24. https://doi.org/10.1016/j.smrv.2015.10.002

Archer, S. N., Laing, E. E., Moller-Levet, C. S., van der Veen, D. R., Bucca, G., Lazar, A. S., Santhi, N., Slak, A., Kabiljo, R., von Schantz, M., Smith, C. P., & Dijk, D.-J. (2014). Mistimed sleep disrupts circadian regulation of the human transcriptome. *Proceedings of the National Academy of Sciences of the United States of America, 111*(6), E682–E691. https://doi.org/10.1073/pnas.1316335111

Astill, R. G., Van der Heijden, K. B., Van Ijzendoorn, M. H., & Van Someren, E. J. (2012). Sleep, cognition, and behavioral problems in school-age children: A century of research meta-analyzed. *Psychological Bulletin, 138*(6), 1109–1138. https://doi.org/10.1037/a0028204

Baglioni, C., Battagliese, G., Feige, B., Spiegelhalder, K., Nissen, C., Voderholzer, U., Lombardo, C., & Riemann, D. (2011). Insomnia as a predictor of depression: A meta-analytic evaluation of longitudinal epidemiological studies. *Journal of Affective Disorders, 135*(1–3), 10–19. https://doi.org/10.1016/j.jad.2011.01.011

Ball, L. J., Palesh, O., & Kriegsfeld, L. J. (2016). The pathophysiologic role of disrupted circadian and neuroendocrine rhythms in breast carcinogenesis. *Endocrine Reviews, 37*(5), 450–466. https://doi.org/10.1210/er.2015-1133

Barclay, N. L., Eley, T. C., Maughan, B., Rowe, R., & Gregory, A. M. (2011). Associations between diurnal preference, sleep quality and externalizing behaviours: A behavioural genetic analysis. *Psychological Medicine, 41*(5), 1029–1040. https://doi.org/10.1017/S0033291710001741

Barger, L. K., Ayas, N. T., Cade, B. E., Cronin, J. W., Rosner, B., Speizer, F. E., & Czeisler, C. A. (2006). Impact of extended-duration shifts on medical errors, adverse events, and attentional failures. *PLOS Medicine, 3*(12), Article e487. https://doi.org/10.1371/journal.pmed.0030487

Bixler, E. O., Papaliaga, M. N., Vgontzas, A. N., Lin, H. M., Pejovic, S., Karataraki, M., Vela-Bueno, A., & Chrousos, G. P. (2009). Women sleep objectively better than men and the sleep of young women is more resilient to external stressors: Effects of age and menopause. *Journal of Sleep Research, 18*(2), 221–228. https://doi.org/10.1111/j.1365-2869.2008.00713.x

Bjørkum, A. A., Carrasco Duran, A., Frode, B., Sinha Roy, D., Rosendahl, K., Birkeland, E., & Stuhr, L. (2021). Human blood serum proteome changes after 6 hours of sleep deprivation at night. *Sleep Science and Practice, 5*(1), Article 14.

Blackwell, T., Yaffe, K., Ancoli-Israel, S., Schneider, J. L., Cauley, J. A., Hillier, T. A., & Fink, H. A. (2006). Poor sleep is associated with impaired cognitive function in older women: The study of osteoporotic fractures. *Journals of Gerontology: Series A, 61*(4), 405–410. https://doi.org/10.1093/gerona/61.4.405

Blakeman, V., Williams, J. L., Meng, Q. J., & Streuli, C. H. (2016). Circadian clocks and breast cancer. *Breast Cancer Research, 18*(1), Article 89. https://doi.org/10.1186/s13058-016-0743-z

Blanchflower, D. G., & Bryson, A. (2021). Unemployment and sleep: Evidence from the United States and Europe. *Economics & Human Biology, 43*, Article 101042. https://doi.org/10.1016/j.ehb.2021.101042

Boomsma, D. I., van Someren, E. J., Beem, A. L., de Geus, E. J., & Willemsen, G. (2008). Sleep during a regular week night: A twin-sibling study. *Twin Research and Human Genetics, 11*(5), 538–545. https://doi.org/10.1375/twin.11.5.538

Borbely, A. A., Daan, S., Wirz-Justice, A., & Deboer, T. (2016). The two-process model of sleep regulation: A reappraisal. *Journal of Sleep Research, 25*(2), 131–143. https://doi.org/10.1111/jsr.12371

Bourke, R., Anderson, V., Yang, J. S., Jackman, A. R., Killedar, A., Nixon, G. M., Davey, M. J., Walker, A. M., Trinder, J., & Horne, R. S. C. (2011). Cognitive and academic functions are impaired in children with all severities of sleep-disordered breathing. *Sleep Medicine, 12*(5), 489–496. https://doi.org/10.1016/j.sleep.2010.11.010

Brink-Kjaer, A., Leary, E. B., Sun, H., Westover, M. B., Stone, K. L., Peppard, P. E., Lane, N. E., Cawthon, P. M., Redline, S., Jennum, P., Sorensen, H. B. D., & Mignot, E. (2022). Age estimation from sleep studies using deep learning predicts life expectancy. *NPJ Digital Medicine, 5*(1), Article 103. https://doi.org/10.1038/s41746-022-00630-9

Bubu, O. M., Andrade, A. G., Umasabor-Bubu, O. Q., Hogan, M. M., Turner, A. D., de Leon, M. J., Ogedegbe, G., Ayappa, I., Jean-Louis, G., Jackson, M. L., Varga, A. W., & Osorio, R. S. (2020). Obstructive sleep apnea, cognition and Alzheimer's disease: A systematic review integrating three decades of multidisciplinary research. *Sleep Medicine Reviews, 50*, Article 101250. https://doi.org/10.1016/j.smrv.2019.101250

Bubu, O. M., Brannick, M., Mortimer, J., Umasabor-Bubu, O., Sebastiao, Y. V., Wen, Y., Schwartz, S., Borenstein, A. R., Wu, Y., Morgan, D., & Anderson, W. D. (2017). Sleep, cognitive impairment, and Alzheimer's disease: A systematic review and meta-analysis. *Sleep, 40*(1), Article zsw032. https://doi.org/10.1093/sleep/zsw032

Bubu, O. M., Kaur, S. S., Mbah, A. K., Umasabor-Bubu, O. Q., Cejudo, J. R., Debure, L., Mullins, A. E., Parekh, A., Kam, K., Osakwe, Z. T., Williams, E. T., Turner, A. D., Glodzik, L., Rapoport, D. M., Ogedegbe, G., Fieremans, E., de Leon, M. J., Ayappa, I., Jean-Louis, G., . . . Osorio, R. S. (2022). Obstructive sleep apnea and hypertension with longitudinal amyloid-beta burden and cognitive changes. *American Journal of Respiratory and Critical Care Medicine, 206*(5), 632–636. https://doi.org/10.1164/rccm.202201-0107LE

Bubu, O. M., Umasabor-Bubu, O. Q., Turner, A. D., Parekh, A., Mullins, A. E., Kam, K., Birckbichler, M. K., Mukhtar, F., Mbah, A. K., Williams, N. J., Rapoport, D. M., de Leon, M., Jean-Louis, G., Ayappa, I., Varga, A. W., Osorio, R. S., & Alzheimer's Disease Neuroimaging Initiative. (2021). Self-reported obstructive sleep apnea, amyloid and tau burden, and Alzheimer's disease time-dependent progression. *Alzheimer's & Dementia*, 17(2), 226–245. https://doi.org/10.1002/alz.12184

Buysse, D. J. (2014). Sleep health: Can we define it? Does it matter? *Sleep, 37*(1), 9–17. https://doi.org/10.5665/sleep.3298

Buysse, D. J., Reynolds, C. F., 3rd, Monk, T. H., Berman, S. R., & Kupfer, D. J. (1989). The Pittsburgh Sleep Quality Index: A new instrument for psychiatric practice and research. *Psychiatry Research, 28*(2), 193–213.

Buysse, D. J., Reynolds, C. F., 3rd, Monk, T. H., Hoch, C. C., Yeager, A. L., & Kupfer, D. J. (1991). Quantification of subjective sleep quality in healthy elderly men and women using the Pittsburgh Sleep Quality Index (PSQI). *Sleep, 14*(4), 331–338.

Cai, H., Liang, J., Liu, Z., Fang, L., Zheng, J., Xu, J., Chen, L., Sun, W., & Zhang, H. (2020). Causal effects of sleep traits on ischemic stroke and its subtypes: A Mendelian randomization study. *Nature and Science of Sleep, 12*, 783–790. https://doi.org/10.2147/NSS.S265946

Caraballo, C., Mahajan, S., Valero-Elizondo, J., Massey, D., Lu, Y., Roy, B., Riley, C., Annapureddy, A. R., Murugiah, K., Elumn, J., Nasir, K., Nunez-Smith, M., Forman, H. P., Jackson, C. L., Herrin, J., & Krumholz, H. M. (2022). Evaluation of temporal trends in racial and ethnic disparities in sleep duration among US adults, 2004–2018. *JAMA Network Open, 5*(4), Article e226385. https://doi.org/10.1001/jamanetworkopen.2022.6385

Cauley, J. A., Blackwell, T. L., Redline, S., Ensrud, K. E., Ancoli-Israel, S., Fink, H. A., Orwoll, E. S., & Stone, K. L. (2014). Hypoxia during sleep and the risk of falls and fractures in older men: The Osteoporotic Fractures in Men Sleep Study. *Journal of the American Geriatric Society, 62*(10), 1853–1859. https://doi.org/10.1111/jgs.13069

Centers for Disease Control and Prevention. (2012). Short sleep duration among workers—United States, 2010. *MMWR Morbidity and Mortality Weekly Report, 61*(16), 281–285.

Charest, J., & Grandner, M. A. (2020). Sleep and athletic performance: Impacts on physical performance, mental performance, injury risk and recovery, and mental health. *Sleep Medicine Clinics, 15*(1), 41–57. https://doi.org/10.1016/j.jsmc.2019.11.005

Chen, X., Wang, R., Zee, P., Lutsey, P. L., Javaheri, S., Alcantara, C., Jackson, C. L., Williams, M. A., & Redline, S. (2015). Racial/ethnic differences in sleep disturbances: The Multi-Ethnic Study of Atherosclerosis (MESA). *Sleep, 38*(6), 877–888. https://doi.org/10.5665/sleep.4732

Chen, Y., Tan, F., Wei, L., Li, X., Lyu, Z., Feng, X., Wen, Y., Guo, L., He, J., Dai, M., & Li, N. (2018). Sleep duration and the risk of cancer: A systematic review and meta-analysis including dose-response relationship. *BMC Cancer, 18*(1), Article 1149. https://doi.org/10.1186/s12885-018-5025-y

Cheng, M., He, H., Wang, D., Xu, L., Wang, B., Ho, K. M., & Chen, W. (2019). Shift work and ischaemic heart disease: Meta-analysis and dose-response relationship. *Occupational Medicine, 69*(3), 182–188. https://doi.org/10.1093/occmed/kqz020

Chennaoui, M., Sauvet, F., Drogou, C., Van Beers, P., Langrume, C., Guillard, M., Gourby, B., Bourrilhon, C., Florence, G., & Gomez-Merino, D. (2011). Effect of one night of sleep loss on changes in tumor necrosis factor alpha (TNF-alpha) levels in healthy men. *Cytokine, 56*(2), 318–324. https://doi.org/10.1016/j.cyto.2011.06.002

Cheong, A. J. Y., Tan, B. K. J., Teo, Y. H., Tan, N. K. W., Yap, D. W. T., Sia, C. H., Ong, T. H., Leow, L. C., See, A., & Toh, S. T. (2022). Obstructive sleep apnea and lung cancer: A systematic review and meta-analysis. *Annals of the American Thorac Society, 19*(3), 469–475. https://doi.org/10.1513/AnnalsATS.202108-960OC

Chepesiuk, R. (2009). Missing the dark: Health effects of light pollution. *Environmental Health Perspectives, 117*(1), A20–A27.

Chung, J., Goodman, M., Huang, T., Bertisch, S., & Redline, S. (2021). Multidimensional sleep health in a diverse, aging adult cohort: Concepts, advances, and implications for research and intervention. *Sleep Health, 7*(6), 699–707. https://doi.org/10.1016/j.sleh.2021.08.005

Clark, I., & Landolt, H. P. (2017). Coffee, caffeine, and sleep: A systematic review of epidemiological studies and randomized controlled trials. *Sleep Medicine Reviews, 31*, 70–78. https://doi.org/10.1016/j.smrv.2016.01.006

Czeisler, C. A., Wickwire, E. M., Barger, L. K., Dement, W. C., Gamble, K., Hartenbaum, N., Ohayon, M. M., Pelayo, R., Phillips, B., Strohl, K., Tefft, B., Rajaratnam, S. M. W., Malhotra, R., Whiton, K., & Hirshkowitz, M. (2016). Sleep-deprived motor vehicle operators are unfit to drive: A multidisciplinary expert consensus statement on drowsy driving. *Sleep Health, 2*(2), 94–99. https://doi.org/10.1016/j.sleh.2016.04.003

Dashti, H. S., Jones, S. E., Wood, A. R., Lane, J. M., van Hees, V. T., Wang, H., Rhodes, J. A., Song, Y., Patel, K., Anderson, S. G., Beaumont, R. N., Bechtold, D. A., Bowden, J., Cade, B. E., Garaulet, M., Kyle, S. D., Little, M. A., Loudon, A. S., Luik, A. I., . . . Saxena, R. (2019). Genome-wide association study identifies genetic loci for self-reported habitual sleep duration supported by accelerometer-derived estimates. *Nature Communications, 10*(1), Article 1100. https://doi.org/10.1038/s41467-019-08917-4

Davies, S. K., Ang, J. E., Revell, V. L., Holmes, B., Mann, A., Robertson, F. P., Cui, N., Middleton, B., Ackermann, K., Kayser, M., Thumser, A. E., Raynaud, F. I., & Skene, D. J. (2014). Effect of sleep deprivation on the human metabolome. *Proceedings of the National Academy of Sciences of the United States of America, 111*(29), 10761–10766. https://doi.org/10.1073/pnas.1402663111

Davis, K. F., Parker, K. P., & Montgomery, G. L. (2004). Sleep in infants and young children: Part one: Normal sleep. *Journal of Pediatric Health Care, 18*(2), 65–71. https://doi.org/10.1016/s0891-5245(03)00149-4

Dawson, D., & Reid, K. (1997). Fatigue, alcohol and performance impairment. *Nature, 388*(6639), Article 235. https://doi.org/10.1038/40775

de Almondes, K. M., Costa, M. V., Malloy-Diniz, L. F., & Diniz, B. S. (2016). Insomnia and risk of dementia in older adults: Systematic review and meta-analysis. *Journal of Psychiatric Research, 77*, 109–115. https://doi.org/10.1016/j.jpsychires.2016.02.021

Desantis, A. S., Diez Roux, A. V., Moore, K., Baron, K. G., Mujahid, M. S., & Nieto, F. J. (2013). Associations of neighborhood characteristics with sleep timing and quality: The Multi-Ethnic Study of Atherosclerosis. *Sleep, 36*(10), 1543–1551. https://doi.org/10.5665/sleep.3054

Dibner, C., Schibler, U., & Albrecht, U. (2010). The mammalian circadian timing system: Organization and coordination of central and peripheral clocks. *Annual Review of Physiology, 72*, 517–549. https://doi.org/10.1146/annurev-physiol-021909-135821

Diekelmann, S., & Born, J. (2010). The memory function of sleep. *Nature Reviews Neuroscience, 11*(2), 114–126. https://doi.org/10.1038/nrn2762

Dijk, D. J., Duffy, J. F., Riel, E., Shanahan, T. L., & Czeisler, C. A. (1999). Ageing and the circadian and homeostatic regulation of human sleep during forced desynchrony of rest, melatonin and temperature rhythms. *Journal of Physiology, 516*(Pt. 2), 611–627.

Dijk, D. J., Groeger, J. A., Stanley, N., & Deacon, S. (2010). Age-related reduction in daytime sleep propensity and nocturnal slow wave sleep. *Sleep*, *33*(2), 211–223.

Ding, G., Li, J., & Lian, Z. (2020). Both short and long sleep durations are associated with cognitive impairment among community-dwelling Chinese older adults. *Medicine*, *99*(13), Article e19667. https://doi.org/10.1097/MD.0000000000019667

Duncan, D. T., Kawachi, I., & Redline, S. (2019). *The social epidemiology of sleep*. Oxford University Press.

Durmer, J. S., & Dinges, D. F. (2005). Neurocognitive consequences of sleep deprivation. *Seminars in Neurology*, *25*(1), 117–129. https://doi.org/10.1055/s-2005-867080

Dzierzewski, J. M., Sabet, S. M., Ghose, S. M., Perez, E., Soto, P., Ravyts, S. G., & Dautovich, N. D. (2021). Lifestyle factors and sleep health across the lifespan. *International Journal of Environmental Research and Public Health*, *18*(12), Article 6626. https://doi.org/10.3390/ijerph18126626

Ebrahim, I. O., Shapiro, C. M., Williams, A. J., & Fenwick, P. B. (2013). Alcohol and sleep I: Effects on normal sleep. *Alcohol: Clinical and Experimental Research*, *37*(4), 539–549. https://doi.org/10.1111/acer.12006

Elkhatib Smidt, S. D., Hitt, T., Zemel, B. S., & Mitchell, J. A. (2021). Sex differences in childhood sleep and health implications. *Annals of Human Biology*, *48*(6), 474–484. https://doi.org/10.1080/03014460.2021.1998624

Fan, M., Sun, D., Zhou, T., Heianza, Y., Lv, J., Li, L., & Qi, L. (2020). Sleep patterns, genetic susceptibility, and incident cardiovascular disease: A prospective study of 385 292 UK biobank participants. *European Heart Journal*, *41*(11), 1182–1189. https://doi.org/10.1093/eurheartj/ehz849

Fan, R., Chen, V., Xie, Y., Yin, L., Kim, S., Albert, P. S., & Simons-Morton, B. (2015). A functional data analysis approach for circadian patterns of activity of teenage girls. *Journal of Circadian Rhythms*, *13*, Article 3. https://doi.org/10.5334/jcr.ac

Fatima, Y., Doi, S. A., & Mamun, A. A. (2016). Sleep quality and obesity in young subjects: A meta-analysis. *Obesity Reviews*, *17*(11), 1154–1166. https://doi.org/10.1111/obr.12444

Ferrie, J. E., Kivimaki, M., Akbaraly, T. N., Singh-Manoux, A., Miller, M. A., Gimeno, D., Kumari, M., Smith, G. D., & Shipley, M. J. (2013). Associations between change in sleep duration and inflammation: Findings on C-reactive protein and interleukin 6 in the Whitehall II Study. *American Journal of Epidemiology*, *178*(6), 956–961. https://doi.org/10.1093/aje/kwt072

Finkel, K. J., Searleman, A. C., Tymkew, H., Tanaka, C. Y., Saager, L., Safer-Zadeh, E., Bottros, M., Selvidge, J. A., Jacobsohn, E., Pulley, D., Duntley, S., Becker, C., & Avidan, M. S. (2009). Prevalence of undiagnosed obstructive sleep apnea among adult surgical patients in an academic medical center. *Sleep Medicine*, *10*(7), 753–758. https://doi.org/10.1016/j.sleep.2008.08.007

Fischer, D., Lombardi, D. A., Marucci-Wellman, H., & Roenneberg, T. (2017). Chronotypes in the US—Influence of age and sex. *PLOS ONE*, *12*(6), Article e0178782. https://doi.org/10.1371/journal.pone.0178782

Foldvary-Schaefer, N. R., & Waters, T. E. (2017). Sleep-disordered breathing. *Continuum*, *23*(4), 1093–1116. https://doi.org/10.1212/01.CON.0000522245.13784.f6

Foley, D. J., Monjan, A. A., Brown, S. L., Simonsick, E. M., Wallace, R. B., & Blazer, D. G. (1995). Sleep complaints among elderly persons: An epidemiologic study of three communities. *Sleep*, *18*(6), 425–432.

Foley, D. J., Vitiello, M. V., Bliwise, D. L., Ancoli-Israel, S., Monjan, A. A., & Walsh, J. K. (2007). Frequent napping is associated with excessive daytime sleepiness, depression, pain, and nocturia in older adults: Findings from the National Sleep Foundation "2003 Sleep in America" poll. *American Journal of Geriatric Psychiatry*, *15*(4), 344–350. https://doi.org/10.1097/01.JGP.0000249385.50101.67

Fritz, J., Huang, T., Depner, C. M., Zeleznik, O. A., Cespedes Feliciano, E. M., Li, W., Stone, K. L., Manson, J. E., Clish, C., Sofer, T., Schernhammer, E., Rexrode, K., Redline, S., Wright, K. P., Jr., & Vetter, C. (2023). Sleep duration, plasma metabolites, and obesity and diabetes: A metabolome-wide association study in US women. *Sleep*, *46*(1), Article zsac226. https://doi.org/10.1093/sleep/zsac226

Fritz, J., Phillips, A. J. K., Hunt, L. C., Imam, A., Reid, K. J., Perreira, K. M., Mossavar-Rahmani, Y., Daviglus, M. L., Sotres-Alvarez, D., Zee, P. S., Patel, S. R., & Vetter, C. (2021). Cross-sectional and prospective associations between sleep regularity and metabolic health in the Hispanic Community Health Study/Study of Latinos. *Sleep*, *44*(4), Article zsaa218. https://doi.org/10.1093/sleep/zsaa218

Full, K. M., Gallo, L. C., Malhotra, A., Bellettiere, J., Kerr, J., Arredondo, E., Stone, K. L., Zaslavsky, L., Lewis, C. E., Lin, X., & Lacrois, A. Z. (2020). Modeling the cardiometabolic benefits of sleep in older women: Exploring the 24-hour day. *Sleep*, *43*(1), Article zsz205. https://doi.org/10.1093/sleep/zsz205

Fuller-Rowell, T. E., Curtis, D. S., El-Sheikh, M., Chae, D. H., Boylan, J. M., & Ryff, C. D. (2016). Racial disparities in sleep: The role of neighborhood disadvantage. *Sleep Medicine, 27–28*, 1–8. https://doi.org/10.1016/j.sleep.2016.10.008

Furihata, R., Hall, M. H., Stone, K. L., Ancoli-Israel, S., Smagula, S. F., Cauley, J. A., Kaneita, Y., Uchiyama, M., & Buysse, D. J.; for the Study of Osteoporotic Fractures (SOF) Research Group. (2017). An aggregate measure of sleep health is associated with prevalent and incident clinically significant depression symptoms among community-dwelling older women. *Sleep, 40*(3), Article zsw075. https://doi.org/10.1093/sleep/zsw075

Galland, B. C., Taylor, B. J., Elder, D. E., & Herbison, P. (2012). Normal sleep patterns in infants and children: A systematic review of observational studies. *Sleep Medicine Reviews, 16*(3), 213–222. https://doi.org/10.1016/j.smrv.2011.06.001

Gao, B., Dwivedi, S., Milewski, M. D., & Cruz, A. I., Jr. (2019). Lack of sleep and sports injuries in adolescents: A systematic review and meta-analysis. *Journal of Pediatric Orthopaedics, 39*(5), e324–e33. https://doi.org/10.1097/BPO.0000000000001306

Garfield, V. (2021). Sleep duration: A review of genome-wide association studies (GWAS) in adults from 2007 to 2020. *Sleep Medicine Reviews, 56*, Article 101413. https://doi.org/10.1016/j.smrv.2020.101413

Gebara, M. A., Siripong, N., DiNapoli, E. A., Maree, R. D., Germain, A., Reynolds, C. F., Kasckow, J. W., Weiss, P. M., & Karp, J. F. (2018). Effect of insomnia treatments on depression: A systematic review and meta-analysis. *Depression and Anxiety, 35*(8), 717–731. https://doi.org/10.1002/da.22776

Gehrman, P. R., Ghorai, A., Goodman, M., McCluskey, R., Barilla, H., Almasy, L., Roenneberg, T., & Bucan, M. (2019). Twin-based heritability of actimetry traits. *Genes, Brain and Behavior, 18*(5), Article e12569. https://doi.org/10.1111/gbb.12569

Goldsmith, J., Zipunnikov, V., & Schrack, J. (2015). Generalized multilevel function-on-scalar regression and principal component analysis. *Biometrics, 71*(2), 344–353. https://doi.org/10.1111/biom.12278

Gottlieb, D. J., Hek, K., Chen, T. H., Watson, N. F., Eiriksdottir, G., Byrne, E. M., Cornelis, M., Warby, S. C., Bandinelli, S., Cherkas, L., Evans, D. S., Grabe, H. J., Lahti, J., Li, M., Lehtimäki, T., Lumley, T., Marciante, K. D., Pérusse, L., Psaty, B. M., . . . Tiemeier, H. (2015). Novel loci associated with usual sleep duration: The CHARGE Consortium genome-wide association study. *Molecular Psychiatry, 20*(10), 1232–1239. https://doi.org/10.1038/mp.2014.133

Gottlieb, D. J., Yenokyan, G., Newman, A. B., O'Connor, G. T., Punjabi, N. M., Quan, S. F., Redline, S., Resnick, H. E., Tong, E. K., Diener-West, M., & Shahar, E. (2010). Prospective study of obstructive sleep apnea and incident coronary heart disease and heart failure: The Sleep Heart Health Study. *Circulation, 122*(4), 352–360. https://doi.org/10.1161/CIRCULATIONAHA.109.901801

Grandner, M. A. (2017). Sleep, health, and society. *Sleep Medicine Clinics, 12*(1), 1–22. https://doi.org/10.1016/j.jsmc.2016.10.012

Grandner, M. A., Williams, N. J., Knutson, K. L., Roberts, D., & Jean-Louis, G. (2016). Sleep disparity, race/ethnicity, and socioeconomic position. *Sleep Medicine, 18*, 7–18. https://doi.org/10.1016/j.sleep.2015.01.020

Guidozzi, F. (2015). Gender differences in sleep in older men and women. *Climacteric, 18*(5), 715–721. https://doi.org/10.3109/13697137.2015.1042451

Hagenauer, M. H., & Lee, T. M. (2012). The neuroendocrine control of the circadian system: Adolescent chronotype. *Frontiers in Neuroendocrinology, 33*(3), 211–229. https://doi.org/10.1016/j.yfrne.2012.04.003

Hale, L., Hill, T. D., & Burdette, A. M. (2010). Does sleep quality mediate the association between neighborhood disorder and self-rated physical health? *Preventive Medicine, 51*(3–4), 275–278. https://doi.org/10.1016/j.ypmed.2010.06.017

Hale, L., Hill, T. D., Friedman, E., Nieto, F. J., Galvao, L. W., Engelman, C. D., Malecki, K. M. C., & Peppard, P. E. (2013). Perceived neighborhood quality, sleep quality, and health status: Evidence from the Survey of the Health of Wisconsin. *Social Science & Medicine, 79*, 16–22. https://doi.org/10.1016/j.socscimed.2012.07.021

Hansen, J. (2017). Night shift work and risk of breast cancer. *Current Environmental Health Reports, 4*(3), 325–339. https://doi.org/10.1007/s40572-017-0155-y

Heath, A. C., Kendler, K. S., Eaves, L. J., & Martin, N. G. (1990). Evidence for genetic influences on sleep disturbance and sleep pattern in twins. *Sleep, 13*(4), 318–335. https://doi.org/10.1093/sleep/13.4.318

Heckler, B., Lee, M., Stone, K., Bauer, C., & Xiao, Q. (2023). Cross-sectional and prospective associations of rest–activity rhythms with body mass index in older men: A novel analysis using harmonic hidden Markov models. *Journal of Biological Rhythms, 38*(1), 87–97. https://doi.org/10.1177/07487304221134163

Higgins, J. S., Michael, J., Austin, R., Akerstedt, T., Van Dongen, H. P., Watson, N., Czeisler, C., Pack, A. I., & Rosekind, M. R. (2017). Asleep at the wheel—The road to addressing drowsy driving. *Sleep*, *40*(2), Article zsx001. https://doi.org/10.1093/sleep/zsx001

Hill, S. M., Belancio, V. P., Dauchy, R. T., Xiang, S., Brimer, S., Mao, L., Hauch, A., Lundberg, P. W., Summers, W., Yuan, L., Frasch, T., & Blask, D. E. (2015). Melatonin: An inhibitor of breast cancer. *Endocrine-Related Cancer*, *22*(3), R183–R204. https://doi.org/10.1530/ERC-15-0030

Hill, T. D., Burdette, A. M., & Hale, L. (2009). Neighborhood disorder, sleep quality, and psychological distress: Testing a model of structural amplification. *Health & Place*, *15*(4), 1006–1013. https://doi.org/10.1016/j.healthplace.2009.04.001

Hill, T. D., Trinh, H. N., Wen, M., & Hale, L. (2016). Perceived neighborhood safety and sleep quality: A global analysis of six countries. *Sleep Medicine*, *18*, 56–60. https://doi.org/10.1016/j.sleep.2014.12.003

Hofman, A., Voortman, T., Ikram, M. A., & Luik, A. I. (2022). Time spent in physical activity, sedentary behavior, and sleep: Associations with self-rated sleep quality in middle-aged and older adults. *Sleep Health*, *8*(6), 701–704. https://doi.org/10.1016/j.sleh.2022.06.009

Hood, S., & Amir, S. (2017). The aging clock: Circadian rhythms and later life. *Journal of Clinical Investigation*, *127*(2), 437–446. https://doi.org/10.1172/JCI90328

Howard, S. K., Rosekind, M. R., Katz, J. D., & Berry, A. J. (2002). Fatigue in anesthesia: Implications and strategies for patient and provider safety. *Anesthesiology*, *97*(5), 1281–1294. https://doi.org/10.1097/00000542-200211000-00035

Hua, J., Zhuang, S., Shen, Y., Tang, X., Sun, H., & Fang, Q. (2021). Exploring the bidirectional associations between short or long sleep duration and lower cognitive function: A 7-year cohort study in China. *Frontiers in Aging Neuroscience*, *13*, Article 727763. https://doi.org/10.3389/fnagi.2021.727763

Huang, T., Zeleznik, O. A., Poole, E. M., Clish, C. B., Deik, A. A., Scott, J. M., Vetter, C., Schernhammer, E. S., Brunner, R., Hale, L., Manson, J. E., Hu, H. B., Redline, S., Tworoger, S. S., & Rexrode, K. M. (2019). Habitual sleep quality, plasma metabolites and risk of coronary heart disease in postmenopausal women. *International Journal of Epidemiology*, *48*(4), 1262–1274. https://doi.org/10.1093/ije/dyy234

International League Against Epilepsy Consortium on Complex Epilepsies. (2014). Genetic determinants of common epilepsies: A meta-analysis of genome-wide association studies. *Lancet Neurology*, *13*(9), 893–903. https://doi.org/10.1016/S1474-4422(14)70171-1

Irwin, M. R. (2019). Sleep and inflammation: Partners in sickness and in health. *Nature Reviews Immunology*, *19*(11), 702–715. https://doi.org/10.1038/s41577-019-0190-z

Irwin, M. R., Olmstead, R., & Carroll, J. E. (2016). Sleep disturbance, sleep duration, and inflammation: A systematic review and meta-analysis of cohort studies and experimental sleep deprivation. *Biological Psychiatry*, *80*(1), 40–52. https://doi.org/10.1016/j.biopsych.2015.05.014

Itani, O., Jike, M., Watanabe, N., & Kaneita, Y. (2017). Short sleep duration and health outcomes: A systematic review, meta-analysis, and meta-regression. *Sleep Medicine*, *32*, 246–256. https://doi.org/10.1016/j.sleep.2016.08.006

Jaehne, A., Loessl, B., Barkai, Z., Riemann, D., & Hornyak, M. (2009). Effects of nicotine on sleep during consumption, withdrawal and replacement therapy. *Sleep Medicine Reviews*, *13*(5), 363–377. https://doi.org/10.1016/j.smrv.2008.12.003

Jaussent, I., Bouyer, J., Ancelin, M. L., Akbaraly, T., Peres, K., Ritchie, K., Besset, A., & Dauvilliers, Y. (2011). Insomnia and daytime sleepiness are risk factors for depressive symptoms in the elderly. *Sleep*, *34*(8), 1103–1110. https://doi.org/10.5665/SLEEP.1170

Jike, M., Itani, O., Watanabe, N., Buysse, D. J., & Kaneita, Y. (2018). Long sleep duration and health outcomes: A systematic review, meta-analysis and meta-regression. *Sleep Medicine Reviews*, *39*, 25–36. https://doi.org/10.1016/j.smrv.2017.06.011

Johns, M. W. (1991). A new method for measuring daytime sleepiness: The Epworth Sleepiness Scale. *Sleep*, *14*(6), 540–545.

Johnson, D. A., Lisabeth, L., Hickson, D., Johnson-Lawrence, V., Samdarshi, T., Taylor, H., & Diez Roux, A. V. (2016). The social patterning of sleep in African Americans: Associations of socioeconomic position and neighborhood characteristics with sleep in the Jackson Heart Study. *Sleep*, *39*(9), 1749–1759. https://doi.org/10.5665/sleep.6106

Johnson, D. A., Simonelli, G., Moore, K., Billings, M., Mujahid, M. S., Rueschman, M., Kawachi, I., Redline, S., Diez Roux, A. V., & Patel, S. R. (2017). The neighborhood social environment and objective measures of sleep in the multi-ethnic study of atherosclerosis. *Sleep, 40*(1), Article zsw016. https://doi.org/10.1093/sleep/zsw016

Johnson, D. A., Thorpe, R. J., McGrath, J. A., Jackson, W. B., & Jackson, C. L. (2018). Black–White differences in housing type and sleep duration as well as sleep difficulties in the United States. *International Journal of Environmental Research and Public Health, 15*(4), Article 564. https://doi.org/10.3390/ijerph15040564

Jonasdottir, S. S., Minor, K., & Lehmann, S. (2021). Gender differences in nighttime sleep patterns and variability across the adult lifespan: A global-scale wearables study. *Sleep, 44*(2), Article zsaa169. https://doi.org/10.1093/sleep/zsaa169

Jones, S. E., Lane, J. M., Wood, A. R., van Hees, V. T., Tyrrell, J., Beaumont, R. N., Jeffries, A. R., Dashti, H. S., Hillsdon, M., Ruth, K. S., Tuke, M. A., Yaghootkar, H., Sharp, S. A., Jie, Y., Thompson, W. D., Harrison, J. W., Dawes, A., Byrne, E. M., Tiemeier, H., . . . Weedon, M. N. (2019). Genome-wide association analyses of chronotype in 697,828 individuals provides insights into circadian rhythms. *Nature Communications, 10*(1), Article 343. https://doi.org/10.1038/s41467-018-08259-7

Jones, S. E., Tyrrell, J., Wood, A. R., Beaumont, R. N., Ruth, K. S., Tuke, M. A., Yaghootkar, H., Hu, Y., Teder-Laving, M., Hayward, C., Roenneberg, T., Wilson, J. F., Del Greco, F., Hicks, A. A., Shin, C., Yun, C.-H., Lee, S. K., Metspalu, A., Byrne, E. M., . . . Weedon, M. N. (2016). Genome-wide association analyses in 128,266 individuals identifies new morningness and sleep duration loci. *PLOS Genetics, 12*(8), Article e1006125. https://doi.org/10.1371/journal.pgen.1006125

Kapur, V., Strohl, K. P., Redline, S., Iber, C., O'Connor, G., & Nieto, J. (2002). Underdiagnosis of sleep apnea syndrome in U.S. communities. *Sleep and Breathing, 6*(2), 49–54. https://doi.org/10.1007/s11325-002-0049-5

Kerr, J., Carlson, J., Godbole, S., Cadmus-Bertram, L., Bellettiere, J., & Hartman, S. (2018). Improving hip-worn accelerometer estimates of sitting using machine learning methods. *Medicine & Science in Sports & Exercise, 50*(7), 1518–1524. https://doi.org/10.1249/MSS.0000000000001578

Kessler, R. C., & Walters, E. E. (1998). Epidemiology of DSM-III-R major depression and minor depression among adolescents and young adults in the National Comorbidity Survey. *Depression and Anxiety, 7*(1), 3–14. https://doi.org/10.1002/(sici)1520-6394(1998)7:1<3::aid-da2>3.0.co;2-f

Kleinbaum, D. G., Kupper, L. L., & Morganstern, H. (1982). Key issues in epidemiologic research: An overview. In *Epidemiologic research: Principles and quantitative methods* (pp. 2–15). Van Nostrand Reinhold.

Kline, C. E., Hillman, C. H., Bloodgood Sheppard, B., Tennant, B., Conroy, D. E., Macko, R. F., Marquez, D. X., Petruzzello, S. J., Powell, K. E., & Erickson, K. I. (2021). Physical activity and sleep: An updated umbrella review of the 2018 Physical Activity Guidelines Advisory Committee report. *Sleep Medicine Reviews, 58*, Article 101489. https://doi.org/10.1016/j.smrv.2021.101489

Knutson, K. L., & von Schantz, M. (2018). Associations between chronotype, morbidity and mortality in the UK Biobank cohort. *Chronobiology International, 35*(8), 1045–1053. https://doi.org/10.1080/07420528.2018.1454458

Kobayashi Frisk, M., Hedner, J., Grote, L., Ekblom, O., Arvidsson, D., Bergstrom, G., Borjesson, M., & Zou, D. (2022). Eveningness is associated with sedentary behavior and increased 10-year risk of cardiovascular disease: The SCAPIS pilot cohort. *Scientific Reports, 12*(1), Article 8203. https://doi.org/10.1038/s41598-022-12267-5

Kothari, V., Cardona, Z., Chirakalwasan, N., Anothaisintawee, T., & Reutrakul, S. (2021). Sleep interventions and glucose metabolism: Systematic review and meta-analysis. *Sleep Medicine, 78*, 24–35. https://doi.org/10.1016/j.sleep.2020.11.035

Kryger, M. H., Roth, T., & Dement, W. C. (2010). *Principles and practice of sleep medicine.* Elsevier Health Sciences.

Kuo, C. Y., Hsiao, H. T., Lo, I. H., & Nikolai, T. (2020). Association between obstructive sleep apnea, its treatment, and Alzheimer's disease: Systematic mini-review. *Frontiers in Aging Neuroscience, 12*, Article 591737. https://doi.org/10.3389/fnagi.2020.591737

Kwok, C. S., Kontopantelis, E., Kuligowski, G., Gray, M., Muhyaldeen, A., Gale, C. P., Peat, G. M., Cleator, J., Chew-Graham, C., Loke, Y. K., & Mamas, M. A. (2018). Self-reported sleep duration and quality and cardiovascular disease and mortality: A dose–response meta-analysis. *Journal of the American Heart Association, 7*(15), Article e008552. https://doi.org/10.1161/JAHA.118.008552

Lam, A., Haroutonian, C., Grummitt, L., Ireland, C., Grunstein, R. R., Duffy, S., D'Rozario, A., & Naismith, S. L. (2021). Sleep-dependent memory in older people with and without MCI: The relevance of sleep microarchitecture, OSA, hippocampal subfields, and episodic memory. *Cerebral Cortex, 31*(6), 2993–3005. https://doi.org/10.1093/cercor/bhaa406

Lam, L. T., & Lam, M. K. (2021). Sleep disorders in early childhood and the development of mental health problems in adolescents: A systematic review of longitudinal and prospective studies. *International Journal of Environmental Research and Public Health, 18*(22), Article 11782. https://doi.org/10.3390/ijerph182211782

Lane, J. M., Liang, J., Vlasac, I., Anderson, S. G., Bechtold, D. A., Bowden, J., Emsley, R., Gill, S., Little, M. A., Luik, A. I., Loudon, A., Scheer, F. A. J. L., Purcell, S. M., Kyle, S. D., Lawlor, D. A., Zhu, X., Redline, S., Ray, D. W., Rutter, M. K., & Saxena, R. (2017). Genome-wide association analyses of sleep disturbance traits identify new loci and highlight shared genetics with neuropsychiatric and metabolic traits. *Nature Genetics, 49*(2), 274–281. https://doi.org/10.1038/ng.3749

Larson, J. S. (1999). The conceptualization of health. *Medical Care Research and Review, 56*(2), 123–136. https://doi.org/10.1177/107755879905600201

Lee, S., Mu, C. X., Wallace, M. L., Andel, R., Almeida, D. M., Buxton, O. M., & Patel, S. R. (2022). Sleep health composites are associated with the risk of heart disease across sex and race. *Scientific Reports, 12*(1), Article 2023. https://doi.org/10.1038/s41598-022-05203-0

Lee, S. W. H., Ng, K. Y., & Chin, W. K. (2017). The impact of sleep amount and sleep quality on glycemic control in Type 2 diabetes: A systematic review and meta-analysis. *Sleep Medicine Reviews, 31*, 91–101. https://doi.org/10.1016/j.smrv.2016.02.001

Leproult, R., Holmback, U., & Van Cauter, E. (2014). Circadian misalignment augments markers of insulin resistance and inflammation, independently of sleep loss. *Diabetes, 63*(6), 1860–1869. https://doi.org/10.2337/db13-1546

Li, J., Somers, V. K., Lopez-Jimenez, F., Di, J., & Covassin, N. (2021). Demographic characteristics associated with circadian rest–activity rhythm patterns: A cross-sectional study. *International Journal of Behavioral Nutrition and Physical Activity, 18*(1), Article 107. https://doi.org/10.1186/s12966-021-01174-z

Li, W., Chen, Z., Ruan, W., Yi, G., Wang, D., & Lu, Z. (2019). A meta-analysis of cohort studies including dose–response relationship between shift work and the risk of diabetes mellitus. *European Journal of Epidemiology, 34*(11), 1013–1024. https://doi.org/10.1007/s10654-019-00561-y

Li, Y., Cai, S., Ling, Y., Mi, S., Fan, C., Zhong, Y., & Shen, Q. (2019). Association between total sleep time and all cancer mortality: Non-linear dose-response meta-analysis of cohort studies. *Sleep Medicine, 60*, 211–218. https://doi.org/10.1016/j.sleep.2019.03.026

Lian, Y., Yuan, Q., Wang, G., & Tang, F. (2019). Association between sleep quality and metabolic syndrome: A systematic review and meta-analysis. *Psychiatry Research, 274*, 66–74. https://doi.org/10.1016/j.psychres.2019.01.096

Liu, J., Richmond, R. C., Anderson, E. L., Bowden, J., Barry, C.-J. S., Dashti, H. S., Daghlas, I. S., Lane, J. M., Kyle, S. D., Vetter, C., Morrison, C. L., Jones, S. E., Wood, A. R., Frayling, T. M., Wright, A. K., Carr, M. J., Anderson, S. G., Emsley, R. A., Ray, D. W., . . . Lawlor, D. A. (2022). The role of accelerometer-derived sleep traits on glycated haemoglobin: A Mendelian randomization study. *Scientific Reports, 14*, Article 14962.

Liu, Y., Wheaton, A. G., Chapman, D. P., Cunningham, T. J., Lu, H., & Croft, J. B. (2016). Prevalence of healthy sleep duration among adults—United States, 2014. *MMWR Morbidity and Mortality Weekly Report, 65*(6), 137–141. https://doi.org/10.15585/mmwr.mm6506a1

Lowrie, J., & Brownlow, H. (2020). The impact of sleep deprivation and alcohol on driving: A comparative study. *BMC Public Health, 20*(1), Article 980. https://doi.org/10.1186/s12889-020-09095-5

Luckhaupt, S. E., Tak, S., & Calvert, G. M. (2010). The prevalence of short sleep duration by industry and occupation in the National Health Interview Survey. *Sleep, 33*(2), 149–159. https://doi.org/10.1093/sleep/33.2.149

Luik, A. I., Zuurbier, L. A., Hofman, A., Van Someren, E. J., & Tiemeier, H. (2013). Stability and fragmentation of the activity rhythm across the sleep–wake cycle: The importance of age, lifestyle, and mental health. *Chronobiology International, 30*(10), 1223–1230. https://doi.org/10.3109/07420528.2013.813528

Lunsford-Avery, J. R., Keller, C., Kollins, S. H., Krystal, A. D., Jackson, L., & Engelhard, M. M. (2020). Feasibility and acceptability of wearable sleep electroencephalogram device use in adolescents: Observational study. *JMIR mHealth uHealth, 8*(10), Article e20590. https://doi.org/10.2196/20590

Luo, L., Buxton, O. M., Gamaldo, A. A., Almeida, D. M., & Xiao, Q. (2021). Opposite educational gradients in sleep duration between Black and White adults, 2004–2018. *Sleep Health, 7*(1), 3–9. https://doi.org/10.1016/j.sleh.2020.10.003

Maglione, J. E., Ancoli-Israel, S., Peters, K. W., Paudel, M. L., Yaffe, K., Ensrud, K. E., & Stone, K. L. (2014). Subjective and objective sleep disturbance and longitudinal risk of depression in a cohort of older women. *Sleep, 37*(7), 1179–1187. https://doi.org/10.5665/sleep.3834

Mai, Q. D., Hill, T. D., Vila-Henninger, L., & Grandner, M. A. (2019). Employment insecurity and sleep disturbance: Evidence from 31 European countries. *Journal of Sleep Research, 28*(1), Article e12763. https://doi.org/10.1111/jsr.12763

Mander, B. A., Marks, S. M., Vogel, J. W., Rao, V., Lu, B., Saletin, J. M., Ancoli-Israel, S., Jagust, W. J., & Walker, M. P. (2015). β-Amyloid disrupts human NREM slow waves and related hippocampus-dependent memory consolidation. *Nature Neuroscience, 18*(7), 1051–1057. https://doi.org/10.1038/nn.4035

Mander, B. A., Winer, J. R., & Walker, M. P. (2017). Sleep and human aging. *Neuron, 94*(1), 19–36. https://doi.org/10.1016/j.neuron.2017.02.004

Manouchehri, E., Taghipour, A., Ghavami, V., Ebadi, A., Homaei, F., & Latifnejad Roudsari, R. (2021). Night-shift work duration and breast cancer risk: An updated systematic review and meta-analysis. *BMC Womens Health, 21*(1), Article 89. https://doi.org/10.1186/s12905-021-01233-4

Marino, C., Andrade, B., Montplaisir, J., Petit, D., Touchette, E., Paradis, H., Côté, S. M., Tremblay, R. E., Szatmari, P., & Boivin, M. (2022). Testing bidirectional, longitudinal associations between disturbed sleep and depressive symptoms in children and adolescents using cross-lagged models. *JAMA Network Open, 5*(8), Article e2227119. https://doi.org/10.1001/jamanetworkopen.2022.27119

Marler, M. R., Gehrman, P., Martin, J. L., & Ancoli-Israel, S. (2006). The sigmoidally transformed cosine curve: A mathematical model for circadian rhythms with symmetric non-sinusoidal shapes. *Statistics in Medicine, 25*(22), 3893–3904. https://doi.org/10.1002/sim.2466

Mason, G. M., Lokhandwala, S., Riggins, T., & Spencer, R. M. C. (2021). Sleep and human cognitive development. *Sleep Medicine Reviews, 57*, Article 101472. https://doi.org/10.1016/j.smrv.2021.101472

Matthews, K. A., Hall, M., & Dahl, R. E. (2014). Sleep in healthy Black and White adolescents. *Pediatrics, 133*(5), e1189–e1196. https://doi.org/10.1542/peds.2013-2399

McHill, A. W., Phillips, A. J., Czeisler, C. A., Keating, L., Yee, K., Barger, L. K., Garaulet, M., Scheer, F. A. J. L., & Klerman, E. B. (2017). Later circadian timing of food intake is associated with increased body fat. *American Journal of Clinical Nutrition, 106*(5), 1213–1219. https://doi.org/10.3945/ajcn.117.161588

Mehra, R., Stone, K. L., Blackwell, T., Ancoli Israel, S., Dam, T. T., Stefanick, M. L., & Redline, S.; for the Osteoporotic Fractures in Men Study. (2007). Prevalence and correlates of sleep-disordered breathing in older men: Osteoporotic fractures in men sleep study. *Journal of the American Geriatric Society, 55*(9), 1356–1364. https://doi.org/10.1111/j.1532-5415.2007.01290.x

Miller, M. A., Kandala, N. B., Kivimaki, M., Kumari, M., Brunner, E. J., Lowe, G. D., Marmot, M. G., & Cappuccio, F. P. (2009). Gender differences in the cross-sectional relationships between sleep duration and markers of inflammation: Whitehall II study. *Sleep, 32*(7), 857–864.

Miller, M. A., Wright, H., Ji, C., & Cappuccio, F. P. (2014). Cross-sectional study of sleep quantity and quality and amnestic and non-amnestic cognitive function in an ageing population: The English Longitudinal Study of Ageing (ELSA). *PLOS ONE, 9*(6), Article e100991. https://doi.org/10.1371/journal.pone.0100991

Mitchell, J. A., Morales, K. H., Williamson, A. A., Huffnagle, N., Ludwick, A., Grant, S. F. A., Dinges, D. F., & Zemel, B. A. (2020). Changes in sleep duration and timing during the middle-to-high school transition. *Journal of Adolescent Health, 67*(6), 829–836. https://doi.org/10.1016/j.jadohealth.2020.04.024

Mogavero, M. P., DelRosso, L. M., Fanfulla, F., Bruni, O., & Ferri, R. (2021). Sleep disorders and cancer: State of the art and future perspectives. *Sleep Medicine Reviews, 56*, Article 101409. https://doi.org/10.1016/j.smrv.2020.101409

Morin, C. M., Colecchi, C., Stone, J., Sood, R., & Brink, D. (1999). Behavioral and pharmacological therapies for late-life insomnia: A randomized controlled trial. *JAMA, 281*(11), 991–999.

Morris, C. J., Purvis, T. E., Hu, K., & Scheer, F. A. (2016). Circadian misalignment increases cardiovascular disease risk factors in humans. *Proceedings of the National Academy of Sciences of the United States of America, 113*(10), E1402–E1411. https://doi.org/10.1073/pnas.1516953113

Morris, C. J., Purvis, T. E., Mistretta, J., Hu, K., & Scheer, F. (2017). Circadian misalignment increases C-reactive protein and blood pressure in chronic shift workers. *Journal of Biological Rhythms, 32*(2), 154–164. https://doi.org/10.1177/0748730417697537

Muzet, A. (2007). Environmental noise, sleep and health. *Sleep Medicine Reviews, 11*(2), 135–142. https://doi.org/10.1016/j.smrv.2006.09.001

National Institutes of Health. (2005). National Institutes of Health state of the science conference statement: Manifestations and management of chronic insomnia in adults, June 13–15, 2005. *Sleep, 28*(9), 1049–1057. https://doi.org/10.1093/sleep/28.9.1049

Netzer, N. C., Stoohs, R. A., Netzer, C. M., Clark, K., & Strohl, K. P. (1999). Using the Berlin Questionnaire to identify patients at risk for the sleep apnea syndrome. *Annals of Internal Medicine, 131*(7), 485–491. https://doi.org/10.7326/0003-4819-131-7-199910050-00002

Nyarko, S. H., Luo, L., Schlundt, D. G., & Xiao, Q. (2023). Individual and neighborhood socioeconomic status and long-term individual trajectories of sleep duration among Black and White adults: The Southern Community Cohort Study. *Sleep, 46*(1), Article zsac225. https://doi.org/10.1093/sleep/zsac225

Ohayon, M. M., Carskadon, M. A., Guilleminault, C., & Vitiello, M. V. (2004). Meta-analysis of quantitative sleep parameters from childhood to old age in healthy individuals: Developing normative sleep values across the human lifespan. *Sleep, 27*(7), 1255–1273.

Ohayon, M., Wickwire, E. M., Hirshkowitz, M., Albert, S. M., Avidan, A., Daly, F. J., Dauvilliers, Y., Ferri, R., Fung, C., Gozal, D., Hazen, N., Krystal, A., Lichstein, K., Mallampalli, M., Plazzi, G., Rawding, R., Scheer, F. A., Somers, V., & Vitiello, M. V. (2017). National Sleep Foundation's sleep quality recommendations: Dirst report. *Sleep Health, 3*(1), 6–19. https://doi.org/10.1016/j.sleh.2016.11.006

Otsuka, Y., Takeshima, O., Itani, O., Matsumoto, Y., & Kaneita, Y. (2022). Associations among alcohol drinking, smoking, and nonrestorative sleep: A population-based study in Japan. *Clocks & Sleep, 4*(4), 595–606. https://doi.org/10.3390/clockssleep4040046

Park, S. Y., Oh, M. K., Lee, B. S., Kim, H. G., Lee, W. J., Lee, J. H., Lim, J.-T., & Kim, J.-Y. (2015). The effects of alcohol on quality of sleep. *Korean Journal of Family Medicine, 36*(6), 294–299. https://doi.org/10.4082/kjfm.2015.36.6.294

Parsey, C. M., & Schmitter-Edgecombe, M. (2019). Using actigraphy to predict the ecological momentary assessment of mood, fatigue, and cognition in older adulthood: mixed-methods study. *JMIR Aging, 2*(1), Article e11331. https://doi.org/10.2196/11331

Partinen, M., Kaprio, J., Koskenvuo, M., Putkonen, P., & Langinvainio, H. (1983). Genetic and environmental determination of human sleep. *Sleep, 6*(3), 179–185. https://doi.org/10.1093/sleep/6.3.179

Paruthi, S., Brooks, L. J., D'Ambrosio, C., Hall, W. A., Kotagal, S., Lloyd, R. M., Malow, B. A., Maski, K., Nichols, C., Quan, S. F., Rosen, C. L., Troester, M. M., & Wise, M. S. (2016). Recommended amount of sleep for pediatric populations: A consensus statement of the American Academy of Sleep Medicine. *Journal of Clinical Sleep Medicine, 12*(6), 785–786. https://doi.org/10.5664/jcsm.5866

Patel, D., Steinberg, J., & Patel, P. (2018). Insomnia in the elderly: A review. *Journal of Clinical Sleep Medicine, 14*(6), 1017–1024. https://doi.org/10.5664/jcsm.7172

Paudel, M. L., Taylor, B. C., Ancoli-Israel, S., Blackwell, T., Stone, K. L., Tranah, G., Redline, S., Cummings, S. R., & Ensrud, K. E.; for the Osteoporotic Fractures in Men (MrOS) Study Group. (2010). Rest/activity rhythms and mortality rates in older men: MrOS Sleep Study. *Chronobiology International, 27*(2), 363–377. https://doi.org/10.3109/07420520903419157

Peeri, N. C., Tao, M. H., Demissie, S., & Nguyen, U. D. T. (2022). Sleep duration, chronotype, and insomnia and the risk of lung cancer: United Kingdom Biobank cohort. *Cancer Epidemiology, Biomarkers & Prevention, 31*(4), 766–774. https://doi.org/10.1158/1055-9965.EPI-21-1093

Pengo, M. F., Won, C. H., & Bourjeily, G. (2018). Sleep in women across the life span. *Chest, 154*(1), 196–206. https://doi.org/10.1016/j.chest.2018.04.005

Posner, A. B., Tranah, G. J., Blackwell, T., Yaffe, K., Ancoli-Israel, S., Redline, S., Leng, Y., Zeitzer, J. M., Chen, D. M., Webber, K. R., & Stone, K. L. (2021). Predicting incident dementia and mild cognitive impairment in older women with nonparametric analysis of circadian activity rhythms in the Study of Osteoporotic Fractures. *Sleep, 44*(10), Article zsab119. https://doi.org/10.1093/sleep/zsab119

Puttonen, S., Viitasalo, K., & Harma, M. (2011). Effect of shiftwork on systemic markers of inflammation. *Chronobiology International, 28*(6), 528–535. https://doi.org/10.3109/07420528.2011.580869

Quan, S. F., Howard, B. V., Iber, C., Kiley, J. P., Nieto, F. J., O'Connor, G. T., Rapoport, D. M., Redline, S., Robbins, J., Samet, J. M., & Wahl, P. W. (1997). The Sleep Heart Health Study: Design, rationale, and methods. *Sleep, 20*(12), 1077–1085.

Quan, S. F., Landrigan, C. P., Barger, L. K., Buie, J. D., Dominguez, C., Iyer, J. M., Majekodunmi, A., Papautsky, E. L., Robbins, R., Shen, B. H., Stephens, J. T., Weaver, M. D., & Czeisler, C. A. (2023). Impact of sleep deficiency on surgical performance: A prospective assessment. *Journal of Clinical Sleep Medicine, 19*(4), 673–683. https://doi.org/10.5664/jcsm.10406

Raikes, A. C., Athey, A., Alfonso-Miller, P., Killgore, W. D. S., & Grandner, M. A. (2019). Insomnia and daytime sleepiness: Risk factors for sports-related concussion. *Sleep Medicine, 58*, 66–74. https://doi.org/10.1016/j.sleep.2019.03.008

Redline, S., Yenokyan, G., Gottlieb, D. J., Shahar, E., O'Connor, G. T., Resnick, H. E., Diener-West, M., Sanders, M. H., Wolf, P. A., Geraghty, E. M., Ali, T., Lebowitz, M., & Punjabi, N. M. (2010). Obstructive sleep apnea-hypopnea and incident stroke: The Sleep Heart Health Study. *American Journal of Respiratory and Critical Care Medicine, 182*(2), 269–277. https://doi.org/10.1164/rccm.200911-1746OC

Richmond, R. C., Anderson, E. L., Dashti, H. S., Jones, S. E., Lane, J. M., Strand, L. B., Brumpton, B., Rutter, M. K., Wood, A. R., Straif, K., Relton, C. L., Munafo, M., Frayling, T. M., Martin, R. M., Saxena, R., Weedon, M. N., Lawlor, D. A., & Smith, G. D. (2019). Investigating causal relations between sleep traits and risk of breast cancer in women: Mendelian randomisation study. *BMJ, 365*, Article l2327. https://doi.org/10.1136/bmj.l2327

Robbins, J., & Gottlieb, F. (1990). Sleep deprivation and cognitive testing in internal medicine house staff. *West Journal of Medicine, 152*(1), 82–86.

Roehrs, T., Burduvali, E., Bonahoom, A., Drake, C., & Roth, T. (2003). Ethanol and sleep loss: A "dose" comparison of impairing effects. *Sleep, 26*(8), 981–985. https://doi.org/10.1093/sleep/26.8.981

Roehrs, T., & Roth, T. (2001). Sleep, sleepiness, and alcohol use. *Alcohol Research & Health, 25*(2), 101–109.

Roenneberg, T., Kuehnle, T., Juda, M., Kantermann, T., Allebrandt, K., Gordijn, M., & Merrow, M. (2007). Epidemiology of the human circadian clock. *Sleep Medicine Reviews, 11*(6), 429–438. https://doi.org/10.1016/j.smrv.2007.07.005

Rogers, T. S., Blackwell, T. L., Lane, N. E., Tranah, G., Orwoll, E. S., Cauley, J. A., Ancoli-Israel, S., Stone, K. L., Cummings, S. R., & Cawthon, P. M. (2017). Rest–activity patterns and falls and fractures in older men. *Osteoporos International, 28*(4), 1313–1322. https://doi.org/10.1007/s00198-016-3874-2

Rogers-Soeder, T. S., Blackwell, T., Yaffe, K., Ancoli-Israel, S., Redline, S., Cauley, J. A., Ensrud, K. E., Paudel, M., Barrett-Connor, E., LeBlanc, E., Stone, K., Lane, N. E., & Tranah, G.; for the Osteoporotic Fractures in Men Study Research Group. (2018). Rest–activity rhythms and cognitive decline in older men: The Osteoporotic Fractures in Men Sleep Study. *Journal of the American Geriatric Society, 66*(11), 2136–2143. https://doi.org/10.1111/jgs.15555

Rollinson, D. C., Rathlev, N. K., Moss, M., Killiany, R., Sassower, K. C., Auerbach, S., & Fish, S. S. (2003). The effects of consecutive night shifts on neuropsychological performance of interns in the emergency department: A pilot study. *Annals of Emergency Medicine, 41*(3), 400–406. https://doi.org/10.1067/mem.2003.77

Rosique-Esteban, N., Papandreou, C., Romaguera, D., Warnberg, J., Corella, D., Martinez-Gonzalez, M. A., Diaz-Lopez, A., Estruch, R., Vioque, J., Aros, F., Garcia-Rios, A., Bueno-Cavanillas, A., Vidal, J., Serra-Majem, L., Sibai, A. A., Tinahones, F. J., Martinez, J. A., Ordovas, J. M., Tur, J. A., . . . Salas-Salvado, J. (2018). Cross-sectional associations of objectively-measured sleep characteristics with obesity and type 2 diabetes in the PREDIMED-Plus trial. *Sleep, 41*(12), Article zsy190. https://doi.org/10.1093/sleep/zsy190

Rusu, A., Ciobanu, D. M., Inceu, G., Craciun, A. E., Fodor, A., Roman, G., & Bala, C. G. (2022). Variability in sleep timing and dietary intake: A scoping review of the literature. *Nutrients, 14*(24), Article 5248. https://doi.org/10.3390/nu14245248

Sauvet, F., Leftheriotis, G., Gomez-Merino, D., Langrume, C., Drogou, C., Van Beers, P., Bourrilhon, C., Florence, G., & Chennaoui, M. (2010). Effect of acute sleep deprivation on vascular function in healthy subjects. *Journal of Applied Physiology, 108*(1), 68–75. https://doi.org/10.1152/japplphysiol.00851.2009

Saz-Lara, A., Luceron-Lucas-Torres, M., Mesas, A. E., Notario-Pacheco, B., Lopez-Gil, J. F., & Cavero-Redondo, I. (2022). Association between sleep duration and sleep quality with arterial stiffness: A systematic review and meta-analysis. *Sleep Health, 8*(6), 663–670. https://doi.org/10.1016/j.sleh.2022.07.001

Scheiermann, C., Gibbs, J., Ince, L., & Loudon, A. (2018). Clocking in to immunity. *Nature Reviews Immunology, 18*(7), 423–437. https://doi.org/10.1038/s41577-018-0008-4

Scheiermann, C., Kunisaki, Y., & Frenette, P. S. (2013). Circadian control of the immune system. *Nature Reviews Immunology, 13*(3), 190–198. https://doi.org/10.1038/nri3386

Schmid, S. M., Hallschmid, M., Jauch-Chara, K., Wilms, B., Lehnert, H., Born, J., & Schultes, B. (2011). Disturbed glucoregulatory response to food intake after moderate sleep restriction. *Sleep, 34*(3), 371–377. https://doi.org/10.1093/sleep/34.3.371

Schrack, J. A., Kuo, P. L., Wanigatunga, A. A., Di, J., Simonsick, E. M., Spira, A. P., Ferrucci, L., & Zipunnikov, V. (2019). Active-to-sedentary behavior transitions, fatigability, and physical functioning in older adults. *Journals of Gerontology: Series A, 74*(4), 560–567. https://doi.org/10.1093/gerona/gly243

Sen, A., Opdahl, S., Strand, L. B., Vatten, L. J., Laugsand, L. E., & Janszky, I. (2017). Insomnia and the risk of breast cancer: The HUNT Study. *Psychosomatic Medicine, 79*(4), 461–468. https://doi.org/10.1097/PSY.0000000000000417

Shantha, G. P. S., Kumar, A. A., Cheskin, L. J., & Pancholy, S. B. (2015). Association between sleep-disordered breathing, obstructive sleep apnea, and cancer incidence: A systematic review and meta-analysis. *Sleep Medicine, 16*(10), 1289–1294. https://doi.org/10.1016/j.sleep.2015.04.014

Shi, L., Chen, S. J., Ma, M. Y., Bao, Y. P., Han, Y., Wang, Y.-M., Shi, J., Vitiello, M. V., & Lu, L. (2018). Sleep disturbances increase the risk of dementia: A systematic review and meta-analysis. *Sleep Medicine Reviews, 40*, 4–16. https://doi.org/10.1016/j.smrv.2017.06.010

Shi, T., Min, M., Sun, C., Zhang, Y., Liang, M., & Sun, Y. (2020). Does insomnia predict a high risk of cancer? A systematic review and meta-analysis of cohort studies. *Journal of Sleep Research, 29*(1), Article e12876. https://doi.org/10.1111/jsr.12876

Shieu, M. M., Zaheed, A., Shannon, C., Chervin, R. D., Conceicao, A., Paulson, H. L., Braley, T. J., & Dunietz, G. L. (2022). Positive airway pressure and cognitive disorders in adults with obstructive sleep apnea: A systematic review of the literature. *Neurology, 99*(4), e334–e346. https://doi.org/10.1212/WNL.0000000000200383

Shockey, T. M., & Wheaton, A. G. (2017). Short sleep duration by occupation group—29 states, 2013–2014. *MMWR Morbidity and Mortality Weekly Report, 66*(8), 207–213. https://doi.org/10.15585/mmwr.mm6608a2

Short, M. A., Gradisar, M., Lack, L. C., Wright, H., & Carskadon, M. A. (2012). The discrepancy between actigraphic and sleep diary measures of sleep in adolescents. *Sleep Medicine, 13*(4), 378–384. https://doi.org/10.1016/j.sleep.2011.11.005

Shou, H., Zipunnikov, V., Crainiceanu, C. M., & Greven, S. (2015). Structured functional principal component analysis. *Biometrics, 71*(1), 247–257. https://doi.org/10.1111/biom.12236

Simonds, J. F., & Parraga, H. (1984). Sleep behaviors and disorders in children and adolescents evaluated at psychiatric clinics. *Journal of Developmental and Behavioral Pediatrics, 5*(1), 6–10.

Simonelli, G., Dudley, K. A., Weng, J., Gallo, L. C., Perreira, K., Shah, N. A., Alcantara, C., Zee, P. C., Ramos, A. R., Llabre, M. M., Sotres-Alvarez, D., Wang, R., & Patel, S. R. (2017). Neighborhood factors as predictors of poor sleep in the Sueno Ancillary Study of the Hispanic Community Health Study/Study of Latinos. *Sleep, 40*(1), Article zsw025. https://doi.org/10.1093/sleep/zsw025

Slavish, D. C., Taylor, D. J., & Lichstein, K. L. (2019). Intraindividual variability in sleep and comorbid medical and mental health conditions. *Sleep, 42*(6), Article zsz052. https://doi.org/10.1093/sleep/zsz052

Slopen, N., Lewis, T. T., & Williams, D. R. (2016). Discrimination and sleep: A systematic review. *Sleep Medicine, 18*, 88–95. https://doi.org/10.1016/j.sleep.2015.01.012

Smagula, S. F., Ancoli-Israel, S., Blackwell, T., Boudreau, R., Stefanick, M. L., Paudel, M. L., Stone, K. L., & Cauley, J. A.; for the Osteoporotic Fractures in Men (MrOS) Research Group. (2015). Circadian rest–activity rhythms predict future increases in depressive symptoms among community-dwelling older men. *American Journal of Geriatric Psychiatry, 23*(5), 495–505. https://doi.org/10.1016/j.jagp.2014.06.007

Spira, A. P., Gamaldo, A. A., An, Y., Wu, M. N., Simonsick, E. M., Bilgel, M., Zhou, Y., Wong, D. F., Ferrucci, L., & Resnick, S. M. (2013). Self-reported sleep and beta-amyloid deposition in community-dwelling older adults. *JAMA Neurology, 70*(12), 1537–1543. https://doi.org/10.1001/jamaneurol.2013.4258

Steinberg, S., de Jong, S., Andreassen, O. A., Werge, T., Borglum, A. D., Mors, O., Mortensen, P. B., Gustafsson, O., Costas, J., Pietilainen, O. P. H., Demontis, D., Papiol, S., Huttenlocher, J., Mattheisen, M., Breuer, R., Vassos, E., Giegling, I., Fraser, G., Walker, N., . . . Stefansson, K.; for the Irish Schizophrenia Genomics Consortium. (2011). Common variants at VRK2 and TCF4 conferring risk of schizophrenia. *Human Molecular Genetics, 20*(20), 4076–4081. https://doi.org/10.1093/hmg/ddr325

Stickgold, R. (2005). Sleep-dependent memory consolidation. *Nature, 437*(7063), 1272–1278. https://doi.org/10.1038/nature04286

Stone, K. L., Ancoli-Israel, S., Blackwell, T., Ensrud, K. E., Cauley, J. A., Redline, S., Hillier, T. A., Schneider, J., Claman, D., & Cummings, S. R. (2008). Actigraphy-measured sleep characteristics and risk of falls in older women. *Archives of Internal Medicine, 168*(16), 1768–1775. https://doi.org/10.1001/archinte.168.16.1768

Stone, K. L., Blackwell, T. L., Ancoli-Israel, S., Barrett-Connor, E., Bauer, D. C., Cauley, J. A., Ensrud, K. E., Hoffman, A. R., Mehra, R., Stefanick, M. L., Varosy, P. D., Yaffe, K., & Redline, S.; Osteoporotic Fractures in Men (MrOS) Study Research Group. (2016). Sleep disordered breathing and risk of stroke in older community-dwelling men. *Sleep, 39*(3), 531–540. https://doi.org/10.5665/sleep.5520

Stone, K. L., Blackwell, T. L., Ancoli-Israel, S., Cauley, J. A., Redline, S., Marshall, L. M., & Ensrud, K. E.; for the Osteoporotic Fractures in Men Study Group (2014). Sleep disturbances and risk of falls in older community-dwelling men: The outcomes of Sleep Disorders in Older Men (MrOS Sleep) Study. *Journal of the American Geriatric Society, 62*(2), 299–305. https://doi.org/10.1111/jgs.12649

Stone, K. L., Ensrud, K. E., & Ancoli-Israel, S. (2008). Sleep, insomnia and falls in elderly patients. *Sleep Medicine, 9*(S1), S18–S22. https://doi.org/10.1016/S1389-9457(08)70012-1

Stone, K. L., & Li, V. (2022). Actigraphy methods and technical issues. In M. H. Kryger, T. Roth, & C. A. Goldstein (Eds.), *Principles and practices of sleep medicine* (pp. 1984–1991). Elsevier.

Stone, K. L., & Xiao, Q. (2018). Impact of poor sleep on physical and mental health in older women. *Sleep Medicine Clinics, 13*(3), 457–465. https://doi.org/10.1016/j.jsmc.2018.04.012

Strausz, S., Ruotsalainen, S., Ollila, H. M., Karjalainen, J., Kiiskinen, T., Reeve, M., Kurki, M., Mars, N., Havulinna, A. S., Luonsi, E., Aly, D. M., Ahlqvist, E., Teder-Laving, M., Palta, P., Groop, L., Magi, R., Makitie, A., Salomaa, V., Bachour, A., . . . Ripatti, S., (2021). Genetic analysis of obstructive sleep apnoea discovers a strong association with cardiometabolic health. *European Respiratory Journal, 57*(5), Article 2003091. https://doi.org/10.1183/13993003.03091-2020

Sun, X., Ye, D., Jiang, M., Qian, Y., & Mao, Y. (2021). Genetically proxied morning chronotype was associated with a reduced risk of prostate cancer. *Sleep, 44*(10), Article zsab104. https://doi.org/10.1093/sleep/zsab104

Taffinder, N. J., McManus, I. C., Gul, Y., Russell, R. C., & Darzi, A. (1998). Effect of sleep deprivation on surgeons' dexterity on laparoscopy simulator. *Lancet, 352*(9135), Article 1191. https://doi.org/10.1016/s0140-6736(98)00034-8

Tan, X., Ciuculete, D. M., Schioth, H. B., & Benedict, C. (2020). Associations between chronotype, MTNR1B genotype and risk of type 2 diabetes in UK Biobank. *Journal of Internal Medicine, 287*(2), 189–196. https://doi.org/10.1111/joim.12994

Tauman, R., Berall, M., Berry, R., Etzioni, T., Shrater, N., Hwang, D., Marai, I., Manthena, P., Rama, A., Speigel, R., Penzel, T., Koren Morag, N., & Pillar, G. (2020). Watch-PAT is useful in the diagnosis of sleep apnea in patients with atrial fibrillation. *Nature and Science of Sleep, 12*, 1115–1121. https://doi.org/10.2147/NSS.S278752

Teixeira, G. P., Guimaraes, K. C., Soares, A., Marqueze, E. C., Moreno, C. R. C., Mota, M. C., & Crispim, C. A. (2022). Role of chronotype in dietary intake, meal timing, and obesity: A systematic review. *Nutrition Reviews, 81*(1), 75–90. https://doi.org/10.1093/nutrit/nuac044

Thakkar, M. M., Sharma, R., & Sahota, P. (2015). Alcohol disrupts sleep homeostasis. *Alcohol, 49*(4), 299–310. https://doi.org/10.1016/j.alcohol.2014.07.019

Thomas, K. S., Bardwell, W. A., Ancoli-Israel, S., & Dimsdale, J. E. (2006). The toll of ethnic discrimination on sleep architecture and fatigue. *Health Psychology, 25*(5), 635–642. https://doi.org/10.1037/0278-6133.25.5.635

Tighe, C. A., Brindle, R. C., Stahl, S. T., Wallace, M. L., Bramoweth, A. D., Forman, D. E., & Buysse, D. J. (2021). Multidimensional sleep health and physical functioning in older adults. *Gerontology and Geriatric Medicine, 7*, Article 23337214211016222. https://doi.org/10.1177/23337214211016222

Torquati, L., Mielke, G. I., Brown, W. J., & Kolbe-Alexander, T. (2018). Shift work and the risk of cardiovascular disease. A systematic review and meta-analysis including dose–response relationship. *Scandinavian Journal of Work, Environment & Health, 44*(3), 229–238. https://doi.org/10.5271/sjweh.3700

Touitou, Y. (2013). Adolescent sleep misalignment: A chronic jet lag and a matter of public health. *Journal of Physiology (Paris), 107*(4), 323–326. https://doi.org/10.1016/j.jphysparis.2013.03.008

Tranah, G. J., Blackwell, T., Ancoli-Israel, S., Paudel, M. L., Ensrud, K. E., Cauley, J. A., Redline, S., Hillier, T. A., Cummings, S. R., & Stone, K. L.; for the Study of Osteoporotic Fractures Research Group. (2010). Circadian activity rhythms and mortality: The study of osteoporotic fractures. *Journal of the American Geriatrics Society, 58*(2), 282–291. https://doi.org/10.1111/j.1532-5415.2009.02674.x

Tranah, G. J., Blackwell, T., Stone, K. L., Ancoli-Israel, S., Paudel, M. L., Ensrud, K. E., Cauley, J. A., Redline, S., Hillier, T. A., Cummings, S. R., & Yaffe, K.; for the SOF Research Group. (2011). Circadian activity rhythms and risk of incident dementia and mild cognitive impairment in older women. *Annals of Neurology, 70*(5), 722–732. https://doi.org/10.1002/ana.22468

Trockel, M. T., Menon, N. K., Rowe, S. G., Stewart, M. T., Smith, R., Lu, M., Kim, P. K., Quinn, M. A., Lawrence, E., Marchalik, D., Farley, H., Normand, P., Felder, M., Dudley, J. C., & Shanafelt, T. D. (2020). Assessment of physician sleep and wellness, burnout, and clinically significant medical errors. *JAMA Network Open*, *3*(12), Article e2028111. https://doi.org/10.1001/jamanetworkopen.2020.28111

Troxel, W. M., Shih, R. A., Ewing, B., Tucker, J. S., Nugroho, A., & D'Amico, E. J. (2017). Examination of neighborhood disadvantage and sleep in a multi-ethnic cohort of adolescents. *Health & Place*, *45*, 39–45. https://doi.org/10.1016/j.healthplace.2017.03.002

Turner, R. W., 2nd, Vissa, K., Hall, C., Poling, K., Athey, A., Alfonso-Miller, P., Gehrels, J.-A., & Grandner, M. A. (2021). Sleep problems are associated with academic performance in a national sample of collegiate athletes. *Journal of American College Health*, *69*(1), 74–81. https://doi.org/10.1080/07448481.2019.1655027

Unruh, M. L., Redline, S., An, M. W., Buysse, D. J., Nieto, F. J., Yeh, J. L., & Newman, A. B. (2008). Subjective and objective sleep quality and aging in the Sleep Heart Health Study. *Journal of the American Geriatrics Society*, *56*(7), 1218–1227. https://doi.org/10.1111/j.1532-5415.2008.01755.x

Van Dongen, H. P., Maislin, G., Mullington, J. M., & Dinges, D. F. (2003). The cumulative cost of additional wakefulness: Dose–response effects on neurobehavioral functions and sleep physiology from chronic sleep restriction and total sleep deprivation. *Sleep*, *26*(2), 117–126. https://doi.org/10.1093/sleep/26.2.117

Van Someren, E. J., Swaab, D. F., Colenda, C. C., Cohen, W., McCall, W. V., & Rosenquist, P. B. (1999). Bright light therapy: Improved sensitivity to its effects on rest–activity rhythms in Alzheimer patients by application of nonparametric methods. *Chronobiology International*, *16*(4), 505–518. https://doi.org/10.3109/07420529908998724

Vetter, C., Devore, E. E., Ramin, C. A., Speizer, F. E., Willett, W. C., & Schernhammer, E. S. (2015). Mismatch of sleep and work timing and risk of Type 2 diabetes. *Diabetes Care*, *38*(9), 1707–1713. https://doi.org/10.2337/dc15-0302

Vgontzas, A. N., Zoumakis, E., Bixler, E. O., Lin, H. M., Follett, H., Kales, A., & Chrousos, G. P. (2004). Adverse effects of modest sleep restriction on sleepiness, performance, and inflammatory cytokines. *Journal of Clinical Endocrinology & Metabolism*, *89*(5), 2119–2126. https://doi.org/10.1210/jc.2003-031562

Vitiello, M. V., Moe, K. E., & Prinz, P. N. (2002). Sleep complaints cosegregate with illness in older adults: Clinical research informed by and informing epidemiological studies of sleep. *Journal of Psychosomatic Research*, *53*(1), 555–559. https://doi.org/10.1016/s0022-3999(02)00435-x

Wallace, M. L., Buysse, D. J., Redline, S., Stone, K. L., Ensrud, K., Leng, Y., Ancoli-Israel, S., & Hall, M. H. (2019). Multidimensional sleep and mortality in older adults: A machine-learning comparison with other risk factors. *Journals of Gerontology: Series A*, *74*(12), 1903–1909. https://doi.org/10.1093/gerona/glz044

Wallace, M. L., Lee, S., Stone, K. L., Hall, M. H., Smagula, S. F., Redline, S., Ensrud, K., Ancoli-Israel, S., & Buysse, D. J. (2022). Actigraphy-derived sleep health profiles and mortality in older men and women. *Sleep*, *45*(4), Article zsac015. https://doi.org/10.1093/sleep/zsac015

Wallace, M. L., Stone, K., Smagula, S. F., Hall, M. H., Simsek, B., Kado, D. M., Redline, S., Vo, T. N., & Buysse, D. J.; Oseoporotic Fractures in Men (MrOS) Study Research Group. (2018). Which sleep health characteristics predict all-cause mortality in older men? An application of flexible multivariable approaches. *Sleep*, *41*(1), Article zsx189. https://doi.org/10.1093/sleep/zsx189

Wallace, M. L., Yu, L., Buysse, D. J., Stone, K. L., Redline, S., Smagula, S. F., Stefanick, M. L., Kritz-Silverstein, D., & Hall, M. H. (2021). Multidimensional sleep health domains in older men and women: An actigraphy factor analysis. *Sleep*, *44*(2), Article zsaa181. https://doi.org/10.1093/sleep/zsaa181

Walsh, C. M., Blackwell, T., Tranah, G. J., Stone, K. L., Ancoli-Israel, S., Redline, S., Paudel, M., Kramer, J. H., & Yaffe, K. (2014). Weaker circadian activity rhythms are associated with poorer executive function in older women. *Sleep*, *37*(12), 2009–2016. https://doi.org/10.5665/sleep.4260

Wang, D., Ruan, W., Chen, Z., Peng, Y., & Li, W. (2018). Shift work and risk of cardiovascular disease morbidity and mortality: A dose–response meta-analysis of cohort studies. *European Journal of Preventive Cardiology*, *25*(12), 1293–1302. https://doi.org/10.1177/2047487318783892

Wang, H., Lane, J. M., Jones, S. E., Dashti, H. S., Ollila, H. M., Wood, A. R., van Hees, V. T., Brumpton, B., Winsvold, B. S., Kantojarvi, K., Palviainen, T., Cade, B. E., Sofer, T., Song, Y., Patel, K., Anderson, S. G., Bechtold, D. A., Bowden, J., Emsley, R., . . . Saxena, R. (2019). Genome-wide association analysis of self-reported daytime sleepiness identifies 42 loci that suggest biological subtypes. *Nature Communications*, *10*(1), Article 3503. https://doi.org/10.1038/s41467-019-11456-7

Wang, J., Tang, H., Duan, Y., Yang, S., & An, J. (2021). Association between sleep traits and lung cancer: A Mendelian randomization study. *Journal of Immunology Research, 2021*, Article 1893882. https://doi.org/10.1155/2021/1893882

Wei, L., Han, N., Sun, S., Ma, X., & Zhang, Y. (2021). Sleep-disordered breathing and risk of the breast cancer: A meta-analysis of cohort studies. *International Journal of Clinical Practice, 75*(11), Article e14793. https://doi.org/10.1111/ijcp.14793

Wesnes, K. A., Walker, M. B., Walker, L. G., Heys, S. D., White, L., Warren, R., & Eremin, O. (1997). Cognitive performance and mood after a weekend on call in a surgical unit. *British Journal of Surgery, 84*(4), 493–495.

Wheaton, A. G., Olsen, E. O., Miller, G. F., & Croft, J. B. (2016). Sleep duration and injury-related risk behaviors among high school students—United States, 2007–2013. *MMWR Morbidity and Mortality Weekly Report, 65*(13), 337–341. https://doi.org/10.15585/mmwr.mm6513a1

Whelehan, D. F., McCarrick, C. A., & Ridgway, P. F. (2020). A systematic review of sleep deprivation and technical skill in surgery. *Surgeon, 18*(6), 375–384. https://doi.org/10.1016/j.surge.2020.01.004

Whinnery, J., Jackson, N., Rattanaumpawan, P., & Grandner, M. A. (2014). Short and long sleep duration associated with race/ethnicity, sociodemographics, and socioeconomic position. *Sleep, 37*(3), 601–611. https://doi.org/10.5665/sleep.3508

Williamson, A. M., & Feyer, A. M. (2000). Moderate sleep deprivation produces impairments in cognitive and motor performance equivalent to legally prescribed levels of alcohol intoxication. *Occupational & Environmental Medicine, 57*(10), 649–655. https://doi.org/10.1136/oem.57.10.649

Wong, A. T. Y., Heath, A. K., Tong, T. Y. N., Reeves, G. K., Floud, S., Beral, V., & Travis, R. C.; on behalf of the Million Women Study. (2021). Sleep duration and breast cancer incidence: Results from the Million Women Study and meta-analysis of published prospective studies. *Sleep, 44*(2), Article zsaa166. https://doi.org/10.1093/sleep/zsaa166

World Health Organization. (1995). *Constitution of the World Health Organization.*

Wright, K. P., Jr., Drake, A. L., Frey, D. J., Fleshner, M., Desouza, C. A., Gronfier, C., & Czeisler, C. A. (2015). Influence of sleep deprivation and circadian misalignment on cortisol, inflammatory markers, and cytokine balance. *Brain, Behavior, and Immunity, 47*, 24–34. https://doi.org/10.1016/j.bbi.2015.01.004

Xiao, L., Huang, L., Schrack, J. A., Ferrucci, L., Zipunnikov, V., & Crainiceanu, C. M. (2015). Quantifying the lifetime circadian rhythm of physical activity: A covariate-dependent functional approach. *Biostatistics, 16*(2), 352–367. https://doi.org/10.1093/biostatistics/kxu045

Xiao, Q., Bauer, C., Layne, T., & Playdon, M. (2021). The association between overnight fasting and body mass index in older adults: The interaction between duration and timing. *International Journal of Obesity, 45*(3), 555–564. https://doi.org/10.1038/s41366-020-00715-z

Xiao, Q., Blot, W. J., & Matthews, C. E. (2019). Weekday and weekend sleep duration and mortality among middle-to-older aged White and Black adults in a low-income southern US cohort. *Sleep Health, 5*(5), 521–527. https://doi.org/10.1016/j.sleh.2019.04.008

Xiao, Q., Derkach, A., Moore, S. C., Zheng, W., Shu, X. O., Gu, F., Caporaso, N. E., Sampson, J. N., & Matthews, C. E. (2017). Habitual sleep and human plasma metabolomics. *Metabolomics, 13*(5), Article 63. https://doi.org/10.1007/s11306-017-1205-z

Xiao, Q., Garaulet, M., & Scheer, F. (2019). Meal timing and obesity: Interactions with macronutrient intake and chronotype. *International Journal of Obesity, 43*(9), 1701–1711. https://doi.org/10.1038/s41366-018-0284-x

Xiao, Q., & Hale, L. (2018). Neighborhood socioeconomic status, sleep duration, and napping in middle-to-old aged US men and women. *Sleep, 41*(7), Article zsy076. https://doi.org/10.1093/sleep/zsy076

Xiao, Q., Lu, J., Zeitzer, J. M., Matthews, C. E., Saint-Maurice, P. F., & Bauer, C. (2022). Rest–activity profiles among U.S. adults in a nationally representative sample: A functional principal component analysis. *International Journal of Behavioral Nutrition and Physical Activity, 19*(1), Article 32. https://doi.org/10.1186/s12966-022-01274-4

Xiao, Q., Matthews, C. E., Playdon, M., & Bauer, C. (2022). The association between rest–activity rhythms and glycemic markers: The US National Health and Nutrition Examination Survey, 2011-2014. *Sleep, 45*(2), Article zsab291. https://doi.org/10.1093/sleep/zsab291

Xiao, Q., Qian, J., Evans, D. S., Redline, S., Lane, N. E., Ancoli-Israel, S., Scheer, F. A. J. L., & Stone, K. L.; for the Osteoporotic Fractures in Men (MrOS) Study Group. (2020). Cross-sectional and prospective associations of rest–activity rhythms with metabolic markers and Type 2 diabetes in older men. *Diabetes Care, 43*(11), 2702–2712. https://doi.org/10.2337/dc20-0557

Xiao, Q., Qian, J., Evans, D. S., Redline, S., Lane, N. E., Ancoli-Israel, S., Scheer, F. A. J. L., & Stone, K. L.; Osteoporotic Fractures in Men (MrOS) Study Group. (2022). Cross-sectional and prospective associations of rest–activity rhythms with circulating inflammatory markers in older men. *Journals of Gerontology: Series A, 77*(1), 55–65. https://doi.org/10.1093/gerona/glab095

Xiao, Q., Sampson, J. N., LaCroix, A. Z., Shadyab, A. H., Zeitzer, J. M., Ancoli-Israel, S., Yaffe, K., & Stone, K. L.; Osteoporotic Fractures in Men (MrOS) Study Group. (2022). Nonparametric parameters of 24-hour rest–activity rhythms and long-term cognitive decline and incident cognitive impairment in older men. Journals of Gerontology: Series A, *77*(2), 250–258. https://doi.org/10.1093/gerona/glab275

Xiao, Q., Shadyab, A. H., Rapp, S. R., Stone, K. L., Yaffe, K., Sampson, J. N., Chen, J.-C., Hayden, K. M., Henderson, V. W., & LaCroix, A. Z. (2022). Rest–activity rhythms and cognitive impairment and dementia in older women: Results from the Women's Health Initiative. *Journal of the American Geriatrics Society, 70*(10), 2925–2937. https://doi.org/10.1111/jgs.17926

Xie, L., Kang, H., Xu, Q., Chen, M. J., Liao, Y., Thiyagarajan, M., O'Donnell, J., Christensen, D. J., Nicholson, C., Iliff, J. J., Takano, T., Deane, R., & Nedergaard, M. (2013). Sleep drives metabolite clearance from the adult brain. *Science, 342*(6156), 373–377. https://doi.org/10.1126/science.1241224

Xu, S. Y., Nelson, S., Kerr, J., Godbole, S., Johnson, E., Patterson, R. E., Rock, C. L., Sears, D. D., Abramson, I., & Natarajan, L. (2019). Modeling temporal variation in physical activity using functional principal components analysis. *Statistics in Bioscience, 11*(2), 403–421.

Xu, W., Tan, C. C., Zou, J. J., Cao, X. P., & Tan, L. (2020). Sleep problems and risk of all-cause cognitive decline or dementia: An updated systematic review and meta-analysis. *Journal of Neurology, Neurosurgery & Psychiatry, 91*(3), 236–244. https://doi.org/10.1136/jnnp-2019-321896

Yaffe, K., Laffan, A. M., Harrison, S. L., Redline, S., Spira, A. P., Ensrud, K. E., Ancoli-Israel, S., & Stone, K. L. (2011). Sleep-disordered breathing, hypoxia, and risk of mild cognitive impairment and dementia in older women. *JAMA, 306*(6), 613–619. https://doi.org/10.1001/jama.2011.1115

Yang, L., Feng, H., Chen, J., Wing, Y. K., Benedict, C., Tan, X., & Zhang, J. (2023). Association of circadian rest–activity rhythms with cardiovascular disease and mortality in Type 2 diabetes. *Diabetes Research and Clinical Practice, 197*, Article 110262. https://doi.org/10.1016/j.diabres.2023.110262

Young, T. (2009). Rationale, design and findings from the Wisconsin Sleep Cohort Study: Toward understanding the total societal burden of sleep disordered breathing. *Sleep Medicine Clinics, 4*(1), 37–46. https://doi.org/10.1016/j.jsmc.2008.11.003

Young, T., Palta, M., Dempsey, J., Skatrud, J., Weber, S., & Badr, S. (1993). The occurrence of sleep-disordered breathing among middle-aged adults. *New England Journal of Medicine, 328*(17), 1230–1235. https://doi.org/10.1056/NEJM199304293281704

Young, T., Shahar, E., Nieto, F. J., Redline, S., Newman, A. B., Gottlieb, D. J., Walsleben, J. A., Finn, L., Enright, P., & Samet, J. M.; Sleep Heart Health Study Research Group. (2002). Predictors of sleep-disordered breathing in community-dwelling adults: The Sleep Heart Health Study. *Archives of Internal Medicine, 162*(8), 893–900.

Yu, J. H., Yun, C. H., Ahn, J. H., Suh, S., Cho, H. J., Lee, S. K., Yoo, H. J., Seo, J. A., Kim, S. G., Choi, K. M., Baik, S. H., Choi, D. S., Shin, C., & Kim, N. H. (2015). Evening chronotype is associated with metabolic disorders and body composition in middle-aged adults. *Journal of Clinical Endocrinology & Metabolism, 100*(4), 1494–1502. https://doi.org/10.1210/jc.2014-3754

Yuan, S., Mason, A. M., Titova, O. E., Vithayathil, M., Kar, S., Chen, J., Li, X., Burgess, S., & Larsson, S. C. (2023). Morning chronotype and digestive tract cancers: Mendelian randomization study. *International Journal of Cancer, 152*(4), 697–704. https://doi.org/10.1002/ijc.34284

Zeitzer, J. M., Blackwell, T., Hoffman, A. R., Cummings, S., Ancoli-Israel, S., & Stone, K.; Osteoporotic Fractures in Men (MrOS) Study Research Group. (2018). Daily patterns of accelerometer activity predict changes in sleep, cognition, and mortality in older men. *Journals of Gerontology: Series A, 73*(5), 682–687. https://doi.org/10.1093/gerona/glw250

Zhang, Y., & Papantoniou, K. (2019). Night shift work and its carcinogenicity. *Lancet Oncology, 20*(10), Article e550. https://doi.org/10.1016/S1470-2045(19)30578-9

CHAPTER

21 Sleep Disorders: Classification and Diagnosis

Jack D. Edinger, Ana I. Fins, *and* Charles M. Morin

Abstract

This chapter reviews classification schemes of sleep disorders and discusses assessment procedures commonly used to derive a diagnosis. Three different classifications, based predominantly on expert opinions and consensus, have evolved in parallel over the last few decades. Two of them are incorporated within larger taxonomies, such as the *International Classification of Diseases* (ICD) from the World Health Organization and the *Diagnostic and Statistical Manual of Mental Disorders* (DSM) from the American Psychiatric Association. A more specialized taxonomy, the *International Classification of Sleep Disorders*, has been developed by sleep medicine and research societies. Historically significant discrepancies have existed among these classification systems. However, increased collaboration among the nosologists charged with the development and refinement of these systems has made significant advances in increasing the concordance of these distinctive taxonomies. Yet the validity and reliability of the disorders listed in these classification schemes remain uneven, with some disorders supported by extensive empirical evidence and ascertained via reliable objective assays and others based primarily on consensus and identified largely by the questionably reliable clinical interview. Despite somewhat uneven evidence supporting the validity and reliability for the disorders these systems describe, they remain widely used by clinicians and researchers. Regardless of the system in use, accurate diagnosis is based on a multilevel assessment including a clinical interview, screening questionnaires and self-monitoring and in some cases laboratory procedures, and ambulatory behavioral assessment devices. Further research is needed to examine the validity and reliability of various sleep disorders and the clinical utility of current taxonomies.

Key Words: sleep disorder, classification, diagnosis, evaluation, taxonomy, nosology

Introduction

Patients who present with sleep/wake disorders are an extremely diverse group of individuals whose complaints represent a range of underlying etiologies, defining clinical symptoms, associated morbidity outcomes, prognoses, and treatment needs. Given the complexity and diversity represented in this population, the need for a nosology that aids clinicians in their diagnostic and treatment efforts with their patients has long been apparent. Since the latter part of the last century, a variety of professional organizations have attempted to address this need through the development of sleep disorder classification systems. In this chapter we consider the evolution and purpose of these classification schemes and review their overall structures and the specific diagnoses they describe. We also consider their clinical utility, degree of similarity and dissimilarity, and the limited evidence regarding the reliability and validity of the specific diagnostic categories they describe.

Although there has been some discordance among the sleep disorder nosologies proposed over the years, each has provided a framework for differentiating among patients with distinctive sleep disorders. As such, the process of differentiating among currently recognized sleep disorder diagnoses is a useful endeavor for those who confront patients with sleep complaints. Given this fact, the latter portion of the chapter provides general guidelines for assessing and diagnosing sleep-disordered patients. Specifically, this discussion considers the use of the clinical interview, structured interview protocols, prospective sleep-monitoring strategies, sleep/wake-focused questionnaires, and methods for assessing sleep/wake functioning in the laboratory and home settings. Also included in this discussion are the challenges that clinicians face when differentiating among some of the more difficult-to-discriminate diagnostic categories. Admittedly, the area of sleep disorder classification and diagnosis remains as much an art as it is a science. As noted in the concluding section of this chapter, research designed to refine and improve current sleep disorder diagnostic systems is very much needed. Thus, this chapter has been structured so as to provide the reader with a critical understanding of the nature, strengths, and salient limitations of our current sleep disorder nosologies and the diagnostic practices that follow from their use.

Sleep Disorder Classification

Evolution and Purpose of Sleep Disorder Classification

Like most other areas of clinical focus, the field of sleep disorder medicine evolved gradually, from early laboratory studies of normal human sleep to studies of various forms of sleep pathology and sleep disorders. In 1930, the German psychiatrist Hans Berger conducted the first electroencephalographic (EEG) studies of human sleep that showed sleep to be a dynamic process involving various patterns of brain-wave and bodily activity that we now use to characterize different sleep stages. In the 1950s, seminal work by Aserinsky and Kleitman (1953, 1955) added to this initial work through their study of rapid-eye-movement (REM) sleep and their linking of this component of the sleep process to dream phenomena. Such research provided the foundation for our current understanding of normal sleep process and structure. However, it was not until the 1960s and 1970s when researchers increasingly began studying individuals with contrasting forms of sleep/wake pathology including those with chronic nighttime sleep difficulties, those with excessive daytime sleepiness, and those with unusual sleep-related behaviors. Only then did the diversity among extant sleep disorders become apparent. Such research, in turn, highlighted the clinical needs of the myriad patients suffering from sleep pathology; thus, during the 1970s, the clinical practice of sleep medicine began taking form.

Once clinical practitioners began specializing in the treatment of patients with varying sleep disorders, the need for a sleep disorder classification system became obvious. As a result, systems for classifying and diagnosing sleep disorders began to appear in the mid- and later 1970s and have continued to evolve over time. As noted by Buysse et al. (2003), these classifications systems serve a number of important and pragmatically useful purposes. At the most basic level, they provide standardized definitions for distinctive sleep disorders and, thus, aid in the description of patients and communication among practitioners charged with their treatment. Likewise, the standard definitions and criteria sets these classifications systems include serve as "anchor points" for researchers and aid in standardizing basic and clinical research concerning the sleep disorders these systems describe. Inasmuch as the assignment of a particular diagnosis implicitly connotes specific treatment needs, these classification systems guide clinicians in their treatment decisions with sleep disorder patients. Furthermore, the assignment of a particular sleep disorder diagnosis may also connote a patient's prognosis to the extent that information about that specific sleep disorder's long-term course is known. Finally, these systems provide the basis for the more mundane task of diagnostic coding required by many third-party payers and healthcare systems for patient billing purposes. Thus, as is the case for other medical and psychiatric nosologies, sleep disorder classification systems serve multiple purposes relevant to research and clinical management.

History and Nature of Previous Sleep Disorder Nosologies

Ideally, a system for differentiating among and diagnosing any set of related medical disorders should be based on clearly defined etiologies. In the absence of unambiguous pathologies, however (as is the case for many sleep disorders), classification schemes typically rely on less compelling factors such as symptom presentation, physiological measurements, clinical utility, expert opinion/experience, and consensus (Buysse et al., 2003). As noted above, the sleep disorder classification systems in use today initially emerged when basic sleep research led to the identification of a heterogeneous array of sleep disorder subtypes. Subsequently, through the empirical study of varying phenotypes and the evolving practice of clinical sleep medicine, the heterogeneity of sleep disorders became increasingly obvious. However, research progress has not occurred at a consistent pace across all recognized sleep disorders. As a consequence, the sleep disorder nosologies developed to date have relied as much on expert opinion/consensus as they have on basic and clinical research evidence. Hence, despite the extensive research devoted to the understanding of distinctive sleep disorders since the 1980s, sleep disorder classification has remained as much an art as it is a science.

To date, several prominent organizations including the World Health Organization (WHO), the American Psychiatric Association (APA), and past and present professional sleep societies have all shown active interest in sleep disorder classification systems. Unfortunately, these organizations historically had limited collaboration in their nosological work, particularly through the earlier years of their efforts. Thus, previous versions of these various nosologies were notably discrepant in the sleep disorders they listed as well as how they viewed their underlying etiologies. As noted later in this chapter, research highlighting this discordance and other deficiencies of the earlier nosologies has led to a gradual convergence of these diagnostic systems over time. Figure 21.1 shows the different lineages of sleep disorder nosologies that have evolved from these organizations from their early stages to the present day. As suggested by the following discussion, these three lines of nosological efforts for many years reflected not only notably different methods for classifying sleep disorders but also differing conceptualizations of sleep disorder pathology in general.

The professional sleep societies were among the earliest to involve themselves in the task of sleep disorder classification at a time when the field of sleep disorder medicine was still in its early stages of evolution. In 1979 the Association of Sleep Disorders Centers (ASDC) published its landmark monograph, the *Diagnostic Classification of Sleep and Arousal Disorders* (Association of Sleep Disorders Centers & Association for the Psychophysiological Study of Sleep, 1979). Within this system, the sleep disorders recognized at the time were divided into four categories based on their presenting symptoms.

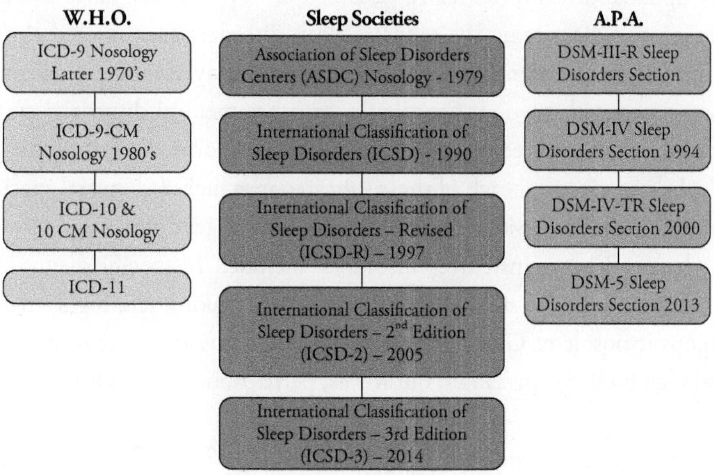

Figure 21.1 The evolution and lineages of sleep disorder nosologies

Note. This figure shows the evolution of sleep disorder classification systems promoted by the World Health Organization, the professional sleep societies, and the American Psychiatric Association. A.P.A. = American Psychiatric Association; DSM = *Diagnostic and Statistical Manual of Mental Disorders* (III = 3rd. ed.; IV = 4th ed.; 5 = fifth ed.; R = revised; TR = text revision); ICD-9 = *International Classification of Diseases* (9–11 = editions; CM = *Clinical Modification*).

Among these were the disorders of initiating and maintaining sleep, the disorders of excessive somnolence, the sleep–wake schedule disorders, and the parasomnias. Given the description of the sleep disorders it provided, this initial ASDC scheme proposed the view that many sleep problems may evolve from a combination of endogenous and exogenous factors and were not necessarily caused solely by biological/medical pathology or environmental/behavioral/lifestyle factors.

Efforts by the WHO were also among the earliest to provide a method or schema for classifying the range of sleep disorders encountered in clinical practice. In the late 1970s, the WHO developed a sleep disorder nosology and incorporated it into the ninth edition of its *International Classification of Diseases* (ICD; WHO, 1977). A number of years later, the WHO presented a somewhat refined version of this classification scheme and subsequently incorporated this updated nosology in its ICD-9 *Clinical Modification* manual (WHO, 1994). Both of these ICD nosologies provided a variety of sleep disorder diagnoses and employed a *scaffold*, in which the range of listed sleep disorders were characterized as either nonorganic (i.e., due largely to exogenous factors) or organic (i.e., "true" endogenous sleep disturbances) in origin. The nonorganic disorders included some subtypes defined largely by chronicity of the complaint (transient vs. persistent), as well as disorders due to phase-shift disruption of the sleep–wake cycle, as associated with shift work or jet lag.

Through the 1980s the ASDC evolved into the American Sleep Disorders Association (ASDA), and this newer organization continued sleep specialists' efforts in the area of sleep disorder classification. As a result of these efforts, the ASDA published the *International Classification of Sleep Disorders* (ICSD) in 1990. This publication, along with the later cosmetically updated revision (ICSD-R; ASDA, 1997), provided a fairly complex system for categorizing and diagnosing the range of sleep disorders encountered clinically. This system grouped sleep disorders into four large categories: dyssomnias; parasomnias; sleep disorders associated with mental, neurologic, or other medical disorders; and proposed sleep disorders. The first three of these four global categories were then divided into a number of subcategories, and each of these subcategories included several specific diagnoses. For example, the "intrinsic sleep disorders" included 13 different specific diagnostic categories, whereas the "extrinsic sleep disorders" included 14 specific diagnoses. Overall, the ICSD included over 80 sleep disorder diagnoses, making it a highly technical and specific diagnostic nosology. Given its specificity, it could be argued that not only was this system developed by sleep specialists, but it was, perhaps, best suited for their use in sleep specialty centers.

Running parallel and somewhat independent to the efforts of the WHO, the ASDC, and the ASDA classification efforts, the APA also involved itself in sleep disorder classification beginning in the 1980s. These early efforts resulted in the APA's sleep disorder nosology first appearing in the *Diagnostic and Statistical Manual of Mental Disorders*, third revised edition (DSM-III-R; APA, 1987). This system, which was continued with minor modifications and improvements in the DSM-IV and subsequent text revision DSM-IV-TR (APA, 1994, 1997), made an essential distinction between the *dyssomnias* (disorders intrinsic to the mechanisms of sleep) and the *parasomnias* (unusual behaviors or events that occur during sleep: sleep terrors, nocturnal seizures, nightmares, and sleepwalking). Within the dyssomnias, the DSM relies primarily upon the presumed etiology of the sleep disturbance to make major diagnostic distinctions (primary vs. secondary to another condition). Primary dyssomnia diagnoses include primary insomnia, breathing-related sleep disorder, narcolepsy, primary hypersomnia, circadian rhythm disorder, and dyssomnia not otherwise specified. Secondary disorders include sleep disorders related to another mental disorder, due to a general medical condition, and substance-induced conditions.

In the later 1990s and early 2000s, the ASDA evolved into the American Academy of Sleep Medicine (AASM) and soon thereafter began work on revising the ICSD/ICSD-R system. Given the complexity of the original ICSD, the panel charged with its revision extended considerable efforts to simplify the scaffold or framework for organizing the range of sleep disorders to be included in the revised manual and, thus, make it more "user-friendly." The ICSD-2 (AASM, 2005) emanating from these efforts borrowed some of its organizational structure from the original ASDC nosology by selecting an organizing scaffold based as much on phenotypic symptom presentation as underlying pathophysiology. Accordingly, the ICSD-2 grouped sleep disorders into the seven major categories of insomnia, sleep-related breathing disorders, hypersomnias of central origin, circadian rhythm sleep disorders, parasomnias, sleep-related movement disorders, and other sleep disorders. Selection of specific disorders and their criteria sets for inclusion in these broad categories was influenced strongly by the previous ASDC and ASDA manuals as well as by the DSM-IV/DSM-IV-TR manuals. To assist clinicians in their diagnostic efforts, the ICSD-2 manual included a section that describes *isolated symptoms* and *normal variants* (e.g., sleep talking, normal short or long sleep patterns) that have minimal clinical significance as well as *unresolved issues* (i.e., conditions that require further study). The panel constructing the ICSD-2 also recognized the ubiquitous nature of sleep/wake difficulties in other medical and psychiatric conditions. Hence, the ICSD-2 included the appendices "Sleep Disorders Associated With Conditions Classifiable Elsewhere" and "Other Psychiatric and Behavioral Disorders Frequently Encountered in the Differential Diagnosis of Sleep Disorders" to limit the excessive assignment of sleep disorder diagnoses to primary medical, neurologic, and psychiatric disorders that commonly give rise to sleep/wake complaints.

During the development of the ICSD-2, the panel in charge of its development engaged in extensive liaison efforts with the WHO concerning the emerging sleep nosology. As a result of these efforts, the WHO agreed to accept the new nosology and incorporate it into its ICD classification system. This development reduced some of the interorganizational disagreement in regard to sleep disorder diagnoses. However, the nosologies in the ICSD-2 and DSM-IV-TR sleep disorder taxonomies represented markedly different conceptions of sleep pathology as well as discrepant approaches toward sleep disorder classification. The ICSD-2 arguably reduced some of the complexity of the ICSD/ICSD-R systems but continued to include a large number of highly specific sleep disorder diagnoses. By contrast, the DSM-IV-TR represented a much less complex approach to sleep disorder classification by including a relatively limited number of more globally defined diagnostic categories.

Empirical Tests of the Previous Sleep Disorder Nosologies

Despite the interest in and efforts devoted to the development of the aforementioned sleep disorder nosologies, there has been a relative paucity of research conducted to examine their levels of concordance in identifying sleep disorder diagnoses, clinician acceptance, overall reliabilities, and validities for sleep disorder classification. The studies that have been conducted have highlighted an unacceptable level of discordance among these systems and have also raised serious questions about their reliabilities and validities for sleep disorder classification. In the end such studies provided the impetus for refinement of these systems as well as for efforts to make them more concordant.

To investigate the concordance among the sleep disorder nosologies, Buysse et al. (1994) compared the diagnoses assigned to 216 patients with insomnia by sleep specialists using the DSM-IV, the original version of the ICSD, and the ICD-10. As might be expected, results of this study showed varied and somewhat discordant diagnostic assignments derived from each classification system. Figure 21.2 shows the variations in diagnostic assignments derived from each system. As the figure shows, the group of 52 patients assigned a DSM-IV diagnosis of primary insomnia was assigned five different

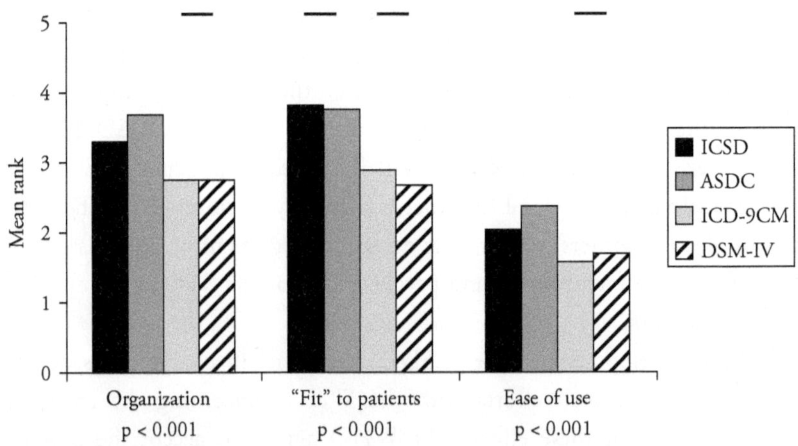

Figure 21.2 Sleep specialists' ratings of sleep disorder nosologies
Note. ASDC = Association of Sleep Disorders Centers; DSM-IV = *Diagnostic and Statistical Manual of Mental Disorders*, 4th ed.; ICD-9CM = *International Classification of Diseases*, 9th ed., *Clinical Modification*; ICSD = *International Classification of Sleep Disorders.*

ICSD diagnoses, with psychophysiological insomnia being the most frequently used ICSD diagnosis. The same group of patients was assigned four different ICD diagnoses, but 85% of the sample was categorized as nonorganic insomnia, a condition reasonably analogous to primary insomnia. Hence, in this study, the ICD appeared more concordant with DSM-IV than did the ICSD. Such a finding is perhaps not surprising since the ICD traditionally has been a global classification scheme like the DSM-IV, whereas the ICSD is much more specific and complex. Thus, use of the ICSD and DSM-IV produced somewhat discordant results when employed with the same patient group.

In another study (Ohayon & Roberts, 2001), 794 adolescents, aged 15–18 years, and 1,447 young adults, aged 19–24 years, were interviewed via telephone and assigned both ICSD and DSM-IV diagnoses using a computer-driven structured interview. Of the subjects who received a DSM-IV diagnosis, 73.2% met criteria for an ICSD diagnosis. In contrast, only 39.8% of subjects who were assigned an ICSD diagnosis also met criteria for a DSM-IV diagnosis. The finding that the DSM-IV criteria yielded a much lower prevalence for sleep disorders than did the ICSD criteria highlights the discordance between these two diagnostic systems. Thus, as was the case with the Buysse et al. study, this study highlighted the marked discordance between the ICSD and DSM systems.

Research concerning the reliability of DSM and ICSD subtypes has been limited and relates primarily to the insomnia spectrum disorders. The limited number of studies conducted (Bertisch et al., 2018; Edinger et al., 1996; Hening et al., 2003; Morin et al., 1994; Ohayon et al., 1999; Schramm et al., 1993) provided reliability data for sleep disorder diagnoses in the DSM or ICSD systems, and these studies collectively included a total sample of only 515 individuals. Two of these studies (Buysse et al., 1994; Schramm et al., 1993) were conducted solely or in part to evaluate the diagnostic reliability of the DSM (DSM-III-R or DSM-IV) insomnia classification system. In the earlier of these studies, Schramm et al. (1993) examined inter-rater reliability among clinicians using a structured interview to diagnose three DSM-III-R insomnia subtypes. In the latter multisite study, Buysse et al. (1994) examined inter-rater reliability among clinicians using standard clinical interviews to identify DSM-IV insomnia diagnoses. Given sample size limitations, only the reliability data for two DSM insomnia diagnoses was reported in this latter study. In a third study, Edinger et al. (1996) reported inter-rater reliability data for two clinicians who reviewed archival data from a small insomnia sample (n = 31) and independently assigned both DSM-III-R and ICSD insomnia diagnoses. In the fourth study, Morin et al. (1994) assessed reliability for ICSD diagnoses by comparing impressions derived from clinical interviews with diagnoses derived independently from sleep history, psychometric evaluations, and available polysomnographic (PSG) findings. The fifth study, by Ohayon et al. (1999), compared a computer-assisted structured interview with impressions of clinical interviewers to determine their agreement for detecting the presence or absence of any ICSD insomnia diagnosis. The final study, by Hening et al. (2003), assessed inter-rater reliability for the diagnosis of restless legs syndrome (RLS) among raters who used a structured interview designed specifically for identifying this condition.

Table 21.1 provides summary data taken from these studies. These data show that the reliability indices for DSM categories and RLS derived from structured interviews are very impressive and suggest highly acceptable reliability of these global diagnoses. In contrast, when such global diagnoses are derived from standard clinical interviews, as was the case in the Buysse et al. (1994) study, reliabilities are less impressive. The remaining studies by Edinger et al. (1996), Morin et al. (1994), and Ohayon et al. (1999) suggest reasonable reliability for ICSD diagnoses; but unfortunately, only the Morin et al. study provided reliability data for any specific ICSD categories. Overall, these data must be considered very limited and incomplete as there is no reliability information about most of the diagnostic categories included in either the prior DSM-IV-TR or ICSD systems. Thus, the reliability data available provides us little guidance in ascertaining which of these approaches to sleep disorder classification may be optimal.

Evidence supporting the validity of past sleep disorder nosologies is also rather limited and unimpressive at this juncture. This state of affairs is likely due, in part, to the fact that establishing the validity of a diagnostic system comprising the entire range of recognized sleep disorders is an extremely challenging task. At a minimum, this task requires a demonstration that the diagnostic system adequately deals with population heterogeneity

Table 21.1 Inter-rater reliability data reported for various insomnia subtypes

Study	Sample	Insomnia subtypes	Reliability index[a]
Schramm et al. (1993): Germany	*N* = 68	Primary Mental disorder Medical	.86 .84 .86
Buysse et al. (1994): 5 US sleep centers	*N* = 216	Primary Mental disorder	.40 .40
Morin et al. (1994): Richmond, VA, USA	*N* = 100	Psychophysiological Mental Hypnotic-dependent Other mixed	.54 .64 .70 .84
Edinger et al. (1996): Durham, NC, USA	*N* = 31	Mixed DSM-III-R Mixed ICSD-90	.71 .68
Ohayon et al. (1999): Palo Alto, CA, and Germany	*N* = 105	ICSD-90 insomnia yes vs. no	.78
Hening et al. (2003): Baltimore, MD, USA	*N* = 75	Restless legs syndrome yes vs. no	.95

[a]Reliability indices shown are all kappa values except the value shown for the Henning et al. study, which reported an intraclass correlation coefficient among three raters.

Note. DSM-III-R = *Diagnostic and Statistical Manual of Mental Disorders*, 3rd ed., rev.; ICSD-90 = 1990 version of the *International Classification of Sleep Disorders*.

by subdividing a diverse group of conditions such as the sleep disorders into "true" or naturally occurring homogenous subgroups. What this statement implies is that careful application of the diagnostic criteria for a particular sleep disorder results in the identification of a unique condition that can be shown to differ in some clinically meaningful manners (e.g., presenting symptoms, underlying pathophysiology, specific treatment needs, prognosis, etc.) from other conditions included in the classification scheme and/or from non-complaining individuals. In addition, under ideal conditions, the diagnostic system manages to minimize the differences among those meeting criteria for the same diagnosis and maximize the differences between individuals or groups that have distinctive sleep disorder diagnoses.

To date, several strategies have been employed to assess the validity of the previous sleep disorder nosologies, but these have almost exclusively focused on the insomnia sections of these systems. One such research strategy used entails the comparison of classification results derived from usual clinical means with those derived from cluster analysis, an empirical procedure designed to group individuals on the basis of common clinical features. Clinicians first assign diagnoses to each patient in a large cohort using data derived from clinical interview, chart review, or other source of pertinent information. Subsequently, subgroups in the cohort are identified empirically by applying a statistical cluster analysis (Milligan, 1980; Tabachnick & Fidell, 1989) to a set of variables considered relevant to the clinical diagnoses of interest. In the case of insomnia, for example, data concerning nature, duration, and frequency of sleep complaint, daytime symptoms, medical history, psychiatric history, age, gender, etc. can be employed in the cluster analysis to identify homogenous subgroups. Once the cluster analysis is completed, the results of the clinical and the empirical classifications can be compared. Ideally, each cluster will be composed mainly of patients sharing a single clinically assigned diagnosis. When this outcome is obtained, the validity of the nosology is supported by the concordance of the empirical and clinical classification results. When the clinical and empirical results disagree, questions about the nosology's validity remain.

Two studies have employed this methodology to test the validity of previous versions of the current-day insomnia nosologies. In the earlier of these studies, Hauri (1983) assessed a group of 99 individuals (89 patients with insomnia and 10 good sleepers) and empirically identified nine discrete groups or clusters as a test of the 1979 ASDC nosology. Only two of the groups identified were totally "pure" (i.e., consisted of only patients with a single ASDC diagnosis), and these clusters respectively were composed of patients with clinically assigned diagnoses of psychophysiological insomnia and childhood-onset insomnia. In a subsequent study, Edinger and colleagues (1996) tested the DSM-III-R and the ICSD systems by comparing cluster analytic results with the clinical classification results for 98 insomnia outpatients. The results obtained showed that none of the 14 empirically derived subgroups (clusters) were composed of only one DSM-III-R or ICSD subtype. Comparisons of clustering results with DSM-III-R diagnoses assigned clinically showed there were three clusters composed of only two clinically identified diagnostic subgroups. Comparisons of the clustering results against the clinically assigned ICSD diagnoses yielded even less promising results, with only two clusters composed of two ICSD diagnostic subgroups. These findings imply that both the more global DSM approach and the more highly specific ICSD system have limited validity for insomnia classification. However, it should be noted that studies employing clustering methods for empirical identification of diagnostic subtypes at best represent proxies to true validity tests since they can be and usually are limited by the variables selected for conducting the cluster analysis. Although such variables are selected for their presumed relevance to the diagnoses in question, it is possible that the sets employed for the studies described were collectively inadequate for assessing the set of disorders in question. Hence, results of such studies should be considered with this limitation in mind.

A somewhat different approach to assessing the validity of insomnia diagnoses was employed by Edinger, Kirby, et al. (2004) as part of their efforts to develop research diagnostic criteria for insomnia disorders. The approach used entailed a systematic literature review to identify the insomnia diagnostic subtypes that have evidence supporting their validity. Evidence supporting the validity of these subtypes was taken from various types of studies, including (1) studies that demonstrated significant difference between one or more insomnia subtypes and normal sleepers/controls, (2) studies that showed differences between two or more insomnia subtypes or between an insomnia subtype and other types of sleep disorders, (3) comparisons showing differences between one or more insomnia subtypes and normative data, and (4) comparisons showing differences in the treatment responsiveness of two or more insomnia subtypes undergoing the same insomnia treatment. From the results of the systematic review, these authors concluded that the best-supported insomnia diagnoses included DSM-IV primary insomnia and insomnia due to a mental disorder as well as the ICSD subtypes psychophysiological insomnia and paradoxical insomnia. However, this sort of literature review admittedly is a "piecemeal approach" toward testing the validity of a classification system as a whole since it considers only a few subtypes at a time, and it does so on a retrospective basis. With this sort of approach, it is not possible to ascertain whether a particular classification scheme is optimal for classifying the array of disorders it considers.

In a more indirect test of validity, Buysse et al. (1997) examined the effect of DSM-IV and ICSD insomnia diagnoses on clinicians' treatment decisions. In this study both sleep specialists and non-specialists were first asked to use both DSM-IV and ICSD criteria to diagnose a series of insomnia sufferers they interviewed. Subsequently they were asked to rate the applicability of a range of treatment/management strategies that might be used to address each patient's complaint. Results of these hypothetical treatment assignments are shown in Figure 21.3. This figure shows the effects of diagnosis on treatment assignments.

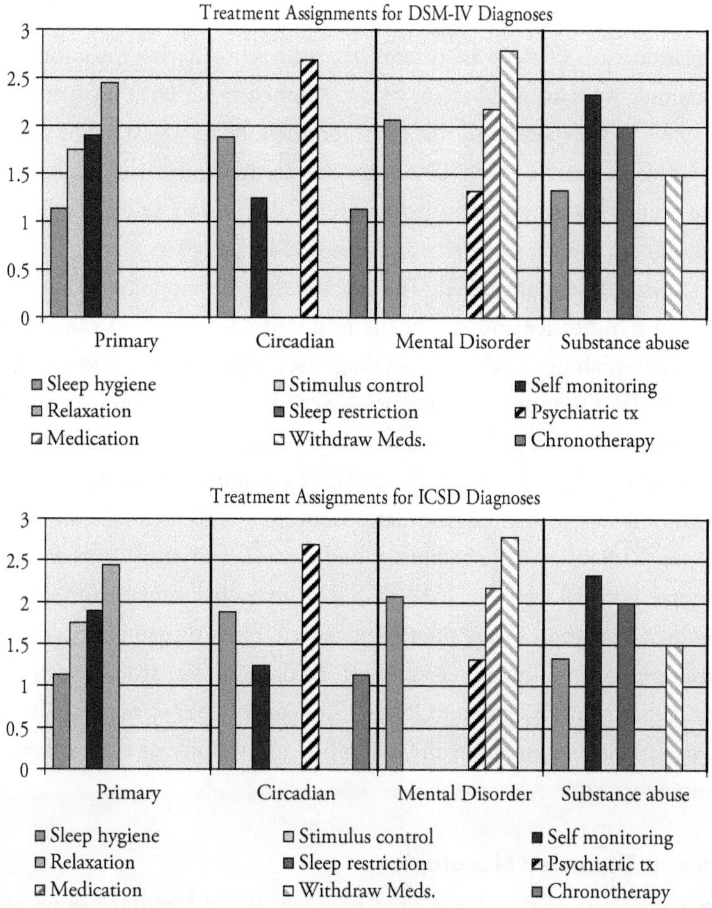

Figure 21.3 Treatment assignments by diagnoses
Note: DSM-IV = *Diagnostic and Statistical Manual of Mental Disorders*, 4th ed.; ICSD = *International Classification of Sleep Disorders*; tx = treatment.

Specifically, this figure shows that the clinicians assigned distinctive combinations of intervention strategies to the distinctive insomnia diagnoses within both the DSM-IV and ICSD nosologies. Admittedly, such findings provide no information about the effectiveness of such treatment matching, but they do connote the potential importance physicians place on specific insomnia diagnoses in their treatment decision-making. Thus, in an indirect manner, such findings provide comment on the validity of these diagnoses for predicting treatment needs and response.

Perhaps the most omnibus test of the ICSD and DSM systems was reported by Edinger et al. (2011). In their study, Edinger and colleagues tested the reliability and validity of the ICSD-2 and DSM-IV-TR insomnia classification systems in a large study sample (N = 352) using a multitrait/multimethod correlational research design. Within this study, three clinical pairs at each of two study sites were asked to use distinctive assessment methods (structured interviews, unstructured interviews, unstructured interviews plus examination of sleep laboratory recordings) to derive insomnia diagnoses in study patients they were assigned to interview. After each patient they interviewed, clinicians were asked to independently rate the goodness of fit of 10 DSM-IV-TR and 37 ICSD-2 insomnia diagnoses using 100-point visual analogue rating scales. Correlations of diagnostic ratings within clinician pairs were then used to assess the reliabilities of the diagnoses examined, whereas correlations across clinician pairs were used to assess the validities of the diagnoses considered. The authors then developed a rating system, based on the statistical significance and size of the resultant reliability and validity coefficients, to evaluate the acceptability of the various diagnoses tested. Results showed that the best-supported DSM-IV-TR insomnia categories were insomnia related to another mental disorder, insomnia due to a general medical condition, breathing-related sleep disorder, and circadian rhythm sleep disorder. The ICSD-2 categories receiving the strongest support were insomnia due to mental disorder, insomnia due to medical condition, obstructive sleep apnea, RLS, idiopathic insomnia, and circadian rhythm sleep disorder–delayed sleep phase type. Surprisingly the DSM-IV-TR primary insomnia diagnosis and most of the related ICSD-2 diagnoses were poorly supported, likely due to their symptom overlap with the various comorbid insomnia subtypes. To date, similar studies with the full sleep disorder nosologies provided in the DSM-IV-TR and ICSD-2 manuals have yet to be conducted, so little is known about the reliability and validity of sleep diagnoses outside of the insomnia sections.

Current Sleep Disorder Nosologies

Despite the limitations of the above-cited research, it did highlight some of the weaknesses of prior efforts to develop universally useful sleep disorder classification schemes. In particular, the studies showing discordance among the previous nosologies created confusion for clinicians and sleep researchers alike. Fortunately, nosologists working with the AASM, the WHO, and the APA recognized the confusion caused by the discordance among the previous diagnostic systems they had developed. As a result, they collectively made increased efforts to collaborate on revisions of the prior diagnostic systems they had provided and to develop consensus about the sleep disorders that should be included in the subsequent current classification scheme. These efforts were readily apparent in the development of the DSM-5 (APA, 2013) and ICSD-3 (AASM, 2014) manuals that currently are available and used for sleep disorder classification and diagnosis. In fact, many of those sleep experts served on workgroups or as advisors in the crafting of these two systems. Moreover, there have been efforts to collaborate with the WHO to encourage its acceptance of the ICSD-3/DSM-5 diagnostic scheme for sleep disorders into the newer ICD version, the ICD-11 (WHO, 2019). These various collaborative efforts have generally been successful and have resulted in reasonably concordant sleep disorder nosologies. Tables 21.2–21.4 display the ICSD-3, DSM-5, and ICD-11 classification schemes for the currently recognized sleep disorders. As can be seen, these systems agree in their listing of six major sleep disorder categories: insomnia disorders, hypersomnolence disorders, sleep-related breathing disorders, circadian rhythm

Table 21.2 *International Classification of Sleep Disorders*, third edition, sleep disorders and *International Classification of Diseases*, 10th revision, *Clinical Modification*, codes

	Insomnia
F51.01	Chronic insomnia disorder
F51.02	Short-term insomnia disorder
F51.09	Other insomnia disorder
	Sleep-related breathing disorders
	Obstructive sleep apnea
G47.33	Obstructive sleep apnea (adult and pediatric)
	Central sleep apnea syndromes
R06.3	Central sleep apnea with Cheyne-Stokes breathing
G47.37	Central sleep apnea due to a medical disorder without Cheyne-Stokes breathing
G47.32	Central sleep apnea due to high-altitude periodic breathing
G47.39	Central sleep apnea due to a medication or substance
G47.31	Primary central sleep apnea
P28.3	Primary central sleep apnea of infancy
P28.4	Primary central apnea of prematurity
G47.39	Treatment-emergent central sleep apnea
	Sleep-related hypoventilation disorders
E66.2	Obesity hypoventilation syndrome
G47.35	Congenital central alveolar hypoventilation syndrome
G47.36	Late-onset central hypoventilation with hypothalamic dysfunction
G47.34	Idiopathic central alveolar hypoventilation
G47.36	Sleep-related hypoventilation due to a medication or substance
G47.36	Sleep-related hypoventilation due to a medical disorder
	Sleep-related hypoxemia disorder
G47.36	Sleep-related hypoxemia
	Central disorders of hypersomnolence
G47.411	Narcolepsy Type 1
G47.419	Narcolepsy Type 2
G47.11	Idiopathic hypersomnia
G47.13	Kleine-Levin syndrome
G47.14	Hypersomnia due to a medical disorder
F11–F19	Hypersomnia due to a medication or substance
F51.13	Hypersomnia associated with a psychiatric disorder
F51.12	Insufficient sleep syndrome
	Circadian rhythm sleep–wake disorders
G47.21	Delayed sleep–wake phase disorder
G47.22	Advanced sleep–wake phase disorder
G47.23	Irregular sleep–wake rhythm disorder
G47.24	Non-24-hour sleep–wake rhythm disorder
G47.26	Shift-work disorder
G47.25	Jet lag disorder
G47.20	Circadian sleep–wake disorder not otherwise specified

Continued

Table 21.2 Continued	
	Parasomnias
	NREM-related parasomnias
G47.51	Confusional arousals
F51.3	Sleepwalking
F51.4	Sleep terrors
G47.59	Sleep-related eating disorder
	REM-related parasomnias
G47.52	REM sleep behavior disorder
G47.53	Recurrent isolated sleep paralysis
F51.5	Nightmare disorder
	Other parasomnias
G47.59	Exploding head syndrome
H53.16	Sleep-related hallucinations
N39.44	Sleep enuresis
G47.54	Parasomnia due to a medical disorder
F11–F19	Parasomnia due to a medication or substance
G47.50	Parasomnia, unspecified
	Sleep-related movement disorders
G25.81	Restless legs syndrome
G47.61	Periodic limb movement disorder
G47.62	Sleep-related leg cramps
G47.63	Sleep-related bruxism
G47.69	Sleep-related rhythmic movement disorder
G47.69	Benign sleep myoclonus of infancy
G47.69	Propriospinal myoclonus at sleep onset
G47.69	Sleep-related movement disorder due to a medical disorder
F11–F19	Sleep-related movement disorder due to a medication or substance
G47.69	Sleep-related movement disorder, unspecified
G47.8	Other sleep disorder

Note. NREM = non-rapid eye movement; REM = rapid eye movement.

sleep-wake disorders, parasomnias, and sleep-related movement disorders. Furthermore, the specific sleep disorder diagnoses listed within each of the major categories are largely concordant as well, although their definitions and criteria vary somewhat across systems. Nonetheless, the congruence among these systems has gone a long way toward facilitating communication among clinicians using these different systems, and it also has provided sleep researchers standard and consistent diagnostic subtypes for their current and future research.

To date, there has been relatively limited research evaluating these systems individually or in comparison to their current or previous counterparts. One study by K. F. Chung et al. (2015) conducted an epidemiological community survey with a sample of 2,011 respondents to examine the prevalence of insomnia disorders using criteria from the DSM-IV, ICD10, ICSD-2, and DSM-5. Results showed prevalence rates of 22.1%, 4.7%, 15.1%, and 10.8%, respectively for DSM-IV, ICD10, ICSD-2, and DSM-5, with the differences in these prevalence rates attributed to discordance between the criteria sets used among the older systems and between these older systems and the newer DSM-5. In another study, Taylor et al. (2018) used a structured interview to assign DSM-5 sleep disorder diagnoses to each individual in a sample of 106 military veterans presenting to participate in a research trial. Inter-rater reliabilities (kappa values) were found to be good to excellent for a range of sleep disorders ascertained including insomnia (1.0), RLS (0.83), nightmare disorder (0.78), obstructive sleep apnea–hypopnea (0.73), hypersomnolence (0.50), and circadian rhythm sleep–wake disorders (0.50). In another study Loddo et al. (2019) had three interviewers conduct independent

Table 21.3 *Diagnostic and Statistical Manual of Mental Disorders*, fifth edition, sleep–wake disorders and *International Classification of Diseases*, 10th revision, *Clinical Modification*, codes

F51.01	Insomnia disorder
F51.11	Hypersomnolence disorder
	Narcolepsy
G47.411	Narcolepsy with cataplexy or hypocretin deficiency (Type 1)
G47.419	Narcolepsy without cataplexy and either without hypocretin deficiency or hypocretin unmeasured
G47.421	Narcolepsy with cataplexy or hypocretin deficiency due to a medical condition
G47.429	Narcolepsy without cataplexy and without hypocretin deficiency due to a medical condition
	Breathing-related sleep disorders
G47.33	Obstructive sleep hypopnea
	Central sleep apnea
G47.31	Idiopathic central sleep apnea
R06.3	Cheyne-Stokes breathing
G47.37	Central sleep apnea comorbid with opioid use
	Sleep-related hypoventilation
G47.31	Idiopathic hypoventilation
G47.35	Congenital central alveolar hypoventilation
G47.36	Comorbid sleep-related hypoventilation
	Circadian rhythm sleep–wake disorders
G47.21	Delayed sleep phase type
G47.22	Advanced sleep phase type
G47.23	Irregular sleep–wake type
G47.24	Non-24-hour sleep–wake type
G47.26	Shift-work type
G47.20	Unspecified type
	Parasomnias
	Non-rapid-eye-movement sleep arousal disorders
F51.3	Sleepwalking type
F51.4	Sleep terror type
F51.5	Nightmare disorder
G47.52	Rapid-eye-movement sleep behavior disorder

Continued

Table 21.3 *Continued*	
G25.81	Restless legs syndrome
	Substance-/medication-induced sleep disorder
F10.182	Alcohol, with mild use disorder
F10.282	Alcohol, with moderate use or severe use disorder
F10.982	Alcohol, without use disorder
F15.982	Caffeine, without use disorder
F12.188	Cannabis, with mild use disorder
F12.288	Cannabis, with moderate or severe use disorder
F12.988	Cannabis, without use disorder
F11.182	Opioid, with mild use disorder
F11.282	Opioid, with moderate or severe use disorder
F11.982	Opioid, without use disorder
F13.182	Sedative, hypnotic, or anxiolytic, with mild use disorder
F13.282	Sedative, hypnotic, or anxiolytic, with moderate or severe use disorder
F13.982	Sedative, hypnotic, or anxiolytic, without use disorder
F15.182	Amphetamine-type substance (or other stimulant) with mild use disorder
F15.282	Amphetamine-type substance (or other stimulant), with moderate or severe use disorder
F15.982	Amphetamine-type substance (or other stimulant), without use disorder
F14.182	Cocaine, with mild use disorder
F14.282	Cocaine, with moderate or severe use disorder
F14.982	Cocaine, without use disorder
F17.208	Tobacco, with moderate or severe use disorder
	Other (or unknown) substance, with mild use disorder
	Other (or unknown)
G47.09	Other specified insomnia disorder
G47.00	Unspecified insomnia disorder
G47.19	Other specified hypersomnolence disorder
G47.10	Unspecified hypersomnolence disorder
G47.8	Other specified sleep–wake disorder
G47.9	Unspecified sleep–wake disorder

interviews with a series of 126 patients to evaluate the reliability of their ICSD-3 arousal disorder diagnostic assignments. Results of this study showed excellent reliability (kappa values) for the diagnoses of confusional arousal (0.89), sleepwalking (0.87), and sleep terrors (0.87). Although promising, further tests of the reliability of the range of diagnoses listed in the three current sleep disorder nosologies are needed. Moreover, tests of the overall validity of these systems have yet to be conducted. Nonetheless, the improved concordance of these systems represents a major step forward in sleep disorder classification and provides a more consistent basis for sleep disorder diagnosis in clinical practice.

Table 21.4 *International Classification of Diseases*, 11th revision, sleep–wake disorders and codes

Insomnia disorders 7A00 Chronic insomnia 7A01 Short-term insomnia 7A0Z Insomnia disorders, unspecified
Hypersomnolence disorders 7A20 Narcolepsy 7A20.0 Narcolepsy, Type 1 7A20.1 Narcolepsy, Type 2 7A20.Z Narcolepsy, unspecified 7A21 Idiopathic hypersomnia 7A22 Kleine-Levin syndrome 7A23 Hypersomnia due to a medical condition 7A24 Hypersomnia due to a medication or substance 7A25 Hypersomnia associated with a mental disorder 7A26 Insufficient sleep syndrome 7A2Y Other specified hypersomnolence disorders 7S2Z Hypersomnolence disorders, unspecified
Sleep-related breathing disorders 7A40 Central sleep apneas 7A40.0 Primary central sleep apnea 7A40.1 Primary central sleep apnea of infancy 7A40.2 Primary central sleep apnea of prematurity 7A40.3 Central sleep apnea due to a medical condition with Cheyne-Stokes breathing 7A40.4 Central sleep apnea due to a medical condition without Cheyne-Stokes breathing 7A40.5 Central sleep apnea due to high-altitude periodic breathing 7A40.6 Central sleep apnea due to a medication or substance 7A40.Y Other specified central sleep apneas 7A40.Z Central sleep apneas, unspecified 7A41 Obstructive sleep apnea 7A42 Sleep-related hypoventilation syndrome 7A42.1 Congenital central alveolar sleep-related hypoventilation 7A42.3 Idiopathic central alveolar hypoventilation 7A42.4 Sleep-related hypoventilation due to a medication or substance 7A42.5 Sleep-related hypoventilation due to medical condition 7A42.6 Sleep-related hypoxemia due to a medical condition 7A42.Y Other specified sleep-related hypoventilation or hypoxemia disorders 7A42.Z Sleep-related hypoventilation or hypoxemia disorders unspecified MD11.4 Sleep-related Cheyne-Stokes respiration 7A4Y Other specified sleep-related breathing disorders 7A4Z Sleep-related breathing disorders, unspecified
Circadian rhythm sleep–wake disorders 7A60 Delayed sleep–wake phase disorder 7A61 Advanced sleep–wake phase disorder 7A62 Irregular sleep–wake rhythm disorder 7A63 Non-24-hour sleep–wake rhythm disorder 7A64 Circadian rhythm sleep–wake disorder, shift-work type 7A65 Circadian rhythm sleep–wake disorder, jet lag type 7A6Z Circadian rhythm sleep–wake disorders, unspecified

Continued

Table 21.4 *Continued*
Sleep-related movement disorders
7A80 Restless legs syndrome
7A81 Periodic limb movement disorder
7A82 Sleep-related leg cramps
7A83 Sleep-related bruxism
7A84 Sleep-related rhythmic movement disorder
7A85 Benign sleep myoclonus of infancy
7A86 Propriospinal myoclonus at sleep onset
7A87 Sleep-related movement disorder due to a medical condition
7A88 Sleep-related movement disorder due to a medication or substance
7B01.0 REM sleep behavior disorder
7A8Y Other specified sleep-related movement disorders
7A8Z Sleep-related movement disorders, unspecified
Parasomnia disorders
7B00 Disorders of arousal from non-REM sleep
7B00.0 Confusional arousals
7B00.1 Sleepwalking disorder
7B00.2 Sleep terrors
7B00.3 Sleep-related eating disorder
7B00.Y Other specified disorders of arousal from non-REM sleep
7B00.Z Disorders of arousal from non-REM sleep, unspecified
7B01 Parasomnias related to REM sleep
7B01.0 REM sleep behavior disorder
7B01.1 Recurrent isolated sleep paralysis
7B01.2 Nightmare disorder
7B01.Y Other specified parasomnias related to REM sleep
7B01.Z Parasomnias related to REM sleep, unspecified
7B02 Other parasomnias
7B02.0 Hypnagogic exploding head syndrome
7B02.1 Sleep-related hallucinations
7B02.2 Parasomnia disorder due to a medical condition
7B02.3 Parasomnia due to a medication or substance
6C00.0 Nocturnal enuresis
7B0Y Other specified parasomnia disorders
7B0Z Parasomnia disorders, unspecified
7B2Y Other specified sleep–wake disorders
7B2Z Sleep–wake disorders, unspecified

Note. REM = rapid eye movement.

Diagnosis

Even with the most reliable and valid classification system, accurate diagnosis of sleep disorders rests upon a comprehensive evaluation. This principle applies to all clinical disorders, but it is particularly true for sleep disorders because sleep is affected by a host of psychological, medical, environmental, and circadian factors. A comprehensive evaluation should include a clinical interview, screening questionnaires, prospective self-monitoring of sleep, laboratory tests (PSG, Multiple Sleep Latency Test [MSLT]), and other ancillary assessment procedures (actigraphy). The diagnosis of some disorders (e.g., insomnia) is based predominantly on clinical assessment, whereas a diagnostic procedure such as PSG is necessary to confirm the presence and severity of other disorders (e.g., sleep apnea). In this section, we discuss the role and limitations of these assessment methods in making a sleep disorder diagnosis. A more detailed description of clinical, ambulatory, and laboratory assessment is presented in the next few chapters.

Role and Limitations of the Clinical Interview

The clinical interview is the most important assessment component for any sleep disorder. Patients with sleep complaints usually report different nighttime and daytime symptoms that may involve difficulties sleeping at night, abnormal behaviors and movements during the sleep period, and undesired or excessive sleepiness during the day. These complaints are not mutually exclusive as a patient may report mixed trouble sleeping at night with excessive sleepiness during the day. The clinical interview may reveal that sleep difficulties are associated with recent stressful life events (e.g., separation), whereas daytime sleepiness may result from disrupted or shortened sleep. A clinical interview is, thus, essential to derive an accurate diagnosis.

The interview should gather detailed information about the nature of the presenting sleep complaint, psychiatric and medical history, use of prescribed and over-the-counter medications as well as other substances, history of alcohol and drug use, psychosocial and family history, and previous treatments and their outcomes. The sleep history is particularly important and should elicit the chief complaint (insomnia, daytime sleepiness, sleepwalking), its duration (acute vs. chronic) and course (recurrent, persistent), as well as information about the patient's typical sleep schedule (bedtime, arising time, naps). A detailed analysis of precipitating, perpetuating, and alleviating factors, as well as perceived daytime impairments is particularly important for a condition such as insomnia. Aside from differential diagnosis, the functional analysis is helpful to derive a case formulation and a treatment plan (Edinger & Carney, 2015; Manber & Carney, 2015; Morin & Espie, 2003).

Several standardized interviews have been developed to gather critical information for making a differential sleep disorder diagnosis. For example, the Structured Clinical Interview for DSM-5 Sleep Disorders was developed to assist in the assessment of sleep disorders. Inter-rater reliability was found to vary from moderate to excellent for six of the nine disorders covered by the interview—insomnia, hypersomnolence, obstructive sleep apnea, circadian rhythm sleep–wake, nightmare, and RLS disorders (Taylor et al., 2018). The Duke Structured Interview for Sleep Disorders (Edinger, Kirby, et al., 2004) is a comprehensive interview that was originally based on ICSD-2 and DSM-IV-TR criteria but since has been updated to provide DSM-5 and ICSD-3 diagnoses; it provides a series of systematic and structured questions around the different disorders and is accompanied by symptom checklists completed by patients. The Insomnia Interview Schedule (Morin, 1993) was designed primarily for individuals suspected of insomnia. It provides a semi-structured format to gather information about the nature, severity, impact, and course of insomnia and includes key questions to guide the functional analysis and rule out other sleep disorders. Those interviews just described are helpful to standardize the assessment process and improve the diagnostic reliability of sleep disorders; however, they are all designed for use by someone who has some knowledge of and experience in sleep medicine.

Because sleep disorder patients are often unaware of some symptoms they display during their sleep, interviewing a patient's bed partner can yield very valuable diagnostic information. The bed partner is likely to provide a more accurate description of some diagnostically important symptoms for certain types of sleep problems. For example, patients with sleep apnea are usually unaware of their snoring or breathing pauses during sleep, two core symptoms of sleep apnea. Likewise, patients suffering from sleepwalking or sleep terrors often have no recollection of these events the next day; the bed partner (or parent) represents an important source of information to describe the nature and timing of occurrence of these abnormal phenomena during sleep. REM behavior disorder is often brought to the attention of clinicians when a spouse or bed partner has been injured as a result of the abrupt and repetitive movements of the limbs during sleep, all unknown to the patient suffering from this condition. Because some patients may underestimate the impact of daytime sleepiness on social or occupational functioning, a significant other, whether sharing the same bed or not, may provide a more accurate evaluation of the significance of this symptom in the context of certain sleep disorders.

The clinical interview may be sufficient in some cases to make a provisional diagnosis and even initiate treatment. For instance, the diagnosis of insomnia, RLS, and circadian disorders is based primarily on clinical history. In other cases, additional assessment and diagnostic procedures are required to rule out several conditions and make a more definitive diagnosis. Even when the diagnosis seems clear after the clinical interview, PSG may be necessary to determine the severity of the sleep disorder and the most appropriate treatment.

Indications for PSG

PSG is considered the gold standard for measuring sleep and is essential to confirm the diagnosis of several disorders such as sleep apnea, periodic limb movements, narcolepsy, and some parasomnias (e.g., REM behavior disorder; Kushida et al., 2005). The main reason for this is that patients are typically unaware of many symptoms of such disorders since they present only during the sleep period. Nocturnal PSG is a procedure that involves continuous monitoring of several electrophysiological parameters (EEG, electromyography, electro-oculography) that are used to distinguish sleep from wakefulness and to quantify the proportion of time spent in different sleep stages throughout the night. Concurrent monitoring of respiration, oxygen saturation, and limb movements allows for detecting and measuring the severity of core symptoms (breathing pauses, leg movements) of selected sleep disorders. PSG can also provide very valuable data to assess the severity of sleep disturbances in insomnia; however, it is not considered an essential procedure for this condition as the diagnosis of insomnia is based on the patient's subjective complaint (Schutte-Rodin et al., 2008). Nonetheless, it can provide useful information to assess the extent of sleep state misperception, a common feature among patients with a diagnosis of insomnia. Sometimes, insomnia is the presenting complaint, but PSG assessment reveals other abnormalities that are diagnostic of another sleep disorder. For instance, increasing evidence suggests that sleep apnea is often comorbid with insomnia (Sweetman et al., 2021).

The MSLT is a daytime laboratory test conducted after a full night of PSG recording. During the MSLT, the patient is offered five 20-minute nap opportunities at 2-hour intervals throughout the day. The average latency to the onset of sleep during these five tests yields an objective measure of daytime sleepiness. Individuals who are well rested and without sleep disorders usually take more than 10 minutes to fall asleep or do not fall asleep at all. A sleep latency shorter than 5 minutes is considered pathological and is associated with significant risks of falling asleep at inappropriate times and places such as while driving. The MSLT should be an integral component of the evaluation whenever daytime alertness is compromised. It is particularly useful to determine the degree of impairment associated with disorders such as sleep apnea and narcolepsy. It is also used to detect daytime REM sleep propensity as conveyed by early-onset REM sleep during MSLT naps, a confirmatory diagnostic marker of narcolepsy (Littner et al., 2005). Patients with narcolepsy enter REM sleep much faster than normal sleepers, and the presence of two or more sleep onset REM episodes during the MSLT is considered diagnostic of narcolepsy. The Maintenance of Wakefulness Test is a related daytime test during which the patient is instructed to try to stay awake rather than to go to sleep; also a measure of excessive daytime sleepiness, this test is not used as frequently as the MSLT.

Nocturnal PSG and daytime MSLT together provide for a comprehensive assessment of sleep disorders. These diagnostic procedures are indicated when the presenting complaint is excessive daytime sleepiness and when symptoms of sleep apnea, narcolepsy, periodic limb movements, and several other conditions are present (Kushida et al., 2005). PSG is not recommended for the routine evaluation of insomnia or circadian disorders. The diagnosis of these conditions is based on a clinical evaluation, sleep diary monitoring, and assessment of rest–activity cycles with actigraphy. The diagnostic value of a single night of PSG for many parasomnias is unclear as these conditions rarely occur on a nightly basis.

The Role of Patient Questionnaires

There is a wide variety of questionnaires that can be completed by patients to complement the clinical evaluation of sleep disorders. Some of these are primarily designed as general screening measures, whereas others are used to evaluate the severity and impact of sleep disorders or to assess the presumed mediating factors of a given disorder (e.g., dysfunctional sleep beliefs in insomnia). Because of the large number of these measures, our present discussion is limited only to a sample of screening measures that can assist clinicians in the diagnosis of selected sleep disorders (see Table 21.5).

Table 21.5 Screening measures for sleep disorders

Insomnia Severity Index (Morin et al., 2011)	Seven-item rating scale used to assess insomnia severity (score range: 0–28; normal <8; subthreshold 8–13; moderate insomnia 14–21; severe 22–28).
Pittsburgh Sleep Quality Index (Buysse et al., 1989)	Nineteen self-rated items assessing sleep quality and disturbances over a 1-month interval. A summary score ranging from 0 to 21 can be derived from seven component scores.
Patient-Reported Outcomes Information System (PROMIS; Buysse et al., 2010)	Self-report questions assessing sleep disturbance (27 items) and sleep-related impairments (16 items). Instrument developed as part of PROMIS, a National Institutes of Health Roadmap initiative.
Epworth Sleepiness Scale (Johns, 1991)	Eight-item self-report questionnaire used to assess subjective sleepiness (score range: 0–24; normal <10).
Stanford Sleepiness Scale (Hoddes et al., 1973)	A single seven-point item rating scale of sleepiness.
Karolinska Sleepiness Scale (Akerstedt & Gillberg, 1990)	A single nine-point item rating scale of state sleepiness.
The STOP-Bang Questionnaire (F. Chung et al., 2008)	Ten-item questionnaire used to assess the risk of sleep apnea (three risk categories from high to low).
Restless Legs Syndrome Scale (Walters et al., 2003)	Ten-item rating scale used to evaluate severity and impact of restless legs syndrome (score range: 0–40; 0–10, mild; 11–20, moderate; 21–30, severe; 31–40, very severe)
Morningness–Eveningness Questionnaire (Horne & Ostberg, 1976)	Nineteen-item questionnaire that provides information about circadian tendencies (score range: 16–86; high scores (59–86) correspond to morning-type, low scores (16–41) correspond to evening-type, and scores from 42 to 58 refer to an intermediate type.

The Insomnia Severity Index is a seven-item scale measuring the severity and impact of insomnia (Morin et al., 2011); it is widely used as a screening as well as an outcome measure in clinical trials. A score of 14 or greater is suggestive of moderate to severe insomnia. The Pittsburgh Sleep Quality Index is a general measure of sleep quality that also screens for several sleep disorders (Buysse et al., 1989). The Epworth Sleepiness Scale (Johns, 1991) is a global and retrospective measure assessing the likelihood (on a 4-point scale) of falling asleep in eight different situations (e.g., sitting and reading, watching TV, driving a car); a score greater than 10 suggests significant sleepiness. Two additional single-item scales can provide useful screening data on daytime sleepiness. The Stanford Sleepiness Scale (Hoddes et al., 1973) is a 7-point Likert scale measuring subjective sleepiness at a specific moment in time. The Karolinska Sleepiness Scale (Akerstedt & Gillberg, 1990) is a similar 9-point state measure of sleepiness. The STOP-Bang Questionnaire is a widely used screening questionnaire assessing the risk of obstructive sleep apnea based on core signs, symptoms, and clinical features of the disorder (snoring, breathing pauses, sleepiness, blood pressure, BMI, age, neck circumference, and gender; F. Chung et al., 2016). The Restless Legs Syndrome Rating Scale is a 10-item scale that measures several nighttime and daytime components of restless legs; it yields a global severity score ranging from mild to very severe (The International Restless Legs Syndrome Study Group, 2003). The Morningness–Eveningness Questionnaire (Horne & Ostberg, 1976) is a 19-item scale that provides information about circadian preferences; it is helpful in the assessment of circadian disorders.

While there are multiple other sleep-related questionnaires, the self-report questionnaires just described provide a cut-point to assess the likelihood of a sleep disorder (e.g., insomnia, RLS, sleep apnea) or the severity of its core symptoms. The diagnostic specificity, sensitivity, and clinical utility of these instruments are quite variable; but in general, these instruments are designed to serve as initial screening assessment devices even before a clinical interview is conducted. It is important to keep in mind, however, that none of these questionnaires have been specifically validated to make a formal diagnosis. As such, they should not be used in isolation as evidence of a sleep disorder diagnosis. Rather, they should be used as complementary tools to the other clinical and laboratory assessment procedures.

Assessment of psychological symptoms may be indicated for patients with some sleep disorders. Although any sleep disorder can be associated with comorbid psychopathology, the prevalence of psychiatric disorders is particularly high among patients with insomnia (Hertenstein et al., 2019) and higher than with any other sleep disorders. Psychopathology is less frequent among patients with sleep apnea, circadian disorders, and even parasomnias such as sleepwalking and night terrors. The most reliable strategy for determining the presence of psychopathology is to incorporate key questions from the Structured Clinical Interview for DSM-5 (APA, 2013) into the clinical interview, along with questions about past psychiatric history and treatment. Also, there are abbreviated interviews for screening for psychiatric disorders (e.g., Primary Care Evaluation for Mental Disorders [PRIME-MD]) which may also serve this purpose. When there is no indication of major psychopathology, a more cost-effective approach is to use brief screening questionnaires that target specific psychological symptoms (e.g., anxiety, depression). Instruments such as the PHQ-9 (nine-item Patient Health Questionnaire; Kroenke et al., 2001) and the GAD-7 (seven-item Generalized Anxiety Disorder; Spitzer et al., 2006) are particularly helpful to screen for depression and anxiety, respectively, although neither of those self-report measures should be used alone to make a diagnosis. Psychometric screening should always be complemented by a clinical interview.

When there is evidence of coexisting sleep and psychiatric disorders, such a finding does not necessarily imply that the sleep disorder is secondary to the concurrent psychiatric condition. For instance, when insomnia is comorbid with depression, the nature and direction of the relationship between those two conditions are not always clear and may actually change over time. A clinical interview is helpful to determine what should be the main focus of treatment, although it is often necessary to target both conditions.

Consideration of the sleep disorder as a comorbid condition will also have implications for treatment in that it connotes that the sleep complaints may warrant independent therapeutic attention.

Other Assessment Methods

Prospective daily sleep diary monitoring can provide useful data for making the diagnosis of some sleep disorders, particularly insomnia and some circadian rhythm disorders (Buysse et al., 2006). A typical sleep diary includes entries for bedtime, arising time, sleep latency, number and duration of awakenings, total sleep time, naps, use of sleep aids, and various indices of sleep quality and daytime functioning (Carney et al., 2012). These data provide information about a patient's sleep schedule, the nature of sleep difficulties, and their frequency and intensity, all of which may vary considerably from a patient's global evaluation obtained during the interview and from PSG assessment. Self-monitoring also offers valuable information about variability in sleep schedules and timing of sleep, two important features for diagnosing circadian rhythm disorders such as advanced and delayed sleep phase syndromes. It may also yield valuable diagnostic information to aid in determining when excessive daytime sleepiness is due to insufficient sleep rather than being the result of other primary sleep disorders. In addition, self-monitoring of the timing of unusual events at night can assist in differentiating between nightmares and sleep terrors.

Several behavioral assessment devices are increasingly used to monitor sleep–wake patterns. Of these, wrist actigraphy is the best-validated device for ambulatory data collection. This activity-based monitoring system uses a microprocessor to record and store wrist movement along with the actual clock time. Data are processed through microcomputer software, and an algorithm is used to estimate sleep and wake based on wrist activity. The presence of motor activity is interpreted as wakefulness, and the absence of activity is interpreted as sleep. This device, as well as other behavioral assessment devices, does not measure sleep stages. Despite this limitation, wrist actigraphy remains a useful assessment procedure for monitoring sleep–wake schedules and provides useful diagnostic information for insomnia and some circadian disorders related to advanced and delayed sleep phases (Smith et al., 2018). More information on actigraphy is available in Chapter 26 of this book.

With continued advances in technology, many forms of wearable devices have been introduced. While many of these monitors utilize similar technology to that used in actigraphy to monitor movement and calculate sleep/wake parameters, others include additional physiological measures such as electrocardiography and plethysmography that can facilitate the identification of symptoms associated with sleep disorders, for example, sleep apnea. Moreover, some of these wearable devices attempt to categorize sleep beyond a sleep/wake dichotomy by attempting to distinguish, for example, light versus deep sleep or REM versus non-REM sleep. Validation data to support these additional sleep classifications with wearable devices is limited, however (de Zambotti et al., 2019). Moreover, de Zambotti et al. (2024) note that most validation studies have been conducted with young and healthy adults, which greatly limits the generalizability of their findings. Contactless devices have also been developed. These do not require that the individual wear the device. Instead, these devices may rely on various forms of infrared detection (e.g., cameras or thermometers to monitor body temperature), bed sensors, sonar/radar detection, or sounds; but their ability to accurately classify sleep is not well established (Ibanez et al., 2019). While Ibanez et al. (2019) caution that contactless devices may be less accurate than those requiring direct contact, Chinoy et al. (2021) noted that both types of devices (e.g., contact and contactless devices), when compared to PSG, perform equally well as or better than actigraphy. Regardless, this area of sleep assessment is in its infancy, and research with a broader range of participants more representative of the population and with a variety of sleep disorders is necessary.

Challenge of Differential Diagnosis

The differential diagnosis of sleep disorders can be quite challenging for clinicians with more limited experience. This is true for most clinical disorders but more so for sleep disorders because sleep is affected by a host of psychological, medical, pharmacological, environmental, and circadian factors. In clinical practice, the differential diagnosis requires a very systematic evaluation to rule in or out the various potential contributing factors for any single sleep disorder.

Even with a systematic assessment, accurate diagnosis may be complicated by several factors. First, there are numerous sleep disorders (more than 70 described in the ICSD-3) with many overlapping symptoms among some of them. For example, a complaint of difficulties initiating sleep at bedtime, a classic symptom of insomnia, may be due to restless legs, an anxiety disorder, or even a circadian-based phase delay disorder. Likewise, difficulty maintaining sleep at night, another common insomnia symptom, may result from periodic limb movements, recurrent nightmares, or even a sleep-related breathing disorder. Thus, the same presenting symptom can be associated with multiple disorders. Another reason that may complicate diagnosis is that patients are not always aware of symptoms occurring during sleep. For example, snoring, breathing pauses, and leg movements during sleep are typically noted by the bed partner, not by the individual with a sleep disorder, hence the importance of interviewing the bed partner whenever feasible.

Not only is the differential diagnosis difficult among sleep disorders, it can also be complicated to distinguish some sleep disorders, such as insomnia disorder, from mental disorders. Because of the extensive comorbidity between insomnia and psychiatric disorders, this challenge usually arises for insomnia comorbid with anxiety (generalized anxiety disorder [GAD]) or depression (dysthymia or major depression). The differential diagnosis is not always clear because several symptoms (e.g., sleep disturbance, fatigue, mood and cognitive problems) overlap among these conditions. For example, excessive worrying is the predominant feature in GAD; this symptom is also present in insomnia disorder, although the main source of worry is limited to poor sleep and its potential consequences, whereas in GAD worrying is about multiple sources (e.g., health, family, work). In depression, the predominant symptoms are sadness and loss of interest. In insomnia disorder, the interest is present, but there is a lack of energy or fatigue, presumably resulting from sleep disturbances, preventing the individual from engaging in potentially pleasurable activities or social interactions. From this discussion, it becomes clear that the clinical interview is critical to derive an accurate diagnosis. In addition to the nature of the symptoms, the history should identify the relative onset and course of each condition in order to determine what is the main diagnosis and what should be the principal focus of treatment. However, this implies that the clinician is able to obtain accurate historical information from the patient. As discussed previously in this chapter, criteria for several sleep disorders were based on expert opinions and consensus, and there has been limited research specifically focused on validating the different diagnostic entities (Edinger et al., 2011) and even less since the publication of the ICSD-3 and DSM-5 diagnostic nosologies. Clearly, additional work is warranted to validate current nosologies of sleep disorders and within each of the major categories to identify specific phenotypes that could be matched to the most relevant treatment alternatives.

Current Limitations and Directions for Future Development and Research

From the discussion presented, it is obvious that the past and current systems for sleep disorder classification have been particularly encumbered by a number of limitations. As noted, these systems have been devised as much on the basis of clinical experience and consensus as on actual empirical evidence. This state of affairs is, at least in part, a result of the uneven knowledge base across the currently recognized sleep disorders; for some conditions much is known about underlying pathophysiological mechanisms, whereas for other conditions little, if any, knowledge is currently available. This situation does not necessarily preclude the possibility that many sleep disorders listed in the current nosologies represent valid entities that can be reliably identified in clinical and research settings. Yet it remains to be determined if this is indeed the case. As noted above, the available literature assessing the reliability and validity of sleep disorders remains rather limited and remarkably unimpressive. In fact, there have been no formal reliability/validity assessments of many of the sleep disorder categories listed in current nosologies nor have there been tests of reliability and validity of these systems as a whole. Specifically, the question remains as to how accurately these systems subdivide the universe of sleep disorders into all sleep disorder subtypes that presumably exist. Thus, much more research is needed that is specifically designed to assess the reliability/validity of many of the sleep disorders individually and of the classification schemes taken as a whole.

Whereas research has improved our existing diagnostic schemes for sleep disorders, there have been some concerted efforts at improving our phenotyping, at least with some of the global sleep disorder categories. Within the area of insomnia classification, for example, Vgontzas et al. (2013) have suggested classifying patients with short (<6 hours/night) and more normal (≥6 hours per night) objective sleep duration. Studies by Vgontzas et al. (Vgontzas, Liao, Bixler, et al., 2009; Vgontzas, Liao, Pejovic, et al., 2009; Vgontzas et al., 2020) and others (Bathgate et al., 2016, 2017) have shown that relative to the longer sleeping insomnia phenotype, those with short sleep duration have greater risk for medical morbidity and a poorer response to cognitive behavioral therapy for insomnia (CBT-I). Van Someren and colleagues have also conducted extensive research concerning insomnia phenotypes with differing forms of symptom presentation and severity. Using a latent class analysis of responses to various questionnaires designed to tap several distinct categories (e.g., arousal, negative affect, childhood trauma, rumination, insomnia response to stress), Van Someren and colleagues identified five distinct subtypes (Blanken et al., 2019). Three of these groups were characterized as exhibiting high pre-sleep arousal. The first of these three subtypes was also characterized by high distress and low subjective happiness. The other two groups with high pre-sleep arousal were identified as exhibiting moderate distress but differed regarding degree of reduced positive affect and reduced positive rumination. Lastly, the fourth and fifth subtypes both exhibited low general distress but differed in their reactivity to insomnia responses after exposure to life events, that is, high reactivity and low reactivity, respectively. Numerous comparisons across the groups were made, and several differences were notable. For example, while differences between sleep onset/sleep maintenance difficulties or early morning awakenings did not distinguish among the groups, developmental onset of sleep difficulties differed across some of the groups. Other differential findings across subtypes included the presence of ICD-10 mental and behavioral disorders, the prevalence of current or lifetime depression, and response to benzodiazepine intake as well as CBT-I. Subtype differences were also observed on objective psychophysiological responses (i.e., evoked response potentials to auditory stimuli). Moreover, differences in depression risk were as great as fivefold across the subtypes. Blanken et al. (2019) also noted that the classification of these subtypes remained stable over time. This line of work suggests that further understanding specific insomnia profiles may enhance insomnia nosology and provide support for tailored interventions that target specific insomnia presentations.

In addition to this work focused on insomnia disorders, there has been interest in improvement of other categories of sleep disorder. Work by the International Restless Legs Syndrome Study Group, for example, has proposed criteria for improving the diagnosis of RLS (Marelli et al., 2015). These criteria, which align more closely to the ICSD-3 than the DSM-5 criteria, provide a more rigorous approach to case ascertainment and a better characterization of patients by specifying clinical significance and course. Noting the recent development of novel therapies and diagnostic tests for sleep apnea, Stuck and Mauer (2017) have advocated integration of the new diagnostic technologies into the diagnosis of those with sleep disordered breathing. Yet significant work and research is required to determine the best definitions and diagnostic procedures for the range of extant sleep disorders.

Ultimately, the challenge for the field of sleep medicine is to develop a diagnostic system that has reliability, validity, and clinical utility. It also seems theoretically important to arrive at a classification scheme that is optimal for classifying the range of sleep disorders encountered in clinical and research settings. Such a system should strike the proper balance between achieving reasonable homogeneity within diagnostic subgroups while accounting for the heterogeneity between those with discrete disorders. In moving the area of sleep disorder classification forward, it will be important to employ methodologies that can simultaneously assess the reliability/validity of individual categories and evaluate the overall effectiveness of the system of diagnostic subtyping. An example of such an approach is the previously mentioned multitrait/multimethod research strategy used by Edinger et al. (2011) for testing the utility of the DSM-IV-TR and ICSD-2 systems for insomnia classification. This approach allows for simultaneous assessment of the reliability, convergent validity, and discriminant validity of each diagnosis. As such, this approach allows assessment of each individual category as well as the overall arrangement of all categories included in the system. With such approaches applied to different segments (i.e., insomnias, hypersomnias, parasomnias, etc.) of existing sleep nosologies, it should eventually be possible to ascertain the optimal system for sleep disorder classification. Of course, such developments will take some time, and currently there is a need for sleep disorder classification/diagnosis in the many clinical venues where patients with sleep/wake complaints present.

References

Akerstedt, T., & Gillberg, M. (1990). Subjective and objective sleepiness in the active individual. *International Journal of Neuroscience*, *52*(1–2), 29–37. https://doi.org/10.3109/00207459008994241

American Academy of Sleep Medicine. (2005). *International classification of sleep disorders* (2nd ed.).

American Academy of Sleep Medicine. (2014). *International classification of sleep disorders* (3rd ed.).

American Psychiatric Association. (1987). *Diagnostic and statistical manual of mental disorders* (3rd ed.).

American Psychiatric Association. (1994). *Diagnostic and statistical manual of mental disorders* (4th ed.).

American Psychiatric Association. (1997). *Diagnostic and statistical manual of mental disorders* (4th ed., text rev.).

American Psychiatric Association. (2013). *Diagnostic and statistical manual of mental disorders* (5th ed.).

American Sleep Disorders Association. (1990). *The international classification of sleep disorders.*

American Sleep Disorders Association. (1997). *The international classification of sleep disorders, revised: Diagnostic and coding manual.*

Aserinsky, E., & Kleitman, N. (1953). Regularly occurring periods of eye motility, and concomitant phenomena, during sleep. *Science*, *118*(3062), 273–274. https://doi.org/10.1126/science.118.3062.273

Aserinsky, E., & Kleitman, N. (1955). Two types of ocular motility occurring in sleep. *Journal of Applied Physiology*, *8*(1), 1–10. https://doi.org/10.1152/jappl.1955.8.1.1

Association of Sleep Disorders Centers & Association for the Psychophysiological Study of Sleep. (1979). Diagnostic classification of sleep and arousal disorders. *Sleep*, *2*, 1–154.

Bathgate, C. J., Edinger, J. D., & Krystal, A. D. (2017). Insomnia patients with objective short sleep duration have a blunted response to cognitive behavioral therapy for insomnia. *Sleep*, *40*(1), Article zsw012. https://doi.org/10.1093/sleep/zsw012

Bathgate, C. J., Edinger, J. D., Wyatt, J. K., & Krystal, A. D. (2016). Objective but not subjective short sleep duration associated with increased risk for hypertension in individuals with insomnia. *Sleep, 39*(5), 1037–1045. https://doi.org/10.5665/sleep.5748

Berger, H. (1930). Ueber das elektroenkephalogramm des menschen. *Journal of Psychology and Neurology, 40*, 160–170.

Bertisch, S. M., Pollock, B. D., Mittleman, M. A., Buysse, D. J., Bazzano, L. A., Gottlieb, D. J., & Redline, S. (2018). Insomnia with objective short sleep duration and risk of incident cardiovascular disease and all-cause mortality: Sleep Heart Health Study. *Sleep, 41*(6), Article zsy047. https://doi.org/10.1093/sleep/zsy047

Blanken, T. F., Benjamins, J. S., Borsboom, D., Vermunt, J. K., Paquola, C., Ramautar, J., Ramautar, J., Dekker, K., Stoffers, D., Wassing, R., Wei, Y., & Van Someren, E. J. W. (2019). Insomnia disorder subtypes derived from life history and traits of affect and personality. *Lancet Psychiatry, 6*(2), 151–163. https://doi.org/10.1016/S2215-0366(18)30464-4

Buysse, D. J., Ancoli-Israel, S., Edinger, J. D., Lichstein, K. L., & Morin, C. M. (2006). Recommendations for a standard research assessment of insomnia. *Sleep, 29*(9), 1155–1173.

Buysse, D. J., Reynolds, C. F., Kupfer, D. J., Thorpy, M. J., Bixler, E., Kales, A., Manfredi, R., Vgontzas, A., Stepanski, E., Roth, T., Hauri, P., & Stapf, D. (1997). Effects of diagnosis on treatment recommendations in chronic insomnia—A report from the APA/NIMH DSM-IV field trial. *Sleep, 20*(7), 542–552.

Buysse, D. J., Reynolds, C. F., 3rd, Kupfer, D., Thorpy, M., Bixler, E., Manfredi, R., Kales, A., Vgontzas, A., Stepanski, E., Roth, T., Hauri, P., & Mesiano, D. (1994). Clinical diagnoses in 216 insomnia patients using the International Classification of Sleep Disorders (ICSD), DSM-IV and ICD-10 categories: A report from the APA/NIMH DSM-IV field trial. *Sleep, 17*(7), 630–637.

Buysse, D. J., Reynolds, C. F., 3rd, Monk, T. H., Berman, S. R., & Kupfer, D. J. (1989). The Pittsburgh Sleep Quality Index: A new instrument for psychiatric practice and research. *Psychiatry Research, 28*(2), 193–213. https://doi.org/10.1016/0165-1781(89)90047-4

Buysse, D. J., Young, T., Edinger, J. D., Carroll, J., & Kotagal, S. (2003). Clinicians' use of the International Classification of Sleep Disorders: Results of a national survey. *Sleep, 26*(1), 48–51.

Buysse, D. J., Yu, L., Moul, D. E., Germain, A., Stover, A., Dodds, N. E., Johnston, K. L., Shablesky-Cade, M. A., & Pilkonis, P. A. (2010). Development and validation of patient-reported outcome measures for sleep disturbance and sleep-related impairments. *Sleep, 33*(6), 781–792. https://doi.org/10.1093/sleep/33.6.781

Carney, C. E., Buysse, D. J., Ancoli-Israel, S., Edinger, J. D., Krystal, A. D., Lichstein, K. L., & Morin, C. M. (2012). The Consensus Sleep Diary: Standardizing prospective sleep self-monitoring. *Sleep, 35*(2), 287–302. https://doi.org/10.5665/sleep.1642

Chinoy, E. D., Cuellar, J. A., Huwa, K. E., Jameson, J. T., Watson, C. H., Bessman, S. C., Hirsch, D. A., Cooper, A. D., Drummond, S. P. A., & Markwald, R. R. (2021). Performance of seven consumer sleep-tracking devices compared with polysomnography. *Sleep, 44*(5), Article zsaa291. https://doi.org/10.1093/sleep/zsaa291

Chung, F., Abudullah, H. R., & Liao, P. (2016). STOP-Bang questionnaire: A practical approach to screen for obstructive sleep apnea. Chest, 149(3), 631–638. https://doi.org/10.1378/chest.15-0903

Chung, K. F., Yeung, W. F., Ho, F. Y., Yung, K. P., Yu, Y. M., & Kwok, C. W. (2015). Cross-cultural and comparative epidemiology of insomnia: The Diagnostic and statistical manual (DSM), International classification of diseases (ICD) and International classification of sleep disorders (ICSD). *Sleep Medicine, 16*(4), 477–482. https://doi.org/10.1016/j.sleep.2014.10.018

de Zambotti, M., Cellini, N., Goldstone, A., Colrain, I. M., & Baker, F. C. (2019). Wearable sleep technology in clinical and research settings. *Medicine & Science in Sports & Exercise, 51*(7), 1538–1557. https://doi.org/10.1249/MSS.0000000000001947

de Zambotti, M., Goldstein, C., Cook, J., Menghini, L., Altini, M., Cheng, P., & Robillard, R. (2024). State of the science and recommendations for using wearable technology in sleep and circadian research. Sleep, 47, 1–31. https://doi.org/10.1093/sleep/zsad325

Edinger, J., Bonnet, M., Bootzin, R., Doghramji, K., Dorsey, C., Espie, C., Jamieson, A. O., McCall, W. V., Morin, C. M., & Stepanski, E. (2004). Derivation of research diagnostic criteria for insomnia: Report of an American Academy of Sleep Medicine work group. *Sleep, 27*(8), 1567–1596.

Edinger, J. D., & Carney, C. E. (2015). *Overcoming insomnia: A cognitive-behavioral approach—Therapist guide*. Oxford University Press.

Edinger, J. D., Fins, A. I., Goeke, J. M., McMillan, D. K., Gersh, T. L., Krystal, A. D., & McCall, W. V. (1996). The empirical identification of insomnia subtypes: A cluster analytic approach. *Sleep, 19*(5), 398–411.

Edinger, J., Kirby, A., Lineberger, M., Loiselle, M., & Wohlgemuth, W. M. (2004). *The Duke structured interview for sleep disorders.* Duke University Medical Center.

Edinger, J. D., Wyatt, J. K., Stepanski, E. J., Olsen, M. K., Stechuchak, K. M., Carney, C. E., Chiang, A., Crisostomo, M. I., Lineberger, M. D., Means, M. K., Radtke, R. A., Wohlgemuth, W. K., & Krystal, A. D. (2011). Testing the reliability and validity of DSM-IV-TR and ICSD-2 insomnia diagnoses. Results of a multitrait-multimethod analysis. *Archives of General Psychiatry, 68*(10), 992–1002. https://doi.org/10.1001/archgenpsychiatry.2011.64

Hauri, P. J. (1983). A cluster analysis of insomnia. *Sleep, 6*(4), 326–338. https://doi.org/10.1093/sleep/6.4.326

Hening, W. A., Allen, R. P., Thanner, S., Washburn, T., Heckler, D., Walters, A. S., & Earley, C. J. (2003). The Johns Hopkins telephone diagnostic interview for the restless legs syndrome: Preliminary investigation for validation in a multi-center patient and control population. *Sleep Medicine, 4*(2), 137–141. https://doi.org/10.1016/s1389-9457(03)00006-6

Hertenstein, E., Feige, B., Gmeiner, T., Kienzler, C., Spiegelhalder, K., Johann, A., Jansson-Fröjmark, M., Palagini, L., Rücker, G., Riemann, D., & Baglioni, C. (2019). Insomnia as a predictor of mental disorders: A systematic review and meta-analysis. *Sleep Medicine Reviews, 43*, 96–105. https://doi.org/10.1016/j.smrv.2018.10.006

Hoddes, E., Zarcone, V., Smythe, H., Phillips, R., & Dement, W. C. (1973). Quantification of sleepiness: A new approach. *Psychophysiology, 10*(4), 431–436.

Horne, J. A., & Ostberg, O. (1976). A self-assessment questionnaire to determine morningness–eveningness in human circadian rhythms. *International Journal of Chronobiology, 4*(2), 97–110.

Ibanez, V., Silva, J., Navarro, E., & Cauli, O. (2019). Sleep assessment devices: Types, market analysis, and a critical view on accuracy and validation. *Expert Review of Medical Devices, 16*(12), 1041–1052. https://doi.org/10.1080/17434440.2019.1693890

Johns, M. W. (1991). A new method for measuring daytime sleepiness: The Epworth Sleepiness Scale. *Sleep, 14*(6), 540–545.

Kroenke, K., Spitzer, R. L., & Williams, J. B. (2001). The PHQ-9: Validity of a brief depression severity measure. *Journal of General Internal Medicine, 16*(9), 606–613. https://doi.org/10.1046/j.1525-1497.2001.016009606.x

Kushida, C. A., Littner, M. R., Morgenthaler, T., Alessi, C. A., Bailey, D., Coleman, J., Jr., Friedman, L., Hirshkowitz, M., Kapen, S., Kramer, M., Lee-Chiong, T., Loube, D. L., Owens, J., Pancer, J. P., & Wise, M. (2005). Practice parameters for the indications for polysomnography and related procedures: An update for 2005. *Sleep, 28*(4), 499–521. https://doi.org/10.1093/sleep/28.4.499

Littner, M. R., Kushida, C., Wise, M., Davila, D. G., Morgenthaler, T., Lee-Chiong, T., Hirshkowitz, M., Loube, D. L., Bailey, D., Berry, R. B., Kapen, S., & Kramer, M. Standards of Practice Committee of the American Academy of Sleep Medicine. (2005). Practice parameters for clinical use of the multiple sleep latency test and the maintenance of wakefulness test. *Sleep, 28*(1), 113–121. https://doi.org/10.1093/sleep/28.1.113

Loddo, G., Vignatelli, L., Zenesini, C., Lusa, F., Sambati, L., Baldelli, L., Favoni, V., Pisani, L. R., Pierangeli, G., Cevoli, S., & Provini, F. (2019). Interobserver reliability of ICSD-3 diagnostic criteria for disorders of arousal in adults. *Sleep and Breathing, 23*(4), 1309–1314. https://doi.org/10.1007/s11325-019-01937-w

Manber, R., & Carney, C. E. (2015). *Treatment plans and interventions for insomnia. A case formulation approach.* Guilford Press.

Marelli, S., Galbiati, A., Rinaldi, F., Giora, E., Oldani, A., Ferini Strambi, L., & Zucconi, M. (2015). Restless legs syndrome/Willis Ekbom disease: New diagnostic criteria according to different nosology. *Archives Italiennes de Biologie, 153*(2–3), 184–193. https://doi.org/10.12871/0003982920152343

Milligan, G. W. (1980). An examination of the effect of six types of error perturbation on fifteen clustering algorithms. *Psychometrika, 45*, 325–342.

Morin, C. M. (1993). *Insomnia: Psychological assessment and management.* Guilford Press.

Morin, C. M., Belleville, G., Belanger, L., & Ivers, H. (2011). The Insomnia Severity Index: Psychometric indicators to detect insomnia cases and evaluate treatment response. *Sleep, 34*(5), 601–608. https://doi.org/10.1093/sleep/34.5.601

Morin, C. M., & Espie, C. A. (2003). *Insomnia. A clinical guide to assessment and treatment.* Springer.

Morin, C. M., Stone, J., McDonald, K., & Jones, S. (1994). Psychological management of insomnia—A clinical replication series with 100 patients. *Behavior Therapy, 25*(2), 291–309. https://doi.org/10.1016/s0005-7894(05)80289-8
Ohayon, M. M., Guilleminault, C., Zulley, J., Palombini, L., & Raab, H. (1999). Validation of the sleep-EVAL system against clinical assessments of sleep disorders and polysomnographic data. *Sleep, 22*(7), 925–930. https://doi.org/10.1093/sleep/22.7.925
Ohayon, M. M., & Roberts, R. E. (2001). Comparability of sleep disorders diagnoses using DSM-IV and ICSD classifications with adolescents. *Sleep, 24*(8), 920–925.
Schramm, E., Hohagen, F., Grasshoff, U., Riemann, D., Hajak, G., Weess, H. G., & Berger, M. (1993). Test–retest reliability and validity of the Structured Interview for Sleep Disorders according to DSM-III-R. *American Journal of Psychiatry, 150*(6), 867–872. https://doi.org/10.1176/ajp.150.6.867
Schutte-Rodin, S., Broch, L., Buysse, D., Dorsey, C., & Sateia, M. (2008). Clinical guideline for the evaluation and management of chronic insomnia in adults. *Journal of Clinical Sleep Medicine, 4*(5), 487–504.
Smith, M. T., McCrae, C. S., Cheung, J., Martin, J. L., Harrod, C. G., Heald, J. L., & Carden, K. A. (2018). Use of actigraphy for the evaluation of sleep disorders and circadian rhythm sleep–wake disorders: An American Academy of Sleep Medicine clinical practice guideline. *Journal of Clinical Sleep Medicine, 14*(7), 1231–1237. https://doi.org/10.5664/jcsm.7230
Spitzer, R. L., Kroenke, K., Williams, J. B., & Lowe, B. (2006). A brief measure for assessing generalized anxiety disorder: The GAD-7. *Archives of Internal Medicine, 166*(10), 1092–1097. https://doi.org/10.1001/archinte.166.10.1092
Stuck, B. A., & Maurer, J. T. (2017). Recent developments in the diagnosis and treatment of obstructive sleep apnea. *Journal of Prosthetic Dentistry, 65*(S1), 13–18.
Sweetman, A., Lack, L., McEvoy, R. D., Smith, S., Eckert, D. J., Osman, A., Carberry, J. C., Wallace, D., Nguyen, P. D., & Catcheside, P. (2021). Bi-directional relationships between co-morbid insomnia and sleep apnea (COMISA). *Sleep Medicine Reviews, 60*, Article 101519. https://doi.org/10.1016/j.smrv.2021.101519
Tabachnick, J. L., & Fidell, L. F. (1989). *Using multivariate statistics*. Harper Collins.
Taylor, D. J., Wilkerson, A. K., Pruiksma, K. E., Williams, J. M., Ruggero, C. J., Hale, W., Mintz, J., Organek, K. M., Nicholson, K. L., Litz, B. T., Young-McCaughan, S., Dondanville, K. A., Borah, E. V., Brundige, A., Peterson, A. L., & Consortium, S. S. (2018). Reliability of the Structured Clinical Interview for DSM-5 sleep disorders module. *Journal of Clinical Sleep Medicine, 14*(3), 459–464. https://doi.org/10.5664/jcsm.7000
The International Restless Legs Syndrome Study Group. (2003). Validation of the International Restless Legs Syndrome Study Group rating scale for restless legs syndrome. Sleep Medicine, 4(2), 121–132. https://doi.org/10.1016/s1389-9457(02)00258-7
Vgontzas, A. N., Fernandez-Mendoza, J., Liao, D., & Bixler, E. O. (2013). Insomnia with objective short sleep duration: The most biologically severe phenotype of the disorder. *Sleep Medicine Reviews, 17*(4), 241–254. https://doi.org/10.1016/j.smrv.2012.09.005
Vgontzas, A. N., Liao, D., Bixler, E. O., Chrousos, G. P., & Vela-Bueno, A. (2009). Insomnia with objective short sleep duration is associated with a high risk for hypertension. *Sleep, 32*(4), 491–497.
Vgontzas, A. N., Liao, D., Pejovic, S., Calhoun, S., Karataraki, M., & Bixler, E. O. (2009). Insomnia with objective short sleep duration is associated with Type 2 diabetes: A population-based study. *Diabetes Care, 32*(11), 1980–1985. https://doi.org/10.2337/dc09-0284
Vgontzas, A. N., Puzino, K., Fernandez-Mendoza, J., Krishnamurthy, V. B., Basta, M., & Bixler, E. O. (2020). Effects of trazodone versus cognitive behavioral therapy in the insomnia with short sleep duration phenotype: a preliminary study. *Journal of Clinical Sleep Medicine, 16*(12), 2009–2019. https://doi.org/10.5664/jcsm.8740
World Health Organization. (1977). *International classification of diseases* (Vol. 1, 9th rev.).
World Health Organization. (1994). *International classification of diseases, clinical modification* (4th ed., 9th rev.). Medicode.
World Health Organization. (1993). *The ICD-10 classification of mental and behavioural disorders.*
World Health Organization. (2019). *ICD-11: International classification of diseases* (11th rev.). https://icd.who.int/

CHAPTER

22 Value-Based Clinical Sleep Medicine: Health Economic Considerations Regarding Insomnia and Obstructive Sleep Apnea

Emerson M. Wickwire

Abstract

In the modern healthcare climate of increasing costs, on the one hand, and limited resources, on the other, economic aspects of sleep medicine have never been more important. In addition to improving health outcomes, sleep disorders treatments are increasingly expected to demonstrate positive economic impact, broadly defined by multiple diverse stakeholders with at times competing interests. Over the past several decades, a growing body of literature has demonstrated substantial costs of untreated sleep disorders borne by patients, payers, employers, and society. More important, recent research has demonstrated that treatment of sleep disorders can result in positive economic impact. The purpose of this chapter is to introduce key health economic concepts as pertains to sleep medicine. Insomnia and obstructive sleep apnea, the two most common sleep disorders among adults, will be considered.

Key Words: sleep, health economics, insomnia, obstructive sleep apnea, cost, payment

Introduction

Insomnia, defined as difficulty initiating and/or maintaining sleep with associated daytime consequence, and obstructive sleep apnea (OSA) are the two most common sleep disorders seen in adult clinical practice. As reviewed in detail elsewhere in this volume, each of these conditions incurs substantial risk for a broad range of adverse health outcomes and diminished quality of life (QOL). Yet beyond these adverse impacts on health, insomnia and OSA each result in dramatic economic costs that are borne by patients, payers, employers, and society (Wickwire, Albrecht, et al., 2019; Wickwire et al., 2015). Surprisingly, relative to the many thousands of studies exploring pathophysiologic, clinical, and epidemiologic aspects of insomnia and OSA, few studies have evaluated the economic aspects of insomnia treatment and OSA treatment. In the modern healthcare climate of rising costs, on the one hand, and limited resources, on the other, such insight is desperately needed by payers, employers, and policymakers to make evidence-based decisions regarding allocation of scarce healthcare resources. Thus, the purpose of this brief chapter is to introduce key health economic concepts pertaining to insomnia and OSA and to highlight very briefly several key issues regarding health economic aspects of treatments for these two common conditions.

Introduction to Health Economic Aspects of Sleep Disorders

Costs of Untreated Sleep Disorders

Broadly speaking, sleep disorder costs can be divided into three categories: direct costs, indirect costs, and health-related QOL (HrQOL). Direct costs include costs of evaluation and management, including provider consultation, follow-up visits, prescription medications, over-the-counter or other sleep aids, medical devices (e.g., positive airway pressure [PAP] machines and equipment or oral appliances for OSA), and novel approaches (e.g., transcranial magnetic stimulation or digital therapeutics for insomnia). Indirect costs include costs unrelated to treatment that are nonetheless attributable to sleep disorders, such as increased healthcare resource utilization (HCRU) for non-sleep conditions, diminished workplace productivity (e.g., absenteeism or presenteeism—when an employee is physically present but produces less work than expected), and increased risk of workplace accidents and errors including motor vehicle crashes (MVCs). It is important to realize that even though total aggregate societal costs are often cited to highlight the staggering costs of sleep disorders, these direct and indirect costs are primarily borne by different stakeholders (Wickwire & Verma, 2018).

A detailed review of costs associated with insomnia and OSA is beyond the scope of this chapter. However, readers will be interested that estimated total costs for insomnia in the United States have ranged from $28.1 billion to $216 billion (Martin et al., 2004; National Commission on Sleep Disorders et al., 1993), with increased direct and indirect costs in each of the domains outlined above. Of note, one study in Quebec used a validated measure of insomnia severity (the Insomnia Severity Index) and found that workplace productivity (i.e., absenteeism and presenteeism) accounted for a staggering >90% of total insomnia-related costs (Daley et al., 2009). In terms of OSA, a 2016 white paper commissioned by the American Academy of Sleep Medicine estimated total society-level costs of OSA to exceed $150 billion per year in the United States alone, including costs associated with lost workplace productivity ($86.9 billion), increased HCRU ($30 billion), MVCs ($26.2 billion), and workplace accidents and injuries ($6.5 billion; American Academy of Sleep Medicine, 2016).

In the context of this chapter, it is important to realize that both insomnia and OSA are highly comorbid with other sleep, medical, and psychiatric disorders. Indeed, each condition can precipitate, exacerbate, or prolong many chronic conditions. For example, sleep specialists are well aware of the relationship between insomnia and risk for depression or OSA and risk for cardiovascular disease (CVD). Even so, from a methodological perspective, disentangling the effects of sleep disorders and these frequent comorbid conditions is highly challenging. Even sophisticated analytic approaches, such as inverse probability of treatment weighting, cannot eliminate the potential for residual confounding. Further, available data sources are limited and generally can be either very detailed (e.g., longitudinal cohort or clinical trials data based on detailed, multimethod serial assessment over many years) or very large (e.g., administrative claims data) but not both. As a result, when presented with data pertaining to costs of untreated sleep disorders, payers and other economic stakeholders are rightfully skeptical that high costs are due to sleep disorders and not the comorbid chronic conditions (e.g., depression and/or CVD), which are independently associated with very high costs. Addressing this important methodological concern is a key challenge for sleep scientists in the future.

HrQOL

Beyond direct and indirect costs, HrQOL is a key economic outcome (Muennig & Bounthavong, 2016; Neumann et al., 2017). HrQOL includes both general as well as disease-specific components, each of which can be measured using validated tools. In general, HrQOL measures subjective satisfaction with life and one's ability to function independently in the world. Common general HrQOL measures include the Patient-Reported Outcomes Measurement Information System (PROMIS®), developed as part of the National Institutes of Health Roadmap (Hanmer et al., 2015), the Short-Form 36 (Ware & Sherbourne, 1992), and the EuroQol-5D (Brooks, 1996). These measures ask about overall subjective satisfaction and function in various general life domains (e.g., ambulation, eyesight, etc.). By contrast, disease-specific measures of HrQOL seek to capture impairments associated with a specific disorder (e.g., fatigue for insomnia or sleepiness for OSA). The Hotel-Dieu-16 is an example of an insomnia-specific measure of HrQOL. The Functional Outcomes of Sleep Questionnaire (Weaver et al., 1997) is one OSA-specific measure.

Another common economic metric to quantify HrQOL is the quality-adjusted life year (QALY). QALYs incorporate both HrQOL and time (i.e., quality [on a 0–1 utility scale] × time [in years]). Thus, although non-monetary, QALYs provide a standardized metric that researchers and decision makers can use to compare return on investment across diverse disease states. As one example, many cost-effectiveness analyses (Mohit & Cohen, 2019) determine cost-effectiveness based on the ratio of cost to quality as measured by QALYs. This metric is known as the *incremental cost-effectiveness ratio*, a metric of value that reflects the cost per QALY. Of course, the value of a QALY is ultimately determined by how much a given stakeholder is willing to pay. Broadly speaking, individual payers, health systems, and other stakeholders determine willingness to pay (WTP) per QALY. In the United States, the rule of thumb is that costs <$50,000 per QALY are considered a marker of cost-effectiveness. Ample evidence gathered over multiple decades demonstrates that untreated insomnia and OSA both worsen HrQOL. Treatments improve HrQOL and are generally considered cost-effective based on inconsistent rules of thumb that vary by country and health system (Wickwire, Albrecht, et al., 2019; Wickwire et al., 2015).

Of course, from a consumer perspective, individual patients do not employ sophisticated measures of HrQOL or analytic frameworks when determining their personal WTP. At the patient level, WTP is based on perceived benefit and costs, individual resources, available alternatives, and so on. Even though patients are a key stakeholder group and often rate the importance of sleep very highly, few empirical studies have sought to determine WTP from the patient perspective for either insomnia or OSA treatment. A single discrete-choice experiment in a West Virginia hospital found that among primary care patients with insomnia (n = 82), WTP was $66.69 for an insomnia treatment that reduced sleep latency (by 10 minutes) and wakefulness after sleep onset (by 15 minutes) and increased total sleep time by 1 hour. For those interested in consumer approaches to healthcare, a review of available direct-to-consumer product and service offerings, as well as their price points and payment terms, can be highly illustrative.

Economic Perspective: Value Is in the Eye of the Beholder

Multiple diverse stakeholders are included in the sleep medicine ecosystem. Patients, payers, providers, health systems, and equipment manufacturers incur different costs (and potentially cost savings or revenues). It is thus not surprising that each perceives the value of sleep differently. Most important, patients value QOL, including increased energy for work or leisure activities, and ease of care experience. Payers value cost savings. Employers value workplace productivity and reduced accident risk. Providers value testing and treatment options that are valid, reliable, and easy to administer. Stakeholder perspectives in sleep medicine are summarized in Table 22.1.

Economic Impact of Insomnia and OSA Treatments

Economic Aspects of Insomnia Treatment

A comprehensive review of the literature found that, overall, both pharmacotherapy and cognitive-behavioral treatment for insomnia (CBTI) were associated with positive economic benefit, including in comorbid conditions (Wickwire et al., 2015). Table 22.2 summarizes several studies that have examined the economic impact of insomnia treatments. Even so, it is important to realize that clinical settings, patient populations, study designs, and outcome measures have varied widely in insomnia economic studies to date.

Table 22.1 Economic perspectives in sleep medicine

Perspective	Perceived value/desired outcome
Patient	Quality of life, ease of treatment experience
Payer	Cost savings (profit)
Employer	Workplace productivity, reduced accident risk
Health system	Revenue (profit), population health
Society	Total costs and health economic outcomes

Table 22.2 Summary of select empirical studies examining economic impact of insomnia treatments

Reference	Sample	Design	Insomnia treatment	Economic outcome	Key findings
(Snedecor et al., 2009)	824 adults	RCT	Eszopiclone	QALY, drug costs	Eszopiclone gained .0137 QALYs at a cost of $91. Incremental cost per QALY was <$6,795.
(Snedecor et al., 2010)	434 adults with depression and comorbid insomnia	RCT	Eszopiclone	QALY, drug costs	Versus PBO+FLX, ESZ+FLX gained .0058 QALYs at a direct cost of $110. Incremental cost per QALY was $19,026.
(Morgan et al., 2004)	410 chronic hypnotic users	RCT	CBTI	QALY, drug costs	Cost per QALY was $9,155 at 6 months. Cost effectiveness was achieved at 4 years.
(McCrae et al., 2014)	84 US adults	RCT	CBTI	Total costs	Both treatment completion and treatment response were associated with reduced costs over 6 months ($249 and $261, respectively).
(Bonin et al., 2014)	151 London adults	RCT	group CBTI	QALY, CBTI costs	Versus education, group CBTI produced no between-group differences in QALYs over 3 months. The likelihood of cost-effectiveness using standard approaches was only 80%.
(Watanabe et al., 2015)	37 patients with refractory depression and insomnia	RCT	CBTI	QALY, CBTI costs	Versus TAU, CBT gained .019 QALYs at a cost of $316. Incremental cost per QALY was $17,121.

Note. Costs have been updated to 2022 US dollars using the inflation calculator provided by the US Bureau of Labor Statistics. (When needed, costs were first translated from international currencies to US dollars in the year of publication, then adjusted for inflation.) CBTI = cognitive behavioral treatment for insomnia; ESZ = eszopiclone; FLX = fluoxetine; PBO = placebo; RCT = randomized controlled trial; QALY = quality-adjusted life year; TAU = treatment as usual.

In general, larger studies have been less likely to include measures of insomnia severity (e.g., instead relying on administrative diagnostic claims as the operational definition of insomnia) and less likely to include nuanced measurement of insomnia treatment-related change (e.g., impact on daytime function; Wickwire & Morin, 2020). These limitations are particularly salient when considering real-world evidence. For example, multiple administrative claims analyses have found insomnia medication treatments to be associated with *increased* future costs (Amari et al., 2022; Wickwire, Amari, et al., 2022; Wickwire, Vadlamani, et al., 2019). Although there are valid reasons why insomnia medications or CBTI could increase costs (e.g., accidents associated with residual sedation from medications or sleepiness resulting from sleep restriction during CBTI), lack of measurement sensitivity to detect economic benefit and economic perspective are both major issues. After all, administrative claims data is unlikely to include measures of workplace productivity, which include the vast majority of insomnia-related costs and are borne entirely by employers. Another key consideration is treatment costs, which are impacted by treatment format (e.g., in-person, group, or digital insomnia care). A number of recent studies have demonstrated positive economic benefit from CBTI approaches, including digital CBTI (Baka et al., 2022; Buntrock et al., 2021; Darden et al., 2021; Sampson et al., 2022) and telephone-based CBTI in chronic pain (Yeung et al., 2022).

Economic Aspects of OSA Treatment

A systematic review of OSA treatments found that 15 of 17 comparisons resulted in positive economic benefit (Wickwire, Albrecht, et al., 2019). More recently, several additional studies have reported positive economic benefit from PAP, including in patients with CVD (Bock et al., 2022; Chhatre et al., 2020; Kirsch et al., 2019). These CVD data is particularly important not only because of the frequent comorbidity of OSA and CVD (Collen et al., 2020) but also because they highlight the importance of patient selection in clinical and health economic research. Two recent reports are illustrative. In a study of older adults with CVD and comorbid OSA, PAP adherence was associated with \$4,477 lower total costs over 12 months (i.e., a 40% reduction; \$6,825 vs. \$11,302, $p < .05$; Bock et al., 2022). In another study of older adult Medicare beneficiaries with CVD and comorbid OSA, high PAP adherence was associated with a 59% reduction in 30-day hospital readmissions (Bailey et al., 2022). Although readmissions were not dollarized in this study, 30-day readmission is a key quality metric of high relevance to patients, payers, and health systems. In the United States, 30-day readmissions are also associated with substantial financial penalties from the Centers for Medicaid and Medicare Services. It should be noted that these two studies employed similar analytic frameworks using administrative claims data. Even so, these results are consistent with prior reports and support future sleep health economic research in different populations using varied study designs, research methodologies, and outcome measures. Table 22.3 summarizes several studies that have examined the economic impact of OSA treatments.

Table 22.3 Summary of select empirical studies examining economic impact of obstructive sleep apnea treatments

Reference	Sample	Design	OSA treatment	Economic outcome	Key findings
(Albarrak et al., 2005)	34 Canadian men (M age = 48 years)	Retrospective cohort study	CPAP	Outpatient visits, physician costs	Versus 1 year prediagnosis, CPAP reduced outpatient visits (1.03 visits) and physician costs $17.22 over 5 years.
(Bahammam et al., 1999)	344 Canadian men (M age = 49 years)	Prospective cohort study	CPAP or BPAP	Physician costs, hospitalizations	Versus 2 years prediagnosis, CPAP adherence was associated with reduced physician costs and hospitalizations over 2 years.
(Bailey et al., 2022)	1,301 US Medicare beneficiaries	Retrospective cohort study	CPAP	30-day hospital readmissions	Versus low adherence, high CPAP adherence was associated with 59% reduction in 30-day readmissions.
(Banno et al., 2006)	414 Canadian men (M age = 49 years)	Retrospective cohort study	CPAP or BPAP	Outpatient visits, physician costs	CPAP was associated with reduced outpatient visits and physician costs ($45.10) over 2 years.
(Bock et al., 2022)	856 US Medicare beneficiaries with CVD and comorbid OSA	Retrospective cohort study	CPAP	Total costs (including inpatient, outpatient, skilled nursing, home health, and DME costs)	Versus low adherence, high CPAP adherence was associated with reduced total costs ($8,261 vs. $13,691, $p < .05$).
(Cai et al., 2012)	15,424 US adults (70% men, M age = 48 years)	Retrospective cohort study	CPAP	Total costs, all-cause and OSA-related hospitalizations	CPAP was associated with reduced total costs ($959 vs. $1,069) and rates of all-cause (19% vs. 24.2%) and OSA-related (8% vs. 11.3%) hospitalizations over 2 years.
(Chhatre et al., 2020)	22,361 US Medicare beneficiaries	Retrospective cohort study	CPAP	Total costs	Versus low adherence, CPAP adherence was associated with reduced total costs.
(de Vries et al., 2019)	86 US adults, 82.3% men in US (M age = 50.7 years)	Multicenter RCT	CPAP, OA	QALY, treatment costs	CPAP was more clinically effective, but OA was more cost-effective over 1 year ($51,558 per QALY gained).

(Hoffman et al., 2010)	248, 99% men, commercial drivers in US (M age = 44 years)	Retrospective cohort study	CPAP or BPAP	Total costs	Versus prediagnosis, CPAP was associated with reduced HCRU costs over 2 years (Year 1: $3,706; Year 2: $4,194).
(Javaheri et al., 2011)	30,719, 43% men in US (M age = 67.1 years)	Retrospective cohort study	CPAP	Costs	Versus those not tested, not clinically diagnosed, and not treated, costs were lowest for those tested, diagnosed, and treated ($7,825/quarter vs. $14,621/quarter).
(Jennum & Kjellberg, 2011)	19,438, 78% men in Denmark	Retrospective cohort study	CPAP, UPPP	Total costs	Neither CPAP nor UPPP reduced HCRU or costs over 2 years.
(Kirsch et al., 2019)	1,098, 63% men in US (M age = 55.7 years)	Retrospective cohort study	CPAP	Acute care HCRU and costs	CPAP adherence was associated with reduced inpatient (RR = 0.92, 95% CI [0.86, 0.98]) and acute care visits (RR = 0.96, 95% CI [0.92, 0.99]).
(McMillan et al., 2015)	278, 79% men in UK (M age = 71 years)	Multicenter RCT	APAP	QALY, treatment costs	APAP was associated with 0.018 QALYs gained and reduced costs $74 over 1 year and was marginally cost-effective.
(Peker et al., 1997)	82, 82% men in Sweden (M age = 55 years)	Retrospective cohort study	CPAP	Hospital costs	CPAP was associated with reduced CVD-related hospitalization costs ($97,651 vs. $13,476) over 2 years.
(Tarasiuk et al., 2004)	740 children <18 years (M age = 5.6 years), 37% boys in Israel	Prospective, longitudinal case–control study	TA	Total costs	CPAP was associated with 32.5% reduced total costs over 1 year.
(Wickwire, Bailey, et al., 2022)	1,921 US Medicare beneficiaries with CVD and comorbid OSA	Retrospective cohort study	CPAP	Inpatient HCRU	High CPAP adherence was associated with 25% reduction in inpatient visits (HR = 0.75, 95% CI [0.57, 0.97]).

Note. Costs have been updated to 2022 US dollars using the inflation calculator provided by the US Bureau of Labor Statistics. (When needed, costs were first translated from international currencies to US dollars in the year of publication, then adjusted for inflation.) APAP = auto-titrating positive airway pressure; BPAP = bilevel positive airway pressure; CI = confidence interval; CPAP = continuous positive airway pressure; CVD = cardiovascular disease; DME = durable medical equipment; HCRU = healthcare resource utilization; HR = hazard ratio; M = mean; OA = oral appliance; OSA = obstructive sleep apnea; QALY = quality-adjusted life year; RCT = randomized controlled trial; RR = risk ratio; TA = tonsillectomy and adenoidectomy; UPPP = uvulopalatopharyngoplasty.

In terms of OSA economics, several issues warrant mention. First, OSA costs include costs of diagnostic testing, which can vary widely (e.g., home sleep apnea test [HSAT]/ auto-titrating positive airway pressure to hospital-based, fully attended polysomnography and separate titration). Broadly speaking, OSA care pathways are understudied in sleep medicine and are influenced by patient, provider, and health system–level characteristics. Second, different stakeholders experience different costs differently. For example, Kim and colleagues (2015) performed an economic analysis of a multi-site OSA clinical trial. From the payer perspective, relative to in-lab management, in-home management was associated with $264 savings over 3 months. However, from the provider perspective, operating margin was reduced ($142 to –$161) and became not profitable during this same period (Kim et al., 2015). Finally, time horizon is an important consideration as costs of insomnia and OSA treatment are front-loaded, but economic benefit can be realized over time.

Transition to Value-Based Care

Healthcare costs increase at an alarming rate. However, as highlighted in this chapter, different costs are borne by different stakeholders. To reduce costs and minimize financial risk, stakeholders engage in cost-shifting. For example, employers and insurance plan sponsors frequently require increased copayments or high-deductible health plans, thereby shifting upfront costs to employees and patients. Figure 22.1 depicts tensions inherent in cost-shifting.

Another approach to financial risk management is to modify payment structures. In the broader healthcare universe, alternative payment models (APMs) have been implemented to accelerate the transition away from fee-for-service (FFS; i.e., from volume-based care to value-based care). The goals of value-based frameworks are to maximize quality and minimize cost. Figure 22.2 presents a continuum of shared risk, ranging from FFS at the most conservative end of the continuum to full population health management at the other. In a traditional FFS model, health providers (e.g., hospitals, durable

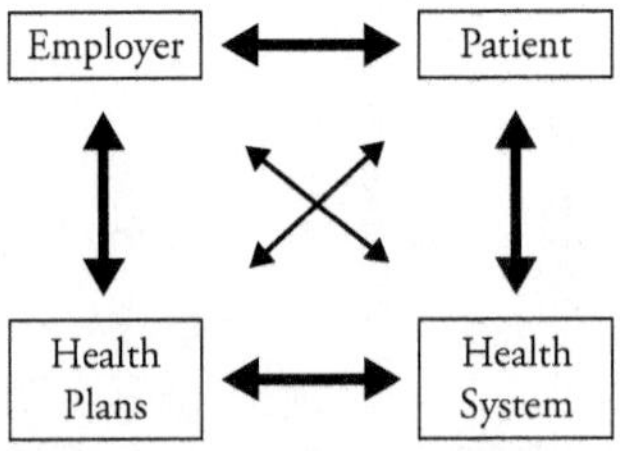

Figure 22.1 Cost-shifting transfers financial risk between stakeholders

Note. Cost-shifting is an approach used by payers, employers, health systems, and patients to reduce costs and minimize financial risk. Each stakeholder seeks to "shift" costs, often up-front costs such as co-pays or deductibles, to another. Figure from Wickwire EM, Verma T. Value and payment in sleep medicine. *J Clin Sleep Med. 2018;14*(5):881–884. Copyright American Academy of Sleep Medicine. Reproduced with permission.

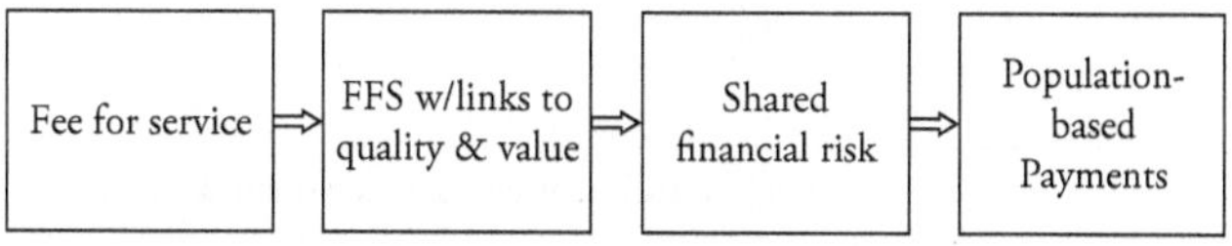

Figure 22.2 Alternate payment models support transition from volume to value

Note. Alternate payment models (APMs) are designed to support the transition from volume-based fee-for-service (FFS) payments to value-based care. Incremental steps transition from exclusive FFS payments to FFS payments with links to quality, then to shared financial risk, and finally to total population health. Interested readers are referred to the excellent white paper published by the Health Care Payment & Learning Action Network at www.hcp-lan.org. Figure from Wickwire EM, Verma T. Value and payment in sleep medicine. *J Clin Sleep Med. 2018;14*(5):881–884. Copyright American Academy of Sleep Medicine. Reproduced with permission.

medical equipment [DME] providers, etc.) receive a pre-negotiated fee for a given service. Although the FFS approach is highly predictable for health providers, FFS models largely commoditize health services, separate billable activities from health outcomes, and do not provide any financial incentives to provide high-quality patient care. The next model on the continuum remains primarily an FFS model but also incorporates a quality metric. To illustrate this approach, a DME provider could receive a fee of $X for PAP masks and resupply, but for each patient who remains adherent to PAP, this fee is increased by 10%. Interested readers are referred to a more detailed discussion using HSAT as an example, including cost-shifting between stakeholders (Wickwire & Verma, 2018). Although APMs are only beginning to emerge in sleep medicine, savvy sleep medicine providers will prepare for bundled payments and shared risk, which are sure to impact the practice of sleep medicine in the future.

Future Research Directions

To maximize impact, sleep scientists seeking to increase the perceived value of the field must adopt several strategies as part of a value-based, sleep health economic research roadmap. First, sleep researchers should include carefully selected economic endpoints in all insomnia and OSA clinical trials and throughout sleep research. Second, given that insomnia and OSA are highly comorbid with a broad range of medical and psychiatric conditions, it is essential to evaluate economic aspects of sleep disorders within comorbid disease subgroups. Although it is methodologically challenging to disentangle the effects of sleep disorders within the context of comorbid disease conditions, such efforts are vital (Wickwire, 2017). Third, to understand the economic impact of sleep disorders, researchers must adopt the diverse perspectives of stakeholders whom we serve, including the employer perspective. After all, the majority of insomnia and OSA-related costs are borne by employers, but very few studies have evaluated economic outcomes from the employer perspective. Fourth, much greater attention needs to be paid to the economic impact of PAP adherence, including economic aspects of interventions designed to improve PAP adherence (Wickwire, 2017; Wickwire, Albrecht, et al., 2019; Wickwire et al., 2013).

Table 22.4 Recommendations for future research	
Domain	Recommendation
Incorporate health economic outcomes	Measure direct and indirect costs of sleep disorders in all clinical trials.
Assess HrQOL	Include measures of generic and disease-specific HrQOL.
Target key subpopulations	Perform health economic analyses among demographic groups, including racial groups, women, older adults, and children.
Investigate comorbid sleep disorders	Evaluate economic impact of insomnia and OSA treatments in key comorbid disease states (e.g., cardiovascular disease, depression).
Increase PAP adherence	Evaluate cost–benefit of interventions to increase treatment adherence, including behavioral approaches, telehealth and remote monitoring, and automated approaches.
Adopt stakeholder perspectives	Consider especially the employer perspective (e.g., study workplace productivity and accident and injury risk).
Consider global impact	Study sleep disorder treatments in various healthcare delivery systems globally.
Compare established treatments	Compare economic effectiveness of established sleep disorder treatments to guide allocation of limited healthcare resources.

Note. HrQOL = health-related quality of life; OSA = obstructive sleep apnea; PAP = positive airway pressure.

Finally, especially given the rapid uptake of telehealth during COVID-19, greater insight into economic aspects of telehealth and remote monitoring is vital. Table 22.4 presents actionable recommendations to advance sleep health economic science.

Conclusions

Sleep disorders including insomnia and OSA incur significant economic costs borne by payers, health systems, industry partners, and other key stakeholders. A small and rapidly expanding scientific literature suggests that diagnosis and treatment of these sleep disorders are associated with positive economic benefit. Sleep researchers should include economic endpoints in all future clinical trials and strive to adopt the economic perspectives of the multiple stakeholders whom we serve. These recommendations will become even more important as economic aspects of care increasingly determine health policy and resource allocation in the future.

References

Albarrak, M., Banno, K., Sabbagh, A. A., Delaive, K., Walld, R., Manfreda, J., & Kryger, M. H. (2005). Utilization of healthcare resources in obstructive sleep apnea syndrome: A 5-year follow-up study in men using CPAP. *Sleep*, *28*(10), 1306–1311.

Amari, D. T., Juday, T., Frech, F. H., Wang, W., Wu, Z., Atkins, N., & Wickwire, E. M. (2022). Falls, healthcare resources and costs in older adults with insomnia treated with zolpidem, trazodone, or benzodiazepines. *BMC Geriatrics*, *22*(1), Article 484. https://doi.org/10.1186/s12877-022-03165-6

American Academy of Sleep Medicine. (2016). *Hidden health crisis costing America billions: Underdiagnosing and undertreating obstructive sleep apnea draining healthcare system*. Frost and Sullivan.

Bahammam, A., Delaive, K., Ronald, J., Manfreda, J., Roos, L., & Kryger, M. H. (1999). Health care utilization in males with obstructive sleep apnea syndrome two years after diagnosis and treatment. *Sleep*, *22*(6), 740–747.

Bailey, M. D., Wickwire, E. M., Somers, V. K., & Albrecht, J. S. (2022). Adherence to continuous positive airway pressure reduces the risk of 30-day hospital readmission among older adults with comorbid obstructive sleep apnea and cardiovascular disease. *Journal of Clinical Sleep Medicine*, *18*(12), 2739–2744. https://doi.org/10.5664/jcsm.10196

Baka, A., van der Zweerde, T., Lancee, J., Bosmans, J. E., & van Straten, A. (2022). Cost-effectiveness of guided internet-delivered cognitive behavioral therapy in comparison with care-as-usual for patients with insomnia in general practice. *Behavioral Sleep Medicine*, *20*(2), 188–203. https://doi.org/10.1080/15402002.2021.1901708

Banno, K., Manfreda, J., Walld, R., Delaive, K., & Kryger, M. H. (2006). Healthcare utilization in women with obstructive sleep apnea syndrome 2 years after diagnosis and treatment. *Sleep*, *29*(10), 1307–1311.

Bock, J. M., Needham, K. A., Gregory, D. A., Ekono, M. M., Wickwire, E. M., Somers, V. K., & Lerman, A. (2022). Continuous positive airway pressure adherence and treatment cost in patients with obstructive sleep apnea and cardiovascular disease. *Mayo Clinic Proceedings: Innovations, Quality & Outcomes*, *6*(2), 166–175. https://doi.org/10.1016/j.mayocpiqo.2022.01.002

Bonin, E. M., Beecham, J., Swift, N., Raikundalia, S., & Brown, J. S. (2014). Psycho-educational CBT-insomnia workshops in the community. A cost-effectiveness analysis alongside a randomised controlled trial. *Behaviour Research and Therapy*, *55*, 40–47. https://doi.org/10.1016/j.brat.2014.01.005

Brooks, R. (1996). EuroQol: The current state of play. *Health Policy (Amsterdam, Netherlands)*, *37*(1), 53–72. https://doi.org/10.1016/0168-8510(96)00822-6

Buntrock, C., Lehr, D., Smit, F., Horvath, H., Berking, M., Spiegelhalder, K., Riper, H., & Ebert, D. D. (2021). Guided internet-based cognitive behavioral therapy for insomnia: Health-economic evaluation from the societal and public health care perspective alongside a randomized controlled trial. *Journal of Medical Internet Research*, *23*(5), Article e25609. https://doi.org/10.2196/25609

Cai, Q., Tan, H., & Singer, J. (2012). Impact of positive airway pressure among obstructive sleep apnea patients. *The American Journal of Managed Care*, *18*(6), e225–e233.

Chhatre, S., Chang, Y. H. A., Gooneratne, N. S., Kuna, S., Strollo, P., & Jayadevappa, R. (2020). Association between adherence to continuous positive airway pressure treatment and cost among Medicare enrollees. *Sleep*, *43*(1), Article zsz188. https://doi.org/10.1093/sleep/zsz188

Collen, J., Lettieri, C., Wickwire, E., & Holley, A. (2020). Obstructive sleep apnea and cardiovascular disease, a story of confounders! *Sleep and Breathing*, *24*, 1299–1313. https://doi.org/10.1007/s11325-019-01945-w

Daley, M., Morin, C. M., LeBlanc, M., Gregoire, J. P., & Savard, J. (2009). The economic burden of insomnia: Direct and indirect costs for individuals with insomnia syndrome, insomnia symptoms, and good sleepers. *Sleep*, *32*(1), 55–64.

Darden, M., Espie, C. A., Carl, J. R., Henry, A. L., Kanady, J. C., Krystal, A. D., & Miller, C. B. (2021). Cost-effectiveness of digital cognitive behavioral therapy (Sleepio) for insomnia: A Markov simulation model in the United States. *Sleep*, *44*(4), Article zsaa223. https://doi.org/10.1093/sleep/zsaa223

de Vries, G. E., Hoekema, A., Vermeulen, K. M., Claessen, J. Q. P. J., Jacobs, W., van der Maten, J., van der Hoeven, J. H., Stegenga, B., Kerstjen, H. A. M., & Wijkstra, P. J. (2019). Clinical- and cost-effectiveness of a mandibular advancement device versus continuous positive airway pressure in moderate obstructive sleep apnea. *Journal of Clinical Sleep Medicine*, *15*(10), 1477–1485. https://doi.org/10.5664/jcsm.7980

Hanmer, J., Feeny, D., Fischhoff, B., Hays, R. D., Hess, R., Pilkonis, P. A., Revicki, D. A., Roberts, M. S., Tsevat, J., & Yu, L. (2015). The PROMIS of QALYs. *Health Qual Life Outcomes*, *13*, Article 122. https://doi.org/10.1186/s12955-015-0321-6

Hoffman, B., Wingenbach, D. D., Kagey, A. N., Schaneman, J. L., & Kasper, D. (2010). The long-term health plan and disability cost benefit of obstructive sleep apnea treatment in a commercial motor vehicle driver population. *Journal of Occupational and Environmental Medicine*, *52*(5), 473–477. https://doi.org/10.1097/JOM.0b013e3181dbc8ab

Javaheri, S., Caref, E. B., Chen, E., Tong, K. B., & Abraham, W. T. (2011). Sleep apnea testing and outcomes in a large cohort of Medicare beneficiaries with newly diagnosed heart failure. *American Journal of Respiratory and Critical Care Medicine*, *183*(4), 539–546. https://doi.org/10.1164/rccm.201003-0406OC

Jennum, P., & Kjellberg, J. (2011). Health, social and economical consequences of sleep-disordered breathing: A controlled national study. *Thorax*, *66*(7), 560–566. https://doi.org/10.1136/thx.2010.143958

Kim, R. D., Kapur, V. K., Redline-Bruch, J., Rueschman, M., Auckley, D. H., Benca, R. M., Foldvary-Schafer, N. R., Iber, C., Zee, P. C., Rosen, C. L., Redline, S., & Ramsey, S. D. (2015). An economic evaluation of home versus laboratory-based diagnosis of obstructive sleep apnea. *Sleep, 38*(7), 1027–1037. https://doi.org/10.5665/sleep.4804

Kirsch, D. B., Yang, H., Maslow, A. L., Stolzenbach, M., & McCall, A. (2019). Association of positive airway pressure use with acute care utilization and costs. *Journal of Clinical Sleep Medicine, 15*(9), 1243–1250. https://doi.org/10.5664/jcsm.7912

Martin, S. A., Aikens, J. E., & Chervin, R. D. (2004). Toward cost-effectiveness analysis in the diagnosis and treatment of insomnia. *Sleep Medicine Reviews, 8*(1), 63–72. https://doi.org/10.1016/j.smrv.2003.08.001

McCrae, C. S., Bramoweth, A. D., Williams, J., Roth, A., & Mosti, C. (2014). Impact of brief cognitive behavioral treatment for insomnia on health care utilization and costs. *Journal of Clinical Sleep Medicine, 10*(2), 127–135. https://doi.org/10.5664/jcsm.3436

McMillan, A., Bratton, D. J., Faria, R., Laskawiec-Szkonter, M., Griffin, S., Davies, R. J., Nunn, A. J., Stradling, J. R., Riha, R. L., & Morrell, M. J. (2015). A multicentre randomised controlled trial and economic evaluation of continuous positive airway pressure for the treatment of obstructive sleep apnoea syndrome in older people: PREDICT. *Health Technology Assessment (Winchester, England), 19*(40), 1–188. https://doi.org/10.3310/hta19400

Mohit, B., & Cohen, J. T. (2019). Trends of cost-effectiveness studies in sleep medicine. *Sleep Medicine, 53*, 176–180. https://doi.org/10.1016/j.sleep.2018.06.001

Morgan, K., Dixon, S., Mathers, N., Thompson, J., & Tomeny, M. (2004). Psychological treatment for insomnia in the regulation of long-term hypnotic drug use. *Health Technology Assessment (Winchester, England), 8*(8), iii–iv, 1–68. https://doi.org/10.3310/hta8080

Muennig, P., & Bounthavong, M. (2016). *Cost-effectiveness analysis in health: A practical approach* (3rd ed.). Jossey-Bass.

National Commission on Sleep Disorders Research. (1993). *Wake up America: A national sleep alert: Report of the National Commission on Sleep Disorders Research.*

Neumann, P. J., Sanders, G. D., Russell, L. B., Siegel, J. E., & Ganiats, T. G. (2017). *Cost-effectiveness in health and medicine* (2nd ed.). Oxford University Press.

Peker, Y., Hedner, J., Johansson, A., & Bende, M. (1997). Reduced hospitalization with cardiovascular and pulmonary disease in obstructive sleep apnea patients on nasal CPAP treatment. *Sleep, 20*(8), 645–653.

Sampson, C., Bell, E., Cole, A., Miller, C. B., Marriott, T., Williams, M., & Rose, J. (2022). Digital cognitive behavioural therapy for insomnia and primary care costs in England: An interrupted time series analysis. *BJGP Open, 6*(2), Article BJGPO.2021.0146. https://doi.org/10.3399/BJGPO.2021.0146

Snedecor, S. J., Botteman, M. F., Bojke, C., Schaefer, K., Barry, N., & Pickard, A. S. (2009). Cost-effectiveness of eszopiclone for the treatment of adults with primary chronic insomnia. *Sleep, 32*(6), 817–824.

Snedecor, S. J., Botteman, M. F., Schaefer, K., Sarocco, P., Barry, N., & Pickard, A. S. (2010). Economic outcomes of eszopiclone treatment in insomnia and comorbid major depressive disorder. *The Journal of Mental Health Policy and Economics, 13*(1), 27–35.

Tarasiuk, A., Simon, T., Tal, A., & Reuveni, H. (2004). Adenotonsillectomy in children with obstructive sleep apnea syndrome reduces health care utilization. *Pediatrics, 113*(2), 351–356.

Ware, J. E., Jr., & Sherbourne, C. D. (1992). The MOS 36-item short-form health survey (SF-36). I. Conceptual framework and item selection. *Medical Care, 30*(6), 473–483.

Watanabe, N., Furukawa, T. A., Shimodera, S., Katsuki, F., Fujita, H., Sasaki, M., Sado, M., & Perlis, M. L. (2015). Cost-effectiveness of cognitive behavioral therapy for insomnia comorbid with depression: Analysis of a randomized controlled trial. *Psychiatry and Clinical Neurosciences, 69*(6), 335–343. https://doi.org/10.1111/pcn.12237

Weaver, T. E., Laizner, A. M., Evans, L. K., Maislin, G., Chugh, D. K., Lyon, K., Smith, P. L., Schwartz, A. R., Redline, S., Pack, A. I., & Dinges, D. F. (1997). An instrument to measure functional status outcomes for disorders of excessive sleepiness. *Sleep, 20*(10), 835–843.

Wickwire, E. M. (2017). Making dollars and sense of SAVE. *Journal of Clinical Sleep Medicine, 13*(5), 765–766. https://doi.org/10.5664/jcsm.6606

Wickwire, E. M., Albrecht, J. S., Towe, M. M., Abariga, S. A., Diaz-Abad, M., Shipper, A. G., Cooper, L. M., Assefa, S. Z., Tom, S. E., & Scharf, S. M. (2019). The impact of treatments for OSA on monetized health economic outcomes: A systematic review. *Chest, 155*(5), 947–961. https://doi.org/10.1016/j.chest.2019.01.009

Wickwire, E. M., Amari, D. T., Juday, T. R., Frech, F., Gor, D., & Malhotra, M. (2022). Incremental health care resource use and costs among adult patients with depression and treated for insomnia with zolpidem, trazodone, or benzodiazepines. *Current Medical Research and Opinion*, *38*(5), 711–720. https://doi.org/10.1080/03007995.2022.2047537

Wickwire, E. M., Bailey, M. D., Somers, V. K., Oldstone, L. M., Srivastava, M. C., Johnson, A. M., Scharf, S. M., & Albrecht, J. S. (2022). CPAP adherence is associated with reduced inpatient utilization among older adult Medicare beneficiaries with pre-existing cardiovascular disease. *Journal of Clinical Sleep Medicine*, *18*(1), 39–45. https://doi.org/10.5664/jcsm.9478

Wickwire, E. M., Lettieri, C. J., Cairns, A. A., & Collop, N. A. (2013). Maximizing positive airway pressure adherence in adults: A common-sense approach. *Chest*, *144*(2), 680–693. https://doi.org/10.1378/chest.12-2681

Wickwire, E. M., & Morin, C. M. (2020). Advancing a value framework for sleep: Update on economic aspects of cognitive-behavioral treatments for insomnia. *Sleep Medicine Reviews*, *54*, Article 101387. https://doi.org/10.1016/j.smrv.2020.101387

Wickwire, E. M., Shaya, F. T., & Scharf, S. M. (2015). Health economics of insomnia treatments: The return on investment for a good night's sleep. *Sleep Medicine Reviews*, *30*, 72–82. https://doi.org/10.1016/j.smrv.2015.11.004

Wickwire, E. M., Vadlamani, A., Tom, S. E., Johnson, A. M., Scharf, S. M., & Albrecht, J. S. (2019). Economic aspects of insomnia medication treatment among Medicare beneficiaries. *Sleep*, *43*(1), Article zsz192. https://doi.org/10.1093/sleep/zsz192

Wickwire, E. M., & Verma, T. (2018). Value and payment in sleep medicine. *Journal of Clinical Sleep Medicine*, *14*(5), 881–884. https://doi.org/10.5664/jcsm.7130

Yeung, K., Zhu, W., McCurry, S. M., Von Korff, M., Wellman, R., Morin, C. M., & Vitiello, M. V. (2022). Cost-effectiveness of telephone cognitive behavioral therapy for osteoarthritis-related insomnia. *Journal of the American Geriatrics Society*, *70*(1), 188–199. https://doi.org/10.1111/jgs.17469

CHAPTER

23

Clinical Assessment of Sleep–Wake Complaints

Jason C. Ong, Colin A. Espie, *and* James K. Wyatt

Abstract

This chapter presents an overview of the assessment of sleep disorders, including the clinical tools and recommendations for how to apply them in a clinical setting. The core components of conducting a clinical interview are reviewed, including how to conduct a functional analysis of the sleep complaint. The sleep diary is the primary self-reported measure to assess sleep/wake patterns, and various formats of sleep diaries are discussed along with the standard parameters collected in diaries. A number of self-report measures are reviewed that can serve to confirm the patient history, provide information about the severity of the sleep condition, or assess the likelihood of comorbid conditions. Considerations for conducting the assessment related to the clinical setting, patient-centered factors, and the integration of emerging technology are also discussed throughout the chapter. Conducting a comprehensive clinical assessment allows the sleep clinician to determine the appropriate diagnosis and set the stage for treatment of the sleep disorder.

Key Words: sleep, assessment, clinical interview, questionnaire, medical history

Introduction

A clinical assessment involves the collection and integration of relevant data from interviews, tests, and behavioral observations for the purpose of determining a diagnosis and/or treatment plan. The assessment of sleep/wake complaints typically begins with one or more of these tools to form a diagnostic impression. For some sleep disorders, such as insomnia, the clinical data is sufficient to determine a diagnosis and formulate a treatment plan. In some cases, the use of wrist actigraphy can provide valuable objective data on longitudinal patterns of sleep and circadian rhythms to clarify the diagnosis and further inform the treatment plan. For other sleep disorders, such as sleep disordered breathing, objective testing with polysomnography (PSG) is required to render an appropriate diagnosis.

In addition to the goal of determining the appropriate diagnosis, a comprehensive assessment should be patient-centered, setting the stage for treatment of the sleep disorder. Assessing the patient's preferred learning method (e.g., oral, demonstrated, written) and any communication barriers (e.g., language problems, hearing or vision deficits, memory problems) can help the clinician determine the most appropriate means of conducting the assessment. Providing expectations to the patient (e.g., what will be covered at this visit vs. follow-up tests) can aid in building rapport with the patient. Allowing patients to respond without interruption and taking time to listen and answer questions can increase satisfaction with the encounter (Lin et al., 2001; Rhoades et al., 2001). Finally, providing appropriate education about the findings of the assessment, explaining the rationale for any additional testing, and instilling hope about the effectiveness of treatment can motivate the patient to adhere to their treatment plan and improve the likelihood of follow-up with the provider (Bell et al., 2002).

For the purposes of this chapter, the outpatient, comprehensive sleep assessment will be reviewed. This approach is recommended for patients presenting for an initial sleep evaluation, for patients requesting a second opinion, and for patients transferring care for a previously diagnosed sleep disorder. Considerations for adapting the assessment for specific referral questions or other settings are discussed. Finally, objective measures such as actigraphy, PSG, and the integration of emerging technologies in the assessment of sleep and future possibilities are briefly covered; and the reader is referred to Chapters 24 and 25 for more detailed discussions of these topics.

Clinical Assessment Tools

Clinical Interview

A semi-structured clinical interview is the primary tool in the assessment of sleep/wake complaints. While there is no "perfect" or definitive sequence to obtaining a patient history, the typical clinical interview for assessing sleep disorders consists of several key areas, which are listed in Box 23.1 and described in this section.

The interview typically begins with the chief complaint or reason for referral. Often, this will involve dissatisfaction with sleep quantity, sleep quality, or sleep patterns; but it could include a primary complaint about daytime functioning and the perceived impact of poor sleep on personal well-being. In some cases, the patient might not have any sleep complaints but present to the clinic due to concerns from a bed partner, family member, or healthcare provider due to medical or psychiatric risk factors. Potential answers range from "My doctor made me come here" to "I fell asleep while driving." These responses should be considered with behavioral observations to help the clinician begin the process of gauging the patient's readiness to engage in the diagnostic and treatment processes. Paying attention to the chief complaint serves as a starting point for directing the interview and interpreting the information collected during the remainder of the interview.

After the chief complaint, an in-depth assessment of the patient's current sleep schedule should be conducted. Specifically, information should be obtained about the bedtime routine, sleep hygiene, and typical bedtime, sleep latency, number and duration of

Box 23.1 Key Areas for Clinical Assessment of Sleep Complaints

Core Components

- Chief complaint or reason for referral, including patient's perception of the sleep problem(s)
- Sleep–wake schedule, including bedtimes and wake times, variability of schedule, problems with sleep initiation or maintenance
- Sleep hygiene
- Daytime functioning, including daytime sleepiness, fatigue, napping, cognitive functioning, and perceived social and emotional sequelae of the sleep problem
- Symptoms of specific sleep disorders
- Previous sleep assessments, diagnoses, and treatment
- Family history, including medical, psychiatric, and sleep problems
- Health habits, including exercise, caffeine, nicotine, alcohol, illicit substances
- Medications, over-the-counter medications, and supplements
- Allergies, including medication, environmental, and food
- Past medical and surgical history, including acute and chronic conditions and recent emergency room visits or hospitalizations
- Psychiatric history

Optional Components

- Functional analysis of sleep
- Physical examination (as appropriate, depending on provider qualifications)

awakenings during the sleep episode, wake time, and total sleep time. Consideration of variability and unpredictability in these sleep–wake characteristics often assists understanding of sleep–wake complaints. It is important to ask about weeknight versus weekend or other non-work or non-school nights, given the common occurrence of people extending their sleep hours on an ad lib schedule. Patients with insomnia may also report worse sleep on school or work nights, given anticipation of functional impairment or other symptoms the next day. To provide context for the current sleep patterns, clinicians should also assess the patient's sleep patterns prior to the onset of the presenting episode of sleep problem. If a bed partner or support person is present at the interview, the clinician can ask about any perceived changes in the patient's sleep patterns since the onset of the problem. Finally, changes over time in the patient's sleep should be explored, including the suddenness of the symptom onset, worsening or stability of the symptoms over time, and any periods of remission or worsening of sleep disturbance.

The next section of the interview assesses daytime functioning, including excessive daytime sleepiness, fatigue, and the impact on interpersonal or occupational/academic functioning. An important aspect of assessing daytime sleepiness is the tendency to take naps along with the frequency, duration, and restorative value of naps. In assessing the impact of sleep disturbance on daytime functioning, questions should include the presence of unintentional naps or inability to stay awake at school or work along with the patient's work or school schedule, noting how sleep-related symptoms vary across the course of the day. Changes in concentration, memory, and mood stability are commonly reported as consequences of many sleep disorders.

Next, clinicians should assess for the presence and severity of symptoms of specific sleep disorders. Symptoms of insomnia, including difficulty falling and/or staying asleep, will typically be reported by the patient during the review of sleep patterns; and the clinician can inquire further about the intensity or severity of these symptoms or evaluate other related symptoms. Similarly, symptoms of circadian rhythm sleep–wake disorders (CRSWDs) will typically be reported in terms of misalignment of the timing of the current sleep period with the desired sleep period. Questions aimed at obstructive sleep apnea (OSA) include loud snoring, witnessed gasping or choking, witnessed pauses in breathing, morning headache or dry mouth, enuresis or nocturia, body position–related worsening of snoring or witnessed apnea, and nasal airway patency when lying down. Hypersomnolence-related questions include daytime sleep attacks, cataplexy, automatic behavior, hypnagogic or hypnopompic hallucinations, and sleep paralysis. Specific symptoms of parasomnias or sleep-related movement disorders include sleepwalking, sleep talking, acting out dreams, jaw clenching or teeth grinding during sleep, and repetitive leg or arm twitching during sleep. Assessment of restless legs syndrome (RLS) includes (1) an irresistible urge to move the legs, typically co-occurring with an unusual sensory component; (2) actual movement of the legs; (3) improvement in symptoms with movement and worsening with immobility; and (4) a time-of-day pattern with worsening of symptoms later in the day or in the early evening hours. If available, having patients complete a questionnaire with a list of these symptoms prior to the clinic visit can facilitate the efficiency of this component of the interview.

At this point, the clinician will likely have enough information to determine a working diagnosis. The other components of the interview aid in making a further differential diagnosis (e.g., relationship with comorbid medical or psychiatric condition) and inform treatment planning. Information about previous sleep evaluations and treatment can reinforce the working diagnosis and help determine a treatment plan based on previous success or failure. For example, alternative treatments might be considered for patients who were previously intolerant of positive airway pressure (PAP). Similarly, cognitive-behavioral therapy for insomnia (CBT-I) might be recommended for patients who previously only used hypnotic medication and did not respond or developed hypnotic dependence. It should be noted that assessment of sleep medications should include both prescription medications as well as over-the-counter medications and health food supplements as these are commonly used by patients as a first step in resolving their sleep disturbance. The medical history includes questions about chronic and acute conditions, major injuries, hospitalizations, and surgeries. The psychiatric history should include questions about mood and anxiety disorders as these can have high comorbidity with many sleep disorders. Information about these medical and psychiatric conditions can elucidate the relationship between the sleep problem and the comorbid condition (i.e., primary vs. secondary) to inform treatment planning, such as the sequence of treatment. Information about the family history can provide further indications of certain sleep disorders that have higher risk within families (e.g., OSA) or a known genetic component (e.g., narcolepsy). Similarly, gathering information about health habits, such as use of nicotine, drugs, or excessive caffeine, can be useful in determining the potential cause of the sleep disturbance and/or potential targets for lifestyle modification. Finally, gathering information about environmental factors such as problems with the temperature of the bedroom, noise, sleep disruption caused by the bed partner, or having any caregiving responsibilities during the night can determine the extent to which these factors impact sleep.

Functional Analysis of Sleep

As part of the clinical interview, a functional analysis can be another useful evaluation tool, especially when primary insomnia is suspected as the main diagnosis. Developed from operant conditioning theory, a functional analysis is a method for identifying causal and maintaining factors associated with an individual's behavior by examining the antecedents that trigger the behavior and the consequences that reinforce the behavior. In clinical practice, conducting functional analyses can help the clinician understand the context of the sleep problem and develop a specific plan for targeting behavior change (see Sturmey, 2020).

In assessing sleep and wake complaints for insomnia, conducting a functional analysis can yield information on processes that may be reinforcing sleep-incompatible behaviors. This can provide a better understanding of the perpetuating factors that are maintaining the insomnia and aid in treatment planning for CBT-I. This can be conducted throughout the clinical interview or at a later session, if the patient is to begin CBT. When assessing sleep hygiene, the clinician can inquire about the pre-sleep routine. There are several areas of inquiry that are relevant when conducting a functional analysis of sleep: (1) pre-sleep routine, (2) sleep environment, (3) experiential avoidance, (4) daytime cognitions, and (5) secondary gain.

First, the functions of the pre-sleep routine should be assessed. For example, is there adequate time for winding down, or does the patient use the bed as a place to process the day's events or plan for tomorrow? Does the patient become apprehensive about sleep as bedtime approaches? Does the patient engage in activities for the sake of trying to fall asleep? Next, it is important to inquire about the stimulus value of the bed and bedroom to determine if conditioned arousal is a factor. Does the patient become anxious or tense when getting into bed? Does the patient sleep better away from home? Many patients with insomnia will also exhibit experiential avoidance, where the patient develops a restricted pattern of thoughts or behaviors that limits the opportunity to test the veracity of the thoughts or the benefits of changing behavior. Inquiry into experiential avoidance might consist of asking patients why they do not get out of bed when they cannot sleep or why they attempt to go to bed early despite not feeling sleepy. In addition to nighttime behaviors, functional analysis should include careful examination of daytime cognitions. For example, how does the patient respond to a night of disturbed sleep? Does the patient engage in automatic thoughts about the consequences of sleep disturbance? Has the patient begun to engage in "safety behaviors" (e.g., restricting daytime behaviors due to insomnia; Harvey, 2002)? Finally, issues related to secondary gain should be explored: the potential reinforcement from missing work, increased attention, or avoidance of social obligations. Does the patient appear to be assuming the sick role? Has the patient recently retired and taken on the new job of solving their sleep problem? Are there family conflicts that might play a role in reinforcing the patient's sleep complaints? The patient may or may not have insight into these issues, so questioning should be careful so as to not implicate an ulterior motive.

Functional analysis can also be applied to other sleep disorders beyond insomnia. For example, is there evidence of secondary gain from hypersomnolence? Is non-adherence to continuous PAP (CPAP) treatment a result of perceived loss of control? Are symptoms of RLS triggered by situational cues? Each of these behaviors can be addressed using the same targeted evaluation and interpretation as in the case of insomnia.

Physical Examination

Although a physical examination is generally included as part of a medical evaluation, there is no clear consensus on the need for a physical examination as part of the clinical evaluation of a sleep patient. First, there is variability in terms of the provider. If the provider is a physician, the physical examination is standard and may add important clinical information to inform diagnosis. For example, a more extensive neurological examination may be indicated for suspected RLS or periodic limb movement disorder. Neck circumference, judging the Mallampati score (visual appraisal of space in the posterior oral airway), assessing nasal airway patency, measuring blood pressure and pulse and respiratory rate, and calculating the body mass index are essential as part of the physical examination for working up a sleep-related breathing disorder. If the provider is a psychologist or other non-physician conducting the clinical evaluation for a specific referral, such as evaluation and treatment of insomnia, the patient should have previously received a physical examination during an office visit with the referring provider or primary care physician in the past few months. Ideally, the sleep clinician should obtain a copy of those results to supplement the clinical assessment of the sleep complaint.

Second, the rise of telehealth evaluations has also changed the notion of a traditional physical examination. Although it might be possible to use synchronous videoconferencing to determine a Mallampati score or to observe a patient measuring their own neck circumference, most telehealth consults do not involve a physical examination. The overall requirements for a physical examination should be based upon the clinical need, provider's background, and modality of evaluation (in-person vs. telehealth).

Self-Report Measures

Self-report measures are another key component of the clinical assessment and generally follow the same areas listed in Box 23.1 to complement the clinical interview. Sleep diaries are the primary self-report measure in the clinical evaluation of sleep disorders. Several sleep-specific validated questionnaires can complement the clinical interview with additional information about the frequency, severity, and intensity of specific sleep symptoms. Validated measures of psychiatric conditions can help determine the presence of comorbid conditions such as depression, anxiety, or post-traumatic stress disorder (PTSD). Finally, measures of health-related quality of life can provide a global assessment of the impact of sleep disorders on the patient's quality of life.

The selection of these measures should be based on the goals of the assessment along with considerations for patient burden to complete the measures. When administered prior to the clinical interview, these can be very useful tools to guide the clinician in directing the interview to relevant domains and more specific lines of questioning. When administered following the clinical interview, measures such as the sleep–wake diary can reveal patterns of sleep disturbance and timing that can assist in differential diagnosis (e.g., insomnia vs. delayed sleep phase). Several recommended and commonly used measures in sleep medicine are reviewed in this section and summarized in Table 23.1.

SLEEP–WAKE DIARIES

Perhaps the most commonly used self-report tool in the assessment of sleep disorders is the daily sleep diary, or sleep log. Sleep diaries are indicated as a practice parameter guideline in the assessment and treatment of insomnia and the CRSWDs (Morgenthaler et al., 2007; Schutte-Rodin et al., 2008). While not indicated as a practice parameter, sleep diaries can also provide valuable information in the appraisal and management of other sleep disorders such as narcolepsy, idiopathic hypersomnolence, and OSA.

There is a variety of sleep diary formats, but most include patient ratings of sleep patterns, sleep continuity, and daytime functioning. Specifically, patients are asked to record the time they get into bed in the evening and the time they get out of bed in the morning, providing a calculation of the total time in bed (TIB). Patients are also asked to estimate the time it takes them to fall asleep after getting into bed, referred to as *sleep onset latency* (SOL). Sleep diaries should also include space for patients to record the number of awakenings during the night and the total time they spent awake during these awakenings, referred to as *wake after sleep onset* (WASO). Patients are also often asked to estimate their total sleep time (TST) each night, or this can be determined by subtracting SOL and WASO from TIB. With respect to daytime functioning, ratings of sleepiness and fatigue and/or the timing and duration of any naps during the day should also be recorded. Finally, a patient-centered sleep diary can include a free-response space for patients to record additional information that may impact sleep, such as unusual stressors of the day, consumption of alcohol, or use of medications for sleep.

Table 23.1 List of recommended sleep questionnaires

Domain assessed	Measure	Author(s)	Population	Description
Multiple sleep domains	Pittsburgh Sleep Quality Index	Buysse et al. (1989)	Adults	A 19-item scale that assesses subjective sleep quality, sleep latency, sleep duration, sleep efficiency, sleep disturbances, use of sleep medications, and daytime dysfunction.
	PROMIS Sleep Disturbance	Buysse et al. (2010)	Adults	Scale consisting of a 27-item bank that measures perceptions of sleep quality, sleep depth, and restfulness of sleep. Can be administered using short form or computer adaptive testing.
	PROMIS Sleep-Related Impairment	Buysse et al. (2010)	Adults	Scale consisting of a 16-item bank that measures perceptions of alertness, sleepiness, and tiredness during usual waking hours and the perceived functional impairments during wakefulness associated with sleep problems or impaired alertness. Can be administered as a short form or using computerized adaptive testing.
	Sleep Habits Survey	Wolfson and Carskadon (1998)	Adolescents	Assesses sleep patterns (e.g., school-night sleep time, weekend bedtime and delay, and number of nights sleeping in same bed) as well as daytime functioning (e.g., accidents/injuries, school performance, depressed mood, daytime sleepiness).
	Children's Sleep Habits Questionnaire	Owens et al. (2000)	Children 4–12 years old	A 45-item scale completed by parents that assesses bedtime resistance, sleep onset delay, sleep duration, sleep anxiety, nighttime awakenings, parasomnias, sleep disordered breathing, and daytime sleepiness.
Daytime sleepiness	Stanford Sleepiness Scale	Hoddes et al. (1973)	Adults	State measure of subjective sleepiness that asks patients to rate sleepiness from "feeling active and alert" to "sleep onset soon."
	Karolinska Sleepiness Scale	Åkerstedt and Gilberg (1990)	Adults	State measure of subjective sleepiness that asks patients to rate sleepiness from "very alert" to "very sleepy."

Continued

Table 23.1 *Continued*

Domain assessed	Measure	Author(s)	Population	Description
	Epworth Sleepiness Scale	Johns (1991)	Adults	An eight-item scale that asks patients to rate their propensity to fall asleep or "doze off" in a variety of common activities that range from passive to active situations. Higher scores represent greater daytime sleepiness.
	Pediatric Daytime Sleepiness Scale	Drake et al. (2003)	Children 11–15 years old	An eight-item scale that asks children to rate sleepiness in common situations (e.g., in class, doing homework), difficulty waking in the morning, and daytime tiredness and grumpiness.
	Functional Outcomes of Sleep Questionnaire	Weaver et al. (1997)	Adults	A 30-item scale that assesses impact of excessive daytime sleepiness on five domains of daily activities (general activity, vigilance, interpersonal relationships, general productivity, and social activities).
Daytime fatigue	Fatigue Severity Scale	Krupp et al. (1989)	Adults	A seven-item scale that assesses fatigue severity.
	Flinders Fatigue Scale	Gradisar et al. (2007)	Adults	Scale assessing fatigue attributed to insomnia.
Chronotype	Morningness–Eveningness Questionnaire	Horne and Östberg (1976)	Adults	A 19-item scale assessing preference toward increased activity in the mornings versus the evenings.
	Munich Chronotype Questionnaire	Roenneberg et al. (2003)	Adults	A 17-item scale assessing habitual sleep timing on workdays and free days.
Insomnia	Insomnia Severity Index	Bastien et al. (2001)	Adults	A seven-item scale that assesses difficulty initiating and maintaining sleep, daytime consequences of poor sleep, and subjective distress about sleep disturbance.
	Sleep Condition Indicator	Espie et al. (2014)	Adults	An eight-item scale assessing nighttime and daytime complaints presenting in insomnia, based upon DSM-5 criteria

	Glasgow Sleep Impact Index	Kyle et al. (2013)	Adults	Generates and assesses the three domains of impairment most salient to the patient presenting with insomnia
	Dysfunctional Attitudes and Beliefs About Sleep Scale	Morin et al. (1993)	Adults	A 30-item scale that assesses beliefs about the causes of insomnia and consequences of insomnia, unrealistic sleep expectations, perceptions of diminished control over sleep, and beliefs about sleep-promoting behaviors.
Obstructive sleep apnea	Berlin Questionnaire	Netzer et al. (1999)	Adults	Screening tool used to identify patients at high risk for sleep apnea. Assesses snoring, daytime sleepiness, and physical/ medical risk factors.
	Pediatric Sleep Questionnaire	Chervin et al. (2000)	Children 2–18 years old	A 22-item scale completed by parents that assesses sleep disordered breathing, daytime sleepiness, and inattention/ hyperactivity.
Restless legs syndrome	International Restless Legs Scale	Allen et al. (2003)	Adults	A 10-item scale that assesses RLS symptom frequency, severity, and impact on sleep, as well as impact of RLS symptoms on daily activity and mood. Sensitive to detect changes in RLS following pharmacological treatment.
Depression	PROMIS Depression Scale	Pilkonis et al. (2011)	Adults	Self-report measure of negative mood (sadness, guilt), views of self (self-criticism, worthlessness), social cognition (loneliness, interpersonal alienation), decreased positive affect and engagement (loss of interest, meaning, and purpose).
	PHQ-9	Kroenke et al. (2001)	Adults	A nine-item scale measuring severity of depression symptoms. Validated as a screening tool as well as measuring clinically meaningful changes in depressive symptoms associated with treatment.
	Geriatric Depression Scale	Yesavage et al. (1982)	Older Adults	A 30-item scale measuring depression in older adults.
Anxiety	PROMIS Anxiety Scale	Pilkonis et al. (2011)	Adults	Self-report measures of fear, anxious thoughts (worry, dread), hyperarousal (tension, restlessness), and somatic symptoms (racing heart, dizziness).

Continued

Table 23.1 *Continued*

Domain assessed	Measure	Author(s)	Population	Description
	State Trait Anxiety Inventory	Spielberger et al. (1970)	Adults	A 40-item scale measuring symptoms of anxiety (feelings of unease, worry, tension) as a state and trait.
	GAD-7	Spitzer et al. 2006	Adults	A seven-item scale assessing symptoms of generalized anxiety disorder. Validated as a screening tool as well as measuring clinically meaningful changes in symptoms of anxiety and worry associated with treatment.
Post-traumatic stress disorder	Nightmare Frequency Questionnaire	Krakow et al. (2002)	Adults	Retrospective measure that asks patients to indicate the number of nights they had nightmares and number of nightmares they had in the past 3 months.
	PSQI- Addendum for PTSD	Germain et al. (2005)	Adults	A 10-item measure to be administered with the PSQI that asks patients to rate frequency of sleep disturbances associated with PTSD.
Health-related quality of life	PROMIS Global-10	Hays et al. (2009)	Adults	A 10-item scale measuring overall health-related quality of life including physical functioning, fatigue, pain, emotional distress, and social health.
	SF-36	Ware et al. (1993)	Adults	A 36-item measure that contains eight dimensions of health and well-being: (1) physical functioning, (2) social functioning, (3) role limitations (physical problems), (4) role limitations (emotional problems), (5) mental health, (6) vitality, (7) pain, and (8) general health perception.

Note. DSM-5 = Diagnostic and Statistical Manual of Mental Disorders, fifth edition; PHQ-9 = nine-item Patient Health Questionnaire; PROMIS = Patient-Reported Outcomes Measurement Information System; PSQI = Pittsburgh Sleep Quality Index; PTSD = post-traumatic stress disorder; RLS = restless legs syndrome; SF-36 = 36-item Short Form.

From these patient-reported variables, additional useful variables can be computed. *Sleep efficiency* (SE) is the percentage of the total time that patients spend in bed that they are asleep. SE is particularly useful in the diagnosis and treatment of insomnia (Spielman et al., 1987). Studies also suggest that markers of circadian phase can be reliably estimated from habitual sleep patterns reported in sleep diaries (Burgess et al., 2003; Wyatt et al., 2006). Thus, clinicians can make recommendations regarding the timing of phototherapy administration without requiring that patients undergo physiological tests of circadian phase, such as dim light melatonin onset (DLMO) assessment (Lewy & Sack, 1989).

Sleep diaries can take many formats. Traditionally, the tabular format is used on which patients note clock times for bedtime and rising time, with each row of the table representing 1 day and each page representing 1 week. Specifically, patients record any naps, unusual stressors, use of medications, bedtime, SOL, number of awakenings, WASO, rising time, and estimated TST after waking in the morning. Then, prior to going to bed, patients provide a rating of their sleepiness and fatigue for the day. An alternative format uses a grid in which patients note sleep patterns by marking off or blacking out boxes that represent units of time. This format can be particularly useful clinically as it provides a quick visual representation of a patient's sleep patterns (e.g., delayed or advanced sleep–wake rhythms) but lacks the ability to derive quantitative data if needed for research purposes. Sleep diaries can be modified to include other variables of interest such as ratings of cognitive and psychophysiological arousal or mood before bedtime. Space can also be provided for patients to record compliance with treatment recommendations, such as implementation of stimulus control techniques in the treatment of insomnia or the use of phototherapy in the treatment of delayed sleep phase syndrome. While clinical settings allow for more flexibility and customization of diaries to fit patient needs and the purpose of the diary, a standard sleep diary is now recommended for research purposes (Carney et al., 2012), which includes set items and instructions for recording estimated sleep parameters such as bedtime, SOL, number of nighttime awakenings, and rise time. Whenever possible, clinicians should consider using this version of the sleep diary for continuity and standardization, which can facilitate generalizability from research findings (see Figure 23.1).

In addition to using sleep diaries during an evaluation, they can be useful to monitor progress with treatment and adherence to treatment recommendations. For example, when using sleep restriction therapy, the average SE over a given week is used to determine the treatment recommendations for the following week. For patients with CRSWDs, adherence to the timing of recommended sleep schedules (e.g., gradual advancement of bedtime and wake time) or timing of light exposure can be gleaned from the sleep diary, particularly when used with actigraphy.

Although many clinical settings still use paper sleep diaries, digital sleep diaries have become more popular as mobile devices have become widespread. Digital data collection of sleep can be more convenient for patients as reminders and push notifications can be

	Consensus Sleep Diary-Core				ID/Name: ______			
	Sample							
Today's date	4/5/11							
1. What time did you get into bed?	10:15 p.m							
2. What time did you try to go to sleep?	11:30 p.m							
3. How long did it take you to fall asleep?	55 min.							
4. How many times did you wake up, not counting your final awakening?	3 times							
5. In total, how long did these awakenings last?	1 hour 10 min.							
6. What time was your final awakening?	6:35 a.m.							
7. What time did you get out of bed for the day?	7:20a.m							
8. How would you rate the quality of your sleep?	☐ Very poor ☒ Poor ☐ Fair ☐ Good ☐ Very good	☐ Very poor ☐ Poor ☐ Fair ☐ Good ☐ Very good	☐ Very poor ☐ Poor ☐ Fair ☐ Good ☐ Very good	☐ Very poor ☐ Poor ☐ Fair ☐ Good ☐ Very good	☐ Very poor ☐ Poor ☐ Fair ☐ Good ☐ Very good	☐ Very poor ☐ Poor ☐ Fair ☐ Good ☐ Very good	☐ Very poor ☐ Poor ☐ Fair ☐ Good ☐ Very good	☐ Very poor ☐ Poor ☐ Fair ☐ Good ☐ Very good
9. Comments (if applicable)	I have a cold							

Figure 23.1 Consensus sleep diary-core

sent to minimize missing data and problems with retrospective recall. Moreover, digital diaries can be programmed to calculate parameters such as TIB and SE and display these to the patient using charts and graphs to help them monitor progress. This can be useful to monitor progress during the course of treatment.

MEASURES OF SLEEP/WAKE SYMPTOMS

Global Measures of Sleep Disturbance

There are several self-reported measures used in the assessment of sleep/wake complaints (see Table 23.1). One of the most commonly used measures of global sleep quality in adults is the Pittsburgh Sleep Quality Index (PSQI; Buysse et al., 1989). The PSQI can be quickly completed by patients in less than 5 minutes and is easily scored and interpreted. The PSQI has 19 items that assess seven domains of sleep: subjective sleep quality, SOL, sleep duration, habitual SE, sleep disturbances, use of sleep medications, and daytime dysfunction. Domain scores are summed to create a total PSQI score, where a score greater than 5 is used to designate "poor sleepers" from "good sleepers" (Buysse et al., 1989). The Sleep Disturbance and Sleep-Related Impairment scales from the Patient-Reported Outcomes Measurement Information System (PROMIS) are validated measures of the nighttime and daytime aspects of sleep disturbance, respectively (Buysse et al., 2010).

One advantage that the PROMIS offers is the use of computer adaptive testing, which allows for a very efficient number of items needed to obtain the appropriate level of sleep disturbance or daytime impairment based on item response theory. This is a more sophisticated psychometric approach than that used in the development of other scales.

For children and adolescents, the Sleep Habits Survey (SHS) can be used to assess sleep patterns and waking activities (Wolfson & Carskadon, 1998). The SHS yields three variables about sleep patterns over the last 2 weeks: school-night sleep time, weekend bedtime delay (difference between weeknight and weekend bedtime), and number of nights sleeping in the same bed. The SHS also yields 10 measures of daytime functioning over the last 6 months including total number of accidents/injuries, number of accidents/injuries related to alcohol or drugs, school performance, depressed mood, daytime sleepiness, satisfaction with sleep quality, circadian phase delay, and chronotype. The Children's Sleep Habits Questionnaire is a parent-completed measure that has been used to assess global sleep quality in younger populations, specifically children ages 4 through 12 years (Owens et al., 2000). Parents are asked to indicate how frequently various sleep symptoms (e.g., child is afraid of sleeping alone, child sleepwalks, child snores loudly, or child has a hard time getting out of bed) happen in a "typical week." A subset of 33 items can also be used to compute a total score which represents overall sleep quality, with higher scores representing poorer sleep quality.

Measures of Daytime Consequences

Measuring daytime symptoms and the extent of functional impairment is needed to determine the impact of the sleep disturbance. Sleepiness is a key daytime symptom characterized by the inability to stay alert and/or maintain wakefulness. Excessive daytime sleepiness is a prominent symptom of sleep-related breathing disorders, disorders of hypersomnolence, and some CRSWDs. The Epworth Sleepiness Scale (ESS) is a widely used measure of excessive daytime sleepiness which evaluates the propensity to fall sleep or "doze off" in eight common situations ranging from passive situations, such as watching TV, to active situations, such as having a conversation with someone (Johns, 1991, 1992). Total scores range from 0 to 24, with higher scores indicative of greater daytime sleepiness; and a cutoff of greater than 10 has been used to distinguish *excessive* daytime sleepiness. Patients with narcolepsy, idiopathic hypersomnolence, and OSA all had significantly higher scores on the ESS than controls (Johns, 1991). With respect to OSA, ESS scores were positively correlated with respiratory disturbance index (RDI) as measured by PSG such that greater severity in apnea was associated with greater daytime sleepiness (Johns, 1991). The ESS has also been found to be sensitive to improvement in sleepiness following CPAP treatment of OSA (Johns, 1992).

Two other commonly used measures of daytime sleepiness are the Stanford Sleepiness Scale and the Karolinska Sleepiness Scale (KSS). The Stanford Sleepiness Scale (Hoddes et al., 1973) asks patients to rate their current level of sleepiness using a 7-point scale. A validation study demonstrated that Stanford Sleepiness scores are sensitive to increased sleepiness following partial sleep deprivation and decreased sleepiness following recovery sleep (Herscovitch & Broughton, 1981). The KSS is a similar scale that asks patients to rate subjective sleepiness on a 9-point scale (Åkerstedt & Gillberg, 1990). Validation studies have found that the scores from the KSS were significantly correlated with sleepiness as measured by electroencephalogram and electro-oculogram (Åkerstedt & Gillberg, 1990; Kaida et al., 2006). In addition, greater KSS scores are associated with decreased performance as measured by tasks of vigilance and reaction time (Gillberg et al., 1994). Both the Stanford Sleepiness Scale and the KSS can be easily completed in less than 1 minute and are ideal for repeated assessment of sleepiness at several time points during the day.

For younger populations, the Pediatric Daytime Sleepiness Scale (PDSS) is an 8-item scale for adolescents (ages 11–15) to rate sleepiness in common situations, difficulty waking in the morning, and daytime symptoms of tiredness and grumpiness (Drake et al., 2003). Higher PDSS scores are associated with poorer school performance, greater anger toward others, and more frequent illness (Drake et al., 2003).

The Functional Outcomes of Sleep Questionnaire (FOSQ) can be used to assess the impact that excessive sleepiness has on daily activities (Weaver et al., 1997). The FOSQ is a 30-item questionnaire that asks patients to rate their level of difficulty performing a variety of activities as a result of sleepiness, and higher scores are indicative of greater difficulty due to excessive daytime sleepiness. Factor analysis of the FOSQ yielded five factors: (1) general activity level, (2) vigilance, (3) impact on intimacy and sexual relationships, (4) general productivity, and (5) impact on social outcomes. Compared to other scales on sleepiness, the FOSQ takes considerably longer to complete (approximately 15 minutes). Thus, patient burden and time constraints should be factored in with the importance of this clinical data.

Fatigue is a distinct concept from sleepiness, characterized by low energy, lethargy, and malaise, compared with *sleepiness*, which is the behavioral tendency to fall asleep. A common measure of the impact of fatigue on daily functioning is the 9-item Fatigue Severity Scale (FSS; Krupp et al., 1989), where a score greater than 36 has been used to distinguish abnormal levels of fatigue (Flachenecker et al., 2002). Increased fatigue as measured by the FSS has been demonstrated in patients with sleep disorders including narcolepsy, OSA, and insomnia (Valko et al., 2008). For patients with insomnia the Flinders Fatigue Scale has proven to be useful in identifying complaints of fatigue that are specifically attributed to the sleep complaint (Gradisar et al., 2007).

Chronotype

The Morningness–Eveningness Questionnaire (MEQ) can be a useful tool in the assessment of circadian preferences and possible circadian misalignment (Horne & Ostberg, 1976). The MEQ is a 19-item questionnaire designed to assess chronotype (e.g., preference toward increased activity and alertness in the mornings vs. the evenings). Respondents answer each item using a 4-point scale, with higher scores representing a "morning type" and lower scores representing an "evening type." The MEQ was initially validated in a student sample and found to correlate with body temperature, a marker of circadian phase (Horne & Ostberg, 1976), and has also been validated in a middle-aged population (Taillard et al., 2004). The Munich Chronotype Questionnaire (MCTQ; 17 items) provides an estimate of the mid-point of sleep on workdays and free days and is particularly useful for indexing social jet lag (Roenneberg et al., 2003; Zavada et al., 2005). The MCTQ correlates well with the MEQ, and both correlate moderately with DLMO (Kantermann et al. 2015). Short-form versions of both scales are available (reduced MEQ [Adan & Almirall, 1991], μMTCQ [Ghotbi et al., 2020]).

MEASURES OF SLEEP DISORDERS

Insomnia Measures

The Insomnia Severity Index (ISI) is a 7-item scale that assesses difficulty initiating and maintaining sleep, daytime consequences of poor sleep, and subjective distress about sleep disturbance that can be used as a brief screening tool in the assessment of insomnia (Bastien et al., 2001). Scores of 8 to 14 are suggestive of subclinical levels of insomnia, scores of 15 to 21 suggest moderately severe clinical insomnia, and scores >22 are suggestive of severe insomnia (Bastien et al., 2001). Thus, the ISI can be used as a valid and efficient screening tool for insomnia, especially when daily sleep log data is not available. In addition, the ISI is sensitive to clinically significant changes in insomnia symptoms following treatment, with a reduction in total score >7 indicating treatment response and a total score <8 indicating treatment remission (Morin et al., 2011).

The Sleep Condition Indicator (SCI; Espie et al., 2014) also evaluates insomnia. The SCI comprises eight items: two quantitative items on sleep continuity (Item 1, Item 2), two qualitative items on sleep satisfaction/dissatisfaction (Item 4, Item 7), two quantitative items on severity (Item 3, Item 8), and two qualitative items on attributed daytime consequences of poor sleep (Item 5, personal functioning; Item 6, daytime performance). The score range of 0 to 32 can be converted to a 10-point scale, offering a user-friendly sleep metric. A score of 16 or less out of 32 (5 out of 10) reflects possible insomnia disorder, and a change of 7 points reflects reliable change. Reference values for age and sex subgroups have been published (Espie et al., 2018), and there is also a validated short-form (2-item) version of the SCI (Luik et al., 2019).

The Glasgow Sleep Impact Index (Kyle et al., 2013) is a specific measure that provides a patient-generated index of concern about the consequences of insomnia. It asks patients to generate and assess three domains of impairment specific to their own individual context and in their own words (e.g., "feeling I can cope during the day," "managing my work responsibilities," "having to rely too much on other people"). These three areas of impairment are then ranked in order of concern (1 to 3, where 1 = the most concerning impairment) and then rated on a visual analogue scale with respect to impact in the past 2 weeks.

Patients are then able to re-rate these specified areas of impairment at post-intervention, which permits evaluation of change on the outcomes that are of greatest importance to the patient.

The Dysfunctional Beliefs and Attitudes about Sleep (DBAS) scale is a 30-item scale that assesses sleep-related cognitions (e.g., distorted beliefs about the amount of sleep needed or the consequences of poor sleep) that are associated with and can often perpetuate insomnia (Morin et al., 1993). The original DBAS includes items to reflect five domains: beliefs about the causes of insomnia, beliefs about the consequences of insomnia, unrealistic sleep expectations, perceptions of diminished control over sleep, and beliefs about sleep-promoting behaviors. A 16-item short form of the DBAS has also been validated and is available to minimize patient burden (Morin et al., 2007). The DBAS can also be used as a treatment planning tool (e.g., identifying target cognitions) and a measure of treatment response to cognitive techniques in CBT-I (Morin et al., 2002).

OSA Questionnaires

The Berlin Questionnaire is a brief screening tool that has been used to identify patients at high risk for having OSA who should receive further evaluation with PSG (Netzer et al., 1999). Items on the Berlin Questionnaire assess sleep-disordered breathing symptoms and risk factors in three categories: snoring, daytime sleepiness, physical and medical risk factors (e.g., history of hypertension, height, weight, and neck circumference). Patients are classified as "high risk" for sleep apnea if they have positive responses in two of three categories. Initially found to have adequate specificity and sensitivity in a primary care population (Netzer et al., 1999), the Berlin Questionnaire scores were only moderately correlated with RDI in a sample of patients presenting to a sleep disorders clinic (Ahmadi et al., 2008). However, sensitivity of the Berlin Questionnaire was significantly improved with the removal of the hypersomnolence items (Ahmadi et al., 2008).

For children and adolescents ages 2 through 18 years, the Pediatric Sleep Questionnaire can be used to assess sleep disordered breathing (e.g., snoring, witnessed apneas, mouth breathing), daytime sleepiness, and inattention/hyperactivity (Chervin et al., 2000). Parents are asked to respond to each question using a yes/no format, and completion of the questionnaire takes about 5 minutes. Validated in a sample of children with OSA as diagnosed by PSG (apnea/hypopnea index >5), the criterion of 8 or more positive responses across domains on the Pediatric Sleep Questionnaire was found to have adequate sensitivity and specificity (Chervin et al., 2000). It should be emphasized that the Pediatric Sleep Questionnaire and Berlin Questionnaire should be used as screening tools and do not eliminate the need for a diagnostic PSG.

RLS

The International Restless Legs Scale (IRLS) is a 10-item scale that assesses the severity of RLS symptoms and impact (Allen et al., 2003). The IRLS consists of two subscales: (1)

the RLS Symptoms subscale, which includes items about severity of discomfort in legs/arms, frequency of RLS symptoms, and impact on sleep, and (2) the RLS Symptoms Impact subscale, which assesses the impact of RLS symptoms on a patient's daily activities and mood. The IRLS has been found to have adequate reliability and validity in a sample of patients with RLS (Walters et al., 2003). In addition, the IRLS appears to be responsive to changes in severity of symptoms following treatment with ropinirole (Abetz et al., 2006). This data suggests that the IRLS may be a useful tool in assessing response to pharmacological treatment for RLS and in identifying the need for additional intervention for patients with RLS.

MEASURES OF PSYCHIATRIC SYMPTOMS

Given the high comorbidity between sleep disorders and mental disorders, it is important to assess psychopathology in addition to sleep-specific symptoms. Although these measures should not be used to diagnose a mental disorder, they can be administered quickly and efficiently as screening tools for psychopathology. The PROMIS can be a particularly useful tool as it includes scales for both depression and anxiety (Pilkonis et al., 2011) in addition to the sleep domains described earlier. The 9-item Patient Health Questionnaire (PHQ-9) is another commonly used measure of depression and has the advantage of being quick to complete and straightforward to score, yielding validated cutoff scores for clinical depression (Kroenke et al., 2001). For older adults, the Geriatric Depression Scale (Yesavage et al., 1982) should be considered a screening tool as it has been validated for this population. Legacy measures such as the Beck Depression Inventory-II (Beck et al., 1996), the State-Trait Anxiety Inventory (Spielberger et al., 1970), and the Beck Anxiety Inventory (Beck et al., 1988) can be considered; but these measures are generally more burdensome to the patient and typically require clinics to pay a fee for using these instruments. The 7-item Generalized Anxiety Disorder scale is increasingly used to screen for generalized anxiety disorder (Spitzer et al., 2006) and may be used in combination with the PHQ-9 because it is similarly formatted.

For patients with frequent and disturbing nightmares, symptoms of PTSD should be assessed. The Nightmare Frequency Questionnaire (NFQ) is a retrospective measure that can be used to quickly assess the frequency of PTSD-related nightmares (Krakow et al., 2002). In a sample of victims of sexual assault, the NFQ showed good test–retest reliability and adequate correlation with prospective dream logs as well as other measures of PTSD-related symptoms (Krakow et al., 2002). In addition to nightmares, patients with PTSD report a variety of other sleep disturbances such as night terrors, nocturnal panic, and parasomnias. The PSQI Addendum for PTSD (PSQI-A) is a 10-item measure that was developed to be administered with the original PSQI to assess these additional PTSD-related sleep disturbances (Germain et al., 2005). The PSQI-A has been shown to have good reliability and convergent validity with other clinical measures of PTSD, and a cutoff score of >4 demonstrated adequate sensitivity and specificity in identifying patients with PTSD (Germain et al., 2005).

Health-Related Quality of Life

Assessment of health-related quality of life can be important in gauging the patient's current state of well-being as well as the impact of the sleep problem on the patient's social and occupational functioning. The PROMIS Global-10 is a 10-item scale that assesses general domains of health and functioning including physical, mental, and social health, along with pain, fatigue, and overall perceived quality of life (Hays et al., 2009). Similar to the other PROMIS scales, the Global-10 can be administered efficiently to minimize patient burden. The Medical Outcomes Study Short Form-36 (Ware & Sherbourne, 1992) is another commonly used questionnaire that provides an indication of well-being across different disorders and can be useful in both research and clinical settings to assess a patient's baseline level as well as a response to treatment.

Putting Together the Clinical Assessment Tools

There are several considerations when deciding how to approach the clinical assessment of sleep. First, the setting of the assessment should be considered. If the assessment is conducted in a specialty sleep clinic, a comprehensive evaluation is likely needed to determine the need for an overnight sleep study, daytime testing, or further evaluation. Such an evaluation might follow a more structured approach where the priority is to ensure accurate diagnosis and to implement recommended treatment(s). This approach might require a longer visit to conduct the initial clinical interview along with a more comprehensive set of self-reported questionnaires to screen for comorbid conditions. If the assessment is conducted in a primary care or other medical clinic (e.g., general neurology clinic, pulmonary clinic), it is likely that efficiency is prioritized and sleep is only one aspect of the evaluation. Therefore, a tailored approach might be favored. The goal in this context is typically to efficiently determine the need for referral for a sleep study, such as in the case of suspected sleep disordered breathing, or to initiate treatment for conditions that can be diagnosed based on clinical information, such as initiating CBT-I. If the assessment is conducted in a mental health clinic, the patient might report symptoms of a sleep disorder that are comorbid with a psychiatric condition. The goal in this setting would be to make a differential diagnosis to determine if further evaluation and treatment of the sleep disorder are warranted. A tailored approach could be conducted here using a clinical interview and relevant self-reported measures, bearing in mind that sleep disorders should be actively treated whenever they present and should not be assumed to be secondary to other conditions. If the mental health provider is qualified to deliver CBT-I and receives referrals for this purpose, then the assessment might include a tailored approach to evaluate readiness for treatment, appraise comorbid psychiatric conditions, and inform treatment planning. Another aspect of the setting is whether the assessment is conducted in-person or via telehealth. If the assessment is conducted using telehealth, clinicians should determine the importance of tools such as the physical exam or further questionnaire data for making a diagnosis. In both cases, clinicians should provide expectations to the patient about the need for further testing (e.g., overnight sleep study) as a follow-up to the clinical visit when relevant.

Clinicians should also be mindful of other factors when putting together the clinical assessment tools. First, some diagnoses primarily require clinical information from the interview, such as insomnia and RLS. Other diagnoses may remain provisional until confirmed by further data collection, such as sleep diaries, wrist actigraphy, overnight PSG, or the Multiple Sleep Latency Test. Thus, the referral question or symptom profile might determine the set of clinical tools to be used. Second, the patient may have been previously diagnosed with a sleep disorder or may have engaged in self-diagnosis. While this can serve as a starting point for evaluation, it does not rule out the possibility of another sleep disorder, and a comprehensive evaluation should still be conducted. For example, insomnia is often comorbid with OSA, and accumulating evidence suggests that both conditions should be treated (Ong et al., 2021). Third, issues of secondary gain and the validity of the patient's information must be kept in mind. For example, a long-haul truck driver has a strong motivation for minimizing complaints of excessive daytime sleepiness or drowsy driving, knowing that their job may be at risk if this was known. Alternatively, a patient who expresses somaticizing, hypochondriacal, or histrionic traits may exaggerate the significance or severity of symptoms. Clinical judgment is often required to gauge the validity of the information given by the patient, and the use of objective measures can be helpful in these situations. Based on these considerations, Table 23.2 provides an example of how to put together the tools for a clinical assessment of sleep/wake disorders in a sleep clinic setting.

Table 23.2 Putting the clinical tools together

Time point	Assessment tools and activities	Considerations
Prior to the clinic visit	• Patient information and chief complaint/reason for referral • Screening questionnaires • Sleep diary	Balance patient burden with information to enhance efficiency of the clinic visit
Clinic visit (in person or telehealth)	• Clinical interview • Physical exam (as appropriate) • Review of self-reported measures • Patient education about the results of the evaluation and next steps	Use a patient-centered approach including use of patient's preferred method of communication, reviewing/confirming any information the patient has already completed, and providing education on the results of the evaluation
Follow-up assessment (as appropriate)	• Schedule overnight PSG and/or MSLT • Sleep diary and/or actigraphy monitoring (1–2 weeks)	Focus on tools needed for differential diagnosis, treatment planning, and outcome evaluation

Note. MSLT = Multiple Sleep Latency Test; PSG = polysomnography.

Conclusion

This chapter provides a description of the tools used in the clinical assessment of sleep/wake complaints. Similar to other medical and psychiatric conditions, the semi-structured clinical interview remains the primary tool along with the sleep diary and other self-report measures that can supplement or validate the patient history. Clinicians should consider several factors when selecting the tools and prioritizing the order of the tools and use clinical judgment when interpreting and synthesizing the information. A comprehensive assessment should lead the clinician to develop a treatment plan or determine the need for further testing prior to initiating treatment.

Future Directions

The process of assessing sleep complaints will continue to evolve as advances are made in science and technology. As discussed in this chapter, the integration of technology into the assessment process is emerging and will likely expand in the future. The rise of telehealth has improved access of sleep medicine to remote locations, including those living in rural areas and those who might not have access to sleep specialty providers (e.g., expertise in narcolepsy, behavioral sleep medicine). However, this also raises questions about licensure and jurisdiction of practice across states, provinces, or countries. The use of digital tools can facilitate collection of patient information and administration of screening questionnaires, which can minimize patient burden. Moreover, this data can be directly linked to the patient's electronic medical records, improving data accuracy and efficiency for the provider to review the information prior to or during the clinic visit. As discussed earlier, digital sleep diaries are becoming more popular and are often requested by patients. Soon, these tools could include data from wearable or other devices that can track biological data. Although consumer devices for monitoring sleep are not yet validated for clinical settings, they could provide opportunities for enhancing the clinical assessment of sleep complaints in the near future.

The rise of personalized medicine and research on phenotypes and endotypes will also push the boundaries of clinical assessment. The accumulated data in electronic medical records allows for the use of "big data" analyses and artificial intelligence to customize the assessment tools and ultimately deliver a more personalized treatment plan. For example, cluster analyses of clinical data collected from people with symptoms of OSA and insomnia have revealed phenotypes that are associated with cardiovascular disease (Ye et al., 2014) as well as those who are more likely to respond to PAP therapy (Pien et al., 2018). Studies such as these could challenge our traditional notion of diagnostic classification of sleep disorders and shift the paradigm on the assessment process. Moving forward, the assessment of sleep/wake complaints will likely be multimodal, and the lines between clinical assessment and objective testing may become blurred.

References

Abetz, L., Arbuckle, R., Allen, R. P., Garcia-Borreguero, D., Hening, W., Walters, A. S., Mavraki, E., & Kirsch, J. M. (2006). The reliability, validity and responsiveness of the International Restless Legs Syndrome Study Group rating scale and subscales in a clinical-trial setting. *Sleep Medicine, 7*(4), 340–349. https://doi.org/10.1016/j.sleep.2005.12.011

Adan, A., & Almirall, H. (1991). Horne & Östberg Morningness–Eveningness Questionnaire: A reduced scale. *Personality and Individual Differences, 12*(3), 241–253.

Ahmadi, N., Chung, S. A., Gibbs, A., & Shapiro, C. M. (2008). The Berlin questionnaire for sleep apnea in a sleep clinic population: Relationship to polysomnographic measurement of respiratory disturbance. *Sleep and Breathing, 12*(1), 39–45. https://doi.org/10.1007/s11325-007-0125-y

Åkerstedt, T., & Gillberg, M. (1990). Subjective and objective sleepiness in the active individual. *International Journal of Neuroscience, 52*(1–2), 29–37. https://doi.org/10.3109/00207459008994241

Allen, R. P., Kushida, C. A., & Atkinson, M. J. (2003). Factor analysis of the International Restless Legs Syndrome Study Group's scale for restless legs severity. *Sleep Medicine, 4*(2), 133–135. https://doi.org/10.1016/S1389-9457(02)00193-4

Bastien, C. H., Vallieres, A., & Morin, C. M. (2001). Validation of the Insomnia Severity Index as an outcome measure for insomnia research. *Sleep Medicine, 2*(4), 297–307.

Beck, A. T., Epstein, N., Brown, G., & Steer, R. A. (1988). An inventory for measuring clinical anxiety: Psychometric properties. *Journal of Consulting and Clinical Psychology, 56*(6), 893–897.

Beck, A. T., Steer, R. A., & Brown, G. K. (1996). *Beck depression inventory (BDI-II)*. Pearson.

Bell, R. A., Kravitz, R. L., Thom, D., Krupat, E., & Azari, R. (2002). Unmet expectations for care and the patient–physician relationship. *Journal of General Internal Medicine, 17*(11), 817–824. https://doi.org/10.1046/j.1525-1497.2002.10319.x

Burgess, H. J., Savic, N., Sletten, T., Roach, G., Gilbert, S. S., & Dawson, D. (2003). The relationship between the dim light melatonin onset and sleep on a regular schedule in young healthy adults. *Behavioral Sleep Medicine, 1*(2), 102–114.

Buysse, D. J., Reynolds, C. F., 3rd, Monk, T. H., Berman, S. R., & Kupfer, D. J. (1989). The Pittsburgh Sleep Quality Index: A new instrument for psychiatric practice and research. *Psychiatry Research, 28*(2), 193–213.

Buysse, D. J., Yu, L., Moul, D. E., Germain, A., Stover, A., Dodds, N. E., . . . Pilkonis, P. A. (2010). Development and validation of patient-reported outcome measures for sleep disturbance and sleep-related impairments. *Sleep, 33*(6), 781–792.

Carney, C. E., Buysse, D. J., Ancoli-Israel, S., Edinger, J. D., Krystal, A. D., Lichstein, K. L., & Morin, C. M. (2012). The consensus sleep diary: Standardizing prospective sleep self-monitoring. *Sleep, 35*(2), 287–302. https://doi.org/10.5665/sleep.1642

Chervin, R. D., Hedger, K., Dillon, J. E., & Pituch, K. J. (2000). Pediatric sleep questionnaire (PSQ): Validity and reliability of scales for sleep-disordered breathing, snoring, sleepiness, and behavioral problems. *Sleep Medicine, 1*(1), 21–32.

Drake, C., Nickel, C., Burduvali, E., Roth, T., Jefferson, C., & Pietro, B. (2003). The pediatric daytime sleepiness scale (PDSS): Sleep habits and school outcomes in middle-school children. *Sleep, 26*(4), 455–458.

Espie, C. A., Farias Machado, P., Carl, J. R., Kyle, S. D., Cape, J., Siriwardena, A. N., & Luik, A. I. (2018). The Sleep Condition Indicator: Reference values derived from a sample of 200 000 adults. *Journal of Sleep Research, 27*(3), Article e12643.

Espie, C. A., Kyle, S. D., Hames, P., Gardani, M., Fleming, L., & Cape, J. (2014). The Sleep Condition Indicator: A clinical screening tool to evaluate insomnia disorder. *BMJ Open, 4*(3), Article e004183. https://doi.org/10.1136/bmjopen-2013-004183

Flachenecker, P., Kumpfel, T., Kallmann, B., Gottschalk, M., Grauer, O., Rieckmann, P., . . . Toyka, K. V. (2002). Fatigue in multiple sclerosis: A comparison of different rating scales and correlation to clinical parameters. *Multiple Sclerosis, 8*(6), 523–526.

Germain, A., Hall, M., Krakow, B., Katherine Shear, M., & Buysse, D. J. (2005). A brief sleep scale for posttraumatic stress disorder: Pittsburgh Sleep Quality Index addendum for PTSD. *Journal of Anxiety Disorders, 19*(2), 233–244.

Ghotbi, N., Pilz, L. K., Winnebeck, E. C., Vetter, C., Zerbini, G., Lenssen, D., Frighetto, G., Salamanca, M., Costa, R., Montagnese, S., & Roenneberg, T. (2020). The μMCTQ: An ultra-short version of the Munich ChronoType Questionnaire. *Journal of Biological Rhythms, 35*(1), 98–110.

Gillberg, M., Kecklund, G., & Akerstedt, T. (1994). Relations between performance and subjective ratings of sleepiness during a night awake. *Sleep, 17*(3), 236–241.
Gradisar, M., Lack, L., Richards, H., Harris, J., Gallasch, J., Boundy, M., & Johnston, A. (2007). The Flinders Fatigue Scale: Preliminary psychometric properties and clinical sensitivity of a new scale for measuring daytime fatigue associated with insomnia. *Journal of Clinical Sleep Medicine, 3*(7), 722–728.
Harvey, A. G. (2002). Identifying safety behaviors in insomnia. *The Journal of Nervous and Mental Disease, 190*(1), 16–21.
Hays, R. D., Bjorner, J. B., Revicki, D. A., Spritzer, K. L., & Cella, D. (2009). Development of physical and mental health summary scores from the Patient-Reported Outcomes Measurement Information System (PROMIS) global items. *Quality of Life Research, 18*(7), 873–880.
Herscovitch, J., & Broughton, R. (1981). Sensitivity of the Stanford Sleepiness Scale to the effects of cumulative partial sleep deprivation and recovery oversleeping. *Sleep, 4*(1), 83–91.
Hoddes, E., Zarcone, V., Smythe, H., Phillips, R., & Dement, W. C. (1973). Quantification of sleepiness: A new approach. *Psychophysiology, 10*(4), 431–436.
Horne, J. A., & Ostberg, O. (1976). A self-assessment questionnaire to determine morningness–eveningness in human circadian rhythms. *International Journal of Chronobiology, 4*(2), 97–110.
Johns, M. W. (1991). A new method for measuring daytime sleepiness: The Epworth Sleepiness Scale. *Sleep, 14*(6), 540–545.
Johns, M. W. (1992). Reliability and factor analysis of the Epworth Sleepiness Scale. *Sleep, 15*(4), 376–381.
Kaida, K., Takahashi, M., Akerstedt, T., Nakata, A., Otsuka, Y., Haratani, T., & Fukasawa, K. (2006). Validation of the Karolinska Sleepiness Scale against performance and EEG variables. *Clinical Neurophysiology, 117*(7), 1574–1581.
Kantermann, T., Sung, H., & Burgess, H. J. (2015). Comparing the Morningness–Eveningness Questionnaire and Munich ChronoType Questionnaire to the dim light melatonin onset. *Journal of Biological Rhythms, 30*(5), 449–453.
Krakow, B., Schrader, R., Tandberg, D., Hollifield, M., Koss, M. P., Yau, C. L., & Cheng, D. T. (2002). Nightmare frequency in sexual assault survivors with PTSD. *Journal of Anxiety Disorders, 16*(2), 175–190.
Kroenke, K., Spitzer, R. L., & Williams, J. B. (2001). The PHQ-9: Validity of a brief depression severity measure. *Journal of General Internal Medicine, 16*(9), 606–613.
Krupp, L. B., LaRocca, N. G., Muir-Nash, J., & Steinberg, A. D. (1989). The Fatigue Severity Scale: Application to patients with multiple sclerosis and systemic lupus erythematosus. *Archives of Neurology, 46*(10), 1121–1123.
Kyle, S. D., Crawford, M. R., Morgan, K., Spiegelhalder, K., Clark, A. A., & Espie, C. A. (2013). The Glasgow Sleep Impact Index (GSII): A novel patient-centred measure for assessing sleep-related quality of life impairment in insomnia disorder. *Sleep Medicine, 14*(6), 493–501.
Lewy, A. J., & Sack, R. L. (1989). The dim light melatonin onset as a marker for circadian phase position. *Chronobiology International, 6*(1), 93–102.
Lin, C. T., Albertson, G. A., Schilling, L. M., Cyran, E. M., Anderson, S. N., Ware, L., & Anderson, R. J. (2001). Is patients' perception of time spent with the physician a determinant of ambulatory patient satisfaction? *Archives of Internal Medicine, 161*(11), 1437–1442.
Luik, A. I., Machado, P. F., Siriwardena, N., & Espie, C. A. (2019). Screening for insomnia in primary care: Using a two-item version of the Sleep Condition Indicator. *British Journal of General Practice, 69*(679), 79–80.
Morgenthaler, T. I., Lee-Chiong, T., Alessi, C., Friedman, L., Aurora, R. N., Boehlecke, B., . . . Standards of Practice Committee of the American Academy of Sleep Medicine. (2007). Practice parameters for the clinical evaluation and treatment of circadian rhythm sleep disorders. An American Academy of Sleep Medicine report. *Sleep, 30*(11), 1445–1459.
Morin, C. M., Belleville, G., Bélanger, L., & Ivers, H. (2011). The Insomnia Severity Index: Psychometric indicators to detect insomnia cases and evaluate treatment response. *Sleep, 34*(5), 601–608.
Morin, C. M., Blais, F., & Savard, J. (2002). Are changes in beliefs and attitudes about sleep related to sleep improvements in the treatment of insomnia? *Behaviour Research and Therapy, 40*(7), 741–752.
Morin, C. M., Stone, J., Trinkle, D., Mercer, J., & Remsberg, S. (1993). Dysfunctional beliefs and attitudes about sleep among older adults with and without insomnia complaints. *Psychology and Aging, 8*(3), 463–467.

Morin, C. M., Vallieres, A., & Ivers, H. (2007). Dysfunctional beliefs and attitudes about sleep (DBAS): Validation of a brief version (DBAS-16). *Sleep, 30*(11), 1547–1554.

Netzer, N. C., Stoohs, R. A., Netzer, C. M., Clark, K., & Strohl, K. P. (1999). Using the Berlin Questionnaire to identify patients at risk for the sleep apnea syndrome. *Annals of Internal Medicine, 131*(7), 485–491.

Ong, J. C., Crawford, M. R., & Wallace, D. M. (2021). Sleep apnea and insomnia: Emerging evidence for effective clinical management. *Chest, 159*(5), 2020–2028.

Owens, J. A., Spirito, A., & McGuinn, M. (2000). The Children's Sleep Habits Questionnaire (CSHQ): Psychometric properties of a survey instrument for school-aged children. *Sleep, 23*(8), 1043–1051.

Pien, G. W., Ye, L., Keenan, B. T., Maislin, G., Bjornsdottir, E., Arnardottir, E. S., . . . Pack, A. I. (2018). Changing faces of obstructive sleep apnea: Treatment effects by cluster designation in the Icelandic sleep apnea cohort. *Sleep, 41*(3), Article zsx201.

Pilkonis, P. A., Choi, S. W., Reise, S. P., Stover, A. M., Riley, W. T., & Cella, D.; PROMIS Cooperative Group. (2011). Item banks for measuring emotional distress from the Patient-Reported Outcomes Measurement Information System (PROMIS®): Depression, anxiety, and anger. *Assessment, 18*(3), 263–283.

Rhoades, D. R., McFarland, K. F., Finch, W. H., & Johnson, A. O. (2001). Speaking and interruptions during primary care office visits. *Family Medicine, 33*(7), 528–532.

Roenneberg, T., Wirz-Justice, A., & Merrow, M. (2003). Life between clocks: Daily temporal patterns of human chronotypes. *Journal of Biological Rhythms, 18*, 80–90.

Schutte-Rodin, S., Broch, L., Buysse, D., Dorsey, C., & Sateia, M. (2008). Clinical guideline for the evaluation and management of chronic insomnia in adults. *Journal of Clinical Sleep Medicine, 4*(5), 487–504.

Spielberger, C. D., Gorsuch, R. L., & Lushene, R. E. (1970). *Manual for the State-Trait Anxiety Inventory.* Consulting Psychologists Press.

Spielman, A. J., Saskin, P., & Thorpy, M. J. (1987). Treatment of chronic insomnia by restriction of time in bed. *Sleep, 10*(1), 45–56.

Spitzer, R. L., Kroenke, K., Williams, J. B., & Lowe, B. (2006). A brief measure for assessing generalized anxiety disorder: The GAD-7. *Archives of Internal Medicine, 166*(10), 1092–1097.

Sturmey, P. (2020). *Functional analysis in clinical treatment.* Academic Press.

Taillard, J., Philip, P., Chastang, J. F., & Bioulac, B. (2004). Validation of Horne and Ostberg morningness–eveningness questionnaire in a middle-aged population of French workers. *Journal of Biological Rhythms, 19*(1), 76–86.

Valko, P. O., Bassetti, C. L., Bloch, K. E., Held, U., & Baumann, C. R. (2008). Validation of the fatigue severity scale in a Swiss cohort. *Sleep, 31*(11), 1601–1607.

Walters, A. S., LeBrocq, C., Dhar, A., Hening, W., Rosen, R., Allen, R. P., . . . International Restless Legs Syndrome Study Group. (2003). Validation of the International Restless Legs Syndrome Study Group rating scale for restless legs syndrome. *Sleep Medicine, 4*(2), 121–132.

Ware, J. E., Jr., & Sherbourne, C. D. (1992). The MOS 36-item short-form health survey (SF-36). I. Conceptual framework and item selection. *Medical Care, 30*(6), 473–483.

Weaver, T. E., Laizner, A. M., Evans, L. K., Maislin, G., Chugh, D. K., Lyon, K., . . . Dinges, D. F. (1997). An instrument to measure functional status outcomes for disorders of excessive sleepiness. *Sleep, 20*(10), 835–843.

Wolfson, A. R., & Carskadon, M. A. (1998). Sleep schedules and daytime functioning in adolescents. *Child Development, 69*(4), 875–887.

Wyatt, J. K., Stepanski, E. J., & Kirkby, J. (2006). Circadian phase in delayed sleep phase syndrome: Predictors and temporal stability across multiple assessments. *Sleep, 29*(8), 1075–1080.

Ye, L., Pien, G. W., Ratcliffe, S. J., Bjornsdottir, E., Arnardottir, E. S., Pack, A. I., . . . Gislason, T. (2014). The different clinical faces of obstructive sleep apnoea: A cluster analysis. *European Respiratory Journal, 44*(6), 1600–1607.

Yesavage, J. A., Brink, T. L., Rose, T. L., Lum, O., Huang, V., Adey, M., & Leirer, V. O. (1982). Development and validation of a geriatric depression screening scale: A preliminary report. *Journal of Psychiatric Research, 17*(1), 37–49.

Zavada, A., Gordijn, M. C., Beersma, D. G., Daan, S., & Roenneberg, T. (2005). Comparison of the Munich Chronotype Questionnaire with the Horne-Ostberg's morningness–eveningness score. *Chronobiology International, 22*(2), 267–278.

CHAPTER 24

Actigraphy and Behavioral Assessments of Sleep and Circadian Disorders

Monica R. Kelly, Nathaniel Yuan, Alexander J. Erickson, *and* Jennifer L. Martin

Abstract

Actigraphy devices can be used to assess sleep/wake patterns in a person's natural sleep environment, which makes this method preferable to single-night in-laboratory assessments for some applications. Actigraphy can be useful in the diagnosis and treatment of multiple sleep disorders. It can inform clinical decision-making and evaluation of treatment effectiveness in cases where multiple nights of assessment are needed. Actigraphy can also be useful in patient populations for whom recall of sleep habits and routines presents a challenge, such as in children or adults with neurocognitive impairments. While the number of consumer products using actigraphy methods to estimate sleep is growing, the accuracy and validity of these devices, especially in patients with sleep disorders, remains unknown and limits their usability in clinical practice.

Key Words: actigraphy, behavioral assessment, sleep, circadian rhythm disorder, consumer device

Introduction

Actigraphy refers to the use of a device containing an accelerometer, typically worn on the wrist like a watch, to measure movement that is categorized as sleep or wake using a mathematical algorithm. Data from actigraphs is processed with specialized software to provide summary statistics that can be used for clinical and research purposes. Research-grade actigraphy software often has the capability to provide raw movement data such as activity counts by epoch as well as daily summaries or weekly averages of sleep–wake variables such as total sleep time (TST) via automated algorithms or via manual scoring (Ancoli-Israel et al., 2015). Consumer-grade wearable devices that also provide movement-based sleep–wake data have become widely available with functional and fashionable designs as well as additional features not available in actigraphs commonly used in research and clinical practice such as heart rate variability and other proprietary metrics (Khosla et al., 2018; Ko et al., 2016).

There are multiple applications for actigraphy in both clinical and research environments given its relative ease of use and low cost relative to other objective sleep monitoring methods. Actigraphy may be used to augment subjective, prospective daily sleep diary paper or digital logs in the assessment of sleep disorders and to evaluate treatment adherence. Actigraphy can also serve as an alternative to in-laboratory polysomnography (PSG) in cases where multiple nights of recording are needed and when sleep disorders such as sleep apnea are not being assessed. This chapter provides an overview of the utility and function of actigraphy, including comparisons between actigraphy and other behavioral assessments as well as best practices and limitations in the use of actigraphy in the evaluation of sleep and circadian disorders.

Validation of Wrist Actigraphy Versus PSG

PSG is the gold-standard measure of objective sleep. However, actigraphy has many advantages over PSG, including low patient burden and total cost as well as the ability to conduct longitudinal assessment of sleep–wake patterns in a patient's normal sleep environment. Since sleep-related symptoms can vary nightly, this can be advantageous as compared to a single night in a sleep laboratory. A limitation of actigraphy is the potential for misclassification of movements during sleep as wake states or of wakeful immobility as sleep. This is especially true in some special populations, including individuals with conditions like sleep disordered breathing (Blackwell et al., 2011) and conditions that include sleep-related movements like Parkinson's disease (Louter et al., 2014). Other limitations include actigraphy's limited ability to categorize sleep stages precisely, even in devices that include additional physiological measures, such as heart rate, that are more commonly available in consumer wearables, as well as difficulties with coverage by some private insurance carriers in some regions.

Validity-focused studies have illustrated comparable results between standard actigraphy and PSG regarding the measurement of TST, with some evidence that actigraphy has lower specificity in being able to identify wake states (Conley et al., 2019; de Souza et al., 2003; Marino et al., 2013). Additionally, the measurement of TST, sleep efficiency (SE), and wake after sleep onset (WASO) in healthy adults has been demonstrated to be comparable between actigraphy and PSG across 29 different studies per a meta-analysis conducted by Conley and colleagues (2019). This consistency appears to wane in the context of adult populations with chronic conditions, with actigraphy studies illustrating evidence of overestimating TST and SE, while underestimating sleep onset latency (SOL; Conley et al., 2019).

While there are studies that compare the accuracy of actigraphy to PSG, it is unlikely that one would replace the other as the two methods provide different types of information and are used for different purposes. This is because actigraphy is one-dimensional versus PSG that benefits from three data sources (electroencephalography, electro-oculography, electromyography [EMG]) to determine wake and sleep. Therefore, actigraphy cannot be held to the same expectations to estimate parameters of sleep as PSG (Ancoli-Israel et al., 2003).

Actigraphy Versus Other Sleep Assessments

While actigraphy cannot be used as a replacement for laboratory PSG in the diagnosis of some sleep disorders, it can be useful in some circumstances. For example, when a patient's presenting complaint involves poor or incongruous sleep and clinical interview suggests fluctuations in daily activity patterns, objective monitoring in the home sleep environment can be more useful than a single night of assessment in the sleep laboratory. The sleep assessment method utilized in a diagnostic assessment depends upon the diagnostic criteria and potential differential diagnoses. Specific recommendations are made in relevant clinical practice guidelines (Smith et al., 2018a). Table 24.1 outlines the pros and cons of various methods of behavioral sleep assessment. As noted above, actigraphy may prove to be most useful when the desired sleep–wake metrics include an objective assessment of sleep habits over the course of several days or weeks with minimal patient burden and lower cost than PSG. However, actigraphy will have less utility when diagnostic assessment requires measurement of sleep architecture or subjective information about a patient's perception of their sleep and related symptoms.

Daily Sleep Diaries and Other Subjective Measures

Sleep diaries, completed on paper or using an electronic device, are a useful clinical and research tool in the evaluation of daily sleep habits, though they are not without limitations. In the assessment and behavioral treatment of insomnia disorder, for example, patient sleep diary data may conflict with actigraphy data in clinically relevant ways. In the evaluation of adherence to a set bedtime, individuals may report an earlier bedtime by as much as an hour versus what is shown by actigraphy data (Carney et al., 2004). Other studies have also noted differences between sleep diary and actigraphy in terms of daytime napping, WASO, and SOL in adults (Lockley et al., 1999), as well as TST, WASO, and SOL in pediatric populations on school days versus non-school days (Mazza et al., 2020). Both younger (Lauderdale et al., 2008) and older adults (Van Den Berg et al., 2008) without sleep complaints have also shown elevated TST on sleep diaries as compared to actigraphy. This data suggests that a combination approach may be necessary in certain populations or when an individual's subjective report of sleep symptoms does not concur with other aspects of their clinical assessment.

In addition to sleep diaries, several self-report measures exist that can be used in tandem with actigraphy (as well as PSG or sleep diaries) to further characterize patient perception of their sleep and/or sleep problems. Commonly used sleep-focused questionnaires include the Pittsburgh Sleep Quality Index (PSQI) for measuring subjective sleep quality (Buysse et al., 1989), the Insomnia Severity Index (ISI) for measuring insomnia symptoms (Bastien et al., 2001), and the Epworth Sleepiness Scale for measuring daytime sleepiness (Johns, 1991). Though some evidence exists, particularly regarding the PSQI, illustrating side-by-side comparisons between these sleep-focused measures and actigraphy (Mollayeva et al., 2016), more research needs to be conducted to better understand

Table 24.1 Comparison of actigraphy versus other methods of sleep assessment

Sleep assessment	Pros	Cons
Actigraphy	Low patient burden Lower cost to administer versus PSG Objective assessment of intra- and inter-daily sleep variability and duration Provide information on daily sleep habits in the home environment Does not rely on patient recall or perceptions	Higher cost to clinician/researcher versus questionnaires/ diary (e.g. devices, maintenance, software) Sleep diary should be collected concurrently for concordance with actigraphy data Does not fully assess sleep architecture
Questionnaires	Low patient burden Lower cost to administer versus actigraphy or PSG Provide retrospective information on daily sleep habits in the home environment	Rely on patient recall or perceptions of their sleep Do not assess sleep architecture
Sleep diaries	Lower patient burden versus actigraphy or PSG Lower cost to administer versus actigraphy or PSG Subjective assessment of intra- and inter-daily sleep variability and duration Provide information on daily sleep habits in the home environment	Rely on patient recall or perceptions of their sleep Require daily completion for validity Do not assess sleep architecture
Commercially available consumer sleep trackers	Low patient burden Objective assessment of intra- and inter-daily sleep variability and duration Do not rely on patient recall or perceptions Provide information on daily sleep habits in the home environment	Moderate to high initial cost to patient (e.g., not reimbursable via insurance) Lack of access to scoring algorithms and raw data; limited validation data Do not fully assess sleep architecture
Laboratory PSG	Gold-standard single-night objective sleep–wake assessment Does not rely on patient recall or perceptions Accurate assessment of sleep architecture	High patient burden (e.g., travel to lab) High cost to clinician/researcher (e.g., staffing, equipment, supplies, maintenance) Lack of information on daily sleep habits in the home environment (e.g., intra- and inter-daily sleep variability and duration) Possible "first night effect" (e.g., patient may demonstrate worse sleep on the first night in an unfamiliar environment)

Note. PSG = polysomnography.

the similarities and differences between these metrics and actigraphy. As was reflected previously regarding actigraphy and PSG, sleep-focused measures and actigraphy are likely not interchangeable and would benefit most from being administered together to get a more encompassing understanding of individual sleep and sleep-related problems.

Commercially Available Activity Trackers

Consumer wearable devices with actigraphy abilities are emerging, although there are multiple challenges in using these devices in clinical or research applications. Additionally, many consumer wearables often provide summary rather than raw data that is scored by proprietary algorithms via lay user-friendly platforms; however, some commercial-grade wearables do allow for access to raw data for research purposes. Common devices include the Fitbit Alta HR ($150; Fitbit Inc., San Francisco, CA), the Oura ring ($399 with additional monthly membership; Oulu, Finland; Altini & Kinnunen, 2021), the Samsung Gear Sport watch ($300; USA), the Jawbone UP3 ($50; Jawbone, San Francisco, CA), and the Apple Watch Series 2 ($299; Cupertino, CA), among others. Many studies compare the accuracy of these to medical-grade actigraphy with mixed conclusions. Of note, there is a Fitbit database which keeps track of publications using Fitbit devices that list >650 abstracts and journal papers (https://www.fitabase.com/research-library).

The consensus is that wearable actigraphy devices seem to have high sensitivity, which is the ability to detect true sleep. Conversely, actigraphy in general is poor at detecting true wake (specificity) and innately limited in identifying motionless awake. Caution must be used when consumer wearable devices predict sleep staging (light sleep vs. deep sleep or N1–N3 vs. rapid-eye-movement [REM] sleep). There are numerous algorithms of various degrees of "high" versus "low" thresholds to estimate PSG sleep staging, based on what is decided for investigation. For example, if one were evaluating a specific therapy on sleep disruption, then it would be best to use an algorithm prioritizing high accuracy in wake detection.

Studies suggest that Fitbit significantly underestimates TST and overestimates WASO. Within sleep staging, Fitbit overestimates stage N1 + N2 sleep (light sleep), while it underestimates stage N3 sleep (Lee et al., 2019). The Oura ring also consistently underestimates TST and overestimates WASO. Furthermore, the Oura ring underestimates REM and light sleep but overestimates deep sleep (Chee et al., 2021). In a 2020 study, the Samsung watch had greater mean differences compared to the Oura ring in the overestimation of TST and SE but profoundly underestimated WASO (Asgari Mehrabadi et al., 2020). When the Jawbone UP3 is compared to the Actiwatch 2 (AW2), these devices appear to not have significantly different estimations of TST, SE, or WASO. The Jawbone UP3 does not accurately measure sleep duration or identify sleep stages during PSG and the Multiple Sleep Latency Test (MSLT; Cook et al., 2018; de Zambotti et al., 2015). In another study of Jawbone vs PSG on women with or without insomnia, Jawbone overestimated TST and SOL and underestimated WASO, with the conclusion that there was a detectable difference if the individual had clinical insomnia (de Zambotti et al., 2015). The Apple Watch when compared to PSG overestimates TST and underestimates WASO, while having no correlation to SOL (Roberts et al., 2020).

As above, there is considerable variability in consumer wearable devices in tracking sleep parameters. To standardize the testing validity when comparing wearable devices across studies, de Zambotti et al. (2019) suggested a systematic method of analysis. Until these wearable devices become both standardized and optimized to population demographics, the determination between wake and sleep is limited. Caution must be used when making clinical decisions based on a wearable device's report of light sleep versus deep sleep or stages of sleep, including REM. At the very least, wearable devices promote awareness about individuals' sleep habits through suggestions of both bedtime and morning alarms.

Strategies to Enhance Precision of Wrist Actigraphy Data

Having a comprehensive instructional session and/or manual for individuals who will be wearing the actigraph device, including instructions on what to do in case of an adverse reaction and contact information for technical support, is crucial to ensuring data is collected in a systematic manner. Individuals should be instructed on how the device collects data (e.g., via movement and light, if applicable) and the extent to which the device is water-resistant versus waterproof. These instructions should reinforce wearing of the device consistently across the relevant time frame or removing it briefly when necessary, as well as awareness of how behaviors (e.g., wearing long-sleeved clothing over a light sensor) may impede data collection.

Regarding an appropriate time frame for data collection, a minimum of 1 week of actigraphy data is beneficial in order to capture sleep–wake patterns on both weekdays and weekends; however, a longer duration of 2 weeks may be best in the case of assessment of some disorders (e.g., circadian rhythm sleep–wake disorders [CRSWDs]; Smith et al., 2018a) or longer for some research protocols.

Either the dominant or non-dominant wrist may be used with equivalent results in adults (Sadeh et al., 1994) or on the legs in infants (Gershoni-Baruch et al., 1994); however, it is customary for many groups to utilize a protocol that instructs adults to wear the actigraph device on their dominant (or at least the same) wrist for consistency and to rule out the possibility that changes from pre- to a post-assessment are not due to simply switching the device from one limb to another.

Clinical Use of Wrist Actigraphy for Patients With Sleep Disorders

Actigraphy can be of significant benefit in a variety of clinical applications, including diagnostic evaluation as well as treatment, and in a range of populations across the developmental spectrum. This includes assessment of sleep and circadian disorders and for cases in which ruling out insufficient sleep opportunity is a necessary part of a thorough diagnostic assessment. The American Academy of Sleep Medicine (AASM) published clinical practice guidelines (Table 24.2) on the use of actigraphy in the assessment of sleep and circadian rhythm disorders in 2018 (Smith et al., 2018a), which were based on a systematic review of available evidence for the use of actigraphy (Smith et al., 2018b). The guidelines suggest that actigraphy may be useful in the diagnosis and evaluation of treatment outcomes for pediatric and adult patients with insomnia disorder or CRSWDs. The guidelines also suggest use of actigraphy in combination with home sleep apnea testing (HSAT) to provide a measure of TST during HSAT in adults as use of estimated TST improves the accuracy of HSAT compared to using total recording time in computing the apnea–hypopnea index. The guidelines also support use of actigraphy prior to the MSLT to confirm that a patient being assessed for central disorders of hypersomnolence gets sufficient sleep in the period of time leading up to the MSLT. Individuals who may be experiencing insufficient sleep due to occupational or other factors may also benefit from use of actigraphy to quantify TST to inform clinical decision-making. Finally, the guidelines recommend *against* the use of actigraphy as an alternative to EMG in the assessment of

Table 24.2 Summary of American Academy of Sleep Medicine clinical practice guidelines for the use of actigraphy in sleep and circadian sleep–wake disorders

	Indication for or against the use of actigraphy	Recommendation by population[a]	
Disorder/syndrome		Pediatric	Adult
Insomnia disorder	Use for diagnostic assessment and estimation of sleep parameters as part of a behavioral intervention	Conditional, For	Conditional, For
Circadian sleep–wake disorder	Use for diagnostic assessment	Conditional, For	Conditional, For
Sleep disordered breathing	Use for integration with a home sleep apnea test for estimation of total sleep time as part of a diagnostic assessment	N/A	Conditional, For
Hypersomnolence	Use for estimation of total sleep time prior to a Multiple Sleep Latency Test as part of a diagnostic assessment	Conditional, For	Conditional, For
Insufficient sleep syndrome	Use for diagnostic assessment to estimate total sleep time	N/A	Conditional, For
Periodic limb movement disorder	Do not use in place of electromyography as part of a diagnostic assessment	Strong, Against	Strong, Against

Note. From Smith et al. (2018a).

[a]For recommendations: strong = the vast majority of patients should receive this assessment as indicated, conditional = most patients should receive this assessment as indicated when determined to be clinically appropriate and in line with the patient's values/preferences. N/A = not addressed in the clinical practice guidelines.

periodic limb movement disorder, a sleep-related movement disorder, due to low accuracy when compared to gold-standard laboratory PSG.

In general, actigraphy should not be used to replace PSG when PSG is clinically indicated for diagnostic purposes; however, actigraphy can provide additional information useful in the assessment of sleep disorders. For example, using actigraphy can improve the validity of the MSLT when used a week prior to testing. Actigraphy can also provide data to support a diagnosis of a sleep disorder for which PSG would not be indicated, particularly disorders that require longitudinal assessment (e.g., CRSWDs). Additionally, populations that may be unable to provide an accurate sleep history or maintain a daily sleep log (e.g., pediatric populations, older adults with cognitive impairment) may benefit from the addition of actigraphy to their sleep evaluation. Following the evaluation phase, actigraphy can serve to assess patient treatment adherence and response to clinical interventions.

In clinical settings, several challenges limit the use of actigraphy. First, and most notably, many payors do not cover actigraphy as a diagnostic tool in the assessment of sleep disorders, despite guidelines that support the clinical utility of actigraphy monitoring. It is sometimes provided as an out-of-pocket service; however, this limits access for lower-income patients. Second, device damage and loss are an additional barrier to use. Since patients wear the devices for extended periods of time (3–14 days), they can be misplaced or lost. This can increase the overall costs of using actigraphy in clinical settings.

Due to the ever-advancing market of wearable electronic devices, there is a plethora of wearable actigraphy devices to estimate sleep parameters. The hardware of movement-tracking sensors has remained relatively unchanged through the years, but the nuances of proprietary algorithm software that interprets the raw data make it challenging to systematically validate and compare. Common actigraphy devices used in research include the AW2 (from Minimiter, which merged with Philips Respironics); the Micromini Motionlogger (from Ambulatory Monitoring, Inc.); the Actiwatch 4/Actiwatch Plus and Motionwatch (from Camntech); GENEactiv (from Activinsights); wActisleep-BT, GTX-BT, GT3X+, GT3X, and Actisleep+ (from Actigraph); Visi Grey Flash (from Stowood); and Somnowatch (from Somnomedics). Philips Respironics was the most common in studies of young children, while Ambulatory Monitoring, Inc., was the most common in studies of infants (Schoch et al., 2021). For children, actigraphy placements utilized both the ankle/calf/leg and arm/wrist. The most used epoch length is 1 minute, but this can range from 1 second to 2 minutes with duration of monitoring from a few hours to 60 days. The most common algorithm applied for infants and young children was that published by Sadeh and colleagues (Acebo et al., 1999), while adult algorithms are provided by the manufacturer (e.g., Philips Respironics, Inc., Bend, OR) or publicly available (Cole et al., 1992). The prices of these research actigraphy products can be up to $3,000 per unit, with devices, interfaces, and software sold separately or as a package. Some devices include features such as high-frequency sampling rate (16–100 Hz) based on multi-axis piezo-electric accelerometers, an event marker button, waterproofing, a rechargeable lithium-ion battery, Bluetooth connectivity, ambient light/lux sensors (range 380–750 nm), and high memory capacity for data collection of up to 4 GB.

Actigraphy in the Diagnosis and Management of Insomnia Disorder

Insomnia disorder, or difficulty initiating or maintaining sleep resulting in daytime functioning impairment, is a diagnosis made on the basis of self-report data, such as from subjective sleep measures (e.g., sleep diary, ISI) in combination with a clinician interview (AASM, 2014). Objective measures of sleep are not required in the diagnostic criteria for insomnia disorder. Utilizing objective assessments such as PSG introduces several variables such as an unfamiliar laboratory environment and multiple sensors on the head, chest, and limbs that can result in an impaired ability to fall or stay asleep that is greater in individuals with insomnia versus good sleepers (Toussaint et al., 1995) and may continue to impair sleep on repeat assessments (Le Bon et al., 2001). Given the elevated burden and cost of PSG, this method is also unable to capture the nightly variability in sleep parameters that is common in individuals with insomnia (Edinger et al., 1991; Vallieres et al., 2005).

The AASM conditionally recommends the use actigraphy in the evaluation of insomnia disorder in adults in cases which may require further assessment (Smith et al., 2018a). For example, in individuals who are poor historians of their personal sleep patterns and unsuccessfully complete a course of cognitive behavioral therapy for insomnia (CBT-I), actigraphy can assess adherence to CBT-I recommendations or rule out possible circadian rhythm disorders. Studies have demonstrated that actigraphy is adequate in comparison to PSG in the assessment of TST, WASO, and SE but is not appropriate for the assessment of SOL (Jean-Louis et al., 2001; Lichstein et al., 2006). The use of actigraphy should not serve as a replacement for standard assessments of insomnia as described above. Given that insomnia is a disorder that is characterized by extended wakefulness while lying in bed, automated scoring algorithms are likely to miscategorize immobile wakefulness as sleep in populations with insomnia disorder. Actigraphy is also able to reliably demonstrate worse sleep in individuals with insomnia as compared to good sleepers (Natale et al., 2009).

Actigraphy in the Diagnosis and Management of CRSWDs

The AASM conditionally recommends the use of actigraphy in the evaluation of CRSWDs in adult and pediatric populations (Smith et al., 2018a). Actigraphy is able to capture an individual's sleep patterns across multiple days with minimal cost and burden compared to PSG as well as with greater detail compared to sleep diaries. This methodology has been effectively utilized to assess circadian rhythms in a variety of patient populations across the life span, from pediatrics (Carskadon et al., 1997) to older adults with neurocognitive disorders (Gehrman et al., 2004), individuals with cancer (Mormont et al., 2000), and shift workers (Lavie et al., 1992). Actigraphy may also be clinically helpful when other diagnostic measures are less available or may not qualify for reimbursement. Cheng and colleagues (2021) published a model that utilizes data from actigraphy to estimate dim light melatonin onset (DLMO) in night shift workers, which may be an alternative to salivary assessment of DLMO to inform the treatment of CRSWD. In the case of CRSWD treatment, actigraphy can assess for an individual's adherence to treatment recommendations or progress in the treatment of phase advance or delay (Nagtegaal et al., 1998), jet lag (Beaumont et al., 2004; Burgess et al., 2003), and shift-work disorder (Kubo et al., 2009). Although several studies have developed models to assess circadian sleep–wake patterns (Luik et al., 2013; Marler et al., 2006; Zeitzer et al., 2018), there is no standardized methodology in the field.

Actigraphy in the Diagnosis of Sleep Disordered Breathing

Actigraphy is not considered a viable alternative to assessment of guideline-based recommendations for the diagnosis of sleep disordered breathing (SDB), including obstructive and central sleep apnea. There is evidence that, in the use of HSAT inclusion of TST in estimating the severity of SDB can improve accuracy, and actigraphy can be used for this purpose. Ideally, actigraphy could be integrated into HSAT devices and provide a reliable estimate of TST (Smith et al., 2018a), improving the accuracy of diagnosis. One limitation is that arousals from sleep during apneas may lead to movements erroneously categorized as wakefulness; however, even with this limitation, actigraphy can improve precision of HSAT.

Actigraphy in the Diagnosis and Management of Hypersomnia and Excessive Daytime Sleepiness

Actigraphy within the context of hypersomnia diagnosis remains an area of growing research, both in establishing diagnoses of hypersomnia and related disorders as well as in examining how actigraphy can aid in the validation of current idiopathic hypersomnia (IH) diagnostic criteria (Trotti, 2019). Though actigraphy has become a potential path for assessing sleep duration and other factors in clarifying hypersomnia diagnosis, Trotti (2019) highlighted multiple gaps in the actigraph validation literature warranting further investigation, including a current lack of validation studies examining actigraphy in home settings for individuals with IH as well as a limited supply of studies with large sample sizes. In light of this, several studies have employed the use of actigraphy in the diagnosis of hypersomnia-related disorders, often in conjunction with other sleep measures such as the MSLT.

In the diagnosis of hypersomnia and related disorders, the MSLT currently stands as the "gold-standard" measure of objective severity of daytime sleepiness, though it has demonstrated questionable test–retest reliability with this diagnostic population as well as high patient burden and expense (Lopez et al., 2017). The MSLT has also been shown to be influenced by multiple factors, particularly a person's recent sleep history (Bradshaw et al., 2007). Though actigraphy is generally not a recommended substitute for the MSLT, evidence exists regarding its utility in informing MSLT interpretation, particularly when deployed prior to MSLTs to better account for the influential role of a patient's recent sleep history (Bradshaw et al., 2007; Kelly et al., 2022). Other smaller-scale studies have found actigraphy to have value in differentiating individuals with hypersomnia from healthy controls as well as certain forms of narcolepsy (Leger et al., 2018; Torstensen et al., 2021).

In comparison to PSG, actigraphy appears to be a generally valid and reliable measure of TST for individuals with hypersomnolence and related sleep disorders like narcolepsy, though there is some evidence of minor underestimation of TST (Alakuijala et al., 2021). Actigraphy can also serve as a concurrent measure when employing subjective sleep measures in cases of hypersomnia and related disorders, given evidence of a discrepancy between subjective and objective sleep measures in this population based on smaller-scale studies (Tomita et al., 2013). Though several studies have been described in this section, much more research in this area is warranted to better establish best practices regarding actigraphy use in the diagnosis and treatment of hypersomnia-related disorders.

Use of Actigraphy in Pediatric Patients

From infancy to childhood, natural sleep behaviors shift, which are prone to disruptions by external factors. These commonly result in sleep issues that parents then relate to their child's healthcare provider. Such complaints of "sleep irregularities" may be a norm for the child's sleep physiology depending on their stage of development but perhaps a social nuance according to the parents' schedule. For example, a frustrated parent complains of a fussy infant waking up too many times a night or a toddler excessively sleeping during the day. When such is questioned and the decision is made to monitor the child's sleep, periods of both day and night must be counted. Daytime sleep accounts for up to 20% of sleep in the first year of life and up to 5% at age 6 (Schoch et al., 2021). By this age, most children in the United States are enrolled in a formal education system (preschool), which sometimes structures a period of naptime. One study of 137 preschool children utilized actigraphy to compare rarely napping children with frequently napping children and showed that there was no difference in total sleep across the 24-hour day (Acebo et al., 2005; Spencer et al., 2016). These findings were consistent with previous research which suggested that short overnight sleep durations were associated with longer naps, as if napping may be a compensatory mechanism for insufficient sleep (Acebo et al., 2005).

For children with suspected behavioral, neurological, or mood disorders, it may be clinically important to examine their sleep to provide guidance for therapy. Actigraphy may be useful for children who do not tolerate sleeping in a lab for PSG. The challenge of monitoring sleep in this population with actigraphy is standardizing the pediatric scoring rules (Meltzer & Westin, 2011), especially considering the varying sleep conditions (sleeping while being carried, in a car, bed sharing; Galland et al., 2014). These periods of sleep in the setting of unintentional background activity may mislead the actigraphy to suggest wakefulness. Several studies of infants, young children, and adolescents have determined that the agreement of sleep diary and actigraphy of starting, ending, and assumed sleep is acceptable (up to a mean disagreement within 30 minutes). However, the actual sleep time and nocturnal wake times between actigraphy and diary data were insufficient (Gnidovec et al., 2002; Sadeh, 1996; Sadeh et al., 1994; Werner et al., 2008). Specifically, parents underestimated the number of night-wakings and overestimated the quality of their children's sleep (Tikotzky & Sadeh, 2001). In adolescents, the subjective sleep duration was longer than objective measures by up to 1 hour if self-estimated and 2.3 hours if parent/guardian-estimated (Holzhausen et al., 2021).

The evaluation of daytime fatigue due to insufficient sleep in the population of teens particularly benefits from the use of actigraphy. Teens carry enough autonomy to choose their sleep schedule (often in the privacy of their own room), which may or may not be what their parents notice and report to the provider. For example, a parent of a sleepy teen can insist on a "normal amount of sleep" on a school day when actually the naturally delayed-sleep-phased individual sleeps hours later after intended sleep time. In this case, actigraphy with ambient light detection can highlight one of the common causes of daytime fatigue in this population.

Similar to adults, medical-grade actigraphy studies on children underestimated TST and overestimated WASO (Meltzer et al., 2012; Spruyt et al., 2011). There are no known objective sleep elements that contribute to a perceived sleep quality. Interestingly TST, SOL, and SE as determined on PSG did not predict a child rating of sleep quality but predicted a marginal effect for WASO for values <30 minutes (So et al., 2021). This provides direction for future areas of study in children for improving tools to track therapies to optimize "healthy" sleep. From an epidemiological study of children, sleep patterns can be economically studied through actigraphy to provide insight on differences based on ethnicity, socioeconomic status, and location. For example, over a 2-year course, young Pacific Island children had poorer sleep patterns than their European counterparts (Vaipuna et al., 2018).

Use of Actigraphy in Patients With Neurocognitive Disabilities

Certain populations require prior planning and interpretation of actigraphy data, especially when data is collected from individuals with movement disorders or cognitive limitations. Those with limited movement, such as in cerebral palsy or motor deficits by stroke, have an overall blunted effect across data. This makes it challenging to determine if an individual is laying still but awake or asleep. Furthermore, one would need to determine which hand or leg the motion device should be attached to. On the other hand, those with neuro-movement disorders such as tremors, akathisia, tardive dyskinesia, and body rocking/swaying in attention-deficit/hyperactivity disorder can mimic the activity level of exercise when they may be resting. One study showed that actigraphy placement with hand tremor (tremor-prominent hand vs. opposite hand) yielded similar nighttime sleep measures (Maglione et al., 2013). Interestingly, an exploration of nocturnal movements in Parkinson's disease using multiple interconnected and synchronized wearable sensors can be used to create a body area network, resulting in three-dimensional information on body motion and position (Zampogna et al., 2020). Another study utilized actigraphy to reveal that movement disorders, in particular parkinsonism (up to 85%), were associated with reduced physical activity and increased sedentary behavior in patients with psychotic disorders (Pieters et al., 2021).

Actigraphy use in nursing homes can help track residents' sleep duration, presence of circadian rhythm disorders, daytime activity, and excessive napping. This highlights areas for improvement on an individual level as well as quality standards among institutions. A study using validated psychometric questionnaires and actigraphy data on nursing home residents with dementia revealed a lesser quality of life versus their home-dwelling counterparts (Olsen et al., 2016).

For those with intellectual disability and autism, the sensory stimulation of a band on the wrist may not be tolerated. Creative solutions such as sewing the actigraphy to a pocket sleeve of the pajamas will provide sufficient nocturnal data.

Conclusions

Wrist actigraphy is a useful technology that can inform clinical practice and enhance the overall understanding of a patient's sleep/wake habits and patterns. This is true in both adult and pediatric patient populations. It cannot generally replace laboratory PSG in the diagnosis of sleep disorders, but appropriate use can inform diagnosis and treatment selection. Consumer products do not currently meet sufficiently high standards for reliability and validity to replace approved devices used in clinical applications.

Future Directions

The following questions, if answered, would enhance the utility of actigraphy for clinical and research applications

1. How can less expensive technologies and/or disposable sensors be used to reduce the cost of actigraphy and increase access to this diagnostic tool?
2. Is the cost–benefit ratio favorable in terms of clinical use of actigraphy, and if so, how can reimbursement be improved?
3. Can actigraphy be used in population-based research to obtain objective estimates of sleep and sleep habits across diverse groups of adults and children?
4. Can the appeal of consumer products be combined with the reliability and accuracy of actigraphs used for clinical/research purposes so that this technology can be used more easily and widely?
5. Can enhanced scoring algorithms be developed that are age-/population-specific using artificial intelligence methods?

Acknowledgments

Supported by Veterans Affairs (VA) Health Services Research & Development Service Research Career Scientist Award RCS 20-191 (J. L. Martin), National Institutes of Health/National Heart Lung Blood Institute K23 HL157754 (M. R. Kelly) and K24 HL143055 (J. L. Martin), and the VA Greater Los Angeles Healthcare System Geriatric Research, Education and Clinical Center.

References

Acebo, C., Sadeh, A., Seifer, R., Tzischinsky, O., Hafer, A., & Carskadon, M. A. (2005). Sleep/wake patterns derived from activity monitoring and maternal report for healthy 1- to 5-year-old children. *Sleep, 28*(12), 1568–1577. https://doi.org/10.1093/sleep/28.12.1568

Acebo, C., Sadeh, A., Seifer, R., Tzischinsky, O., Wolfson, A. R., Hafer, A., & Carskadon, M. A. (1999). Estimating sleep patterns with activity monitoring in children and adolescents: How many nights are necessary for reliable measures? *Sleep, 22*(1), 95–103.

Alakuijala, A., Sarkanen, T., Jokela, T., & Partinen, M. (2021). Accuracy of actigraphy compared to concomitant ambulatory polysomnography in narcolepsy and other sleep disorders. *Frontiers in Neurology, 12*, Article 629709. https://doi.org/10.3389/fneur.2021.629709

Altini, M., & Kinnunen, H. (2021). The promise of sleep: A multi-sensor approach for accurate sleep stage detection using the Oura ring. *Sensors, 21*(13), Article 4302. https://doi.org/10.3390/s21134302

American Academy of Sleep Medicine. (2014). *International classification of sleep disorders* (3rd ed.).

Ancoli-Israel, S., Cole, R., Alessi, C., Chambers, M., Moorcroft, W., & Pollak, C. P. (2003). The role of actigraphy in the study of sleep and circadian rhythms. *Sleep, 26*(3), 342–392. https://doi.org/10.1093/sleep/26.3.342

Ancoli-Israel, S., Martin, J. L., Blackwell, T., Buenaver, L., Liu, L., Meltzer, L. J., Sadeh, A., Spira, A. P., Taylor, D., Owens, J., & Smith, M. (2015). The SBSM guide to actigraphy monitoring: Clinical and research applications. *Journal of Behavioral Sleep Medicine, 13*(S1), S4–S38.

Asgari Mehrabadi, M., Azimi, I., Sarhaddi, F., Axelin, A., Niela-Vilén, H., Myllyntausta, S., Stenholm, S., Dutt, N., Liljeberg, P., & Rahmani, A. M. (2020). Sleep tracking of a commercially available smart ring and smartwatch against medical-grade actigraphy in everyday settings: Instrument validation study. *JMIR Mhealth Uhealth, 8*(10), Article e20465. https://doi.org/10.2196/20465

Bastien, C. H., Vallieres, A., & Morin, C. M. (2001). Validation of the Insomnia Severity Index as an outcome measure for insomnia research. *Sleep Medicine, 2*(4), 297–307.

Beaumont, M., Batejat, D., Pierard, C., Van Beers, P., Denis, J. B., Coste, O., Doireau, P., Chauffard, F., French, J., & Lagarde, D. (2004). Caffeine or melatonin effects on sleep and sleepiness after rapid eastward transmeridian travel. *Journal of Applied Physiology, 96*(1), 50–58. https://doi.org/10.1152/japplphysiol.00940.2002

Blackwell, T., Ancoli-Israel, S., Redline, S., Stone, K. L., & Osteoporotic Fractures in Men Study Group. (2011). Factors that may influence the classification of sleep–wake by wrist actigraphy: The MrOS Sleep Study. *Journal of Clinical Sleep Medicine, 7*(4), 357–367. https://doi.org/10.5664/JCSM.1190

Bradshaw, D. A., Yanagi, M. A., Pak, E. S., Peery, T. S., & Ruff, G. A. (2007). Nightly sleep duration in the 2-week period preceding multiple sleep latency testing. *Journal of Clinical Sleep Medicine, 3*(6), 613–619. https://www.ncbi.nlm.nih.gov/pubmed/17993043

Burgess, H. J., Crowley, S. J., Gazda, C. J., Fogg, L. F., & Eastman, C. I. (2003). Preflight adjustment to eastward travel: 3 days of advancing sleep with and without morning bright light. *Journal of Biological Rhythms, 18*(4), 318–328. https://doi.org/10.1177/0748730403253585

Buysse, D. J., Reynolds, C. F. I., Monk, T. H., Berman, S. R., & Kupfer, D. J. (1989). The Pittsburgh Sleep Quality Index: A new instrument for psychiatric practice and research. *Psychiatry Research, 28*(2), 193–213.

Carney, C. E., Lajos, L. E., & Waters, W. F. (2004). Wrist actigraph versus self-report in normal sleepers: Sleep schedule adherence and self-report validity. *Behavioral Sleep Medicine, 2*(3), 134–143. https://doi.org/10.1207/s15402010bsm0203_2

Carskadon, M. A., Acebo, C., Richardson, G. S., Tate, B. A., & Seifer, R. (1997). An approach to studying circadian rhythms of adolescent humans. *Journal of Biological Rhythms, 12*(3), 278–289. https://doi.org/10.1177/074873049701200309

A systematic review and meta-analysis. *Sleep Medicine Reviews, 25*, 52–73. https://doi.org/10.1016/j.smrv.2015.01.009

Mormont, M. C., Waterhouse, J., Bleuzen, P., Giacchetti, S., Jami, A., Bogdan, A., Lellouch, J., Misset, J. L., Touitou, Y., & Levi, F. (2000). Marked 24-h rest/activity rhythms are associated with better quality of life, better response, and longer survival in patients with metastatic colorectal cancer and good performance status. *Clinical Cancer Research, 6*(8), 3038–3045. https://www.ncbi.nlm.nih.gov/pubmed/10955782

Nagtegaal, J. E., Kerkhof, G. A., Smits, M. G., Swart, A. C., & Van Der Meer, Y. G. (1998). Delayed sleep phase syndrome: A placebo-controlled cross-over study on the effects of melatonin administered five hours before the individual dim light melatonin onset. *Journal of Sleep Research, 7*(2), 135–143. https://doi.org/10.1046/j.1365-2869.1998.00102.x

Natale, V., Plazzi, G., & Martoni, M. (2009). Actigraphy in the assessment of insomnia: A quantitative approach. *Sleep, 32*(6), 767–771. https://doi.org/10.1093/sleep/32.6.767

Olsen, C., Pedersen, I., Bergland, A., Enders-Slegers, M. J., Jøranson, N., Calogiuri, G., & Ihlebæk, C. (2016). Differences in quality of life in home-dwelling persons and nursing home residents with dementia—A cross-sectional study. *BMC Geriatrics, 16*, Article 137. https://doi.org/10.1186/s12877-016-0312-4

Pieters, L. E., Deenik, J., Tenback, D. E., van Oort, J., & van Harten, P. N. (2021). Exploring the relationship between movement disorders and physical activity in patients with schizophrenia: An actigraphy study. *Schizophrenia Bulletin, 47*(4), 906–914. https://doi.org/10.1093/schbul/sbab028

Roberts, D. M., Schade, M. M., Mathew, G. M., Gartenberg, D., & Buxton, O. M. (2020). Detecting sleep using heart rate and motion data from multisensor consumer-grade wearables, relative to wrist actigraphy and polysomnography. *Sleep, 43*(7), Article zsaa045. https://doi.org/10.1093/sleep/zsaa045

Sadeh, A. (1996). Evaluating night wakings in sleep-disturbed infants: A methodological study of parental reports and actigraphy. *Sleep, 19*(10), 757–762.

Sadeh, A., Sharkey, K. M., & Carskadon, M. A. (1994). Activity-based sleep–wake identification: An empirical test of methodological issues. *Sleep, 17*(3), 201–207. https://doi.org/10.1093/sleep/17.3.201

Schoch, S. F., Kurth, S., & Werner, H. (2021). Actigraphy in sleep research with infants and young children: Current practices and future benefits of standardized reporting. *Journal of Sleep Research, 30*(3), Article e13134. https://doi.org/10.1111/jsr.13134

Smith, M. T., McCrae, C. S., Cheung, J., Martin, J. L., Harrod, C. G., Heald, J. L., & Carden, K. A. (2018a). Use of actigraphy for the evaluation of sleep disorders and circadian rhythm sleep–wake disorders: An American Academy of Sleep Medicine clinical practice guideline. *Journal of Clinical Sleep Medicine, 14*(7), 1231–1237. https://doi.org/10.5664/jcsm.7230

Smith, M. T., McCrae, C. S., Cheung, J., Martin, J. L., Harrod, C. G., Heald, J. L., & Carden, K. A. (2018b). Use of actigraphy for the evaluation of sleep disorders and circadian rhythm sleep–wake disorders: An American Academy of Sleep Medicine systematic review, meta-analysis, and GRADE assessment. *Journal of Clinical Sleep Medicine, 14*(7), 1209–1230. https://doi.org/10.5664/jcsm.7228

So, C. J., Palmer, C. A., Gonzalez, R. D., Bower, J. L., Lau, S., & Alfano, C. A. (2021). Which objective sleep elements predict children's perceptions of good sleep quality? A preliminary investigation based on polysomnography and actigraphy. *Sleep Health, 7*(1), 65–71. https://doi.org/10.1016/j.sleh.2020.07.001

Spencer, R. M. C., Campanella, C., de Jong, D. M., Desrochers, P., Root, H., Cremone, A., & Kurdziel, L. B. F. (2016). Sleep and behavior of preschool children under typical and nap-promoted conditions. *Sleep Health, 2*(1), 35–41. https://doi.org/10.1016/j.sleh.2015.12.009

Spruyt, K., Gozal, D., Dayyat, E., Roman, A., & Molfese, D. L. (2011). Sleep assessments in healthy school-aged children using actigraphy: Concordance with polysomnography. *Journal of Sleep Research, 20*(1, Pt. 2), 223–232. https://doi.org/10.1111/j.1365-2869.2010.00857.x

Tikotzky, L., & Sadeh, A. (2001). Sleep patterns and sleep disruptions in kindergarten children. *Journal of Clinical and Child Psychology, 30*(4), 581–591.

Tomita, S., Kitajima, T., Mekata, T., Tscuchiya, A., Sano, W., Esaki, Y., Marina, H., Fujita, S., & Iwata, N. (2013). Comparison of sleep diary and actigraphy to evaluate total sleep time in hypersomnia patients. *Sleep and Biological Rhythms, 11*, 65–73. https://doi.org/10.1111/sbr.12004

Torstensen, E. W., Pickering, L., Kornum, B. R., Wanscher, B., Baandrup, L., & Jennum, P. J. (2021). Diagnostic value of actigraphy in hypersomnolence disorders. *Sleep Medicine, 85*, 1–7. https://doi.org/10.1016/j.sleep.2021.06.033

Toussaint, M., Luthringer, R., Schaltenbrand, N., Carelli, G., Lainey, E., Jacqmin, A., Muzet, A., & Macher, J. P. (1995). First-night effect in normal subjects and psychiatric inpatients. *Sleep, 18*(6), 463–469. https://doi.org/10.1093/sleep/18.6.463

Trotti, L. M. (2019). Are we there yet? Getting closer to certainty in idiopathic hypersomnia diagnosis. *Journal of Clinical Sleep Medicine, 15*(4), 539–540. https://doi.org/10.5664/jcsm.7706

Vaipuna, T. F. W., Williams, S. M., Farmer, V. L., Meredith-Jones, K. A., Richards, R., Galland, B. C., Te Morenga, L., & Taylor, R. W. (2018). Sleep patterns in children differ by ethnicity: Cross-sectional and longitudinal analyses using actigraphy. *Sleep Health, 4*(1), 81–86. https://doi.org/10.1016/j.sleh.2017.10.012

Vallieres, A., Ivers, H., Bastien, C. H., Beaulieu-Bonneau, S., & Morin, C. M. (2005). Variability and predictability in sleep patterns of chronic insomniacs. *Journal of Sleep Research, 14*(4), 447–453. https://doi.org/10.1111/j.1365-2869.2005.00480.x

Van Den Berg, J. F., Van Rooij, F. J., Vos, H., Tulen, J. H., Hofman, A., Miedema, H. M., Neven, A. K., & Tiemeier, H. (2008). Disagreement between subjective and actigraphic measures of sleep duration in a population-based study of elderly persons. *Journal of Sleep Research, 17*(3), 295–302. https://doi.org/10.1111/j.1365-2869.2008.00638.x

Werner, H., Molinari, L., Guyer, C., & Jenni, O. G. (2008). Agreement rates between actigraphy, diary, and questionnaire for children's sleep patterns. *Archives of Pediatric and Adolescent Medicine, 162*(4), 350–358.

Zampogna, A., Manoni, A., Asci, F., Liguori, C., Irrera, F., & Suppa, A. (2020). Shedding light on nocturnal movements in Parkinson's disease: Evidence from wearable technologies. *Sensors, 20*(18), Article 5171. https://doi.org/10.3390/s20185171

Zeitzer, J. M., Blackwell, T., Hoffman, A. R., Cummings, S., Ancoli-Israel, S., & Stone, K.; Osteoporotic Fractures in Men Study Research Group. (2018). Daily patterns of accelerometer activity predict changes in sleep, cognition, and mortality in older men. *Journals of Gerontology, Series A, 73*(5), 682–687. https://doi.org/10.1093/gerona/glw250

CHAPTER

25 Polysomnography and Emerging Technologies to Evaluate Sleep Disorders

Thomas Penzel, Ingo Fietze, Martin Glos, Lisa Rosenblum, *and* Matthew Salanitro

Abstract

Sleep is a sensitive process with a huge amount of regulatory and restorative functions. If an individual suffers from problems during sleep, it could impair daytime functioning. For this reason, individuals suspected of having a sleep disorder should be assessed in an environment where external and internal influencing factors can be controlled. Furthermore, they should be recorded with clinically validated devices that can accurately extract sleep parameters. In this chapter, the gold standard method for recording sleep and its simplified version will be explained in detail, covering what, how, and why each measure is needed. Following this, the authors will delve into the latest emerging technologies that evaluate sleep. These future technologies could potentially pave the way for faster diagnosis of sleep disorders through automatic scoring of sleep studies. In addition, they could substantially reduce the pressure of waiting lists for sleep studies due to the affordability of the devices. By the end of this chapter, the current standards of practice, recent advancements, and state-of-the-art technologies used in the evaluation of sleep disorders will have been discussed.

Key Words: assessment, evaluation, polysomnography, device, technology

Introduction

Sleep is a sensitive process with a huge amount of regulatory and restorative functions. For this reason, sleep should be assessed in an environment where external and internal influencing factors can be controlled. For instance, noise, light, smell, and extreme temperatures are known to affect a subject's sleep. This assessment typically occurs in a sleep laboratory that contains multiple bedrooms that all have noise protection, constant temperature settings, and control of luminance. Furthermore, there are no timepieces in each room, and an option to call a nurse or supervising staff should be available.

Polysomnography (PSG) is the gold standard for sleep recording, it consists of recording physiological signals such as brain activity, heart rate, blood oxygen levels, breathing, and eye and leg movements continuously throughout the night. PSG is used in parallel with video and sound recording to capture all physiological and pathophysiological conditions of the subject. While there are other methods of measuring sleep such as home sleep testing (HST) and home sleep apnea testing (HSAT), PSG is the predominant method used in sleep laboratories. PSG is perceived as the reference measurement technique to objectively quantify sleep and all related physiological parameters. It is common for all other emerging technologies to be evaluated and validated against it.

Sleep Laboratory

Most sleep laboratories are equipped with a PSG recording device, an infrared-sensitive video camera, a room microphone, and a patient alarm button to request help from a sleep technician or nurse during the night if needed. Usually, several sleeping rooms are used in parallel and together with a supervision room. The supervision room, therefore, typically contains multiple computers for PSG recordings, video monitoring recordings, patient alarm indicators, and vital sign alarms (e.g., electrocardiogram [ECG] or oxygen). During the night, two sleep technicians should be present to monitor the recordings so that one person can help the other. For instance, if one technician is busy with a patient, the other can still monitor the remaining patients (Troester et al., 2023).

Sleep laboratories are commonly used to monitor the progression of sleep over the course of the night. However, they can also be used during the daytime to monitor naps and to investigate conditions that cause individuals to fall asleep during the daytime. These daytime investigations include not only a period of sleep but possibly also tasks like driving simulators, reaction time tests, specific tests to check for the latency to fall asleep during daytime (e.g., multiple sleep latency tests), and for the ability to stay awake (e.g., maintenance of wakefulness test; Carskadon, 1986; Littner et al., 2005). This means that the sleep laboratory is more than just a bedroom; it also contains other furniture. For example, during vigilance testing, a comfortable chair to rest on may be an additional and useful piece of furniture. For other cognitive tests, it is very common to use pen and paper, so a small table is useful.

Digital sleep recordings are usually stored in a company's proprietary data format. However, sleep centers tend to cooperate and exchange digital sleep recordings for either scientific purposes, obtaining a second opinion, or quality assurance. For this reason, a standard data format for storing raw signals of digital sleep recordings became popular (Kemp et al., 1992). This was developed as part of a European Union–funded project and therefore received the name *European Data Format* (EDF). The advanced version is called EDF+, and that contains definitions that are more restricted. In addition, EDF+ has the ability to store annotations like sleep stages and other events in the same data file, which is not available in EDF (Kemp & Olivan, 2003). A competing data format is *Digital Imaging and Communications in Medicine* (DICOM), and they recently added to their comprehensive image storing definitions a neurophysiological signal storing definition (Bidgood & Horii, 1992; Halford et al., 2021).

PSG

The recording of physiological signals in the sleep lab by PSG is fairly standardized today (Troester et al., 2023). Since sleep is regulated by activity within the brain, the recording of the brain waves by electroencephalogram (EEG) is the first port of call. EEG is the preferred measurement as there are no localized areas of the brain where sleep occurs; therefore, an overall recording of brain activity is important for sleep recording. The output presents us with specific waves and patterns that help classify sleep stages into light sleep and deep sleep. In the beginning, a consensus-based standard manual for the recording and scoring was written by a group of experts which was chaired by two people, Rechtschaffen and Kales (1968). Their manual required only one EEG lead to record and score sleep. This was the EEG lead C4-A1 (central C4–reference A1) from a 10–20-electrode placement system (American Electroencephalographic Society, 1991). Later the C3-A2 lead was integrated as a backup. This EEG lead was a kind of compromise to detect waves and patterns sufficiently. However, in order to precisely detect the waves such as alpha and delta, frontal (e.g., F4) and occipital (e.g., O2) leads serve better. These were only integrated when digital sleep recordings were introduced. Before this, the number of leads could be problematic. According to the current standard manual for the recording and scoring of sleep (from the American Academy of Sleep Medicine [AASM]; Troester et al., 2023), it is recommended to record F4-M1, C4-M1, and O2-M1. The placement of the reference electrode was moved from A1 to M1 for practical reasons and to improve the accuracy of recordings.

In addition to the EEG, it is essential to record eye movements and muscle tone. The electro-oculogram (EOG) records eye movements by making use of the eye as an electrical dipole. The signal contains the eye movements and frontal components of the EEG. One electrode is placed 1 centimeter below the left eye at the outer cantus (the position is called *E1*) and the other is placed 1 centimeter above the right eye at the other outer cantus (called *E2*). Both electrodes are referenced to M2. If M2 fails, M1 is an equally good alternative. The position of E1 and E2 makes it possible to differentiate the eye movement output; it can range from rapid blinks when awake, slow eye movements when falling asleep, to rapid eye movements during rapid-eye-movement (REM) sleep.

The third signal is collected by the electromyogram (EMG), which monitors and records muscle tone. The muscles on the face are very well controlled, and EMG can pick up even the most sensitive of changes in muscle tone. Typically, muscle tone declines from wakefulness to sleep and is lowest during REM sleep. Therefore, EMG serves as a good indicator of reaching REM sleep. The electrodes are placed under the chin, and activity is recorded by referencing one electrode against the other one. According to the AASM guidelines, three electrodes are used in order to have one electrode as a reserve. Chin 1 and Chin 2 are below the chin, and chin Z is centered above the chin. It is not uncommon that one electrode loosens during the course of the night in terms of contact. Therefore,

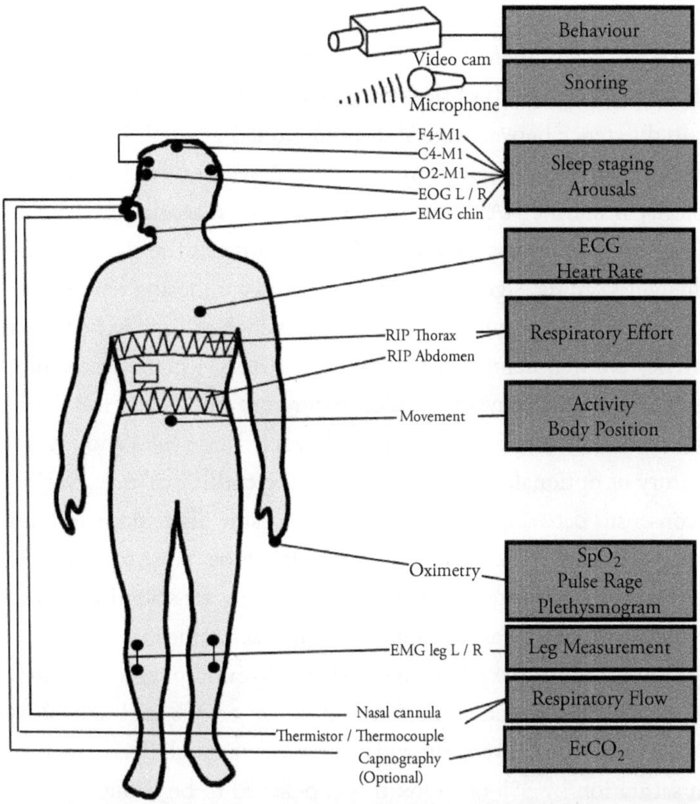

Figure 25.1 An illustration of sensor placement for standard polysomnography

Note. F4 = Frontal lobe position 4; C4 = Central lobe position 4; O2 = Occipital lobe position 2; M1 = Left mastoid; EOG = Electrooculogram; L / R = left and right; EMG = Electromyogram; ECG = Electrocardiogram; SpO_2 = Oxygen saturation; RIP = Respiratory Inductance Plethysmography; $EtCO_2$ = End-tidal carbon dioxide.

it is very useful to have a backup electrode. See Figure 25.1 for an illustration of sensor placement for standard PSG.

Sleep Scoring Manual

The rules created by Rechtschaffen and Kales for visually scoring sleep stages remained the standard recommendation for decades. The AASM announced an update of the sleep scoring rules in conjunction with many additions and published the first version in 2007: *The AASM Manual for Scoring of Sleep and Associated Events* (Iber et al., 2007). The AASM manual has been regularly updated to accommodate new knowledge, evidence, and techniques. Every 5 years major updates are planned, with smaller updates made whenever needed. This is specified in the procedural notes of the AASM manual. The current version is 3 and was published in 2023 (Troester et al., 2023). Since then it has refined many rules in order to remove ambiguity, improve the scoring reliability, and improve speed of completion. Other amendments were related to the introduction of digital technology regarding the transitional needs of sleep medicine.

The main difference between the above-mentioned manuals is that the manual published by Rechtschaffen and Kales was primarily developed for scoring sleep in young, healthy subjects, while the AASM manual is devoted to scoring healthy and disturbed sleep for all age groups, across all known sleep disorders. The AASM manual contains advice for digital recording, signal categorization, and composing reports on sleep parameters. With this, the most popular sleep parameters such as time in bed, total sleep time, and sleep latency are well defined. In addition, the AASM manual contains chapters on arousal rules, cardiac rules, movement rules, respiratory rules, and HSAT rules in order to diagnose patients with the appropriate sleep disorder. These rules and recommendations, being mandatory or optional, are mostly based on scientific evidence. When this was not available, a consensus between experts was achieved using discussions and multiple voting rounds. Some people argue that the AASM manual comes close to American reimbursement rules. This means some recommendations not only are scientifically based but present compromises with healthcare authorities—when scientific evidence is not completely clear. One prominent example of this is the debate around oxygen desaturation. Should desaturation events be counted from 3% and above or 4% and above? Typically, this results in an A and a B type of recommendation in the manual. Recommendation A refers to a drop in saturation by 3% or more; this is believed to be enough desaturation to fit the criteria of a respiratory event such as a hypopnea. Recommendation B is considered as "acceptable" within the manual. Here, a respiratory event can be identified when there is a drop in saturation by 4% or more. Recommendation A is more inclusive when scoring respiratory events, which is why it is more widely used. Some patients may not reach desaturation of 4% yet still experience hypopneas. As a consequence of this ambiguity, other initiatives have tried to create alternative sleep scoring manuals. These may contain variable-length epochs, cyclic alternating patterns, and other event definitions. However, none of these initiatives published a final alternative scoring manual. There has been a recent movement toward automated sleep staging. However, this research is still ongoing. The goal is to reduce all limitations that are produced by visual sleep staging such as time-consuming efforts, reliability, and consistency in scoring (Penzel, 2022).

PSG With More Than EEG, EOG, EMG

The remainder of this chapter refers to the current version of the AASM manual when discussing the rules, terminology, and specifications of scoring sleep and associated events (Troester et al., 2023).

PSG has evolved from being primarily a research tool to a vital clinical diagnostic method, especially with the recognition of sleep-disordered breathing as a significant health risk (Hirshkowitz, 2016). This shift made the recording of respiration, cardiac events, and movement even more critical in PSG studies. Newly published papers, backed by medical societies, established definitions for arousals, respiratory event scoring, and movement event scoring. These definitions were then condensed into recommendations for recording and scoring, which became key chapters in the *AASM Manual for the Scoring of Sleep and Associated Events*. To stay aligned with advancements and adjusted definitions, the manual is revised every five years. As a result, the latest version offers a comprehensive overview of the current physiological functions monitored during PSG, along with the sensor technologies used to capture them. A summary of this can be seen in Table 25.1. The table also links to HST and new emerging technologies.

Respiration is measured by assessing the airflow from the nose and mouth. The most accurate measurement of respiration is achieved using a pneumotachograph. However, this device requires a full-face mask, which is heavily weighted and difficult to handle. Therefore, indirect methods are preferred, for instance, a combination of thermal sensors (thermistors or thermocouples) and pressure sensors (also denoted as nasal prongs). Previous research has indicated that sleep-related breathing disorders feature not only impaired airflow but also respiratory effort (Kushida et al., 2005). Thus, it became mandatory to record respiratory effort in addition to airflow. Respiratory effort is best shown by changes in intrathoracic pressure. Intrathoracic pressure is quantitatively assessed by esophageal pressure recording. However, this method is invasive due to using a thin catheter inside the esophagus with a piezo pressure tip. Consequently, this is not well tolerated by sleeping subjects; again, indirect methods are preferred. The next best method for intrathoracic pressure is respiratory inductive plethysmography (RIP) belts. Other indirect methods like piezo sensor belts, impedance measurement, or diaphragm EMG have proven to be inferior to RIP. Accordingly, RIP is recommended in the AASM manual. Respiratory events are scored as apneas and hypopneas when airflow amplitude changes and the duration of the event is longer than 10 seconds. These events are further scored as being obstructive or central, depending on the presence of increased respiratory effort. A diagnosis of sleep apnea is made if more than five apnea/hypopnea events per hour of sleep are found. This number is called the Apnea/Hypopnea Index (AHI), and the findings are specified as AHI >5/hour. If the amplitude criteria for airflow do not meet the minimum value to score an apnea or hypopnea event but central nervous arousals are still associated with the changes in airflow, then these events are called *respiratory-related arousals* (RERAs; Fietze et al., 1999). An increased respiratory effort may reflect an increased resistance of the upper airways, which does not result in a hypopnea or apnea event, according to the airflow amplitude criteria. See Figure 25.2 for an example of an obstructive apnea event found in a PSG recording.

The effect of respiration can be observed in blood gas changes—oxygen (O_2) and carbon dioxide (CO_2) in the blood. The direct continuous measurement of blood gases is still very difficult and expensive. Due to this, pulse oximetry (oxygen saturation [SpO_2]) in the periphery (typically a finger) is used as an estimate of blood oxygenation, and the

Table 25.1 Sleep recording thought from physiology to technical implementation in polysomnography (PSG), home sleep testing systems, and wearables

Physiology	**Sensors, recording**	**PSG**	**PSG** scoring	**Home sleep testing (HST) (medical certified)**	**Wearables for sleep (consumer devices)**
Electroencephalogram (EEG), electro-oculogram, electromyogram (EMG)	Electrical brain activity, gel electrodes, dry electrodes	Integral part of PSG	Sleep stages, arousal	Single EEG for driver vigilance, insomnia screening	Rarely used in caps during sleep
Respiration: airflow	Thermo-sensors, nasal pressure sensors, microphone sound	Integral part of PSG	Apnea and hypopnea	Home sleep apnea testing (HSAT)	Not used
Respiration: effort	Esophageal sensor, respiratory inductive plethysmography (RIP), piezo belts, microphone sound, ballistocardiogram	Integral part of PSG: RIP	Obstructive central apnea and hypopnea, snoring	HSAT: RIP belts, piezo belts	Piezo belts, mainly sports-related, ballistocardiogram for sleep apnea estimation
Oxygen SaO_2, SpO_2	Photoplethysmography (PPG), pulse oximetry (SpO_2), transcutaneous O_2 (SaO_2)	Integral part of PSG	Desaturation	HSAT always with PPG for desaturation and pulse rate, sometimes respiration estimation, PPG exploitation as peripheral arterial tonometry	PPG is popular, SpO_2 value, pulse rate, sleep apnea estimation
Carbon dioxide (CO_2)	End-tidal CO_2, transcutaneous CO_2	Only for hypoventilation recording	Hypoventilation, hypercapnia, respiratory rate	Not available	Not available
Movement of limbs	Electrical muscle activity EMG, ballistocardiogram	Integral part of PSG	Periodic limb movements during sleep, periodic limb movement disorder, restless legs syndrome	Rarely used for HSTs	Not used in wearables

Actigraphy	Wrist-worn accelerometer, ballistocardiogram, radar technology	Rarely used	Not included in PSG scoring	Actigraphy can be a home test device by itself, see Chapter 27	Sleep estimation, sometimes sleep stages, and respiration estimation
Electrocardiogram (ECG)	ECG, ballistocardiogram	ECG is integral part of PSG	Heart rate and arrhythmia estimation	HSAT uses sometimes heart rate, sometimes respiration estimation	Arrhythmia detection (e.g., Apple watch), heart rate recording
Blood pressure	Sphygmomanometry, finger PPG, pulse transit time (PTT)	Rarely used	Hypertension during sleep and apnea	If used in HSAT, then as an additional device, few exceptions with integrated PTT	Not used in sleep wearables
Body temperature	Rectal probe, skin buttons, ear sensors	Rarely used, only in circadian research	Sleep regulation	Not used in home sleep tests	Not evaluated in sleep wearables
Body position	Gravity sensors, switch-based sensors, video	Integral part of PSG	Modifier for sleep disordered breathing	HSAT: gravity sensors or switch-based sensors	Rarely used

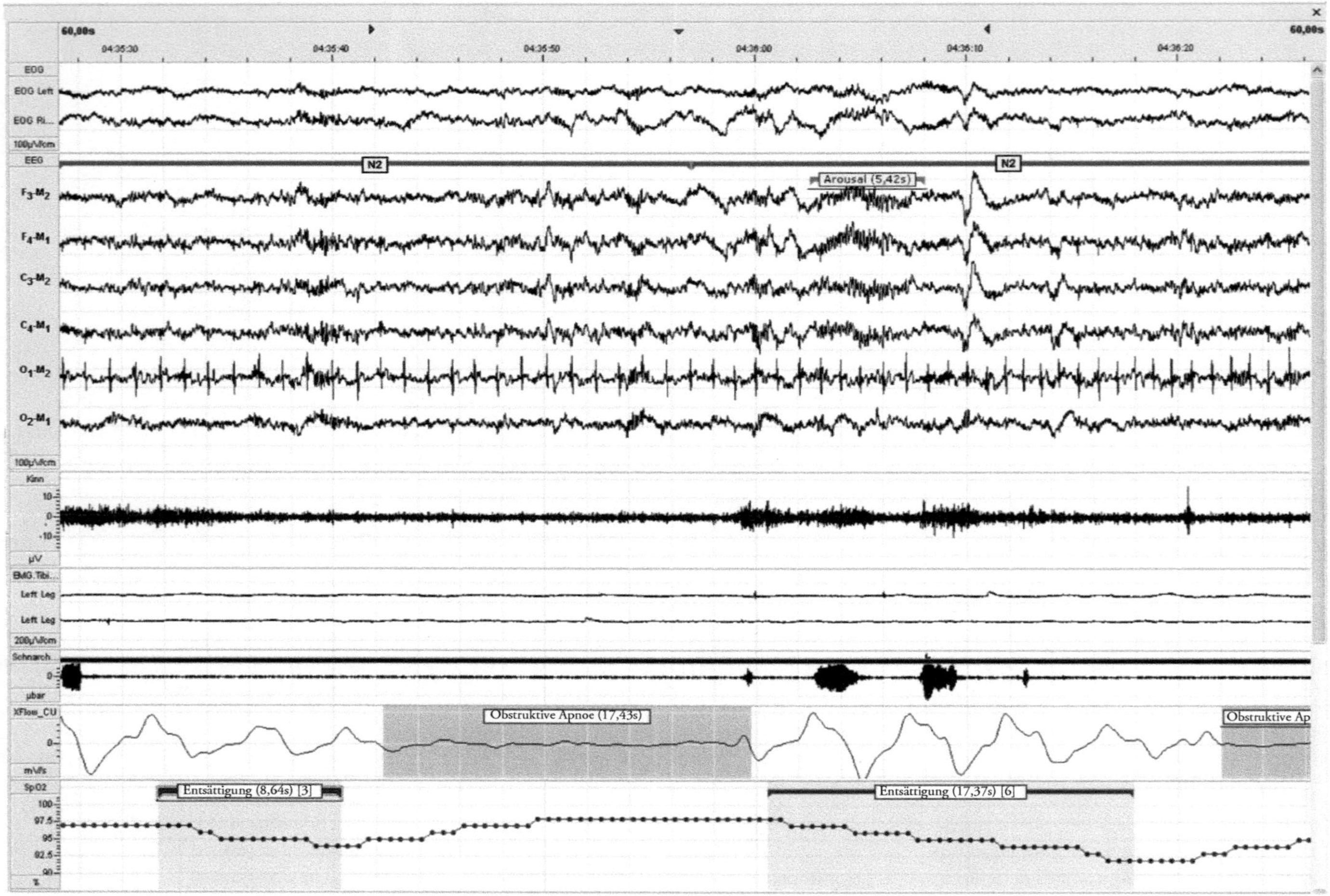

Figure 25.2 A 60-second screenshot of a sleep recording containing electroencephalogram, electro-oculogram, electromyogram, and respiratory channels configured according to American Academy of Sleep Medicine recommendations

Note. This screenshot displays an example of sleep stage N2, snoring, and an obstructive apnea accompanied by a desaturation event. The event is terminated by respiratory arousal.

measurement devices are at a very low cost today. Pulse oximetry is an excellent example of how technology drives medical use and applications. It is becoming more common for consumers to buy portable devices that contain pulse oximetry, and, of course, these new emerging devices must be validated against PSG before they can be used in confidence within a medical setting. Current available research has shown that portable pulse oximetry devices such as finger rings may be useful as a preliminary diagnosis of sleep breathing disorders. However, this technology is extremely new, and we could expect that in the near future, these devices could be as reliable as PSG when scoring respiratory events (Ma et al., 2018; Miller et al., 2022).

On the other hand, CO_2 monitoring may be even more important due to CO_2 excess having a stronger drive on respiration compared to lack of oxygen. However, in practice, CO_2 monitoring is only recommended for hypoventilation quantification, due to the high device costs and difficulties in handling the measurement apparatus. CO_2 recording requires a facial mask (as end-tidal side-stream concentration measurement), and the alternative transcutaneous CO_2 recording requires expensive and sensitive heated electrodes to be placed on the skin.

Sound recording is regarded as part of respiratory signal monitoring when it is used for recording snoring. It usually impresses the patients when their snoring sound recordings are played back to them the next morning during the physician's interview. Sound recording is also useful for the detection of pavor nocturnus, bruxism, and nocturnal talking. The technology for recording snoring sounds differs a lot between PSG devices. The AASM manual requires a simplified recording of sounds similar to EMG signals. This only produces a loudness assessment with no audible sounds due to the low sampling frequency. The reason is that the video monitoring of the sleeping person is usually supplemented by a room microphone; this means that the recording can give a good replay of nocturnal sounds and snoring if needed. A few specific PSG devices provide a full high-quality sound recording similar to a music recording. In every case of using video and sound recording, privacy issues need to be cleared with the patient or volunteer before the night recording. More recent microphone sensors allow us to detect respiratory flow and snoring and to estimate respiratory effort (Glos et al., 2018; Sabil et al., 2019). These sensors can distinguish inspiratory and expiratory sounds with an additional sensor. In addition, they can estimate the intrathoracic pressure if the sensors are placed on the suprasternal notch.

Video monitoring is a common technique used in overnight sleep studies for a number of reasons—mainly to provide context to disturbances or arousals shown in the signals of sleep recordings. If an arousal appears, then the sleep technician can refer to the video to see if the arousal was caused by the patient moving. This is commonly paired with sound in order to provide further context to the disturbance in the signals. Another advantage of using video monitoring in the sleep lab is that it can serve as a live feed to the night staff. In this context, it is possible to see if a patient leaves their bed or behaves in such a way that requires the assistance of the night staff.

For the diagnosis of movement disorders during sleep, placement of EMG electrodes had been defined for limb movement recordings in the early standard of practice papers; these were integrated into the AASM manual. Besides the electrode placement, well-defined scoring criteria had been established to score single and periodic leg movements. The criteria are so well defined that automatic scoring has been developed and can be used for this kind of evaluation reliably. Visual scoring is still needed in order to eliminate artifacts and other reasons for movements such as apnea events. Twitches and bruxism events are also part of movement quantification during sleep.

An actigraphy device on the wrist, a bedside movement sensor, or sensors underneath the mattress are alternative and indirect methods for movement recording. These signals all relate to body movement during sleep but do not reflect the electrical muscle activity as the EMG does. Not only do bedside and mattress sensors pick up major body movements, but they can also detect smaller movements related to respiration or even heartbeat. If a sensor is placed under the mattress, the resulting signal is called a *ballistocardiogram*. This kind of sensor is sometimes used with HSAT and with wearables.

Changes in body position occur frequently during the night, and usually, these changes are associated with an arousal. These can be observed in EEG activity. Over the course of the night, young, healthy subjects tend to experience on average 23 arousals/awakenings associated with body position changes (Basner, 2008). These changes are so short that the sleeping subject does not become aware of the positional change. Recording of body position is clinically important for some disorders, especially sleep-related breathing disorders, as they can modify the number of arousals during the night. For example, if a subject experiences the majority of apnea events when lying supine, this is positional apnea. More precisely, if AHI <5/hour in lateral positions and AHI >5/hour in the supine position, this is positional sleep apnea. Positional apnea may require a different treatment modality and therefore stresses the importance of body position recordings (Omobomi & Quan, 2018).

Sleep apnea has been linked with the risk of developing acute cardiovascular consequences such as myocardial infarction or stroke. For this reason, monitoring and recording vital signs in the sleep laboratory became essential. Cardiac activity measured by the ECG is regarded as the key vital sign to be monitored overnight using a one-channel ECG lead. In addition to measuring cardiac activity, a low heart rate alarm is usually configured in the PSG system to inform the sleep technicians and nurses if they need to take action. The ECG can also be used to track respiratory movement if the electrodes are placed along a heart vector. This specific ECG lead is called *Eindhoven II*, and it is the recommended measurement due to its placement of ECG electrodes. With the use of this single-channel ECG recording, it is possible to detect severe bradycardia, severe tachycardia, and asystolic pauses. However, arrhythmia detection and classification cannot be recorded with a single-channel ECG. Only an estimate of arrhythmia occurrence is possible.

It is well recognized that both sympathetic tone and parasympathetic tone increase with hypoxia and sleep apnea events. There are no direct biosignals to record sympathetic or parasympathetic tone with PSG. However, it is possible to gain related information indirectly. For instance, heart rate is a good mirror of these activities; with a waxing and waning of heart rate it is possible to observe the course of each apnea event. This is called a *cyclical variation of heart rate*. In addition, heart rate changes characteristically with sleep stages, which means heart rate variability can even be used to estimate sleep stages to some extent in a normal healthy person. A large body of sleep research is devoted to heart rate variability during sleep and sleep disorders.

In terms of cardiac consequences, it is of considerable interest to track blood pressure continuously during sleep. However, the traditional method of recording arterial blood pressure values is using sphygmomanometry. This results in an instantaneous systolic, diastolic, and mean blood pressure value, which is not a continuous signal. Alternative systems were developed to create continuous noninvasive blood pressure monitoring such as finger photoplethysmography. These devices can estimate blood pressure from pulse transit time beat to beat. Finger photoplethysmography is a technique that has been around since the 1970s (Imholz et al., 1993). An uncomfortable cuff is placed on the finger, which is inflated to keep the transmural pressure at zero; and with this measurement principle the cuff pressure equals the blood pressure in the finger. If the finger is placed at heart level, then the cuff can produce a precise estimate of blood pressure. However, due to discomfort, this technique is not regularly used. Another method of measuring blood pressure is by calculating pulse transit time (PTT). PTT makes use of the principle that blood pressure is inversely related to blood vessel stiffness. The stiffer a blood vessel, the faster a pressure wave travels from the heart to the periphery. If the time delay of the pressure wave from the heart to the finger is precisely determined, then, together with calibration, it is possible to estimate blood pressure with acceptable accuracy (Gehring et al., 2018).

Circadian sleep research has informed us that body temperature changes are strongly associated with the wake/sleep continuum. Therefore, it is essential to measure body temperature throughout the night. The optimal method to record core body temperature is with a rectal probe. However, this is not comfortable; and therefore, other means have been developed such as skin temperature. Detailed research has shown that skin temperature is regulated in a different manner compared to core body temperature (Van Someren, 2006). Core body and skin body temperature work together in the regulation of temperature, so it makes sense to record both, in order to better understand the physiological mechanisms of sleep regulation. Unfortunately, the corresponding recording devices are expensive, and the clinical consequences are not linked to sleep disorder diagnostic requirements. Due to this, the recording of body temperature has not become mandatory for PSG. The recording of body temperature remains limited to specific clinical studies for the detection of sleep–wake rhythm disorders or research studies that investigate modifications of sleep environment, such as room conditions and mattresses, or overall sleep quality and sleep regulation.

The following measurements are rarely used and are optional:

Electrodermal activity (EDA) measures skin impedance and sweating. These signals reflect sympathetic and parasympathetic activities. The sympathetic and parasympathetic tone changes with sleep stages and with sleep disorders. Therefore, related biosignals are a subject of continuous investigation. So far, there are no standardized reliable sensors and recording equipment for EDA technology, which means this parameter has not become a standard for PSG recordings.

Esophageal and gastric pH recordings are used to study gastroesophageal reflux during sleep. Reflux events disturb sleep, and affected patients wake up right after a reflux event. During sleep, the clearance of reflux in the esophagus lasts double the duration compared to daytime reflux. This is due to the body position and the reduced muscle activity during sleep. Recording pH dropping events can be objectively quantified by measuring the clearance and possible treatment effects.

Additional EEG leads are recommended for patients with the suspicion of epileptic seizures and other neurological disorders during sleep. Specifically, patients with hypersomnia and parasomnias tend to receive additional EEG leads according to the 10–20 system for electrode placement in order to check for focal and unusual brain activations (American Electroencephalographic Society, 1991). Neurophysiological EEG interpretation skills are required to score and interpret a full EEG recording under these circumstances.

Ambulatory Techniques

HST

HST is the general term for any device that allows one to record sleep at home. The Scandinavian countries use home PSG a lot. Home PSG, also denoted as *unattended* PSG, follows the same requirements in terms of sensor and scoring rules as PSG, described above. The difference is that the sleeping room is not controlled, and neither are the conditions; and there is no possibility for intervention. This means that if a sensor or electrode falls off, then this cannot be fixed during the night. Therefore, the setup of a home PSG requires skilled technical expertise to apply the device either at the home of the person or at a sleep center. In the case of receiving the device at the sleep center, the subject is sent home with all sensors attached. HST also includes devices with fewer or simplified EEG leads. The main purpose of these devices is to quantify and objectify insomnia and hypersomnia complaints. Sensor development on these simplified devices has reached the point where EEG, EOG, and EMG sensors are now self-applicable. Some devices use a frontal EEG application and then try to decompose the mixed signal from the forehead into EEG, EOG, and EMG components (Ehlert et al., 1998; Fietze et al., 2015). Others try a grid of flexible printed electrodes around the ear for EEG recording (Da Silva Souto et al., 2021). HST is still under development and adapts to new physiological knowledge and new sensor technologies. All these devices are certified as medical devices and are used for clinical purposes by sleep physicians and sleep experts. Moving sleep studies from the lab to the home will increase the ecological validity of the output. The patient will be in their natural bedroom environment with fewer disturbing electrodes, which ultimately allows the possibility of gathering more naturalistic sleep data.

HSAT

One of the most common sleep problems is sleep disordered breathing. The class of HST device used for the specific purpose of diagnosing sleep disordered breathing is the HSAT. This is a subset of home PSG due to its needing fewer sensors. Since no EEG, EOG, or EMG is needed, sensors can be applied at home by the patient or a spouse just before going to bed. The use of HSAT is increasing every day in comparison to in-lab PSG recordings, specifically for the diagnosis of sleep disordered breathing (Hirshkowitz, 2016). An alternative term is *out of center recording* or *polygraphy* (Collop et al., 2011). The configuration of these devices is built on the knowledge obtained from PSG recordings, as explained above.

For sleep disordered breathing diagnosis, six diagnostic criteria are needed: sleep or wake, respiratory effort, respiratory flow, oxygen saturation, pulse or heart rate, and body position (Shokoueinejad et al., 2017). These six sensors are the universally agreed minimum set of sensors and signals for HSAT (Qaseem et al., 2014). For sleep or wake, a detailed sleep stage scoring is not required. Indeed, it would be preferable to know whether a patient is in light sleep, deep sleep, or REM sleep. However, for diagnostic purposes and for initiating therapy, this has no relevance. Positional sleep apnea can be identified using HSAT devices, while RERA events cannot be identified due to the lack of EEG sensors. Without these sensors, it is impossible to reliably identify arousal events. Sensor technologies and scoring options are summarized in Table 25.1. Some HSAT devices offer some flexibility in terms of sensor configuration. There are devices that can record snoring and speech during sleep in high quality, like MP3 music recording. Other HSAT devices have the option to record limb movements. This is very useful to distinguish between sleep apnea–related movements and pure limb movement activities. Another type of HSAT device exploits the ECG and pulse wave analysis for PTT to estimate blood pressure continuously. Some devices rely on indirect measurement of respiratory flow and effort by a sophisticated analysis of other signals. A popular example is peripheral arterial tonometry, which derives much information (apnea, hypopnea, oxygen saturation, pulse rate, non-REM and REM sleep) from a patented finger sensor. This creates a pretreated pulse wave signal for further analysis (Schnall et al., 2022).

In Scandinavia, a different device has been developed and used for many decades to monitor sleep disordered breathing. The technology is known as the *ballistocardiogram*. The ballistocardiogram is a contactless technology that uses a sensor pad below the bed linen. The sensor pad typically contains one or multiple sensors that can pick up the movements of the body when sleeping. Large movements reflect position changes and are typical of wakefulness. Respiration and the heartbeat also cause movements at a much lower amplitude. A much more sensitive sensor pad is required to detect these. A higher number of sensors inside the pad may help to better distinguish coarse movements, respiratory movements, and heartbeat-related movements. A few to mention are foils and stripes. These have been developed to be placed in the bed, and they can differ in size from small (pillow size) to large (full bed size). Recent technological developments have converted the concept of the ballistocardiogram into an even more comfortable sensor device. For instance, radar wave technology placed next to the bed can also record body movements (Alizadeh et al., 2019). These signals can be split into the components of coarse movements, respiratory movements, and heartbeat-related movements. Several companies have released their own HSAT devices, which mainly differ in terms of algorithms and user interface. Nevertheless, all of these devices need to be validated against PSG in order to be certified as medical devices according to Food and Drug Administration or Medical Device Reporting regulations.

Emerging Technologies: Wearables and Sleep Apps

Sleep recording technologies like PSG and HST are becoming smaller, smarter, less power-consuming, more digital, and more precise (Khosla et al., 2018). These improvements all benefit the medical diagnosis of sleep disorders (Behar et al., 2013). The ballistocardiogram is a master example of sensor technology becoming more portable and comfortable for the user (Zhao et al., 2021). In some cases, consumer technology can outperform medical devices and offer more options. For instance, smartphones can serve not only as video streaming or gaming devices but also as health tools. Counting steps and observing sleep were among the first applications in the "quantify yourself" domain. Sensors such as audio recording and exploiting the built-in three-axis accelerometers were the sensor basis for quantifying sleep with a simple smartphone. The first sleep apps recorded movement when placed under a pillow and provided the user with a curve about deep sleep, light sleep, and wake times (Behar et al., 2013).

Besides movement and the more comprehensive ballistocardiogram, the other popular set of signals used in wearables are derived from pulse waves. These signals are easily recorded on the wrist or on a finger with optical technology. Pulse rate and heart rate give the same result if there are no cardiac arrhythmias. The optical signal recording can give even more than just pulse rate. Smartwatches and finger rings with integrated pulse recording can calculate oxygen saturation if light-emitting diodes with appropriate wavelengths are used (Zhao et al., 2022).

The combination of recording pulse waves with movement can be very useful. These are common functions of smartwatches and finger rings to track sleep. According to Table 25.1, these smartwatches can estimate total sleep time, sleep stage, and sleep apnea.

The quality of the estimation depends on the quality of the software, whether appropriate expertise was consulted, and whether validation studies against PSG have been performed. Unfortunately, these performance details are not transparent, either to the consumers, users, medical staff, or the scientific community. Another severe limitation of the new emerging devices is that the recorded data is usually not available to the user but remains in a proprietary cloud. Only congregated data is given to the user. This restricts access to the raw data, which makes it impossible to check for artifacts and to edit results if the device was taken off for a period of time (De Zambotti et al., 2019).

Conclusions

PSG is both a historic and up-to-date reference tool to study sleep and related disorders. During recent decades, the role of PSG in clinical work and in the field of sleep medicine has changed substantially. With this increased recognition, PSG and sleep centers have spread all over the world and are used frequently for clinical diagnosis. As time has gone on, knowledge in the field has increased and so have technical innovations so that now it is possible clinically to diagnose disorders with much simpler and more focused systems, like HST or HSAT (Zancanella et al., 2022). As a result, PSG is not always needed. These advancements have led sleep medicine down the path of becoming more efficient.

Future Directions

Consumer technology has advanced the public knowledge of sleep. It has taught the public how to take care of their sleep, similar to how the public has learned how to take care of their nutritional diets. However, in the case of sleep, all clinical measurements of sleep will need to continue to be backed up by precise physiology-based technology. This means new emerging wearable devices that measure sleep must be validated against PSG before they can be considered to be used in clinical populations.

References

Alizadeh, M., Shaker, G., De Almeida, J. C. M., Morita, P. P., & Safavi-Naeini, S. (2019). Remote monitoring of human vital signs using mm-wave FMCW radar. *IEEE Access*, *7*, 54958–54968.

American Electroencephalographic Society. (1991). American Electroencephalographic Society guidelines for standard electrode position nomenclature. *Journal of Clinical Neurophysiology*, *8*(2), 200–202.

Basner, M. (2008). Nocturnal aircraft noise exposure increases objectively assessed daytime sleepiness. *Somnologie*, *12*, 110–117. https://doi.org/10.1007/s11818-008-0338-8

Behar, J., Roebuck, A., Domingos, J. S., Gederi, E., & Clifford, G. D. (2013). A review of current sleep screening applications for smartphones. *Physiological Measurement*, *34*, R29–R46. https://doi.org/10.1088/0967-3334/34/7/R29

Bidgood, W. D., Jr., & Horii, S. C. (1992). Introduction to the ACR-NEMA DICOM standard. *Radiographics*, *12*, 345–355.

Carskadon, M. A. (1986). Guidelines for the Multiple Sleep Latency Test (MSLT): A standard measure of sleepiness. *Sleep*, *9*(4), 519–524.

Collop, N. A., Tracy, S. L., Kapur, V., Mehra, R., Kuhlmann, D., Fleishman, S. A., & Ojile, J. M. (2011). Obstructive sleep apnea devices for out-of-center (OOC) testing: Technology evaluation. *Journal of Clinical Sleep Medicine*, *7*(5), 531–548.

Da Silva Souto, C. F., Pätzold, W., Wolf, K. I., Paul, M., Matthiesen, I., Bleichner, M. G., & Debener, S. (2021). Flex-printed ear-EEG sensors for adequate sleep staging at home. *Frontiers in Digital Health, 3*, Article 688122 https://doi.org/10.3389/fdgth.2021.688122

De Zambotti, M., Cellini, N., Goldstone, A., Colrain, I. M., & Baker, F. C. (2019). Wearable sleep technology in clinical and research settings. *Medicine and Science in Sports and Exercise, 51*(7), 1538–1557.

Ehlert, I., Danker-Hopfe, H., Höller, L., von Rickenbach, P., Baumgart-Schmitt, R., & Herrmann, W. M. (1998). A comparison between EEG-recording and scoring by QUISI version 1.0 and standard PSG with visual scoring. *Somnologie, 2*, 104–116.

Fietze, I., Penzel, T., Partinen, M., Sauter, J., Küchler, G., Suvoro, A., & Hein, H. (2015). Actigraphy combined with EEG compared to polysomnography in sleep apnea patients. *Physiological Measurement, 36*, 385–396. https://doi.org/10.1088/0967-3334/36/3/385

Fietze, I., Quispe-Bravo, S., Schiller, W., Röttig, J., Penzel, T., Baumann, G., & Witt, C. (1999). Respiratory arousals in mild obstructive sleep apnea syndrome. *Sleep, 22*(5), 583–589. https://doi.org/10.1093/sleep/22.5.583

Gehring, J., Gesche, H., Drewniok, G., Küchler, G., & Patzak, A. (2018). Nocturnal blood pressure fluctuations measured by using pulse transit time in patients with severe obstructive sleep apnea syndrome. *Sleep and Breathing, 22*, 337–343. https://doi.org/10.1007/s11325-017-1555-9

Glos, M., Sabil, A., Jelavic, K. S., Schöbel, C., Fietze, I., & Penzel, T. (2018). Characterization of respiratory events in obstructive sleep apnea using suprasternal pressure monitoring. *Journal of Clinical Sleep Medicine, 14*, 359–369.

Halford, J. J., Clunie, D. A., Brinkmann, B. H., Krefting, D., Rémi, J., Rosenow, F., Husain, A., Fürbass, F., Ehrenberg, J. A., & Winkler, S. (2021). Standardization of neurophysiology signal data into the DICOM® standard. *Clinical Neurophysiology, 132*(4), 993–997. https://doi.org/10.1016/j.clinph.2021.01.019

Hirshkowitz, M. (2016). Polysomnography challenges. *Sleep Medicine Clinics, 11*, 403–411. https://doi.org/10.1016/j.jsmc.2016.07.002

Iber, C., Ancoli-Israel, S., Chesson, A., & Quan, S. F.; for the American Academy of Sleep Medicine. (2007). *The AASM manual for the scoring of sleep and associated events: Rules. Terminology and Technical Specifications.* American Academy of Sleep Medicine.

Imholz, B. P. M., Langewouters, G. J., van Montfrans, G. A., Parati, G., van Goudoever, J., Wesseling, K. H., Wieling, W., & Mancia, G. (1993). Feasibility of ambulatory, continuous 24-hour finger arterial pressure recording. *Hypertension, 21*, 65–73.

Kemp, B., & Olivan, J. (2003). European data format "plus" (EDF+), an EDF alike standard format for the exchange of physiological data. *Clinical Neurophysiology, 114*(9), 1755–1761.

Kemp, B., Värri, A., Rosa, A. C., Nielsen, K. D., & Gade, J. (1992). A simple format for exchange of digitized polygraphic recordings. *Electroencephalography and Clinical Neurophysiology, 82*(5), 391–393.

Khosla, S., Deak, M. C., Gault, D., Goldstein, C. A., Hwang, D., Kwon, Y., O'Hearn, D., Schutte-Rodin, S., Yurcheshen, M., Rosen, I. M., & Kirsch, D. B. (2018). Consumer sleep technology: An American Academy of Sleep Medicine position statement. *Journal of Clinical Sleep Medicine, 14*(5), 877–880.

Kushida, C. A., Littner, M. R., Morgenthaler, T., Alessi, C. A., Bailey, D., Coleman, J., Jr., Friedman, L., Hirshkowitz, M., Kapen, S., Kramer, M., Lee-Chiong, T., Loube, D. L., Owens, J., Pancer, J. P., & Wise, M. (2005). Practice parameters for the indications for polysomnography and related procedures: An update for 2005. *Sleep, 28*(4), 499–523.

Littner, M. R., Kushida, C., Wise, G., Davila, D., Morgenthaler, T., Lee-Chiong, T., Hirshkowitz, M., Loube, D. L., Bailey, D., Berry, R. B., Kapen, S., & Kramer, M.; Standards of Practice Committee of the American Academy of Sleep Medicine. (2005). Practice parameters for clinical use of the multiple sleep latency test and the maintenance of wakefulness test. *Sleep, 28*(1), 113–121.

Ma, J. R., Huang, J. J., Chen, Q., Wu, H. T., Xiao, K. L., & Zhang, Y. T. (2018). Value of pulse oximetry watch for diagnosing pediatric obstructive sleep apnea/hypopnea syndrome. *Acta Oto-Laryngologica, 138*(2), 175–179.

Miller, D. J., Sargent, C., & Roach, G. D. (2022). A validation of six wearable devices for estimating sleep, heart rate and heart rate variability in healthy adults. *Sensors, 22*(16), Article 6317.

Omobomi, O., & Quan, S. F. (2018). Positional therapy in the management of positional obstructive sleep apnea—A review of the current literature. *Sleep and Breathing, 22*, 297–304. https://doi.org/10.1007/s11325-017-1561-y

Penzel, T. (2022). Sleep scoring moving from visual scoring towards automated scoring. *Sleep*, *45*, Article zsac190. https://doi.org/10.1093/sleep/zsac190

Qaseem, A., Dallas, P., Owens, D. K., Starkey, M., Holty, J. E., & Shekelle, P.; Clinical Guidelines Committee of the American College of Physicians. (2014). Diagnosis of obstructive sleep apnea in adults: A clinical practice guideline from the American College of Physicians. *Annals of Internal Medicine*, *161*(3), 210–220. https://doi.org/10.7326/M12-3187

Rechtschaffen, A., & Kales, A. (1968). *A manual of standardized terminology, techniques and scoring system for sleep stages of human subjects*. UCLA Brain Information Service/Brain Research Institute.

Sabil, A., Glos, M., Günther, A., Schöbel, C., Veauthier, C., Fietze, I., & Penzel, T. (2019). Comparison of apnea detection using oronasal thermal airflow sensor, nasal pressure transducer, respiratory inductance plethysmography and tracheal sound sensor. *Journal of Clinical Sleep Medicine*, *15*, 285–292.

Schnall, R. P., Sheffy, J., & Penzel, T. (2022). Peripheral arterial tonometry—PAT technology. *Sleep Medicine Reviews*, *61*, Article 101566. https://doi.org/10.1016/j.smrv.2021.101566

Shokoueinejad, M., Fernandez, C., Carroll, E., Wang, F., Levin, J., Rusk, S., Glattard, N., Mulchrone, A., Zhang, X., Xie, A., Teodorescu, M., Dempsey, J., & Webster, J. (2017). Sleep apnea: A review of diagnostic sensors, algorithms, and therapies. *Physiological Measurement*, *38*, R204–R252.

Troester, M. M., Quan, S. F., Berry, R. B., Plante, D.T., Abreu, A. R., Alzoubaidi, M., Bandyopadhyay, A., DelRosso, L., Ebben, M., Kwon, Y., Mao., M. M., Munir, S. S., Pressman, M. R., Rodriguez, A. J., Ryals, S., So, J. Y., Vaughn, B., & Thomas, S. M.; for the American Academy of Sleep Medicine. (2023). *The AASM manual for the scoring of sleep and associated events: Rules, terminology and technical specifications* (Version 3). American Academy of Sleep Medicine.

Van Someren, E. J. W. (2006). Mechanisms and functions of coupling between sleep and temperature rhythms. *Progress in Brain Research*, *153*, 309–324.

Zancanella, E., do Prado, L. F., de Carvalho, L. B., Machado Júnior, A. J., Crespo, A. N., & do Prado, G. F. (2022). Home sleep apnea testing: An accuracy study. *Sleep and Breathing*, *26*(1), 117–123.

Zhao, R., Xue, J., Dong, X. S., Zhi, H., Chen, J., Zhao, L., Zhang, X., Li, J., Penzel, T., & Han, F. (2021). Screening for obstructive sleep apnea using a contact-free system compared with polysomnography. *Journal of Clinical Sleep Medicine*, *17*(5), 1075–1082. https://doi.org/10.5664/jcsm.9138

Zhao, R., Xue, J., Zhang, X., Peng, M., Li, J., Zhou, B., Zhao, L., Penzel, T., Kryger, M., Dong, X. S., Gao, Z., & Han, F. (2022). Comparison of ring pulse oximetry using reflective photoplethysmography and PSG in the detection of OSA in Chinese adults: A pilot study. *Nature and Science of Sleep*, *14*, 1427–1436. https://doi.org/10.2147/NSS.S367400

SECTION 5

Disorders of Sleep and Circadian Function: Management and Treatment

CHAPTER

26 Insomnia I: Conceptualization and Etiology

Hannah Scott, Philip Gehrman, *and* Michael Perlis

Abstract

The present chapter reviews the past and current theoretical conceptualizations of insomnia. As straightforward as it may seem, the definition of insomnia is complex and has evolved considerably over time. Several attempts have been made to refine the definition in terms of descriptive and diagnostic types and subtypes of insomnia. Alongside this pursuit, there have been advancements in understanding insomnia etiology and pathophysiology, resulting in 15 major human models of insomnia. The present chapter reviews (1) the definition of insomnia, (2) the major theoretical perspectives regarding the etiology and pathophysiology of insomnia, (3) the current evidence and implications of each perspective, and (4) promising directions for future research to better understand insomnia pathophysiology and its successful treatment.

Key Words: insomnia, diagnostic criterion, model, cognitive, behavioral, neuropsychological

Introduction

Decades of research have been dedicated toward explaining how the universal experience of a "bad night's sleep" can evolve into a self-perpetuating clinical sleep disorder. As the prominent characteristics of insomnia are becoming increasingly understood, the diagnostic criteria have also become more refined. Several prominent etiological theories have also emerged which focus on one or more of the proposed behavioral, cognitive, neurophysiological, biological, and social determinants of insomnia. The prior edition of this chapter discussed nine such models. These models included the hyperarousal model and traditional behavioral and cognitive models, which have dominated the theoretical perspectives on insomnia for decades. Since the prior edition, multiple complementary and integrated models have emerged: the metacognitive model, the neurobiological model, the REM sleep instability model, and the fully integrated parallel process model. Evidence that supports or challenges these models has also continued to accrue at a rapid rate. The present chapter provides a timely review of (1) past and current definitions for insomnia, (2) past and current theoretical perspectives on the etiology of insomnia, and (3) the state of evidence for and implications of each theoretical perspective. These efforts are made toward outlining critical directions for future research to further our understanding about the development, maintenance, and successful treatment of insomnia.

Conceptualization of Insomnia

Contrary to the colloquial use of the term *insomnia* by the general population, insomnia in the clinical sense does not simply mean "a bad night's sleep." There are two manuals that outline diagnostic criteria for insomnia: the *Diagnostic and Statistical Manual of Mental Disorders*, fifth edition, and the *International Classification of Sleep Disorders*, third edition (ICSD-3; American Academy of Sleep Medicine, 2014; American Psychiatric Association, 2013). The overarching criteria are consistent across both manuals. To meet a diagnosis for insomnia disorder, the patient must report difficulties initiating or maintaining sleep, that these occur despite adequate sleep opportunity, and that daytime impairments accompany these difficulties. Typically, patients report fatigue, difficulties with attention and memory, irritability, anxiety about sleep, and reduced quality of life (Buysse et al., 2007; Riedel & Lichstein, 2000). The sleep difficulties and daytime symptoms must be present at least three times per week for at least three months. See Chapter 27 for in-depth discussion about the diagnosis and assessment of insomnia.

The current diagnostic criteria differ from past definitions in three major ways. First, there is no longer a differentiation between primary insomnia and secondary insomnia. *Primary insomnia* was the term used when an individual had disturbed sleep but otherwise was free of other medical or psychiatric disorders that could be negatively impacting sleep. The presence of these comorbidities led to the use of the term *secondary insomnia*, which presumed that the insomnia was the result of the concurrent conditions and would be unresponsive to targeted insomnia treatment. This distinction is no longer made, owing to a large series of studies showing that secondary insomnia was responsive to targeted treatment and to a degree that was often the same as observed with primary insomnia (Currie et al., 2000; Edinger et al., 1996; Lichstein et al., 2000; McCrae & Lichstein, 2001; Quesnel et al., 2003; Stepanski & Rybarczyk, 2006). More, when insomnia is comorbid with other health conditions, its resolution can often help treat the comorbidity, as is the case with many psychiatric disorders (Cheng et al., 2019; Hertenstein et al., 2022; Leerssen et al., 2022; Mason et al., 2022). Further, delineating between primary and secondary insomnia is often an impossible exercise. Second, "non-restorative sleep," in the absence of sleep continuity difficulties, is no longer considered a form of insomnia. Third, the ICSD-3 provides a quantitative threshold for frequency of sleep difficulties (must occur at least three times per week) and has modified the chronicity threshold from 1 month to 3 months.

When operationalizing the diagnostic criteria to assess for insomnia, there are notable complexities to the criteria that warrant mentioning here. While there are quantitative thresholds for the frequency and chronicity of insomnia symptoms, there is no consensus for a sleep difficulty threshold (i.e., degree of "difficulty" initiating or maintaining or waking too early from sleep). In research contexts, a duration-based threshold of ≥30 minutes for sleep latency, wake after sleep onset, and early morning awakenings is often applied for methodological and data interpretation purposes (Edinger et al., 2004; Roth & Drake, 2006), but this is not necessarily the case in clinical practice. Moreover, there is no criterion with respect to sleep duration, although patients with insomnia in clinical practice often report shorter than average sleep (Perlis et al., 2000; Sweetman et al., 2020; van de Laar et al., 2015). Additionally, aside from general agreement about the typical daytime impairments that occur with insomnia (e.g., fatigue, irritability, difficulties concentrating), there is no consensus about instruments or thresholds for assessing impairment. Consensus is needed on the operationalization of the criteria for insomnia.

Subtyping Insomnia

Beyond the general diagnostic criteria, there have been several attempts to further classify this heterogenous sleep disorder into subtypes. Such distinctions are typically based on the type of sleep difficulty (presenting complaint), phenotypic traits (clinical profile), or chronicity of symptoms.

By Type of Sleeping Difficulty

Historically, the first edition of the ICSD included subtypes for *initial* (difficulties initiating sleep at the beginning of the sleep period), *middle* (difficulties maintaining sleep during the sleep period), and *late insomnia* (waking earlier than desired). With these distinctions, it follows that each of these subtypes may occur due to different mechanistic factors and may thus require different treatment regimens for maximal therapeutic effects. While these subtypes are reliably reported by patients, they appear to be temporally unstable. Hohagen et al. (1994) found that 50% of patients with insomnia reported a change in sleeping difficulty pattern during a 4-month interval. Pillai et al. (2015), in a longitudinal study ($N = 954$), showed that sleep initiation and maintenance complaints tend to be unstable over the course of 1 year in up to 40% of patients. In addition to such fundings, multiple studies have found that the incidence of, or type of, insomnia varies greatly from night to night (Bei et al., 2016; Buysse et al., 2010; Perlis et al., 2010; Vallières et al., 2005). It may be the case that type of insomnia, when it changes, is of clinical relevance to the extent that it signals a change in biopsychosocial milieu in which the insomnia occurs. Such changes may yet have relevance for treatment.

By Clinical Presentation (Phenotype)

The ICSD-3 describes three phenotypes of insomnia: psychophysiological insomnia, paradoxical insomnia, and idiopathic insomnia. These phenotypes are used as descriptors of this insomnia but do not bear on diagnosis.

Psychophysiological insomnia is characterized by heightened cortical and somatic arousal when attempting sleep, a physiological response that perpetuates the sleeping difficulties (Perlis et al., 1997). These patients can sleep markedly better in other settings (i.e., *reverse first night effect*; Hauri & Olmstead, 1989; Riedel et al., 2001). It is theorized that these patients may have conditioned insomnia, a phenomenon that will be discussed further below with respect to the four-factor model of insomnia.

Paradoxical insomnia is characterized by large differences between self-reported and objectively assessed sleep (Castelnovo et al., 2019). A key feature of the diagnostic criteria for insomnia disorder is that the sleeping difficulties are based on self-report: There is no criterion for objectively assessed sleeping difficulties (e.g., via polysomnography [PSG] recording). This said, large differences between self-reported and objectively assessed sleeping difficulties may suggest an altered sleep/wake arousal system. There are multiple proposed causes for this phenomenon, but a prevailing finding is that patients with this subtype may have greater arousal during sleep—when assessed via more precise neuroimaging or electroencephalographic (EEG) spectral analysis techniques than traditional sleep scoring—compared to patients without this subtype (Andrillon et al., 2019; Li et al., 2022).

Idiopathic insomnia is characterized by the early onset of sleeping difficulties, typically in infancy or early childhood (Espie et al., 2012). Such sleeping difficulties are often stable and unremitting over the patient's life span. Genetic or congenital factors may predispose the patient to develop this insomnia subtype, which may alter the sleep and/or arousal systems, although no such biomarkers have been found.

In recent years, a fourth phenotype has been proposed: *insomnia with objectively estimated short sleep duration* (≤6 hours as defined typically from a single night of PSG data; Vgontzas et al., 2013). There is some evidence suggesting that such individuals have poorer daytime function (Fernandez-Mendoza et al., 2010; Fernandez-Mendoza et al., 2020) and/or have more significant medical and psychiatric comorbidity than patients with insomnia without objectively estimated short sleep duration (Fernandez-Mendoza et al., 2012; Vgontzas et al., 2009, 2010). Not all studies, however, show this form of insomnia to be more consequential (Fernandez-Mendoza et al., 2012; Lovato et al., 2021; Vgontzas et al., 2009, 2010). Since this subtype has been typically defined from the first night of PSG data, this effect may be a proxy measure for those patients who have more severe insomnia on more nights per week. Alternatively, this effect may be a reliable index that the patient is not meeting their sleep need.

There are many questions remaining with respect to these phenotypes for insomnia. More specifically, there are no standard assessment criteria for each phenotype, potentially leading to the inconsistencies seen across research studies. The specificity of each phenotype between individuals is also unclear: In practice, patients tend to exhibit a degree of multiple types (psychophysiological with some degree of paradoxical insomnia), so the categories may not be discrete. More stable, discrete phenotypes may be found in affect and personality traits (Blanken et al., 2019). As phenotyping efforts continue, it remains to be shown that treatment outcome varies by one or more of the insomnia phenotypes. This evidence is needed to justify the use of subtyping insomnia by clinical presentation for clinical practice.

By Chronicity

In a sense, the subtyping of insomnia could involve consideration of the stages from good sleep to chronic insomnia. In the case of *acute insomnia* (termed *short-term insomnia* in the ICSD-3), the insomnia symptoms are present for less than the 3-month threshold required to diagnose *chronic insomnia* but are still severe and stressful to the patient. If these symptoms persist beyond 3 months, then chronic insomnia can be diagnosed. Therefore, acute insomnia is conceptualized as a transitional stage between good/"normal" sleep and clinically significant chronic insomnia, potentially with its own underlying pathology. Multiple etiological models of insomnia have theorized about the defining features of acute versus chronic insomnia and how the transition from acute to chronic may or may not occur, as will be discussed below.

Summary

While experiencing insomnia symptoms on occasion is universal, insomnia as a clinical disorder severely affects the patient's daytime functioning and quality of life over a prolonged period, sometimes decades. There is good evidence that persistent insomnia exists as a risk factor for new-onset medical and/or psychiatric disorders (de Almondes et al., 2016; Neckelmann et al., 2007; Taylor et al., 2003) and may serve to exacerbate others (Bubu et al., 2017; Pigeon et al., 2008). Thus, the prevalence and consequences of insomnia strongly suggest that it should not go undiagnosed and untreated. This said, there are notable complications in conceptualizing and assessing the disorder, including in defining sleep "difficulties" and operationalizing daytime impairment. Multiple subtypes of insomnia have been proposed, though there is little evidence to date that this is relevant for treatment choice or outcome. Additional research is required to better define and assess insomnia subtypes and to elucidate their potential utility for clinical practice. What is apparent, however, is that insomnia is a heterogeneous, complex disorder, with multiple potential pathways from which it can emerge and perpetuate.

Etiology of Insomnia

In this section, we review several of the major etiologic models of insomnia (also summarized in Table 26.1) that continue to have a lasting effect on the assessment and treatment of insomnia. It is important to note that there are several models of insomnia not described here, particularly emerging models for which research is ongoing. Additionally, there are several animal models of insomnia with important implications for the biological

Table 26.1 Overview of the theoretical models of insomnia

Models	Key points	References
Hyperarousal models		
Earliest perspectives	- Insomnia results from increased physiological arousal.	(Monroe, 1967; Riemann et al., 2010)
Caffeine model	- Caffeine-induced arousal as an arousal model of insomnia.	(Bonnet & Arand, 1992)
Behavioral models		
Stimulus control model	- Insomnia results from stimulus dys-control.	(Bootzin, 1972)
Three-factor model	- Transition from good sleep to chronic insomnia via the influence of predisposing, precipitating, and perpetuating factors.	(Spielman et al., 1987)
Four-factor model extension	- Chronic insomnia persists due to conditioned arousal.	(Perlis et al., 2005)
Cognitive models		
Earliest perspectives	- The worry and rumination cycle underlies insomnia.	(Morin, 1993)
Cognitive model	- Selective attention, distorted perception of daytime impairments, and safety behaviors are primary mediators for insomnia.	(A. G. Harvey, 2002a)
Sleep interfering–interpreting process model	- Delineates processes which interfere with sleep and processes which predispose the individual to distorted perceptions about sleep.	(Lundh & Broman, 2000)
Metacognitive model	- Emphasizes the role of metacognitions in the maintenance of insomnia.	(Ong et al., 2012)
Microanalytic model	- Outlines three levels of arousal: cognitive, emotional, and physiological.	(Morin, 1993)
Neuropsychological models		
Neurocognitive model	- Cortical arousal central to insomnia. - Relevance of sensory and information processing during and around NREM sleep.	(Perlis et al., 1997; Perlis, Merica, et al., 2001)
Psychobiological inhibition model	- Inability to inhibit wakefulness, rather than hyperarousal underlies insomnia. - Emphasizes the attention–intention–effort pathway.	(Espie, 2002; Espie et al., 2006)
Neurobiological model	- Insomnia as a sleep–wake regulation disorder, characterized by wake-like activity during sleep.	(Buysse et al., 2011)
REM sleep instability model	- Instability of REM sleep as a major contributor to insomnia.	(Riemann et al., 2012)
Parallel process model	- Integrates the above perspectives into one conceptual framework.	(Perlis et al., 2005)

Note. NREM = non-rapid-eye-movement; REM = rapid-eye-movement.

underpinnings of insomnia (Belfer et al., 2021; Cano et al., 2008; Seugnet et al., 2009), which are not discussed here.

Hyperarousal Model

DESCRIPTION

One of the earliest and most prominent theoretical perspectives on the etiology and pathophysiology of insomnia is the hyperarousal model (Monroe, 1967; Riemann et al., 2010). Hyperarousal is a broad construct and has been defined in various ways, from a generalized trait to a momentary phenomenon experienced when attempting sleep. At the core of the hyperarousal model is the concept that the patient experiences an elevated level of physiological arousal that is incompatible with sleep, resulting in the observed sleep continuity difficulties. This fundamental principle has provided a robust framework for the development of several etiological theories of insomnia, which theorize how hyperarousal develops and maintains insomnia over time.

One experimental model of hyperarousal, referred to as the *caffeine model of insomnia*, uses repeated dosing with caffeine to mimic the physiological arousal that is presumed to be characteristic of insomnia. In addition to elevated somatic arousal, this model may exert its effects by modulating adenosine levels in ways which alter sleep–wake homeostasis. Accordingly, the model has high face validity. In the first evaluation of this model (Bonnet & Arand, 1992), 400 mg of caffeine was provided to good sleeper subjects three times daily for 7 days. Caffeine administration increased whole-body metabolic rate, reduced total sleep time and sleep efficiency, and increased sleep latency, wake after sleep onset, and diurnal sleep ability (i.e., daytime sleepiness) as measured by the Multiple Sleep Latency Test. In contrast to patients with insomnia, these subjects did not complain of daytime fatigue. Further, the effects on metabolism and sleep continuity were reduced by the end of the week. Together, these findings suggested that caffeine-induced hyperarousal may simulate acute but not chronic insomnia, potentially due to caffeine tolerance. Such findings may suggest that sustained hyperarousal over prolonged periods (years in the case of chronic insomnia) may not be possible and/or that dietary use of caffeine and/or adenosine modulation may not be the mechanism by which insomnia is perpetuated over time.

STATE OF THE EVIDENCE

Many investigations have sought to identify a biomarker of physiological arousal (Bonnet & Arand, 2010). This has included the use of basic psychophysiological measures (e.g., EEG), whole-body metabolic rate, heart rate variability, neuroendocrine measures, and functional neuroimaging. Broadly speaking, there is reliable evidence that patients with insomnia exhibit elevated levels of somatic arousal. While stress is a well-known trigger for insomnia, research into physiological stress (i.e., cortisol) as a marker of insomnia has produced varied findings (Chen et al., 2017; Dodds et al., 2017; Mikoteit et al., 2017;

Riemann et al., 2002; Xia et al., 2013). There is also evidence against the notion that patients with insomnia have a generally heightened state of arousal versus good sleepers (i.e., hyperarousal as a trait-like phenomenon). Further, an important assumption of the hyperarousal model is that physiological arousal and sleep are mutually exclusive: One cannot be asleep and have elevated arousal. There is a growing body of evidence that refutes this assumption (Kay & Buysse, 2017). This said, the phenomenon of interest may be related to heightened arousal when attempting sleep and/or an inability to downregulate neurophysiological activity (Riemann et al., 2010).

IMPLICATIONS FOR RESEARCH AND PRACTICE

Even after >50 years of research, many important questions about hyperarousal remained unanswered. There is a need for formal evaluations regarding (1) how hyperarousal develops, (2) reliable markers of hyperarousal for the assessment and treatment of insomnia, and (3) the minimum magnitude of hyperarousal required to disrupt sleep continuity. In practice, a reliable biomarker of hyperarousal could lead to a point-of-care test that could be implemented as part of routine care. Such a test has already been trialed in insomnia (Chen et al., 2017). Given that almost 40% of patients do not fully remit after cognitive behavioral therapy for insomnia (CBT-I; Miller et al., 2014; Okajima et al., 2011; Trauer et al., 2015), a hyperarousal test that could predict treatment responsiveness warrants investigation.

Behavioral Models

All behavioral models of insomnia share a common proposition: that behaviors, often made to recover from poor sleep, underlie the persistence (perpetuation) of sleep continuity disturbance.

STIMULUS CONTROL MODEL

Description

Originally described by Bootzin (1972), stimulus control is based on the instrumental conditioning perspective that one stimulus may elicit a variety of responses, depending on the conditioning history. When a stimulus is always paired with a single behavior (a simple conditioning history), there is a high probability that the stimulus will yield only one response. When a stimulus is paired with a variety of behaviors (a complex conditioning history), there is a low probability that the stimulus will yield only one response. In patients with insomnia, the stimuli normally associated with sleep (e.g., bed, bedroom, bedtime) are frequently paired with behaviors other than sleep. This results in a low probability that the typically sleep-inducing stimuli will yield sleep.

One of the ways in which patients with insomnia can develop a complex conditioning history pertains to how the individual responds to a poor night's sleep. To cope with nocturnal wakefulness, individuals may engage in behaviors such as viewing their smartphone, watching television, reading, and working in the bed or bedroom. These coping behaviors may appear to the patient to be intuitive and reasonable as they may serve as distractors and as such curtail anxiety and worry about sleeplessness. More, such behaviors may appear to hasten the reinitiation of sleep. This said, such behaviors also promote (or reinforce) a complex conditioning history and stimulus "dys-control," whereby sleep-related stimuli no longer elicit sleep and sleepiness.

State of the Evidence

As derived from this model, stimulus control therapy (SCT) is one of the most widely used and endorsed behavioral treatments for insomnia owing to its well-established and robust efficacy (Engle-Friedman et al., 1992; Morin et al., 1999; Zwart & Lisman, 1979). Yet, the success of the therapy does not necessarily mean that stimulus dys-control is responsible for the development and maintenance of insomnia. In fact, one investigation found that the reverse of stimulus control instructions also improved sleep continuity (i.e., counter-control instructions; Davies et al., 1986). Whether SCT is efficacious through addressing stimulus dys-control has yet to be demonstrated. Other potential factors (proximal consequences of SCT) include reduced time in bed awake, diminished sleep effort, the prevention of micro-sleeps, and the promotion of full wakefulness when it may result in a greater homeostatic prime for subsequent sleep. With respect to the last point, there is preliminary evidence that diurnal and nocturnal wakefulness have different effects on sleep homeostasis (Klerman et al., 2019; Münch et al., 2010).

Implications for Research and Practice

Given that SCT manipulates many factors, dismantling studies are warranted to determine which components underlie its efficacy. Aside from addressing stimulus dys-control via limiting bedroom activities to sleep and sex, stimulus control instructions also include going to bed only when sleepy, leaving the bedroom when awake, getting up at the same time every morning irrespective of how much sleep is obtained, and not napping during the day. Any of these additional instructions may account for the efficacy of SCT through addressing other pathogenic factors such as sleep scheduling irregularity, conditioned wakefulness, and/or sleep homeostasis dysregulation. Experimental studies to disentangle these components to SCT may also yield new evidence about the stimulus control model.

THREE-FACTOR (THREE-P) MODEL

Description

Originally proposed by Spielman et al. (1987), the three-factor model describes the trajectory from initial onset (acute insomnia) to a self-perpetuating form of insomnia (chronic insomnia). The factors that are central to this model are framed in terms of three classes of variables: predisposing, precipitating, and perpetuating variables. The model takes a diathesis–stress perspective to describe how existing vulnerabilities (predisposing) and a stressor (precipitating) interact to cause insomnia, with the third factor (perpetuating) describing how the resultant acute condition persists over time.

Predisposing factors are the factors which determine an individual's preexisting vulnerability to developing insomnia. These may include biological (e.g., elevated basal activity of the sympathetic nervous system, hyperreactivity), psychological (e.g., tendency to worry or ruminate), and social factors (e.g., work and social demands, compatibility of sleep schedule with bed partner's schedule; C. Harvey et al., 2014; LeBlanc et al., 2009).

Precipitating factors are events which initially trigger sleep difficulties. More often than not, these factors are related to negative life events (i.e., significant threats to the quantity or quality of one's life; Bastien et al., 2004). Precipitating factors may also include positive life events to the extent that they represent significant life changes (i.e., a change from the known to the unknown). All such triggers may produce sleeplessness via elevated levels of autonomic arousal. Beyond this, there are likely a raft of other factors that may promote insomnia via physical discomfort and/or through the transient dysregulation of the circadian and/or homeostatic control of sleep.

Perpetuating factors are behaviors which the individual adopts to cope with sleeplessness and sleep loss but actually reinforces such problems (Ellis et al., 2021). These behaviors are thought to include staying in bed when unable to sleep and/or extending sleep opportunity in order to recover lost sleep (Spielman et al., 1987). The former behavior is central to the stimulus control model, while the latter behavior is the primary focus of the three-factor model. Extending sleep opportunity can include napping, going to bed earlier, or getting out of bed later. To some extent, these behaviors can allow for the recovery of lost sleep, but they lead to a mismatch between sleep opportunity (time spent in bed) and sleep ability (how long the individual can sleep for). When sleep opportunity exceeds sleep ability, the individual's sleep efficiency will decrease, and they may experience nonconsolidated sleep (polyphasic sleep).

An update of this model (the four-factor model) included the addition of a fourth factor (a fourth "P"): *Pavlovian conditioning* (Perlis et al., 2005). This factor describes an independent perpetuating factor for insomnia whereby the experience of spending prolonged periods of time awake in bed can result in sleep-related cues becoming conditioned stimuli for the automatic, physiological response of wakefulness or arousal, rather than the "normal" response of sleepiness and sleep. This phenomenon is best illustrated by the common patient report of suddenly feeling "wide awake" when they enter the sleep environment. The conditioning factor may, in and of itself, perpetuate the insomnia ad infinitum, irrespective of whether the precipitating and/or the other perpetuating factors have resolved. See an illustration of the temporal course of chronic insomnia with the revised model in Figure 26.1.

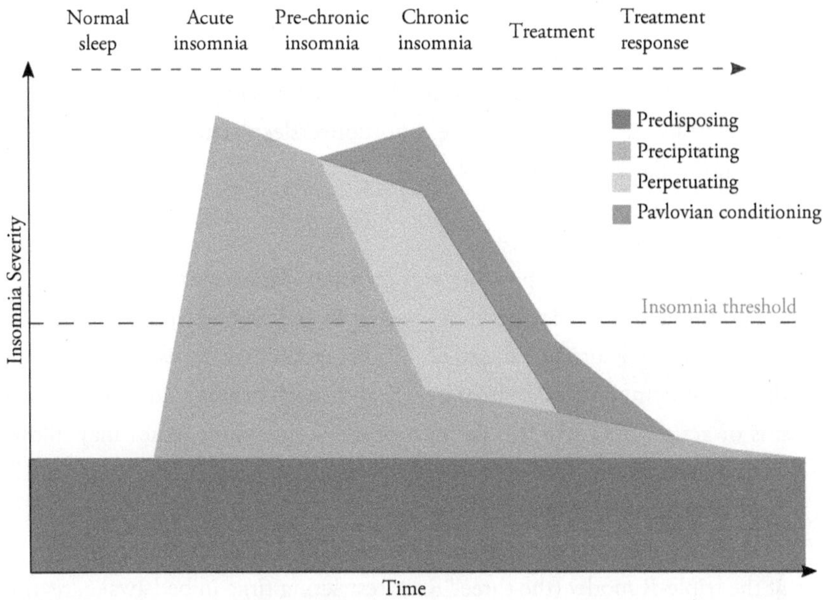

Figure 26.1 The time course of the development and resolution of insomnia according to the four-factor etiological model

State of the Evidence

As with the stimulus control model, some of the most compelling evidence for the three-factor model is the efficacy of the behavioral therapy derived from the model. Sleep restriction therapy (SRT) is widely regarded as a highly efficacious treatment that produces large and enduring changes in insomnia symptoms (Edinger et al., 2021; Maurer et al., 2021). It is worthwhile noting, however, that dismantling studies to estimate the relative contribution of SRT to the efficacy of CBT-I are lacking. Of the few that exist, one study found that patients randomized to receive behavioral treatment components alone had more rapid, but less durable, gains than those who received only cognitive treatment components (A. G. Harvey et al., 2014). Finally, there is some evidence to suggest that the restriction of time in bed, over regularization of the sleep opportunity, is the component of SRT that most contributes to treatment outcome (Maurer et al., 2018, 2020).

Prospective studies have been conducted to test the central tenet of the three-factor model (Ellis et al., 2014, 2021; Morin et al., 2009; Perlis et al., 2021). That is, sleep extension is the factor responsible for the transition from acute to chronic insomnia. One of these studies found that patients who developed chronic insomnia did not differ from those who recovered from acute insomnia with respect to time in bed. Another study found that time in bed does not mediate the effects of CBT-I on insomnia symptoms (Parsons et al., 2021). Thus, it may be that sleep extension (increased sleep opportunity to recover lost sleep) is not the factor that serves to perpetuate insomnia. Instead, it may be a more subtle scenario: The reduction in sleep ability that occurs with acute insomnia coupled with the failure to "naturally" restrict sleep opportunity sets into place the mismatch between sleep ability and opportunity that maintains insomnia over the long term. This scenario may also set the stage for the conditioned sleeplessness that appears to occur with chronic insomnia (Perlis et al., 2021).

Implications for Research and Practice

Several avenues for research are possible and ongoing. Three such areas include natural history studies (to identify the factors that predispose, precipitate, and perpetuate chronic insomnia; Fernandez-Mendoza et al., 2021; Walker et al., 2022), dismantling studies (to identify the active components of treatment), and mechanistic studies (to identify the mechanisms of action for CBT-I). Clarification regarding these issues may allow us to increase treatment response, diminish the risk for recurrence (as an adjuvant to traditional CBT-I), or prophylactically to prevent episodes of insomnia.

With respect to the mechanisms of action for CBT-I, this has recently been framed in terms of the triple-R model (the three "Rs"): restricting time in bed awake, regularizing timing of sleep and wake, and reconditioning sleep-related stimuli as strong associates for (if not conditioned stimuli for) sleepiness and sleep (Maurer et al., 2018). These components of therapy are thought to be the core of CBT-I treatment and the factors responsible for cognitive, behavioral, and physiologic or neurophysiologic change. Mechanistic trials are ongoing (Maurer et al., 2020, 2022). Further investigations are required to test this model, particularly with respect to the temporal pattern of changes in physiological, cognitive, and behavioral factors.

Cognitive Models

All cognitive models of insomnia share a common proposition: that maladaptive cognitions about insomnia symptoms contribute to the arousal that maintains the sleep disturbance.

EARLY COGNITIVE PERSPECTIVES

Description

Early cognitive theories largely pertained to the role of worry and rumination and maladaptive beliefs in the development and maintenance of insomnia. These theories are summarized below.

Individuals prone to *worry and rumination* may operate at higher basal levels of cognitive arousal such that they are more likely to develop hyperarousal and acute insomnia (Dorsey & Bootzin, 1997). These individuals may also be more reactive to life stressors in terms of an exaggerated cognitive response. In addition, worry and rumination may serve as perpetuating factors of insomnia (Ellis et al., 2021). This may occur when the inability to sleep itself and the consequences of sleep loss become targets of cognitive activity, fueling further worry and the worry further fueling the insomnia (Morin, 1993).

Cognitive arousal may also act as a precipitating factor for insomnia, whereby a stressor (i.e., a stressful life event) initiates an increase in cognitive activities such as problem-solving that, during the day, are adaptive and can serve as active coping strategies. During the night, these same processes interfere with initiation of sleep. As sleep is disrupted, the resultant sleepiness and/or sleep loss may impair cognitive function and decrease the probability of effective problem-solving while increasing the likelihood of rumination and worry, thus setting the stage for a cycle of persistent cognitive activation and insomnia.

Attitudes and beliefs about sleep also appear to moderate the effects of worry on sleep (Morin et al., 1993, 2002). For example, if an individual believes that sleeping for 8 hours is necessary, then, when faced with the prospect of getting less than 8 hours of sleep, the individual will be more prone to worry. This, in turn, may lead to insomnia.

State of the Evidence

Several studies have supported the role of worry and rumination in the development and maintenance of insomnia. Patients with chronic insomnia tend to display personality factors related to trait worry (Dorsey & Bootzin, 1997; Kales et al., 1983), suggesting that this trait is a predisposing factor for insomnia. Additionally, although there are no longitudinal studies to demonstrate this shift in the transition from acute to chronic insomnia, empirical data supports the hypothesis that worry in chronic insomnia is often "worry about sleep." For instance, studies that sample thought content around sleep onset in chronic insomnia patients (A. G. Harvey, 2000; Kuisk et al., 1989) and studies that differentiate between good and poor sleepers' pre-sleep cognitions (Smith et al., 2001) show that the content of worry is indeed sleep-focused in patients with insomnia.

There is also evidence to support the role of attitudes and beliefs about sleep. Patients with insomnia tend to endorse more dysfunctional beliefs and attitudes about sleep and believe them to a stronger degree than good sleepers (Morin et al., 1993). The successful treatment of insomnia via CBT-I is also associated with reductions in the endorsement of these beliefs about sleep (Edinger et al., 2001; Morin et al., 2002; Parsons et al., 2021).

Implications for Research and Practice

Longitudinal studies are needed to assess trait-level worry and rumination as predictive factors of insomnia onset, which may lead to novel avenues for insomnia prevention. While addressing and challenging these cognitions as part of cognitive therapy is not efficacious as a stand-alone therapy, their resolution is associated with stronger treatment durability and may thus be important for remission minimization.

COGNITIVE MODEL OF INSOMNIA

Description

Proposed by Harvey in 2002, the cognitive model of insomnia expands upon these earlier perspectives to theorize how the transition from acute to chronic insomnia occurs and how chronic insomnia is maintained (A. G. Harvey, 2002a). The theory proposes that the initial worry and rumination inherent to acute insomnia can trigger arousal and distress, leading to selective attention and monitoring of sleep-related threats (conditions that may precipitate an incidence of, or worsening of, insomnia), distorted perceptions about deficits to functioning, and, ultimately, real daytime impairments. Further, the initial cognitive activity is exacerbated by dysfunctional beliefs and safety behaviors. Each model component is described below, and the process is illustrated in Figure 26.2.

Excessive negatively toned cognitive activity are thoughts, worries, and ruminations about getting enough sleep and the impact of poor sleep on health and functioning.

Arousal and *distress* refer to the physiological (sympathetic nervous system activation) and emotional responses to the cognitive activity.

Selective attention and monitoring result from the arousal and distress, whereby attention becomes narrowly focused on sleep-related threats. These threats include internal cues (e.g., sensations associated with arousal and distress) and external cues (e.g., sleep-inconducive environmental stimuli). Detection of threats provides further reason to worry and ruminate, further fueling the initial cognitive activity, arousal, and distress and reinforcing the monitoring behavior. This self-perpetuating cycle occurs automatically and is usually outside of conscious awareness.

Distorted perception of deficit occurs due to selective attention and monitoring being a 24/7 phenomenon, whereby during the day, the individual is more sensitive to noticing the consequences of poor sleep. These consequences may include fatigue and daytime impairments because of the sleep continuity disturbance, as well as random cues which are misattributed to the sleep problem. This distorted perception leads to an exaggeration of the degree of sleep-related impairment. In combination with the other model components, this can lead to real deficits to sleep and daytime functioning.

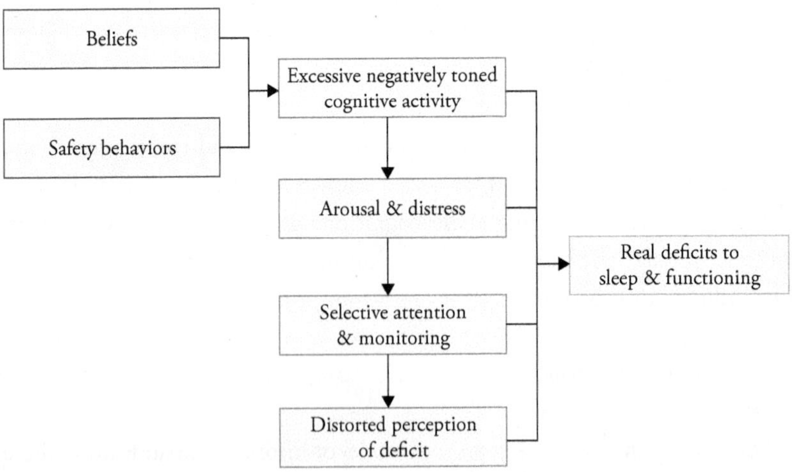

Figure 26.2 The cognitive model of insomnia

Beliefs that contribute to the cognitive activity include unrealistic expectations about an individual's sleep ability and overestimating the negative consequences of a poor night's sleep.

Safety behaviors are counterproductive strategies used to cope with the insomnia symptoms. These behaviors include trying to stop thinking or to stop racing thoughts (i.e., thought control) and avoiding daytime activities in line with their beliefs about the negative consequences of sleep loss. Such avoidance may only reinforce worry and cognitive arousal and may result in additional worries as to the growing impact of the insomnia on increasing domains of life.

State of the Evidence

Consistent with this cognitive model, studies have found that patients with insomnia excessively monitor their sleeping environment, selectively attend to sleep-related stimuli (Semler & Harvey, 2004a, 2004b), and engage in daytime safety behaviors (A. G. Harvey, 2002b). The relative contribution of these cognitive factors to the perpetuation and discontinuation of insomnia warrants investigation.

As with the behavior-focused models, evidence for this model can be derived from efficacy for its associated treatments. Cognitive therapy for insomnia is focused on addressing dysfunctional beliefs, cognitive distortions, and safety behaviors (Hiller et al., 2015; Sunnhed et al., 2022). This therapy is efficacious when used in combination with behavioral therapies for the treatment of insomnia (Edinger et al., 2021). It appears to be less efficacious as a stand-alone treatment, although one study found that 6 months after treatment completion cognitive therapy alone was superior to behavior therapy alone on rates of insomnia remission (A. G. Harvey et al., 2014). Nonetheless, addressing cognitive factors over the course of therapy tends to result in greater reductions in insomnia symptoms.

Implications for Research and Practice

More dismantling studies are warranted to examine (1) the relative efficacy of the various forms of cognitive therapy, (2) the relative contribution of cognitive therapy to CBT-I outcomes viz. sleep continuity, and (3) treatment benefits beyond efficacy to highlight its benefits for promoting adherence and preventing relapse.

SLEEP INTERFERING—INTERPRETING PROCESS MODEL

Description

Proposed by Lundh and Broman (2000), this model proposes two types of psychological processes that underlie the maintenance of insomnia: sleep-interfering processes and sleep-interpreting processes.

Sleep-interfering processes are the cognitive processes that affect emotional, cognitive, or physiological arousal which interfere with sleep. Most theories of insomnia focus on these processes, which include arousability, sensitivity, worrying, and conflicts with others.

Sleep-interpreting processes represent the unique components of this model, which have been built upon in subsequent cognitive models. These cognitive processes concern how an individual perceives, interprets, and responds to their sleep, influencing their vulnerability to insomnia symptoms. Such processes include attributions of poor sleep and daytime functioning, beliefs about sleep and consequences of sleep loss, and perfectionism as a personality trait.

The *sleep-interpreting processes*, and the interaction of the two processes, may explain much about the experience of insomnia, particularly the discordances between illness severity and daytime dysfunction (i.e., the phenomenon that "some suffer a lot from a little and some suffer a little from a lot"; Boyle et al., 2021).

State of the Evidence

The best evidence for this model is that several sleep-interfering and sleep-interpreting factors have been found to precipitate and perpetuate insomnia, as illustrated in evidence discussed in other models of insomnia. There is less evidence for the potential bidirectional relationships between processes, particularly with respect to insomnia subtypes. Natural history studies are warranted to examine whether sleep-interfering or sleep-interpreting factors occur first in the transition from acute to chronic insomnia. Mechanistic studies are needed to assess the extent to which specific factors within these domains account for illness severity, response to treatment, duration of remission, or the incidence of relapse.

Implications for Research and Practice

The consideration of sleep-interfering and sleep-interpreting processes as distinct and interactive components underlying insomnia has important clinical implications. It is perhaps the case that the processes are best addressed via different therapeutic approaches. Sleep-interfering processes may be best targeted through behavioral therapies (stimulus control and sleep restriction), whereas sleep-interpreting processes may be the target for cognitive therapies. Research is required to test this prediction. Further, it is likely true that both processes will need to be addressed, to various degrees, with any given individual.

METACOGNITIVE MODEL

Description

Proposed by Ong et al. (2012), the metacognitive model of insomnia is based on the principles of mindfulness and acceptance. The model expands upon the prior cognitive models to explain how metacognitive processes contribute to cognitive arousal.

The model proposes that there are two levels of arousal central to the perpetuation of insomnia and of relevance for its treatment. *Primary arousal* refers to the cognitive activity which directly interferes with sleep. This concept is similar to the sleep-interfering process (Lundh & Broman, 2000) and includes distorted perception of deficits and excessive negatively toned cognitive activity (A. G. Harvey, 2002a). *Secondary arousal* refers to how an individual relates to cognitions about sleep (i.e., the metacognitive component), which can indirectly interfere with sleep. This concept is similar to the sleep-interpreting process described by Lundh and Broman and includes selective attention and bias described by Harvey. In a sense, secondary arousal can amplify the effects of primary arousal. If, for example, an individual is particularly rigid in their beliefs about the consequences of sleep loss, then their beliefs will have a greater impact on their arousal levels when attempting sleep, further exacerbating the insomnia. Thus, the metacognitive model uniquely posits metacognitions (i.e., secondary arousal) as an explicitly distinct, addressable factor underlying insomnia. It follows that secondary arousal is a potential target for intervention to treat the insomnia, using cognitive therapies (namely, mindfulness and acceptance).

State of the Evidence

In brief, mindfulness therapy has the end goal of having the individual be a nonjudgmental observer of their thoughts, particularly when experiencing sleeplessness. Research is mounting with respect to the efficacy of mindfulness therapy for the treatment of insomnia. From the limited evidence available, this therapy appears to result in modest improvements in insomnia symptoms (Ong et al., 2009, 2014; Perini et al., 2021; Rash et al., 2019). Much research remains to be done to test this therapy and the mechanism of action theorized by this model.

Implications for Research and Practice

Owing to the limited evidence to date, there is no recommendation for the use of mindfulness for the treatment of insomnia (Edinger et al., 2021). Perhaps the promise of this therapy, as an adjuvant to CBT-I, is in its potential to augment patient adherence, treatment response, and remission and/or as a prophylactic measure against relapse.

MICROANALYTIC MODEL

Description

Proposed by Morin (1993), the microanalytic model theorizes that four factors account for the maintenance of insomnia over time: arousal, dysfunctional cognitions, consequences, and maladaptive habits.

Arousal, according to this model, refers to the emotional, cognitive, and physiological types of arousal.

Dysfunctional cognitions refer to worry, rumination, and unrealistic expectations about sleep and sleep loss.

Consequences refer to the negative outcomes that occur with insomnia, such as fatigue, mood disturbances, and social discomfort.

Maladaptive habits refer to behaviors such as excessive time in bed, irregular sleep–wake schedules, and napping. These behaviors presumably occur in relation to the effort to recover lost sleep.

Central to this model is the idea that these components have bidirectional relationships with one another and that, together, they create the "cycle of insomnia" (Morin, 1993). That is, insomnia is a self-reinforcing phenomenon whereby each occurrence of insomnia has consequences on cognitions and behaviors which increase the likelihood of insomnia reoccurring. Without intervention to break the cycle, insomnia can thus continue unabated.

State of the Evidence

While the subtype and severity of insomnia can change over time, insomnia does appear to be an unrelenting disorder (Morin et al., 2009, 2020). One study has shown that untreated chronic insomnia can persist for up to 5 years, supporting the "cycle of insomnia" notion (Morin et al., 2020). Indeed, this theoretical model has been supported by (and has shaped) most contemporary insomnia research and clinical practice.

Implications for Research and Practice

The clear therapeutic implication of this model is that the treatment of insomnia may benefit from adopting a multicomponent approach to break the insomnia cycle. Not surprisingly, the model was introduced along with the first delineation of a multicomponent cognitive-behavioral approach to the treatment of insomnia (Morin, 1993). Prior to this, there were no published treatment manuals, and most clinical researchers and clinicians adopted either a cognitive or a behavioral approach. This said, the microanalytic model stresses the importance of dysfunctional cognitions and serves as the foundational rationale for their assessment and treatment in the context of CBT-I. As with other models, natural history studies will be required to examine whether dysfunctional beliefs mediate or moderate the transition from acute to chronic insomnia. More, mechanistic studies will be needed to assess the extent to which these cognitions account for illness severity, response to treatment, duration of remission, or the incidence of relapse.

Neuropsychological Models

All models of insomnia within this domain share a common proposition: Insomnia has a neurobiological component which underlies and maintains sleep continuity disturbance.

NEUROCOGNITIVE MODEL

Description

Proposed by Perlis et al. (1997), the neurocognitive model emphasizes the need to specifically (1) delineate the concept of hyperarousal into three types, cortical (e.g., brain activity), cognitive (e.g., worry and rumination vs. perception and recall), and somatic arousal (e.g., autonomic activity/peripheral nervous system activity); (2) focus on cognition in neuropsychological terms; and (3) assess brain activity in terms of beta- and/or gamma-frequency EEG activity. The guiding hypothesis is that, in chronic insomnia, heightened cortical arousal (as measured by increased beta/gamma EEG activity) exerts its deleterious effects via three processes: enhanced sensory processing, enhanced information processing, and enhanced long-term memory formation.

Enhanced sensory processing results in greater detection of endogenous and exogenous stimuli around sleep onset and during non-rapid-eye-movement (NREM) sleep, directly interfering with sleep continuity.

Enhanced information processing of stimuli and the formation of short-term memories for stimulating events around sleep onset and during NREM sleep results in the blurring of boundaries between sleep and wake.

Enhanced long-term memory formation results in greater recollection of stimulating events around sleep onset and during NREM sleep, which underlies the discrepancy between objectively estimated sleep continuity and an individual's retrospective recall of their sleep.

The neurocognitive model is an extension of the three-factor and four-factor behavioral models. It posits that acute insomnia occurs due to predisposing and precipitating factors and that chronic insomnia is maintained via perpetuating factors. Like the three-factor model, chronic insomnia is perpetuated by the instrumental conditioning that occurs with sleep extension. Like the four-factor model, classical conditioning serves as a perpetuating factor for chronic insomnia whereby the repeated pairing of sleep-related stimuli with cortical arousal ultimately causes the sleep-related stimuli to elicit (or maintain) higher than usual levels of cortical arousal (prior to and/or coexistent with the normal levels of peri-sleep onset and/or NREM brain activity).

State of the Evidence

There is evidence to suggest that patients with insomnia, compared to good sleepers, exhibit increased cortical arousal when assessed using measures such as quantitative EEG (Merica et al., 1998; Merica & Gaillard, 1992; Perlis, Smith, Andrews, et al., 2001; Spiegelhalder et al., 2012). There is also limited evidence that patients with insomnia tend to exhibit increased sensory or information processing (Kertesz & Cote, 2011; Yang & Lo, 2007), an attenuation of the normal mesograde amnesia of sleep (Perlis, Smith, Orff, et al., 2001), and an association between sleep state misperception and objective measures of cortical arousal or evoked response potential abnormalities (Krystal et al., 2002; Nofzinger et al., 2000).

Implications for Research and Practice

It remains to be shown that there is a conditioned aspect to the "insomnia response" (i.e., neurocognitive processing is "condition-able") and that altered neurocognitive processing has clear *neurobiological substrates* (e.g., altered activity in specific brain regions or the occurrence of local neuronal wakefulness) and *functional consequences* (sleep continuity disturbance and sleep state misperception). If true, then the neurocognitive model may provide some insight into the potential mechanisms of action of existing therapies. For example, SRT might work through deepening sleep (sleep pressure–related attenuation of beta/gamma activity), which may, in turn, augment the normal mesograde amnesia of sleep. Further, more intensive forms of sleep restriction may therefore be helpful to promote counterconditioning, such as intensive sleep retraining (Harris et al., 2012; Lack et al., 2019). This therapy repeatedly pairs the sleeping environment with the experience of falling asleep quickly: a process which may assist counterconditioning.

PSYCHOBIOLOGIC INHIBITION MODEL

Description

Proposed by Espie et al. (2006), the psychobiologic inhibition model takes a counterposition to the hyperarousal model. This model instead theorizes that psychophysiological insomnia is due to the failure to "de-arouse," rather than heightened arousal.

This model makes two assumptions about good sleep: that it is ensured by automaticity (sleep as an involuntary process governed by homeostatic and circadian regulation) and plasticity (sleep as flexible to real-world circumstances). With the occurrence of stressful life events, physiological and psychological hyperarousal can and does occur in some people, but the insomnia is perpetuated in all patients by the failure to de-arouse (Espie, 2023). In acute insomnia, the inhibition of de-arousal interferes with the normal homeostatic and circadian regulation of sleep. The insomnia is then either resolved or perpetuated based on whether the stressor resolves or the individual attends to the insomnia symptoms. This shift of attention from the life stressor to the insomnia symptoms is thought to be the first of three critical events that transition acute insomnia to a chronic condition. The three events are referred to as the attention–intention–effort (A–I–E) pathway, as described below.

When *attention* is drawn selectively toward sleep-related cues, the very process of attending to an otherwise automatic process prevents perceptual disengagement.

The individual then makes the explicit *intention* to sleep since they are now attending to the lack of sleep, which further inhibits the normal downregulation of arousal.

The intention to fall asleep triggers *effort* to sleep, which serves only to further inhibit sleep-related de-arousal.

Taken together, A–I–E factors may serve to perpetuate insomnia ad infinitum. See Figure 26.3 for a graphical illustration of this model.

State of the Evidence

The central tenet of the model, that insomnia is associated with the inhibition of sleep-related de-arousal rather than hyperarousal, represents a substantial paradigm shift regarding the pathophysiology of insomnia. This is true not only from a psychological and behavioral vantage point but also from a neurobiological perspective as it is possible (if not

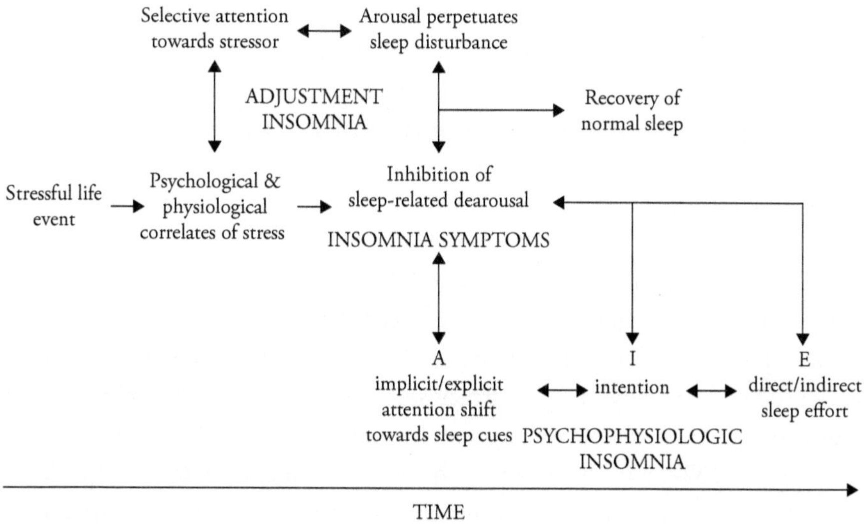

Figure 26.3 The pathway for development of adjustment insomnia, insomnia symptoms, and psychophysiological insomnia, according to the psychobiologic inhibition model of insomnia

likely) that "hyperarousal" and "the inhibition of de-arousal" have different neurobiological substrates. Further research is required to test the model's proposed causal mechanism. That is, data is needed to show that "hyperarousal" and "the inhibition of de-arousal" are legitimately different constructs and how they may be differently relevant with respect to the etiology and pathophysiology of insomnia. For example, it may be that one, some, or all three forms of hyperarousal are relevant for the incidence of acute insomnia and that chronic sleep continuity disturbance occurs in association with the inhibition of de-arousal. More, the former condition may be a part of the "flight-or-fight" response, while the latter condition may develop via conditioning and/or neuroadaptation. For a commentary regarding the relevance of the difference between the two constructs, please refer to the work of Marques et al. (2015). Multiple experiments have been conducted to test the A–I–E model, however, particularly the concept of sleep-related attention (Harris et al., 2015). These studies have generally found that insomnia is associated with a differential sleep-related attentional bias on measures such as dot-probe and the Posner task. The role of this attentional bias in the development and maintenance of insomnia warrants further investigation.

Implications for Research and Practice

This model may help to explain the efficacy of existing insomnia treatments. Any intervention that potentiates sleep-related de-arousal or promotes the disengagement of attention, intention, and effort should, according to this model, help to restore normal sleep. SRT may help to reinstate sleep automaticity by increasing homeostatic pressure and overcoming the effects of increased attention, intention, or effort. Similarly, SCT may strengthen adaptive and automatic bed-sleep de-arousal associations. Finally, relaxation, distraction, and imagery methods may reduce worry about sleep; and paradoxical intention methods may refocus the A–I–E pathway away from sleep preoccupation. This model is also consistent with approaches that aim to retrain attentional mechanisms (e.g., mindfulness).

NEUROBIOLOGICAL MODEL

Description

Proposed by Buysse et al. (2011), the neurobiological model of insomnia focuses on changes in sleep–wake regulation within the central nervous system. More specifically, the authors posit that insomnia is "a disorder of sleep–wake regulation characterized by persistent wake-like activity in neural structures during NREM sleep, resulting in simultaneous and regionally specific waking and sleeping neuronal activity patterns" (Buysse et al., 2011, pp. 132–133). The wake-like brain activity during NREM sleep is thought to occur in the prefrontal and parietal cortices, the paralimbic cortex, the thalamus, and the hypothalamic–brainstem arousal centers. Localized activation within these regions (local wakefulness) is expected to be associated with increased awareness of the external environment. Put differently, insomnia is defined as a hybrid state (part sleep and part wakefulness) that occurs due to local variations in sleep depth and results in some degree of sensory and information processing during NREM sleep. This may explain phenomena such as sleep state misperception (i.e., paradoxical insomnia) since the localized wakefulness responsible for the perception of wake may be undetected by traditional PSG sleep staging. The model does not offer an explanation regarding how the neurobiologically based hybrid state comes into existence.

State of the Evidence

This model is informed by the evidence for the two-process model of sleep regulation (Borbély, 1982; Borbely et al., 2016) and supported by recent findings regarding the "sleep switch" and localized sleep (Andrillon et al., 2019; Saper et al., 2001). Further research is required to test the proposed mechanism, potentially via neuroimaging in between-group and within-group models. Extending such paradigms cross-sectionally and longitudinally could explain how abnormal sleep–wake regulation manifests during the transition from good sleep to chronic insomnia.

Implications for Research and Practice

According to this model, therapies to minimize or eliminate local wakefulness may be particularly efficacious for treating insomnia. Whether existing treatments achieve this outcome is yet to be determined. CBT-I may accomplish this by increasing homeostatic pressure for sleep, and pharmacotherapy using benzodiazepines and benzodiazepine receptor agonists may accomplish this by modulating central nervous system gamma-aminobutyric acid activity. Techniques to increase regional brain activity during wakefulness or to decrease such activity during sleep warrant further investigation. One such possibility may be via the therapeutic use of transcranial electrical stimulation or transcranial magnetic stimulation.

REM SLEEP INSTABILITY MODEL

Description

Riemann et al. (2012) proposed that insomnia may be due to instability during rapid-eye-movement (REM) sleep. This instability may occur as macro- and/or micro-awakenings during REM sleep, the sleep stage with the greatest neurophysiological activation. The authors proposed that dysfunction in the limbic and paralimbic brain regions may lead to greater brain activation and greater sensitivity to arousal and fragmentation of REM sleep, leading to complaints of waking from sleep. Additionally, persistent awakenings during REM sleep are more likely to be perceived as wakefulness compared to NREM sleep, contributing to the sleep difficulty reports. The model, as with the neurobiological model, does not explain how REM sleep instability occurs nor how it is associated with incident insomnia or the transition from acute to chronic insomnia.

State of the Evidence

Several studies point to increased REM sleep fragmentation in patients with insomnia compared to control participants, a difference which seems to be attenuated with the effective treatment of the insomnia (Van Someren, 2021; Wassing et al., 2019). These differences are largely observed at the microstructural level using quantitative EEG techniques for more precise identification of changes in brain activity during REM sleep. The use of such techniques in natural history studies to examine how and when REM sleep instability manifests during the transition from good sleep to chronic insomnia is warranted.

Implications for Research and Practice

The future implications of this model include the development of pharmacotherapies to reduce REM sleep fragmentation. Indeed, this model may help explain the efficacy of CBT-I. SRT may work by increasing REM sleep drive, which in turn may reduce sensitivity to arousal and consolidate REM sleep.

PARALLEL PROCESS MODEL

Description

This model was proposed to represent each core component from the existing models of insomnia within one integrated framework (see Figure 26.4; Perlis et al., 2005). Pertinent features of this model include the suggestion that all identified factors are (to one degree or another) contributory, that the cognitive behavioral and the neurocognitive–neurobiological domains represent "two sides of the same coin," and that acute insomnia

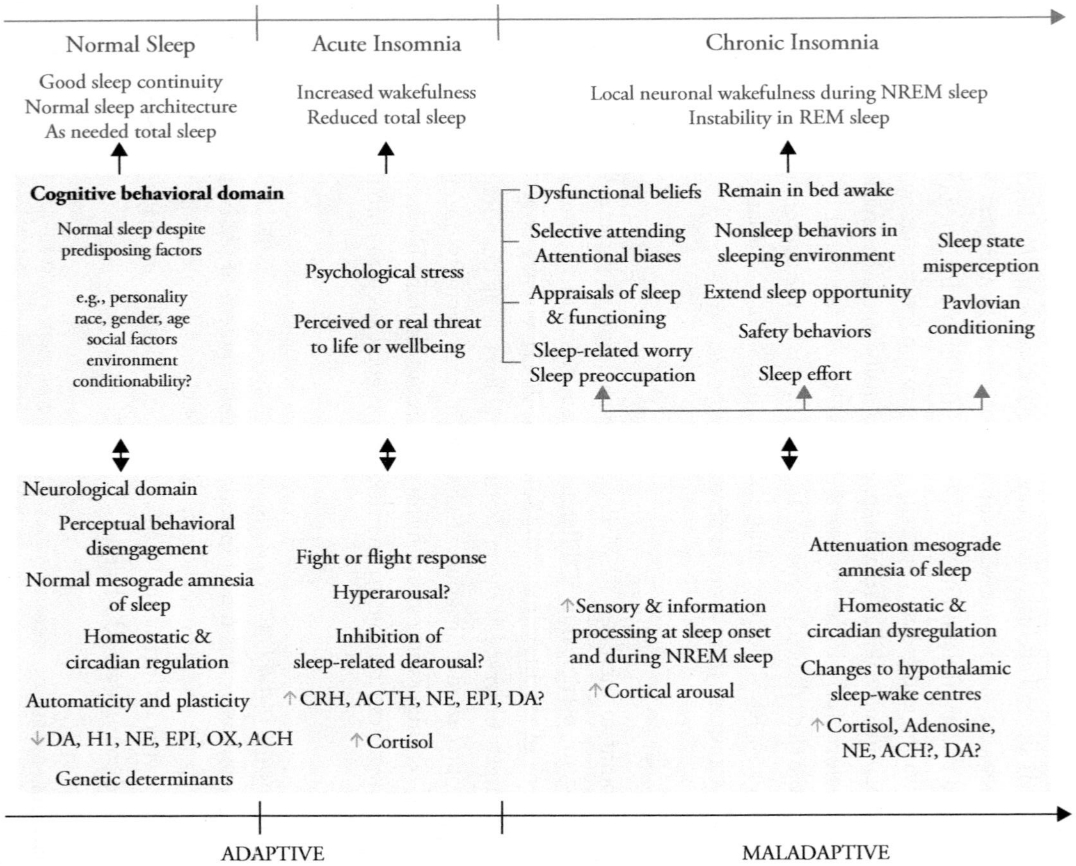

Figure 26.4 The parallel process model of insomnia, integrating existing models under one conceptual framework

Note. ACH = acetylcholine; ACTH = adrenocorticotropic hormone; CRH = corticotropin releasing hormone; DA = dopamine; EPI = epinephrine; NE = norepinephrine; NREM = non-rapid-eye-movement; OX = oxytocin; REM = rapid-eye-movement.

is possibly an adaptive response (a part of the flight-or-fight response, a necessary override to the normal homeostatic and circadian regulation of sleep and wakefulness).

More specifically, the model proposes that good sleep is observable as good sleep continuity, normal sleep architecture, and "as needed" total sleep (i.e., enough sleep to meet sleep need). Under the cognitive behavioral domain, good sleep occurs despite the presence of predisposing factors which make the individual more prone to an acute insomnia response. Under the neurobiological domain, good sleep is evident in (and fostered by) homeostatic sleep drive and circadian rhythm regulation, sleep automaticity and plasticity, and perceptual disengagement and the mesograde amnesia of sleep.

When a perceived or actual stress occurs, the individual may experience increased wakefulness and reduced total sleep. This form of sleeplessness may be a systemic part of the fight-or-flight response, mediated by both the cognitive behavioral (psychological stress) and the neurological domains (hyperarousal and/or inhibition of sleep-related dearousal). While the insomnia response likely has short-term deleterious effects, it likely has adaptive value by allowing (or enforcing) sleeplessness when it is not safe to sleep. This concept was nicely encapsulated by Art Spielman in 1991: "no matter how important sleep may be, it was adaptively deferred when the lion entered the cave" (Spielman & Glovinsky, 1991, p. 3).

The system's response becomes maladaptive when it persists and results in abnormal cognitions (e.g., dysfunctional beliefs, selective attention, sleep-related worry, and preoccupations) and behaviors (e.g., remaining in bed awake, safety behaviors, sleep effort), which in turn only serve to perpetuate sleeplessness. This maladaptive response is mirrored by marked changes in the neurobiological domain. These changes include increased sensory and information processing during NREM sleep, fragmentation of REM sleep, localized wakefulness during sleep and other alterations to cortical arousal, and dysregulation of homeostatic sleep drive and the circadian system. Such changes at both levels may foster sleep state misperception and the development of the conditioned insomnia response and underlie the "cycle of insomnia."

State of the Evidence

The synthesis of the predisposing, precipitating, and perpetuating factors of insomnia under one conceptual model makes the shortcomings of our current theories of insomnia easier to identify. For example, even within the integrated model, the two-process model of sleep–wake regulation is largely in the periphery, and socioecological issues as risk factors (Grandner, 2014, 2019) for the development of both acute and chronic insomnia are remarkably lacking. Finally, there is the enormous challenge of assessing the various factors concurrently so that their relative conceptual utility can be assessed.

Implications for Research and Practice

It is hoped that the practice of synthesizing existing models into one conceptual framework will stimulate new research ideas and potential clinical interventions.

Future Directions

Evidence is accruing that supports multiple models, but substantial work remains before the claim can be made that the etiology and pathophysiology of insomnia are "known." Some important future directions needed to advance the field include the following.

1. Insomnia is a heterogeneous disorder with multiple pathways that lead to multiple presentations of what is diagnosed as, essentially, the same disorder. Given that one accepts the "subtypes of insomnia" are of relevance, greater consideration is warranted for which etiologic model(s) of insomnia applies to each proposed insomnia subtype. While some models propose multiple pathways to insomnia (e.g., three-factor model, psychobiologic inhibition model), other models specify mechanisms underpinning the disorder (e.g., REM instability). Exploring which pathways are most explanatory for proposed subtypes may lead to the refinement of subtype criteria and potentially the identification of new distinct subtypes.
2. For the models that do not specifically indicate it, how is it that the putative mechanisms that underlie insomnia come to be (e.g., what is the etiology of the pathophysiology?). For example, if cortical arousal and/or the failure to inhibit wakefulness and/or the incidence of "wake-on" neuronal activity during NREM sleep undergirds the incidence and severity of chronic insomnia, how do such aberrant states "become the norm."
3. The relative contributions of homeostatic sleep drive (specifically, drives for NREM and REM sleep) and circadian rhythm processes need to be addressed within the existing and new models. The use of sleep monitoring technologies to estimate sleep and circadian factors may be ideal to elucidate how these processes may underlie sleeping continuity difficulties.
4. Critical gaps remain in the proposed etiologic framework for insomnia. For example, a social–ecological model of insomnia is remarkably lacking. Existing theories in other areas of health and sleep health may provide useful foundations for the development of such models (Grandner, 2014, 2019). Next steps would then be to develop an integrated biopsychosocial model of insomnia, as has been done for depression (Garcia-Toro & Aguirre, 2007), diabetes (Peyrot et al., 1999), and even obstructive sleep apnea (Crawford et al., 2014).
5. Another example of a critical gap pertains to the concept of sleep need. It is presumed that sleep need likely falls within 7–9 hours for most adults,

but sleep need varies between individuals. New and existing theories need to "factor in" the concept of sleep need (no matter how complicated its measurement may be). Such information may critically inform how we conceptualize the etiology and pathophysiology of insomnia.

Conclusion

In summary, insomnia is a highly prevalent clinical disorder that, once chronic, often persists for years, if not decades. Many, sometimes competing, models of etiology and pathophysiology have been proposed that approach insomnia from a diversity of perspectives. The most recent models argue that insomnia can be understood only through integration across theoretical perspectives. According to this view, insomnia is not a behavioral, cognitive, neurophysiological, or social phenomenon but rather a clinical state with characteristics across each domain. It is not a matter of which theoretical perspective is correct but rather which model(s) is most relevant for each given individual.

It is likely that there are multiple pathways to insomnia given the heterogeneity of this disorder, so the ultimate goals of future research will be to identify which pathway is implicated for any given individual. These efforts could lead to clinical treatments that are personalized to the individual such that it targets the unique constellation of physiological, behavioral, and cognitive factors at play. To reach this goal, new-generation models are needed that approach insomnia from a multidisciplinary, integrated perspective.

References

American Academy of Sleep Medicine. (2014). *International classification of sleep disorders* (3rd ed.).

American Psychiatric Association. (2013). *Diagnostic and statistical manual of mental disorders* (5th ed.).

Andrillon, T., Windt, J., Silk, T., Drummond, S. P. A., Bellgrove, M. A., & Tsuchiya, N. (2019). Does the mind wander when the brain takes a break? Local sleep in wakefulness, attentional lapses and mind-wandering. *Frontiers in Neuroscience, 13*, Article 949. https://doi.org/10.3389/fnins.2019.00949

Bastien, C. H., Vallières, A., & Morin, C. M. (2004). Precipitating factors of insomnia. *Behavioral Sleep Medicine, 2*(1), 50–62.

Bei, B., Wiley, J. F., Trinder, J., & Manber, R. (2016). Beyond the mean: A systematic review on the correlates of daily intraindividual variability of sleep/wake patterns. *Sleep Medicine Reviews, 28*, 108–124. https://doi.org/10.1016/j.smrv.2015.06.003

Belfer, S. J., Bashaw, A. G., Perlis, M. L., & Kayser, M. S. (2021). A *Drosophila* model of sleep restriction therapy for insomnia. *Molecular Psychiatry, 26*(2), 492–507.

Blanken, T. F., Benjamins, J. S., Borsboom, D., Vermunt, J. K., Paquola, C., Ramautar, J., Dekker, K., Stoffers, D., Wassing, R., Wei, Y., & Van Someren, E. J. W. (2019). Insomnia disorder subtypes derived from life history and traits of affect and personality. *The Lancet Psychiatry, 6*(2), 151–163. https://doi.org/10.1016/S2215-0366(18)30464-4

Bonnet, M. H., & Arand, D. (1992). Caffeine use as a model of acute and chronic insomnia. *Sleep, 15*(6), 526–536.

Bonnet, M. H., & Arand, D. L. (2010). Hyperarousal and insomnia: State of the science. *Sleep Medicine Reviews, 14*(1), 9–15. https://doi.org/10.1016/j.smrv.2009.05.002

Bootzin, R. R. (1972). Stimulus control treatment for insomnia. *Proceedings of the American Psychological Association, 7*, 395–396.

Borbély, A. A. (1982). A two process model of sleep regulation. *Human Neurobiology, 1*(3), 195–204.

Borbely, A. A., Daan, S., Wirz-Justice, A., & Deboer, T. (2016). The two-process model of sleep regulation: A reappraisal. *Journal of Sleep Research*, *25*(2), 131–143. https://doi.org/10.1111/jsr.12371

Boyle, J. T., Vargas, I., Rosenfield, B., Grandner, M. A., & Perlis, M. L. (2021). Insomnia severity and degree of dysfunction: What is to be learned when these domains are discordant? *Behavioral Sleep Medicine*, *20*(2), 164–172. https://doi.org/10.1080/15402002.2021.1895794

Bubu, O. M., Brannick, M., Mortimer, J., Umasabor-Bubu, O., Sebastião, Y. V., Wen, Y., Schwartz, S., Borenstein, A. R., Wu, Y., & Morgan, D. (2017). Sleep, cognitive impairment, and Alzheimer's disease: A systematic review and meta-analysis. *Sleep*, *40*(1), Article zsw032.

Buysse, D. J., Cheng, Y., Germain, A., Moul, D. E., Franzen, P. L., Fletcher, M., & Monk, T. H. (2010). Night-to-night sleep variability in older adults with and without chronic insomnia. *Sleep Medicine*, *11*(1), 56–64. https://doi.org/10.1016/j.sleep.2009.02.010

Buysse, D. J., Germain, A., Hall, M., Monk, T. H., & Nofzinger, E. A. (2011). A neurobiological model of insomnia. *Drug Discovery Today: Disease Models*, *8*(4), 129–137.

Buysse, D. J., Thompson, W., Scott, J., Franzen, P. L., Germain, A., Hall, M., Moul, D. E., Nofzinger, E. A., & Kupfer, D. J. (2007). Daytime symptoms in primary insomnia: A prospective analysis using ecological momentary assessment. *Sleep Medicine*, *8*(3), 198–208. https://doi.org/10.1016/j.sleep.2006.10.006

Cano, G., Mochizuki, T., & Saper, C. B. (2008). Neural circuitry of stress-induced insomnia in rats. *Journal of Neuroscience*, *28*(40), 10167–10184.

Castelnovo, A., Ferri, R., Punjabi, N. M., Castronovo, V., Garbazza, C., Zucconi, M., Ferini-Strambi, L., & Manconi, M. (2019). The paradox of paradoxical insomnia: A theoretical review towards a unifying evidence-based definition. *Sleep Medicine Reviews*, *44*, 70–82.

Chen, I. Y., Jarrin, D. C., Ivers, H., & Morin, C. M. (2017). Investigating psychological and physiological responses to the Trier Social Stress Test in young adults with insomnia. *Sleep Medicine*, *40*, 11–22.

Cheng, P., Kalmbach, D. A., Tallent, G., Joseph, C. L., Espie, C. A., & Drake, C. L. (2019). Depression prevention via digital cognitive behavioral therapy for insomnia: A randomized controlled trial. *Sleep*, *42*(10), Article zsz150.

Crawford, M. R., Espie, C. A., Bartlett, D. J., & Grunstein, R. R. (2014). Integrating psychology and medicine in CPAP adherence—New concepts? *Sleep Medicine Reviews*, *18*(2), 123–139. https://doi.org/10.1016/j.smrv.2013.03.002

Currie, S. R., Wilson, K. G., Pontefract, A. J., & deLaplante, L. (2000). Cognitive-behavioral treatment of insomnia secondary to chronic pain. *Journal of Consulting and Clinical Psychology*, *68*(3), 407–416.

Davies, R., Lacks, P., Storandt, M., & Bertelson, A. D. (1986). Countercontrol treatment of sleep-maintenance insomnia in relation to age. *Psychology and Aging*, *1*(3), 233–238.

de Almondes, K. M., Costa, M. V., Malloy-Diniz, L. F., & Diniz, B. S. (2016). Insomnia and risk of dementia in older adults: Systematic review and meta-analysis. *Journal of Psychiatric Research*, *77*, 109–115.

Dodds, K. L., Miller, C. B., Kyle, S. D., Marshall, N. S., & Gordon, C. J. (2017). Heart rate variability in insomnia patients: A critical review of the literature. *Sleep Medicine Reviews*, *33*, 88–100.

Dorsey, C. M., & Bootzin, R. R. (1997). Subjective and psychophysiologic insomnia: An examination of sleep tendency and personality. *Biological Psychiatry*, *41*(2), 209–216.

Edinger, J. D., Arnedt, J. T., Bertisch, S. M., Carney, C. E., Harrington, J. J., Lichstein, K. L., Sateia, M. J., Troxel, W. M., Zhou, E. S., Kazmi, U., Heald, J. L., & Martin, J. L. (2021). Behavioral and psychological treatments for chronic insomnia disorder in adults: An American Academy of Sleep Medicine clinical practice guideline. *Journal of Clinical Sleep Medicine*, *17*(2), 255–262. https://doi.org/10.5664/jcsm.8986

Edinger, J. D., Bonnet, M. H., Bootzin, R. R., Doghramji, K., Dorsey, C. M., Espie, C. A., Jamieson, A. O., McCall, W. V., Morin, C. M., & Stepanski, E. J. (2004). Derivation of research diagnostic criteria for insomnia: Report of an American Academy of Sleep Medicine work group. *Sleep*, *27*(8), 1567–1596.

Edinger, J. D., Fins, A. I., Sullivan, R. J., Marsh, G. R., Dailey, D. S., & Young, M. (1996). Comparison of cognitive-behavioral therapy and clonazepam for treating periodic limb movement disorder. *Sleep*, *19*(5), 442–444.

Edinger, J. D., Wohlgemuth, W. K., Radtke, R. A., Marsh, G. R., & Quillian, R. E. (2001). Does cognitive-behavioral insomnia therapy alter dysfunctional beliefs about sleep? *Sleep*, *24*(5), 591–599.

Ellis, J. G., Perlis, M. L., Bastien, C. H., Gardani, M., & Espie, C. A. (2014). The natural history of insomnia: Acute insomnia and first-onset depression. *Sleep*, *37*(1), 97–106.

Ellis, J. G., Perlis, M. L., Espie, C. A., Grandner, M. A., Bastien, C. H., Barclay, N. L., Altena, E., & Gardani, M. (2021). The natural history of insomnia: Predisposing, precipitating, coping, and perpetuating factors over the early developmental course of insomnia. *Sleep, 44*(9), Article zsab095.

Engle-Friedman, M., Bootzin, R. R., Hazlewood, L., & Tsao, C. (1992). An evaluation of behavioral treatments for insomnia in the older adult. *Journal of Clinical Psychology, 48*(1), 77–90.

Espie, C. A. (2002). Insomnia: Conceptual issues in the development, persistence, and treatment of sleep disorders in adults. *Annual Review of Psychology, 53*, 215–243.

Espie, C. A. (2023). Revisiting the psychobiological inhibition model: A conceptual framework for understanding and treating insomnia using cognitive and behavioural therapeutics (CBTx). *Journal of Sleep Research, 32*(6), Article e13841.

Espie, C. A., Barrie, L. M., & Forgan, G. S. (2012). Comparative investigation of the psychophysiologic and idiopathic insomnia disorder phenotypes: Psychologic characteristics, patients' perspectives, and implications for clinical management. *Sleep, 35*(3), 385–393.

Espie, C. A., Broomfield, N. M., MacMahon, K. M., Macphee, L. M., & Taylor, L. M. (2006). The attention–intention–effort pathway in the development of psychophysiologic insomnia: A theoretical review. *Sleep Medicine Reviews, 10*(4), 215–245.

Fernandez-Mendoza, J., Bourchtein, E., Calhoun, S., Puzino, K., Snyder, C. K., He, F., Vgontzas, A. N., Liao, D., & Bixler, E. (2021). Natural history of insomnia symptoms in the transition from childhood to adolescence: Population rates, health disparities, and risk factors. *Sleep, 44*(3), Article zsaa187.

Fernandez-Mendoza, J., Calhoun, S., Bixler, E. O., Pejovic, S., Karataraki, M., Liao, D., Vela-Bueno, A., Ramos-Platon, M. J., Sauder, K. A., & Vgontzas, A. N. (2010). Insomnia with objective short sleep duration is associated with deficits in neuropsychological performance: A general population study. *Sleep, 33*(4), 459–465.

Fernandez-Mendoza, J., He, F., Puzino, K., Amatrudo, G., Calhoun, S., Liao, D., Vgontzas, A. N., & Bixler, E. (2020). Insomnia with objective short sleep duration is associated with cognitive impairment: A first look at cardiometabolic contributors to brain health. *Sleep, 44*(1), Article zsaa150. https://doi.org/10.1093/sleep/zsaa150

Fernandez-Mendoza, J., Vgontzas, A. N., Liao, D., Shaffer, M. L., Vela-Bueno, A., Basta, M., & Bixler, E. O. (2012). Insomnia with objective short sleep duration and incident hypertension: The Penn State cohort. *Hypertension, 60*(4), 929–935. https://doi.org/10.1161/HYPERTENSIONAHA.112.193268

Garcia-Toro, M., & Aguirre, I. (2007). Biopsychosocial model in depression revisited. *Medical Hypotheses, 68*(3), 683–691.

Grandner, M. A. (2014). Addressing sleep disturbances: An opportunity to prevent cardiometabolic disease? *International Review of Psychiatry, 26*(2), 155–176. https://doi.org/10.3109/09540261.2014.911148

Grandner, M. A. (2019). Social-ecological model of sleep health. In M. A. Grandner (Ed.), *Sleep and health* (pp. 45–53). Elsevier.

Harris, J., Lack, L., Kemp, K., Wright, H., & Bootzin, R. (2012). A randomized controlled trial of intensive sleep retraining (ISR): A brief conditioning treatment for chronic insomnia. *Sleep, 35*(1), 49–60. https://doi.org/10.5665/sleep.1584

Harris, K., Spiegelhalder, K., Espie, C. A., MacMahon, K. M., Woods, H. C., & Kyle, S. D. (2015). Sleep-related attentional bias in insomnia: A state-of-the-science review. *Clinical Psychology Review, 42*, 16–27. https://doi.org/10.1016/j.cpr.2015.08.001

Harvey, A. G. (2000). Pre-sleep cognitive activity: A comparison of sleep-onset insomniacs and good sleepers. *British Journal of Clinical Psychology, 39*(3), 275–286.

Harvey, A. G. (2002a). A cognitive model of insomnia. *Behaviour Research and Therapy, 40*(8), 869–893.

Harvey, A. G. (2002b). Identifying safety behaviors in insomnia. *The Journal of Nervous and Mental Disease, 190*(1), 16–21.

Harvey, A. G., Bélanger, L., Talbot, L., Eidelman, P., Beaulieu-Bonneau, S., Fortier-Brochu, É., Ivers, H., Lamy, M., Hein, K., Soehner, A. M., Mérette, C., & Morin, C. M. (2014). Comparative efficacy of behavior therapy, cognitive therapy, and cognitive behavior therapy for chronic insomnia: A randomized controlled trial. *Journal of Consulting and Clinical Psychology, 82*(4), 670–683. https://doi.org/10.1037/a0036606

Harvey, C., Gehrman, P., & Espie, C. (2014). Who is predisposed to insomnia: A review of familial aggregation, stress-reactivity, personality and coping style. *Sleep Medicine Reviews, 18*(3), 237–247.

Hauri, P. J., & Olmstead, E. M. (1989). Reverse first night effect in insomnia. *Sleep, 12*(2), 97–105.

Hertenstein, E., Trinca, E., Wunderlin, M., Schneider, C. L., Züst, M. A., Fehér, K. D., Su, T., VanStraten, A., Berger, T., & Baglioni, C. (2022). Cognitive behavioral therapy for insomnia in patients with mental disorders and comorbid insomnia: A systematic review and meta-analysis. *Sleep Medicine Reviews, 62*, Article 101597.

Hiller, R. M., Johnston, A., Dohnt, H., Lovato, N., & Gradisar, M. (2015). Assessing cognitive processes related to insomnia: A review and measurement guide for Harvey's cognitive model for the maintenance of insomnia. *Sleep Medicine Reviews, 23*, 46–53.

Hohagen, F., Käppler, C., Schramm, E., Riemann, D., Weyerer, S., & Berger, M. (1994). Sleep onset insomnia, sleep maintaining insomnia and insomnia with early morning awakening—Temporal stability of subtypes in a longitudinal study on general practice attenders. *Sleep, 17*(6), 551–554.

Kales, A., Caldwell, A. B., Soldatos, C. R., Bixler, E. O., & Kales, J. D. (1983). Biopsychobehavioral correlates of insomnia: II. Pattern specificity and consistency with the Minnesota Multiphasic Personality Inventory. *Psychosomatic Medicine, 45*(4), 341–356.

Kay, D. B., & Buysse, D. J. (2017). Hyperarousal and beyond: New insights to the pathophysiology of insomnia disorder through functional neuroimaging studies. *Brain Sciences, 7*(3), Article 23.

Kertesz, R. S., & Cote, K. A. (2011). Event-related potentials during the transition to sleep for individuals with sleep-onset insomnia. *Behavioral Sleep Medicine, 9*(2), 68–85. https://doi.org/10.1080/15402002.2011.557989

Klerman, E. B., Hilaire, M., Perlis, M., Hilditch, C. J., McHill, A., Rahman, S. A., & Czeisler, C. A. (2019, August 25–29). *Effect of time-of-day and prior wake on electroencephalographic delta and beta power in 10-min naps during 30 continuous hours of 90-minute "days"* [Paper presentation]. XVI European Biological Rhythms Society Congress, Lyon, France.

Krystal, A. D., Edinger, J. D., Wohlgemuth, W. K., & Marsh, G. R. (2002). NREM sleep EEG frequency spectral correlates of sleep complaints in primary insomnia subtypes. *Sleep, 25*(6), 626–636.

Kuisk, L. A., Bertelson, A. D., & Walsh, J. K. (1989). Presleep cognitive hyperarousal and affect as factors in objective and subjective insomnia. *Perceptual and Motor Skills, 69*(3–2), 1219–1225.

Lack, L., Scott, H., & Lovato, N. (2019). Intensive sleep retraining treatment of insomnia. *Sleep Medicine Clinics, 14*(2), 245–252. https://doi.org/10.1016/j.jsmc.2019.01.005

LeBlanc, M., Mérette, C., Savard, J., Ivers, H., Baillargeon, L., & Morin, C. M. (2009). Incidence and risk factors of insomnia in a population-based sample. *Sleep, 32*(8), 1027–1037.

Leerssen, J., Lakbila-Kamal, O., Dekkers, L. M., Ikelaar, S. L., Albers, A. C., Blanken, T. F., Lancee, J., Van Der Lande, G. J., Maksimovic, T., & Mastenbroek, S. E. (2022). Treating insomnia with high risk of depression using therapist-guided digital cognitive, behavioral, and circadian rhythm support interventions to prevent worsening of depressive symptoms: A randomized controlled trial. *Psychotherapy and Psychosomatics, 91*(3), 168–179.

Li, Y., Zou, G., Shao, Y., Yao, P., Liu, J., Zhou, S., Hu, S., Xu, J., Guo, Y., & Gao, J.-H. (2022). Sleep discrepancy is associated with alterations in the salience network in patients with insomnia disorder: An EEG-fMRI study. *NeuroImage: Clinical, 35*, Article 103111.

Lichstein, K. L., Wilson, N. M., & Johnson, C. T. (2000). Psychological treatment of secondary insomnia. *Psychology and Aging, 15*(2), 232–240.

Lovato, N., Micic, G., & Lack, L. (2021). Sleep misestimation among older adults suffering from insomnia with short and normal objective sleep duration and the effects of cognitive behavior therapy. *Sleep, 44*(5), Article zsaa250.

Lundh, L.-G., & Broman, J.-E. (2000). Insomnia as an interaction between sleep-interfering and sleep-interpreting processes. *Journal of Psychosomatic Research, 49*(5), 299–310.

Marques, D. R., Allen Gomes, A., Clemente, V., Santos, J. M., & Castelo-Branco, M. (2015). Hyperarousal and failure to inhibit wakefulness in primary insomnia: "Birds of a feather"? *Sleep and Biological Rhythms, 13*(3), 219–228.

Mason, E. C., Grierson, A. B., Sie, A., Sharrock, M. J., Li, I., Chen, A. Z., & Newby, J. M. (2022). Co-occurring insomnia and anxiety: A randomized controlled trial of internet CBT for insomnia vs. internet CBT for anxiety. *Sleep, 46*(2), Article zsac205.

Maurer, L. F., Espie, C. A., & Kyle, S. D. (2018). How does sleep restriction therapy for insomnia work? A systematic review of mechanistic evidence and the introduction of the triple-R model. *Sleep Medicine Reviews, 42*, 127–138.

Maurer, L. F., Espie, C. A., Omlin, X., Emsley, R., & Kyle, S. D. (2022). The effect of sleep restriction therapy for insomnia on sleep pressure and arousal: A randomized controlled mechanistic trial. *Sleep, 45*(1), Article zsab223. https://doi.org/10.1093/sleep/zsab223

Maurer, L. F., Espie, C. A., Omlin, X., Reid, M. J., Sharman, R., Gavriloff, D., Emsley, R., & Kyle, S. D. (2020). Isolating the role of time in bed restriction in the treatment of insomnia: A randomised, controlled, dismantling trial comparing sleep restriction therapy with time in bed regularisation. *Sleep, 43*(11), Article zsaa096. https://doi.org/10.1093/sleep/zsaa096

Maurer, L. F., Schneider, J., Miller, C. B., Espie, C. A., & Kyle, S. D. (2021). The clinical effects of sleep restriction therapy for insomnia: A meta-analysis of randomised controlled trials. *Sleep Medicine Reviews, 58*, Article 101493. https://doi.org/10.1016/j.smrv.2021.101493

McCrae, C. S., & Lichstein, K. L. (2001). Secondary insomnia: Diagnostic challenges and intervention opportunities. *Sleep Medicine Reviews, 5*(1), 47–61.

Merica, H., Blois, R., & Gaillard, J. M. (1998). Spectral characteristics of sleep EEG in chronic insomnia. *European Journal of Neuroscience, 10*(5), 1826–1834.

Merica, H., & Gaillard, J. M. (1992). The EEG of the sleep onset period in insomnia: A discriminant analysis. *Physiology & Behavior, 52*, 199–204.

Mikoteit, T., Pawlowski, M., Seiffert, N., Seelig, E., Bilz, S., Hatzinger, M., & Holsboer-Trachsler, E. (2017). Heart rate variability during sleep distinguishes between insomnia and normal sleep. *Sleep Medicine, 40*, e223–e224.

Miller, C. B., Espie, C. A., Epstein, D. R., Friedman, L., Morin, C. M., Pigeon, W. R., Spielman, A. J., & Kyle, S. D. (2014). The evidence base of sleep restriction therapy for treating insomnia disorder. *Sleep Medicine Reviews, 18*(5), 415–424. https://doi.org/10.1016/j.smrv.2014.01.006

Monroe, L. J. (1967). Psychological and physiological differences between good and poor sleepers. *Journal of Abnormal Psychology, 72*(3), 255–264.

Morin, C. M. (1993). *Insomnia: Psychological assessment and management.* Guilford Press.

Morin, C. M., Bélanger, L., LeBlanc, M., Ivers, H., Savard, J., Espie, C. A., Mérette, C., Baillargeon, L., & Grégoire, J.-P. (2009). The natural history of insomnia: A population-based 3-year longitudinal study. *Archives of Internal Medicine, 169*(5), 447–453.

Morin, C. M., Blais, F., & Savard, J. (2002). Are changes in beliefs and attitudes about sleep related to sleep improvements in the treatment of insomnia? *Behaviour Research and Therapy, 40*(7), 741–752.

Morin, C. M., Hauri, P. J., Espie, C. A., Spielman, A. J., Buysse, D. J., & Bootzin, R. R. (1999). Nonpharmacologic treatment of chronic insomnia. *Sleep, 22*(8), 1134–1156.

Morin, C. M., Jarrin, D. C., Ivers, H., Merette, C., LeBlanc, M., & Savard, J. (2020). Incidence, persistence, and remission rates of insomnia over 5 years. *JAMA Network Open, 3*(11), Article e2018782. https://doi.org/10.1001/jamanetworkopen.2020.18782

Morin, C. M., Stone, J., Trinkle, D., Mercer, J., & Remsberg, S. (1993). Dysfunctional beliefs and attitudes about sleep among older adults with and without insomnia complaints. *Psychology and Aging, 8*(3), 463–467.

Münch, M., Silva, E. J., Ronda, J. M., Czeisler, C. A., & Duffy, J. F. (2010). EEG sleep spectra in older adults across all circadian phases during NREM sleep. *Sleep, 33*(3), 389–401. https://doi.org/10.1093/sleep/33.3.389

Neckelmann, D., Mykletun, A., & Dahl, A. A. (2007). Chronic insomnia as a risk factor for developing anxiety and depression. *Sleep, 30*(7), 873–880.

Nofzinger, E. A., Price, J. C., Meltzer, C. C., Buysse, D. J., Villemagne, V. L., Miewald, J. M., Sembrat, R. C., Steppe, D. A., & Kupfer, D. J. (2000). Towards a neurobiology of dysfunctional arousal in depression: The relationship between beta EEG power and regional cerebral glucose metabolism during NREM sleep. *Psychiatry Research: Neuroimaging, 98*(2), 71–91.

Okajima, I., Komada, Y., & Inoue, Y. (2011). A meta-analysis on the treatment effectiveness of cognitive behavioral therapy for primary insomnia. *Sleep and Biological Rhythms, 9*(1), 24–34. https://doi.org/10.1111/j.1479-8425.2010.00481.x

Ong, J. C., Manber, R., Segal, Z., Xia, Y., Shapiro, S., & Wyatt, J. K. (2014). A randomized controlled trial of mindfulness meditation for chronic insomnia. *Sleep, 37*(9), 1553–1563.

Ong, J. C., Shapiro, S. L., & Manber, R. (2009). Mindfulness meditation and cognitive behavioral therapy for insomnia: A naturalistic 12-month follow-up. *Explore, 5*(1), 30–36.

Ong, J. C., Ulmer, C. S., & Manber, R. (2012). Improving sleep with mindfulness and acceptance: A metacognitive model of insomnia. *Behaviour Research and Therapy, 50*(11), 651–660.

Parsons, C. E., Zachariae, R., Landberger, C., & Young, K. S. (2021). How does cognitive behavioural therapy for insomnia work? A systematic review and meta-analysis of mediators of change. *Clinical Psychology Review, 86*, Article 102027.

Perini, F., Wong, K. F., Lin, J., Hassirim, Z., Ong, J. L., Lo, J., Ong, J. C., Doshi, K., & Lim, J. (2021). Mindfulness-based therapy for insomnia for older adults with sleep difficulties: A randomized clinical trial. *Psychological Medicine, 53*(3), 1038–1048.

Perlis, M., Aloia, M., Millikan, A., Boehmler, J., Smith, M., Greenblatt, D., & Giles, D. (2000). Behavioral treatment of insomnia: A clinical case series study. *Journal of Behavioral Medicine, 23*(2), 149–161.

Perlis, M., Giles, D., Mendelson, W., Bootzin, R., & Wyatt, J. (1997). Psychophysiological insomnia: The behavioural model and a neurocognitive perspective. *Journal of Sleep Research, 6*(3), 179–188.

Perlis, M. L., Merica, H., Smith, M. T., & Giles, D. E. (2001). Beta EEG activity and insomnia. *Sleep Medicine Reviews, 5*(5), 365–376.

Perlis, M. L., Morales, K. H., Vargas, I., Posner, D. A., Grandner, M. A., Muench, A. L., Seewald, M. W., Gooneratne, N. S., Kloss, J. D., & Gencarelli, A. M. (2021). The natural history of insomnia: Does sleep extension differentiate between those that do and do not develop chronic insomnia? *Journal of Sleep Research, 30*(5), Article e13342.

Perlis, M. L., Smith, M. T., Andrews, P. J., Orff, H., & Giles, D. E. (2001). Beta/gamma EEG activity in patients with primary and secondary insomnia and good sleeper controls. *Sleep, 24*(1), 110–117.

Perlis, M. L., Smith, M. T., Orff, H. J., Andrews, P. J., & Giles, D. E. (2001). The mesograde amnesia of sleep may be attenuated in subjects with primary insomnia. *Physiology & Behavior, 74*(1–2), 71–76.

Perlis, M. L., Smith, M. T., & Pigeon, W. R. (2005). Etiology and pathophysiology of insomnia. *Principles and Practice of Sleep Medicine, 4*, 714–725.

Perlis, M. L., Swinkels, C. M., Gehrman, P. R., Pigeon, W. R., Matteson-Rusby, S. E., & Jungquist, C. R. (2010). The incidence and temporal patterning of insomnia: A pilot study. *Journal of Sleep Research, 19*(1, Pt. 1), 31–35. https://doi.org/10.1111/j.1365-2869.2009.00768.x

Peyrot, M., McMurry, J. F., Jr., & Kruger, D. F. (1999). A biopsychosocial model of glycemic control in diabetes: Stress, coping and regimen adherence. *Journal of Health and Social Behavior, 40*(2), 141–158.

Pigeon, W. R., Hegel, M., Unützer, J., Fan, M.-Y., Sateia, M. J., Lyness, J. M., Phillips, C., & Perlis, M. L. (2008). Is insomnia a perpetuating factor for late-life depression in the IMPACT cohort? *Sleep, 31*(4), 481–488.

Pillai, V., Roth, T., & Drake, C. L. (2015). The nature of stable insomnia phenotypes. *Sleep, 38*(1), 127–138. https://doi.org/10.5665/sleep.4338

Quesnel, C., Savard, J., Simard, S., Ivers, H., & Morin, C. M. (2003). Efficacy of cognitive-behavioral therapy for insomnia in women treated for nonmetastatic breast cancer. *Journal of Consulting and Clinical Psychology, 71*(1), 189–200.

Rash, J. A., Kavanagh, V. A., & Garland, S. N. (2019). A meta-analysis of mindfulness-based therapies for insomnia and sleep disturbance: Moving towards processes of change. *Sleep Medicine Clinics, 14*(2), 209–233.

Riedel, B. W., & Lichstein, K. L. (2000). Insomnia and daytime functioning. *Sleep Medicine Reviews, 4*(3), 277–298.

Riedel, B. W., Winfield, C. F., & Lichstein, K. L. (2001). First night effect and reverse first night effect in older adults with primary insomnia: Does anxiety play a role? *Sleep Medicine, 2*(2), 125–133.

Riemann, D., Klein, T., Rodenbeck, A., Feige, B., Horny, A., Hummel, R., Weske, G., Al-Shajlawi, A., & Voderholzer, U. (2002). Nocturnal cortisol and melatonin secretion in primary insomnia. *Psychiatry Research, 113*(1–2), 17–27.

Riemann, D., Spiegelhalder, K., Feige, B., Voderholzer, U., Berger, M., Perlis, M., & Nissen, C. (2010). The hyperarousal model of insomnia: A review of the concept and its evidence. *Sleep Medicine Reviews, 14*(1), 19–31. https://doi.org/10.1016/j.smrv.2009.04.002

Riemann, D., Spiegelhalder, K., Nissen, C., Hirscher, V., Baglioni, C., & Feige, B. (2012). REM sleep instability—A new pathway for insomnia? *Pharmacopsychiatry, 45*(5), 167–176.

Roth, T., & Drake, C. (2006). Defining insomnia: The role of quantitative criteria: Comment on Lineberger MD; Carney CE; Edinger JD et al. Defining insomnia: quantitative criteria for insomnia severity and frequency. *Sleep, 29*(4), 424–425.

Saper, C. B., Chou, T. C., & Scammell, T. E. (2001). The sleep switch: Hypothalamic control of sleep and wakefulness. *Trends in Neurosciences*, *24*(12), 726–731.

Semler, C. N., & Harvey, A. G. (2004a). An investigation of monitoring for sleep-related threat in primary insomnia. *Behaviour Research and Therapy*, *42*(12), 1403–1420.

Semler, C. N., & Harvey, A. G. (2004b). Monitoring for sleep-related threat: A pilot study of the Sleep Associated Monitoring Index (SAMI). *Psychosomatic Medicine*, *66*(2), 242–250.

Seugnet, L., Suzuki, Y., Thimgan, M., Donlea, J., Gimbel, S. I., Gottschalk, L., Duntley, S. P., & Shaw, P. J. (2009). Identifying sleep regulatory genes using a *Drosophila* model of insomnia. *Journal of Neuroscience*, *29*(22), 7148–7157.

Smith, M., Perlis, M., Carmody, T., Smith, M., & Giles, D. (2001). Presleep cognitions in patients with insomnia secondary to chronic pain. *Journal of Behavioral Medicine*, *24*(1), 93–114.

Spiegelhalder, K., Regen, W., Feige, B., Holz, J., Piosczyk, H., Baglioni, C., Riemann, D., & Nissen, C. (2012). Increased EEG sigma and beta power during NREM sleep in primary insomnia. *Biological Psychology*, *91*(3), 329–333.

Spielman, A. J., Caruso, L. S., & Glovinsky, P. B. (1987). A behavioral perspective on insomnia treatment. *Psychiatric Clinics of North America*, *10*(4), 541–553. https://doi.org/10.1016/s0193-953x(18)30532-x

Spielman, A. J., & Glovinsky, P. B. (1991). The varied nature of insomnia. In P. J. Hauri (Ed.), *Case studies in insomnia* (pp. 1–15). Springer.

Stepanski, E. J., & Rybarczyk, B. (2006). Emerging research on the treatment and etiology of secondary or comorbid insomnia. *Sleep Medicine Reviews*, *10*(1), 7–18.

Sunnhed, R., Hesser, H., Andersson, G., Carlbring, P., Lindner, P., Harvey, A. G., & Jansson-Fröjmark, M. (2022). Mediators of cognitive therapy and behavior therapy for insomnia disorder: A test of the processes in the cognitive model. *Journal of Consulting and Clinical Psychology*, *90*(9), 696–708.

Sweetman, A., Lovato, N., Micic, G., Scott, H., Bickley, K., Haycock, J., Harris, J., Gradisar, M., & Lack, L. (2020). Do symptoms of depression, anxiety or stress impair the effectiveness of cognitive behavioral therapy for insomnia? A chart-review of 455 patients with chronic insomnia. *Sleep Medicine*, *75*, 401–410. https://doi.org/10.1016/j.sleep.2020.08.023

Taylor, D. J., Lichstein, K. L., & Durrence, H. H. (2003). Insomnia as a health risk factor. *Behavioral Sleep Medicine*, *1*(4), 227–247.

Trauer, J. M., Qian, M. Y., Doyle, J. S., Rajaratnam, S. M., & Cunnington, D. (2015). Cognitive behavioral therapy for chronic insomnia: A systematic review and meta-analysis. *Annals of Internal Medicine*, *163*(3), 191–204. https://doi.org/10.7326/M14-2841

Vallières, A., Ivers, H., Bastien, C. H., Beaulieu-Bonneau, S., & Morin, C. M. (2005). Variability and predictability in sleep patterns of chronic insomniacs. *Journal of Sleep Research*, *14*(4), 447–453. https://doi.org/10.1111/j.1365-2869.2005.00480.x

van de Laar, M., Pevernagie, D., van Mierlo, P., & Overeem, S. (2015). Psychiatric comorbidity and aspects of cognitive coping negatively predict outcome in cognitive behavioral treatment of psychophysiological insomnia. *Behavioral Sleep Medicine*, *13*(2), 140–156. https://doi.org/10.1080/15402002.2013.845781

Van Someren, E. J. W. (2021). Brain mechanisms of insomnia: New perspectives on causes and consequences. *Physiological Reviews*, *101*(3), 995–1046. https://doi.org/10.1152/physrev.00046.2019

Vgontzas, A. N., Fernandez-Mendoza, J., Liao, D., & Bixler, E. O. (2013). Insomnia with objective short sleep duration: The most biologically severe phenotype of the disorder. *Sleep Medicine Reviews*, *17*(4), 241–254. https://doi.org/10.1016/j.smrv.2012.09.005

Vgontzas, A. N., Liao, D., Pejovic, S., Calhoun, S., Karataraki, M., Basta, M., Fernández-Mendoza, J., & Bixler, E. O. (2010). Insomnia with short sleep duration and mortality: The Penn State cohort. *Sleep*, *33*(9), 1159–1164. https://doi.org/10.1093/sleep/33.9.1159

Vgontzas, A. N., Liao, D., Pejovic, S., Calhoun, S., Karataraki, M., & Bixler, E. O. (2009). Insomnia with objective short sleep duration is associated with Type 2 diabetes: A population-based study. *Diabetes Care*, *32*(11), 1980–1985.

Walker, J. L., Vargas, I., Drake, C. L., Ellis, J. G., Muench, A., & Perlis, M. L. (2022). The natural history of insomnia: High sleep reactivity interacts with greater life stress to predict the onset of acute insomnia. *Sleep*, *45*(9), Article zsac149.

Wassing, R., Lakbila-Kamal, O., Ramautar, J. R., Stoffers, D., Schalkwijk, F., & Van Someren, E. J. (2019). Restless REM sleep impedes overnight amygdala adaptation. *Current Biology*, *29*(14), 2351–2358.

Xia, L., Chen, G.-H., Li, Z.-H., Jiang, S., & Shen, J. (2013). Alterations in hypothalamus–pituitary–adrenal/thyroid axes and gonadotropin-releasing hormone in the patients with primary insomnia: a clinical research. *PLOS ONE, 8*(8), Article e71065.

Yang, C.-M., & Lo, H.-S. (2007). ERP evidence of enhanced excitatory and reduced inhibitory processes of auditory stimuli during sleep in patients with primary insomnia. *Sleep, 30*(5), 585–592.

Zwart, C. A., & Lisman, S. A. (1979). Analysis of stimulus control treatment of sleep-onset insomnia. *Journal of Consulting and Clinical Psychology, 47*(1), 113–118.

CHAPTER

27 Insomnia II: Behavioral and Physiological Assessment

Célyne H. Bastien, Jason G. Ellis, Florence Lambert-Beaudet, Alexandre Rudziavic Provençal, *and* Elham Garmroudinezhad-Rostami

Abstract

This chapter is focused on the different assessment methods used to characterize insomnia, complement its evaluation and, enhance diagnostic accuracy. Besides subjective measures, physiological assessment methods, the most popular being polysomnography, are introduced as well as more refined neurophysiological techniques such as quantitative electroencephalography, neuroimaging, and event-related potentials. A table describing the most commonly used techniques of assessments presents the advantages and disadvantages of each of them. In addition, to compare results obtained from individuals suffering from insomnia to those obtained from good sleepers, this chapter provides a review of the most recent literature while, at times, considering that different subtypes of insomnia exist. As such, some references will be made to different subtypes throughout the chapter. This chapter also briefly reports on the use of the different assessment methods in individuals affected by other sleep disorders. Finally, two tables listing influential research studies related to the neurophysiological assessment techniques complete the chapter.

Key Words: insomnia, assessment, subjective sleep, objective sleep, device, polysomnography, power spectral analysis, neuroimaging, event-related potential

Introduction

Although research and clinical guidelines are regularly updated, the assessment of insomnia proves to be challenging. The evaluation and diagnosis of this disorder are based primarily on clinical history (Sateia et al., 2000). As mentioned in this book, insomnia is multidimensional and multifaceted. The *Diagnostic and Statistical Manual of Mental Disorders*, fifth edition (American Psychiatric Association, 2013), now suggests insomnia is not to be considered as a "secondary" disorder and that insomnia as a disorder can be comorbid with another sleep, medical, or psychological/psychiatric disorder or not (*insomnia without comorbidity* [ICW], previously called *primary insomnia*). Still, like many other sleep disorders, insomnia comprises a spectrum of complaints reflecting dissatisfaction with the quality, duration, or efficiency of sleep. Unlike many other sleep disorders (e.g., apnea, rapid-eye-movement [REM] sleep behavior disorder, nocturnal myoclonus), insomnia is first reported by the individual themselves, as the individual is "aware" of their problem. Nonetheless, and contrary to most other sleep disorders, insomnia does not require objective verification. In that regard, several subjective, behavioral, and physiological approaches are available to characterize the disorder, complement its evaluation, and improve diagnostic accuracy. This chapter summarizes the assessment methods available for the evaluation of insomnia, with an emphasis on neurophysiological approaches.

Assessment Methods and Technologies

A detailed clinical history/assessment of the patient's subjective complaint will greatly benefit or even depend on complementary data from more systematic sources such as subjective, behavioral, physiological, and neurophysiological assessments. In Table 27.1, all assessment methods/techniques reviewed throughout this chapter are presented, along with their respective advantages and disadvantages.

The Essential of the Subjective Assessment: The "Sleep Diary"

Sleep-onset insomnia and sleep-maintenance insomnia are typically defined by a latency to sleep onset and/or time awake after sleep onset greater than 30 minutes, with corresponding sleep efficiency lower than 85%. Likewise, early-morning awakening can be operationalized by a complaint of waking up earlier (more than 30 minutes) than desired, with an inability to go back to sleep and before total sleep time (TST) reaches 6.5 hours. These criteria, while largely arbitrary (Lichstein et al., 2003), are useful to quantitatively operationalize the definition of insomnia. In that regard, sleep diary monitoring is an invaluable tool to document the perceived severity of insomnia and to examine treatment progress. Monitoring can be done on paper, by phone in, with an electronic recorder (personal digital assistant [PDA]), or on a computer-accessible secure site. A sleep diary usually requires self-recording of bedtime and arising time for at least 2 consecutive weeks, along with estimates of sleep-onset latency (SOL), number and duration of awakenings, TST, and several indices of sleep quality from the previous night (Krystal et al., 2019). Other indices linked to the severity of sleep difficulties can be derived using estimates provided by the sleep diary. For example, sleep efficiency (SE) can be obtained by dividing TST by total time in bed. Daily morning estimates of sleep parameters such as SOL or wake after sleep onset yield a reliable and valid index of insomnia, even though they do not reflect absolute values obtained from polysomnography (PSG; Coates et al., 1982). By tracking sleep over several consecutive nights, a sleep diary is more likely to capture the night-to-night variability that often characterizes the sleep of individuals with chronic insomnia; as such, it may yield a more representative sample of a patient's sleep than 1 or 2 nights of PSG.

Despite some limitations, the sleep diary remains a standard assessment procedure in insomnia research. When diaries are used with the different subtypes of insomnia, it

Table 27.1 Types of assessments with their advantages and disadvantages

Type of assessment	Type of tools	Advantages	Disadvantages
Subjective measure	Sleep diaries	• Document the perceived severity of insomnia • Monitor treatment progress • Representative sample of a patient's sleep	• Subjective data
	Wrist actigraphy	• Objective data • Unobtrusive measures of rest–activity cycle • Ecological (in the patient's home environment). • Sensitive to treatment effect among individuals with IWC	• Equivocal validity for estimating more discrete variables • Accuracy of the device and validity of the algorithms still need to be improved
Behavioral devices	Sleep assessment Device/ sleep monitoring	• Corresponds relatively well to PSG evaluations	• Underestimates wakefulness
	Switch-activated clock	• Objective measure of sleep latency	• Questionable if it is the inability to produce a behavioral response or the retrieval of consciousness that determines sleep onset
Physiological measures	PSG	• Comprehensive data on sleep continuity and sleep architecture • Detection of other sleep disorders • Identify different subtypes of insomnia • Provide qualitative information about atypical EEG features • Objective data to complement the patient's subjective report • Useful to ascertain the extent of sleep recuperation • Quantify or qualify the effects of the different treatment components • Portable devices are ecological and can provide a sample of sleep from home on multiple days	• Not indicated for routine clinical evaluation of insomnia • In lab recordings may not provide a valid sample of a patient's typical sleep at home

Continued

Table 27.1 *Continued*

Type of assessment	Type of tools	Advantages	Disadvantages
	Nightcap/REMview	• Best when total sleep time, total wake time, and sleep efficiency (percentage) are used as outcomes measures in clinical trials	
	Power spectral analysis	• Distinguish insomnia sufferers from normal sleepers and other psychopathology • Might explain a part of insomnia sufferers' experience	• Has not been linked to the severity of sleep difficulties yet
Neurophysiological measures	Neuroimaging measures	• Noninvasive investigations • Detection of subtle anatomical and morphological changes • Good spatial resolution (CNS abnormalities and EEG activity during sleep) • Clarify the pathophysiology of different sleep disorders and point toward effective treatment strategies • Assess and compare the effects of treatments on brain functions • PET: More accurate measure of whole-brain activity during wakefulness and NREM sleep	• Individuals are required to sleep in an unusual environment • SPECT: Lack of spatial resolution relative to other neuroimaging techniques • Expensive
	Event-related potentials	• Extremely useful to sleep researchers for the daytime assessment of the impact of sleep disruption and the determination of CNS functions during sleep • Complement neuropsychological assessment • Investigate cognitive functions or information processing during wake or sleep • Direct measure and precise timing of cortical arousal and dynamic neural mechanisms • Complementary to behavioral measures in performance studies • Insensitive to language differences (unlike neuropsychological testing)	• Special setup for recordings (e.g., Faraday room) • Specialized, expensive equipment and sophisticated methodology

Note. CNS = central nervous system; EEG = electroencephalography; IWC = insomnia without comorbidity; NREM = non-rapid-eye-movement; PET = positron emission tomography; PSG = polysomnography; SPECT = single-photon-emission computed tomography.

has been shown that the sleep of individuals with psychophysiological insomnia is subject to extensive night-to-night variability and is seemingly unpredictable. In that regard, Vallières et al. (2005) have shown that three types of sleep patterns are usually found among individuals with insomnia: Type 1, 2 bad nights followed by a good night; Type 2, 3 bad nights followed by a good night; and Type 3, unpredictable patterns. Sometimes, sleep unexpectedly improves for individuals with insomnia in a novel environment because the conditioned arousal that prevents sleep in the home is not present. Predictability in patterns has also been confirmed in a clinical population (Laroche et al., 2024).

In treatment studies, the sleep diary is an irreplaceable tool. Not only does it reflect the impact (efficacy) of the treatment (either during its course or pre- to post-comparisons) or some of its components (e.g., with the introduction of sleep restriction, decreased sleep-onset time, or wake after sleep-onset time, increased SE), it can be used to identify if medication or alcohol was used on a given night, if an event was linked to any peculiar sleep difficulties on 1 night, or even if the treated individual complied with treatment procedures (adherence; Krystal et al., 2019). In addition, of all the available measures, the sleep diary is the least expensive.

Behavioral Devices

Several behavioral assessment devices have been designed to obtain more objective and relatively unobtrusive measures of sleep in the patient's home environment. One of them is wrist actigraphy, which is increasingly used in sleep research (see Figure 27.1 for a picture of watches and actigraph) and is considered to have satisfactory reliability with PSG as well as being useful for assessing response to therapy in patients with insomnia (Krystal et al., 2019; Morgenthaler et al., 2007). The actigraph is a small motion sensor device usually worn on the wrist (alternatively, waist or ankle). It records motor activity continuously for longer periods. Thus, it provides the general rest–activity cycle of an individual. Algorithms have been developed to estimate sleep–wake parameters based on the presence (wake) or absence (sleep) of movement. It is recommended to record at least three consecutive 24-hour periods (Littner, Kushida, et al., 2003) in order to obtain valid comparisons with other sleep assessment techniques. Studies with healthy adults have shown that data obtained from this device for global measures of sleep duration and total wake time correlates highly with PSG data. However, the validity of actigraphy is more equivocal for estimating more discrete variables such as SOL, wake after sleep onset, and number of awakenings (Ancoli-Israel et al., 2003). A study by Tonetti et al. (2008), comparing two types of actigraphy, underlines that compared to PSG, sleep onset is the least often reliably scored variable, a great underestimation being observed with actigraphs. The best way to use actigraphy as an assessment for insomnia is to use the combination of TST, SOL, and the number of awakenings (Natale et al., 2009). Pre- and post-treatment actigraphy data comparisons have shown that this device is sensitive to treatment among individuals suffering from ICW (Vallières & Morin, 2003). Even if it is not indicated for

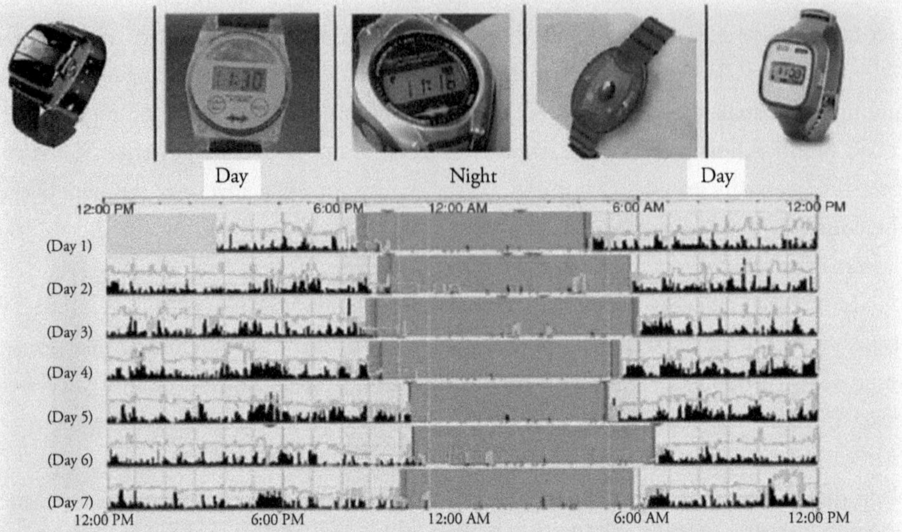

	Start time	End time	Onset latency	Efficiency	WASO	#Wake bouts	Sleep time
DAY 1	11:26:00 PM	6:04:00 AM	22.00	63.24	90.00	31	308.00
DAY 2	11:15:00 PM	6:58:00 AM	21.00	77.94	85.00	33	378.00
DAY 3	9:56:00 PM	5:05:00 AM	15.00	61.22	88.00	31	341.00
DAY 4	11:04:00 PM	6:40:00 AM	3.00	78.45	81.00	26	375.00
DAY 5	1:35:00 AM	8:48:00 AM	37.00	72.41	84.00	34	349.00
DAY 6	12:06:00 AM	8:23:00 AM	18.00	70.93	131.00	49	366.00
DAY 7	11:16:00 PM	6:59:00 AM	2.00	79.32	91.00	38	372.00
Average (n)	*	*	17.60	73.93	97.65	36.49	388.14
Std dev (n–1)	*	*	15.51	6.38	26.57	8.68	46.05

Figure 27.1 Watch and data activity plots

Note. Watches and actigraphs are depicted at the top of the figure. In the middle panel, actigraphy recordings of daytime and nighttime activities are displayed for 7 consecutive days. Finally, data from actigraphy recordings are reported for the individual suffering from insomnia without comorbidity, as shown from the low sleep efficiency (below 85%) and long duration of time spent awake after sleep onset (mean of 97.65 minutes) more than 3 nights a week. Based on Figure 204.8 of the Chapter Assessment of Insomnia, by Perlis, Vargas, Grandner, Bastien, Posner & Spielman (in mem), 2021. Principle and Practices of Sleep Medicine. 7th Edition.

the routine evaluation of insomnia or other sleep disorders, actigraphy still represents a useful addition to other assessment methods (Smith et al., 2018). In a recent systematic review, actigraphy was shown to provide consistent objective data for patients with suspected or diagnosed insomnia (Smith et al., 2018). Also, compared to PSG, the use of actigraphy over several nights has been shown to be a valid indicator of sleep (Withrow et al., 2019). Paquet et al. (2007, p. 1362) pointed out that actigraphy might not be recommended in "clinical populations with fragmented sleep or in situations where the sleep–wake cycle is challenged, such as jet lag and shift work." Smith et al. (2018) in their review also suggested that it is a reliable measure for many sleep disorders and circadian rhythm disorders except periodic limb movement disorders, in both pediatric and adult populations. Overall, the recent literature suggests that actigraphy can detect unique sleep patterns from patients' subjective estimates associated with specific sleep disorders and that it can have as much as 97% accuracy compared to PSG, while not interfering with sleep like PSG could (Sadeh, 2011; Smith et al., 2018; Xu & Lian, 2022). Despite its unobtrusive nature, additional research is necessary to improve the accuracy of this device and the validity of the algorithms.

Physiological Methods

Several physiological methods are available to complement self-reports of sleep complaints. Along with PSG (either in the lab or ambulatory), which remains the gold standard for sleep assessment, autonomic arousal measures can be used to circumscribe the physiological bases of insomnia. These measures are described in this next section.

PSG

A standard (PSG) sleep montage includes electroencephalographic (EEG; minimal central and occipital leads), electro-oculographic (EOG), and electromyographic (EMG) indices (Iber et al., 2007; Rechtschaffen & Kales, 1968). These physiological indices are measured through electrodes applied to the scalp (EEG), around the eyes (EOG), and on the chin (EMG). Signals coming from the electrodes are then amplified, and the data is recorded for later offline analysis. An example of such a signal is depicted in Figure 27.2. Such a montage provides comprehensive data on sleep continuity (sleep latency, time awake after sleep onset, sleep time) and sleep architecture (percentage of time spent in different non-REM (NREM) and REM sleep stages, latency to REM sleep, number of cycles, stage shifts, and awakenings). Additional measures (e.g., airflow, tidal volume, oxygen saturation, and anterior tibialis EMG) are increasingly used by laboratories in order to detect other sleep disorders such as sleep apnea or periodic limb movement disorder. PSG also provides data on effort parameters and body position parameters, as well as on sleep scoring, arousal events, and respiratory events (Iber et al., 2007).

On a day-to-day basis, PSG is not indicated for the routine clinical evaluation of insomnia (Littner, Hirshkowitz, et al., 2003; Reite et al., 1995). Still, it is most useful to rule out the presence of other sleep disorders that might contribute to the insomnia complaint (Riemann, Espie, et al., 2023). In addition, PSG can be particularly helpful if subtypes of insomnia are under study and especially in the case of paradoxical insomnia. For example, our own laboratory has developed a set of diagnostic criteria for this peculiar subtype, criteria that specify that this diagnosis can only be confirmed after subjective–objective discrepancies have been observed following 2 consecutive nights of recording (Bastien, Guimond, et al., 2008). Furthermore, PSG can provide precious qualitative information about atypical EEG features (e.g., alpha–delta sleep) observed in some forms of insomnia. An important limitation of PSG is that it may not provide a valid sample of a patient's typical sleep at home and that only 1 night of recording must be interpreted with caution (Williams et al., 2016). Indeed, the sleep of otherwise good sleepers is more

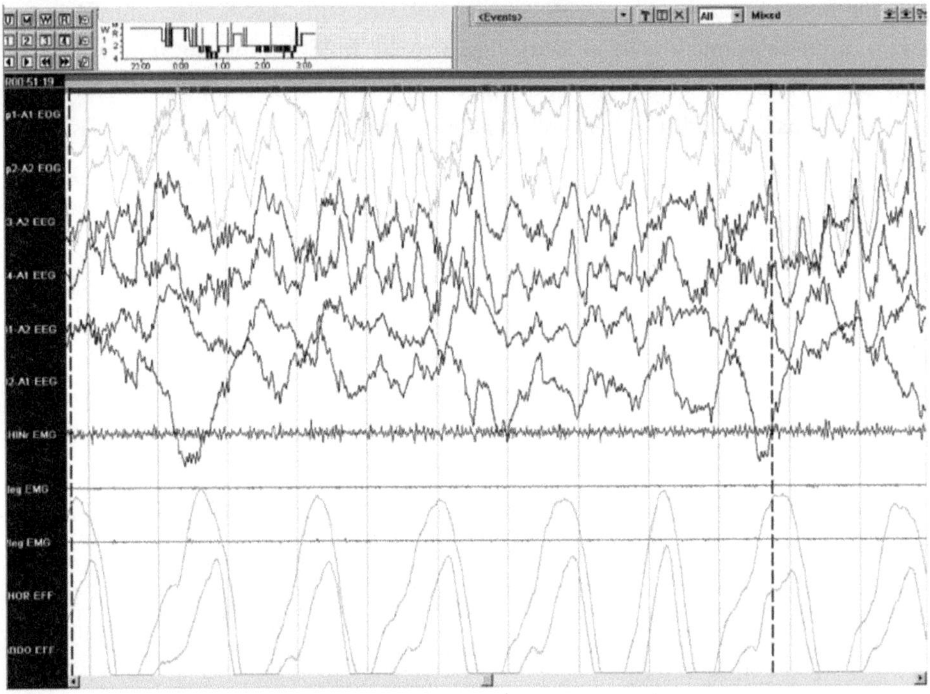

Figure 27.2 Signals (channels) recorded which are often those used for scoring sleep stages and detecting some sleep disorders

Note. In this figure, electro-oculography (EOG) corresponds to Fp1 and Fp2 (left and right eyes, respectively); electroencephalography (EEG) corresponds to C3, C4, O1 and O2; electromyographic (EMG) activity from the right chin (CHINr), left and right tibialis for leg movements (Lleg and Rleg, respectively); thoracic (THOR) and abdominal (ABDO) bands for respiratory efforts. Tibialis and respiratory efforts are used for obtaining indexes for PLMS and apnea/hypopnea. The individual is in Stage S3 (eye movement following the EEG—slow-wave sleep and delta waves; low EMG), and the hypnogram of the night is depicted in the white box at the top of the figure.

disrupted during their first night of recording in the sleep laboratory (i.e., *first-night effect*), whereas the sleep of individuals with insomnia may actually improve in the laboratory (i.e., *reverse first-night effect*). Interestingly, depending on the subtype of insomnia as paradoxical insomnia sufferers do not show a pronounced first-night effect (Saint-Hilaire & Bastien, 2017). For this reason, it is recommended to conduct more than 1 night of PSG to minimize this effect. Also, ambulatory recording may attenuate the effect of the sleep laboratory (Wohlgemuth et al., 1999). It is to be expected that a single night of PSG evaluation will not provide a completely valid sample of a patient's sleep problem. However, it has the incomparable advantage of yielding objective data to complement the patient's subjective report.

PSG is becoming a standard practice in insomnia research. As such, screening PSG is recommended in epidemiological and treatment effectiveness studies, while it is essential in mechanism/evaluation studies as well as in treatment efficacy studies (Buysse et al.,

2006). Insomnia protocols typically conduct 2 or 3 consecutive nights of PSG recordings for pre- and post-treatment comparisons. The first night is usually an adaptation/screening night. Then, a standard sleep montage is used on the second and third nights in the absence of other sleep disorders on the first night. Some laboratories are also beginning to use PSG (either in the lab or ambulatory) at mid-treatment to quantify or qualify the effects of the different treatment components. For example, PSG could be indicated to study the consolidation of sleep after sleep restriction is introduced. Another insomnia research protocol might require sleep deprivation. In this instance, PSG would prove to be most useful to ascertain the extent of sleep recuperation. Several parameters, such as SOL, number and duration of awakenings, and TST, can be used as indicators of insomnia severity or as endpoints in treatment outcome studies. SE, which is recognized as being a very informative indicator of treatment efficacy, is then derived from recorded parameters. Additional PSG information, such as percent of time spent in the different sleep stages and the number of arousals and spontaneous events (e.g., K-Complexes and spindles), may also prove to be useful to complete a basic physiological picture of insomnia complaints.

Modest differences in the macrostructure of sleep are usually observed between insomnia complainers and noncomplainers. Complainers' objective measures reveal that they tend to spend more time in Stage NREM1, spend less time in Stage NREM3, and display more frequent stage shifts through the night (Coates et al., 1982; Hauri & Fisher, 1986; Reynolds et al., 1984). More recently, differences in Stage NREM2 were also observed (Wei et al., 2017), this stage of sleep displaying frequent transitions to lighter sleep (NREM1), which could be indicative of an instability of the EEG of insomnia individuals. Regarding the general microstructure of sleep and phasic events, one study conducted by Wauquier et al. (1995) compared the occurrence of well-defined spontaneous K-Complexes during 5 minutes of both ascending and descending Stage 2 in patients suffering from generalized epilepsy, insomnia, narcolepsy, and obstructive sleep apnea, compared to control participants. The authors observed a lower occurrence of K-Complexes in sleep disordered individuals compared to controls. Although their results were limited to ascending and descending phases of Stage 2 sleep, this group difference may be a true group difference while still restricted to the time during state transition. More recently, our group has compared the occurrence and density of both spontaneous K-Complexes and sleep spindles during Stage 2, subdivided into the early and late portions of the night. Our results showed that the occurrence and density of both phasic events were similar in individuals with psychophysiological insomnia and good sleeper controls (Bastien, St-Jean, Turcotte, Morin, Lavallée, & Carrier, 2009; Bastien, St-Jean, Turcotte, Morin, Lavallée, Carrier, & Forget, 2009). Altogether, results from phasic event studies generally suggest that sleep-protection mechanisms appear intact in individuals with insomnia.

Good sleepers think about sleep only when they lack it. Individuals with insomnia, even if they set everything into motion to facilitate sleep, perceive they do not get enough or any at all. Although some individuals do really have objective low SE, others do not. Perlis et al. (1997) suggest that individuals with insomnia tend to perceive they are awake more often than good sleepers, even when PSG-defined sleep is observed. This difference between the objective (PSG, actigraphy, etc.) and subjective (sleep diary) measures is called *misperception of sleep*, and it can also affect the perceived daytime functioning of these individuals (Means et al., 2003; Semler & Harvey, 2005). In that regard, about 73% of the time individuals with insomnia claim that they are awake when they are in fact sleeping, while only about 45%–50% of the time good sleepers make this claim (Perlis et al., 1997). However, the subjective–objective discrepancy relative to sleep perception varies according to sleep stage, number of study nights, and method of awakening (Perlis et al., 1997). It is also well documented that individuals with insomnia have a tendency to overestimate the time they take to fall asleep and to underestimate their TST in comparison to PSG measures (Bastien et al., 2014; Coates et al., 1982; Crönlein et al., 2019; Means et al., 2003; Tang & Harvey, 2005; Te Lindert et al., 2020). Commonly, it has been reported that individuals with insomnia overestimate their SOL by about 10 to 45 minutes while underestimating their TST by 30 to 45 minutes (Perlis et al., 1997). Conversely, good sleepers are usually quite accurate at estimating their SOL and TST (Perlis et al., 1997). Good sleepers even tend to overestimate their TST (Tang & Harvey, 2005; Van Den Berg et al., 2008). These discrepancies appear to be a function of the sleep setting (home vs. laboratory) and of psychological/personality characteristics (e.g., more discrepancies among depressed subjects; Means et al., 2003). Interestingly, individuals with insomnia taking hypnotics or psychotropic drugs are less likely to say they were awake while they were asleep (Mendelson, 1993, 1995). One might then ask whether individuals with insomnia have "lighter" sleep (i.e., can be more easily awoken by external stimuli such as tones). One study, from Mendelson et al. (1986), compared arousal thresholds in individuals with subjective insomnia and good sleepers by presenting either tones or one's own name while participants were asleep. Surprisingly, the two groups had similar auditory arousal thresholds suggesting that "subjective poor sleep is not necessarily 'light sleep' " (p. 267). Furthermore, in both groups, the auditory arousal threshold was found to be lower for the participant's own name than for tones. This last observation suggests that information processing does occur during sleep, at least to some extent. Another study, by Haynes et al. (1985), also investigated arousal thresholds in individuals with sleep-onset insomnia or paradoxical insomnia and good sleepers. All three groups showed again similar auditory arousal thresholds with the exception that those with sleep-onset insomnia took longer to fall back asleep following the tones than the other two groups. The results from these two studies suggest that arousal thresholds are similar between those with insomnia and good sleepers and that insomnia cannot be explained by differences in arousal threshold.

However, sleep recordings of subjectively defined insomnia sufferers sometime shows significant overlap with that of good sleepers. In this regard, some individuals with insomnia complaints may show better physiological sleep than those without complaints, and, conversely, some good sleepers may show more sleep impairments than those with insomnia during laboratory recordings. These overlaps might explain some of the group discrepancies between objective (PSG) and subjective (diary) measures introduced earlier (i.e., overestimation of time awake and underestimation of sleep time). Another study, by Riemann and colleagues (2010), suggests a model for insomnia that describes hyperarousal as having a role in the pathophysiology of insomnia. In fact, there is significant evidence which indicates that higher levels of hyperarousal during sleep may lead to sleep difficulties and that this is what contributes to symptoms of insomnia. On another note, PSG could lead to helpful data for assessment as it can measure short sleep durations, which has been said to be one of the most biologically severe types of insomnia, due to cortical arousal and activation of the stress system, resulting in a higher risk of hypertension (Vgontzas et al., 2013).

More detailed analyses of the objective–subjective discrepancies have been conducted by researchers by varying the criterion used to define sleep onset and by examining the perception of sleep at different moments during the night. For example, the best concordance between subjective reports and objective measures of SOL is obtained when sleep onset is defined as the first epoch of Stage 2 and followed by 15 minutes of uninterrupted sleep (Hauri & Olmstead, 1983). Coates et al. (1983) reported that a greater percentage of individuals with insomnia claimed to be awake after the first spindle, while a greater percentage of good sleepers reported being drowsy at that time.

The complaint of fatigue is often associated with insomnia. Although some individuals with insomnia report excessive daytime sleepiness, a more thorough investigation reveals that instead of true physiological sleepiness, these individuals characteristically experience mental and physical fatigue. The Multiple Sleep Latency Test (MSLT) is frequently used as a diagnostic tool for many sleep disorders (e.g., excessive daytime sleepiness, apnea). That said, results from the insomnia population remain somewhat equivocal. While some reports indicate that daytime sleepiness appears comparable among individuals with chronic insomnia and good sleepers as observed with findings from the MSLT (Lichstein et al., 1994; Stepanski et al., 1988), others find that individuals with insomnia took longer to fall asleep during the MSLT (Bonnet & Arand, 1995). Nonetheless, excessive daytime sleepiness is more common among individuals with insomnia also suffering from another medical (e.g., pain) or sleep disorders (e.g., periodic limb movements, sleep-related breathing disorders).

Besides PSG, other physiological devices have been designed but have not been extensively used in either clinical or research settings. For example, the Nightcap was initially designed for monitoring the sleep of astronauts during prolonged space flights (Stickgold & Hobson, 1999). This device has two channels, providing ambulatory PSG through a headband monitor, and distinguishes wake, REM sleep, and NREM sleep on the basis of eye movements and body movements. Its successor, a similar device called the REMview, has been used to evaluate treatment response among individuals with insomnia (Kushida et al., 2003). Results from Edinger et al. (2004) suggested that the REMview's performance, compared to that of PSG, actigraphy, and the PDA electronic sleep log, is best when TST, total wake time, and SE (percentage) are used as outcomes measures in clinical trials. Recently, many new devices have been created and advertised to measure sleep. These wearable digital devices (also known as *wearable sleep-trackers* or *personal monitoring devices*) measure sleep 24/7 by extracting information about different biosignals (e.g., heart rate [HR]) but provide little guidance as to how to accurately assess the data they provide. They hold promise but should be used with care in sleep research and clinical sleep medicine as they tend to overestimate sleep duration in normal sleepers, with far worse accuracy in insomnia patients (De Zambotti et al., 2019; Krystal et al., 2019).

Although PSG is the gold standard in sleep research and is indicated to identify most sleep disorders, its application with insomnia remains limited. In addition, current EEG technology may not be sensitive enough to detect subtle brain wave patterns that may account for a subjective sense of wakefulness but are scored as physiological sleep. Studies using spectral analysis (described later) have begun to uncover the physiological basis of subjective sleep perception in insomnia. Other physiological measures, not used routinely in insomnia research, can still provide useful information, especially considering that insomnia has been linked to a general arousal state in those individuals. This is the case of autonomic arousal measures.

Autonomic Arousal Measures

More than 40 years ago, the hypothesis that insomnia individuals were more physiologically aroused than good sleepers was tested with the use of autonomic arousal measures. Several studies have since compared individuals with insomnia and normal sleepers on such measures as well as on cortisol, adrenocorticotropic hormone (ACTH), and melatonin secretion rate, as well as core body temperature.

One of the earliest reports, by Monroe (1967), observed that poor sleepers showed higher vasoconstriction rates and basal skin resistance, a tendency for increased HR and pulse volume, and higher rectal temperatures. In this classic study, between-group differences were observed both at the peri-onset of sleep as well as in sleep. A few years later, a study conducted by Johns et al. (1971) collected urine samples four times a day over a period of 72 hours (morning, afternoon, evening, overnight) from male medical students who were either good or poor sleepers. Those individuals reporting poor sleep exhibited greater adrenocortical secretion during both the day and the night than those self-defined as good sleepers. Another study, by Freedman (1986), observed higher muscle tone and HR and lower finger temperatures at sleep onset and during sleep in those with sleep-onset insomnia compared to controls. Other studies, conducted by Adam et al. (1986) and Bonnet and Arand (1995, 1998), have shown that individuals with insomnia display faster HR, elevated body temperature, higher frontalis and chin muscle tension, increased body movements, and greater basal skin resistance during sleep as well as during the pre-sleep period, compared to controls. During both day and night, Bonnet and Arand (1995) have observed that insomnia was associated with higher levels of metabolic rate. Increased 24-hour cortisol and ACTH secretion, reflecting higher hypothalamic–pituitary–adrenal axis activation, also appear to be present in individuals with chronic insomnia (Vgontzas et al., 2001). Riemann et al. (2002) compared cortisol and melatonin secretion (7:00 p.m. until 9:00 a.m.) in those with ICW and good sleepers. Although individuals with insomnia showed a lower melatonin secretion at all testing times compared to good sleepers, cortisol secretion was similar in both groups. A very recent systematic review and case–control study by Dressle et al. (2022) combining results from 20 studies (449 individuals with insomnia and 357 good sleepers) yielded only a moderately higher level of cortisol in those with insomnia compared to good sleepers.

Increased HR was also observed in individuals with sleep-onset insomnia before and after they were exposed to pre-sleep cognitive stressors (mental arithmetic tasks) on 2 study nights (Haynes et al., 1981). Although HR was similar in both groups on the first experimental night, strangely enough, the good sleepers had an increase in HR following the stressor on the second experimental night. In addition, increased sleep latency was observed in good sleepers, while decreased sleep latency was observed in individuals with insomnia. It is possible that the stressor acted as a disrupter to the rumination reported by those with insomnia, thus allowing them to fall asleep more quickly (Haynes et al., 1981). In 2011, Spiegelhalder and colleagues observed that while a lower reduction in wake to sleep HR was observed in individuals with insomnia, compared to good sleepers, resting state HR was similar between groups. Based on these results, the authors suggest that it is possible that increased rates in cardiovascular morbidity and mortality usually associated with insomnia might be mediated by a lower wake-to-sleep HR reduction and alterations in HRV variables. More recently, observing contradictory results in HR studies involving those with insomnia, Dodds et al. (2017) conducted a review to shed some light on the HR activity in this group of patients. Their systematic review revealed that the heightened HR variability in insomnia individuals compared to good sleepers was not supported by empirical evidence and that more longitudinal studies were needed.

Generally, cross-sectional studies suggest that autonomic arousal is more elevated in individuals with insomnia than in good sleepers. Whether arousal is a consequence or cause of insomnia, however, remains to be determined.

Neurophysiological Methods

Several neurophysiological methods are available to quantify or qualify sleep complaints. Quantitative techniques such as power spectral analysis (PSA) and high-resolution brain assessment techniques such as event-related potentials (ERPs) and neuroimaging are used to examine the neurophysiological bases of insomnia. These techniques are expensive, time-consuming, and require specialized equipment as well as qualified technicians specially trained to operate the equipment and interpret the results. Therefore, they are not used routinely for diagnostic purposes, but they can be useful to corroborate sleep complaints and specify cortical activation in individuals with insomnia. Selected research studies on PSA are presented in Table 27.2, while studies pertaining to ERPs and neuroimaging are presented in Table 27.3.

Quantitative EEG: PSA

Since PSG could not explain why only half of individuals with insomnia differed from controls in terms of TST, SOL, and other traditional PSG variables, attention has focused on quantitative EEG (QEEG), a finer grained measure of EEG. Although the techniques employed in QEEG are not diagnostic or routine clinical tools, they have been used in research for decades. QEEG is most often used to study brain changes related to Alzheimer's, Parkinson's, migraines, and epilepsy (Caviness et al., 2015; Ferreira et al., 2016). An increasing number of researchers find this method useful in the diagnosis of attention-deficit/hyperactivity disorder (Barry et al., 2007; Ochojska et al., 2021); various mental dysfunctions, including depressive and schizophrenic syndromes (Walkowiak, 2015; Wiśniewska et al., 2016); and addictions (Verrusio et al., 2015). More interestingly, they have been shown to be useful in supporting clinical observations in insomnia, and it is in this perspective that PSA, the most often used QEEG, is presented in the following section.

From EEG recordings, it is possible to apply techniques aimed at describing the microstructure of sleep. As such, PSA is performed by computing Fast Fourier transforms (FFTs), which reveals the frequency and amplitude of the sine wave constituents in the analyzed portion of the EEG. Results are pooled by averaging the data in specified frequency bands, usually defined as slow waves (0–1 Hz), delta (1–4 Hz), theta (4–7 Hz), alpha (7–11 Hz), sigma (11–14 Hz), beta1 (14–20 Hz), beta2 (20–35 Hz), gamma (35–60 Hz), and omega (60–125 Hz). The results of the FFT tell us about the power (square microvolts), which corresponds to the square of the amplitude, in each of the specified frequency bands. Data may be presented as such (absolute power) or as the proportion of the power in a frequency band relative to the sum of the power in all frequency bands (relative power). PSA values can be related to the degree of cortical activation in a way that elevated powers in fast frequency bands reflect increased activity, whereas an increase in a slower band presupposes less activity.

Table 27.2 Studies on power spectral analysis

Authors	Year	Objective	Participants	Methods	Sleep stages studied	Results	Interpretation
Studies comparing insomnia sufferers to controls							
Hall et al.	2007	To evaluate relationships between psychological stress, sleep, and physiological arousal in IWC	• 30 chronic IWC (18 women, 12 men), mean age 30.2 (8.6) years	• 3 PSG recording nights in laboratory • Recordings at central and occipital bilateral sites • Computation of relative powers in the delta and beta bands	Stages 1–4	Higher levels of perceived stress correlated with decreased delta power and increased beta power	Stress is associated with QEEG measures of arousal

Krystal et al.	2002	To study the relationship of NREM frequency spectral indexes with sleep time underestimation and to compare subjective and objective IWC subtypes with normal controls	• 30 IWC, sleep maintenance insomnia only (18 women, 12 men), mean age 54.9 (10.4) years
			  • 18 objective IWC
			  • 12 subjective IWC
			• 20 healthy subjects (12 women, 8 men), mean age 53.5 (10.4) years
				• Single night of ambulatory PSG recording
				• PSA at C3 on epochs free of movements, artifacts, arousals, or transitions between stages
				• Computation of absolute and relative powers
					NREM and REM of the entire night	• Subjective IWC presented lower delta and greater alpha, sigma, and beta NREM EEG activity compared to controls	Diminished delta and increased alpha, sigma, and beta EEG relative spectral powers correlate with sleep complaints

Lamarche & Ogilvie	1997	To compare psychophysiological insomnia sufferers, psychiatric insomnia sufferers, and controls on PSA at the SOP	• 6 psychophysiological insomnia sufferers (3 women, 3 men), mean age 27.8 (10.3) years • 6 psychiatric insomnia sufferers (one or more elevation [>1 SD] at the MMPI-2; 3 women, 3 men), mean age 31.5 (10.2) years • 6 controls (4 women, 2 men), mean age 27.8 (9.6) years	• 2 consecutive nights of laboratory PSG recording • PSA on data of both nights at SOP • Computation of absolute and relative powers for each quartile of SOP	SOP: wake, Stages 1 and 2	• Less alpha in the first part of SOP, less delta in the last quartile, and higher relative beta during wakefulness in psychophysiological insomnia sufferers compared to the other groups	Psychophysiological insomnia sufferers have higher cortical arousal than controls and psychiatric insomnia sufferers at SOP

Continued

Table 27.2 *Continued*

Authors	Year	Objective	Participants	Methods	Sleep stages studied	Results	Interpretation
Merica et al.	1998	To determine if spectral characteristics of insomnia sufferers differ from healthy subjects	• 20 IWC (12 women, 8 men; 17 psychophysiological, 3 idiopathic), mean age 30.2 (10.9) years • 19 healthy subjects (10 women, 9 men), mean age 25.3 (4.0) years	• 3 nights of PSG recordings • PSA on Night 2 at F4 • Computation of relative power	First four complete NREM–REM cycles	• In NREM, IWC presented higher levels of beta power and lower levels below the beta band • IWC presented lower levels in the delta and theta bands in REM • Delayed delta peak in IWC	IWC is characterized by a slow-wave deficiency and excessive hyperarousal
Perlis, Kehr, et al.	2001	To evaluate in terms of cycle, stage, and time elapsed from sleep onset the temporal distribution of beta activity	Mean age: 37.5 (10.7) years, 66% female: 1. IWC (n = 9) 2. Insomnia comorbid to major depressive disorder (n = 9) 3. Good sleepers (n = 9)	• Minimum of 2 nights of PSG recordings • PSA on Night 1 • Computation of relative powers: mean values by site	Stages 1 and 2, SWS and REM for Sleep Cycles 1–3	• IWC presented the highest levels of beta1, beta2, and gamma activity and the lowest levels of omega activity • In Stages 1 and 2, IWC presented more beta1 • In REM and SWS, IWC presented more beta2 • In Stage 2 and SWS, IWC presented more gamma activity	Results support the hyperactivation theory of insomnia
Perlis, Smith, et al.	2001	To evaluate the high-frequency activity found in IWC around sleep onset and NREM sleep, its possible association with subjective and PSG estimates, and the difference between comorbid and not insomnia	Mean age: 37.5 (10.7) years, 66% female: 1. IWC (n = 9) 2. Insomnia comorbid with major depressive disorder (n = 9) 3. Good sleepers (n = 9)	• Minimum of 2 nights of PSG recordings • PSA on Night 1 • Computation of mean beta relative powers	NREM of Cycles 1–3	• IWC presented more beta1, beta2, and gamma activity compared to comorbid insomnia and controls • More beta activity is associated with larger discrepancies between objective and subjective TST	• For IWC supports difficulty in disengaging from cognitive processes around sleep onset and during NREM sleep • High-frequency EEG interferes with sleep quantity and quality perception

Studies implying treatment for insomnia							
Bastien et al.	2003	To compare sleep microstructure of older adults suffering from chronic insomnia, using BZ on a usual basis or medication-free, and good sleepers.	• 15 IWC using BZ (8 women, 7 men), mean age 30.2 (10.9) years • 15 IWC drug-free (7 women, 8 men), mean age 30.2 (10.9) years • 16 self-defined good sleepers (7 women, 9 men), mean age 25.3 (4.0) years	• 3 PSG recording nights in laboratory • PSA at C3 on Night 2 only • Computation of absolute powers	NREM of the first 4 sleep cycles	• In IWC BZ use showed less delta power in Cycles 2 and 3, less theta power in Cycles 1–3, more beta1 activity in Cycles 3 and 4, and less delta and theta activity in Stage 2 compared to controls • In IWC BZ use had lower delta and theta levels in Cycle 2, higher beta1 level in Cycle 4, and lower theta level in Stage 2 compared to drug-free IWC	BZ use does not normalize sleep of insomnia sufferers
Cervena et al.	2004	To evaluate modifications in PSG and sleep EEG power densities after 8 weeks of CBT-I	• 9 psychophysiological IWC (7 women, 2 men), mean age 47 (9.7) years	• 2 PSG recording nights in laboratory at baseline and after treatment • PSA at C3 on the second night of baseline and after treatment • Computation of absolute and relative powers	N/A	After treatment, absolute and relative slow-wave activity in NREM increased, theta and alpha bands increased in absolute power but decreased in relative power, sigma and beta decreased in relative power; in REM, absolute beta power increased	CBT-I has an effect on CNS hyperarousal during sleep and reinforces the cortical synchronization and sleep pressure to maintain sleep longer

Continued

Table 27.2 *Continued*

Authors	Year	Objective	Participants	Methods	Sleep stages studied	Results	Interpretation
Jacobs et al.	1993	To evaluate the effects of a behavioral intervention for insomnia on CNS activity in sleep-onset insomnia sufferers	• 12 IWC (7 women, 5 men), mean age 37.8 (9.1) years • 14 normal sleepers (PSG SOL ≤15 minutes; 9 women, 5 men), mean age 36.9 (7.4) years	• 2 nights of ambulatory PSG recording at a 1-week interval, pre- and post-treatment • PSA on data of Night 2 • Computation of relative powers	Wake (eyes open and closed) and Stage 1	• IWC had greater beta percent total power in the beta range in the eye closed condition at pre-test • At post-treatment, this variable was significantly lower in IWC but still higher compared to the control group	Multifactor behavioral intervention may reduce pre-sleep CNS arousal

Note. BZ = benzodiazepines; CBT-I = cognitive behavioral therapy for insomnia; CNS = central nervous system; EEG = electroencephalography; IWC = insomnia without comorbidity; MMPI = Minnesota Multiphasic Personality Inventory; N/A = not available; NREM = non-rapid-eye-movement; PSA = power spectral analysis; PSG = polysomnography; QEEG = quantitative electroencephalography; REM = rapid eye movement; SD = standard deviation; SOL = sleep onset latency; SOP = sleep onset period; SWS = slow-wave sleep; TST = total sleep time.

Table 27.3 Studies on event-related potentials and neuroimaging

Authors	Year	Objective	Participants	Methods	Sleep stages studied	Results	Interpretation
Studies comparing insomnia sufferers to controls							
Smith et al.	2002	To provide preliminary data on regional cerebral activity in subjects with IWC compared to good sleeper controls	• 5 IWC (all women), mean age 37.8 (12.1) years • 4 good sleepers (all women), mean age 34.5 (11.9)	• 3 PSG recording nights in laboratory: Night 1 = adaptation to PSG, Night 2 = PSG evaluation, Night 3 = PSG + SPECT scan	First NREM sleep cycle	• IWC showed a pattern of decreased rCBF over all regions; the largest and most significant reductions compared to good sleepers are localized in the basal ganglia, the frontal medial cortex, the occipital cortex, and the parietal cortex	Contradicts the hyperarousal theory of insomnia; IWC might be associated with abnormal CNS activity during NREM sleep
Nofzinger et al.	2004	To investigate the neurobiological basis of poor sleep and daytime fatigue in insomnia	• 7 IWC (4 women, 3 men), mean age 34.2 (8.9) years • 20 healthy subjects (13 women, 7 men), mean age 32.6 (8.4) years	• 3 nights of PSG recording: Night 1 = adaptation to PSG, Night 2 = PSG evaluation + PET scan during the morning, Night 3 = PSG + PET scan	Wake and NREM sleep	IWC showed increased global cerebral glucose metabolism compared with control subjects during both waking and NREM sleep, a smaller decrease in relative metabolism from wakefulness to NREM sleep, and reduced relative metabolism in the prefrontal cortex while awake	IWC is associated with greater brain metabolism; daytime fatigue may reflect decreased activity in the prefrontal cortex resulting from inefficient sleep

Continued

Table 27.3 *Continued*

Authors	Year	Objective	Participants	Methods	Sleep stages studied	Results	Interpretation
Kay et al.	2019	To examine the effects of acute sleep restriction on cerebral glucose metabolism during NREM sleep in IWC when compared to good sleepers	• 17 IWC (11 women, 6 men), mean age 40 (7) years • 19 good sleepers (9 women, 10 men), mean age 36 (9) years	• Acute sleep restriction protocol for 1 night • 2 NREM PET scans in laboratory • 4 nights of PSG in laboratory	NREM	Lack of reduction in global glucose metabolism in the brain during recovery NREM sleep when compared to good sleepers	Sleep restriction may not increase global sleep drive processes but might increase more regional sleep drive processes
Drummond et al.	2013	To compare neural correlates of performance during working memory tasks in IWC to good sleepers	• 25 IWC (12 women, 13 men), mean age 32.2 (7.2) years • 25 good sleepers (12 women, 13 men), mean age 32.4 (7.1) years	• 2 nights of PSG in the laboratory • 1 fMRI scan while completing an *n*-back task		Lower deactivation of the middle frontal gyrus, posterior cingulate, and orbital frontal gyrus when increasing task difficulty for IWC	Incapacity to deactivate the default mode network may cause lower working memory performance
Huang et al.	2012	To examine the functional connectivity of the amygdala in IWC	• 10 IWC • 10 good sleepers	• 1 resting state MRI scan • 1 fMRI scan		• Decreased functional connectivity between the amygdala and insula, striatum, and thalamus • Increased functional connectivity between the amygdala and the premotor cortex as the sensorimotor cortex • Positive correlation of the connectivity between the amygdala and the premotor cortex and the total PSQI score	• Supports the hypothesis of a dysfunctional emotional circuit • Seems to cause an adaptive response to a perceived internal threat

Winkelman et al.	2008	To assess GABA levels in IWC	• 8 IWC (8 women), mean age 37.3 (8.1) years • 16 good sleepers (7 women, 9 men), mean age 37.6 (4.5) years	• Actigraphy • PSG • ^{1}H-MRS	Wake	• Average GABA level is about 30% lower in IWC when compared to good sleepers	• Lower GABA levels support the hyperarousal model • Seems to lead to an incapacity to regulate cortical arousal
Devoto et al.	2003	To evaluate the hyperarousal hypothesis while controlling for the quality of sleep in the preceding night	• 11 IWC (7 women, 4 men), mean age 22 (4) years • 11 good sleepers (5 women, 6 men), mean age 21 (1) years	• P300 recorded in the laboratory in the morning after a good night and a bad night of sleep	Wake	-In IWC P300 amplitude is significantly higher after a bad night and lower after a good night compared to good sleepers	Supports the hyperarousal theory; hyperarousal in IWC is not a stable individual characteristic but is associated with the poor quality of nocturnal sleep
Sforza & Haba-Rubio	2006	To investigate if pre-sleep to post-sleep ERPs differ in insomnia sufferers and whether these changes are affected by the severity of subjective and objective sleep alterations	• 15 psychophysiological IWC (10 women, 5 men), mean age 43.5 (9.4) years • 13 healthy subjects (7 women, 6 men) mean age 40.2 (6.4) years	• 2 nights of PSG recordings: Night 1 = adaptation to PSG, Night 2 = PSG evaluation • ERPs before going to bed on Night 2 and after waking up in the morning	Wake	• No differences between groups for N1, P2, or P3 amplitude • One negative significant correlation between a smaller N1 in the morning relative to that seen pre-sleep with the amount of Stage 1 sleep, the number of stage changes, and the number of awakenings during the night in the insomnia group	Factors other than sleep alterations might affect ERPs

Continued

Table 27.3 *Continued*

Authors	Year	Objective	Participants	Methods	Sleep stages studied	Results	Interpretation
Yang & Lo	2007	To examine the processing of auditory information during sleep in insomnia sufferers through the recording of ERPs during different sleep stages	• 15 IWC (9 women, 6 men), mean age 35.3 (12.4) years • 15 good sleepers (10 women, 5 men), mean age 34.3 (12.9) years	• 2 nights of PSG recordings: Night 1 = adaptation to PSG, Night 2 = PSG evaluation + ERPs during the night	All sleep stages	IWC showed larger N1 and smaller P2 to rare tones and smaller N350 to standard tones than controls during the first 5 minutes of continuous Stage 2 sleep	Supports the hyperactivation theory of insomnia
Bastien, St-Jean et al.	2008	To compare ERPs in chronic psychophysiological insomnia sufferers without comorbidities and good sleepers during multiple recordings	• 15 psychophysiological IWC (5 women, 10 men), mean age 46.3 (7.6) years • 16 good sleepers (10 women, 6 men), mean age 36.8 (10.2) years	• 4 nights of PSG recordings: Night 1 = adaptation, Night 2 = PSG evaluation, Nights 3–4 = ERPs recorded in the evening and upon awakening, with sleep-onset recordings on Night 4	Wake and sleep onset	• The amplitude of N1 was larger in IWC than good sleepers in the morning and the evening; while the amplitude of N350 was larger in good sleepers than in IWC at sleep onset, the amplitude of P2 was greater in IWC than in GS at that time	Supports the hyperactivation theory of insomnia; greater cortical arousal in psychophysiological insomnia especially in the morning; difficulties disengaging from wake processes and some inability at initiating normal sleep processes in IWC compared to good sleepers

Studies implying treatment for insomnia							
Smith et al.	2005	To evaluate whether behavior therapy might be associated with normalization in brain function	• 4 IWC (all women), mean age 34.5 (12) years.	• SPECT scan during NREM sleep before and after behavior therapy	NREM sleep	• IWC showed a significant increase in CBF in the basal ganglia after treatment	In IWC, sleep therapy may be associated with a reversal in cerebral deactivation (see Smith et al., 2002)
Altena et al.	2008	To investigate functional brain activation in insomnia and the modifications after non-medicated sleep therapy	• 21 IWC (17 women, 4 men), mean age 61 (6.2) years • 12 healthy controls • (9 women, 3 men), mean age 60 (8.2) years	• fMRI scanning during the performance of a category and a letter fluency task • Sleep therapy for 6 weeks		IWC showed less activation than controls in certain regions during the performance of both tasks; after treatment, the activation was restored in both tasks	Insomnia interferes in a reversible way with activation of the prefrontal cortex during daytime task performance

Note. CNS = central nervous system; ERPs = event-related potentials; fMRI = functional magnetic resonance imaging; GABA = gamma-aminobutyric acid; ^{1}H-MRS = proton magnetic resonance spectroscopy; IWC = insomnia without comorbidity; NREM = non-rapid-eye-movement; PET = positron emission tomography; PSG = polysomnography; PSQI = Pittsburgh Sleep Quality Inventory; rCBF = regional cerebral blood flow; SPECT = single-photon-emission computed tomography.

PSA PARTICULARITIES IN INDIVIDUALS WITH INSOMNIA

Sleep-Onset Period

The model of insomnia that suggested a conditioned aroused state at bedtime (see Perlis et al., 1997, for a neurocognitive model of insomnia) inspired many authors to perform PSA during the sleep-onset period (SOP). It was found that during wakefulness, individuals with insomnia have significantly more beta activity and less alpha activity than normal sleepers, translating into higher activation in the former group (Freedman, 1986). In individuals with IWC and sleep-maintenance IWC, this higher beta activity continues during sleep onset (Merica et al., 1998 [see Table 27.2 for more details on this study]; Merica & Gaillard, 1992), although less delta activity was found in sleep-maintenance insomnia (Merica & Gaillard, 1992). Therefore, the hypothesis of cortical hyperarousal at bedtime, when those with insomnia are subject to rumination, is supported by research findings in individuals with sleep-onset or sleep-maintenance difficulties.

As for individuals with psychophysiological insomnia, compared to normal sleeper controls and individuals with insomnia and psychiatric conditions, they show less delta absolute power at the end of the SOP and therefore seem more cortically activated. Furthermore, less deactivation, expressed by stable alpha levels, is found in individuals with psychophysiological insomnia across the SOP, preventing them from falling asleep. Moreover, higher relative beta activity (i.e., higher activation) is present during wakefulness in individuals with psychophysiological insomnia compared to the other groups. Altogether, these results converge toward higher cortical arousal in individuals with psychophysiological insomnia at the SOP (Lamarche & Ogilvie, 1997; see Table 27.2).

Sleep Period

Higher beta activity is maintained during Stage 1 and REM sleep of individuals with sleep-onset insomnia compared to good sleepers (Freedman, 1986). In IWC, elevated beta1 activity is found in Stages 1 and 2, elevated beta2 activity in REM and slow-wave sleep (SWS), and finally elevated gamma activity in Stage 2 and SWS (Perlis, Kehr, et al., 2001; see Table 27.2). Those suffering from IWC show increased beta activity in REM and NREM as well as lower levels of power in frequency bands below the beta band in NREM. Much less attention has been dedicated to frequency bands below beta. First, cortical hyperarousal may be characterized not just by beta activity but also by activity in higher and lower frequency bands. Second, lower delta activity in individuals with insomnia may indicate decreased hyperpolarization of thalamocortical neurons during NREM sleep. However, because patients with insomnia have less N3 (dominated by delta activity; Baglioni et al., 2014), lower delta activity during NREM sleep may possibly be connected to the ratio of N3 and N2 during the NREM period analyzed (Zhao et al., 2021). In REM, individuals with insomnia present lower power in the delta and theta bands. Thus, individuals with IWC are characterized by a slow-wave deficiency and excessive hyperarousal (Merica et al., 1998). Such changes may coexist with either decreased thalamocortical hyperpolarization during N3 or a shorter duration of N3 relative to N2 during the NREM period (Zhao et al., 2021).

Higher beta activity in IWC is a recurrent result that indubitably translates into higher activation, but does it have other implications? It appears that more beta activity is associated with larger discrepancies between objective and subjective TST (Perlis, Smith, et al., 2001; see Table 27.2). Having higher beta activity during sleep would induce the impression of being awake, and sleep misperception is mostly associated with subjective/paradoxical insomnia. Indeed, in individuals with subjective insomnia, decreased delta and increased alpha, sigma, and beta relative spectral powers correlate with sleep complaints (Krystal et al., 2002; see Table 27.2). Higher levels of perceived stress are also associated with higher cortical activity expressed by decreased delta power and increased beta power in NREM of individuals with chronic insomnia (Hall et al., 2007; for more details on this study, see Table 27.2).

Wake

Congruent with what was found during the SOP and sleep, more beta and less alpha activity are found in individuals with insomnia with sleep-onset difficulties compared to controls (Freedman, 1986). A majority of studies have shown higher-frequency power in the beta and gamma range (Colombo et al., 2016; Corsi-Cabrera et al., 2016; Kwan et al., 2018; Wolynczyk-Gmaj & Szelenberger, 2011). In those with insomnia, after a 20-minute period of auditory ERP recordings, a decrease in delta power was observed while an increase was found in normal sleeper controls. In addition, beta power increased more in those with insomnia than in controls. Again, individuals with insomnia presented a higher level of cortical activity (Kronholm et al., 2007). However, results were affected by the fatigue induced by the ERP task, and distinctions between groups' raw scores were unknown. EEG information obtained during resting-state wakefulness revealed co-occurring increases in theta activity, which have been linked to daytime sleepiness. Individuals with insomnia appear to have considerable and robust declines in delta power during NREM sleep. Thus, insomnia disorders may be caused by abnormal activation of wake-promoting and sleep-promoting brain regions during the day and at night (Zhao et al., 2021).

IMPACT OF SLEEP-PROMOTING MEDICATION

Researchers have investigated the effect of hypnotics on PSA in those with insomnia. Benzodiazepine users, compared to controls, are more activated since they present less delta power in Cycles 2 and 3, less theta power in Cycles 1–3, more beta1 activity in Cycles 3 and 4, and less delta and theta activity in Stage 2. Compared to drug-free individuals with insomnia, benzodiazepine users are again more activated as shown by the lower delta and theta levels in Cycle 2, a higher beta1 level in Cycle 4, and a lower theta level in Stage 2. These results suggest that benzodiazepine use does not normalize sleep microstructure (Bastien et al., 2003; see Table 27.2 for more details). Benzodiazepine users showed significantly increased sigma activity and decreased delta and theta activity during the night compared to good sleepers (Manconi et al., 2017; Marzano et al., 2008; Poyares et al., 2004). However, medication status had a substantial effect on theta activity only during wakefulness (Zhao et al., 2021).

As for zolpidem, a short-acting nonbenzodiazepine hypnotic, it increases the power density in the delta band, therefore decreasing cerebral activity, in individuals with insomnia (Declerck et al., 1992; Monti et al., 2000). Zolpidem suppressed power in the theta and alpha bands (4–11.0 Hz). Power density was also enhanced within the sigma frequency range at 11.5–15.0 Hz (1-Hz bins data; Lundahl et al., 2012). Other classes of medication, such as selective serotonin reuptake inhibitors, have also been studied in insomnia by means of PSA (e.g., Nowell et al. 1999). Nevertheless, not all research concludes that changes occur in the sleep microstructure of individuals with insomnia when medication is taken. In addition, the observed changes are not significantly related to objective and subjective sleep improvements. Microarchitectural changes also remain to be documented in conjunction with dual orexin receptor antagonists, this new class of medication for insomnia targeting orexin (Muench et al. 2022).

IMPACT OF A NON-MEDICATION TREATMENT ON PSA

Whereas studies have failed to find consistent signs of sleep quality improvements in the PSA of individuals with insomnia using sleep aids, other treatments have been shown to be effective at reducing high EEG activity. Jacobs et al. (1993; see Table 27.2) studied the effect of a multifactor behavioral intervention for insomnia. They observed individuals with insomnia had greater beta power in wake prior to treatment. However, at post-treatment, the beta activity was significantly lower but still higher compared to a healthy control group. They concluded that the intervention may reduce pre-sleep central nervous system (CNS) arousal. Furthermore, Cervena et al. (2004) evaluated the impact of a cognitive behavioral therapy for insomnia (CBT-I) as described in Table 27.2. At post-treatment, in NREM, absolute and relative slow-wave activity powers increased, theta and alpha bands increased in absolute power but decreased in relative power, and sigma as well as beta decreased in relative power. In REM, only absolute beta power increased. These signs of reduced activity led the authors to suggest that CBT-I has an effect on CNS hyperarousal during sleep and reinforces cortical synchronization and sleep pressure to maintain sleep longer. These promising results may explain why improvements from non-medication treatment tend to last longer than those made from hypnotics and could inspire future research.

Kwan et al. (2022) evaluated the effect of a neurofeedback protocol for reducing cortical arousal in those with insomnia compared to CBT-I. The neurofeedback group showed decreases in beta waves and increases in theta and alpha waves in various areas of the EEG, indicating lower cortical arousal. This study confirmed that neurofeedback training could alleviate some insomnia symptoms by reducing cortical hyperarousal in patients, despite the limited effect in reducing cognitive dysfunction compared to CBT-I (Kwan et al., 2022).

PSA studies in insomnia, however, have limits. Among technical issues, the sample size is sometimes small, some studies use ambulatory devices and others laboratory recordings, the recording sites are often limited to C3, the analyzed period does not cover the entire night, and, in some cases, it might include arousals or artifacts. Also, the definition of the frequency bands slightly varies across studies. Moreover, the inclusion and exclusion criteria for those with insomnia differ (e.g., some studies recruiting only those with sleep-onset or -maintenance insomnia), making comparisons between studies more challenging.

Nonetheless, PSA appears to distinguish those with insomnia from normal sleepers and those with other psychopathologies. It further supports the hypothesis of a difficulty for those with insomnia in disengaging from cognitive processes near sleep onset and during NREM sleep. Consequently, a high level of EEG activity is maintained throughout the night and, in turn, translates into misperception of sleep quantity and reports of poor sleep quality. The relation between high cortical activity and sleep misperception illustrates that, combined with subjective sleep measures, PSA might explain a part of the individual's experience of insomnia. As such, further studies are needed to clarify the origins and consequences of the elevated cortical activity in insomnia as well as the other possible contributing factors (laboratory environment, stress, depression symptoms, etc.). PSA in other sleep disorders, such as sleep apnea (Dumont et al., 2007; El-Mekkawy et al., 2022; Greneche et al. 2008; Mullins et al., 2021), narcolepsy (Ferri et al., 2005; Kathami et al., 2007), or restless legs syndrome (Hornyak et al., 2005), have also been studied; and comparisons with insomnia may enhance our comprehension and differentiation of these disorders and of the individuals' sleep complaints. PSA might also be a useful tool to automate PSG sleep stage scoring; work to this effect has already been conducted using animal models (Kohtoh et al., 2008).

PSA can also be useful to study another component of sleep which is often not adequately described in objective studies: sleep quality. This concept is often measured as the number of arousals, NREM Stages N1 and N3, while we know that the duration of N1 (and its percentage) has increased with the American Academy of Sleep Medicine (AASM) scoring criteria (Iber et al. 2007). In fact, the AASM requirement to change NREM sleep stage to NREM1 following an arousal all but invalidates NREM1 time as a measure of sleep depth. Because of this rule, NREM1 time adds little beyond the arousal index; there is an excellent correlation between NREM1 percentage and the arousal index (Qanash et al., 2017). Interscorer agreements are also the lowest for all NREM stages (Younes et al., 2018). Odds ratio products (ORPs) are derived from PSA, range from 0 to 2.5 (deepest sleep to wake scores), and are indexes of objective sleep quality as they reflect the depth of sleep within each 30-second epoch of all sleep stages (Younes et al., 2015, 2022). In fact, they have been shown to be very reliable and able to differentiate between patterns of sleep apnea to quantify severity while linking the ORP index to clinical outcomes (Penner et al., 2019). Furthermore, there might be two phenotypes in short-sleep duration insomnia (Younes et al., 2022), the most detrimental insomnia phenotype according to some authors (Vgontzas, Liao, Bixler, et al., 2009; Vgontzas, Liao, Pejovic, et al., 2009; Vgontzas et al., 2010, 2013). Understanding sleep quality on a depth scale is much more devoted to the understanding of clinical profiles than gross PSG recordings. As part of the artificial intelligence (AI) era, ORPs might be the next generation of indexes which will be needed to disentangle the subjective and objective sleep of individuals with insomnia, linking both to clinical outcomes.

Neuroimaging Measures

The development of neuroimaging measures has provided an important tool for non-invasive investigation allowing for the detection of subtle anatomical or morphological changes associated with sleep disorders. These techniques, while not providing the temporal resolution of QEEG, can provide a better spatial resolution to identify CNS abnormalities and to examine the relationship between EEG activity and changes in activity within cortical and subcortical areas of the brain during sleep. Some preliminary studies of diverse sleep disorders have suggested that neuroimaging methods have the potential to clarify brain function and the pathophysiology of insomnia in a manner not accessible to PSG, as well as to point us toward effective treatment strategies. However, up to now, there have been very few neuroimaging studies specific to those with insomnia due to methodological difficulties that can limit the use of these techniques. It can be quite challenging to catch clinical manifestations of sleep disorders during the scanning session since they are often unpredictable, variable, and transient. Moreover, the individuals are often required to sleep in a very unusual environment (the scanner) while the experimenter tries to capture tomographs during sleep or during specific sleep stages. Nonetheless, some studies have recently been conducted using neuroimaging techniques.

SINGLE-PHOTON EMISSION COMPUTED TOMOGRAPHIC METHOD

The single-photon emission computed tomographic (SPECT) method allows the visualization of cerebral metabolism by analyzing the signal emitted by a short-lived radioactive tracer injected intravenously before scanning. This technique was used in order to assess cerebral activity during the first NREM cycle among individuals with insomnia. It was found that those individuals, compared to good sleepers, have decreased cerebral blood flow in the frontal medial, occipital, and parietal cortices, with a profound deactivation in the basal ganglia (Smith et al., 2002). These results indicate that individuals with IWC are hypometabolic rather than hypermetabolic when compared to good sleepers (see Table

27.3 for more details on this study). The decreased cerebral perfusion found in those with insomnia appears to contradict the proposed hyperarousal theory of insomnia. However, only a 2-minute window of perfusion during the first NREM cycle was sampled, so it remains possible that subjects with insomnia are more aroused over the entirety of NREM sleep. This argument could also be supported by Perlis, Kehr et al.'s (2001) study that showed a more pronounced increase of beta EEG activity in the latter portion of the night in those with insomnia. While this study suggests the feasibility of a neuroimaging technique in combination with traditional PSG, the results remain difficult to interpret in light of methodological restrictions. The effects of behavior therapy on cerebral blood flow during NREM sleep have also been evaluated using SPECT. Since behavior therapy has been recognized as an effective treatment for insomnia (Morin, 2004), a reversal, after treatment, of the previously reported patterns of cerebral deactivation could be expected. Indeed, when comparing post- to pre-treatment, a significant increase in cerebral blood flow was found in the basal ganglia (Smith et al., 2005; see Table 27.3). Sadly, most of the studies using SPECT were conducted in the early 2000s and have not been replicated since.

POSITRON EMISSION TOMOGRAPHY

Positron emission tomography (PET) represents another imaging technique with a more accurate measure of whole-brain activity that can be used during wakefulness as well as during sleep. It involves the injection (usually into the blood circulation) of a short-lived radioactive tracer isotope which decays by emitting a positron, chemically incorporated into a metabolically active molecule. This technique demonstrated that individuals with insomnia show increased global cerebral glucose metabolism when compared with control subjects during both wake and NREM sleep (Kay et al., 2019; Nofzinger et al., 2004; see Table 27.3). Individuals with insomnia also appear to present a smaller decrease than control participants in relative metabolism from wakefulness to NREM sleep states in the ascending reticular activating system, hypothalamus, thalamus, insular cortex, amygdala, hippocampus, and anterior cingulate and medial prefrontal cortices (Kay et al., 2019; Nofzinger et al., 2004). During wakefulness, individuals with insomnia show relative hypometabolism in bilateral prefrontal, left hemispheric superior temporal, parietal, and occipital cortices; the thalamus; hypothalamus; and brainstem reticular formation compared to good-sleeping individuals. Since this pattern has also been observed in healthy good sleepers following sleep deprivation (Thomas et al., 2000), this suggests those with insomnia are chronically sleep-deprived and that their sleep is associated with increased brain metabolism. An inability to fall asleep could also be related to an abnormal progression of brain activity from wake to sleep states, in which there would be a failure of arousal mechanisms to decline in activity. Moreover, the subjective daytime fatigue experienced by individuals with insomnia may reflect decreased activity in the prefrontal cortex resulting from inefficient sleep. Using the PET technique has also allowed researchers to suggest the presence of interacting neural networks, including a general arousal system (ascending reticular formation and hypothalamus), an emotion-regulating system (hippocampus, amygdala, and anterior cingulate cortex), and a cognitive system (prefrontal cortex) in the neurobiology of insomnia.

FUNCTIONAL MAGNETIC RESONANCE IMAGING

One of the most recently developed forms of neuroimaging has been used to replicate the prefrontal hypoactivation in individuals with insomnia. Functional magnetic resonance imaging (fMRI) measures the hemodynamic response related to neural activity in the brain. Using this technique, it was found that individuals with insomnia show less activation than controls in the left medial prefrontal cortex and left inferior frontal gyrus when completing performance tasks (Altena et al., 2008). A pre- and post-treatment comparison also revealed that a 6-week treatment might partly restore the activation in those areas (see Table 27.3 for more details on this study). It was concluded that insomnia interferes in a reversible way with activation of the prefrontal cortex during daytime task performance. A more recent study explained this effect on performance by what seems to be a failure to deactivate regions from the default mode network (i.e., middle frontal gyrus, posterior cingulate, and orbital frontal gyrus), which would prohibit individuals with insomnia from disengaging from irrelevant tasks (Drummond et al., 2013). This technique also showed the connectivity between the amygdala and the premotor cortex increased positively with the intensity of insomnia symptoms (Huang et al., 2012). This suggests a hyper-reactivity to threats, which is consistent with the hyperarousal model of insomnia. On another note, fMRI was also used to examine the sleep spindle firing neuronal network (Shao et al., 2021). It appears that the anterior cingulate area is also a region which can be quite activated in the absence of sleep spindles, suggesting again that lack of inhibition or sleep protection (which some authors consider hyperarousal) is one of the components underpinning insomnia disorder.

LOW-RESOLUTION BRAIN ELECTROMAGNETIC TOMOGRAPHY

Low-resolution brain electromagnetic tomography is another noninvasive method that allows the mapping of current density measures according to a standard brain atlas, in order to localize electrical activity in the brain. Using this technique, it was found that individuals with IWC show less current density in cerebral regions involved in affect and cognitive performance (i.e., orbitofrontal, medial prefrontal, and anterior cingulate cortices) relative to normal controls (Szelenberger & Niemcewizc, 2001). Furthermore, the differences observed in these brain regions between the control group and those with insomnia were associated with insomnia severity.

STRUCTURAL IMAGING

Structural neuroimaging techniques, such as functional magnetic resonance spectroscopy (MRS), have been used to characterize brain differences in individuals with insomnia.

MRS is a noninvasive technique that estimates the concentration of certain molecules in the brain. Winkelman et al. (2008) found that global gamma-aminobutyric acid (GABA) levels were significantly lower in those with IWC. Since GABA is an inhibitory neurotransmitter, lower GABA levels may lead to an incapacity to regulate cortical arousal, which falls in line with the hyperarousal model of insomnia. Some studies also have used MRI to showcase structural brain changes associated with insomnia; but they have shown contradictory results, and very few studies have been replicated (O'Byrne et al., 2014).

In summary, neuroimaging methods have contributed to reveal both a hypermetabolism in certain brain regions related to the arousal system and a hypometabolism in specific areas that could suggest a chronic sleep deprivation in individuals with insomnia. However, the few studies using neuroimaging techniques have shown some contradictory results and are rarely replicated. While there are currently no clinical indications for any of these neuroimaging techniques, they hold considerable promise for unraveling the neurocircuitry and metabolic pathways of insomnia in the immediate future and in helping with diagnosis and treatment planning in the future. Neuroimaging studies performed on a vast and heterogeneous insomnia population could reveal if the different clinical presentations of this disorder (with or without comorbidity) share a common neurobiological basis. They could also help classify the different subtypes based on their underlying pathophysiology. Finally, preliminary studies show that neuroimaging techniques are useful to assess and compare the effects of different types of treatment on brain functions. These methods present many advantages and could help further our understanding of clinical sleep disorders. However, more studies need to be conducted before these techniques can be systematically applied in the routine assessment and management of patients with sleep disorders.

ERPs

ERPs are the electrical responses of the brain to sensory stimulation (visual, somatosensory, olfactive, nociceptive, or auditive) that reflect how the brain "processes and classifies" environmental stimuli. An external physical stimulus or internal psychological event elicits small-amplitude changes in the EEG, therefore providing a means to "probe" the extent of processing within the nervous system during sleep. The high temporal resolution of ERPs (about one-tenth of a millisecond) makes it a useful tool to precisely measure, in true time, all aspects of information processing. ERP components can be simply classified according to their latencies: Early components (<80 ms approximately) typically reflect sensory processing, those around 100 ms are sensitive to arousal and attention, and later components are thought to reflect higher-order CNS processing related to cognitive functions such as attention, vigilance, memory, and inhibition of information processing in wake and sleep (Colrain & Campbell, 2007). In the ERP nomenclature, the latency and amplitude of the successive peaks are used to name the different components: *N* refers to a negative wave and *P* to a positive wave. As such, *N100* would refer to a negative wave appearing 100 ms after stimulus onset.

Information processing of external stimuli remains present during sleep, although reduced relative to wakefulness. Since it is impossible for individuals to respond verbally or behaviorally while they are sleeping, the study of information processing during sleep is limited. ERPs can be extremely useful to sleep researchers for the daytime assessment of the impact of sleep disruption and determination of CNS function during sleep (Colrain & Campbell, 2007). QEEG studies have suggested that CNS hyperarousal is associated with insomnia; ERPs offer a means to directly evaluate the concept of cortical activation. The ERPs protocol used in sleep studies is the oddball paradigm (a train of auditory stimuli containing a frequent standard tone as well as a deviant tone, which occurs less frequently). Participants can be instructed to pay attention to the auditory stimulation (target stimuli generating a P300), or they can be asked to simply ignore the stimulations. While only a handful of studies have used ERPs to evaluate information processing among those with insomnia, there are some promising results. It was found that individuals with insomnia, relative to good sleepers, have shorter response latency during wakefulness, higher P300 amplitude immediately before sleep onset, and smaller N350 amplitude, which is usually associated with the inhibition of environmental stimuli, during the initial part of Stage 2 sleep (Hull, 1993). It was also found that poor sleepers have a larger N1 and a smaller P2 than good sleepers during wakefulness (Loewy & Bootzin, 1998; Loewy et al., 1999). While N1 represents arousal, the P2 component usually reflects inhibitory processes. This reveals that individuals with sleep disturbances are more vigilant during wakefulness. However, this cortical activation appears to persist during sleep. It was reported that individuals with insomnia show larger N1 and smaller P2 to rare tones as well as smaller N350 to standard tones than controls during the first 5 minutes of continuous Stage 2 sleep (Yang & Lo, 2007; see Table 27.3 for more information).

Could poor sleep quality in insomnia be associated with daytime measures of ERPs? It has been reported that the P300 amplitude recorded after a perceived good night is smaller in those with insomnia relative to controls (DeVoto et al., 2003; see Table 27.3). However, it was found that the P300 amplitude is higher among those with insomnia compared to good sleepers after a perceived poor night of sleep. This supports the hypothesis of cortical hyperarousal among those with insomnia. Larger P300 amplitudes have also been observed among individuals with insomnia on their worst night of sleep (assessed with overnight actigraphy), which could suggest hyperarousal in this group before and after the worst night of sleep (DeVoto et al., 2005). Other objective sleep parameters can also be linked to the amplitudes and latencies of ERP components (Turcotte & Bastien, 2009). Indeed, as the amplitude of N1 and P2 increases before going to sleep in those with insomnia, sleep quality on the following night seems to decrease. In a reverse manner, the sleep quality of the previous night appears to be linked to the ERPs' amplitude recorded on the following morning. Thus, hyperactivation and inhibition deficits present in those with insomnia appear to be directly associated with poorer sleep quality.

A study found that ERPs recorded prior to going to sleep do not differ between individuals with insomnia and controls for N1, P2, or P3 amplitude. However, the N1 amplitude differences (smaller N1 in the morning relative to that seen pre-sleep) seem to be linked with the amount of Stage 1 sleep, the number of stage changes, and the number of awakenings during the night in individuals with insomnia (Sforza & Haba-Rubio, 2006; see Table 27.3). Another study, by Bastien, St-Jean, et al. (2008), assessing chronic psychophysiological insomnia reported hyperarousal in this group upon awakening in the morning (greater N1 amplitude) as well as inhibition deficits at sleep onset (smaller N350). Therefore, it was suggested both processes, cortical arousal and inhibition deficits, are underlying neurophysiological mechanisms of chronic insomnia (see Table 27.3 for more details on this study). Bastien et al. (2013) observed afterward inhibitory deficits in REM sleep (especially in P2) in individuals with paradoxical insomnia, inhibitory deficits which might be related to the misperception of sleep, or wake, depending on the position held by the researcher. These results also appeared to be in line with the REM sleep instability hypothesis set forward by Riemann and colleagues (2012). Just recently, Feige and colleagues (2021) provided more empirical evidence to the REM sleep instability hypothesis by showing that P2 was smaller in REM sleep in individuals with insomnia compared to good sleeper controls but only in phasic REM, not in tonic REM. Moreover, this reduced P2 amplitude was negatively associated with the misperception of sleep. It is also well known that K-Complexes can be spontaneous or evoked (Bastien & Campbell, 1992). A study by Forget et al. (2011) specifically compared spontaneous K-Complexes to evoked ones and replicated earlier results by Bastien and colleagues (Bastien, Ladouceur, & Campbell, 2000; Bastien, St-Jean, Turcotte, Morin, Lavallée, & Carrier, 2009; Bastien, St-Jean, Turcotte, Morin, Lavallée, Carrier, & Forget, 2009). They found that spontaneous and evoked K-Complexes appear to be sleep-protective mechanisms and do not differ between good sleepers and individuals with insomnia (Forget et al., 2011).

These results suggest the presence of an increased cortical arousal level in those with insomnia not only while they are awake but also while they are asleep. Results also support the utility of ERPs as a tool to investigate cognitive functions or information processing during wake or sleep. Contrary to PSA, they provide a direct measure and precise timing of cortical arousal and dynamic neural mechanisms. Individuals with insomnia can also present subtle cognitive deficits that do not always emerge in neuropsychological tests. Therefore, ERPs can be used to complement behavioral measures in performance studies. However, repeated recordings are recommended to capture the variability linked to sleep quality and, hence, to cortical activity.

Conclusion

As mentioned earlier, the patient's subjective complaint(s) and history are the essential foundation for the diagnosis of insomnia. In this chapter, we have described a wide range of behavioral, physiological, and neurophysiological associated measures. These measures/

techniques are useful to conduct sophisticated sleep assessments and to complement the clinical history. Besides PSG, these technologies are still infrequently used for clinical or research purposes, often because they are not readily available and are costly. Although there is no doubt that these evaluation tools can provide a better understanding of the nature and pathophysiology of insomnia, more work is nonetheless needed. These promising techniques could also be helpful in guiding the choice of appropriate treatments, whether pharmacological or not. They open an array of new opportunities to advance our understanding of brain organization in individuals with insomnia.

Future Directions

Future studies should investigate how using available technologies and other clinical characteristics can enlighten us with regard to the severity of the disorder or the development of a comorbidity. For example, sleep patterns on multiple nights from the sleep diary can be informative regarding the presence of an undiagnosed comorbidity (e.g., anxiety, depression). Some EEG graphoelements (sleep spindles or K-Complexes) could also be used as predictors of severity or quality of sleep. One can also ask whether AI would be helpful in disentangling different subtypes of insomnia or even those at risk of developing insomnia. Would it be of interest to study the depth of sleep, this latter being linked to the severity or clinical sleep quality reported by insomnia patients? Could we model the study of sleep depth on what is observed with patients suffering from obstructive sleep apnea (Penner et al., 2019)? Moreover, looking at objective sleep measures, whichever they may be, could this potentially inform us on the success or failure of treatment, whether behavioral, cognitive, or pharmaceutical? These questions remain unanswered while being of current interest.

References

Adam, K., Tomeny, M., & Oswald, I. (1986). Physiological and psychological differences between good and poor sleepers. *Journal of Psychiatric Research, 20*, 301–316.

Altena, E., Van Der Merf, Y. D., Sanz-Arigita, E.J., Voorn, T. A., Rombouts, S. A., Kuijer, J. P., & Van Someren, E. J. W. (2008). Prefrontal hypoactivation and recovery in insomnia. *Sleep, 31*(9), 1271–1276.

American Psychiatric Association. (2013). *Diagnostic and statistical manual of mental disorders* (5th ed.).

Ancoli-Israel, S., Cole, R., Alessi, C., Chambers, M., Moorcroft, W., & Pollak, C. P. (2003). The role of actigraphy in the study of sleep and circadian rhythms. *Sleep, 26*, 342–392.

Baglioni, C., Regen, W., Teghen, A., Spiegelhalder, K., Feige, B., Nissen, C., & Riemann, D. (2014). Sleep changes in the disorder of insomnia: A meta-analysis of polysomnographic studies. *Sleep Medicine Reviews, 18*(3), 195–213.

Barry, R. J., Clarke, A. R., Johnstone, S. J., Magee, C. A., & Rushby, J. A. (2007). EEG differences between eyes-closed and eyes-open resting conditions. *Clinical Neurophysiology, 118*(12), 2765–2773.

Bastien, C., & Campbell, K. (1992). The evoked K-Complex: All-or-none phenomenon? *Sleep, 15*(3), 236–245. https://doi.org/10.1093/sleep/15.3.236

Bastien, C. H., Ceklic, T., St-Hilaire, P., Desmarais, F., Pérusse, A. D., Lefrançois, J., & Pedneault-Drolet, M. (2014). Insomnia and sleep misperception. *Pathologie-Biologie, 62*(5), 241–251.

Bastien, C. H., Guimond, S., Lemelin, S., St-Jean, G., & Turcotte, I. (2008a). Signs of insomnia in borderline personality individuals. *Journal of Clinical Sleep Medicine, 4*(5), 462–470.

Bastien, C. H., Ladouceur, C., & Campbell, K. B. (2000). EEG characteristics prior to and following the evoked K-Complex. *Canadian Journal of Experimental Psychology/Revue canadienne de psychologie expérimentale*, *54*(4), 255–265. https://doi.org/10.1037/h0087345
Bastien, C. H., Leblanc, M., Carrier, J., & Morin, C.M. (2003). Sleep EEG power spectra insomnia and chronic use of benzodiazepines. *Sleep*, *26*(3), 313–317.
Bastien, C. H., St-Jean, G., Turcotte, I., Morin, C. M., & Carrier, J. (2008b). Chronic psychophysiological insomnia: Hyperarousal and/or inhibition deficits? An ERPs investigation. *Sleep*, *31*(6), 887–898.
Bastien, C. H., St-Jean, G., Turcotte, I., Morin, C. M., Lavallée, M., & Carrier, J. (2009). Sleep spindles in chronic psychophysiological insomnia. *Journal of Psychosomatic Research*, *66*, 59–65.
Bastien, C. H., St-Jean, G., Turcotte, I., Morin, C.M., Lavallée, M., Carrier, J., & Forget, D. (2009). Spontaneous K-Complexes in chronic psychophysiological insomnia. *Journal of Psychosomatic Research*, *67*, 117–125.
Bastien, C. H., Turcotte, I., St-Jean, G., Morin, C. M., & Carrier, J. (2013). Information processing varies between insomnia types: Measures of N1 and P2 during the night. *Behavioral Sleep Medicine*, *11*(1), 56–72.
Bonnet, M. H., & Arand, D. L. (1995). 24-Hour metabolic rate in insomniacs and matched normal sleepers. *Sleep*, *18*, 581–588.
Bonnet, M. H., & Arand, D. L. (1998). HR variability in insomniacs and matched normal sleepers. *Psychosomatic Medicine*, *60*, 610–615.
Buysse, D. J., Ancoli-Israel, S., Edinger, J. D., Lichstein, K. L., & Morin, C. M. (2006). Recommendations for a standard research assessment of insomnia. *Sleep*, *29*(9), 1155–1173.
Carney, C. E., Buysse, D. J., Ancoli-Israel, S., Edinger, J. D., Krystal, A. D., Lichstein, K. L., & Morin, C. M. (2012). The consensus sleep diary: Standardizing prospective sleep self-monitoring. *Sleep*, *35*(2), 287–302.
Caviness, J. N., Hentz, J. G., Belden, C. M., Shill, H. A., Driver-Dunckley, E. D., Sabbagh, M. N., Powell, J. J., & Adler, C. H. (2015). Longitudinal EEG changes correlate with cognitive measure deterioration in Parkinson's disease. *Journal of Parkinson's Disease*, *5*(1), 117–124. https://doi.org/10.3233/JPD-140480
Cervena, K., Dauvilliers, Y., Espa, F., Touchon, J., Matousek, M., Billiard, M., & Besset, A. (2004). Effect of cognitive behavioural therapy for insomnia on sleep architecture and sleep EEG power spectra in psychophysiological insomnia. *Journal of Sleep Research*, *13*(4), 385–393.
Coates, T. J., Killen, J. D., George, J., Marchini, E., Silverman, S., & Thoresen, C. (1982). Estimating sleep parameters: A multitrait–multimethod analysis. *Journal of Consulting and Clinical Psychology*, *50*, 345–352.
Coates, T. J., Killen, J. D., Silverman, S., George, J., Marchini, E., Hamilton, S., & Thoresen, C. E. (1983). Cognitive activity, sleep disturbance, and stage specific differences between recorded and reported sleep. *Psychophysiology*, *20*, 243–250.
Colombo, M. A., Ramautar, J. R., Wei, Y., Gomez-Herrero, G., Stoffers, D., Wassing, R., Benjamins, J. S., Tagliazucchi, E., van der Werf, Y. D., Cajochen, C., & Van Someren, E. J. W. (2016). Wake high-density electroencephalography spatio spectral signatures of insomnia. *Sleep*, *39*(5), 1015–1027.
Colrain, I. M., & Campbell, K. B. (2007). The use of evoked potentials in sleep research. *Sleep Medicine Review*, *11*(4), 277–293. https://doi.org/10.1016/j.smrv.2007.05.001
Corsi-Cabrera, M., Rojas-Ramos, O. A., & del Río-Portilla, Y. (2016). Waking EEG signs of non-restoring sleep in primary insomnia patients. *Clinical Neurophysiology*, *127*(3), 1813–1821.
Crönlein, T., Lehner, A., Schüssler, P., Geisler, P., Rupprecht, R., & Wetter, T. C. (2019). Changes in subjective–objective sleep discrepancy following inpatient cognitive behavior therapy for insomnia. *Behavior Therapy*, *50*(5), 994–1001.
Declerck, A. C., Ruwe, F., O'Hanlon, J. F., & Wauquier, A. (1992). Effects of zolpidem and flunitrazepam on nocturnal sleep of women subjectively complaining of insomnia. *Psychopharmacology*, *106*(4), 497–501.
Devoto, A., Manganelli, S., Lucidi, F., Lombardo, C., Russo, P. M., & Violani, C. (2005). Quality of sleep and P300 amplitude in primary insomnia: A preliminary study. *Sleep*, *28*(7), 859–863.
Devoto, A., Violani, C., Lucidi, F., & Lombardo, C. (2003). P300 amplitude in subjects with primary insomnia is modulated by their sleep quality. *Journal of Psychosomatic Research*, *54*, 3–10.
De Zambotti, M., Cellini, N., Goldstone, A., Colrain, I. M., & Baker, F. C. (2019). Wearable sleep technology in clinical and research settings. *Medicine and Science in Sports and Exercise*, *51*(7), 1538–1557.
Dodds, K. L., Miller, C. B., Kyle, S. D, Marshall, N. S., & Gordon, C. J. (2017). Heart rate variability in insomnia patients: A critical review of the literature. *Sleep Medicine Reviews*, *33*, 88–100. https://doi.org/10.1016/j.smrv.2016.06.004

Dressle, R. J., Feige, B., Spiegelhalder, K., Schmucker, C., Benz, F., Mey, N. C., & Riemann, D. (2022). HPA axis activity in patients with chronic insomnia: A systematic review and meta-analysis of case-control studies. *Sleep Medicine Reviews, 62*, Article 101588. https://doi.org/10.1016/j.smrv.2022.101588

Drummond, S. P., Walker, M., Almklov, E., Campos, M., Anderson, D. E., & Straus, L. D. (2013). Neural correlates of working memory performance in primary insomnia. *Sleep, 36*(9), 1307–1316.

Dumont, M., Jurysta, F., Lanquart, J. P., Noseda, A., van de Borne, P., & Linkowski, P. (2007). Scale-free dynamics of the synchronization between sleep EEG power bands and the high frequency component of HR variability in normal men and patients with sleep apnea–hypopnea syndrome. *Clinical Neurophysiology, 118*(12), 2752–2764.

Edinger, J. D., Means, M. K., Stechuchak, M., & Olsen, M. K. (2004). A pilot study of inexpensive sleep-assessment devices. *Behavioral Sleep Medicine, 2*(1), 41–49.

El-Makkawy, L., El Salmawy, D., Basheer, M. A., Maher, E., & Nada, M. M. (2022). Screening of non-restorative sleep by quantitative EEG. *Egyptian Journal of Neurology, Psychiatry and Neurosurgery, 58*(11), Article 11.

Feige, B., Baglioni, C., Boehm, P., Heinrich, A., Trumm, S., Benz, F., Nissen, C., Domschke, K., Frase, L., & Riemann, D. (2021). Event-related potentials in insomnia reflect altered perception of sleep. *Sleep, 44*(10), Article zsab137. https://doi.org/10.1093/sleep/zsab137

Ferreira, D., Jelic, V., Cavallin, L., Oeksengaard, A. R., Snaedal, J., Høgh, P., Andersen, B. B., Naik, M., Engedal, K., Westman, E., & Wahlund, L. O. (2016). Electroencephalography is a good complement to currently established dementia biomarkers. *Dementia and Geriatric Cognitive Disorders, 42*(1–2), 80–92.

Ferri, R., Miano, S., Bruni, O., Vankova, J., Nevsimalova, S., Vandi, S., Montagna, P., Ferini-Strambi, & Plazzi, G. (2005). NREM sleep alterations in narcolepsy/cataplexy. *Clinical Neurophysiology, 116*(11), 2675–2684.

Forget, D., Morin, C. M., & Bastien, C. H. (2011). The role of the spontaneous and evoked K-Complex in good-sleeper controls and in individuals with insomnia. *Sleep, 34*(9), 1251–1260. https://doi.org/10.5665/SLEEP.1250

Freedman, R. R. (1986). EEG power spectra in sleep-onset insomnia. *Electroencephalography and Clinical Neurophysiology, 63*, 408–413.

Greneche, J., Krieger, J., Erhardt, C., Bonnefond, A., Eschenlauer, A., Muzet, A., & Tassi, P. (2008). EEG spectral power and sleepiness during 24h of sustained wakefulness in patients with obstructive sleep apnea syndrome. *Clinical Neurophysiology, 119* (2), 418–428.

Hall, M., Thayer, J. F., Germain, A., Moul, D., Vasko, R., Puhl, M., Miewald, J., & Buysse, D. J. (2007). Psychological stress is associated with heightened physiological arousal during NREM sleep in primary insomnia. *Behavioural Sleep Medicine, 5*(3), 178–193.

Hauri, P. J., & Fisher, J. (1986). Persistent psychophysiologic (learned) insomnia. *Sleep, 9*, 38–53.

Hauri, P. J., & Olmstead, E. (1983). What is the moment of sleep onset for insomniacs? *Sleep, 6*, 10–15.

Haynes, S. N., Adams, A., & Franzen, M. (1981). The effects of presleep stress on sleep-onset insomnia. *Journal of Abnormal Psychology, 90*(6), 601–606.

Haynes, S. N., Fitzgerald, G., Shute, G., & O'Meary, M. (1985). Responses of psychophysiologic and subjective insomniacs to auditory stimuli during sleep: A replication and extension. *Journal of Abnormal Psychology, 94*(3), 338–345.

Hornyak, M., Feige, B., Voderholzer, U., & Riemann, D. (2005). Spectral analysis of sleep EEG in patients with restless legs syndrome. *Clinical Neurophysiology, 116*(6), 1265–1272.

Huang, Z., Liang, P., Jia, X., Zhan, S., Li, N., Ding, Y., Lu, J., Wang, Y., & Li, K. (2012). Abnormal amygdala connectivity in patients with primary insomnia: Evidence from resting state fMRI. *European Journal of Radiology, 81*(6), 1288–1295.

Hull, J. S. (1993). *Event-related potentials during the wake/sleep transition in adults with and without primary insomnia* (Publication No. 9417834) [Doctoral dissertation], University of Southern Mississippi]. ProQuest Dissertations.

Iber, C., Ancoli-Israel, S., Chesson, A., & Quan, S. F. (2007). *The AASM manual for the scoring of sleep and associated events: Rules, terminology and technical specifications*. American Academy of Sleep Medicine.

Jacobs, G. D., Benson, H., & Friedman, R. (1993). Home-based central nervous system assessment of a multifactor behavioural intervention for chronic sleep onset insomnia. *Behaviour Therapy, 24*(1), 159–174.

Johns, M. W., Gay, T. J., Masterton, J. P., & Bruce, D. W. (1971). Relationship between sleep habits, adrenocortical activity and personality. *Psychosomatic Medicine, 33*(6), 499–508.

Kathami, R., Landolt, H. P., Achermann, P., Retey, J. V., Werth, E., Mathis, J., & Bassetti, C. L. (2007). Insufficient non-REM sleep intensity in narcolepsy-cataplexy. *Sleep, 30*(8), 980–989.

Kay, D. B., Karim, H. T., Hasler, B. P., James, J. A., Germain, A., Hall, M. H., Franzen, P. L., Price, J. C., Nofzinger, E. A., & Buysse, D. J. (2019). Impact of acute sleep restriction on cerebral glucose metabolism during recovery non-rapid eye movement sleep among individuals with primary insomnia and good sleeper controls. *Sleep Medicine, 55*, 81–91.

Kohtoh, S., Taguchi, Y., Matsumoto, N., Wada, M., Huang, Z. L., & Urade, Y. (2008). Algorithm for sleep scoring in experimental animals based on fast Fourier transform power spectrum analysis of the electroencephalogram. *Sleep and Biological Rhythms, 6*(3), 163–171.

Kronholm, E., Virkkala, J., Kärki, T., Karjaleinen, P., Lang, H., & Hämälaïnen, H. (2007). Spectral power and fractal dimension: Methodological comparison in a sample of normal sleepers and chronic insomniacs. *Sleep and Biological Rhythms, 5*(4), 239–250.

Krystal, A. D., Edinger, J. D., Wohlgemuth, W. K., & Marsh, G. R. (2002). NREM sleep EEG frequency spectral correlates of sleep complaints in primary insomnia subtypes. *Sleep, 25*, 630–640.

Krystal, A. D., Prather, A. A., & Ashbrook, L. H. (2019). The assessment and management of insomnia: An update. *World Psychiatry, 18*(3), 337–352.

Kushida, C. A., Kuo, T. F., Manber, R., Cardell, C., Behari, S., Hyde, P., & Dement, W. (2003). Polysomnographic and REMview assessment of treatment outcomes in patients with insomnia. *Sleep, 26*, Article S292.

Kwan, Y., Baek, C., Chung, S., Kim, T. H., & Choi, S. (2018). Resting-state quantitative EEG characteristics of insomniac patients with depression. *International Journal of Psychophysiology, 124*, 26–32.

Kwan, Y., Yoon, S., Suh, S., & Choi, S. (2022). A randomized controlled trial comparing neurofeedback and cognitive-behavioral therapy for insomnia patients: Pilot study. *Applied Psychophysiology and Biofeedback, 47*, 95–106.

Lamarche, C. H., & Ogilvie, R. D. (1997). Electrophysiological changes during the sleep onset period of psychophysiological insomniacs, psychiatric insomniacs and normal sleepers. *Journal of Sleep Research and Sleep Medicine, 20*(9), 724–733.

Laroche, D., Ivers, H., Bastien, C. H., & Vallières, A. (2024). Predictability of sleep in insomnia: Sleep patterns of patients from a sleep psychology clinic. *Journal of Sleep Research, 26*, e14369. https://doi.org/10.1111/jsr.14369. Epub ahead of print.

Lichstein, K. L., Durrence, H. H., Taylor, D. J., Bush, A. J., & Riedel, B. W. (2003). Quantitative criteria for insomnia. *Behaviour Research and Therapy, 41*(4), 427–445.

Lichstein, K. L., Wilson, N. M., Noe, S. L., Aguillard, R. N., & Bellur, S. N. (1994). Daytime sleepiness in insomnia: Behavioral, biological and subjective indices. *Sleep, 17*(8), 693–702.

Littner, M., Hirshkowitz, M., Kramer, M., Kapen, S., Anderson, W. M., Bailey, D., Berry, R. B., Davila, D., Johnson, S., Kushida, C., Loube, D. I., Wise, M., & Woodson, B. T.; American Academy of Sleep Medicine, & Standards of Practice Committee (2003). Practice parameters for using polysomnography to evaluate insomnia: An update. *Sleep, 26*(6), 754–760.

Littner, M., Kushida, C. A., Anderson, W. M., Bailey, D., Berry, R. B., Davila, D. G., Hirshkowitz, M., Kapen, S., Kramer, M., Loube, D., Wise, M., & Johnson, S. F. (2003). Practice parameters for the role of actigraphy in the study of sleep and circadian rhythms: An update for 2002. *Sleep, 26*(3), 337–341.

Loewy, D. H., & Bootzin, R. (1998). Event-related potentials measures of information processing in insomniacs at bedtime and during sleep. *Sleep, 21*, Article 98.

Loewy, D. H., Burdik, R. S., Al-Shajlawi, A., Franzen, P., & Bootzin, R. (1999). Enhanced information processing at the peri-sleep onset period in insomniacs as measured by event-related potentials. *Sleep, 22*, Article S152.

Lundahl, J., Deacon, S., Maurice, D., & Staner, L. (2012). EEG spectral power density profiles during NREM sleep for gaboxadol and zolpidem in patients with primary insomnia. *Journal of Psychopharmacology, 26*(8), 1081–1087.

Manconi, M., Ferri, R., Miano, S., Maestri, M., Bottasini, V., Zucconi, M., & Ferini-Strambi, L. (2017). Sleep architecture in insomniacs with severe benzodiazepine abuse. *Clinical Neurophysiology, 128*(6), 875–881.

Marzano, C., Ferrara, M., Sforza, E., & De Gennaro, L. (2008). Quantitative electroencephalogram (EEG) in insomnia: A new window on pathophysiological mechanisms. *Current Pharmaceutical Design, 14*(32), 3446–3455.

Means, M. K., Edinger, J. D., Glenn, D. M., & Fins, A. I. (2003). Accuracy of sleep perceptions among insomnia sufferers and normal sleepers. *Sleep Medicine, 4*, 285–296.

Mendelson, W. B. (1993). Pharmacologic alteration of the perception of being awake or asleep. *Sleep, 16*(7), 641–646.

Mendelson, W. B. (1995). Effects of flurazepam and zolpidem on the perception of sleep in insomniacs. *Sleep, 18*(2), 92–96.

Mendelson, W. B., James, S. P., Garnett, D., Sack, D. A., & Rosenthal, N. E. (1986). A psychophysiological study of insomnia. *Psychiatry Research, 19*, 267–284.

Merica, H., Blois, R., & Gaillard, J.-M. (1998). Spectral characteristics of sleep EEG in chronic insomnia. *European Journal of Neuroscience, 10*, 1826–1834.

Merica, H., & Gaillard, J. (1992). The EEG of the sleep onset period in insomnia: A discriminant analysis. *Physiology and Behavior, 52*, 199–204.

Monroe, L. J. (1967). Psychological and physiological differences between good and poor sleepers. *Journal of Abnormal Psychology, 72*(3), 255–264.

Monti, J. M., Alvariño, F., & Monti, D. (2000). Conventional and power spectrum analysis of the effects of zolpidem on sleep EEG in patients with chronic primary insomnia. *Sleep, 23*(8), 1075–1084.

Morgenthaler, T., Alessi, C., Friedman, L., Owens, J., Kapur, V., Boehlecke, B., Brown, T., Chesson, A. Jr., Coleman, J., Lee-Chiong, T., Pancer, J., & Swick, T. J.; Standards of Practice Committee & American Academy of Sleep Medicine. (2007). Practice parameters for the use of actigraphy in the assessment of sleep and sleep disorders: An update for 2007. *Sleep, 30*(4), 519–529.

Morin, C. M. (2004). Cognitive-behavioral approaches to the treatment of insomnia. *Journal of Clinical Psychiatry, 65*(16), 33–40.

Muench, A., Vargas, I., Grandner, M. A., Ellis, J. G., Posner, D., Bastien, C. H., Drummond, S. P., & Perlis, M. L. (2022). We know CBT-I works, now what? *Faculty Opinions, 11*, Article 4. https://doi.org/10.12703/r/11-4

Mullins, A. E., Kim, J. W., Wong, K. K. H., Bartlett, D. J., Vakulin, A., Dijk, D.-J., Marshall, N. S., Grunstein, R. R., & D'Rozario, A. L. (2021). Sleep EEG microstructure is associated with neurobehavioural impairment after extended wakefulness in obstructive sleep apnea. *Sleep and Breathing, 25*, 347–354.

Natale, V., Plazzi, G., & Martoni, M. (2009). Actigraphy in the assessment of insomnia: A quantitative approach. *Sleep, 32*(6), 767–771.

Nofzinger, E. A., Buysse, D. J., Germain, A., Price, J. C., Miewald, J. M., & Kupfer, D. J. (2004). Functional neuroimaging evidence for hyperarousal in insomnia. *American Journal of Psychiatry, 161*(11), 2126–2128.

Nowell, P. D., Reynolds, C. F., Buysse, D. J., Dew, M. A., & Kupfer, D. J. (1999). Paroxetine in the treatment of primary insomnia: Preliminary clinical and electroencephalogram sleep data. *Journal of Clinical Psychiatry, 60*(2), 89–95.

O'Byrne, J. N., Berman, R. M., Gouin, J. P., & Dang-Vu, T. T. (2014). Neuroimaging findings in primary insomnia. *Pathologie Biologie, 62*(5), 262–269. https://doi.org/10.1016/j.patbio.2014.05.013

Ochojska, D. B., Dejnowicz-Velitchkov, A., & Kopańska, M. (2021). Diagnosing ADHD using QEEG and planning EEG-biofeedback (neurofeedback) therapy—Pilot studies. *Medycyna Ogolna i Nauki o Zdrowiu, 27*(2), 205–212.

Paquet, J., Kawinska, A., & Carrier, J. (2007). Wake detection capacity of actigraphy during sleep. *Sleep, 30*(10), 1362–1369.

Penner, C. G., Gerardy, B., Ryan, R., &Williams, M. (2019). The odds ratio product (an objective sleep depth measure): Normal values, repeatability, and change with CPAP in patients with OSA. *Journal of Clinical Sleep Medicine, 15*(8), 1155–1163.

Perlis, M. L., Giles, D. E., Mendelson, W. B., Bootzin, R. R., & Wyatt, J. K. (1997). Psychophysiological insomnia: The behavioural model and a neurocognitive perspective. *Journal of Sleep Research, 5*(3), 179–188.

Perlis, M. L., Kehr, E. L., Smith, M. T., Andrews, P. J., Orff, H., & Giles, D. E. (2001). Temporal and stagewise distribution of high frequency EEG activity in patients with primary and secondary insomnia and good sleeper controls. *Journal of Sleep Research, 10*, 93–104.

Perlis, M. L., Merica, H., Smith, M. T., & Giles, D. E. (2001). Beta EEG activity and insomnia. *Sleep Medicine Reviews, 5*(5), 365–376.

Perlis, M. L., Smith, M. T., Andrews, P. J., Orff, H., & Giles, D. (2001). Beta/gamma EEG activity in patients with primary and secondary insomnia and good sleeper controls. *Sleep, 24*, 110–117.

Poyares, D., Guilleminault, C., Ohayon, M. M., & Tufik, S. (2004). Chronic benzodiazepine usage and withdrawal in insomnia patients. *Journal of Psychiatric Research, 38*(3), 327–334.

Qanash, S., Giannouli, E., & Younes, M. (2017). Assessment of intervention-related changes in non-rapid-eye-movement sleep depth: Importance of sleep depth changes within Stage 2. *Sleep Medicine, 40*, 84–93.

Rechtschaffen, A., & Kales, A. (1968). *A manual of standardized terminology, techniques, and scoring system for sleep stage scoring of human subjects*. US Department of Health, Education and Welfare.

Reite, M., Buysse, D., Reynolds, C., & Mendelson, W. (1995). The use of polysomnography in the evaluation of insomnia. *Sleep, 18*, 58–70.

Reynolds, C. F., 3rd, Taska L. S., Sewitch D. E., Restifo K., Coble P. A., & Kupfer D. J. (1984). Persistent psychophysiologic insomnia: Preliminary research diagnostic criteria and EEG sleep data. *American Journal of Psychiatry, 141*, 804–805.

Riemann, D., Espie, C. A., Altena, E., Arnardottir, E. S., Baglioni, C., Bassetti, C. L. A., Bastien, C. H., Berzina, N., Bjorvatn, B., Dikeos, D., Dolenc Groselj, L., Ellis, J. G., Garcia-Borreguero, D., Geoffroy, P. A., Gjerstad, M., Gonçalves, M., Hertenstein, E., Hoedlmoser, K., Hion, T., . . . Spiegelhalder, K. (2023). The European Insomnia Guideline: An update on the diagnosis and treatment of insomnia. *Journal of Sleep Research, 32*(6), e14035. https://doi.org/10.1111/jsr.14035

Riemann, D., Klein, T., Rodenbeck, A., Feige, B., Horny, A., Hummel, R., Weske, G., Al-Shajlawi, A., & Voderholzer, U. (2002). Nocturnal cortisol and melatonin secretion in primary insomnia. *Psychiatry Research, 113*(1–2), 17–27.

Riemann, D., Spiegelhalder, K., Feige, B., Voderholzer, U., Berger, M., Perlis, M., & Nissen, C. (2010). The hyperarousal model of insomnia: A review of the concept and its evidence. *Sleep Medicine Reviews, 14*(1), 19–31.

Riemann, D., Spiegelhalder, K., Nissen, C., Hirscher, V., Baglioni, C., & Feige, B. (2012). REM sleep instability—A new pathway for insomnia? *Pharmacopsychiatry, 45*(5), 167–176.

Sadeh, A. (2011). The role and validity of actigraphy in sleep medicine: an update. *Sleep Medicine Reviews, 15*(4), 259–267.

Saint-Hilaire, P., & Bastien, C. H. (2017). Sleep misperception and first night effect in laboratory. *International Journal of Psychiatry, 2*(2), 1–10.

Sateia, M. J., Doghramji, K., Hauri, P. J., & Morin, C. M. (2000). Evaluation of chronic insomnia. An American Academy of Sleep Medicine review. *Sleep, 23*(2), 243–308.

Semler, C. N., & Harvey, A. G. (2005). Misperception of sleep can adversely affect daytime functioning in insomnia. *Behaviour Research and Therapy, 43*(7), 843–856.

Sforza, E., & Haba-Rubio, J. (2006). Event-related potentials in patients with insomnia and sleep-related breathing disorders: Evening-to-morning changes. *Sleep, 29*, 805–813.

Shao, Y., Zou, G., Tabarak, S., Chen, J., Gao, X., Yao, P., Liu, J., Li, Y., Xiong, N., Pan, W., Ma, M., Zhou, S., Xu, J., Ma, Y., Deng, J., Sun, Q., Bao, Y., Sun, W., Shi, J., . . . Sun, H. (2021). Spindle-related brain activation in patients with insomnia disorder: An EEG-fMRI study. *Research Square*. https://doi.org/10.21203/rs.3.rs-422001/v1

Smith, M. T., McCrae, C. S., Cheung, J., Martin, J. L., Harrod, C. G., Heald, J. L., & Carden, K. A. (2018). Use of actigraphy for the evaluation of sleep disorders and circadian rhythm sleep–wake disorders: An American Academy of Sleep Medicine Systematic review, meta-analysis, and GRADE assessment. *Journal of Clinical Sleep Medicine, 14*(7), 1209–1230.

Smith, M. T., Perlis, M. L., Chengazi, V. U., Pennington, J., Soeffing, J., Ryan, J. M., & Giles, D. E. (2002). Neuroimaging of NREM sleep in primary insomnia: A Tc-99-HMPAO single photon emission computed tomography study. *Sleep, 25*, 325–335.

Smith, M. T., Perlis, M. L., Chengazi, V. U., Soeffing, J., & McCann, U. (2005). NREM sleep cerebral blood flow before and after behavior therapy for chronic primary insomnia: Preliminary single photon emission computed tomography (SPECT) data. *Sleep Medicine, 6*(1), 93–94.

Spiegelhalder, K., Fuchs, L., Ladwig, J., Kyle, S. D, Nissen, C., Voderholzer, U., Feige, B., & Riemann, D. (2011). Heart rate and heart rate variability in subjectively reported insomnia. *Journal of Sleep Research, 20*(1, Pt. 2), 137–145. https://doi.org/10.1111/j.1365-2869.2010.00863.x

Stepanski, E., Zorick, F., Roehrs, T., Young, D., & Roth, T. (1988). Daytime alertness in patients with chronic insomnia compared with asymptomatic control subjects. *Sleep, 11*, 54–60.

Stickgold, R., & Hobson, J. A. (1999). REM sleep and sleep efficiency are reduced during space flight. *Sleep, 22*, Article S82.

Szelenberger, W., & Niemcewicz, S. (2001). Event-related current density in primary insomnia. *Acta Neurobiologiae Experimentalis (Wars)*, *61*, 299–308.

Tang, N. K. Y., & Harvey, A. G. (2005). Time estimation ability and distorted perception of sleep in insomnia. *Behavioral Sleep Medicine*, *3*, 134–150.

Te Lindert, B. H. W., Blanken, T. F., van der Meijden, W. P., Dekker, K., Wassing, R., van der Werf, Y. D., Ramautar, J. R., & Van Someren, E. J. W. (2020). Actigraphic multi-night home-recorded sleep estimates reveal three types of sleep misperception in insomnia disorder and good sleepers. *Journal of Sleep Research*, *29*(1), Article e12937. https://doi.org/10.1111/jsr.12937

Thomas, M., Sing, H., Belenky, G., Holcomb, H., Mayberg, H., Dannals, R., Wagner, H., Thorne, D., Popp, K., Rowland, L., Welsh, A., Balwinski, S., & Redmond, D. (2000). Neural basis of alertness and cognitive performance impairments during sleepiness, I: Effects of 24h of sleep deprivation on waking human regional brain activity. *Journal of Sleep Research*, *9*, 335–352.

Tonetti, L., Pasquini, F., Fabbri, M., Belluzzi, M., & Natale, V. (2008). Comparison of two different actigraphs with polysomnography in healthy young subjects. *Chronobiology International*, *25*(1), 145–153.

Turcotte, I., & Bastien, C. H. (2009). Is sleep quality linked to ERPs N1 and P2 in psychophysiological insomnia sufferers? *International Journal of Psychophysiology*, *72*, 314–322.

Vallières, A., Ivers, H., Bastien, C. H., Beaulieu-Bonneau, S., & Morin, C. M. (2005). Variability and predictability in sleep patterns of chronic insomniacs. *Journal of Sleep Research*, *14*, 447–453.

Vallières, A., & Morin, C. M. (2003). Actigraphy in the assessment of insomnia. *Sleep*, *26*(7), 902–906.

Van Den Berg, J. F., Van Rooij, F. J., Vos, H., Tulen, J. H., Hofman, A., Miedema, H. M., Neve, A. K., & Tiemeier, H. (2008). Disagreement between subjective and actigraphic measures of sleep duration in a population-based study of elderly persons. *Journal of Sleep Research*, *17*(3), 295–302.

Verrusio, W., Ettorre, E., Vicenzini, E., Vanacore, N., Cacciafesta, M., & Mecarelli, O. (2015). The Mozart effect: A quantitative EEG study. *Consciousness and Cognition*, *35*, 150–155.

Vgontzas, A. N., Bixler, E. O., Lin, H. M., Prolo, P., Mastorakos, G., Vela-Bueno, A., Kales, A., & Chrousos, G. P. (2001). Chronic insomnia is associated with nyctohemeral activation of the hypothalamic–pituitary–adrenal axis: Clinical implications. *Journal of Clinical Endocrinology and Metabolism*, *86*(8), 3787–3794.

Vgontzas, A. N., Fernandez-Mendoza, J., Liao, D., & Bixler, E. O. (2013). Insomnia with objective short sleep duration: The most biologically severe phenotype of the disorder. *Sleep Medicine Reviews*, *17*(4), 241–254.

Vgontzas, A. N., Liao, D., Bixler, E. O., Chrousos, G. P., & Vela-Bueno, A. (2009). Insomnia with objective short sleep duration is associated with a high risk for hypertension. *Sleep*, *32*(4), 491–497. https://doi.org/10.1093/sleep/32.4.491

Vgontzas, A. N., Liao, D., Pejovic, S., Calhoun, S., Karataraki, M., Basta, M., Fernández-Mendoza, J., & Bixler, E. O. (2010). Insomnia with short sleep duration and mortality: The Penn State cohort. *Sleep*, *33*(9), 1159–1164. https://doi.org/10.1093/sleep/33.9.1159

Vgontzas, A. N., Liao, D., Pejovic, S., Calhoun, S., Karataraki, M., & Bixler, E. O. (2009). Insomnia with objective short sleep duration is associated with Type 2 diabetes: A population-based study. *Diabetes Care*, *32*(11), 1980–1985. https://doi.org/10.2337/dc09-0284

Walkowiak, H. (2015). EEG biofeedback: Characteristics, application, opinions of specialists. *Educational Studies*, *36*, 307–325.

Wauquier, A., Aloe, L., & Declerck, A. K. (1995). K-Complexes: Are they signs of arousal or sleep protective? *Journal of Sleep Research*, *4*, 138–143.

Wei, Y., Colombo, M. A., Ramautar, J. R., Blanken, T. F., van der Werf, Y. D., Spiegelhalder, K., Feige, B., Riemann, D., & Van Someren, E. J. W. (2017). Sleep stage transition dynamics reveal specific Stage 2 vulnerability in insomnia. *Sleep*, *40*(9), Article zsx117. https://doi.org/10.1093/sleep/zsx117

Williams, S. G., Wickwire, E. M., & York, C. (2016). A snapshot in time: Subjective–objective discrepancies during in-lab polysomnography. *Journal of Clinical Sleep Medicine*, *12*(11), 1437–1438.

Winkelman, J. W., Buxton, O. M., Jensen, J. E., Benson, K. L., O'Connor, S. P., Wang, W., & Renshaw, P. F. (2008). Reduced brain GABA in primary insomnia: Preliminary data from 4T proton magnetic resonance spectroscopy (^{1}H-MRS). *Sleep*, *31*(11), 1499–1506.

Wiśniewska, M., Gmitrowicz, A., & Pawełczyk, N. (2016). Application of QEEG in psychiatry considering the developmental population. *Psychiatria i Psychologia Kliniczna*, *16*, 188–193.

Withrow, D., Roth, T., Koshorek, G., & Roehrs, T. (2019). Relation between ambulatory actigraphy and laboratory polysomnography in insomnia practice and research. *Journal of Sleep Research*, *28*(4), Article e12854.

Wohlgemuth, W. K., Edinger, J. D., Fins, A. I., & Sullivan, R. J. (1999). How many nights are enough? The short-term stability of sleep parameters in elderly insomniacs and normal sleepers. *Psychophysiology, 36*, 233–244.

Wolynczyk-Gmaj, D., & Szelenberger, W. (2011). Waking EEG in primary insomnia. *Acta Neurobiologiae Experimentalis, 71*(3), 387–392.

Xu, X., & Lian, Z. (2022). Objective sleep assessments for healthy people in environmental research: A literature review. *Indoor Air, 32*(5), e13034. https://doi.org/10.1111/ina.13034

Yang, C.-M., & Lo, H.-S. (2007). ERP evidence of enhanced excitatory and reduced inhibitory processes of auditory stimuli during sleep in patients with primary insomnia. *Sleep, 30*, 585–592.

Younes, M., Gerardy, B., Pack A. I., Kuna, S. T., Castro-Diehl, C., & Redline, S. (2022). Sleep architecture based on sleep depth and propensity: Patterns in different demographics and sleep disorders and association with health outcomes. *Sleep. 45*(6), Article zsac059. https://doi.org/10.1093/sleep/zsac059

Younes, M., Kuna, S. T., Pack, A. I., Walsh, J. K., Kushida, C. A., Staley, B., & Pien, G. W. (2018). Reliability of the American Academy of Sleep Medicine rules for assessing sleep depth in clinical practice. *Journal of Clinical Sleep Medicine, 14*(2), 205–213.

Younes, M., Ostrowski, M., Soiferman, M., Younes, H., Younes, M., Raneri, J., & Hanly, P. (2015). Odds ratio product of sleep EEG as a continuous measure of sleep state. *Sleep, 38*(4), 641–654. https://doi.org/10.5665/sleep.4588

Zhao, W., Van Someren, E., Li, C., Chen, X., Gui, W., Tian, Y., Liu, Y., & Lei, X. (2021). EEG spectral analysis in insomnia disorder: A systematic review and meta-analysis. *Sleep Medicine Reviews, 59*, Article 101457. https://doi.org/10.1016/j.smrv.2021.101457

CHAPTER

28 Cognitive Behavioral Therapies for Insomnia: Current Status and Challenges Ahead

Charles M. Morin *and* Simon D. Kyle

Abstract

This chapter summarizes the current status of cognitive behavioral therapies for insomnia (CBT-I). After presenting a conceptual model of insomnia, the core therapeutic components of CBT-I are described along with other emerging therapies such as mindfulness, acceptance and commitment therapy, and intensive sleep retraining. The authors present a summary of the evidence that has led CBT-I to be recognized as the treatment of choice in current clinical practice guidelines. Potential mechanisms of changes are discussed, as well as the emerging literature on digital therapies. The authors conclude with some practical and clinical considerations that should guide therapists in the implementation of CBT-I. Given that CBT-I is still underutilized and that not all patients actually respond to CBT-I, recommendations for future research are made with reference to the design of more personalized therapies and greater deployment of digital therapies to improve access to insomnia treatment.

Key Words: cognitive behavioral therapy, insomnia, treatment, efficacy, clinical trial

Introduction

Insomnia is a prevalent condition that affects all segments of the population but more frequently women, middle-aged and older adults, and patients with comorbid medical and psychiatric disorders. Insomnia can present as a disorder (about 10% of adults) or as a symptom (25%–30%). Chronic insomnia is associated with a significant impact on quality of life and with long-term adverse consequences including increased risk of depression, hypertension, and accidents (Kyle et al., 2010; Morin et al., 2015; Morin & Jarrin, 2022).

Of the different treatment modalities for insomnia (i.e., psychological, pharmacological, and complementary and alternative therapies), cognitive-behavioral therapy (CBT) is currently recognized as the treatment of choice by several medical and sleep organizations (Edinger et al., 2021a; Qaseem et al., 2016; Riemann et al., 2017). This chapter summarizes the current state of evidence on CBT for insomnia (CBT-I). After a brief overview of the typical trajectory of care for insomnia, we present the rationale and a conceptual model of insomnia and describe CBT core clinical components, as well as other emerging psychological and behavioral therapies. Evidence about efficacy—magnitude, durability, and generalizability of treatment effects—is reviewed as well as presumed mechanisms of change. We then review the evidence about different treatment delivery methods and, more specifically, digital CBT-I and other forms of low-intensity treatment delivery methods. The benefits and limitations of combining CBT-I and medication are discussed, and we conclude with clinical and practical considerations that should guide clinicians in the management of insomnia.

Current Treatment Practices

Despite its high prevalence and negative impact, insomnia often remains unrecognized and untreated. Barriers to treatment may be related to both patients' and clinicians' perceptions, including concerns about the use of medication and drug dependency, the lack of information about alternative treatments (i.e., CBT), low priority given to insomnia when comorbid with another medical or psychiatric condition, and various beliefs about insomnia or its treatment (Araujo et al., 2017; Cheung et al., 2014, 2016). Most individuals who eventually initiate treatment for sleep disturbances do so without professional consultation and often resort to over-the-counter medications or alternative remedies (herbal or dietary supplements) with unknown risks and benefits (Morin et al., 2006). When insomnia is brought to professional attention, typically to a primary care physician, treatment is often limited to generic sleep hygiene advice of limited benefit or sedative medications, including hypnotics and off-label antidepressants (Everitt et al., 2014). A recent study in Switzerland found that just 1% of patients with insomnia who presented to primary care were provided access to CBT (Maire et al., 2020). If and when a patient eventually reaches a clinician with CBT-I expertise, usually a behavioral sleep medicine specialist, it may have been preceded by a long journey of rather frustrating experiences.

A Conceptual Model of Insomnia

Based on the well-known Spielman conceptual model (Spielman & Glovinsky, 1991), the development and maintenance of insomnia are the result of several predisposing, precipitating, and perpetuating factors. Risk factors that may predispose to insomnia include female sex, older age, poor mental health, a personal or family history of insomnia, an anxiety-prone personality style, and several others (LeBlanc et al., 2009). Acute insomnia is often precipitated by stressful life events (e.g., death of a loved one, breakup of a relationship, financial problems, loss of a job), but most people resume normal sleep once the initial triggering event has faded away or the person has adjusted to its more persisting nature. For some people, perhaps those with increased vulnerability, sleep disturbances may persist even after the initial precipitating event is no longer a contributing factor (Spielman & Glovinsky, 1991). For example, a person may develop acute insomnia due to pain after a motor vehicle accident. After a few months, the pain may no longer be a contributing factor even though the sleep problem persists; at this point in time, behavioral and cognitive factors play a salient role in perpetuating sleep disturbances. For instance, bedrest and daytime napping may have been helpful initially to cope with the pain and the sequelae of the accident; however, over time those behaviors exacerbate and perpetuate sleep disturbances. At the psychological or cognitive level, that person may have been worrying initially about whether the pain would become chronic and prevent them from going back to work; now, the worrying is about being unable to sleep and about its negative consequences on daytime functioning, which feeds into the vicious insomnia cycle. This example illustrates how behavioral and cognitive factors are almost always instrumental in perpetuating insomnia over time; also, it highlights the importance of addressing those factors for the effective management of chronic insomnia. There are several other conceptual models of insomnia, complementary to this one, that have been proposed over recent decades, each with its specificities; for more information, see other sources (Espie, 2002; Harvey, 2005; Morin & Espie, 2003).

Based on the Spielman conceptualization of insomnia, the most relevant targets of CBT include psychological, behavioral, and cognitive factors that perpetuate or exacerbate sleep disturbances. Such features may involve counterproductive sleep scheduling, sleep habits (e.g., spending excessive amounts of time in bed), conditioning, hyperarousal, unhelpful sleep-related beliefs and excessive worry about sleep, and inadequate sleep hygiene practices.

Description of CBTs

CBT-I typically involves one or more behavioral interventions (e.g., sleep restriction, stimulus control, relaxation), a cognitive intervention (e.g., standard cognitive restructuring), and an educational component (e.g., sleep hygiene). Additional interventions along the third wave of CBT, such as mindfulness-based therapy or acceptance and commitment therapy (ACT), may also be used singly or combined with some behavioral procedures. This section provides a brief synopsis of the core therapeutic components usually comprised under the label of CBT-I, as well as some emerging therapies. More detailed descriptions of those procedures with clinical guidance for their implementation are available in several published treatment manuals (Baglioni et al., 2022; Edinger & Carney, 2014; Harvey & Buysse, 2017; Manber & Carney, 2015; Morin & Espie, 2003).

Sleep Restriction

Many individuals with insomnia are inclined to increase the time they spend in bed simply to rest or increase the opportunity for sleep. Although this strategy may be effective in the short term, in the long run it is more likely to result in fragmented, irregular, and poor-quality sleep because there is a mismatch between sleep need and sleep opportunity. Sleep restriction therapy (SRT) consists of curtailing the amount of time spent in bed as close as possible to the actual amount of time asleep (Spielman et al., 1987). That sleep window is subsequently adjusted on the basis of sleep efficiency (ratio of total sleep time to time in bed × 100%) for a given period, usually 1 week. For example, if a person reports sleeping an average of 6 hours per night out of 8 hours spent in bed, the initial prescribed sleep window (i.e., from initial bedtime to final arising time) would be 6 hours (see Figure 28.1). The subsequent sleep window is increased by 15 to 20 minutes for a given week when sleep efficiency exceeds 85%, it is decreased by the same amount when sleep efficiency is lower than 80%, and it is kept stable when sleep efficiency falls between 80% and 85%. Adjustments are made weekly until optimal sleep duration is achieved, which delivers optimal functioning during wakefulness. It is important to note that there is significant variation in how SRT is delivered across protocols and trials (Kyle et al., 2015). Changes to the prescribed sleep window can be made at the beginning of the night (i.e., postponing bedtime), at the end of the sleep period (i.e., advancing arising time), or at both ends. This can be based on the type of sleep problem (sleep-onset insomnia or early morning awakening) and on patients' preference.

Sleep compression, a variation of sleep restriction, consists of reducing time in bed more gradually than with sleep restriction and was principally developed for those with reduced sleep need. Other variations may involve changing the time in bed on the basis of a moving average of the sleep efficiency (e.g., the past 3–5 days) or changing it on a weekly basis regardless of changes in sleep efficiency (Lichstein et al., 2001). To minimize excessive daytime sleepiness, the prescribed time in bed should not be less than 5 hours

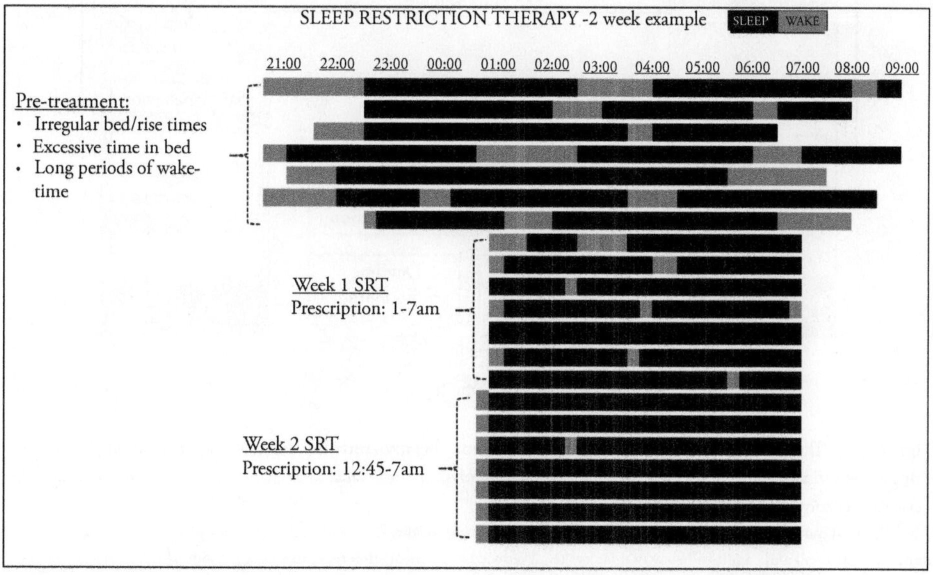

Figure 28.1 Patient example showing 7-day baseline sleep diary and the first 2 weeks of sleep restriction therapy (SRT)

Note. SRT restricts time in bed to match baseline sleep duration, while subsequent changes to time in bed are made based on sleep efficiency thresholds (e.g., increasing time in bed by 15 minutes if sleep efficiency exceeds 85%).

per night, regardless of the reported initial sleep duration. This caution is particularly important for those whose jobs require operating motor vehicles or who have duties in which drowsiness may be a danger to the patient or others. Studies show that objective sleep duration is decreased, on average, by between 50 and 90 minutes during the first 2–3 weeks of treatment. For this reason, sleep restriction should also be avoided or should be used cautiously with patients who need to drive or operate heavy equipment and with those who are already excessively sleepy during the day. Sleep restriction should also be avoided in patients with a history of seizures, certain parasomnias (e.g., sleepwalking), and manic or hypomanic episodes (as in bipolar disorder) because it may lower the threshold for, or exacerbate, these conditions.

Sleep restriction is hypothesized to work by restricting time in bed awake, regularizing the timing of sleep and wake, and reconditioning the association between sleep and the bedroom (see Figure 28.2). Partial sleep loss during early treatment potentiates sleepiness at bedtime, which reduces pre-sleep arousal and obviates sleep effort, leading to reduced

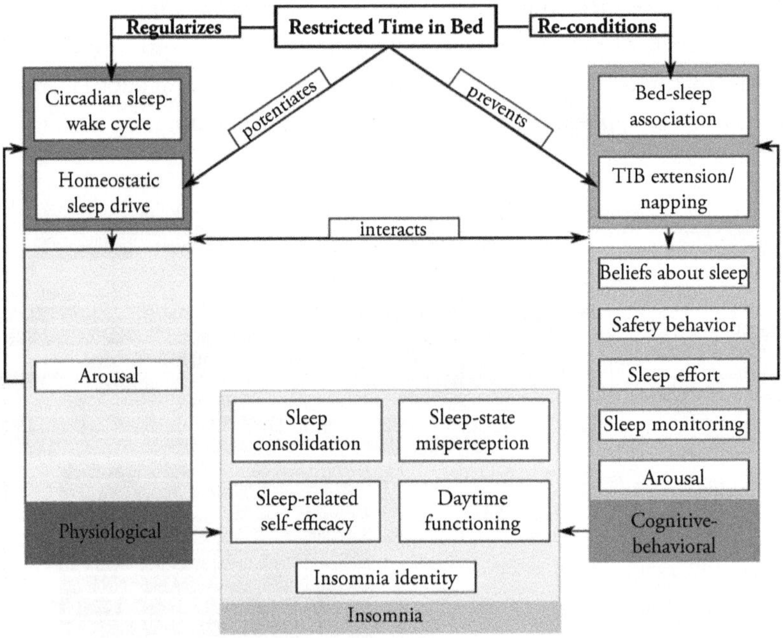

Figure 28.2 The Triple-R model posits that sleep restriction therapy exerts its treatment effects by doing three key things: restricting time in bed awake, regularizing timing of sleep and wake, and reconditioning the association between bedroom factors and sleep.

Note. Targeted modification of these key processes subsequently drives a cascade of change in subsidiary physiological (e.g., diminished arousal) and cognitive behavioral factors (e.g., reduced sleep effort) that serve to weaken insomnia maintenance factors and restore normal sleep. Interaction between cognitive behavioral and physiological pathways improves sleep consolidation, reduces subjective–objective sleep discrepancy, and ensures that sleep-related psychological agency (which in insomnia serves to disrupt sleep) surrenders to the two-process model of sleep–wake regulation. Consequently, those with insomnia will have a positive sleep experience that enhances sleep self-efficacy. With continued experience of predictable and restorative sleep, alongside sleep window extension and improved daytime function, the insomnia identity is challenged and ultimately revised. TIB = time in bed. Reproduced with permission from Maurer, Espie & Kyle, 2018 Sleep Medicine Reviews.

sleep onset, consolidated sleep during the night, and improved sleep quality (Maurer et al., 2022). Delaying sleep attempt has also been shown to increase circadian phase angle (sleep-onset time relative to dim-light melatonin onset), suggesting that a potential mechanism of SRT, at least for some patients, is to time sleep opportunity at a more conducive circadian phase (Maurer et al., 2021). Increased sleep depth and reduced sleep–wake variability from night to night may also have important psychological consequences, such as challenging unhelpful beliefs about sleep, decreasing sleep preoccupation, and enhancing feelings of mastery and self-efficacy. While sleep restriction is effective, it is considered the most challenging aspect of CBT due to the acute effects of restricted sleep opportunity. Controlled and uncontrolled evidence shows that SRT increases daytime sleepiness and reduces psychomotor vigilance during the first few weeks of treatment (Kyle et al., 2014). Hence, it is important to inform patients about these potential consequences so that they can adequately prepare (e.g., find alternative transport arrangements during early implementation, recruit the support of family members).

Stimulus Control Therapy

Stimulus control therapy (Bootzin et al., 1991) involves five relatively straightforward instructions designed to strengthen the temporal (bedtime) and environmental (bed and bedroom) stimuli with rapid sleep onset and to establish a regular circadian sleep–wake rhythm.

- Go to bed only when sleepy—not just fatigued but sleepy.
- Get out of bed when unable to sleep (e.g., after 20 minutes), go to another room, and return to bed only when sleep is imminent.
- Curtail all sleep-incompatible activities: no eating, watching television, using electronic devices, or planning or problem-solving in bed.
- Arise at a regular time every morning regardless of the amount of sleep achieved.
- Avoid daytime napping.

Persons with insomnia often develop apprehension around bedtime and the bedroom and come to associate this period of the day and environment with the frustration of being unable to sleep. Over time, the pre-sleep rituals usually associated with relaxation and sleep become cues for worrying and wakefulness. In addition, many insomnia patients display counterproductive sleep habits that emerge as a means of coping with sleep disturbances. For example, poor sleep at night can lead to daytime napping or sleeping late on weekends in an attempt to catch up on lost sleep. Individuals might lie in bed for prolonged periods trying to force sleep, only to find themselves becoming more awake. Stimulus control procedures are designed to recreate a positive association between pre-sleep rituals and the bedroom environment.

Stimulus control instructions appear quite simple; however, the challenge for clinicians is to foster strict adherence with these instructions. Several consultations held on a weekly or biweekly basis are often necessary to assist patients in implementing these behavioral changes. Stimulus control instructions can be combined with sleep restriction, for example, by having patients stay up until they are sleepy and it is at least their prescribed bedtime ("threshold time for bed"; Morin & Espie, 2003). Also, the stimulus control instruction to avoid napping can be modified to allow a short mid-afternoon nap in the early phase of sleep restriction, particularly in older adults or those who are overly sleepy with the nighttime sleep restriction. Caution with the instruction of getting out of bed at night when unable to sleep is also indicated for older adults using hypnotic medication who may be at greater risk for falls.

Relaxation-Based Interventions

Because stress, tension, and anxiety are common contributing factors to sleep disturbances, relaxation is probably the most commonly used intervention for insomnia. This treatment aims to reduce arousal at bedtime or upon nighttime awakening. Among the different relaxation interventions, some methods (e.g., progressive muscle relaxation, autogenic training) focus on reducing somatic arousal, whereas attention-focusing procedures (e.g., imagery training, thought stopping) target mental arousal in the form of worries, intrusive thoughts, or a racing mind (Lichstein, 1988). Biofeedback is designed to train patients to control some physiologic parameters (e.g., tension) through visual or auditory feedback; despite its popularity in the 1980s and 1990s, this method is used infrequently today.

Most relaxation procedures are equally effective for treating insomnia. Selection of a particular method should be based on the subtype of arousal (somatic vs. mental) interfering with sleep, although these often overlap, and the patient's preference. There is no formal contraindication to using relaxation, but some patients might have a paradoxical response and become more anxious when trying to relax. The most critical issue is to encourage daily practice of the selected method for at least 2 to 4 weeks. The focus should be on reducing arousal rather than on inducing sleep. The selected relaxation method should be practiced out of bed, especially if the patient is also using stimulus control therapy. Professional guidance is often necessary during initial training.

Cognitive Therapy

Cognitive therapy for insomnia seeks to alter sleep-disruptive cognitions (e.g., unhelpful beliefs, expectations) and maladaptive cognitive processes (e.g., excessive self-monitoring, worrying) through Socratic questioning and behavioral experiments (Bélanger et al., 2006; Harvey, 2002; Harvey et al., 2007; Morin, 1993). The basic premise of this approach is that appraisal of a given situation (sleeplessness) can trigger negative thoughts and emotions (anxiety) that are incompatible with sleep. For example, worries about the consequences of sleep loss on the next day's performance can lead to further arousal and more sleep disturbance, thus forming a vicious cycle. Likewise, a person may engage in self-monitoring (e.g., clock watching to check how many hours are left in the night) and safety activities (e.g., trying to stop thinking), which can prolong the nocturnal awakenings (Harvey, 2002).

Cognitive therapy is designed to short-circuit the self-fulfilling nature of this vicious cycle through verbal interventions and behavioral homework. Some therapeutic targets for cognitive restructuring include unrealistic expectations ("I must get 8 hours of sleep every night"), faulty causal attributions ("My insomnia is entirely caused by a biochemical imbalance"), and amplification of the consequences of insomnia ("After a poor night's sleep, I can't function the next day"). There are several key messages to communicate to patients in the context of cognitive therapy (see Table 28.1).

In addition to these verbal interventions, behavioral experiments can be quite powerful to change a person's beliefs about sleep and insomnia. For example, if a patient is convinced that bed rest is a good strategy to conserve energy, a behavioral experiment is designed to test the validity of this belief: The patient is instructed to engage specifically in this strategy (bed rest) on a day following insomnia and, on another day, to engage in the opposite behavior, such as performing a series of activities designed to generate energy

Table 28.1 Examples of cognitive interventions to change unhelpful beliefs about sleep

Key principles	Beliefs and attitudes to promote (examples)
Keep realistic expectations	There are individual differences in sleep needs; not everyone needs 8 hours. A shortcut, but more consolidated sleep periods are more refreshing/satisfying than a longer but fragment sleep period.
Never "try" to sleep	Whenever you try to force sleep, it generates more performance anxiety. The best you can do is to create circumstances that are conducive to sleep.
Examine all potential causes of insomnia	There is rarely just one cause of insomnia (pain, menopause); insomnia is often caused by both biological and behavioral factors. Try to focus on those that you can change.
Do not give too much importance to sleep	Sleep is important to both physical and mental health. Although it occupies about one-third of your life, don't let sleep drive your entire life.
Avoid dramatizing the consequences of sleep difficulties	Insomnia may be an unpleasant experience, but it is not dangerous!!! Excessive worrying about sleeplessness and its potential consequences may be more detrimental to health than insomnia itself.
Develop tolerance to the effects of sleep loss	Insomnia clearly affects quality of life and produces fatigue and daytime impairments, but you can still enjoy life despite these daytime limitations.

after a poor night's sleep (e.g., exercising, meeting with friends, doing errands). For each experiment, the patient is asked to monitor (on an hourly basis) several parameters such as fatigue, energy level, etc. In most instances, patients come back with the experience that energy was much better on those days that they were active. Such homework can be quite effective to change a person's belief about ways to preserve or generate energy in the context of insomnia (Harvey et al., 2007). Additional cognitive strategies may be useful in treating insomnia. For instance, paradoxical intention is a procedure designed to eliminate performance anxiety. In the context of insomnia, any attempt to control or induce sleep voluntarily is likely to generate performance anxiety and to delay sleep onset. With paradoxical intention, the patient is instructed to remain passively awake and to give up any effort (intention) to fall asleep.

As bedtime is often a prime time for thinking, planning, and worrying, another helpful cognitive procedure involves a method known as "time out for worrying." To minimize worrying and mental activity interfering with sleep, patients are instructed to set aside a time and a place (other than bedtime and the bedroom) to write down thoughts or worries and plans for the next day. This sort of exercise needs to be repeated daily to produce benefits, and if excessive worrying persists at bedtime or while awake at night, the patient is instructed to get out of bed and put down in writing the nature of the worries and intrusive thoughts. Imagery techniques can also be useful to block out such unwanted nocturnal thoughts (Harvey & Payne, 2002).

Mindfulness-Based Interventions

Developed through meditation, mindfulness is a method based on awareness in the present moment, without judgment. One of the most common mindfulness programs used in healthcare today is mindfulness-based stress reduction (MBSR). Despite some variability in its implementation, this intervention usually involves eight weekly group therapy sessions and a 1-day silent retreat. Participants learn various meditation practices including breathing meditation, body scan, sitting meditation, hatha yoga, and walking meditation. Daily personal meditation is expected. The program teaches principles of nonjudging, beginner's mind, trust, nonstriving, acceptance, and letting go (Kabat-Zinn, 2013). MBSR has been used with various health conditions to reduce stress and symptoms, enhance calmness, and improve quality of life. As used in the context of insomnia, the goal is to reduce stress and psychophysiological arousal.

Mindfulness-based therapy for insomnia is an intervention that integrates behavioral procedures such as sleep restriction and stimulus control therapy into MBSR (Ong et al., 2014; Ong & Sholtes, 2010). The mindfulness principles are believed to complement the conventional behavioral therapies and to replace the need for cognitive therapy. For example, nonstriving is consistent with relinquishing the counterproductive desire to actively control sleep. Also, mindfulness encourages a nonjudgmental observation of one's thoughts as mental events, and this is believed to improve clarity of thought and calmness, thereby reducing arousal (Ong et al., 2008).

Acceptance Therapy

ACT is part of the third wave of CBT. While its foundation may seem a bit paradoxical with standard CBT-I (e.g., a patient may be asked to stay in bed rather than leaving the bed when unable to sleep), it seeks to increase the patient's acceptance and willingness to experience the conditioned physiological and psychological discomfort commonly associated with not sleeping. Such acceptance may paradoxically be instrumental in lessening the mental and physiological nocturnal arousal, thus promoting a state of rest and sleepiness, rather than struggle and wakefulness. Although there are some common assumptions with MBSR and cognitive therapy principles, the methods of ACT to overcome the psychological discomfort or distress that comes with insomnia are different. ACT aims to develop and expand behavioral and psychological flexibility, that is, the ability to stay in contact with the present moment more fully and based on what the situation offers. In addition, ACT relates the processes of acceptance and attention to the processes of commitment and behavior change (Hayes et al., 2011). Individuals first learn to accept their challenges and then commit to resolving them with behavioral change strategies. Preliminary and uncontrolled evidence suggests that ACT may be an effective strategy for treating insomnia (El Rafihi-Ferreira et al., 2022) and in those who are unresponsive to CBT (Hertenstein et al., 2014) by shifting focus away from the sleep problem and efforts to control it to the acceptance of the associated thoughts and feelings. This method is potentially useful for patients who do not comply or do not achieve optimal treatment response to standard CBT, although additional controlled studies are needed to compare against standard CBT-I and to determine who is a good candidate for this therapy.

Intensive Sleep Retraining

Intensive sleep retraining (ISR) is a brief and intensive in-laboratory procedure that utilizes sleep deprivation in combination with repeated sleep-onset opportunities to promote the ability to fall asleep via a counter-conditioning process (Lack et al., 2019; Mair et al., 2022). This procedure involves multiple (>40 trials) and short (<5-minute) sleep opportunities, typically every 30 minutes over a 24-hour period. Patients are awakened shortly after they fall asleep to preserve a strong homeostatic sleep drive. In addition, they are not allowed to sleep between the repeated trials. The rationale behind this intervention is that rapid sleep onset on repeated trials, facilitated by a strong homeostatic sleep drive, leads to a reconditioning of the person's ability to fall asleep quickly. Preliminary results about its efficacy are promising (Lack et al., 2019). Although ISR is fairly demanding in human resources because of the supervision required for implementation in the sleep laboratory, a recent study has demonstrated its feasibility using a smartphone-delivered protocol (Mair et al., 2022). This treatment, which seems best implemented under supervision in a clinical setting, may represent an alternative intervention especially for patients who do not respond to more standard CBT-I.

Sleep Hygiene Education

Sleep hygiene education is intended to provide basic information about lifestyle (diet, exercise, substance use) and environmental factors (light, noise, temperature) that might either interfere with or promote better sleep (Hauri, 1997). It can also include general sleep-facilitating recommendations, such as allowing enough time to relax before bedtime, avoiding clock watching, and maintaining a regular sleep schedule. Some of these instructions overlap with other behavioral procedures. Sleep hygiene guidelines include the following:

- Avoid stimulants (e.g., caffeine, nicotine) for several hours before bedtime.
- Avoid alcohol around bedtime because it fragments sleep.
- Exercise regularly (especially in late afternoon or early evening).
- Allow at least a 1-hour period to unwind before bedtime.
- Keep the bedroom environment quiet, dark, and comfortable.
- Maintain a regular sleep schedule.
- Remove electronic devices from the bedroom.

While it may be helpful for mild insomnia, sleep hygiene education is rarely sufficient for more severe insomnia. A didactic approach can also be used to provide basic information about normal sleep, individual differences in sleep needs, and changes in sleep physiology with aging. This information is very useful to help some patients distinguish clinical insomnia from normal (age-related) sleep disturbances. Such knowledge can prevent excessive worry and concern, which can themselves lead to clinical insomnia; however, sleep hygiene is not recommended as a monotherapy and should always be delivered alongside evidence-based treatment components (Edinger et al., 2021b).

Evidence Base for CBT-I: State-of-the-Art

Multiple meta-analyses show that CBT-I is effective at reducing global insomnia symptom severity as well as key sleep diary parameters, including sleep latency, wake time after sleep onset, and sleep efficiency (see Figure 28.3). Robust treatment effects in the self-report domain have been observed across a range of delivery formats, including individual and group therapy as well as self-help, telehealth, and app-based or digital intervention (Edinger et al., 2021b; Riemann et al., 2017). While CBT improves sleep quality and self-reported sleep continuity, it has small and typically nonsignificant effects on sleep duration (van Straten et al., 2018). Moreover, meta-analysis suggests that CBT-I has no effect or very modest effects on polysomnography (PSG) and actigraphy-defined sleep (Mitchell et al., 2019), although some studies have shown some improvements in PSG-defined sleep

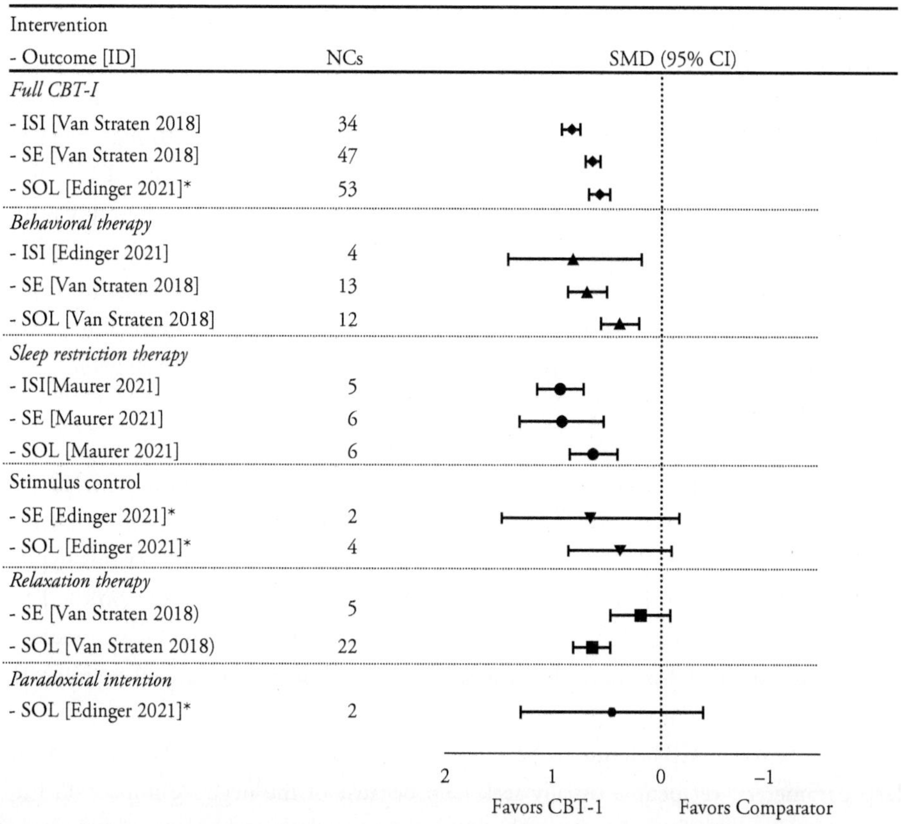

Figure 28.3 Overview of standardized mean differences for insomnia severity and sleep diary–derived sleep efficiency, and sleep onset latency across cognitive behavioral therapy for insomnia and its components

Note. Standardized mean differences (SMDs) and 95% confidence intervals were derived from meta-analyses (ID presented in form of the first author and the year of publication) or manually calculated with data provided by the meta-analysis (marked with an asterisk). When more than one meta-analysis provided relevant outcome data, we included the meta-analysis that was based on a higher number of comparisons or provided outcome data in SMD format. CBT-I = cognitive behavioral therapy for insomnia; CI = confidence interval; ISI = insomnia severity index; NCs = number of comparisons; SE = sleep efficiency; SOL = sleep onset latency. Reproduced with permission from Maurer and Kyle (2022).

parameters (Morin et al., 1999). More research is needed, especially during active treatment, incorporating serial measurement of sleep physiology in the home environment (Maurer et al., 2020). Effect sizes are strongest for global insomnia symptom severity, and efficacy does not appear to be moderated by baseline factors such as age, comorbidity, or hypnotic medication use. Most trials have assessed multicomponent CBT, but a small number of studies have interrogated single-component treatment strategies. Sleep restriction, stimulus control, and relaxation therapy have been assessed as single components in meta-analysis (see Figure 28.3), with the strongest and most consistent effects being observed for sleep restriction. Indeed, effect sizes for the insomnia severity index (ISI) from six trials were similar in magnitude for SRT (g = 0.93) compared to multicomponent CBT (g = 0.82). Prospective studies comparing SRT to multicomponent CBT, while not powered to appraise non-inferiority, do not show clear differences in insomnia outcomes (Drake et al., 2019; Epstein et al., 2012; Krieger et al., 2019), suggesting that sleep restriction may be one of the most active and critical components of CBT-I. In support of this, a recent component network meta-analysis of 80 studies found that SRT was the most effective treatment component in reducing insomnia severity and improving sleep parameters (Steinmetz et al., 2024). More work is needed to establish (1) the comparative efficacy of *specific* cognitive and behavioral therapies; (2) optimal *sequencing* of components; and (3) whether systematic *tailoring* of treatment to patient phenotype can enhance outcomes.

One suggested phenotype—insomnia with objective short sleep duration—is hypothesized to be associated with poorer response to CBT-I (Vgontzas et al., 2013), but results are conflicting (Bathgate et al., 2017; Rochefort et al., 2019) and often based on post hoc analyses. In the largest (n = 642) preregistered moderation test of this hypothesis, actigraphy-defined sleep duration did not moderate treatment effects on the ISI at 6 months following SRT (Kyle et al., 2023). Future studies are needed where recruited samples are enriched for short sleep duration at baseline to adequately examine this hypothesis.

The efficacy of CBT tends to be judged based on global insomnia symptoms and sleep parameters, yet people usually seek help because of the negative impact on functioning and quality of life (Morin et al., 2006). Meta-analysis and large randomized controlled trials (RCTs) show that CBT has reliable, though relatively modest, effects on quality of life and other daytime symptoms, like cognitive failures, fatigue, relationship functioning, and work productivity (Alimoradi et al., 2022; Benz et al., 2020; Espie et al., 2019). Modest effects may be attributed to the limited focus on daytime functioning within therapy, the limited effects of CBT on objective sleep parameters, and/or the use of generic measures to appraise health-related quality of life (e.g., the Short Form-36, EuroQol-5D), which may lack sensitivity to insomnia and its treatment. In one study of digital CBT-I (n = 1,711; Espie et al., 2019), a patient-centered measure, the Glasgow Sleep Impact Index (Kyle et al., 2013), showed markedly larger between-group effects (d = 1.4) relative to a generic measure of health-related quality of life (Patient-Reported Outcomes Measurement Information System-10; d = 0.3). Measuring important life domains unique to each individual, and in the patient's own language, may be a more valid and sensitive approach to appraising the effects of insomnia treatment.

Health-related quality of life is also an important outcome because it is used by healthcare systems, alongside healthcare costs, to determine if a treatment is cost-effective (the incremental cost-effectiveness ratio) and therefore worth investing in. Relatively few studies have formally and systematically assessed the cost-effectiveness of CBT-I in clinical trials (Natsky et al., 2020), and findings have been mixed, in part because generic utility measures do not appear sensitive (Baka et al., 2022). More work is needed in this area, especially within routine care settings so that healthcare costs can be reliably quantified, alongside broader societal costs like work-related productivity loss and out-of-pocket spending on over-the-counter medications. Uncontrolled data from a large implementation study of digital CBT-I in primary care suggested that treatment may lead to savings of £70 (approximately 90 US$) per user, chiefly through reduction in primary care visits and prescriptions (Sampson et al., 2022). If these results were to be scaled up, digital CBT-I may save £20 million (approximately 26M US$) per year in England; however, controlled evidence with sufficient long-term follow-up (12 months plus horizon) is required to accurately appraise the health economics of digital insomnia treatment.

The vast majority of early insomnia treatment trials have focused on insomnia in the absence of comorbidity, despite such samples being unrepresentative of the insomnia population at large. In recent years, given the strong association between insomnia and poor mental and physical health, researchers have asked whether treating insomnia in the context of comorbidity influences outcomes relevant to the comorbid disorder. Randomized trials and meta-analyses show that treating insomnia through CBT drives reduction in anxiety and depressive symptoms in clinical and nonclinical populations (Gee et al., 2019; Hertenstein et al., 2022) and may even prevent incident and recurrent depression (Irwin et al., 2022). Intriguingly, in two head-to-head comparisons of CBT-I versus CBT for depression or anxiety, the former improved depression and anxiety symptoms to the same degree as the latter yet had larger effects on sleep (Blom et al., 2015; Mason et al., 2022). Generalized effects of CBT-I have also been observed for other mental health outcomes (Hertenstein et al., 2022), pain (Selvanathan et al., 2021), and cancer-related symptoms (Squires et al., 2022), suggesting that insomnia may be causally involved in the maintenance of these comorbidities. More implementation studies of insomnia treatment within clinical services are needed to ensure that scientific findings adequately translate to healthcare systems (Harvey, 2022).

In contrast to treatment efficacy, there has been limited focus on the possibility that CBT-I is associated with side effects (Kyle et al., 2011). A recent systematic review of all published CBT-I trials found that only 7% of RCTs adequately reported on measurement of adverse events, and even fewer used appropriate measurement (Condon et al., 2021). A similar conclusion was reached by the recent American Academy of Sleep Medicine task force review (Edinger et al., 2021b). More work is needed to understand potential adverse effects of CBT components. In a controlled trial comparing online CBT-I to sleep hygiene control, participants in the CBT-I arm were more likely to report excessive sleepiness, fatigue, irritability, headaches, poor memory and concentration, and reduced motivation (Espie et al., 2019), effects that were attributed to behavioral treatment components. Work by other groups has further localized these effects to behavioral strategies, showing that (1) behavioral therapy leads to significantly more side effects than cognitive therapy, particularly for sleepiness and fatigue (Sunnhed et al., 2020), and (2) SRT is the treatment component most commonly identified by patients as causing side effects during CBT-I (Kaldo et al., 2015). It is important to note that side effects might be perceived as worse when using online CBT-I due to the lack of therapist guidance. Through restriction of sleep opportunity, SRT engenders mild sleep deprivation (Maurer et al., 2020) which manifests in enhanced sleepiness and impaired vigilance during acute treatment (Kyle et al., 2014; Maurer et al., 2021, 2022). Importantly, a minority of patients also report concerns with driving during SRT implementation (Kyle et al., 2011), although a recent trial did not find any increase in falls, road traffic accidents, or falling asleep while driving during SRT relative to sleep hygiene (Kyle et al., 2023). Other work has also shown that insomnia, in and of itself, may increase the risk of road accidents (Morin, Altena, et al., 2020). Nevertheless, the overall evidence highlights the importance of communicating the risks of daytime sleepiness to participants during treatment and to adapt time in bed where necessary. Furthermore, because side effects of SRT (and stimulus control therapy) may affect patient experience of treatment (Chan et al., 2017; Krieger et al., 2019; Parsons et al., 2021) and may undermine clinical benefit (Vincent & Lewycky, 2009), the field should develop and test countermeasures that aim to support patients during treatment.

How Does CBT-I Work?

CBTs were developed by clinical researchers to target specific insomnia maintenance factors. Treatment strategies have been informed by clinical observation, theory, and developments in clinical science. However, despite the success of CBT-I, there has been relatively limited empirical testing of its mechanisms. One early review focused on pre-to-post changes in putative mediators in the context of randomized trials. CBT was associated with reduction in napping and time in bed, bedtime and rise time variability, cognitive arousal and dysfunctional beliefs and attitudes about sleep, and increased sleep-related self-efficacy (Schwartz & Carney, 2012). A recent systematic review evaluated trials where putative mediators were formally assessed using mediation analysis (Parsons et al., 2021). There was evidence that change in dysfunctional beliefs about sleep and markers of (cognitive) arousal—though not time in bed—were associated with treatment outcome; however, a major limitation of the literature is that mediators and outcomes were typically assessed at the same time, precluding assessment of temporal precedence and therefore causal ordering. Similar observations were made for studies of single-component SRT (Maurer et al., 2018).

A range of designs and methodologies are clearly required to advance understanding of the active ingredients and treatment mechanisms of CBT-I. For example, in a randomized controlled dismantling trial, Maurer and colleagues (2020) compared sleep restriction with a dismantled control arm (time in bed regularization) in order to isolate the role of time in bed restriction in driving both clinical and mechanistic outcomes. Compared to simple regularization of time in bed, sleep restriction led to greater reduction of insomnia severity and improvements in quality of life. Sleep restriction also increased evening sleepiness, reduced pre-sleep arousal, consolidated sleep, potentiated electroencephalographic delta power, and decreased beta power during non-rapid-eye-movement sleep. Similar designs could be applied to other components of CBT-I, especially since trials of multicomponent intervention packages (which vary in component composition, dose, and order) make it difficult to link specific treatment strategies to mechanistic change. However, the interaction between components of CBT-I should also be appraised in dedicated studies since synergistic effects may also be important for specific subgroups of patients. On the other hand, an interesting possibility is that behavioral treatments may have effects that extend beyond their proximal and circumscribed targets. For example, following a dismantling study of CBT, comparing behavior therapy and cognitive therapy to the full CBT intervention, analyses of mediators indicated that the behavioral processes (e.g., time in bed, variability in sleep schedule) mediated outcome for behavior therapy but not cognitive therapy, whereas the cognitive processes (e.g., worry, unhelpful beliefs, sleep monitoring) mediated outcome in both behavior therapy and cognitive therapy (Harvey et al., 2017). This may mean that relatively brief and focused treatments can address multiple insomnia maintenance factors (and patient phenotypes) and, due to their simplicity, have the potential to be scaled up and deployed in clinical settings (e.g., primary care) for maximum patient benefit. A final reflection is that while mediation analysis is an important tool in the search for mechanisms, exclusive focus on linear, unidirectional (and singular) mediators may not sufficiently capture the complexity, bidirectionality, and idiographic trajectories of treatment processes. Advances in understanding mechanisms may also depend, therefore, on developments in individual network dynamic approaches (cf. Hofmann et al., 2020).

Combined CBT-I and Medication

Although CBT is recognized as the treatment of choice, there may be instances where CBT and medication can play a complementary role in the management of insomnia. A combined approach should, in principle, optimize outcome by capitalizing on the more rapid effects of medication and the more sustained benefits of CBT. The evidence, however, is not as clear on whether adding medication enhances final outcomes or not.

Fewer than 10 controlled studies have evaluated the differential and combined effects of CBT and pharmacologic therapies for insomnia (see, e.g., Jacobs et al., 2004; Milby et al., 1993; Morin et al., 1999, 2009; Morin, Edinger, et al., 2020; Sivertsen et al., 2006; Wu et al., 2006). Collectively, those studies have shown that CBT is at least as effective as benzodiazepine (i.e., temazepam, triazolam) and non-benzodiazepine medications (i.e., zolpidem, zopiclone) in the short term (3–8 weeks) and more effective in the long term (6–24 months). When used singly, medication produces rapid improvements, but these benefits are quickly lost after drug discontinuation. Conversely, sleep improvements obtained with CBT take longer, but they are also well sustained even after treatment. There is generally a slight additive effect of combined approaches relative to medication alone but not necessarily relative to CBT alone. In terms of speed of therapeutic effects, medication may have a boosting effect early in treatment when added to CBT, but this initial advantage tends to disappear by the sixth or eighth week of treatment (Morin et al., 2014). Finally, while CBT produces larger benefits than medication in reducing insomnia symptoms and improving sleep continuity parameters (i.e., sleep latency, wake after sleep onset, sleep efficiency), one small open trial reported that trazodone was more effective than CBT-I for increasing total sleep time, an improvement that was greater among patients with objective short sleep duration (Vgontzas et al., 2020).

Sometimes it may be preferable to provide treatment sequentially rather than concomitantly. One study comparing four treatment sequences found that first-stage therapy with either behavior therapy or zolpidem produced equivalent percentages of responders (behavior therapy, 45.5%; zolpidem, 49.7%) and remitters (behavior therapy, 38.03%; zolpidem, 30.3%) (Morin, Edinger, et al., 2020). For patients who did not remit with their initial treatment, second-stage therapy increased the proportion of responders for the two conditions starting with behavior therapy (behavior therapy to zolpidem, 40.6% to 62.7%; behavior therapy to cognitive therapy, 50.1% to 68.2%), but no significant increase was obtained following zolpidem treatment. A significant increase in percentage of remitters was observed in two of the four sequences (behavior therapy to zolpidem, 38.1% to 55.9%; zolpidem to trazodone, 31.4% to 49.4%). Of significant interest, treatment sequences that involved cognitive therapy or trazodone as second-stage therapy yielded better outcomes for patients with comorbid insomnia, perhaps due to the broader and more transdiagnostic feature of those treatments (i.e., cognitive therapy and trazodone).

Because of the mediating role of psychological factors in chronic insomnia, behavioral and attitudinal changes appear essential to sustain improvements in sleep patterns. When behavioral and drug therapies are combined, patients' attributions of the initial benefits may be critical in determining long-term outcomes. Attribution of therapeutic benefits to the medication alone, without integration of self-management skills, can place a patient at greater risk for insomnia recurrence after the drug is discontinued. In addition, there is a risk that medication might undermine the patient's effort and motivation to implement behavioral changes in sleep habits and sleep scheduling. Thus, despite the intuitive appeal of combining therapies, it is not entirely clear when, how, and for whom combining CBT and medication is indicated. Additional research is needed to examine optimal methods for combining or integrating these therapies.

Clinical and Practical Considerations

The management of insomnia disorder with CBT poses several challenges to both patients and clinicians, and several clinical and practical issues must be considered when planning treatment. First, patient's acceptance of CBT-I is a sine qua non of treatment engagement. If a patient is expecting a "quick fix" and is reluctant to invest time and effort in exploring potential psychological and behavioral issues contributing to insomnia, CBT cannot be forced on them. Patients (and clinicians not familiar with CBT) need to understand that CBT-I does not work like a medication, hence the importance of taking time to explain the rationale underlying CBT-I. Another issue directly related to treatment acceptability is about treatment adherence. The success of CBT-I depends largely on the patient's willingness to comply with the recommended behavioral and cognitive changes. Direct and ongoing therapist guidance is often a critical factor to facilitate optimal treatment adherence for a successful outcome.

CBT is not a formula or recipe derived from a cookbook. Of course, it involves core therapeutic components, but they must be adapted to each patient. Treatment must be individualized to the specific characteristics and comorbidities of each patient. Since more than half of patients with insomnia present a comorbid medical (e.g., pain) or psychiatric disorder (e.g., depression), such coexisting conditions cannot be ignored. Rather, treatment implementation may need to be adapted and take those comorbidities into consideration. Such adaptations have been made for patients with comorbid cancer, pain, and depression.

Many patients come to therapy for insomnia after they have been using different types of hypnotic medications or other products intended to promote sleep. With prolonged usage, many patients feel dependent and unable to discontinue their use. This type of patient presents a particular challenge and will often require that a clinician works with the prescribing physician or a pharmacist to design an appropriate withdrawal/tapering schedule. Whether discontinuation of the medication should occur before, during, or after CBT-I is an issue that requires examining the patient's level of anxiety and self-efficacy regarding this endeavor. A systematic and time-limited tapering schedule has proved successful with long-term users of benzodiazepines for insomnia (Morin et al., 2004).

Refinements to CBT and Future Research

Given that CBT-I is still not accessible for the vast majority of people with insomnia, the key priority has to be to make evidence-based treatment more accessible. In this regard, digital therapies and scalable models of brief CBT within primary care settings (or low-intensity psychological therapy programs; Clark, 2018) may help address dissemination and access issues (Espie, 2009; Morin, 2017; Riemann et al., 2022). Moreover, from a scientific perspective, rigorously testing and demonstrating the benefits of CBT-I in terms of cost–utility will be important in convincing decision makers that insomnia treatment is worth investing in (Wickwire & Morin, 2020).

While CBT is effective, a sizable proportion of patients do not remit or do not achieve a clinically meaningful response, and for some patients, initial clinical benefits are not sustained over long-term follow-up (van der Zweerde et al., 2019). There is clearly room for improvement. At least two lines of enquiry may help refine CBT-I. The first involves adding treatment components that specifically address circadian disruption. For example, there is preliminary evidence from small trials that adding a "circadian rhythm support" intervention (comprising management of light exposure, temperature, and physical activity) may yield improved outcomes (Dekker et al., 2020; Leerssen et al., 2022). This may be especially important for insomnia comorbid with mental health problems. A recent trial in postpartum insomnia (n = 114) also found that light–dark therapy (light therapy on awakening and minimizing artificial light exposure in the evening) reduced insomnia severity to a similar level as CBT, although a combined treatment was not tested (Verma et al., 2020). Formally integrating monitored exercise interventions (Lowe et al., 2019) or novel brain stimulation paradigms (e.g., electrical or acoustic) may potentiate clinical gains, but appropriately powered trials are needed to assess whether improvement can be demonstrated beyond the "standard" CBT-I protocol. In the context of treating comorbid insomnia, some studies have also shown that adding a therapeutic component that targets cancer-related symptoms, such as fatigue, enhances treatment outcomes (Savard et al., 2005).

The second approach is to make treatment more precise and dynamic (Espie et al., 2014). That is, the field should assess the utility of tailoring treatments to patient-specific psychobiological features. When it comes to treating insomnia, there is probably no one-size-fits-all, and more research is needed, first, to validate reliable insomnia phenotypes and, second, to test whether some phenotypes respond better to specific treatment. While still theoretical at this stage, such an approach could include baseline profiling of sleep physiology, hyperarousal, circadian phase and light sensitivity, environmental variables (e.g., patterning and composition of light exposure), and psychological factors, from which personalized cognitive, behavioral, and circadian therapies could be prescribed. Matching of sleep and circadian modules to diverse sleep phenotypes and patient preference has recently been tested in the context of severe mental illness (Harvey et al., 2021). Several preliminary studies have also examined treatment response as a function of objective sleep duration among insomnia patients (Bathgate et al., 2017; Rochefort et al., 2019; Vgontzas et al., 2020); this line of research warrants further investigation. Finally, developments in digital technology may support the implementation of CBT-I strategies in real time and better detect non-engagement and/or non-response, leading to the rapid deployment of personalized intervention or the introduction of alternative therapeutic strategies (Forsell et al., 2019).

Conclusions

In this chapter, we described core components of CBT-I and summarized the evidence supporting this approach for the management of insomnia disorder. Looking back over recent decades, the field has moved a long way from some generic sleep hygiene guidelines to a well-defined and well-accepted clinical treatment with few adverse effects. CBT-I is now recognized in clinical practice guidelines as the treatment of choice for insomnia disorder. It took many RCTs to raise CBT-I to its current status, but even with this level of recognition, CBT-I is still not very well known and remains clearly underutilized in clinical practice.

Despite this tremendous progress achieved in the last few decades, there are still quite a few challenges ahead to optimize treatment outcomes and to make this therapeutic approach mainstream. First, there is still an important proportion of patients treated with CBT-I who do not achieve remission or an adequate treatment response. Additional research is needed to develop reliable phenotypes of insomnia and validate treatment algorithms that match phenotypes to treatment strategies. Second, while we have an effective treatment, with much evidence to support it, there is still a huge gap between the evidence base and current clinical practices. Despite its acceptance and recognition in the field, CBT-I has not reached wide implementation in clinical practice. Is this strictly a matter of not having enough competent CBT-I therapists? Probably not. Digital CBT-I is certainly one solution to reduce this gap and make treatment more accessible and available/affordable. While this technology can clearly broaden the reach of CBT-I, many patients with severe insomnia and comorbidities are likely to continue requiring guidance from a live therapist to assist them with treatment implementation.

Acknowledgments

Preparation of this chapter was supported in part by grants from the Canadian Institutes of Health Research to Charles M. Morin (Grants 483689, 483692, 83000212). Simon D. Kyle is supported by the National Institute for Health and Care Research (NIHR) Oxford Health Biomedical Research Centre; Health Technology Assessment Programme (Ref. 16/84/01); Programme Grants for Applied Research (Ref. 203667); and Efficacy and Mechanisms Evaluation Programme (Ref. 131789). The views expressed are those of the authors and not necessarily those of the National Health Service, the NIHR, or the Department of Health.

References

Alimoradi, Z., Jafari, E., Brostrom, A., Ohayon, M. M., Lin, C. Y., Griffiths, M. D., Blom, K., Jernelov, S., Kaldo, V., & Pakpour, A. H. (2022). Effects of cognitive behavioral therapy for insomnia (CBT-I) on quality of life: A systematic review and meta-analysis. *Sleep Medicine Reviews*, *64*, Article 101646. https://doi.org/10.1016/j.smrv.2022.101646

Araujo, T., Jarrin, D. C., Leanza, Y., Vallieres, A., & Morin, C. M. (2017). Qualitative studies of insomnia: Current state of knowledge in the field. *Sleep Medicine Reviews*, *31*, 58–69. https://doi.org/10.1016/j.smrv.2016.01.003

Baglioni, C., Espie, C. A., & Riemann, D. (Eds.). (2022). *Cognitive-Behavioural Therapy for Insomnia (CBT-I) across the life span: Guidelines and clinical protocols for health professionals*. John Wiley & Sons.

Baka, A., van der Zweerde, T., Lancee, J., Bosmans, J. E., & van Straten, A. (2022). Cost-effectiveness of guided internet-delivered cognitive behavioral therapy in comparison with care-as-usual for patients with insomnia in general practice. *Behavioral Sleep Medicine*, *20*(2), 188–203. https://doi.org/10.1080/15402002.2021.1901708

Bathgate, C. J., Edinger, J. D., & Krystal, A. D. (2017). Insomnia patients with objective short sleep duration have a blunted response to cognitive behavioral therapy for insomnia. *Sleep*, *40*(1), Article zsw012. https://doi.org/10.1093/sleep/zsw012

Bélanger, L., Savard, J., & Morin, C. M. (2006). Clinical management of insomnia using cognitive therapy. *Behavioral Sleep Medicine*, *4*(3), 179–198. https://doi.org/10.1207/s15402010bsm0403_4

Benz, F., Knoop, T., Ballesio, A., Bacaro, V., Johann, A. F., Rücker, G., Feige, B., Riemann, D., & Baglioni, C. (2020). The efficacy of cognitive and behavior therapies for insomnia on daytime symptoms: A systematic review and network meta-analysis. *Clinical Psychology Review, 80*, Article 101873. https://doi.org/10.1016/j.cpr.2020.101873

Blom, K., Jernelöv, S., Kraepelien, M., Bergdahl, M. O., Jungmarker, K., Ankartjärn, L., Lindefors, N., & Kaldo, V. (2015). Internet treatment addressing either insomnia or depression, for patients with both diagnoses: A randomized trial. *Sleep, 38*(2), 267–277. https://doi.org/10.5665/sleep.4412

Bootzin, R. R., Epstein, D., & Wood, J. M. (1991). Stimulus control instructions. In P. Hauri (Ed.), *Case studies in insomnia* (pp. 19–28). Plenum Press.

Chan, C., West, S., & Glozier, N. (2017). Commencing and persisting with a web-based cognitive behavioral intervention for insomnia: A qualitative study of treatment completers. *Journal of Medical Internet Research, 19*(2), Article e37. https://doi.org/10.2196/jmir.5639

Cheung, J. M., Bartlett, D. J., Armour, C. L., Glozier, N., & Saini, B. (2014). Insomnia patients' help-seeking experiences. *Behavioral Sleep Medicine, 12*(2), 106–122. https://doi.org/10.1080/15402002.2013.764529

Cheung, J. M., Bartlett, D. J., Armour, C. L., Laba, T. L., & Saini, B. (2016). To drug or not to drug: A qualitative study of patients' decision-making processes for managing insomnia. *Behavioral Sleep Medicine, 18*, 1–26. https://doi.org/10.1080/15402002.2016.1163702

Clark, D. M. (2018). Realizing the mass public benefit of evidence-based psychological therapies: The IAPT program. *Annual Review of Clinical Psychology, 14*, 159–183. https://doi.org/10.1146/annurev-clinpsy-050817-084833

Condon, H. E., Maurer, L. F., & Kyle, S. D. (2021). Reporting of adverse events in cognitive behavioural therapy for insomnia: A systematic examination of randomised controlled trials. *Sleep Medicine Reviews, 56*, Article 101412. https://doi.org/10.1016/j.smrv.2020.101412

Dekker, K., Benjamins, J. S., Maksimovic, T., Filardi, M., Hofman, W. F., van Straten, A., & Van Someren, E. J. W. (2020). Combined internet-based cognitive-behavioral and chronobiological intervention for insomnia: A randomized controlled trial. *Psychotherapy and Psychosomatics, 89*(2), 117–118. https://doi.org/10.1159/000503570

Drake, C. L., Kalmbach, D. A., Arnedt, J. T., Cheng, P., Tonnu, C. V., Cuamatzi-Castelan, A., & Fellman-Couture, C. (2019). Treating chronic insomnia in postmenopausal women: A randomized clinical trial comparing cognitive-behavioral therapy for insomnia, sleep restriction therapy, and sleep hygiene education. *Sleep, 42*(2), Article zsy217. https://doi.org/10.1093/sleep/zsy217

Edinger, J. D., Arnedt, J. T., Bertisch, S. M., Carney, C. E., Harrington, J. J., Lichstein, K. L., Sateia, M. J., Troxel, W. M., Zhou, E. S., Kazmi, U., Heald, J. L., & Martin, J. L. (2021a). Behavioral and psychological treatments for chronic insomnia disorder in adults: An American Academy of Sleep Medicine clinical practice guideline. *Journal of Clinical Sleep Medicine, 17*(2), 255–262. https://doi.org/10.5664/jcsm.8986

Edinger, J. D., Arnedt, J. T., Bertisch, S. M., Carney, C. E., Harrington, J. J., Lichstein, K. L., Sateia, M. J., Troxel, W. M., Zhou, E. S., Kazmi, U., Heald, J. L., & Martin, J. L. (2021b). Behavioral and psychological treatments for chronic insomnia disorder in adults: An American Academy of Sleep Medicine systematic review, meta-analysis, and GRADE assessment. *Journal of Clinical Sleep Medicine, 17*(2), 263–298. https://doi.org/10.5664/jcsm.8988

Edinger, J. D., & Carney, C. E. (2014). *Overcoming insomnia: A cognitive-behavioral approach—Therapist guide*. Oxford University Press.

El Rafihi-Ferreira, R., Morin, C. M., Hasan, R., Brasil, I. S., Zago Ribeiro, J. H. J., & Cecilia Toscanini, A. (2022). A pilot randomized controlled trial (RCT) of acceptance and commitment therapy versus cognitive behavioral therapy for chronic insomnia. *Behavioral Sleep Medicine, 21*(2), 193–207. https://doi.org/10.1080/15402002.2022.2071272

Epstein, D. R., Sidani, S., Bootzin, R. R., & Belyea, M. J. (2012). Dismantling multicomponent behavioral treatment for insomnia in older adults: A randomized controlled trial. *Sleep, 35*(6), 797–805. https://doi.org/10.5665/sleep.1878

Espie, C. A. (2002). Insomnia: Conceptual issues in the development, persistence, and treatment of sleep disorder in adults. *Annual Review of Psychology, 53*, 215–243. https://doi.org/10.1146/annurev.psych.53.100901.135243

Espie, C. A. (2009). "Stepped care": A health technology solution for delivering cognitive behavioral therapy as a first line insomnia treatment. *Sleep, 32*(12), 1549–1558. http://www.ncbi.nlm.nih.gov/entrez/query.fcgi?cmd=Retrieve&db=PubMed&dopt=Citation&list_uids=20041590

Espie, C. A., Emsley, R., Kyle, S. D., Gordon, C., Drake, C. L., Siriwardena, A. N., Cape, J., Ong, J. C., Sheaves, B., Foster, R., Freeman, D., Costa-Font, J., Marsden, A., & Luik, A. I. (2019). Effect of digital cognitive behavioral therapy for insomnia on health, psychological well-being, and sleep-related quality of life: A randomized clinical trial. *JAMA Psychiatry, 76*(1), 21–30. https://doi.org/10.1001/jamapsychiatry.2018.2745

Espie, C. A., Kyle, S. D., Gehrman, P., Ong, J., & Hames, P. (2014). Tailoring CBT for insomnia to specific needs: A personalised behavioural medicine approach. In C. Bassetti, Z. Dogas, & P. Peigneux (Eds.), *ESRS European Sleep Medicine Textbook* (pp. 193–206). European Sleep Research Society (ESRS).

Everitt, H., McDermott, L., Leydon, G., Yules, H., Baldwin, D., & Little, P. (2014). GPs' management strategies for patients with insomnia: A survey and qualitative interview study. *The British Journal of General Practice, 64*(619), e112–e119. https://doi.org/10.3399/bjgp14X677176

Forsell, E., Jernelöv, S., Blom, K., Kraepelien, M., Svanborg, C., Andersson, G., Lindefors, N., & Kaldo, V., . . . Kaldo, V. (2019). Proof of concept for an adaptive treatment strategy to prevent failures in internet-delivered CBT: A single-blind randomized clinical trial with insomnia patients. *American Journal of Psychiatry, 176*(4), 315–323. https://doi.org/10.1176/appi.ajp.2018.18060699

Gee, B., Orchard, F., Clarke, E., Joy, A., Clarke, T., & Reynolds, S. (2019). The effect of non-pharmacological sleep interventions on depression symptoms: A meta-analysis of randomised controlled trials. *Sleep Medicine Reviews, 43*, 118–128. https://doi.org/10.1016/j.smrv.2018.09.004

Harvey, A. G. (2002). A cognitive model of insomnia. *Behaviour Research and Therapy, 40*(8), 869–893. https://doi.org/10.1016/s0005-7967(01)00061-4

Harvey, A. G. (2005). A cognitive theory and therapy for chronic insomnia. *Journal of Cognitive Psychotherapy, 19*(1), 41–59. https://doi.org/10.1891/jcop.19.1.41.66332

Harvey, A. G. (2022). Treating sleep and circadian problems to promote mental health: Perspectives on comorbidity, implementation science and behavior change. *Sleep, 45*(4), Article zsac026. https://doi.org/10.1093/sleep/zsac026

Harvey, A. G., & Buysse, D. J. (2017). *Treating sleep problems: A transdiagnostic approach*. Guilford Press.

Harvey, A. G., Dong, L., Belanger, L., & Morin, C. M. (2017). Mediators and treatment matching in behavior therapy, cognitive therapy and cognitive behavior therapy for chronic insomnia. *Journal of Consulting and Clinical Psychology, 85*(10), 975–987. https://doi.org/10.1037/ccp0000244

Harvey, A. G., Dong, L., Hein, K., Yu, S. H., Martinez, A. J., Gumport, N. B., Smith, F. L., Chapman, A., Lisman, M., Mirzadegan, I. A., Mullin, A. C., Fine, E., Dolsen, E. A., Gasperetti, C. E., Bukosky, J., Alvarado-Martinez, C. G., Kilbourne, A. M., Rabe-Hesketh, S., & Buysse, D. J. (2021). A randomized controlled trial of the Transdiagnostic Intervention for Sleep and Circadian Dysfunction (TranS-C) to improve serious mental illness outcomes in a community setting. *Journal of Consulting and Clinical Psychology, 89*(6), 537–550. https://doi.org/10.1037/ccp0000650

Harvey, A. G., & Payne, S. (2002). The management of unwanted pre-sleep thoughts in insomnia: Distraction with imagery versus general distraction. *Behaviour Research and Therapy, 40*(3), 267–277. https://doi.org/10.1016/S0005-7967(01)00012-2

Harvey, A. G., Sharpley, A. L., Ree, M. J., Stinson, K., & Clark, D. M. (2007). An open trial of cognitive therapy for chronic insomnia. *Behaviour Research and Therapy, 45*(10), 2491–2501. https://doi.org/10.1016/j.brat.2007.04.007

Hauri, P. J. (1997). Can we mix behavioral therapy with hypnotics when treating insomniacs? *Sleep, 20*(12), 1111–1118.

Hayes, S., Strosahl, K., & Wilson, K. (2011). *Acceptance and commitment therapy: The process and practice of mindful change* (2nd ed.). Guilford Press.

Hertenstein, E., Thiel, N., Lüking, M., Külz, A. K., Schramm, E., Baglioni, C., Spiegelhalder, K., Riemann, D., & Nissen, C. (2014). Quality of life improvements after acceptance and commitment therapy in nonresponders to cognitive behavioral therapy for primary insomnia. *Psychotherapy and Psychosomatics, 83*(6), 371–373. https://doi.org/10.1159/000365173

Hertenstein, E., Trinca, E., Wunderlin, M., Schneider, C. L., Züst, M. A., Fehér, K. D., Su, T., Straten, V. A., Berger, T., Baglioni, C., Johann, A., Spiegelhalder, K., Riemann, D., Feige, B., & Nissen, C. (2022). Cognitive behavioral therapy for insomnia in patients with mental disorders and comorbid insomnia: A systematic review and meta-analysis. *Sleep Medicine Reviews, 62*, Article 101597. https://doi.org/10.1016/j.smrv.2022.101597

Hofmann, S. G., Curtiss, J. E., & Hayes, S. C. (2020). Beyond linear mediation: Toward a dynamic network approach to study treatment processes. *Clinical Psychology Review, 76*, Article 101824. https://doi.org/10.1016/j.cpr.2020.101824

Irwin, M. R., Carrillo, C., Sadeghi, N., Bjurstrom, M. F., Breen, E. C., & Olmstead, R. (2022). Prevention of incident and recurrent major depression in older adults with insomnia: A randomized clinical trial. *JAMA Psychiatry, 79*(1), 33–41. https://doi.org/10.1001/jamapsychiatry.2021.3422

Jacobs, G. D., Pace-Schott, E. F., Stickgold, R., & Otto, M. W. (2004). Cognitive behavior therapy and pharmacotherapy for insomnia: A randomized controlled trial and direct comparison. *Archives of Internal Medicine, 164*(17), 1888–1896. https://doi.org/10.1001/archinte.164.17.1888

Kabat-Zinn, J. (2013). *Full catastrophe living: Using the wisdom of your body and mind to face stress, pain, and illness* (rev. ed.). Bantam Books.

Kaldo, V., Jernelöv, S., Blom, K., Ljótsson, B., Brodin, M., Jörgensen, M., Kraepelien, M., Rück, C., & Lindefors, N. (2015). Guided internet cognitive behavioral therapy for insomnia compared to a control treatment—A randomized trial. *Behaviour Research and Therapy, 71*, 90–100. https://doi.org/10.1016/j.brat.2015.06.001

Krieger, T., Urech, A., Duss, S. B., Blättler, L., Schmitt, W., Gast, H., Bassetti, C., & Berger, T. (2019). A randomized controlled trial comparing guided internet-based multi-component treatment and internet-based guided sleep restriction treatment to care as usual in insomnia. *Sleep Medicine, 62*, 43–52. https://doi.org/10.1016/j.sleep.2019.01.045

Kyle, S. D., Aquino, M. R., Miller, C. B., Henry, A. L., Crawford, M. R., Espie, C. A., & Spielman, A. J. (2015). Towards standardisation and improved understanding of sleep restriction therapy for insomnia disorder: A systematic examination of CBT-I trial content. *Sleep Medicine Reviews, 23*, 83–88. https://doi.org/10.1016/j.smrv.2015.02.003

Kyle, S. D., Crawford, M. R., Morgan, K., Spiegelhalder, K., Clark, A. A., & Espie, C. A. (2013). The Glasgow Sleep Impact Index (GSII): A novel patient-centered measure for assessing sleep-related quality of life impairment in insomnia disorder. *Sleep Medicine, 14*(6), 493–501. https://doi.org/10.1016/j.sleep.2012.10.023

Kyle, S. D., Espie, C. A., & Morgan, K. (2010). ". . . Not just a minor thing, it is something major, which stops you from functioning daily": quality of life and daytime functioning in insomnia. *Behavioral Sleep Medicine, 8*(3), 123–140. https://doi.org/10.1080/15402002.2010.487450

Kyle, S. D., Miller, C. B., Rogers, Z., Siriwardena, A. N., MacMahon, K. M., & Espie, C. A. (2014). Sleep restriction therapy for insomnia is associated with reduced objective total sleep time, increased daytime somnolence, and objectively impaired vigilance: Implications for the clinical management of insomnia disorder. *Sleep, 37*(2), 229–237. https://doi.org/10.5665/sleep.3386

Kyle, S. D., Morgan, K., Spiegelhalder, K., & Espie, C. A. (2011). No pain, no gain: An exploratory within-subjects mixed-methods evaluation of the patient experience of sleep restriction therapy (SRT) for insomnia. *Sleep Medicine, 12*(8), 735–747. https://doi.org/10.1016/j.sleep.2011.03.016

Kyle, S. D., Siriwardena, A. N., Espie, C. A., Yang, Y., Petrou, S., Ogburn, E., Begum, N., Maurer, L. F., Robinson, B., Gardner, C., Lee, V., Armstrong, S., Pattinson, J., Mort, S., Temple, E., Harris, V., Yu, L. M., Bower, P., & Aveyard, P. (2023). Clinical and cost-effectiveness of nurse-delivered sleep restriction therapy for insomnia in primary care (HABIT): A pragmatic, superiority, open-label, randomised controlled trial. *The Lancet*, 402(10406), 975–987. https://doi.org/10.1016/S0140-6736(23)00683-9

Lack, L., Scott, H., & Lovato, N. (2019). Intensive sleep retraining treatment of insomnia. *Sleep Medicine Clinics, 14*(2), 245–252. https://doi.org/10.1016/j.jsmc.2019.01.005

LeBlanc, M., Mérette, C., Savard, J., Ivers, H., Baillargeon, L., & Morin, C. M. (2009). Incidence and risk factors of insomnia in a population-based sample. *Sleep, 32*(8), 1027–1037. http://www.ncbi.nlm.nih.gov/entrez/query.fcgi?cmd=Retrieve&db=PubMed&dopt=Citation&list_uids=19725254

Leerssen, J., Lakbila-Kamal, O., Dekkers, L. M. S., Ikelaar, S. L. C., Albers, A. C. W., Blanken, T. F., Lancee, J., van der Lande, G. J. M., Maksimovic, T., Mastenbroek, S. E., Reesen, J. E., van de Ven, S., van der Zweerde, T., Foster-Dingley, J. C., & Van Someren, E. J. W. (2022). Treating insomnia with high risk of depression using therapist-guided digital cognitive, behavioral, and circadian rhythm support interventions to prevent worsening of depressive symptoms: A randomized controlled trial. *Psychotherapy and Psychosomatics, 91*(3), 168–179. https://doi.org/10.1159/000520282

Lichstein, K. L. (1988). *Clinical relaxation strategies.* Wiley.

Lichstein, K. L., Riedel, B. W., Wilson, N. M., Lester, K. W., & Aguillard, R. N. (2001). Relaxation and sleep compression for late-life insomnia: A placebo-controlled trial. *Journal of Consulting and Clinical Psychology, 69*(2), 227–239.

Lowe, H., Haddock, G., Mulligan, L. D., Gregg, L., Fuzellier-Hart, A., Carter, L. A., & Kyle, S. D. (2019). Does exercise improve sleep for adults with insomnia? A systematic review with quality appraisal. *Clinical Psychology Review, 68*, 1–12. https://doi.org/10.1016/j.cpr.2018.11.002

Mair, A., Scott, H., & Lack, L. (2022). Intensive sleep retraining treatment for insomnia administered by smartphone in the home: An uncontrolled pilot study. *Journal of Clinical Sleep Medicine, 18*(6), 1515–1522. https://doi.org/10.5664/jcsm.9892

Maire, M., Linder, S., Dvořák, C., Merlo, C., Essig, S., Tal, K., Del Giovane, C., Syrogiannouli, L., Duss, S. B., Heinzer, R., Nissen, C., Bassetti, C. L. A., & Auer, R., . . . Auer, R. (2020). Prevalence and management of chronic insomnia in Swiss primary care: Cross-sectional data from the "Sentinella" practice-based research network. *Journal of Sleep Research, 29*(5), Article e13121. https://doi.org/10.1111/jsr.13121

Manber, R., & Carney, C. E. (2015). *Treatment plans and interventions for insomnia. A case formulation approach.* Guilford Press.

Mason, E. C., Grierson, A. B., Sie, A., Sharrock, M. J., Li, I., Chen, A. Z., & Newby, J. M. (2022). Co-occurring insomnia and anxiety: A randomized controlled trial of internet CBT for insomnia vs. internet CBT for anxiety. *Sleep, 46*(2), Article zsac205. https://doi.org/10.1093/sleep/zsac205

Maurer, L. F., Espie, C. A., Omlin, X., Emsley, R., & Kyle, S. D. (2022). The effect of sleep restriction therapy for insomnia on sleep pressure and arousal: A randomized controlled mechanistic trial. *Sleep, 45*(1), Article zsab223. https://doi.org/10.1093/sleep/zsab223

Maurer, L. F., Espie, C. A., & Kyle, S. D. (2018). How does sleep restriction therapy for insomnia work? A systematic review of mechanistic evidence and the introduction of the Triple-R model. *Sleep Medicine Reviews*, 42, 127–138. https://doi.org/10.1016/j.smrv.2018.07.005

Maurer, L. F., Espie, C. A., Omlin, X., Reid, M. J., Sharman, R., Gavriloff, D., Emsley, R., & Kyle, S. D. (2020). Isolating the role of time in bed restriction in the treatment of insomnia: A randomized, controlled, dismantling trial comparing sleep restriction therapy with time in bed regularization. *Sleep, 43*(11), Article zsaa096. https://doi.org/10.1093/sleep/zsaa096

Maurer, L. F., Ftouni, S., Espie, C. A., Bisdounis, L., & Kyle, S. D. (2021). The acute effects of sleep restriction therapy for insomnia on circadian timing and vigilance. *Journal of Sleep Research, 30*(4), Article e13260. https://doi.org/10.1111/jsr.13260

Milby, J. B., Williams, V., Hall, J. N., Khuder, S., McGill, T., & Wooten, V. (1993). Effectiveness of combined triazolam–behavioral therapy for primary insomnia. *American Journal of Psychiatry, 150*(8), 1259–1260. https://doi.org/10.1176/ajp.150.8.1259

Mitchell, L. J., Bisdounis, L., Ballesio, A., Omlin, X., & Kyle, S. D. (2019). The impact of cognitive behavioural therapy for insomnia on objective sleep parameters: A meta-analysis and systematic review. *Sleep Medicine Reviews, 47*, 90–102. https://doi.org/10.1016/j.smrv.2019.06.002

Morin, C. M. (1993). *Insomnia: Psychological assessment and management.* Guilford Press.

Morin, C. M. (2017). Issues and challenges in implementing clinical practice guideline for the management of chronic insomnia. *Journal of Sleep Research, 26*(6), 673–674. https://doi.org/10.1111/jsr.12639

Morin, C. M., Altena, E., Ivers, H., Merette, C., LeBlanc, M., Savard, J., & Philip, P. (2020). Insomnia, hypnotic use, and road collisions: A population-based, 5-year cohort study. *Sleep, 43*(8), Article zsaa032. https://doi.org/10.1093/sleep/zsaa032

Morin, C. M., Bastien, C., Guay, B., Radouco-Thomas, M., LeBlanc, J., & Vallières, A. (2004). Randomized clinical trial of supervised tapering and cognitive behavior therapy to facilitate benzodiazepine discontinuation in older adults with chronic insomnia. *American Journal of Psychiatry, 161*(2), 332–342. https://doi.org/10.1176/appi.ajp.161.2.332

Morin, C. M., Beaulieu-Bonneau, S., Ivers, H., Vallieres, A., Guay, B., Savard, J., & Merette, C. (2014). Speed and trajectory of changes of insomnia symptoms during acute treatment with cognitive-behavioral therapy, singly and combined with medication. *Sleep Medicine, 15*(6), 701–707. https://doi.org/10.1016/j.sleep.2014.02.004

Morin, C. M., Colecchi, C., Stone, J., Sood, R., & Brink, D. (1999). Behavioral and pharmacological therapies for late-life insomnia: A randomized controlled trial. *Journal of the American Medical Association, 281*(11), 991–999. https://doi.org/10.1001/jama.281.11.991

Morin, C. M., Drake, C. L., Harvey, A. G., Krystal, A. D., Manber, R., Riemann, D., & Spielgelhalder, K. (2015). Insomnia disorder. *Nature Reviews Disease Primers, 1*, Article 15026. https://doi.org/10.1038/nrdp.2015.26

Morin, C. M., Edinger, J. D., Beaulieu-Bonneau, S., Ivers, H., Krystal, A. D., Guay, B., Bélanger, L., Cartwright, A., Simmons, B., Lamy, M., & Busby, M. (2020). Effectiveness of sequential psychological and medication therapies for insomnia disorder: A randomized clinical trial. *JAMA Psychiatry, 77*(11), 1–9.

Morin, C. M., & Espie, C. A. (2003). *Insomnia: A clinical guide to assessment and treatment*. Kluwer Academic/Plenum.

Morin, C. M., & Jarrin, D. C. (2022). Epidemiology of insomnia: Prevalence, course, risk factors, and public health burden. *Sleep Medicine Clinics, 17*(2), 173–191. https://doi.org/10.1016/j.jsmc.2022.03.003

Morin, C. M., LeBlanc, M., Daley, M., Grégoire, J. P., & Mérette, C. (2006). Epidemiology of insomnia: Prevalence, self-help treatments, consultations, and determinants of help-seeking behaviors. *Sleep Medicine, 7*(2), 123–130. https://doi.org/10.1016/j.sleep.2005.08.008

Morin, C. M., Vallières, A., Guay, B., Ivers, H., Savard, J., Mérette, C., Bastien, C., & Baillargeon, L. (2009). Cognitive behavioral therapy, singly and combined with medication, for persistent insomnia: A randomized controlled trial. *Journal of the American Medical Association, 301*(19), 2005–2015. https://doi.org/10.1001/jama.2009.682

Natsky, A. N., Vakulin, A., Chai-Coetzer, C. L., Lack, L., McEvoy, R. D., Lovato, N., Sweetman, A., Gordon, C. J., Adams, R. J., & Kaambwa, B. (2020). Economic evaluation of cognitive behavioural therapy for insomnia (CBT-I) for improving health outcomes in adult populations: A systematic review. *Sleep Medicine Reviews, 54*, Article 101351. https://doi.org/10.1016/j.smrv.2020.101351

Ong, J. C., Manber, R., Segal, Z., Xia, Y., Shapiro, S., & Wyatt, J. K. (2014). A randomized controlled trial of mindfulness meditation for chronic insomnia. *Sleep, 37*(9), 1553–1563. https://doi.org/10.5665/sleep.4010

Ong, J. C., Shapiro, S. L., & Manber, R. (2008). Combining mindfulness meditation with cognitive-behavior therapy for insomnia: A treatment-development study. *Behavior Therapy, 39*(2), 171–182. https://doi.org/10.1016/j.beth.2007.07.002

Ong, J. C., & Sholtes, D. (2010). A mindfulness-based approach to the treatment of insomnia. *Journal of Clinical Psychology, 66*(11), 1175–1184. https://doi.org/10.1002/jclp.20736

Parsons, C. E., Zachariae, R., Landberger, C., & Young, K. S. (2021). How does cognitive behavioural therapy for insomnia work? A systematic review and meta-analysis of mediators of change. *Clinical Psychology Review, 86*, Article 102027. https://doi.org/10.1016/j.cpr.2021.102027

Qaseem, A., Kansagara, D., Forciea, M. A., Cooke, M., & Denberg, T. D. (2016). Management of chronic insomnia disorder in adults: A clinical practice guideline from the American College of Physicians. *Annals of Internal Medicine, 165*, 125–133. https://doi.org/10.7326/M15-2175

Riemann, D., Baglioni, C., Bassetti, C., Bjorvatn, B., Dolenc Groselj, L., Ellis, J. G., Espie, C. A., Garcia-Borreguero, D., Gjerstad, M., Gonçalves, M., Hertenstein, E., Jansson-Fröjmark, M., Jennum, P. J., Leger, D., Nissen, C., Parrino, L., Paunio, T., Pevernagie, D., Verbraecken, J., . . . Spiegelhalder, K. (2017). European guideline for the diagnosis and treatment of insomnia. *Journal of Sleep Research, 26*(6), 675–700. https://doi.org/10.1111/jsr.12594

Riemann, D., Benz, F., Dressle, R. J., Espie, C. A., Johann, A. F., Blanken, T. F., Leerssen, J., Wassing, R., Henry, A. L., Kyle, S. D., Spiegelhalder, K., & Van Someren, E. J. W. (2022). Insomnia disorder: State of the science and challenges for the future. *Journal of Sleep Research, 31*(4), Article e13604. https://doi.org/10.1111/jsr.13604

Rochefort, A., Jarrin, D. C., Belanger, L., Ivers, H., & Morin, C. M. (2019). Insomnia treatment response as a function of objectively measured sleep duration. *Sleep Medicine, 56*, 135–144. https://doi.org/10.1016/j.sleep.2019.01.016

Sampson, C., Bell, E., Cole, A., Miller, C. B., Marriott, T., Williams, M., & Rose, J. (2022). Digital cognitive behavioural therapy for insomnia and primary care costs in England: An interrupted time series analysis. *BJGP Open, 6*(2), Article BJGPO.2021.0146. https://doi.org/10.3399/BJGPO.2021.0146

Savard, J., Simard, S., Ivers, H., & Morin, C. M. (2005). Randomized study on the efficacy of cognitive-behavioral therapy for insomnia secondary to breast cancer, part I: Sleep and psychological effects. *Journal of Clinical Oncology, 23*, 6083–6096. https://doi.org/10.1200/JCO.2005.09.548

Schwartz, D. R., & Carney, C. E. (2012). Mediators of cognitive-behavioral therapy for insomnia: A review of randomized controlled trials and secondary analysis studies. *Clinical Psychology Review, 32*(7), 664–675. https://doi.org/10.1016/j.cpr.2012.06.006

Selvanathan, J., Pham, C., Nagappa, M., Peng, P. W. H., Englesakis, M., Espie, C. A., Morin, C. M., & Chung, F. (2021). Cognitive behavioral therapy for insomnia in patients with chronic pain—A systematic review and meta-analysis of randomized controlled trials. *Sleep Medicine Reviews, 60,* Article 101460. https://doi.org/10.1016/j.smrv.2021.101460

Sivertsen, B., Omvik, S., Pallesen, S., Bjorvatn, B., Havik, O. E., Kvale, G., Nielsen, G. H., & Nordhus, I. H. (2006). Cognitive behavioral therapy vs zopiclone for treatment of chronic primary insomnia in older adults: A randomized controlled trial. *Journal of the American Medical Association, 295*(24), 2851–2858. https://doi.org/10.1001/jama.295.24.2851

Spielman, A. J., & Glovinsky, P. B. (1991). The varied nature of insomnia. In P. Hauri (Ed.), *Case studies in insomnia* (pp. 1–15). Plenum Press.

Spielman, A. J., Saskin, P., & Thorpy, M. J. (1987). Treatment of chronic insomnia by restriction of time in bed. *Sleep, 10*(1), 45–56. http://www.ncbi.nlm.nih.gov/pubmed/3563247

Squires, L. R., Rash, J. A., Fawcett, J., & Garland, S. N. (2022). Systematic review and meta-analysis of cognitive-behavioural therapy for insomnia on subjective and actigraphy-measured sleep and comorbid symptoms in cancer survivors. *Sleep Medicine Reviews, 63,* Article 101615. https://doi.org/10.1016/j.smrv.2022.101615

Sunnhed, R., Hesser, H., Andersson, G., Carlbring, P., Morin, C. M., Harvey, A. G., & Jansson-Frojmark, M. (2020). Comparing internet-delivered cognitive therapy and behavior therapy with telephone support for insomnia disorder: A randomized controlled trial. *Sleep, 43*(2), Article zsz245. https://doi.org/10.1093/sleep/zsz245

Steinmetz, L., Simon, L., Feige, B., Riemann, D., Johann, A. F., Ell, J., Ebert, D. D., Baumeister, H., Benz, F., & Spiegelhalder, K. (2024). Network meta-analysis examining efficacy of components of cognitive-behavioral therapy for insomnia. *Clinical Psychology Review,* 114, 102507. https://doi.org/10.1016/j.cpr.2024.102507

van der Zweerde, T., Bisdounis, L., Kyle, S. D., Lancee, J., & van Straten, A. (2019). Cognitive behavioral therapy for insomnia: A meta-analysis of long-term effects in controlled studies. *Sleep Medicine Reviews, 48,* Article 101208. https://doi.org/10.1016/j.smrv.2019.08.002

van Straten, A., van der Zweerde, T., Kleiboer, A., Cuijpers, P., Morin, C. M., & Lancee, J. (2018). Cognitive and behavioral therapies in the treatment of insomnia: A meta-analysis. *Sleep Medicine Reviews, 38,* 3–16. https://doi.org/10.1016/j.smrv.2017.02.001

Verma, S., Rajaratnam, S. M. W., Davey, M., Wiley, J. F., & Bei, B. (2020). Cognitive behavioural therapy and light dark therapy for maternal postpartum insomnia symptoms: Protocol of a parallel-group randomised controlled efficacy trial. *Frontiers in Global Women's Health, 1,* Article 591677. https://doi.org/10.3389/fgwh.2020.591677

Vgontzas, A. N., Fernandez-Mendoza, J., Liao, D., & Bixler, E. O. (2013). Insomnia with objective short sleep duration: The most biologically severe phenotype of the disorder. *Sleep Medicine Reviews, 17*(4), 241–254. https://doi.org/10.1016/j.smrv.2012.09.005

Vgontzas, A. N., Puzino, K., Fernandez-Mendoza, J., Krishnamurthy, V. B., Basta, M., & Bixler, E. O. (2020). Effects of trazodone versus cognitive behavioral therapy in the insomnia with short sleep duration phenotype: A preliminary study. *Journal of Clinical Sleep Medicine, 16*(12), 2009–2019. https://doi.org/10.5664/jcsm.8740

Vincent, N., & Lewycky, S. (2009). Logging on for better sleep: RCT of the effectiveness of online treatment for insomnia. *Sleep, 32,* 807–815.

Wickwire, E. M., & Morin, C. M. (2020). Advancing a value framework for sleep: Update on economic aspects of cognitive-behavioral treatments for insomnia. *Sleep Medicine Reviews, 54,* Article 101387. https://doi.org/10.1016/j.smrv.2020.101387

Wu, R., Bao, J., Zhang, C., Deng, J., & Long, C. (2006). Comparison of sleep condition and sleep-related psychological activity after cognitive-behavior and pharmacological therapy for chronic insomnia. *Psychotherapy and Psychosomatics, 75*(4), 220–228. https://doi.org/10.1159/000092892

CHAPTER

29 Parasomnias I: Nightmares

Serena Scarpelli, Valentina Alfonsi, *and* Luigi De Gennaro

Abstract

Nightmare disorder is a rapid-eye-movement (REM) parasomnia provoking disturbing oneiric activity and significant distress. This chapter provides a comprehensive overview of the diagnostic criteria and definition of this sleep disorder. The authors reviewed findings on neural correlates of nightmares, also examining the changes over the life span. They describe the most common comorbid psychiatric conditions, such as post-traumatic stress disorder, depression, suicidality, anxious state, and personality disorders. Also, the effectiveness of the different therapeutic strategies to treat this parasomnia is discussed. Finally, they propose a reflection on the potential functional role of nightmares. Based on the view that nightmares may represent a reliable index of individuals' well-being, the authors believe that this field of research deserves further investigation, concluding with suggestions for future studies.

Key Words: nightmare, disturbing dream, sleep, PTSD, mental health

Introduction

Nightmare is defined as mental sleep activity characterized by intense negative emotions associated with contents such as threats to survival, security, physical integrity, or self-esteem. This peculiar kind of oneiric activity has been recognized as a clinical entity for centuries. The *Diagnostic and Statistical Manual of Mental Disorders*, fifth edition (DSM-5; American Psychiatric Association, 2013), and the *International Classification of Sleep Disorders*, third edition (American Academy of Sleep Medicine [AASM], 2014), consider nightmare disorder a rapid-eye-movement (REM) parasomnia with a "repeated occurrence of extended, extremely dysphoric, and well-remembered dreams that usually involve efforts to avoid threats to survival, security, or physical integrity and that generally occur during the second half of the major sleep episode." (DSM-5; American Psychiatric Association, 2013, p. 404). Nightmare sufferers should experience clinically significant distress or impairment. It has been estimated that this disorder affects approximately 4%–8% of the population (American Psychiatric Association, 2013; Levin & Nielsen, 2009; Nielsen & Zadra, 2000) and seems to occur more frequently in women than in men (Li et al., 2010; Munezawa et al., 2011; Sandman et al., 2013; Schredl, 2010; Wiechers et al., 2011). Notably, there are no strict frequency criteria, albeit the DSM-5 manual recommends considering a mild nightmare disorder as less than one episode per week, a moderate disorder as one or more episodes per week but less than nightly, and a severe disorder as nightly episodes (American Psychiatric Association, 2013). Moreover, concerning duration, an acute episode lasts 1 month or less, a subacute episode lasts at least 1 month but less than 6 months, and chronic nightmares last for 6 months or longer (American Psychiatric Association, 2013).

It should be noted that the previous diagnostic manual (DSM-IV; American Psychiatric Association, 1994) described this disturbance as "repeated awakenings from the major sleep period or naps with a detailed recall of extended and extremely frightening dreams," (DSM-IV; American Psychiatric Association, 1994, p. 631) while in the new manual the awakening from sleep is no longer a necessary diagnostic criterion for nightmare disorder (DSM-5; American Psychiatric Association, 2013). Along this vein, some authors tend to use a broader definition, including dreams with different dysphoric emotions that do not immediately awaken the subject (Blagrove et al., 2004; Robert & Zadra, 2014; Spoormaker & Van Den Bout, 2006; Zadra & Donderi, 2000). In this view, both bad dreams and nightmares would be characterized by frightening emotions and, to some extent, would overlap (Blagrove et al., 2004). In fact, findings on the "awakening criterion" are conflicting. Some investigations suggested a relationship between awakenings and the degree of distress associated with the oneiric activity (Zadra & Donderi, 2000). Also, direct awakening appeared to be linked to higher scores of psychopathologies and post-traumatic complaints assessed by the Symptom Checklist-90 (Schreuder et al., 2000). Conversely, another study revealed no association between unpleasant dreams and awakenings (Kellner et al., 1992). Regardless of the presence of awakenings, some findings showed that frightening dreams are a reliable well-being index (Blagrove et al., 2004), as also described in recent pandemic studies revealing that nightmares were greater during the pandemic and that the COVID-19 subjects were more affected than controls (Scarpelli, De Santis, Alfonsi et al., 2022; Scarpelli, Nadorff, et al., 2022).

Fear is the prevalent emotion appearing in nightmares, with a percentage ranging from 65% to 85% (Robert & Zadra, 2014); but also sadness and anger have been identified (Köthe & Pietrowsky, 2001; Robert & Zadra, 2014). Subjects can feel these negative emotions during the oneiric episode, upon awakening from the unpleasant dream, or during the nightmare recall. Some authors suggest that nightmares are related to fear-dysfunction disorders, namely, phobias, anxiety disorder, and, in general, low psychological well-being (Zadra & Donderi, 2000). Indeed, recurring nightmares are linked to many mental disturbances, sleep fragmentation, insomnia, and daytime dysfunction, also provoking tiredness, lack of energy, concentration deficit, and worry about sleep (Cattarius & Schlarb, 2016; Krakow, 2006; Lancee & Schrijnemaekers, 2013). Anxiety, mood alterations (Blagrove et al., 2004; Levin & Fireman, 2002), suicide (Nadorff et al., 2011; Sandman et al., 2017; Sjöström et al., 2009), and poor academic performance (Schultz et al., 2021; Wiechers et al., 2011) are exacerbated by nightmares.

Significantly, nightmare disorder is frequently associated with post-traumatic stress disorder (PTSD; Germain, 2013; see in this section below).

On the other hand, idiopathic nightmares, without a known cause and apparently unrelated to adverse events, should be considered (Nielsen & Levin, 2007). The existing literature suggests that many factors could cause idiopathic nightmares, for example, hereditary variables (Coolidge et al., 2010), psychological distress (Klůzová Kráčmarová & Plháková, 2015), alexithymic personality (Callaghan & Tottenham, 2016), schizoid personality (Hartmann, 1984), and poor sleep hygiene (Germain & Nielsen, 2003). Notably, both idiopathic and post-traumatic nightmares may be due to a vulnerability elicited by adverse experiences. In this respect, some authors have hypothesized that these two kinds of nightmares could be placed along a continuum based on the degree of severity of the stressful events (Nielsen, 2017).

Moreover, disturbed dreams could be elicited by some drugs and pharmacological treatments (Pagel, 2010). Specifically, benzodiazepines and some antidepressants provoking REM sleep suppression seem to induce nightmares (Pagel, 1996). Disordered dreaming could also be a secondary effect of the REM sleep rebound after the interruption of REM-suppressant drugs (Coupland et al., 1996; Pagel, 1996). However, frequent nightmares appear also during the withdrawal from REM sleep–suppressant medications (e.g., cannabis, cocaine, and opiates; Wade et al., 2006); and the underlying mechanisms of altered dreaming, in this case, are less clear. Dopamine agonists and amphetamines may also induce nightmares by stimulating dopamine receptors. For instance, levodopa is recognized to cause nightmares along with a wide range of neuropsychiatric effects (Lin & Ziegler, 1976). Furthermore, some evidence highlighted that even during pharmacologic treatment for smoking cessation, nightmares increase (Ebbert et al., 2015). Specifically, varenicline, a partial agonist binding with high affinity and selectivity at $\alpha 4\beta 2$ neuronal nicotinic acetylcholine receptors that stimulates dopamine release, has frequent nightmares among its side effects. However, a recent study suggests having higher nightmares could result from the significant increase in the number of awakenings during pharmacological treatment. In fact, the authors showed significant correlations between dream recall rate and sleep fragmentation measures, underlining that varenicline cannot be considered a direct cause of altered dreams (Polini et al., 2017).

Concerning the differential diagnosis, nightmares should not be confused with night terrors (sleep terrors or pavor nocturnus). Some specific features help the distinction between these two sleep phenomena: (a) nightmares have a high visual vividness and complicated plots that are lacking in night terrors; (b) night terrors are not well remembered since they are often followed by amnesia and are associated with confusional arousal; (c) night terrors usually occur during slow-wave sleep; and (d) during sleep terrors individuals feel intense fear accompanied by specific physiological alterations, such as tachycardia, sweating, and mydriasis (C. Fisher et al., 1970; Hefez et al., 1987; Nielsen & Levin, 2007).

Clinical interviews (e.g., Structured Clinical Interview for DSM-5; American Psychiatric Association, 2013) along with prospective logs may be considered the best methods to establish a differential diagnosis. Moreover, the assessment of specific nightmares features (i.e., frequency and distress) can be obtained by different standardized instruments. Among the main tools there are (a) the Mannheim Dream Questionnaire (Schredl et al., 2014), (b) the Nightmare Frequency Questionnaire (Krakow et al., 2002), (c) the Nightmare Distress Questionnaire (Belicki, 1992), (d) the Pittsburgh Sleep Quality Index–Addendum (Germain et al., 2005), (e) the Disturbing Dream and Nightmare Severity Index (Bolstad et al., 2021), (f) a subscale of the SLEEP-50 assessing nightmare distress (Lancee et al., 2010), (g) the Nightmare Effects Questionnaire (Schlarb et al., 2016), and (h) the Van Dream Anxiety Scale (Ağargün et al., 1999). The number of items and the constructs measured by each questionnaire are detailed in Table 29.1.

It is worth noting that all these questionnaires are retrospective measures. On the one hand, they are considered the best choice to assess nightmare frequency and distress since they represent the simplest and quickest strategy. On the other hand, these instruments are more prone to memory biases (Zadra & Donderi, 2000). Indeed, nightmares retrospectively investigated may be underestimated when compared to daily dream logs obtained immediately after awakenings (Zadra & Donderi, 2000).

Neural Correlates of Nightmares

Historically, the neurobiological bases of dreaming have been studied through different approaches (i.e., neuropsychological, neuroimaging, neurochemical and electrophysiological; for a review, see Scarpelli, Gorgoni, et al., 2019). Although there is a growing scientific literature on the neural correlates of dream recall, research on the brain mechanism of nightmares is still scarce and inconclusive.

Some neuropsychological studies explored specific cognitive functions among nightmare sufferers, providing hypotheses on the functioning of different brain regions in these patients. For instance, some findings suggest that nightmares are linked to a deficit in executive function and emotional regulation, specifically reflecting an executive deficit in regulating arousal (Levin & Nielsen, 2009). Accordingly, impaired executive functions have been shown in people with frequent nightmares, as highlighted by their performance on different neuropsychological tasks (Simor et al., 2012). Patients showed slower performance on the Emotional Stroop and the Emotional Go/NoGo task and higher perseveration on Verbal Fluency than controls (Simor et al., 2012). A more recent study confirmed more significant perseveration errors among nightmare patients during this latter task (Carr et al., 2017).

Nevertheless, nightmare sufferers reported fewer errors than controls on the Color-Word Stroop, suggesting better functioning on tasks involving dorsolateral prefrontal and

Table 29.1 Standardized Questionnaires to Assess Nightmare Features

Instruments	Items (n)	NM-related features
MADRE	21	NM frequency NM distress Recurring NM related to waking life NM frequency during childhood
NFQ	2	NM frequency
NDQ	13	NM distress NM effects on sleep and well-being
PSQI-A	10	NM frequency Emotions NM-related Time of night associated with NM
DDNSI	5	NM frequency and chronicity NM severity and intensity Awakenings NM-related
SLEEP-50	50	NM presence/absence Awakenings NM-related Memory/orientation problems NM-related Physical effects NM-related
NEQ	21	NM frequency Physical effects NM-related Emotions NM-related NM interpretation Terrifying scenes
VDAS	17	NM frequency NM effects on sleep Emotions NM-related NM distress Memory/concentration problem NM-related

Note. DDNSI = Disturbing Dream and Nightmare Severity Index; MADRE = Mannheim Dream Questionnaire; NDQ = Nightmare Distress Questionnaire; NEQ = Nightmare Effects Questionnaire; NFQ = Nightmare Frequency Questionnaire; NM = nightmare; PSQI-A = Pittsburgh Sleep Quality Index–Addendum; VDAS = Van Dream Anxiety Scale.

dorsal-anterior cingulate regions. Moreover, in a sample of frequent nightmares, nightmare distress appeared to be related to lower frontal activity during a negative picture-viewing task (Marquis et al., 2019). Overall, these findings suggest that frontal regulatory deficit may be viewed as a neural correlate of nightmares (Carr et al., 2020). This would also implicate a potential overlap between brain mechanisms responsible for nightmare experience during sleep and distress during wakefulness among nightmare sufferers (Carr et al., 2020).

Polysomnography (PSG) is considered the gold-standard method for studying the electrophysiological bases of oneiric activity (Scarpelli et al., 2015). Multiple investigations identified the electrophysiological (EEG) correlates of dream recall by using provoked awakenings associated with PSG recordings of one or more sleep nights. Individuals are awakened to explore the EEG oscillations predicting the presence/absence of a dream recall (e.g., Marzano et al., 2011; Scarpelli, Bartolacci, et al., 2020; Scarpelli et al., 2017; Siclari et al., 2017) or to evaluate the relationship between specific qualitative features and sleep EEG patterns (Scarpelli, D'Atri, et al., 2020). However, studies on the EEG correlates of nightmares are still lacking.

Actually, nightmares do not frequently occur in a laboratory setting, and some studies highlighted that dream contents recorded at home have a greater emotional load than those reported in a laboratory (Domhoff & Kamiya, 1964; Sándor et al., 2015; Weisz & Foulkes, 1970). Indeed, nightmares have been detected with a low incidence range from 1% to 10% (C. Fisher et al., 1970; Hefez et al., 1987; Mellman et al., 1997; Woodward et al., 1996). Hence, some authors conclude that the best strategy to study nightmares is to provide home recordings or, in an unfamiliar setting, to repeat PSG recordings for more days to promote the participants' adaptation (Spoormaker et al., 2006).

Starting from some neuropsychological findings, it has been hypothesized that the impairment of prefrontal and frontolimbic functions so that the individual is unable to regulate emotional activation during REM sleep is one of the crucial aspects of disturbed dreaming (Maquet et al., 2005). It is worth noting that REM sleep is associated with activation of the specific emotional network (i.e., amygdala, ventromedial prefrontal cortex; Desseilles et al., 2011; Maquet et al., 2005) and has been repeatedly linked to emotional processing during sleep (Nishida et al., 2009; Scarpelli, Bartolacci, et al., 2019). Indeed, REM sleep is implicated in the consolidation of fear (Marshall et al., 2014) and the modulation of emotional reactivity (Alger et al. 2015). Along this vein, some evidence revealed REM-specific alterations in nightmare sufferers, such as longer REM latency, increased skipping of early REM periods and cycle length, and more frequent REM periods (Nielsen et al., 2010).

From a neurophysiological point of view, some authors suggested that noradrenergic systems are inappropriately active during REM sleep, especially in PTSD nightmare sufferers; and this would provoke the REM sleep fragmentation and dysfunctional sleep–dependent emotional processing (Richards et al., 2020), eliciting distressing oneiric scenarios (Woodward et al., 2018). Considering heart rate as a proxy measure of noradrenergic activity, two investigations revealed a heart rate increase during REM sleep among nightmare sufferers (C. Fisher et al., 1970; Nielsen & Zadra, 2005). These results could index the physiological response to the fear. Consistently, a recent investigation confirmed that activation of the autonomic nervous system might be linked to nightmares (Paul et al., 2019). Specifically, the authors revealed increased heart rate frequency, breathing cycle length, electrodermal responses, and REM density (i.e., the rate of rapid eye movements during REM sleep), showing increased autonomic activity in people suffering from nightmares (Paul et al., 2019). However, other findings did not find increased heart rate before nightmare arousal but relative stability in the sleep preceding the awakening (Phelps et al., 2018; Richards et al., 2023). The authors also showed that nightmare awakenings could frequently occur during non-REM (NREM) sleep (Phelps et al., 2018; Richards et al., 2023).

In addition, some EEG findings highlighted the presence of slow frontal and central theta activity during REM sleep in a group of nightmare recallers (Marquis et al., 2017). Further studies reported evidence for reduced slow-wave sleep and greater intra-sleep wakefulness (Simor et al., 2012), increased alpha power during REM sleep, and higher levels of EEG desynchronization in NREM sleep of students with frequent nightmares (Simor et al., 2013). In other words, as shown for dream recall frequency (e.g., Scarpelli, Bartolacci, et al., 2020; Scarpelli et al., 2017; Siclari et al., 2017), higher autonomic and electrophysiological activation may provide the physiological background to the nightmare occurrence (C. Fisher et al., 1970; Nielsen & Zadra, 2005). This is consistent with the self-reported experience of greater emotional and physical activations during the nightmare occurrence and is partly consistent with the idea that subjects who are more prone to nightmares have specific trait-like features that steadily cause a general increase in sensitivity (Carr & Nielsen, 2017). In this regard, Carr and colleagues (2020) found that nightmare participants, during the picture-viewing task, reported a greater level of emotional arousal regardless of the picture's emotional valence. In other words, nightmare sufferers may have a trait of "sensory-processing sensitivity," promoting increased emotional reactivity (Aron & Aron, 1997).

Nightmares During the Life Span

The abovementioned studies on nightmare sufferers have been conducted on young adults (e.g., C. Fisher et al., 1970; Nielsen et al., 2010; Marquis et al., 2017; Paul et al., 2019). However, in parallel with dreaming, sparse evidence suggests that nightmares also change during the life span.

Several findings underlined that disturbing dreams are pretty common among children, from pre-school age to pre-adolescence (Hawkins & Williams, 1992; Muris et al., 2000; Salzarulo & Chevalier, 1983; Simonds & Parraga, 1982). Some studies showed frequent bad dreams during the first years of life (Simard et al., 2008). In particular, idiopathic nightmares seem very widespread among children and more prevalent in the female gender (Nielsen et al., 2019). A study investigating children's dream activity through parent reports revealed that nightmare frequency was greater in cases of abuse history and family problems occurring at 0–4 years (Lereya et al., 2017). Therefore, this evidence supports the hypothesis that idiopathic nightmares—as a consequence of such adverse events—could share pathophysiological mechanisms with PTSD-related nightmares (Nielsen et al., 2019).

Additionally, some investigations assessed the relationship between nightmare disorder and other sleep problems during childhood (Salzarulo & Chevalier, 1983). Children aged 6–10 years showed more frightening dreams than those in different age ranges. Nightmares are also more frequent in children with circadian rhythm alterations during the first year of life than in normal sleepers (Salzarulo & Chevalier, 1983). However, while some evidence highlighted that sleeplessness symptoms are factors predicting the presence of bad dreams in young children, a longitudinal study on disturbing dreams, evaluated by parents at 29 months, 41 months, 50 months, 5 years, and 6 years, did not show a relationship between sleep loss and frightened oneiric activity (Simard et al., 2008). In other words, this latter investigation suggests that such a relationship between nightmares and insomnia would appear later during development. Accordingly, comorbidity between nightmares and insomnia symptoms has been found during adolescence (Besiroglu et al., 2005; Ohayon et al., 1997).

The relationship between nightmares and mental well-being seems to be confirmed in childhood. Children with emotional disturbances, such as separation anxiety (Nielsen et al., 2000) or difficult temperament during infancy (Morrell & Steele, 2003; Sadeh & Anders, 1993), report a high rate of disturbing dreams (Nielsen et al., 2000; Mindell & Barrett, 2002). Simard et al. (2008) showed that the best predictor of nightmares was the presence of disturbing dreams at the preceding age, suggesting that this may be a stable trait of subjects. Namely, bad dreams at 29 months predict disturbing dreams at 5–6 years (e.g., starting school), a period of life characterized by multiple environmental requests that may result in higher stress. Hence, the children's susceptibility to stress at 29 months can interact with stressful life changes (Simard et al., 2008).

Distinguishing nightmares from sleep terrors (night terrors or pavor nocturnus) during childhood is crucial (AASM, 2014). Night terrors could occur during childhood from the age of 1.5 years, in association with confusional arousals and sleepwalking, and tend to resolve by puberty (Castelnovo et al., 2018; Laberge et al., 2000). During the night terror episode, the child shows a more intense fear than during a nightmare and appears inconsolable, not responsive, and shaken. As for adults, children cannot remember the episode (Ophoff et al., 2018). Although some authors hypothesized that night terrors are related to a great anxiety level (LaBerge et al., 2000) or significant adverse events (Rosen et al., 1995) during wakefulness, other findings suggest that sleep terrors may be associated just with poor sleep hygiene (Ophoff et al., 2018). Nevertheless, since the impossibility of having direct access to dreaming while the subject is experiencing a sleep terror, no studies have investigated the oneiric activity associated with this phenomenon.

A few studies have explored nightmares and bad dreams in older adults. Many findings reported a general decline in recall frequency during aging for nightmares (Salvio et al., 1992; Schredl, 2008; Schredl & Goritz, 2015). Schredl and Göritz (2015) analyzed the changes in dream recall rate and nightmare frequency in a sample with a large age range (16–89 years of age), over 3 years. They found a reduction during aging, confirming findings from previous cross-sectional studies (Schredl, 2008, 2009; Stepansky et al., 1998). We could hypothesize that the reduction of strain and pressure in the lifestyle of older adults could explain this phenomenon (Schredl & Goritz, 2015) since the nightmares are usually elicited by stressful factors (Schredl, 2003). This could also be consistent with the continuity hypothesis positing that oneiric contents would reflect the dreamer's current thoughts, concerns, and salient experiences during the waking state (Hall & Nordby, 1972; for a review, see Scarpelli, Alfonsi, et al., 2022). Other authors hypothesized that age-related changes in dream recall might result from age-related changes in dream saliency. Namely, older adults could be less interested in their oneiric materials (Cohen & MacNeilage, 1974).

Although the prevalence of nightmares in the elderly is just equal to 4% (Salvio et al., 1992), older adults who suffer from anxiety disorders frequently report nightmares (Mallon et al., 2000; Nadorff et al., 2014; Potvin et al., 2014), showing, once again, a continuity between sleep and waking experiences (Hall & Nordby, 1972). In particular, Nadorff and colleagues (2014) showed a significant relationship between generalized anxiety disorder (GAD) and disturbing dream frequency in the elderly. Furthermore, older adults with GAD reported more bad dreams than healthy older subjects (Mallon et al., 2000).

Although the literature on nightmares during the life span is extensive and constantly growing, specific investigations exploring neural correlates are missing. Therefore, it is necessary to plan future studies in which the evidence mentioned above can be substantiated by objective findings on the neural correlates underlying nightmares during the different life periods.

Nightmares, PTSD, and Other Mental Complaints

The current literature considers replicative nightmares as the hallmark of PTSD (Germain, 2013). PTSD is a mental disorder that may occur in subjects who have experienced a traumatic event (e.g., war, accident, terrorist attack, natural disaster, etc.). Patients with PTSD have three categories of symptoms lasting more than 1 month: (a) intrusion, or re-experiencing the traumatic event with intrusive memories and thoughts; (b) avoidance of cues trauma-related; and (c) hyperarousal, typically expressed as insomnia or increased tension. Nightmares are included in the "intrusion" cluster along with flashbacks (AASM, 2014) and, generally, concern themes, sensations, or emotions linked to the trauma.

PTSD-related nightmares affect more than 50% of trauma-exposed adults (Krakow et al., 2002; Narrow et al., 2013), with a frequency as high as six nightmares per week

(Krakow et al., 2002). Unlike idiopathic nightmares, trauma-related nightmares rarely occur among children (Narrow et al., 2013).

Several pieces of evidence highlight that nightmare frequency is associated with PTSD severity (Hinton et al., 2013; Kilpatrick et al., 1998; Pigeon et al., 2013; Schreuder et al., 2000; van Liempt et al., 2013). Nightmares are associated with higher severity of PTSD symptoms at baseline, as shown by an investigation of 80 veterans (Pigeon et al., 2013). Van Liempt et al. (2013) also found that nightmare frequency predicts greater severity of PTSD at a 6-month follow-up. Interestingly, having frequent nightmares before being exposed to a traumatic event represents a risk factor for developing more severe PTSD symptoms (Bryant et al., 2010; Kobayashi et al., 2008; van Liempt et al., 2013). In this view, PTSD and nightmares show a two-way relationship in which nightmares strengthen PTSD symptoms and PTSD, in turn, provokes nightmares.

Frequent nightmares in PTSD patients are more challenging to resolve than idiopathic nightmares. They may occur for 40–50 years after the traumatic event (Guerrero & Crocq, 1994; Kaup et al., 1994) and significantly reduce people's quality of life (Detweiler et al., 2012). Post-traumatic nightmares provoke severe arousal, sleep fragmentation, and more elevated helplessness and lack of control than idiopathic nightmares (Wittmann & De Dassel, 2015). In fact, post-traumatic nightmares are related to sleepiness, daytime impairment, and a high risk of suicide (Lancee & Schrijnemaekers, 2013; Sjöström et al., 2009). The vulnerability of nightmare sufferers to report suicidal ideas or attempts is highly worrying (Panagioti et al., 2012; Sjöström et al., 2009). Sjöstrom et al. (2009) showed that nightmare disorder increases suicidality fivefold. Also, findings on PTSD subjects revealed that they report suicidal ideation with a greater incidence than those without PTSD (Panagioti et al., 2012).

Although post-traumatic nightmares and suicidality have some common factors, such as hopelessness and a sense of defeat (Littlewood et al., 2016), the mechanisms underlying the relationship between suicidality and nightmares are not entirely understood (Weber et al., 2020).

It should be considered that comorbid psychiatric disorders could mediate the relationship between PTSD, nightmares, and suicidal ideation (Weber et al., 2020). Indeed, a recent study among veterans found that the association between suicide attempts and nightmares disappeared after controlling for psychiatric disorders (Bishop et al., 2020).

Frequent nightmares are associated with various mental illnesses. Anxiety and depression are often accompanied by nightmares (Blagrove et al., 2004; Levin & Fireman, 2002; Mume, 2009; van Schagen et al., 2017). However, results on depression are conflicting since some findings have shown that PTSD patients with recurrent nightmares had lower levels of depression than PTSD patients without post-traumatic nightmares (Ohayon et al., 1997).

Recent investigations revealed a relationship between frequent nightmares and psychosis (H. L. Fisher et al., 2014; Thompson et al., 2015). Nightmares could also represent a risk factor for psychotic disorders (Mume, 2009; Sheaves et al., 2015) but also borderline personality disorders (Lerey et al., 2017; Semiz et al., 2008; Simor et al., 2010). Moreover, it has been hypothesized that people with neuroticism as a personality factor are more prone to develop nightmares (Blagrove et al., 2004; Schredl et al., 2003; Zadra & Donderi, 2000). Actually, the general psychopathology and this personality trait are highly intercorrelated (Zadra & Donderi, 2000). Nevertheless, it is worth noting that most of the existing studies were carried out by retrospective methods (i.e., interviews, questionnaires) that, as previously mentioned, could be affected by memory biases. Hence, we cannot rule out that individuals with a high level of neuroticism are more likely to recall and report their nightmares.

Interestingly, some findings showed an association between drug use and nightmares. Namely, drugs could be assumed to cope with the nightmare distress or increase patient sleep quality (Simpson et al., 2012; Spoormaker et al., 2006; Vandrey et al., 2014).

Notably, recurring nightmares often coexist with other sleep disorders, such as night terrors (Ohayon et al., 1999), sleep disordered breathing (Krakow, Melendrez, et al., 2001), and especially insomnia (Cattarius & Schlarb, 2016; Krakow, 2006; Lancee & Schrijnemaekers, 2013; Lancee et al., 2010). Indeed, 70% of patients with a relevant nightmare condition reported comorbid insomnia (Krakow, 2006). It should be underlined that nightmares and insomnia could share some pathophysiological mechanisms, such as physiological and psychological hyperarousal (Simor et al., 2012). In other words, an arousal predisposition could represent a risk factor for both sleep disorders (M. L. Rogers et al., 2017).

Another issue to consider is the significant increase of nightmares reported during the pandemic among both healthy subjects (e.g., Scarpelli, Alfonsi, Mangiaruga et al., 2021) and patients with COVID-19 (Scarpelli, Nadorff, et al., 2022a). Additionally, individuals suffering from long-COVID-19 syndrome reported higher sleep alterations and increased nightmare rate than subjects with "short COVID" (Scarpelli, De Santis, et al., 2022). Moreover, patients with severe diseases who need to be admitted to intensive care units (ICUs) showed a high risk of experiencing PTSD symptoms (Shaw et al., 2009). Specifically, survivors of severe COVID-19 and treated in an ICU reported poor sleep (Kaseda & Levine, 2020) along with frequent nightmares and hallucinations (Eklind et al., 2023; J. P. Rogers et al., 2020; Saif & Pick, 2021). It should be highlighted that these problems could also impair their quality of life after discharge, negatively impacting the recovery process of patients (Rousseau et al., 2021; Weidman et al., 2022).

Overall, the high prevalence of nightmares in subjects affected by mental diseases and their influence on well-being and daily functioning deserve attention. Further studies should clarify the role of chronic nightmares in different psychopathologies to potentially consider them for prognosis and provide a specific and independent treatment when appropriate.

Which Functional Role for Nightmares?

In the previous paragraphs, we have stated that nightmares are frequently comorbid with many clinical conditions, such as depression, anxiety, personality disorders, and PTSD. Along this view, nightmares would have mainly a pathological meaning. Freud (1900) supported the idea that nightmares are equivalent to anxiety dreams aimed at suppressing unacceptable unconscious impulses. It is still unclear whether nightmares are simply symptomatic of an underlying clinical condition or whether they play some homeostatic or cognitive and emotional function. Several theories have been proposed to explain some adaptive advantages of nightmares, suggesting that they may be implicated in emotional responses over time (C. Fisher et al., 1970; Nielsen & Levin, 2007; Revonsuo, 2000; Walker & van der Helm, 2009; Wright & Koulack, 1987).

In general, dream activity appears to be involved in emotional regulation and memory consolidation (Scarpelli, Bartolacci, et al., 2019b). It is well known that stressors during waking can be incorporated into dream scenarios and converted into unpleasant oneiric emotions (Malinowski & Horton, 2014). In this regard, the disruption–avoidance–adaptation theory (Wright & Koulack, 1987) posited that oneiric activity oscillates between mastery and avoidance functions. Dreaming could reflect a kind of emotional problem-solving that helps solve disturbing waking events. Nevertheless, the so-called avoidance dreams would provoke sleep fragmentation, and the lack of sleep continuity would prevent any form of the traumatic memories' adaptation. The authors suggest that the oscillation between mastery and avoidance persists until stress adaptation is obtained (Wright & Koulack, 1987).

Similarly, desomatization (C. Fisher et al., 1970) and mood regulatory (Kramer, 1993) theories hypothesize that nightmares have some role in emotional processing. In particular, C. Fisher et al. (1970) reported that nightmares spontaneously reported in the laboratory were featured by lower autonomic activation during REM sleep, and this arousal was limited to the last minutes before the awakening. The authors speculated that REM dreaming represents a way to modulate anxiety and desomatizing physiological responses. This would preserve REM sleep and contribute to the mastery of traumatic experiences. This process may differ from the repetitive-traumatic patterns in which the trauma-related emotions steadily remain without any adaptation. Indeed, when the anxiety overcomes a certain limit, the REM desomatization process breaks down, allowing autonomic activation. In parallel, a neurophysiologic explanation (Walker & van der Helm, 2009) highlighted that the decreased aminergic activity during REM sleep promotes the downregulation of emotion, allowing decoupling of mnestic traces from their related autonomic reactions (Pace-Schott, & Hobson, 2002).

A novel approach tried to explain nightmares based on the stress acceleration hypothesis of mental illness (Nielsen, 2017). This model posits that adverse events occurring during infantile amnesia (around 3 years) increase vulnerability to mental disturbances, representing a sensitive time window for emotional development. Early experienced negative situations could accelerate the neural and behavioral maturation of the emotional network responsible for fear memories' extinction and expression. Therefore, the disruption of infantile amnesia would expose individuals to memories typically forgotten, impacting later emotions. The alterations of sleep and waking emotional regulation would lead to less effective fear extinction processes. This would implicate an abnormal REM sleep function in regulating fear extinction, increasing the risk of developing nightmares. According to the idea that nightmares are the expression of a dysfunctional fear-memory extinction process (Nielsen & Levin, 2007), some authors reported that at the neural level the network, including the amygdala, hippocampus, and medial prefrontal cortex, would appear altered, resulting in an abnormally intense activation of fear. Dreaming may help remove the fear-memory components from their episodic context and recombine them into a new context without aversive elements. Nevertheless, nightmares, especially those with repetitive contents, disrupt this mechanism, preventing the possibility of creating new extinction memories.

More directly, the evolutionary theory of threat simulation (Revonsuo, 2000) suggests that the role of dreaming and nightmares is to promote the creation of a virtual—but realistic—environment for facing threatening situations. Namely, oneiric activity can be considered simulations that, if repeated, increase the probability of successfully coping with real adverse situations during the waking state. The authors speculate that this mechanism is highly activated when subjects are exposed to severe traumatic events. In this view, nightmares may contribute to promoting mood regulation, expressing a coping mechanism for stress. Nightmare frequency and intensity are related to waking stress as well as increasing coping efforts (Picchioni et al., 2002). Accordingly, nightmares and dream activity increased during the pandemic (Scarpelli, Alfonsi, et al., 2021) and after other adverse events (e.g., earthquake; Tempesta et al., 2013).

Overall, nightmares could be placed along a spectrum of severity based on frequency and level of distress. In some form, they may have an adaptive role in metabolizing, down-regulating, and coping with emotions triggered by adverse or traumatic events. In light of the existing literature, it may be speculated that when nightmares are repetitive, intrusive, and distressing they reflect the failure/interruption of emotional regulation/depotentiation processes (Walker & van der Helm, 2009). In other words, nightmares that are neither too frequent nor too severe may be those that play some functional role.

Therapeutic Strategies

As mentioned in the previous paragraph, nightmare disorder could provoke high daytime distress and persist for decades (Schreuder et al., 2000). Unfortunately, many patients remain untreated or inappropriately treated. Indeed, among adults who complained of clinically significant nightmares, only one in three shared this problem with a healthcare professional (Nadorff et al., 2015). Nevertheless, the existing literature reports multiple therapeutic strategies to face the nightmare disorder.

The first approach to treating nightmares was represented by desensitization and exposure therapy, both based on the principles of extinction and inhibitory learning (Kellner et al., 1992). The desensitization, associated with muscular relaxation techniques, requires nightmare sufferers to imagine the disturbing oneiric scenario without modifying it and trying to relax themself when they experience tension or distress. In exposure therapy, the subject should imagine the nightmare in its original form but without any relaxation exercise (Kunze et al., 2017). Albeit these methods elicited greater arousal in patients during treatment, their effectiveness appears similar to the imagery rehearsal therapy (IRT; Kellner et al., 1992; Krakow, Hollifield, et al., 2001; Kunze et al., 2017).

IRT is considered the first-choice strategy to treat nightmare disorder by the Oxford Centre for Evidence-Based Medicine (Cranston et al., 2011) and the AASM (Morgenthaler et al., 2018). It consists in rescripting the nightmare's plot and is very effective at reducing chronic nightmares within 6–12 weeks of therapy (Germain et al., 2004; Kellner et al., 1992; Krakow, Hollifield, et al., 2001). This technique allows nightmare sufferers to change the recurrent disturbing dream by removing unpleasant components and including mastery or more neutral items (Kellner et al., 1992). The patients learn and rehearse the new oneiric scenes a couple of times every day. A meta-analysis revealed this method's large pre-post within-subject effect size for nightmare frequency (Hansen et al., 2013). Moreover, IRT reduces PTSD severity (Hansen et al., 2013) and increases sleep quality (Casement & Swanson, 2012). IRT has moderate effects also on patients with other mental health complaints (Van Schagen et al., 2015), and this amelioration remains stable over time (Van Schagen et al., 2016). Importantly, IRT among psychiatric patients reduces suicidal ideation (Ellis et al., 2019). This intervention is also effective during childhood and adolescence (Simard & Nielsen, 2009). IRT could be a multicomponent treatment including psychoeducation, sleep diaries, and relaxation exercises (Lancee et al., 2010). Also, recording nightmares every morning seems to reduce nightmare rate and distress (Lancee et al., 2010).

Additionally, lucid dreaming induction seems to be a potentially helpful therapy for decreasing nightmares (Holzinger et al., 2015; Rak et al., 2015; Spoormaker & Van Den Bout, 2006; Zadra & Pihl, 1997). Recent literature highlights that lucid dreams could be considered a sort of coping strategy to face frightening components of dream experience (Scarpelli, Alfonsi, D'Anselmo, et al., 2021; Schiappa et al., 2018). Along this vein, lucid dream therapy is a cognitive technique that allows patients to learn to be aware of and modify their mental sleep activity during their nightmares through daily exercises (Spoormaker et al., 2006; Zadra & Pihl, 1997). In other words, while IRT provides a narrative change of dreaming during wakefulness, lucid dreaming induction aims to modify the oneiric scenes when the subject is still asleep. Becoming aware of controlling one's own oneiric activity may help improve nightmare disorder and sleep-related disturbances. In a study carried out on 32 veterans suffering from PTSD, 82% of subjects were frequently aware of nightmares, but only 24% could control the oneiric scenario (Harb et al., 2017).

Another approach to treating nightmare parasomnia is represented by cognitive therapy on dysfunctional beliefs (Harvey et al., 2005). Specifically, nightmares could also be described in insomnia patients, so an intervention targeting nightmares has been incorporated into the cognitive behavioral therapy for insomnia protocol (Casement & Swanson, 2012). Indeed, nightmare sufferers often ruminate and catastrophize on the consequences of their parasomnia, resulting in worse sleep quality. Ameliorating negative beliefs has been shown as effective (Kunze et al., 2017), as well as the use of paradoxical intention, encouraging subjects to have nightmares (Spoormaker, 2008). More recently, eye movement desensitization and reprocessing (EMDR; Shapiro, 1989) has been applied for treating post-traumatic nightmares, which have been considered as expressions of adverse events not correctly processed and stored in a dysfunctional manner. This approach elicits the recall of distressing oneiric contents while activating a bilateral sensory input (e.g., tapping or side-to-side eye movement). This procedure would reduce the vividness of imagery, producing emotional and physiological changes resulting in a relaxing response and decreased autonomic response. EMDR has been administered to patients with PTSD with promising results (Cusack et al., 2016; Silver et al., 1995). A study involving 83 Vietnam veterans with PTSD showed a greater reduction of nightmare severity obtained by EMDR than other interventions (e.g., relaxation training, biofeedback), also at a follow-up assessment (Silver et al., 1995).

Finally, pharmacological treatment has been mentioned by the AASM as an additional therapy for nightmares and other PTSD symptoms (Aurora et al., 2010). Although the neurophysiological and neurochemical bases of nightmares are still unknown, the most used medications to treat nightmares aim to increase noradrenergic tone (Arnsten et al., 2015; Raskind et al., 2000). In particular, prazosin, a central nervous system alpha-1 adrenoreceptor antagonist, may be used, albeit a recent trial did not show significant effects after treatment (Raskind et al., 2018). Also, antidepressants and antipsychotics are proposed as possible pharmacotherapy for nightmares (El-Solh, 2018); nevertheless, the findings about the effectiveness of these agents on nightmare severity are not always consistent, and the AASM does not consider these interventions among the first choice.

Furthermore, some preliminary findings suggest that cannabis use in adults could help in nightmare reduction (Conroy & Arnedt, 2014; Garcia & Salloum, 2015; Gates et al., 2014). On the one hand, cannabis could decrease the hyperarousal in people with PTSD, albeit, commonly, cannabis promotes sleep fragmentation (Gates et al., 2014). The synthetic endocannabinoid receptor agonist nabilone seems effective at reducing post-traumatic nightmares (Fraser, 2009; Passie et al., 2012). A single double-blind, placebo-controlled study by Jetly and colleagues (2015) showed that treatment with nabilone was linked to important reductions in nightmare severity and improved overall PTSD symptom severity. However, side effects such as dizziness, headaches, dry mouth, lightheadedness, and rare case of psychosis have been found (Cameron et al., 2014). Overall, most studies on medications are still carried out without a placebo in double-blinded investigations, and most psychotherapeutic strategies were tested without a nonrandomized or control/waiting list group. Further investigations should be conducted to fill this gap and explore the effectiveness of the above-mentioned intervention for nightmare disorder.

Conclusions and Future Directions

Here, we provided a comprehensive overview of the literature about nightmare disorder. Nevertheless, the current literature is far from exhaustive and homogeneous. We highlighted that the criteria to diagnose this parasomnia have changed over time, giving different importance to awakenings.

Empirical evidence on sleep architecture and EEG patterns, as well as neuropsychological data, are inconsistent and too scarce to allow researchers to draw definitive conclusions about nightmares' brain correlates and their changes during the life span. As for studies on dreaming activity, some findings point out that an electrophysiological milieu characterized by higher activation may predict nightmares (e.g., C. Fisher et al., 1970; Simor et al., 2013).

Although recurring nightmares are strictly related to PTSD, we emphasized that chronic nightmares also characterize different mental illnesses impairing individual well-being. In light of this, several strategies have been proposed to treat nightmares, from cognitive behavioral standard approaches to new methods such as lucid dream induction or EMDR. Many of them deserve further systematic investigations to determine their effectiveness in different populations.

Finally, we provided an update about the functional theories on nightmares, suggesting that, to some extent, the presence of frightening dreams has some role in the emotional regulation processes. However, empirical studies supporting the functional theories on nightmares are still lacking.

It is worth noting that the study of nightmares has critical methodological limitations, such as the intrinsic difficulty of direct access to oneiric activity, the problem of eliciting nightmares in a laboratory setting, and the difficulty of obtaining reliable relations between waking events and nightmare contents.

Since nightmares and oneiric changes over time could represent a reliable index of mental well-being, this research field deserves further investigation. Future research should be directed to the following:

- Assess the relationship between nightmares' features and psychopathological conditions or personality traits, also focusing on systematic evaluation of therapeutic approaches.
- Obtain objective neurophysiological measures using PSG recordings in the laboratory or at-home recordings.
- Comparatively, investigate the relationship between nightmares' features and sleep macro- and micro-structural patterns among different nightmare sufferers (e.g., idiopathic nightmares vs. post-traumatic nightmares).

References

Ağargün, M. Y., Kara, H., Bilici, M., Çilli, A. S., Telci, M., Semiz, Ü. B., & Başoğlu, C. (1999). The Van Dream Anxiety Scale: A subjective measure of dream anxiety in nightmare sufferers. *Sleep and Hypnosis, 1*(4), 204–211.

Alger, S. E., Chambers, A. M., Cunningham, T., & Payne, J. D. (2015). The role of sleep in human declarative memory consolidation. In P. Meerlo, R. Benca, & T. Abel (Eds.), *Sleep, neuronal plasticity and brain function. Current topics in behavioral neurosciences* (Vol. 25, pp. 269–306). Springer. https://doi.org/10.1007/7854_2014_341

American Academy of Sleep Medicine. (2014). *International classification of sleep disorders* (3rd ed.).

American Psychiatric Association. (1994). *Diagnostic and statistical manual of mental disorders* (4th ed.).

American Psychiatric Association. (2013). *Diagnostic and statistical manual of mental disorders* (5th ed.).

Arnsten, A. F., Raskind, M. A., Taylor, F. B., & Connor, D. F. (2015). The effects of stress exposure on prefrontal cortex: Translating basic research into successful treatments for post-traumatic stress disorder. *Neurobiology of Stress, 1*, 89–99. https://doi.org/10.1016/j.ynstr.2014.10.002

Aron, E. N., & Aron, A. (1997). Sensory-processing sensitivity and its relation to introversion and emotionality. *Journal of Personality and Social Psychology, 73*(2), Article 345. https://doi.org/10.1037/0022-3514.73.2.345

Aurora, R. N., Zak, R. S., Auerbach, S. H., Casey, K. R., Chowdhuri, S., Karippot, A., Maganti, R. K., Ramar, K., Kristo, D. A., Bista, S. R., Lamm, C. I., Timothy, I., &Morgenthaler, T. I. (2010). Best practice guide for the treatment of nightmare disorder in adults. *Journal of Clinical Sleep Medicine, 6*(4), 389–401. https://doi.org/10.5664/jcsm.27883

Belicki, K. (1992). Nightmare frequency versus nightmare distress: Relations to psychopathology and cognitive style. *Journal of Abnormal Psychology, 101*(3), 592–597. https://doi.org/10.1037/0021-843X.101.3.592

Besiroglu, L., Agargun, M. Y., & Inci, R. (2005). Nightmares and terminal insomnia in depressed patients with and without melancholic features. *Psychiatry Research, 133*(2–3), 285–287. https://doi.org/10.1016/j.psychres.2004.12.001

Bishop, T. M., Walsh, P. G., Ashrafioun, L., Lavigne, J. E., & Pigeon, W. R. (2020). Sleep, suicide behaviors, and the protective role of sleep medicine. *Sleep Medicine, 66*, 264–270. https://doi.org/10.1016/j.sleep.2019.07.016

Blagrove, M., Farmer, L., & Williams, E. (2004). The relationship of nightmare frequency and nightmare distress to wellbeing. *Journal of Sleep Research, 13*, 129–136. https://doi.org/10.1111/j.1365-2869.2004.00394.x

Bolstad, C. J., Szkody, E., & Nadorff, M. R. (2021). Factor analysis and validation of the Disturbing Dreams and Nightmare Severity Index. *Dreaming, 31*(4), 329–341. https://doi.org/10.1037/drm0000178

Bryant, R. A., Creamer, M., O'Donnell, M., Silove, D., & McFarlane, A. C. (2010). Sleep disturbance immediately prior to trauma predicts subsequent psychiatric disorder. *Sleep, 33*(1), 69–74. https://doi.org/10.1093/sleep/33.1.69

Callaghan, B. L., & Tottenham, N. (2016). The neuro-environmental loop of plasticity: A cross-species analysis of parental effects on emotion circuitry development following typical and adverse caregiving. *Neuropsychopharmacology, 41*(1), 163–176. https://doi.org/10.1038/npp.2015.204

Cameron, C., Watson, D., & Robinson, J. (2014). Use of a synthetic cannabinoid in a correctional population for posttraumatic stress disorder–related insomnia and nightmares, chronic pain, harm reduction, and other indications: A retrospective evaluation. *Journal of Clinical Psychopharmacology, 34*(5), 559–564. https://doi.org/10.1097/JCP.0000000000000180

Carr, M., & Nielsen, T. (2017). A novel differential susceptibility framework for the study of nightmares: Evidence for trait sensory processing sensitivity. *Clinical Psychology Review, 58*, 86–96. https://doi.org/10.1016/j.cpr.2017.10.002

Carr, M., Saint-Onge, K., Blanchette-Carrière, C., Paquette, T., & Nielsen, T. (2017). Elevated perseveration errors on a verbal fluency task in frequent nightmare recallers: A replication. *Journal of Sleep Research, 27*, Article e12644. https://doi.org/10.1111/jsr.12644

Carr, M., Summers, R., Bradshaw, C., Newton, C., Ellis, L., Johnston, E., & Blagrove, M. (2020). Frontal brain activity and subjective arousal during emotional picture viewing in nightmare sufferers. *Frontiers in Neuroscience, 14*, Article 585574. https://doi.org/10.3389/fnins.2020.585574

Casement, M. D., & Swanson, L. M. (2012). A meta-analysis of imagery rehearsal for post-trauma nightmares: Effects on nightmare frequency, sleep quality, and posttraumatic stress. *Clinical Psychology Review, 32*, 566–574. https://doi.org/10.1016/j.cpr.2012.06.002

Castelnovo, A., Lopez, R., Proserpio, P., Nobili, L., & Dauvilliers, Y. (2018). NREM sleep parasomnias as disorders of sleep-state dissociation. *Nature Reviews Neurology, 14*(8), 470–481. https://doi.org/10.1038/s41582-018-0030-y

Cattarius, B. G., & Schlarb, A. A. (2016). Gegenseitige beeinflussung von eltern und babys in ihrem schlafverhalten. Der heimliche blick ins schlafzimmer [Mutual influence of parents and babies on their sleep behaviour. A look behind closed doors]. *Somnologie, 20*, 189–198. https://doi.org/10.1007/s11818-016-0064-6

Cohen, D. B., & MacNeilage, P. F. (1974). A test of the salience hypothesis of dream recall. *Journal of Consulting and Clinical Psychology, 42*(5), 699–703.

Conroy, D. A., & Arnedt, J. T. (2014). Sleep and substance use disorders: An update. *Current Psychiatry Reports, 16*(10), Article 487. https://doi.org/10.1007/s11920-014-0487-3

Coolidge, F. L., Segal, D. L., Coolidge, C. M., Spinath, F. M., & Gottschling, J. (2010). Do nightmares and generalized anxiety disorder in childhood and adolescence have a common genetic origin? *Behavior Genetics, 40*(3), 349–356. https://doi.org/10.1007/s10519-009-9310-z

Coupland, N. J., Bell, C. J., & Potokar, J. P. (1996). Serotonin reuptake inhibitor withdrawal. *Journal of Clinical Psychopharmacology, 16*(5), 356–362. https://doi.org/10.1097/00004714-199610000-00003

Cranston, C. C., Davis, J. L., Rhudy, J. L., & Favorite, T. K. (2011). Replication and expansion of "best practice guide for the treatment of nightmare disorder in adults." *Journal of Clinical Sleep Medicine, 7*, 549–553.

Cusack, K., Jonas, D. E., Forneris, C. A., Wines, C., Sonis, J., Middleton, J. C., Feltner, C., Brownley, K. A., Olmsted, K. R., Greenblatt, A., Weil, A., & Gaynes, B. N. (2016). Psychological treatments for adults with posttraumatic stress disorder: A systematic review and meta-analysis. *Clinical Psychology Review, 43*, 128–141. https://doi.org/10.1016/j.cpr.2015.10.003

Desseilles, M., Dang-Vu, T. T., Sterpenich, V., & Schwartz, S. (2011). Cognitive and emotional processes during dreaming: A neuroimaging view. *Consciousness and Cognition, 20*(4), 998–1008. https://doi.org/10.1016/j.concog.2010.10.005

Detweiler, M. B., Arif, S., Candelario, J., Altman, J., Murphy, P. F., Halling, M. H., Vesudeva, S., & Detweiler, J. G. (2012). Salem VAMC–US Army Fort Bragg Warrior Transition Clinic telepsychiatry collaboration: 12-month operation clinical perspective. *Telemedicine and e-Health, 18*(2), 81–86. https://doi.org/10.1089/tmj.2011.0064

Domhoff, B., & Kamiya, J. (1964). Problems in dream content study with objective indicators: A comparison of home and laboratory dream reports. *Archives of General Psychiatry, 11*(5), 519–524. https://doi.org/10.1001/archpsyc.1964.01720290067008

Ebbert, J. O., Hughes, J. R., West, R. J., Rennard, S. I., Russ, C., McRae, T. D., Treadow, J., Yu, C. R., Dutro, M. P., & Park, P. W. (2015). Effect of varenicline on smoking cessation through smoking reduction: A randomized clinical trial. *JAMA, 313*(7), 687–694. https://doi.org/10.1001/jama.2015.280

Eklind, S., Olby, K., & Åkerman, E. (2023). The intensive care unit diary—A significant complement in the recovery after intensive care. A focus group study. *Intensive and Critical Care Nursing, 74*, Article 103337. https://doi.org/10.1016/j.iccn.2022.103337

Ellis, T. E., Rufino, K. A., & Nadorff, M. R. (2019). Treatment of nightmares in psychiatric inpatients with imagery rehearsal therapy: An open trial and case series. *Behavioral Sleep Medicine, 17*, 112–123. https://doi.org/10.1080/15402002.2017.1299738

El-Solh, A. A. (2018). Management of nightmares in patients with posttraumatic stress disorder: Current perspectives. *Nature and Science of Sleep, 10*, 409–420. https://doi.org/10.2147/NSS.S166089

Fisher, C., Byrne, J., Edwards, A., & Kahn, E. (1970). A psychophysiological study of nightmares. *Journal of the American Psychoanalytic Association, 18*(4), 747–782. https://doi.org/10.1177/000306517001800401

Fisher, H. L., Lereya, S. T., Thompson, A., Lewis, G., Zammit, S., & Wolke, D. (2014). Childhood parasomnias and psychotic experiences at age 12 years in a United Kingdom birth cohort. *Sleep, 37*(3), 475–482. https://doi.org/10.5665/sleep.3478

Fraser, G. A. (2009). The use of a synthetic cannabinoid in the management of treatment-resistant nightmares in posttraumatic stress disorder (PTSD). *CNS Neuroscience & Therapeutics, 15*(1), 84–88. https://doi.org/10.1111/j.1755-5949.2008.00071.x

Freud, S. (1900). *The interpretation of dreams*. Basic Books.

Garcia, A. N., & Salloum, I. M. (2015). Polysomnographic sleep disturbances in nicotine, caffeine, alcohol, cocaine, opioid, and cannabis use: A focused review. *American Journal on Addictions, 24*(7), 590–598. https://doi.org/10.1111/ajad.12291

Gates, P. J., Albertella, L., & Copeland, J. (2014). The effects of cannabinoid administration on sleep: A systematic review of human studies. *Sleep Medicine Reviews, 18*(6), 477–487. https://doi.org/10.1016/j.smrv.2014.02.005

Germain, A. (2013). Sleep disturbances as the hallmark of PTSD: Where are we now? *American Journal of Psychiatry, 170*(4), 372–382. https://doi.org/10.1176/appi.ajp.2012.12040432

Germain, A., Hall, M., Krakow, B., Shear, M. K., & Buysse, D. J. (2005). A brief sleep scale for posttraumatic stress disorder: Pittsburgh Sleep Quality Index Addendum for PTSD. *Journal of Anxiety Disorders, 19*(2), 233–244. https://doi.org/10.1016/j.janxdis.2004.02.001

Germain, A., Krakow, B., Faucher, B., Zadra, A., Nielsen, T., Hollifield, M., Warner, T., & Koss, M. (2004). Increased mastery elements associated with imagery rehearsal treatment for nightmares in sexual assault survivors with PTSD. *Dreaming, 14*, 195–206. https://doi.org/10.1037/1053-0797.14.4.195

Germain, A., & Nielsen, T. (2003). Impact of imagery rehearsal treatment on distressing dreams, psychological distress, and sleep parameters in nightmare patients. *Behavioral Sleep Medicine, 1*(3), 140–154. https://doi.org/10.1207/S15402010BSM0103_2

Guerrero, J., & Crocq, M. A. (1994). Sleep disorders in the elderly: Depression and post-traumatic stress disorder. *Journal of Psychosomatic Research, 38*, 141–150. https://doi.org/10.1016/0022-3999(94)90144-9

Hall, C. S., & Nordby, V. J. (1972). *The individual and his dreams.* New American Library.

Hansen, K., Höfling, V., Kröner-Borowik, T., Stangier, U., & Steil, R. (2013). Efficacy of psychological interventions aiming to reduce chronic nightmares: A meta-analysis. *Clinical Psychology Review, 33*, 146–155. https://doi.org/10.1016/j.cpr.2012.10.012

Harb, G. C., Greene, J. L., Dent, K. M., & Ross, R. J. (2017). 1077 Lucid dreaming in veterans with PTSD: Non-nightmare dreams and nightmares. *Sleep, 40*, Article A401. https://doi.org/10.1093/sleepj/zsx050.1076

Hartmann, E. (1984). *The nightmare: The psychology and the biology of terrifying dreams.* Basic Books.

Harvey, A. G., Tang, N. K. Y., & Browning, L. (2005). Cognitive approaches to insomnia. *Clinical Psychology Review, 25*, 593–611. https://doi.org/10.1016/j.cpr.2005.04.005

Hawkins, C., & Williams, T. I. (1992). Nightmares, life events and behaviour problems in preschool children. *Child: Care, Health and Development, 18*(2), 117–128. https://doi.org/10.1111/j.1365-2214.1992.tb00346.x

Hefez, A., Metz, L., & Lavie, P. (1987). Long-term effects of extreme situational stress on sleep and dreaming. *American Journal of Psychiatry, 144*(3), 344–347.

Hinton, D. E., Field, N. P., Nickerson, A., Bryant, R. A., & Simon, N. (2013). Dreams of the dead among Cambodian refugees: Frequency, phenomenology, and relationship to complicated grief and posttraumatic stress disorder. *Death Studies, 37*(8), 750–767. https://doi.org/10.1080/07481187.2012.692457

Holzinger, B., Klösch, G., & Saletu, B. (2015). Studies with lucid dreaming as add-on therapy to gestalt therapy. *Acta Neurologica Scandinavica, 131*, 355–363. https://doi.org/10.1111/ane.12362

Jetly, R., Heber, A., Fraser, G., & Boisvert, D. (2015). The efficacy of nabilone, a synthetic cannabinoid, in the treatment of PTSD-associated nightmares: A preliminary randomized, double-blind, placebo-controlled cross-over design study. *Psychoneuroendocrinology, 51*, 585–588. https://doi.org/10.1016/j.psyneuen.2014.11.002

Kaseda, E. T., & Levine, A. J. (2020). Post-traumatic stress disorder: A differential diagnostic consideration for COVID-19 survivors. *The Clinical Neuropsychologist, 34*(7–8), 1498–1514. https://doi.org/10.1080/13854046.2020.1811894

Kaup, B. A., Ruskin, P. E., & Nyman, G. (1994). Significant life events and PTSD in elderly World War II veterans. *American Journal of Geriatric Psychiatry, 2*(3), 239–243. https://doi.org/10.1097/00019442-199400230-00008

Kellner, R., Neidhardt, J., Krakow, B., & Pathak, D. (1992). Changes in chronic nightmares after one session of desensitization or rehearsal instructions. *American Journal of Psychiatry, 149*, 659–663.

Kilpatrick, D. G., Resnick, H. S., Freedy, J. R., Pelcovitz, D., Resick, P., Roth, S., & van der Kolk, B. (1998). The posttraumatic stress disorder field trial: Evaluation of the PTSD construct: Criteria A through E. *DSM-IV Sourcebook, 4*, 803–844.

Klůzová Kráčmarová, L., & Plháková, A. (2015). Nightmares and their consequences in relation to state factors, absorption, and boundaries. *Dreaming, 25*(4), 312–320. https://doi.org/10.1037/a0039712

Kobayashi, I., Sledjeski, E. M., Spoonster, E., Fallon, W. F., Jr., & Delahanty, D. L. (2008). Effects of early nightmares on the development of sleep disturbances in motor vehicle accident victims. *Journal of Traumatic Stress, 21*(6), 548–555. https://doi.org/10.1002/jts.20368

Köthe, M., & Pietrowsky, R. (2001). Behavioral effects of nightmares and their correlations to personality patterns. *Dreaming, 11*, 43–52. https://doi.org/10.1023/a:1009468517557

Krakow, B. (2006). Nightmare complaints in treatment-seeking patients in clinical sleep medicine settings: Diagnostic and treatment implications. *Sleep, 29*, 1313–1319. https://doi.org/10.1093/sleep/29.10.1313

Krakow, B., Hollifield, M., Johnston, L., Koss, M., Schrader, R., Warner, T. D., Tandberg, D., Lauriello, J., McBride, L., Cutchen, D., Cheng, D., Emmons, S., Germain, A., Melendrez, D., Sandoval, D., & Prince, H. (2001). Imagery rehearsal therapy for chronic nightmares in sexual assault survivors with posttraumatic stress disorder: A randomized controlled trial. *JAMA, 286*, 537–545. https://doi.org/10.1001/jama.286.5.537

Krakow, B., Melendrez, D., Pedersen, B., Johnston, L., Hollifield, M., Germain, A., Koss, M., Warner, T. D., & Schrader, R. (2001). Complex insomnia: Insomnia and sleep-disordered breathing in a consecutive series of crime victims with nightmares and PTSD. *Biological Psychiatry, 49*(11), 948–953. https://doi.org/10.1016/s0006-3223(00)01087-8

Krakow, B., Schrader, R., Tandberg, D., Hollifield, M., Koss, M. P., Yau, C. L., & Cheng, D. T. (2002). Nightmare frequency in sexual assault survivors with PTSD. *Journal of Anxiety Disorders, 16*(2), 175–190. https://doi.org/10.1016/S0887-6185(02)00093-2

Kramer, M. (1993). The selective mood regulatory function of dreaming: An update and revision. In A. Moitt, M. Kramer, & R. Hofmann (Eds.), *The functions of dreaming* (pp. 139–196). State University of New York Press.

Kunze, A. E., Arntz, A., Morina, N., Kindt, M., & Lancee, J. (2017). Efficacy of imagery rescripting and imaginal exposure for nightmares: A randomized wait-list controlled trial. *Behaviour Research and Therapy, 97*, 14–25. https://doi.org/10.1016/j.brat.2017.06.005

Laberge, L., Tremblay, R. E., Vitaro, F., & Montplaisir, J. (2000). Development of parasomnias from childhood to early adolescence. *Pediatrics, 106*(1), 67–74. https://doi.org/10.1542/peds.106.1.67

Lancee, J., & Schrijnemaekers, N. C. M. L. (2013). The association between nightmares and daily distress. *Sleep and Biological Rhythms, 11*, 14–19. https://doi.org/10.1111/j.1479-8425.2012.00586.x

Lancee, J., Spoormaker, V. I., & van den Bout, J. (2010). Cognitive-behavioral self-help treatment for nightmares: A randomized controlled trial. *Psychotherapy and Psychosomatics, 79*(6), 371–377. https://doi.org/10.1159/000320894

Lereya, S. T., Winsper, C., Tang, N. K., & Wolke, D. (2017). Sleep problems in childhood and borderline personality disorder symptoms in early adolescence. *Journal of Abnormal Child Psychology, 45*(1), 193–206. https://doi.org/10.1007/s10802-016-0158-4

Levin, R., & Fireman, G. (2002). Nightmare prevalence, nightmare distress, and self-reported psychological disturbance. *Sleep, 25*, 205–212.

Levin, R., & Nielsen, T. (2009). Nightmares, bad dreams, and emotion dysregulation: A review and new neurocognitive model of dreaming. *Current Directions in Psychological Science, 18*, 84–88. http://dx.doi.org/10.1111/j.1467-8721.2009.01614.x

Li, S. X., Zhang, B., Li, A. M., & Wing, Y. K. (2010). Prevalence and correlates of frequent nightmares: A community-based 2-phase study. *Sleep, 33*, 774–780. https://doi.org/10.1093/sleep/33.6.774

Lin, J. T.-Y., & Ziegler, D. K. (1976). Psychiatric symptoms with initiation of carbidopa-levodopa treatment. *Neurology, 26*(7), 699–699. https://doi.org/10.1212/WNL.26.7.699

Littlewood, D. L., Gooding, P. A., Panagioti, M., & Kyle, S. D. (2016). Nightmares and suicide in posttraumatic stress disorder: The mediating role of defeat, entrapment, and hopelessness. *Journal of Clinical Sleep Medicine, 12*(3), 393–399. https://doi.org/10.5664/jcsm.5592

Malinowski, J., & Horton, C. L. (2014). Evidence for the preferential incorporation of emotional waking-life experiences into dreams. *Dreaming, 24*(1), 18–31. https://doi.org/10.1037/a0036017

Mallon, L., Broman, J. E., & Hetta, J. (2000). Sleeping difficulties in relation to depression and anxiety in elderly adults. *Nordic Journal of Psychiatry, 54*(5), 355–360. https://doi.org/10.1080/080394800457192

Maquet, P., Ruby, P., Maudoux, A., Albouy, G., Sterpenich, V., Dang-Vu, T., Desserilles, M., Boly, M., Perrin, F., Peigneux, P., & Laureys, S. (2005). Human cognition during REM sleep and the activity profile within frontal and parietal cortices: A reappraisal of functional neuroimaging data. *Progress in Brain Research, 150*, 219–227, 595. https://doi.org/10.1016/S0079-6123(05)50016-5

Marquis, L. P., Julien, S. H., Baril, A. A., Blanchette-Carrière, C., Paquette, T., Carr, M., Soucy, J. P., Montplasir, J., & Nielsen, T. (2019). Nightmare severity is inversely related to frontal brain activity during waking state picture viewing. *Journal of Clinical Sleep Medicine, 15*(2), 253–264. https://doi.org/10.5664/jcsm.7628

Marquis, L. P., Paquette, T., Blanchette-Carrière, C., Dumel, G., & Nielsen, T. (2017). REM sleep theta changes in frequent nightmare recallers. *Sleep, 40*(9), Article zsx110. https://doi.org/10.1093/sleep/zsx110

Marshall, A. J., Acheson, D. T., Risbrough, V. B., Straus, L. D., & Drummond, S. P. (2014). Fear conditioning, safety learning, and sleep in humans. *Journal of Neuroscience, 34*(35), 11754–11760. https://doi.org/10.1523/JNEUROSCI.0478-14.2014

Marzano, C., Ferrara, M., Mauro, F., Moroni, F., Gorgoni, M., Tempesta, D., Cipolli, C., & De Gennaro, L. (2011). Recalling and forgetting dreams: theta and alpha oscillations during sleep predict subsequent dream recall. *Journal of Neuroscience, 31*, 6674–6683. https://doi.org/10.1523/JNEUROSCI.0412-11.2011

Mellman, T. A., Nolan, B., Hebding, J., Kulick-Bell, R., & Dominguez, R. (1997). A polysomnographic comparison of veterans with combat-related PTSD, depressed men, and non-ill controls. *Sleep, 20*(1), 46–51. https://doi.org/10.1093/sleep/20.1.46

Mindell, J. A., & Barrett, K. M. (2002). Nightmares and anxiety in elementary-aged children: Is there a relationship? *Child: Care, Health and Development, 28*(4), 317–322. https://doi.org/10.1046/j.1365-2214.2002.00274.x

Morgenthaler, T. I., Auerbach, S., Casey, K. R., Kristo, D., Maganti, R., Ramar, K., Zak, R., & Kartje, R. (2018). Position paper for the treatment of nightmare disorder in adults: An American Academy of Sleep Medicine position paper. *Journal of Clinical Sleep Medicine, 14*, 1041–1055. https://doi.org/10.5664/jcsm.7178

Morrell, J., & Steele, H. (2003). The role of attachment security, temperament, maternal perception, and care-giving behavior in persistent infant sleeping problems. *Infant Mental Health Journal, 24*(5), 447–468. https://doi.org/10.1002/imhj.10072

Mume, C. O. (2009). Nightmare in schizophrenic and depressed patients. *European Journal of Psychiatry, 23*(3), 177–183. https://doi.org/10.4321/s0213-61632009000300006

Munezawa, T., Kaneita, Y., Osaki, Y., Kanda, H., Ohtsu, T., Suzuki, H., Minowa, M., Suzuki, K., Higuchi, S., Mori, J., & Ohida, T. (2011). Nightmare and sleep paralysis among Japanese adolescents: A nationwide representative survey. *Sleep Medicine, 12*, 56–64. https://doi.org/10.1016/j.sleep.2010.04.015

Muris, P., Merckelbach, H., Gadet, B., & Moulaert, V. (2000). Fears, worries, and scary dreams in 4- to 12-year-old children: Their content, developmental pattern, and origins. *Journal of Clinical Child Psychology, 29*(1), 43–52. https://doi.org/10.1207/S15374424jccp2901_5

Nadorff, M. R., Nadorff, D. K., & Germain, A. (2015). Nightmares: Under-reported, undetected, and therefore untreated. *Journal of Clinical Sleep Medicine, 11*(7), 747–750. https://doi.org/10.5664/jcsm.4850

Nadorff, M. R., Nazem, S., & Fiske, A. (2011). Insomnia symptoms, nightmares, and suicidal ideation in a college student sample. *Sleep, 34*, 93–98. https://doi.org/10.1093/sleep/34.1.93

Nadorff, M. R., Porter, B., Rhoades, H. M., Greisinger, A. J., Kunik, M. E., & Stanley, M. A. (2014). Bad dream frequency in older adults with generalized anxiety disorder: Prevalence, correlates, and effect of cognitive behavioral treatment for anxiety. *Behavioral Sleep Medicine, 12*(1), 28–40. https://doi.org/10.1080/15402002.2012.755125

Narrow, W. E., Clarke, D. E., Kuramoto, S. J., Kraemer, H. C., Kupfer, D. J., Greiner, L., & Regier, D. A. (2013). DSM-5 field trials in the United States and Canada, Part III: Development and reliability testing of a cross-cutting symptom assessment for DSM-5. *American Journal of Psychiatry, 170*(1), 71–82. https://doi.org/10.1176/appi.ajp.2012.12071000

Nielsen, T. (2017). The stress acceleration hypothesis of nightmares. *Frontiers in Neurology, 8*, Article 201. https://doi.org/10.3389/fneur.2017.00201

Nielsen, T., Carr, M., Picard-Deland, C., Marquis, L. P., Saint-Onge, K., Blanchette-Carrière, C., & Paquette, T. (2019). Early childhood adversity associations with nightmare severity and sleep spindles. *Sleep Medicine, 56*, 57–65. https://doi.org/10.1016/j.sleep.2019.03.004

Nielsen, T. A., Laberge, L., Paquet, J., Tremblay, R. E., Vitaro, F., & Montplaisir, J. (2000). Development of disturbing dreams during adolescence and their relation to anxiety symptoms. *Sleep, 23*(6), 1–10. https://doi.org/10.1093/sleep/23.6.1

Nielsen, T., & Levin, R. (2007). Nightmares: A new neurocognitive model. *Sleep Medicine Reviews, 11*, 295–310. https://doi.org/10.1016/j.smrv.2007.03.004

Nielsen, T. A., Paquette, T., Solomonova, E., Lara-Carrasco, J., Popova, A., & Levrier, K. (2010). REM sleep characteristics of nightmare sufferers before and after REM sleep deprivation. *Sleep Medicine, 11*(2), 172–179. https://doi.org/10.1016/j.sleep.2008.12.018

Nielsen, T., & Zadra, A. (2000). Dreaming disorders. In M. Kryger, T. Roth, & W. Dement (Eds.), *Principles and practice of sleep medicine* (3rd ed., pp. 753–772). W. B. Saunders.

Nielsen, T. A., & Zadra, A. (2005). Nightmares and other common dream disturbances. In M. H. Kryger, T. Roth, & W. C. Dement (Eds.), *Principles and practice of sleep medicine* (4th ed., pp. 926–935). W.B. Saunders.

Nishida, M., Pearsall, J., Buckner, R. L., & Walker, M. P. (2009). REM sleep, prefrontal theta, and the consolidation of human emotional memory. *Cerebral Cortex, 19*(5), 1158–1166. https://doi.org/10.1093/cercor/bhn155

Ohayon, M. M., Morselli, P. L., & Guilleminault, C. (1997). Prevalence of nightmares and their relationship to psychopathology and daytime functioning in insomnia subjects. *Sleep, 20*(5), 340–348. https://doi.org/10.1093/sleep/20.5.340

Ohayon, M. M., Guilleminault, C., & Priest, R. G. (1999). Night terrors, sleepwalking, and confusional arousals in the general population: Their frequency and relationship to other sleep and mental disorders. *Journal of Clinical Psychiatry, 60*(4), Article 12808. https://doi.org/10.4088/jcp.v60n0413

Ophoff, D., Slaats, M. A., Boudewyns, A., Glazemakers, I., Van Hoorenbeeck, K., & Verhulst, S. L. (2018). Sleep disorders during childhood: A practical review. *European Journal of Pediatrics, 177*(5), 641–648. https://doi.org/10.1007/s00431-018-3116-z

Pace-Schott, E. F., & Hobson, J. A. (2002). The neurobiology of sleep: Genetics, cellular physiology and subcortical networks. *Nature Reviews Neuroscience, 3*(8), 591–605. https://doi.org/10.1038/nrn895

Pagel, J. F. (1996). Pharmacological alteration of sleep and dreams—A clinical framework for utilizing the electrophysiological and sleep stage effects of psychoactive medications. *Human Psychopharmacology: Clinical and Experimental, 11*(3), 217–223. https://doi.org/10.1002/(SICI)1099-1077(199605)11:3<217::AID-HUP790>3.0.CO;2-0

Pagel, J. F. (2010). Drugs, dreams, and nightmares. *Sleep Medicine Clinics, 5*(2), 277–287. https://doi.org/10.1016/j.jsmc.2010.01.007

Panagioti, M., Gooding, P. A., & Tarrier, N. (2012). A meta-analysis of the association between posttraumatic stress disorder and suicidality: The role of comorbid depression. *Comprehensive Psychiatry, 53*(7), 915–930. https://doi.org/10.1016/j.comppsych.2012.02.009

Passie, T., Emrich, H. M., Karst, M., Brandt, S. D., & Halpern, J. H. (2012). Mitigation of post-traumatic stress symptoms by cannabis resin: A review of the clinical and neurobiological evidence. *Drug Testing and Analysis, 4*(7–8), 649–659. https://doi.org/10.1002/dta.1377

Paul, F., Alpers, G. W., Reinhard, I., & Schredl, M. (2019). Nightmares do result in psychophysiological arousal: A multimeasure ambulatory assessment study. *Psychophysiology, 56*(7), Article e13366. https://doi.org/10.1111/psyp.13366

Phelps, A. J., Kanaan, R. A., Worsnop, C., Redston, S., Ralph, N., & Forbes, D. (2018). An ambulatory polysomnography study of the post-traumatic nightmares of post-traumatic stress disorder. *Sleep, 41*(1), zsx188. https://doi.org/10.1093/sleep/zsx188

Picchioni, D., Goeltzenleucher, B., Green, D. N., Convento, M. J., Crittenden, R., Hallgren, M., & Hicks, R. A. (2002). Nightmares as a coping mechanism for stress. *Dreaming, 12*(3), 155–169. https://doi.org/10.1023/A:1020118425588

Pigeon, W. R., Campbell, C. E., Possemato, K., & Ouimette, P. (2013). Longitudinal relationships of insomnia, nightmares, and PTSD severity in recent combat veterans. *Journal of Psychosomatic Research, 75*(6), 546–550. https://doi.org/10.1016/j.jpsychores.2013.09.004

Polini, F., Principe, R., Scarpelli, S., Clementi, F., & De Gennaro, L. (2017). Use of varenicline in smokeless tobacco cessation influences sleep quality and dream recall frequency but not dream affect. *Sleep Medicine, 30*, 1–6. https://doi.org/10.1016/j.sleep.2016.11.002

Potvin, O., Lorrain, D., Belleville, G., Grenier, S., & Préville, M. (2014). Subjective sleep characteristics associated with anxiety and depression in older adults: A population-based study. *International Journal of Geriatric Psychiatry, 29*(12), 1262–1270. https://doi.org/10.1002/gps.4106

Rak, M., Beitinger, P., Steiger, A., Schredl, M., & Dresler, M. (2015). Increased lucid dreaming frequency in narcolepsy. *Sleep, 38*, 787–792. https://doi.org/10.5665/sleep.4676

Raskind, M. A., Dobie, D. J., Kanter, E. D., Petrie, E. C., Thompson, C. E., & Peskind, E. R. (2000). The α1-adrenergic antagonist prazosin ameliorates combat trauma nightmares in veterans with posttraumatic stress disorder: A report of 4 cases. *Journal of Clinical Psychiatry, 61*(2), 129–133.

Raskind, M. A., Peskind, E. R., Chow, B., Harris, C., Davis-Karim, A., Holmes, H. A., Hart, K. L., McFall, M., Mellman, T. A., Reist, C., Romesser, J., Rosenheck, R., Shih, M. C., Stein, M. B., Swift, R., Gleason, T., Lu, Y., & Huang, G. D. (2018). Trial of prazosin for post-traumatic stress disorder in military veterans. *New England Journal of Medicine, 378*(6), 507–517. https://doi.org/10.1056/NEJMoa1507598

Revonsuo, A. (2000). The reinterpretation of dreams: An evolutionary hypothesis of the function of dreaming. *Behavioral and Brain Sciences, 23*(6), 877–901.

Richards, A., Kanady, J. C., & Neylan, T. C. (2020). Sleep disturbance in PTSD and other anxiety-related disorders: An updated review of clinical features, physiological characteristics, and psychological and neurobiological mechanisms. *Neuropsychopharmacology, 45*(1), 55–73. https://doi.org/10.1038/s41386-019-0486-5

Richards, A., Woodward, S. H., Baquirin, D. P. G., Yack, L. M., Metzler, T. J., Udupa, N. S., Staggs, E. J., & Neylan, T. C. (2023). The sleep physiology of nightmares in veterans with psychological trauma: Evaluation of a dominant model using participant-applied electroencephalography in the home environment. *Journal of Sleep Research, 32*(2), Article e13639. https://doi.org/10.1111/jsr.13639

Robert, G., & Zadra, A. (2014). Thematic and content analysis of idiopathic nightmares and bad dreams. *Sleep, 37*(2), 409–417. https://doi.org/10.5665/sleep.3426

Rogers, J. P., Chesney, E., Oliver, D., Pollak, T. A., McGuire, P., Fusar-Poli, P., Zandi, M. S., Lewis, G., & David, A. S. (2020). Psychiatric and neuropsychiatric presentations associated with severe coronavirus infections: A systematic review and meta-analysis with comparison to the COVID-19 pandemic. *Lancet Psychiatry, 7*(7), 611–627. https://doi.org/10.1016/S2215-0366(20)30203-0

Rogers, M. L., Schneider, M. E., Tucker, R. P., Law, K. C., Anestis, M. D., & Joiner, T. E. (2017). Overarousal as a mechanism of the relation between rumination and suicidality. *Journal of Psychiatric Research, 92*, 31–37. https://doi.org/10.1016/j.jpsychires.2017.03.024

Rosen, G., Mahowald, M. W., & Ferber, R. (1995). Sleepwalking, confusional arousals, and sleep terrors in the child. In R. Ferber, & M. Kryger (Eds.), *Principles and practice of sleep medicine in the child* (pp. 45–53). W. B. Saunders.

Rousseau, A. F., Minguet, P., Colson, C., Kellens, I., Chaabane, S., Delanaye, P., Cavalier, E., Chase, J. G., Lambermont, B., & Misset, B. (2021). Post-intensive care syndrome after a critical COVID-19: Cohort study from a Belgian follow-up clinic. *Annals of Intensive Care, 11*(1), Article 118. https://doi.org/10.1186/s13613-021-00910-9

Sadeh, A., & Anders, T. F. (1993). Infant sleep problems: Origins, assessment, interventions. *Infant Mental Health Journal, 14*(1), 17–34. https://doi.org/10.1002/1097-0355(199321)14:1<17::AID-IMHJ2280140103>3.0.CO;2-Q

Saif, A., & Pick, A. (2021). Polyneuropathy following COVID-19 infection: The rehabilitation approach. *BMJ Case Reports, 14*(5), Article e242330. https://doi.org/10.1136/bcr-2021-242330

Salvio, M.-A., Wood, J. M., Schwartz, J., & Eichling, P. S. (1992). Nightmare prevalence in the healthy elderly. *Psychology and Aging, 7*(2), 324–325. https://doi.org/10.1037/0882-7974.7.2.324

Salzarulo, P., & Chevalier, A. (1983). Sleep problems in children and their relationship with early disturbances of the waking–sleeping rhythms. *Sleep, 6*(1), 47–51. https://doi.org/10.1093/sleep/6.1.47

Sandman, N., Valli, K., Kronholm, E., Ollila, H. M., Revonsuo, A., Laatikainen, T., & Paunio, T. (2013). Nightmares: Prevalence among the Finnish general adult population and war veterans during 1972–2007. *Sleep, 36*, 1041–1050. https://doi.org/10.5665/sleep.2806

Sandman, N., Valli, K., Kronholm, E., Vartiainen, E., Laatikainen, T., & Paunio, T. (2017). Nightmares as predictors of suicide: An extension study including war veterans. *Scientific Reports, 7*, Article 44756. https://doi.org/10.1038/srep44756

Sándor, P., Szakadát, S., Kertész, K., & Bódizs, R. (2015). Content analysis of 4 to 8 year-old children's dream reports. *Frontiers in Psychology, 6*, Article 534. https://doi.org/10.3389/fpsyg.2015.00534

Scarpelli, S., Alfonsi, V., D'Anselmo, A., Gorgoni, M., Musetti, A., Plazzi, G., De Gennaro, L., & Franceschini, C. (2021). Dream activity in narcoleptic patients during the COVID-19 lockdown in Italy. *Frontiers in Psychology, 12*, Article 1907. https://doi.org/10.3389/fpsyg.2021.681569

Scarpelli, S., Alfonsi, V., Gorgoni, M., & De Gennaro, L. (2022). What about dreams? State of the art and open questions. *Journal of Sleep Research, 31*(4), Article e13609. https://doi.org/10.1111/jsr.13609

Scarpelli, S., Alfonsi, V., Mangiaruga, A., Musetti, A., Quattropani, M. C., Lenzo, V., Freda, M. F., Lemmo, D., Vegni, E., Borghi, L., Saita, E., Cattivelli, R., Castelnuovo, G., Plazzi, G., De Gennaro, L., & Franceschini, C. (2021). Pandemic nightmares: Effects on dream activity of the COVID-19 lockdown in Italy. *Journal of Sleep Research, 30*(5), Article e13300. https://doi.org/10.1111/jsr.13300

Scarpelli, S., Bartolacci, C., D'Atri, A., Camaioni, M., Annarumma, L., Gorgoni, M., Cloos, C., Ferrara, M., & De Gennaro, L. (2020). Electrophysiological correlates of dream recall during REM sleep: Evidence from multiple awakenings and within-subjects design. *Nature and Science of Sleep, 12*, Article 1043. https://doi.org/10.2147/NSS.S279786

Scarpelli, S., Bartolacci, C., D'Atri, A., Gorgoni, M., & De Gennaro, L. (2019). The functional role of dreaming in emotional processes. *Frontiers in Psychology, 10*, Article 459. https://doi.org/10.3389/fpsyg.2019.00459

Scarpelli, S., D'Atri, A., Bartolacci, C., Gorgoni, M., Mangiaruga, A., Ferrara, M., & De Gennaro, L. (2020). Dream recall upon awakening from non-rapid eye movement sleep in older adults: Electrophysiological pattern and qualitative features. *Brain Sciences, 10*(6), Article 343. https://doi.org/10.3390/brainsci10060343

Scarpelli, S., D'Atri, A., Gorgoni, M., Ferrara, M., & De Gennaro, L. (2015). EEG oscillations during sleep and dream recall: State-or trait-like individual differences? *Frontiers in Psychology, 6*, Article 605. https://doi.org/10.3389/fpsyg.2015.00605

Scarpelli, S., D'Atri, A., Mangiaruga, A., Marzano, C., Gorgoni, M., Schiappa, C., Ferrara, M., & De Gennaro, L. (2017). Predicting dream recall: EEG activation during NREM sleep or shared mechanisms with wakefulness? *Brain Topography, 30*(5), 629–638. https://doi.org/10.1007/s10548-017-0563-1

Scarpelli, S., De Santis, A., Alfonsi, V., Gorgoni, M., Morin, C. M., Espie, C., Merikanto, I., Chung, F., Penzel, T., Bjorvatn, B., Dauvilliers, Y., Holzinger, B., Wing, Y. K., Partinen, M., Plazzi, G., & De Gennaro, L. (2022). The role of sleep and dreams in long-COVID. *Journal of Sleep Research, 32*(3), Article e13789. https://doi.org/10.1111/jsr.13789

Scarpelli, S., Gorgoni, M., D'Atri, A., Ferrara, M., & De Gennaro, L. (2019). Structural and functional differences in brain mechanisms of dream recall. In H. C. Dringenberg (Ed.), *Handbook of sleep research. Handbook of behavioral neuroscience* (Vol. 30, pp. 269–281). Academic Press. https://doi.org/10.1016/B978-0-12-813743-7.00018-9

Scarpelli, S., Nadorff, M. R., Bjorvatn, B., Chung, F., Dauvilliers, Y., Espie, C. A., Inoue, Y., Matsui, K., Merikanto, I., Morin, C. M., Penzel, T., Sieminski, M., Fang, H., Macêdo, T., Mota-Rolim, S. A., Leger, D., Plazzi, G., Chan, N. Y., Partinen, M., . . . De Gennaro, L. (2022). Nightmares in people with COVID-19: Did coronavirus infect our dreams? *Nature and Science of Sleep, 14*, 93–108. https://doi.org/10.2147/NSS.S344299

Schiappa, C., Scarpelli, S., D'Atri, A., Gorgoni, M., & De Gennaro, L. (2018). Narcolepsy and emotional experience: A review of the literature. *Behavioral and Brain Functions, 14*(1), Article 19. https://doi.org/10.1186/s12993-018-0151-x

Schlarb, A. A., Zschoche, M., & Schredl, M. (2016). Der Nightmare Effects Questionnaire (NEQ). Pilotstudie zu ersten psychometrischen kennwerten bei jugendlichen und jungen erwachsenen [The Nightmare Effects Questionnaire (NEQ). A pilot study on the first psychometric characteristics among adolescents and young adults]. *Somnologie, 20*, 251–257. https://doi.org/10.1007/s11818-016-0086-0

Schredl, M. (2003). Effects of state and trait factors on nightmare frequency. *European Archives of Psychiatry and Clinical Neuroscience, 253*(5), 241–247. https://doi.org/10.1007/s00406-003-0438-1

Schredl, M. (2008). Dream recall frequency in a representative German sample. *Perceptual and Motor Skills, 106*(3), 699–702. https://doi.org/10.2466/pms.106.3.699-702

Schredl, M. (2009). Recall frequency of positive and negative dreams in a representative German sample. *Perceptual and Motor Skills, 108*(3), 677–680. https://doi.org/10.2466/pms.108.3.677-680

Schredl, M. (2010). Nightmare frequency and nightmare topics in a representative German sample. *European Archives of Psychiatry and Clinical Neuroscience, 260*, 565–570. https://doi.org/10.1007/s00406-010-0112-3

Schredl, M., Berres, S., Klingauf, A., Schellhaas, S., & Göritz, A. S. (2014). The Mannheim Dream questionnaire (MADRE): Retest reliability, age and gender effects. *International Journal of Dream Research, 7*(2), 141–147. https://doi.org/10.11588/ijodr.2014.2.16675

Schredl, M., & Göritz, A. S. (2015). Changes in dream recall frequency, nightmare frequency, and lucid dream frequency over a 3-year period. *Dreaming, 25*(2), 81–87. https://doi.org/10.1037/a0039165

Schredl, M., Landgraf, C., & Zeiler, O. (2003). Nightmare frequency, nightmare distress and neuroticism. *North American Journal of Psychology, 5*, 345–350.

Schreuder, B. J., Kleijn, W. C., & Rooijmans, H. G. (2000). Nocturnal re-experiencing more than forty years after war trauma. *Journal of Traumatic Stress, 13*(3), 453–463. https://doi.org/10.1023/A:1007733324351

Schultz, J. H., Forsberg, J. T., Harb, G., & Alisic, E. (2021). Prevalence and characteristics of posttraumatic nightmares in war-and conflict-affected students. *Nature and Science of Sleep, 13*, 423–433. https://doi.org/10.2147/NSS.S282967

Semiz, U. B., Basoglu, C., Ebrinc, S., & Cetin, M. (2008). Nightmare disorder, dream anxiety, and subjective sleep quality in patients with borderline personality disorder. *Psychiatry and Clinical Neurosciences, 62*(1), 48–55. https://doi.org/10.1111/j.1440-1819.2007.01789.x

Shapiro, F. (1989). Eye movement desensitization: A new treatment for post-traumatic stress disorder. *Journal of Behavior Therapy and Experimental Psychiatry, 20*(3), 211–217. https://doi.org/10.1016/0005-7916(89)90025-6

Shaw, R. J., Harvey, J. E., Bernard, R., Gunary, R., Tiley, M., & Steiner, H. (2009). Comparison of short-term psychological outcomes of respiratory failure treated by either invasive or non-invasive ventilation. *Psychosomatics, 50*(6), 586–591. https://doi.org/10.1016/S0033-3182(09)70860-6

Sheaves, B., Onwumere, J., Keen, N., Stahl, D., & Kuipers, E. (2015). Nightmares in patients with psychosis: The relation with sleep, psychotic, affective, and cognitive symptoms. *Canadian Journal of Psychiatry/La Revue Canadienne de Psychiatrie, 60*(8), 354–361. https://doi.org/10.1177/070674371506000804

Siclari, F., Baird, B., Perogamvros, L., Bernardi, G., LaRocque, J. J., Riedner, B., Boly, M., Postle, B. R., & Tononi, G. (2017). The neural correlates of dreaming. *Nature Neuroscience, 20*(6), 872–878. https://doi.org/10.1038/nn.4545

Silver, S. M., Brooks, A., & Obenchain, J. (1995). Treatment of Vietnam War veterans with PTSD: A comparison of eye movement desensitization and reprocessing, biofeedback, and relaxation training. *Journal of Traumatic Stress, 8*(2), 337–342. https://doi.org/10.1007/BF02109568

Simard, V., & Nielsen, T. (2009). Adaptation of imagery rehearsal therapy for nightmares in children: A brief report. *Psychotherapy: Theory, Research, Practice, Training, 46*, 492–497. https://doi.org/10.1037/a0017945

Simard, V., Nielsen, T. A., Tremblay, R. E., Boivin, M., & Montplaisir, J. Y. (2008). Longitudinal study of preschool sleep disturbance: The predictive role of maladaptive parental behaviors, early sleep problems, and child/mother psychological factors. *Archives of Pediatrics & Adolescent Medicine, 162*(4), 360–367. https://doi.org/10.1001/archpedi.162.4.360

Simonds, J. F., & Parraga, H. (1982). Prevalence of sleep disorders and sleep behaviors in children and adolescents. *Journal of the American Academy of Child & Adolescent Psychiatry, 21*(4), 383–388. https://doi.org/10.1016/S0002-7138(09)60942-0

Simor, P., Bódizs, R., Horváth, K., & Ferri, R. (2013). Disturbed dreaming and the instability of sleep: Altered nonrapid eye movement sleep microstructure in individuals with frequent nightmares as revealed by the cyclic alternating pattern. *Sleep, 36*(3), 413–419. https://doi.org/10.5665/sleep.2462

Simor, P., Csoka, S., & Bodizs, R. (2010). Nightmares and bad dreams in patients with borderline personality disorder: Fantasy as a coping skill? *European Journal of Psychiatry, 24*(1), 28–37. https://doi.org/10.4321/s0213-61632010000100004

Simor, P., Horváth, K., Gombos, F., Takács, K. P., & Bódizs, R. (2012). Disturbed dreaming and sleep quality: Altered sleep architecture in subjects with frequent nightmares. *European Archives of Psychiatry and Clinical Neuroscience, 262*(8), 687–696. https://doi.org/10.1007/s00406-012-0318-7

Simpson, T. L., Stappenbeck, C. A., Varra, A. A., Moore, S. A., & Kaysen, D. (2012). Symptoms of posttraumatic stress predict craving among alcohol treatment seekers: Results of a daily monitoring study. *Psychology of Addictive Behaviors, 26*(4), 724–733. https://doi.org/10.1037/a0027169

Sjöström, N., Hetta, J., & Waerna, M. (2009). Persistent nightmares are associated with repeat suicide attempt: A prospective study. *Psychiatry Research, 170*, 208–211. https://doi.org/10.1016/j.psychres.2008.09.006

Spoormaker, V. I. (2008). A cognitive model of recurrent nightmares. *International Journal of Dream Research, 1*, 15–22. https://doi.org/10.11588/heidok.00008436

Spoormaker, V. I., Schredl, M., & Van Den Bout, J. (2006). Nightmares: From anxiety symptom to sleep disorder. *Sleep Medicine Reviews, 10*(1), 19–31. https://doi.org/10.1016/j.smrv.2005.06.001

Spoormaker, V. I., & Van Den Bout, J. (2006). Lucid dreaming treatment for nightmares: A pilot study. *Psychotherapy and Psychosomatics, 75*, 389–394. https://doi.org/10.1159/000095446

Stepansky, R., Holzinger, B., Schmeiser-Rieder, A., Saletu, B., Kunze, M., & Zeitlhofer, J. (1998). Austrian dream behavior: Results of a representative population survey. *Dreaming, 8*(1), 23–30. https://doi.org/10.1023/B:DREM.0000005912.77493.d6

Tempesta, D., Curcio, G., De Gennaro, L., & Ferrara, M. (2013). Long-term impact of earthquakes on sleep quality. *PLOS ONE, 8*(2), Article e55936. https://doi.org/10.1371/journal.pone.0055936

Thompson, A., Lereya, S. T., Lewis, G., Zammit, S., Fisher, H. L., & Wolke, D. (2015). Childhood sleep disturbance and risk of psychotic experiences at 18: UK birth cohort. *British Journal of Psychiatry, 207*(1), 23–29. https://doi.org/10.1192/bjp.bp.113.144089

Vandrey, R., Babson, K. A., Herrmann, E. S., & Bonn-Miller, M. O. (2014). Interactions between disordered sleep, posttraumatic stress disorder, and substance use disorders. *International Review of Psychiatry*, *26*(2), 237–247. https://doi.org/10.3109/09540261.2014.901300

Van Liempt, S., van Zuiden, M., Westenberg, H., Super, A., & Vermetten, E. (2013). Impact of impaired sleep on the development of PTSD symptoms in combat veterans: A prospective longitudinal cohort study. *Depression and Anxiety*, *30*(5), 469–474. https://doi.org/10.1002/da.22054

Van Schagen, A. M., Lancee, J., De Groot, I. W., Spoormaker, V. I., & Van Den Bout, J. (2015). Imagery rehearsal therapy in addition to treatment as usual for patients with diverse psychiatric diagnoses suffering from nightmares: A randomized controlled trial. *Journal of Clinical Psychiatry*, *76*, e1105–e1113. https://doi.org/10.4088/jcp.14m09216

Van Schagen, A. M., Lancee, J., Spoormaker, V. I., & Van Den Bout, J. (2016). Long-term treatment effects of imagery rehearsal therapy for nightmares in a population with diverse psychiatric disorders. *International Journal of Dream Research*, *9*, 67–70. https://doi.org/10.11588/ijodr.2016.1.24953

Van Schagen, A. M., Lancee, J., Swart, M., Spoormaker, V. I., & Van Den Bout, J. (2017). Nightmare disorder, psychopathology levels, and coping in a diverse psychiatric sample. *Journal of Clinical Psychology*, *73*, 65–75. https://doi.org/10.1002/jclp.22315

Wade, D. T., Makela, P. M., House, H., Bateman, C., & Robson, P. (2006). Long-term use of a cannabis-based medicine in the treatment of spasticity and other symptoms in multiple sclerosis. *Multiple Sclerosis Journal*, *12*(5), 639–645. https://doi.org/10.1177/1352458505070618

Walker, M. P., & van Der Helm, E. (2009). Overnight therapy? The role of sleep in emotional brain processing. *Psychological Bulletin*, *135*(5), 731–748. https://doi.org/10.1037/a0016570

Weber, F. C., Norra, C., & Wetter, T. C. (2020). Sleep disturbances and suicidality in posttraumatic stress disorder: An overview of the literature. *Frontiers in Psychiatry*, *11*, Article 167. https://doi.org/10.3389/fpsyt.2020.00167

Weidman, K., LaFond, E., Hoffman, K. L., Goyal, P., Parkhurst, C. N., Derry-Vick, H., Schenck, E., & Lief, L. (2022). Post–intensive care unit syndrome in a cohort of COVID-19 survivors in New York City. *Annals of the American Thoracic Society*, *19*(7), 1158–1168. https://doi.org/10.1513/AnnalsATS.202104-520OC

Weisz, R., & Foulkes, D. (1970). Home and laboratory dreams collected under uniform sampling conditions. *Psychophysiology*, *6*(5), 588–596. https://doi.org/10.1111/j.1469-8986.1970.tb02247.x

Wiechers, S., Schlarb, A. A., Urschitz, M. S., Eggebrecht, E., Schlaud, M., & Poets, C. F. (2011). Sleep problems and poor academic performance in primary school children. *Somnologie*, *15*, 243–248. https://doi.org/10.1007/s11818-011-0535-8

Wittmann, L., & De Dassel, T. (2015). Posttraumatic nightmares: From scientific evidence to clinical significance. In M. Kramer & M. L. Glucksman (Eds.), *Dream research. Contributions to clinical practice* (pp. 135–148). Routledge.

Woodward, S. H., Bliwise, D. L., Friedman, M. J., & Gusman, F. D. (1996). First night effects in posttraumatic stress disorder inpatients. *Sleep*, *19*(4), 312–317. https://doi.org/10.1093/sleep/19.4.312

Woodward, S. H., Michell, G., & Santerre, C. (2018). The psychophysiology of PTSD nightmares. In E. Vermetten, A. Germain, & T. Neylan (Eds.), *Sleep and combat-related post traumatic stress disorder* (pp. 233–242). Springer. https://doi.org/10.1007/978-1-4939-7148-0_20

Wright, J., & Koulack, D. (1987). Dreams and contemporary stress: A disruption–avoidance–adaptation model. *Sleep*, *10*(2), 172–179.

Zadra, A., & Donderi, D. C. (2000). Nightmares and bad dreams: Their prevalence and relationship to well-being. *Journal of Abnormal Psychology*, *109*(2), Article 273. https://doi.org/10.1037//0021-843X.109.2.273

Zadra, A. L., & Pihl, R. O. (1997). Lucid dreaming as a treatment for recurrent nightmares. *Psychotherapy and Psychosomatics*, *66*(1), 50–55. https://doi.org/10.1159/000289106

CHAPTER

30 Parasomnias II: Rapid-Eye-Movement Sleep Behavior Disorder

Alex Iranzo

Abstract

Rapid-eye-movement (REM) sleep behavior disorder (RBD) is characterized by nightmares and vigorous manifestations (e.g., prominent body jerking, yelling, punching) in REM sleep with excessive electromyographic activity. Diagnosis requires video-polysomnography evaluating the mentalis and flexor digitorum superficialis muscle activity plus audiovisual analysis of the manifestations occurring in REM sleep. Accurate diagnosis is important as the idiopathic form of RBD (IRBD) represents an early manifestation of the synucleinopathies Parkinson's disease, dementia with Lewy bodies, and multiple system atrophy and because other conditions (e.g., severe obstructive sleep apnea) may present with nightmares and abnormal sleep behaviors. Patients with IRBD are candidates to receive neuroprotective therapy to stop the ongoing neurodegenerative process and develop parkinsonism and dementia. Clonazepam and melatonin improve the RBD symptomatology.

Key Words: idiopathic RBD, video-polysomnography, synuclein, Parkinson's disease, dementia, Lewy body, multiple system atrophy, neuroprotection, melatonin, clonazepam

Introduction

Parasomnias are events or experiences that consist of abnormal behaviors, unpleasant dreams, and altered perceptions that occur during sleep or in transitions between sleep and wakefulness (American Academy of Sleep Medicine, 2014). They are clinical disorders that can lead to injuries, sleep fragmentation, health problems, legal issues, psychosocial problems, and neurodegeneration. They can affect the patient's sleep as well as the bed partner's and relatives' sleep quality. The *International Classification of Sleep Disorders* divides the parasomnias into those associated with rapid-eye-movement (REM) sleep, those associated with non-REM (NREM) sleep (also known as *disorders of arousal*), and a third group called *other parasomnias* which includes, for example, enuresis. REM-related parasomnias include REM sleep behavior disorder (RBD), recurrent isolated sleep paralysis, and nightmare disorder (American Academy of Sleep Medicine, 2014). In this chapter I will focus on the idiopathic and secondary forms of RBD.

The Concept of RBD

As the name indicates, RBD is a parasomnia that occurs during REM sleep. It is characterized by abnormal vocal and motor behaviors, nightmares, and absence of muscle atonia, all occurring during REM sleep. RBD indicates dysfunction of the lower brainstem nuclei (subcoeruleus nucleus in the pons and magnocellularis nucleus in the medulla oblongata) that modulate physiological muscle atonia during REM sleep. There is an idiopathic form (IRBD; in subjects without associated neurological diseases) and a secondary form that is linked to the use of some medications and to neurological disorders such as limbic encephalitis, stroke, multiple sclerosis, and neurodegenerative diseases (American Academy of Sleep Medicine, 2014; Iranzo et al., 2016).

IRBD

The idiopathic form is not a simple parasomnia but, in most cases, constitutes the first manifestation of a neurodegenerative disease such as Parkinson's disease (PD), dementia with Lewy bodies (DLB), and multiple system atrophy (MSA) before the onset of parkinsonism and dementia (American Academy of Sleep Medicine, 2014). These three diseases are designated *synucleinopathies* since neuropathology demonstrates abnormal synuclein deposits in the neurons and glial cells. Of note, IRBD also receives the terms *primary* and *isolated* in the medical literature.

Epidemiology

For unknown reasons, IRBD is much more common in males (70%–80%) than in females (20%–30%). Sex hormone levels are normal in males with IRBD relative to age- and sex-matched controls. With very few exceptions, IRBD appears in people over 50 years of age, and the mean age at presentation in sleep centers is between 65 and 70 years (Fernández-Arcos et al., 2016). The diagnosis of RBD requires the use of polysomnography (PSG) with synchronized audiovisual recording (V-PSG) showing increased muscle activity in REM sleep linked to abnormal manifestations (American Academy of Sleep Medicine, 2014). Epidemiological studies where the diagnosis of RBD was confirmed by V-PSG have shown that the prevalence of the idiopathic form in the general population over 60 years of age is between 0.25% and 1% (Cicero, Giuliano, Luna, et al., 2021). These prevalence studies with V-PSG confirmation have been conducted in China, South Korea, Japan, Spain, Italy, Czech Republic, Switzerland, and Denmark (Buskova et al., 2016; Chiu et al., 2000; Cicero, Giuliano, Sgroi, et al., 2021; Fedorova et al., 2020; Haba-Rubio et al., 2018; Kang et al., 2013; Pujol et al., 2017; Sasai-Sakuma et al., 2020). Large epidemiological studies performed in the general population where the estimation of RBD was only made by validated RBD questionnaires (without the confirmation by V-PSG) showed a much higher prevalence, up to 10% (Ma et al., 2016, 2017; Wong et al., 2016). This is due to the occurrence of other sleep disorders that mimic RBD symptomatology (false positives) that are also characterized by vigorous sleep behaviors and fearful dreams. These RBD mimics are sleepwalking, sleep terrors, severe obstructive sleep apnea, periodic limb movement disorder, severe hypoglycemia, peduncular hallucinosis, sleep-related hypermotor epilepsy, and post-traumatic stress disorder (Gaig et al., 2017; Iranzo & Santamaria, 2005; Iranzo et al., 2016; Montini et al., 2021; Muñoz-Lopetegi et al., 2021). IRBD is an underdiagnosed condition because (1) many patients sleeping alone are not aware of experiencing abnormal behaviors during sleep (false negatives by clinical history) and (2) patients and their relatives do not know that having motor and vocal manifestations during sleep can be a pathological phenomenon. In the end, these subjects do not go to the doctor seeking medical advice and remain underdiagnosed.

Associations

Publications where RBD was confirmed by V-PSG have identified some environmental risk factors for RBD. They include smoking, head injury, former participation as an occupation in football (soccer), pesticide exposure, solvent exposure, and farming (Collia et al., 2023; Postuma, Montplaisir, et al., 2012). All these factors (except smoking) are also risk factors that predispose to PD. Antidepressant use is also associated with the occurrence of RBD (Postuma et al., 2013). Non-motor and non-cognitive symptomatology of PD and DLB, namely orthostatic hypotension, constipation, depression, and hyposmia, are more common in IRBD than in the general population (American Academy of Sleep Medicine, 2014). Neuroimaging and electrophysiological studies have revealed abnormalities way beyond the nuclei that regulate REM sleep in the brainstem, involving the nigrostriatal system, the cortex, the limbic system, and the peripheral autonomic system (Jiménez-Jiménez et al., 2021a; Miglis, Adler, et al., 2021). Genetic abnormalities such as GBA mutations occur in approximately 10% of the cases and are more common than in the community (Gámez-Valero et al., 2018; Honeycutt et al., 2019). As mentioned before, IRBD represents in most of the patients an early manifestation of the synucleinopathies PD, DLB, and MSA (Iranzo et al., 2016).

Pathophysiology

The pathophysiology of RBD lies in the dysfunction of the nucleus subcoeruleus (also termed the *sublaterodorsal nucleus* in rodents and *perilocus-alpha* in cats) in the pons and the magnocellularis nucleus (also termed *gigantocellularis*) in the medulla oblongata (Iranzo 2018). In normal conditions, these two nuclei are responsible during normal REM sleep for inhibiting the motor neurons of the brainstem (the ones that originate the cranial nerves) and of the anterior horn of the spinal cord (the ones that originate the peripheral nerves), causing muscle atonia. This is known from animal models in which these nuclei were impaired by electrolytic lesions or by genetic manipulation inactivating the transport of glutamate and glycine. The afferents from these two nuclei, especially those coming from the limbic system (mainly the amygdala and the anterior cingulate gyrus), the posterior hypothalamus (where the neurons that synthesize hypocretin are located), and the motor cortex, are also involved in some way or another. Of note, the dreams in IRBD are nightmares which have an emotional content (implicating the limbic system), and IRBD patients can speak and gesticulate as if they were awake (implicating the motor cortex and Broca's area). Postmortem neuropathological studies in IRBD patients who died demonstrate neuronal loss plus synuclein deposits within the subcoeruleus and magnocellularis nuclei (Iranzo et al., 2013). The main neurotransmitters involved in the pathophysiology of RBD are glutamate, gamma-aminobutyric acid, and glycine. However, the involvement of other systems, such as the cholinergic, serotonergic, and hypocretinergic systems, and melatonin may also be relevant in the pathophysiology of RBD. For example, antidepressants such as clomipramine and venlafaxine may precipitate the occurrence of RBD or may worsen its symptomatology due to serotoninergic and anticholinergic effects (Postuma et al., 2013).

Clinical Characteristics

RBD is characterized by unpleasant dreams plus abnormal motor and vocal manifestations in sleep that represent dream-enacting. They occur in REM sleep. Interestingly, in a study from our center involving 203 IRBD patients confirmed by V-PSG, 70% reported sleeping well and having no sleep problems, 44% were not aware of displaying abnormal behaviors at night, and 7% did not recall unpleasant dreams (Fernández-Arcos et al., 2016). This is in contrast to bed partner's or other reliable informants' reports that witness abnormal sleep behaviors.

The dreams usually have an unpleasant content that includes arguments, fights, chases, robberies, animal attacks (e.g., by horses, donkeys, bulls, dogs, snakes), and falls off of cliffs. In the dream, the subject is usually the one being attacked for no reason other than the aggressors' viciousness. The dreamer usually does not recognize the faces of the aggressors, but sometimes they are familiar people (e.g., a relative, a friend, an ex-boss) or scary and creeping monsters. The context may be set in situations or places in the subject's past (e.g., home town, former job), the subject's home (e.g., while some robbers enter the home to steal), or neutral locations (e.g., a street, a forest). Occasionally, in the dream there is a comic content or an exciting participation in a football (soccer) game. While normal REM sleep dreams are long and bizarre, RBD patients report a very brief content (a situation) that is mainly the report of a summary rather than a complex and long plot. When an IRBD patient is awakened in REM sleep, they may or may not remember at that moment the dream content.

Abnormal behaviors during sleep are usually referred by the bed partner. Up to 50% of patients would not see a physician if it were not for the bed partner's observations. This is because many patients report that they sleep well and are not aware of their abnormal sleep behaviors. In these cases, the history should be taken with the bed partner or another reliable observer. Patients during REM sleep may scream, moan, sob, cry, talk (the content can or cannot be understood), swear, or shout profanity or foul language. Sometimes they may laugh, sing, or even bark. Movements include gesticulations, slapping, punching, kicking, and, less frequently, biting, sitting up in bed, and jumping or falling out of bed. Only very rarely do they get out of bed and wander around the room or the house, and this situation is indicative of impending cognitive impairment (the ambulation probably represents a confusional state rather than a motor manifestation that occurs in REM sleep). It is not uncommon for the patients to knock objects off the bedside table or hit the person accompanying them, injuring them or injuring themselves. These behaviors can cause injuries such as hematomas, lacerations, ecchymosis, incisions, bruises, fractures (rib, extremities, scapular, vertebral), and even subdural hematomas, which have been described after sudden falls from the bed. Due to these violent behaviors, it is not rare for bed partners to go to sleep in another room or to sleep in a separate bed. There are cases in which the subjects tie themselves to the bed, sleep on the floor, put parapets with towels on radiators near the bed, or place chairs, mattresses, cushions, and pillows on the floor to cushion possible falls. Occasionally they may present complex and elaborate behaviors as if they were giving a speech, arguing, or calling out to someone. Unlike patients with NREM parasomnias, subjects with IRBD have their eyes closed when they are dream-enacting during REM sleep. Family members report that there are nights when there are no motor disturbances. However, the lack of atonia occurs almost every night, although its intensity and expressivity can be variable, even between different REM phases of the same night. The last REM sleep stage occurs around 5:00–7:00 a.m. and is usually the longest and when behaviors are more common and vigorous. Of note, antidepressants reduce REM sleep time, and some patients taking these medications do not show REM sleep in some nights, thus improving REM sleep symptomatology (absence of REM sleep indicates the obvious disappearance of RBD symptomatology). It should be considered that antidepressants also increase the muscular activity in REM sleep, and therefore, the clinical symptomatology of RBD might be aggravated if REM sleep appears during the night.

Diagnosis

An accurate and correct diagnosis of IRBD is crucial because it carries a high risk of an eventual evolving synucleinopathy (American Academy of Sleep Medicine, 2014; Cesari et al., 2022; Puligheddu et al., 2023). The diagnosis of IRBD requires (1) chronic history of vigorous behaviors during sleep, (2) V-PSG demonstration of REM sleep with increased electromyographic (EMG) activity, (3) absence of overt motor and cognitive complaints, (4) unremarkable neurological examination, and (5) normal brain magnetic resonance imaging (MRI) excluding structural lesions (e.g., ischemic, hemorrhagic, demyelinating plaques, neoplasms, cavernomas, abscesses, inflammatory lesions) damaging the structures that modulate REM sleep (Figures 30.1 and 30.2).

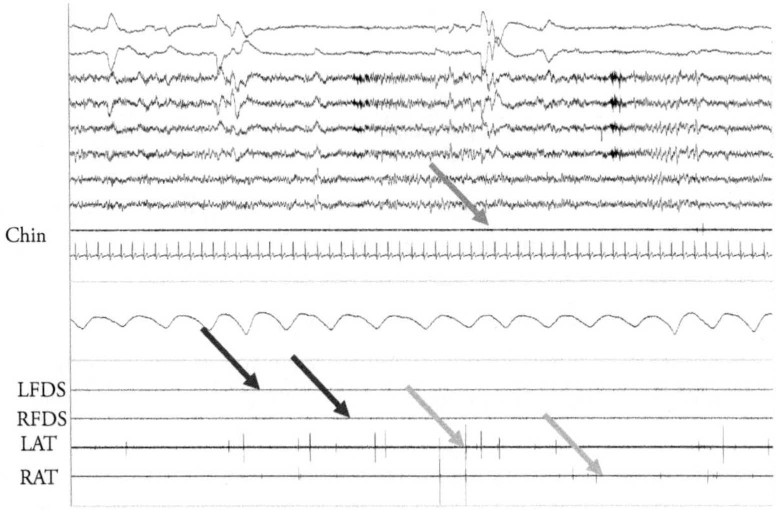

Figure 30.1 Thirty seconds of normal rapid-eye-movement sleep
Note. There is atonia in the mentalis muscle in the chin (blue arrow) and in the upper limbs (red arrows). In the lower limbs there are small twitches that are not related to movement and are normal (green arrows). LAT = left anterior tibialis; LFDS = left flexor digitorum superficialis; RAT = right anterior tibialis; RFDS = right flexor digitorum superficialis.

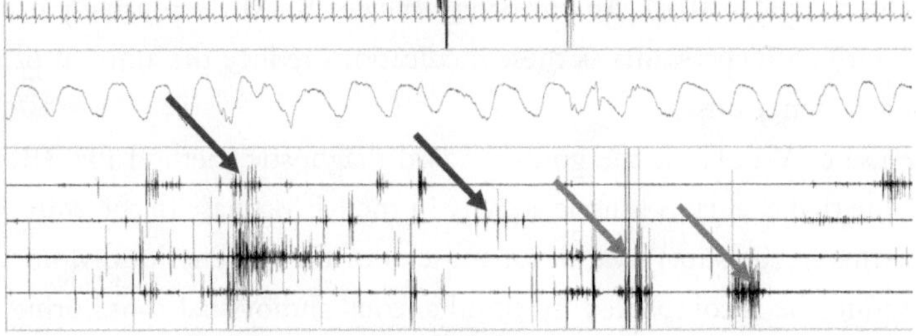

Figure 30.2 Thirty seconds of rapid-eye-movement sleep behavior disorder
Note. There is excessive phasic (intermittent) electromyographic activity in the mentalis muscle in the chin (blue arrow), in the upper limbs (red arrows), and in the lower limbs (green arrows).

The American Academy of Sleep Medicine established in 2014 the following diagnostic criteria for RBD that must be met:

A. Repeated episodes of sleep-related vocalization and/or complex motor behaviors.
B. Behaviors are documented by PSG to occur during REM sleep or, based on a clinical history of dream enactment, are presumed to occur during REM sleep.
C. PSG demonstrates REM sleep without atonia.
D. The disturbance is not better explained by another sleep disorder, mental disorder, medication, or substance abuse.

However, in point C ("PSG demonstrates REM sleep without atonia") it was not stated where the EMG has to be measured; neither was the exact meaning of "REM sleep without atonia" defined. There was no indication when the EMG activity in REM sleep is considered "excessive" or "increased" or "augmented" for RBD to be diagnosed as no cutoffs of EMG activity were provided to define what is normal and what is abnormal. The Sleep Innsbruck Barcelona group, using visual/manual quantification of the EMG activity in 3-second mini-epochs of REM sleep, concluded that the diagnosis of RBD can be made with very high accuracy and sensitivity when the phasic (transient) and tonic (sustained) EMG activity in REM sleep is greater than 32% of the entire REM sleep period measured simultaneously in the mentalis (in the chin) and both flexor digitorum superficialis muscles (in the forearms; Frauscher, Iranzo, et al., 2012). This method is based on the Lapierre and Montplaisir (1992) quantitative scoring system of EMG in the mentalis. However, video-recording of abnormal behaviors in REM sleep is essential to diagnose RBD in a small subset of patients with EMG values within the normal range. Moreover, in one study V-PSG had to be repeated in 16% of the cases for the diagnosis of RBD because of insufficient REM sleep or EMG artifacts from coexistent apneas (Fernández-Arcos et al., 2016). Absent or insufficient REM sleep usually occurs in subjects treated with antidepressants as these medications reduce the amount of REM sleep and increase its latency onset.

For the use of V-PSG, as the gold-standard diagnostic method for RBD, the ideal setup is the one that evaluates muscle activity in the REM phase in the chin muscles and in both forearms in the superficial flexor muscles of the fingers. Ideally, nocturnal PSG recordings should be accompanied by simultaneous audiovisual monitoring to see and hear abnormal behaviors during REM sleep without atonia. In the diagnostic V-PSG, about 66% of the abnormal manifestations are minor/simple jerks, 9% are major manifestations, 22% are complex, and only 1% are violent.

As pointed out, it is accepted that current diagnosis of RBD requires documentation of excessive EMG activity using V-PSG. But V-PSG is expensive, is not available in all centers, and in some cases must be repeated; and the manual/visual quantification of EMG activity is time-consuming and requires training and expertise. Thus, one of the current challenges is to find out an easier, faster, and more reliable diagnostic methodology. Experts have proposed several alternatives, namely automatic analysis of the EMG activity, actigraphy, analysis of audiovisual recordings, and questionnaires. A challenging option is to study the patients outside the sleep laboratory in their own home environment with automated three-dimensional video analysis of body movements or other systems.

Available validated questionnaires and single questions for the diagnosis of IRBD are sensitive (Frauscher, Ehrmann, et al., 2012; Postuma, Arnulf, et al., 2012; Stiasny-Kolster et al., 2007), but their specificity is moderate or low due to misidentification of individuals with IRBD mimics (false positives; Stefani et al., 2023). They can be used in the general population or in large cohorts as a first diagnostic step before the implementation of V-PSG in positive cases.

Differential Diagnosis

V-PSG is necessary for the diagnosis of IRBD because other entities may present with complex sleep behaviors (NREM parasomnias, obstructive apneas, sleep hypermotor epilepsy, periodic limb movement disorder, nocturnal visual hallucinations, confusional states, nocturnal hypoglycemia) mimicking RBD. In these mimics, V-PSG shows REM sleep with atonia. We must keep in mind that RBD can coexist, by chance, with other sleep disturbances such as obstructive apneas, periodic limb movements, and very rarely non-REM parasomnias. The V-PSG will help to identify these coexistent disorders in a patient with true IRBD.

OBSTRUCTIVE SLEEP APNEA

There is a group of patients with severe obstructive sleep apnea who, in addition to the typical symptoms of sleep apnea (e.g., snoring and hypersomnia), also report the same dream-enacting behaviors (e.g., punching, assaulting the bed partner, falling out of bed, shouting) and unpleasant dreams (e.g., being attacked and chased) occurring in IRBD (Iranzo & Santamaria, 2005). As with IRBD, these patients are commonly unaware of their actions and may be self-injured, and the condition is more frequent in men, with a mean age at presentation of 60 years. PSG with synchronized audiovisual recording excludes RBD showing REM sleep with intact muscle atonia and is diagnostic of severe obstructive sleep apnea demonstrating that the reported abnormal sleep behaviors only occur during apnea-induced agitated arousals, in both NREM sleep and REM sleep. These patients usually show more than 50 apneas per hour of sleep. While clonazepam is not effective and may increase the severity and number of apneas, continuous positive airway pressure eliminates the abnormal sleep behaviors, unpleasant dreams, snoring, and hypersomnia. Of note, IRBD and obstructive sleep apnea may coexist in the same person by chance because the latter is common in the general population, particularly in the elderly.

SLEEPWALKING AND SLEEP TERRORS

Subjects with these NREM parasomnias may report similar unpleasant dreams and dream-enacting behaviors as those seen in IRBD (American Academy of Sleep Medicine, 2014). Unpleasant dreams involve aggression, threat, fear, adversity, and the need to escape from someone or something. Sleep talking, yelling, crying, sitting up in bed, manipulating objects, walking, and performing complex activities like texting or getting dressed are frequent. Behaviors may be reckless or violent, resulting in injuries. In comparison to IRBD, behaviors are more elaborated and complex, leaving the bed is much more frequent, and the episodes are performed with the eyes open, predominate in the first half of the night, are longer in duration, are favored by sleep deprivation, and are triggered by physical contact and noise. Positive family history is common in NREM sleep parasomnias but not in IRBD. The key feature to distinguish NREM sleep parasomnias from IRBD is that the former usually starts during childhood or adolescence. However, in a few cases with NREM sleep parasomnias, the onset may be after the age of 30, and persistence after the age of 50 may occur but is exceptional. PSG with audiovisual recording demonstrates normal REM sleep with muscle atonia and elaborated behaviors emerging abruptly from NREM sleep. As in IRBD, clonazepam is effective for the treatment of the NREM sleep parasomnias. RBD may coexist in a few persons with NREM sleep parasomnias, a condition termed *parasomnia overlap disorder* (American Academy of Sleep Medicine, 2014).

SLEEP-RELATED HYPERMOTOR EPILEPSY

In most cases, a careful clinical history can distinguish IRBD from this form of epilepsy (Montini et al., 2021). Characteristic sleep behaviors include dystonic postures, bimanual or bipedal movements, wandering, and running. However, patients may also display sleep behaviors typically seen in IRBD like screaming, body jerking, kicking, and semi-purposeful movements that may be vigorous. The age at onset is usually during childhood and adolescence but may be after the age of 40. In contrast to IRBD, unpleasant dreams are not frequent, episodes occur almost nightly and several times per night, events are relatively stereotyped within a patient, consciousness may be retained, and seizures during wakefulness may occur. Positive family history is frequent in nocturnal frontal lobe epilepsy but not in IRBD. V-PSG shows normal REM sleep with atonia and may or may not detect interictal and ictal discharges during NREM sleep. Carbamazepine usually improves the condition.

PERIODIC LIMB MOVEMENT DISORDER IN SLEEP

Patients with severe periodic limb movements in sleep report the same dream-enacting behaviors (e.g., kicking, punching, talking, groaning) and unpleasant dreams (e.g., attacked and chased by someone) seen in IRBD (Gaig et al., 2017). As with IRBD, behaviors may result in injuries, most patients are men, and the mean age at diagnosis is in the fifth decade. Patients are usually unaware of their actions but may report disruptive sleep. Restless legs syndrome is rare and when it occurs is of mild intensity and not the main referral complaint. V-PSG with audiovisual recording shows REM sleep with intact muscle atonia plus gross periodic leg movements in NREM sleep that also involve the upper limbs and trunk. These movements are associated with arousals where vocalizations and dream-enacting behaviors occur. Dopaminergic agents decrease the frequency and intensity of both sleep behaviors and unpleasant dreams and do not result in the emergence of restless legs syndrome.

HYPOGLYCEMIA

A few patients with diabetes may show very low levels of glucose at night that may awaken the subject and cause prolonged episodes of agitation and vocalizations without dream recall (Muñoz-Lopetegi et al., 2021). Restoration of glucose levels at night resolves the problem.

CONFUSIONAL AROUSALS IN THE ELDERLY

Individuals with advanced age and cognitive impairment may present nocturnal awakenings where they wander around the house disoriented with the eyes open (American Academy of Sleep Medicine, 2014).

VISUAL HALLUCINATIONS

Some patients, particularly those with associated cognitive impairment, are not able to distinguish a dream from visual hallucinations occurring during darkness when patients are falling asleep (American Academy of Sleep Medicine, 2014).

NIGHTMARE DISORDER

Patients display extreme dysphoric and well-remembered dreams that usually involve threat to survival, security, or physical integrity (American Academy of Sleep Medicine, 2014). Dream-enacting behaviors are absent. On awakening from the nightmare, the subject is fully oriented and alert and recalls the dream. These repetitive nightmares cause clinically significant distress, mood disturbance, and impaired interpersonal and social function. The extreme form is post-traumatic stress disorder where nightmares arise following an emotional trauma.

DISSOCIATIVE STATES AND MALINGERING

Patients with these two different disorders may report very vivid dreams involving fear and threat associated with elaborated sleep behaviors (e.g., fighting, wandering, running) that sometimes may last more than 30 minutes. V-PSG with audiovisual recording demonstrates that the reported abnormal behaviors arise from wakefulness.

Importance

Patients with IRBD have no overt motor or cognitive complaints, and neurological examination and brain MRI are unremarkable. However, there are five lines of evidence indicating that IRBD is an early stage of the synucleinopathies PD, DLB, and MSA. In this scenario the brainstem nuclei that govern REM sleep are already damaged before the brain regions that produce dementia and parkinsonism are clinically affected. These are the five following lines of evidence supporting that IRBD is a synucleinopathy:

1. There is a synucleinopathy-based RBD mouse model where IRBD progresses to parkinsonism, depression, gastrointestinal dysmotility, and olfactory dysfunction with time. This model consists of the injection of synuclein fibrils into the sublaterodorsal tegmental nucleus (the equivalent of the subcoeruleus in humans) that propagates to the substantia nigra pars compacta, olfactory bulb, enteral neuroplexus, and dorsal motor nucleus of the vagus nerve, inducing clinical symptomatology (Shen et al., 2020).
2. Patients with IRBD show clinical and subclinical alterations that are typical of PD, DLB, and MSA, indicating that the neurological damage is widespread beyond the brainstem nuclei that modulate REM sleep (Jiménez-Jiménez et al., 2021a; Miglis, Adler, et al., 2021; Box 30.1). Patients with IRBD frequently present with loss of smell, depression, neuropsychological alterations in tests despite having no cognitive complaints, minimal parkinsonian signs (hypomimia, decreased gait swinging, mild hypophonia, mild bradykinesia in upper limbs without rigidity and tremor), and dysautonomic manifestations (constipation, orthostatic hypotension, impotence in males). Neuroimaging techniques show indirect evidence of loss of dopaminergic neurons in the substantia nigra (deficit of the dopamine transporter [DAT] in the putamen measured by DAT imaging with single-photon emission computed tomography [DAT-SPECT]), iron accumulation (hyperechogenicity of the substantia nigra measured by transcranial sonography), and activation of microglia (measured by positron emission tomography using specific tracers for these nerve cells), which are typical postmortem findings in the substantia nigra of patients with PD. In addition, cholinergic cortical dysfunction is demonstrated by neuroimaging. Some features worsen with time (motor function, cognitive function, DAT-SPECT striatal uptake, EMG activity in REM sleep), while others do not (smell function, constipation, orthostatic hypotension, echogenicity of the substantia nigra).
3. Clinical follow-up of patients shows that over time most of them end up being clinically diagnosed in life with PD, DLB, and, more rarely, MSA. This was first described in 1996 by Schenck and colleagues in Minnesota.

Box 30.1 Coexisting Abnormalities in Polysomnography-Confirmed Patients with Idiopathic REM Sleep Behavior Disorder

1. Clinical symptoms and signs
   - Subtle parkisonian signs (reduced arm swinging, mild bradykinesia, hypophonia, hypomimia, deficits in dual-tasking, impaired rhythm skills, abnormal speech, abnormal gait initiation, postural tremor)
   - Olfactory deficit
   - Color vision impairment
   - Taste loss
   - Autonomic abnormalities (constipation, increased colonic volume, orthostatic hypotension, impaired 24-hour blood pressure, sudomotor abnormalities, urinary symptoms, erectile dysfunction, higher baseline pupil diameter and decreased rod-transient pupillary light reflex amplitude, low blink rates plus dampened pupil constriction and dilation responses)
   - Depression
   - Emotion dysregulation
   - Apathy
     - Fatigue
     - Anxiety
   - Alexithymia
   - Reward insensitivity
   - Pareidolic responses
   - Dysregulation of the sleep–wake cycle
   - Minor hallucinations
   - Abnormal horizontal anti-saccades
   - Abnormal smooth pursuit
2. Neuropsychological deficits in the visuospatial, executive, and memory domains
3. Electrophysiological abnormalities
   - Electroencephalographic slowing in frontal, temporal, and occipital regions during wakefulness and rapid-eye-movement (REM) sleep
   - Decreased intracortical facilitation determined by transcranial magnetic stimulation
   - Electroencephalography showing slow oscillations with low amplitude, long duration, and shallow slope in non-REM sleep
   - Spindles show lower power
   - Decreased sleep cyclic alternating pattern
   - Reduced heart rate variability
   - Increased muscle sympathetic nerve activity and impaired baroreflex control
   - Impaired somatosensory function
   - Esophageal motor impairment
   - Retinal nerve fiber layer thinning with higher vascularization of the deep capillary plexus
   - Abnormal vestibular evoked myogenic potentials
   - Reduced P300 amplitude
   - Abnormal prepulse modulation and enhanced auditory startle reflex
4. Neuroimaging abnormalities
   - Reduced striatal presynaptic dopaminergic uptake
   - Substantia nigra hyperechogenicity
   - Elevated iron content in the substantia nigra

Increased free water in the substantia nigra

Substantia nigra loss of dorsolateral nigral hyperintensity

Loss of the nigrosome-1 sign in the substantia nigra

Substantia nigra microglia activation

Basal ganglia connectivity dysfunction

Altered connectivity between the left substantia nigra with the left putamen and the right occipital lobe

Reduced neuromelanin signal intensity in the coeruleus/subcoeruleus area

Brainstem raphe hypoechogenicity

Disrupted posterior functional brain connectivity

Altered resting-state thalamo-occipital functional connectivity

Impaired left posterior insular cortex functional connectivity

Altered functional connectivity within the limbic striatum

Impaired structural connectivity in brainstem nuclei including subcoeruleus nucleus, medullary reticular formation, and posterior cortical regions

Decreased fractional anisotropy and increased mean diffusivity in the midbrain and pontine nuclei that regulate REM sleep

Hyperperfusion in the pons and right hippocampus and hypoperfusion in the frontal lobe

Hypometabolism in the occipital and cerebellar regions

Abnormal metabolic network characterized by increased activity in the pons and hippocampus and decreased activity in occipital and temporal areas

Increased gray matter density in the hippocampus

Decreased gray matter volume in the frontal, temporal, parietal, and occipital cortices as well as increased gray matter volume in the cerebellum posterior lobe, putamen, and thalamus

Right hippocampal atrophy

Cerebellar atrophy and the hot cross bun sign in conventional brain magnetic resonance imaging

Cortical thinning progression in bilateral superior parietal and precuneus, the right cuneus, the left occipital pole, and lateral orbitofrontal gyri

Small pineal gland volume

Macular ganglion cell complex thinning in the retina

Enlarged perivascular space in centrum semiovale, basal ganglia, substantia nigra, and brainstem

Impaired cortical blood flow microcirculation

Neocortical cholinergic denervation

Increased cholinergic innervation in the bulbar reticular formation, pontine coeruleus/subcoeruleus complex, tegmental periaqueductal gray, and mesopontine cholinergic nuclei

Cholinergic (parasympathetic) gut denervation

Decreased metaiodobenzylguanidine uptake

Altered sensorimotor cortex noradrenergic function

Noradrenergic thalamic denervation

Reduced noradrenergic nerve terminals originating in the locus coeruleus

Altered noradrenergic neurotransmission in the primary sensorimotor cortex

5. Biological abnormalities

Misfolded synuclein in the cerebrospinal fluid, olfactory mucosa, and skin

Aggregates of phosphorylated synuclein in the autonomic nerve fibers that innervate the colon, salivary glands, and skin

Exosomes containing synuclein in the blood
Reduced intraepidermal nerve fiber density
MicroRNA 19b is downregulated in the serum
Longitudinal deregulation of 12 microRNAs (let-7c-5p, miR-19b-3p, miR-140, miR-22-3p, miR-221-3p, miR-24-3p, miR-25-3p, miR-29c-3p, miR-361-5p, miR-425-5p, miR-4505, and miR-451a)
Presence of single-nucleotide polymorphisms SCARB2 and MAPT
Presence of GBA gene variants
Genetic variants of the 3′ and 5′ untranslated region of alpha-synuclein
Altered expression of the clock genes (Per2 and 3, Bmal1, and Nr1d1)
Increased TNF-α and IL-10 and reduced IL-6/IL-10 and IL-8/IL-10 in the plasma
$CD4^+$ T-cell dysregulation characterized by lower TBX21, STAT3, and STAT4 and higher FOXP3 transcription factor expression
Abnormal proteomic expression in the serum
Abnormal gut microbiota in stool samples
Reduction in serum levels of dopamine β-hydroxylase and vitamin D binding protein
Hypomethylation of intron 1 of the synuclein gene in leukocytes
Rare coding variants in BST1 and rare noncoding variants in LAMP3 genes
Increased expression of CD11b and decreased HLA-DR expression in blood monocytic cells
Increased classical monocytes and mature natural killer cells in blood
Abnormal lipoprotein and glycosylated protein profiles in the serum
Increased serum allantoin (a major oxidation product of uric acid)
Increased transferrin sialylation
Risk loci are SNCA, GBA, TMEM175, INPP5F, and SCARB2

In our sleep disorder center in Barcelona, we estimated that, in a cohort of 174 IRBD patients, at 5 years, the conversion rate to one of these three synucleinopathies was 35%, 75% at 10 years, and 92% at 14 years from the diagnosis of IRBD with V-PSG (Iranzo et al., 2014). In a large multicenter study involving 1,280 PSG-confirmed IRBD patients from 24 centers, the overall conversion rate from IRBD diagnosis to an overt neurodegenerative syndrome was 6.3% per year, with 73.5% converting after 12-year follow-up (Postuma et al., 2019).

4 The few neuropathological studies of patients who died with the diagnosis of IRBD confirmed by V-PSG or who were initially diagnosed with IRBD (also demonstrated by V-PSG) and before dying developed dementia and/or parkinsonism (and were therefore diagnosed during their lifetime with PD, DLB, or MSA) showed widespread central nervous system synucleinopathy and neuronal loss (Iranzo et al., 2013). In IRBD patients who developed cognitive impairment, besides widespread Lewy bodies containing synuclein, neuropathology also shows extensive beta-amyloid, tau, phospho-tau, and TDP43 deposits. However, in these patients synuclein pathology predominates when compared with Alzheimer's disease pathology and TDP43.

5. In living individuals with IRBD, biopsies of tissues (stomach, colon, submandibular salivary gland, labial salivary glands, parotid gland, and skin) demonstrate in their nerve terminals the presence of phosphorylated synuclein in 25%–89% of subjects using immunohistochemistry, whereas this abnormal protein is only found in 0%–5% of controls. Using the real-time quaking-induced conversion technique, abnormal misfolded synuclein can be detected in the cerebrospinal fluid (sensitivity between 64% and 93%, specificity between 90% and 98%), skin (sensitivity between 66% and 97%, specificity between 87% and 100%), and olfactory mucosa (sensitivity of 44% and specificity of 90%; Al-Qassabi et al., 2021; Antelmi et al., 2017; Concha-Marambio et al., 2023; Doppler et al., 2017, 2022; Fernández-Arcos et al., 2018; Iranzo et al., 2018, 2021, 2023; Kuzkina et al., 2023; Miglis, Zitser, et al., 2021; Poggiolini et al., 2022; Shin et al., 2022; Sprenger et al., 2015; Stefani et al., 2021; Vilas et al., 2016; Table 30.1).

Course and Prognosis

Longitudinal studies have shown that most IRBD patients will be diagnosed with a synucleinopathy (PD, DLB, MSA) with time (Iranzo et al., 2013, 2014, 2016; Postuma et al., 2019; Schenck et al., 1996). Predictors of short-term of conversion are age, abnormal quantitative motor testing, abnormal DAT-SPECT in the putamen, hyposmia, color vision abnormalities, mild cognitive impairment, and increased muscular activity in the mentalis during REM sleep (Miglis, Adler, et al., 2021). Approximately 48% of patients with IRBD will be diagnosed with sporadic PD, another 48% with DLB, and the remaining 4% with MSA (both cerebellar and parkinsonian forms equally; Iranzo et al., 2016). Patients who remain with IRBD after more than 10 years of follow-up frequently show hyposmia, abnormal DAT-SPECT, and altered neuropsychological tests, indicating that the underlying neurodegenerative process exists and does not represent a pure isolated form (Iranzo et al., 2017).

IRBD patients without neurobehavioral complaints who have abnormal neuropsychological testing are at risk of developing mild cognitive impairment. Patients diagnosed with IRBD who develop mild cognitive impairment (subjects with subjective cognitive complaints demonstrated on neuropsychological tests but without dementia and maintaining activities of daily living) are usually diagnosed with DLB after a few years. These DLB patients often show rigid-akinetic parkinsonism and visual hallucinations. Patients with IRBD who develop hallucinations during wakefulness during the darkness (usually in bed while going to sleep) are prone to develop DLB, as are those who experience reversible delirium and confusional states while admitted to a hospital for any circumstance. Also, patients with IRBD who report occasional nocturnal wandering are prone

Table 30.1 Studies evaluating the presence of abnormal synuclein in subjects with IRBD

Tissue	Procedure	Method	Patients (n)	Controls (n)	Adequate material (%)	Sensitivity (%)	Specificity (%)
Colon	Biopsy	IH	20	22	82	24	100
Submandibular gland	Biopsy	IH	21	26	54	89	100
Salivary glands	Biopsy	IH	62	33	100	50	97
Parotid	Biopsy	IH	1	10	100	100	30
Skin	Biopsy	IH	12	55	100	75	100
Skin	Biopsy	IH	18	20	100	56	100
Skin	Biopsy	IH	25	18	100	64	100
Skin	Biopsy	IH	28	21	100	82	100
Stomach	Biopsy	IH	4	3	100	80	100
Esophagus	Biopsy	IH	1	0	100	100	Not applicable
Olfactory mucosa	Nasal brush	RT-QuIC	63	59	100	44	90
Cerebrospinal fluid	Lumbar puncture	RT-QuIC	52	40	100	90	90
Cerebrospinal fluid	Lumbar puncture	RT-QuIC	45	55	100	64	96
Cerebrospinal fluid	Lumbar puncture	RT-QuIC	88	40	100	75	97
Skin	Biopsy	RT-QuIC	91	41	100	77	98
Skin	Biopsy	RT-QuIC	38	23	100	97	87
Skin	Biopsy	IH	38	23	100	66	100
Cerebrospinal fluid	Cerebrospinal fluid	RT-QuIC	29	50	100	93	98

Note. IH = immunohistochemistry; IRBD = idiopathic rapid-eye-movement sleep behavior disorder; RT-QuIC = real-time quaking-induced conversion.

to be diagnosed with DLB. Patients who develop PD present the rigid-akinetic profile, and resting tremor may be present in a few patients after several years of parkinsonism. The pattern of PD that evolves from IRBD consists of advanced age, rigid-akinetic type, orthostatic hypotension, and cognitive impairment. If a patient with IRBD shows atrophy of the cerebellum, the hot cross bun, or the putaminal rim on brain MRI, they are usually diagnosed with MSA after a few years. Normosmia in IRBD indicates conversion to either PD, DLB, or MSA. Hyposmia indicates conversion to PD or DLB but not MSA. Orthostatic hypotension, constipation, and depression are nonspecific as they indicate conversion to either PD, DLB, or MSA.

Secondary RBD

RBD occurs in the setting of several neurological conditions (e.g., PD, multiple sclerosis, narcolepsy, Machado-Joseph disease) as one of their symptoms (Box 30.2). In some of these conditions RBD is distinctive and common, and it has been incorporated in the current diagnostic criteria (e.g., DLB) or considered as one of the red flags of the disease (e.g., MSA). The occurrence of RBD in these conditions implies direct or indirect dysfunction of the lower brainstem nuclei that modulate REM sleep atonia. In secondary RBD, the content of the dreams and the abnormal sleep manifestations are the same as those seen in the idiopathic form (Iranzo et al., 2005). The diagnosis of RBD in the setting of a neurological condition is made in the same fashion as in IRBD. In this chapter we briefly review RBD in the setting of PD, DLB, MSA, narcolepsy, and anti-IgLON5 disease.

RBD in Patients with PD

PD is a neurodegenerative disorder characterized by neuronal loss and synuclein in the substantia nigra and many other structures of the nervous system (Diaconu et al., 2021). RBD is common among PD patients because in these diseases both cell loss and synuclein pathology are common within the neuronal structures that regulate REM sleep atonia in the lower brainstem. RBD occurs in sporadic PD and in PD linked to genetic mutations. RBD occurs in PD patients whether treated or untreated with dopaminergic agents. RBD is seen in 25%–60% of patients with sporadic PD, antedating the onset of parkinsonism in 20% of them. In the remaining sporadic patients, RBD manifests after the onset of parkinsonism and after the start of therapy with dopaminergic agents. RBD is more frequent in advanced versus early PD. The frequency of RBD increases significantly over time in PD. In sporadic PD, the presence of PD is associated with cognitive impairment, the rigid-akinetic motor subtype, older age, male predominance, autonomic dysfunction, and cognitive impairment. Interestingly, during the RBD episodes the movements are faster, stronger, and smoother than those seen when the PD patient was awake. Similarly, speech during RBD is more intelligible, better articulated, and louder than during wakefulness.

Box 30.2 Conditions Associated With Polysomnography-Confirmed REM sleep behavior disorder

1. Neurodegenerative diseases
   - Parkinson disease
   - Parkinsonism linked to Parkin 2 gene mutations
   - Parkinsonism linked to LRRK2 gene mutations
   - Parkinsonism linked to gamma-aminobutyric acid gene mutations
   - Carriers of the p.A53T alpha-synuclein gene mutation
   - Dementia with Lewy bodies
   - Multiple system atrophy
   - Mild cognitive impairment
   - Pure autonomic failure
   - Alzheimer's disease
   - Progressive supranuclear palsy
   - Guadalupean parkinsonism
   - Corticobasal degeneration
   - Frontotemporal dementia
   - DJ-1 mutations and parkinsonism–dementia–amyotrophic lateral sclerosis complex
   - Amyotrophic lateral sclerosis
   - Neurodegeneration with brain accumulation Type 1
   - Dentatorubropallidoluysian atrophy
   - Huntington disease
   - Spinocerebellar ataxia Type 2
   - Spinocerebellar ataxia Type 3
   - Spinocerebellar ataxia Type 31
   - Wilson disease
   - Fatal familial insomnia
   - Creutzfeldt-Jakob disease
2. Autoimmune disorders
   - Narcolepsy with cataplexy
   - Limbic encephalitis associated with antibodies to voltage-gated potassium channels/LIG-1
   - Anti-N-methyl-D-aspartate receptor encephalitis
   - Anti-Ma1 encephalitis
   - Anti-Ma2 encephalitis
   - CASPR2-related Morvan syndrome
   - Guillain-Barré syndrome
   - Paraneoplastic cerebellar degeneration
   - Pediatric acute-onset neuropsychiatric syndrome
   - Anti-IgLON5 disease
3. Other neurological conditions
   - Myotonic dystrophy Type 2
   - Autism
   - Attention-deficit hyperactivity disorder
   - Tourette's syndrome
   - Arnold-Chiari malformation
   - Smith-Magenis syndrome
   - Moebius syndrome
   - Essential tremor
   - Focal brainstem lesions (stroke, cavernoma, tumor, multiple sclerosis plaques)
4. Medications
   - Antidepressants
   - Beta-blockers

RBD also occurs in PD patients linked to Parkin 2 mutations, but in the setting of this condition RBD-related clinical manifestations are usually mild. RBD occurs in PD associated with LRRK2 G2019S mutations, where parkinsonism onset precedes RBD onset. RBD was not detected in one PARK 6 family, an autosomal recessive disorder that manifests as early-onset PD with a particularly mild progression.

RBD in Patients with MSA

MSA is a neurodegenerative disease clinically characterized by parkinsonism, dysautonomia, and cerebellar syndrome in any combination (Iranzo et al., 2005). Most, if not all, patients have RBD. The findings that brainstem cell loss and glial cytoplasmatic inclusions containing synuclein are consistently widespread and severe in MSA may explain the high prevalence of RBD in this disease. RBD is currently considered a red flag for the diagnosis of MSA. In our first published case series comprising 26 consecutive MSA cases with RBD free of psychoactive drugs, 77% of the patients were unaware of their abnormal behaviors, which were only noticed by bed partners. Recall of unpleasant dreams was absent in 35% of the patients. Like in PD, RBD-related movements are faster, stronger, and smother than during wakefulness. RBD may be the first symptom of MSA. In our series, RBD onset antedated parkinsonian and cerebellar onset in 35 of 67 (52%) patients by a mean of 7 years (range 1–38 years). MSA is eventually diagnosed in only a few subjects with the initial diagnosis of IRBD (most of them are diagnosed with PD and DLB), probably because in the general population MSA is much rarer than PD and DLB.

RBD in Patients with DLB

DLB is the second most common cause of neurodegenerative dementia after Alzheimer's disease (Fernández-Arcos et al., 2019). In patients with DLB, neuronal loss and Lewy bodies are found in the brainstem, limbic system, and neocortex. DLB is characterized by dementia, parkinsonism, recurrent visual hallucinations, and fluctuations in cognition and alertness. DLB is diagnosed if dementia precedes or appears within 1 year before the onset of parkinsonism. Since RBD is common in DLB and not in Alzheimer's disease, RBD has been incorporated as one of the core clinical criteria of DLB at the same level as parkinsonism, hallucinations, and fluctuations.

RBD occurs in 50% of the patients with DLB, and for unknown reasons it is more common in males than in females. Around 70% of them are not aware of displaying dream-enacting behaviors, and in about 65% the parasomnia precedes the onset of cognitive impairment. When compared with DLB patients without RBD, those with RBD are predominantly male and have shorter duration of dementia, earlier onset of parkinsonism and visual hallucinations, and less Alzheimer's disease–related pathology on autopsy. For RBD diagnosis, the sensitivity of the Mayo Sleep Questionnaire is 50%, specificity is 67%, positive predictive value is 83%, and negative predictive value is 28%. False-positive RBD cases according to clinical history and the Mayo Sleep Questionnaire had hallucinatory-like behaviors, severe obstructive sleep apnea, and prominent periodic limb movements in sleep (Fernández-Arcos et al., 2019).

RBD in Narcolepsy Type 1 (With Cataplexy)

Narcolepsy Type 1 is a condition of probable autoimmune basis clinically characterized by excessive daytime sleepiness, cataplexy, sleep-related hallucinations, sleep paralysis, and fragmented nocturnal sleep (Antelmi et al., 2020). Narcolepsy Type 1 is due to the loss of the neurons in the hypothalamus that synthesize hypocretin (also called *orexin*). Hypocretin is a peptide that promotes wakefulness and prevents the onset of REM sleep. Hypocretin innervates many areas in the brain, including the brainstem and limbic system structures that modulate REM sleep. Consequently, it can be speculated that the absence of hypocretin in narcolepsy Type 1 produces an imbalance of these structures leading to RBD. While RBD occurs in about 30%–60%% of patients with narcolepsy Type 1 (associated with cataplexy), it is very rare in subjects with narcolepsy Type 2 (without cataplexy). In narcolepsy Type 1, RBD can occur in all ages, particularly in narcoleptics older than 50 years. However, RBD has been described in children with narcolepsy Type 1. In a very few cases, RBD is the first clinical manifestation of the disease prior to the appearance of hypersomnia and cataplexy. In most of the patients, the severity of RBD is mild or moderate, but in a few cases the severity may be severe in patients who display elaborate complex behaviors in bed.

RBD in Anti-IgLON5 Disease

This disease is a neurological condition initially described at our institution in 2014 (Gaig et al., 2019; Sabater et al., 2014). It affects adults of both sexes, with a median age of about 60 years at presentation. The disease is identified when the serum and cerebrospinal fluid contain antibodies against the neuronal protein IgLON5. There is a strong HLA association with HLA-DRB1*10:01 and HLA-DQB1*05:01 alleles. Neuropathology shows a unique pattern defined by tau deposits in the brainstem and hypothalamus impairing the nuclei that regulate sleep. Patients may display a wide variability of sleep symptoms (restless and unrefreshed sleep, nocturia, abnormal behaviors during sleep, insomnia, and hypersomnia), bulbar symptomatology, motor neuron disease–like movement disorders, and cognitive impairment in various combinations. PSG shows abnormal sleep architecture (where conventional stages are difficult to recognize), obstructive sleep apnea, stridor, purposeful behaviors in NREM sleep, and RBD.

In anti-Iglon5 disease, RBD occurs in more than 50% of the cases and is usually not severe. RBD in this disease is characterized by excessive tonic and phasic muscular activity in the mentalis and all four limbs associated with face, neck, limb, or body jerks. Abnormal movements occurring in NREM sleep are more complex and elaborated that those seen in REM sleep in the same patient. In this condition RBD is related to neuronal loss and tau deposits in the magnocellularis, while the locus subcoeruleus is intact.

Treatment

Once RBD has been diagnosed, one of the goals is to reduce the frequency and intensity of the vigorous motor manifestations and the unpleasant dreams (Aurora et al., 2010; Jiménez-Jiménez et al., 2021b). RBD manifestations can be violent and potentially dangerous for the patient and the bed partner. Thus, one of the main recommendations is to establish a safe environment for sleeping. The treatment of concomitant sleep disorders such as obstructive sleep apnea and avoiding therapy with beta-blockers and antidepressants may produce some benefit.

Medical treatment should be initiated with clonazepam (0.25–2 mg before bedtime) or melatonin (3–12 mg before bedtime) when (1) there is a risk of injury due to the vigorous behaviors; (2) the nightmares bother the patient, making them suffer; and (3) the vigorous behaviors bother the bed partner, not allowing them to sleep. Some patients do not require treatment because the intensity of the behaviors is mild. In contrast, there are IRBD patients in whom clonazepam and melatonin are not effective or cannot be administered because of side effects. In these cases, it seems that there are no other solid pharmacologically effective options. There are case reports, however, showing therapeutic benefit with the use of agomelatine (melatonin receptor agonist), ramelteon (melatonin receptor agonist), levodopa, pramipexol, rotigotine, safinamide, sodium oxybate, zopiclone, clozapine, cannabidiol, gabapentin, levetiracetam, carbamazepine, desipramine, imipramine, fluvoxamine, paroxetine, trazodone, vortioxetine, bupropion and donepezil, memantine, rivastigmine, and yi gan-san (Aurora et al., 2010; Jiménez-Jiménez et al., 2021b).

Conclusions and Recommendations for Future Research

IRBD represents an early feature of an impending neurodegenerative synucleinopathy, and the diagnosis needs V-PSG confirmation of REM with atonia linked to abnormal manifestations. Treatment is effective only with melatonin and clonazepam, but some patients are refractory and there is potential risk of injuries.

A first upcoming challenge is to provide an alternative to V-PSG for the diagnosis of RBD. But this new method must be reliable, accurate, easy, fast, not expensive, and widely available. A second upcoming challenge is the implementation of a neuroprotective clinical trial in subjects with IRBD to prevent the onset of parkinsonism and dementia. Many biological targets may be chosen such as anti-inflammatory medications or drugs that interfere with iron metabolism or the function of mitochondria and lysosomes. Another option is to apply passive or active immunotherapy against synuclein to block its transfer through the nervous system. A third upcoming challenge is to identify an effective symptomatic therapy for RBD symptomatology in subjects in whom clonazepam and melatonin are not effective or are associated with side effects.

References

Al-Qassabi, A., Tsao, T. S., Racolta, A., Kremer, T., Cañamero, M., Belousov, A., Santana, M. A., Beck, R. C., Zhang, H., Meridew, J., Pugh, J., Lian, F., Robida, M. D., Ritter, M., Czech, C., Beach, T. G., Pestic-Dragovich, L., Taylor, K. I., Zago, W., ... Postuma, R. B. (2021). Immunohistochemical detection of synuclein pathology in skin in idiopathic rapid eye movement sleep behavior disorder and parkinsonism. *Movement Disorders, 36*(4), 895–904. https://doi.org/10.1002/mds.28399

American Academy of Sleep Medicine. (2014). *International classification of sleep disorders* (3rd ed.).

Antelmi, E., Donadio, V., Incensi, A., Plazzi, G., & Liguori, R. (2017). Skin nerve phosphorylated α-synuclein deposits in idiopathic REM sleep behavior disorder. *Neurology, 88*(22), 2128–2131. https://doi.org/10.1212/WNL.0000000000003989

Antelmi, E., Pizza, F., Franceschini, C., Ferri, R., & Plazzi, G. (2020). REM sleep behavior disorder in narcolepsy: A secondary form or an intrinsic feature? *Sleep Medicine Reviews, 50,* Article 101254. https://doi.org/10.1016/j.smrv.2019.101254

Aurora, R. N., Zak, R. S., Maganti, R. K., Auerbach, S. H., Casey, K. R., Chowdhuri, S., Karippot, A., Ramar, K., Kristo, D. A., Morgenthaler, T. I., Standards of Practice Committee, & American Academy of Sleep Medicine. (2010). Best practice guide for the treatment of REM sleep behavior disorder (RBD). *Journal of Clinical Sleep Medicine, 6*(1), 85–95.

Buskova, J., Ibarburu, V., Sonka, K., & Ruzicka, E. (2016). Screening for REM sleep behavior disorder in the general population. *Sleep Medicine, 24,* Article 147. https://doi.org/10.1016/j.sleep.2016.07.003

Cesari, M., Heidbreder, A., St. Louis, E. K., Sixel-Döring, F., Bliwise, D. L., Baldelli, L., Bes, F., Fantini, M. L., Iranzo, A., Knudsen-Heier, S., Mayer, G., McCarter, S., Nepozitek, J., Pavlova, M., Provini, F., Santamaria, J., Sunwoo, J. S., Videnovic, A., Högl, B., ... Stefani, A. (2022). Video-polysomnography procedures for diagnosis of rapid eye movement sleep behavior disorder (RBD) and the identification of its prodromal stages: Guidelines from the International RBD Study Group. *Sleep, 45*(3), Article zsab257. https://doi.org/10.1093/sleep/zsab257

Chiu, H. K. F., Wing, Y. K., Lam, L. C. W., Li, S. W., Lum, C. M., Leung, T., & Ho, C. K. (2000). Sleep-related injury in the elderly—An epidemiological study in Hong Kong. *Sleep, 23,* 513–517.

Cicero, C. E., Giuliano, L., Luna, J., Zappia, M., Preux, P. M., & Nicoletti, A. (2021). Prevalence of idiopathic REM behavior disorder: A systematic review and meta-analysis. *Sleep, 44*(6), Article zsaa294. https://doi.org/10.1093/sleep/zsaa294

Cicero, C. E., Giuliano, L., Sgroi, R., Squillaci, R., Terravecchia, C., Vancheri, E., Todaro, V., Reitano, P., Rizzo, S., Luca, A., Mostile, G., Paradisi, V., Zappia, M., Nicoletti, A., & Italian Society of General Medicine of Catania Study Group. (2021). Prevalence of isolated RBD in the city of Catania, Italy: A population-based study. *Journal of Clinical Sleep Medicine, 17*(11), 2241–2248. https://doi.org/10.5664/jcsm.9416

Collia, A., Iranzo, A., Serradell, M., Muñoz-Lopetegi, A., Mayà, G., Santamaría, J., Sánchez-Valle, R., & Gaig, C. (2023). Former participation in professional football as an occupation in patients with isolated REM sleep behaviour disorder leading to a synucleinopathy: A case–control study. *Journal of Neurology, 270*(6), 3234–3242. https://doi.org/10.1007/s00415-023-11591-8

Concha-Marambio, L., Weber, S., Farris, C. M., Dakna, M., Lang, E., Wicke, T., Ma, Y., Starke, M., Ebentheuer, J., Sixel-Döring, F., Muntean, M. L., Schade, S., Trenkwalder, C., Soto, C., & Mollenhauer, B. (2023). Accurate detection of α-synuclein seeds in cerebrospinal fluid from isolated rapid eye movement sleep behavior disorder and patients with Parkinson's disease in the DeNovo Parkinson (DeNo Pa) cohort. *Movement Disorders, 38*(4), 567–578. https://doi.org/10.1002/mds.29329

Diaconu, Ş., Falup-Pecurariu, O., Ţînţ, D., & Falup-Pecurariu, C. (2021). REM sleep behaviour disorder in Parkinson's disease (Review). *Experimental and Therapeutic Medicine, 22*(2), Article 812. https://doi.org/10.3892/etm.2021.10244

Doppler, K., Jentschke, H. M., Schulmeyer, L., Vadasz, D., Janzen, A., Luster, M., Höffken, H., Mayer, G., Brumberg, J., Booij, J., Musacchio, T., Klebe, S., Sittig-Wiegand, E., Volkmann, J., Sommer, C., & Oertel, W. H. (2017). Dermal phospho-alpha-synuclein deposits confirm REM sleep behaviour disorder as prodromal Parkinson's disease. *Acta Neuropathologica, 133*(4), 535–545. https://doi.org/10.3892/etm.2021.10244

Doppler, K., Mammadova, S., Kuzkina, A., Reetz, K., Michels, J., Hermann, W., Sommerauer, M., Volkmann, J., Oertel, W. H., Janzen, A., & Sommer, C. (2022). Association between probable REM sleep behavior disorder and increased dermal alpha-synuclein deposition in Parkinson's disease. *Parkinsonism & Related Disorders, 99,* 58–61. https://doi.org/10.1016/j.parkreldis.2022.05.010

Fedorova, T. D., Knudsen, K., Sommerauer, M., Svendsen, K. B., Otto, M., & Borghammer, P. (2020). A screening-based method for identifying patients with REM sleep behaviour disorder in a Danish community setting. *Journal of Parkinson's Disease, 10*(3), 1249–1253. https://doi.org/10.3233/JPD-202020
Fernández-Arcos, A., Iranzo, A., Serradell, M., Gaig, C., & Santamaria, J. (2016). The clinical phenotype of idiopathic Rapid Eye Movement sleep behavior disorder at presentation: A study in 203 consecutive patients. *Sleep, 39*(1), 121–132. https://doi.org/10.5665/sleep.5332
Fernández-Arcos, A., Morenas-Rodríguez, E., Santamaria, J., Sánchez-Valle, R., Lladó, A., Gaig, C., Lleó, A., & Iranzo, A. (2019). Clinical and video-polysomnographic analysis of rapid eye movement sleep behavior disorder and other sleep disturbances in dementia with Lewy bodies. *Sleep, 42*(7), Article zsz086. https://doi.org/10.1093/sleep/zsz086
Fernández-Arcos, A., Vilaseca, I., Aldecoa, I., Serradell, M., Tolosa, E., Santamaría, J., Gelpi, E., & Iranzo, A. (2018). Alpha-synuclein aggregates in the parotid gland of idiopathic REM sleep behavior disorder. *Sleep Medicine, 52,* 14–17. https://doi.org/10.1016/j.sleep.2018.08.003
Frauscher, B., Ehrmann, L., Zamarian, L., Auer, F., Mitterling, T., Gabelia, D., Brandauer, E., Delazer, M., Poewe, W., & Högl, B. (2012). Validation of the Innsbruck REM sleep behavior disorder inventory. *Movement Disorders, 27*(13), 1673–1678. https://doi.org/10.1002/mds.25223
Frauscher, B., Iranzo, A., Gaig, C., Gschliesser, V., Guaita, M., Raffelseder, V., Ehrmann, L., Sola, N., Salamero, M., Tolosa, E., Poewe, W., Santamaria, J., Högl, B., & SINBAR (Sleep Innsbruck Barcelona) Group. (2012). Normative EMG values during REM sleep for the diagnosis of REM sleep behavior disorder. *Sleep, 35*(6), 835–847. https://doi.org/10.5665/sleep.1886
Gaig, C., Iranzo, A., Cajochen, C., Vilaseca, I., Embid, C., Dalmau, J., Graus, F., & Santamaria, J. (2019). Characterization of the sleep disorder of anti-IgLON5 disease. *Sleep, 42*(9), Article zsz133. https://doi.org/10.1093/sleep/zsz133
Gaig, C., Iranzo, A., Pujol, M., Perez-Diaz, H., & Santamaria, J. (2017). Periodic limb movements during sleep mimicking REM sleep behavior disorder: A new form of periodic limb movement disorder. *Sleep, 40*(3), Article zsw063. https://doi.org/10.1093/sleep/zsw063
Gámez-Valero, A., Iranzo, A., Serradell, M., Vilas, D., Santamaria, J., Gaig, C., Álvarez, R., Ariza, A., Tolosa, E., & Beyer, K. (2018). Glucocerebrosidase gene variants are accumulated in idiopathic REM sleep behavior disorder. *Parkinsonism & Related Disorders, 50,* 94–98. https://doi.org/10.1016/j.parkreldis.2018.02.034
Haba-Rubio, J., Frauscher, B., Marques-Vidal, P., Toriel, J., Tobback, N., Andries, D., Preisig, M., Vollenweider, P., Postuma, R., & Heinzer, R. (2018). Prevalence and determinants of rapid eye movement sleep behavior disorder in the general population. *Sleep, 41*(2), Article zsx197. https://doi.org/10.1093/sleep/zsx197
Honeycutt, L., Montplaisir, J. Y., Gagnon, J. F., Ruskey, J., Pelletier, A., Gan-Or, Z., & Postuma, R. B. (2019). Glucocerebrosidase mutations and phenoconversion of REM sleep behavior disorder to parkinsonism and dementia. *Parkinsonism & Related Disorders, 65,* 230–233. https://doi.org/10.1016/j.parkreldis.2019.04.016
Iranzo, A. (2018). The REM sleep circuit and how its impairment leads to REM sleep behavior disorder. *Cell and Tissue Research, 373*(1), 245–266. https://doi.org/10.1007/s00441-018-2852-8
Iranzo, A., Borrego, S., Vilaseca, I., Martí, C., Serradell, M., Sánchez-Valle, R., Kovacs, G. G., Valldeoriola, F., Gaig, C., Santamaria, J., Tolosa, E., & Gelpi, E. (2018). α-Synuclein aggregates in labial salivary glands of idiopathic rapid eye movement sleep behavior disorder. *Sleep, 41*(8), Article zsy101. https://doi.org/10.1093/sleep/zsy101
Iranzo, A., Fairfoul, G., Ayudhaya, A. C. N., Serradell, M., Gelpi, E., Vilaseca, I., Sanchez-Valle, R., Gaig, C., Santamaria, J., Tolosa, E., Riha, R. L., & Green, A. J. E. (2021). Detection of α-synuclein in CSF by RT-QuIC in patients with isolated rapid-eye-movement sleep behaviour disorder: A longitudinal observational study. *The Lancet. Neurology, 20*(3), 203–212. https://doi.org/10.1016/S1474-4422(20)30449-X
Iranzo, A., Fernández-Arcos, A., Tolosa, E., Serradell, M., Molinuevo, J. L., Valldeoriola, F., Gelpi, E., Vilaseca, I., Sánchez-Valle, R., Lladó, A., Gaig, C., & Santamaría, J. (2014). Neurodegenerative disorder risk in idiopathic REM sleep behavior disorder: Study in 174 patients. *PLOS One, 9*(2), Article e89741. https://doi.org/10.1371/journal.pone.0089741
Iranzo, A., Mammana, A., Muñoz-Lopetegi, A., Dellavalle, S., Mayà, G., Rossi, M., Serradell, M., Baiardi, S., Arqueros, A., Quadalti, C., Perissinotti, A., Ruggeri, E., Cano, J. S., Gaig, C., & Parchi, P. (2023). Misfolded α-synuclein assessment in skin and CSF by RT-QuIC in isolated REM sleep behavior disorder. *Neurology, 100*(18), e1944–e1954. https://doi.org/10.1212/WNL.0000000000207147

Iranzo, A., & Santamaria, J. (2005). Severe obstructive sleep apnea/hypopnea mimicking REM sleep behavior disorder. *Sleep, 28*(2), 203–206. https://doi.org/10.1093/sleep/28.2.203.

Iranzo, A., Santamaria, J., Rye, D. B., Valldeoriola, F., Martí, M. J., Muñoz, E., Vilaseca, I., & Tolosa, E. (2005). Characteristics of idiopathic REM sleep behavior disorder and that associated with MSA and PD. *Neurology, 65*(2), 247–252. https://doi.org/10.1212/01.wnl.0000168864.97813.e0

Iranzo, A., Santamaria, J., & Tolosa, E. (2016). Idiopathic rapid eye movement sleep behaviour disorder: Diagnosis, management, and the need for neuroprotective interventions. *The Lancet. Neurology, 15*(4), 405–419. https://doi.org/10.1016/S1474-4422(16)00057-0

Iranzo, A., Stefani, A., Serradell, M., Martí, M. J., Lomeña, F., Mahlknecht, P., Stockner, H., Gaig, C., Fernández-Arcos, A., Poewe, W., Tolosa, E., Högl, B., Santamaria, J., & SINBAR (Sleep Innsbruck Barcelona) group (2017). Characterization of patients with longstanding idiopathic REM sleep behavior disorder. *Neurology, 89*(3), 242–248. https://doi.org/10.1212/WNL.0000000000004121

Iranzo, A., Tolosa, E., Gelpi, E., Molinuevo, J. L., Valldeoriola, F., Serradell, M., Sanchez-Valle, R., Vilaseca, I., Lomeña, F., Vilas, D., Lladó, A., Gaig, C., & Santamaria, J. (2013). Neurodegenerative disease status and post-mortem pathology in idiopathic rapid-eye-movement sleep behaviour disorder: An observational cohort study. *The Lancet. Neurology, 12*(5), 443–453. https://doi.org/10.1016/S1474-4422(13)70056-5

Jiménez-Jiménez, F. J., Alonso-Navarro, H., García-Martín, E., & Agúndez, J. A. G. (2021a). Neurochemical features of REM sleep behaviour disorder. *Journal of Personalized Medicine, 11*(9), Article 880. https://doi.org/10.3390/jpm11090880

Jiménez-Jiménez, F. J., Alonso-Navarro, H., García-Martín, E., & Agúndez, J. A. G. (2021b). Current treatment options for REM sleep behaviour disorder. *Journal of Personalized Medicine, 11*(11), Article 1204. https://doi.org/10.3390/jpm11111204

Kang, S. H., Yoon, I.-Y., Lee, S. D., Han, J. W., Kim, T. H., & Kim, K. W. (2013). REM sleep behavior disorder in the Korean elderly population: Prevalence and clinical characteristics. *Sleep, 36*(8), 1147–1152. https://doi.org/10.5665/sleep.2874

Kuzkina, A., Panzer, C., Seger, A., Schmitt, D., Rößle, J., Schreglmann, S. R., Knacke, H., Salabasidou, E., Kohl, A., Sittig, E., Barbe, M., Berg, D., Volkmann, J., Sommer, C., Oertel, W. H., Schaeffer, E., Sommerauer, M., Janzen, A., & Doppler, K. (2023). Dermal real-time quaking-induced conversion is a sensitive marker to confirm isolated rapid eye movement sleep behavior disorder as an early α-Synucleinopathy. *Movement Disorders, 38*(6), 1077–1082. https://doi.org/10.1002/mds.29340

Lapierre, O., & Montplaisir, J. (1992). Polysomnographic features of REM sleep behavior disorder: Development of a scoring method. *Neurology, 42*(7), 1371–1374. https://doi.org/10.1212/wnl.42.7.1371

Ma, J. F., Hou, M. M., Tang, H. D., Gao, X., Liang, L., Zhu, L. F., Zhou, Y., Zha, S. Y., Cui, S. S., Du, J. J., Li, G., Liu, J., & Chen, S. D. (2016). REM sleep behavior disorder was associated with Parkinson's disease: A community-based study. *BMC neurology*, 16, Article 123. https://doi.org/10.1186/s12883-016-0640-1

Ma, J. F., Qiao, Y., Gao, X., Liang, L., Liu, X. L., Li, D. H., Tang, H. D., & Chen, S. D. (2017). A community-based study of risk factors for probable rapid eye movement sleep behavior disorder. *Sleep Medicine, 30*, 71–76. https://doi.org/10.1016/j.sleep.2016.06.027

Miglis, M. G., Adler, C. H., Antelmi, E., Arnaldi, D., Baldelli, L., Boeve, B. F., Cesari, M., Dall'Antonia, I., Diederich, N. J., Doppler, K., Dušek, P., Ferri, R., Gagnon, J. F., Gan-Or, Z., Hermann, W., Högl, B., Hu, M. T., Iranzo, A., Janzen, A., … Oertel, W. H. (2021). Biomarkers of conversion to α-synucleinopathy in isolated rapid-eye-movement sleep behaviour disorder. *The Lancet. Neurology, 20*(8), 671–684. https://doi.org/10.1016/S1474-4422(21)00176-9

Miglis, M. G., Zitser, J., Schneider, L., During, E., Jaradeh, S., Freeman, R., & Gibbons, C. H. (2021). Cutaneous α-synuclein is correlated with autonomic impairment in isolated rapid eye movement sleep behavior disorder. *Sleep, 44*(12), Article zsab172. https://doi.org/10.1093/sleep/zsab172

Montini, A., Loddo, G., Baldelli, L., Cilea, R., & Provini, F. (2021). Sleep-related hypermotor epilepsy vs disorders of arousal in adults: A step-wise approach to diagnosis. *Chest, 160*(1), 319–329. https://doi.org/10.1016/j.chest.2021.01.059

Muñoz-Lopetegi, A., Pujol, M., Giménez, M., Gaig, C., Brieva, L., & Santamaria, J. (2021). Abnormal sleep behavior caused by hypoglycemia. *Sleep Medicine, 85*, 268–270. https://doi.org/10.1016/j.sleep.2021.07.029

Poggiolini, I., Gupta, V., Lawton, M., Lee, S., El-Turabi, A., Querejeta-Coma, A., Trenkwalder, C., Sixel-Döring, F., Foubert-Samier, A., Pavy-Le Traon, A., Plazzi, G., Biscarini, F., Montplaisir, J., Gagnon, J. F., Postuma, R. B., Antelmi, E., Meissner, W. G., Mollenhauer, B., Ben-Shlomo, Y., … Parkkinen, L. (2022).

Diagnostic value of cerebrospinal fluid alpha-synuclein seed quantification in synucleinopathies. *Brain*, *145*(2), 584–595. https://doi.org/10.1093/brain/awab431

Postuma, R. B., Arnulf, I., Högl, B., Iranzo, A., Miyamoto, T., Dauvilliers, Y., Oertel, W., Ju, Y. E., Puligheddu, M., Jennum, P., Pelletier, A., Wolfson, C., Leu-Semenescu, S., Frauscher, B., Miyamoto, M., Cochen De Cock, V., Unger, M. M., Stiasny-Kolster, K., Fantini, M. L., & Montplaisir, J. Y. (2012). A single-question screen for rapid eye movement sleep behavior disorder: A multicenter validation study. *Movement Disorders*, *27*(7), 913–916. https://doi.org/10.1002/mds.25037

Postuma, R. B., Gagnon, J. F., Tuineaig, M., Bertrand, J. A., Latreille, V., Desjardins, C., & Montplaisir, J. Y. (2013). Antidepressants and REM sleep behavior disorder: Isolated side effect or neurodegenerative signal?. *Sleep*, *36*(11), 1579–1585. https://doi.org/10.5665/sleep.3102

Postuma, R. B., Iranzo, A., Hu, M., Högl, B., Boeve, B. F., Manni, R., Oertel, W. H., Arnulf, I., Ferini-Strambi, L., Puligheddu, M., Antelmi, E., Cochen De Cock, V., Arnaldi, D., Mollenhauer, B., Videnovic, A., Sonka, K., Jung, K. Y., Kunz, D., Dauvilliers, Y., ... Pelletier, A. (2019). Risk and predictors of dementia and parkinsonism in idiopathic REM sleep behaviour disorder: A multicentre study. *Brain*, *142*(3), 744–759. https://doi.org/10.1093/brain/awz030

Postuma, R. B., Montplaisir, J. Y., Pelletier, A., Dauvilliers, Y., Oertel, W., Iranzo, A., Ferini-Strambi, L., Arnulf, I., Hogl, B., Manni, R., Miyamoto, T., Mayer, G., Stiasny-Kolster, K., Puligheddu, M., Ju, Y., Jennum, P., Sonka, K., Santamaria, J., Fantini, M. L., ... Wolfson, C. (2012). Environmental risk factors for REM sleep behavior disorder: A multicenter case-control study. *Neurology*, *79*(5), 428–434. https://doi.org/10.1212/WNL.0b013e31825dd383

Pujol, M., Pujol, J., Alonso, T., Fuentes, A., Pallerola, M., Freixenet, J., Barbé, F., Salamero, M., Santamaría, J., & Iranzo, A. (2017). Idiopathic REM sleep behavior disorder in the elderly Spanish community: A primary care center study with a two-stage design using video-polysomnography. *Sleep Medicine*, *40*, 116–121. https://doi.org/10.1016/j.sleep.2017.07.021

Puligheddu, M., Figorilli, M., Congiu, P., Lecca, R., Casaglia, E., Tamburrino, L., Orrù, R., Meloni, F., & Ferri, R. (2023). Quantification of REM sleep without atonia: A review of study methods and meta-analysis of their performance for the diagnosis of RBD. *Sleep Medicine Reviews*, *68*, Article 101745. https://doi.org/10.1016/j.smrv.2023.101745

Sabater, L., Gaig, C., Gelpi, E., Bataller, L., Lewerenz, J., Torres-Vega, E., Contreras, A., Giometto, B., Compta, Y., Embid, C., Vilaseca, I., Iranzo, A., Santamaría, J., Dalmau, J., & Graus, F. (2014). A novel non-rapid-eye movement and rapid-eye-movement parasomnia with sleep breathing disorder associated with antibodies to IgLON5: A case series, characterisation of the antigen, and post-mortem study. *The Lancet. Neurology*, *13*(6), 575–586. https://doi.org/10.1016/S1474-4422(14)70051-1

Sasai-Sakuma, T., Takeuchi, N., Asai, Y., Inoue, Y., & Inoue, Y. (2020). Prevalence and clinical characteristics of REM sleep behavior disorder in Japanese elderly people. *Sleep*, *43*(8), Article zsaa024. https://doi.org/10.1093/sleep/zsaa024

Schenck, C. H., Bundlie, S. R., & Mahowald, M. W. (1996). Delayed emergence of a parkinsonian disorder in 38% of 29 older men initially diagnosed with idiopathic rapid eye movement sleep behaviour disorder. *Neurology*, *46*(2), 388–393. https://doi.org/10.1212/wnl.46.2.388

Shen, Y., Yu, W. B., Shen, B., Dong, H., Zhao, J., Tang, Y. L., Fan, Y., Yang, Y. F., Sun, Y. M., Luo, S. S., Chen, C., Liu, F. T., Wu, J. J., Xiao, B. G., Yu, H., Koprich, J. B., Huang, Z. L., & Wang, J. (2020). Propagated α-synucleinopathy recapitulates REM sleep behaviour disorder followed by parkinsonian phenotypes in mice. *Brain*, *143*(11), 3374–3392. https://doi.org/10.1093/brain/awaa283

Shin, C., Kim, S. I., Park, S. H., Shin, J. H., Lee, C. Y., Yang, H. K., Lee, H. J., Kong, S. H., Suh, Y. S., Kim, H. J., & Jeon, B. (2022). Sensitivity of detecting alpha-synuclein accumulation in the gastrointestinal tract and tissue volume examined. *Journal of Movement Disorders*, *15*(3), 264–268. https://doi.org/10.14802/jmd.22042

Sprenger, F. S., Stefanova, N., Gelpi, E., Seppi, K., Navarro-Otano, J., Offner, F., Vilas, D., Valldeoriola, F., Pont-Sunyer, C., Aldecoa, I., Gaig, C., Gines, A., Cuatrecasas, M., Högl, B., Frauscher, B., Iranzo, A., Wenning, G. K., Vogel, W., Tolosa, E., & Poewe, W. (2015). Enteric nervous system α-synuclein immunoreactivity in idiopathic REM sleep behavior disorder. *Neurology*, *85*(20), 1761–1768. https://doi.org/10.1212/WNL.0000000000002126

Stefani, A., Iranzo, A., Holzknecht, E., Perra, D., Bongianni, M., Gaig, C., Heim, B., Serradell, M., Sacchetto, L., Garrido, A., Capaldi, S., Sánchez-Gómez, A., Cecchini, M. P., Mariotto, S., Ferrari, S., Fiorini, M., Schmutzhard, J., Cocchiara, P., Vilaseca, I., ... SINBAR (Sleep Innsbruck Barcelona) group (2021).

Alpha-synuclein seeds in olfactory mucosa of patients with isolated REM sleep behaviour disorder. *Brain, 144*(4), 1118–1126. https://doi.org/10.1093/brain/awab005

Stefani, A., Serradell, M., Holzknecht, E., Gaig, C., Ibrahim, A., Marrero, P., Cesari, M., Pérez-Carbonell, L., Brandauer, E., Fernández-Arcos, A., Bergmann, M., Matos, N., Santamaria, J., Högl, B., Iranzo, A., & Sleep Innsbruck Barcelona (SINBAR) group (2023). Low specificity of rapid eye movement sleep behavior disorder questionnaires: Need for better screening methods. *Movement Disorders, 38*(6), 1000–1007. https://doi.org/10.1002/mds.29407

Stiasny-Kolster, K., Mayer, G., Schäfer, S., Möller, J. C., Heinzel-Gutenbrunner, M., & Oertel, W. H. (2007). The REM sleep behavior disorder screening questionnaire—A new diagnostic instrument. *Movement Disorders, 22*(16), 2386–2393. https://doi.org/10.1002/mds.21740

Vilas, D., Iranzo, A., Tolosa, E., Aldecoa, I., Berenguer, J., Vilaseca, I., Martí, C., Serradell, M., Lomeña, F., Alós, L., Gaig, C., Santamaria, J., & Gelpi, E. (2016). Assessment of α-synuclein in submandibular glands of patients with idiopathic rapid-eye-movement sleep behaviour disorder: A case-control study. *The Lancet. Neurology, 15*(7), 708–718. https://doi.org/10.1016/S1474-4422(16)00080-6

Wong, J. C., Li, J., Pavlova, M., Chen, S., Wu, A., Wu, S., & Gao, X. (2016). Risk factors for probable REM sleep behavior disorder: A community-based study. *Neurology, 86*(14), 1306–1312. https://doi.org/10.1212/WNL.0000000000002414

CHAPTER

31 Parasomnias III: Sleep Terrors and Somnambulism

Antonio Zadra *and* Francesca Siclari

Abstract

Sleepwalking (somnambulism) and sleep terrors constitute two of the most frequent and impressive non-rapid-eye-movement (NREM) sleep parasomnias. This chapter discusses the clinical presentation, etiology, polysomnographic findings, diagnostic considerations, prevalence, and treatment options associated with these two parasomnias. Sleepwalking and sleep terrors share many characteristics. Most episodes arise from slow-wave sleep and are characterized by relative unresponsiveness to external stimuli, mental confusion, motor activation, and variable retrograde amnesia. Episodes can be precipitated by factors that intensify or fragment sleep. Factors suggested as being operant include abnormal sleep physiology, elevated psychopathology, and genetics. Laboratory evidence suggests that NREM parasomnias may reflect the simultaneous interplay between states of sleep and wakefulness. While a variety of treatments have been recommended, well-designed controlled clinical trials are lacking.

Key Words: sleepwalking, somnambulism, sleep terrors, parasomnia, genetics, treatment

Introduction

Parasomnias are undesirable physical, behavioral, or experiential phenomena that occur during entry into sleep, within sleep, or during partial arousals from sleep (American Academy of Sleep Medicine [AASM], 2014). This chapter focuses on two prototypic non-rapid-eye-movement (NREM) sleep parasomnias, namely sleepwalking (somnambulism) and sleep terrors. A summary and comparison of the main features of NREM and rapid-eye-movement (REM) sleep parasomnias are presented in Table 31.1.

Although disorders of arousal vary along dimensions of emotional, autonomic, and motor activation, they nevertheless share a number of characteristics. NREM parasomnias are common in children and tend to decrease in frequency with age. Episodes generally arise out of slow-wave sleep (SWS; Stage N3) but also from lighter N2 sleep. Consequently, NREM parasomnias tend to take place in the first third of the night when SWS is predominant. Symptoms and manifestations of the disorders of arousal can be considered along a spectrum, but most episodes are characterized by misperception and relative unresponsiveness to external stimuli, mental confusion, simple to complex

Table 31.1 Comparison of Common Features of Rapid-Eye-Movement (REM) and Non-REM Sleep Parasomnias

	Confusional arousal	Somnambulism	Sleep terrors	Nightmares	RBD
Time of night	First third to half of the sleep period	First third to half of the sleep period	First third to half of the sleep period	Last half of the sleep period	Last half of the sleep period
Sleep stage	SWS	SWS	SWS	REM	REM without atonia
Associated activity	May sit up in bed	Simple to complex movements; possible ambulation	Sits, screams; agitated motor activity	Movements are rare and limited	Behavior that correlates with dream content
Duration	1–15 minutes	1–30 minutes	1–10 minutes	3–20 minutes	1–10 minutes
Autonomic activation	Low	Low to moderate	Moderate to extreme	None to moderate	Low to moderate
Recall for the event	Variable amnesia for the event	Variable amnesia for the event	Variable amnesia for the event	Vivid and detailed dream recall	Vivid and detailed dream recall
Full awakening	Uncommon	Uncommon	Uncommon	Common	Common
State after event	Confused/disoriented	Confused/disoriented	Confused/disoriented	Fully awake and functional	Fully awake and functional
Arousal threshold	High	High	High	Low	Low
Reduced in sleep laboratory	Yes	Yes	Yes	Yes	No
PSG findings	Partial arousals from SWS	Partial arousals from SWS	Partial arousals from SWS	REM	Excessive EMG during REM
Potential for injury/violence	Yes	Yes	Yes	No	Yes

Note. EMG = electromyography; PSG = polysomnography; RBD = REM sleep behavior disorder; SWS = slow-wave sleep.

behaviors, perceived threat, and variable retrograde amnesia. Conditions that intensify sleep such as sleep deprivation and neuroleptics or medications with depressive central nervous system effects can facilitate or precipitate NREM parasomnias in predisposed individuals. Factors that fragment sleep, including sleep disordered breathing, stress, and environmental or endogenous stimuli, can have similar effects. Finally, a common genetic component is suspected as people with an arousal disorder often have a positive family history for one or more of the NREM parasomnias.

Sleepwalking

Clinical Features

That people sometimes engage in complex ambulatory behaviors during sleep has been known for centuries. For example, Shakespeare's *Macbeth* contains a widely known episode of somnambulism during which a guilt-ridden Lady Macbeth tries to wash imaginary bloodstains from her hands while speaking of the crimes she and her husband have committed. Interestingly, this early 17th-century depiction of somnambulism is consistent with the medical view that existed until the mid-1960s which held that sleepwalking represented a dissociative state related to dreaming. As detailed below, a growing number of findings suggest that Shakespeare's depiction of sleepwalking may not have been that far off the mark.

The symptoms and manifestations that characterize sleepwalking can vary greatly both within and across patients. A sleepwalker's emotional expression can range from happy, neutral, or calm to extremely agitated (Clé et al., 2019). Similarly, actual behavioral manifestations can range from clumsy or simple and isolated actions such as suddenly sitting up in bed, pointing at a wall, and walking about a room to surprisingly complex behaviors such as rearranging furniture, cooking or eating, getting dressed, playing a musical instrument, and reenacting daytime activities (Oudiette et al., 2011). The sleepwalker's eyes are usually open throughout an episode, but they may appear to have a glassy stare. Sleepwalkers may spontaneously return to bed or eventually lie down to sleep elsewhere. Given the heterogeneous nature of sleepwalking episodes, their duration can vary from a few seconds to dozens of minutes.

While influential initial reports suggested that sleepwalkers were most often unconscious or could not recall any mental content associated with parasomnia episodes (Broughton, 1968; Jacobson et al., 1965), it is now acknowledged that the level of consciousness during NREM parasomnia episodes is more variable, especially in adults (Castelnovo et al., 2021; Cataldi et al., 2024; Siclari, 2024). In fact, that patients suffering from sleepwalking can and do recall at least portions of their episodes upon awakening has been known for decades (Montplaisir & Demers, 1983; Schenck & Mahowald, 1995). One retrospective study (Oudiette et al., 2009) of patients with a history of sleepwalking and/or sleep terrors found that 71% recalled short, unpleasant dreamlike mentations and that patients' reported mentation was often congruent with the observed behaviors during an episode, suggesting that sleepwalking may represent acting out of dreamlike mentations. Similarly, one investigation (Zadra et al., 2019) of 165 sleepwalkers referred to a sleep disorders clinic for chronic somnambulism revealed that the three factors rated by the greatest proportion of sleepwalkers as "often" or "always" precipitating their episodes were stress (71% of all patients), bad dreams and nightmares (47%), and dreams in general (35%). In a laboratory study, patients with a history of sleepwalking and sleep terrors reported conscious experiences with dream-like content 56% of the time when immediately interviewed after their parasomnia episodes (Cataldi et al., 2024). It is not surprising then that somnambulistic behaviors are construed by many patients as being motivated by an intrinsic sense of urgency or underlying reason that accounts for their actions during actual episodes. It should also be noted that auditory, visual, and tactile hallucinations, including hallucinatory pain, can be present during episodes (Bušková & Sonka, 2014; Siclari et al., 2020).

Such reports raise important questions as to the role that phenomenological contents play in how somnambulistic episodes are experienced and unfold. In addition, these findings suggest that somnambulism should not be assumed to necessarily reflect automatic behaviors in the pure sense of the term and that morning recall of sleepwalking episodes may be greater than generally believed. Clinicians and researchers may gain valuable information by investigating these dimensions of sleepwalkers' experiences.

Whereas the occurrence of sleepwalking in children is frequently viewed as a relatively benign condition, somnambulism in adults can result in serious injury to the sleeper or others (see Siclari et al., 2010, for a review). Adults suffering from somnambulism often consult due to a history of aggressive and/or injurious behavior during sleep or after suffering a serious injury, having attacked a bed partner during an episode, or both (Moldofsky et al., 1995; Schenck et al., 1989). Sexual behaviors occur in 10%–15% of regular adult sleepwalkers and can lead to sex-related violence (Dubessy et al., 2017). Other reported behaviors in extreme cases include driving motor vehicles, suspected suicide, and even homicide, raising fundamental questions as to the medico-forensic implications of these acts (Cartwright, 2004; Cramer Bornemann & Mahowald, 2017; Pressman, 2007; Siclari et al., 2010; Stallman & Bari, 2017).

Etiology

Sleepwalking and sleep terrors have been conceptualized as "disorders of arousal" (Broughton, 1968) because of the autonomic and motor arousal which drives the patient toward a state of partial wakefulness from sleep. The traditional idea of somnambulism as a disorder of arousal might be too conceptually restrictive, however; and a more comprehensive view including the idea of simultaneous interplay between states of sleep and wakefulness is likely warranted (Zadra et al., 2013). Exact pathophysiological mechanisms of somnambulism remain unclear, but several general factors have been proposed, including a dysfunction in SWS regulation, psychopathology, and genetics.

Dysfunction in SWS Regulation

Recent conceptualizations of sleepwalking (Castelnovo et al., 2018; Zadra et al., 2013) suggest that the disorder reflects a dysfunction in the regulation of SWS. One of the more robust features of the otherwise preserved sleep architecture in sleepwalkers as compared to age-matched controls is the lack of NREM sleep continuity, as reflected by an increased number of spontaneous awakenings and electroencephalographic (EEG) arousals occurring out of SWS, even on nights without episodes (Gaudreau et al., 2000; Lopez et al., 2018; Pilon et al., 2008). Relatedly, when compared to controls, sleepwalkers display more frequent slow EEG activity patterns during their SWS, and the number of SWS arousals has been used to successfully discriminate the polysomnographies (PSGs) of sleepwalkers from those of controls (Lopez et al., 2018).

Sleepwalkers also show an atypical decrease in slow-wave activity (SWA) during their first sleep cycles (Gaudreau et al., 2000; Guilleminault et al., 2001) and a different time course of delta activity decay across the night (Espa et al., 2000). Sleepwalkers' frequent awakenings from SWS may thus interfere with the normal buildup of SWA, especially during the first two sleep cycles when most of their awakenings from SWS occur. Further evidence for sleepwalkers' disturbance in SWS consolidation comes from studies showing that sleepwalkers display an increased cyclic alternating pattern (CAP) rate (Guilleminault et al., 2006; Zucconi et al., 1995), an endogenous rhythm considered to be a measure of NREM instability.

Sleepwalkers' fragmentation of NREM sleep may thus reflect a milder manifestation of their presumed arousal dysfunction. NREM sleep instability and arousal oscillation may thus represent typical microstructural features of parasomniacs' NREM sleep and play a role in triggering sleepwalkers' abnormal motor episodes.

When compared to baseline recordings, sleep deprivation (with recovery sleep being initiated in the morning) significantly increases the number of SWS awakenings in sleepwalkers but not in controls (Blanchette-Carrière et al., 2024; Pilon et al., 2008). Sleepwalkers may thus be particularly vulnerable to increased homeostatic sleep pressure following sleep deprivation when sleep is initiated at a circadian time of increasing wake propensity. When compared to controls, sleepwalkers have increased arousal thresholds in REM, but not NREM, sleep, which may reflect a compensatory homeostatic mechanism in reaction to NREM sleep fragmentation (Pilon et al., 2012).

While early studies suggested that hypersynchronous delta waves (HSDs), usually described as continuous high-voltage (>150 μV) delta waves, characterize the SWS EEG of patients with sleepwalking/sleep terrors, especially prior to episode onset, more recent studies of HSD prior to sleepwalking episodes have shown that HSD occurs in the SWS of normal controls and has low specificity for the diagnosis of NREM parasomnias

(Pilon et al., 2006; Pressman, 2004). HSD, however, may be related to expression of the homeostatic process underlying sleep regulation, particularly of delta activity during NREM sleep.

Spectral analysis of sleep EEG signals prior to behavioral episodes in patients with sleepwalking and/or sleep terrors indicates that the onset of a parasomnia is likely to be preceded by an increase in low delta power (0.25–2.0Hz; Jaar et al., 2010; Perrault et al., 2014) and/or beta power within 30 seconds prior to an episode (Cataldi et al., 2022; Januszko et al., 2016).

Taken together, these processes may reflect cortical reactions to activation of arousal systems. This interpretation is supported by the observation that parasomnia episodes are preceded by autonomic nervous system activity (tachycardia and peripheral vasoconstriction), which sets in before episode onset (Ledard et al., 2020). However, one should note that these EEG and autonomous nervous system changes are not necessarily specific to parasomnia episodes. For instance, a recent study (Cataldi et al., 2022) found an increase in SWA and beta power in frontal and central brain regions, reminiscent of HSD, not only immediately prior to parasomnia episodes but also to the same extent before normal awakenings out of SWS, without behavioral manifestations of parasomnias.

Finally, one EEG-based functional brain connectivity study (Desjardins et al., 2017) of 27 sleepwalkers who experienced a somnambulistic episode during SWS found decreased functional local connectivity for lower-frequency bands (delta) in parietal and occipital regions, together with increased connectivity for higher-frequency bands (alpha and beta) in large-scale frontoparietal networks, in the 20 seconds preceding the episodes. This data suggests that somnambulistic episodes are preceded by brain processes characterized by the coexistence of arousal and deep sleep and are in line with evidence from brain imaging and intracerebral electrode studies showing that sleepwalking might result from an imbalance between sleep and wakefulness (Nobili et al., 2011; Terzaghi et al., 2009).

Turning to postarousal EEG activity, one landmark study (Schenck et al., 1998) described three postarousal EEG patterns that characterize most SWS arousals in adults with sleepwalking/sleep terrors. These patterns, subsequently found to also characterize somnambulistic events (Zadra et al., 2004), suggest that sleepwalkers are caught between NREM sleep and full EEG arousal and are thus not fully awake during their episodes (as translated clinically by their apparent lack of awareness or insight) nor fully asleep (as revealed behaviorally by their capacity to interact with others and to navigate their immediate environment).

Finally, it should be noted that compared to normal awakenings out of SWS, parasomnia episodes in sleepwalkers contain higher SWA and lower beta activity in frontal and central brain regions (Cataldi et al., 2022). This may be related to the fact that somnambulistic episodes occur on a background of abnormally high SWA compared to normal awakenings, with SWA persisting after episode onset. As recently suggested, the occurrence of parasomnia episodes may therefore be consequent to an abnormally timed engagement of arousal systems (Cataldi et al., 2022).

Psychopathology

Traditionally, the presence of somnambulism (with or without concomitant sleep terrors) in adulthood has been viewed as a sign of major psychopathology (A. Kales, Soldatos, Caldwell, et al., 1980). In early childhood, the occurrence of somnambulism can be associated with separation anxiety (Petit et al., 2007). Epidemiologic evidence suggests a higher prevalence of psychopathology among adult patients with arousal disorders (Ohayon et al., 1999), and psychopathology has been reported in subgroups of adolescents with sleep terrors and/or sleepwalking (Gau & Soong, 1999). Epidemiological findings further reveal that almost 50% of adults with arousal disorders report having experienced a stressful event in the past 12 months (e.g., divorce or separation from a spouse, bereavement) and that they are significantly more likely than controls to describe their lives as being highly stressful (Ohayon et al., 1999). However, several studies have shown that many adult patients do not suffer from psychiatric disorders, including from clinically elevated levels of anxiety and depression, nor do they necessarily present with highly disturbed personality traits (Guilleminault et al., 2005; Labelle et al., 2013; Schenck et al., 1989). When psychopathology is present in sleepwalkers, it is more likely to be associated with a higher frequency of nightmares, with potentially injurious behaviors enacted during somnambulistic episodes, and with a negative family history for sleepwalking (Labelle et al., 2013).

Genetic Predisposition

A strong genetic component to somnambulism has been well documented. About 80% of somnambulistic patients have at least one family member affected by this parasomnia, and the prevalence of somnambulism is higher in children of parents with a history of sleepwalking (Hori & Hirose, 1995; A. Kales, Soldatos, Bixler, et al., 1980). One twin study of over 300 pairs found that monozygotic (MZ) twins are concordant for the disorder six times as often as dizygotic (DZ) twins (Barkwin, 1970). A population-based twin study (Hublin et al., 1997) of 1,045 MZ and 1,899 DZ pairs showed a considerable genetic effect in adulthood sleepwalking, although the effect in childhood sleepwalking was not as pronounced. Genetic contributions to sleepwalking have also been documented in a large cohort of youth aged between 8 and 22 years (Chiba et al., 2021). Unfortunately, few molecular genetic studies have attempted to identify genes that may predispose to somnambulism. One group (Lecendreux et al., 2003) described an association between familial sleepwalkers and the HLA DQB1*05 and *04 alleles, but the functional significance of this finding remains unclear. Another promising candidate is the ADA gene as adenosine and the ADA enzyme play an important role in the homeostatic regulation of NREM sleep. However, one recent study of a large cohort of adult sleepwalkers failed to find a strong association between ADA variants and sleepwalking (Fournier et al., 2021).

Other Findings

Until recently, daytime somnolence or impairment in daytime functioning was not considered as part of the clinical picture associated with sleepwalking. However, a growing number of studies, including on the Multiple Sleep Latency Test (the gold standard in objective assessment of excessive daytime sleepiness) and the Epworth Sleepiness Scale, indicate that excessive daytime somnolence may represent an important characteristic of the disorder (Desautels et al., 2013; Lopez et al., 2014; Oudiette et al., 2009). Studies using transcranial magnetic stimulation and brain imaging have also documented daytime functioning anomalies in sleepwalkers (Oliviero et al., 2007), thereby supporting the idea that clinical considerations should not be limited to patients' sleep.

A single-photon emission computed tomographic investigation of a sleepwalking episode recorded from a 16-year-old man with a history of somnambulism revealed an increase of 25% in regional cerebral blood flow (rCBF) in the posterior cingulate and anterior cerebellum compared to SWS without episodes (Bassetti et al., 2000). The authors suggest that variations in the motor and emotional manifestations of sleepwalking may be related to different activation patterns of the cingulate cortex as it modulates behavior in response to emotional processes. A decrease in rCBF in frontoparietal associative cortices was also noted in comparison to the wakefulness pattern of normal subjects. Since this pattern occurs in normal SWS, this finding suggests that the brain is indeed sleeping during somnambulism. These pilot findings have been complemented by case reports of intracerebral recordings in epileptic patients displaying confusional arousals (Terzaghi et al., 2012), which have confirmed the simultaneous presence of sleep signals (slow oscillations, spindles) in frontoparietal associative areas, the hippocampus, and the thalamus and of wake-like brain activity in other brain areas, including the cingulate, sensorimotor, orbitofrontal, and lateral temporal cortices. Taken together, these observations support the notion that sleepwalking is a dissociated state consisting of motor arousal and persisting mind sleep.

Finally, a structural magnetic resonance imaging study (Heidbreder et al., 2017) of 14 patients with NREM parasomnia found reduced gray matter volumes in the left dorsal posterior (BA23) and posterior midcingulate (BA24) cortices compared to controls. Since these brain areas project to the spinal cord and primary motor cortex and are involved in multisensory orientation, the authors postulate that the gray matter volume reduction in the posterior midcingulate cortex may explain the contrasting activation states of the motor and cingulate cortices, which likely give rise to the kinds of fixed motor patterns frequently encountered in NREM parasomnias. Indeed, sleepwalkers have been shown to display enhanced motor automation compared to controls during wakefulness (Kannape et al., 2017). However, a tendency toward more automatic behaviors in sleepwalkers, if true, would only explain part of the clinical picture since, as detailed above, somnambulism can also feature a variety of goal-directed (non-automatic) behaviors performed in relation to oneiric experiences.

Studies also suggest that adult sleepwalkers may lack nociception during their episodes, including self-injurious events (e.g., only realizing the extent of their episode-related injuries upon awakening the next morning; Lopez et al., 2015). Findings of nociceptive dysregulation during somnambulism add to the view of sleepwalking as a dissociated brain state.

Finally, it is important to note that disorders of arousal can be triggered by medication, including sedatives/hypnotics (zolpidem), neuroleptics, lithium, minor tranquilizers, stimulants, and antihistamines (Stallman et al., 2018).

Assessment and Differential Diagnosis

Key assessment issues that should be covered during the clinical history for somnambulism and sleep terrors are presented in Box 31.1.

Diagnosis of sleepwalking can often be made based on a detailed clinical history, including complete description of the time course and content of sleep-related behaviors (Zadra et al., 2013). Given that variable retrograde amnesia can characterize somnambulistic episodes, descriptive information from family members or a bed partner can be particularly valuable. Similarly, home video recording can also be helpful in characterizing behavioral manifestations. It should be noted, however, that sleepwalking and sleep terrors can co-occur and that the two conditions are sometimes difficult to differentiate.

Box 31.1 Key Assessment Features During a Clinical Interview for Non-Rapid-Eye-Movement Parasomnias

- Age at onset
- Timing of the episode during the sleep period
- Episode frequency and duration
- Detailed description of the episode, including behavioral manifestations, affect, and mentation during and after the event
- Responsiveness to external stimuli during the event
- Level of consciousness or awareness when awakened from an episode
- Memory for the event
- Precipitating or triggering factors
- Sleep–wake pattern and sleep environment
- Symptoms of daytime sleepiness
- Symptoms of other sleep disorders
- Familial history for non-rapid-eye-movement parasomnias and other sleep disorders
- Medical, psychiatric, and neurological history
- Medication and substance use

When case presentations involve violent or injurious behaviors, excessive daytime sleepiness, or associated medical or neurological conditions, more extensive evaluations, including overnight PSG with an expanded EEG montage, may be required. Continuous audiovisual monitoring is indispensable to document behavioral manifestations and to correlate monitored events with PSG parameters. Sleep laboratory investigations can be useful in ruling out other disorders (e.g., nocturnal seizures, episodic nocturnal wandering, REM sleep behavior disorder [RBD]) or in identifying primary sleep-related disorders (e.g., sleep disordered breathing, periodic limb movement disorder) that might underlie the parasomnia, but no validated sleep protocol exists to directly confirm the diagnosis of sleepwalking.

The principal difficulty in diagnosing sleepwalking directly with PSG is that behavioral events rarely occur in the laboratory. In addition, when partial episodes do develop, they are usually less complex than what is described for the patient's home environment. Some PSG features (e.g., HSD) have been proposed as indirect evidence supporting the diagnosis, and while some of these variables show poor sensitivity and specificity for NREM parasomnias (Pilon et al., 2006; Pressman, 2007), other PSG-related markers appear more promising (Lopez et al., 2018).

Sleepwalking can be secondary to sleep respiratory events, including obstructive sleep apnea and upper airway resistance syndrome, or other sleep disorders such as periodic limb movements in sleep. An association between sleepwalking/sleep terrors and sleep disordered breathing has been described in several studies (Espa et al., 2002; Goodwin et al., 2004). Treatment of the precipitating sleep disorder (e.g., continuous positive airway pressure for sleep disordered breathing) can result in a disappearance of the disorder of arousal.

Somnambulism needs to be distinguished from RBD. RBD is characterized by intermittent loss of REM sleep atonia and by the appearance of elaborate motor activity associated with dream mentation during REM sleep. Patients often have a vivid recall of the dreams that appear to correlate with observed behaviors. RBD can also be distinguished from NREM parasomnias by its usual occurrence during the second half of the night and by the absence of mental confusion upon awakening. However, some patients may have behavioral manifestations during both REM and NREM sleep, with RBD occurring in combination with a disorder of arousal. This condition is known as *parasomnia overlap disorder* (Schenck et al., 1997).

Disorders of arousal and focal seizures with altered awareness also share several clinical similarities, including sudden onset, unresponsiveness, and retrograde amnesia. In addition, these conditions are all sensitive to factors that deepen sleep, such as sleep deprivation. Nocturnal frontal lobe epilepsy can be particularly difficult to differentiate from NREM parasomnias. Complex partial seizures usually involve repetitive stereotypic behaviors, and patients rarely return to bed. Epileptic seizures may occur in any sleep stage throughout the sleep period. Similar seizure activity may occur during daytime wakefulness.

Based on clinical and experimental data, factors described as facilitating or precipitating somnambulistic episodes in predisposed individuals have been grouped into two categories: factors that deepen sleep (e.g., increased SWS following sleep deprivation) and factors that fragment sleep (e.g., stress, arousing stimuli). Several studies have shown that sleep deprivation significantly increases the frequency and complexity of somnambulistic events recorded in the laboratory (Joncas et al., 2002; Zadra et al., 2008). The probability of recording an episode can be further increased by combining sleep deprivation with the factors that fragment sleep, namely, presentation of auditory stimuli during patients' recovery sleep (Pilon et al., 2008).

These results support the hypothesis that via its homeostatic pressure for increased SWS, sleep deprivation facilitates the occurrence of somnambulistic episodes in predisposed individuals and that this effect can be greatly augmented by incorporating forced arousals. Sleepwalkers' heightened sensitivity to the effects of sleep deprivation is further supported by findings suggestive of atypical autonomic activation during their recovery SWS (Scavone et al., 2021) as well as brain imaging studies revealing post–sleep deprivation local reductions in CBF in inferior temporal regions (Dang-Vu et al., 2015) as well as increased executive impairments (flexibility and commission errors; Labelle et al., 2015).

Medico-Legal Considerations

As previously described, the clinical presentation of somnambulism can include instances of violent behaviors toward others. Recent decades have seen increasing numbers of legal cases involving sleep-related violence, and sleepwalking represents a significant cause of sleep-related injury. However, there is considerable debate regarding the validity of scientific evidence sometimes presented to support a sleepwalking defense (Cartwright, 2004; Pressman et al., 2009, 2014). For instance, whereas alcohol is reported by some as increasing the possibility of sleepwalking, a review of this literature indicates that there is no actual scientific support for such a statement (Pressman, 2019; Pressman et al., 2007). A detailed account of forensic aspects of sleep disorders is presented in Chapter 46.

Prevalence and Developmental Aspects

Sleepwalking is more common in childhood than in adulthood as most children will experience, at least temporarily, one or more of the NREM sleep parasomnias during childhood or early adolescence. However, childhood somnambulism is typically benign (and nonviolent) and usually does not require any intervention. The prevalence of sleepwalking is around 3% in toddlers, steadily increases to about 11% at ages 7 and 8, and reaches approximately 13% at age 12 (Petit et al., 2007; Stallman & Kohler, 2016). The prevalence of sleepwalking rapidly decreases during adolescence to reach about 2%–4% in adulthood (Hublin et al., 1997; Ohayon et al., 1999, 2012). Most children thus outgrow the disorder during adolescence, although it may persist into adulthood in up to 25% of cases. Sleepwalking can also appear de novo in adults, and some evidence suggests that adult-onset sleepwalking may be more frequent in people presenting with a clear psychiatric history or with the presence of complex or comorbid sleep disorders (e.g., Hublin, et al., 1997; Labelle et al., 2013; Lam et al., 2009).

Several prospective longitudinal studies of children (Laberge et al., 2000; Petit et al., 2015) revealed high rates of co-occurrence for sleepwalking and sleep terrors. In addition, children with sleep terrors can develop sleepwalking at a later age, and the two parasomnias can occur within the same episode (e.g., sleep terror followed by sleepwalking).

Prevention and Treatment Options

Treatment is often unnecessary when the episodes are benign and not associated with potential injury. In this case, reassuring the patient/family about the benign nature of the episodes and demystifying the events is often sufficient. However, attention should be paid to potential precipitating factors, such as sleep deprivation, stress, and environmental disturbances, so that such factors can be avoided. When patients present with a history of agitated somnambulism or sleep terrors, precautions should be taken to ensure a safe sleep environment. Preventative measures can include the removal of obstructions in the bedroom, securing windows, sleeping on the ground floor, installing locks or alarms on outside doors, covering windows with heavy curtains, using a nightlight, placing barriers in stairways, and removing all sharp or otherwise dangerous objects.

Properly powered, controlled clinical trials for the treatment of somnambulism are lacking. Traditionally, benzodiazepines, especially clonazepam and diazepam, as well as tricyclic antidepressants (e.g., imipramine) have been used for the treatment of somnambulism (Drakatos et al., 2018; Irfan et al., 2021); but they do not always result in adequate control of sleepwalking, and discontinuation of the medication can result in the disorder's reappearance, sometimes in more severe form. These treatments should always include instructions on sleep hygiene, avoidance of sleep deprivation, and stress management. The most frequently recommended non-pharmacological treatment for adult somnambulism is hypnosis as a large number of descriptive studies and case reports have reported on the treatment's efficacy (Harris & Grunstein, 2009; Stallman & Kohler, 2016). In children, the preferred treatment for somnambulism consists of a behavioral technique called *anticipatory* or *scheduled awakening*. Parents keep a diary of their child's episodes and determine the approximate time at which the episodes typically occur. They will then awaken their child about 15–20 minutes before the episode's typical time of occurrence for a period of 1 month. Based on several case reports, it appears that this simple intervention can yield rapid results and that benefits are maintained for several months after the end of the treatment (Durand & Mindell, 1999; Frank et al., 1997).

Clinical Variants

Sleep-Related Eating Disorder

According to the *International Classification of Sleep Disorders* (ICSD-3; AASM, 2014), sleep-related eating disorder (SRED), which is classified under the "NREM Parasomnia" section, consists of recurrent episodes of involuntary eating and drinking during arousal from sleep with problematic consequences. Episodes, which are typically both frequent and chronic, tend to occur during partial arousals from NREM sleep during the first third of the night and are characterized by varying degrees of awareness and subsequent recall (Howell et al., 2009; Winkelman, 1998). Patients may consume inedible food (e.g., cigarettes, frozen meat) during SRED episodes, indicating altered cognition. PSG studies have associated SRED with a variety of underlying sleep disorders, the most frequent of which is sleepwalking (Schenck et al., 1993; Winkelman, 1998).

Although SRED can affect both sexes and all ages, it is most common in young adult women, particularly in those with a history of current or past eating disorder. SRED affects up to 4% of college students (Winkelman et al., 1999) and can result in a variety of adverse consequences, including health problems and considerable weight gain (Schenck et al., 1993). SRED can also occur in association with medications such as zolpidem and sodium oxybate (Merino et al., 2022).

When comorbid sleep disorders are present (e.g., restless legs syndrome, obstructive sleep apnea), treatment should focus on their control. Although based on limited evidence, medications reported as being effective for the treatment of SRED include topiramate, an anticonvulsant, and dopaminergic agents (Irfan et al., 2021).

Sleep-Related Abnormal Sexual Behavior

Sleep-related abnormal sexual behavior (SRASB) consists of inappropriate sexual activities occurring during sleep, in a state of altered awareness (Andersen et al., 2007; Schenck et al., 2007). Other terms proposed for these episodes include *sexsomnia* and *sleep sex*. SRASB can range from sexual vocalizations or sexualized bodily movements to violent masturbation or sexual assaults and may be markedly different from behaviors normally initiated during the patient's waking state (Andersen et al., 2007; Dubessy et al., 2017; Schenck et al., 2007).

According to the ICSD-3 (AASM, 2014), SRASB is classified in the "Disorders of Arousal" section as a clinical subtype of confusional arousal. Disorders of arousal, and sleepwalking in particular, are the most frequent sleep disorders associated with SRASB, although they could also occur in association with RBD or NREM complex partial seizures (Andersen et al., 2007; Schenck et al., 2007). As detailed in a thorough review, however (Schenck et al., 2007), a wide range of sleep-related disorders may be associated with SRASB.

SRASB may give rise to a variety of negative emotions and cognitions including feelings of embarrassment, guilt, shame, or depression; it often carries interpersonal consequences and has important clinical and forensic implications.

The use of clonazepam, sometimes in association with psychotherapy or stress management, or paroxetine has been reported to be effective for the treatment SRASB (Dubessy et al., 2017; Schenck et al., 2007). When associated sleep disorders are present, their treatment should be prioritized.

Sleep Terrors

Clinical Features

Historically, sleep terrors have been confused with nightmares, a distinct REM sleep parasomnia (see Table 31.1 for comparison of the main features of NREM and REM sleep parasomnias and Chapter 29 for details on nightmares). Sleep terrors arise out of SWS, typically within 90 minutes after sleep onset, and are characterized by a loud piercing scream or cry for help, intense autonomic activation (e.g., sweating, flushing of the skin, mydriasis, tachycardia, rapid breathing), inconsolability, and overwhelming fear or acute panic. On rarer occasions, this initial terror can be followed by complex behavioral manifestations such as leaving the bed, fleeing the room, or thrashing around. Behaviors can also be violent, resulting in self-injury or property damage. These more extreme episodes can result in considerable distress for family members of affected patients. The duration of sleep terrors is usually relatively short, often from under a minute to a few minutes. Attempting to console or awaken an individual during a sleep terror can prolong or intensify the episode. Once the sleep terror episode has subsided, the person usually does not fully awaken, returns to sleep, and remains partially or completely amnesic for the event the following day.

If questioned immediately following an episode, patients may report distinct recollections of immediate threats from which they were trying to escape. Precipitating imagery, ranging from a brief frightening image or thought to more elaborate dreamlike mentation has been noted, particularly in adults (Cataldi et al., 2024; Oudiette et al., 2009; Siclari et al., 2024). Some patients predominantly experience sleep terrors characterized by the illusion of choking. They typically awake from sleep with the impression that they have swallowed a specific object (avocado, ping-pong ball, spoon) that is stuck in their throat (Flamand et al., 2015). Although choking can also occur as a manifestation of sleep-related seizures with temporal lobe onset, patients with this type of sleep terror have a history of NREM parasomnias and no manifestations of seizures.

Etiology

Many parasomniacs present a history of both somnambulism and sleep terrors, and, as previously described, these two NREM parasomnias share many common features. Not surprisingly, factors considered as being operant in the pathophysiology of sleep terrors are similar to those previously described for sleepwalking. Consequently, they are only presented summarily below.

Although many studies have shown that NREM parasomnias can occur in otherwise mentally healthy individuals (Labelle et al., 2013; Schenck & Mahowald, 2000), sleep terrors in adulthood have been described in relation to psychopathology and personality disorders (J. D. Kales et al., 1980). Epidemiological findings indicate that individuals reporting sleep terrors are twice as likely as sleepwalkers, 5 times more likely than controls to meet diagnostic criteria for a *Diagnostic and Statistical Manual of Mental Disorders* (fourth edition) mood disorder, and about 3.5 times more likely than sleepwalkers or controls to report a history of mental disorders, including mood and anxiety disorders (Ohayon et al., 1999).

As is true for somnambulism, genetic factors play a major role. MZ twins are more concordant than DZ twins for sleep terrors (Nguyen et al., 2008), and sleep terrors are more frequent in children for whom one or both parents have a sleepwalking history than in children with non-affected parents (Petit et al., 2015). This data and the clinical similarities between these two parasomnias suggest a common genetic predisposition and similar pathophysiological mechanisms.

EEG Findings Prior to and During Episodes

When compared to controls, children and adults with sleep terrors or a mixture of disorders of arousal (e.g., sleep terrors and sleepwalking) show an increased number of arousals during SWS as well as alterations in the number of CAP cycles and rates (Bruni et al., 2008; Espa et al., 2002). As detailed previously, similar findings have been reported in relation to sleepwalking. In addition, the three main postarousal EEG patterns identified by Schenck et al. (1998) and described in the previous section on sleepwalking also apply to sleep terrors.

Differential Diagnosis

Diagnosis of sleep terrors can often be made based on a detailed clinical history, including complete description of the time course and content of sleep-related behaviors. As with sleepwalking, descriptive information from family members or a bed partner and the use of home video recording can be particularly valuable in characterizing behavioral manifestations.

Sleep terrors need to be distinguished from nightmare disorder, complex partial seizures, and nocturnal panic attacks. See corresponding section on sleepwalking for the differentiation between NREM parasomnias and RBD.

Nightmares are vivid and disturbing mental experiences that generally occur during REM sleep and often result in awakening. They can be distinguished from sleep terrors by their usual occurrence during the second half of the night, when REM is most prominent, and by the recall of detailed dream content. The degree of automatic activation (e.g., palpitations and dyspnea) is much greater during sleep terrors, and there is an absence of mental confusion upon awakening from a nightmare as opposed to a sleep terror. Actual screaming or other intense vocalizations which can characterize sleep terrors are rare during nightmares.

Disorders of arousal and complex partial epileptic seizures share several clinical similarities and precipitating factors. Complex partial seizures may occur in any sleep stage throughout the sleep period and usually involve repetitive stereotypic behaviors. Sleep terrors and seizures may coexist in the same person.

Approximately 50% of all patients with panic disorder have nocturnal panic attacks, which are characterized by intense fear or discomfort accompanied by cognitive and physical symptoms of arousal. These attacks are comparable to panic attacks experienced in the daytime, and they may sometimes be clinically similar to sleep terrors. Nocturnal panic attacks usually occur in late Stage 2 or early Stage 3 sleep, and, unlike many sleep terrors, patients do not become physically agitated or aggressive during the panic attack (Craske & Tsao, 2005). Immediately after a nocturnal panic attack, patients are oriented, can vividly recall their attack, and usually have difficulty returning to sleep (i.e., suffer from insomnia); these features differ from those observed in patients with sleep terrors.

Assessment

Given the similarities in pathophysiological processes believed to underlie disorders of arousal, most of the assessment considerations described in relation to sleepwalking also apply for sleep terrors. As has been shown with sleepwalking, the occurrence of sleep terrors in both children and adult populations can be secondary to sleep respiratory events, including obstructive sleep apnea and upper airway resistance syndrome, or other sleep disorders. Treatment of the precipitating sleep disorder may result in a disappearance of sleep terror episodes.

Prevalence and Developmental Aspects

Reported incidence estimates for sleep terrors are wide-ranging, partly due to important variations in the age range studied, sampling methods, and definitions used. Further, parents and patients may not differentiate between nightmares and sleep terrors. The overall prevalence of sleep terrors in children ranges from 1% to 18%, with a peak prevalence between ages 5 and 7 (Moreno, 2015; Petit et al., 2007, 2015). Persistent sleep terrors can be related to separation anxiety or other stressors, such as having one's parents divorce. One parent-based investigation (Nguyen et al., 2008) of 390 pairs of MZ and DZ twins assessed at 10 months and 30 months revealed a prevalence of sleep terrors of 36.9% at 18 months and 19.7% at 30 months, with no notable gender differences. By age 11, approximately 35% of children with sleep terrors will also experience episodes of somnambulism (Laberge et al., 2000). As is the case with somnambulism and confusional arousals, sleep terrors tend to resolve during adolescence and do not display a gender difference. The prevalence in the general adult population is about 2.2%, shows no significant gender differences, and declines gradually with age to about 1% at 65 years of age and older (Ohayon et al., 1999).

Treatment Options

The scheduled awakening technique, previously described for the management of sleepwalking, has also been shown to be effective in the treatment of sleep terrors in children. In adults, when the episodes are not associated with injury potential, treatment is often unnecessary. If a treatment is needed, the same pharmacological and non-pharmacological approaches as for somnambulism can be tried.

Conclusions

While the exact mechanisms which give rise to NREM parasomnias remain unclear, considerable progress has been made in documenting their associated factors and identifying key variables involved in their etiology. Although the precise mode of inheritance for disorders of arousal remains to be specified, a genetic contribution has been well documented, and compelling evidence indicates that disorders of arousal are related to a dysregulation in maintaining stable and consolidated NREM sleep. Continued work in the fields of genetics and PSG, including spectral analyses and the use of high-density EEG, likely represent the most promising venues to elucidate our understanding of these sleep disorders.

In addition, a growing body of work on phenomenological aspects of somnambulism and sleep terrors indicates that dreamlike conscious experiences are frequent during parasomnia episodes and may include rich perceptual, cognitive, and affective dimensions. Although these features are not systematically explored in clinical practice, they are so characteristic of these disorders that they may help in establishing the diagnosis of arousal disorders (Siclari et al., 2020).

Sleep research in recent decades has revealed that sleep is not a global phenomenon that uniformly affects all brain regions at the same time, but that instead it occurs and is regulated locally (Siclari & Tononi, 2017). Using appropriate neuroimaging techniques, it has become possible to relate regional patterns of brain activity to dream contents (Horikawa et al., 2013; Siclari et al., 2018). Although methodologically challenging, applying some of these noninvasive techniques to the study of sleepwalking not only may pave the way toward a better understanding of disorders of arousal, but hopefully will also clarify how local sleep patterns relate to changes in consciousness, environmental (dis) connection, and cognition (Siclari, 2024). A recent laboratory study for instance showed that confusional arousals associated with conscious experiences were preceded by similar local brain activity patterns as dreams in healthy individuals (Cataldi et al., 2024). Unlike most sleep disorders, the diagnosis of sleepwalking and sleep terrors is still primarily based on the patient's clinical history. The development of an investigative protocol that would allow researchers and clinicians to establish a PSG-based diagnosis for disorders of arousal remains central. This issue is especially important given the growing number of medico-legal cases of sleep-related violence. It appears particularly important in this context to go beyond standard sleep scoring, which simplifies sleep architecture in both the spatial as well as the temporal domains (only a few electrodes are typically used, and scoring is performed on long [30-second] epochs). A recent study focusing on sleep microstructure instead of macrostructure showed, for instance, that the presence of slow EEG activity during microarousals can help distinguish PSGs of sleepwalkers from those of healthy controls (Lopez et al., 2018).

Finally, while a variety of non-pharmacological as well as pharmacological treatments have been recommended for long-term management of somnambulism and sleep terrors, well-designed controlled clinical trials are needed to guide and support treatment decisions.

Future Directions

1. What role does NREM instability play in the pathophysiology of NREM parasomnias?
2. Why do common genetic and pathophysiological factors give rise to sleepwalking in some individuals and sleep terrors in others?
3. How do regional patterns of brain activity relate to conscious experiences associated with somnambulistic episodes and sleep terrors (degree of consciousness, hallucinations, amnesia, and environmental disconnection)?
4. Is the activation of arousal systems in NREM parasomnia episodes the cause (trigger) or the consequence of dreamlike experiences reported by patients?
5. Can a validated investigative protocol be developed that will allow researchers and clinicians to establish a PSG-based diagnosis for sleepwalking and sleep terrors?
6. What are the neurobiological predictors of pharmacological and non-pharmacological treatment responses in patients suffering from disorders of arousal?
7. To what extent can brain imaging and clinical trials help us understand possible neurotransmitter dysfunctions in NREM parasomnias?

References

American Academy of Sleep Medicine. (2014). *International classification of sleep disorders* (3rd ed.).

Andersen, M. L., Poyares, D., Alves, R. S., Skomro, R., & Tufik, S. (2007). Sexsomnia: Abnormal sexual behavior during sleep. *Brain Research Reviews, 56*(2), 271–282. https://doi.org/10.1016/j.brainresrev.2007.06.005

Barkwin, H. (1970). Sleepwalking in twins. *Lancet, 2*, 446–447.

Bassetti, C., Vella, S., Donati, F., Wielepp, P., & Weder, B. (2000). SPECT during sleepwalking. *Lancet, 356*(9228), 484–485. https://doi.org/10.1016/S0140-6736(00)02561-7

Blanchette-Carrière, C., Montplaisir, J., Boucetta, S., Desautels, A., & Zadra, A. (2024). Differential effects of sleep deprivation on sleepwalking: Role of demographic and clinical profiles. *Sleep medicine*, *121*, 144–150. https://doi.org/10.1016/j.sleep.2024.06.016

Broughton, R. J. (1968). Sleep disorders: Disorders of arousal? *Science*, *159*, 1070–1078.

Bruni, O., Ferri, R., Novelli, L., Finotti, E., Miano, S., & Guilleminault, C. (2008). NREM sleep instability in children with sleep terrors: The role of slow wave activity interruptions. *Clinical Neurophysiology*, *119*(5), 985–992. https://doi.org/10.1016/j.clinph.2008.01.015

Bušková, J., & Sonka, K. (2014). Adult NREM parasomnia associated with lancinating throat pain. *Journal of Clinical Sleep Medicine*, *10*(8), 925–926. https://doi.org/10.5664/jcsm.3974

Cartwright, R. (2004). Sleepwalking violence: A sleep disorder, a legal dilemma, and a psychological challenge. *American Journal of Psychiatry*, *161*(7), 1149–1158. http://www.ncbi.nlm.nih.gov/entrez/query.fcgi?cmd=Retrieve&db=PubMed&dopt=Citation&list_uids=15229043

Castelnovo, A., Loddo, G., Provini, F., Miano, S., & Manconi, M. (2021). Mental activity during episodes of sleepwalking, night terrors or confusional arousals: Differences between children and adults. *Nature and Science of Sleep*, *13*, 829–840. https://doi.org/10.2147/nss.S309868

Castelnovo, A., Lopez, R., Proserpio, P., Nobili, L., & Dauvilliers, Y. (2018). NREM sleep parasomnias as disorders of sleep-state dissociation. *Nature Reviews Neurology*, *14*(8), 470–481. https://doi.org/10.1038/s41582-018-0030-y

Cataldi, J., Stephan, A. M., Haba-Rubio, J., & Siclari, F. (2024). Shared EEG correlates between non-REM parasomnia experiences and dreams. *Nature Communications*, *15*, 3906. https://doi.org/10.1038/s41467-024-48337-7

Cataldi, J., Stephan, A. M., Marchi, N. A., Haba-Rubio, J., & Siclari, F. (2022). Abnormal timing of slow wave synchronization processes in non-rapid eye movement sleep parasomnias. *Sleep*, *45*(7), Article zsac111. https://doi.org/10.1093/sleep/zsac111

Chiba, Y., Phillips, O. R., Takenoshita, S., Ollila, H. M., Hallmayer, J. F., Nishino, S., & Singh, M. K. (2021). Genetic and demographic predisposing factors associated with pediatric sleepwalking in the Philadelphia Neurodevelopmental Cohort. *Journal of Neurological Sciences*, *430*, Article 119997. https://doi.org/10.1016/j.jns.2021.119997

Clé, M., Maranci, J. B., Weyn Banningh, S., Lanfranchi, J., Vidailhet, M., & Arnulf, I. (2019). Smiling asleep: A study of happy emotional expressions during adult sleep. *Journal of Sleep Research*, *28*(4), Article e12814. https://doi.org/10.1111/jsr.12814

Cramer Bornemann, M. A., & Mahowald, M. W. (2017). Legal topics in sleep medicine. In M. Kryger, T. Roth, & W. C. Dement (Ed.), *Principles and practice of sleep medicine* (6th ed., pp. 653–660). Elsevier.

Craske, M. G., & Tsao, J. C. (2005). Assessment and treatment of nocturnal panic attacks. *Sleep Medicine Reviews*, *9*(3), 173–184. https://doi.org/10.1016/j.smrv.2004.11.003

Dang-Vu, T. T., Zadra, A., Labelle, M. A., Petit, D., Soucy, J. P., & Montplaisir, J. (2015). Sleep deprivation reveals altered brain perfusion patterns in somnambulism. *PLOS ONE*, *10*(8), Article e0133474. https://doi.org/10.1371/journal.pone.0133474

Desautels, A., Zadra, A., Labelle, M. A., Dauvilliers, Y., Petit, D., & Montplaisir, J. (2013). Daytime somnolence in adult sleepwalkers. *Sleep Medicine*, *14*(11), 1187–1191. https://doi.org/10.1016/j.sleep.2013.04.029

Desjardins, M., Carrier, J., Lina, J. M., Fortin, M., Gosselin, N., Montplaisir, J., & Zadra, A. (2017). EEG functional connectivity prior to sleepwalking: Evidence of interplay between sleep and wakefulness. *Sleep*, *40*(4), Article zsx024. https://doi.org/10.1093/sleep/zsx024

Drakatos, P., Marples, L., Muza, R., Higgins, S., Gildeh, N., Macavei, R., Dongol, E. M., Nesbitt, A., Rosenzweig, I., Lyons, E., d'Ancona, G., Steier, J., Williams, A. J., Kent, B. D., & Leschziner, G. (2018). NREM parasomnias: A treatment approach based upon a retrospective case series of 512 patients. *Sleep Medicine*, *53*, 181–188. https://doi.org/10.1016/j.sleep.2018.03.021

Dubessy, A. L., Leu-Semenescu, S., Attali, V., Maranci, J. B., & Arnulf, I. (2017). Sexsomnia: A specialized non-REM parasomnia? *Sleep*, *40*(2), Article zsw043. https://doi.org/10.1093/sleep/zsw043

Durand, V. M., & Mindell, J. A. (1999). Behavioral intervention for childhood sleep terrors. *Behavior Therapy*, *30*(4), 705–715. https://doi.org/10.1016/S0005-7894(99)80034-3

Espa, F., Dauvilliers, Y., Ondze, B., Billiard, M., & Besset, A. (2002). Arousal reactions in sleepwalking and night terrors in adults: The role of respiratory events. *Sleep*, *25*(8), 871–875. https://www.ncbi.nlm.nih.gov/pubmed/12489893

Espa, F., Ondze, B., Deglise, P., Billiard, M., & Besset, A. (2000). Sleep architecture, slow wave activity, and sleep spindles in adult patients with sleepwalking and sleep terrors. *Clinical Neurophysiology, 111*(5), 929–939. https://doi.org/10.1016/s1388-2457(00)00249-2

Flamand, M., Herlin, B., Leu-Semenescu, S., Attali, V., Launois, C., & Arnulf, I. (2015). Choking during sleep: Can it be expression of arousal disorder? *Sleep Medicine, 16*(11), 1441–1447. https://doi.org/10.1016/j.sleep.2015.03.023

Fournier, S., Dauvilliers, Y., Warby, S. C., Labrecque, M., Zadra, A., Boucetta, S., El Gewely, M., Kaddioui, H., Lopez, R., Montplaisir, J. Y., Bareke, E., Tétreault, M., & Desautels, A. (2021). Does the adenosine deaminase (ADA) gene confer risk of sleepwalking? *Journal of Sleep Research, 31*(4), Article e13537. https://doi.org/10.1111/jsr.13537

Frank, N. C., Spirito, A., Stark, L., & Owens-Stively, J. (1997). The use of scheduled awakenings to eliminate childhood sleepwalking. *Journal of Pediatric Psychology, 22*(3), 345–353. https://doi.org/10.1093/jpepsy/22.3.345

Gau, S.-F., & Soong, W.-T. (1999). Psychiatric comorbidity of adolescents with sleep terrors or sleepwalking: A case–control study. *Australian & New Zealand Journal of Psychiatry, 33*(5), 734–739.

Gaudreau, H., Joncas, S., Zadra, A., & Montplaisir, J. (2000). Dynamics of slow-wave activity during the NREM sleep of sleepwalkers and control subjects. *Sleep, 23*(6), 755–760.

Goodwin, J. L., Kaemingk, K. L., Fregosi, R. F., Rosen, G. M., Morgan, W. J., Smith, T., & Quan, S. F. (2004). Parasomnias and sleep disordered breathing in Caucasian and Hispanic children—The Tucson children's assessment of sleep apnea study. *BMC Medicine, 2*(1), Article 14. https://doi.org/10.1186/1741-7015-2-14

Guilleminault, C., Kirisoglu, C., Bao, G., Arias, V., Chan, A., & Li, K. K. (2005). Adult chronic sleepwalking and its treatment based on polysomnography. *Brain, 128*(Pt. 5), 1062–1069.

Guilleminault, C., Kirisoglu, C., da Rosa, A. C., Lopes, C., & Chan, A. (2006). Sleepwalking, a disorder of NREM sleep instability. *Sleep Medicine, 7*(2), 163–170. https://doi.org/10.1016/j.sleep.2005.12.006

Guilleminault, C., Poyares, D., Aftab, F. A., & Palombini, L. (2001). Sleep and wakefulness in somnambulism: A spectral analysis study. *Journal of Psychosomatic Research, 51*(2), 411–416. https://doi.org/10.1016/s0022-3999(01)00187-8

Harris, M., & Grunstein, R. R. (2009). Treatments for somnambulism in adults: Assessing the evidence. *Sleep Medicine Reviews, 13*(4), 295–297. https://doi.org/10.1016/j.smrv.2008.09.003

Heidbreder, A., Stefani, A., Brandauer, E., Steiger, R., Kremser, C., Gizewski, E. R., Young, P., Poewe, W., Högl, B., & Scherfler, C. (2017). Gray matter abnormalities of the dorsal posterior cingulate in sleep walking. *Sleep Medicine, 36*, 152–155. https://doi.org/10.1016/j.sleep.2017.05.007

Hori, A., & Hirose, G. (1995). Twin studies on parasomnias. *Sleep Research Online, 24A*, Article 324.

Horikawa, T., Tamaki, M., Miyawaki, Y., & Kamitani, Y. (2013). Neural decoding of visual imagery during sleep. *Science, 340*(6132), 639–642. https://doi.org/10.1126/science.1234330

Howell, M. J., Schenck, C. H., & Crow, S. J. (2009). A review of nighttime eating disorders. *Sleep Medicine Reviews, 13*(1), 23–34. https://doi.org/10.1016/j.smrv.2008.07.005

Hublin, C., Kaprio, J., Partinen, M., Heikkila, K., & Koskenvuo, M. (1997). Prevalence and genetics of sleepwalking: A population-based twin study. *Neurology, 48*(1), 177–181.

Irfan, M., Schenck, C. H., & Howell, M. J. (2021). NonREM disorders of arousal and related parasomnias: An updated review. *Neurotherapeutics, 18*(1), 124–139. https://doi.org/10.1007/s13311-021-01011-y

Jaar, O., Pilon, M., Carrier, J., Montplaisir, J., & Zadra, A. (2010). Analysis of slow-wave activity and slow-wave oscillations prior to somnambulism. *Sleep, 33*(11), 1511–1516. https://doi.org/10.1093/sleep/33.11.1511

Jacobson, A., Kales, A., & Zweig, J. R. (1965). Somnambulism: All-night electroencephalographic studies. *Science, 148*, 975–977.

Januszko, P., Niemcewicz, S., Gajda, T., Wołyńczyk-Gmaj, D., Piotrowska, A. J., Gmaj, B., Piotrowski, T., & Szelenberger, W. (2016). Sleepwalking episodes are preceded by arousal-related activation in the cingulate motor area: EEG current density imaging. *Clinical Neurophysiology, 127*(1), 530–536. https://doi.org/10.1016/j.clinph.2015.01.014

Joncas, S., Zadra, A., Paquet, J., & Montplaisir, J. (2002). The value of sleep deprivation as a diagnostic tool in adult sleepwalkers. *Neurology, 58*(6), 936–940.

Kales, A., Soldatos, C. R., Bixler, E. O., Ladda, R. L., Charney, D. S., Weber, G., & Schweitzer, P. K. (1980). Hereditary factors in sleepwalking and night terrors. *British Journal of Psychiatry, 137*, 111–118.

Kales, A., Soldatos, C. R., Caldwell, A. B., Kales, J. D., Humphrey, F. J., 2nd, Charney, D. S., & Schweitzer, P. K. (1980). Somnambulism. Clinical characteristics and personality patterns. *Archives of General Psychiatry, 37*(12), 1406–1410.

Kales, J. D., Kales, A., Soldatos, C. R., Caldwell, A. B., Charney, D. S., & Martin, E. D. (1980). Night terrors. Clinical characteristics and personality patterns. *Archives of General Psychiatry, 37*(12), 1413–1417.

Kannape, O. A., Perrig, S., Rossetti, A. O., & Blanke, O. (2017). Distinct locomotor control and awareness in awake sleepwalkers. *Current Biology, 27*(20), R1102–R1104. https://doi.org/10.1016/j.cub.2017.08.060

Labelle, M. A., Dang-Vu, T. T., Petit, D., Desautels, A., Montplaisir, J., & Zadra, A. (2015). Sleep deprivation impairs inhibitory control during wakefulness in adult sleepwalkers. *Journal of Sleep Research, 24*(6), 658–665. https://doi.org/10.1111/jsr.12315

Labelle, M. A., Desautels, A., Montplaisir, J., & Zadra, A. (2013). Psychopathologic correlates of adult sleepwalking. *Sleep Medicine, 14*(12), 1348–1355. https://doi.org/10.1016/j.sleep.2013.05.023

Laberge, L., Tremblay, R. E., Vitaro, F., & Montplaisir, J. (2000). Development of parasomnias from childhood to early adolescence. *Pediatrics, 106*(1, Pt. 1), 67–74.

Lam, S. P., Fong, S. Y., Yu, M. W., Li, S. X., & Wing, Y. K. (2009). Sleepwalking in psychiatric patients: Comparison of childhood and adult onset. *Australian & New Zealand Journal of Psychiatry, 43*, 426–430. https://doi.org/10.1080/00048670902817703

Lecendreux, M., Bassetti, C., Dauvilliers, Y., Mayer, G., Neidhart, E., & Tafti, M. (2003). HLA and genetic susceptibility to sleepwalking. *Molecular Psychiatry, 8*(1), 114–117.

Ledard, N., Artru, E., Colmenarez Sayago, P., Redolfi, S., Golmard, J. L., Carrillo-Solano, M., & Arnulf, I. (2020). Adrenergic reactions during N3 sleep arousals in sleepwalking and sleep terrors: The chicken or the egg? *Journal of Sleep Research, 29*(6), Article e12946. https://doi.org/10.1111/jsr.12946

Lopez, R., Jaussent, I., & Dauvilliers, Y. (2014). Objective daytime sleepiness in patients with somnambulism or sleep terrors. *Neurology, 83*(22), 2070–2076. https://doi.org/10.1212/WNL.0000000000001019

Lopez, R., Jaussent, I., & Dauvilliers, Y. (2015). Pain in sleepwalking: A clinical enigma. *Sleep, 38*(11), 1693–1698. https://doi.org/10.5665/sleep.5144

Lopez, R., Shen, Y., Chenini, S., Rassu, A. L., Evangelista, E., Barateau, L., Jaussent, I., & Dauvilliers, Y. (2018). Diagnostic criteria for disorders of arousal: A video-polysomnographic assessment. *Annals of Neurology, 83*(2), 341–351. https://doi.org/10.1002/ana.25153

Merino, D., Gérard, A. O., Van Obberghen, E. K., Ben Othman, N., Ettore, E., Giordana, B., Viard, D., Rocher, F., Destere, A., Benoit, M., & Drici, M. D. (2022). Medications as a trigger of sleep-related eating disorder: A disproportionality analysis. *Journal of Clinical Medicine, 11*(13), Article 3890. https://doi.org/10.3390/jcm11133890

Moldofsky, H., Gilbert, R., Lue, F. A., & MacLean, A. W. (1995). Sleep-related violence. *Sleep, 18*(9), 731–739.

Montplaisir, J., & Demers, L. (1983). Le somnambulisme [Somnambulism]. *Union Medicale du Canada, 112*(7), 619–623.

Moreno, M. A. (2015). Sleep terrors and sleepwalking: Common parasomnias of childhood. *JAMA Pediatrics, 169*(7), Article 704. https://doi.org/10.1001/jamapediatrics.2014.2140

Nguyen, B. H., Perusse, D., Paquet, J., Petit, D., Boivin, M., Tremblay, R. E., & Montplaisir, J. (2008). Sleep terrors in children: A prospective study of twins. *Pediatrics, 122*(6), e1164–e1167. https://doi.org/10.1542/peds.2008-1303

Nobili, L., Ferrara, M., Moroni, F., De Gennaro, L., Russo, G. L., Campus, C., Cardinale, F., & De Carli, F. (2011). Dissociated wake-like and sleep-like electro-cortical activity during sleep. *Neuroimage, 58*(2), 612–619. https://doi.org/10.1016/j.neuroimage.2011.06.032

Ohayon, M. M., Guilleminault, C., & Priest, R. G. (1999). Night terrors, sleepwalking, and confusional arousals in the general population: Their frequency and relationship to other sleep and mental disorders. *Journal of Clinical Psychiatry, 60*(4), 268–276.

Ohayon, M. M., Mahowald, M. W., Dauvilliers, Y., Krystal, A. D., & Leger, D. (2012). Prevalence and comorbidity of nocturnal wandering in the U.S. adult general population. *Neurology, 78*(20), 1583–1589. https://doi.org/10.1212/WNL.0b013e3182563be5

Oliviero, A., Della Marca, G., Tonali, P. A., Pilato, F., Saturno, E., Dileone, M., Rubino, M., & Di Lazzaro, V. (2007). Functional involvement of cerebral cortex in adult sleepwalking. *Journal of Neurology, 254*(8), 1066–1072. https://doi.org/10.1007/s00415-006-0489-0

Oudiette, D., Constantinescu, I., Leclair-Visonneau, L., Vidailhet, M., Schwartz, S., & Arnulf, I. (2011). Evidence for the re-enactment of a recently learned behavior during sleepwalking. *PLOS ONE, 6*(3), Article e18056. https://doi.org/10.1371/journal.pone.0018056

Oudiette, D., Leu, S., Pottier, M., Buzare, M. A., Brion, A., & Arnulf, I. (2009). Dreamlike mentations during sleepwalking and sleep terrors in adults. *Sleep, 32*(12), 1621–1627.

Perrault, R., Carrier, J., Desautels, A., Montplaisir, J., & Zadra, A. (2014). Electroencephalographic slow waves prior to sleepwalking episodes. *Sleep Medicine, 15*(12), 1468–1472. https://doi.org/10.1016/j.sleep.2014.07.020

Petit, D., Pennestri, M. H., Paquet, J., Desautels, A., Zadra, A., Vitaro, F., Tremblay, R. E., Boivin, M., & Montplaisir, J. (2015). Childhood sleepwalking and sleep terrors: A longitudinal study of prevalence and familial aggregation. *JAMA Pediatrics, 169*(7), 653–658. https://doi.org/10.1001/jamapediatrics.2015.127

Petit, D., Touchette, E., Tremblay, R. E., Boivin, M., & Montplaisir, J. (2007). Dyssomnias and parasomnias in early childhood. *Pediatrics, 119*(5), e1016–e1025. https://doi.org/10.1542/peds.2006-2132

Pilon, M., Desautels, A., Montplaisir, J., & Zadra, A. (2012). Auditory arousal responses and thresholds during REM and NREM sleep of sleepwalkers and controls. *Sleep Medicine, 13*(5), 490–495. https://doi.org/10.1016/j.sleep.2011.10.031

Pilon, M., Montplaisir, J., Zadra, A., Pilon, M., Montplaisir, J., & Zadra, A. (2008). Precipitating factors of somnambulism: Impact of sleep deprivation and forced arousals. *Neurology, 70*(24), 2284–2290.

Pilon, M., Zadra, A., Joncas, S., & Montplaisir, J. (2006). Hypersynchronous delta waves and somnambulism: Brain topography and effect of sleep deprivation. *Sleep, 29*(1), 77–84. https://doi.org/10.1093/sleep/29.1.77

Pressman, M. R. (2004). Hypersynchronous delta sleep EEG activity and sudden arousals from slow-wave sleep in adults without a history of parasomnias: Clinical and forensic implications. *Sleep, 27*(4), 706–710.

Pressman, M. R. (2007). Factors that predispose, prime and precipitate NREM parasomnias in adults: Clinical and forensic implications. *Sleep Medicine Reviews, 11*(1), 5–30; discussion 31–33. https://doi.org/10.1016/j.smrv.2006.06.003

Pressman, M. R. (2019). The neurophysiological and neurochemical effects of alcohol on the brain are inconsistent with current evidence based models of sleepwalking. *Sleep Medicine Reviews, 43*, 92–95. https://doi.org/10.1016/j.smrv.2018.10.003

Pressman, M. R., Mahowald, M. W., Schenck, C. H., & Bornemann, M. C. (2007). Alcohol-induced sleepwalking or confusional arousal as a defense to criminal behavior: A review of scientific evidence, methods and forensic considerations. *Journal of Sleep Research, 16*(2), 198–212. https://doi.org/10.1111/j.1365-2869.2007.00586.x

Pressman, M. R., Mahowald, M., Schenck, C., Bornemann, M. C., Banerjee, D., Howell, M., Buchanan, P., & Avidan, A. (2014). Spectral EEG analysis and sleepwalking defense: Unreliable scientific evidence. *Journal of Clinical Sleep Medicine, 10*(1), 111–112. https://doi.org/10.5664/jcsm.3380

Pressman, M. R., Mahowald, M. W., Schenck, C. H., Bornemann, M. C., Montplaisir, J. Y., Zadra, A., Pilon, M., Grunstein, R., Buchanan, P. R., & Tachibana, N. (2009). Sleep-related automatism and the law. *Medicine, Science, and the Law, 49*(2), 139–143.

Scavone, G., Baril, A.-A., Montplaisir, J., Carrier, J., Desautels, A., & Zadra, A. (2021). Autonomic modulation during baseline and recovery sleep in adult sleepwalkers. *Frontiers in Neurology, 12*, Article 680596. https://doi.org/10.3389/fneur.2021.680596

Schenck, C. H., Arnulf, I., & Mahowald, M. W. (2007). Sleep and sex: What can go wrong? A review of the literature on sleep related disorders and abnormal sexual behaviors and experiences. *Sleep, 30*(6), 683–702.

Schenck, C. H., Boyd, J. L., & Mahowald, M. W. (1997). A parasomnia overlap disorder involving sleepwalking, sleep terrors, and REM sleep behavior disorder in 33 polysomnographically confirmed cases. *Sleep, 20*(11), 972–981. https://doi.org/10.1093/sleep/20.11.972

Schenck, C. H., Hurwitz, T. D., O'Connor, K. A., & Mahowald, M. W. (1993). Additional categories of sleep-related eating disorders and the current status of treatment. *Sleep, 16*(5), 457–466.

Schenck, C. H., & Mahowald, M. W. (1995). A polysomnographically documented case of adult somnambulism with long-distance automobile driving and frequent nocturnal violence: Parasomnia with continuing danger as a noninsane automatism? *Sleep, 18*(9), 765–772.

Schenck, C. H., & Mahowald, M. W. (2000). On the reported association of psychopathology with sleep terrors in adults. *Sleep, 23*(4), 1–2. https://doi.org/10.1093/sleep/23.4.1

Schenck, C. H., Milner, D. M., Hurwitz, T. D., Bundlie, S. R., & Mahowald, M. W. (1989). A polysomnographic and clinical report on sleep-related injury in 100 adult patients. *American Journal of Psychiatry, 146*(9), 1166–1173.

Schenck, C. H., Pareja, J. A., Patterson, A. L., & Mahowald, M. W. (1998). Analysis of polysomnographic events surrounding 252 slow-wave sleep arousals in thirty-eight adults with injurious sleepwalking and sleep terrors. *Journal of Clinical Neurophysiology, 15*(2), 159–166.

Siclari, F. (2024). Consciousness in non-REM parasomnia episodes. *Journal of Sleep Research, 1*, e14275. https://doi: 10.1111/jsr.14275

Siclari, F., Bernardi, G., Cataldi, J., & Tononi, G. (2018). Dreaming in NREM sleep: A high-density EEG study of slow waves and spindles. *Journal of Neuroscience, 38*(43), 9175–9185. https://doi.org/10.1523/JNEUROSCI.0855-18.2018

Siclari, F., Khatami, R., Urbaniok, F., Nobili, L., Mahowald, M. W., Schenck, C. H., Cramer Bornemann, M. A., & Bassetti, C. L. (2010). Violence in sleep. *Brain, 133*(Pt. 12), 3494–3509. https://doi.org/10.1093/brain/awq296

Siclari, F., & Tononi, G. (2017). Local aspects of sleep and wakefulness. *Current Opinion in Neurobiology, 44*, 222–227. https://doi.org/10.1016/j.conb.2017.05.008

Siclari, F., Valli, K., & Arnulf, I. (2020). Dreams and nightmares in healthy adults and in patients with sleep and neurological disorders. *Lancet Neurology, 19*(10), 849–859. https://doi.org/10.1016/s1474-4422(20)30275-1

Stallman, H. M., & Bari, A. (2017). A biopsychosocial model of violence when sleepwalking: Review and reconceptualisation. *BJPsych Open, 3*(2), 96–101. https://doi.org/10.1192/bjpo.bp.116.004390

Stallman, H. M., & Kohler, M. (2016). Prevalence of sleepwalking: A systematic review and meta-analysis. *PLOS ONE, 11*(11), Article e0164769. https://doi.org/10.1371/journal.pone.0164769

Stallman, H. M., Kohler, M., & White, J. (2018). Medication induced sleepwalking: A systematic review. *Sleep Medicine Reviews, 37*, 105–113. https://doi.org/10.1016/j.smrv.2017.01.005

Terzaghi, M., Sartori, I., Tassi, L., Didato, G., Rustioni, V., LoRusso, G., Manni, R., Nobili, L., Terzaghi, M., Sartori, I., Tassi, L., Didato, G., Rustioni, V., LoRusso, G., Manni, R., & Nobili, L. (2009). Evidence of dissociated arousal states during NREM parasomnia from an intracerebral neurophysiological study. *Sleep, 32*(3), 409–412.

Terzaghi, M., Sartori, I., Tassi, L., Rustioni, V., Proserpio, P., Lorusso, G., Manni, R., & Nobili, L. (2012). Dissociated local arousal states underlying essential clinical features of non-rapid eye movement arousal parasomnia: An intracerebral stereo-electroencephalographic study. *Journal of Sleep Research, 21*(5), 502–506. https://doi.org/10.1111/j.1365-2869.2012.01003.x

Winkelman, J. W. (1998). Clinical and polysomnographic features of sleep-related eating disorder. *Journal of Clinical Psychiatry, 59*(1), 14–19.

Winkelman, J. W., Herzog, D. B., & Fava, M. (1999). The prevalence of sleep-related eating disorder in psychiatric and non-psychiatric populations. *Psychological Medicine, 29*(6), 1461–1466. https://doi.org/10.1017/s0033291799008272

Zadra, A., Desautels, A., Petit, D., & Montplaisir, J. (2013). Somnambulism: Clinical aspects and pathophysiological hypotheses. *Lancet Neurology, 12*(3), 285–294. https://doi.org/10.1016/S1474-4422(12)70322-8

Zadra, A., Pilon, M., Desautels, A., & Montplaisir, J. (2019). Stress, dreams and sleep deprivation as precipitating factors for sleepwalking. *Sleep Medicine, 64*(S1), S436.

Zadra, A., Pilon, M., Joncas, S., Rompre, S., & Montplaisir, J. (2004). Analysis of postarousal EEG activity during somnambulistic episodes. *Journal of Sleep Research, 13*(3), 279–284.

Zadra, A., Pilon, M., Montplaisir, J., Zadra, A., Pilon, M., & Montplaisir, J. (2008). Polysomnographic diagnosis of sleepwalking: Effects of sleep deprivation. *Annals of Neurology, 63*(4), 513–519.

Zucconi, M., Oldani, A., Ferini-Strambi, L., & Smirne, S. (1995). Arousal fluctuations in non-rapid eye movement parasomnias: The role of cyclic alternating pattern as a measure of sleep instability. *Journal of Clinical Neurophysiology, 12*(2), 147–154.

CHAPTER

32 Circadian Rhythm Sleep–Wake Disorders I: Advanced and Delayed Phase Disorders

Leon C. Lack, Gorica Micic, *and* Nicole Lovato

Abstract

Delayed sleep–wake phase disorder (DSWPD) is debilitating and the most common circadian rhythm disorder. It is defined as having a sleep pattern delayed by at least 2–3 hours from conventional timing, with great difficulty sleeping at conventional sleep times despite the frequent desire to do so. It is assumed to be caused by a delay of the endogenous circadian rhythm. Although it has its own diagnostic criteria, it lies on a continuum spanning from intermediate to moderate and extreme evening chronotypes to DSWPD and to non-24-hour phase disorder. This continuum is mainly driven by endogenous circadian period length varying from just over 24 hours to an extreme of 25 hours. Behavioral, psychological, and societal variables also contribute to the difficulty adhering to conventional sleep times. The recent novel findings of many DSWPD patients who do not have a substantial circadian rhythm delay suggest the contribution of non-circadian factors to the intransigence of a late timed sleep period; there is considerable evidence of the association of mental and physical health risks with the apparent inability to synchronize with the earth's 24-hour period of rotation. Advanced sleep–wake phase disorder is defined as having a sleep pattern timed earlier than desired or conventional. Attempts to delay bedtime to a more conventional time are difficult and result in reduced total sleep time since wake times remain early. This condition is relatively rare, affecting 0.0%–0.33% of the population, and infrequently presents for treatment.

Key Words: sleep–wake phase, circadian rhythm disorder, sleep pattern, health risk, treatment, sleep time, circadian rhythm

Introduction

The subtitle of this chapter, "Advanced and Delayed Phase Disorders," lists two polar opposite circadian rhythm disorders. The intent of the title was for this second edition to update the same chapter from the first edition of the *Oxford Handbook of Sleep and Sleep Disorders*. Advanced sleep–wake phase disorder (ASWPD), as it is now titled, is distinguished by an earlier than normal or desired sleep pattern. Earlier than desired onset of sleepiness as well as earlier than desired final awakening from sleep are the major symptoms. For example, preferred sleep period may be from 11:00 p.m. to 7:00 a.m., but the individual struggles to stay awake beyond 9:00 p.m. and falls asleep quickly at early bedtimes (8:00–9:00 p.m.). Awakenings start occurring early in the morning, and a time is reached past which resuming sleep is very difficult and rare (e.g., 3:00–4:00 a.m.). Deliberately forcing oneself to stay awake until later, to delay sleep timing, usually does not result in a later wake time but results instead in reduced amount of sleep. Delayed sleep–wake phase disorder (DSWPD) presents the opposite problem, later than preferred sleep onset and wake-up times (e.g., 2:00 a.m. and 11:00 a.m.). Attempting a more conventional sleep timing (e.g., 11:00 p.m.–7:00 a.m.) results in a long time to fall asleep and reduced total sleep if a more conventional wake-up time is successfully enforced in order to meet social/work commitments.

Although the advanced and delayed phase disorders have equal weight in the title, they will not be given equal weight in this chapter. DSWPD will lead off and be the main focus. Compared to DSWPD, ASWPD is rare. In a large population survey (N = 7,700) more than 30 years ago, no one who participated in the survey fit the *International Classification of Sleep Disorders* (ICSD) definition of ASWPD (Schrader et al., 1993). More recently in the operation of a sleep disorders clinic over a 9-year period with 2,422 new patients, only 8 (0.33%) had indication of advanced sleep phase and only 1 (0.04%) met the full criteria of ASWPD (Curtis et al., 2019). Probably as a result of this rarity, there has been little investigation of ASWPD and few reports of treatment. The last clinical practice guidelines regarding ASWPD (Auger et al., 2015) could provide no new update on clinical treatments following the previous guidelines published in 2007 (Morgenthaler et al., 2007). We will include a short discussion of ASWPD at the end of the chapter. However, we will now deal with the more prevalent and debilitating DSWPD, sometimes referred to as *extreme evening types* or *night owls*.

The "Problems" With Night Owls

Owls are beautiful creatures with sensitive, piercing eyes and binocular vision. They fly silently at night to prey effectively on generally troublesome vermin, playing an important ecological role in the natural environment. We have no problem with them. However, there may be problems for the human sort of night owl. *Night owl* for the purposes of this article is simply a colloquialism for humans who spend much of their waking life at night. Another term for this group is *evening type* (Horne & Ősterberg, 1976). This group can be defined by their later-than-normal sleep–wake patterns. Typically evening types go to bed after midnight and tend to wake up late (after about 9:00 a.m., especially on weekends; Lack et al., 2009). Variability in their sleep timing is a distinguishing feature. If employed in a conventional 9:00 a.m. to 5:00 p.m. daytime job or a student in school, evening types struggle to get to sleep before midnight on weeknights (even if they go to bed earlier) and find it difficult to awake early enough in the morning to get to work/school on time. Usually, they experience some sleep loss on weeknights. On weekends or "free" days without early commitments, evening types tend to go to bed later but sleep in the next morning noticeably later (9:00 a.m. to noon). This "sleep-in" is partly to recover sleep lost on work/weeknights and because it coincides with the later timing of their "body clock." Evening types can adjust to night-shift work readily and are more commonly employed in the hospitality industry due to their preference to work during the late hours. Across holiday periods with reduced daytime commitments, evening types show a consistently late sleep period (e.g., 2:00 a.m.–10:00 a.m.) but usually an adequate amount and quality of sleep.

Evening types can also be distinguished by their attitudinal and behavioral preferences for different times across the day. They feel slow and lethargic and experience reduced competence in the first few hours after awakening. They feel progressively better across the waking hours, to reach their best feelings and productivity in the late evening, often in the last few hours before their intended bedtime (Kerkhof, 1998). Understandably they find the mornings aversive but evenings pleasurable. It is likely that behavioral choice to sleep late is reinforced by the avoidance of their typical morning aversive experiences, and delayed bedtime is reinforced by the prolongation of their rewarding evening times. Thus, behavioral tendencies and preferences are likely contributors to the late sleep patterns of evening types (Lovato et al., 2023).

Extending the evening wake period to a later time will expose evening types to phase-delaying evening light and exacerbate their already delayed circadian rhythms. In addition, sleeping in later given the opportunity on "free" or low-commitment days (e.g., weekends) will remove them from the phase-advancing effects of morning light, resulting in a net phase delay on those "sleep-in" mornings. This results in difficulties getting to sleep on Sunday and Monday nights and increased tiredness the following week (Taylor et al., 2008). This delay in the timing of sleep on weekends or "free days" has been termed *social jet lag* and is taken as an indicator of a delayed endogenous circadian rhythm (Roenneberg & Merrow, 2007).

Humans Are Diurnal

Owls (our feathered friends) are nocturnal animals whose evolution through natural selection has placed their optimal or adaptive period of wakefulness and activity during the night. Humans, on the other hand, evolved as diurnal animals, presumably because being wakeful during the day had advantages over being wakeful during the night. Our vision is not nearly as sensitive in the dark as that of owls or larger, potentially dangerous, human predators. Our hearing is not as sharp, nor smell as keen. We would be in danger of accident or attack if we roamed afield at night. Ancestors who were awake and active during the night would have been at a selective disadvantage and would have had lower survival chances. Probably for these reasons we have developed a mechanism to ensure that our ancestors did not prowl the plains of Africa at night. This mechanism ensured that our wakefulness occurred during the day and our necessary sleep occurred at night, opposite to the owl that is awake at night and sleeps during the day.

Body Clock Control of Sleep

The mechanism ensuring a wakeful day and night sleep is the circadian rhythm or "body clock." It can be illustrated in its operation by many different physiological and behavioral measures (Czeisler et al., 1980). Despite the generalization that humans are "warm-blooded" and maintain constant core body temperature, that is not strictly the case. When all other influences on body temperature (e.g., exercise, environmental temperature, sleep, meals, etc.) are removed, slight but regular 24-hour cyclic variations in core temperature remain (approximately 0.4°C). This is called the *endogenous circadian rhythm*. Circadian (*circa* = about, *dian* = day) rhythms are approximately 24 hours in period length, the time taken to complete one full cycle (e.g., from maximum value to minimum and back to the maximum value again). For example, in humans who sleep at conventional times at night (11:00 p.m.–7:00 a.m.) the endogenous core temperature rhythm reaches its maximum at about 7:00 p.m. and its minimum at about 5:00 a.m. (Dijk et al., 1992; Lack & Lushington, 1996). Virtually all other physiological measures taken across the 24-hour period also show endogenous circadian rhythms but not necessarily reaching maximum at the same time. For example, by instructions from the central clock (the suprachiasmatic nucleus in the hypothalamus of the brain), melatonin begins secreting into the bloodstream from the pineal gland in the brain about 1–2 hours before typical sleep onset. This time, referred to as the *dim light melatonin onset* (DLMO), is another commonly used marker for the timing of the circadian system. At whatever times these various measures reach their maximums, these times remain similar from day to day and stay synchronized with each other. A few examples are shown in Figure 32.1.

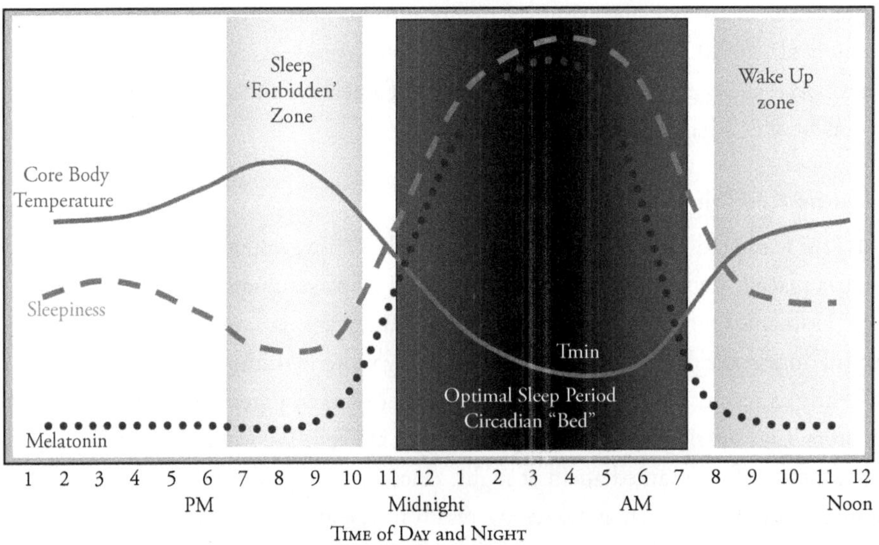

Figure 32.1 For a typical good sleeper regularly sleeping from about 11:00 p.m. to 7:00 a.m., three estimated circadian rhythms are illustrated: core body temperature, plasma or salivary melatonin concentration, and the circadian contribution to sleepiness or sleep propensity. Note that the optimal circadian sleep period is bracketed by two alert zones: the sleep "forbidden" zone in the early evening and the "wake-up" zone in the late morning.

This whole complex of circadian rhythms has a strong influence on the times across the 24-hour period when we are most alert and other times most sleepy (Lack & Lushington, 1996). The rhythms in the conventionally timed sleeper (11:00 p.m.–7:00 a.m.) create the time of maximum alertness between about 6:00 and 9:00 p.m. and the time of maximum sleepiness about 4:00 to 6:00 a.m. (Gradisar & Lack, 2004). However, in the evening type ("night owl") the rhythms are delayed, with maximum alertness around 9:00 p.m.–midnight and maximum sleepiness about 9:00–11:00 a.m. (Lack et al., 2009).

Critical Role of Circadian Rhythm Period Length

If evening types are late sleepers because of a late timed (delayed) circadian rhythm, how does the circadian rhythm become delayed from conventional timing? One answer to this question involves the period length of circadian rhythms. Implied by the term *circadian*, the period length is about 24 hours. This means that they cycle at about the same rate as the rotation of the earth, allowing our sleep–wake pattern to synchronize with night/day alternation. However, *about* is the critical word here. They are not exactly 24 hours in length. Several laboratory studies have carefully measured the endogenous circadian period length of normally entrained good sleepers (sleeping well at conventional times) compared to those with circadian rhythm disorders. In good sleepers the average period length is about 24.2 hours, ranging from 23.9 to 24.4 hours (Duffy et al., 2001). If this is extrapolated to the general population, it appears that most of us have intrinsic circadian period lengths slightly longer than 24 hours, and very few have exactly 24 hours or shorter. In the study above only 1 out of 17 healthy young men (6%) had a period length of less than 24 hours, and he was the most morning type in the sample. This means that most of us would tend to start the next circadian cycle a little bit later (0.2 hours or 12 minutes) each day and, therefore, have a slight tendency to become delayed with respect to the official clock time based on the earth's precise 24-hour rotation. It turns out that evening types have a longer period length at 24.3 hours (Duffy et al., 2001). Therefore, evening types have a tendency to delay about 18 minutes each day rather than 12 minutes, making the weekend "sleep-in," although helpful in paying off sleep debt, a strongly phase-delaying effect exacerbating their already delayed rhythms (Taylor et al., 2008).

Recently our research studies measured the intrinsic period lengths of both the melatonin and core body temperature rhythms in those with DSWPD compared with normal good sleepers (Micic et al., 2016). The point at which the amount of delay becomes a disorder rather than just a normal evening type person is somewhat arbitrary and dependent on how difficult it is to shift back earlier to more conventional sleeping hours and the impact of the delay on the individual's daily functioning. We found longer circadian period lengths in sufferers of DSWPD (Micic et al., 2016). They had circadian period lengths averaging 24.5 hours. In other words, they tend to delay 30 minutes each day. Presumably that more extreme tendency to delay contributes to their later sleep times and greater difficulty shifting back to a more conventionally timed sleep–wake pattern.

In summary, evening types have longer than normal intrinsic circadian rhythm period lengths, and those with DSWPD, whose sleep pattern is even later, have even longer period lengths. Therefore, having a longer than normal circadian period length with a stronger than normal tendency to delay with respect to the 24-hour earth's rotation would be an obvious contributor to their delayed sleep–wake pattern and the difficulties associated with trying to align with societal norms.

Changing the Timing of the "Body Clock"

The good news is that the timing of the circadian rhythm can be altered, a bit like resetting our clocks by an hour when we go onto or come off daylight savings time each year. Considerable research has shown that the strongest circadian clock resetting tool (*zeitgeber*) in humans is the visual exposure to light at appropriate times (Czeisler et al., 1989; Dawson et al., 1993). The mechanism by which retinal light stimulation has direct effects on the timing of the circadian clock is well understood (for a recent review, see Blume et al., 2019). The duration, intensity, and wavelength of the light all affect the strength of rhythm retiming. But probably the most important feature of the light is the circadian phase during which the light is presented (Duffy & Czeisler, 2009). Briefly, if light is presented at, or just before, one's normal wake-up time (around the time of the core body temperature minimum and for 1–3 hours after that), the effect will be to shift the timing earlier (phase advance) by as much as 10–100 minutes depending on intensity (>200 lux more effective), duration (longer more effective), and wavelength (blue/green more effective than amber/red; H. R. Wright et al., 2004). To maintain a stable, albeit later timed, circadian rhythm and not continue to drift later in clock time, an evening type must effectively phase-advance about 18 minutes each day, and those with DSWPD phase-advance about 30 minutes each day. Presumably they can do this by getting exposed to enough ambient light in the late morning and middle of the day when ambient light is likely to be at its peak. The previously mentioned study of DSWPD individuals also found a subsample of people ($n = 4$) whose sleep timing tended to drift later every day (non-24-hour circadian disorder; Micic et al., 2016). This subsample of people had circadian period lengths of about 25 hours. To retain a stable sleep–wake pattern they would have to phase-advance about an hour each day, which was presumably beyond the capacity of their daily light exposure to achieve.

In a premodern environment, before the advent of bright indoor lighting, our experience of light was more determined by the natural light/dark cycle (i.e., sunlight during the day and relatively dark at night with only low-intensity, orange-rich light from a candle or fire). This had the effect of strongly entraining our circadian rhythms and corralling our sleep period into the night. Unavoidable exposure to outdoor light in the morning would put the brakes on the tendency for our rhythms to drift later and tend to push our sleep period back into the night. Light in the late afternoon/early evening would delay any early timed rhythm into the night. An experiment that exposed young adults to a premodern lighting environment (summertime camping out in the mountains) found their circadian rhythms phase-advanced by about 2 hours, especially for those who were evening types. At their mountain camp the young adults slept well from 11:00 p.m. to 7:00 a.m. when compared to their delayed sleep timing of 12:30–8:00 a.m. at home (K. P. Wright et al., 2013). The fact that the timing of our sleep period is in the last half of the dark night period, even when camping out with no appreciable light in the evening, probably arises from the longer-than-24-hour period length of our circadian rhythm that allows our body clock timing and sleep period to drift later into the night until it meets the morning light at sunrise. In our modern environment, evening electric light exposure and the ability to extend sleep in the morning in a quiet, darkened bedroom will result in taking the "brakes off" the tendency to delay. This results in the delay of our body clocks on the order of 30–50 minutes over a weekend of sleep-ins (Taylor et al., 2008; K. P. Wright et al., 2013; Yang et al., 2001). This will, however, reignite the difficulty faced by evening types in getting to sleep Sunday night early enough to get adequate sleep before the start of the next working week.

The Puzzling "Non-Circadian" DSWPD

Extensive circadian research has established that for normally entrained, good sleepers the evening "sleep-forbidden-zone" (Lavie, 1986) of the circadian system inhibiting sleep onset is timed to end at about the typical DLMO time and 8 hours before the endogenous minimum of core body temperature, Tmin. These normal phase angles are also evident in typical DSWPD patients with comparable delays of 3–4 hours in endogenous circadian timing, the endogenous sleep propensity rhythm, and typical sleep times. However, this arrangement is not true for all those who are clinically diagnosed with DSWPD on the basis of delayed sleep pattern. There are patients who do not exhibit this expected delay in the endogenous circadian rhythms and, therefore, have been termed *non-circadian* DSWPD. They have been found in 33%–56% of carefully diagnosed clinical samples (Micic et al., 2021; Murray et al., 2017; Sletten et al., 2018). In these non-circadian patients the timing of their endogenous melatonin and core body temperature rhythms is within the normal range of normally entrained good sleepers. However, their typical sleep times and endogenous sleep propensity rhythms are about 3 hours later than would be normally expected according to their endogenous circadian rhythms (Micic et al., 2021). These non-circadian DSWPD patients apparently do not feel sleepy nor can they fall asleep until 4 hours after their DLMO (instead of 2 hours for good sleepers) and just 4 hours before their Tmin instead of 6 hours normally.

Non-circadian DSWPD patients' sleep timing may still be governed by their circadian rhythms, just timed at a later circadian phase than normal. Therefore, the label *non-circadian* may be a misnomer; they simply may have a later phase angle (i.e., greater delay of sleep propensity rhythm relative to circadian rhythms).

The clinical implications for treatment are important. Firstly, if these patients are, indeed, circadian-determined DSWPD, they may be treatable with the same chronobiologic tools recommended for "circadian" DSWPD (e.g., morning bright light, early evening low-dose melatonin, etc.). Whether their circadian timing can be affected by these chronobiologic tools needs to be tested. Secondly, whether the timing of the phase–response curves for these tools has the same relationship to their endogenous circadian measures or, instead, to their relatively delayed sleep–wake cycle is a fascinating and important clinical question that needs investigation. The phase–response curve, showing the magnitude and direction of phase change to a pulse of light in normally entrained good sleepers, on the average, shows an inflection point close to the timing of the nadir of the core body temperature rhythm, Tmin, determining the change from delay to advance (Czeisler et al., 1989; Dawson et al., 1993). Only a few hours' difference in the timing of the light from 2–3 hours before Tmin to 1–3 hours following Tmin results in the maximum phase delay or the maximum phase advance, respectively, of the endogenous circadian rhythm. The optimal light treatment for "circadian" DSWPD, based on the average response in samples of normally entrained people would administer a high-intensity 2–3-hour light pulse weighted to the blue end of the visible light spectrum starting from about the typical wake time on commitment days (weekdays) of 9:00 a.m. at about their Tmin. In non-circadian DSWPD if the phase–response curve inflection point is also at Tmin, optimal phase-advance would be achieved with the light pulse beginning in the middle of the typical sleep period when Tmin occurs. However, if the inflection point is relative to the typical sleep period, optimal phase-advance treatment would result from the light pulse administered 4 hours later. In this case a light pulse in the middle of the sleep period could produce a counterproductive maximal phase-delay and worsen the disorder. Therefore, effective treatment of these common non-circadian DSWPD patients requires the establishment of their phase–response curve to light. Is it linked to their endogenous circadian rhythm as the normal phase–response curve or to their delayed sleep–wake pattern or nonexistent?

Recently, an international group of circadian rhythm clinical researchers (Abbott et al., 2023) suggested a "neutral terminology" of DSWPD *Type 1* and *Type 2* instead of *circadian* and *non-circadian*, respectively. This is to acknowledge that the circadian system is multidimensional, and at present we have "limited understanding of the heterogeneity of the pathophysiology of DSWPD" (Abbott et al., 2023). For example, in addition to the likely role of longer circadian period length elaborated above, they point out apparently contradictory evidence of both an increased light sensitivity in DSWPD, especially Type 1, and a decreased melanopic light sensitivity, particularly in more extreme DSWPD with a tendency to "free run" (non-24-hour circadian rhythm sleep wake disorder). Since those with non-24-hour disorder appear to have an even longer period length than those with DSWPD (Micic et al., 2021), their increased tendency to delay is less controlled by a reduced melanopic light sensitivity to light following awakenings, thus leading more frequently to free-running. In the spirit of this commentary (Abbott et al., 2023), this speculation about DSWPD phenotypes needs to be resolved by further research on the circadian sensitivity to light pulses, as suggested above, by studies to establish the phase–response curves for these DSWPD Types 1 and 2. These will be challenging and expensive studies but ultimately definitive for determining the most effective chronobiologic treatment for clinically diagnosed DSWPD.

Another recent report (Lack et al., 2023) has also suggested significant comorbidity between DSWPD and conditioned sleep-onset insomnia. Sleep-onset insomnia becomes conditioned from frequent experiences of frustration and anxiety associated with unsuccessful attempts initiating sleep when earlier than normal bedtimes are attempted, as on weeknights. This sleep-onset insomnia may at least partly explain the DSWPD Type 2 arising more from a behavioral/psychological factor than a delayed circadian rhythm. Of course, the resultant delayed exposure to evening light and morning light from sleeping in on the weekends is likely to delay circadian rhythms and is consistent with some small delay evident in Type 2 DSWPD compared with normal entrained good sleepers (Micic et al., 2021).

Evidence of Problems With Eveningness

Eveningness has been associated with a myriad of problems and challenges, namely poor mental health and impacts on physical health and lifestyle. In addition to difficulties with sleep initiation leading to insufficient sleep and daytime impairments, eveningness is associated with poorer mental health outcomes (increased depression, anxiety, bipolar disorder, seasonal affective disorder, psychotic disorders, addictive disorders, attention-deficit/hyperactivity disorder, and eating disorders), academic and occupational challenges, unhealthy lifestyle behaviors, and chronic health conditions (Dewald et al., 2010; Hasler et al., 2012; Nagane et al., 2011; Partonen, 2023; Preckel et al., 2011; Toomey et al., 2015). These associations may be due to the misalignment between the internal biological clock and societal demands, leading to chronic sleep deprivation and disruption of circadian rhythms (Antypa et al., 2016; Merikanto et al., 2015; Park et al., 2015). Some studies have identified genetic variants associated with eveningness that are also linked to an increased risk of depression (Toomey et al., 2015). However, more research is needed to fully understand the complex relationship between genetics, chronotype, and depression.

Anxiety disorders are also linked with eveningness whereby physiological arousal, measured by increased heart rate and systolic blood pressure and decreased heart rate variability, is increased in night owls, both at rest and during acute stress (Roeser et al., 2012). Irregularity of melatonin rhythms (i.e., circadian misalignment) has also been associated with psychosomatic complaints, including anxiety (Nagane et al., 2011).

Circadian misalignment and psychiatric problems overlap, likely due to negative thinking patterns, rumination, and overthinking linked with both. When individuals with eveningness experience sleep problems, they may have more extended periods of rumination during the evening while attempting sleep onset, thus exacerbating their symptoms. People with an eveningness preference also might experience higher levels of stress due to difficulties in adapting to early-morning schedules or feeling out of sync with societal expectations. This increased stress can contribute to the development or exacerbation of anxiety symptoms which are characterized by an overamplification of the threat and an underappraisal of one's own ability to cope. Contributing to this stress, eveningness may impact social interactions and relationships whereby social jet lag and misalignment can lead to feelings of isolation or difficulty in maintaining social connections, potentially contributing to aggravation of psychiatric difficulties through lack of social supports (Walsh et al., 2022).

Correlational studies suggest a link between eveningness and various physical health conditions, namely metabolic disorders and cardiovascular health. Some studies have found associations between eveningness and an increased risk of metabolic disorders such as obesity, Type 2 diabetes, and metabolic syndrome. Cardiovascular health, including hypertension, cardiovascular disease, and adverse cardiac events, has been linked with eveningness (Partonen, 2023). A recent population study confirmed elevated cardiovascular and metabolic disease markers associated with evening chronotypes and those with social jet lag (Sladek et al., 2023). It is hypothesized that the misalignment between the internal circadian rhythm and social/environmental factors may disrupt metabolic processes and contribute to these health issues. Sleep disturbances, including inadequate sleep duration and poor sleep quality, often experienced by evening types, can also contribute to these associations. Reduced physical activity may also be contributing to these physical health issues. Evening types tend to be less physically active, report poorer perceived health in general, and have a lower tolerance threshold to pain compared to morning and intermediate types (Jankowski, 2013).

Personality differences, namely increased neuroticism and lower conscientiousness, might predispose individuals to eveningness and altered unhelpful thinking patterns and behaviors that lead to challenges (Futenma et al., 2023; Micic et al., 2017; Wilhelmsen-Langeland et al., 2014). DSWPD patients score higher on scales of neuroticism and significantly lower on conscientiousness, extraversion, and agreeableness compared to normal sleepers. As an extension of these findings, Micic et al. (2017) found a continuum in virtually all these personality dimensions from normal controls, Type 2 DSWPD (non-circadian), and Type 1 DSWPD to non-24-hour sleep–wake disorder (N24SWD). Furthermore, greater circadian and sleep phase delays were highly correlated with the psychological measures of neuroticism, introversion, less agreeableness, and less conscientiousness as well as higher depression scores on depression, anxiety, and stress scales (Micic et al., 2017). These findings form the view that instead of circadian delay and psychological impairments being independent in our DSWPD sample, they lay on a continuum of DSWPD severity reflected in sleep delay, circadian delay, psychological impairments, and distress.

These findings raise important questions regarding the development of the sleep disorder and specific traits. That is, do personality characteristics lead to poor sleep behaviors (e.g., low conscientiousness leading to procrastination of bedtime and wake time) and eventually to more extreme eveningness and DSWPD, or does the development of eveningness and DSWPD arise more from endogenous circadian factors (e.g., longer period lengths) and subsequently lead to the development of these personality traits? Qualitative studies indicate that individuals' sleeping difficulties could have implications for their self-image as society tends to consider individuals with delayed sleep characteristics as being "lazy" and "unmotivated." Perhaps through uncertainty, self-blame, and self-defeat, patients take on this identity in response to their problems (Micic et al., 2017; Van den Berg et al., 2018; Wilhelmsen-Langeland et al., 2014). Future prospective studies of the development of eveningness, DSWPD, and N24SWD and the outcomes of treatment studies are necessary to understand the bidirectionality of circadian rhythms and mental health/personality factors.

Given consistent personality differences between evening types and intermediate types, assessment of personality factors may be warranted to implement appropriate therapies and develop effective long-term treatments for those with varying degrees of the tendency to fall behind the timing of earth's rotation (evening types, DSWPD, and N24SWD).

Not surprisingly, the timing misalignment experienced by night owls can also have negative consequences in academic and occupational settings. Studies have found that eveningness is associated with lower academic performance, increased school dropout rates, and decreased work productivity (Dewald et al., 2010). A meta-analysis of cognitive ability and academic performance found consistently worse academic achievement and performance in evening types than morning types (Preckel et al., 2011). These difficulties may arise from suboptimal functioning and alertness during early-morning classes or work shifts, which are typically designed to cater to morning-oriented individuals. Lower academic performance may also arise from a generally reduced ability to attend and remember information because of chronic sleep loss, particularly on week (school) days (Lack, 1986). The previously mentioned mental and physical health problems would also contribute to impaired academic performance (Preckel et al., 2011). Interestingly, the same meta-analysis suggests that the lower academic performance of evening types does not come from lower cognitive ability. If anything, the evening types showed somewhat higher intelligence and cognitive ability. This suggests that evening types underachieve for their ability and holds the promise that if the circadian rhythms and sleeping patterns of evening types can be normalized with treatment, their academic success and other psychological difficulties may be substantially improved.

It is important to note that while eveningness may be associated with increased problems and challenges in some individuals, it does not mean that all evening-oriented people will experience problems or that these problems are exclusive to evening types. Often, these challenges are complex and multifactorial conditions influenced by various biological, genetic, environmental, and psychological factors. Additionally, eveningness is not inherently negative as it may offer advantages in certain situations, such as creative work or evening-oriented activities and permanent night shift, especially in the context of our modern 24/7 society.

Possible Role of Inadequate Sleep?

Inadequate sleep when forced morning awakenings are necessary is a prominent feature of DSWPD (Merikanto et al., 2015). Lack of sufficient sleep can have a range of negative effects on cognitive functioning, mood, attention, and overall well-being (Saxvig et al., 2013; Wilhelmsen-Langeland et al., 2019). Objective measures of sleep such as actigraphy and polysomnography show that individuals with DSWPD often have a delayed timing of sleep onset, resulting in a shorter total sleep time when they need to wake up early. This delayed sleep onset can lead to insufficient sleep duration and partial sleep deprivation, which can further exacerbate the disorder. Chronic sleep deprivation may also have long-term health consequences, including an increased risk of cardiovascular diseases, metabolic disorders, and mental health issues.

Successful implementation of chronobiologic treatments (e.g., chrono- and bright light therapy) that aim to reset the circadian rhythm to a more conventional pattern often results in improved sleep onset and duration. This indicates that the inadequate sleep experienced by individuals with DSWPD is a consequence of the misalignment of their circadian rhythm. Whether this treatment to rectify their circadian timing and improve total sleep time will eventually ameliorate the behavioral, personality, and social/psychological difficulties associated with DSWPD remains an important empirical question (Richardson et al., 2018).

DSWPD Treatment Effects

The primary goal of treatment for DSWPD is to help individuals establish a more desired, earlier-timed sleep–wake schedule that aligns with their daily activities, allows more adequate total sleep, and improves daytime function and their quality of life. While treatment approaches can be successful at shifting sleep temporarily or more permanently to a desired sleep time, the effectiveness varies among individuals.

Treatments of light therapy, chronotherapy, sleep schedule adjustment, and evening melatonin administration can help shift the sleep–wake pattern. Successful treatment of DSWPD can help ameliorate the problems associated with eveningness. By aligning sleep timing with the desired schedule, individuals may experience improved total sleep time and daytime functioning (e.g., greater alertness in the morning, better academic or work performance, and enhanced overall well-being; Merikanto et al., 2015; Richardson et al., 2018). Treatment can also benefit comorbid conditions such as depression, anxiety, or other mental health issues that may be exacerbated by DSWPD (Coleman & Cain, 2019; Kivela et al., 2018; Van den Berg et al., 2018; Walsh et al., 2022). There is evidence that bright light therapy for DSWPD shifts self-reported scores on the Morningness–Eveningness Questionnaire toward morningness (Burgess et al., 2018). However, the ability to maintain the shifted schedule long-term may depend on various factors, including individual preferences, personality characteristics (e.g., conscientiousness), lifestyle, and environmental/social constraints.

The response to treatment and the ability to shift to an intermediate sleep preference can vary among individuals. Factors such as the severity of DSWPD, adherence to treatment recommendations, individual biological characteristics (e.g., circadian period length), and external factors (e.g., social commitments, work or school requirements) can influence the success of treatment outcomes. Some individuals may achieve long-term changes in sleep timing, but relapse is common. Relapse prevention may require ongoing management or adjustments to maintain the desired sleep–wake schedule (Micic et al., 2019). Treatment should be tailored to individual needs, considering their preferences, lifestyle, and specific challenges.

Other Treatments for DSWPD

Established by considerable research evidence, morning bright light and early-evening melatonin administration, based on their zeitgeber strengths, are the two most recommended treatments for advancing the circadian rhythms of DSWPD. However, for more extreme delay cases of DSWPD (including N24SWD), an opposite strategy has been recommended with some clinical success. Chronotherapy was first suggested by Czeisler et al. (1981) and Weitzman et al. (1981) for the treatment of delayed sleep phase syndrome and consisted of delaying six or seven consecutive bedtimes by 3 hours on each occasion until the target sleep timing is achieved. At that point the patient is to keep a consistent lights-out time and lights-on wake time in the mornings. A follow-up case series also suggested its efficacy (Ito et al., 1993). However, these early studies had small numbers of patients and no control or comparison conditions and were resource-intensive in order to monitor adherence either in the laboratory/hospital or at home. The most recent clinical practice guidelines (Auger et al. 2015) did not mention chronotherapy for DSWPD for lack of any further research. New technology including wearable devices and nearable sensors with mobile phone apps to relay daily information of sleep timing to clinicians may make it more feasible to restart much needed research into the efficacy of chronotherapy for DSWPD.

In addition to recommended chronotherapeutic treatments, more recent evidence and clinical observations suggest that cognitive behavioral therapy for insomnia (CBT-I) as an adjunct therapy can be beneficial for individuals with DSWPD (Gradisar et al., 2011; Richardson et al., 2016). CBT-I is a non-pharmacological approach that focuses on addressing the underlying behavioral and cognitive factors contributing to insomnia and sleep-related issues. Several case studies and clinical reports have described positive outcomes with CBT-I in individuals with DSWPD. These reports suggest that CBT-I techniques, such as sleep schedule adjustment, stimulus control therapy, and sleep hygiene education, can help shift the sleep–wake schedule to a more desired timing and improve overall sleep quality.

Although limited in number, some small-scale studies have explored the effectiveness of CBT-I in DSWPD. These studies have demonstrated promising results in terms of improving sleep timing, sleep quality, and daytime functioning. For example, CBT-I led to significant improvements in sleep onset latency, sleep efficiency, and total sleep time in adolescents with DSWPD (Gradisar et al., 2011).

Some studies have examined the combination of CBT-I with other interventions, such as bright light therapy or chronotherapy, for the treatment of DSWPD (Danielsson et al., 2016; Gradisar et al., 2011). These integrated approaches have shown positive outcomes in terms of advancing sleep–wake timing and improving overall sleep parameters. Guidelines often recommend CBT-I as a potential treatment option for DSWPD. While the evidence base for CBT-I in DSWPD is still emerging, there are clearly potential benefits of applying CBT-I techniques to help individuals with DSWPD adjust their sleep–wake schedules and improve sleep quality (Danielsson et al., 2016; Gradisar et al., 2011; Micic et al., 2019; Wilhelmsen-Langeland et al., 2014).

While light and melatonin administration have a substantial evidence base as circadian zeitgebers, other possible zeitgebers seem to be emerging. Establishing consistent mealtimes and a regular eating pattern may help synchronize the body's internal clock and promote better sleep–wake regulation. Some studies suggest that carefully timed intake of caffeine may help regulate circadian rhythms (Burke et al., 2015), which could be beneficial for individuals with DSWPD. However, these studies are not specific to DSWPD and include a variety of participants with different sleep patterns. Further experimental trials testing their zeitgeber strength are sorely needed. Stimulants such as caffeine, nicotine, and alcohol can interfere with sleep quality and disrupt circadian rhythms. Individuals with DSWPD may be more sensitive to the effects of these substances and may have a preference for them in the latter part of the day. Limiting or avoiding their consumption in the latter half of the day, especially in the evening or close to bedtime, may help promote better sleep and improve overall sleep–wake patterns.

While the timing of food, exercise, and stimulants can be beneficial for managing DSWPD, it is important to note that these are not first-line or stand-alone treatments. These strategies should be part of a comprehensive approach that includes other established interventions; a comprehensive, tailored approach that includes appropriate sleep–wake scheduling, light exposure, melatonin administration, and other behavioral interventions should, at this stage, be the primary focus for treating DSWPD.

ASWPD

Although this is classed as one of the circadian sleep–wake disorders, it may be misleading to consider it a "disorder." It is defined as earlier than desired or conventional sleep onset and wake times. Should we attach the label *disorder* to a difficulty with matching our desired sleep times or failure to conform to the conventional or average sleep times? If it results in losing sleep and suffering the daytime effects of chronic partial sleep deprivation, such is often the case with DSWPD, the term *disorder* would be more appropriate. However, loss of sleep is usually not experienced in ASWPD unless bedtime is delayed to a much later time than normal for that person (e.g., 11:00 p.m.) but wake-up time still occurs soon after their normal wake time (e.g., 5:00 a.m.). Their desire to stay up later than normal may be motivated by social or entertainment reasons and be understandable, but should their difficulty in doing so be considered a disorder in the sense of it being a pathology that should be treated? Nevertheless, if we have tools that can address conditions that people have considered to be a difficulty for them, the information about these tools can readily be shared. Our main point in raising this "diagnostic" or definition issue is to depathologize the condition and discuss ways in which the timing of our body's circadian rhythms can be manipulated, not just to treat a "disorder" but to maximize well-being and quality of life.

The latest practice parameters for circadian sleep disorders (Auger et al., 2015) noted the lack of additional research on ASWPD since the previous practice parameters (Morgenthaler et al., 2007) and that the earlier publication had included studies of individuals who did not strictly meet the diagnostic criteria for ASWPD. Yet, as Morgenthaler et al. (2007) note, the amount of phase-advance of the sleep period compared to desired or normal required to meet the ASWPD criteria, especially given its rarity, can be relaxed if a suspected phase-advance of circadian rhythm is causing some sleep impairment. This seems to be the case in some studies of those with sleep maintenance insomnia, especially early morning awakening insomnia in which sleep is terminated spontaneously well before intended with consequent inadequate total sleep amount (Campbell et al., 1993; Lack & Wright, 1993; Lack et al., 2005). These studies found a conventional bedtime (e.g., 11:00 p.m.) but an early final wake time (e.g., 5:00 a.m.) with inability to resume sleep. Generally, these studies found earlier than normal circadian phase markers, suggesting that, before treatment, the early termination of sleep may have arisen from the early timed circadian rhythm. All three studies used evening bright light therapy and found improvements in total sleep time and efficiency with significant phase-delays of circadian markers.

Although these patients would not have met the ASWPD criteria requiring an advanced sleep onset time, their sleep disorder appeared to arise from an advanced circadian rhythm, which, when delayed by evening bright light treatment, resulted in improvements of sleep and daytime functioning. A more appropriate disorder classification may be *advanced circadian rhythm phase difficulties*. At present, it seems that if an advanced circadian individual succumbs to early sleepiness and has a bedtime earlier than 8:00 p.m. but gets adequate sleep by spontaneous awakening at 3:00 a.m., they meet the criterion of ASWPD. However, if they manage to stay awake until 10:00 p.m. and spontaneously awake at 4:00 a.m. getting less than adequate sleep (e.g. 6 hours), they do not have ASWPD but have, instead, early morning awakening insomnia. This classification ignores the fact that their sleeping difficulty is mainly driven by an advanced circadian rhythm and would be more appropriately treated if chronobiologic tools are included. Of course, advanced circadian phase and early morning awakening insomnia can co-occur, in which the early awakening can be associated with frustration and lead to a conditioned arousal response. In that case CBT-I, particularly bedtime restriction therapy, may be helpful in extinguishing the learned arousal response. The most appropriate treatments arise from the most accurate assessment of the causes of the problem, not the superficial symptoms of the problem. This raises the issue of assessing the timing of the endogenous circadian rhythm.

Can the Endogenous Circadian Rhythm Timing Be Readily and Reliably Assessed?

If an advanced circadian rhythm is suspect, it becomes necessary to confirm it using either of the generally accepted circadian phase markers of DLMO and Tmin. Then the newly (yet-to-be) established phase–response curves to the timing of light or melatonin administration can be used to effect optimal phase-advancing or -delaying treatment.

Unfortunately, these circadian phase markers (DLMO and Tmin) are time-consuming, expensive, and not readily available. Therefore, they are not clinically practical or justifiable. What is generally collected in clinical practice are sleep–wake diaries completed each morning over at least a full week as representative of the individual's typical sleep pattern and timing. Studies have shown this information about average sleep onset times, wake times, and mid-sleep timing to be significantly associated with gold-standard circadian phase measures of DLMO and Tmin, with correlations on the order of .60–.88 (Lovato et al., 2016). Other studies have reported similar correlations between sleep diary parameters and DLMO (Burgess & Eastman, 2005; Crowley et al., 2006; Keijzer et al., 2014). Although estimates are within 1.5 hours of the "gold-standard" phase measures for about 75% of the sample, larger errors for some patients could result in problematic treatment outcomes. For example, if the estimated Tmin from sleep diary information is 2:00 a.m., then a bright blue/green light pulse from midnight to 2:00 a.m. would be recommended for maximal phase-delay. However, if, in fact, Tmin was as early as midnight, then this light "treatment" following the Tmin would produce a phase-advance and exacerbate the difficulty of early sleep and awakening. Therefore, more accurate but practical, noninvasive measures of DLMO and Tmin are a desirable aim. This would be particularly important for identifying the common DSWPD "non-circadian" Type 2, whose circadian phase markers will be considerably earlier than estimated from diaries or actigraphy measures.

What has become practical through their popularity and widespread adoption is the objective measurement of activity using wrist actigraphy (e.g., Fitbits, Garmins, Apple watches, Samsung watches, etc.). Based on actigraphy, these devices can objectively determine the onsets and offsets of the major nocturnal sleep periods without relying on the subjective estimates by individuals hopefully recorded each morning in sleep diaries. Studies have shown significant correspondence (mean absolute error of 1 hour) between measured DLMO and that predicted from models based on objective wrist actigraphy in wearable devices (Huang et al., 2021). Furthermore, the technology in these wearable devices is improving quickly, and many now include additional sensors for heart rate, oxygen saturation, electrodermal activity, skin temperature, etc. The combination of all available sensors in mathematical models may be able to provide improved estimates of endogenous gold-standard circadian phase estimates (DLMO and Tmin). Their accuracy could become comparable to the small, spontaneous intraindividual variation in the gold-standard measures of 21–37-minute mean absolute differences from night to night (Lushington et al., 1997; Selmaoui & Touitou, 2003). Such research to improve circadian phase measurement would be a welcome contribution to improving best practice in the treatment of circadian rhythm disorders.

Treatment Suggestions

DSWPD

1. Determine baseline sleep period timing for the patient. Presently, the most practical method is a sleep diary or wearable device providing objective information of sleep timing. From a typical 2-week period of sleep timing data, calculate the average sleep onset and wake-up times for both week-/workdays and weekend/free days.
2. Decide with the patient their preferred or target sleep timing that best suits their lifestyle needs, commitments, and total sleep need. The focus should be on the preferred wake-up times on week-/workdays in order to obtain sufficient sleep to meet regular work/school/family commitments. For example, if on most days commitments start at 9:00 a.m. and a 7:30 wake-up time provides just enough time to meet that commitment time and sleep need is 8 hours of sleep to feel rested, then a sleep onset time of 11:30 p.m. and bedtime of 11:00 p.m. would be preferred. Calculate the time difference of this preferred target with present sleep timing.
3. Decide with the patient whether advancing or delaying sleep timing is the best direction for retiming their body clock to this target time. If present sleep timing is more than 5–6 hours later than the target timing, then delaying with chronotherapy may be the most effective treatment if it is practically feasible for the patient. For the more common difference of less than 5 hours, phase-advance treatment is probably the more efficient.

For Phase-Advance Treatment

1. Start light administration and initial wake-up time at the average wake-up time on week-/workdays. (Although this is likely to be several hours after Tmin for the non-circadian Type 2 DSWPD, it will be immediately after Tmin for the circadian Type 1 DSWPD patients.) Therefore, this timing of light will capture all DSWPD patients on the phase-advance side of the phase–response curve.) The light should be of sufficient intensity (e.g., >300 melanopic lux) starting at wake-up time for at least 2 hours, longer if possible. (Melanopic lux is the value measured with a photometer adjusted down by the melanopic ratio, the percentage of the light source spectrum coinciding with the circadian-sensitive, melanopic, or blue/green part of the visible spectrum. See further information at https://luminusdevices.zendesk.com/hc/en-us/articles/4409868024461-What-is-the-Melanopic-Ratio-1.) Outdoor sunlight, if available, would be the most effective source of light. Schedule activities outside as soon as possible after scheduled wake-up time. Avoid the use of sunglasses if possible. Caffeine upon awakening may help the circadian phase-advance and would help motivate outside activities (e.g., walking the dog, gardening, having breakfast, etc.). These suggestions may be more feasible if treatment starts on the weekend or free days.
2. Advance (shift earlier) wake-up time and the start of light exposure by 20 minutes (or whatever incremental shift can be managed) each consecutive morning until the target sleep timing is achieved.
3. After achieving the target sleep times, continue with the timing of wake-up time and light exposure at the target times for at least 2 weeks. Length of bright light exposure following wake-up time may then be gradually reduced depending on the maintenance of target sleep timing.
4. For deciding bedtimes follow the CBT-I instructions for stimulus control therapy to go to bed only when sleepiness becomes evident. If sleep onset does not occur within about 15 minutes, get out of bed and wait for sleepiness again before returning to bed, etc. (This procedure may result in a few initial nights of reduced amount of sleep, but the mounting sleep pressure will help ensure quicker sleep onsets on subsequent nights and a gradual recovery of sleep debt. These instructions address the likely comorbidity of DSWPD and sleep onset insomnia [Morris et al., 1990] by reconditioning the bed environment with quick sleep onsets rather than long, frustrating delays when trying to fall asleep.)

5. Administer low-dose (1–2 mg), quick-release pure melatonin 3–6 hours before desired bedtime. At evening meal time (e.g., 6:00–7:00 p.m.) would be convenient and close to optimal timing.
6. Avoid caffeine in the second half of the day and bright blue light in the last 3 hours before bedtime. Wear blue-blocking glasses or provide dim ambient light. If computer screens are used before bed, blue-light blocking software (e.g., F.lux, nightshift or night mode on most modern devices) can minimize shorter-wavelength light automatically without the need of blue blocking glasses (e.g., https://en.wikipedia.org/wiki/F.lux).

For Phase-Delay Treatment (Chronotherapy)

1. Compared to typical bedtime, delay bedtime by 2 hours on each consecutive sleep period until the target bedtime is achieved. In most cases this can be achieved over a 9-day period starting on one weekend and finishing at the end of the following weekend. This would most probably require a week of leave from work/school or other daytime responsibilities since sleep will occupy the daytimes in the intervening week.
2. Get outdoor sunshine for 1–3 hours prior to each bedtime. This will facilitate the circadian delay. Normally one would expect a spontaneous delay from the longer period lengths of DSWPD patients in the order of up to an hour. The required 2-hour delay of circadian rhythms can be achieved by adding bright light prior to bedtime and Tmin.
3. When the target sleep period is reached, it is very important to maintain stability with the help of melatonin in the early evening and switching the bright light exposure to the morning immediately after wake-up time.
4. Using a fail-safe alarm (loud and out of reach to require exiting the bed) to ensure awakening at the target wake-up time is important.

This chronotherapy process is illustrated in Figure 32.2. For an extremely delayed DSWPD patient it shows a pretreatment sleep period from 6:00 a.m. to 2:00 p.m. Then bedtime delays by 2 hours each subsequent night. The cartoon suns indicate bright light exposure prior to bedtime to facilitate the delay process. The sunglasses indicate avoidance of sunshine following sleep, also to facilitate delay. On the sixth treatment day 2 mg of melatonin can be taken at bedtime (6:00 p.m.) to facilitate further delay. Then 1 mg quick-release melatonin can be taken at meal time (6:00–7:00 p.m.) to help stabilize the circadian rhythm and desired sleep timing from 11:00 p.m. to 7:00 a.m. Most importantly, bright light should now be avoided in the evening but presented instead at wake-up

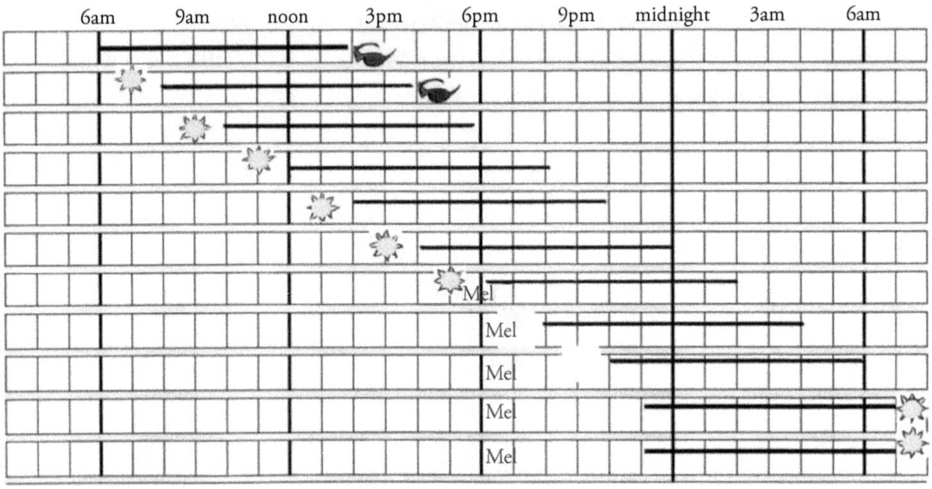

Figure 32.2 The figure illustrates an example of chronotherapy delay for the treatment of extreme DSWPD. Over a 10-day period bedtimes are delayed each sleep period by 2 hours until the target bedtime (in this case, 11:00 p.m.) is reached. Bright light visual stimulation (e.g., outside sunshine or light therapy glasses during inclement weather) is recommended in the hours before bedtime (as indicated by the sun cartoon) to facilitate the delay, and avoidance of bright light (indicated by the dark glasses cartoon) is recommended after awakening. When the target bedtimes are achieved, light stimulation needs to occur only at wake-up time. Low-dose (1 mg), immediate-release melatonin (Mel) can be ingested in the early evening at meal time to help maintain circadian timing at the target time.

time (7:00–9:00 a.m.). Continued use of low-dose melatonin in the early evening and morning light therapy may be necessary to maintain stability.

Attention to Psychological Factors in the Treatment of DSWPD

All of the above treatment suggestions have been directed at circadian rhythm retiming and behavioral changes to support them. However, in an earlier section, "Problems with Night Owls," we suggested that the experiences of those with DSWPD result in an aversion to mornings and an attraction to evenings that could produce significant treatment barriers for implementing the above treatment suggestions. Therefore, for either the phase-advance or phase-delay treatment for DSWPD, maintaining the target bed and wake times is critical for long-term improvement. The motivation for this consistent behavior will tend to be undermined by the long-established conditioned avoidance of mornings and extension of the evenings. Changing the valences of these times would be a helpful adjunct treatment. If the mornings can be made more attractive with the addition of regular enjoyable activities and social commitments, it will increase the motivation to stick to regular earlier wake times. Over time the mornings may become more attractive in general and less dependent on the artificial construction of enjoyable activities. If it is possible to shift some of the previously enjoyed evening activities (e.g., chatting digitally with friends and relatives, playing computer games with remotely located competitors, etc.) to the morning hours, that might help to shift the positive valence of the evenings to the morning period, making it easier to adhere to the circadian retiming suggestions.

ASWPD

Whether a patient has met the latest ICSD-3 criteria for ASWPD including advanced bedtimes and wake times or only advanced wake times, both cases have been shown to have advanced circadian rhythms and should be treatable with chronobiologic and behavioral treatments. Although phase-advancing chronotherapy has been suggested with anecdotal single-case success and is the logical converse of delayed chronotherapy for DSWPD, the apparent rarity of individuals with period lengths much less than 24 hours makes it unlikely to be the most efficient direction of phase change. Therefore, only the phase-delay therapy for ASWPD will be summarized here.

1. Collect 2 consecutive typical weeks of either sleep diary or actigraphy from wearable devices. Calculate average baseline sleep onset and wake-up time.
2. Decide with the patient their preferred bedtimes and wake-up times to suit their lifestyle and achieve adequate total sleep time.
3. Administer bright (>300 melanopic lux) light for 2–3 hours before typical bedtime in the visual field of the patient for 2 consecutive nights.
4. Administer 2 mg sustained-release melatonin at bedtime on each of these 2 nights.
5. If the target bedtime is later (as will be the case for those with undesirably early bedtimes), continue with the light and melatonin administration but delay the bedtime by 30 minutes for the next 2 nights. Continue the 30-minute delays of bedtime, light, and melatonin every 2 nights until the target bedtime is achieved. For those already at their target bedtime but with earlier than desired wake-up times, continue with light and melatonin administration as described in Points 3 and 4 above.
6. Once the target bedtime is achieved, continue with the pre-bed light and melatonin administration for at least another week.
7. If, after the above treatment, final wake-up time has not delayed enough to provide an adequate amount of total sleep, it probably indicates some early-morning awakening conditioned insomnia. CBT-I could then be used to address this factor and could involve sleep education about the normalcy of awakenings during sleep, relaxation skill to help the resumption of sleep, and instructions to exit the bed and start the day if sleep is not resumed within about 15–20 minutes.
8. If undesirably early awakenings continue, administration of low-dose (0.5–1.0 mg), quick-release melatonin taken at that early awakening time may work better to resume sleep and further delay the body clock than the 2-mg sustained-release preparation taken at initial bedtime.

References

Abbott, S. M., Phillips, A. J., Reid, K. J., Cain, S. W., & Zee, P. C. (2023). What's in a name? delayed by any other name is still a circadian disorder: A call for improved nomenclature for delayed sleep–wake phase disorder subtypes. *Sleep*, *46*(11), Article zsad222. https://doi.org/10.1093/sleep/zsad222

Antypa, N., Vogelzangs, N., Meesters, Y., Schoevers, R., & Penninx, B. W. (2016). Chronotype associations with depression and anxiety disorders in a large cohort study. *Depression and Anxiety*, *33*(1), 75–83. https://doi.org/10.1002/da.22422

Auger, R. R., Burgess, H. J., Emens, J. S., Deriy, L. V., Thomas, S. M., & Sharkey, K. M. (2015). Clinical practice guideline for the treatment of intrinsic circadian rhythm sleep–wake disorders: Advanced sleep–wake phase disorder (ASWPD), delayed sleep–wake phase disorder (DSWPD), non-24-hour sleep–wake rhythm disorder (N24SWD), and irregular sleep–wake rhythm disorder (ISWRD). An update for 2015: An American Academy of Sleep Medicine clinical practice guideline. *Journal of Clinical Sleep Medicine*, *11*(10), 1199–1236. https://doi.org/10.5664/jcsm.5100

Blume, C., Garbazza, C., & Spitschan, M. (2019). Effects of light on human circadian rhythms, sleep and mood. *Somnologie*, *23*(3), 147–156. https://doi.org/10.1007/s11818-019-00215-x

Burgess, H. J., & Eastman, C. I. (2005). The dim light melatonin onset following fixed and free sleep schedules. *Journal of Sleep Research*, *14*(3), 229–237.

Burgess, H. J., Kikyo, F., Valdespino-Hayden, Z., Rizvydeen, M., Kimura, M., Pollack, M. H., Hobfoll, S. E., Rajan, K. B., Zalta, A. K., & Burns, J. W. (2018). Do the Morningness–Eveningness Questionnaire and Munich ChronoType Questionnaire change after morning light treatment? *Sleep Science and Practice*, *2*, Article 12. https://doi.org/10.1186/s41606-018-0031-1

Burke, T. M., Markwald, R. R., McHill, A. W., Chinoy, E. D., Snider, J. A., Bessman, S. C., Jung, C. M., O'Neill, J. S., & Wright, K. P., Jr. (2015). Effects of caffeine on the human circadian clock in vivo and in vitro. *Science Translational Medicine*, *7*(305), Article 305ra146. https://doi.org/10.1126/scitranslmed.aac5125

Campbell, S. S., Dawson, D., & Anderson, M. W. (1993). Alleviation of sleep maintenance insomnia with timed exposure to bright light. *Journal of the American Geriatrics Society*, *41*(8), 829–836. http://www.ncbi.nlm.nih.gov/pubmed/8340561

Coleman, M. Y., & Cain, S. W. (2019). Eveningness is associated with greater subjective cognitive impairment in individuals with self-reported symptoms of unipolar depression. *Journal of Affective Disorders*, *256*, 404–415.

Crowley, S. J., Acebo, C., Fallone, G., & Carskadon, M. A. (2006). Estimating dim light melatonin onset (DLMO) phase in adolescents using summer or school-year sleep/wake schedules. *Sleep*, *29*(12), 1632–1641. https://doi.org/10.1093/sleep/29.12.1632

Curtis, B. J., Ashbrook, L. H., Young, T., Finn, L. A., Fu, Y. H., Ptacek, L. J., & Jones, C. R. (2019). Extreme morning chronotypes are often familial and not exceedingly rare: The estimated prevalence of advanced sleep phase, familial advanced sleep phase, and advanced sleep–wake phase disorder in a sleep clinic population. *Sleep*, *42*(10), Article zsz149. https://doi.org/10.1093/sleep/zsz148

Czeisler, C., Kronauer, R., Allan, J., Duffy, J., Jewett, M., Brown, E., & Ronda, J. (1989). Bright light induction of strong (type 0) resetting of the human circadian pacemaker. *Science*, *244*, 1328–1333.

Czeisler, C., Richardson, G., Coleman, R., Zimmerman, J., Moore-Ede, M., Dement, W., & Weitzman, E. (1981). Chronotherapy: Resetting the circadian clocks of patients with delayed sleep phase insomnia. *Sleep*, *4*(1), 1–21.

Czeisler, C. A., Weitzman, E., Moore-Ede, M. C., Zimmerman, J. C., & Knauer, R. S. (1980). Human sleep: Its duration and organization depend on its circadian phase. *Science*, *210*(4475), 1264–1267.

Danielsson, K., Jansson-Frojmark, M., Broman, J. E., & Markstrom, A. (2016). Cognitive behavioral therapy as an adjunct treatment to light therapy for delayed sleep phase disorder in young adults: A randomized controlled feasibility study. *Behavioral Sleep Medicine*, *14*(2), 212–232. https://doi.org/10.1080/15402002.2014.981817

Dawson, D., Lack, L., & Morris, M. (1993). Phase resetting of the human circadian pacemaker with use of a single pulse of bright light. *Chronobiological International*, *10*(2), 94–102.

Dewald, J. F., Meijer, A. M., Oort, F. J., Kerkhof, G. A., & Bogels, S. M. (2010). The influence of sleep quality, sleep duration and sleepiness on school performance in children and adolescents: A meta-analytic review. *Sleep Medicine Reviews*, *14*(3), 179–189. https://doi.org/10.1016/j.smrv.2009.10.004

Dijk, D.-J., Duffy, J. F., & Czeisler, C. A. (1992). Circadian and sleep/wake dependent aspects of subjective alertness and cognitive performance. *Journal of Sleep Research, 1*, 112–117.
Duffy, J. F., & Czeisler, C. A. (2009). Effect of light on human circadian physiology. *Sleep Medicine Clinics, 4*(2), 165–177. https://doi.org/10.1016/j.jsmc.2009.01.004
Duffy, J. F., Rimmer, D. W., & Czeisler, C. A. (2001). Association of intrinsic circadian period with morningness–eveningness, usual wake time, and circadian phase. *Behavioral Neuroscience, 115*(4), 895–899.
Futenma, K., Takaesu, Y., Komada, Y., Shimura, A., Okajima, I., Matsui, K., Tanioka, K., & Inoue, Y. (2023). Delayed sleep–wake phase disorder and its related sleep behaviors in the young generation. *Frontiers in Psychiatry, 14*, Article 1174719. https://doi.org/10.3389/fpsyt.2023.1174719
Gradisar, M., Dohnt, H., Gardner, G., Paine, S., Starkey, K., Menne, A., Slater, A., Wright, H., Hudson, J. L., Weaver, E., & Trenowden, S. (2011). A randomized controlled trial of cognitive-behavior therapy plus bright light therapy for adolescent delayed sleep phase disorder. *Sleep, 34*(12), 1671–1680. https://doi.org/10.5665/sleep.1432
Gradisar, M., & Lack, L. (2004). Relationships between the circadian rhythms of finger temperature, core temperature, sleep latency and subjective sleepiness. *Journal of Biological Rhythms, 19*(2), 157–163.
Hasler, B. P., Smith, L. J., Cousins, J. C., & Bootzin, R. R. (2012). Circadian rhythms, sleep, and substance abuse. *Sleep Medicine Reviews, 16*(1), 67–81. https://doi.org/10.1016/j.smrv.2011.03.004
Horne, J., & Östberg, O. (1976). A self-assessment questionnaire to determine morningness–eveningness in human circadian rhythms. *International Journal of Chronobiology, 4*, 97–110.
Huang, Y., Mayer, C., Cheng, P., Siddula, A., Burgess, H. J., Drake, C., Goldstein, C., Walch, O., & Forger, D. B. (2021). Predicting circadian phase across populations: A comparison of mathematical models and wearable devices. *Sleep, 44*(10), Article zsab126. https://doi.org/10.1093/sleep/zsab126
Ito, A., Ando, K., Hayakawa, T., Iwata, T., Kayukawa, Y., Ohta, T., & Kasahara, Y. (1993). Long-term course of adult patients with delayed sleep phase syndrome. *Psychiatry and Clinical Neurosciences, 47*(3), 563–567. https://doi.org/10.1111/j.1440-1819.1993.tb01800.x
Jankowski, K. S. (2013). Morning types are less sensitive to pain than evening types all day long. *European Journal of Pain, 17*(7), 1068–1073. https://doi.org/10.1002/j.1532-2149.2012.00274.x
Keijzer, H., Smits, M. G., Duffy, J. F., & Curfs, L. M. (2014). Why the dim light melatonin onset (DLMO) should be measured before treatment of patients with circadian rhythm sleep disorders. *Sleep Medicine Reviews, 18*(4), 333–339. https://doi.org/10.1016/j.smrv.2013.12.001
Kerkhof, G. A. (1998). The 24-hour variation of mood differs between morning- and evening-type individuals. *Perceptual and Motor Skills, 86*(1), 264–266.
Kivela, L., Papadopoulos, M. R., & Antypa, N. (2018). Chronotype and psychiatric disorders. *Current Sleep Medicine Reports, 4*(2), 94–103. https://doi.org/10.1007/s40675-018-0113-8
Lack, L. (1986). Delayed sleep and sleep loss in university students. *Journal of American College Health, 35*(3), 105–110.
Lack, L., Bailey, M., Lovato, N., & Wright, H. (2009). Chronotype differences in circadian rhythms of temperature, melatonin and sleepiness as measured in a modified constant routine protocol. *Nature and Science of Sleep, 1*, 1–7.
Lack, L., & Lushington, K. (1996). The rhythms of human sleep propensity and core body temperature. *Journal of Sleep Research, 5*, 1–11.
Lack, L., & Wright, H. (1993). The effect of evening bright light in delaying the circadian rhythms and lengthening the sleep of early morning awakening insomniacs. *Sleep, 16*(3), 436–443.
Lack, L., Wright, H., Kemp, K., & Gibbon, S. (2005). The treatment of early-morning awakening insomnia with 2 evenings of bright light. *Sleep, 28*(5), 616–623.
Lack, L. C., Micic, G., & Lovato, N. (2023). Circadian aspects in the aetiology and pathophysiology of insomnia. *Journal of Sleep Research, 32*(6), Article e13976. https://doi.org/10.1111/jsr.13976
Lavie, P. (1986). Ultrashort sleep-waking schedule. III. "Gates" and "forbidden zones" for sleep. *Electroencephalography and Clinical Neurophysiology, 63*, 414–425.
Lovato, N., Micic, G., Gradisar, M., Ferguson, S. A., Burgess, H. J., Kennaway, D. J., & Lack, L. (2016). Can the circadian phase be estimated from self-reported sleep timing in patients with delayed sleep wake phase disorder to guide timing of chronobiologic treatment? *Chronobiology International, 33*(10), 1376–1390. https://doi.org/10.1080/07420528.2016.1220386
Lovato, N., Phillips, A. J. K., Micic, G., Lack, L., & Cain, S. W. (2023). Delayed sleep-phase type. In C. A. Kushida (Ed.), *Encyclopedia of sleep & circadian rhythms* (2nd ed., pp. 606–611). Academic Press.

Lushington, K., Pollard, K., Lack, L., Kennaway, D., & Dawson, D. (1997). Daytime melatonin administration in elderly good and poor sleepers: Effects on core body temperature and sleep latency. *Sleep*, *20*(12), 1135–1144.

Merikanto, I., Kronholm, E., Peltonen, M., Laatikainen, T., Vartiainen, E., & Partonen, T. (2015). Circadian preference links to depression in general adult population. *Journal of Affective Disorders*, *188*, 143–148. https://doi.org/10.1016/j.jad.2015.08.061

Micic, G., Lovato, N., Ferguson, S. A., Burgess, H. J., & Lack, L. (2021). Circadian tau differences and rhythm associations in delayed sleep–wake phase disorder and sighted non-24-hour sleep-wake rhythm disorder. *Sleep*, *44*(1), Article zsaa132. https://doi.org/10.1093/sleep/zsaa132

Micic, G., Lovato, N., Gradisar, M., Burgess, H. J., Ferguson, S. A., & Lack, L. (2016). Circadian melatonin and temperature taus in delayed sleep–wake phase disorder and non-24-hour sleep–wake rhythm disorder patients: An ultradian constant routine study. *Journal of Biological Rhythms*, *31*(4), 387–405. https://doi.org/10.1177/0748730416650069

Micic, G., Lovato, N., Gradisar, M., & Lack, L. C. (2017). Personality differences in patients with delayed sleep–wake phase disorder and non-24-h sleep-wake rhythm disorder relative to healthy sleepers. *Sleep Medicine*, *30*, 128–135. https://doi.org/10.1016/j.sleep.2016.04.002

Micic, G., Richardson, C., Cain, N., Reynolds, C., Bartel, K., Maddock, B., & Gradisar, M. (2019). Readiness to change and commitment as predictors of therapy compliance in adolescents with delayed sleep-wake phase disorder. *Sleep Medicine*, *55*, 48–55. https://doi.org/10.1016/j.sleep.2018.12.002

Morgenthaler, T., Alessi, C., Friedman, L., Owens, J., Kapur, V., Boehlecke, B., Brown, T., Chesson, A., Coleman, J., Lee-Chiong, T., Pancer, J., & Swick, T. J. (2007). Practice parameters for the use of actigraphy in the assessment of sleep and sleep disorders: An update for 2007. *Sleep*, *30*(4), 519–529.

Morris, M., Lack, L., & Dawson, D. (1990). Sleep-onset insomniacs have delayed temperature rhythms. *Sleep*, *13*(1), 1–14.

Murray, J. M., Sletten, T. L., Magee, M., Gordon, C., Lovato, N., Bartlett, D. J., Kennaway, D. J., Lack, L. C., Grunstein, R. R., Lockley, S. W., & Rajaratnam, S. M.; Delayed Sleep on Melatonin Study Group. (2017). Prevalence of circadian misalignment and its association with depressive symptoms in delayed sleep phase disorder. *Sleep*, *40*(1), Article zsw002. https://doi.org/10.1093/sleep/zsw002

Nagane, M., Suge, R., & Watanabe, S. (2011). Relationship between psychosomatic complaints and circadian rhythm irregularity assessed by salivary levels of melatonin and growth hormone. *Journal of Circadian Rhythms*, *9*, Article 9. https://doi.org/10.1186/1740-3391-9-9

Park, C. I., An, S. K., Kim, H. W., Koh, M. J., Namkoong, K., Kang, J. I., & Kim, S. J. (2015). Relationships between chronotypes and affective temperaments in healthy young adults. *Journal of Affective Disorders*, *175*, 256–259. https://doi.org/10.1016/j.jad.2015.01.004

Partonen, T. (2023). Extreme chronotype, regardless of misalignment, links to cardiovascular disease risks. *Sleep*, *46*(6), Article zsad081. https://doi.org/10.1093/sleep/zsad081

Preckel, F., Lipnevich, A. A., Schneider, S., & Roberts, R. D. (2011). Chronotype, cognitive abilities, and academic achievement: A meta-analytic investigation. *Learning and Individual Differences*, *21*(5), 483–492.

Richardson, C., Cain, N., Bartel, K., Micic, G., Maddock, B., & Gradisar, M. (2018). A randomised controlled trial of bright light therapy and morning activity for adolescents and young adults with delayed sleep–wake phase disorder. *Sleep Medicine*, *45*, 114–123. https://doi.org/10.1016/j.sleep.2018.02.001

Richardson, C. E., Gradisar, M., & Barbero, S. C. (2016). Are cognitive "insomnia" processes involved in the development and maintenance of delayed sleep wake phase disorder? *Sleep Medicine Reviews*, *26*, 1–8. https://doi.org/10.1016/j.smrv.2015.05.001

Roenneberg, T., & Merrow, M. (2007). Entrainment of the human circadian clock. *Cold Spring Harbor Symposia on Quantitative Biology*, *72*, 293–299. https://doi.org/10.1101/sqb.2007.72.043

Roeser, K., Obergfell, F., Meule, A., Vogele, C., Schlarb, A. A., & Kubler, A. (2012). Of larks and hearts—Morningness/eveningness, heart rate variability and cardiovascular stress response at different times of day. *Physiology & Behavior*, *106*(2), 151–157. https://doi.org/10.1016/j.physbeh.2012.01.023

Saxvig, I. W., Wilhelmsen-Langeland, A., Pallesen, S., Vedaa, O., Nordhus, I. H., Sorensen, E., & Bjorvatn, B. (2013). Objective measures of sleep and dim light melatonin onset in adolescents and young adults with delayed sleep phase disorder compared to healthy controls. *Journal of Sleep Research*, *22*(4), 365–372. https://doi.org/10.1111/jsr.12030

Schrader, H., Bovim, G., & Sand, T. (1993). The prevalence of delayed and advanced sleep phase syndromes. *Journal of Sleep Research*, *2*, 51–55.

Selmaoui, B., & Touitou, Y. (2003). Reproducibility of the circadian rhythms of serum cortisol and melatonin in healthy subjects: A study of three different 24-h cycles over six weeks. *Life Sciences, 73*(26), 3339–3349. https://doi.org/10.1016/j.lfs.2003.05.007

Sladek, M., Klusacek, J., Hamplova, D., & Sumova, A. (2023). Population-representative study reveals cardiovascular and metabolic disease biomarkers associated with misaligned sleep schedules. *Sleep, 46*(6), Article zsad037. https://doi.org/10.1093/sleep/zsad037

Sletten, T. L., Magee, M., Murray, J. M., Gordon, C. J., Lovato, N., Kennaway, D. J., Gwini, S. M., Bartlett, D. J., Lockley, S. W., Lack, L. C., Grunstein, R. R., & Rajaratnam, S. M. W.; Delayed Sleep on Melatonin Study Group. (2018). Efficacy of melatonin with behavioural sleep–wake scheduling for delayed sleep–wake phase disorder: A double-blind, randomised clinical trial. *PLOS Medicine, 15*(6), Article e1002587. https://doi.org/10.1371/journal.pmed.1002587

Taylor, A., Wright, H., & Lack, L. (2008). Sleeping-in on the weekend delays circadian phase and increases sleepiness the following week. *Sleep and Biological Rhythms, 6*, 172–179.

Toomey, R., Panizzon, M. S., Kremen, W. S., Franz, C. E., & Lyons, M. J. (2015). A twin-study of genetic contributions to morningness–eveningness and depression. *Chronobiology International, 32*(3), 303–309. https://doi.org/10.3109/07420528.2014.971366

Van den Berg, J. F., Kivela, L., & Antypa, N. (2018). Chronotype and depressive symptoms in students: An investigation of possible mechanisms. *Chronobiology International, 35*(9), 1248–1261. https://doi.org/10.1080/07420528.2018.1470531

Walsh, N. A., Repa, L. M., & Garland, S. N. (2022). Mindful larks and lonely owls: The relationship between chronotype, mental health, sleep quality, and social support in young adults. *Journal of Sleep Research, 31*(1), Article e13442. https://doi.org/10.1111/jsr.13442

Weitzman, E. D., Czeisler, C. A., Coleman, R. M., Spielman, A. J., Zimmerman, J. C., & Dement, W. (1981). Delayed sleep phase syndrome: A chronobiological disorder with sleep-onset insomnia. *Archives of General Psychiatry, 38*, 137–146.

Wilhelmsen-Langeland, A., Saxvig, I. W., Johnsen, E. H., Marszalek, M. A., Wiig Andersen, M. I., Saetre, V. K., Lundervold, A. J., Vedaa, O., Nordhus, I. H., Pallesen, S., & Bjorvatn, B. (2019). Patients with delayed sleep–wake phase disorder show poorer executive functions compared to good sleepers. *Sleep Medicine, 54*, 244–249. https://doi.org/10.1016/j.sleep.2018.10.035

Wilhelmsen-Langeland, A., Saxvig, I. W., Pallesen, S., Nordhus, I. H., Vedaa, O., Sorensen, E., & Bjorvatn, B. (2014). The personality profile of young adults with delayed sleep phase disorder. *Behavioral Sleep Medicine, 12*(6), 481–492. https://doi.org/10.1080/15402002.2013.829063

Wright, H. R., Lack, L. C., & Kennaway, D. J. (2004). Differential effects of light wavelength in phase advancing the melatonin rhythm. *Journal of Pineal Research, 36*, 140–144.

Wright, K. P., Jr., McHill, A. W., Birks, B. R., Griffin, B. R., Rusterholz, T., & Chinoy, E. D. (2013). Entrainment of the human circadian clock to the natural light–dark cycle. *Current Biology, 23*(16), 1554–1558. https://doi.org/10.1016/j.cub.2013.06.039

Yang, C.-M., Spielman, A. J., D'Ambrosio, P., Serizawa, S., Nunes, J., & Birnbaum, J. (2001). A single dose of melatonin prevents the phase delay associated with a delayed weekend sleep pattern. *Sleep, 24*(3), 272–281.

CHAPTER

33 Circadian Rhythm Sleep–Wake Disorders II: Shift Work, Irregular, and Non-24-Hour Sleep–Wake Rhythm Disorders

Diane B. Boivin *and* Philippe Boudreau

Abstract

This chapter reviews the epidemiology, diagnosis, physiopathology, and treatment of shift-work disorder irregular and non-24-hour sleep–wake rhythm disorders. Shift-work disorder is caused by self-selected behavioral changes due to an atypical work schedule, whereas the other disorders are presumably caused by an intrinsic malfunction of the endogenous circadian timing system. The clinical management of these disorders requires long periods of investigation and observation. Various countermeasures such as improved light/dark exposure, sleep management, and careful use of hypnotics and stimulants when needed can be considered in shift workers with severe sleep–wake disturbances. For the other disorders, therapeutic decisions should seek to consolidate sleep at night; and a multimodal approach is suggested, although no clear guidelines are available. Exogenous melatonin or melatonin agonists are recommended for free-running patients with blindness. In all cases, a careful review of sleep hygiene is important as maladaptive behaviors are frequent.

Key Words: shift work disorder, circadian rhythm, sleep, alertness, sleepiness

Introduction

According to the *International Classification of Sleep Disorders*, 3rd edition (ICSD-3; American Academy of Sleep Medicine, 2014), the disorders described in this review are part of a broader category defined as *circadian rhythm sleep–wake disorders* (CRSWDs). These disorders are characterized by at least one of three situations: (1) a dysfunctional circadian system, (2) a circadian system misaligned with the environment, or (3) an alteration in circadian entrainment. In these situations, various rhythms within the circadian system are misaligned with the environmental light/dark cycle and can also be desynchronized between each other. This chapter reviews the epidemiology, diagnosis, physiopathology, and treatment of three CRSWDs: shift-work disorder and irregular and non-24-hour sleep–wake rhythm disorders, based on the ICSD-3.

Shift-Work Disorder

Shift work is vital in industries requiring 24-hour coverage, as in emergency services, to allow for continuous production. In a publication covering approximately 1.2 billion workers from 41 countries, the International Labour Organization and the European Foundation for the Improvement of Living and Working Conditions estimate that between 10% and 30% of workers are undertaking night shifts at least once a month (Eurofound & International Labour Organization, 2019). In North America, it was reported that 12%–13% of working adults are scheduled on rotating or regular night shifts (Rydz et al., 2020; Yong et al., 2017). While women represent roughly half of the shift working population, they are more likely to work part-time, experience work–life conflicts, and devote more hours to unpaid work (Eurofound & International Labour Organization, 2019).

Atypical work is defined as work scheduled outside of conventional weekday hours. A wide variety of atypical work rosters exist and often include work shifts covering the night period; a combination of day, evening, or night shifts (i.e., rotating shifts); shifts with an early morning start; or long periods of work extending into the night. All of these schedules have in common that work hours can overlap with the worker's habitual nocturnal sleep period.

Staying awake all or part of the night and trying to sleep during the day is not physiological in humans. Circadian adaptation to a night-oriented schedule is a gradual and generally incomplete process. Without specific intervention to reset the endogenous circadian system, it is estimated that only ~25% of workers show substantial circadian adaptation to night schedules (Boudreau et al., 2013; Folkard, 2008). Moreover, workers usually return to a conventional day-oriented sleep–wake schedule during rest days to maintain a social life and to enjoy their family, reinforcing a day-oriented schedule. Working on atypical schedules leads to chronic irregular and disrupted sleep–wake behavior, conflicting circadian time cues, and circadian disturbances. These conditions also create performance and alertness impairments at work (Anvekar et al., 2021; Behrens et al., 2019; Boivin, Boudreau, & Tremblay, 2012; Boudreau et al., 2013; Chellappa et al., 2019; Wilson et al., 2019; Zhao et al., 2021), with an increased risk of accidents and incidents at work and while commuting home (Anderson et al., 2018; Fischer et al., 2017; Kecklund & Axelsson, 2016; Lee et al., 2016; Liang et al., 2019). Individual tolerance to shift work varies greatly in the population. When patients present severe impairments with symptoms of sleepiness and insomnia related to their work schedule, a diagnosis of shift-work disorder (SWD) can be considered.

Epidemiology

The prevalence of SWD is estimated to be between 10% and 38% in rotating and night-shift workers (ICSD-3). In a recent meta-analysis of 29 original studies with various shift types, the prevalence of SWD among shift workers was estimated to be 26.5% (Pallesen et al., 2021). The diagnostic criteria of the ICSD-3 are more stringent than those of prior versions such that prior prevalence estimates can be lower. The ICSD-3 requires a reduction in total sleep time caused by the work schedule, a longer symptom duration (3 months vs. 1 month), and a longer observation period (14 vs. 7 days). Considering that approximately one out of four shift workers is affected, the prevalence of SWD in the general population is estimated to be about 2% to 5%, which is substantial.

Diagnosis

The core symptoms of SWD are complaints of insomnia and excessive sleepiness associated with the recurrent work schedule, especially if it overlaps with the usual nocturnal sleep period. These symptoms should cause clinically significant distress or impairment in mental, physical, social, occupational, or other important areas of functioning. To meet the ICSD-3 diagnostic criteria, these core symptoms must be accompanied by a reduction in total sleep time (no minimal duration specified) and be present for at least 3 months. A thorough examination of the sleep–wake pattern in relation to the work schedule is essential to diagnose SWD. The use of a sleep diary and ideally an actigraphy monitoring device is advised to document the sleep–wake pattern over at least 14 successive work and rest days. Finally, the disturbances should not be better explained by another current sleep disorder such as narcolepsy or respiratory sleep disorders, medical or neurological disorder, mental disorder, medication use, poor sleep hygiene, or substance use.

Insomnia symptoms are most frequently reported during days with night, early-morning, or rotating shifts. Following night shifts, insomnia consists mainly of difficulties maintaining sleep during the daytime, leading to late-morning or early-afternoon awakenings. Falling asleep in the morning after a night shift is quite easy since both the circadian and homeostatic processes maximally promote sleep at this time. On the other hand, sleep-onset insomnia and difficulty awakening in the morning may be experienced by workers in association with early-morning shifts. Overall, fragmentation of the main sleep episode is frequently observed, and sleep quality is perceived as unsatisfactory. Subjective scales, such as the Insomnia Severity Index (Morin et al., 2011), can help to assess the degree of sleep disturbances, with a score ≥10 being considered clinically relevant. Polysomnography is not necessary to diagnose SWD but can be used to exclude other sleep disorders. Daily sleep deprivation of 1 to 4 hours can be observed in SWD (Akerstedt & Wright, 2009; Savarese & Di Perri, 2020), leading to a cumulative sleep debt during a succession of shifts. This is reflected by a reduction in rapid-eye-movement and Stage 2 sleep, whereas slow-wave sleep remains mostly unaffected (Akerstedt & Wright, 2009). Moreover, free time is often used to recover from acute and chronic sleep debt, which often disrupts family and social life.

Excessive sleepiness usually occurs during work periods overlapping nighttime hours and is generally greatest in the middle and late night. Decreases in mental capacity, alertness, and performance and a peak in sleepiness often coincide with the circadian nadir at the end of the night and can compromise occupational safety. Patients with SWD are at risk of falling asleep involuntarily during their work and behind the wheel when commuting home in the morning. The Epworth Sleepiness Scale can be administered in clinical settings to assess the degree of self-reported sleepiness, with a score >10 being considered clinically significant (Johns, 1991). Although not systematically evaluated, the Multiple Sleep Latency Test and Maintenance of Wakefulness Test can be used to investigate sleepiness in patients suspected of SWD (Krahn et al., 2021). Patients suffering from SWD may demonstrate excessive sleepiness on the Multiple Sleep Latency Test scheduled during the habitual time of the work shift (Savarese & Di Perri, 2020). However, the diagnosis value of such a test done at night remains unclear. The Bergen Shift Work Sleep Questionnaire (Flo et al., 2012) and the Shift Work Disorder questionnaire (Barger et al., 2012) can be used to aid in the diagnosis of SWD, although they were both developed and validated in the context of the ICSD-2.

Pathophysiology

Atypical work schedules force abrupt and recurrent alterations of the sleep–wake cycle. As a result, the sleep–wake pattern is abruptly shifted, or even inverted, relative to its habitual daily schedule on rest days, which results in its recurrent misalignment with the endogenous circadian system. Undertaking sleep at inappropriate endogenous circadian phases leads to reduced sleep duration and quality, whereas sustaining wakefulness during the habitual sleep period leads to increased sleepiness, especially when it is combined with prolonged periods of awakening. Simulated night-shift experiments and field-based studies with shift workers both indicate that the endogenous circadian system is resistant to adaptation to a night-oriented schedule, as determined by a lack of substantial phase shifts in rhythms of melatonin, cortisol, and body temperature (Boudreau et al., 2013; Crowley et al., 2004; M. A. Jensen, Garde, et al., 2016; M. A. Jensen et al., 2020; Kosmadopoulos et al., 2024). The circadian profiles of melatonin and cortisol rhythms can also be distorted as a result of distorted behavioral and light exposure (Boivin & James, 2002b; Dijk et al., 2012; M. A. Jensen, Hansen, et al., 2016; McIntyre et al., 1989; Rahman et al., 2013; Razavi et al., 2019; Touitou et al., 1990; Zeitzer et al., 2000). Environmental light exposure prevents, or at least slows down, circadian adaptation to a night-oriented schedule.

A state of misalignment between the sleep–wake cycle and the circadian system is observed not only for rhythms controlled by the central circadian pacemaker (e.g., core body temperature, melatonin, cortisol) but also for rhythms controlled by peripheral circadian clocks (e.g., circadian clock gene expression in peripheral tissues). As various levels of the circadian system can be affected differently, working nights can create a state of desynchrony between several body rhythms.

Disturbed rhythms of clock gene expression in peripheral blood mononuclear cells (PBMCs) (Cuesta et al., 2017; Resuehr et al., 2019), blood cells (Skene et al., 2018), hair follicle cells (Akashi et al., 2010; Bescos et al., 2018; Hattammaru et al., 2019), and oral mucosa cells (Koshy et al., 2019), as well as transcriptomic rhythms in PBMCs (Kervezee et al., 2018; Resuehr et al., 2019) were reported following night shifts. In addition, altered metabolite rhythms were observed when working nights (Kervezee et al., 2019; Rotter et al., 2018; Skene et al., 2018) and could contribute to the increased risk of metabolic disorders reported in shift-working populations.

Circadian misalignment induced by atypical work schedules is the main cause but not the only contributor to SWD. Individual variability in tolerance for and adaptation to shift work is probably the key discriminant between people who will or will not develop SWD. These factors may affect the degree of sleepiness and performance impairment experienced by workers, as well as their ability to sleep during the day. Several individual and occupational factors have been associated with an increased risk of SWD, but more longitudinal studies are needed to establish causal relationships between these factors and the risk of developing SWD.

A recent systematic review explored individual factors that are associated with SWD in healthcare workers (Booker et al., 2018). From high-quality studies that used validated SWD questionnaires, the authors concluded that older workers, with more shift-work experience, were more likely to present SWD, a finding that was corroborated by others (Sack et al., 2007a; Saksvik et al., 2011), although the effect of age on shift workers' tolerance (not SWD) may increase with age or follow a U-shaped association (Ritonja et al., 2019). Higher score on hardiness, defined as a general resilience and reaction to stress and illness, was a key protective factor.

The chronotype, a measure of the individual preference in the timing of sleep and daily activities, was associated with sleep-related impartments (Booker et al., 2018) and may impact the propensity to develop SWD. In a field study of 76 police officers, increased evening preference was correlated with longer sleep duration during a series of night shifts, whereas morning preference was associated with longer sleep duration during morning shifts (Kervezee et al., 2021). Aligning individual preferences with the work schedule was shown to improve sleep and well-being (Vetter et al., 2015).

Being married and having children were associated with greater risks of sleep impairments when working atypical shifts (Booker et al., 2018), although it is not clear whether this led to an increased risk of SWD. Since the time devoted to domestic and familial obligations is generally higher in women, it is plausible that gender issues affect the risk of developing SWD, although only weak or nonconclusive gender differences were found in the prevalence of SWD (Booker et al., 2018; Sack et al., 2007a).

Lifestyle factors, such as high body mass index, alcohol intake, and smoking, have not been associated with SWD (Booker et al., 2018), although caffeine intake can deteriorate sleep if taken too close to bedtime. A genetic predisposition to SWD is generally not reported (Sack et al., 2007a; Saksvik et al., 2011; Thun et al., 2016), but one study reported an association between susceptibility to SWD and a *PER1* polymorphism

(Taniyama et al., 2015). Psychological, psychiatric, or other sleep-related disorders known to affect sleep, circadian rhythms, or alertness levels may increase the risk of developing SWD.

At the occupational level, shift type is the main contributing factor to SWD. Maximal circadian misalignment and desynchronization unsurprisingly occur during night shifts, and schedules involving more night work lead to higher odds of developing SWD. In a 2-year prospective study of more than 1,000 shift-working nurses, Waage et al. (2021) reported that workers with and without SWD were working on average 33.9 and 12.9 night shifts per year at baseline, respectively. They also observed that moving from a day to a night schedule (odds ratio [OR] = 4.75) or increasing the number of yearly night shifts (OR = 2.95, increase by >10 nights/year) were the strongest predictors of developing SWD. Other scheduling factors affect the well-being of shift workers and may affect the risk of developing SWD, including the shift start times, the number of consecutive hours and shifts worked (Blum & Zeitzer, 2021), the speed and direction of rotation (Waage et al., 2021), and the perceived control over the work schedule (Bambra et al., 2008).

Treatment

As SWD is primarily caused by a misalignment between the sleep–wake cycle and the endogenous circadian system, different treatment options were proposed to facilitate circadian adaptation, improve sleep, and reduce sleepiness in shift workers. Considering the important interindividual variability and the various factors contributing to the development of SWD, these treatment options should be viewed as complementary, and a multilevel approach is recommended.

PHOTOTHERAPY

A proposed strategy is to facilitate circadian adaptation through timed bright light exposure (i.e., phototherapy). Indeed, light is the most powerful circadian synchronizer and can shift the endogenous circadian system to different internal biological times. The resetting effect of light is phase-dependent, such that exposure to light in the late evening and early night delays circadian rhythms, whereas exposure in the late night and early morning advances rhythms (Czeisler et al., 1989; Khalsa et al., 2003; Minors et al., 1991). The habitual strategy for night-shift workers is to favor circadian adaptation by delaying their circadian system. This is achieved by exposing themselves to bright light in the evening and the first half of the night using a phototherapy lamp and avoiding or shielding themselves from light in the early morning using sunglasses. Studies conducted in the laboratory and in the field demonstrated that such strategies can promote complete or partial circadian adaptation to night-shift work (Boivin, Boudreau, & Tremblay, 2012; Boivin & James, 2002a; Crowley et al., 2003; Lammers-van der Holst et al., 2021; Shechter et al., 2020). However, there are very few studies on strategic light–dark interventions in real shift workers in their natural field conditions, even fewer if we consider only those with reliable circadian assessment (Boivin et al., 2021). Moreover, a given light–dark strategy can be successful for a given group of workers (Boivin, Boudreau, James, & Kin, 2012; Boivin & James, 2002a; James et al., 2004) but not for another one (Boivin, Boudreau, & Tremblay, 2012). These inconsistencies underline the inadequacy of directly extrapolating results collected in artificial, highly controlled environments to natural work environments where numerous sources of counterproductive light exposure are interacting. Photic resetting of the endogenous circadian system to a night-oriented schedule requires multiple days, so interventions based on strategic light–dark exposure might only be beneficial for particular work rosters with long sequences of night shifts, rather than irregular or fast-rotating schedules. Such approaches can also lead to large interindividual variabilities considering the difficulties of reliably assessing circadian phase in ambulatory settings.

Maintaining a partial circadian adaptation throughout work and rest days may be an alternative to complete circadian adaptation. By maintaining a delayed sleep period during rest days (e.g., 3:00–11:00 a.m.), the circadian nadir of alertness could, in theory, be maintained during the first half of the daytime sleep period. Consequently, nighttime sleepiness would be reduced and daytime sleep improved on days of night-shift work. Although partial circadian adaptation was tested in healthy subjects during simulated night shifts (Chapdelaine et al., 2012; Crowley et al., 2004; Smith et al., 2009), studies in real shift workers are lacking.

Aside from its circadian effect, light at night and during the day can exert a direct alerting effect in humans (Cajochen, 2007; Lok et al., 2018) depending on its intensity (Cajochen et al., 2000) and spectral composition (Figueiro et al., 2016; Rahman et al., 2014). The alerting effect of light follows an exponential dose–response curve, such that half of the maximum alerting response to the bright light (9,100 lux) can be obtained with relatively normal ambient light exposure (100 lux; Cajochen et al., 2000). Blue-enriched light was reported to have a stronger alerting effect than white large-spectrum light (Figueiro et al., 2009; Rahman et al., 2014; Viola et al., 2008), especially when administered at night (Rahman et al., 2013). It can improve nocturnal sustained attention and sleepiness (Aarts et al., 2020; Motamedzadeh et al., 2017; Sletten et al., 2017, 2021; van Woerkom, 2021). Light at night was also reported to improve daytime sleep duration (Boivin, Boudreau, James, & Kin, 2012; Sasseville & Hebert, 2010) and quality (Figueiro & Pedler, 2020), although this effect is inconsistent across studies (H. I. Jensen et al., 2016; Kazemi et al., 2019; Rahman et al., 2013).

BEHAVIORAL INTERVENTIONS

Several behavioral interventions were proposed to improve the health and well-being of SWD patients, including education on sleep hygiene, planned napping, and diet.

Behavioral approaches that can be used to maximize sleep are generally referred to as sleep hygiene. Sleep hygiene education is beneficial for most patients with symptoms of insomnia (Stepanski & Wyatt, 2003) and should also be offered to shift workers with specific recommendations for them (Shriane et al., 2020). Bright light from the environment should be avoided in the hours before going to sleep, but if unavoidable, sunglasses should be used, ideally those blocking blue light. A predictable bedtime routine should be put in place, including, for example, a shower and quiet activities favoring relaxation. Smartphones should be avoided, especially in the bedroom. The bedroom itself should be a dark, cool, and quiet environment reserved for sleep. The sleeper should avoid looking at the time while sleeping but can set an alarm to go off at the desired wake time. The sleep schedule should be kept as regular as possible. Sleep following a night shift may be more beneficial when planned in the evening rather than in the morning as it would reduce time awake in the second half of the night (W. J. Cheng et al., 2022; Chinoy et al., 2016; Isherwood et al., 2020; Santhi et al., 2008). However, this strategy might not work for everyone as some individuals might have difficulty sleeping prior to a night shift, thus increasing their risk of severe sleep deprivation and extended waking while at work.

Cognitive behavioral therapy for insomnia is the recommended first choice for treating chronic insomnia (Qaseem et al., 2016; Riemann et al., 2017). A version adapted to shift workers appears beneficial to improve sleep and well-being of shift workers and SWD patients (Jarnefelt et al., 2012, 2020; Peter et al., 2019), and further studies are on their way (Retzer et al., 2021).

Planned napping is an effective approach to reduce sleep deprivation and maintain an adequate daily sleep duration (Morgenthaler et al., 2007). It is more beneficial and safer to prevent the accumulation of a significant sleep debt than to wait for drowsiness to appear at inopportune moments. Short naps of 20–120 minutes can be planned before work shifts in anticipation of a decrease in alertness in the hours to come. Recuperative short naps can also be planned during the work shifts if possible and necessary. However, the use of naps can temporarily reduce alertness and performance, a phenomenon known as *sleep inertia*, with levels usually returning to normal within 30 minutes following awakening (Hilditch & McHill, 2019).

Food intake should be limited at night. A sustaining meal can be taken in the evening, but at night, fasting or light and healthy food choices should be preferred. It was shown that restricting food intake during the daytime can prevent glucose intolerance typically observed in night-shift workers (Chellappa et al., 2021).

HYPNOTICS AND STIMULANTS

Hypnotics can be considered to treat SWD. Hypnotics with a short half-life such as triazolam and zopiclone were suggested to promote daytime sleep in SWD (Morgenthaler et al., 2007). However, a 2014 Cochrane systematic review reports that daytime sleep duration was not significantly improved in shift workers following the administration of zopiclone (Liira et al., 2014). Longer-acting hypnotics may also cause safety issues as residual sedation may be carried over during the night shift. A recent double-blind placebo-controlled randomized clinical trial studied the use of suvorexant, a dual orexin/hypocretin receptor antagonist (DORA), in 19 real shift workers with self-reported daytime sleep difficulties (Zeitzer et al., 2020). Compared to placebo, the authors reported a 2.16-hour increase in daytime sleep duration measured by actigraphy by the end of the 2-week treatment period with a 20-mg dose prior to the daytime sleep period.

Melatonin, a hormone secreted by the pineal gland at night, can be administered exogenously to promote sleep in the daytime. The American Academy of Sleep Medicine recommends the use of exogenous melatonin before bedtime to improve daytime sleep quality and duration in night-shift workers (Morgenthaler et al., 2007). A 2014 Cochrane systematic review and meta-analysis thoroughly summarized the main findings on the use of exogenous melatonin to improve shift workers' sleep (Liira et al., 2014). Melatonin (1 to 10 mg) taken 10 to 60 minutes before daytime sleep following night shifts can increase sleep duration by about 25 minutes compared to placebo. However, melatonin had only a limited effect on nighttime performance and alertness levels (Boivin et al., 2021; Sack et al., 2007a). As demonstrated in the laboratory, properly timed exogenous melatonin administration can promote circadian adaptation, but results in real shift workers are inconclusive (Boivin et al., 2021).

Stimulants can also be used in SWD. Caffeine can enhance alertness and performance during night shifts (Liira et al., 2014) and following sleep loss (Irwin et al., 2020). It has limited adverse effects but can impair daytime sleep. Thus, caffeine should be limited to the first half of a night shift, avoided at least 6 hours before bedtime, and taken in reasonable quantity (<400 mg; P. Cheng & Drake, 2019).

Modafinil and armodafinil are wake-promoting agents approved by the US Food and Drug Administration for patients with sleepiness caused by shift work. Administered in the evening before the night shift, modafinil (200 mg) and armodafinil (50–150 mg) were shown to reduce objective and subjective nighttime sleepiness but have been associated with adverse events, including headache, nausea, and some cases of severe skin reaction (Liira et al., 2014). Although sleepiness is reduced by these wake-promoting agents, sleep latencies during the Multiple Sleep Latency Test and driving performance in the morning were not normalized in more recent studies (Savarese & Di Perri, 2020).

Irregular Sleep–Wake Rhythm Disorder

Irregular sleep–wake rhythm disorder (ISWRD) is characterized by the lack of a clear diurnal sleep–wake cycle (ICSD-3). The patient or caregiver reports that sleep episodes are fragmented into irregularly distributed sleep bouts across the 24-hour day. ISWRD is associated with symptoms of insomnia or excessive sleepiness that occur irregularly throughout the 24-hour day. This disorder has important negative consequences on caregivers whose sleep is constantly disrupted at night.

Epidemiology

Cases of ISWRD in the general population are very rare, and the exact prevalence is unknown (ICSD-3). ISWRD is more common in patients with neurodegenerative disorders, with neurodevelopmental disorders, or following a traumatic brain injury (Steele et al., 2021). In older adults, ISWRD is often comorbid with medical conditions such as Alzheimer's disease, Parkinson's disease, and Huntington's disease. A greater prevalence is observed in institutionalized populations, and ISWRD is also a common cause of institutionalization. ISWRD was observed in children with medical conditions such as the autism spectrum, Angelman syndrome, and Smith-Magenis syndrome. It was reported in psychiatric conditions such as schizophrenia (Abbott & Zee, 2015). No gender difference or familial pattern has been reported, although genetic factors might be involved in sleep–wake disturbances in Alzheimer's disease (Sack et al., 2007b).

Diagnosis

A history of an irregular sleep–wake pattern accompanied by periods of insomnia at night or excessive daytime sleepiness for at least 3 months is essential for diagnosing ISWRD (ICSD-3). Accordingly, this disorder is characterized by the appearance of multiple naps randomly distributed across the 24-hour day, with the longest daily sleep episode, usually less than 4 hours, often occurring between 2:00 and 6:00 a.m. (American Psychiatric Association, 2013). The presence of at least three sleep bouts (typically of 2–4 hours) per 24-hour period must be documented using a sleep diary or with continuous actigraphy monitoring over a minimum observation period of 7 days, preferably 14 days. The total sleep time over a 24-hour period may be normal compared to a population of the same age. ISWRD should not be better explained by another sleep disorder, medical condition, medication use, or substance abuse. A polysomnographic sleep recording is not required to diagnose ISWRD but can help to exclude other sleep disorders.

The use of circadian markers such as body temperature, melatonin, or cortisol secretion can be helpful to document the dampening, disruption, or loss of circadian rhythmicity corresponding to the dysregulation of the sleep–wake cycle. However, the endogenous nature of these rhythms might be masked by the disrupted rest–activity cycle and quite difficult to assess in field conditions. Patients with ISWRD should be differentiated from those with poor sleep hygiene and those who voluntarily adopt an irregular schedule of sleep and light exposure, such as shift workers.

Pathophysiology

A dampening, dysregulation, or loss of the circadian regulation of sleep and wakefulness could lead to sleep fragmentation and loss of its nighttime consolidation in patients with ISWRD. In healthy individuals, sleep is regulated by the interaction of a homeostatic and a circadian process. The homeostatic process increases and decreases sleep propensity as a function of time awake or time asleep, respectively. The circadian process promotes sleep and wakefulness as a function of time of day and is dependent on the action of the circadian system on sleep and arousal centers. If the circadian process is dampened or lost, sleep and wakefulness become governed solely by the homeostatic process, leading to short and irregular sleep bouts, independently of the time of day. In animals with lesions of the suprachiasmatic nucleus (SCN), the central circadian clock (Edgar et al., 1993; Mistlberger, 2005), the rest–activity cycle becomes arrhythmic and fragmented across the 24-hour day. Similar findings were reported in human cases of presumed SCN lesions (Cohen & Albers, 1991; Schwartz et al., 1986).

Different etiology can partially or totally affect the circadian regulation of sleep. Brain trauma or developmental abnormalities may directly affect the central circadian system, its inputs or outputs, and lead to ISWRD (Abbott & Zee, 2015; Steele et al., 2021). A significant loss of SCN neurons has been observed postmortem in certain neurodegenerative diseases, such as Alzheimer's disease, and may account for the disruption of the sleep–wake cycle (Sack et al., 2007b; Swaab et al., 1985). In postmortem brain tissues, a loss of rhythmic expression of pineal clock genes (Wu et al., 2006), as well as a desynchronization between the central SCN clock and non-SCN brain oscillators (Cermakian et al., 2011) were reported. Sleep and circadian disturbances can contribute to the progression of the disease (Van Erum et al., 2018). In Alzheimer's disease, factors other than SCN tissue degeneration can further disorganize the sleep–wake cycle (Fernandez et al., 2021). With age, a reduction in retinal sensitivity to light combined with a decrease in light exposure could contribute to the onset of sleep disturbances and nocturnal restlessness. In institutionalized elderly patients, a reduction in exposure to external synchronizing agents, such as environment light, social interactions, and physical activity can contribute to ISWRD.

Non-circadian causes are also possible, and the etiology of ISWRD is likely multifactorial. For instance, poor sleep hygiene and a chaotic household could be contributing factors.

Treatment

The American Academy of Sleep Medicine updated its clinical practice guidelines for the treatment of ISWRD in 2015 (Auger et al., 2015). Elderly patients with dementia can benefit from the use of phototherapy but should avoid sleep-promoting medications and oral melatonin as they can increase the risk of falls and may have adverse effects on mood, respectively. Since these guidelines were published, recent evidence suggests that newer hypnotics such as DORAs could be safe (Murphy et al., 2020), although experimental testing in these populations is needed. Children and adolescents with neurologic disorders can benefit from strategically timed administration of oral melatonin or melatonin agonists. Other treatment options were considered by the task force for ISWRD, including regular sleep–wake schedule, strategic darkness exposure, and wake-promoting medications; but no recommendation was made due to the lack of supporting data.

Overall, therapeutic decisions should seek to consolidate sleep at night. Patients could benefit from a multimodal approach, which includes minimizing time in bed during the day, increasing daytime physical activity and social interactions, enhancing exposure to bright light in the morning, implementing a bedtime routine, and reducing noise and light disturbances at night. Such a mixed modality treatment was recommended for elderly patients with dementia in the prior American Academy of Sleep Medicine guidelines (Morgenthaler et al., 2007) as it showed small improvement toward nighttime sleep consolidation in two separate populations of elderly patients with dementia (Alessi et al., 2005; McCurry et al., 2005). However, the most recent guidelines do not provide a recommendation for such mixed modality approaches as these two studies were excluded due to a lack of ISWRD diagnosis or missing critical outcome measures (Auger et al., 2015).

Non-24-Hour Sleep–Wake Rhythm Disorder

Non-24-hour sleep–wake rhythm disorder (N24SWD) is described as a chronic deviation of the sleep–wake cycle from the conventional 24-hour day. It occurs when the circadian system fails to entrain to the 24-hour terrestrial days and appears to free-run according to its own intrinsic rhythmicity. It manifests as a progressive daily shift, usually a delay, of the main sleep episode, slowly drifting in and out of phase with the earth light–dark cycle. Cyclic bouts of severe insomnia and excessive sleepiness are observed when patients try to sleep or stay awake at inappropriate circadian phases. N24SWD is frequent in patients with complete loss of sight but was also reported in sighted individuals.

Epidemiology

N24SWD is commonly observed in up to 63% of populations with complete loss of sight and no light perception (Abbott, 2019), with symptoms occurring at any age and often coinciding with vision loss, even when this loss is congenital.

In sighted people, this disorder is rare, but its exact prevalence is unknown. Case series of sighted individuals with N24SWD show a strong male predominance (between 72% and 86% of cases), and in most cases, symptoms usually appear before the age of 30 (Hayakawa et al., 2005; Malkani et al., 2018; Uchiyama & Lockley, 2015). In a large case series, 28% of the 57 patients had a premorbid psychiatric condition, such as mood disorder, schizophrenia, obsessive–compulsive disorder, or mental retardation (Hayakawa et al., 2005). An additional 34% of patients developed a major depression following N24SWD. In the same study, delayed sleep–wake phase disorder (DSWPD) was also diagnosed in 26% of the patients who eventually developed N24SWD. Moreover, adult patients with a DSWPD can develop N24SWD following chronotherapy treatments (Oren & Wehr, 1992). Almost all N24SWD patients report a history of disturbed social functioning as a result of being unable to comply with a regular school or work schedule (Uchiyama & Lockley, 2015). A few cases have also been reported following traumatic brain injuries (Boivin et al., 2003; Eliott et al., 1971; O'Neill et al., 2014).

Diagnosis

The N24SWD diagnosis is based on a history of insomnia and excessive daytime sleepiness alternating with asymptomatic episodes over the course of at least 3 months (ICSD-3). A sleep diary or continuous actigraphy monitoring over a minimum period of 14 days is essential to document the progressive shift of the main sleep period. However, a longer monitoring period is highly preferable. Indeed, if the 14-day observation period is scheduled when patients are sleeping in phase with their endogenous circadian system, the diagnosis can be missed. Patients with N24SWD usually delay their sleep period to match their free-running circadian system. Patients with blindness usually have shorter daily shifts than sighted ones (Flynn-Evans et al., 2014; Hayakawa et al., 2005), such that the monitoring period should be even longer. In approximately half of the patients, significant abrupt delays, qualified as "jumps," were observed when the sleep period occurred in the daytime (Abbott, 2019). The use of circadian markers such as dim light melatonin onset or urinary 6-sulfatoxy-melatonin excretion can help document the free course of the circadian system. Symptoms should not be better explained by another condition such as another sleep disorder, a medical condition, or substance abuse.

Symptoms typically follow a predictable pattern. Subsequent to an asymptomatic phase, the patient starts reporting difficulties falling asleep and a progressively delayed sleep schedule. Gradually, the patient experiences excessive daytime sleepiness and frequent daytime napping. Eventually, these symptoms subside with the recurrence of an asymptomatic phase. The duration of these asymptomatic/symptomatic phases can be shorter (e.g., ~3.6-week cycle for a 25-hour circadian period) or longer (e.g., ~4 months for a 24.2-hour circadian period) depending on the patient's intrinsic circadian period. Therefore, depending on the time of clinical assessment, an N24SWD patient could appear to have insomnia, excessive daytime sleepiness, or an advanced or delayed sleep–wake phase disorder. These two latter disorders are characterized by a tendency to fall asleep and wake up at abnormally early or late times, respectively, compared to societal norms. The important criteria for the differential diagnosis of N24SWD is the inability to maintain a stable sleep–wake pattern aligned with the terrestrial 24-hour day. Attempts to adopt a conventional sleep schedule lead to the appearance of severe and recurrent sleep and alertness disturbances. During these unsuccessful attempts, patients may develop an addiction to alcohol, sedatives, hypnotics, and stimulants, which in turn may worsen their sleep and alertness problems (Uchiyama & Lockley, 2015).

When patients have flexibility in the timing of their work or social activities, they can follow their natural tendency to free-run and avoid symptoms of insomnia and excessive sleepiness.

Pathophysiology

In the general population, the average endogenous circadian period is about 24.2 hours, with a narrow distribution (Czeisler et al., 1999; Gronfier et al., 2007). Sex differences were observed with an average period shorter in women versus men (24.09 vs. 24.19 hours) and a greater percentage of women with a period shorter than 24 hours (35% vs. 14%; Duffy et al., 2011). Other individual factors such as racial differences can affect the circadian period (Eastman et al., 2015, 2017). As the circadian period is not exactly 24 hours, the circadian system needs to be continuously realigned to the terrestrial day, in a process called *circadian entrainment*. In humans as in other animal species, light is the most potent synchronizer of endogenous circadian rhythms. Light information is received by the image-forming rod and cone photoreceptors but also by intrinsically photosensitive retinal ganglion cells expressing the photopigment melanopsin (Hughes et al., 2012). The light information from these three specialized cell types is integrated into the latter, and conveyed to the SCN via a direct monosynaptic pathway, the retinohypothalamic track (Foster, 2021).

In sighted healthy individuals, the circadian system is continuously realigned and entrained to the environment. However, in patients with blindness and no light perception, the photic information cannot reach the SCN, and the endogenous circadian system follows its own intrinsic period and free-runs relative to the environment. Most patients with N24SWD drift by going to bed later every day instead of earlier, supporting the observation that the circadian period is usually longer than 24 hours. Symptoms thus depend on when the patients try to sleep or stay awake relative to their endogenous circadian system.

Some patients with blindness can perceive light as a circadian synchronizer, as evidenced by its melatonin-suppressing effect at night, and can thus be entrained by light (Czeisler et al., 1995). This is presumably the case for nearly 50% of patients with blindness (Uchiyama & Lockley, 2015). The circadian system of persons with low vision but some light perception and intact photosensitive retinal ganglion cells or with cortical blindness could still be responsive to light (Flynn-Evans et al., 2014). Some patients with blindness could also manage to adjust their circadian system to the environment because their intrinsic circadian period is very close to a 24-hour rhythm. Under these circumstances, nonphotic synchronizers, such as the rest–activity cycle, the rhythm of food intake, physical activity, or social interactions, could be sufficient (Emens et al., 2005).

In sighted patients with N24SWD, causes are usually more complex and less well identified. It was reported that the average length of the sleep–wake cycle in sighted N24SWD patients was close to 25 hours based on actigraphy monitoring (Hayakawa et al., 2005), whereas it was closer to 24 hours in patients with blindness. However, in most of these studies, the endogenous circadian period is not formally measured but rather inferred from the sleep–wake cycle length, thus suffering from masking effects. It has been proposed that the 24-hour terrestrial day falls outside of the range of circadian entrainment in sighted N24SWD patients or that they require stronger synchronizers to entrain, although this has not been experimentally demonstrated. Alternatively, N24SWD could be related to an inability to respond to light or microtraumas to the SCN. Episodes of relative coordination to the 24-hour day were reported when patients are transiently in and out of phase, with environmental synchronizers too weak to fully entrain them to the geophysical environment (Figures 33.1 and 33.2; Boivin et al., 2004). An abnormal phase angle was observed between the endogenous circadian system and sleep schedule in patients with N24SWD (Boivin et al., 2003; Uchiyama et al., 2000). Weaker sleep homeostatic pressure, leading to prolonged wake periods and late exposure to light during the delay portion of the phase–response curve to light, is also possible. In patients with psychiatric comorbidities, social isolation, behavioral problems, and poor sleep hygiene could disturb light–dark exposure and contribute to the free-running of their sleep–wake cycle (Blum & Zeitzer, 2021). In a recent study, low light exposure was identified as a main contributor to the appearance of N24SWD in schizophrenic patients (Skeldon et al., 2022).

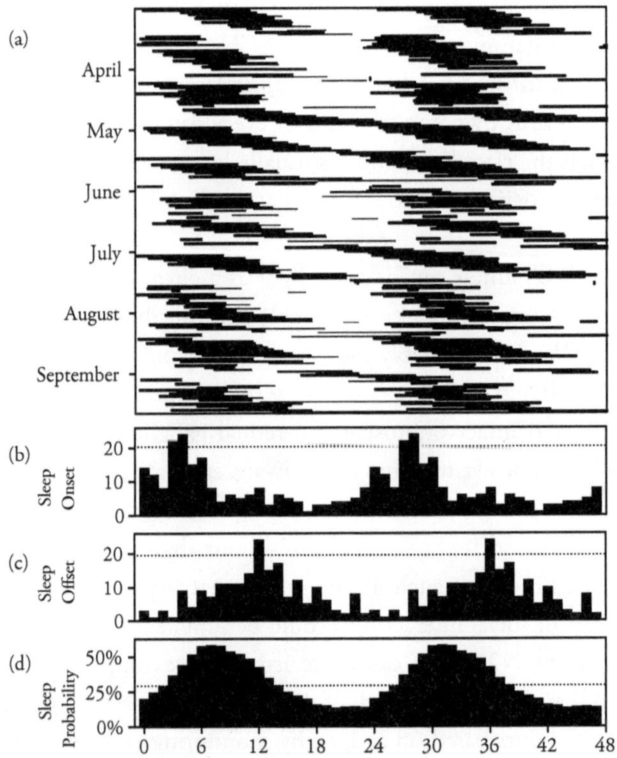

Figure 33.1 Sleep–wake cycle in a case of N24SWD
Note. Panel A: Sleep episodes are shown as black bars and are double-plotted for clarity. Sleep times were confirmed by wrist actigraphy recording and analyzed by a software-derived algorithm (AW-64 monitor and Sleepwatch software; Mini-Mitter, Bend, OR, USA). Frequency of temporal distribution of sleep onset (B) and sleep offset (C) throughout the day, as determined from sleep logs and plotted in 1-hour bins. Within panels B and C, dotted lines represent the upper limit of the 95% confidence interval (mean + 2 standard deviations) describing the number of observations. (D) Percent probability of the patient being asleep at particular times of day. The dotted line represents the median value of this probability. Figure from Boivin et al. (2004). Association between delayed sleep phase and hypernyctohemeral syndroms: A case study. *Sleep*, *27*(3), 417–421, by permission of Oxford University Press.

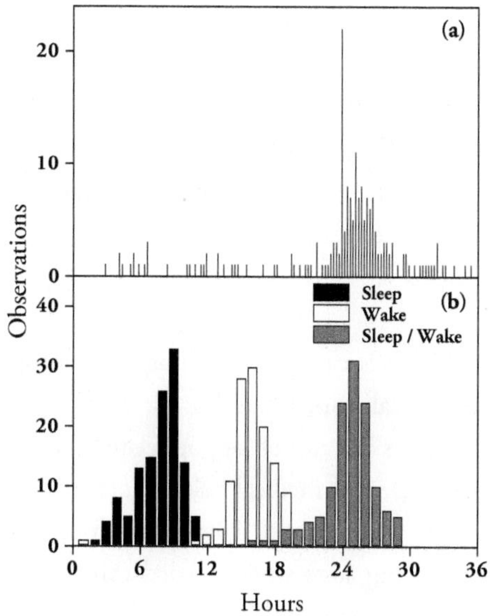

Figure 33.2 Distribution of sleep–wake cycle length in a case of N24SWD

Note. Panel A: A sleep–wake cycle is defined as a sleep episode, reported as a main sleep episode by the patient, immediately followed by a waking episode. Analyses excluded sleep episodes reported as naps. Descriptive statistics were used to determine the duration of our patient's sleep–wake cycles. Panel B: Sleep–wake cycles (hatched) with mean duration withing 1 standard deviation of the initial mean cycle length were included; associated wake periods (white) and sleep periods (black) were plotted with a 60-minute resolution. The sharp peak at 24 hours observed in panel A was interpreted as being the result of relative coordination to the environment and was thus excluded from these last analyses. Figure from Boivin et al. (2004). Association between delayed sleep phase and hypernyctohemeral syndroms: A case study. *Sleep*, 27(3), 417–421, by permission of Oxford University Press.

Treatment

For patients with blindness, properly timed administration of exogenous melatonin or melatonin agonists is the treatment recommended by the American Academy of Sleep Medicine to entrain the circadian system to the 24-hour day (Abbott & Zee, 2015). Administration of exogenous melatonin (3–10 mg) should be scheduled 1 hour before bedtime until the patient reaches entrainment, which usually occurs after 3–9 weeks (Zee et al., 2013). As the exact timing of the circadian system is unknown in N24SWD patients, it is likely that it will take a few weeks of melatonin administration before reaching the correct circadian phase of ingestion. Once synchronization occurs, a smaller dose (≤0.5 mg) could be administered to maintain circadian entrainment.

Tasimelteon, a selective agonist for the melatonin receptors MT1 and MT2, is the first drug approved in the United States and in the European Union for the treatment of N24SWD in patients with blindness. A randomized, double-blind, placebo-controlled clinical trial demonstrated that entrainment occurred in 20% of the patients after 26 weeks of treatment with tasimelteon compared to 3% of those treated with placebo, though the authors report that a longer treatment period may be more effective (Lockley et al., 2015). Interestingly, a greater rate of entrainment, 67% of patients, was reported in those treated with melatonin (0.5–10 mg) for 3.7 to 11.6 weeks in a small meta-analysis of three studies (Auger et al., 2015).

For sighted patients, no clear recommendations were made because of a lack of evidence (Auger et al., 2015). Some case reports showed re-entrainment with properly timed phototherapy and/or melatonin administration. Treatment success probably depends on the underlying cause of N24SWD. According to a recent review (Abbott, 2019), it is suggested to wait until the appearance of an asymptomatic phase occurring at conventional times of day before starting active treatments.

Conclusion

In susceptible individuals, SWD is caused by self-imposed abrupt shifts in the timing of behavioral rhythms due to atypical work schedules. Circadian misalignment combined with sleep–wake disturbances increases the risk of fatigue-related incidents and, over time, could be main contributors to the increased medical risks reported in shift-working populations. Various countermeasures such as improved light–dark exposure, sleep management, and careful use of hypnotics and stimulants when needed can be considered. In comparison, ISWRD and N24SWD are presumably caused by an intrinsic malfunction of the endogenous circadian timing system, although behavioral factors can aggravate sleep–wake disturbances. Comorbid medical or psychiatric conditions can also exist with these disorders and should be treated. Overall, therapeutic decisions should seek to consolidate sleep at night, and a multimodal approach is suggested, although no clear guidelines are available for sighted patients. For patients with blindness and N24SWD, properly timed administration of exogenous melatonin or melatonin agonists is the treatment of choice. The clinical management of CRSWDs usually requires long periods of investigation and observation. In all cases, a careful review of sleep hygiene is important as maladaptive behaviors are often superimposed.

Future Directions

The ability to reliably and easily assess circadian phase remains a challenge for the clinical management of CRSWDs. Whether derived from melatonin, cortisol, or core body temperature, the assessment of circadian phase is subjected to important masking effects in field conditions. Another challenge is the heterogeneity of clinical presentation in which intrinsic and extrinsic factors often interact. Finally, most of our current knowledge on circadian rhythms and physiology is based on data collected predominantly in Caucasian men. Improving inclusiveness in research is essential to adapt our clinical management to individual sensitivities. Thus, future studies should address the following questions:

- What are the most reliable and direct ways to assess circadian phase in field conditions?
- What are the respective roles of intrinsic and extrinsic factors in the etiology of CRSWDs?
- What individual factors affect the susceptibility to CRSWDs and responses to treatment?

References

Aarts, M. P. J., Hartmeyer, S. L., Morsink, K., Kort, H. S. M., & de Kort, Y. A. W. (2020). Can special light glasses reduce sleepiness and improve sleep of nightshift workers? A placebo-controlled explorative field study. *Clocks Sleep*, *2*(2), 225–245. https://doi.org/10.3390/clockssleep2020018

Abbott, S. M. (2019). Non-24-hour sleep–wake rhythm disorder. *Neurologic Clinics*, *37*(3), 545–552. https://doi.org/10.1016/j.ncl.2019.03.002

Abbott, S. M., & Zee, P. C. (2015). Irregular sleep–wake rhythm disorder. *Sleep Medicine Clinics*, *10*(4), 517–522. https://doi.org/10.1016/j.jsmc.2015.08.005

Akashi, M., Soma, H., Yamamoto, T., Tsugitomi, A., Yamashita, S., Yamamoto, T., Nishida, E., Yasuda, A., Liao, J. K., & Node, K. (2010). Noninvasive method for assessing the human circadian clock using hair follicle cells. *Proceedings of the National Academy of Sciences of the United States of America*, *107*(35), 15643–15648. https://doi.org/10.1073/pnas.1003878107

Akerstedt, T., & Wright, K. P., Jr. (2009). Sleep loss and fatigue in shift work and shift work disorder. *Sleep Medicine Clinics*, *4*(2), 257–271. https://doi.org/10.1016/j.jsmc.2009.03.001

Alessi, C. A., Martin, J. L., Webber, A. P., Cynthia Kim, E., Harker, J. O., & Josephson, K. R. (2005). Randomized, controlled trial of a nonpharmacological intervention to improve abnormal sleep/wake patterns in nursing home residents. *Journal of the American Geriatric Society*, *53*(5), 803–810. https://doi.org/10.1111/j.1532-5415.2005.53251.x

American Academy of Sleep Medicine. (2014). *International classification of sleep disorders* (3rd ed.).

American Psychiatric Association. (2013). *Diagnostic and statistical manual of mental disorders* (5th ed.).

Anderson, C., Ftouni, S., Ronda, J. M., Rajaratnam, S. M. W., Czeisler, C. A., & Lockley, S. W. (2018). Self-reported drowsiness and safety outcomes while driving after an extended duration work shift in trainee physicians. *Sleep*, *41*(2), Article zsx195. https://doi.org/10.1093/sleep/zsx195

Anvekar, A. P., Nathan, E. A., Doherty, D. A., & Patole, S. K. (2021). Effect of shift work on fatigue and sleep in neonatal registrars. *PLOS ONE*, *16*(1), Article e0245428. https://doi.org/10.1371/journal.pone.0245428

Auger, R. R., Burgess, H. J., Emens, J. S., Deriy, L. V., Thomas, S. M., & Sharkey, K. M. (2015). Clinical practice guideline for the treatment of intrinsic circadian rhythm sleep–wake disorders: Advanced sleep–wake phase disorder (ASWPD), delayed sleep–wake phase disorder (DSWPD), non-24-hour sleep–wake rhythm disorder (N24SWD), and irregular sleep–wake rhythm disorder (ISWRD). An update for 2015: An American Academy of Sleep Medicine clinical practice guideline. *Journal of Clinical Sleep Medicine*, *11*(10), 1199–1236. https://doi.org/10.5664/jcsm.5100

Bambra, C. L., Whitehead, M. M., Sowden, A. J., Akers, J., & Petticrew, M. P. (2008). Shifting schedules: The health effects of reorganizing shift work. *American Journal of Preventive Medicine*, *34*(5), 427–434. https://doi.org/10.1016/j.amepre.2007.12.023

Barger, L. K., Ogeil, R. P., Drake, C. L., O'Brien, C. S., Ng, K. T., & Rajaratnam, S. M. (2012). Validation of a questionnaire to screen for shift work disorder. *Sleep*, *35*(12), 1693–1703. https://doi.org/10.5665/sleep.2246

Behrens, T., Burek, K., Pallapies, D., Kosters, L., Lehnert, M., Beine, A., Wichert, K., Kantermann, T., Vetter, C., Bruning, T., & Rabstein, S. (2019). Decreased psychomotor vigilance of female shift workers after working night shifts. *PLOS ONE*, *14*(7), Article e0219087. https://doi.org/10.1371/journal.pone.0219087

Bescos, R., Boden, M. J., Jackson, M. L., Trewin, A. J., Marin, E. C., Levinger, I., Garnham, A., Hiam, D. S., Falcao-Tebas, F., Conte, F., Owens, J. A., Kennaway, D. J., & McConell, G. K. (2018). Four days of simulated shift work reduces insulin sensitivity in humans. *Acta Physiologica*, *223*(2), Article e13039. https://doi.org/10.1111/apha.13039

Blum, D. J., & Zeitzer, J. M. (2021). Irregular sleep–wake, non-24-hour sleep–wake, jet lag, and shift work sleep disorders. In E. H. During & C. A. Kushida (Eds.), *Clinical sleep medicine—A comprehensive guide for mental health and other medical professionals* (pp. 245–271). American Psychiatric Association.

Boivin, D. B., Boudreau, P., James, F. O., & Kin, N. M. (2012). Photic resetting in night-shift work: Impact on nurses' sleep. *Chronobiology International*, *29*(5), 619–628. https://doi.org/10.3109/07420528.2012.675257

Boivin, D. B., Boudreau, P., & Tremblay, G. M. (2012). Phototherapy and orange-tinted goggles for night-shift adaptation of police officers on patrol. *Chronobiology International*, *29*(5), 629–640. https://doi.org/10.3109/07420528.2012.675252

Boivin, D. B., Caliyurt, O., James, F. O., & Chalk, C. (2004). Association between delayed sleep phase and hypernyctohemeral syndromes: A case study. *Sleep*, *27*(3), 417–421. https://doi.org/10.1093/sleep/27.3.417

Boivin, D. B., & James, F. O. (2002a). Circadian adaptation to night-shift work by judicious light and darkness exposure. *Journal of Biological Rhythms*, *17*(6), 556–567. https://doi.org/10.1177/0748730402238238

Boivin, D. B., & James, F. O. (2002b). Phase-dependent effects of room light exposure in a 5-h advance of the sleep–wake cycle: Implications for jet lag. *Journal of Biological Rhythms*, *17*(3), 266–276. https://doi.org/10.1177/074873040201700310

Boivin, D. B., James, F. O., Santo, J. B., Caliyurt, O., & Chalk, C. (2003). Non-24-hour sleep–wake syndrome following a car accident. *Neurology*, *60*(11), 1841–1843. https://doi.org/10.1212/01.wnl.0000061482.24750.7c

Booker, L. A., Magee, M., Rajaratnam, S. M. W., Sletten, T. L., & Howard, M. E. (2018). Individual vulnerability to insomnia, excessive sleepiness and shift work disorder amongst healthcare shift workers. A systematic review. *Sleep Medicine Reviews*, *41*, 220–233. https://doi.org/10.1016/j.smrv.2018.03.005

Boudreau, P., Dumont, G. A., & Boivin, D. B. (2013). Circadian adaptation to night shift work influences sleep, performance, mood and the autonomic modulation of the heart. *PLOS ONE*, *8*(7), Article e70813. https://doi.org/10.1371/journal.pone.0070813

Cajochen, C. (2007). Alerting effects of light. *Sleep Medicine Reviews*, *11*(6), 453–464.

Cajochen, C., Zeitzer, J. M., Czeisler, C. A., & Dijk, D.-J. (2000). Dose–response relationship for light intensity and ocular and electroencephalographic correlates of human alertness. *Behavioural Brain Research*, *115*(1), 75–83. https://doi.org/10.1016/S0166-4328(00)00236-9

Cermakian, N., Lamont, E. W., Boudreau, P., & Boivin, D. B. (2011). Circadian clock gene expression in brain regions of Alzheimer's disease patients and control subjects. *Journal of Biological Rhythms*, *26*(2), 160–170. https://doi.org/10.1177/0748730410395732

Chapdelaine, S., Paquet, J., & Dumont, M. (2012). Effects of partial circadian adjustments on sleep and vigilance quality during simulated night work. *Journal of Sleep Research*, *21*(4), 380–389. https://doi.org/10.1111/j.1365-2869.2012.00998.x

Chellappa, S. L., Morris, C. J., & Scheer, F. (2019). Effects of circadian misalignment on cognition in chronic shift workers. *Scientific Reports*, *9*(1), Article 699. https://doi.org/10.1038/s41598-018-36762-w

Chellappa, S. L., Qian, J., Vujovic, N., Morris, C. J., Nedeltcheva, A., Nguyen, H., Rahman, N., Heng, S. W., Kelly, L., Kerlin-Monteiro, K., Srivastav, S., Wang, W., Aeschbach, D., Czeisler, C. A., Shea, S. A., Adler, G. K., Garaulet, M., & Scheer, F. (2021). Daytime eating prevents internal circadian misalignment and glucose intolerance in night work. *Science Advances*, *7*(49), Article eabg9910. https://doi.org/10.1126/sciadv.abg9910

Cheng, P., & Drake, C. (2019). Shift work disorder. *Neurologic Clinics*, *37*(3), 563–577. https://doi.org/10.1016/j.ncl.2019.03.003

Cheng, W. J., Hang, L. W., Kubo, T., Vanttola, P., & Huang, S. C. (2022). Impact of sleep timing on attention, sleepiness, and sleep quality among real-life night shift workers with shift work disorder: A cross-over clinical trial. *Sleep*, *45*(4), Article zsac034. https://doi.org/10.1093/sleep/zsac034

Chinoy, E. D., Harris, M. P., Kim, M. J., Wang, W., & Duffy, J. F. (2016). Scheduled evening sleep and enhanced lighting improve adaptation to night shift work in older adults. *Occupational & Environmental Medicine*, *73*(12), 869–876. https://doi.org/10.1136/oemed-2016-103712

Cohen, R. A., & Albers, H. E. (1991). Disruption of human circadian and cognitive regulation following a discrete hypothalamic lesion: A case study. *Neurology*, *41*(5), 726–729. https://doi.org/10.1212/wnl.41.5.726

Crowley, S. J., Lee, C., Tseng, C. Y., Fogg, L. F., & Eastman, C. I. (2003). Combinations of bright light, scheduled dark, sunglasses, and melatonin to facilitate circadian entrainment to night shift work. *Journal of Biological Rhythms*, *18*(6), 513–523. https://doi.org/10.1177/0748730403258422

Crowley, S. J., Lee, C., Tseng, C. Y., Fogg, L. F., & Eastman, C. I. (2004). Complete or partial circadian re-entrainment improves performance, alertness, and mood during night-shift work. *Sleep*, *27*(6), 1077–1087. https://doi.org/10.1093/sleep/27.6.1077

Cuesta, M., Boudreau, P., Cermakian, N., & Boivin, D. B. (2017). Rapid resetting of human peripheral clocks by phototherapy during simulated night shift work. *Scientific Reports*, *7*(1), Article 16310. https://doi.org/10.1038/s41598-017-16429-8

Czeisler, C. A., Duffy, J. F., Shanahan, T. L., Brown, E. N., Mitchell, J. F., Rimmer, D. W., Ronda, J. M., Silva, E. J., Allan, J. S., Emens, J. S., Dijk, D. J., & Kronauer, R. E. (1999). Stability, precision, and near-24-hour period of the human circadian pacemaker. *Science, 284*(5423), 2177–2181. http://www.ncbi.nlm.nih.gov/pubmed/10381883

Czeisler, C. A., Kronauer, R., Allan, J., Duffy, J., Jewett, M., Brown, E., & Ronda, J. (1989). Bright light induction of strong (Type 0) resetting of the human circadian pacemaker. *Science, 244*(4910), 1328–1333. https://doi.org/10.1126/science.2734611

Czeisler, C. A., Shanahan, T. L., Klerman, E. B., Martens, H., Brotman, D. J., Emens, J. S., Klein, T., & Rizzo, J. F., 3rd. (1995). Suppression of melatonin secretion in some blind patients by exposure to bright light. *New England Journal of Medicine, 332*(1), 6–11. https://doi.org/10.1056/NEJM199501053320102

Dijk, D. J., Duffy, J. F., Silva, E. J., Shanahan, T. L., Boivin, D. B., & Czeisler, C. A. (2012). Amplitude reduction and phase shifts of melatonin, cortisol and other circadian rhythms after a gradual advance of sleep and light exposure in humans. *PLOS ONE, 7*(2), Article e30037. https://doi.org/10.1371/journal.pone.0030037

Duffy, J. F., Cain, S. W., Chang, A. M., Phillips, A. J., Munch, M. Y., Gronfier, C., Wyatt, J. K., Dijk, D. J., Wright, K. P., Jr., & Czeisler, C. A. (2011). Sex difference in the near-24-hour intrinsic period of the human circadian timing system. *Proceedings of the National Academy of Sciences of the United States of America, 108*(S3), 15602–15608. https://doi.org/10.1073/pnas.1010666108

Eastman, C. I., Suh, C., Tomaka, V. A., & Crowley, S. J. (2015). Circadian rhythm phase shifts and endogenous free-running circadian period differ between African-Americans and European-Americans. *Scientific Reports, 5*, Article 8381. https://doi.org/10.1038/srep08381

Eastman, C. I., Tomaka, V. A., & Crowley, S. J. (2017). Sex and ancestry determine the free-running circadian period. *Journal of Sleep Research, 26*(5), 547–550. https://doi.org/10.1111/jsr.12521

Edgar, D. M., Dement, W. C., & Fuller, C. A. (1993). Effect of SCN lesions on sleep in squirrel monkeys: Evidence for opponent processes in sleep–wake regulation. *Journal of Neuroscience, 13*(3), 1065–1079. https://www.ncbi.nlm.nih.gov/pubmed/8441003

Eliott, A. L., Mills, J. N., & Waterhouse, J. M. (1971). A man with too long a day. *Journal of Physiology, 212*(2), 30P–31P. https://www.ncbi.nlm.nih.gov/pubmed/5548010

Emens, J. S., Lewy, A. J., Lefler, B. J., & Sack, R. L. (2005). Relative coordination to unknown "weak zeitgebers" in free-running blind individuals. *Journal of Biological Rhythms, 20*(2), 159–167. https://doi.org/10.1177/0748730404273294

Eurofound & International Labour Organization. (2019). *Working conditions in a global perspective*. Publications Office of the European Union. http://eurofound.link/ef18066

Fernandez, F. X., Kaladchibachi, S., & Negelspach, D. C. (2021). Resilience in the suprachiasmatic nucleus: Implications for aging and Alzheimer's disease. *Experimental Gerontology, 147*, Article 111258. https://doi.org/10.1016/j.exger.2021.111258

Figueiro, M. G., Bierman, A., Plitnick, B., & Rea, M. S. (2009). Preliminary evidence that both blue and red light can induce alertness at night. *BMC Neuroscience, 10*(1), Article 105. https://doi.org/10.1186/1471-2202-10-105

Figueiro, M. G., & Pedler, D. (2020). Red light: A novel, non-pharmacological intervention to promote alertness in shift workers. *Journal of Safety Research, 74*, 169–177. https://doi.org/10.1016/j.jsr.2020.06.003

Figueiro, M. G., Sahin, L., Wood, B., & Plitnick, B. (2016). Light at night and measures of alertness and performance: Implications for shift workers. *Biological Research for Nursing, 18*(1), 90–100. https://doi.org/10.1177/1099800415572873

Fischer, D., Lombardi, D. A., Folkard, S., Willetts, J., & Christiani, D. C. (2017). Updating the "risk index": A systematic review and meta-analysis of occupational injuries and work schedule characteristics. *Chronobiology International, 34*(10), 1423–1438. https://doi.org/10.1080/07420528.2017.1367305

Flo, E., Bjorvatn, B., Folkard, S., Moen, B. E., Gronli, J., Nordhus, I. H., & Pallesen, S. (2012). A reliability and validity study of the Bergen Shift Work Sleep Questionnaire in nurses working three-shift rotations. *Chronobiology International, 29*(7), 937–946. https://doi.org/10.3109/07420528.2012.699120

Flynn-Evans, E. E., Tabandeh, H., Skene, D. J., & Lockley, S. W. (2014). Circadian rhythm disorders and melatonin production in 127 blind women with and without light perception. *Journal of Biological Rhythms, 29*(3), 215–224. https://doi.org/10.1177/0748730414536852

Folkard, S. (2008). Do permanent night workers show circadian adjustment? A review based on the endogenous melatonin rhythm. *Chronobiology International, 25*(2), 215–224. https://doi.org/10.1080/07420520802106835

Foster, R. G. (2021). Fundamentals of circadian entrainment by light. *Lighting Research & Technology, 53*(5), 377–393. https://doi.org/10.1177/14771535211014792

Gronfier, C., Wright, K. P., Jr., Kronauer, R. E., & Czeisler, C. A. (2007). Entrainment of the human circadian pacemaker to longer-than-24-h days. *Proceedings of the National Academy of Sciences of the United States of America, 104*(21), 9081–9086. https://doi.org/10.1073/pnas.0702835104

Hattammaru, M., Tahara, Y., Kikuchi, T., Okajima, K., Konishi, K., Nakajima, S., Sato, K., Otsuka, K., Sakura, H., Shibata, S., & Nakaoka, T. (2019). The effect of night shift work on the expression of clock genes in beard hair follicle cells. *Sleep Medicine, 56*, 164–170. https://doi.org/10.1016/j.sleep.2019.01.005

Hayakawa, T., Uchiyama, M., Kamei, Y., Shibui, K., Tagaya, H., Asada, T., Okawa, M., Urata, J., & Takahashi, K. (2005). Clinical analyses of sighted patients with non-24-hour sleep–wake syndrome: A study of 57 consecutively diagnosed cases. *Sleep, 28*(8), 945–952. https://doi.org/10.1093/sleep/28.8.945

Hilditch, C. J., & McHill, A. W. (2019). Sleep inertia: Current insights. *Nature and Science of Sleep, 11*, 155–165. https://doi.org/10.2147/NSS.S188911

Hughes, S., Hankins, M. W., Foster, R. G., & Peirson, S. N. (2012). Melanopsin phototransduction: Slowly emerging from the dark. *Progress in Brain Research, 199*, 19–40. https://doi.org/10.1016/B978-0-444-59427-3.00002-2

Irwin, C., Khalesi, S., Desbrow, B., & McCartney, D. (2020). Effects of acute caffeine consumption following sleep loss on cognitive, physical, occupational and driving performance: A systematic review and meta-analysis. *Neuroscience & Biobehavioral Reviews, 108*, 877–888. https://doi.org/10.1016/j.neubiorev.2019.12.008

Isherwood, C. M., Chinoy, E. D., Murphy, A. S., Kim, J. H., Wang, W., & Duffy, J. F. (2020). Scheduled afternoon-evening sleep leads to better night shift performance in older adults. *Occupational & Environmental Medicine, 77*(3), 179–184. https://doi.org/10.1136/oemed-2019-105916

James, F. O., Walker, C. D., & Boivin, D. B. (2004). Controlled exposure to light and darkness realigns the salivary cortisol rhythms in night shift workers. *Chronobiology International, 21*(6), 961–972. https://doi.org/10.1081/cbi-200035944

Jarnefelt, H., Harma, M., Sallinen, M., Virkkala, J., Paajanen, T., Martimo, K. P., & Hublin, C. (2020). Cognitive behavioural therapy interventions for insomnia among shift workers: RCT in an occupational health setting. *International Archives of Occupational and Environmental Health, 93*(5), 535–550. https://doi.org/10.1007/s00420-019-01504-6

Jarnefelt, H., Lagerstedt, R., Kajaste, S., Sallinen, M., Savolainen, A., & Hublin, C. (2012). Cognitive behavioral therapy for shift workers with chronic insomnia. *Sleep Medicine, 13*(10), 1238–1246. https://doi.org/10.1016/j.sleep.2012.10.003

Jensen, H. I., Markvart, J., Holst, R., Thomsen, T. D., Larsen, J. W., Eg, D. M., & Nielsen, L. S. (2016). Shift work and quality of sleep: Effect of working in designed dynamic light. *International Archives of Occupational and Environmental Health, 89*(1), 49–61. https://doi.org/10.1007/s00420-015-1051-0

Jensen, M. A., Garde, A. H., Kristiansen, J., Nabe-Nielsen, K., & Hansen, Å. M. (2016). The effect of the number of consecutive night shifts on diurnal rhythms in cortisol, melatonin and heart rate variability (HRV): A systematic review of field studies. *International Archives of Occupational and Environmental Health, 89*(4), 531–545. https://doi.org/10.1007/s00420-015-1093-3

Jensen, M. A., Hansen, A. M., Kristiansen, J., Nabe-Nielsen, K., & Garde, A. H. (2016). Changes in the diurnal rhythms of cortisol, melatonin, and testosterone after 2, 4, and 7 consecutive night shifts in male police officers. *Chronobiology International, 33*(9), 1280–1292. https://doi.org/10.1080/07420528.2016.1212869

Jensen, M. A., Kjærgaard, J. B., Petersen, J. D., Hansen, Å. M., Kristiansen, J., & Garde, A. H. (2020). The urinary 6-sulfatoxymelatonin level after three different work schedules with 2, 4 and 7 consecutive night shifts among Danish police officers. *Chronobiology International, 37*(9–10), 1400–1403. https://doi.org/10.1080/07420528.2020.1807560

Johns, M. W. (1991). A new method for measuring daytime sleepiness: The Epworth Sleepiness Scale. *Sleep, 14*(6), 540–545. https://doi.org/10.1093/sleep/14.6.540

Kazemi, R., Alighanbari, N., & Zamanian, Z. (2019). The effects of screen light filtering software on cognitive performance and sleep among night workers. *Health Promotion Perspectives, 9*(3), 233–240. https://doi.org/10.15171/hpp.2019.32

Kecklund, G., & Axelsson, J. (2016). Health consequences of shift work and insufficient sleep. *BMJ, 355*, Article i5210. https://doi.org/10.1136/bmj.i5210

Kervezee, L., Cermakian, N., & Boivin, D. B. (2019). Individual metabolomic signatures of circadian misalignment during simulated night shifts in humans. *PLOS Biology, 17*(6), Article e3000303. https://doi.org/10.1371/journal.pbio.3000303

Kervezee, L., Cuesta, M., Cermakian, N., & Boivin, D. B. (2018). Simulated night shift work induces circadian misalignment of the human peripheral blood mononuclear cell transcriptome. *Proceedings of the National Academy of Sciences of the United States of America, 115*(21), 5540–5545. https://doi.org/10.1073/pnas.1720719115

Kervezee, L., Gonzales-Aste, F., Boudreau, P., & Boivin, D. B. (2021). The relationship between chronotype and sleep behavior during rotating shift work: A field study. *Sleep, 44*(4), Article zsaa225. https://doi.org/10.1093/sleep/zsaa225

Khalsa, S. B. S., Jewett, M. E., Cajochen, C., & Czeisler, C. A. (2003). A phase response curve to single bright light pulses in human subjects. *Journal of Physiology, 549*(3), 945–952.

Koshy, A., Cuesta, M., Boudreau, P., Cermakian, N., & Boivin, D. B. (2019). Disruption of central and peripheral circadian clocks in police officers working at night. *FASEB Journal, 33*(6), 6789–6800. https://doi.org/10.1096/fj.201801889R

Kosmadopoulos, A., Boudreau, P., Kervezee, L., & Boivin, D. B. (2024). Circadian adaptation of melatonin and cortisol in police officers working rotating shifts. *Journal of Biological Rhythms, 39*(1), 49–67. https://doi.org/10.1177/07487304231196280

Krahn, L. E., Arand, D. L., Avidan, A. Y., Davila, D. G., DeBassio, W. A., Ruoff, C. M., & Harrod, C. G. (2021). Recommended protocols for the Multiple Sleep Latency Test and Maintenance of Wakefulness Test in adults: Guidance from the American Academy of Sleep Medicine. *Journal of Clinical Sleep Medicine, 17*(12), 2489–2498. https://doi.org/10.5664/jcsm.9620

Lammers-van der Holst, H. M., Wyatt, J. K., Horowitz, T. S., Wise, J. C., Wang, W., Ronda, J. M., Duffy, J. F., & Czeisler, C. A. (2021). Efficacy of intermittent exposure to bright light for treating maladaptation to night work on a counterclockwise shift work rotation. *Scandinavian Journal of Work, Environment & Health, 47*(5), 356–366. https://doi.org/10.5271/sjweh.3953

Lee, M. L., Howard, M. E., Horrey, W. J., Liang, Y., Anderson, C., Shreeve, M. S., O'Brien, C. S., & Czeisler, C. A. (2016). High risk of near-crash driving events following night-shift work. *Proceedings of the National Academy of Sciences of the United States of America, 113*(1), 176–181. https://doi.org/10.1073/pnas.1510383112

Liang, Y., Horrey, W. J., Howard, M. E., Lee, M. L., Anderson, C., Shreeve, M. S., O'Brien, C. S., & Czeisler, C. A. (2019). Prediction of drowsiness events in night shift workers during morning driving. *Accident Analysis & Prevention, 126*, 105–114. https://doi.org/10.1016/j.aap.2017.11.004

Liira, J., Verbeek, J. H., Costa, G., Driscoll, T. R., Sallinen, M., Isotalo, L. K., & Ruotsalainen, J. H. (2014). Pharmacological interventions for sleepiness and sleep disturbances caused by shift work. *Cochrane Database of Systematic Reviews, 8*, CD009776. https://doi.org/10.1002/14651858.CD009776.pub2

Lockley, S. W., Dressman, M. A., Licamele, L., Xiao, C., Fisher, D. M., Flynn-Evans, E. E., Hull, J. T., Torres, R., Lavedan, C., & Polymeropoulos, M. H. (2015). Tasimelteon for non-24-hour sleep–wake disorder in totally blind people (SET and RESET): Two multicentre, randomised, double-masked, placebo-controlled phase 3 trials. *Lancet, 386*(10005), 1754–1764. https://doi.org/10.1016/S0140-6736(15)60031-9

Lok, R., Smolders, K., Beersma, D. G. M., & de Kort, Y. A. W. (2018). Light, alertness, and alerting effects of white light: A literature overview. *Journal of Biological Rhythms, 33*(6), 589–601. https://doi.org/10.1177/0748730418796443

Malkani, R. G., Abbott, S. M., Reid, K. J., & Zee, P. C. (2018). Diagnostic and treatment challenges of sighted non-24-hour sleep–wake disorder. *Journal of Clinical Sleep Medicine, 14*(4), 603–613. https://doi.org/10.5664/jcsm.7054

McCurry, S. M., Gibbons, L. E., Logsdon, R. G., Vitiello, M. V., & Teri, L. (2005). Nighttime insomnia treatment and education for Alzheimer's disease: A randomized, controlled trial. *Journal of the American Geriatric Society, 53*(5), 793–802. https://doi.org/10.1111/j.1532-5415.2005.53252.x

McIntyre, I. M., Norman, T. R., Burrows, G. D., & Armstrong, S. M. (1989). Human melatonin suppression by light is intensity dependent. *Journal of Pineal Research, 6*(2), 149–156.

Minors, D. S., Waterhouse, J. M., & Wirz-Justice, A. (1991). A human phase–response curve to light. *Neuroscience Letters, 133*(1), 36–40. https://doi.org/10.1016/0304-3940(91)90051-T

Mistlberger, R. E. (2005). Circadian regulation of sleep in mammals: Role of the suprachiasmatic nucleus. *Brain Research Reviews, 49*(3), 429–454. https://doi.org/10.1016/j.brainresrev.2005.01.005

Morgenthaler, T. I., Lee-Chiong, T., Alessi, C., Friedman, L., Aurora, R. N., Boehlecke, B., Brown, T., Chesson, A. L., Jr., Kapur, V., Maganti, R., Owens, J., Pancer, J., Swick, T. J., Zak, R., & Standards of Practice Committee of the American Academy of Sleep Medicine. (2007). Practice parameters for the clinical evaluation and treatment of circadian rhythm sleep disorders. An American Academy of Sleep Medicine report. *Sleep, 30*(11), 1445–1459. https://doi.org/10.1093/sleep/30.11.1445

Morin, C. M., Belleville, G., Belanger, L., & Ivers, H. (2011). The Insomnia Severity Index: Psychometric indicators to detect insomnia cases and evaluate treatment response. *Sleep, 34*(5), 601–608. https://doi.org/10.1093/sleep/34.5.601

Motamedzadeh, M., Golmohammadi, R., Kazemi, R., & Heidarimoghadam, R. (2017). The effect of blue-enriched white light on cognitive performances and sleepiness of night-shift workers: A field study. *Physiology & Behavior, 177*, 208–214. https://doi.org/10.1016/j.physbeh.2017.05.008

Murphy, P., Kumar, D., Zammit, G., Rosenberg, R., & Moline, M. (2020). Safety of lemborexant versus placebo and zolpidem: Effects on auditory awakening threshold, postural stability, and cognitive performance in healthy older participants in the middle of the night and upon morning awakening. *Journal of Clinical Sleep Medicine, 16*(5), 765–773. https://doi.org/10.5664/jcsm.8294

O'Neill, B., Gardani, M., Findlay, G., Whyte, T., & Cullen, T. (2014). Challenging behaviour and sleep cycle disorder following brain injury: A preliminary response to agomelatine treatment. *Brain Injury, 28*(3), 378–381. https://doi.org/10.3109/02699052.2013.865264

Oren, D. A., & Wehr, T. A. (1992). Hypernyctohemeral syndrome after chronotherapy for delayed sleep phase syndrome. *New England Journal of Medicine, 327*(24), Article 1762. https://doi.org/10.1056/NEJM199212103272417

Pallesen, S., Bjorvatn, B., Waage, S., Harris, A., & Sagoe, D. (2021). Prevalence of shift work disorder: A systematic review and meta-analysis. *Frontiers in Psychology, 12*, Article 638252. https://doi.org/10.3389/fpsyg.2021.638252

Peter, L., Reindl, R., Zauter, S., Hillemacher, T., & Richter, K. (2019). Effectiveness of an online CBT-I intervention and a face-to-face treatment for shift work sleep disorder: A comparison of sleep diary data. *International Journal of Environmental Research and Public Health, 16*(17), Article 3081. https://doi.org/10.3390/ijerph16173081

Qaseem, A., Kansagara, D., Forciea, M. A., Cooke, M., Denberg, T. D., & Clinical Guidelines Committee of the American College of Physicians. (2016). Management of chronic insomnia disorder in adults: A clinical practice guideline from the American College of Physicians. *Annals of Internal Medicine, 165*(2), 125–133. https://doi.org/10.7326/M15-2175

Rahman, S. A., Flynn-Evans, E. E., Aeschbach, D., Brainard, G. C., Czeisler, C. A., & Lockley, S. W. (2014). Diurnal spectral sensitivity of the acute alerting effects of light. *Sleep, 37*(2), 271–281.

Rahman, S. A., Shapiro, C. M., Wang, F., Ainlay, H., Kazmi, S., Brown, T. J., & Casper, R. F. (2013). Effects of filtering visual short wavelengths during nocturnal shiftwork on sleep and performance. *Chronobiology International, 30*(8), 951–962. https://doi.org/10.3109/07420528.2013.789894

Razavi, P., Devore, E. E., Bajaj, A., Lockley, S. W., Figueiro, M. G., Ricchiuti, V., Gauderman, W. J., Hankinson, S. E., Willett, W. C., & Schernhammer, E. S. (2019). Shift work, chronotype, and melatonin rhythm in nurses. *Cancer Epidemiology Biomarkers & Prevention, 28*(7), 1177–1186. https://doi.org/10.1158/1055-9965.EPI-18-1018

Resuehr, D., Wu, G., Johnson, R. L., Jr., Young, M. E., Hogenesch, J. B., & Gamble, K. L. (2019). Shift work disrupts circadian regulation of the transcriptome in hospital nurses. *Journal of Biological Rhythms, 34*(2), 167–177. https://doi.org/10.1177/0748730419826694

Retzer, L., Feil, M., Reindl, R., Richter, K., Lehmann, R., Stemmler, M., & Graessel, E. (2021). Anonymous online cognitive behavioral therapy for sleep disorders in shift workers—A study protocol for a randomized controlled trial. *Trials, 22*(1), Article 539. https://doi.org/10.1186/s13063-021-05437-9

Riemann, D., Baglioni, C., Bassetti, C., Bjorvatn, B., Dolenc Groselj, L., Ellis, J. G., Espie, C. A., Garcia-Borreguero, D., Gjerstad, M., Goncalves, M., Hertenstein, E., Jansson-Frojmark, M., Jennum, P. J., Leger, D., Nissen, C., Parrino, L., Paunio, T., Pevernagie, D., Verbraecken, J., . . . Spiegelhalder, K. (2017). European guideline for the diagnosis and treatment of insomnia. *Journal of Sleep Research, 26*(6), 675–700. https://doi.org/10.1111/jsr.12594

Ritonja, J., Aronson, K. J., Matthews, R. W., Boivin, D. B., & Kantermann, T. (2019). Working Time Society consensus statements: Individual differences in shift work tolerance and recommendations for research and practice. *Industrial Health, 57*(2), 201–212. https://doi.org/10.2486/indhealth.SW-5

Rotter, M., Brandmaier, S., Covic, M., Burek, K., Hertel, J., Troll, M., Bader, E., Adam, J., Prehn, C., Rathkolb, B., Hrabe de Angelis, M., Grabe, H. J., Daniel, H., Kantermann, T., Harth, V., Illig, T., Pallapies, D., Behrens, T., Bruning, T., . . . Wang-Sattler, R. (2018). Night shift work affects urine metabolite profiles of nurses with early chronotype. *Metabolites, 8*(3), Article 45. https://doi.org/10.3390/metabo8030045

Rydz, E., Hall, A. L., & Peters, C. E. (2020). Prevalence and recent trends in exposure to night shiftwork in Canada. *Annals of Work Exposures and Health, 64*(3), 270–281. https://doi.org/10.1093/annweh/wxaa001

Sack, R. L., Auckley, D., Auger, R. R., Carskadon, M. A., Wright, K. P., Jr., Vitiello, M. V., Zhdanova, I. V., & American Academy of Sleep Medicine. (2007a). Circadian rhythm sleep disorders: Part I, Basic principles, shift work and jet lag disorders. An American Academy of Sleep Medicine review. *Sleep, 30*(11), 1460–1483. https://doi.org/10.1093/sleep/30.11.1460

Sack, R. L., Auckley, D., Auger, R. R., Carskadon, M. A., Wright, K. P., Jr., Vitiello, M. V., Zhdanova, I. V., & American Academy of Sleep Medicine. (2007b). Circadian rhythm sleep disorders: Part II, Advanced sleep phase disorder, delayed sleep phase disorder, free-running disorder, and irregular sleep–wake rhythm. An American Academy of Sleep Medicine review. *Sleep, 30*(11), 1484–1501. https://doi.org/10.1093/sleep/30.11.1484

Saksvik, I. B., Bjorvatn, B., Hetland, H., Sandal, G. M., & Pallesen, S. (2011). Individual differences in tolerance to shift work—A systematic review. *Sleep Medicine Reviews, 15*(4), 221–235. https://doi.org/10.1016/j.smrv.2010.07.002

Santhi, N., Aeschbach, D., Horowitz, T. S., & Czeisler, C. A. (2008). The impact of sleep timing and bright light exposure on attentional impairment during night work. *Journal of Biological Rhythms, 23*(4), 341–352. https://doi.org/10.1177/0748730408319863

Sasseville, A., & Hebert, M. (2010). Using blue-green light at night and blue-blockers during the day to improves adaptation to night work: A pilot study. *Progress in Neuro-Psychopharmacology and Biological Psychiatry, 34*(7), 1236–1242. https://doi.org/10.1016/j.pnpbp.2010.06.027

Savarese, M., & Di Perri, M. C. (2020). Excessive sleepiness in shift work disorder: A narrative review of the last 5 years. *Sleep and Breathing, 24*(1), 297–310. https://doi.org/10.1007/s11325-019-01925-0

Schwartz, W. J., Busis, N. A., & Hedley-Whyte, E. T. (1986). A discrete lesion of ventral hypothalamus and optic chiasm that disturbed the daily temperature rhythm. *Journal of Neurology, 233*(1), 1–4. https://doi.org/10.1007/BF00313981

Shechter, A., Quispe, K. A., Mizhquiri Barbecho, J. S., Slater, C., & Falzon, L. (2020). Interventions to reduce short-wavelength ("blue") light exposure at night and their effects on sleep: A systematic review and meta-analysis. *Sleep Advances, 1*(1), Article zpaa002.

Shriane, A. E., Ferguson, S. A., Jay, S. M., & Vincent, G. E. (2020). Sleep hygiene in shift workers: A systematic literature review. *Sleep Medicine Reviews, 53*, Article 101336. https://doi.org/10.1016/j.smrv.2020.101336

Skeldon, A. C., Dijk, D. J., Meyer, N., & Wulff, K. (2022). Extracting circadian and sleep parameters from longitudinal data in schizophrenia for the design of pragmatic light interventions. *Schizophrenia Bulletin, 48*(2), 447–456. https://doi.org/10.1093/schbul/sbab124

Skene, D. J., Skornyakov, E., Chowdhury, N. R., Gajula, R. P., Middleton, B., Satterfield, B. C., Porter, K. I., Van Dongen, H. P. A., & Gaddameedhi, S. (2018). Separation of circadian- and behavior-driven metabolite rhythms in humans provides a window on peripheral oscillators and metabolism. *Proceedings of the National Academy of Sciences of the United States of America, 115*(30), 7825–7830. https://doi.org/10.1073/pnas.1801183115

Sletten, T. L., Ftouni, S., Nicholas, C. L., Magee, M., Grunstein, R. R., Ferguson, S., Kennaway, D. J., O'Brien, D., Lockley, S. W., & Rajaratnam, S. M. W. (2017). Randomised controlled trial of the efficacy of a blue-enriched light intervention to improve alertness and performance in night shift workers. *Occupational and Environmental Medicine, 74*(11), 792–801. https://doi.org/10.1136/oemed-2016-103818

Sletten, T. L., Raman, B., Magee, M., Ferguson, S. A., Kennaway, D. J., Grunstein, R. R., Lockley, S. W., & Rajaratnam, S. M. W. (2021). A blue-enriched, increased intensity light intervention to improve alertness and performance in rotating night shift workers in an operational setting. *Nature and Science of Sleep, 13*, 647–657. https://doi.org/10.2147/NSS.S287097

Smith, M. R., Fogg, L. F., & Eastman, C. I. (2009). Practical interventions to promote circadian adaptation to permanent night shift work: Study 4. *Journal of Biological Rhythms, 24*(2), 161–172. https://doi.org/10.1177/0748730409332068

Steele, T. A., St Louis, E. K., Videnovic, A., & Auger, R. R. (2021). Circadian rhythm sleep–wake disorders: A contemporary review of neurobiology, treatment, and dysregulation in neurodegenerative disease. *Neurotherapeutics, 18*(1), 53–74. https://doi.org/10.1007/s13311-021-01031-8

Stepanski, E. J., & Wyatt, J. K. (2003). Use of sleep hygiene in the treatment of insomnia. *Sleep Medicine Reviews, 7*(3), 215–225. https://doi.org/10.1053/smrv.2001.0246

Swaab, D. F., Fliers, E., & Partiman, T. S. (1985). The suprachiasmatic nucleus of the human brain in relation to sex, age and senile dementia. *Brain Research, 342*(1), 37–44. https://doi.org/10.1016/0006-8993(85)91350-2

Taniyama, Y., Yamauchi, T., Takeuchi, S., & Kuroda, Y. (2015). PER1 polymorphism associated with shift work disorder. *Sleep and Biological Rhythms, 13*(4), 342–347.

Thun, E., Le Hellard, S., Osland, T., Bjorvatn, B., Moen, B., Magerøy, N., Steen, V., Giddaluru, S., Brattbakk, H.-R., & Pallesen, S. (2016). Circadian clock gene variants and insomnia, sleepiness, and shift work disorder. *Sleep and Biological Rhythms, 14*(1), 55–62.

Touitou, Y., Motohashi, Y., Reinberg, A., Touitou, C., Bourdeleau, P., Bogdan, A., & Auzeby, A. (1990). Effect of shift work on the night-time secretory patterns of melatonin, prolactin, cortisol and testosterone. *European Journal of Applied Physiology and Occupational Physiology, 60*(4), 288–292. http://www.ncbi.nlm.nih.gov/pubmed/2357985

Uchiyama, M., & Lockley, S. W. (2015). Non-24-hour sleep–wake rhythm disorder in sighted and blind patients. *Sleep Medicine Clinics, 10*(4), 495–516. https://doi.org/10.1016/j.jsmc.2015.07.006

Uchiyama, M., Okawa, M., Shibui, K., Kim, K., Tagaya, H., Kudo, Y., Kamei, Y., Hayakawa, T., Urata, J., & Takahashi, K. (2000). Altered phase relation between sleep timing and core body temperature rhythm in delayed sleep phase syndrome and non-24-hour sleep–wake syndrome in humans. *Neuroscience Letters, 294*(2), 101–104. https://doi.org/10.1016/s0304-3940(00)01551-2

Van Erum, J., Van Dam, D., & De Deyn, P. P. (2018). Sleep and Alzheimer's disease: A pivotal role for the suprachiasmatic nucleus. *Sleep Medicine Reviews, 40*, 17–27. https://doi.org/10.1016/j.smrv.2017.07.005

van Woerkom, M. (2021). A quasi-experimental study into the effects of naps and therapy glasses on fatigue and well-being. *Journal of Nursing Management, 29*(3), 562–571. https://doi.org/10.1111/jonm.13172

Vetter, C., Fischer, D., Matera, J. L., & Roenneberg, T. (2015). Aligning work and circadian time in shift workers improves sleep and reduces circadian disruption. *Current Biology, 25*(7), 907–911. https://doi.org/10.1016/j.cub.2015.01.064

Viola, A. U., James, L. M., Schlangen, L. J., & Dijk, D.-J. (2008). Blue-enriched white light in the workplace improves self-reported alertness, performance and sleep quality. *Scandinavian Journal of Work, Environment & Health, 34*(4), 297–306.

Waage, S., Pallesen, S., Moen, B. E., Vedaa, O., Thun, E., Vikanes Buchvold, H., Blytt, K. M., Harris, A., & Bjorvatn, B. (2021). Changes in work schedule affect the prevalence of shift work disorder among Norwegian nurses—A two year follow-up study. *Chronobiology International, 38*(6), 924–932. https://doi.org/10.1080/07420528.2021.1896535

Wilson, M., Permito, R., English, A., Albritton, S., Coogle, C., & Van Dongen, H. P. A. (2019). Performance and sleepiness in nurses working 12-h day shifts or night shifts in a community hospital. *Accident Analysis & Prevention, 126*, 43–46. https://doi.org/10.1016/j.aap.2017.09.023

Wu, Y. H., Fischer, D. F., Kalsbeek, A., Garidou-Boof, M. L., van der Vliet, J., van Heijningen, C., Liu, R. Y., Zhou, J. N., & Swaab, D. F. (2006). Pineal clock gene oscillation is disturbed in Alzheimer's disease, due to functional disconnection from the "master clock." *FASEB Journal, 20*(11), 1874–1876. https://doi.org/10.1096/fj.05-4446fje

Yong, L. C., Li, J., & Calvert, G. M. (2017). Sleep-related problems in the US working population: Prevalence and association with shiftwork status. *Occupational & Environmental Medicine, 74*(2), 93–104. https://doi.org/10.1136/oemed-2016-103638

Zee, P. C., Attarian, H., & Videnovic, A. (2013). Circadian rhythm abnormalities. *Continuum, 19*(1), 132–147. https://doi.org/10.1212/01.CON.0000427209.21177.aa

Zeitzer, J. M., Dijk, D. J., Kronauer, R., Brown, E., & Czeisler, C. (2000). Sensitivity of the human circadian pacemaker to nocturnal light: Melatonin phase resetting and suppression. *Journal of Physiology, 526*(Pt. 3), 695–702. https://doi.org/10.1111/j.1469-7793.2000.00695.x

Zeitzer, J. M., Joyce, D. S., McBean, A., Quevedo, Y. L., Hernandez, B., & Holty, J. E. (2020). Effect of suvorexant vs placebo on total daytime sleep hours in shift workers: A randomized clinical trial. *JAMA Network Open, 3*(6), Article e206614. https://doi.org/10.1001/jamanetworkopen.2020.6614

Zhao, X. C., Han, K. Y., Gao, Y. Y., Li, N., Wang, L., Yu, L. L., Song, M., & Wang, X. Y. (2021). Effects of shift work on sleep and cognitive function among male miners. *Psychiatry Research, 297*, Article 113716. https://doi.org/10.1016/j.psychres.2021.113716

CHAPTER

34 Sleep-Related Breathing Disorders I: Physiology and Etiology

Danny J. Eckert

Abstract

The spectrum of sleep-related breathing disorders ranges from snoring to obstructive and central sleep apnea through to obesity hypoventilation syndrome. Each of these different manifestations of sleep disordered breathing is unique, and the underlying pathophysiological causes can vary markedly between individuals. However, there are common and often overlapping pathophysiological features across the sleep disordered breathing spectrum. This brief chapter describes the latest knowledge on upper airway and respiratory physiology and the control of breathing and the key changes that occur during sleep. The different etiologies of sleep disordered breathing and the key mechanisms that contribute to the underlying pathophysiology are also highlighted.

Key Words: sleep disordered breathing, upper airway physiology, respiratory physiology, lung, phenotype, endotype, control of breathing, pathophysiology

Introduction

Sleep-related breathing disorders include snoring, central sleep apnea (CSA), obstructive sleep apnea (OSA), and obesity hypoventilation syndrome (OHS) (Figure 34.1A). While the perpetuating physiological and clinical factors, manifestations, and consequences of each form of sleep disordered breathing vary, there are common underlying features. This chapter provides an overview of upper airway anatomy and physiology, the control of breathing, the changes that occur in upper airway physiology and control of breathing during sleep, the spectrum of sleep-related breathing disorders, and the latest knowledge on underlying pathophysiology including sleep apnea endotypes. Finally, key unanswered questions and future research directions for this topic are highlighted.

Upper Airway Anatomy and Physiology

The human upper airway is a complex multifunctional structure that serves important functions such as swallowing, speech, and breathing. These tasks require a malleable structure capable of achieving rapid, dynamic changes in shape and size. Accordingly, the upper airway is comprised of over 25 pairs of muscles and lacks bony rigid support. Given

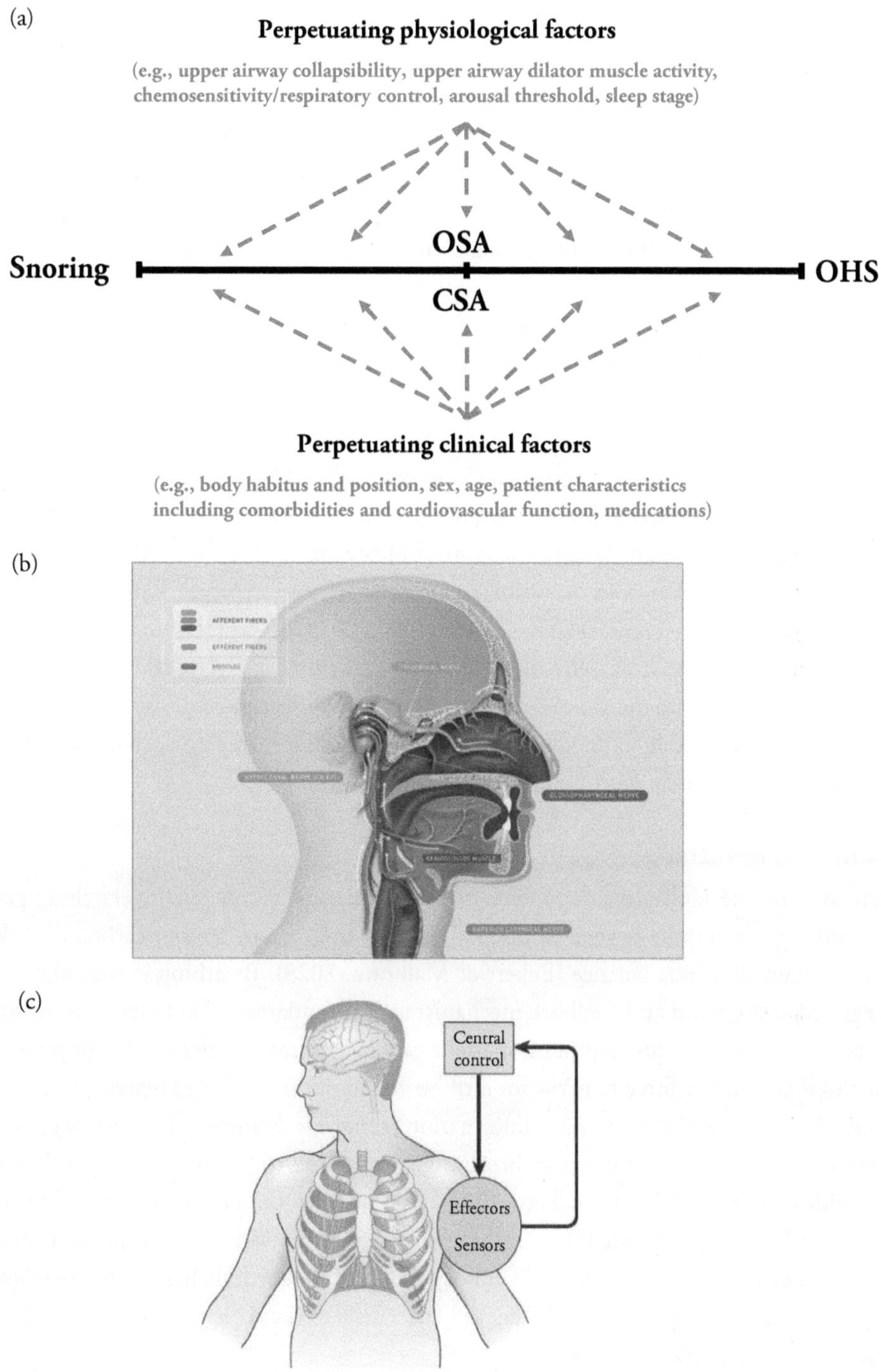

Page 1.

Figure 34.1 Sleep-related breathing disorders

Note. Panel A: Schematic of the spectrum of sleep-related breathing disorders. Includes examples of some of the perpetuating physiological and clinical factors that can contribute to the different manifestations of sleep disordered breathing. Note that this is dynamic and in addition to night-to-night variation in sleep disordered breathing severity, which can occur with transient changes in the perpetuating factors, there is the potential to shift between the different types of sleep-related breathing disorders over time. However, this is less well defined. Panel B: Schematic of the upper airway and key upper airway dilator muscle reflex inputs. From Osman et al. (2023). Panel C: Schematic overview of the fundamental elements of the control of the breathing system. CSA = central sleep apnea; OHS = obesity hypoventilation syndrome; OSA = obstructive sleep apnea. This figure was originally published in *Principles and Practice of Sleep Medicine*, 7th ed., Vol. 1, Eckert, D. J., Respiratory physiology: Understanding the control of ventilation pp. 245–251, Copyright Elsevier (2022).

the multiple functional requirements of the upper airway and reliance on muscles, the motor control of the pharyngeal muscles is arguably the most complex of all the muscles in the human body. For example, during quiet breathing, there are at least five different patterns of drive to the largest and most studied upper airway dilator muscle, the genioglossus (Saboisky et al., 2006). The genioglossus is a fan-shaped muscle located at the base of the tongue and plays a crucial role in maintaining airway patency (Figure 34.1B; Eckert & Malhotra, 2023). The different patterns of drive that the genioglossus receives during quiet breathing include some neurons that are activated at a constant level throughout the breathing cycle, termed *tonic* drive; others that only fire during either inspiration or expiration; and others that fire throughout the breathing cycle but vary their rate of activity during inspiration or expiration (Saboisky et al., 2006). The genioglossus muscle receives input from the hypoglossal motor nucleus via the hypoglossal nerve from a variety of central sites that are involved in the control of breathing (Eckert & Malhotra, 2023) as well as reflex feedback from exquisitely sensitive mechanoreceptors located throughout the pharyngeal airway (Figure 34.1B; Carberry et al., 2015, 2022; Horner, Innes, Holden, & Guz, 1991; Osman et al., 2023). While these structural characteristics and complex motor patterns facilitate the various required functions of the upper airway, they also render the airway vulnerable to unwanted narrowing and collapse during sleep in susceptible individuals when muscle motor control changes.

Control of Breathing

Facilitated by the multiple components of the respiratory system, the overarching goal of breathing is to supply oxygen to the body tissues and organs, remove carbon dioxide, and maintain acid–base balance (Eckert & Malhotra, 2023). Breathing is controlled via integrated feedforward and feedback mechanisms. The fundamental key elements include (1) brainstem neurons for respiratory pattern generation (*central control*), (2) respiratory muscles that generate force to allow for airflow in and out of the lungs (*effectors*), and (3) inputs that relay respiratory sensory information (*sensors*) to brainstem respiratory control centers to allow for adjustments in breathing in response to the prevailing physiological conditions (Figure 34.1C; Eckert, 2022). The primary center for central respiratory control of breathing is located within the medulla, which also receives important input from the pons. Within the ventral respiratory group of the medulla lies the *pre-Botzinger complex*, which is believed to be the central "pacemaker" that controls breathing regulation (Smith et al., 1991).

Impairment to any one of the fundamental elements that controls breathing can lead to breathing problems. However, there are multiple additional protective compensatory inputs to breathing that can be activated to maintain breathing and blood gas levels within acceptable levels despite impairment to key elements that mediate control of breathing. For instance, there is a greater cortical contribution to breathing with increasing age and in those with chronic obstructive pulmonary disease compared to healthy young people during wakefulness (Nguyen et al., 2018). However, compensatory mechanisms such as the cortical contribution to breathe and inputs from touch, temperature, pain, emotional stimuli, and movement that can provide strong inputs to breathing during wakefulness are either markedly downregulated or absent during sleep. Thus, breathing problems associated with impairment in the respiratory system often only emerge, or get worse, during sleep (Eckert, 2022).

Chemical Control of Breathing

Chemical control is the most important mediator of breathing during both wakefulness and sleep. All cells in the human body can modulate their activity in response to extreme changes in chemical stimuli. However, certain cells are exquisitely sensitive to very small changes in chemical stimuli and as such are termed *chemoreceptors*. These neurons can regulate breathing directly or have projections to central control of breathing sites.

Central Versus Peripheral Chemoreceptors

There are chemoreceptors located centrally within the brainstem as well as peripherally at the bifurcation of the common carotid arteries (Dempsey & Smith, 2014). The retrotrapezoid nucleus, which is located on the ventral surface of the medulla, is believed to be particularly important for central chemoreception (Guyenet et al., 2010; Wang et al., 2013). It has major projections to key respiratory control centers (Rosin et al., 2006; Takakura et al., 2006). The central chemoreceptors respond to changes in carbon dioxide via pH-sensitive mechanisms detected via the extracellular fluid, whereby carbon dioxide diffuses across the blood–brain barrier to increase hydrogen ion concentration in the cerebrospinal fluid (Eckert, 2022). Central chemoreceptors can take up to a minute to respond to changes in chemical stimuli via this process. As highlighted below, chemoreceptor response delays are critically important in contributing to cyclical breathing instability during sleep (Eckert, 2023; Eckert, Jordan, et al., 2007).

The peripherally located chemoreceptors respond to changes in oxygen, carbon dioxide, and hydrogen ions (Dempsey & Smith, 2014). Detection of these stimuli is capable of modulating breathing quickly within one to two breaths. In addition, recent advances in knowledge indicate that the carotid bodies respond to a wide range of other stimuli including potassium, noradrenaline, temperature, glucose, insulin, and immune-related cytokines (Dempsey & Smith, 2014; Kumar & Prabhakar, 2012). Repetitive exposure to hypoxia can cause plasticity changes within the carotid bodies that can contribute to increased vulnerability to breathing instability during sleep (Dempsey & Smith, 2014; Kumar & Prabhakar, 2012). While, the peripheral chemoreceptors are important for moment-to-moment modulation of breathing, the strongest input to breathing while awake is via the aforementioned central chemoreceptors.

While the central and peripheral chemoreceptors are distinct structures and have different response characteristics, there appears to be complex interconnectivity in their function (Dempsey & Smith, 2014; Dempsey et al., 2012; Kumar & Prabhakar, 2012; Smith et al., 2015). For instance, the activity of the central chemoreceptors is interdependent on the activity of the peripheral chemoreceptors and vice versa. This link has been described as a "hyper additive model" (Dempsey & Smith, 2014; Dempsey et al., 2012; Eckert, 2022; Kumar & Prabhakar, 2012; Smith et al., 2015).

Changes That Occur in Upper Airway Physiology and Control of Breathing During Sleep

There are major changes in upper airway physiology and the control of breathing that occur during sleep. The abrupt transition from alpha to theta brain waves (wakefulness to sleep) is accompanied by major reductions in pharyngeal muscle reflex control and upper airway and respiratory pump muscle activity (Shea et al., 1999; Trinder et al., 1992; Worsnop et al., 1998). These changes contribute to increased upper airway resistance and reductions in breathing (Pierce et al., 2007; Worsnop et al., 1998). In addition, the independent wakefulness drive to breathe and behavioral influences are removed at sleep onset (Skatrud & Berssenbrugge, 1983). Chemosensitivity also decreases (Dunai et al., 1996; Eckert, 2022). Consequently, breathing is inherently unstable during the electroencephalography-defined transition from wakefulness to sleep. Indeed, pauses in breathing with the onset of sleep are common, even in people who do not have a clinical sleep-related breathing disorder. Thus, sleep onset affects all the key components that mediate respiratory control which contributes to "sleep state instability."

The reduction in key excitatory inputs to breathe that occurs with sleep onset continues into stable sleep. The ability to compensate for the respiratory loading that accompanies sleep-induced airway narrowing is also reduced during stable sleep compared to wakefulness (Amatoury et al., 2018; Wiegand et al., 1988). In addition, down regulation in chemosensitivity occurs beyond the sleep onset period whereby ventilatory responses to hypoxia are reduced during N2 and slow-wave sleep compared to wakefulness. Indeed, marked reductions in oxygen are required to stimulate breathing during sleep (Berthon-Jones & Sullivan, 1982; Douglas, White, Weil, Pickett, Martin, et al., 1982). As a result of these collective physiological changes, chemical control of breathing, and in particular carbon dioxide, becomes the dominant driver of breathing during sleep. However, ventilatory responses to increased levels of carbon dioxide are also reduced during sleep compared to wakefulness, albeit to a lesser extent than hypoxia (Douglas, White, Weil, Pickett, & Zwillich, 1982).

Accordingly, minute ventilation remains lower during stable sleep compared to wakefulness, and we can tolerate lower levels of minute ventilation and higher levels of carbon dioxide versus wakefulness. Depending on the prevailing metabolic conditions, minute ventilation is reduced by 1–2 liters/minute, and partial pressure of carbon dioxide in the blood increases by approximately 3–8 mm Hg during stable sleep (Skatrud et al., 1988).

In healthy individuals, breathing is quite regular during stable non-rapid-eye movement (REM) sleep. However, upper airway muscle activity and collapsibility are sleep stage–dependent (Carberry et al., 2016). Pharyngeal muscle activity is greatest during deep sleep, reduces during N2 sleep, and is lower still during light N1 and REM sleep. Compensatory upper airway reflex responses are also inhibited during sleep, especially in REM (Eckert, McEvoy, et al., 2007). Periods of active eye movements during REM sleep are associated with further marked inhibition of pharyngeal dilator muscle activity and tidal volume (Eckert, Malhotra, Lo, et al., 2009; Wiegand et al., 1988).

Finally, given the reliance on carbon dioxide levels to maintain breathing during sleep, if carbon dioxide levels fall below a critical level, known as the *apnea threshold*, breathing ceases. The apnea threshold is approximately 2–6 mm Hg below the stable sleep carbon dioxide level. Given the typical sleep-related reductions in breathing and the accompanying 3–8-mm Hg rise in carbon dioxide levels, the apnea threshold is typically quite similar to the wakefulness carbon dioxide level (Dempsey, 2005; Meza et al., 1998; Skatrud & Dempsey, 1983). The difference between the apnea threshold and the wakefulness carbon dioxide level varies between individuals and across disease states and is often termed the *carbon dioxide reserve*. The reduction in carbon dioxide required to cause breathing cessation is importantly dependent on the peripheral chemoreceptors (Smith et al., 2007).

The Spectrum of Sleep-Related Breathing Disorders

As highlighted in Figure 34.1A and described in detail below, the sleep-related breathing disorders spectrum includes snoring, CSA, OSA, and OHS. The section below outlines the contributing pathophysiological and clinical factors, the different manifestations, and the consequences of each form of sleep disordered breathing as well as the common underlying features.

Snoring

In susceptible individuals, with the sleep-related changes in upper airway physiology and the control of breathing, snoring can occur. Specifically, snoring arises as a result of airflow limitation and increased work of breathing due to airflow turbulence and tissue vibration of upper airway soft tissues and structures (Pevernagie et al., 2010). The vibration of airway tissues under these conditions creates the characteristic sounds of snoring that can vary considerably between individuals in intensity and duration and can occur during both inspiration and expiration depending on the characteristics of the airway. Alcohol is a potent vasodilator which, along with potential central nervous depressant effects on upper airway muscle tone and sensory processing, can lead to increased nasal resistance and, thus, increased work of breathing and snoring during sleep (Eckert, Elgar, et al., 2010). Other environmental and physiological factors that cause nasal congestion can also contribute to snoring (Kohler et al., 2007).

The prevalence of regular snoring in the general population has been challenging to define as most existing epidemiological studies rely on either self-reports or bed partner reports of snoring frequency and/or intensity, which may be unreliable. For example, a meta-analysis reported a wide range of snoring prevalence of 2%–83% in men and 1%–71% in women (Chan et al., 2012). However, a recent report objectively monitored nightly snoring in a global sample of over 12,000 participants (~90% male) over an approximately 6-month period in the home using an under-the-mattress sleep sensor (Lechat et al., 2024). This technology provided an estimate of the average percentage of sleep time spent snoring per night. Approximately 30%, 15%, and 5% of the study population snored for an average of >10%, 20%, and 30% per night, respectively (Lechat et al., 2024).

While snoring in the absence of accompanying blood gas disturbances may be considered the mildest form of a sleep-related breathing disorder, there are potential adverse consequences. Physiologically, partial upper airway obstruction that occurs with snoring increases negative intrathoracic pressure swings and transmural pressure pre- and afterloads on the heart. This increase in the work of breathing may elicit brief awakenings from sleep (cortical arousals) and cause sleep disruption as well as accompanying blood pressure surges. Indeed, in the recent study led by Lechat and colleagues (2024), multiple blood pressure recordings were made throughout the 6-month recording period, and regular snoring was associated with a nearly twofold increased odds ratio of having uncontrolled hypertension. This finding was independent of the more severe form of sleep disordered breathing, OSA. The tissue vibrations that occur with snoring may also be injurious to the upper airway and surrounding tissues, including the carotid arteries (Amatoury et al., 2006; Cho et al., 2011). Loud snoring may also directly affect sleep quality, both that of the individual snoring and, of course, that of the bed partner. Most hypopnea events, which reflect partial airway obstruction, are also typically accompanied by snoring. Consequently most, but not all, individuals with the more severe form of sleep disordered breathing, OSA, frequently snore loudly on most nights.

OSA

Further along the sleep-related breathing disorder severity spectrum, OSA is characterized by repetitive upper airway narrowing or collapse during sleep that results in blood gas disturbances (i.e., hypoxemia and hypercapnia) and sleep disruption. OSA is estimated to affect nearly one billion people globally (Benjafield et al., 2019; Lechat et al., 2022) and is associated with a range of health and safety consequences including adverse cardiometabolic outcomes, depression, cognitive impairment, and increased risk of motor vehicle and occupational accidents and injury (Heinzer et al., 2015; Teran-Santos et al., 1999; Yaggi et al., 2005). The risk of OSA, sometimes referred to as *clinical phenotypes*, increases with age and obesity and is estimated to be two to three times more common in men versus women (Young et al., 2004). However, the sex-specific prevalence gap narrows post-menopause. OSA is also very common in conjunction with certain comorbid conditions including cardiometabolic disease (Tietjens et al., 2019). While these are common clinical phenotypes associated with OSA, the pathogenesis of OSA varies considerably between individuals, as do the clinical features. For example, approximately half of all people diagnosed with OSA are not obese (Gray et al., 2017). Thus, as highlighted in the "OSA Endotypes" section below, in the absence of anatomical risk factors associated with obesity, other mechanisms must play a key role in the pathogenesis of OSA in non-obese people.

OSA Endotypes

Recent advances in knowledge of the different mechanisms that contribute to OSA have identified four key pathophysiological traits, or OSA *endotypes* (Figure 34.2; Altree et al., 2021; Eckert, 2018; Eckert et al., 2013; Pepin et al., 2022). The term *pathophysiological phenotype* has been used to describe the different mechanisms that contribute to OSA pathogenesis (Altree et al., 2021; Eckert, 2018; Eckert et al., 2013). However, as highlighted in the section above, the term *phenotype* can also encompass the different clinical manifestations and consequences of disease. Thus, *endotype* is technically the more appropriate term to define disease mechanisms and is therefore used throughout this chapter.

There are at least four key OSA endotypes that contribute to OSA pathogenesis (Figure 34.2). The first and most important contributor is impaired pharyngeal anatomy or a collapsible upper airway (Eckert, 2018; Eckert et al., 2013). However, most people with OSA (~70%) also have impairments in one or more non-anatomical endotypes which importantly contribute to their OSA pathogenesis. These include impaired pharyngeal muscle function, waking up too easily to minor airway narrowing disturbances (a low respiratory arousal threshold), and unstable control of breathing (high loop gain). The relative contribution of each of these OSA endotypes varies from person to person, and thus, as outlined below, there is considerable interindividual heterogeneity in OSA pathogenesis. The interindividual variability in OSA pathogenesis has important implications for OSA therapy (Pepin et al., 2022).

Increased Upper Airway Collapsibility

Impaired pharyngeal anatomy or increased upper airway collapsibility during sleep is a common feature of OSA pathogenesis for everyone with OSA (Eckert et al., 2013). Major risk factors for increased upper airway collapsibility are obesity, restricted craniofacial shape (e.g., retrognathia) and size, supine posture, and rostral fluid shifts, which can increase pharyngeal collapsibility especially in people with cardiometabolic disease (Altree & Eckert, 2022; Neelapu et al., 2017). However, the magnitude of pharyngeal anatomical variability varies markedly between people with OSA. Approximately 20% of people with OSA have a major anatomical problem whereby their airway consistently closes during sleep with positive airway pressure in excess of +2 cmH_2O. Most people with

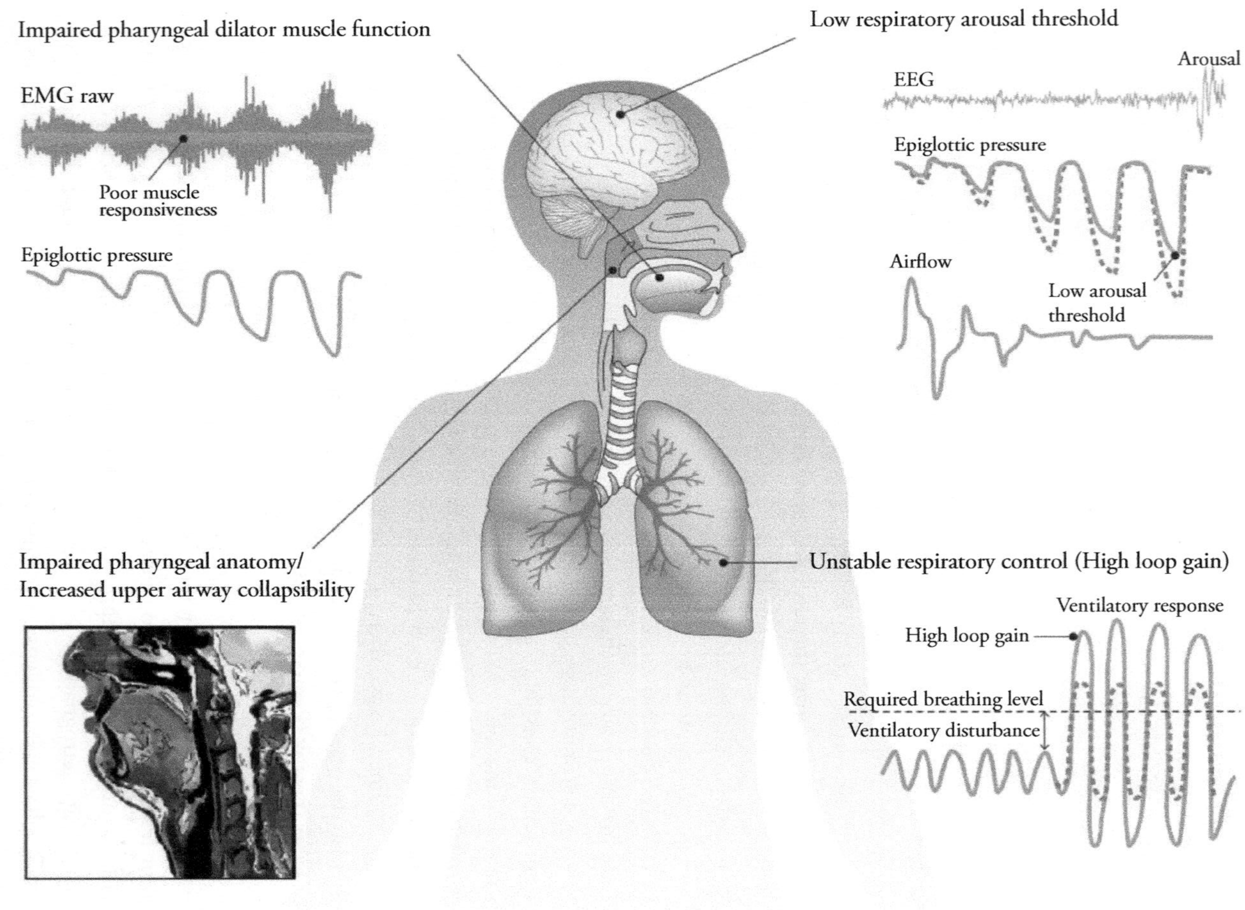

Figure 34.2 Schematic of the different endotypes that contribute to obstructive sleep apnea
Note. From Eckert and Yaggi (2022). Copyright © 2022 by the American Thoracic Society. Refer to the text for further detail.

OSA (~60%) have a moderately collapsible upper airway in which the airway closes at or near 0 cmH_2O. The remaining approximately 20% of people with OSA require suction pressure (between –2 and –5 cmH_2O) to close their airway during sleep. This level of pharyngeal anatomical compromise is equivalent to many people without OSA (Eckert et al., 2013). People with mild anatomical compromise are protected from OSA as they either do not have major impairment in any of the non-anatomical traits such as high loop gain/unstable control of breathing (Eckert et al., 2013) or have excellent pharyngeal dilator muscle responsiveness during sleep (Sands et al., 2014). The opposite is also true whereby everyone with mild anatomical impairment and OSA has impairment in one or more of the non-anatomical endotypes (Eckert et al., 2013).

Structurally, anatomical factors such as short mandible length are associated with increased risk of OSA in men (Chi et al., 2011). OSA is also very common in adults with smaller upper airway bony dimensions (Neelapu et al., 2017). Increased length of the upper airway, which is more common in men than women, and a more inferior hyoid position are also associated with increased risk of OSA (Genta, Schorr, et al., 2014; Malhotra et al., 2002; Neelapu et al., 2017).

Functionally, adipose tissue deposition surrounding the pharyngeal airway and directly within the pharyngeal muscles, and in particular the tongue, leads to airway crowding (Eckert, 2018; Kim et al., 2014). These factors increase the propensity for upper airway collapse during sleep when protective neuromuscular compensatory mechanisms are reduced. Upper airway collapsibility is also body position–dependent. Indeed, upper airway collapsibility is greatest in the supine position when gravitational forces tend to retract the mandible and major airway dilator muscles posteriorly to reduce airway size versus the lateral position and when the neck is flexed as opposed to extended (Joosten et al., 2015; Ong et al., 2011; Walsh et al., 2008). Gravity-related fluid redistribution from the lower limbs where fluid tends to accumulate after a day of activity toward the tissues surrounding the upper airway when moving to the supine position in the evening may also play a role in increasing upper airway collapsibility during sleep (L. H. White & Bradley, 2013). Abdominal obesity, which is common in men, lowers resting lung volume and reduces caudal traction on the structures surrounding the pharyngeal airway, which also increases the propensity for pharyngeal collapse (Stadler et al., 2009; Tong et al., 2019).

Impaired Pharyngeal Dilator Muscle Function

As highlighted, there are multiple pairs of muscles that surround the pharynx which require complex motor control organization to facilitate the key functional tasks of the upper airway, of which breathing is one. Given the multiple functional requirements of the upper airway, there are pharyngeal muscles that play a key role in airway dilation; some stiffen the airway, while others can constrict the airway, which is important for swallowing. In the context of breathing, key upper airway dilator muscles such as the genioglossus and tensor palatini receive respiration-related drive from brainstem pattern generator neurons, mechanoreceptors in the pharynx that respond to rapid changes in airway pressure (Figure 34.1B), and chemoreceptor inputs that respond to blood gas changes, in particular changes in carbon dioxide (Carberry et al., 2015; Eckert, Saboisky, et al., 2010; Horner, Innes, Murphy, & Guz, 1991; Lo et al., 2006). As discussed, upper airway dilator muscle activity is also sleep stage–dependent, with higher levels of drive to the genioglossus during slow-wave sleep and lowest levels during REM sleep, particularly when active eye movements are present (Carberry et al., 2016; Eckert, Malhotra, Lo, et al., 2009). Changes in pharyngeal muscle activity across sleep stages are accompanied by corresponding changes in the propensity for upper airway collapse (Carberry et al., 2016). Accordingly, these physiological changes may explain, at least in part, why OSA severity is reduced in slow-wave sleep and worse in lighter stages of sleep and REM sleep (Ratnavadivel et al., 2009).

Given the multiple inputs to the upper airway dilator muscles, there are several points of potential failure in dilator muscle function which can contribute to OSA pathogenesis. For example, over one-third of people with OSA have impaired dilator muscle responsiveness during sleep (Eckert, 2018; Eckert et al., 2013). These people are unable to increase neural drive to the dilator muscles in response to the respiratory stimuli that accompany airway narrowing during sleep such as hypercapnia and negative pharyngeal pressure (Eckert et al., 2013). Accordingly, the only way these individuals can reactivate their pharyngeal dilator muscles and restore adequate airflow is via a change in state (i.e., an arousal from sleep). The reasons why one-third of people with OSA are unable to activate their dilator muscles during sleep are unclear but may include an inherited predisposition, upper airway inflammation, and edema or neuropathy from upper airway trauma that accompanies repetitive airway narrowing and closure in untreated OSA (Saboisky, Butler, et al., 2012; Saboisky, Stashuk, et al., 2012). Some people may have impaired dilator muscle reflex function due to functional impairment in the brainstem neurons that control dilator muscle reflexes due to central nervous system lesions caused by pathological disease processes such as multiple sclerosis (Hensen et al., 2022). Regardless of the underlying cause, inability to recruit the airway dilator muscles during sleep combined with an anatomically vulnerable airway are key contributors to OSA pathogenesis. In others, the dilator muscles may adequately respond to the respiratory stimuli that accompany airway narrowing and closure during sleep. However, the increased drive may be ineffective to restore airflow. This may be due to altered pharyngeal muscle mechanics secondary to fat deposition, more easily fatigable muscles, or poorly coordinated muscle contraction (Dotan et al., 2013, 2015; Eckert, Lo, et al., 2011; Saboisky, Butler, et al., 2012). Negative effort dependence may also play a role whereby, despite increased drive to the airway dilators, drive to the pump muscles is greater (Genta, Owens, et al., 2014). This results in a situation where the upper airway is effectively sucked closed with increased respiratory drive that occurs during airway narrowing and closure.

Low Respiratory Arousal Threshold

While knowledge of the mechanisms that contribute to arousal from sleep during respiratory events continues to evolve (Amatoury et al., 2018), increased ventilatory drive or effort to breathe is believed to be a key surrogate that triggers cortical arousal under these conditions (Carter & Eckert, 2021). The level of ventilatory drive that elicits an arousal from sleep differs from person to person and between sleep stages (Eckert et al., 2013; Eckert & Younes, 2014; Gleeson et al., 1990; Younes, 2004). However, approximately one-third of people with OSA consistently wake up to relatively small changes in airway narrowing/ventilatory drive. This is known as a *low respiratory arousal threshold*, defined as waking up to negative intrathoracic pressure swings of only 0 to −15 cmH_2O (Eckert, Owens, et al., 2011). As many as 85% of people with OSA who are not obese may have a low respiratory arousal threshold (Gray et al., 2017).

A low respiratory arousal threshold endotype may contribute to OSA pathogenesis via several mechanisms. Firstly, if arousal occurs too easily to minor airway-narrowing events, this may prevent other compensatory mechanisms which are less destabilizing for sleep from being activated. This includes activation of upper airway dilator muscles, which need sufficient time and respiratory stimuli (i.e., carbon dioxide and negative airway pressure) to counterbalance the reduced ventilation in response to the increased level of ventilatory drive. The sleep fragmentation that occurs with repetitive arousals in someone with a low arousal threshold endotype also prevents progression into deeper stages of sleep where respiratory events are rare due to the accompanying beneficial ventilatory changes associated with deep sleep. These beneficial effects include a transiently increased threshold for arousal and increased upper airway dilator muscle activity (Carberry et al., 2016; Jordan et al., 2009; Ratnavadivel et al., 2009; Saboisky et al., 2010). Indeed, even in lighter sleep stages, pharyngeal dilator muscle responses are often sufficient to counteract increased ventilatory drive and prevent arousal in people with higher arousal thresholds, whereas awakenings occur prior to compensatory dilator muscle responses in those with low arousal thresholds (Eckert & Younes, 2014; Younes et al., 2007). Arousals also transiently increase breathing (Jordan et al., 2003), which, upon the return to sleep, can lower blood carbon dioxide levels to below the apnea threshold. In addition to breathing cessation, reductions in carbon dioxide levels can reduce drive to the pharyngeal dilator muscles and trigger breathing inability and a cycle of hyperventilation and apnea, typical of OSA (Iber et al., 1986; Younes, 2004).

Ventilatory Control Instability—High Loop Gain

Loop gain is a term used in the engineering field to characterize the sensitivity of a system controlled by feedback loops. This concept has been applied to breathing to describe the ventilatory control feedback system. For instance, when ventilation is reduced in response to airway narrowing, there is an increase in blood carbon dioxide levels. This blood gas change is first sensed by the peripheral chemoreceptors, which trigger an increased ventilatory response, the magnitude of which is dependent on the sensitivity of the ventilatory control system, which varies between individuals. In addition to chemosensitivity, or controller gain, loop gain is influenced by plant gain, which reflects the effectiveness of the respiratory system and tissues to alter blood gases. Physiological factors that can increase plant gain, and therefore loop gain, include reduced lung volume. This reduces the capacity to eliminate carbon dioxide from the lungs and, thus, increases carbon dioxide tension in the pulmonary capillaries. People with disproportionately large breathing responses to relatively small breathing disturbances/changes in blood gases have high loop gain. High loop gain is an important non-anatomical contributor to OSA (Eckert, 2018). People with high loop gain are vulnerable to breathing instability and repetitive upper airway obstruction as their breathing control system is too sensitive and inherently unstable. Indeed, as breathing rapidly oscillates between high and low levels, drive to the airway dilator muscles may transiently fall, leading to pharyngeal airway narrowing and repetitive collapse (Eckert et al., 2013). High loop gain plays a key role in OSA pathophysiology in over one-third of people with OSA (Eckert et al., 2013; Wellman et al., 2004).

CSA

Less than 1% of the adult population aged over 40 are estimated to have CSA, which is characterized by centrally mediated cessation of breathing (Donovan & Kapur, 2016). Like OSA, CSA tends to be even more common in men than women. Unlike OSA, however, daytime sleepiness and obesity are less common characteristic features of CSA (Donovan & Kapur, 2016). Unstable control of breathing/high loop gain underpins the different manifestations of CSA (Eckert, Jordan, et al., 2007; Eckert, Malhotra, & Jordan, 2009). For example, in addition to OSA, central and mixed obstructive/central breathing disturbances are common in people with heart failure (Orr et al., 2021; Randerath et al., 2017). While the mechanisms remain incompletely understood, the pathology related to heart failure including increased sympathetic activity is associated with heightened chemosensory and, thus, high loop gain, which fuels central breathing instability during sleep. In very severe cases, this manifests as Cheyne-Stokes breathing with the classical crescendo and decrescendo pattern. The cycle length between each breathing disturbance in Cheyne-Stokes breathing tends to be long (~1 minute or more). This reflects the increased circulation delay that accompanies heart failure. CSA can also be caused by other medical conditions that impact central nervous system integrity that either directly or indirectly impact the mechanisms responsible for control of breathing. These include neurological conditions such as multiple sclerosis, particularly when brainstem lesions are involved (Braley et al., 2012; Eckert, 2023; Lin et al., 2017). Another example is a rare but serious congenital condition, congenital central hypoventilation syndrome. This condition is characterized by the presence of a PHOX2B mutation (Antic et al., 2006) which is associated with profound impairment of chemosensitivity and central respiratory control

(Paton et al., 1989), necessitating breathing support during sleep. With the ascent to altitude, if you go high enough, everyone will eventually develop central breathing instability characterized by central respiratory events. This is due to the transient changes in chemosensitivity and control of breathing (D. P. White et al., 1987). Conversely, while at lower doses opioid medications such as morphine may actually lower loop gain and stabilize breathing during sleep in people with sleep disordered breathing who have high loop gain (Martins et al., 2020), with high enough doses or longer-term cumulative use, central breathing suppression/apnea is common due to opioid-induced impairment in central drive and respiratory control (Eckert & Yaggi, 2022). Finally, others develop CSA for no apparent pathological reason, termed *idiopathic CSA*. These individuals may have inherently high loop gain which predisposes them to CSA breathing instability (Xie et al., 1995).

OHS

OHS is defined by the combination of obesity, sleep disordered breathing, and daytime hypercapnia (arterial carbon dioxide tension ≥45 mm Hg) that is present in the absence of an alternative neuromuscular, mechanical, or metabolic explanation for the hypoventilation (Masa et al., 2019; Mokhlesi et al., 2008). While OHS is often undiagnosed, its prevalence may be as high as 10%–20% in obese people with OSA and up to ~0.4% in the general adult population (Chau et al., 2012; Masa et al., 2019).

Obesity and its accompanying consequences, such as reduced lung volume, impairs pharyngeal anatomy through the local accumulation of adipose tissue and places extra demand on the respiratory pump muscles (Kim et al., 2014; Li et al., 2012; Messineo & Eckert, 2020; Stadler et al., 2009). However, in some people, compensatory pharyngeal muscle activation can be robust enough to keep the airway open during sleep and prevent OSA despite compromised pharyngeal anatomy (Sands et al., 2014). However, in OHS this is not the case, and the opposite occurs whereby marked, sustained hypoventilation occurs during sleep. This is because with the loss of protective wakefulness mechanisms, the individual is no longer able to sufficiently overcome the mechanical burden to breathe that is placed on the respiratory system due to obesity, which is often severe in people with OHS. Why some morbidly obese people develop OHS and others do not is not known. Mechanistically, obesity tends to increase loop gain due to high plant gain secondary to decreased lung volume from obesity as smaller lung stores of blood gases will produce greater fluctuations in alveolar gas tensions to relatively small changes in breathing (Bokov et al., 2016; Hudgel et al., 1998; Messineo & Eckert, 2020; Peppard et al., 2009). However, in OHS, overall loop gain is likely to be low due to blunted chemosensitivity. On average, people who are obese also tend to have a high respiratory arousal threshold (Edwards et al., 2014). In people with OHS, this combination likely explains the prolonged sleep hypoventilation and accompanying blood gas disturbances.

Conclusions

There are different manifestations of sleep-related breathing disorders which range from snoring, CSA and OSA, to OHS. While the underlying pathophysiological and clinical features and consequences of each form of sleep disordered breathing vary, there are common key features. Recent advances in knowledge of upper airway and respiratory physiology, including the development of sleep apnea endotyping concepts, have shed new light on the underlying mechanisms and offer promise for novel tailored therapeutic solutions.

Future Directions

Despite recent advances in knowledge and understanding, there are multiple important unanswered research questions on the pathophysiology and consequences of sleep-related breathing disorders that are priorities for future research directions. Some of these key questions include the following:

- How can we better define and quantify snoring and its potential health impacts at scale?
- What are the mechanistic origins of increased loop gain and breathing instability in the various manifestations of CSA?
- What are the precise mechanisms that contribute to impaired pharyngeal muscle function during sleep?
- How can we best develop clinically scalable tools to accurately estimate sleep-related breathing disorder endotypes to inform clinical decision-making?
- Why do some morbidly obese people develop OHS while others with comparable body habitus do not?

Acknowledgments

D. J. Eckert is supported by a National Health and Medical Research Council of Australia Leadership Fellowship (1196261). He has received research grants from Apnimed, Bayer, Takeda, Eli Lilly, and Invicta Medical and has served as a consultant/advisor for Bayer, Takeda, Apnimed, Invicta Medical, and Mosanna.

References

Altree, T. J., Chung, F., Chan, M. T. V., & Eckert, D. J. (2021). Vulnerability to postoperative complications in obstructive sleep apnea: Importance of phenotypes. *Anesthesia and Analgesia, 132*(5), 1328–1337. https://doi.org/10.1213/ANE.0000000000005390

Altree, T. J., & Eckert, D. J. (2022). Obstructive sleep apnea endotypes and their postoperative relevance. *International Anesthesiology Clinics, 60*(2), 1–7. https://doi.org/10.1097/AIA.0000000000000357

Amatoury, J., Howitt, L., Wheatley, J. R., Avolio, A. P., & Amis, T. C. (2006). Snoring-related energy transmission to the carotid artery in rabbits. *Journal of Applied Physiology, 100*(5), 1547–1553. https://doi.org/10.1152/japplphysiol.01439.2005

Amatoury, J., Jordan, A. S., Toson, B., Nguyen, C., Wellman, A., & Eckert, D. J. (2018). New insights into the timing and potential mechanisms of respiratory-induced cortical arousals in obstructive sleep apnea. *Sleep, 41*(11), Article zsy160. https://doi.org/10.1093/sleep/zsy160

Antic, N. A., Malow, B. A., Lange, N., McEvoy, R. D., Olson, A. L., Turkington, P., Windisch, W., Samuels, M., Stevens, C. A., Berry-Kravis, E. M., & Weese-Mayer, D. E. (2006). PHOX2B mutation-confirmed congenital central hypoventilation syndrome: Presentation in adulthood. *American Journal of Respiratory and Critical Care Medicine*, *174*(8), 923–927.

Benjafield, A. V., Ayas, N. T., Eastwood, P. R., Heinzer, R., Ip, M. S. M., Morrell, M. J., Nunez, C. M., Patel, S. R., Penzel, T., Pépin, J.-L., Peppard, P. E., Sinha, S., Tufik, S., Valentine, K., & Malhotra, A. (2019). Estimation of the global prevalence and burden of obstructive sleep apnoea: A literature-based analysis. *Lancet Respiratory Medicine*, *7*(8), 687–698. https://doi.org/10.1016/S2213-2600(19)30198-5

Berthon-Jones, M., & Sullivan, C. E. (1982). Ventilatory and arousal responses to hypoxia in sleeping humans. *American Review of Respiratory Disease*, *125*(6), 632–639. https://doi.org/10.1164/arrd.1982.125.6.632

Bokov, P., Essalhi, M., & Delclaux, C. (2016). Loop gain in severely obese women with obstructive sleep apnoea. *Respiratory Physiology & Neurobiology*, *221*, 49–53. https://doi.org/10.1016/j.resp.2015.11.003

Braley, T. J., Segal, B. M., & Chervin, R. D. (2012). Sleep-disordered breathing in multiple sclerosis. *Neurology*, *79*(9), 929–936. https://doi.org/10.1212/WNL.0b013e318266fa9d

Carberry, J. C., Burke, P. G. R., Osman, A. M., Juge, L., Toson, B., Gandevia, S. C., Butler, J. E., Bilston, L. E., & Eckert, D. J. (2022). Regional genioglossus reflex responses to negative pressure pulses in people with obstructive sleep apnea. *Journal of Applied Physiology*, *133*(3), 755–765. https://doi.org/10.1152/japplphysiol.00083.2021

Carberry, J. C., Hensen, H., Fisher, L. P., Saboisky, J. P., Butler, J. E., Gandevia, S. C., & Eckert, D. J. (2015). Mechanisms contributing to the response of upper-airway muscles to changes in airway pressure. *Journal of Applied Physiology*, *118*(10), 1221–1228. https://doi.org/10.1152/japplphysiol.01103.2014

Carberry, J. C., Jordan, A. S., White, D. P., Wellman, A., & Eckert, D. J. (2016). Upper airway collapsibility (Pcrit) and pharyngeal dilator muscle activity are sleep stage dependent. *Sleep*, *39*(3), 511–521.

Carter, S. G., & Eckert, D. J. (2021). Effects of hypnotics on obstructive sleep apnea endotypes and severity: Novel insights into pathophysiology and treatment. *Sleep Medicine Reviews*, *58*, Article 101492. https://doi.org/10.1016/j.smrv.2021.101492

Chan, C. H., Wong, B. M., Tang, J. L., & Ng, D. K. (2012). Gender difference in snoring and how it changes with age: Systematic review and meta-regression. *Sleep and Breathing*, *16*(4), 977–986. https://doi.org/10.1007/s11325-011-0596-8

Chau, E. H., Lam, D., Wong, J., Mokhlesi, B., & Chung, F. (2012). Obesity hypoventilation syndrome: A review of epidemiology, pathophysiology, and perioperative considerations. *Anesthesiology*, *117*(1), 188–205. https://doi.org/10.1097/ALN.0b013e31825add60

Chi, L., Comyn, F. L., Mitra, N., Reilly, M. P., Wan, F., Maislin, G., Chmiewski, L., Thorne-FitzGerald, M. D., Victor, U. N., Pack, A. I., & Schwab, R. J. (2011). Identification of craniofacial risk factors for obstructive sleep apnoea using three-dimensional MRI. *European Respiratory Journal*, *38*(2), 348–358. https://doi.org/10.1183/09031936.00119210

Cho, J. G., Witting, P. K., Verma, M., Wu, B. J., Shanu, A., Kairaitis, K., Amis, T. C., & Wheatley, J. R. (2011). Tissue vibration induces carotid artery endothelial dysfunction: A mechanism linking snoring and carotid atherosclerosis? *Sleep*, *34*(6), 751–757. https://doi.org/10.5665/SLEEP.1042

Dempsey, J. A. (2005). Crossing the apnoeic threshold: Causes and consequences. *Experimental Physiology*, *90*(1), 13–24.

Dempsey, J. A., & Smith, C. A. (2014). Pathophysiology of human ventilatory control. *European Respiratory Journal*, *44*(2), 495–512. https://doi.org/10.1183/09031936.00048514

Dempsey, J. A., Smith, C. A., Blain, G. M., Xie, A., Gong, Y., & Teodorescu, M. (2012). Role of central/peripheral chemoreceptors and their interdependence in the pathophysiology of sleep apnea. *Advances in Experimental Medicine and Biology*, *758*, 343–349. https://doi.org/10.1007/978-94-007-4584-1_46

Donovan, L. M., & Kapur, V. K. (2016). Prevalence and characteristics of central compared to obstructive sleep apnea: Analyses from the Sleep Heart Health Study cohort. *Sleep*, *39*(7), 1353–1359. https://doi.org/10.5665/sleep.5962

Dotan, Y., Pillar, G., Schwartz, A. R., & Oliven, A. (2015). Asynchrony of lingual muscle recruitment during sleep in obstructive sleep apnea. *Journal of Applied Physiology*, *118*(12), 1516–1524. https://doi.org/10.1152/japplphysiol.00937.2014

Dotan, Y., Pillar, G., Tov, N., Oliven, R., Steinfeld, U., Gaitini, L., Odeh, M., Schwartz, A. R., & Oliven, A. (2013). Dissociation of electromyogram and mechanical response in sleep apnoea during propofol anaesthesia. *European Respiratory Journal*, *41*(1), 74–84. https://doi.org/10.1183/09031936.00159611

Douglas, N. J., White, D. P., Weil, J. V., Pickett, C. K., Martin, R. J., Hudgel, D. W., & Zwillich, C. W. (1982). Hypoxic ventilatory response decreases during sleep in normal men. *American Review of Respiratory Disease, 125*(3), 286–289.

Douglas, N. J., White, D. P., Weil, J. V., Pickett, C. K., & Zwillich, C. W. (1982). Hypercapnic ventilatory response in sleeping adults. *American Review of Respiratory Disease, 126*(5), 758–762.

Dunai, J., Wilkinson, M., & Trinder, J. (1996). Interaction of chemical and state effects on ventilation during sleep onset. *Journal of Applied Physiology, 81*(5), 2235–2243.

Eckert, D. J. (2018). Phenotypic approaches to obstructive sleep apnoea—New pathways for targeted therapy. *Sleep Medicine Reviews, 37*, 45–59. https://doi.org/10.1016/j.smrv.2016.12.003

Eckert, D. J. (2022). Respiratory physiology: Understanding the control of ventilation. In M. H. Kryger, T. Roth, & C. A. Goldstein (Eds.), *Principles and practice of sleep medicine* (7th ed., Vol. 1, pp. 245–251). Elsevier.

Eckert, D. J. (2023). Central sleep apnea due to other medical disorders—Not Cheyne-Stokes. In C. A. Kushida (Ed.), *Encyclopedia of sleep and circadian rhythms* (2nd ed., pp. 84–95). Academic Press.

Eckert, D. J., Elgar, N. J., McEvoy, R. D., & Catcheside, P. G. (2010). Alcohol alters sensory processing to respiratory stimuli in healthy men and women during wakefulness. *Sleep, 33*(10), 1389–1395.

Eckert, D. J., Jordan, A. S., Merchia, P., & Malhotra, A. (2007). Central sleep apnea: Pathophysiology and treatment. *Chest, 131*(2), 595–607.

Eckert, D. J., Lo, Y. L., Saboisky, J. P., Jordan, A. S., White, D. P., & Malhotra, A. (2011). Sensorimotor function of the upper-airway muscles and respiratory sensory processing in untreated obstructive sleep apnea. *Journal of Applied Physiology, 111*(6), 1644–1653. https://doi.org/10.1152/japplphysiol.00653.2011

Eckert, D. J., & Malhotra, A. (2023). Control of breathing. In M. H. Kryger, A. Y. Avidan, & C. Goldstein (Eds.), *Atlas of clinical sleep medicine* (3rd ed., pp. 56–63). Elsevier.

Eckert, D. J., Malhotra, A., & Jordan, A. S. (2009). Mechanisms of apnea. *Progress in Cardiovascular Diseases, 51*(4), 313–323. https://doi.org/10.1016/j.pcad.2008.02.003

Eckert, D. J., Malhotra, A., Lo, Y. L., White, D. P., & Jordan, A. S. (2009). The influence of obstructive sleep apnea and gender on genioglossus activity during rapid eye movement sleep. *Chest, 135*(4), 957–964.

Eckert, D. J., McEvoy, R. D., George, K. E., Thomson, K. J., & Catcheside, P. G. (2007). Genioglossus reflex inhibition to upper-airway negative-pressure stimuli during wakefulness and sleep in healthy males. *Journal of Physiology, 581*(Pt. 3), 1193–1205. https://doi.org/10.1113/jphysiol.2007.132332

Eckert, D. J., Owens, R. L., Kehlmann, G. B., Wellman, A., Rahangdale, S., Yim-Yeh, S., White, D. P., & Malhotra, A. (2011). Eszopiclone increases the respiratory arousal threshold and lowers the apnoea/hypopnoea index in obstructive sleep apnoea patients with a low arousal threshold. *Clinical Science, 120*(12), 505–514. https://doi.org/10.1042/CS20100588

Eckert, D. J., Saboisky, J. P., Jordan, A. S., White, D. P., & Malhotra, A. (2010). A secondary reflex suppression phase is present in genioglossus but not tensor palatini in response to negative upper airway pressure. *Journal of Applied Physiology, 108*(6), 1619–1624.

Eckert, D. J., White, D. P., Jordan, A. S., Malhotra, A., & Wellman, A. (2013). Defining phenotypic causes of obstructive sleep apnea. Identification of novel therapeutic targets. *American Journal of Respiratory and Critical Care Medicine, 188*(8), 996–1004. https://doi.org/10.1164/rccm.201303-0448OC

Eckert, D. J., & Yaggi, H. K. (2022). Opioid use disorder, sleep deficiency, and ventilatory control: Bidirectional mechanisms and therapeutic targets. *American Journal of Respiratory and Critical Care Medicine, 206*(8), 937–949. https://doi.org/10.1164/rccm.202108-2014CI

Eckert, D. J., & Younes, M. K. (2014). Arousal from sleep: Implications for obstructive sleep apnea pathogenesis and treatment. *Journal of Applied Physiology, 116*(3), 302–313. https://doi.org/10.1152/japplphysiol.00649.2013

Edwards, B. A., Eckert, D. J., McSharry, D. G., Sands, S. A., Desai, A., Kehlmann, G., Bakker, J. P., Genta, P. R., Owens, R. L., White, D. P., Wellman, A., & Malhotra, A. (2014). Clinical predictors of the respiratory arousal threshold in patients with obstructive sleep apnea. *American Journal of Respiratory and Critical Care Medicine, 190*(11), 1293–1300. https://doi.org/10.1164/rccm.201404-0718OC

Genta, P. R., Owens, R. L., Edwards, B. A., Sands, S. A., Eckert, D. J., Butler, J. P., Loring, S. H., Malhotra, A., Jackson, A. C., White, D. P., & Wellman, A. (2014). Influence of pharyngeal muscle activity on inspiratory negative effort dependence in the human upper airway. *Respiratory Physiology & Neurobiology, 201*, 55–59. https://doi.org/10.1016/j.resp.2014.07.005

Genta, P. R., Schorr, F., Eckert, D. J., Gebrim, E., Kayamori, F., Moriya, H. T., Malhotra, A., & Lorenzi-Filho, G. (2014). Upper airway collapsibility is associated with obesity and hyoid position. *Sleep*, *37*(10), 1673–1678. https://doi.org/10.5665/sleep.4078

Gleeson, K., Zwillich, C. W., & White, D. P. (1990). The influence of increasing ventilatory effort on arousal from sleep. *American Review of Respiratory Disease*, *142*(2), 295–300.

Gray, E. L., McKenzie, D. K., & Eckert, D. J. (2017). Obstructive sleep apnea without obesity is common and difficult to treat: Evidence for a distinct pathophysiological phenotype. *Journal of Clinical Sleep Medicine*, *13*(1), 81–88.

Guyenet, P. G., Stornetta, R. L., & Bayliss, D. A. (2010). Central respiratory chemoreception. *Journal of Comparative Neurology*, *518*(19), 3883–3906. https://doi.org/10.1002/cne.22435

Heinzer, R., Vat, S., Marques-Vidal, P., Marti-Soler, H., Andries, D., Tobback, N., Mooser, V., Preisig, M., Malhotra, A., Waeber, G., Vollenweider, P., Tafti, M., & Haba-Rubio, J. (2015). Prevalence of sleep-disordered breathing in the general population: The HypnoLaus study. *Lancet Respiratory Medicine*, *3*(4), 310–318. https://doi.org/10.1016/S2213-2600(15)00043-0

Hensen, H. A., Carberry, J. C., Krishnan, A. V., Osman, A. M., Mosch, A. H., Toson, B., Tay, K. L., & Eckert, D. J. (2022). Impaired pharyngeal reflex responses to negative pressure: A novel cause of sleep apnea in multiple sclerosis. *Journal of Applied Physiology*, *132*(3), 815–823. https://doi.org/10.1152/japplphysiol.00240.2021

Horner, R. L., Innes, J. A., Holden, H. B., & Guz, A. (1991). Afferent pathway(s) for pharyngeal dilator reflex to negative pressure in man: A study using upper airway anaesthesia. *Journal of Physiology*, *436*, 31–44.

Horner, R. L., Innes, J. A., Murphy, K., & Guz, A. (1991). Evidence for reflex upper airway dilator muscle activation by sudden negative airway pressure in man. *Journal of Physiology*, *436*(1), 15–29. https://doi.org/10.1113/jphysiol.1991.sp018536

Hudgel, D. W., Gordon, E. A., Thanakitcharu, S., & Bruce, E. N. (1998). Instability of ventilatory control in patients with obstructive sleep apnea. *American Journal of Respiratory and Critical Care Medicine*, *158*(4), 1142–1149. https://doi.org/10.1164/ajrccm.158.4.9712105

Iber, C., Davies, S. F., Chapman, R. C., & Mahowald, M. M. (1986). A possible mechanism for mixed apnea in obstructive sleep apnea. *Chest*, *89*(6), 800–805. https://doi.org/10.1378/chest.89.6.800

Joosten, S. A., Edwards, B. A., Wellman, A., Turton, A., Skuza, E. M., Berger, P. J., & Hamilton, G. S. (2015). The effect of body position on physiological factors that contribute to obstructive sleep apnea. *Sleep*, *38*(9), 1469–1478. https://doi.org/10.5665/sleep.4992

Jordan, A. S., Eckert, D. J., Catcheside, P. G., & McEvoy, R. D. (2003). Ventilatory response to brief arousal from non-rapid eye movement sleep is greater in men than in women. *American Journal of Respiratory and Critical Care Medicine*, *168*(12), 1512–1519.

Jordan, A. S., White, D. P., Lo, Y.-L., Wellman, A., Eckert, D. J., Yim-Yeh, S., Eikermann, M., Smith, S. A., Stevenson, K. E., & Malhotra, A. (2009). Airway dilator muscle activity and lung volume during stable breathing in obstructive sleep apnea. *Sleep*, *32*(3), 361–368. https://doi.org/10.1093/sleep/32.3.361

Kim, A. M., Keenan, B. T., Jackson, N., Chan, E. L., Staley, B., Poptani, H., Torigian, D. A., Pack, A. I., & Schwab, R. J. (2014). Tongue fat and its relationship to obstructive sleep apnea. *Sleep*, *37*(10), 1639–1648. https://doi.org/10.5665/sleep.4072

Kohler, M., Bloch, K. E., & Stradling, J. R. (2007). The role of the nose in the pathogenesis of obstructive sleep apnoea and snoring. *European Respiratory Journal*, *30*(6), 1208–1215. https://doi.org/10.1183/09031936.00032007

Kumar, P., & Prabhakar, N. R. (2012). Peripheral chemoreceptors: Function and plasticity of the carotid body. *Comprehensive Physiology*, *2*(1), 141–219. https://doi.org/10.1002/cphy.c100069

Lechat, B., Naik, G., Appleton, S., Manners, J., Scott, H., Nguyen, D. P., Escourrou, P., Adams, R., Catcheside, P., & Eckert, D. J. (2024). Regular snoring is associated with uncontrolled hypertension. *NPJ Digital Medicine*, *7*(1), 38. https://doi.org/10.1038/s41746-024-01026-7

Lechat, B., Naik, G., Reynolds, A., Aishah, A., Scott, H., Loffler, K. A., Vakulin, A., Escourrou, P., McEvoy, R. D., Adams, R. J., Catcheside, P. G., & Eckert, D. J. (2022). Multinight prevalence, variability, and diagnostic misclassification of obstructive sleep apnea. *American Journal of Respiratory and Critical Care Medicine*, *205*(5), 563–569. https://doi.org/10.1164/rccm.202107-1761OC

Li, Y., Lin, N., Ye, J., Chang, Q., Han, D., & Sperry, A. (2012). Upper airway fat tissue distribution in subjects with obstructive sleep apnea and its effect on retropalatal mechanical loads. *Respiratory Care*, *57*(7), 1098–1105. https://doi.org/10.4187/respcare.00929

Lin, M., Krishnan, A. V., & Eckert, D. J. (2017). Central sleep apnea in multiple sclerosis: A pilot study. *Sleep & Breathing, 21*(3), 691–696. https://doi.org/10.1007/s11325-016-1442-9

Lo, Y. L., Jordan, A. S., Malhotra, A., Wellman, A., Heinzer, R. C., Schory, K., Dover, L., Fogel, R. B., & White, D. P. (2006). Genioglossal muscle response to CO_2 stimulation during NREM sleep. *Sleep, 29*(4), 470–477.

Malhotra, A., Huang, Y., Fogel, R. B., Pillar, G., Edwards, J. K., Kikinis, R., Loring, S. H., & White, D. P. (2002). The male predisposition to pharyngeal collapse: Importance of airway length. *American Journal of Respiratory and Critical Care Medicine, 166*(10), 1388–1395.

Martins, R. T., Carberry, J. C., Wang, D., Rowsell, L., Grunstein, R. R., & Eckert, D. J. (2020). Morphine alters respiratory control but not other key obstructive sleep apnoea phenotypes: A randomised trial. *European Respiratory Journal, 55*(6), Article 1901344. https://doi.org/10.1183/13993003.01344-2019

Masa, J. F., Pepin, J. L., Borel, J. C., Mokhlesi, B., Murphy, P. B., & Sanchez-Quiroga, M. A. (2019). Obesity hypoventilation syndrome. *European Respiratory Review, 28*(151), Article 180097. https://doi.org/10.1183/16000617.0097-2018

Messineo, L., & Eckert, D. J. (2020). Pathogenesis of sleep apnea. In A. Tulaimat (Ed.), *Obesity hypoventilation syndrome: Physiologic principles and clinical practice* (pp. 55–66). Elsevier.

Meza, S., Mendez, M., Ostrowski, M., & Younes, M. (1998). Susceptibility to periodic breathing with assisted ventilation during sleep in normal subjects. *Journal of Applied Physiology, 85*(5), 1929–1940.

Mokhlesi, B., Kryger, M. H., & Grunstein, R. R. (2008). Assessment and management of patients with obesity hypoventilation syndrome. *Proceedings of the American Thoracic Society, 5*(2), 218–225. https://doi.org/10.1513/pats.200708-122MG

Neelapu, B. C., Kharbanda, O. P., Sardana, H. K., Balachandran, R., Sardana, V., Kapoor, P., Gupta, A., & Vasamsetti, S. (2017). Craniofacial and upper airway morphology in adult obstructive sleep apnea patients: A systematic review and meta-analysis of cephalometric studies. *Sleep Medicine Reviews, 31*, 79–90. https://doi.org/10.1016/j.smrv.2016.01.007

Nguyen, D. A. T., Boswell-Ruys, C. L., McBain, R. A., Eckert, D. J., Gandevia, S. C., Butler, J. E., & Hudson, A. L. (2018). Inspiratory pre-motor potentials during quiet breathing in ageing and chronic obstructive pulmonary disease. *Journal of Physiology, 596*(24), 6173–6189. https://doi.org/10.1113/JP275764

Ong, J. S., Touyz, G., Tanner, S., Hillman, D. R., Eastwood, P. R., & Walsh, J. H. (2011). Variability of human upper airway collapsibility during sleep and the influence of body posture and sleep stage. *Journal of Sleep Research, 20*(4), 533–537. https://doi.org/10.1111/j.1365-2869.2011.00925.x

Orr, J. E., Ayappa, I., Eckert, D. J., Feldman, J. L., Jackson, C. L., Javaheri, S., Khayat, R. N., Martin, J. L., Mehra, R., Naughton, M. T., Randerath, W. J., Sands, S. A., Somers, V. K., & Badr, M. S. (2021). Research priorities for patients with heart failure and central sleep apnea. An official American Thoracic Society research statement. *American Journal of Respiratory and Critical Care Medicine, 203*(6), e11–e24. https://doi.org/10.1164/rccm.202101-0190ST

Osman, A. M., Mukherjee, S., Altree, T. J., Delbeck, M., Gehring, D., Hahn, M., Lang, T., Xing, C., Muller, T., Weimann, G., & Eckert, D. J. (2023). Topical potassium channel blockage improves pharyngeal collapsibility: A translational, placebo-controlled trial. *Chest, 163*(4), 953–965. https://doi.org/10.1016/j.chest.2022.11.024

Paton, J. Y., Swaminathan, S., Sargent, C. W., & Keens, T. G. (1989). Hypoxic and hypercapnic ventilatory responses in awake children with congenital central hypoventilation syndrome. *American Review of Respiratory Disease, 140*(2), 368–372. https://doi.org/10.1164/ajrccm/140.2.368

Pepin, J. L., Eastwood, P., & Eckert, D. J. (2022). Novel avenues to approach non-CPAP therapy and implement comprehensive obstructive sleep apnoea care. *European Respiratory Journal, 59*(6), Article 2101788. https://doi.org/10.1183/13993003.01788-2021

Peppard, P. E., Ward, N. R., & Morrell, M. J. (2009). The impact of obesity on oxygen desaturation during sleep-disordered breathing. *American Journal of Respiratory and Critical Care Medicine, 180*(8), 788–793. https://doi.org/10.1164/rccm.200905-0773OC

Pevernagie, D., Aarts, R. M., & De Meyer, M. (2010). The acoustics of snoring. *Sleep Medicine Reviews, 14*(2), 131–144. https://doi.org/10.1016/j.smrv.2009.06.002

Pierce, R., White, D., Malhotra, A., Edwards, J. K., Kleverlaan, D., Palmer, L., & Trinder, J. (2007). Upper airway collapsibility, dilator muscle activation and resistance in sleep apnoea. *European Respiratory Journal, 30*(2), 345–353.

Randerath, W., Verbraecken, J., Andreas, S., Arzt, M., Bloch, K. E., Brack, T., Buyse, B., De Backer, W., Eckert, D. J., Grote, L., Hagmeyer, L., Hedner, J., Jennum, P., La Rovere, M. T., Miltz, C., McNicholas, W. T., Montserrat, J., Naughton, M., Pepin, J. L., . . . Levy, P. (2017). Definition, discrimination, diagnosis and treatment of central breathing disturbances during sleep. *European Respiratory Journal, 49*(1), Article 1600959. https://doi.org/10.1183/13993003.00959-2016

Ratnavadivel, R., Chau, N., Stadler, D., Yeo, A., McEvoy, R. D., & Catcheside, P. G. (2009). Marked reduction in obstructive sleep apnea severity in slow wave sleep. *Journal of Clinical Sleep Medicine, 5*(6), 519–524.

Rosin, D. L., Chang, D. A., & Guyenet, P. G. (2006). Afferent and efferent connections of the rat retrotrapezoid nucleus. *Journal of Comparative Neurology, 499*(1), 64–89. https://doi.org/10.1002/cne.21105

Saboisky, J., Eckert, D., & Malhotra, A. (2010). Stable breathing through deeper sleeping. *Thorax, 65*(2), 95–96.

Saboisky, J. P., Butler, J. E., Fogel, R. B., Taylor, J. L., Trinder, J. A., White, D. P., & Gandevia, S. C. (2006). Tonic and phasic respiratory drives to human genioglossus motoneurons during breathing. *Journal of Neurophysiology, 95*(4), 2213–2221.

Saboisky, J. P., Butler, J. E., Gandevia, S. C., & Eckert, D. J. (2012). Functional role of neural injury in obstructive sleep apnea. *Frontiers in Neurology, 3*, Article 95. https://doi.org/10.3389/fneur.2012.00095

Saboisky, J. P., Stashuk, D. W., Hamilton-Wright, A., Carusona, A. L., Campana, L. M., Trinder, J., Eckert, D. J., Jordan, A. S., McSharry, D. G., White, D. P., Nandedkar, S., David, W. S., & Malhotra, A. (2012). Neurogenic changes in the upper airway of patients with obstructive sleep apnea. *American Journal of Respiratory and Critical Care Medicine, 185*(3), 322–329. https://doi.org/10.1164/rccm.201106-1058OC

Sands, S. A., Eckert, D. J., Jordan, A. S., Edwards, B. A., Owens, R. L., Butler, J. P., Schwab, R. J., Loring, S. H., Malhotra, A., White, D. P., & Wellman, A. (2014). Enhanced upper-airway muscle responsiveness is a distinct feature of overweight/obese individuals without sleep apnea. *American Journal of Respiratory and Critical Care Medicine, 190*(8), 930–937. https://doi.org/10.1164/rccm.201404-0783OC

Shea, S. A., Edwards, J. K., & White, D. P. (1999). Effect of wake–sleep transitions and rapid eye movement sleep on pharyngeal muscle response to negative pressure in humans. *Journal of Physiology, 520*(Pt. 3), 897–908.

Skatrud, J. B., & Berssenbrugge, A. D. (1983). Effect of sleep state and chemical stimuli on breathing. *Progress in Clinical and Biological Research, 136*, 87–95.

Skatrud, J. B., & Dempsey, J. A. (1983). Interaction of sleep state and chemical stimuli in sustaining rhythmic ventilation. *Journal of Applied Physiology, 55*(3), 813–822.

Skatrud, J. B., Dempsey, J. A., Badr, S., & Begle, R. L. (1988). Effect of airway impedance on CO_2 retention and respiratory muscle activity during NREM sleep. *Journal of Applied Physiology, 65*(4), 1676–1685.

Smith, C. A., Blain, G. M., Henderson, K. S., & Dempsey, J. A. (2015). Peripheral chemoreceptors determine the respiratory sensitivity of central chemoreceptors to CO_2: Role of carotid body CO_2. *Journal of Physiology, 593*(18), 4225–4243. https://doi.org/10.1113/JP270114

Smith, C. A., Chenuel, B. J., Henderson, K. S., & Dempsey, J. A. (2007). The apneic threshold during non-REM sleep in dogs: Sensitivity of carotid body vs. central chemoreceptors. *Journal of Applied Physiology, 103*(2), 578–586.

Smith, J. C., Ellenberger, H. H., Ballanyi, K., Richter, D. W., & Feldman, J. L. (1991). Pre-Botzinger complex: A brainstem region that may generate respiratory rhythm in mammals. *Science, 254*(5032), 726–729.

Stadler, D. L., McEvoy, R. D., Sprecher, K. E., Thomson, K. J., Ryan, M. K., Thompson, C. C., & Catcheside, P. G. (2009). Abdominal compression increases upper airway collapsibility during sleep in obese male obstructive sleep apnea patients. *Sleep, 32*(12), 1579–1587.

Takakura, A. C., Moreira, T. S., Colombari, E., West, G. H., Stornetta, R. L., & Guyenet, P. G. (2006). Peripheral chemoreceptor inputs to retrotrapezoid nucleus (RTN) CO_2-sensitive neurons in rats. *Journal of Physiology, 572*(Pt. 2), 503–523. https://doi.org/10.1113/jphysiol.2005.103788

Teran-Santos, J., Jimenez-Gomez, A., & Cordero-Guevara, J. (1999). The association between sleep apnea and the risk of traffic accidents. Cooperative Group Burgos-Santander. *New England Journal of Medicine, 340*(11), 847–851.

Tietjens, J. R., Claman, D., Kezirian, E. J., De Marco, T., Mirzayan, A., Sadroonri, B., Goldberg, A. N., Long, C., Gerstenfeld, E. P., & Yeghiazarians, Y. (2019). Obstructive sleep apnea in cardiovascular disease: A review of the literature and proposed multidisciplinary clinical management strategy. *Journal of the American Heart Association, 8*(1), Article e010440. https://doi.org/10.1161/JAHA.118.010440

Tong, J., Juge, L., Burke, P. G., Knapman, F., Eckert, D. J., Bilston, L. E., & Amatoury, J. (2019). Respiratory-related displacement of the trachea in obstructive sleep apnea. *Journal of Applied Physiology, 127*(5), 1307–1316. https://doi.org/10.1152/japplphysiol.00660.2018

Trinder, J., Whitworth, F., Kay, A., & Wilkin, P. (1992). Respiratory instability during sleep onset. *Journal of Applied Physiology, 73*(6), 2462–2469.

Walsh, J. H., Maddison, K. J., Platt, P. R., Hillman, D. R., & Eastwood, P. R. (2008). Influence of head extension, flexion, and rotation on collapsibility of the passive upper airway. *Sleep, 31*(10), 1440–1447.

Wang, S., Shi, Y., Shu, S., Guyenet, P. G., & Bayliss, D. A. (2013). Phox2b-expressing retrotrapezoid neurons are intrinsically responsive to H^+ and CO_2. *Journal of Neuroscience, 33*(18), 7756–7761. https://doi.org/10.1523/JNEUROSCI.5550-12.2013

Wellman, A., Jordan, A. S., Malhotra, A., Fogel, R. B., Katz, E. S., Schory, K., Edwards, J. K., & White, D. P. (2004). Ventilatory control and airway anatomy in obstructive sleep apnea. *American Journal of Respiratory and Critical Care Medicine, 170*(11), 1225–1232.

White, D. P., Gleeson, K., Pickett, C. K., Rannels, A. M., Cymerman, A., & Weil, J. V. (1987). Altitude acclimatization: Influence on periodic breathing and chemoresponsiveness during sleep. *Journal of Applied Physiology, 63*(1), 401–412.

White, L. H., & Bradley, T. D. (2013). Role of nocturnal rostral fluid shift in the pathogenesis of obstructive and central sleep apnoea. *Journal of Physiology, 591*(5), 1179–1193. https://doi.org/10.1113/jphysiol.2012.245159

Wiegand, L., Zwillich, C. W., & White, D. P. (1988). Sleep and the ventilatory response to resistive loading in normal men. *Journal of Applied Physiology, 64*(3), 1186–1195.

Worsnop, C., Kay, A., Pierce, R., Kim, Y., & Trinder, J. (1998). Activity of respiratory pump and upper airway muscles during sleep onset. *Journal of Applied Physiology, 85*(3), 908–920.

Xie, A., Rutherford, R., Rankin, F., Wong, B., & Bradley, T. D. (1995). Hypocapnia and increased ventilatory responsiveness in patients with idiopathic central sleep apnea. *American Journal of Respiratory and Critical Care Medicine, 152*(6, Pt. 1), 1950–1955.

Yaggi, H. K., Concato, J., Kernan, W. N., Lichtman, J. H., Brass, L. M., & Mohsenin, V. (2005). Obstructive sleep apnea as a risk factor for stroke and death. *New England Journal of Medicine, 353*(19), 2034–2041.

Younes, M. (2004). Role of arousals in the pathogenesis of obstructive sleep apnea. *American Journal of Respiratory and Critical Care Medicine, 169*(5), 623–633.

Younes, M., Ostrowski, M., Atkar, R., Laprairie, J., Siemens, A., & Hanly, P. (2007). Mechanisms of breathing instability in patients with obstructive sleep apnea. *Journal of Applied Physiology, 103*(6), 1929–1941. https://doi.org/10.1152/japplphysiol.00561.2007

Young, T., Skatrud, J., & Peppard, P. E. (2004). Risk factors for obstructive sleep apnea in adults. *JAMA, 291*(16), 2013–2016.

CHAPTER

35 Sleep-Related Breathing Disorders II: Clinical Management

Amy M. Sawyer, Alexa J. Watach, Bruno Saconi, *and* Lindsey Clark

Abstract

Sleep disordered breathing refers to a spectrum of disorders that feature breathing pauses during sleep. The most common disorder is obstructive sleep apnea (OSA), characterized by episodes of partial (hypopnea) and complete (apnea) occlusions of upper airway, resulting in oxygen desaturation and sleep fragmentation. This chapter reviews the epidemiology, diagnosis, and treatment of sleep-related breathing disorders, specifically OSA. First, the clinical features and symptoms are presented. The pathophysiology of OSA is described and the related comorbidities. Risk factors are discussed. Approaches to the clinical evaluation of OSA are reviewed, followed by treatment options. As positive airway pressure (PAP) is the primary treatment for OSA, PAP-associated outcomes and adherence to treatment are discussed.

Key Words: sleep disordered breathing, sleep apnea, obstructive sleep apnea, diagnosis, treatment, positive airway pressure, adherence, oral appliance, upper airway surgery

Sleep disordered breathing (SDB) refers to a spectrum of disorders that feature breathing pauses during sleep. The most common disorder is obstructive sleep apnea (OSA), characterized by frequent episodes of partial (hypopnea) and complete (apnea) occlusions of the upper airway, resulting in oxygen desaturation and sleep fragmentation. OSA occurs in nearly one billion middle-aged adults globally (Benjafield et al., 2019). Although OSA is highly prevalent, the condition is frequently unrecognized and undiagnosed (Lyons et al., 2020). The economic burden of undiagnosed OSA is high, particularly when societal costs are considered such as those associated with impaired work performance, absenteeism, and occupational/motor vehicle accidents (Lyons et al., 2020). Because OSA is associated with comorbidities like cardiovascular disease, obesity, and metabolic disease, healthcare utilization and costs are excessive when OSA remains undiagnosed. The health-related cost burden for undiagnosed OSA in the United States in 2015 was estimated to be $150 billion; if undiagnosed OSA was identified and treated, a net projected savings of $100 billion was estimated (Frost & Sullivan, 2016). Treatment of OSA is a cost-savings opportunity at both the individual and societal levels (Wickwire et al., 2019).

Epidemiology

Pathogenesis

The pathogenesis of OSA has been linked to four key causes: (1) impaired/abnormal anatomy (primary cause) and three non-anatomical factors, (2) impaired dilator muscle activity, (3) low respiratory arousal, and (4) ventilatory control instability (i.e., high loop gain; Eckert, 2018). OSA is primarily caused by narrowing or collapse of the upper airway because of anatomical and physiological abnormalities. Locations of airway narrowing include the nose, retropalatal region, retroglossal region, or, less commonly, hypoglossal region. The airway obstruction results in either absent (apnea) or reduced (hypopnea) ventilation, despite ongoing respiratory efforts. As a result, hypoxemia and hypercapnia develop that further stimulate respiratory effort. The increased respiratory drive yields no result due to the lack of spontaneous airway opening, so the patient arouses from sleep and the obstruction terminates. After the airway reopens, hyperventilation occurs to correct the blood gas disturbances that developed during the respiratory events. The patient then returns to sleep until another obstruction develops (Eckert, 2018). Repetitive arousals result in significant sleep fragmentation, which may cause excessive daytime sleepiness and neuropsychological deficits that increase the risk for injury and accidents in patients with OSA. Although not fully understood, the underlying pathogenesis of OSA is multifactorial and may vary considerably between individuals (Eckert, 2018; see Chapter 34 for further information on the physiology and etiology of sleep-related breathing disorders).

UPPER AIRWAY ANATOMY

Most patients with OSA have an anatomically smaller cross-sectional area of the upper airway than normal controls that contributes to increased airway collapsibility (Eckert, 2018; Woodson & Franco, 2007). The cross-sectional area of the upper airway decreases as lung volume decreases, leading to increased SDB (Jordan et al., 2014). Anatomic factors, such as increasing airway length, can render the upper airway more susceptible to collapse (Abramson et al., 2010). Other anatomic features that predispose to upper airway narrowing in patients with OSA include retrognathia, reduced cricomental space, micrognathia, and atypical craniofacial anatomy associated with genetic disorders. As well, soft tissue accumulation in and around the upper airway (e.g., fat accumulation, tonsillar hypertrophy) and abdominal obesity result in pharyngeal narrowing that predisposes the upper airway to collapsibility. Nasal obstruction, particularly if variable such as with rhinitis, and fluid excess states, such as congestive heart failure or renal disease, also influence upper airway resistance and collapsibility of the upper airway (McNicholas & Pevernagie, 2022).

UPPER AIRWAY DILATOR MUSCLE ACTIVITY

The interaction between compromised upper airway anatomy and a diminished ability of the upper airway dilator muscles to maintain a patent airway during sleep is central to

OSA pathogenesis. During wakefulness, patients with OSA appear to compensate for an anatomically compromised upper airway by increasing upper airway dilator muscle activity to maintain airway patency. During the onset of sleep, upper airway dilator activity is decreased, in both OSA patients and controls. The genioglossus muscle of the tongue, the largest and most extensively studied upper airway dilator muscle in humans, has higher activity in patients with OSA compared with normal controls. This neuromuscular compensation while awake may be lost or substantially attenuated in sleep, leading to complete or near-complete pharyngeal collapse in patients with OSA (Horner, 2012).

AROUSAL FROM SLEEP

Arousal can be a lifesaving event if it opens the airway to terminate apneas as a last resort. The arousal threshold, or respiratory neuromechanical drive or pressure that is present immediately before an electroencephalogram (EEG)–defined cortical arousal, if low, can be dangerous. Low arousal threshold is associated with a marked hyperventilatory response, which may contribute to apnea pathogenesis. Arousals may increase the severity of the disorder by promoting greater ventilatory instability (Eckert et al., 2009).

VENTILATORY CONTROL STABILITY

Hypersensitive ventilatory control is a predominant non-anatomical cause of OSA (Eckert, 2018). Predisposition to apnea occurs with recurrent cycles of hyperventilation and hypoventilation that vary based on sleep stage and is related to loop gain. Loop gain is the negative feedback loop for regulating ventilation that is responsive to ventilatory disturbance (McNicholas & Pevernagie, 2022). For example, high loop gain occurs following an apnea with the respective increase in the magnitude of ventilation, ventilatory instability, and, thus, an increased likelihood of a recurrent apnea. Ventilatory control stability is also influenced by chemoresponsivity such that hypoventilation similarly increases the likelihood for subsequent, recurring apnea.

Associated Factors

SEX DIFFERENCES IN CLINICAL FEATURES

The male-to-female ratio of OSA is estimated to be 2:1 in the general population (Franklin & Lindberg, 2015). Males are at greater risk for severe OSA compared to females, but this difference in risk is attenuated in postmenopausal females (Lyons et al., 2020). Underdiagnosis of OSA in females may also, in part, explain the prevalence differences. Underreporting, or absence, of classic OSA symptoms in women is a contributing factor. Certain symptoms are more commonly reported in women with OSA, such as nocturnal choking, daytime fatigue, reflux, nocturia, enuresis, memory impairment, morning headache, insomnia, and mood disturbance (Basoglu & Tasbakan, 2018). Thus, women present with atypical symptoms compared to men, which heightens the risk of misdiagnosis, or underdiagnosis, of OSA in women (Schiza & Bouloukaki, 2020). This has implications for the predictive accuracy of commonly employed OSA screening tools that only address typical OSA symptoms.

Other important sex differences in OSA severity and comorbidities have been reported. OSA is less severe in women regarding the mean total number of apneic events, duration of apneic events, and less severe oxygen desaturations with apneic events. Fewer awakenings, longer sleep latency, and increased slow-wave sleep by polysomnography (PSG) are consistent in women compared to men with OSA (Schiza & Bouloukaki, 2020). Importantly, women demonstrate more rapid-eye-movement (REM)–related apnea events, which is a potential explanation for higher risk for all-cause mortality and cardiovascular events in women with untreated OSA (Bonsignore et al., 2021). Consequently, although OSA is less severe in women, its consequences are similar or worse than those in men.

DISPARITIES IN OSA

Black and Hispanic adults experience more severe and greater prevalence of OSA and related comorbidities (X. Chen et al., 2015, Dudley & Patel, 2016; Redline et al., 2014; Thornton et al., 2022). The greater prevalence and severity of OSA among Black adults is primarily among older and younger age groups (Dudley & Patel, 2016; Thornton et al., 2022). OSA is also more frequently undiagnosed and untreated among Asian, Black, and Hispanic adults (Johnson et al., 2022). The high rate of undiagnosed OSA is of significant concern due to the higher prevalence of cardiovascular and metabolic comorbidities in Black and Hispanic adults (Jackson et al., 2015, 2020; Olafiranye et al., 2013). Evidence also suggests there is a positive association between OSA and socioeconomic status (Etindele Sosso & Matos, 2021). Lower socioeconomic status is also associated with poorer sleep quality and short sleep duration, which may contribute to the underdiagnosis of OSA in this subpopulation (Guglielmi et al., 2019). Disadvantaged neighborhoods and neighborhood poverty, including higher prevalence of adverse environmental exposures, likely contribute to risk disparities in OSA (Johnson et al., 2022).

Clinical Features

The classic signs and symptoms for OSA include loud snoring, breathing pauses during sleep, and excessive daytime sleepiness (Stansbury & Strollo, 2015). Various clinical OSA phenotypes or clusters have been identified based on symptom presentation and comorbidities. For example, only a portion (37.7%) of people with OSA present with excessive daytime sleepiness, while others are clustered on disturbed sleep (33.5%) or minimally symptomatic (28.8%; Keenan et al., 2018). A broad range of symptoms and signs is observed in patients with OSA, including differences in clinical presentation by sex. Identifying the clinical features of OSA is crucial for diagnosis and treatment as well as identification of comorbidities associated with the disorder.

NOCTURNAL SYMPTOMS

A common reason for referral and evaluation of OSA is the occurrence of nocturnal obstructive symptoms, such as snoring, snorting, gasping, choking, and witnessed apneas, which are the hallmark symptoms of OSA because they reflect the basic pathophysiology underlying the disorder—a critical narrowing of the upper airway. These symptoms are often underappreciated by the patient, who may only be aware of them because of their bed partner's report. Snoring, a particularly disturbing symptom for bed partners, is a robust predictor of OSA (Sowho et al., 2020).

Although most patients with OSA have little difficulty in initiating sleep, they may report sleep-maintenance insomnia, which likely reflects the sleep-disturbing effect of frequent arousals (Ong et al., 2021). Other nocturnal symptoms of OSA include nocturia, enuresis, diaphoresis, restless sleep, and impotence. Comorbid sleep disorders, such as insomnia and restless legs syndrome, are common in OSA and may impact differential diagnosis and evaluation of response to OSA treatment (Verbraecken, 2022).

DAYTIME SYMPTOMS

Excessive daytime sleepiness is a common symptom of OSA, which is likely influenced by sleep fragmentation due to recurrent arousals with recurring apneic events. Other daytime symptoms in patients with OSA include fatigue, decreased concentration, memory impairment, personality changes, morning nausea, morning headaches, and depression (Verbraecken, 2022). OSA is associated with impaired cognition and performance, including worse performance with attention, executive functions, and impaired memory in those with OSA compared to healthy controls (Caporale et al., 2021).

COMORBIDITIES

OSA is commonly comorbid with other cardiovascular disease, metabolic disease, and Type 2 diabetes (Bonsignore et al., 2019). OSA is a significant, independent predictor for hypertension (Sands-Lincoln et al., 2013), including resistant hypertension and essential hypertension, with a dose–response relationship with OSA severity (Hou et al., 2018). The Joint National Committee on Prevention, Detection, Evaluation, and Treatment of high blood pressure recognized OSA as the first secondary cause of high blood pressure (Chobanian et al., 2003). Other conditions related to OSA are increasingly reported in the literature including cerebrovascular disease, depression, and chronic obstructive pulmonary disease, with varied distribution by sex (Bonsignore et al., 2019).

Risk Factors

OBESITY

Obesity is a main epidemiologic risk factor of OSA, with increases in body mass index (BMI), accumulation of adipose tissue, and increased neck circumference as strong predictors (Eckert et al., 2009). Obesity is common in individuals with OSA, particularly upper-body obesity. BMI is significantly associated with increased risk of OSA and is linearly associated with OSA severity (Deng et al., 2014). Recent evidence indicates that the relationship between obesity and OSA severity is modified by age and is sex-specific for men (Y. Liu et al., 2021). Waist–hip ratio and neck circumference as common anthropometric markers of obesity are also predictors of OSA.

AGE

Age is an important risk factor for OSA (Senaratna et al., 2017). The prevalence of OSA increases with age for both men and women. In older adults, any OSA defined by an apnea–hypopnea index (AHI) of ≥5 events per hour is highly prevalent in some studies, but severe OSA defined by AHI ≥30 events per hour is less prevalent (Senaratna et al., 2017). Deng and colleagues (2014) identified that in men age was associated with OSA severity in those younger than 40 years, whereas in women age was associated with OSA severity in one age group, 45–53 years of age. BMI was associated with OSA severity in both males and females across all age groups (Deng et al., 2014).

SEX AS A BIOLOGICAL FEATURE

Male sex is a primary risk factor for OSA. Sex differences in upper airway anatomy and function (Eckert et al., 2009), fat and its distribution (Basoglu & Tasbakan, 2018), control of ventilation, and hormonal status (Eckert et al., 2009) have been suggested to account for a higher male risk of OSA.

MENOPAUSE

Menopause is a significant risk factor for OSA in women. A higher prevalence of OSA in postmenopausal women has been observed compared to premenopausal women (Jehan et al., 2017). Non-obese women and those without hormone replacement therapy who experience earlier menopause by surgical menopause are at higher risk for OSA, suggesting that abrupt hormonal changes are important to the risk of OSA in women (Huang et al., 2018).

OTHER FACTORS

Craniofacial abnormalities can alter the mechanical properties of the upper airway and increase its propensity to collapse. Genetics have been increasingly supported as a risk factor for OSA. OSA is found to be heritable in families; however, there is limited evidence on specific gene variants (Mukherjee et al., 2018). Whole-genome scans in the Cleveland Family Study have demonstrated genetic factors underlying susceptibility to OSA, with 40% of variability in AHI explained by shared genetic factors (Mukherjee et al., 2018). Alcohol consumption has also been suggested to induce or worsen pharyngeal collapse in OSA. A meta-analysis demonstrated that any alcohol consumption compared to no alcohol or higher amounts of alcohol compared to lower amounts of alcohol increases the likelihood of OSA by 25% (Simou et al., 2018).

Assessment

Comprehensive Clinical Evaluation

A detailed sleep and medical history and physical examination are required for patients suspected of having OSA. Symptoms such as loud snoring, excessive daytime sleepiness, witnessed apnea, or gasping and the presence of obesity, retrognathia, and hypertension may drive the clinical suspicion of OSA, particularly in male patients. When performing physical examination, clinicians should assess for obesity and signs of upper airway narrowing. Morphometric parameters such as BMI >30 kg/m^2, increased neck circumference (>17 inches in men, >16 inches in women), and oral abnormalities such as macroglossia and a narrow oropharynx may suggest the presence of OSA (Epstein et al., 2009).

When interviewing a patient with suspected OSA, it is important to also interview the bed partner, whose description of witnessed nocturnal apneas and snoring provides important additional information to assist in the diagnosis of OSA (Luyster, 2017). The partner's input is also valuable in the identification of the patient's daytime symptoms and functioning. It is common for the patient to report a lesser degree of functional impairment than that observed by the partner, due to factors such as habituation to the symptoms, neurocognitive impairment, and/or denial (Bhat et al., 2016).

CLINICAL PREDICTION MODELS

While not recommended for establishing diagnoses of OSA, clinical tools, questionnaires, and prediction algorithms may help providers in non-sleep-clinic settings to identify patients at increased risk for OSA (Kapur et al., 2017). For example, a simple tool such as the Epworth Sleepiness Scale (ESS) may be used during an office visit to assess the propensity for daytime sleepiness (Johns, 1991). An ESS score of >10 (score range 0–24) is associated with increasing levels of excessive daytime sleepiness (Johns, 2000).

The belief that the evaluation of combined clinical features may improve diagnostic accuracy has led to the development of clinical prediction models or screening tools. Typically, these models evaluate witnessed breathing abnormality during sleep (snoring, apneas, choking, and/or gasping) and anthropomorphic variables (BMI, waist circumference, and/or neck circumference). For moderate to severe OSA, these clinical prediction models have overall high sensitivities (77%–93%) but relatively low specificities (28%–44%) and as yet are not recommended to diagnose OSA in adults in the absence of a sleep study (Chiu et al., 2017; Kapur et al., 2017). Self-reported questionnaires are useful screening tools to simplify the clinical assessment of patients, such as the Multivariable Apnea Prediction Index (Maislin et al., 1995), the Berlin Questionnaire (Netzer et al., 1999), and the STOP-Bang questionnaire (**s**noring, **t**iredness during daytime, **o**bserved apnea, and high blood **p**ressure combined with **B**MI, **a**ge >50, **n**eck size, and **g**ender = male; Chung et al., 2016; Table 35.1).

PSG

Overnight attended PSG is the "gold standard" for the diagnosis of SDB. PSG includes multiple, simultaneous physiological measures: electrocardiograph (ECG), EEG, electro-oculogram, electromyogram of the chin and anterior tibialis muscles, pulse oximetry, air-flow by nasal cannula pressure transducer, respiratory effort, body position, and snoring intensity. A trained technologist with oversight from a sleep physician scores the PSG using standard scoring guidelines (Berry et al., 2020), and the scored record is interpreted by the sleep physician to diagnose and characterize the severity of the disordered breathing.

Table 35.1 The STOP-Bang questionnaire

Question	Response
Snoring? Do you **Snore Loudly** (loud enough to be heard through closed doors or your bed-partner elbows you for snoring at night)?	Yes No
Tired? Do you often feel **Tired, Fatigued,** or **Sleepy** during the daytime (such as falling asleep during driving or talking to someone)?	Yes No
Observed? Has anyone **Observed** you **Stop Breathing** or **Choking/Gasping** during your sleep?	Yes No
Pressure? Do you have or are you being treated for **High Blood Pressure**?	Yes No
Body Mass Index more than 35 kg/m²?	Yes No
Age older than 50 years?	Yes No
Neck size large? (Measured around Adam's apple) For male, is your shirt collar 17 inches/43 cm or larger? For female, is your shirt collar 16 inches/41 cm or larger?	Yes No
Gender = Male?	Yes No
Scoring Criteria: **For general population Low risk of OSA:** Yes to 0–2 questions **Intermediate risk of OSA:** Yes to 3–4 questions **High risk of OSA:** Yes to 5–8 questions or Yes to 2 or more of 4 STOP questions + male gender or Yes to 2 or more of 4 STOP questions + BMI >35 kg/m² or Yes to 2 or more of 4 STOP questions + neck circumference (17"/43 cm in male, 16"/41cm in female)	

Note. Reproduced with permission. Proprietary to University Health Network. www.stopbang.ca. Modified from Chung et al. (2008, 2012, 2014).

While current practice relies on a single-night diagnostic PSG study, night-to-night variability in respiratory variables exists and contributes to misdiagnosis and misclassification of patients with suspected OSA (Roeder et al., 2020). Factors that may contribute to the night-to-night variability of the respiratory variables in PSG studies include time spent in the supine position where AHI is typically higher, alcohol and drug consumption, and variability in sleep stage distribution, particularly REM sleep (Roeder et al., 2020). It is also known that people experience disturbed sleep when sleeping in a new environment, in what is known as the *first-night effect* (Agnew et al., 1966). These alterations to sleep architecture include shorter total sleep time, reduced sleep efficiency and REM sleep, and longer REM sleep latencies (Agnew et al., 1966; Byun et al., 2019). Thus, REM sleep may be underrepresented by in-laboratory sleep studies.

The in-laboratory *split-night* PSG study, a combination of diagnostic study (i.e., PSG only) and a titration study (i.e., PSG + positive airway pressure treatment [PAP]), is a commonly used, cost-effective approach for OSA diagnosis and treatment recommendations. In this protocol, a minimum of 2 hours is devoted to diagnosis and 3 hours for PAP titration on a single-night recording. If moderate to severe OSA (i.e., AHI ≥15 per hour) is evident for at least 2 hours of PSG recording time, PAP is initiated and titrated to the level required to eliminate disordered breathing in the latter part of the night (Kapur et al., 2017). Split-night studies accurately diagnose OSA in adults with uncomplicated, moderate to severe OSA and have the potential to improve efficiency of care by replacing two separate PSG studies, one as diagnostic and one as treatment trial conducted on two separate laboratory nights (Kapur et al., 2017).

HOME-BASED SLEEP STUDIES

PSG studies are costly and generally require the facilities of a sleep laboratory and a trained technician, and patients may encounter long wait times for diagnostic PSGs. In this context, home sleep apnea tests (HSAT) are a common clinical alternative because HSATs are accurate, cost-effective, and a convenient alternative to in-lab PSGs (Fields et al., 2016; Kuna et al., 2011). Current guidelines recommend HSATs for OSA diagnoses in uncomplicated adults who present with signs and symptoms indicative of increased risk of moderate to severe OSA (Kapur et al., 2017).

Some of the disadvantages of using HSAT include the absence of a technician when the study is conducted at home and variations in the physiologic sleep parameters being collected based on HSAT type. While Type II HSATs collect the same parameters as the in-lab PSG, Type III devices do not include EEGs and therefore do not provide sleep stages or sleep fragmentation. Type III HSAT devices include a minimum of two respiratory variables (e.g., effort, airflow), oxygen saturation, and cardiac monitoring (e.g., heart rate, ECG; Kapur et al., 2017). A technically adequate HSAT must include a minimum of 4 hours of concurrently measured pulse oximetry and airflow data. It should be noted that patients presenting with significant comorbidities (e.g., heart failure, cardiorespiratory disease) are recommended to undergo full PSG studies in a sleep lab (Kapur et al., 2017).

DEFINITIONS OF RESPIRATORY EVENTS

Definition and classification of disordered breathing events are shown in Table 35.2. Apneas and hypopneas are classified as obstructive if there is accompanying respiratory effort. The number of apneas and hypopneas per hour of sleep (AHI) is most commonly

Table 35.2 Definitions of respiratory events

Types of events	
Obstructive	Continued effort to breathe during abnormal breathing.
Central	No effort to breathe during abnormal breathing.
Mixed	Both obstructive and central features. The event generally begins as a central event and ends with effort to breathe without airflow.
Breathing events	
Apnea	AASM definition: A clear decrease (>90%) from baseline in the amplitude of a valid measure of breathing during sleep lasting ≥10 seconds.
Hypopnea	A reduction in airflow associated with an EEG arousal or oxygen desaturation. No consensus in definition. AASM definition: A clear amplitude reduction of a validated measure of breathing during sleep (≥30% drop from baseline) lasting ≥10 seconds that is associated with either an oxygen desaturation of ≥3% or an arousal or ≥4% oxygen desaturation (acceptable). The criteria used for scoring must be specified on PSG report. Centers for Medicare and Medicaid Services (CMS) definition: An abnormal respiratory event with a ≥30% reduction in thoracoabdominal movement or airflow as compared to baseline lasting ≥10 seconds and with a ≥4% oxygen desaturation.
Respiratory effort-related arousals (RERAs)	AASM definition: Sequences of breaths which must last for at least 10 seconds and are characterized by increasing respiratory effort or by progressively negative nasal pressure (diagnostic study) leading to arousal from sleep. No consensus on clinical definition.
Indices of sleep disordered breathing	
Apnea–hypopnea index	Shared definition by AASM and CMS: Number of apneas and hypopneas per hour of total sleep time.
Apnea index	Number of apneas per hour of total sleep time.
Hypopnea index	Number of hypopneas per hour of total sleep time.
RERA index	Number of RERAs per hour of total sleep time.
Respiratory disturbance index	AASM definition: Number of apneas, hypopneas, and RERAs per hour of total sleep time. CMS definition: Number of apneas per hour of total sleep time.

Note. AASM = American Academy of Sleep Medicine; EEG = electroencephalography; PSG = polysomnography. Adapted with permission from Berry et al. (2020); Centers for Medicare and Medicaid Services (2008).

used to determine the severity of OSA (Centers for Medicare & Medicaid Services, 2008). While obstructive hypopneas are distinguished from apneas when establishing OSA diagnosis, such a distinction is not significant in routine clinical practice (J. L. Yu et al., 2021). Currently, there is no uniformly employed definition of hypopnea, which can result in considerable variability in the reported AHI (Berry et al., 2022). Despite recent efforts to establish 3% as the threshold for hypopneas, oxygen desaturations of 3% or 4% and specific criteria for arousals are commonly accepted for the definition of hypopnea (Berry et al., 2020, 2022).

Respiratory effort–related arousal (RERA) refers to a series of breaths characterized by an increasing respiratory effort, which leads to an arousal from sleep but does not meet the criteria for an apnea or hypopnea. RERAs can appear without a significant number of apneas and hypopneas but still produce fatigue and excessive daytime sleepiness in what is historically known as *upper airway resistance syndrome* (UARS; Guilleminault et al., 1993). However, current practice guidelines discourage the use of the term *UARS* as a distinct diagnosis because the condition is subsumed under the OSA diagnosis given the shared pathophysiology (Sateia, 2014).

DIAGNOSTIC CRITERIA

The diagnosis of OSA requires the combined assessment of relevant clinical features and the objective demonstration of abnormal breathing during sleep as assessed by a sleep study. According to the third edition of the *International Classification of Sleep Disorders* (ICSD-3; American Academy of Sleep Medicine, 2014), the individual must fulfill criteria A and B or satisfy criterion C (Table 35.3).

While OSA was initially diagnosed based on the AHI, and such an index is still used for establishing OSA severity, the ICSD-3 uses the American Academy of Sleep Medicine definition of respiratory disturbance index (RDI) as the actual OSA diagnostic criterion (American Academy of Sleep Medicine, 2014; Centers for Medicare & Medicaid Services, 2008). Based on the frequency of abnormal respiratory events during sleep, OSA is characterized as mild, moderate, or severe (Epstein et al., 2009):

- Mild: AHI or RDI ≥5 and <15 events per hour
- Moderate: AHI or RDI ≥15 and ≤30 events per hour
- Severe: AHI or RDI >30 events per hour

DIFFERENTIAL DIAGNOSIS

OSA should be distinguished from isolated snoring. People with isolated snoring will not exhibit obstructive respiratory events and do not present other symptoms such as sleepiness, fatigue, or impaired daytime performance. Sleepiness should not be considered a diagnostic criterion if it can be explained by other factors, such as medication adverse effects, alcohol or substance use, narcolepsy, idiopathic hypersomnia, and insufficient

Table 35.3 Diagnostic criteria according to the *International Classification of Sleep Disorders*, third edition
A. The presence of one or more of the following: 1. The patient complains of sleepiness, nonrestorative sleep, fatigue, or insomnia symptoms. 2. The patient wakes with breath holding, gasping, or choking. 3. The bed partner or other observer reports habitual snoring, breathing interruptions, or both during the patient's sleep. 4. The patient has been diagnosed with hypertension, a mood disorder, cognitive dysfunction, coronary artery disease, stroke, congestive heart failure, atrial fibrillation, or Type 2 diabetes mellitus.
B. Polysomnography (PSG) or out-of-center sleep testing (OCST)[a] demonstrates: 1. Five or more predominantly obstructive respiratory events[b] (obstructive and mixed apneas, hypopneas, or respiratory effort–related arousals [RERAs])[c] per hour of sleep during a PSG or per hour of monitoring (OCST).[a]
C. PSG or OCST1 demonstrates: 1. Fifteen or more predominantly obstructive respiratory events (apneas, hypopneas, or RERAs)[c] per hour of sleep during a PSG or per hour of monitoring (OCST).[a]

[a]OCST commonly underestimates the number of obstructive respiratory events per hour as compared to PSG because actual sleep time, as determined by electroencephalography (EEG), is often not recorded. The term *respiratory event index* may be used to denote event frequency based on monitoring time rather than total sleep time.

[b]Respiratory events defined according to the most recent version of the American Academy of Sleep Medicine's *Manual for the Scoring of Sleep and Associated Events* (Berry et al., 2020).

[c]RERAs and hypopnea events based on arousals from sleep cannot be scored using OCST because arousals by EEG criteria cannot be identified.

sleep. Chronic hypoventilation syndromes can be distinguished from OSA by the failure of the partial pressure of carbon dioxide to return to the normal level when awake or after relief of the upper airway obstruction by PAP treatment (American Academy of Sleep Medicine, 2014). OSA is distinguished from central sleep apnea (CSA) by the existence of respiratory efforts during the apnea and hypopnea events. In CSA, periods of apnea/hypopnea are associated with absent or reduced respiratory effort, and an increase in respiratory effort is associated with an increase in ventilation.

Treatment

There are various treatment options for OSA, ranging from lifestyle changes to invasive surgical interventions. Table 35.4 provides an overview of the most common treatment options which are discussed in this chapter.

Adjunct/Lifestyle Changes

For milder cases of OSA, lifestyle changes are recommended for treatment. These include weight reduction (diet, exercise, pharmacotherapy, or bariatric surgery), limiting or quitting alcohol consumption and smoking, use of nasal decongestants or allergy medications, and positional therapy (Benoist et al., 2017; Currie et al., 2021; Gaisl et al., 2019; Hudgel

Table 35.4 Obstructive sleep apnea treatment options

Adjunct/lifestyle changes
Weight reduction
Limiting or quitting alcohol and smoking
Nasal decongestants or allergy medications
Positional therapy
Positive airway pressure (PAP) therapy
Continuous PAP
Autotitrating PAP
Bilevel PAP
Oral appliances
Tongue-retaining devices
Mandibular advancement devices
Surgical intervention
Phase I surgeries Adenotonsillectomy, nasal, palatal, tongue, maxillary expansion
Phase II surgery Maxillomandibular advancement
Additional surgeries Hypoglossal nerve stimulation Tracheostomy
Alternative therapies Myofunctional therapies; pharmacologic

et al., 2018; Kuna et al., 2021; H. T. Liu et al., 2016; Mitchell et al., 2014; Nguyen et al., 2021; Randerath et al., 2011, 2021).

Weight reduction improves OSA by reducing the volume of the upper airway soft tissues that are strongly associated with apneic events (Wang et al., 2020). As little as a 5% weight loss can help reduce obstructive events, but ideally >10% weight loss is necessary to reduce severe OSA (Georgoulis et al., 2022). For individuals with extreme obesity, there is growing popularity for bariatric surgery as a more permanent treatment, with data from a national cohort study indicating OSA remission was obtained in 59.2% of patients who underwent bariatric surgery (Currie et al., 2021).

Further, reducing or eliminating alcohol consumption is strongly recommended as alcohol causes the muscles in the upper airway to relax leading to obstruction and apneic events (Burgos-Sanchez et al., 2020; Simou et al., 2018; Yang et al., 2022). Evidence on the relationship between smoking and OSA is less clear. The effects of smoking cessation on OSA have not been well studied, but it is hypothesized that smoking cessation may improve OSA due to reductions in upper airway edema (Deleanu et al., 2016; Hsu et al.,

2019; Krishnan et al., 2014; Pataka et al., 2022). Additionally, to modify patency of the upper airway, use of nasal decongestants or allergy medications has been shown to significantly reduce OSA severity and improve oxygen saturation during sleep (An et al., 2019; Nguyen et al., 2021).

Positional therapy can also be effective for patients; however, AHI in the non-supine position should be <5–10 events per hour for it to be of benefit (Joosten et al., 2014). Positional therapy has been found to be effective in reducing AHI by approximately 54% and can reduce the amount of time spent sleeping in the supine position by 84% (Ravesloot et al., 2017). Optimal positioning to achieve >80% reduction in AHI is >30 degrees lateral rotation with >70 mm of cervical vertebrae support with head tilting and a >20-mm elevation of the scapula (Lee et al., 2009). Various devices have been utilized or developed for positional therapy, including the use of a tennis ball sewn or pinned to the back of sleepwear, pillows or wedges, backpacks, and position alarms (Srijithesh et al., 2019).

If these adjunct/lifestyle changes do not improve OSA or if OSA is moderate to severe, additional treatments are recommended. If an individual with moderate to severe OSA also has these associated lifestyle factors, lifestyle changes should be recommended in combination with additional therapies such as PAP therapy, oral appliances, and surgery (Chirinos et al., 2014; Hudgel et al., 2018; Jordan et al., 2014). Of these, PAP is often the first-line treatment as the overall efficacy of other treatments tends to fall short when compared to PAP (Iftikhar et al., 2017; Jordan et al., 2014).

PAP Therapy

Since its development in 1981 (Sullivan et al., 1981), PAP therapy has become the "gold-standard" treatment for OSA (Epstein et al., 2009; Jordan et al., 2014; Patil et al., 2019a). PAP is delivered by a small machine at the bedside that compresses room air to deliver pressurized air to the airway. The air that is delivered to the upper airway acts as a pneumatic splint to keep the airway from collapsing during sleep, thereby reducing the number of obstructive events that occur during sleep. The air travels from the machine, through tubing, to a mask that covers the nose or nose and mouth, with the mask held in place with elasticized headgear.

There are various mask styles for patients to choose from, such as nasal pillows, nasal masks, and full-face (i.e., oronasal) masks. Ideally, the patient should select a mask style that feels most comfortable. There are often fewer side effects, better treatment efficacy (i.e., lower residual AHI), and increased adherence with nasal compared with oronasal interfaces (Andrade et al., 2018; L. Y. Chen et al., 2022; Rowland et al., 2018). This data suggests that, for the routine initiation of PAP therapy in adults with OSA, clinicians should generally use nasal-style mask interfaces over oronasal interfaces (Andrade et al., 2018; Patil et al., 2019b; Rowland et al., 2018). However, individual patient factors or preferences can vary. Optimally, a mask should be selected that maximizes tolerability, minimizes side effects, and optimizes efficacy and adherence.

Clinical side effects of PAP therapy can include air leakage from around the mask; skin irritation; congestion; dryness of the nose, mouth, or eyes; aerophagy; and claustrophobia (Ghadiri & Grunstein, 2020). Heated humidification added to the device is favorable for reducing adverse side effects, such as dry nose/mouth, nose bleeds, sore throat, congestion, headaches/sinus pain, and nasal discharge, but does not improve PAP adherence, sleepiness, or quality of life (QoL) compared to no humidification (Hu et al., 2022; Patil et al., 2019b).

FORMS OF PAP PRESSURE DELIVERY

Modes of PAP include continuous positive airway pressure (CPAP), autotitrating PAP (APAP), and bilevel PAP (BPAP).

CPAP

CPAP delivers PAP at a constant pressure throughout the night. CPAP has been shown to significantly reduce the AHI and improve various outcomes, such as daytime sleepiness, QoL, and blood pressure (Patil et al., 2019a; additional details below in section "Treatment Response Outcomes Associated with PAP"). CPAP has traditionally been recognized and used as the simplest, best-studied device; however, APAP has become increasingly popular due to its noninferior performance for both clinical effectiveness and patient-reported outcomes (PROs; Bloch et al., 2018; Patil et al., 2019b) CPAP devices also have a pressure-relief setting that reduces the pressure at onset of exhalation. This setting provides a more natural breathing pattern throughout the night and therefore can be used to improve tolerance of CPAP.

APAP

APAP is set to a pressure range and automatically adjusts pressure requirements in response to obstructive events and acute and chronic changes that can affect effective pressure requirements such as body position, weight changes, or alcohol consumption. As such, APAP devices have become increasingly popular due to their flexibility in providing the most effective treatment to patients over time wherein weight gain or lifestyle changes may necessitate varied pressure to effectively treat OSA. The APAP device does this by defining "normal" airflow for a given patient and adjusting the pressure/delivering additional pressure when the flow is restricted (Pavwoski & Shelgikar, 2017). To date, meta-analyses demonstrate a lack of clinically significant differences in treatment adherence and outcomes between CPAP and APAP (Patil et al., 2019b). However, APAP may not be appropriate for individuals with congestive heart failure, lung disease such as chronic obstructive pulmonary disease, obesity hypoventilation syndrome, lack of snoring, or CSA (Morgenthaler et al., 2008).

BPAP

First developed in the 1990s, bilevel pressure provides independent adjustment of the pressure delivered during inspiration (inspiratory positive airway pressure) and exhalation (expiratory positive airway pressure) to reduce the work of breathing and offer greater comfort to the patient. This applies to all BPAP devices including flexible, modified, and auto-adjusting BPAP (Patil et al., 2019a). BPAP devices are often used for patients with higher pressure requirements than can be provided by CPAP or APAP devices as BPAP facilitates the tolerance of higher pressures by making exhalation easier (Pavwoski & Shelgikar, 2017). In addition to the administration of high-pressure volumes, BPAP is often prescribed for patients with accompanying hypoventilation, often in combination with obesity or neuromuscular disease (Patil et al., 2019a; Selim et al., 2012). During the inspiratory cycle, the high-level pressure battles the inspiratory flow limitations of the upper airway, yielding a greater tidal volume and treating sleep-related hypoventilation (Morgenthaler et al., 2008).

CLINICAL PRACTICE GUIDELINE RECOMMENDATIONS FOR OSA TREATED WITH PAP

The American Academy of Sleep Medicine recommends the following for the treatment of adult OSA with PAP (Patil et al., 2019a): PAP should be used, compared to no therapy, to treat OSA in adults with excessive sleepiness, impaired sleep-related QoL, and comorbid hypertension (Recommendations 1–3). Further recommendations include the following:

4. PAP therapy should be initiated using APAP at home or in-lab PAP titration in adults with no significant comorbidities.
5. Use either CPAP or APAP for ongoing treatment of OSA in adults.
6. Use CPAP or APAP over BPAP in the routine treatment of adults with OSA.
7. Educational interventions should be given with initiation of PAP therapy in adults with OSA.
8. Behavioral and/or troubleshooting interventions should be given during the initial period of PAP therapy.
9. Employ PAP use tele-monitoring-guided interventions during the initial period of PAP therapy.

MONITORING OF PAP USE

Although PAP is the most efficacious treatment, its effectiveness can be severely limited due to non-adherence. Studies have shown that patients make the decision to adhere to therapy (defined as ≥4 hours/night on 70% of nights; Centers for Medicare & Medicaid Services, 2016) during the first week of treatment, and this early usage pattern is associated with long-term use (Weaver & Grunstein, 2008). Therefore, clinical practice guidelines recommend a variety of educational, behavioral, supportive, and troubleshooting interventions to encourage PAP use in adults with OSA (Aardoom et al., 2020; Patil et al., 2019a). Patients should be clinically evaluated within the first 31–90 days of treatment, and if PAP therapy has been well tolerated, annual visits thereafter are considered sufficient (Epstein et al., 2009).

TREATMENT RESPONSE OUTCOMES ASSOCIATED WITH PAP TREATMENT

Clinical outcomes and PROs associated with PAP treatment have been systematically examined in observational studies, clinical trials, and meta-analyses. Clinical outcomes are healthcare provider–reported/measured outcomes, whereas PROs are reported/measured by patients about how they are feeling and functioning (Weinfurt & Reeve, 2022). The combination of these outcomes, whether in practice or research, permits a comprehensive evaluation of the baseline disease state and, when reassessed with treatment, the treatment response. Repeated intervals of outcome assessment during treatment is strongly recommended in OSA patients treated with PAP as a quality metric (Lloyd et al., 2022) and due to the heterogeneity of the sleep disorder, including symptom subtypes (i.e., phenotypes; Allen et al., 2020; Keenan et al., 2018; Mazzotti et al., 2019; Pien et al., 2018) and heterogeneous patient experience of the disorder (Pevernagie et al., 2021). This approach is also consistent with precision medicine or precision healthcare that aims to ensure that the right patient receives the optimal treatment at the right time based on disease and treatment response characteristics (Light et al., 2019; Zinchuk et al., 2017).

Since the inception of PAP as an OSA treatment, both clinical outcomes and PROs have been evaluated as treatment response outcomes. Sleepiness is the most commonly assessed outcome due to its consistent association with OSA, with the prevalence of sleepiness estimated at 40.5% to 58% of adults with OSA (Lal et al., 2021). Other outcomes associated with OSA and PAP treatment response include QoL and function, cognitive performance, mood, cardiovascular and metabolic outcomes, motor vehicle crashes, and mortality outcomes. With evaluation of consistent outcomes in observational studies and randomized controlled trials, meta-analyses (Labarca, Dreyse, et al., 2020; Labarca et al., 2018; Patil et al., 2019b; J. Yu et al., 2017) provide the field with high-level summary evidence to address the question, what outcomes improve with PAP treatment? Table 35.5 provides summary results of a recent systematic review and meta-analysis (Patil et al., 2019b) that underpin the American Academy of Sleep Medicine clinical practice guidelines for PAP treatment of OSA (Patil et al., 2019a).

SLEEPINESS

Sleepiness as a PRO, commonly referred to as *subjective sleepiness*, improves with PAP treatment of at least 1 month (range 4–12 months) with clinically meaningful decrements of ≥2 points on the ESS in sleepy adults with OSA treated with PAP compared to control conditions (weighted mean difference = –2.71; 95% confidence interval [CI; –3.27, –2.15]; Patil et al., 2019b). Even among PAP-treated adults with OSA who are not

Table 35.5 Outcomes with positive airway pressure (PAP) treatment in obstructive sleep apnea: summary of meta-analysis results from randomized controlled trials of PAP versus control conditions

Outcome	Measure	Type	Summary result[a]	Quality
Sleepiness				
Subjective sleepiness	ESS	PRO	↓	Moderate
Wakefulness	Osler test	Clinical	↑	High
Sleep latency	MSLT	Clinical	–	Moderate
Quality of life				
Sleep-related function	FOSQ, SAQLI	PRO	↑	Moderate
Mental function	SF-36		–	Moderate
Physical function	SF-36		–	High
Vitality	SF-36		–	High
Cognitive and performance				
Δ Executive function	Shifting-Trail Making B, Cogscreen Shifting Attention Task Updating PASAT-1, -1.2, -2, -3, -4, Sustained Working Memory Fluid Reasoning-Block Design, Executive Maze	Clinical	–	Moderate
Δ Processing speed	DSST, 8-Choice Reaction Time, Trail Making A Reaction Time		–	High
Δ Attention and vigilance	PVT Reaction Time, PVT Lapses, Rapid Visual Information Processing, SteerClear, Cogscreen Pathfinder Number Test Total Time, Cogscreen Shifting Attention Task		–	High
Δ Memory	Digit Span Backwards, Weschler Memory Scale, Benton Visual Reaction Test, Verbal Recall, Word Pair Memory Recall, WMS-R Visual Reproduction, Buschke Selective Reminding Test-Sum Recall		–	High
Δ Intelligence	Performance IQ Decrement, Weschler Adult Intelligence Scale		–	Low
Mood				
Anxiety	HADS-Anxiety	PRO	–	High
Depression	HADS-Depression	PRO	–	High

Cardiovascular—Blood pressure				
Δ SBP, Nighttime	24-hour ambulatory BP[b]	Clinical	↓	Moderate
Δ DBP, Nighttime	24-hour ambulatory BP[b]		↓	Moderate
Δ SBP, Daytime	24-hour ambulatory BP[b]		↓	Moderate
Δ DBP, Daytime	24-hour ambulatory BP[b]		↓	Moderate
Δ SBP, 24-hour	24-hour ambulatory BP[b]		↓	Moderate
Δ DBP, 24-hour	24-hour ambulatory BP[b]		↓	Moderate
Δ Mean BP, 24-hour	24-hour ambulatory BP[b]		↓	High
Cardiovascular events				
Composite events[c]	Incident or recurring	Clinical	–	Moderate
Left ventricular ejection fraction				
% Δ LVEF	Echocardiography or ventriculography	Clinical	–	Moderate
Metabolic				
Fasting blood sugar	Fasting glucose (millimoles per liter)	Clinical	–	High
HbA1C	HbA1c (percentage)		–	
Motor vehicle crashes				
Driving proficiency (percentage), obstacles hit	SteerClear Simulator	Clinical	–	Moderate
			–	
Mortality				
All-cause mortality	Medical record, death registry	Clinical	–	Moderate

Note. BP = blood pressure; Δ = change; DBP = diastolic blood pressure; DSST = Digit Symbol Substitution Test; ESS = Epworth Sleepiness Scale; FOSQ = Functional Outcomes of Sleep Questionnaire; HADS = Hospital Anxiety and Depression Scale; HbA1c = hemoglobin A1C; LVEF = left ventricular ejection fraction; MSLT = Multiple Sleep Latency Test; PASAT = Paced Auditory Serial Addition Test; PRO = patient-reported outcome; PVT = Psychomotor Vigilance Task; SAQLI = Sleep Apnea Quality of Life Questionnaire; SBP = systolic blood pressure; SF-36 = Short Form Health Survey; WMS-R = Wechsler Memory Scale Revised;

[a]Directional result reported as clinically significant based on task force–defined criteria from Patil et al. (2019b, p. 305).

[b]Majority of randomized controlled trials employed this measure of the outcome.

[c]Varying event components included.

sleepy at baseline (ESS ≤10) when compared to control conditions, ESS scores improve by approximately 1 point (Patil et al., 2019b). The improvement of ESS scores in nonsleepy adults with OSA may still be perceived by patients, particularly as improvements in other outcomes like sleep-related function may be complementary in response. The improvement of sleepiness with PAP is also consistent in older adults (>65 years) with a weighted mean difference of –2.62 (95% CI [–3.30, –1.93]) by ESS compared to control (Labarca, Saavedra et al., 2020). When measuring sleep objectively, propensity to fall asleep is evaluated as a clinical outcome by the Multiple Sleep Latency Test. There is no difference in sleep propensity between PAP-treated adults and control conditions, but the clinical outcome of wakefulness by the Osler Test improves with PAP compared to control (Patil et al., 2019b). High-level evidence indicates that sleepiness improves with PAP, which drives the strong recommendation for baseline and repeated clinical assessments of sleepiness PROs after initiating PAP treatment (Patil et al., 2019a). Studies also indicate that subjective sleepiness at 3 months of treatment is associated with PAP dose. Greater improvements in subjective sleepiness occur with at least 4 hours of PAP use per night (Weaver et al., 2007), with more patients normalizing their subjective sleepiness ratings with at least 5 hours of treatment per night (Antic et al., 2011); but residual sleepiness is present in some patients regardless of treatment use hours (Antic et al., 2011; Weaver et al., 2007). In these cases, clinical evaluation of other contributing causes of daytime sleepiness is indicated (see Lal et al., 2021, for detailed discussion). From the patient value perspective, improvement in sleepiness with treatment of OSA is often a reason for patients, or their partner/family, to seek diagnosis and have expectation for improvement with treatment. Addressing sleepiness PROs by clinicians should be incorporated in the clinical interview with patients both at diagnosis and with PAP treatment.

QOL AND SLEEP-RELATED FUNCTION

QoL and sleep-related function are PROs that are commonly evaluated in research studies in adults with PAP-treated OSA but may not be commonly used in practice. QoL PROs are assessed with generic measures which permit cross-disease/disorder comparisons (Pevernagie et al., 2021). The Short Form Health Survey, or SF-36 (shorter versions are available, such as SF-12 and SF-20), is one measure of QoL that includes a total QoL score, a physical component score (PCS), a mental component score (MCS), and a vitality score that is often reported for OSA treatment studies. Recent meta-analyses of randomized controlled trials (RCTs) comparing at least 1 month of PAP treatment (range 1–48 months) and control conditions consistently show that PCS and vitality scores improve; but these improvements are small, and MCS improvement is negligible (Kuhn et al., 2017; Patil et al., 2019b; Timkova et al., 2020). Total QoL scores also do not improve with PAP treatment to a clinically meaningful degree. The challenge with interpreting these summary results from high-quality evidence is the heterogeneity between studies for duration of treatment, adjustment for confounding factors, and sample populations.

While some individual trials have demonstrated that PAP improves QoL, improvements are likely to be small based on effect sizes (Timkova et al., 2020).

Due to the prevalence of sleepiness as a presenting symptom of OSA, several disease-specific or health-related QoL (HRQoL) tools evaluate sleep-related functions across domains such as social/relationship function, emotional function, and productivity, including the Functional Outcomes of Sleep Questionnaire (FOSQ and short-form FOSQ-10; Chasens et al., 2009; Weaver, Laizner, et al., 1997), the Calgary Sleep Apnea Quality of Life Index (SAQLI; Flemons & Reimer, 2002), and the Quebec Sleep Questionnaire (QSQ; Lacasse et al., 2004). Though other HRQoL measures have been reported recently (Pevernagie et al., 2021), a recent evidence summary included the FOSQ and SAQLI as PROs due to the relatively consistent use of these measures in clinical trials published to date. HRQoL summary score outcomes do improve with at least 1 month of PAP treatment when compared to control conditions (Patil et al., 2019b). Similarly, in older adults, HRQoL improvements by QSQ assessment were identified after at least 3 months of PAP treatment compared to control conditions, including for every HRQoL domain (changes in hypersomnolence, diurnal symptoms, nocturnal symptoms, emotions, and social interaction; Labarca, Saavedra, et al., 2020). Cautious interpretation of the effects of PAP in older adults (>65 years) is acknowledged because of study heterogeneity, publication bias, and the overall low quality of evidence summarized in the meta-analysis. Limited evidence does suggest that a PAP dose response may exist for HRQoL outcomes, with total FOSQ score and activity domains improving with more PAP use per night in the first 3 months of treatment (Antic et al., 2011; Weaver et al., 2007). These exploratory results are based on a relatively small sample and indicate 7 hours/night of PAP use may be necessary to maximize total FOSQ score improvement with PAP (Weaver et al., 2007). Clinicians should discuss sleep-related functional impairments at diagnosis (i.e., baseline) and incorporate patient-reported improvements for these patient-valued HRQoL outcomes with PAP treatment after at least 3 months of treatment and follow-up visits thereafter (Lloyd et al., 2022).

COGNITION AND PERFORMANCE

Cognition and performance clinical outcomes do not significantly improve with PAP treatment based on pooled data from RCTs that compared at least 1 month of PAP treatment (range 1–12 months) to control conditions (Patil et al., 2019b). The domains included in the meta-analysis were executive function, processing speed, attention and vigilance, memory, and intelligence. While the quality of evidence was low to high, depending on the cognitive performance outcome, the domain outcome results most frequently associated with OSA and PAP treatment (attention and vigilance, memory, and processing speed) were evaluated with high-level evidence that indicates negligible improvements (Patil et al., 2019b). Studies did not include adults with comorbid impairments (i.e., mild cognitive impairment, dementia), but all OSA severity groups, defined by AHI, were included. It is therefore unknown if PAP treatment of OSA among certain subpopulations, such as those with high hypoxic burden, those with high neuroinflammatory predisposition (all hypothesized mechanisms for neurocognitive impairments in OSA; X. Liu et al., 2020), or those with comorbidities such as mild cognitive impairment or stroke, may benefit from PAP treatment. Some studies do suggest PAP benefits for specific cognitive and performance outcomes in select subpopulations, but duration of treatment is an important consideration for determining if cognitive and performance outcomes improve (Lal et al., 2022).

MOOD

Mood PROs associated with PAP treatment in OSA include depression and anxiety. Based on a limited set of RCTs (n = 5) of PAP for at least 1 month compared to control conditions with follow-up at 1–4 years, mood outcomes assessed by the Hospital Anxiety and Depression Scale (HADS; Zigmond & Snaith, 1983) demonstrate small improvements with PAP. Clinically meaningful improvement based on a score improvement/difference of 2 points was not, however, found in a meta-analysis of clinical trials (Patil et al., 2019b). The included trials did not enroll OSA adults with baseline mood disturbances or disorders, either anxiety or depression; and there were not strict inclusion criteria for the severity of OSA based on AHI. A recent secondary analysis of data from the Sleep Apnoea Cardiovascular Endpoint trial that enrolled and randomized patients with moderate to severe OSA and cardiovascular disease to PAP or usual care with follow-up data for 3.7 years identified reduced depression cases in the PAP group compared to usual care, with greater effects in patients with baseline depression symptoms using the HADS tool. Anxiety cases did not differ (Zheng et al., 2019). An accompanying pooled analysis of other RCTs (Zheng et al., 2019) confirmed prior meta-analysis results (Patil et al., 2019b) with small positive effects for PAP compared to controls for depression but not for anxiety in adults with OSA and cardiovascular disease. In older adults (>65 years) treated with PAP compared to control conditions, depression measured by HADS data was pooled in a meta-analysis with improvement at follow-up (3–12 months) on PAP with a change score of –0.94 (95% CI [0.25, 1.64]; Labarca, Saavedra, et al., 2020). There may be subgroups of PAP-treated OSA patients who have mood improvements with treatment, but general OSA clinical populations are not likely to have clinically meaningful mood improvements with PAP.

CARDIOVASCULAR FUNCTION

Cardiovascular clinical and survival outcomes have garnered much attention over recent years. This is because observational studies have consistently identified worse cardiovascular outcomes, such as blood pressure, heart failure, and composite event endpoints, with OSA. Meta-analysis of observational studies, in fact, confirms that cardiovascular event rate risk is reduced with PAP compared to controls with a 54% relative risk reduction

(0.46; 95% CI [0.32, 0.66]; Patil et al., 2019b). Data from 11 observational studies (N = 6,357 adults with OSA, n = 2,865 treated with CPAP) with high heterogeneity suggest cardiovascular event risk may be reduced with PAP treatment (Patil et al., 2019b). RCTs comparing PAP treatment to control conditions for cardiovascular outcomes have not, however, demonstrated risk reduction, event reduction, or improved clinical outcomes for most cardiovascular endpoints. Several meta-analyses have demonstrated similar findings (Labarca, Dreyse, et al., 2020; Patil et al., 2019b; Yu et al., 2017). The exception to this conclusion is for blood pressure. PAP treatment does improve daytime and nighttime systolic and diastolic blood pressure as well as 24-hour mean blood pressure in all OSA patients, with significant effects in hypertensive and treatment-resistant hypertensive patients with OSA (Patil et al., 2019b). For all adults with OSA, PAP treatment effects for mean 24-hour blood pressure compared to controls had a weighted mean difference of –2.63 (95% CI [–3.86, –1.39]); and among hypertensive adults with OSA treated with PAP compared to controls, pooled analyses show a difference of –2.16 (95% CI [–3.59, –0.72]; Patil et al., 2019b). Contemporary evidence suggests that cardiovascular events may be associated with the sleepy OSA phenotype (Mazzotti et al., 2019), though others have not similarly found this association (Trzepizur et al., 2022). Until future trials address sleepiness, it is not possible to determine if the sleepy OSA phenotype is a critical feature in untoward cardiovascular outcomes and to determine the effect of PAP treatment. PAP adherence in clinical trials is also a potential explanation for the unexpected, contrasting results between observational and RCT effects of PAP on cardiovascular endpoints (Sawyer et al., 2021), though post hoc analyses of clinical trial data have not consistently demonstrated that "better adherers experience better cardiovascular outcomes."

METABOLIC FUNCTION

Metabolic clinical outcomes, including fasting blood sugar and glycosylated hemoglobin (HbA1c), have been examined in predominantly male, obese adults with moderate to severe OSA. RCT samples included in meta-analysis were heterogeneous in terms of no diabetes (n = 5) or Type 2 diabetes mellitus present (n = 3). Blood glucose assessments before and after PAP for 6–12 weeks demonstrate no clinically meaningful improvement in blood glucose (weighted mean difference = –0.06; 95% CI [–0.24, 0.12]; Patil et al., 2019b). Similarly, HbA1c did not improve after PAP when usage ranged from 3.6 to 5.4 hours/night (Patil et al., 2019b). Labarca and colleagues' meta-analysis of six RCTs demonstrated similar findings in adults with OSA and Type 2 diabetes for fasting glucose or HbA1c (Labarca et al., 2018). This meta-analysis also confirmed no improvement in fasting glucose or HbA1c when more versus less PAP usage was examined (≤ vs. >4 hours/night; Labarca et al., 2018). While summary treatment trial data indicates that CPAP does not improve metabolic clinical outcomes, observational studies consistently link OSA and metabolic disorders, including Type 2 diabetes and metabolic syndrome

(Gleeson & McNicholas, 2022). Longer-term studies of PAP effects on metabolic clinical outcomes are needed.

HEALTHCARE UTILIZATION AND COSTS

Healthcare utilization and healthcare costs with and without PAP treatment have recently been reported (Kirsch et al., 2019; Walter et al., 2017). Although Patil and colleagues (2019b) reported no effect of PAP on readmissions based on a narrative summary of two published studies, recent studies suggest that healthcare utilization and healthcare costs are reduced with PAP treatment in OSA samples (Berezin et al., 2023; Kirsch et al., 2019) and OSA with comorbidity samples (Sterling, Cistulli, et al., 2022; Sterling, Pépin, et al., 2022). More PAP usage, or adherence, significantly reduces healthcare resource consumption and healthcare costs when compared to less PAP usage, or non-adherence (Sterling, Cistulli, et al., 2022; Sterling, Pépin, et al., 2022; Walter et al., 2017).

ACCIDENTS

Sleepiness of OSA has been a promulgating factor for examining the associated risk of motor vehicle accidents, occupational accidents, and occupational driving accidents (Garbarino, Durando, et al., 2016; Garbarino, Guglielmi, et al., 2016). While driving simulator findings do not consistently show improvements in driving proficiency with PAP in OSA populations (Patil et al., 2019b), these studies may not fully represent driving behavior and reactions that lead to motor vehicle accidents (Bonsignore et al., 2021). Untreated OSA is a risk factor for motor vehicle accidents (Bonsignore et al., 2021; Walia et al., 2019); PAP treatment reduces the risk of motor vehicle accidents (Karimi et al., 2015; Walia et al., 2019). Both Europe and Australia have recently implemented regulations to reduce motor vehicle accidents associated with OSA and sleepiness (for review, see McNicholas, 2021).

Adherence to CPAP Treatment

PAP ADHERENCE: IS IT A PROBLEM?

Adherence to PAP treatment was first described as a clinically important problem in the 1990s by four different research teams (Engleman et al., 1994, 1996; Kribbs et al., 1993; Reeves-Hoche et al., 1994; Weaver, Kribbs, et al., 1997) that led the field to understand four main points:

- Subjective reporting of PAP adherence overestimates daily use by approximately 1 hour/night (Engleman et al., 1996).
- Pattern of early PAP use, defined as consistent and inconsistent use, is associated with longer-term PAP adherence (Kribbs et al., 1993; Weaver, Kribbs, et al., 1997).

- Treatment side effects and/or challenges with the device and mask are associated with lower adherence (Engleman et al., 1996).
- Average PAP adherence is less than sleep duration (i.e., the recommended treatment interval or "dose"; Reeves-Hoche et al., 1994).

The average objective PAP use per night reported across these early studies is 4.8 hours/night using endpoint data at 3–6 months. Since these earliest studies of relatively small clinical sleep cohorts, the findings have been replicated in larger studies (Aloia et al., 2007; Budhiraja et al., 2007). Without a scientifically defined threshold for PAP adherence, US third-party payers instituted an expert opinion–based adherence threshold of >4 hours/night to support treatment payment. Though subsequent studies have identified that higher use thresholds equate to better clinical outcomes and PROs (Antic et al., 2011; Weaver et al., 2007) and skepticism exists in the field for the policy-defined adherence threshold, this threshold has been repeatedly used in research studies such that less is understood about other usage thresholds that could better inform clinicians, patients, and policymakers. It is poignant to acknowledge that with a 4-hour/night PAP usage threshold, a large proportion of total sleep time remains untreated. Based on a 7-hour/night average sleep duration of adults worldwide (Coutrot et al., 2022) and an adherence criterion of 4 hours/night, 43% of total sleep time is estimated to be untreated, as OSA acutely recurs based on PAP withdrawal studies (Filtness et al., 2012; Kohler et al., 2011; Young et al., 2013). Furthermore, when a 4-hour/night criterion has been employed in studies, 29%–83% of samples are defined as not adherent to CPAP treatment (Weaver & Grunstein, 2008). Also poignant is evidence that shows decisions to abandon treatment, or minimally use PAP, are established very early in the treatment period (i.e., by Day 2–4 of treatment) and that low use in the first week of treatment is highly predictive of longer-term use (Aloia et al., 2007; Weaver, Kribbs, et al., 1997). The relative prevalence of PAP non-adherence for one of the most prevalent sleep disorders is recognized as a major public health problem that healthcare providers are challenged to manage with patients in everyday practice.

FACTORS ASSOCIATED WITH PAP ADHERENCE

Factors associated with PAP adherence have been extensively reported in the literature (Table 35.6). Studies of patient-level factors and family/partner-level factors are best researched to date relative to their association with PAP adherence, whereas few studies have examined practice-level, community-level, or society-level factors of influence on PAP adherence. Some patient-level characteristic factors, like AHI and BMI, are weakly associated with PAP adherence. Characteristic factors are also not readily modifiable or amenable to intervention. Patient subpopulations may be identified as potentially at risk for PAP non-adherence by such factors; but interindividual variance is high, and studies have demonstrated interaction effects among factors of influence on PAP adherence (see

Table 35.6 Factors associated with better positive airway pressure adherence

Patient level (directionality)	Family/partner level (directionality)	Practice level (directionality)	Community level (directionality)	Societal level (directionality)
Age (older)	Relationship (↑ quality, ↑ stability)	Outreach for troubleshooting (early [vs. none, delayed])	Neighborhood (non-URM, ↑ SES)	Payer model (PAP use as a qualifier for PAP payment)
Sex (male)	Partner engagement (more)	Wait time (none/minimal to PAP after diagnosis)		
Race (White)	Living status (cohabit [vs. live alone])			
SES (↑)	Referral (self [vs. spouse])			
AHI[a] (higher)				
ESS[a] (higher)				
BMI[a] (lower)				
Coping (active, problem-solving)				
Self-efficacy[b] (↑)				
Early PAP use (consistent and/or ↑)				
Claustrophobia (+)				
Nasal volume (↓)				

Note. AHI = apnea–hypopnea index; BMI = body mass index; ESS = Epworth Sleepiness Scale; PAP = positive airway pressure; SES = socioeconomic status; URM = underrepresented minority.

[a]Weak association with conflicting results.

[b]When measured after some PAP use/experience.

Weaver, 2022, for review). Risk identification studies are limited to date and have not been well tested in population-based samples for external validity. Thus, the utility of the associated factors evidence has largely underpinned the design of intervention strategies to promote PAP adherence.

PAP ADHERENCE INTERVENTIONS

PAP adherence interventions have been tested in rigorous studies that provide an evidence base to guide practice approaches and recommendations (Patil et al., 2019a). Several recent meta-analyses of PAP adherence interventions inform "best practices" for adults newly initiated on PAP treatment for OSA (Aardoom et al., 2020; Askland et al., 2020; Labarca et al., 2021; Patil et al., 2019b). It is important to note that most PAP adherence interventions have only been tested in new, naive PAP patients; few studies have addressed the needs of patients who have previously failed, or rejected, PAP treatment; and even fewer intervention studies have tested long-term interventions or the effects of short-term interventions on long-term PAP adherence (i.e., beyond 12 months). As OSA is a chronic sleep disorder and the associated comorbidities are also chronic, addressing PAP adherence over a longer time horizon is critical. Most intervention studies have included predominantly homogenous samples in terms of race, ethnicity, sex, and gender. This also limits the applicability of these interventions in diverse populations or specific subpopulations.

With these caveats in mind, interventions that improve PAP adherence are broadly categorized as educational, troubleshooting/supportive, behavioral, and tele-monitoring/tele-management. Most tested approaches are, in fact, multicomponent in content; and few published interventions are adequately described to support replication or the design/execution of implementation studies such that application in everyday practice settings can be addressed. While these are recognized limitations of the PAP adherence intervention RCT evidence, summarized effects (Patil et al., 2019b) show that patients who are newly initiated on PAP treatment have better adherence outcomes when, at a minimum, disease- and treatment-specific education is provided at the outset of treatment. Larger effects on PAP adherence outcomes are found with supportive/troubleshooting, tele-monitoring/tele-management, and behavioral intervention approaches (Patil et al., 2019b; Figure 35.1).

Educational Interventions

Educational interventions tested in trials demonstrate small effects on PAP adherence, yet patient education is a mainstay of introducing new treatments with the expectation that behavior will change (Bandura 1977, 2004). Education approaches were delivered by various formats including video, group training, personalized sessions that addressed PSG results and baseline symptoms, and using different message framing (positive vs. negative). Thus, the summarized effect of educational interventions by Patil and colleagues

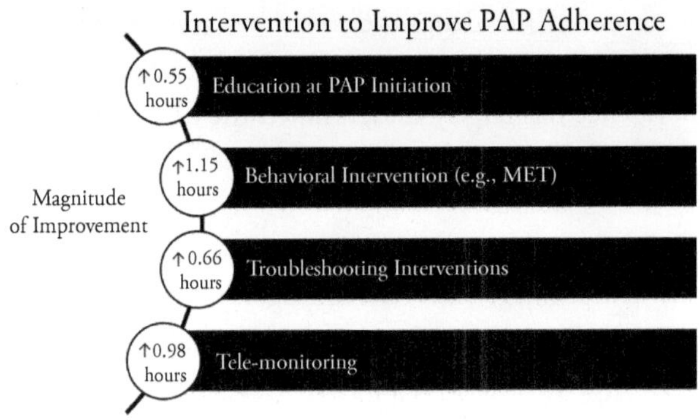

Figure 35.1 Positive airway pressure (PAP) adherence interventions and their estimated improvement for PAP adherence

Note. MET = motivational enhancement therapy. Reprinted from *Sleep Medicine Clinics* 16(2021):125–144, Sawyer AM, Wallace DM, Buenevar LF, Watach AJ, Blase A, Saconi B, Patel SR, Kuna ST, Punjabi NM, Where to Optimizing Adherence in Large-scale Trials of Continuous Positive Airway Pressure (p. 132) with permission from Elsevier.

(2019b) does not provide support for any specific approach for educating patients in order to improve PAP adherence. Other meta-analysts (Askland et al., 2020) have conducted sensitivity analyses that provide some practical insights for structuring education to improve PAP adherence. Some key points for clinicians interested in designing education for patients who are newly initiated on PAP include the following:

- OSA and PAP education will ideally be delivered
  - over a shorter, rather than extended, period of time at the time a diagnosis is established and treatment initiated:
    - ≤4 week delivery interval better than >4 week delivery interval (Askland et al., 2020)
  - with more than one contact session:
    - >1 contact session better than single contact session (Askland et al., 2020)
  - with session being longer in duration:
    - >60 minutes better than ≤60-minute session (Askland et al., 2020)

Troubleshooting/Supportive Interventions

Troubleshooting/supportive interventions tested in clinical trials include patient education plus additional support delivered to patients using varied modalities (e.g., phone calls, home visits, computer-based interactions) in the early phase of treatment, with intervention delivery triggered by patient outreach in most trials (Patil et al., 2019b). Because early PAP use is associated with longer-term use (Budhiraja et al., 2007) and qualitative study results have highlighted the value that patients place on navigating PAP treatment challenges with expert clinicians or expert peer patients (Broström et al., 2010, 2021;

Chou et al., 2021; Luyster et al., 2016), the summarized findings for troubleshooting/supportive interventions are not surprising such that PAP adherence is nearly 45 minutes greater at follow-up (1 month–1 year) when these interventions are delivered compared to usual care conditions (Patil et al., 2019b). Interestingly, Askland and colleagues' (2020) meta-analysis includes sensitivity analyses that address relevant clinical questions about delivering supportive interventions: human or automated, scheduled or ad hoc. Albeit with heterogeneity across the included subgroup studies, human contact resulted in better PAP adherence as opposed to automated-only contact when each was compared to usual care conditions. When ad hoc human contact for support/troubleshooting was compared to control, the effect on PAP adherence was less than for when scheduled human contact for support/troubleshooting was compared to control (Askland et al., 2020). Thus, for clinical programs that offer troubleshooting and supportive interventions as part of OSA/PAP care, regularly scheduling outreach to new PAP users may result in better PAP adherence. The interval during early PAP treatment for delivering troubleshooting and supportive intervention is not well understood, but consistent with the American Academy of Sleep Medicine practice guidelines, this type of clinical intervention should be at least concentrated in the first 3 months of PAP use, and troubleshooting needs should be addressed at all follow-up visits with healthcare providers (Patil et al., 2019a).

Behavioral Interventions

Behavioral interventions for PAP adherence have included motivational enhancement therapy, cognitive behavioral therapy, and tailored behavioral approaches, all of which have been delivered in various ways, including group, individual, and peer-to-peer, and for varying durations of exposure. As well, behavioral interventions include education plus a behavioral strategy. When PAP adherence outcomes are summarized at 1 month to 1 year, odds of achieving at least 4 hours/night of PAP use are 21% greater with behavioral interventions compared to usual care (Patil et al., 2019b). When behavioral intervention trials were examined with sensitivity analyses by Askland and colleagues (2020), duration of <4 weeks or ≥4 weeks, number of contacts for intervention delivery, and duration of contact did not bear influence on the positive effects on PAP adherence of behavioral therapy. Considering the evidence that demonstrates the relationships between disease cognitions (Sawyer et al., 2011; Stepnowsky et al., 2002), self-efficacy (Aloia et al., 2005; Sawyer et al., 2011; Saconi et al., 2020; Ye et al., 2012), and decisional balance (Aloia et al., 2005) with PAP adherence, the impact of behavioral interventions is expectedly positive. As identified by Crawford and colleagues (2014), these psychological and cognitive constructs in combination with theoretically derived behavioral variables account for 11%–58% of variance in PAP use, and thus are opportunistic for improving a behavioral outcome like PAP adherence. While behavioral approaches are efficacious for PAP adherence, translating these approaches to everyday practice is challenging. In large part, this is due to limited resources for delivering behavioral interventions in practice settings.

Tele-Monitoring and Tele-Management Interventions

Tele-monitoring and tele-management interventions are strategies that rely on the flow of objective PAP use data from individual PAP devices to industry cloud-based repositories that are accessible to patients and providers 24/7. Accessible data supports using real-time data as a source of feedback and reflection for patients and as a clinical indicator for providers to readily identify patients who are struggling to use PAP. Pooled data from clinical trials using tele-monitoring intervention strategies, that were notably heterogeneous, indicates that tele-monitoring has positive effects on PAP adherence when compared to usual care with approximately 1 hour/night better adherence at 2–3 months (Patil et al., 2019b). In a separate meta-analysis, Aardoom and colleagues (2020) examined electronic interventions (eHealth) for PAP adherence that included clinical trials of tele-management intervention approaches that use information and communication technologies to guide and deploy interventions. Whether these strategies were added to usual care or replaced usual care, PAP adherence improved by about 30 minutes/night (Aardoom et al., 2020). The applicability of tele-monitoring and/or tele-management approaches in the context of busy clinical practice settings is appealing for both patients and providers. The longer-term effects on PAP adherence of these approaches are not known. Current practice recommendations include tele-monitoring of PAP use from the outset of treatment, and follow-up clinical encounters should address objective PAP use data on a consistent basis (Patil et al., 2019a) such that shared decision-making between healthcare providers and patients is prioritized (Watach et al., 2021).

Oral Appliances

Oral appliances are an effective alternative treatment for individuals with mild to moderate OSA, those who cannot tolerate PAP, and persons with craniofacial factors related to their OSA, such as a shallow mandibular plane angle (Ramar et al., 2015; Randerath et al., 2011). Similar to PAP, these devices are designed to keep the airway open through manipulating the facial anatomy to bring the lower jaw forward or hold the tongue in a different position in order to keep the throat open.

Clinical practice guidelines for oral appliances in the treatment of OSA recommend the following (Ramar et al., 2015):

1. Prescription of oral appliances, rather than no therapy, for patients who request treatment of primary snoring (without OSA).
2. Qualified dentists use custom, titratable appliances over non-custom devices.
3. Prescription of oral appliances for patients who are intolerant of PAP therapy or prefer alternate therapy, rather than no treatment.
4. Qualified dentists provide oversight of oral appliance therapy to survey for dental-related side effects or occlusal changes and reduce their incidence.

5. Sleep physicians conduct follow-up sleep testing to improve or confirm treatment efficacy for patients fitted with oral appliances.
6. Sleep physicians and qualified dentists instruct patients treated with oral appliances for OSA to return for periodic office visits.

The most common oral appliances are tongue-retaining devices, which apply suction to keep the tongue in a protruded position, and mandibular advancement devices (MADs), which mechanically move the mandible forward over time to a protruded position to prevent upper airway collapse (Ramar et al., 2015). Meta-analyses of 34 RCTs indicate that oral appliances can significantly reduce the AHI, RDI, or respiratory event index (REI) across all levels of OSA severity (Ramar et al., 2015). In weighted analyses, the mean reduction in AHI with oral appliance compared to no oral appliance was 13.60 events/hour (95% CI [–15.25, –11.95]; Ramar et al., 2015). However, mean reductions in AHI are still 6.24 events/hour (95% CI [8.14, 4.43]) greater with PAP compared to oral appliances (n = 15 RCTs; Ramar et al., 2015). Further, there is no statistically significant difference between oral appliances and PAP in the percentage of mild OSA patients achieving their target AHI/RDI/REI (<5/<10/>50% reduction), but, for patients with moderate to severe OSA, the odds of achieving target AHI are significantly greater with PAP (Ramar et al., 2015).

Oral appliances are equivalent to PAP such that they significantly reduce daytime sleepiness and improve QoL compared to no treatment and reduce daytime sleepiness and improve QoL (Ramar et al., 2015). Further, adherence with oral appliances is reportedly better than with PAP, but these findings must be interpreted cautiously as oral appliance adherence is often reported subjectively compared to objective PAP adherence measures (Ramar et al., 2015). Recently, advancements in technology have been made wherein thermosensors can assist in tracking of objective adherence to oral appliances, but data on these devices is currently limited (Sutherland & Cistulli, 2019).

DEVICE TYPES

MADs

MADs, also known as *mandibular advancement splints* or *mandibular repositing appliances*, are the most commonly used oral appliances. They can be designed as a one- or two-piece device, with two-piece devices allowing for more mandibular movement and a greater range of settings, leading them to be more comfortable and often more accepted. There is a very low-quality body of evidence that one type of device is more effective than the other in reducing AHI and improving lowest oxygen saturation (Bartolucci et al., 2021).

As the most common appliance, most research on the efficacy of oral appliances has centered on MADs, especially in comparison with PAP treatment. While PAP therapy is considered superior due to demonstrating higher decreases in AHI, in mild to moderate OSA MADs are considered an effective treatment, with AHI values close to the normal range and similar impacts on excessive daytime sleepiness as compared to PAP (Pattipati et al., 2022; Randerath et al., 2021). Compared with MADs, PAP is associated with significantly larger decreases in AHI (mean difference = –5.83; 95% CI [–8.85, –2.81]; $p < .01$) and improved lowest oxygen saturation (mean difference = 0.72; 95% CI [0.51, 0.94]; $p < .01$). However, this meta-analytic data found no statistically significant difference in ESS between PAP and MAD groups (mean difference = 0.23; 95% CI [–0.24, 0.70]; $p = .34$; Pattipati et al., 2022) A different meta-analysis concluded that MADs are effective at reducing daytime sleepiness by 1.7 points (95% CI [1.1, 2.3]) on the ESS, but PAP revealed even larger reductions (2.5 points [2.0, 2.9]; Bratton et al., 2015).

Additional recent meta-analytic data indicates that good responders to MAD include those with a lower baseline AHI (95% CI [–7.23, –1.89]; $p < .00001$), younger age (95% CI [–4.55, –1.62]; $p < .00001$), lower BMI (95% CI [–2.80, –1.11]; $p < .00001$), smaller neck circumference (95% CI [–1.57, –0.52]; $p < .00001$), and those of female sex (95% CI [0.56, 0.91]; $p = .006$; H. Chen et al., 2020). Therefore, these characteristics should be considered when prescribing MADs for OSA.

Tongue-Retaining Devices

Tongue-retaining devices use a suction cavity to anteriorly displace the tongue. Though these devices are less common and less well studied, they can be an appropriate treatment option for individuals who are edentulous as MADs require adhesion to the teeth for effective placement. Tongue-retaining devices can effectively reduce AHI by 53% (33.6 ± 21.1/hour to 15.8 ± 16.0/hour), improve lowest oxygen saturation (LSAT; 79.8 ± 17.5% to 83.9 ± 8.6%), ESS (10.8 ± 4.8 to 8.2 ± 4.5), and oxygen desaturation index (ODI; 29.6 ± 32.1 to 12.9 ± 8.7; Chang et al., 2017). However, compared to PAP, they are less effective at reducing obstructive events (Banhiran et al., 2020).

PRESCRIPTION OF ORAL APPLIANCES

While PAP remains the superior and more effective treatment (Ramar et al., 2015), oral appliances are undoubtedly better than no treatment. In addition to the usual assessment procedures for OSA, the evaluation for candidacy for oral appliance treatment should include a thorough dental history and an oral evaluation to determine if there is sufficient dentition to wear the device (Remmers et al., 2013). Additional tests to evaluate the upper airway might include video endoscopy, drug-induced sleep endoscopy, and remotely controlled mandibular protrusion assessment to assisting in predicting the most effective mandibular protrusion position (Remmers et al., 2013).

Surgical Treatment

Surgical treatment of OSA is most often considered if less invasive therapies have not been effective or are not appropriate options for the patient. For OSA caused by anatomical structures and improper tone of the airway, upper airway surgeries aimed at reducing the degree of obstruction are often indicated. Surgical options are categorized into Phases I and II (Riley et al., 1993). This phasing was developed based on decreasing risk of over-operating as well as postoperative risk, utilization of more conservative approaches, decreased hospital stay, less trauma and pain, and better patient acceptance (Riley et al., 1993). In Phase I, surgeries include nasal surgeries to remove polyps or straighten a deviated septum, palatal surgeries including the removal of tissues, and tongue-based surgeries (Pavwoski & Shelgikar, 2017). Phase II surgery is more invasive, is commonly referred to as *maxillomandibular advancement* (jaw surgery), and is often only used for individuals whose OSA could not be resolved with Phase I surgeries (Pavwoski & Shelgikar, 2017). Outside of these classifications, hypoglossal nerve stimulation is an emerging effective treatment, and tracheostomy can be used but is often reserved for life-threatening/severe situations.

Surgical procedures for treating OSA are most often performed by a "sleep surgeon," such as an otolaryngologist or oral and maxillofacial surgeon with specialized training and expertise in upper airway surgery. The American Academy of Sleep Medicine recently published practice recommendations for the surgical referral of patients with OSA (Kent et al., 2021). Referral to a sleep surgeon is recommended as part of the patient-oriented discussion of alternative treatment options for the following:

1. Patients who are intolerant or unaccepting of PAP.
2. Patients who are intolerant or unaccepting of PAP and have obesity (Class II/III, BMI ≥35), wherein referral to a bariatric surgeon is also recommended.
3. Patients with OSA, BMI <40 kg/m^2, and persistent inadequate PAP adherence due to pressure-related side effects.
4. Patients with major upper airway anatomic abnormalities, after initial recommendation and trial of PAP therapy.

PHASE I SURGERIES

Adenotonsillectomy

Adenotonsillar hypertrophy is the most common cause of pediatric OSA, making adenotonsillectomy the first-line treatment for pediatric OSA (Bhattacharjee et al., 2010). This treatment, which involves the surgical removal of the tonsils and adenoids, is less commonly used for adults as tonsil hypertrophy is rarely the leading or sole cause of OSA in adults. However, for adults with tonsillar hypertrophy, meta-analytic data demonstrates that tonsillectomy reduced AHI by 65.2% (from 40.5 ± 28.9/hour to 14.1 ± 17.1/hour), LSAT improved from 77.7 ± 11.9% to 85.5 ± 8.2%, and daytime sleepiness as measured by the ESS decreased from 11.6 ± 3.7 to 6.1 ± 3.9 (Camacho et al., 2016). A more recent retrospective study of 151 tonsillectomies demonstrated similar but slightly less powerful results, reporting a success rate of 47.6% after tonsillectomy, with success defined as a >50% reduction of the AHI and a total AHI of <20 post-surgery. In this study, average

ESS score was only reduced by 0.69, which was not statistically significant (Sjöblom et al., 2022).

Nasal Surgery

Nasal obstruction can be caused by bone, cartilage, or hypertrophy of tissues (Carvalho et al., 2012). Nasal reconstruction is often not curative for OSA but rather serves as an adjunct therapy to increase airflow at the turbinates, septum, and alar valve; eliminate alar collapse; and resolve bony deformities that can make PAP intolerable. As such, nasal surgeries can facilitate comfort with PAP and thereby improve PAP adherence by decreasing resistance and improving flow dynamics that may contribute to sensations of nasal stuffiness and claustrophobia (Camacho, Riaz, et al., 2015; Ishii et al., 2015; J. Wu et al., 2017).

Palatal Surgery

The primary approach to address this easily collapsible area of the airway is uvulopalatopharyngoplasty (UPPP), which is one of the most common surgeries for OSA and is often applied with other techniques such as tonsillectomy (Stuck et al., 2018). UPPP removes excess tissue from the soft palate and pharynx, including the tonsils, uvula, and excessive pharyngeal tissue. Evidence across 47 studies suggests that the reduction in the frequency of respiratory events and success/response rates ranges from 35% to 95.2% (Stuck et al., 2018). In addition to the varied effectiveness, efficacy of this surgical treatment declines over time (He et al., 2019) Baseline BMI, lowest arterial oxygen saturation, and proportion of sleep time with oxygen saturation <90% are predictive for long-term UPPP response and therefore should be considered when selecting an appropriate surgical treatment option (He et al., 2019). A variety of other palatal procedures also exist to treat OSA, including, but not limited to, suspension palatoplasty (pulling the palatopharyngeus muscle to the pterygomandibular raphe for suspension of the soft palate; Li et al., 2018), z-palatoplasty (widening of the palate; Friedman et al., 2004), and soft-palate implant surgery, also known as *pillar procedure* (Neruntarat, 2011; Nordgård et al., 2006).

Tongue-Based Surgery

In OSA, the tongue can contribute to obstructive events if it collapses backward during sleep or if the base of the tongue is exceptionally large. As such, a variety of surgical procedures have been developed to remedy tongue-based obstructions, including transoral robotic surgery (TORS) glossectomy, radiofrequency ablation (RFA) of the tongue, and midline glossectomy (Shah & Thaler, 2020). Additional procedures to reposition the tongue can include genioglossus advancement, hyoid suspension, and maxillary–mandibular advancements, as well as upper airway stimulation of the hypoglossal nerve that can alleviate tongue-based obstructions (Shah & Thaler, 2020).

TORS was originally developed for the treatment of oropharyngeal cancers but has also been adapted for sleep surgery in the treatment of OSA (Miller et al., 2017). TORS has been used successfully for the treatment of OSA, effectively reducing AHI and improving lowest oxygen saturation, ESS score, and snoring visual analogue scale (VAS; Miller et al., 2017; Thaler et al., 2016). Though upper airway stimulation has proven superior in its effectiveness (Huntley et al., 2019; J. L. Yu et al., 2019), select patients may still be better suited for TORS based on not meeting pre-surgical criteria for upper airway stimulation, which often include a combination of AHI, BMI, and endoscopic results assessing airway anatomy. Particularly, upper airway stimulation is not an option for patients with concentric or predominantly lateral collapse (J. L. Yu et al., 2019). Therefore, TORS may be a suitable option for these patients.

RFA uses radiofrequency energy to produce volumetric shrinkage of the tongue size to alleviate tongue base obstructions (Farrar et al., 2008). Shown to shrink tongue tissues, this technique requires multiple treatments to allow time for healing and shrinkage. RFA has been shown to produce a 31% reduction in short-term (<12 months; odds ratio [OR] = 0.69, 95% CI [0.61, 0.77]) and a 45% reduction (OR = 0.55, 95% CI [0.45, 0.72]) in long-term (>24 months) RDI levels, but short-term results for the lowest oxygen saturations failed to demonstrate any improvement (OR = 1.03, 95% CI [0.88, 1.20]; Farrar et al., 2008). Further, this procedure resulted in a 31% reduction in short-term ESS (OR = 0.69, 95% CI [0.63, 0.75]), which was maintained beyond 12 months. These findings were more recently replicated in a 2015 meta-analysis of 20 studies indicating significant reductions in RDI, ESS, and VAS snoring and increase in lowest oxygen saturation (Baba et al., 2015).

There are also numerous techniques for tongue-based resection, but most include modifications of the midline glossectomy (Shah & Thaler, 2020). This procedure was first described in 1991 and was completed using a CO_2 laser (Fujita et al., 1991). This procedure involved an anterior dissection followed by microdirect laryngoscopy for the tongue-based resection. The procedure was later expanded to include lingualplasty by excising bilateral wedges of tongue tissue adjacent to the midline resection (Woodson & Fujita, 1992). In a review of 18 articles inclusive of 522 patients pre- and post-op, this procedure (alone or in combination with lingualplasty or submucosal minimally invasive lingual excision) demonstrated significant improvement in AHI (48.1 ± 22.01 to 19.05 ± 15.46, $p < .0001$), ESS (11.41 ± 4.38 to 5.66 ± 3.29, $p < .0001$), snoring VAS (9.08 ± 1.21 to 3.14 ± 2.41, $p < .0001$), and LSAT (76.67 ± 10.58 to 84.09 ± 7.90, $p < .0001$; Murphey et al., 2015). Surgical success rate was 59.6% (95% CI [53.0%, 65.9%]), and surgical cure was achieved in 22.5% (95% CI [11.26%, 36.26%]) of cases (Murphey et al., 2015).

Overall, tongue-based surgeries have been performed using a variety of techniques and tools, including traditional diathermy and other tools such as lasers, radiofrequency probes, and coblation plasma technology (Dorrity et al., 2016; Robinson et al., 2003).

The varied techniques discussed above have a positive impact on the reduction of AHI with minimal surgical complications (Dorrity et al., 2016).

Maxillary Expansion Surgery

Maxillary expansion techniques include surgically assisted rapid maxillary expansion, distraction osteogenesis maxillary expansion, and segmental Le Fort I osteotomy (Randerath et al., 2022). These procedures are used to expand the nasal cavity, nasal floor, and palate. The expansion allows for a higher tongue position, which is suspected to contribute to the opening of the airway, and may increase tension on the muscle attached to the palate, thereby assisting in the reduction of upper airway collapses (Buck et al., 2016; Randerath et al., 2022). Meta-analyses indicate that maxillary expansion, compared to pre-surgery, can significantly improve AHI (24.3 ± 27.5, 95% CI [15.3, 33.3], to 9.9 ± 13.7, 95% CI [5.4, 14.4], events/hour) and lowest oxygen desaturation (84.3 ± 8.1%, 95% CI [81.7, 87.0], to 86.9 ± 5.6%, 95% CI [85.1, 88.7]) for adults with OSA (Abdullatif et al., 2016).

PHASE II SURGERY

Maxillomandibular Advancement

When the more conservative treatments do not achieve the desired objectives, a more aggressive approach is used that moves the lower jaw and midface forward (Zhou et al., 2021). Maxillomandibular advancement (MMA) increases the dimension of the upper airway while also improving the stability and tension of the pharyngeal soft tissue. This is typically achieved through Le Fort I osteotomy of the maxilla and bilateral sagittal split osteotomies of the mandible (Pirklbauer et al., 2011; Q. Wu et al., 2019, Zhou et al., 2021). A more comprehensive list of various MMA-based surgical treatment methods is provided by Zhou and colleagues (2021). Overall, this surgical procedure is the most widely studied and efficacious surgical therapy for OSA (Awad et al., 2019). It should be noted that this procedure warrants overnight intensive care unit monitoring, and therefore less invasive treatments should be first considered (Kent et al., 2021; Ravesloot et al., 2019).

Success rates range from 52% to 100%, depending on criteria defined by investigators (Pirklbauer et al., 2011). In a systematic review, 17/18 studies reported ≥80% success post-MMA, with success defined based on a variety of AHI or RDI improvements in pre- and postoperative PSG results (Pirklbauer et al., 2011). In the study reporting the lowest success rate, two different success criteria were examined: AHI <10/hour; and, ≥50% AHI improvement and AHI between 10–20/hour (Blumen et al., 2009). Successful cases were 52% or 80%, respectively by the criteria applied (Blumen et al., 2009). Given that all but one study reported a success rate ≥80%, it is evident that this treatment is highly successful at resolving OSA. This treatment has shown to be effective, even in the long term (Pirklbauer et al., 2011). In a cohort of 30 adults, 46.7% obtained an AHI <5 and 83.4% had an AHI ≤15 events/hour, approximately 6.5 years after MMA (Boyd et al., 2015).

The maxillomandibular complex is advanced a minimum of 10 mm to successfully treat OSA (Pirklbauer et al., 2011). As such, facial aesthetics should be discussed with the patient prior to the procedure, with anticipated changes associated with degree of advancement. Candidacy for MMA is increasingly more individualized and based on patient phenotyping; clinical evaluations such as age, comorbidities, and dentofacial anatomy; and PSG evaluation (S. Y. Liu et al., 2019). Advancements in technology including virtual surgical planning and three-dimensional printing have further aided in pre-surgical planning (Jandali & Barrera, 2020).

ADDITIONAL SURGICAL PROCEDURES

Hypoglossal Nerve Stimulation

Evidence for hypoglossal nerve stimulation (HNS) as a treatment for OSA is relatively new (introduced in 2014 for the treatment of OSA) and limited; as such, it is not currently recommended to be used as first-line treatment (Randerath et al., 2022). This pacemaker-like device consists of three components: (1) a respiratory sensing lead that is implanted between the intercostal muscles in the fourth or fifth intercostal space, (2) a stimulator, and (3) a stimulation lead, implanted submentally in branches of the hypoglossal nerve (see Figure 35.2).

A variety of devices have been approved for clinical use, including mono-/unilateral and bilateral stimulation mechanisms. With both types, when the stimulator is activated during inspiration, the device stimulates the hypoglossal nerve and moves the tongue to a more anterior position, opening the pharyngeal airway and maintaining patency. There are also external components to the device including a "remote" which allows the patient to activate the generator and a programmer that allows providers to adjust

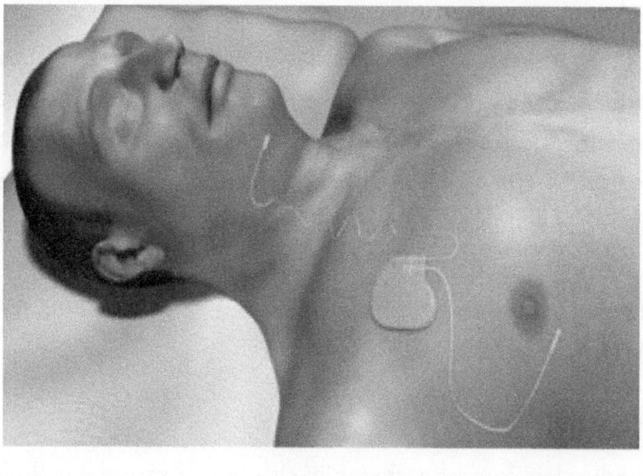

Figure 35.2 Hypoglossal nerve stimulation components: the inspire system (Maple Grove, MN, USA)
Note. Image retrieved from Mashaqi et al. (2021) and reproduced under a CC BY license (http://creativecommons.org/licenses/by/4.0/).

settings noninvasively. The battery life of the device is approximately 7–10 years (Hassan & Kaplish, 2021). Additional description of these intricate functions and mechanisms of HNS devices is beyond the scope of this chapter, but the authors recommend an extensive review by Mashaqi and colleagues (2021) for more technical details.

The US Food and Drug Administration has established stringent eligibility criteria for placement of this device, with the procedure only indicated in patients ≥18 years of age, intolerant of PAP, with moderate to severe OSA, BMI <35 kg/m^2, and absence of complete concentric palatal collapse (Hassan & Kaplish, 2021). Further, before the device can be implanted, drug-induced endoscopy is required to be performed by an otolaryngologist who has undergone manufacturer-specific certification training (Hassan & Kaplish, 2021).

An analysis of six prospective studies with 200 patients found, at 12 months, that HNS demonstrated significant reductions in AHI, ODI, and ESS pre- and post-surgery, with mean differences of -17.51 (95% CI [-20.69, -14.34]), -13.73 (95% CI [-16.87, -10.58]), and -4.42 (95% CI [-5.39, -3.44]), respectively (Certal et al., 2015). Further, AHI was reduced from pre-procedure by 50%–57% and ODI by 48%–52% (Certal et al., 2015). While results regarding its effectiveness have been promising and patient satisfaction has been high (Hofauer et al., 2019), much research is underway to identify traits predictive of a good response to treatment (Suurna et al., 2021).

As invasive HNS has begun to be accepted as a treatment alternative to PAP, transcutaneous electrical stimulation (TES) of the upper airway is also being "revived" and investigated as a noninvasive alternative. As such, a meta-analysis of 20 interventional trails found that AHI was reduced by 24.9 events/hour (95% CI [–28.5, –21.2]) in HNS (χ^2 79%, I^2 82%) and by 16.5 events/hour (95% CI [–25.1, –7.8]) in TES (χ^2 7%, I^2 43%; both $p < .001$), indicating that both invasive and transcutaneous stimulation reduce OSA severity, with invasive stimulation being superior (Ratneswaran et al., 2021).

Tracheostomy

Tracheostomy is another surgical procedure that successfully resolves OSA, nearly entirely, reducing AHI from 73.0 ± 27.1/hour to 0.2 ± 1.2/hour (Camacho, Certal, et al., 2014). Namely, this procedure is so effective because the upper airway anatomy that causes obstructions is bypassed entirely. With this procedure, the surgeon makes an opening in the neck and inserts a metal or plastic tube that aids with breathing. Air is able to pass in and out of the lungs, bypassing the blockages in the upper airway and throat. Due to the significant amount of lifestyle changes that accompany this procedure, it is often a surgery of last resort (Camacho, Certal, et al., 2014).

Alternative Therapies

A variety of alternative, less common, therapies also exist. Examples include myofunctional therapies focused on training the movement, strength, and activation of the upper airway, pharyngeal, and tongue muscles (Camacho, Certal et al., 2015); muscle stimulation therapies through electrical stimulation of the tongue in awake patients (Baptista et al., 2021); and pharmacological therapies targeting upper airway muscle activity, carbonic anhydrase activity, and arousal thresholds (sedatives and hypnotics; Randerath et al., 2022). While these types of therapies have been less well tested and are not commonly recommended, there is potential for them to emerge as promising therapies.

Treatment Summary

At present, PAP remains the first-line, gold-standard treatment for OSA. Advances in medicine have revealed numerous promising treatments, some of which have been described above. As our understanding of clinical phenotypes and the need for individualized therapy advances, combination therapies may be increasingly utilized to target specific outcomes in varied OSA phenotypes.

Conclusion

Sleep-related breathing disorders, in particular OSA, are highly prevalent, commonly undiagnosed or underrecognized, and associated with untoward outcomes and higher comorbidity risks. Screening for signs and symptoms and the history and physical are recommended for identifying adults requiring diagnosis by PSG or HSAT. Treatment options are predicated on the severity of OSA and patient preferences. PAP is the gold-standard treatment with evidence for efficacy, but effectiveness is sometimes limited by non-adherence. Other treatment options including lifestyle modification, oral appliances, or surgical options may be the best fit for patients who struggle to use PAP or refuse PAP treatment or who have mild to moderate OSA as compared to moderate to severe OSA.

Future Directions

Key questions that need to be addressed include the following:

1. Will sex-specific OSA screening approaches improve the likely underdiagnosis of OSA in young and middle-aged females?
2. What is the clinical utility of symptom phenotypes for effective treatment decision-making related to risk reduction of OSA and its associated comorbidities?
3 Are specific symptom phenotypes at greater risk for untoward OSA and associated comorbidity outcomes? Do symptom phenotypes and associated risks vary by subpopulation (e.g., sex, BMI, age)?
4. What are the critical elements of a precision medicine/health model of OSA?
5. Do long-term delivery of treatment adherence interventions improve/sustain PAP use?
6. What combination treatment strategies are most efficacious and effective and for whom?

References

Aardoom, J. J., Loheide-Niesmann, L., Ossebaard, H. C., & Riper, H. (2020). Effectiveness of eHealth interventions in improving treatment adherence for adults with obstructive sleep apnea: Meta-analytic review. *Journal of Medical Internet Research*, *22*(2), Article e16972.

Abdullatif, J., Certal, V., Zaghi, S., Song, S. A., Chang, E. T., Gillespie, M. B., & Camacho, M. (2016). Maxillary expansion and maxillomandibular expansion for adult OSA: A systematic review and meta-analysis. *Journal of Cranio-Maxillofacial Surgery*, *44*(5), 574–578.

Abramson, Z., Susarla, S., August, M., Troulis, M., & Kaban, L. (2010). Three-dimensional computed tomographic analysis of airway anatomy in patients with obstructive sleep apnea. *Journal of Oral and Maxillofacial Surgery*, *68*(2), 354–362.

Agnew, H. W., Jr., Webb, W. B., & Williams, R. L. (1966). The first night effect: An EEG study of sleep. *Psychophysiology*, *2*(3), 263–266.

Allen, A. H., Beaudin, A. E., Fox, N., Raneri, J. K., Skomro, R. P., Hanly, P. J., Mazzotti, D. R., Keenan, B. T., Smith, E. E., Goodfellow, S. D., & Ayas, N. T. (2020). Symptom subtypes and cognitive function in a clinic-based OSA cohort: A multi-centre Canadian study. *Sleep Medicine*, *74*, 92–98.

Aloia, M. S., Arnedt, J. T., Stanchina, M., & Millman, R. P. (2007). How early in treatment is PAP adherence established? Revisiting night-to-night variability. *Behavioral Sleep Medicine*, *5*, 229–240.

Aloia, M. S., Arnedt, J. T., Stepnowsky, C., Hecht, J., & Borrelli, B. (2005). Predicting treatment adherence in obstructive sleep apnea using principles of behavior change. *Journal of Clinical Sleep Medicine*, *1*, 346–353.

American Academy of Sleep Medicine. (2014). *International classification of sleep disorders* (3rd ed.).

An, Y., Li, Y., Kang, D., Sharama-Adhikari, S. K., Xu, W., & Han, D. (2019). The effects of nasal decongestion on obstructive sleep apnoea. *American Journal of Otolaryngology*, *40*(1), 52–56.

Andrade, R. G. S., Viana, F. M., Nascimento, J. A., Drager, L. F., Moffa, A., Brunoni, A. R., Genta, P. R., & Lorenzi-Filho, G. (2018). Nasal vs oronasal CPAP for OSA treatment: A meta-analysis. *Chest*, *153*(3), 665–674.

Antic, N. A., Catcheside, P., Buchan, C., Hensley, M., Naughton, M., Rowland, S., Williamson, B., Windler, S., & McEvoy, R. D. (2011). The effect of CPAP on normalizing daytime sleepiness, quality of life, and neurocognitive function in patients with moderate to severe OSA. *Sleep*, *34*, 111–119.

Askland, K., Wright, L., Wozniak, D. R., Emmanuel, T., Caston, J., & Smith, I. (2020). Educational, supportive and behavioural interventions to improve usage of continuous positive airway pressure machines in adults with obstructive sleep apnoea. *Cochrane Database of Systematic Reviews*, *4*(4), Article CD007736.

Awad, M., Gouveia, C., Zaghi, S., Camacho, M., & Liu, S. Y. (2019). Changing practice: Trends in skeletal surgery for obstructive sleep apnea. *Journal of Cranio-Maxillofacial Surgery*, *47*(8), 1185–1189.

Baba, R. Y., Mohan, A., Metta, V. V., & Mador, M. J. (2015). Temperature controlled radiofrequency ablation at different sites for treatment of obstructive sleep apnea syndrome: A systematic review and meta-analysis. *Sleep and Breathing*, *19*(3), 891–910.

Bandura, A. (1977). Self-efficacy: Toward a unifying theory of behavioral change. *Psychological Reviews*, *84*, 191–215.

Bandura, A. (2004). Health promotion by social cognitive means. *Health Education & Behavior*, *31*(2), 143–164.

Banhiran, W., Durongphan, A., Keskool, P., Chongkolwatana, C., & Metheetrairut, C. (2020). Randomized crossover study of tongue-retaining device and positive airway pressure for obstructive sleep apnea. *Sleep and Breathing*, *24*(3), 1011–1018.

Baptista, P. M., Martínez Ruiz de Apodaca, P., Carrasco, M., Fernandez, S., Wong, P. Y., Zhang, H., Hassaan, A., & Kotecha, B. (2021). Daytime neuromuscular electrical therapy of tongue muscles in improving snoring in individuals with primary snoring and mild obstructive sleep apnea. *Journal of Clinical Medicine*, *10*(9), Article 1883.

Bartolucci, M. L., Bortolotti, F., Corazza, G., Incerti Parenti, S., Paganelli, C., & Alessandri Bonetti, G. (2021). Effectiveness of different mandibular advancement device designs in obstructive sleep apnoea therapy: A systematic review of randomised controlled trials with meta-analysis. *Journal of Oral Rehabilitation*, *48*(4), 469–486.

Basoglu, O. K., & Tasbakan, M. S. (2018). Gender differences in clinical and polysomnographic features of obstructive sleep apnea: A clinical study of 2827 patients. *Sleep and Breathing*, *22*(1), 241–249.

Benjafield, A. V., Ayas, N. T., Eastwood, P. R., Heinzer, R., Ip, M. S. M., Morrell, M. J., Nunez, C. M., Patel, S. R., Penzel, T., Pépin, J. L., Peppard, P. E., Sinha, S., Tufik, S., Valentine, K., & Malhotra, A. (2019). Estimation of the global prevalence and burden of obstructive sleep apnoea: A literature-based analysis. *Lancet Respiratory Medicine, 7*(8), 687–698.

Benoist, L., de Ruiter, M., de Lange, J., & de Vries, N. (2017). A randomized, controlled trial of positional therapy versus oral appliance therapy for position-dependent sleep apnea. *Sleep Medicine, 34*, 109–117.

Berezin, L., Nagappa, M., Poorzargar, K., Saripella, A., Ariaratnam, J., Butris, N., Englesakis, M., & Chung, F. (2023). The effectiveness of positive airway pressure therapy in reducing postoperative adverse outcomes in surgical patients with obstructive sleep apnea: A systematic review and meta-analysis. *Journal of Clinical Anesthesia, 84*, Article 110993.

Berry, R., Quan, S., Abreu, A., Bibbs, M., DelRosso, L., Harding, S., Mao, M.-M., Plante, D., Pressman, M., Troester, M., & Vaughn, B.; American Academy of Sleep Medicine. (2020). *The AASM manual for the scoring of sleep and associated events: Rules, terminology and technical specifications* (Version 2.6). American Academy of Sleep Medicine.

Berry, R. B., Abreu, A. R., Krishnan, V., Quan, S. F., Strollo, P. J., & Malhotra, R. K. (2022). A transition to the American Academy of Sleep Medicine–recommended hypopnea definition in adults: Initiatives of the Hypopnea Scoring Rule Task Force. *Journal of Clinical Sleep Medicine, 18*(5), 1419–1425.

Bhat, S., Upadhyay, H., DeBari, V. A., Ahmad, M., Polos, P. G., & Chokroverty, S. (2016). The utility of patient-completed and partner-completed Epworth Sleepiness Scale scores in the evaluation of obstructive sleep apnea. *Sleep and Breathing, 20*(4), 1347–1354.

Bhattacharjee, R., Kheirandish-Gozal, L., Spruyt, K., Mitchell, R. B., Promchiarak, J., Simakajornboon, N., Kaditis, A. G., Splaingard, D., Splaingard, M., Brooks, L. J., Marcus, C. L., Sin, S., Arens, R., Verhulst, S. L., & Gozal, D. (2010). Adenotonsillectomy outcomes in treatment of obstructive sleep apnea in children: A multicenter retrospective study. *American Journal of Respiratory and Critical Care Medicine, 182*(5), 676–683.

Bloch, K. E., Huber, F., Furian, M., Latshang, T. D., Lo Cascio, C. M., Nussbaumer-Ochsner, Y., Senn, O., Russi, E. W., Kohler, M., Schoch, O. D., Turk, A., Imhof, E., Laube, I., Matthews, F., & Thurnheer, R. (2018). Autoadjusted versus fixed CPAP for obstructive sleep apnoea: A multicentre, randomised equivalence trial. *Thorax, 73*(2), 174–184.

Blumen, M. B., Buchet, I., Meulien, P., Hausser Hauw, C., Neveu, H., & Chabolle, F. (2009). Complications/adverse effects of maxillomandibular advancement for the treatment of OSA in regard to outcome. *Otolaryngology–Head and Neck Surgery, 141*(5), 591–597.

Bonsignore, M. R., Baiamonte, P., Mazzuca, E., Castrogiovanni, A., & Marrone, O. (2019). Obstructive sleep apnea and comorbidities: A dangerous liaison. *Multidisciplinary Respiratory Medicine, 14*, Article 8.

Bonsignore, M. R., Randerath, W., Schiza, S., Verbraecken, J., Elliott, M. W., Riha, R., Barbe, F., Bouloukaki, I., Castrogiovanni, A., Deleanu, O., Goncalves, M., Leger, D., Marrone, O., Penzel, T., Ryan, S., Smyth, D., Teran-Santos, J., Turino, C., & McNicholas, W. T. (2021). European Respiratory Society statement on sleep apnoea, sleepiness and driving risk. *European Respiratory Journal, 57*(2), Article 2001272.

Boyd, S. B., Walters, A. S., Waite, P., Harding, S. M., & Song, Y. (2015). Long-term effectiveness and safety of maxillomandibular advancement for treatment of obstructive sleep apnea. *Journal of Clinical Sleep Medicine, 11*(7), 699–708.

Bratton, D. J., Gaisl, T., Schlatzer, C., & Kohler, M. (2015). Comparison of the effects of continuous positive airway pressure and mandibular advancement devices on sleepiness in patients with obstructive sleep apnoea: A network meta-analysis. *Lancet Respiratory Medicine, 3*(11), 869–878.

Broström, A., Fridlund, B., Fossum, B., Pakpour, A., Nilsen, P., & Ulander, M. (2021). Communication during the initial visit to a CPAP clinic practitioners' experiences of facilitators and barriers when talking to patients with obstructive sleep apnea. *Journal of Sleep Research, 30*(4), Article e13244.

Broström, A., Nilsen, P. Johansson, P., Ulander, M., Strömberg, A., Svanborg, E., & Fridlund, B. (2010). Putative facilitators and barriers for adherence to CPAP treatment in patients with obstructive sleep apnea syndrome: A qualitative content analysis. *Sleep Medicine, 11*(2), 126–130.

Buck, L. M., Dalci, O., Darendeliler, M. A., & Papadopoulou, A. K. (2016). Effect of surgically assisted rapid maxillary expansion on upper airway volume: A systematic review. *Journal of Oral and Maxillofacial Surgery, 74*(5), 1025–1043.

Budhiraja, R., Parthasarathy, S., Drake, C. L., Roth, T., Sharief, I., Budhiraja, P., & Saunders, V. (2007). Early CPAP use identifies subsequent adherence to CPAP therapy. *Sleep, 30*, 320–324.

Burgos-Sanchez, C., Jones, N. N., Avillion, M., Gibson, S. J., Patel, J. A., Neighbors, J., Zaghi, S., & Camacho, M. (2020). Impact of alcohol consumption on snoring and sleep apnea: A systematic review and meta-analysis. *Otolaryngology–Head and Neck Surgery, 163*(6), 1078–1086.

Byun, J. H., Kim, K. T., Moon, H. J., Motamedi, G. K., & Cho, Y. W. (2019). The first night effect during polysomnography, and patients' estimates of sleep quality. *Psychiatry Research, 274*, 27–29.

Camacho, M., Certal, V., Abdullatif, J., Zaghi, S., Ruoff, C. M., Capasso, R., & Kushida, C. A. (2015). Myofunctional therapy to treat obstructive sleep apnea: A systematic review and meta-analysis. *Sleep, 38*(5), 669–675.

Camacho, M., Certal, V., Brietzke, S. E., Holty, J. E., Guilleminault, C., & Capasso, R. (2014). Tracheostomy as treatment for adult obstructive sleep apnea: A systematic review and meta-analysis. *Laryngoscope, 124*(3), 803–811.

Camacho, M., Li, D., Kawai, M., Zaghi, S., Teixeira, J., Senchak, A. J., Brietzke, S. E., Frasier, S., & Certal, V. (2016). Tonsillectomy for adult obstructive sleep apnea: A systematic review and meta-analysis. *Laryngoscope, 126*(9), 2176–2186.

Camacho, M., Riaz, M., Capasso, R., Ruoff, C. M., Guilleminault, C., Kushida, C. A., & Certal, V. (2015). The effect of nasal surgery on continuous positive airway pressure device use and therapeutic treatment pressures: A systematic review and meta-analysis. *Sleep, 38*(2), 279–286.

Caporale, M., Palmeri, R., Corallo, F., Muscarà, N., Romeo, L., Bramanti, A., Marino, S., & Lo Buono, V. (2021). Cognitive impairment in obstructive sleep apnea syndrome: A descriptive review. *Sleep and Breathing, 25*(1), 29–40.

Carvalho, B., Hsia, J., & Capasso, R. (2012). Surgical therapy of obstructive sleep apnea: A review. *Neurotherapeutics, 9*(4), 710–716.

Centers for Medicare & Medicaid Services. (2008). *Decision memo for continuous positive airway pressure (CPAP) therapy for obstructive sleep apnea (OSA)* (CAG-00093R2). Retrieved January 23, 2022, from https://www.cms.gov/medicare-coverage-database/view/ncacal-decision-memo.aspx?proposed=N&NCAId=204

Centers for Medicare & Medicaid Services. (2016). *Positive airway pressure (PAP) devices: Complying with documentation & coverage requirements.*

Certal, V. F., Zaghi, S., Riaz, M., Vieira, A. S., Pinheiro, C. T., Kushida, C., Capasso, R., & Camacho, M. (2015). Hypoglossal nerve stimulation in the treatment of obstructive sleep apnea: A systematic review and meta-analysis. *Laryngoscope, 125*(5), 1254–1264.

Chang, E. T., Fernandez-Salvador, C., Giambo, J., Nesbitt, B., Liu, S. Y., Capasso, R., Kushida, C. A., & Camacho, M. (2017). Tongue retaining devices for obstructive sleep apnea: A systematic review and meta-analysis. *American Journal of Otolaryngology, 38*(3), 272–278.

Chasens, E. R., Ratcliffe, S. J., & Weaver, T. E. (2009). Development of the FOSQ-10: A short version of the functional outcomes of sleep questionnaire. *Sleep, 32*(7), 915–919.

Chen, H., Eckert, D. J., van der Stelt, P. F., Guo, J., Ge, S., Emami, E., Almeida, F. R., & Huynh, N. T. (2020). Phenotypes of responders to mandibular advancement device therapy in obstructive sleep apnea patients: A systematic review and meta-analysis. *Sleep Medicine Reviews, 49*, Article 101229.

Chen, L. Y., Chen, Y. H., Hu, S. W., Lin, M. T., Lee, P. L., Chiang, A. A., & Tu, Y. K. (2022). In search of a better CPAP interface: A network meta-analysis comparing nasal masks, nasal pillows and oronasal masks. *Journal of Sleep Research, 31*(6), Article e13686.

Chen, X., Wang, R., Zee, P., Lutsey, P. L., Javaheri, S., Alcántara, C., Jackson, C. L., Williams, M. A., & Redline, S. (2015). Racial/ethnic differences in sleep disturbances: The Multi-Ethnic Study of Atherosclerosis (MESA). *Sleep, 38*(6), 877–888.

Chirinos, J. A., Gurubhagavatula, I., Teff, K., Rader, D. J., Wadden, T. A., Townsend, R., Foster, G. D., Maislin, G., Saif, H., Broderick, P., Chittams, J., Hanlon, A. L., & Pack, A. I. (2014). CPAP, weight loss, or both for obstructive sleep apnea. *New England Journal of Medicine, 370*(24), 2265–2275.

Chiu, H. Y., Chen, P. Y., Chuang, L. P., Chen, N. H., Tu, Y. K., Hsieh, Y. J., Wang, Y. C., & Guilleminault, C. (2017). Diagnostic accuracy of the Berlin Questionnaire, STOP-BANG, STOP, and Epworth Sleepiness Scale in detecting obstructive sleep apnea: A bivariate meta-analysis. *Sleep Medicine Reviews, 36*, 57–70.

Chobanian, A. V., Bakris, G. L., Black, H. R., Cushman, W. C., Green, L. A., Izzo, J. L., Jr., Jones, D. W., Materson, B. J., Oparil, S., Wright, J. T., Jr., & Roccella, E. J. (2003). Seventh report of the Joint National Committee on Prevention, Detection, Evaluation, and Treatment of High Blood Pressure. *Hypertension, 42*(6), 1206–1252.

Chou, M. S. H., Ting, N. C. H., El-Turk, N., Harrington, Z., & Dobler, C. C. (2021). Treatment burden experienced by patients with obstructive sleep apnoea using continuous positive airway pressure therapy. *PLOS ONE, 16*(6), Article e0252915.

Chung, F., Abdullah, H. R., & Liao, P. (2016). STOP-Bang Questionnaire: A practical approach to screen for obstructive sleep apnea. *Chest, 149*(3), 631–638.

Chung, F., Subramanyam, R., Liao, P., Sasaki, E., Shapiro, C., & Sun, Y. (2012). High STOP-Bang score indicates a high probability of obstructive sleep apnoea. *British Journal of Anaesthesiology, 108*(5), 768–775.

Chung, F., Yang, Y., Brown, R., & Liao, P. (2014). Alternative scoring models of STOP-Bang questionnaire improve specificity to detect undiagnosed obstructive sleep apnea. *Journal of Clinical Sleep Medicine, 10*(9), 951–958.

Chung, F., Yegneswaran, B., Liao, P., Chung, S. A., Vairavanathan, S., Islam, S., Khajehdehi, A., &Shapiro, C. M. (2008). STOP questionnaire: A tool to screen patients for obstructive sleep apnea. *Anesthesiology, 108*(5), 812–821.

Coutrot, A., Lazar, A. S., Richards, M., Manley, E., Wiener, J. M., Dalton, R. C., Hornberger, M., & Spiers, H. J. (2022). Reported sleep duration reveals segmentation of the adult life-course into three phases. *Nature Communications, 13*(1), Article 7697.

Crawford, M. R., Espie, C. A., Bartlett, D. J., & Grunstein, R.R. (2014). Integrating psychology and medicine in CPAP adherence – New concepts? *Sleep Medicine Reviews, 18*(2), 123–139. https://doi.org/10.1016/j.smrv.2013.03.002

Currie, A. C., Kaur, V., Carey, I., Al-Rubaye, H., Mahawar, K., Madhok, B., Small, P., McGlone, E. R., & Khan, O. A. (2021). Obstructive sleep apnea remission following bariatric surgery: A national registry cohort study. *Surgery for Obesity and Related Diseases, 17*(9), 1576–1582.

Deleanu, O. C., Pocora, D., Mihălcuţă, S., Ulmeanu, R., Zaharie, A. M., & Mihălţan, F. D. (2016). Influence of smoking on sleep and obstructive sleep apnea syndrome. *Pneumologia, 65*(1), 28–35.

Deng, X., Gu, W., Li, Y., Liu, M., & Gao, X. (2014). Age-group-specific associations between the severity of obstructive sleep apnea and relevant risk factors in male and female patients. *PLOS ONE, 9*(9), Article e107380.

Dorrity, J., Wirtz, N., Froymovich, O., & Hamlar, D. (2016). Genioglossal advancement, hyoid suspension, tongue base radiofrequency, and endoscopic partial midline glossectomy for obstructive sleep apnea. *Otolaryngologic Clinics of North America, 49*(6), 1399–1414.

Dudley, K. A., & Patel, S. R. (2016). Disparities and genetic risk factors in obstructive sleep apnea. *Sleep Medicine, 18*, 96–102.

Eckert, D. J. (2018). Phenotypic approaches to obstructive sleep apnoea—New pathways for targeted therapy. *Sleep Medicine Reviews, 37*, 45–59.

Eckert, D. J., Malhotra, A., & Jordan, A. S. (2009). Mechanisms of apnea. *Progress in Cardiovascular Diseases, 51*(4), 313–323.

Engleman, H. M., Asgari-Jirandeh, N., McLeod, A. L., Ramsay, C. F., Deary, I. J., & Douglas, N. J. (1996). Self-reported use of CPAP and benefits of CPAP therapy. *Chest, 109*, 1470–1476.

Engleman, H. M., Martin, S. E., & Douglas, N. J. (1994). Compliance with CPAP therapy in patients with the sleep apnoea/hypopnoea syndrome. *Thorax, 49*, 263–266.

Epstein, L. J., Kristo, D., Strollo, P. J., Jr., Friedman, N., Malhotra, A., Patil, S. P., Ramar, K., Rogers, R., Schwab, R. J., Weaver, E. M., & Weinstein, M. D. (2009). Clinical guideline for the evaluation, management and long-term care of obstructive sleep apnea in adults. *Journal of Clinical Sleep Medicine, 5*(3), 263–276.

Etindele Sosso, F. A., & Matos, E. (2021). Socioeconomic disparities in obstructive sleep apnea: A systematic review of empirical research. *Sleep and Breathing, 25*(4), 1729–1739.

Farrar, J., Ryan, J., Oliver, E., & Gillespie, M. B. (2008). Radiofrequency ablation for the treatment of obstructive sleep apnea: A meta-analysis. *Laryngoscope, 118*(10), 1878–1883.

Fields, B. G., Behari, P. P., McCloskey, S., True, G., Richardson, D., Thomasson, A., Korom-Djakovic, D., Davies, K., & Kuna, S. T. (2016). Remote ambulatory management of veterans with obstructive sleep apnea. *Sleep, 39*(3), 501–509.

Filtness, A. J., Reyner, L. A., & Horne, J. A. (2012). One night's CPAP withdrawal in otherwise compliant OSA patients: Marked driving impairment but good awareness of increased sleepiness. *Sleep and Breathing, 16*(3), 865–871.

Flemons, W. W., & Reimer, M. A. (2002). Measurement properties of the Calgary Sleep Apnea Quality of Life Index. *American Journal of Respiratory and Critical Care Medicine, 165*(2), 159–164.

Franklin, K. A., & Lindberg, E. (2015). Obstructive sleep apnea is a common disorder in the population—A review on the epidemiology of sleep apnea. *Journal of Thoracic Disease, 7*(8), 1311–1322.

Friedman, M., Ibrahim, H. Z., Vidyasagar, R., Pomeranz, J., & Joseph, N. J. (2004). Z-palatoplasty (ZPP): A technique for patients without tonsils. *Otolaryngology–Head and Neck Surgery, 131*(1), 89–100.

Frost & Sullivan. (2016). *Hidden health crisis costing America billions. Underdiagnosing and undertreating obstructive sleep apnea draining healthcare system*. American Academy of Sleep Medicine.

Fujita, S., Woodson, B. T., Clark, J. L., & Wittig, R. (1991). Laser midline glossectomy as a treatment for obstructive sleep apnea. *Laryngoscope, 101*(8), 805–809.

Gaisl, T., Haile, S. R., Thiel, S., Osswald, M., & Kohler, M. (2019). Efficacy of pharmacotherapy for OSA in adults: A systematic review and network meta-analysis. *Sleep Medicine Reviews, 46*, 74–86.

Garbarino, S., Durando, P., Guglielmi, O., Dini, G., Bersi, F., Fornarino, S., Toletone, A., Chiorri, C., & Magnavita, N. (2016). Sleep apnea, sleep debt and daytime sleepiness are independently associated with road accidents. A cross-sectional study on truck drivers. *PLOS ONE, 11*(11), Article e0166262.

Garbarino, S., Guglielmi, O., Sanna, A., Mancardi, G. L., & Magnavita, N. (2016). Risk of occupational accidents in workers with obstructive sleep apnea: Systematic review and meta-analysis. *Sleep, 39*(6), 1211–1218.

Georgoulis, M., Yiannakouris, N., Kechribari, I., Lamprou, K., Perraki, E., Vagiakis, E., & Kontogianni, M. D. (2022). Dose–response relationship between weight loss and improvements in obstructive sleep apnea severity after a diet/lifestyle interventions: Secondary analyses of the "MIMOSA" randomized clinical trial. *Journal of Clinical Sleep Medicine, 18*(5), 1251–1261.

Ghadiri, M., & Grunstein, R. R. (2020). Clinical side effects of continuous positive airway pressure in patients with obstructive sleep apnoea. *Respirology, 25*(6), 593–602.

Gleeson, M., & McNicholas, W. T. (2022). Bidirectional relationships of comorbidity with obstructive sleep apnoea. *European Respiratory Review, 31*(164), Article 210256.

Guglielmi, O., Lanteri, P., & Garbarino, S. (2019). Association between socioeconomic status, belonging to an ethnic minority and obstructive sleep apnea: A systematic review of the literature. *Sleep Medicine, 57*, 100–106.

Guilleminault, C., Stoohs, R., Clerk, A., Cetel, M., & Maistros, P. (1993). A cause of excessive daytime sleepiness. The upper airway resistance syndrome. *Chest, 104*(3), 781–787.

Hassan, F., & Kaplish, N. (2021). Hypoglossal nerve stimulator: A novel treatment approach for OSA—Overview of treatment, including diagnostic and patient criteria and procedural terminology codes. *Chest, 160*(4), 1406–1412.

He, M., Yin, G., Zhan, S., Xu, J., Cao, X., Li, J., & Ye, J. (2019). Long-term efficacy of uvulopalatopharyngoplasty among adult patients with obstructive sleep apnea: A systematic review and meta-analysis. *Otolaryngology–Head and Neck Surgery, 161*(3), 401–411.

Hofauer, B., Steffen, A., Knopf, A., Hasselbacher, K., & Heiser, C. (2019). Patient experience with upper airway stimulation in the treatment of obstructive sleep apnea. *Sleep and Breathing, 23*(1), 235–241.

Horner, R. L. (2012). Neural control of the upper airway: integrative physiological mechanisms and relevance for sleep disordered breathing. *Comprehensive Physiology, 2*(1), 479–535.

Hou, H., Zhao, Y., Yu, W., Dong, H., Xue, X., Ding, J., Xing, W., & Wang, W. (2018). Association of obstructive sleep apnea with hypertension: A systematic review and meta-analysis. *Journal of Global Health, 8*(1), Article 010405.

Hsu, W. Y., Chiu, N. Y., Chang, C. C., Chang, T. G., & Lane, H. Y. (2019). The association between cigarette smoking and obstructive sleep apnea. *Tobacco Induced Diseases, 17*, Article 27.

Hu, Y., Zhang, Z., Fang, F., Yang, J., Ma, J., Hu, S., & Guan, J. (2022). Effects of heated humidification on positive airway pressure side effects in patients with obstructive sleep apnoea: A meta-analysis. *Sleep and Breathing, 27*(1), 67–75.

Huang, T., Lin, B. M., Redline, S., Curhan, G. C., Hu, F. B., & Tworoger, S. S. (2018). Type of menopause, age at menopause, and risk of developing obstructive sleep apnea in postmenopausal women. *American Journal of Epidemiology, 187*(7), 1370–1379.

Hudgel, D. W., Patel, S. R., Ahasic, A. M., Bartlett, S. J., Bessesen, D. H., Coaker, M. A., Fiander, P. M., Grunstein, R. R., Gurubhagavatula, I., Kapur, V. K., Lettieri, C. J., Naughton, M. T., Owens, R. L., Pepin, J. L., Tuomilehto, H., & Wilson, K. C. (2018). The role of weight management in the treatment of adult obstructive sleep apnea. An official American Thoracic Society clinical practice guideline. *American Journal of Respiratory and Critical Care Medicine, 198*(6), e70–e87.

Huntley, C., Topf, M. C., Christopher, V., Doghramji, K., Curry, J., & Boon, M. (2019). Comparing upper airway stimulation to transoral robotic base of tongue resection for treatment of obstructive sleep apnea. *Laryngoscope, 129*(4), 1010–1013.

Iftikhar, I. H., Bittencourt, L., Youngstedt, S. D., Ayas, N., Cistulli, P., Schwab, R., Durkin, M. W., & Magalang, U. J. (2017). Comparative efficacy of CPAP, MADs, exercise-training, and dietary weight loss for sleep apnea: A network meta-analysis. *Sleep Medicine, 30*, 7–14.

Ishii, L., Roxbury, C., Godoy, A., Ishman, S., & Ishii, M. (2015). Does nasal surgery improve OSA in patients with nasal obstruction and OSA? A meta-analysis. *Otolaryngology–Head and Neck Surgery, 153*(3), 326–333.

Jackson, C. L., Redline, S., & Emmons, K. M. (2015). Sleep as a potential fundamental contributor to disparities in cardiovascular health. *Annual Review of Public Health, 36*, 417–440.

Jackson, C. L., Walker, J. R., Brown, M. K., Das, R., Jones, N. L. (2020). A workshop report on the causes and consequences of sleep health disparities. *Sleep, 43*(8), Article zsaa037.

Jandali, D., & Barrera, J. E. (2020). Recent advances in orthognathic surgery. *Current Opinion in Otolaryngology & Head and Neck Surgery, 28*(4), 246–250.

Jehan, S., Zizi, F., Pandi-Perumal, S. R., Wall, S., Auguste, E., Myers, A. K., Jean-Louis, G., & McFarlane, S. I. (2017). Obstructive sleep apnea and obesity: Implications for public health. *Sleep Medicine and Disorders, 1*(4), Article 00019.

Johns, M. W. (1991). A new method for measuring daytime sleepiness: The Epworth Sleepiness Scale. *Sleep, 14*(6), 540–545.

Johns, M. W. (2000). Sensitivity and specificity of the Multiple Sleep Latency Test (MSLT), the Maintenance of Wakefulness Test and the Epworth Sleepiness Scale: Failure of the MSLT as a gold standard. *Journal of Sleep Research, 9*(1), 5–11.

Johnson, D. A., Ohanele, C., Alcántara, C., & Jackson, C. L. (2022). The need for social and environmental determinants of health research to understand and intervene on racial/ethnic disparities in obstructive sleep apnea. *Clinics in Chest Medicine, 43*(2), 199–216.

Joosten, S. A., O'Driscoll, D. M., Berger, p. J., & Hamilton, G. S. (2014). Supine position related obstructive sleep apnea in adults: Pathogenesis and treatment. *Sleep Medicine Reviews, 18*(1), 7–17.

Jordan, A. S., McSharry, D. G., & Malhotra, A. (2014). Adult obstructive sleep apnoea. *Lancet, 383*(9918), 736–747.

Kapur, V. K., Auckley, D. H., Chowdhuri, S., Kuhlmann, D. C., Mehra, R., Ramar, K., & Harrod, C. G. (2017). Clinical practice guideline for diagnostic testing for adult obstructive sleep apnea: An American Academy of Sleep Medicine clinical practice guideline. *Journal of Clinical Sleep Medicine, 13*(3), 479–504.

Karimi, M., Hedner, J., Häbel, H., Nerman, O., & Grote, L. (2015). Sleep apnea–related risk of motor vehicle accidents is reduced by continuous positive airway pressure: Swedish Traffic Accident Registry data. *Sleep, 38*(3), 341–349.

Keenan, B. T., Kim, J., Singh, B., Bittencourt, L., Chen, N. H., Cistulli, P. A., Magalang, U. J., McArdle, N., Mindel, J. W., Benediktsdottir, B., Arnardottir, E. S., Prochnow, L. K., Penzel, T., Sanner, B., Schwab, R. J., Shin, C., Sutherland, K., Tufik, S., Maislin, G., . . . Pack, A. I. (2018). Recognizable clinical subtypes of obstructive sleep apnea across international sleep centers: A cluster analysis. *Sleep, 41*(3), Article zsx214.

Kent, D., Stanley, J., Aurora, R. N., Levine, C., Gottlieb, D. J., Spann, M. D., Torre, C. A., Green, K., & Harrod, C. G. (2021). Referral of adults with obstructive sleep apnea for surgical consultation: An American Academy of Sleep Medicine clinical practice guideline. *Journal of Clinical Sleep Medicine, 17*(12), 2499–2505.

Kirsch, D. B., Yang, H., Maslow, A. L., Stolzenbach, M., & McCall, A. (2019). Association of positive airway pressure use with acute care utilization and costs. *Journal of Clinical Sleep Medicine, 15*(9), 1243–1250.

Kohler, M., Stoewhas, A. C., Ayers, L., Senn, O., Bloch, K. E., Russi, E. W., & Stradling, J. R. (2011). Effects of continuous positive airway pressure therapy withdrawal in patients with obstructive sleep apnea: A randomized controlled trial. *American Journal of Respiratory and Critical Care Medicine, 184*(10), 1192–1199.

Kribbs, N. B., Pack, A. I., Kline, L. R., Smith, P. L., Schwartz, A. R., Schubert, N. M., Redline, S., Henry, J. N., Getsy, J. E., & Dinges, D. F. (1993). Objective measurement of patterns of nasal CPAP use by patients with obstructive sleep apnea. *American Reviews in Respiratory Diseases, 147*, 887–895.

Krishnan, V., Dixon-Williams, S., & Thornton, J. D. (2014). Where there is smoke . . . there is sleep apnea: Exploring the relationship between smoking and sleep apnea. *Chest, 146*(6), 1673–1680.

Kuhn, E., Schwarz, E. I., Bratton, D. J., Rossi, V. A., & Kohler, M. (2017). Effects of CPAP and mandibular advancement devices on health-related quality of life in OSA: A systematic review and meta-analysis. *Chest, 151*(4), 786–794.

Kuna, S. T., Gurubhagavatula, I., Maislin, G., Hin, S., Hartwig, K. C., McCloskey, S., Hachadoorian, R., Hurley, S., Gupta, R., Staley, B., & Atwood, C. W. (2011). Noninferiority of functional outcome in ambulatory management of obstructive sleep apnea. *American Journal of Respiratory and Critical Care Medicine, 183*(9), 1238–1244.

Kuna, S. T., Reboussin, D. M., Strotmeyer, E. S., Millman, R. P., Zammit, G., Walkup, M. P., Wadden, T. A., Wing, R. R., Pi-Sunyer, F. X., Spira, A. P., & Foster, G. D. (2021). Effects of weight loss on obstructive sleep apnea severity. Ten-year results of the Sleep AHEAD Study. *American Journal of Respiratory and Critical Care Medicine, 203*(2), 221–229.

Labarca, G., Dreyse, J., Drake, L., Jorquera, J., & Barbe, F. (2020). Efficacy of continuous positive airway pressure (CPAP) in the prevention of cardiovascular events in patients with obstructive sleep apnea: Systematic review and meta-analysis. *Sleep Medicine Reviews, 52*, Article 101312.

Labarca, G., Reyes, T., Jorquera, J., Dreyse, J., & Drake, L. (2018). CPAP in patients with obstructive sleep apnea and Type 2 diabetes mellitus: Systematic review and meta-analysis. *Clinical Respiratory Journal, 12*(8), 2361–2368.

Labarca, G., Saavedra, D., Dreyse, J., Jorquera, J., & Barbe, F. (2020). Efficacy of CPAP for improvements in sleepiness, cognition, mood, and quality of life in elderly patients with OSA: Systematic review and meta-analysis of randomized controlled trials. *Chest, 158*(2), 751–764.

Labarca, G., Schmidt, A., Dreyse, J., Jorquera, J., & Barbe, F. (2021). Telemedicine interventions for CPAP adherence in obstructive sleep apnea patients: Systematic review and meta-analysis. *Sleep Medicine Reviews, 60*, Article 101543.

Lacasse, Y., Bureau, M. P., & Sériès, F. (2004). A new standardised and self-administered quality of life questionnaire specific to obstructive sleep apnoea. *Thorax, 59*(6), 494–499.

Lal, C., Ayappa, I., Ayas, N., Beaudin, A. E., Hoyos, C., Kushida, C. A., Kaminska, M., Mullins, A., Naismith, S. L., Osorio, R. S., Phillips, C. L., Parekh, A., Stone, K. L., Turner, A. D., & Varga, A. W. (2022). The link between obstructive sleep apnea and neurocognitive impairment: An official American Thoracic Society workshop report. *Annals of the American Thoracic Society, 19*(8), 1245–1256.

Lal, C., Weaver, T. E., Bae, C. J., & Strohl, K. P. (2021). Excessive daytime sleepiness in obstructive sleep apnea. Mechanisms and clinical management. *Annals of the American Thoracic Society, 18*(5), 757–768.

Lee, J. B., Park, Y. H., Hong, J. H., Lee, S. H., Jung, K. H., Kim, J. H., Yi, H., & Shin, C. (2009). Determining optimal sleep position in patients with positional sleep-disordered breathing using response surface analysis. *Journal of Sleep Research, 18*(1), 26–35.

Li, H. Y., Lee, L. A., Kezirian, E. J., & Nakayama, M. (2018). Suspension palatoplasty for obstructive sleep apnea—A preliminary study. *Scientific Reports, 8*(1), Article 4224.

Light, M., Owens, R. L., Schmickl, C. N., & Malhotra, A. (2019). Precision medicine for obstructive sleep apnea. *Sleep Medicine Clinics, 14*(3), 391–398.

Liu, H. T., Lin, Y. C., Kuan, Y. C., Huang, Y. H., Hou, W. H., Liou, T. H., & Chen, H. C. (2016). Intranasal corticosteroid therapy in the treatment of obstructive sleep apnea: A meta-analysis of randomized controlled trials. *American Journal of Rhinology & Allergy, 30*(3), 215–221.

Liu, S. Y., Awad, M., Riley, R., & Capasso, R. (2019). The role of the revised Stanford protocol in today's precision medicine. *Sleep Medicine Clinics, 14*(1), 99–107.

Liu, X., Ma, Y., Ouyang, R., Zeng, Z., Zhan, Z., Lu, H., Cui, Y., Dai, Z., Luo, L., He, C., Li, H., Zong, D., & Chen, Y. (2020). The relationship between inflammation and neurocognitive dysfunction in obstructive sleep apnea syndrome. *Journal of Neuroinflammation, 17*(1), Article 229.

Liu, Y., Zou, J., Qian, Y., Xu, H., Zhu, H., Meng, L., Guan, J., Yi, H., & Yin, S. (2021). The association between obesity indices and obstructive sleep apnea is modified by age in a sex-specific manner. *Sleep and Breathing, 25*(1), 189–197.

Lloyd, R., Morgenthaler, T. I., Donald, R., Gray, D. D., Lewin, D., Revana, A., Schutte-Rodin, S., & Trotti, L. M. (2022). Quality measures for the care of adult patients with obstructive sleep apnea: 2022 update after measure maintenance. *Journal of Clinical Sleep Medicine, 18*(11), 2673–2680.

Luyster, F. S. (2017). Impact of obstructive sleep apnea and its treatments on partners: A literature review. *Journal of Clinical Sleep Medicine, 13*(3), 467–477.

Luyster, F. S., Dunbar-Jacob, J., Aloia, M. S., Martire, L. M., Buysse, D. J., & Strollo, P. J. (2016). Patient and partner experiences with obstructive sleep apnea and CPAP treatment: A qualitative analysis. *Behavioral Sleep Medicine, 14*(1), 67–84.

Lyons, M. M., Bhatt, N. Y., Pack, A. I., & Magalang, U. J. (2020). Global burden of sleep-disordered breathing and its implications. *Respirology, 25*(7), 690–702.

Maislin, G., Pack, A. I., Kribbs, N. B., Smith, P. L., Schwartz, A. R., Kline, L. R., Schwab, R. J., & Dinges, D. F. (1995). A survey screen for prediction of apnea. *Sleep, 18*(3), 158–166.

Mashaqi, S., Patel, S. I., Combs, D., Estep, L., Helmick, S., Machamer, J., & Parthasarathy, S. (2021). The hypoglossal nerve stimulation as a novel therapy for treating obstructive sleep apnea—A literature review. *International Journal of Environmental Research and Public Health, 18*(4), Article 1642.

Mazzotti, D. R., Keenan, B. T., Lim, D. C., Gottlieb, D. J., Kim, J., & Pack, A. I. (2019). Symptom Subtypes of obstructive sleep apnea predict incidence of cardiovascular outcomes. *American Journal of Respiratory and Critical Care Medicine, 200*(4), 493–506.

McNicholas, W. T. (2021). Sleepiness behind the wheel and the implementation of European driving regulations. *Sleep Medicine Clinics, 16*(3), 533–543.

McNicholas, W. T., & Pevernagie, D. (2022). Obstructive sleep apnea: Transition from pathophysiology to an integrative disease model. *Journal of Sleep Research, 31*(4), Article e13616.

Miller, S. C., Nguyen, S. A., Ong, A. A., & Gillespie, M. B. (2017). Transoral robotic base of tongue reduction for obstructive sleep apnea: A systematic review and meta-analysis. *Laryngoscope, 127*(1), 258–265.

Mitchell, L. J., Davidson, Z. E., Bonham, M., O'Driscoll, D. M., Hamilton, G. S., & Truby, H. (2014). Weight loss from lifestyle interventions and severity of sleep apnoea: A systematic review and meta-analysis. *Sleep Medicine, 15*(10), 1173–1183.

Morgenthaler, T. I., Aurora, R. N., Brown, T., Zak, R., Alessi, C., Boehlecke, B., Chesson, A. L., Jr., Friedman, L., Kapur, V., Maganti, R., Owens, J., Pancer, J., & Swick, T. J. (2008). Practice parameters for the use of autotitrating continuous positive airway pressure devices for titrating pressures and treating adult patients with obstructive sleep apnea syndrome: An update for 2007. An American Academy of Sleep Medicine report. *Sleep, 31*(1), 141–147.

Mukherjee, S., Saxena, R., & Palmer, L. J. (2018). The genetics of obstructive sleep apnoea. *Respirology, 23*(1), 18–27.

Murphey, A. W., Kandl, J. A., Nguyen, S. A., Weber, A. C., & Gillespie, M. B. (2015). The effect of glossectomy for obstructive sleep apnea: A systematic review and meta-analysis. *Otolaryngology–Head and Neck Surgery, 153*(3), 334–342.

Neruntarat, C. (2011). Long-term results of palatal implants for obstructive sleep apnea. *European Archives of Oto-Rhino-Laryngology, 268*(7), 1077–1080.

Netzer, N. C., Stoohs, R. A., Netzer, C. M., Clark, K., & Strohl, K. P. (1999). Using the Berlin Questionnaire to identify patients at risk for the sleep apnea syndrome. *Annals of Internal Medicine, 131*(7), 485–491.

Nguyen, D. K., Liang, J., & Durr, M. (2021). Topical nasal treatment efficacy on adult obstructive sleep apnea severity: A systematic review and meta-analysis. *International Forum of Allergy & Rhinology, 11*(2), 153–161.

Nordgård, S., Stene, B. K., & Skjøstad, K. W. (2006). Soft palate implants for the treatment of mild to moderate obstructive sleep apnea. *Otolaryngology–Head and Neck Surgery, 134*(4), 565–570.

Olafiranye, O., Akinboboye, O., Mitchell, J. E., Ogedegbe, G., & Jean-Louis, G. (2013). Obstructive sleep apnea and cardiovascular disease in Blacks: A call to action from the Association of Black Cardiologists. *American Heart Journal, 165*(4), 468–476.

Ong, J. C., Crawford, M. R., & Wallace, D. M. (2021). Sleep apnea and insomnia: Emerging evidence for effective clinical management. *Chest, 159*(5), 2020–2028.

Pataka, A., Kotoulas, S., Kalamaras, G., Tzinas, A., Grigoriou, I., Kasnaki, N., & Argyropoulou, P. (2022). Does smoking affect OSA? What about smoking cessation? *Journal of Clinical Medicine, 11*(17), Article 5164.

Patil, S. P., Ayappa, I. A., Caples, S. M., Kimoff, R. J., Patel, S. R., & Harrod, C. G. (2019a). Treatment of adult obstructive sleep apnea with positive airway pressure: An American Academy of Sleep Medicine clinical practice guideline. *Journal of Clinical Sleep Medicine, 15*(2), 335–343.

Patil, S. P., Ayappa, I. A., Caples, S. M., Kimoff, R. J., Patel, S. R., & Harrod, C. G. (2019b). Treatment of adult obstructive sleep apnea with positive airway pressure: An American Academy of Sleep Medicine systematic review, meta-analysis, and GRADE assessment. *Journal of Clinical Sleep Medicine, 15*(2), 301–334.

Pattipati, M., Gudavalli, G., Zin, M., Dhulipalla, L., Kolack, E., Karki, M., Devarakonda, P. K., & L. Yoe, L. (2022). Continuous positive airway pressure vs mandibular advancement devices in the treatment of obstructive sleep apnea: An updated systematic review and meta-analysis. *Cureus, 14*(1), Article e21759.

Pavwoski, P., & Shelgikar, A. V. (2017). Treatment options for obstructive sleep apnea. *Neurology: Clinical Practice, 7*(1), 77–85.

Pevernagie, D., Bauters, F. A., & Hertegonne, K. (2021). The role of patient-reported outcomes in sleep measurements. *Sleep Medicine Clinics, 16*(4), 595–606.

Pien, G. W., Ye, L., Keenan, B. T., Maislin, G., Björnsdóttir, E., Arardottir, E. S., Benediktsdottir, B., Gislason, T., & Pack, A. I. (2018). Changing faces of obstructive sleep apnea: Treatment effects by cluster designation in the Icelandic sleep apnea cohort. *Sleep, 41*(3), Article zsx201.

Pirklbauer, K., Russmueller, G., Stiebellehner, L., Nell, C., Sinko, K., Millesi, G., & Klug, C. (2011). Maxillomandibular advancement for treatment of obstructive sleep apnea syndrome: A systematic review. *Journal of Oral and Maxillofacial Surgery, 69*(6), e165–e176.

Ramar, K., Dort, L. C., Katz, S. G., Lettieri, C. J., Harrod, C. G., Thomas, S. M., & Chervin, R. D. (2015). Clinical practice guideline for the treatment of obstructive sleep apnea and snoring with oral appliance therapy: An update for 2015. *Journal of Clinical Sleep Medicine, 11*(7), 773–827.

Randerath, W., de Lange, J., Hedner, J., Ho, J., Marklund, M., Schiza, S., Steier, J., & Verbraecken, J. (2022). Current and novel treatment options for obstructive sleep apnoea. *ERJ Open Research, 8*(2), Article 00126-2022.

Randerath, W. J., Verbraecken, J., Andreas, S., Bettega, G., Boudewyns, A., Hamans, E., Jalbert, F., Paoli, J. R., Sanner, B., Smith, I., Stuck, B. A., Lacassagne, L., Marklund, M., Maurer, J. T., Pepin, J. L., Valipour, A., Verse, T., & Fietze, I. (2011). Non-CPAP therapies in obstructive sleep apnoea. *European Respiratory Journal, 37*(5), 1000–1028.

Randerath, W., J. Verbraecken, J., de Raaff, C. A. L., Hedner, J., Herkenrath, S., Hohenhorst, W., Jakob, T., Marrone, O., Marklund, M., McNicholas, W. T., Morgan, R. L., Pepin, J. L., Schiza, S., Skoetz, N., Smyth, D., Steier, J., Tonia, T., Trzepizur, W., van Mechelen, P. H., & Wijkstra, P. (2021). European Respiratory Society guideline on non-CPAP therapies for obstructive sleep apnoea. *European Respiratory Review, 30*(162), Article 210200.

Ratneswaran, D., Guni, A., Pengo, M. F., Al-Sherif, M., He, B., Cheng, M. C., Steier, J., & Schwarz, E. I. (2021). Electrical stimulation as a therapeutic approach in obstructive sleep apnea—A meta-analysis. *Sleep and Breathing, 25*(1), 207–218.

Ravesloot, M. J. L., de Raaff, C. A. L., van de Beek, M. J., Benoist, L. B. L., Beyers, J., Corso, R. M., Edenharter, G., den Haan, C., Heydari Azad, J., Ho, J. T. F., Hofauer, B., Kezirian, E. J., van Maanen, J. P., Maes, S., Mulier, J. P., Randerath, W., Vanderveken, O. M., Verbraecken, J., Vonk, P. E., . . . de Vries, N. (2019). Perioperative care of patients with obstructive sleep apnea undergoing upper airway surgery: A review and consensus recommendations. *JAMA Otolaryngology–Head and Neck Surgery, 145*(8), 751–760.

Ravesloot, M. J. L., White, D., Heinzer, R., Oksenberg, A., & Pépin, J. L. (2017). Efficacy of the new generation of devices for positional therapy for patients with positional obstructive sleep apnea: A systematic review of the literature and meta-analysis. *Journal of Clinical Sleep Medicine, 13*(6), 813–824.

Redline, S., Sotres-Alvarez, D., Loredo, J., Hall, M., Patel, S. R., Ramos, A., Shah, N., Ries, A., Arens, R., Barnhart, J., Youngblood, M., Zee, P., & Daviglus, M. L. (2014). Sleep-disordered breathing in Hispanic/Latino individuals of diverse backgrounds. The Hispanic Community Health Study/Study of Latinos. *American Journal of Respiratory and Critical Care Medicine, 189*(3), 335–344.

Reeves-Hoche, M. K., Meck, R., & Zwillich, C. W. (1994). Nasal CPAP: An objective evaluation of patient compliance. *American Journal of Respiratory & Critical Care Medicine, 149*, 149–154.

Remmers, J., Charkhandeh, S., Grosse, J., Topor, Z., Brant, R., Santosham, P., & Bruehlmann, S. (2013). Remotely controlled mandibular protrusion during sleep predicts therapeutic success with oral appliances in patients with obstructive sleep apnea. *Sleep, 36*(10), 1517–1525, 1525a.

Riley, R. W., Powell, N. B., & Guilleminault, C. (1993). Obstructive sleep apnea syndrome: A surgical protocol for dynamic upper airway reconstruction. *Journal of Oral and Maxillofacial Surgery, 51*(7), 742–747; discussion 748–749.

Robinson, S., Lewis, R., Norton, A., & McPeake, S. (2003). Ultrasound-guided radiofrequency submucosal tongue-base excision for sleep apnoea: A preliminary report. *Clinical Otolaryngology and Allied Sciences, 28*(4), 341–345.

Roeder, M., Bradicich, M., Schwarz, E. I., Thiel, S., Gaisl, T., Held, U., & Kohler, M. (2020). Night-to-night variability of respiratory events in obstructive sleep apnoea: A systematic review and meta-analysis. *Thorax, 75*(12), Article 1095.

Rowland, S., Aiyappan, V., Hennessy, C., Catcheside, P., Chai-Coezter, C. L., McEvoy, R. D., & Antic, N. A. (2018). Comparing the efficacy, mask leak, patient adherence, and patient preference of three different CPAP interfaces to treat moderate–severe obstructive sleep apnea." *Journal of Clinical Sleep Medicine, 14*(1), 101–108.

Saconi, B., Yang, H., Watach, A. J., & Sawyer, A. M. (2020). Coping processes, self-efficacy, and CPAP use in adults with obstructive sleep apnea. *Behavioral Sleep Medicine, 18*(1), 68–80.

Sands-Lincoln, M., Grandner, M., Whinnery, J., Keenan, B. T., Jackson, N., & Gurubhagavatula, I. (2013). The association between obstructive sleep apnea and hypertension by race/ethnicity in a nationally representative sample. *Journal of Clinical Hypertension (Greenwich), 15*(8), 593–599.

Sateia, M. J. (2014). International classification of sleep disorders-third edition: Highlights and modifications. *Chest, 146*(5), 1387–1394.

Sawyer, A. M., Canamucio, A., Moriarty, H., Weaver, T. E., Richards, K. C., & Kuna, S. T. (2011). Do cognitive perceptions influence CPAP use? *Patient Education and Counseling, 85*(1), 85–91.

Sawyer, A. M., Wallace, D. M., Buenaver, L. F., Watach, A. J., Blase, A., Saconi, B., Patel, S. R., Kuna, S. T., & Punjabi, N. M. (2021). Where to next for optimizing adherence in large-scale trials of continuous positive airway pressure? *Sleep Medicine Clinics, 16*(1), 125–144.

Schiza, S. E., & Bouloukaki, I. (2020). Does gender matter: Sex-specific aspects of symptoms, outcome, and therapy of obstructive sleep apnea. *Current Opinion in Pulmonary Medicine, 26*(6), 642–649.

Selim, B. J., Junna, M. R., & Morgenthaler, T. I. (2012). Therapy for sleep hypoventilation and central apnea syndromes. *Current Treatment Options in Neurology, 14*(5), 427–437.

Senaratna, C. V., Perret, J. L., Lodge, C. J., Lowe, A. J., Campbell, B. E., Matheson, M. C., Hamilton, G. S., & Dharmage, S. C. (2017). Prevalence of obstructive sleep apnea in the general population: A systematic review. *Sleep Medicine Reviews, 34*, 70–81.

Shah, R. R., & Thaler, E. R. (2020). Base of tongue surgery for obstructive sleep apnea in the era of neurostimulation. *Otolaryngologic Clinics of North America, 53*(3), 431–443.

Simou, E., Britton, J., & Leonardi-Bee, J. (2018). Alcohol and the risk of sleep apnoea: A systematic review and meta-analysis. *Sleep Medicine, 42*, 38–46.

Sjöblom, H. M., Nahkuri, M., Suomela, M., Jero, J., & Piitulainen, J. M. (2022). Treatment of sleep apnoea with tonsillectomy: A retrospective analysis using long-term follow-up data. *European Archives of Oto-Rhino-Laryngology, 279*(7), 3727–3732.

Sowho, M., Sgambati, F., Guzman, M., Schneider, H., & Schwartz, A. (2020). Snoring: A source of noise pollution and sleep apnea predictor. *Sleep, 43*(6) Article zsz305.

Srijithesh, P. R., Aghoram, R., Goel, A., & Dhanya, J. (2019). Positional therapy for obstructive sleep apnoea. *Cochrane Database of Systematic Reviews, 5*(5), Article CD010990.

Stansbury, R. C., & Strollo, P. J. (2015). Clinical manifestations of sleep apnea. *Journal of Thoracic Disease, 7*(9), E298–E310.

Stepnowsky, C. J., Marler, M. R., & Ancoli-Israel, S. (2002). Determinants of nasal CPAP compliance. *Sleep Medicine, 3*, 239–247.

Sterling, K. L., Cistulli, P. A., Linde-Zwirble, W., Malik, A., Benjafield, A. V., Malhotra, A., Cole, K. V., Emami, H., Woodford, C., More, S., Armitstead, J. P., Nunez, C. M., Reutrakul, S., & Pépin, J. L. (2022). Association between positive airway pressure therapy adherence and health care resource utilization in patients with obstructive sleep apnea and Type 2 diabetes in the United States. *Journal of Clinical Sleep Medicine, 19*(3), 563–571.

Sterling, K. L., Pépin, J. L., Linde-Zwirble, W., Chen, J., Benjafield, A. V., Cistulli, P. A., Cole, K. V., Emami, H., Woodford, C., Armitstead, J. P., Nunez, C. M., Wedzicha, J. A., & Malhotra, A. (2022). Impact of positive airway pressure therapy adherence on outcomes in patients with obstructive sleep apnea and chronic obstructive pulmonary disease. *American Journal of Respiratory and Critical Care Medicine, 206*(2), 197–205.

Stuck, B. A., Ravesloot, M. J. L., Eschenhagen, T., de Vet, H. C. W., & Sommer, J. U. (2018). Uvulopalatopharyngoplasty with or without tonsillectomy in the treatment of adult obstructive sleep apnea—A systematic review. *Sleep Medicine, 50*, 152–165.

Sullivan, C. E., Issa, F. G., Berthon-Jones, M., & Eves, L. (1981). Reversal of obstructive sleep apnoea by continuous positive airway pressure applied through the nares. *Lancet, 1*(8225), 862–865.

Sutherland, K., & Cistulli, P. A. (2019). Oral appliance therapy for obstructive sleep apnoea: State of the art. *Journal of Clinical Medicine, 8*(12), Article 2121.

Suurna, M. V., Jacobowitz, O., Chang, J., Koutsourelakis, I., Smith, D., Alkan, U., D'Agostino, M., Boon, M., Heiser, C., Hoff, P., Huntley, C., Kent, D., Kominsky, A., Lewis, R., Maurer, J. T., Ravesloot, M. J., Soose, R., Steffen, A., Weaver, E. M. . . . Ishman, S. L. (2021). Improving outcomes of hypoglossal nerve stimulation therapy: Current practice, future directions, and research gaps. Proceedings of the 2019 International Sleep Surgery Society Research Forum. *Journal of Clinical Sleep Medicine, 17*(12), 2477–2487.

Thaler, E. R., Rassekh, C. H., Lee, J. M., Weinstein, G. S., & O'Malley, B. W., Jr. (2016). Outcomes for multilevel surgery for sleep apnea: Obstructive sleep apnea, transoral robotic surgery, and uvulopalatopharyngoplasty. *Laryngoscope, 126*(1), 266–269.

Thornton, J. D., Dudley, K. A., Saeed, G. J., Schuster, S. T., Schell, A., Spilsbury, J. C., & Patel, S. R. (2022). Differences in symptoms and severity of obstructive sleep apnea between Black and White patients. *Annals of the American Thoracic Society, 19*(2), 272–278.

Timkova, V., Nagyova, I., Reijneveld, S. A., Tkacova, R., van Dijk, J. P., & Bültmann, U. (2020). Quality of life of obstructive sleep apnoea patients receiving continuous positive airway pressure treatment: A systematic review and meta-analysis. *Heart & Lung, 49*(1), 10–24.

Trzepizur, W., Blanchard, M., Ganem, T., Balusson, F., Feuilloy, M., Girault, J. M., Meslier, N., Oger, E., Paris, A., Pigeanne, T., Racineux, J. L., Sabil, A., Gervès-Pinquié, C., & Gagnadoux, F. (2022). Sleep apnea–specific hypoxic burden, symptom subtypes, and risk of cardiovascular events and all-cause mortality. *American Journal of Respiratory and Critical Care Medicine, 205*(1), 108–117.

Verbraecken, J. (2022). More than sleepiness: Prevalence and relevance of nonclassical symptoms of obstructive sleep apnea. *Current Opinion in Pulmonary Medicine, 28*(6), 552–558.

Walia, H. K., Thompson, N. R., Pascoe, M., Faisal, M., Moul, D. E., Katzan, I., Mehra, R., & Foldvary-Schaefer, N. (2019). Effect of positive airway pressure therapy on drowsy driving in a large clinic-based obstructive sleep apnea cohort. *Journal of Clinical Sleep Medicine, 15*(11), 1613–1620.

Walter, R. J., Hagedorn, S. I., & Lettieri, C. J. (2017). Impact of diagnosing and treating obstructive sleep apnea on healthcare utilization. *Sleep Medicine, 38*, 73–77.

Wang, S. H., Keenan, B. T., Wiemken, A., Zang, Y., Staley, B., Sarwer, D. B., Torigian, D. A., Williams, N., Pack, A. I., & Schwab, R. J. (2020). Effect of weight loss on upper airway anatomy and the apnea-hypopnea index. The importance of tongue fat. *American Journal of Respiratory and Critical Care Medicine, 201*(6), 718–727.

Watach, A., Hwang, D., & Sawyer, A. (2021). Personalized and patient-centered strategies to improve positive airway pressure adherence in patients with obstructive sleep apnea. *Patient Preferences and Adherence, 15*, 1557–1570.

Weaver, T. E. (2022). Best predictors of continuous positive airway pressure adherence. *Sleep Medicine Clinics, 17*(4), 587–595.

Weaver, T. E., & Grunstein, R. R. (2008). Adherence to continuous positive airway pressure therapy: The challenge to effective treatment. *Proceedings of the American Thoracic Society, 5*, 173–178.

Weaver, T. E., Kribbs, N. B., Pack, A. I., Kline, L. R., Chugh, D. K., Maislin, G., Smith, P. L., Schwartz, A. R., Schubert, N. M., Gillen, K. A., & Dinges, D. F. (1997). Night-to-night variability in CPAP use over first three months of treatment. *Sleep, 20*, 278–283.

Weaver, T. E., Laizner, A., Evans, L. K., Maislin, G., Chugh, D. K., Lyons, K., Smith, P. L., Schwartz, A. R., Redline, S., Pack, A. I., & Dinges, D. F. (1997). An instrument to measure functional status outcomes for disorders of excessive sleepiness. *Sleep, 20*, 835–843.

Weaver, T. E., G. Maislin, G., Dinges, D. F., Bloxham, T., George, C. F. P., & Greenberg, H., Kader, G., Mahowald, M., Younger, J., & Pack, A. I. (2007). Relationship between hours of CPAP use and achieving normal levels of sleepiness and daily functioning. *Sleep, 30*, 711–719.

Weinfurt, K. P., & Reeve, B. B. (2022). Patient-reported outcome measures in clinical research. *JAMA, 328*(5), 472–473.

Wickwire, E. M., Albrecht, J. S., Towe, M. M., Abariga, S. A., Diaz-Abad, M., Shipper, A. G., Cooper, L. M., Assefa, S. Z., Tom, S. E., & Scharf, S. M. (2019). The impact of treatments for OSA on monetized health economic outcomes: A systematic review. *Chest, 155*(5), 947–961.

Woodson, B. T., & Franco, R. (2007). Physiology of sleep disordered breathing. *Otolaryngologic Clinics of North America, 40*(4), 691–711.

Woodson, B. T., & Fujita, S. (1992). Clinical experience with lingualplasty as part of the treatment of severe obstructive sleep apnea. *Otolaryngology–Head and Neck Surgery, 107*(1), 40–48.

Wu, J., Zhao, G., Li, Y., Zang, H., Wang, T., Wang, D., & Han, D. (2017). Apnea–hypopnea index decreased significantly after nasal surgery for obstructive sleep apnea: A meta-analysis. *Medicine (Baltimore), 96*(5), Article e6008.

Wu, Q., Wang, Y., Wang, P., Xiang, Z., Ye, B., & Li, J. (2019). The inverted-L ramus osteotomy versus sagittal split ramus osteotomy in maxillomandibular advancement for the treatment of obstructive sleep apnea patients: A retrospective study. *Journal of Cranio-Maxillofacial Surgery, 47*(12), 1839–1847.

Yang, S., Guo, X., Liu, W., Li, Y., & Liu, Y. (2022). Alcohol as an independent risk factor for obstructive sleep apnea. *Irish Journal of Medical Science, 191*(3), 1325–1330.

Ye, L., Pack, A. I., Maislin, G., Dinges, D., Hurley, S., McCloskey, S., & Weaver, T. E. (2012). Predictors of continuous positive airway pressure use during the first week of treatment. *Journal of Sleep Research, 21*, 419–426.

Young, L. R., Taxin, Z. H., Norman, R. G., Walsleben, J. A., Rapoport, D. M., & Ayappa, I. (2013). Response to CPAP withdrawal in patients with mild versus severe obstructive sleep apnea/hypopnea syndrome. *Sleep, 36*(3), 405–412.

Yu, J., Zhou, Z., McEvoy, R. D., Anderson, C. S., Rodgers, A., Perkovic, V., & Neal, B. (2017). Association of positive airway pressure with cardiovascular events and death in adults with sleep apnea: A systematic review and meta-analysis. *JAMA, 318*(2), 156–166.

Yu, J. L., Liu, Y., Tangutur, A., Arnold, M., Seay, E. G., Schwartz, A. R., & Dedhia, R. C. (2021). Influence of apnea vs hypopnea predominance in predicting mean therapeutic positive airway pressures among patients with obstructive sleep apnea. *Journal of Clinical Sleep Medicine, 17*(11), 2171–2178.

Yu, J. L., Mahmoud, A., & Thaler, E. R. (2019). Transoral robotic surgery versus upper airway stimulation in select obstructive sleep apnea patients. *Laryngoscope, 129*(1), 256–258.

Zheng, D., Xu, Y., You, S., Hackett, M. L., Woodman, R. J., Li, Q., Woodward, M., Loffler, K. A., Rodgers, A., Drager, L. F., Lorenzi-Filho, G., Wang, X., Quan, W. W., Tripathi, M., Mediano, O., Ou, Q., Chen, R., Liu, Z., Zhang, X. . . . Anderson, C. S. (2019). Effects of continuous positive airway pressure on depression and anxiety symptoms in patients with obstructive sleep apnoea: Results from the sleep apnoea cardiovascular endpoint randomised trial and meta-analysis. *EClinicalMedicine, 11*, 89–96.

Zhou, A., Li, H., Wang, X., Zhang, J., Zhang, Y., He, J., & Liu, S. (2021). Preliminary comparison of the efficacy of several surgical treatments based on maxillomandibular advancement procedures in adult patients with obstructive sleep apnoea: A systematic review and network meta-analysis. *European Archives of Otorhinolaryngology, 278*(2), 543–555.

Zigmond, A. S., & Snaith, R. P. (1983). The hospital anxiety and depression scale. *Acta Psychiatrica Scandinavica, 67*(6), 361–370.

Zinchuk, A. V., Gentry, M. J., Concato, J., & Yaggi, H. K. (2017). Phenotypes in obstructive sleep apnea: A definition, examples and evolution of approaches. *Sleep Medicine Reviews, 35*, 113–123.

CHAPTER

36 Narcolepsies and Other Central Hypersomnolence Disorders

Yves Dauvilliers *and* Lucie Barateau

Abstract

Central hypersomnolence disorders correspond to numerous etiologies of patients with a complaint of excessive daytime sleepiness, excessive quantity of sleep (i.e., hypersomnia), or sleep inertia (i.e., alteration in vigilance following waking up). Hypersomnolence significantly interferes with several aspects of life, including negative social and professional impacts. Several steps of evaluation of these patients are required to explore sleep, sleepiness, and hypersomnia; to quantify the severity of the condition; and to achieve a diagnosis of central hypersomnolence disorder. Hence, clinical interviews, questionnaires, sleep diaries, polysomnography, the Multiple Sleep Latency Test, the Maintenance of Wakefulness Test, continuous 24-hour polysomnography recording, and additional tests in particular circumstances (measurement of hypocretin-1 in cerebrospinal fluid, HLA DQB1*06:02 genotyping, and brain magnetic resonance imaging) allow the definitive diagnosis of central hypersomnolence disorders. This chapter details the clinical signs, laboratory investigations, pathophysiology, management, and some perspectives on most etiologies of central hypersomnolence disorder as reported in the revised *International Classification of Sleep Disorders*, third edition: narcolepsy Type I and Type II; idiopathic hypersomnia; Kleine-Levin syndrome; insufficient sleep syndrome; and hypersomnia due to a medical disorder, due to a medication or substance, or associated with a psychiatric disorder.

Key Words: narcolepsy, idiopathic hypersomnia, cataplexy, MSLT, sleep onset, REM period, depression

Introduction

Sleepiness, defined as the propensity to enter in sleep, is a normal behavioral and physiological state after a prolonged wakefulness period. However, excessive daytime sleepiness (EDS) is pathological and defined as the propensity to fall asleep at inappropriate times. However, where is the limit? EDS is also a common symptom in the general population and is one of the primary symptoms of sleep disorders but is not a disease per se (Pérez-Carbonell et al., 2022). EDS may correspond to several phenotypes with unplanned daytime naps that could be irresistible or not, short or long, refreshing or not, according to the underlying etiology. EDS may also vary in severity, from the inability to stay awake in monotonous situations to unwanted naps during active conditions with a semiautomatic continuation of behavior consequence. Some subjects may also sleep all night and day without any feeling of restoration, with sleep inertia symptoms during their rare waking episodes.

Many epidemiological studies have been performed on the prevalence of EDS in the general population (Bixler et al., 2005; Lugaresi et al., 1983; Ohayon et al., 2002; Perez-Carbonell et al., 2022). Globally, the prevalence varies from 4% to 20%, with huge variabilities between studies due to differences in populations, age, sex, associated conditions, and study design. Hence, the endpoint of studies may rely on a response to a simple yes/no question or use a frequency of EDS per week or a questionnaire. Based on a large volume of literature, severe EDS affects 5% of the general population, and 10%–15% suffer from moderate EDS. However, the absence of a consistent definition of EDS results in an unacceptable variability for proper prevalence, related to these various associated factors. Unlike insomnia symptoms, EDS has not been sex-related in many studies except in the elderly, where there is a higher prevalence for men, probably related to sleep apnea syndromes (Hays et al., 1996; Tsuno et al., 2007). We can also observe important variations between countries (Ohayon et al., 2002).

An excessive quantity of sleep and sleep inertia are other sleep symptoms frequently associated with EDS. The frequency of an excessive duration of nighttime sleep (often defined as >9 hours) is 8.4% in the general population, with a higher prevalence in women than in men (9.2% vs. 7.6%) and with a large age effect (decreasing until 65 years old and increasing thereafter; Ohayon et al., 2012, 2013). Excessive nighttime sleep is associated with significant daytime consequences in 1.6% of those studied. Sleep inertia is defined by major difficulties in waking up in the morning or after a nap with frequent re-entries into sleep, reduced vigilance, and impaired performance, lasting from a few minutes to hours, with "sleep drunkenness" being its extreme manifestation. Due to the lack of a standardized definition of sleep inertia, there is no robust data on its prevalence. However, a large study reported a non-restorative prolonged sleep episode in 1.2% of the general population (Ohayon et al., 2013).

Hypersomnolence has serious impacts on work performance and quality of life and is associated with increased accidents at work or while driving. Few studies have reported that hypersomnolence affects work activities and social and/or marital life and exhibits a negative socioeconomic impact (Ohayon et al., 1997). Cognitive function impairments such as memory alterations and difficulties in learning tasks were also frequently reported in patients with EDS, with an established relationship between memory performance and sleep restriction per se (Foley et al., 2001; Ohayon et al., 1997). The impact of EDS was amplified for night-shift workers (including medical residents), with the poorest job performance occurring during the night shift. Hence, night-shift workers, being frequently sleepy subpopulations, have a significantly higher chance of industrial and medical accidents during the night and following sleep deprivation.

Several studies revealed that 3% to 6% of drivers reported being regularly sleepy at the wheel, with a higher rate of traffic accidents for these subjects (Masa et al., 2000).

The risk of a motor vehicle crash is at least twice as high in the population with severe or moderate daytime sleepiness than in the population without. The highest rate of car accidents occurs in the early morning hours, a time associated with the greatest level of estimated EDS.

We estimated the risk of mortality for EDS in community-dwelling elderly and established, after several adjustments, that EDS was associated with a significant 33% increased risk of mortality (95% confidence interval [CI; 1.13, 1.61]; Empana et al., 2009). Therefore, at least in the elderly, EDS might be independently associated with both total and cardiovascular mortality. Other studies have reported that long sleep durations were related to increased mortality (Rockwood et al., 2001). A large Finnish cohort with a 22-year follow-up of subjects categorized as short (<7 hours), average, or long (>8 hours) sleepers confirmed such associations between extreme sleepers and higher risk of mortality (Hublin et al., 2007).

Although poor nocturnal sleep could be suspected as an etiology of EDS, it is frequently the cardinal symptom of many sleep disorders, as reported in the current *International Classification of Sleep Disorders*, third edition (ICSD-3; American Academy of Sleep Medicine [AASM], 2014). Central disorders of hypersomnolence are defined by a persistent complaint of EDS occurring every day for at least 3 months (AASM, 2005; Dauvilliers, 2006). In recent years, sleep medicine has benefited from the impact of research on hypersomnolence (especially medications) and is now developing as a field particularly in industrialized countries. Nevertheless, hypersomnolence continues to be insufficiently recognized.

The approach we propose in this chapter is, first, to detail how to evaluate patients with central hypersomnolence and, second, to describe hypersomnolence syndromes under several headlines: narcolepsy Type 1 and Type 2; idiopathic hypersomnia (IH); Kleine-Levin syndrome; insufficient sleep syndrome; and hypersomnia due to a medical disorder, due to a medication or substance, or associated with a psychiatric disorder.

Evaluation of Hypersomnolence

Several steps of evaluation are required to achieve a final diagnosis of central hypersomnolence disorder.

Clinical Evaluation

The physician's first step is to thoroughly interview the patient and bed partner (often useful since many problems are denied or over-reported by patients) to determine sleep habits and sleep hygiene, to differentiate EDS and fatigue, and to obtain detailed information on sleep quantity and sleep quality including the duration and quality of the nocturnal sleep period, the number and duration of daytime naps, the refreshing characteristics of those sleep episodes, and the method of awakening (Dauvilliers & Billiard, 2006; Shen et al., 2006). We would emphasize that differentiating EDS and fatigue, even though sometimes difficult, is always necessary for the evaluation. EDS as previously reported is defined by an urge to sleep, with an aggravation by rest and with an improvement by sleep. In contrast to EDS, fatigue fails to lead to rapid onset of sleep during daytime naps. Fatigue is also a prevalent complex phenomenon characterized by impairment in concentration and memory, lack of motivation, and an impression of low energy, with all such conditions partially improved by rest. As acute fatigue frequently occurs in healthy subjects under certain conditions, only chronic fatigue is considered a pathological symptom. Chronic fatigue is commonly reported in patients affected with insomnia, with a wide range of medical and psychiatric disorders, but may also coexist with EDS in particular conditions.

The age at onset of EDS, the existence of circumstances at its onset (e.g., a psychological factor, infectious trigger, vaccination), and factors that led to exacerbation or improvement of symptoms need to be reviewed. The severity of the condition helps in differentiating the etiology of hypersomnia. Several self-questionnaires may be used to quantify the severity of the complaint, such as the well-known Epworth Sleepiness Scale (a score >10 indicates a complaint of EDS; Johns, 1991), the Stanford Sleepiness Scale (Hoddes et al., 1973), the Karolinska Sleepiness Scale (Akerstedt & Gillberg, 1990; evaluates EDS at one moment), and/or visual analog scales.

Once the complaint of EDS is detailed, questions about daily sleep–wake schedules (including the usual bedtime and estimated time to sleep onset and offset), the presence or absence of cataplexy, hypnagogic or hypnopompic hallucinations, sleep paralysis, automatic behaviors (that occur when a patient performs routine activities and fights against EDS), snoring, nocturia, headache, discomfort of the extremities during periods of inactivity, and/or repetitive nocturnal agitation need to be considered systematically (Dauvilliers & Billiard, 2006; Guilleminault & Brooks, 2001). Finally, both current and past medication use and other substance intake as well as a psychiatric assessment are of major interest in a context of hypersomnolence.

Objective Assessment

Objective measures of EDS involve polysomnographic (PSG) techniques (recording of electroencephalogram, electro-oculogram, electromyogram, electrocardiogram, leg movements, and/or respiratory parameters) during nocturnal sleep and the Multiple Sleep Latency Test (MSLT) during the day.

The MSLT consists of five nap opportunities, scheduled at 2-hour intervals, starting 1.5 to 3 hours after awakening (Carskadon et al., 1986). Subjects need to discontinue psychotropic medications at least 2 weeks (depending on the half-life) before the date of the test. Subjects are asked to lie in a quiet, darkened, comfortable bedroom during the test and are instructed not to resist sleep. Each test is terminated after a 15-minute sleep period, or after 20 minutes if the patient does not fall asleep. According to standardized guidelines, the MSLT is the best scientifically validated objective test to detect and quantify the level of EDS in several clinical conditions but also in normal subjects under sleep restriction (Arand et al., 2005; Benbadis et al., 1999). The variables of interest are sleep latency and rapid-eye-movement (REM) sleep latency. When sleep latency is below 8 minutes, it indicates EDS, while it is considered normal if sleep occurs after 10 minutes, with caution for interpretation in between, depending on the clinical status of the patients (AASM, 2005; Billiard & Dauvilliers, 2001). REM latencies below 15 minutes may also be pathological, indicating the presence of sleep-onset REM periods (SOREMP). The presence of at least two SOREMPs on the MSLT, although not highly specific and sensitive, is generally considered to be abnormal and indicative of narcolepsy as the cause of hypersomnolence (American Academy of Sleep Medicine, 2005; see Figure 36.1).

Another test to evaluated EDS/wakefulness is the Maintenance of Wakefulness Test (MWT; Arand et al., 2005). The patient is seated comfortably in bed, with low lighting placed behind with instructions to try to stay awake. During four daytime 40-minute sessions, the patient is asked to stay awake for as long as possible (Arand et al., 2005; Doghramji et al., 1997). The test ends after one epoch (>15 seconds) of any stage of sleep, indicating an insufficient ability to fight against sleep. A mean sleep latency at 30.4 ± 11.2 minutes for normal controls and latency below 19 minutes (limit of 95% CI) is considered abnormal (Arand et al., 2005; Doghramji et al., 1997). The MWT is rarely used as a real test of sleepiness but rather to measure the effectiveness of treatment, especially for research or legal purposes, particularly in cases of driver's license suspension.

Despite normative values for the MSLT and MWT, the interpretation of results from these tests is not absolute, and they correlate poorly with self-reported measures (e.g., Epworth Sleepiness Scale). Therefore, the interpretation of these tests should always be undertaken in the clinical context, with additional investigations sometimes required depending on the particular clinical suspicion.

Several psychomotor tests, based on reaction time such as the Psychomotor Vigilance Task (PVT) and the Oxford Sleep Resistance Test (OSLER), are sometimes used to evaluate performance decrements due to EDS/errors in vigilance (Dinges & Kribbs, 1991). The PVT is a 5- or 10-minute reaction time task in which the subject has to press a button as rapidly as possible whenever a stimulus appears in the window of the device. This test quantifies the response latency in milliseconds to the stimulus, with such data being validated against other tests such as the MSLT in normal controls and sleep-deprived volunteers. The OSLER test consists of four 40-minute-long trials during which there are multiple light-emitting diode signal presentations. The subject needs to respond to each signal with a simple button press. The trials are ended after 40 minutes or after a failure response, meaning a failure to maintain wakefulness. The application of such tools and tests helps to evaluate fatigue, sleepiness, and vigilance; but normative data is limited, except for the PVT, so above all they cannot be proposed for the assessment of the etiology of chronic hypersomnia.

A continuous PSG recording for at least 24 hours on an ad libitum sleep–wake protocol would be necessary to confirm an excessively long nocturnal sleep, especially in the

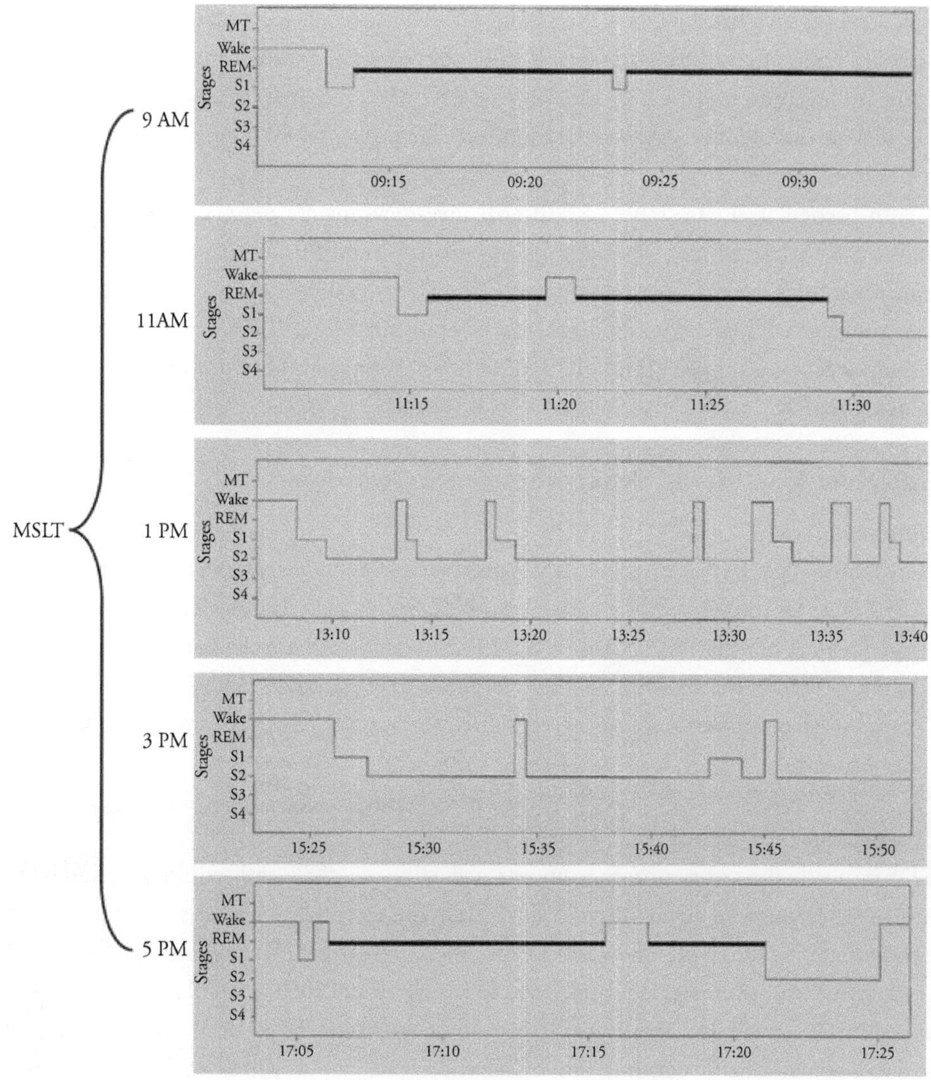

Figure 36.1 Multiple Sleep Latency Test in a patient affected with narcolepsy type 1

Note. Latencies to sleep onset are between 2 and 5 minutes, with three sleep-onset REM periods noted. MSLT = Multiple Sleep Latency Test; REM = rapid eye movement. Reprinted, with permission, from Figure 31.3. Billiard, M., & Dauvilliers, Y. Narcolepsy. In M. Billiard (Ed.), *Sleep, physiology, investigations and medicine* (pp. 403–428), Springer Nature.

case of IH. Such a continuous PSG recording allows for the documentation of a major sleep episode at night (more than 10 hours) and a daytime sleep episode (at least one nap of more than 1 hour), but this procedure still requires standardization and validation before being used routinely (Evangelista et al., 2018, 2021). Actigraphy may also be useful in assessing extended nocturnal sleep in patients with hypersomnolence, when applied in ambulatory care over long periods and under natural conditions. However, despite being well accepted and less expensive than PSG, actigraphy may overestimate sleep and underestimate wakefulness during the day. Finally, sleep inertia, another important hypersomnolence symptom, may be quantified by the PVT (Evangelista et al., 2022). Indeed, this test may be useful for the characterization, management, and follow-up of sleep inertia in patients with IH.

In particular circumstances, additional investigations are necessary to ascertain the etiology of hypersomnia, especially in atypical cases and/or suspicion of hypersomnia associated with neurological conditions (Dauvilliers, 2006). These tests comprise the measurement of hypocretin-1 (Hcrt-1) in cerebrospinal fluid (CSF), the presence of the human leukocyte antigen (HLA) DQB1*06:02 genotype, and brain magnetic resonance imaging (MRI).

Etiologies for Chronic Hypersomnolence Disorders

Narcolepsy Type I

Narcolepsy Type 1 (NT1), previously named *narcolepsy with cataplexy*, is a rare neurological disorder (0.026% of the general population) characterized by EDS and cataplexy (Dauvilliers et al., 2007; Ohayon et al., 2002). Narcolepsy affects teenagers and young adults and persists throughout the lifetime (Barateau et al., 2022; Dauvilliers et al., 2001). Symptoms may get worse following their first occurrence, but they may also improve in older patients.

CLINICAL CHARACTERISTICS

EDS is usually the first symptom to appear, occurring mainly in early adulthood, and is the most severe symptom (Dauvilliers et al., 2001). The essential characteristics of such sleep episodes are that they are often irresistible, short (less than 15–20 minutes), frequently associated with dreaming, refreshing, and followed by a normal wakeful state (Dauvilliers et al., 2007). Severe sleepiness can also lead to unconscious micro-sleep episodes or lapses and to a semiautomatic continuation of behavior, with inappropriate words in a conversation or continuing to act somewhat automatically but out-of-topic, commonly known as *automatic behaviors*.

Cataplexy is a sudden loss of voluntary muscular tone, without any alteration of consciousness, triggered by strong emotive reactions such as laughter, repartee, and surprise but almost never stress, fear, or physical effort (Dauvilliers et al., 2007, 2014). Cataplexy is specific to narcolepsy and is the best diagnostic marker for the NT1 disease. The clinician should inquire specifically about incomplete forms of cataplexy (limited to facial muscles or to the upper or lower limbs, with dysarthria, facial flickering, head dropping, or unlocking of the knees) since the patient does not necessarily perceive them as pathological. The duration of cataplexy varies from a second to less than 2 minutes. Its frequency varies from fewer than one episode per year to several episodes per day. Cataplexy worsens with poor sleep and fatigue.

Disrupted nocturnal sleep (DNS) is the third most common symptom in NT1, after EDS and cataplexy, ranging from 30% to 95%, depending on the definition. A few years ago, international experts characterized DNS clinically and by PSG and found that patients' descriptions and PSG characterizations are different from the typical features of insomnia (Maski et al., 2022). Patients experience fragmented nocturnal sleep and instability of both wake and sleep, with inappropriate and sudden shifts between these states.

Sleep paralysis is characterized by an inability to move the limbs or the head either at sleep onset or upon awakening. Dreamlike auditory, visual, or tactile hallucinations occurring at sleep onset (hypnagogic) or upon awakening (hypnopompic) may also suggest narcolepsy. Sleep-related hallucinations and sleep paralysis are not specific to narcolepsy, being reported at least once by 20% of the general population (Ohayon, 2000); but they are more severe and more frequently reported in over 50% of patients with narcolepsy.

The severity of symptoms of narcolepsy may be assessed by validated self-report questionnaires to monitor and optimize disease management (Dauvilliers et al., 2017). Several other features (e.g., a higher body mass index, parasomnias including sleep talking, and REM sleep behavior disorder) may be observed in narcolepsy but are of less diagnostic value (Dauvilliers et al., 2007; Kotagal et al., 2004).

Finally, depression and altered quality of life are reported in up to 50% of cases (Dauvilliers et al., 2009). A recent case–control study reported that depression, depressive symptoms, suicidal thoughts, and suicide risk were frequent in patients with NT1, especially those without treatment, and were associated with NT1 severity. Depressive symptoms and suicidal thoughts improved after NT1 management (Barateau et al., 2020). Based on a large observational French study of central disorders of hypersomnolence, including narcolepsy with cataplexy, without cataplexy, and IH, we previously confirmed a high frequency of depressive symptoms and the major impact of central hypersomnias on health-related quality of life, especially in patients with cataplexy (Dauvilliers et al., 2009). The high frequency of depressive symptoms supports the hypothesis of an endogenous depression, and narcolepsy shares with major depression a reduced nighttime REM sleep latency and increased REM sleep pressure and sleep fragmentation.

OBJECTIVE ASSESSMENT

The diagnosis of narcolepsy with cataplexy requires a clinical assessment and nocturnal PSG recording followed by an MSLT. The aim of the nighttime PSG is to eliminate other causes of daytime sleepiness and to assess for the presence of sufficient sleep (at least 6 hours) before the MSLT. The MSLT should document a mean sleep onset latency of less than 8 minutes and two or more sleep-onset REM periods (SOREMPs). A SOREMP (within 15 minutes of sleep onset) during the previous nocturnal PSG can replace one of the SOREMPs on the MSLT (Figure 36.1). Alternatively, CSF Hcrt-1 levels <110 pg/ml or one-third of mean normal control values are proposed as a highly specific (and definitive) and sensitive criterion in sporadic cases with clear-cut cataplexy (Box 36.1).

Box 36.1 Diagnostic Criteria for Narcolepsy Type 1: A and B

A. The patient experiences daily episodes of an irresistible need to sleep or sleep attacks for at least 3 months.
B. The presence of one or two of the following elements:
   - Well-defined cataplexy and a mean sleep latency of ≤8 minutes and at least two sleep-onset rapid-eye-movement periods (SOREMPs) on a Multiple Sleep Latency Test (MSLT) performed according to standardized technique. A SOREMP (within 15 minutes of sleep onset) during the previous nocturnal polysomnography can replace one of the SOREMPs on the MSLT.
   - Hypocretin-1 level in the cerebrospinal fluid ≤110 pg/ml or <1/3 of the average values obtained in normal subjects with the same standardized immunoreactivity assay.

Note. From American Academy of Sleep Medicine (2014).

Hcrt-1 levels must be determined in duplicate by direct I^{125} radioimmunoassay (Phoenix Pharmaceuticals, Belmont, CA), then all values back-referenced to the Stanford reference samples (Stanford University Center for Narcolepsy, Palo Alto, CA). CSF Hcrt-1 levels ≤110 pg/ml are considered low, those between 110 and 200 pg/ml intermediate, and those >200 pg/ml normal. All patients with low CSF Hcrt-1 levels are considered NT1 patients, even if they report no cataplexy (around 10%–20% of cases; Figure 36.2).

The diagnosis of narcolepsy is reinforced by the presence of the HLA DQB1*06:02 alleles, found in 92% to 97% of Caucasian narcoleptics and only 20% of the general population; however, the HLA typing was removed in the ICSD-3 from the diagnostic criteria of NT1 (see Figure 36.2).

PHYSIOPATHOLOGY

Recent insights in pathophysiology have demonstrated that NT1 is due to the loss of hypocretin/orexin neurons. Hcrt-1 and -2 are neurotransmitters exclusively synthesized by a population of neurons in the hypothalamus (60,000–80,000 neurons in humans; Dauvilliers et al., 2007; Peyron et al., 2000). These neurons are active during wakefulness and stimulate hypocretin receptors 1 and 2 located in some brain areas: the cortex, thalamus, hypothalamus, and brainstem, producing norepinephrine, dopamine, serotonin, and histamine, allowing for the maintenance of vigilance. Earlier findings in animal models revealed that deficient hypocretin transmission causes narcolepsy, with a mutation of the gene coding Hcrt receptor 2 present in the canine narcolepsy model (Lin et al., 1999). Only one mutation of the gene coding for preprohypocretin has been reported in one atypical and severe case of human narcolepsy (Peyron et al., 2000). The loss of hypocretin/orexin neurons in humans induces sleepiness, instability of wakefulness and sleep states, and cataplexy where positive emotions relayed through the amygdala and prefrontal cortex activate circuits in the dorsal part of the pontine tegmentum that

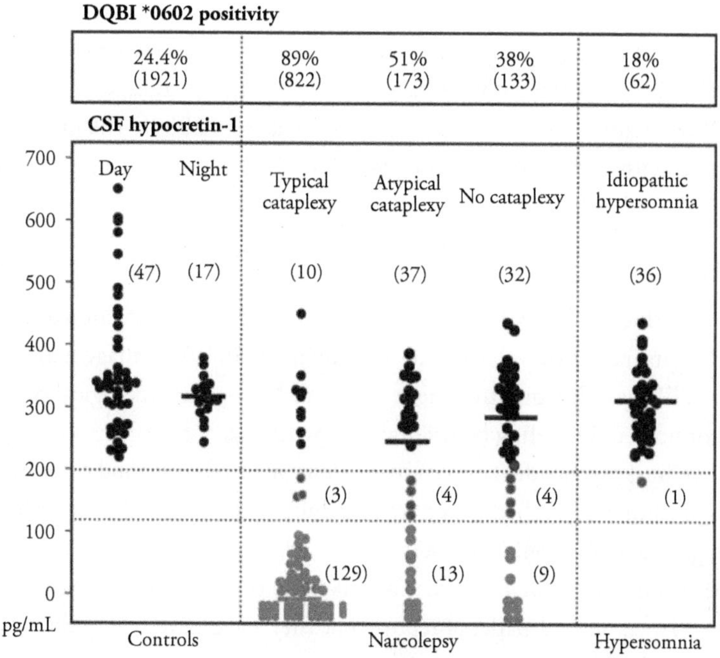

Figure 36.2 HLA DQB1*06:02 positivity and cerebrospinal fluid (CSF) hypocretin-1 levels among narcolepsy subjects with and without cataplexy or idiopathic hypersomnia and controls

Note. Each point represents the concentration of CSF hypocretin-1 in a subject. The cutoffs for normal (>200 pg/ml) and low (<110 pg/ml) hypocretin-1 levels. Median values are shown as a horizontal bar for each group. The percentage of HLA DQB1*06:02 positivity and the total number of subjects with CSF hypocretin-1 levels are noted for each condition. HLA DQB1*06:02 positivity is high in narcoleptics with typical cataplexy and slightly increased in narcoleptics with atypical cataplexy. CSF hypocretin-1 levels are undetectable in most narcoleptic with cataplexy subjects, while the values are clearly higher in other conditions. Reprinted, with permission, Fig. 3. Dauvilliers, Y., Arnulf, I., & Mignot, E. (2007). Narcolepsy with cataplexy. *Lancet, 369*(9560), 499–511.

are responsible for the loss of muscle tone. The exact cause of this neuronal loss is still unknown, but an autoimmune hypothesis is strongly suspected, involving genetic and environmental factors. A familial form of narcolepsy with cataplexy is observed in only 2%–5% of cases (Mignot et al., 2001). More than 95% of patients with NT1 carry the HLA DQB1*06:02 allele, a major histocompatibility complex Class II allele, compared to 25% of the general population. Other genes involved in the immune response are also associated with narcolepsy, such as the gene encoding the alpha chain of the T cell receptor. Studies have shown a link between NT1 and infection with the H1N1 influenza virus, as well as a vaccine against this virus (Pandemrix®), widely used in Europe during the 2009 pandemic (Sarkanen et al., 2018). The autoimmune or inflammatory process is probably transient and focal, which would explain why no antibodies have been discovered. However, recently, hypocretin-specific $CD4^+$ lymphocytes have been detected in the blood of NT1 patients (Latorre et al., 2018; Luo et al., 2018).

NT1 may rarely present as part of other medical conditions: brain lesions caused by tumor, multiple sclerosis, encephalitis, cerebral ischemia, head trauma, and neurodegeneration located in the posterior hypothalamus, the mesencephalon, and the pons (Arnulf et al., 2002; Baumann et al., 2007; Nishino & Kanbayashi, 2005). The medical condition produces narcolepsy with cataplexy and low CSF Hcrt-1 levels to confirm the diagnosis (ICSD-3; AASM, 2014).

MANAGEMENT

The current treatment of narcolepsy is only symptomatic, despite recent major advances in understanding its mechanisms (Barateau & Dauvilliers, 2019). Management strategies are codified in NT1, with lifelong treatment required. Non-pharmacological strategies must always be considered, including behavioral and psychosocial treatment strategies (Bassetti et al., 2021). Thus, psychoeducation of the patient, maintaining good sleep hygiene, with a regular nighttime sleep schedule, short scheduled naps across the day, physical activity, and weight control, should be systematically added to the pharmacological interventions. Patients can learn to predict situations likely to trigger cataplexy attacks and behave accordingly. Hence, several patients report that they have fewer cataplectic attacks after they have learned to better control their emotional response. Joining a patient organization is a source of exchange and support and promotes better disease acceptance and treatment adherence. Among medication options, a single drug can target several symptoms, or multiple medications may be used to treat each specific symptom. Considering the unique pathophysiology of NT1, Hcrt replacement therapy is the most interesting alternative in the future, and Hcrt receptor-2 agonists are very promising candidates to treat narcolepsy (Evans et al., 2022). A third possibility would be to prevent the destruction of Hcrt neurons by immunomodulatory agents, at the onset of NT1, to modify its clinical course. However, attempts to use such therapies on uncontrolled case studies, and with small numbers of patients, have shown often disappointing results.

Symptomatic treatments are the main recommended strategy, with a good evidence level (level A): psychostimulants to manage EDS, antidepressant agents for cataplexy, and sodium oxybate for both symptoms (Barateau et al., 2022). This last drug can also improve disrupted nocturnal sleep. The European Medicines Agency and the US Food and Drug Administration have approved most of these drugs (i.e., psychostimulants and sodium oxybate), but others are used off-label, based on their recognized utility by expert consensus, for example, antidepressant agents for cataplexy. Recent reviews have provided the details of recommended management strategies in narcolepsy: European Sleep Research Society and American Academy of Sleep Medicine guidelines (Bassetti et al., 2021; Maski et al., 2021). First-line medications should be wake-promoting agents/psychostimulants such as modafinil, armodafinil (not available in Europe), pitolisant, solriamfetol, or sodium oxybate. Modafinil and armodafinil increase the extracellular concentration of dopamine by blocking its transporter. Pitolisant is a wake-promoting agent that activates histamine neurons, acting as a selective histamine H3 receptor inverse agonist. Solriamfetol is a phenylalanine derivative with dopaminergic and noradrenergic activity. Oxybate stimulates gamma-aminobutyric acid (GABA) B receptors, modulating effects on GABAergic, noradrenergic, and dopaminergic neurons, as well as on thalamocortical neurons. This drug is taken at night and promotes slow-wave sleep, so it also has an effect on nocturnal sleep, cataplexy and EDS, with a maximum effect on these two last symptoms after a few weeks. A second-line medication is methylphenidate, but this has a low level of evidence; and amphetamines are third-line therapy for EDS because of their potential risk of abuse and serious psychiatric and cardiovascular adverse effects. To manage cataplexy, sodium oxybate and pitolisant are the first-line strategies. Antidepressants (selective serotonin and dual serotonin and noradrenalin reuptake inhibitors) are widely used, are very efficient, and have few side effects; but this is based on expert consensus only because randomized controlled trials are lacking. Drugs with efficacy for cataplexy also reduce hypnagogic hallucinations and sleep paralysis. The treatment of disturbed nocturnal sleep can be managed with sodium oxybate, showing a clear reduction in the number of nighttime awakenings with increased slow-wave sleep, making this drug a first-line treatment for narcoleptic patients with disturbed nighttime sleep. Recently, different compositions of sodium oxybate (e.g., low-salt and long-acting formulations) have been developed to treat narcolepsy.

Narcolepsy Type 2

Narcolepsy type 2 (NT2), previously named *narcolepsy without cataplexy*, was initially considered a phenotypic variant of narcolepsy with cataplexy but is now separated as a different diagnostic entity in the ICSD-3 (AASM, 2014). The prevalence of NT2 when compared to NT1 is still a subject of controversy, initially considered at a ratio from 2–3 NT2 to 10 NT1 (Barateau et al., 2022; Dauvilliers et al., 2007); but more recent data argues for a considerably higher frequency of NT2 in the general population (Mignot et al., 2006).

CLINICAL CHARACTERISTICS

Apart from the presence of cataplexy, the clinical diagnostic criteria are similar to those of narcolepsy with cataplexy, with similar sleep episode characteristics and frequent associated REM abnormalities such as hypnagogic hallucinations and sleep paralysis (Dauvilliers et al., 2007; Box 36.2).

OBJECTIVE ASSESSMENT

PSG followed by the MSLT are required to confirm the diagnosis of NT2, reporting identical PSG and MSLT criteria as in NT1 (i.e., the presence of a mean sleep onset latency of <8 minutes and two or more SOREMPs; AASM, 2005). A SOREMP (within 15 minutes of sleep onset) during the previous nocturnal PSG can replace one of the SOREMPs on

Box 36.2 Diagnostic Criteria for Narcolepsy Type 2: A, B, C, D, and E Are Required

A. The patient experiences daily episodes of an irresistible need to sleep or sleep attacks for at least 3 months.
B. On a Multiple Sleep Latency Test (MSLT) performed according to standardized technique, the mean sleep latency is ≤8 minutes, and there are at least two sleep-onset rapid-eye-movement periods (SOREMPs). A SOREMP (within 15 minutes of sleep onset) during the previous nocturnal polysomnography can replace one of the SOREMPs on the MSLT.
C. There is no cataplexy.
D. Either the hypocretin-1 level in the cerebrospinal fluid has not been measured or the hypocretin-1 level measured by immunoreactivity is >110 pg/ml or >1/3 of the average values obtained in normal subjects with the same standardized assay.
E. The hypersomnolence or the results of the MSLT are not better explained by other causes such as sleep insufficiency, obstructive sleep apnea syndrome, delayed sleep phase, or the effect of medication or substances or their withdrawal.

Note. If cataplexy appears later or if hypocretin-1 levels measured subsequently are ≤110 pg/ml, the disorder should be reclassified as narcolepsy Type 1. From American Academy of Sleep Medicine (2014).

the MSLT. In addition, the hypersomnolence or the results of the MSLT in NT2 must not be better explained by other causes such as sleep insufficiency, obstructive sleep apnea syndrome, delayed sleep phase, or the effect of medication or substances or their withdrawal. In NT2, the association with HLA DQB1*06:02 is weaker (around 40%–50% of cases), and the CSF Hcrt-1 level is >110 pg/mL by definition (Figure 36.2).

PHYSIOPATHOLOGY

The pathophysiology of NT2 is unclear, with partial loss of hypocretin neurons in some cases and a low association with HLA DQB1*06:02 (Dauvilliers et al., 2007). There is no available natural model comparable to the narcoleptic–cataplectic dog. NT2 is a heterogeneous condition, and knowledge of its pathophysiology is limited.

NT2 can also occur as part of other medical conditions and in these cases is referred to as *symptomatic* or *secondary* narcolepsy. Cases of secondary narcolepsy have been reported in patients with brain lesions located in the posterior hypothalamus, the mesencephalon, and the pons (Nishino & Kanbayashi, 2005). Brain lesions may be caused by tumor, multiple sclerosis, encephalitis, cerebral ischemia, head trauma, and neurodegeneration (Arnulf et al., 2002; Baumann et al., 2007; Nishino & Kanbayashi, 2005). In NT2, the medical condition produces narcolepsy in the absence of cataplexy, with normal CSF Hcrt-1 levels.

MANAGEMENT

The management of EDS, fragmented nocturnal sleep, and REM sleep deregulation (hypnogogic hallucinations and sleep paralysis) in NT2 relies on the same strategy as in NT1.

IH

IH is an orphan disorder with an unknown prevalence but is probably rarer than NT1. For a long time, IH has been confused with narcolepsy, and it remains a relatively poorly defined condition due to the absence of specific symptoms such as cataplexy or sleep apnea (Aldrich, 1996). It is characterized by EDS, prolonged nighttime sleep duration, and sleep inertia. The age at onset varies from childhood to early adulthood (Bassetti & Aldrich, 1997; Billiard & Dauvilliers, 2001; Dauvilliers, Bogan, et al., 2022), and there is a female predominance. Family cases are frequent, in the range from 25% to 60%, without any clear mode of inheritance proposed.

CLINICAL CHARACTERISTICS

Patients complain of EDS, fewer irresistible sleep attacks than in narcolepsy but of longer duration, and non-refreshing naps (i.e., not restoring normal vigilance). In the former classification of sleep disorders, two clinical forms were distinguished: one with prolonged total sleep time (more than 11 hours per 24 hours) and one with normal total sleep time (between 6 and 11 hours per 24 hours; AASM, 2005). Nighttime sleep is always of good quality with excellent efficiency. It is sometimes difficult to differentiate the clinical form with prolonged sleep time from non-pathological "long sleepers." Prolonged sleep time does not improve sleepiness in this disorder, unlike in long sleepers. While it is important to screen for this disorder, it should not be overdiagnosed.

The diagnosis of IH requires a thorough clinical interview. Patients report daily excessive sleepiness and unwanted naps that are longer (more than 1 hour) and less irresistible than in narcolepsy and that are non-refreshing irrespective of their duration. Awakening after nighttime or daytime sleep is laborious, with frequent difficulties in reacting adequately to external stimuli upon awakening for up to 3 hours; that is the state referred to as *sleep drunkenness* or *sleep inertia*. Episodes of automatic behavior can occur during this drowsy state, especially in the morning, with frequent amnesia following these episodes (Dauvilliers, Bogan, et al., 2022). Associated REM abnormalities such as hypnagogic hallucinations and sleep paralysis are less frequent and less severe in IH patients compared to people with narcolepsy. An instrument (Idiopathic Hypersomnia Severity Scale) has been validated in IH specifically, opening a path to better assessment of symptoms, impact, and response to treatment (Dauvilliers et al., 2019).

The psychosocial and professional consequences of IH appear similar to those found in narcolepsy (Broughton et al., 1978; Dauvilliers et al., 2009). Depressive symptoms were noted in 15%–25% of patients with IH. Mood changes not qualifying for the diagnosis of affective disorder may precede or follow the onset of EDS and may evolve independently. Neurological and psychological evaluations are necessary and have to be normal to exclude differential diagnoses of other hypersomnolence disorders (ICSD-3; AASM, 2014; Box 36.3).

Box 36.3 Diagnostic Criteria for Idiopathic Hypersomnia: A, B, C, D, E, and F Are Required

A. The patient experiences daily episodes of an irresistible need to sleep or daytime sleep attacks for at least 3 months.
B. There is no cataplexy.
C. A standardized Multiple Sleep Latency Test (MSLT) shows fewer than two sleep-onset rapid-eye-movement (REM) periods (SOREMPs) or no SOREMPs if REM sleep latency on the preceding nocturnal polysomnography is ≤15 minutes.
D. The presence of at least one of the following:
   1. The MSLT shows a mean sleep latency of ≤8 minutes.
   2. The total sleep time over 24 hours is ≥660 minutes (usually 12–14 hours) on a 24-hour polysomnography (performed after correction of chronic sleep deprivation) or by wrist actigraphy with a sleep diary (averaged over a period of at least 7 days performed without sleep restriction).
E. Sleep insufficiency has been excluded (if necessary, by the absence of improvement of sleepiness after an adequate attempt of increased time in bed, preferably confirmed by at least 1 week of wrist actigraphy).
F. Hypersomnolence or MSLT findings are not better explained by the presence of other sleep disorders, other medical or psychiatric disorders, or the effects of medications or substances or their withdrawal.

Note. From American Academy of Sleep Medicine (2014).

OBJECTIVE ASSESSMENT

Diagnostic criteria are currently being reconsidered by experts. It is essential for the diagnosis (1) to eliminate any sleep deprivation and any other cause that may explain the phenotype (e.g., narcolepsy, periodic leg movement disorder, sleep apnea syndrome) and (2) to objectify the disorder using validated tests. PSG followed by MSLT is needed to assess objective EDS and to ascertain the diagnosis. PSG demonstrates normal sleep except for its prolonged duration in a subpopulation. Sleep efficiency is usually above 90%, with normal proportions of non-REM and REM sleep, and the micro-arousal index is <10/hour.

The MSLT typically demonstrates a mean sleep latency of less than 8 minutes with fewer than two SOREMPs (ICSD-3; AASM, 2014; Bassetti & Aldrich, 1997; Billiard & Dauvilliers, 2001). However, the MSLT procedure requires that the patient is woken up early. To evidence abnormally long sleeping hours, a continuous 24-hour to 48-hour PSG recording may be necessary to observe long nocturnal sleep (more than 10 hours asleep) and long daytime naps (more than 1 hour; Evangelista et al., 2018). An extended sleep time of more than 19 hours during a continuous 32-hour PSG ("bedrest protocol") is a better criterion in terms of specificity and sensitivity but is not part of the current classification criteria. If performed, brain imaging is normal. HLA genotyping is not useful, and hypocretin levels are normal in CSF (Figure 36.2). Brain computed tomographic scans and/or MRI are of interest in these conditions to exclude the possibility of hypersomnia associated with a neurological disorder (Dauvilliers, Bogan, et al., 2022).

The evolution of IH is still unknown, but as with NT2, some patients experience spontaneous improvement or even recovery, hence the importance of repeating tests during follow-up and occasionally trying to stop medication. Other patients may remain stable or change phenotype to NT2.

PHYSIOPATHOLOGY

The etiology of IH is currently unknown, and no biological biomarker has been discovered. There is no available natural model of IH.

MANAGEMENT

Non-pharmacologic approaches have a role in management of IH. Behavioral treatments and sleep hygiene could be also proposed but are of limited effect, especially in IH with long sleep time (Bassetti & Aldrich, 1997; Billiard & Dauvilliers, 2001). Naps are always long, non-restorative, and therefore non-useful for these patients, with the absence of the possibility of normal alertness for the rest of the day.

Management strategies have been largely derived from expert consensus, due to a lack of disease-specific assessments and the reliance on case series and rare randomized controlled studies. Guidelines recommend treatment with off-label medications. Modafinil, which was approved for IH until 2011 in Europe, is the most commonly used treatment and improved sleepiness in two recent randomized placebo-controlled trials. Same alerting agents are used to manage IH as in narcolepsy. Recently, low-sodium oxybate showed reduced daytime sleepiness and sleep inertia and improved daily functioning in a placebo-controlled, double-blind, randomized withdrawal study; this drug was approved in the United States for IH (Dauvilliers, Arnulf, et al., 2022). The choice of pharmacotherapy should be guided by symptom profile, age, comorbidities (e.g., depressive symptoms, cardiovascular problems), and concomitant medications (e.g., oral contraceptives; Arnulf et al., 2023). Further research on IH is needed to support treatment algorithms.

Kleine-Levin Syndrome

Kleine-Levin syndrome (KLS) is a rare condition affecting young people in their second decade of life, with an estimated prevalence of 2–5 cases per million. It is characterized by recurrent episodes of severe hypersomnia lasting 10 days on average, which can occur every 1–12 months. During these episodes, patients may sleep for up to 16 hours per day. They may also exhibit cognitive troubles, hyperphagia, or hypersexuality, as well as behavioral and psychiatric disturbances. Episodes are often triggered by factors such as infections, head trauma, or alcohol. The disorder affects young people (teenagers) and more males than females. The episodes are typically separated by weeks or months, during which normal sleep patterns are resumed (Arnulf et al., 2005, 2008; Dauvilliers et al., 2002).

The underlying pathophysiology of KLS remains unclear, but some studies suggest a primary hypothalamic dysfunction mediated by immune mechanisms. During episodes, functional brain imaging reveals abnormal metabolism with changes in several brain regions, including the thalamus, hypothalamus, mesial temporal, and frontal lobes. Although diagnostic criteria are only clinically defined, a 24-hour PSG test may reveal prolonged total sleep time during episodes.

The diagnosis of KLS therefore is primarily clinical, and differential diagnosis must distinguish recurrent hypersomnia from other etiologies of hypersomnolence, including obstructive sleep apnea syndrome or narcolepsy. In order to confirm hypersomnia and to exclude epilepsy and organic pathology, electroencephalographic and PSG recordings as well as brain MRI are required (Arnulf et al., 2008). The etiology of recurrent hypersomnia remains elusive, although most symptoms could be seen as a hypothalamic dysfunction (Lopez et al., 2015). Recent data also suggests links between KLS, circadian regulation, and bipolar disorder and indicates that the *TRANK1* polymorphisms in conjunction with reported birth difficulties may predispose to KLS (Ambati et al., 2021). Recurrent hypersomnia results in major disturbances in social and family life. The evolution throughout life is favorable in most cases, with a progressive disappearance of symptoms after 10 years' duration (Arnulf et al., 2008).

Treatment options for KLS are limited and mostly based on case reports or open-label trials. Stimulants such as modafinil may be used during an episode, but they can induce paradoxical agitation and are of limited efficacy. Prophylactic treatments with mood stabilizers (e.g., lithium carbonate) or antiepileptics (e.g., sodium valproate) may be effective at reducing the frequency and duration of episodes (Arnulf et al., 2005), but no randomized controlled trials have been performed to test such therapies. The prognosis is often good, with spontaneous resolution of symptoms after 10 years. As such, pharmacological management is not always necessary, especially when episodes are infrequent and do not have a major impact on the patient's social life. Resting in a safe and stress-free environment during an episode is advised.

Other "Central Disorders of Hypersomnolence"

Four other categories of central disorders of hypersomnolence are listed in the ICSD-3 (AASM, 2014).

Hypersomnia Due to a Medical Disorder

A medical condition may produce EDS in the absence of cataplexy and without any effect of treatment of the underlying condition (AASM, 2014). Sleep at night is often fragmented by frequent awakenings of variable duration. The MSLT is needed to differentiate objective EDS from fatigue and to document a mean sleep latency of less than 8 minutes and fewer than two SOREMPs. If the criteria for narcolepsy are met, the diagnosis becomes NT1 or NT2 due to a medical condition

A variety of neurological disorders including neurodegenerative affections (Alzheimer's disease, Parkinson's disease), stroke (in the thalamic or mesencephalic levels), encephalitis, and genetic disorders (Niemann-Pick type C, Norrie disease, Prader-Willi syndrome, myotonic dystrophy, etc.) may provoke hypersomnolence (Dauvilliers et al., 2007; Guilleminault et al., 1993; Laberge et al., 2009). In such associations, the main etiologies of chronic hypersomnolence need first to be excluded, such as sleep apnea syndromes, periodic leg movements, and the side effects of drugs (Pérez-Carbonell et al., 2022).

Post-traumatic hypersomnia is also frequently reported in a context of brain injury. It occurs mainly in cases of severe head trauma, with hypersomnia occurring 6 to 18 months after the trauma (Baumann et al., 2007; Guilleminault et al., 2000). EDS has been associated with variable degrees of other symptoms such as headaches, memory loss, and lack of concentration. The evolution of the disorder depends on the location and the extent of the initial lesions. In addition, other pain conditions such as neuropathic pain may be responsible for fragmented nighttime sleep resulting in EDS. A detailed medical history of the patient will clarify the cause of EDS.

In addition to neurological disorders, hypersomnolence may develop several months after many acute infections, including infectious mononucleosis, Guillain-Barré syndrome, pneumonia, hepatitis, or Whipple's disease (Guilleminault & Mondini, 1986). In that context, hypersomnolence frequently mimics IH symptoms. An encephalitic process and/or an elevation of inflammatory cytokines may play a pathogenic role in sleep/wake modifications. PSG examinations in infectious diseases are rare, except for the Gambian form of human African trypanosomiasis, which is due to the injection of trypanosomes by tsetse flies (Buguet et al., 2001). The latter parasitic disease is a frequent cause of severe hypersomnia in western Africa (*Trypanosoma brucei gambiense*) and eastern Africa (*Trypanosoma brucei rhodesiense*; Buguet et al., 2001). However, the possibility of trypanosomiasis needs to be assessed in travelers and individuals migrating from Africa with EDS who may export the disease to the Western world.

Finally, hypersomnolence associated with metabolic or endocrine disorders, such as diabetes, hepatic encephalopathy, hypothyroidism, and acromegaly, and even frequently associated with sleep-related breathing and periodic limb movement (PLM) disorders, is rarely reported.

Hypersomnia Due to a Medication or Substance or as a Result of Stimulant Withdrawal

Hypersomnolence secondary to sedative–hypnotic drug or stimulant withdrawal is easily recognized during a clinical interview. Numerous medications are potentially responsible for EDS, such as hypnotic, anxiolytic, antidepressant, neuroleptic, antihistaminic, antiepileptic (except for lamotrigine), and anti-parkinsonism drugs. Alcohol presents sedative or stimulant effects that depend on dosage and individual susceptibility (Drummond et al., 1998; Roehrs & Roth, 2001). Acute alcohol consumption may delay or contrarily advance sleep induction, with REM sleep postponed to the second half of the night and slow-wave sleep increased in the first half. Discontinuation of alcohol consumption is often reported to be followed by a REM sleep rebound and sometimes REM sleep without atonia. Patients with chronic alcohol use and abuse sleep poorly, with a reduced amount of REM sleep, and their sleep is composed almost exclusively of non-REM sleep.

The interview should eliminate such drug–sleep interactions. In the case of drug-induced hypersomnolence, a careful and progressive withdrawal and/or substitution must be undertaken. However, the relationship between the current use of drugs and the complaint of EDS is not always easy to ascertain (Dauvilliers, 2006). Dosing of drugs, drug–drug interactions, liver or renal impairments, and individual susceptibility may explain the large variability in the EDS phenotype. Diagnosis is clinical, but blood or urine drug screens may be of interest in particular cases.

Hypersomnia Associated With a Psychiatric Disorder

This broad entity, previously named *nonorganic hypersomnia condition* in the ICSD-II, refers to many etiologies associated with hypersomnia such as depressive disorder, seasonal affective disorder (SAD), abnormal personality traits, and conversion episodes.

In this case, the patient has a psychiatric condition, and the mean sleep latency on the MSLT is less than 8 minutes. If hypersomnolence complaint is frequent in the context of mood disorders, it is rarely confirmed objectively, and the sleep latency on the MSLT is often normal. Differentiating between psychiatric hypersomnolence and a central hypersomnolence disorder with comorbid psychiatric symptoms is a challenge for sleep specialists and psychiatrists. The current diagnostic tools are limited in this regard, and further research is necessary.

Patients affected with both psychiatric and sleep disorders mainly reported insomnia complaints (and fatigue) instead of EDS. In contrast, in particular patients, especially those with atypical depression, a complaint of EDS may be noted. The latter condition should be always considered as an important differential diagnosis of IH as patients may present with mood changes that do not qualify for the diagnosis of affective disorders (*Diagnostic and Statistical Manual of Mental Disorders*, fifth edition; American Psychiatric Association, 2013). In addition, patients may have had EDS before the appearance of mood changes, and clinical manifestations may evolve independently. EDS may also be a precursor, symptom, or adverse effect of depression. The complaint of EDS in that condition mainly mimics the sleepiness characteristics of IH with long sleep time, except that it may vary from day to day and is often associated with poor and fragmented sleep at night (Billiard et al., 1994; Nofzinger et al., 1991; Vgontzas et al., 2000). These patients may spend a large amount of time in bed and acknowledge much time resting but awake (clinophilia). Therefore, insomnia and EDS are frequently associated in this category.

Clinicians need to resolve both insomnia and EDS because of the risk of depression onset, worsening of depressive symptoms, and relapse of depression after response to antidepressant treatment.

Hypersomnolence associated with SAD is considered a clinical subtype of this category. SAD is characterized by the fall and winter recurrence of depressive episodes associated with hypersomnia, fatigue, loss of energy, carbohydrate craving, change in appetite, and weight gain, with remission of symptoms in spring and summer (Rosenthal et al., 1984). Sleep recordings of SAD patients confirm the presence of hypersomnolence and show reduced slow-wave sleep during symptomatic episodes. Many hypotheses exist regarding its pathogenic mechanisms, including circadian phase shifting, abnormal pineal melatonin secretion, and abnormal serotonin synthesis. Light therapy is a natural, noninvasive, effective method of treatment. Light therapy every morning for 14 days seems to be an effective treatment, with a significant mood improvement (57%), increased sleep efficiency, decreased sleep latency, decreased slow-wave sleep latency, and increased sleep spindles in the first hour of sleep (Ibatoullina et al., 1997). However, bright light treatment may be insufficient for the more severely ill patients.

PSG studies in hypersomnolence with mood disorders are rare. However, in most studies the MSLT failed to demonstrate short mean sleep latency when compared to normal controls, even though up to 25% of these patients may have abnormal MSLT results (Billiard et al., 1994; Nofzinger et al., 1991; Plante, 2017). In addition, REM sleep is often absent during daytime naps in depressed patients, and 24-hour continuous PSG has revealed a lower total sleep time, an excess of Stage 1 sleep, and a decrease of Stage 3 in patients with a complaint of hypersomnolence associated with mood disorder in comparison to IH patients (Billiard et al., 1994; Nofzinger et al., 1991). Hence, hypersomnia in patients with associated mood disorders is rarely objective, and therefore the daytime complaint appears more related to fatigue, lack of interest, and decreased energy inherent in the depressed condition rather than an increase in sleep propensity or REM sleep propensity.

Finally, chronic fatigue syndrome characterized by persistent or relapsing fatigue that does not resolve with sleep or rest may mimic symptoms of hypersomnolence (Prins et al., 2006; Shen et al., 2006). The subjective experience of "feeling tired" or "fatigued" is the main complaint in the clinical evaluation; however, patients also frequently report complaints of myalgia, anxiety, fever, headaches, and cognitive alterations, with a continuum with the fibromyalgia syndrome. Subjects affected with chronic fatigue preferred the sedentary situations. Chronic fatigue syndrome is not a cause of chronic hypersomnia but a differential diagnosis (Fukuda et al., 1994). However, as already reported, some patients and/or practitioners may have difficulties in clearly distinguishing excessive sleepiness from fatigue. PSG–MSLT studies in chronic fatigue syndrome show reduced sleep efficiency, may document alpha intrusion into the sleep electroencephalogram, and exclude abnormal mean sleep latency on the daytime sessions. There is no clear effective treatment option for chronic fatigue syndrome; however, cognitive behavioral therapy, exercise therapy, antidepressants, and alternative medicines are frequently proposed to manage that condition.

Insufficient Sleep Syndrome

The clinician should consider various differential diagnoses for hypersomnolence, and of these, insufficient sleep syndrome is the most significant. Behaviorally induced insufficient sleep syndrome is a disorder occurring in individuals who fail to obtain sufficient nocturnal sleep required to support normally alert wakefulness (AASM, 2014). Such individuals are chronically sleep-deprived of their own will, without necessarily being aware of it. Such a situation is increasing in our modern technologically inclined societies. As the sleep debt develops, the individual starts suffering from EDS in the afternoon, in the evening, or after meals. Patients typically report that they sleep 5–6 hours nightly on weekdays and 9 hours on the weekends. They have difficulty rising in the morning and sometimes experience sleep drunkenness–like episodes (Carskadon & Dement, 1981; Van Dongen et al., 2003). Work and cognitive performance may be impaired. The patient may also complain about increasing levels of subjective fatigue, mood deterioration, muscular pain, gastrointestinal unrest, and visual disturbances. Children may exhibit hyperactivity rather than sleepiness. Symptoms disappear on weekends and during the holidays. Sleep diaries and actigraphy may be helpful to precisely determine sleep–wake schedules with naps and to verify longer nighttime sleep on weekends (Dauvilliers, 2006). The diagnosis is generally made during the interview. However, in case of a suspected associated pathology, such as respiratory disturbances during sleep, a PSG recording may be indicated. In the case of insufficient sleep syndrome, this recording will show a good sleep efficiency (above 90%) and short sleep latency, indicative of a sleep rebound (AASM, 2014).

To accurately diagnose the patient, the clinician should determine the patient's sleep patterns during weekdays and weekends, through various means such as clinical interview, sleep logs, or actigraphy if necessary. Symptoms may resolve when total sleep time is extended during holidays or weekends, especially in individuals who are known to be long sleepers. However, these individuals may still be sleep-deprived. Shift workers may also experience excessive daytime sleepiness and sometimes have a phenotype similar to NT2. Other sleep disorders such as obstructive sleep apnea, PLM disorder, or circadian rhythm disorders (e.g., delayed sleep phase disorder) should also be ruled out to accurately diagnose the cause of EDS.

Finally, and as suggested above, hypersomnolence may also be observed in many other sleep and circadian disorders. Sleep-related breathing disorders are one of the most frequent etiologies of EDS, which may vary from falling asleep in relaxing situations to a major symptom responsible for car or work-related accidents (Young et al., 1993). Questioning patients and bed partners on associated symptoms such as loud snoring, obesity, headaches, hypertension, fatigue in the morning, nocturia, reduced libido, and witnessed episodes of apnea will provide information for the clinical suspicion of sleep-related breathing disorders. Movement disorders related to rest and sleep have been divided into two syndromes, restless legs syndrome and PLMs during sleep. PLMs are a common finding in various sleep disorders, such as restless legs syndrome, insomnia, narcolepsy, and sleep apnea syndrome, but also in physiological aging. Nocturnal sleep disturbances and/or complaints of EDS are frequently reported in these conditions. A clinical interview of patients and bed partners should address symptoms such as nocturnal agitation and discomfort of the extremities during periods of inactivity that are relieved with movement. PSG will confirm the presence of PLMs. However, the relationship between PLM disorder and EDS is subject to debate (Nicolas et al., 1998). Circadian rhythm sleep disorders may lead to insomnia but also to EDS or both (Wagner, 1996). In particular cases of shift workers, both insufficient sleep and circadian disruptions can lead to a frequent complaint of EDS. A thorough characterization of the daily schedule is always required in the determination of the etiology of chronic hypersomnia. A sleep diary may be helpful to precisely assess the regularity of the sleep–wake schedule.

Conclusions

Hypersomnolence as a symptom has been historically underrecognized, underappreciated, and understudied. Hypersomnolence disorders are associated with high expense and utilization of healthcare. The consequences of hypersomnolence on quality of life and socioeconomic burden are poorly acknowledged. The identification of phenotypes of hypersomnolence is useful and is required to classify patients into the different diagnostic categories as proposed in the ICSD-3. However, except for NT1, there is a lack of knowledge and understanding of the precise underlying neurobiological causes of hypersomnolence, and therefore an uncertainty as to whether these disorders, as we currently define them, are real disease entities. Recently, European experts have suggested a different approach, with a new consistent, complaint-driven, hierarchical classification for central disorders of hypersomnolence (Lammers et al., 2020).

There is a pressing need to identify biomarkers and to increase our understanding of the neurobiology of hypersomnolence to better diagnose and treat patients. However, due to the multiple dimensions of EDS resulting from the balance between the capacity to stay awake and the propensity to fall asleep, to date, there is no gold-standard measurement and no quantifiable biological marker of excessive sleepiness. Clinicians use several methods to explore sleep and wakefulness, to distinguish hypersomnia or sleepiness from fatigue, to confirm the existence of these symptoms, and to diagnose between the different etiologies of hypersomnolence. There is no doubt that progress has been made in the recognition of the different etiologies of hypersomnolence. However, a tendency to overdiagnose sleep disordered breathing, insufficient sleep syndrome, psychiatric-associated conditions, and drug use in patients with EDS still persists. As several of the other causes of chronic hypersomnolence are rare, insufficiently recognized, and poorly defined, especially for the IH condition, there is a need to further develop sleep laboratory investigations to assess the correct diagnosis of chronic hypersomnia.

Recent insights into pathophysiology have demonstrated that NT1 is caused by the early loss of hypothalamic neurons producing hypocretin, a wakefulness-associated neurotransmitter that can be measured in the CSF. A better understanding of the other causes of central hypersomnolence is also needed. Patients need to be diagnosed earlier and more effectively to optimize diagnosis and proposed personalized and precision medicine, at the pharmacological level but also with a global approach taking into account patients' educational, social, and professional needs.

Future Directions

- We need better gold-standard measurement and quantifiable biological markers of the different components of hypersomnolence: EDS, hypersomnia, and sleep inertia.
- We need to improve and revise the criteria used to diagnose central hypersomnolence disorders, to better define real disease categories, for both clinical and research purposes.
- The degree of individualization and overlap between the different central disorders of hypersomnolence, in terms of both pathophysiology and diagnostic features, should be further examined.
- We need to better understand the precise underlying neurobiological causes of central hypersomnolence disorders, other than NT1.
- Patients need to be diagnosed earlier and to receive rapid management with personalized and precision medicine.

References

Akerstedt, T., & Gillberg, M. (1990). Subjective and objective sleepiness in the active individual. *International Journal of Neurosciences, 52*(1–2), 29–37.

Aldrich, M. S. (1996). The clinical spectrum of narcolepsy and idiopathic hypersomnia. *Neurology, 46*, 393–401.

Ambati, A., Hillary, R., Leu-Semenescu, S., Ollila, H. M., Lin, L., During, E. H., Farber, N., Rico, T. J., Faraco, J., Leary, E., Goldstein-Piekarski, A. N., Huang, Y. S., Han, F., Sivan, Y., Lecendreux, M., Dodet, P., Honda, M., Gadoth, N., Nevsimalova, S., . . . Mignot, E. J. (2021). Kleine-Levin syndrome is associated with birth difficulties and genetic variants in the *TRANK1* gene loci. *Proceedings of the National Academy of Sciences of the United States of America, 118*(12), Article e2005753118. https://doi.org/10.1073/pnas.2005753118

American Academy of Sleep Medicine. (2005). *International classification of sleep disorders. Diagnostic and coding manual* (2nd ed.).

American Academy of Sleep Medicine. (2014). *International classification of sleep disorders* (3rd ed.).

American Psychiatric Association. (2013). *Diagnostic and statistical manual of mental disorders* (5th ed.).

Arand, D., Bonnet, M., Hurwitz, T., Mitler, M., Rosa, R., & Sangal, R. B. (2005). The clinical use of the MSLT and MWT. *Sleep, 28*(1), 123–144.

Arnulf, I., Konofal, E., Merino-Andreu, M., Houeto, J. L., Mesnage, V., Welter, M. L., . . . Agid, Y. (2002). Parkinson's disease and sleepiness: An integral part of PD. *Neurology, 58*, 1019–1024.

Arnulf, I., Lin, L., Gadoth, N., File, J., Lecendreux, M., Franco, P., . . . Mignot, E. (2008). Kleine-Levin syndrome: A systematic study of 108 patients. *Annals of Neurology, 63*(4), 482–493.

Arnulf, I., Rico, T. J., & Mignot, E. (2012). Diagnosis, disease course, and management of patients with Kleine-Levin syndrome. *Lancet Neurology, 11*, 918–928.

Arnulf, I., Thomas, R., Roy, A., & Dauvilliers, Y. (2023). Update on the treatment of idiopathic hypersomnia: Progress, challenges, and expert opinion. *Sleep Medicine Reviews, 69*, Article 101766.

Arnulf, I., Zeitzer, J. M., File, J., Farber, N., & Mignot, E. (2005). Kleine-Levin syndrome. A systematic review of 186 cases in the literature. *Brain, 128*(Pt. 12), 2763–2776.

Barateau, L., & Dauvilliers, Y. (2019). Recent advances in treatment for narcolepsy. *Therapeutic Advances in Neurological Disorders, 12*, Article 1756286419875622.

Barateau, L., Lopez, R., Chenini, S., Pesenti, C., Rassu, A. L., Jaussent, I., & Dauvilliers, Y. (2020). Depression and suicidal thoughts in untreated and treated narcolepsy: Systematic analysis. *Neurology, 95*(20), e2755–e2768.

Barateau, L., Pizza, F., Plazzi, G., & Dauvilliers, Y. (2022). Narcolepsy. *Journal of Sleep Research, 31*(4), Article e13631.

Bassetti, C., & Aldrich, M. S. (1997). Idiopathic hypersomnia. A series of 42 patients. *Brain, 120*, 1423–1435.

Bassetti, C. L. A., Kallweit, U., Vignatelli, L., Plazzi, G., Lecendreux, M., Baldin, E., Dolenc-Groselj, L., Jennum, P., Khatami, R., Manconi, M., Mayer, G., Partinen, M., Pollmächer, T., Reading, P., Santamaria, J., Sonka, K., Dauvilliers, Y., & Lammers, G. J. (2021). European guideline and expert statements on the management of narcolepsy in adults and children. *Journal of Sleep Research, 28*(9), 2815–2830. https://doi.org/10.1111/ene.14888

Baumann, C. R., Werth, E., Stocker, R., Ludwig, S., & Bassetti, C. L. (2007). Sleep–wake disturbances 6 months after traumatic brain injury: A prospective study. *Brain, 130*(Pt. 7), 1873–1883.

Benbadis, S. R., Mascha, E., Perry, M. C., Wolgamuth, B. R., Smolley, L. A., & Dinner, D. S. (1999). Association between the Epworth Sleepiness Scale and the Multiple Sleep Latency Test in a clinical population. *Annals of Internal Medicine, 130*(4, Pt. 1), 289–292.

Billiard, M., & Dauvilliers, Y. (2001). Idiopathic hypersomnia. *Sleep Medicine Reviews, 5*, 349–358.

Billiard, M., Dolenc, L., Aldaz, C., Ondze, B., & Besset, A. (1994). Hypersomnia associated with mood disorders. A new perspective. *Journal of Psychosomatic Research, 38*, 41–47.

Bixler, E. O., Vgontzas, A. N., Lin, H. M., Calhoun, S. L., Vela-Bueno, A., & Kales, A. (2005). Excessive daytime sleepiness in a general population sample: The role of sleep apnea, age, obesity, diabetes, and depression. *Journal of Clinical Endocrinology and Metabolism, 90*, 4510–4515.

Broughton, R., Nevsimalova, S., & Roth, B. (1978). The socioeconomic effects (including work, education, recreation and accidents) of idiopathic hypersomnia. *Sleep Research, 7*, 217.

Buguet, A., Bourdon, L., Bouteille, B., Cespuglio, R., Vincendeau, P., Radomski, M. W., & Dumas, M. (2001). The duality of sleeping sickness: Focusing on sleep. *Sleep Medicine Reviews, 5*, 139–153.

Carskadon, M. A., & Dement, W. C. (1981). Cumulative effects of sleep restriction on daytime sleepiness. *Psychophysiology, 18*, 107–113.

Carskadon, M. A., Mitler, M. M., & Roth, T. (1986). Guidelines for the Multiple Sleep Latency Test (MSLT): A standard measure of sleepiness. *Sleep, 9*, 519–524.

Dauvilliers, Y. (2006). Differential diagnosis in hypersomnia. *Current Neurology and Neuroscience Reports, 6*, 156–162.

Dauvilliers, Y., Arnulf, I., Foldvary-Schaefer, N., Morse, A. M., Šonka, K., Thorpy, M. J., Mignot, E., Chandler, P., Parvataneni, R., Black, J., Sterkel, A., Chen, D., Skobieranda, F., & Bogan, R. K. (2022). Safety and efficacy of lower-sodium oxybate in adults with idiopathic hypersomnia: A Phase 3, placebo-controlled, double-blind, randomised withdrawal study. *Lancet Neurology, 21*(1), 53–65.

Dauvilliers, Y., Arnulf, I., & Mignot, E. (2007). Narcolepsy with cataplexy. *Lancet, 369*(9560), 499–511.

Dauvilliers, Y., Beziat, S., Pesenti, C., Lopez, R., Barateau, L., Carlander, B., Luca, G., Tafti, M., Morin, C. M., Billiard, M., & Jaussent, I. (2017). Measurement of narcolepsy symptoms: The Narcolepsy Severity Scale. *Neurology, 88*(14), 1358–1365. https://doi.org/10.1212/WNL.0000000000003787

Dauvilliers, Y., & Billiard, M. (2006). Chronic hypersomnia. *Sleep Medicine Clinics, 1*, 79–88.

Dauvilliers, Y., Bogan, R. K., Arnulf, I., Scammell, T. E., St Louis, E. K., & Thorpy, M. J. (2022). Clinical considerations for the diagnosis of idiopathic hypersomnia. *Sleep Medicine Reviews, 66*, Article 101709.

Dauvilliers, Y., Evangelista, E., Barateau, L., Lopez, R., Chenini, S., Delbos, C., Beziat, S., & Jaussent, I. (2019). Measurement of symptoms in idiopathic hypersomnia: The Idiopathic Hypersomnia Severity Scale. *Neurology, 92*(15), e1754–e1762. https://doi.org/10.1212/WNL.0000000000007264
Dauvilliers, Y., Mayer, G., Lecendreux, M., Neidhart, E., Peraita-Adrados, R., Sonka, K., Billiard, M., &Tafti, M. (2002). Kleine-Levin syndrome: An autoimmune hypothesis based on clinical and genetic analyses. *Neurology, 59,* 1739–1745.
Dauvilliers, Y., Montplaisir, J., Molinari, N., Carlander, B., Ondze, B., Besset, A., & Billiard, M. (2001). Age at onset of narcolepsy in two large populations of patients in France and Quebec. *Neurology, 57*(11), 2029–2033.
Dauvilliers, Y. A., Paquereau, J., Bastuji, H., Drouot, X., Weil, J. S., & Viot-Blanc V. (2009). Psychological health in central hypersomnias: The French Harmony Study. *Journal of Neurology, Neurosurgery and Psychiatry, 80*(6), 636–641.
Dauvilliers, Y., Siegel, J. M., Lopez, R., Torontali, Z. A., & Peever, J. H. (2014). Cataplexy—Clinical aspects, pathophysiology and management strategy. *Nature Reviews Neurology, 10,* 386–395.
Dinges, D. F., & Kribbs, N. B. (1991). Performing while sleepy. Effects of experimentally induced sleepiness. In T. M. Monk (Ed.), *Sleep, sleepiness and performance* (pp. 97–128). Chichester, UK: John Wiley and Sons.
Doghramji, K., Mitler, M. M., Sangal, R. B., Shapiro, C., Taylor, S., Walsleben, J., . . . Youakim, J. M. (1997). A normative study of the Maintenance of Wakefulness Test (MWT). *Electroencephalography and Clinical Neurophysiology, 103*(5), 554–562.
Drummond, S. P., Gillin, J. C., Smith, T. L., & DeModena, A. (1998). The sleep of abstinent pure primary alcoholic patients. Natural course and relationship to relapse. *Alcoholism Clinical and Experimental Research, 22,* 1796–1802.
Empana, J. P., Dauvilliers, Y., Dartigues, J. F., Ritchie, K., Gariepy, J., Jouven, X., . . . Ducimetiere, P. (2009). Excessive daytime sleepiness is an independent risk indicator for cardiovascular mortality in community-dwelling elderly: The three city study. *Stroke, 40,* 1219–1224.
Evangelista, E., Lopez, R., Barateau, L., Chenini, S., Bosco, A., Jaussent, I., & Dauvilliers, Y. (2018). Alternative diagnostic criteria for idiopathic hypersomnia: A 32-hour protocol. *Annals of Neurology, 83,* 235–247.
Evangelista, E., Rassu, A. L., Barateau, L., Lopez, R., Chenini, S., Jaussent, I., & Dauvilliers, Y. (2021). Characteristics associated with hypersomnia and excessive daytime sleepiness identified by extended polysomnography recording. *Sleep, 44*(5), Article zsaa264.
Evangelista, E., Rassu, A. L., Lopez, R., Biagioli, N., Chenini, S., Barateau, L., Jaussent, I., & Dauvilliers, Y. (2022). Sleep inertia measurement with the psychomotor vigilance task in idiopathic hypersomnia. *Sleep, 45*(1), Article zsab220.
Evans, R., Kimura, H., Alexander, R., Davies, C. H., Faessel, H., Hartman, D. S., Ishikawa, T., Ratti, E., Shimizu, K., Suzuki, M., Tanaka, S., Yukitake, H., Dauvilliers, Y., & Mignot, E. (2022). Orexin 2 receptor–selective agonist danavorexton improves narcolepsy phenotype in a mouse model and in human patients. *Proceedings of the National Academy of Sciences of the United States of America, 119*(35), Article e2207531119.
Foley, D., Monjan, A., Masaki, K., Ross, W., Havlik, R., White, L., & Launer, L. (2001). Daytime sleepiness is associated with 3-year incident dementia and cognitive decline in older Japanese-American men. *Journal of American Geriatric Society, 49,* 1628–1632.
Fukuda, K., Strauss, S. E., Hickie, I., Sharpe, M. C., Dobbins, J. G, & Komaroff, A. (1994). The chronic fatigue syndrome: A comprehensive approach to its definition and study. International Chronic Fatigue Syndrome Study Group. *Annals of Internal Medicine, 121,* 953–959.
Guilleminault, C., & Brooks, S. N. (2001). Excessive daytime sleepiness. A challenge for the practising neurologist. *Brain, 124*(Pt. 8), 1482–1491.
Guilleminault, C., & Mondini, S. (1986). Mononucleosis and chronic daytime sleepiness. A long-term follow-up study. *Archives of Internal Medicine, 146*(7), 1333–1335.
Guilleminault, C., Quera-Salva, M. A., & Goldberg, M. P. (1993). Pseudo-hypersomnia and pre-sleep behaviour with bilateral paramedian thalamic lesions. *Brain, 116,* 1549–1563.
Guilleminault, C., Yuen, K. M., Gulevich, M. G., Karadeniz, D., Leger, D., & Philip, P. (2000). Hypersomnia after head-neck trauma: A methodological dilemma. *Neurology, 54,* 653–659.
Hays, J. C., Blazer, D. G., & Foley, D. J. (1996). Risk of napping: Excessive daytime sleepiness and mortality in an older community population. *Journal of the American Geriatrics Society, 44*(6), 693–698.

Hoddes, E., Zarcone, V., Smythe, H., Phillips, R., & Dement, W. C. (1973). Quantification of sleepiness: A new approach. *Psychophysiology, 10*, 431–436.

Hublin, C., Partinen, M., Koskenvuo, M., & Kaprio, J. (2007). Sleep and mortality: A population-based 22-year follow-up study. *Sleep, 30*, 1245–1253.

Ibatoullina, E., Praschak-Rieder, N., & Kasper, S. (1997). Severe atypical symptoms without depression in SAD: Effects of bright light therapy. *Journal of Clinical Psychiatry, 58*, 495.

Johns, M. W. (1991). A new method for measuring daytime sleepiness: The Epworth Sleepiness Scale. *Sleep, 14*, 540–545.

Kotagal, S., Krahn, L. E., & Slocumb, N. (2004). A putative link between childhood narcolepsy and obesity. *Sleep Medicine, 5*(2), 147–150.

Laberge, L., Bégin, P., Dauvilliers, Y., Beaudry, M., Laforte, M., Jean, S., & Mathieu, J. (2009). A polysomnographic study of daytime sleepiness in myotonic dystrophy type 1. *Journal of Neurology, Neurosurgery and Psychiatry, 19*(6), 397–402.

Lammers, G. J., Bassetti, C. L. A., Dolenc-Groselj, L., Jennum, P. J., Kallweit, U., Khatami, R., Lecendreux, M., Manconi, M., Mayer, G., Partinen, M., Plazzi, G., Reading, P. J., Santamaria, J., Sonka, K., & Dauvilliers, Y. (2020). Diagnosis of central disorders of hypersomnolence: A reappraisal by European experts. *Sleep Medicine Reviews, 52*, Article 101306. https://doi.org/10.1016/j.smrv.2020.101306

Latorre, D., Kallweit, U., Armentani, E., Foglierini, M., Mele, F., Cassotta, A., Jovic, S., Jarrossay, D., Mathis, J., Zellini, F., Becher, B., Lanzavecchia, A., Khatami, R., Manconi, M., Tafti, M., Bassetti, C. L., & Sallusto, F. (2018). T cells in patients with narcolepsy target self-antigens of hypocretin neurons. *Nature, 562*, 63–68. https://doi.org/10.1038/s41586-018-0540-1

Lin, L., Faraco, J., Li, R., Kadotani, H., Rogers, W., Lin, X., . . . Mignot, E. (1999). The sleep disorder canine narcolepsy is caused by a mutation in the hypocretin (orexin) receptor 2 gene. *Cell, 98*, 365–376.

Lopez, R., Barateau, L., Chenini, S., & Dauvilliers, Y. (2015). Preliminary results on CSF biomarkers for hypothalamic dysfunction in Kleine-Levin syndrome. *Sleep Medicine, 16*, 194–196.

Lugaresi, E., Cirignotta, F., Zucconi, M., Mondini, S., Lenzi, P. L., & Coccagna, G. (1983). Good and poor sleepers: An epidemiological survey of the San Marino population. In C. Guilleminault & E. Lugaresi (Eds.), *Sleep/wake disorders: Natural history, epidemiology, and long-term evolution* (pp. 1–12). Raven Press.

Luo, G., Ambati, A., Lin, L., Bonvalet, M., Partinen, M., Ji, X., Maecker, H. T., & Mignot, E. J. (2018). Autoimmunity to hypocretin and molecular mimicry to flu in Type 1 narcolepsy. *Proceedings of the National Academy of Sciences of the United States of America, 115*(52), E12323–E12332.

Masa, J. F., Rubio, M., & Findley, L. J. (2000). Habitually sleepy drivers have a high frequency of automobile crashes associated with respiratory disorders during sleep. *American Journal of Respiratory and Critical Care Medicine, 162*(4, Pt. 1), 1407–1412.

Maski, K., Mignot, E., Plazzi, G., & Dauvilliers, Y. (2022). Disrupted nighttime sleep and sleep instability in narcolepsy. *Journal of Clinical Sleep Medicine, 18*(1), 289–304.

Maski, K., Trotti, L. M., Kotagal, S., Robert Auger, R., Rowley, J. A., Hashmi, S. D., & Watson, N. F. (2021). Treatment of central disorders of hypersomnolence: An American Academy of Sleep Medicine clinical practice guideline. *Journal of Clinical Sleep Medicine : JCSM : official publication of the American Academy of Sleep Medicine, 17*(9), 1881–1893. https://doi.org/10.5664/jcsm.9328

Mignot, E., Lin, L., Finn, L., Lopes, C., Pluff, K., Sundstrom, M. L., & Young, T. (2006). Correlates of sleep-onset REM periods during the Multiple Sleep Latency Test in community adults. *Brain, 129*(Pt. 6), 1609–1623.

Mignot, E., Lin L., Rogers, W., Honda, Y., Qiu, X., Lin, X., . . . Risch, N. (2001). Complex HLA-DR and -DQ interactions confer risk of narcolepsy–cataplexy in three ethnic groups. *American Journal of Human Genetics, 68*(3), 686–699.

Nicolas, A., Lesperance, P., & Montplaisir, J. (1998). Is excessive daytime sleepiness with periodic leg movements during sleep a specific diagnostic category? *European Neurology, 40*, 22–26.

Nishino, S., & Kanbayashi, T. (2005). Symptomatic narcolepsy, cataplexy and hypersomnia, and their implications in the hypothalamic hypocretin/orexin system. *Sleep Medicine Reviews, 9*(4), 269–310.

Nofzinger, E. A., Thase, M. E., Reynolds, C. F., 3rd, Himmelhoch, J. M., Mallinger, A., Houck, P., & Kupfer, D. J. (1991). Hypersomnia in bipolar depression. A comparison with narcolepsy using the Multiple Sleep Latency Test. *American Journal of Psychiatry, 148*, 1177–1181.

Ohayon, M. M. (2000). Prevalence of hallucinations and their pathological associations in the general population. *Psychiatry Research, 97*(2–3), 153–164.

Ohayon, M. M., Caulet, M., Philip, P., Guilleminault, C., & Priest, R. (1997). How sleep and mental disorders are related to complaints of daytime sleepiness. *Archives of Internal Medicine, 157*, 2645–2652.

Ohayon, M. M., Dauvilliers, Y., & Reynolds, C. F. (2012). Operational definitions and algorithms for excessive sleepiness in the general population: Implications for DSM-5 nosology. *Archives of General Psychiatry, 69*(1), 71–79.

Ohayon, M. M., Priest, R. G., Zulley, J., Smirne, S., & Paiva, T. (2002). Prevalence of narcolepsy symptomatology and diagnosis in the European general population. *Neurology, 58*(12), 1826–1833.

Ohayon, M. M., Reynolds, C. F., & Dauvilliers, Y. (2013). Excessive sleep duration and quality of life. *Annals of Neurology, 73*(6), 785–794.

Pérez-Carbonell, L., Mignot, E., Leschziner, G., & Dauvilliers, Y. (2022). Understanding and approaching excessive daytime sleepiness. *Lancet, 400*(10357), 1033–1046.

Peyron, C., Faraco, J., Rogers, W., Ripley, B., Overeem, S., Charnay, Y., . . . Mignot, E. (2000). A mutation in a case of early onset narcolepsy and a generalized absence of hypocretin peptides in human narcoleptic brains. *Nature Medicine, 6*, 991–997.

Plante, D. (2017). Sleep propensity in psychiatric hypersomnolence: A systematic review and meta-analysis of multiple sleep latency test findings. *Sleep Medicine Reviews, 31*, 48–57.

Prins, J. B., van der Meer, J. W., & Bleijenberg, G. (2006). Chronic fatigue syndrome. *Lancet, 367*(9507), 346–355.

Rockwood, K., Davis, H. S., Merry, H. R., MacKnight, C., & McDowell, I. (2001). Sleep disturbances and mortality: Results from the Canadian Study of Health and Aging. *Journal of American Geriatric Society, 49*, 639–641.

Roehrs, T., & Roth, T. (2001). Sleep, sleepiness, sleep disorders and alcohol use and abuse. *Sleep Medicine Reviews, 5*, 287–297.

Rosenthal, N. E., Sack, D. A., Gillin, J. C., Lewy, A. J., Goodwin, F. K., Davenport, Y., . . . Wehr, T. A. (1984). Seasonal affective disorder. A description of the syndrome and preliminary findings with light therapy. *Archives of General Psychiatry, 41*, 72–80.

Sarkanen, T. O., Alakuijala, A. P. E., Dauvilliers, Y. A., & Partinen, M. M. (2018). Incidence of narcolepsy after H1N1 influenza and vaccinations: Systematic review and meta-analysis. *Sleep Medicine Reviews, 38*, 177–186.

Shen, J., Barbera, J., & Shapiro, C. M. (2006). Distinguishing sleepiness and fatigue: Focus on definition and measurement. *Sleep Medicine Reviews, 10*(1), 63–76.

Tsuno, N., Jaussent, I., Dauvilliers, Y., Touchon, J., Ritchie, K., & Besset, A. (2007). Determinants of excessive daytime sleepiness in a French community-dwelling elderly population. *Journal of Sleep Research, 16*, 364–371.

US Modafinil in Narcolepsy Multicenter Study Group. (2000). Randomized trial of modafinil as a treatment for the excessive daytime somnolence of narcolepsy. *Neurology, 54*, 1166–1175.

Van Dongen, H. P., Maislin, G., Mullington, J. M., & Dinges, D. F. (2003). The cumulative cost of additional wakefulness: Dose–response effects on neurobehavioral functions and sleep physiology from chronic sleep restriction and total sleep deprivation. *Sleep, 26*, 117–126.

Vgontzas, A. N., Bixler, E. O., Kales, A., Criley, C., & Vela-Bueno, A. (2000). Differences in nocturnal and daytime sleep between primary and psychiatric hypersomnia: Diagnostic and treatment implications. *Psychosomatic Medicine, 62*(2), 220–226.

Wagner, D. R. (1996). Disorders of the circadian sleep–wake cycle. *Neurology Clinics, 14*(3), 651–670.

Young, T., Palta, M., Dempsey, J., Skatrud, J., Weber, S., & Badr, S. (1993). The occurrence of sleep-disordered breathing among middle-aged adults. *New England Journal of Medicine, 328*, 1230–1235.

CHAPTER

37 Restless Legs Syndrome and Periodic Limb Movement Disorder

Raquel Martín, Celia García-Malo, Elisa Gamo, Alejandro Herrero, Sofía Romero, Alba García, *and* Diego García-Borreguero

Abstract

Restless legs syndrome (RLS) is a common sleep disorder that is characterized by an urgent need to move the legs; it causes sleep problems and mood changes, and its pathophysiology is not well understood, although there are associated factors such as iron deficiency. The clinical diagnosis is based on diagnostic criteria, although it is important to make a good differential diagnosis. Non-pharmacological treatment and treatment of exacerbating factors should always be included; pharmacological treatment is indicated when symptoms cause discomfort despite non-pharmacological treatment. Currently the first line of treatment is alpha-delta 2 ligands and dopamine agonists (DAs), using the former whenever possible. In the case of refractory RLS, opioids or benzodiazepines can be used. Studies have also shown the efficacy of dipyridamole and perampanel. The "augmentation phenomenon" is an iatrogenic worsening of the severity of symptoms related to DAs, so it is recommended to use them at the lowest possible dose and for the shortest time and to prioritize long-acting DAs. Management also includes iron replacement therapy, investigation of the use of drugs that may exacerbate RLS, non-pharmacological treatment, and, where appropriate, DA withdrawal. Periodic limb movement disorder is sometimes the motor manifestation of RLS, although it is nonspecific and can be seen in other conditions; diagnosis is made by polysomnography, with a periodic limb movement index of >5/hour in children or >15/hour in adults in addition to sleep problems. Its treatment is not well studied, but replacement iron therapy and pharmacological treatment, similar to RLS, are usually indicated.

Key Words: augmentation, iron replacement, periodic limb movement, restless legs syndrome, sleep movement disorder, treatment, Willis-Ekbom disease

Restless Legs Syndrome

Restless legs syndrome (RLS), also known as Willis-Ekbom disease (WED), is a common sensorimotor sleep disorder that has an estimated prevalence of between 5% and 15% of the adult population (Ohayon et al., 2016). It is characterized by an urgent need to move the legs, sometimes associated with unpleasant sensations in the lower limbs. Symptoms characteristically appear or worsen at rest, are transitorily relieved with movement, and follow a circadian pattern whereby they worsen during the afternoon and evening. RLS causes difficulties falling asleep, nocturnal awakenings, and mood changes, such as depression and/or anxiety. Patients with RLS often have periodic movements of sleep (PLMS; Manconi et al., 2021).

While the pathophysiology of RLS is not completely known, research has provided some insight into factors that play important roles, in particular decreased iron in the central nervous system despite normal systemic iron parameters, dysregulation of the dopaminergic and thalamic systems, and alteration of the circadian rhythm and/or alteration in sensory input from A-delta fibers or even from the microvasculature of the lower limbs.

Numerous risk factors are associated with the disease, including systemic iron deficiency, peripheral neuropathy, impaired kidney function, spinal cord disease, pregnancy, multiple sclerosis, and movement disorders such as Parkinson's disease and essential tremor. However, iron deficiency is the most common factor associated with RLS; not only does it have important therapeutic implications, but it is also an independent risk factor, unrelated to anemia, which has not been independently associated with an increased risk of developing RLS.

Familial RLS is common, with up to 60% of RLS patients having a positive family history (Ondo & Jankovic, 1996), a high rate of concordance between twins, and an inheritance pattern that suggests an autosomal dominant model. However, to date no specific causal genetic mutation has been identified, despite the existence of several variants of several genes associated with RLS risk, the strongest candidates being variants of PTPRD, BTBD9, and MEIS1 (Jiménez-Jiménez et al., 2018).

The diagnosis of RLS is clinical and based on criteria developed by the International Restless Legs Syndrome Study Group. The presence of all five criteria are required for a positive RLS diagnosis:

1 An urge to move the legs usually, but not always, accompanied by, or felt to be caused by, uncomfortable and unpleasant sensations in the legs.
2. The urge to move the legs and any accompanying unpleasant sensations begin or worsen during periods of rest or inactivity such as lying down or sitting.
3. The urge to move the legs and any accompanying unpleasant sensations are partially or totally relieved by movement, such as walking or stretching, at least as long as the activity continues.
4. The urge to move the legs and any accompanying unpleasant sensations during rest or inactivity only occur in the evening or night or are worse at night than during the day.
5. The occurrence of the above features is not solely accounted for as symptoms primary to another medical or a behavioral condition (e.g., myalgia, venous stasis, leg edema, arthritis, leg cramps, positional discomfort, and habitual foot tapping).

The differential diagnosis of RLS is broad and includes myalgias, leg edema, venous stasis, arthritis, leg cramps, positional discomfort, akathisia, and volitional movements (Wijemanne & Ondo, 2017).

Clinical factors that support the diagnosis of RLS are a positive family history, PLMS, and a positive response to dopaminergic agents. Some biological markers such as reduced iron echogenicity in the substantia nigra (Garcia-Malo, Novo-Ponte, et al., 2021) have also been studied in investigational settings to support clinical diagnosis (discussed further in the following section).

Management

In recent years, the general approach to RLS treatment has changed following the recognition and increased awareness of a devasting complication related to the use of dopaminergic agents called *augmentation* (see below, "Augmentation"). There have also been greater investigations into RLS pathophysiology, underlying the crucial role of brain iron deficiency (BID).

It is also important to remind physicians that the course of this disorder is not linear since exacerbations and remissions may occur. It is, therefore, mandatory to ensure a close follow-up of RLS patients as increases or reductions of RLS treatment could be needed.

The treatment algorithm of RLS is complex and must be individualized based on a risk–benefit balance. Non-pharmacological treatment and treatment of exacerbating factors should always be included. Depending on the discomfort of symptoms, the clinician should consider adding pharmacological treatment. Due to the pathophysiology of this disorder, iron levels should always be checked and supplemented when necessary.

Non-Pharmacological Treatment

Non-pharmacological treatment is essential in all patients suffering from RLS and may help to reduce the dose of pharmacological treatment, helping to avoid adverse effects such as augmentation. Although non-pharmacologic therapy should be generally considered a first-line treatment, unfortunately, there is no strong evidence supporting its efficacy. It is unclear to what extent benefits are due to individual interventions, placebo responses, or publication bias (Harrison et al., 2019). Preliminary studies on each of these suggest that high-quality randomized controlled trials may be warranted to support and verify the data presented. Non-pharmacological treatments include the following:

- Proper sleep hygiene with a regular sleep schedule, avoiding sleep deprivation.
- Regular exercise.
- Stretching and massaging the legs before bed or when discomfort begins or cold baths/showers before bed.
- Reduction or elimination of substances such as nicotine, alcohol, and caffeine.

- Pneumatic compression devices have been shown to improve RLS symptom severity, sleep, and quality of life in RLS patients (Eliasson & Lettieri, 2007).
- Near-infrared light therapy based on generating nitric oxide in the endothelium to maintain vasodilation through monochromatic light with a wavelength of 890 nm.
- Alternative medicines include the following (Bega & Malkani, 2016):
- Mind and body practices such as acupuncture, massage, meditation, movement therapies, relaxation techniques, tai chi, and yoga.
- Natural products such as Chinese herbals, valerian vitamins, minerals, and probiotics.

CORRECT EXACERBATING FACTORS

Of the numerous risk factors associated with RLS, iron deficiency is the most prominent. However, in this section, our focus is exclusively on drugs that may worsen RLS symptoms. Some drugs acting as dopamine blockers can contribute to the exacerbation of RLS symptoms: prokinetics, antipsychotics, vestibular sedatives, antihistamines, and antidepressants are the most common (Garcia-Malo, Romero-Peralta, & Cano-Pumarega, 2021).

In daily practice, the patient's current medications must be carefully evaluated and discontinuation of dopaminergic blockers considered individually by assessing the risks and benefits and any comorbidities.

Iron Replacement Therapy in RLS

The role of iron in RLS has been studied for many years. Magnetic resonance imaging studies in RLS patients have shown BID, with low iron deposits in the substantia nigra (SN; R. Allen, 2004); other studies have also shown low cerebrospinal fluid iron levels. Decreased SN iron stores have also been observed in autopsy specimens, as well as in studies using transcranial sonography of the SN (R. P. Allen et al., 2018; Garcia-Malo et al., 2019; Trotti & Becker, 2019). It is also important to address iron metabolism and its relationship with RLS as a circadian pattern has been shown whereby serum iron nadirs start around 8:00 p.m. to midnight, at the peak time of RLS symptom severity. Iron is a cofactor of tyrosine hydroxylase, an enzyme responsible for dopamine production (Trotti & Becker, 2019). Brain iron deposits cannot be predicted by peripheral iron parameters (Garcia-Malo, Novo-Ponte, et al., 2021); furthermore, BID can be present despite normal peripheral iron deposits.

According to current guidelines, the decision about whether to use iron replacement therapy (IRT) or not is strictly determined by serum iron parameters and not by iron levels in the central nervous system. This will likely change in the future as transcranial sonography could prove its utility in the quantification of BID and might help decide which patients could benefit most from IRT, check whether the treatment has been effective for correcting BID, and assess what occurs in those patients who do not respond to

IRT (Garcia-Malo et al., 2019). However, checking systemic iron parameters before indicating IRT is mandatory as the defined cutoff points ensure the safety of the treatment, minimizing the risk of iron overload (R. P. Allen et al., 2018; Garcia-Malo, Miranda, Novo Ponte, et al., 2020). IRT is recommended if transferrin saturation is <45% and serum ferritin is <300 μg/l (Garcia-Malo et al., 2008).

In addition to obtaining systemic iron values, it is important to assess C-reactive protein, erythrocyte sedimentation rate, serum levels of electrolytes, kidney and liver function markers, and thyroid hormone levels as all these parameters are relevant in the evaluation of RLS. It is important to be aware that serum ferritin can be falsely high due to chronic or inflammatory processes (Garcia-Malo et al., 2008).

There are two options available for IRT, oral and intravenous (IV), and the decision on which to use should be individually determined. IV iron replacement is usually preferred if any of the following characteristics are present:

- Any contraindication for oral iron replacement, previous treatment failure, or intolerance to oral iron.
- Personal history of intestinal iron malabsorption or kidney disease.
- A quick response is needed.
- Serum ferritin is <75 μg/l.

Among all IV iron formulations available, ferric carboxymaltose (FCM) is the most effective and safest in RLS. The recommended dose is 1,000 mg of FCM, which can be administered in a single dose or two doses of 500 mg 5–7 days apart (R. P. Allen et al., 2018). Among oral preparations, ferrous sulfate is the most studied in RLS and is recommended at doses of 325 mg (65 mg of elemental iron) given twice a day with 100 mg of vitamin C also twice a day. This combination has been shown to be possibly effective (level C evidence) for treating RLS in patients with serum ferritin <75 μg/l and possibly not effective (level C evidence) in those with serum ferritin >75 μg/l (R. P. Allen et al., 2018).

Following IRT it is important to assess serum iron parameters 3 months after oral iron supplementation and 8 weeks after IV iron infusion (R. P. Allen et al., 2018).

Symptomatic Pharmacological Treatment

Symptomatic pharmacological treatment is indicated when IRT has not been effective or cannot be administered and the patient has moderate or severe symptoms despite non-pharmacological treatment. It can be administered in combination with FeIV since the latter usually does not show efficacy until at least 6–8 weeks. The latest treatment guidelines published in 2016 (García-Borreguero et al., 2016) distinguish between first-line drugs indicated in de novo patients and drugs indicated in refractory RLS (Buchfuhrer, 2021; Winkelman, 2022).

FIRST-LINE TREATMENT

Dopamine agonists (DAs) or alpha delta-2 ligands ($\alpha 2\delta$ ligands) are indicated as first-line treatment in untreated patients (García-Borreguero et al., 2016). Although both drugs have shown efficacy in the short and long term, the only blinded randomized study comparing a DA (pramipexole 0.25 mg or 0.5 mg) and $\alpha 2\delta$ ligands (pregabalin 300 mg) in the long term showed that gabapentin was superior (R. P. Allen et al., 2014). DAs are responsible for two pharmacological complications: augmentation of RLS symptoms and impulse control disorder. While $\alpha 2\delta$ ligands have an anxiolytic and sedative effect (Wanner et al., 2019). For these reasons, treatment with $\alpha 2\delta$ ligands should be tried first when not contraindicated (Buchfuhrer, 2021; Winkelman, 2022). If this treatment is ineffective or poorly tolerated, switching to a DA is recommended (Buchfuhrer, 2021; García-Borreguero et al., 2016; Garcia-Malo, Peralta, & García-Borreguero, 2020; Winkelman, 2022), while being cautious to minimize the risk of augmentation (see "Augmentation" section below).

$\alpha 2\delta$ Ligands

The $\alpha 2\delta$ ligands indicated as the first-line treatment of RLS are gabapentin, pregabalin, and gabapentin enacarbil. The mechanism of action is thought to involve glutamate receptors decreasing glutamatergic transmission (Garcia-Malo et al., 2008). The main conditions that may be aggravated by the use of these drugs are obesity and its complications, severe depression, gait instability, respiratory failure, and substance abuse (Buchfuhrer, 2021; Winkelman, 2022). In these situations, DAs may be preferred over $\alpha 2\delta$ ligands. The main adverse effects of $\alpha 2\delta$ ligands are dizziness, unsteadiness, drowsiness, cognitive disturbances, weight gain, and depression. Table 37.1 summarizes the recommended doses of $\alpha 2\delta$ ligands for RLS.

Dopaminergic Agents

Non-ergot DAs are indicated for RLS treatment. It has been suggested that the increase in brain dopamine levels alters neural circuits and leads to a decrease in glutamatergic transmission (Garcia-Malo et al., 2008). Pramipexole and ropinirole are administered once or twice a day, and rotigotine is administered only once a day. They are approved at far lower doses than in Parkinson's disease, to minimize the possibility of augmentation (discussed below, "Augmentation") and impulse control disorder. Impulse control disorder occurs in 6%–17% of patients treated with DAs. Every patient with RLS should be interviewed about impulse control disorder symptoms before being prescribed a DA and at each visit. When impulse control disorder is present, the DA dose should be reduced or progressively discontinued (Buchfuhrer, 2021; Winkelman, 2022). In addition to these side effects, DAs can cause nausea, light-headedness, daytime sleepiness, nasal stuffiness, constipation, insomnia, orthostatic hypotension, and leg edema (Garcia-Malo et al., 2008; Garcia-Malo, Peralta, & García-Borreguero, 2020). Details of dosage and administration are summarized in Table 37.1.

Table 37.1 Details of dosage and administration: The dose should be adjusted according to patient comorbidities and age

Preparation	Initial dose	Titration	Usual effective daily dose	Recommended time of administration
α2δ Ligands				
Gabapentin	300 mg	Increase 300 mg/day every 2°3 days	900–2,400 mg	2 hours before bedtime
Pregabalin	75 mg	Increase 75 mg/day every 2–3 days	140–450 mg	2 hours before bedtime
Gabapentin enacarbil	600 mg	Double the dose every 7 days	600–1200 mg	5:00–7:00 p.m.
Dopaminergic agonists				
Pramipexol immediate release	0.125 mg	Double the dose every 4–7 days	0.18–0.54 mg	2–3 hours before bedtime
Ropinirole immediate release	0.25 mg	Double the dose after 2 days, then increase 0.5 mg every 7 days	2 mg	1–3 hours before bedtime
Rotigotine	1 mg	Increase 1 mg/day every week	2 mg	Replace it every day, preferably at the same time
Opioids				
Oxycodone	5–10 mg	Increase 25%–50% doses	10–30 mg	
Methadone	2.5–5 mg	Increase every 7 days	5–20 mg	

REFRACTORY RLS

Refractory RLS is considered when RLS symptoms do not respond to first-line treatments in monotherapy. In these cases, in addition to checking iron stores and minimizing exacerbating factors, it is recommended to add a second-line drug (Buchfuhrer, 2021; Winkelman, 2022). Low-potency opioids and benzodiazepines are among the second-line drugs recommended by clinical guidelines.

- *Opioids*. Methadone and oxycodone are the main opioids recommended for the second-line treatment of RLS (Silber et al., 2018; Silver et al., 2011). There is insufficient evidence for the use of other opioids. Long-acting formulations are preferred as these patients could present symptoms throughout the day. The most feared side effects are tolerance and dependence, which must be monitored at each visit. However, the doses prescribed for RLS treatment are usually lower than for chronic pain (see Table 37.1 for recommended doses). Other side effects are sedation, depression and anxiety, constipation, nausea, urinary retention, cognitive dysfunction, and induced respiratory depression or central sleep apnea (Buchfuhrer, 2021; Garcia-Malo, Peralta, & García-Borreguero, 2020; Winkelman, 2022). Patients on long-term therapy should undergo periodic clinical and polysomnographic (PSG) evaluations due to the risk of developing sleep apnea (Walters et al., 2001). Dosage and administration are summarized in Table 37.1.
- *Benzodiazepines*. Benzodiazepines, despite a lack of evidence, are considered a treatment option for RLS in practice guidelines. However, based on their side effects, their chronic use is discouraged (Carlos et al., 2017).

EMERGING TREATMENTS

In recent years, interest in other targets for the treatment of RLS, such as adenosine and glutamate, has increased, with some studies showing positive results with dipyridamole and perampanel (Garcia-Malo et al., 2008; Garcia-Malo, Peralta, & García-Borreguero, 2020).

- *Dipyridamole*. Dipyridamole is a nonselective inhibitor of nucleoside transporter, which increases extracellular adenosine. It is hypothesized that it could reduce the hypoadenosinergic state seen in BID mouse models. García-Borreguero et al. (2021) published a prospective open-label trial and a placebo-controlled crossover study proving clinical benefit as well as improvement in PSG parameters. In the placebo-controlled trial, the mean dose was 218 ± 33.1 mg/day, and the main side effects were abdominal distension, dizziness, diarrhea, and asthenia.

- *Perampanel.* It is hypothesized that perampanel, a non-competitive selective antagonist at the postsynaptic α-amino-3-hydroxy-5-methyl-4-isoxazolepropionic acid glutamate receptor, could reduce glutamatergic overstimulation in the central nervous system described in RLS patients. The only study published is a prospective open trial in 22 subjects that shows that perampanel improves the severity of symptoms and some PSG parameters after 8 weeks of treatment ($p < .001$). The mean dose was 3.8 ± 1.2 mg/day. The main side effects were dizziness, somnolence, headache, and irritability (García-Borreguero et al., 2017).

Augmentation

Augmentation, first described in 1996 following levodopa/carbidopa treatment of RLS, is a worsening of RLS severity in patients undergoing treatment with dopaminergic drugs. Symptoms have an earlier or faster onset, are more severe compared to baseline, and can spread to other body regions; and the effect of medication on symptoms is shorter. Augmentation may be considered an iatrogenic effect of DA use. Although some investigations relate it exclusively to long-term use, usually after 6 months, it can be observed in shorter periods (García-Borreguero et al., 2016).

The prevalence of augmentation varies across studies due to the differences in populations studied, the diagnostic criteria included, the length of follow-up, or the drugs used and has been reported to be between 42% and 68% in some long-term studies (García-Borreguero et al., 2017).

Diagnostic Criteria for Augmentation

To increase the sensitivity and awareness about augmentation, different study groups have tried to define diagnostic criteria. This is challenging because the paradoxical response to DA treatment needs to be identified: Patients who develop augmentation seem to need higher doses to improve RLS symptoms but later suffer from a worsening of symptoms (García-Borreguero et al., 2016).

Augmentation must be distinguished from tolerance, end-of-dose rebound, the natural progression of RLS, fluctuations of disease severity, and worsening because of exacerbating factors (Ellmerer et al., 2020).

In 2016, a combined task force developed guidelines for the prevention and management of augmentation (García-Borreguero et al., 2016). Four questions were proposed to assist in identifying augmentation in patients who have been undergoing treatment for at least 6 months.

1. Do RLS/WED symptoms appear earlier than when the drug was first started?
2. Are higher doses of the drug now needed, or do you need to take the medicine earlier, to control the RLS/WED symptoms compared to the original effective dose?
3. Has the intensity of symptoms worsened since starting the medication?
4. Have symptoms spread to other parts of the body (e.g., arms) since starting the medication?

An affirmative answer to any of these questions warrants further investigation of augmentation (García-Borreguero et al., 2016).

Risk Factors for Augmentation

Several studies have investigated why certain patients develop augmentation. An observational community study established that those who have more frequent or intense symptoms before treatment initiation, comorbid asthma, older age, or longer treatment duration are more likely to develop augmentation ($p < .05$). These findings should be interpreted carefully as this association may be a consequence of higher doses in patients with severe symptoms (Geyer & Bogan, 2017).

Another broadly studied risk factor is low serum ferritin levels. Low ferritin serum levels have been related to a higher probability of developing augmentation in patients with RLS in contrast to those with higher levels of ferritin. This has been explained by the role of the iron-dependent enzyme in dopamine synthesis. Other risk factors include prior tolerance to levodopa, positive family history of RLS, and lack of follow-up. Recently, impulse control disorder and the presence of one addictive behavior have been confirmed as risk factors.

A high score on alexithymia questionnaires or lower education rates have been reported in those developing augmentation; however, these results must be interpreted carefully (Heim et al., 2021). Whether differences in PLMS index or suggested immobilization test score can predict augmentation has also been assessed; but results vary enormously, and further research is needed (García-Borreguero et al., 2016).

Management

As augmentation phenomena consist of an iatrogenic effect related to DA use, the avoidance of these drugs prevents the occurrence of this complication. However, as described previously, DAs are useful and effective and are still recommended when the severity of RLS symptoms requires their use. When DAs are necessary, the global recommendations to prevent augmentation are as follows:

1. Long-acting DAs are preferred over short-acting DAs.
2. Use the lowest effective dose of DAs.
3. Use DAs for the shortest time.

Other recommendations to prevent augmentation are as follows:

1. Investigate iron parameters periodically, and indicate IRT if necessary (R. P. Allen et al., 2018; García-Borreguero, 2015).
2. Review any other medical conditions or the use of drugs that may trigger or exacerbate RLS symptoms (e.g., antidepressants, prokinetic agents, antipsychotics, vestibular sedatives, or antihistamines).
3. Investigate sleep hygiene and other lifestyle conditions that may worsen RLS symptoms (e.g., caffeine intake, sleep deprivation, sedentarism).

When augmentation phenomena are detected, the first recommendation is to correct iron deficiency according to the guidelines (R. P. Allen et al., 2018; Garcia-Malo, Miranda, Romero Peralta, et al., 2020), then investigate the use of drugs that may exacerbate RLS symptoms and recommend their cessation and implement non-pharmacological treatment.

Secondly, in the case of mild augmentation, dividing the total DA dose could be useful, with the first dose before symptom onset and the second dose after. It is important to maintain the total dose stable and reduce it whenever possible (García-Borreguero, 2015). If the patient is on short-acting DAs, the third step consists of switching to a long-acting DA by initially using the equivalent dose. Rotigotine is the preferred DA as its transdermal absorption makes drug levels in the blood more stable (García-Borreguero, 2015).

As the objective is to decrease or even cease DA use, it is recommended to associate DA treatment with other drugs that are effective for RLS but have no risk of augmentation. Because of their safety profile, $\alpha 2\delta$ ligands would be the first option. In more severe cases or when the patient shows no response to $\alpha 2\delta$ ligands or does not tolerate a dose, opioids should be considered (García-Borreguero, 2015). An intermediate step would be to consider other effective drugs such as dipyridamole or perampanel.

Once symptom severity is controlled, the total DA dose should be progressively decreased. The abrupt withdrawal of DAs is not recommended due to the risk of developing dopaminergic dysregulation syndrome (Figure 37.1).

Periodic Limb Movement Disorder

Periodic limb movement disorder (PLMD) involves documentation of PLMS using PSG with a periodic limb movement (PLM) index of >5/hour in children or >15/hour in

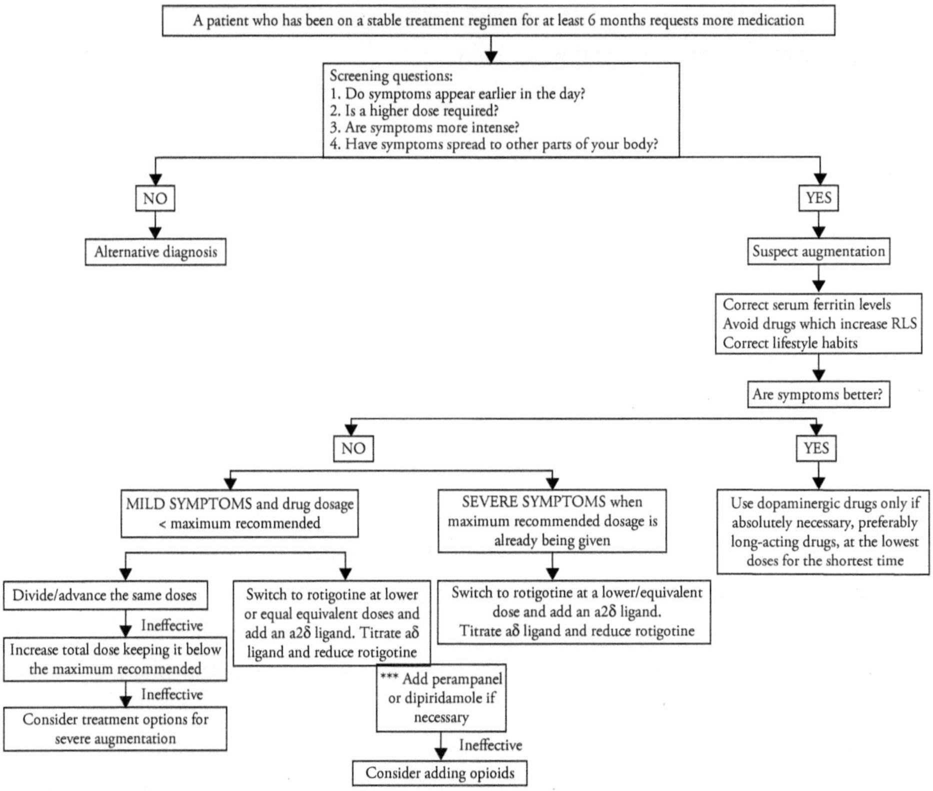

Figure 37.1 Summary of detection and management of augmentation phenomena
Note. RLS = restless legs syndrome. Reprinted from *Encyclopedia of Sleep and Circadian Rhythms*, 2nd Edition, with permission from Elsevier.

adults in addition to insomnia, sleep fragmentation, or daytime fatigue or somnolence. If PLMS are registered on PSG, sleep and other medical or neurological conditions such as RLS, narcolepsy, or rapid-eye-movement (REM) sleep behavior disorder (RBD) should be ruled out (Garcia-Malo, Peralta, & García-Borreguero, 2020).

Management

Even when PLMD and RLS share several pathophysiological and genetic characteristics, the former requires specific attention, treatment, and management. There are insufficient studies evaluating the treatment of PLMD (Winkelman et al., 2016). Currently, no treatment is indicated for isolated PLMS without RLS or PLMD; this could, however, change in the future as recent investigations have correlated isolated PLMS with an increase in vascular risk, including cardiovascular and cerebrovascular disease (Garcia-Malo, Peralta, & García-Borreguero, 2020). More controlled clinical trials must be undertaken to help elucidate if treating isolated PLMS has any positive impact on reducing blood pressure levels or enhances cardiovascular risk and, therefore, life expectancy (Figorilli et al., 2017; Silvani, 2019).

As in RLS, there should be special caution with the use of certain drugs, like antidepressants, that may exacerbate PLMS (Kolla et al., 2018).

IRT

IRT should be considered in the same cases as in RLS.

Symptomatic Pharmacological Treatment

DOPAMINERGIC AGONISTS

Pramipexole, rotigotine, and ropinirole have proven to have high efficacy at reducing PLMS. Some observations reported that treating PLMS with DAs may lead to complications in the long term in the form of augmentation phenomena (Santamaria et al., 2003).

A2Δ LIGANDS

$\alpha 2\delta$ ligands such as pregabalin (330 mg/day) and gabapentin (600–1800 mg/day; García-Borreguero et al., 2013) are also considered safe, well tolerated, and effective for PLMD (Garcia-Malo et al., 2008; Garcia-Malo, Peralta, & García-Borreguero, 2020).

BENZODIAZEPINES

On the other hand, there is little evidence of the efficacy of clonazepam (which appears to have an acute effect more on insomnia than on PLMS), melatonin (which seems to show a reduction in PLMS, PLM index, and arousal associated with PLMS), valproic acid (which does not seem to have a therapeutic effect on PLMS), and selegiline (which, on the contrary, has shown efficacy in the treatment of the disorder; Aurora et al., 2012).

On the other hand, there is little evidence for the efficacy of clonazepam (which appears to have an acute effect more on insomnia than on PLMS), melatonin (which seems to show a reduction in PLMS, PLM index, and arousal associated with PLMS), valproic acid (which does not seem to have a therapeutic effect on PLMS), and selegiline (which, on the contrary, has shown efficacy in the treatment of the disorder; Aurora et al., 2012).

An alternative treatment approach can be the benzodiazepine clonazepam (0.5–1 mg/day), which in various open studies has been shown to reduce the total number of PLMs during wakefulness and REM sleep and PLMS associated with arousals but not a decrease in the PLM index (Horiguchi et al., 1992). However, PLMD comorbid with RBD has been related to a deficient therapeutic response to the administration of clonazepam as a single medication (Lee et al., 2021). Furthermore, benzodiazepines are not exempt from risk or side effects such as drowsiness, dizziness, mental confusion, muscle relaxation, depression, morning sedation, memory impairment, and tolerance.

OPIOIDS

As in RLS, opioids like oxycodone (11 mg/day) could be useful for PLMD (Trenkwalder et al., 2013).

OTHER AGENTS

Although evidence is not too clear, some reports have exposed certain benefits from the γ-aminobutyric acid B agonist receptor baclofen (Guilleminault & Flagg, 1984). Patients frequently develop tolerance to this drug. An open clinical trial with PLMD without RLS patients showed that melatonin (3 mg) significantly reduced PLMs, PLM index, PLMs with arousals, and PLM arousal index, suggesting a contribution of the circadian timing system in the pathophysiology of PLMD (Kunz & Bes, 2001). There is mention of other options for PLMD treatment such as safinamide (Liguori et al., 2018) and subcutaneous apomorphine (Haba-Rubio et al., 2003). Selegiline was examined in one Level V study in patients with PLMD, reporting a substantial decrease in the number of PLMs per hour of total sleep time (Grewal et al., 2002). Some additional agents lack clinical support, such as magnesium (Marshall et al., 2019) and erythropoietin (Aurora et al., 2012).

As in RLS, special care is required with the use of certain drugs, like antidepressants, that may exacerbate PLMS (Kolla et al., 2018).

References

Allen, R. (2004). Dopamine and iron in the pathophysiology of restless legs syndrome (RLS). *Sleep Medicine*, *5*(4), 385–391. https://doi.org/10.1016/j.sleep.2004.01.012

Allen, R. P., Chen, C., García-Borreguero, D., Polo, O., DuBrava, S., Miceli, J., Knapp, L., & Winkelman, J. W. (2014). Comparison of pregabalin with pramipexole for restless legs syndrome. *New England Journal of Medicine*, *370*(7), 621–631. https://doi.org/10.1056/nejmoa1303646

Allen, R. P., Picchietti, D. L., Auerbach, M., Cho, Y. W., Connor, J. R., Earley, C. J., García-Borreguero, D., Kotagal, S., Manconi, M., Ondo, W., Ulfberg, J., & Winkelman, J. W. (2018). Evidence-based and consensus clinical practice guidelines for the iron treatment of restless legs syndrome/Willis-Ekbom disease in adults and children: An IRLSSG task force report. *Sleep Medicine*, *41*, 27–44. https://doi.org/10.1016/j.sleep.2017.11.1126

Aurora, R. N., Kristo, D. A., Bista, S. R., Rowley, J. A., Zak, R. S., Casey, K. R., Lamm, C. I., Tracy, S. L., & Rosenberg, R. S. (2012). Update to the AASM clinical practice guideline: "The treatment of restless legs syndrome and periodic limb movement disorder in adults—An update for 2012: Practice parameters with an evidence-based systematic review and meta-analyses." *Sleep*, *35*(8), 1037. https://doi.org/10.5665/sleep.1986

Bega, D., & Malkani, R. (2016). Alternative treatment of restless legs syndrome: An overview of the evidence for mind–body interventions, lifestyle interventions, and neutraceuticals. *Sleep Medicine*, *17*, 99–105. https://doi.org/10.1016/j.sleep.2015.09.009

Buchfuhrer, M. (2021). *Clinician's manual on restless legs syndrome*. Springer https://doi.org/10.1007/978-3-319-31373-3_5

Carlos, K., Prado, G. F., Teixeira, C. D. M., Conti, C., de Oliveira, M. M., Prado, L. B. F., & Carvalho, L. B. C. (2017). Benzodiazepines for restless legs syndrome. *Cochrane Database of Systematic Reviews*, *2017*(3), CD006939. https://doi.org/10.1002/14651858.CD006939.pub2

Eliasson, A. H., & Lettieri, C. J. (2007). Sequential compression devices for treatment of restless legs syndrome. *Medicine*, *86*(6), 317–323. https://doi.org/10.1097/MD.0b013e31815b1319

Ellmerer, P., Heim, B., Stefani, A., Peball, M., Werkmann, M., Holzknecht, E., Bergmann, M., Brandauer, E., Sojer, M., Zamarian, L., Delazer, M., Seppi, K., Högl, B., Poewe, W., & Djamshidian, A. (2020). Augmentation in restless legs syndrome: An eye tracking study on emotion processing. *Annals of Clinical and Translational Neurology*, *7*(9), 1620–1627. https://doi.org/10.1002/acn3.51144

Figorilli, M., Puligheddu, M., Congiu, P., & Ferri, R. (2017). The clinical importance of periodic leg movements in sleep. *Current Treatment Options in Neurology*, *19*(3), Article 10. https://doi.org/10.1007/s11940-017-0446-5

Garca-Borreguero, D. (2015). Dopaminergic augmentation in restless legs syndrome/Willis-Ekbom disease: Identification and management. *Sleep Medicine Clinics, 10*(3), 287–292. https://doi.org/10.1016/j.jsmc.2015.05.020

García-Borreguero, D., Cano, I., & Granizo, J. J. (2017a). Treatment of restless legs syndrome with the selective AMPA receptor antagonist perampanel. *Sleep Medicine, 34*, 105–108. https://doi.org/10.1016/j.sleep.2017.03.012

García-Borreguero, D., Garcia-Malo, C., Granizo, J. J., & Ferre, S. (2021). A randomized, placebo-controlled crossover study with dipyridamole for restless legs syndrome. *Movement Disorders, 36*(10), 2387–2392. https://doi.org/10.1002/mds.28668

García-Borreguero, D., Kohnen, R., Silber, M. H., Winkelman, J. W., Earley, C. J., Högl, B., Manconi, M., Montplaisir, J., Inoue, Y., & Allen, R. P. (2013). The long-term treatment of restless legs syndrome/Willis-Ekbom disease: Evidence-based guidelines and clinical consensus best practice guidance: A report from the International Restless Legs Syndrome Study Group. *Sleep Medicine, 14*(7), 675–684. https://doi.org/10.1016/j.sleep.2013.05.016

García-Borreguero, D., Silber, M. H., Winkelman, J. W., Högl, B., Bainbridge, J., Buchfuhrer, M., Hadjigeorgiou, G., Inoue, Y., Manconi, M., Oertel, W., Ondo, W., Winkelmann, J., & Allen, R. P. (2016). Guidelines for the first-line treatment of restless legs syndrome/Willis-Ekbom disease, prevention and treatment of dopaminergic augmentation: A combined task force of the IRLSSG, EURLSSG, and the RLS-foundation. *Sleep Medicine, 21*, 1–11. https://doi.org/10.1016/j.sleep.2016.01.017

Garcia-Malo, C., Cano-Pumarega, I., Anguizola, S., Garcia, R., Romero Peralta, S., Botta, L., Novo Ponte, S., Boi, S., & García-Borreguero, D. (2021). Special considerations for treatment of sleep-related movement disorders. In *Reference module in neuroscience and biobehavioral psychology*. https://doi.org/10.1016/B978-0-12-822963-7.00148-1

Garcia-Malo, C., Miranda, C., Novo Ponte, S., Romero Peralta, S., Cano-Pumarega, I., Boi, S., Martínez Vidal, V., Anguizola, S., Botta, L., & García-Borreguero, D. (2020). Low risk of iron overload or anaphylaxis during treatment of restless legs syndrome with intravenous iron: A consecutive case series in a regular clinical setting. *Sleep Medicine, 74*, 48–55. https://doi.org/10.1016/j.sleep.2020.06.002

Garcia-Malo, C., Miranda, C., Romero Peralta, S., Cano-Pumarega, I., Novo Ponte, S., & García-Borreguero, D. (2020). Iron replacement therapy in restless legs syndrome. *Current Treatment Options in Neurology, 22*(4), Article 11. https://doi.org/10.1007/s11940-020-0617-7

Garcia-Malo, C., Novo-Ponte, S., Castro-Villacañas Farzamnia, A., Boi, S., Miranda Castillo, C., Romero Peralta, S., Martínez Vidal, V., Botta, L., Anguizola, S., Cano-Pumarega, I., & García-Borreguero, D. (2021a). Correlation between systemic iron parameters and substantia nigra iron stores in restless legs syndrome. *Sleep Medicine, 85*, 191–195. https://doi.org/10.1016/j.sleep.2021.07.027

Garcia-Malo, C., Peralta, S. R., & García-Borreguero, D. (2020). Restless legs syndrome and other common sleep-related movement disorders. *Continuum: Lifelong Learning in Neurology, 26*(4), 963–987. https://doi.org/10.1212/CON.0000000000000886

Garcia-Malo, C., Romero-Peralta, S., & Cano-Pumarega, I. (2021). Restless legs syndrome—Clinical features. *Sleep Medicine Clinics, 16*(2), 233–247. https://doi.org/10.1016/j.jsmc.2021.02.002

Garcia-Malo, C., Wanner, V., Miranda, C., Romero Peralta, S., Agudelo, L., Cano-Pumarega, Granizo, J. J., & García-Borreguero, D. (2019). Quantitative transcranial sonography of the substantia nigra as a predictor of therapeutic response to intravenous iron therapy in restless legs syndrome. Sleep Medicine, 66, 123–129. https://doi.org/10.1016/j.sleep.2019.09.020

Geyer, J., & Bogan, R. (2017). Identification and treatment of augmentation in patients with restless legs syndrome: Practical recommendations. *Postgraduate Medicine, 129*(7), 667–675. https://doi.org/10.1080/00325481.2017.1360747

Grewal, M., Hawa, R., & Shapiro, C. (2002). Treatment of periodic limb movements in sleep with selegiline HCl. *Movement Disorders, 17*(2), 398–401. https://doi.org/10.1002/mds.10082

Guilleminault, C., & Flagg, W. (1984). Effect of baclofen on sleep-related periodic leg movements. *Annals of Neurology, 15*(3), 234–239. https://doi.org/10.1002/ana.410150304

Haba-Rubio, J., Staner, L., Cornette, F., Lainey, E., Luthringer, R., Krieger, J., & Macher, J. P. (2003). Acute low single dose of apomorphine reduces periodic limb movements but has no significant effect on sleep arousals: A preliminary report. *Neurophysiologie Clinique/Clinical Neurophysiology, 33*(4), 180–184. https://doi.org/10.1016/S0987-7053(03)00056-X

Harrison, E. G., Keating, J. L., & Morgan, P. E. (2019). Non-pharmacological interventions for restless legs syndrome: A systematic review of randomised controlled trials. *Disability and Rehabilitation, 41*(17), 2006–2014. https://doi.org/10.1080/09638288.2018.1453875

Heim, B., Ellmerer, P., Stefani, A., Heidbreder, A., Brandauer, E., Högl, B., Seppi, K., & Djamshidian, A. (2021). Birds of a feather flock together: Disadvantageous decision making in augmented restless legs syndrome patients with and without impulse control disorders. *Brain Sciences, 11*(3), Article 383. https://doi.org/10.3390/brainsci11030383

Horiguchi, J., Inami, Y., Sasaki, A., Nishimatsu, O., & Sukegawa, T. (1992). Periodic leg movements in sleep with restless legs syndrome: Effect of clonazepam treatment. *Psychiatry and Clinical Neurosciences, 46*(3), 727–732. https://doi.org/10.1111/j.1440-1819.1992.tb00548.x

Jiménez-Jiménez, F. J., Alonso-Navarro, H., García-Martín, E., & Agúndez, J. A. G. (2018). Genetics of restless legs syndrome: An update. *Sleep Medicine Reviews, 39*, 108–121. https://doi.org/10.1016/j.smrv.2017.08.002

Kolla, B. P., Mansukhani, M. P., & Bostwick, J. M. (2018). The influence of antidepressants on restless legs syndrome and periodic limb movements: A systematic review. *Sleep Medicine Reviews, 38*, 131–140. https://doi.org/10.1016/j.smrv.2017.06.002

Kunz, D., & Bes, F. (2001). Exogenous melatonin in periodic limb movement disorder: An open clinical trial and a hypothesis. *Sleep, 24*(2), 183–187. https://doi.org/10.1093/sleep/24.2.183

Lee, H. J., Choi, H., & Yoon, I. Y. (2021). Age of diagnosis and comorbid PLMD predict poor response of REM behavior disorder to clonazepam. *Journal of Geriatric Psychiatry and Neurology, 34*(2), 142–149. https://doi.org/10.1177/0891988720915517

Liguori, C., Mercuri, N. B., Stefani, A., & Pierantozzi, M. (2018). Effective treatment of restless legs syndrome by safinamide in Parkinson's disease patients. *Sleep Medicine, 41*, 113–114. https://doi.org/10.1016/j.sleep.2017.09.017

Manconi, M., García-Borreguero, D., Schormair, B., Videnovic, A., Berger, K., Ferri, R., & Dauvilliers, Y. (2021). Restless legs syndrome. *Nature Reviews Disease Primers, 7*(1), Article 80. https://doi.org/10.1038/s41572-021-00311-z

Marshall, N. S., Serinel, Y., Killick, R., Child, J. M., Raisin, I., Berry, C. M., Lallukka, T., Wassing, R., Lee, R. W., Ratnavadivel, R., Vedam, H., Grunstein, R., Wong, K. K., Hoyos, C. M., Cayanan, E. A., Comas, M., Chapman, J. L., & Yee, B. J. (2019). Magnesium supplementation for the treatment of restless legs syndrome and periodic limb movement disorder: A systematic review. *Sleep Medicine Reviews, 48*, Article 101218. https://doi.org/10.1016/j.smrv.2019.101218

Ohayon, M. M., Bagai, K., Roberts, L. W., Walters, A. S., & Milesi, C. (2016). Refining duration and frequency thresholds of restless legs syndrome diagnosis criteria. *Neurology, 87*(24), 2546–2553. https://doi.org/10.1212/WNL.0000000000003386

Ondo, W., & Jankovic, J. (1996). Restless legs syndrome: Clinicoetiologic correlates. *Neurology, 47*(6), 1435–1441. https://doi.org/10.1212/WNL.47.6.1435

Santamaria, J., Iranzo, A., & Tolosa, E. (2003). Development of restless legs syndrome after dopaminergic treatment in a patient with periodic leg movements in sleep. *Sleep Medicine, 4*(2), 153–155. https://doi.org/10.1016/S1389-9457(02)00153-3

Silber, M. H., Becker, P. M., Buchfuhrer, M. J., Earley, C. J., Ondo, W. G., Walters, A. S., & Winkelman, J. W. (2018). The appropriate use of opioids in the treatment of refractory restless legs syndrome. *Mayo Clinic Proceedings, 93*(1), 59–67. https://doi.org/10.1016/j.mayocp.2017.11.007

Silvani, A. (2019). Sleep disorders, nocturnal blood pressure, and cardiovascular risk: A translational perspective. *Autonomic Neuroscience: Basic and Clinical, 218*, 31–42. https://doi.org/10.1016/j.autneu.2019.02.006

Silver, N., Allen, R. P., Senerth, J., & Earley, C. J. (2011). A 10-year, longitudinal assessment of dopamine agonists and methadone in the treatment of restless legs syndrome. *Sleep Medicine, 12*(5), 440–444. https://doi.org/10.1016/j.sleep.2010.11.002

Trenkwalder, C., Beneš, H., Grote, L., García-Borreguero, D., Högl, B., Hopp, M., Bosse, B., Oksche, A., Reimer, K., Winkelmann, J., Allen, R. P., & Kohnen, R. (2013). Prolonged release oxycodone–naloxone for treatment of severe restless legs syndrome after failure of previous treatment: A double-blind, randomised, placebo-controlled trial with an open-label extension. *The Lancet Neurology, 12*(12), 1141–1150. https://doi.org/10.1016/S1474-4422(13)70239-4

Trotti, L. M., & Becker, L. A. (2019). Iron for the treatment of restless legs syndrome. *Cochrane Database of Systematic Reviews, 2019*(1), CD007834. https://doi.org/10.1002/14651858.CD007834.pub3

Walters, A. S., Winkelmann, J., Trenkwalder, C., Fry, J. M., Kataria, V., Wagner, M., Sharma, R., Hening, W., & Li, L. (2001). Long-term follow-up on restless legs syndrome patients treated with opioids. *Movement Disorders*, *16*(6), 1105–1109. https://doi.org/10.1002/mds.1214

Wanner, V., Garcia Malo, C., Romero, S., Cano-Pumarega, I., & García-Borreguero, D. (2019). Non-dopaminergic vs. dopaminergic treatment options in restless legs syndrome. *Advances in Pharmacology*, *84*, 187–205. https://doi.org/10.1016/bs.apha.2019.02.003

Wijemanne, S., & Ondo, W. (2017). Restless legs syndrome: Clinical features, diagnosis and a practical approach to management. *Practical Neurology*, *17*(6), 444–452. https://doi.org/10.1136/practneurol-2017-001762

Winkelman, J. W. (2022). Treating severe refractory and augmented restless legs syndrome. *Chest*, *162*(3), 693–700. https://doi.org/10.1016/j.chest.2022.05.014

Winkelman, J. W., Blackwell, T., Stone, K., Ancoli-Israel, S., Tranah, G. J., & Redline, S.; Osteoporotic Fractures in Men (MrOS) Study Research Group. (2016). Genetic associations of periodic limb movements of sleep in the elderly for the MrOS Sleep Study. *Sleep Medicine*, *16*(11), 1360–1365. https://doi.org/10.1016/j.sleep.2015.07.017

SECTION 6

Disorders of Sleep and Circadian Function: Life Span Issues and Special Populations

CHAPTER

38 Sleep-Related Problems in Childhood and Adolescence

Liat Tikotzky, Michal Kahn, Michael Gradisar, *and* Oliviero Bruni

Abstract

Pediatric sleep problems are very common and may negatively impact various aspects of child development, spanning physical, socio-emotional, behavioral, cognitive, and academic domains. Moreover, sleep problems in children often have a major impact on family relationships and functioning and may lead to significant parental fatigue, stress, and low mood. Numerous intrinsic and extrinsic factors may influence the development of sleep problems and their maintenance, ranging from genetic vulnerability, prematurity, medical problems, and neurodevelopmental disorders to behavioral and socio-environmental factors, such as poor sleep hygiene, ineffective parental sleep-related behaviors, and exposure to academic, social, or family stressors. Given the high prevalence of pediatric sleep problems and associated harmful consequences, assessment of these problems by primary child healthcare providers should be included in any medical or mental health evaluation. Fortunately, there are various evidenced-based effective behavioral and medical interventions that are used to treat specific pediatric sleep disturbances. This chapter describes common sleep disorders in infants, children, and adolescents, including insomnia, parasomnias, circadian problems, sleep-related movement disorders, and obstructive sleep apnea. Current evidence regarding the phenomenology, etiology, assessment, and evidence-based treatment options is addressed pertaining to each disorder. Finally, open questions in the field of pediatric sleep problems are presented, highlighting areas warranting future research.

Key Words: pediatric sleep, childhood sleep disorder, insomnia, parasomnia, circadian problem, movement disorder, sleep apnea, assessment, sleep intervention

Introduction

Childhood sleep problems are very common and are among the most frequent concerns parents present to healthcare professionals. It is estimated that up to 50% of children experience a sleep problem at some point during childhood (Carter et al., 2014; Honaker & Meltzer, 2016; Owens, 2008), and these problems are significantly associated with children's cognitive, socio-emotional, and behavioral difficulties, as well as with children's physical health and family well-being (El-Sheikh & Kelly, 2017; Gregory & Sadeh, 2012; Spruyt, 2019). The high prevalence of pediatric sleep problems and their implications for daytime functioning underscore the importance of familiarizing child-care specialists with normal sleep development and with the assessment and management of pediatric sleep disorders (Meltzer et al., 2021; Sadeh, 2005). Importantly, the manifestation of sleep disturbances changes across childhood, and therefore the diagnosis and treatment of these problems should be considered in a developmental context (Mindell & Owens, 2015; Owens & Mindell, 2011).

This chapter will delineate the assessment of pediatric sleep problems and will review common child and adolescent sleep disorders including insomnia, nighttime fears, parasomnias, circadian problems, and physiological sleep disorders, such as movement disorders and obstructive sleep apnea (OSA). We will specifically address the phenomenology and presentation of these disorders across childhood, factors affecting their expression, and evidence-based treatment options.

Assessment of Pediatric Sleep Problems

Given the high prevalence of pediatric sleep problems and their potential maladaptive consequences, assessment of these problems should be part of any medical or psychiatric child evaluation. Assessments of pediatric sleep problems in clinical settings should include a thorough clinical interview with the parents and—when applicable—with the child. Additional assessment tools consist of subjective measures, such as validated sleep questionnaires and sleep diaries, and objective measures such as actigraphy, videosomnography, and polysomnography (PSG). Each method has its advantages and limitations, and the choice of which tools to use depends largely on the specific assessment questions.

The clinical interview is a basic and necessary component of the assessment procedure, which is needed to determine diagnosis and to develop a personalized intervention program (Mindell & Owens, 2015; Sadeh & Anders, 1993). The interview should cover a detailed description of the present sleep problem and its history, symptoms of other sleep disorders, characteristics of the sleeping environment (e.g., noise, television in bedroom, co-sleeping), parental practices and sleep-related behaviors (e.g., soothing methods, limit-setting), evening and bedtime routines (e.g., consistency of bedtime routine), napping, and prior attempts to treat the problem. Collecting information about parental sleep-related cognitions and expectations may be of value as these are likely to influence parental sleep-related behaviors. Moreover, attention should be drawn to the family's cultural background and its possible impact on parents' perceptions of child sleep–wake patterns and problems. Beyond sleep-related information, the interview should also address the child's developmental, temperamental, psycho-social, and medical history, as well as their current daytime functioning. An evaluation of exposure to family stressors (e.g., marital conflict, poor socioeconomic situation) or stressful events in the environment (e.g., natural disaster, war) is also critical, as is assessment of the parents' emotional functioning (e.g., depressive symptoms) and the quality of the parent–child relationship (e.g., attachment security, separation anxiety, emotional availability). While these factors might not all directly impact sleep, they may have an influence on factors associated with sleep problems such as the child's arousal level and the parents' bedtime and nighttime soothing behaviors. An example of an interview format that provides detailed questions regarding various aspects of sleep and related domains can be found in Mindell and Owens' (2015) *Clinical Guide to Pediatric Sleep* (online Appendix B).

In addition to a comprehensive clinical interview, the assessment of children's sleep problems may include more structured sleep questionnaires. Sleep questionnaires offer a simple and effective way to obtain information on sleep patterns, sleep-related behaviors, and behavioral and physiological sleep disorders. There are many validated questionnaires that can be used to assess sleep among infants, children, and adolescents (Sen & Spruyt, 2020; Spruyt & Gozal, 2011). Some of the most widely used questionnaires that have good psychometric properties include the Brief Infant Sleep Questionnaire (Mindell et al., 2019; Sadeh, 2004), designed to assess sleep in early childhood (0–3 years); the Children's Sleep Habit Questionnaire (Owens et al., 2000), originally developed for children aged 4–10 years; the Sleep Disturbance Scale for Children (Bruni et al., 1996), which evaluates sleep disturbances in school-age children and adolescents; the Pediatric Sleep Questionnaire (Chervin et al., 2000), aimed at measuring sleep-related breathing disorders in children 2–18 years old; and the Sleep Habits Survey (Wolfson et al., 2003), which assesses sleep in adolescents (grades 9–12).

Sleep diaries, usually completed for 1–2 weeks, can provide a detailed and more specific day-to-day assessment of sleep duration and quality (e.g., sleep-onset latency, sleep duration, night-wakings) and sleep-related behaviors (e.g., bedtime routine, settling practices, etc.). In comparison to questionnaires, sleep diaries are less likely to be biased by memory recall. However, parents may find it difficult to complete them over extended periods. Moreover, parents can reliably report their children's bedtime behaviors and sleep schedule, but they are less accurate reporters of sleep quality measures such as the number and length of awakenings because of their restricted knowledge about the child's night-wakings once the child has developed nighttime self-soothing capacities (Belanger et al., 2014; Hall, Live, et al., 2015; Sadeh, 1996; Tikotzky & Sadeh, 2001; Tikotzky & Volkovich, 2019). School-aged children and adolescents can be directly involved in reporting on their own sleep, and these reports seem to be reliable (Gaina et al., 2004; Short et al., 2017).

The assessment of pediatric sleep problems may also include objective sleep measures such as actigraphy, videosomnography, and PSG. The actigraph is a small wristwatch-like device that yields body movement data which is translated into sleep–wake measures based on a computerized scoring algorithm. Actigraphy enables continuous monitoring of sleep for extended periods in the child's natural environment. In clinical practice, actigraphy is particularly recommended for the assessment of circadian sleep disorders and it may also be useful for the assessment of insomnia and treatment response, especially when the parent or child cannot provide reliable reports of their sleep. Limitations of actigraphy include artifacts resulting from externally induced movements and its inability to discriminate between sleep stages. In addition, actigraphy cannot be used to assess behavioral aspects of sleep that occur at bedtime such as settling difficulties, and it cannot discriminate between signaled and unsignaled awakenings (Hall, Live, et al., 2015; Sadeh, 2011, 2015; Tikotzky & Volkovich, 2019). These aspects, as well as other sleep disorders such as night terrors, can be captured with videosomnography. Whereas in the past the scoring of videosomnography was labor-intensive and thus limited in utility, recent developments allowing for auto-scoring of videosomnographic data have substantially increased the cost-effectiveness of this method (Kahn et al., 2021; Kahn & Gradisar, 2022). Still, some parents may be reluctant to use video recording because of privacy issues.

All the above-described methods are appropriate and usually sufficient for the assessment of behavioral sleep problems in children. However, when a physiological sleep disorder, such as OSA or restless legs syndrome (RLS), is suspected, PSG is recommended (Sadeh, 2015). This multiparameter method (including brain activity, eye movements, muscle activity, etc.) provides the most detailed and accurate information on aspects such as sleep architecture, arousals, breathing patterns, and leg movements during sleep.

Insomnia in Children

Childhood insomnia, usually manifested as difficulties initiating and/or maintaining sleep, is a very common problem, with prevalence rates ranging between 10% and 30% across childhood (Armstrong et al., 2014; Blader et al., 1997; de Zambotti et al., 2018; Mindell et al., 2006; Stein et al., 2001). Differences in prevalence rates may be explained by the specific assessment methods and diagnostic criteria that are used, for example, strict *Diagnostic and Statistical Manual of Mental Disorders*, fifth edition (DSM–5), criteria versus more broadly defined insomnia symptoms (Dewald-Kaufmann et al., 2019; Mindell et al., 2006).

When left untreated, insomnia tends to persist over time (Fernandez-Mendoza et al., 2022; Sivertsen et al., 2017) and may have a myriad of negative short- and long-term outcomes (Aslund et al., 2018; Bayer et al., 2007; Insana et al., 2013; Lunsford-Avery et al., 2021; Sadeh et al., 2014; Tikotzky et al., 2015; Williamson et al., 2020). Therefore, early assessment and intervention may be beneficial not only for improving sleep but also for alleviating the broader negative impact insomnia may have on children and their parents.

Diagnostic Criteria

The second edition of the *International Classification of Sleep Disorders* (ICSD-2; American Academy of Sleep Medicine, 2005) differentiated between two types of behavioral insomnia of childhood—the *sleep-onset association* type (difficulties falling asleep and resuming sleep in the absence of the caregiver's assistance) and the *limit-setting* type (the child's persistent refusal to go to sleep and the caregiver's difficulty setting appropriate limits necessary for facilitating sleep). However, this differentiation was removed in the third edition of the manual (ICSD-3; American Academy of Sleep Medicine, 2014), and so has the division between behavioral insomnia of childhood and adult insomnia. Thus, the present diagnostic category of *chronic insomnia disorder* refers to both adults and children. The main criterion (criterion A) specifies that the patient reports or the patient's parents or caregiver observes one or more of the following: (1) difficulty initiating sleep, (2) difficulty maintaining sleep, (3) waking up earlier than desired, (4) resistance to going to bed on appropriate schedule, and (5) difficulty sleeping without parent or caregiver intervention. Naturally, Criteria 4 and 5 are mainly relevant to children. Additional diagnostic criteria include observed or reported daytime dysfunction (e.g., fatigue, sleepiness, mood disturbance/irritability) and presence of the sleep problems despite adequate sleep opportunities. Finally, sleep disturbances should occur at least three times per week, should be present for at least 3 months, and cannot be explained by another sleep disorder. Similar to the ICSD-3, there are no separate diagnostic criteria for child and adult chronic insomnia in the DSM-5, which specifies that in children sleep-onset and night-waking problems may manifest as difficulties initiating sleep and returning to sleep without caregiver intervention. Note that according to both the ICSD and the DSM nosologies, insomnia in children typically involves the child's reliance on parental assistance to transition from wakefulness to sleep. When this help is not provided, the child's difficulties in initiating sleep may be manifested in behaviors such as crying and bedtime refusal. Thus, insomnia in children occurs in the context of parent–child interactions and family dynamics; and therefore, interventions for these disorders usually focus on changing both parents' and children's sleep-related behaviors.

Although the ICSD and DSM do not differentiate between early childhood insomnia and insomnia in older children, in the following sections we separate the discussion for early childhood insomnia (infants, toddlers, and preschoolers), insomnia in school-age children, and insomnia in adolescence because of age-specific developmental issues and the different characteristics of working with parents as the agents of change in early childhood compared with more direct work with the older child or adolescent.

Insomnia in Early Childhood

The diagnosis of early childhood insomnia is usually not considered for infants under the age of 6 months because frequent night-wakings are the rule rather the exception during the first months of life. However, around the age of 6 months most infants develop consolidated sleep and acquire nocturnal self-soothing capacities, that is, the ability to transition independently from wakefulness to sleep (Anders et al., 1992; Henderson et al., 2010, 2011). Those who do not develop this ability may be considered as presenting a sleep problem if meeting the above-mentioned ICSD or DSM criteria (Mindell & Owens, 2015). Importantly, beyond these criteria, the diagnosis of insomnia in young children depends largely on the subjective experience and expectations of the parents (Sadeh & Anders, 1993; Tikotzky & Sadeh, 2010). For instance, infant awakenings could be experienced as more challenging when they cause significant disruption to the parents' sleep and/or considerable emotional distress. It should also be noted that studies based on objective recording of infant sleep (actigraphy or videosomnography) demonstrate that in the absence of medical issues, the main factor discriminating between infants who "sleep through the night" and infants with insomnia is the capacity of the "good sleepers" to resume sleep without signaling to their parents following natural night-wakings (Anders, 1994; Mindell & Owens, 2015; Tikotzky & Sadeh, 2010).

Various physiological (maturation, health problems, temperament), environmental (culture, stress), parental (psychopathology, cognitions), and parent–infant relationship (attachment, bedtime interactions) factors may influence the development of sleep–wake patterns and insomnia in young children. These different factors and the dynamic and ongoing interactions between them have been described in the groundbreaking transactional model of infant sleep developed by Sadeh and Anders (1993; see Figure 38.1).

The development of insomnia in young children could be influenced and exacerbated by intrinsic physiological and medical factors such as genetic vulnerability, prematurity, breathing problems, and allergies (Newton et al., 2020). Neurodevelopmental conditions (e.g., autism spectrum disorder [ASD], Down syndrome) and "difficult" temperament have also been associated with early childhood insomnia (MacDuffie et al.,

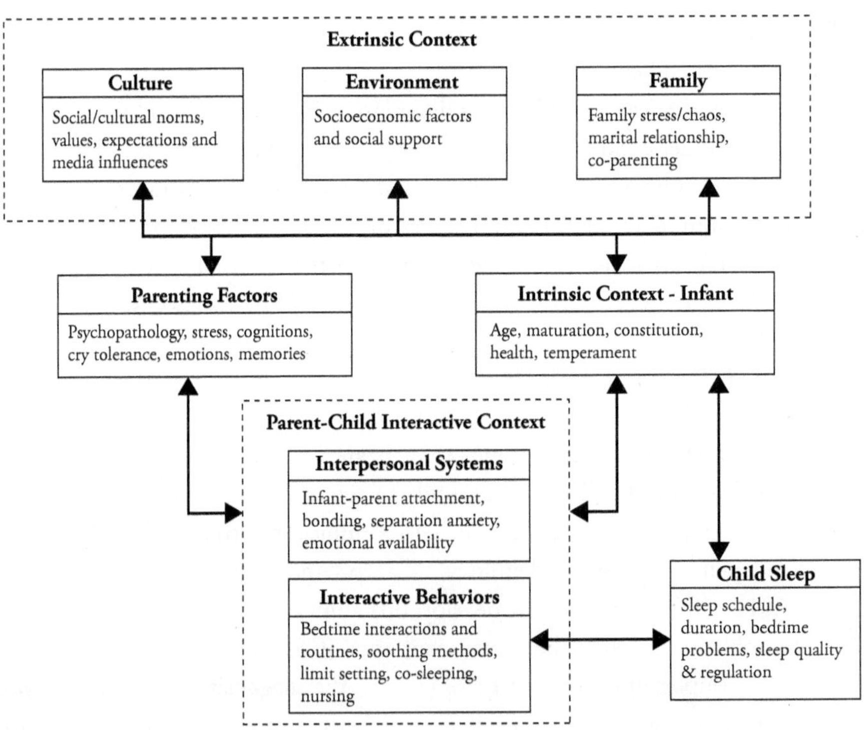

Figure 38.1 A transactional model of child sleep
Note. Adapted from Sadeh and Anders (1993).

2020; Morales-Munoz et al., 2020; Yau et al., 2019). However, the most prominent and persistent findings regarding factors contributing to the development of early childhood insomnia are related to the role of parental involvement in the bedtime settling process (Burnham et al., 2002; DeLeon & Karraker, 2007; Goodlin-Jones et al., 2001; Messayke et al., 2020; Mindell et al., 2010; Morrell & Cortina-Borja, 2002; Newton et al., 2020; Philbrook & Teti, 2016; Sadeh et al., 2009; Schlarb et al., 2020; Tikotzky & Sadeh, 2009; Yu et al., 2017; Zreik et al., 2020). Infants who fall asleep at bedtime while receiving significant help from their parents are less likely to develop self-soothing skills and more likely to develop a night-waking problem, in comparison to infants who fall asleep by themselves or with minimal parental assistance. When parents are actively involved in soothing their infants to sleep, infants may learn to associate falling asleep with parental support (*sleep-onset association*) and thus are less likely to develop the self-soothing capacities that are necessary for achieving consolidated nighttime sleep (Camerota et al., 2019; Sadeh et al., 2010; Tikotzky, 2017). For example, In a recent longitudinal study, parental presence at sleep onset and greater frequency of parent settling activities at 1 month of age predicted less regulated infant sleep, assessed using sleep diaries at 6 and 12 months (Henderson et al., 2020). Voltaire and Teti (2018) differentiated through direct observations between non-distress-initiated interventions (i.e., interventions initiated by parents in response to a calm infant awakening or during infant sleep) and distress-initiated interventions (e.g., in response to infant crying). These authors found that non-distress-initiated parental interventions (rather than distress-initiated interventions) during the first 3 months of life predicted worse infant sleep outcomes, as reported by parents, across the first 9 months in infants who were sleeping in a separate room.

Another aspect of parental bedtime behavior that is linked with children's sleep–wake patterns is parental consistency during bedtime routines. Evidence from both cross-sectional (Jones & Ball, 2014; Mindell et al., 2015; Wilson et al., 2015) and longitudinal (Koulouglioti et al., 2014; Staples et al., 2015) studies demonstrates that a consistent bedtime routine is associated with earlier bedtimes, shorter sleep latency, less bedtime resistance, longer nighttime sleep duration, and better caregiver-reported sleep quality (Mindell & Williamson, 2018).

Parental behaviors during the settling process and during the night seem to be influenced by parents' cognitions (e.g., expectations, interpretations, perceptions) and emotions. Indeed, increasing evidence suggests that parental sleep-related cognitions are an important factor to consider in the development of infant sleep problems (Cook et al., 2017; Golik et al., 2013; N. Johnson & McMahon, 2008; Morrell & Steele, 2003; Sadeh et al., 2007; Tikotzky & Sadeh, 2009). It seems that parents who are more likely to attribute distress to infant night-wakings and who report more concerns regarding limiting parental nighttime involvement are more likely to get actively involved in soothing the infant to sleep, which in turn is associated with more night-waking problems (Morrell & Steele, 2003; Tikotzky & Sadeh, 2009). Relatedly, more infant night-waking problems and higher parental nighttime involvement have also been associated with maternal anxiety related to separation from the child (Scher, 2008; Scher & Blumberg, 1999) and with higher parental sensitivity to infant crying (Kahn et al., 2018; Kahn, Livne-Karp, et al., 2020; Sadeh et al., 2016).

Overall, these findings imply that parents have an important role in the development of infant nocturnal self-soothing capacities and in the development of early childhood insomnia. Therefore, behavioral interventions for early childhood insomnia usually focus on changing parental sleep-related cognitions and behaviors, to ameliorate children's sleep problems (Mindell et al., 2006; Tikotzky & Sadeh, 2010).

TREATMENT OF INSOMNIA IN INFANTS AND TODDLERS

Behavioral interventions for early childhood insomnia are recommended after adequate assessment has been conducted, ruling out physiological and medical problems that may influence night-waking problems (e.g., breathing problems, allergies), which should be treated separately if present. Extensive research demonstrates the effectiveness of these interventions in treating early childhood insomnia (Gradisar et al., 2016; Hall, Hutton, et al., 2015; Kahn, Juda-Hanael, et al., 2020; Meltzer & Mindell, 2014; Mindell et al., 2006; Sadeh, 1994) and in reducing maternal sleep disturbances and depressive symptoms (Gradisar et al., 2016; Hall et al., 2015; Hiscock et al., 2007, 2008). Behavioral infant sleep interventions are largely based on psychological learning theory and focus on providing parents with skills on how to modify or limit their sleep-related interactions with their infant. These changes are expected to foster children's ability to fall asleep independently at bedtime and after waking up at night, thus promoting consolidated sleep. The most common interventions include parent education, extinction-based techniques, scheduled awakenings, positive routine, and bedtime fading (Mindell & Owens, 2015; Sadeh, 2005).

Sleep Education

Sleep education focuses on providing parents with information about infant sleep development (e.g., developmental changes in sleep duration, circadian rhythms, night feeding), safe sleeping, positive bedtime routines, and age-appropriate behavioral strategies to promote sleep consolidation and self-soothing. Providing parents with this information is the main component in prevention programs during pregnancy and the early postpartum period and is usually incorporated in treatment programs for early childhood insomnia. Early studies on the effects of parental education programs in the perinatal period on the development of infant sleep patterns and problems have shown positive effects on settling to sleep, night-wakings, and sleep duration (Kerr et al., 1996; Stremler et al., 2006; Wolfson et al., 1992). However, two recent large randomized controlled trials (RCTs) failed to find differences or found only small differences that were not clinically significant between psychoeducation and control (Galland et al., 2017; Santos et al., 2019).

Additional research is needed to determine which content should be included in these interventions and what would be the optimal timing of delivery to increase their efficacy.

Extinction-Based Techniques

These methods share the rationale that parental active participation in the sleep context should be reduced to improve infant sleep, but they differ in the level of parental involvement maintained during the intervention. According to *unmodified extinction* (also known as *cry it out* or *systematic ignoring*), parents should put the infant in bed drowsy but awake and then refrain from intervening until a predetermined morning wake-up time. This method is meant to facilitate learning that nighttime signaling behavior does not provoke parental attention, which may lead to the ceasing of signaling behavior and to the development of self-soothing skills (France & Hudson, 1990; Rickert & Johnson, 1988). Importantly, unmodified extinction is not commonly recommended nowadays because of the abrupt cessation of parental help and the distress it may cause both infants and parents (Tikotzky & Sadeh, 2010; Whittall et al., 2021). Accordingly, more gradual extinction techniques have been developed to ease the process for parents and infants. One common gradual technique is known in the literature as *graduated extinction* or *checking*. This intervention gradually limits parental involvement in soothing the infant to sleep but at the same time allows parents to assure the infant about their presence (Ferber, 1985; Sadeh, 2005). Unlike standard extinction, after parents leave the room, they are guided to briefly visit the infant—if they are crying and protesting—in fixed brief intervals (e.g., every 5 minutes) or in gradually increasing intervals. The aim of this visit is to consistently convey that the parent is there to protect and reassure the infant but expects the infant to fall asleep independently. The efficacy of the checking technique in improving infant sleep has been demonstrated in several RCTs (Gradisar et al., 2016; Hall, Hutton, et al., 2015; Hiscock et al., 2007; Kahn, Juda-Hanael, et al., 2020). For instance, Gradisar and colleagues (2016) compared this method to bedtime fading and a sleep education control group in 43 infants aged 6–16 months. The checking group showed the largest decrease in parental reports of number of awakenings and wake after sleep onset.

Another related technique is *parental presence*. This method guides parents to sleep in the child's room on a separate mattress (or to feign sleep) for 1–2 weeks and to implement the checking intervention from within the infant's room (Sadeh, 1994). The intervention is based on the premise that the mere presence of the parent in the infant's room would reassure the child, especially when the child's sleep problems are related to separation anxiety. The parent can leave the room after the infant has learned to fall asleep in the parent's presence, and then standard checking from outside the room could continue to be implemented. An even more gradual variation of this technique, known as *camping out*, guides parents to initially remain at close physical proximity to the infant's crib and provide some help such as patting the infant or singing. After the infant learns to fall asleep in the crib with this sort of help, the parents may gradually reduce their involvement and move farther away from the crib, until eventually leaving the room. These more gradual intervention approaches may have the benefit of being better accepted by parents as many of them do not wish to be away from their child while the child is crying or shows signs of distress (Kahn, Juda-Hanael, et al., 2020; Whittall et al., 2021). Three RCTs compared these more gradual interventions involving parental presence in the child's room to standard checking and found similar improvement in infant sleep at post-treatment (Kahn, Juda-Hanael, et al., 2020; Matthey & Črnčec, 2012; Sadeh, 1994). However, Kahn, Juda-Hanael, et al. (2020) found that infant separation anxiety moderated treatment effect. In the standard checking group, a reduction in infant nighttime wakefulness was significant only for infants with low baseline separation anxiety but not for infants with high separation anxiety. In contrast, in the parental presence intervention, significant reductions in nighttime wakefulness were found for infants with both initial low and high separation anxiety. These findings highlight the importance of extending research on the role of treatment moderators and predictors in the field of pediatric sleep interventions.

It is worth noting that all behavioral interventions that guide parents to modify their soothing behaviors typically involve some level of infant crying at the start of the intervention because of the introduced changes to the infants' usual routine. Tolerating infant crying during the intervention process is difficult for many parents because crying is a triggering stimulus that elicits strong physiological and emotional responses. Additionally, many parents fear that ignoring infant signals and crying could be harmful to the child (Etherton et al., 2016; Whittall et al., 2021). Although concerns have also been raised in the theoretical literature regarding the emotional consequences of behavioral sleep interventions (Blunden et al., 2016; Etherton et al., 2016; McKenna et al., 2007), no empirical evidence of harm on child mental health and attachment security as a result of these interventions has yet been able to confirm these propositions (Gradisar et al., 2016; Price et al., 2012). Nevertheless, some parents may still be concerned about the safety of extinction-based interventions or feel that they would be too difficult for them to implement. Therefore, parental concerns and sleep-related cognitions should be addressed and given full attention, to facilitate parental cooperation with the intervention and to help parents make informed decisions about the intervention they choose to implement (Daws & Sutton, 2020; Tikotzky & Sadeh, 2010).

Scheduled Awakenings

This method is aimed at improving sleep consolidation, without requiring parents to reduce their nighttime involvement. Scheduled awakenings may be helpful if the child's awakenings occur at relatively constant times during the night. Unlike extinction-based approaches, in this approach parents are asked to awaken the child about 15–30 minutes before their typical awakening and to sooth them as usual (e.g., feeding, rocking). When spontaneous awakenings become less frequent, the interval between scheduled awakenings can be gradually increased. Several small studies have found this approach to be effective (Johnson & Lerner, 1985; Rickert & Johnson, 1988). However, sleep improvement may take more time compared to extinction-based methods. Also, it may be difficult for parents to comply with this intervention, which requires them to wake up during the night and initiate the child's awakenings (Rickert & Johnson, 1988).

Consistent Bedtime Routines

This method focuses primarily on the bedtime process, instead of reducing parental involvement and night-waking behaviors. Bedtime routines are predictable and pleasant/calming activities that occur in the time preceding lights out, such as bathing, massage, reading a story, and singing (Mindell & Williamson, 2018). A consistent implementation of these activities for as many nights a week as possible is a critical element of this intervention. Positive bedtime routines are thought to exert their positive influence on sleep through providing the infant with a sense of predictability, calmness, and security, thereby reducing the physiological and emotional arousal that frequently accompany bedtime difficulties and resistance. This process is supposed to facilitate the child's transition between wakefulness and sleep (Fiese et al., 2021). In one RCT, mothers of children aged 7–36 months with perceived sleep problems were assigned to either a bedtime routine or a control condition. The bedtime routine group showed significant reductions in maternal reports of sleep-onset latency and in the frequency and duration of nighttime awakenings compared to the control group 2 weeks post-intervention (Mindell et al., 2009).

Bedtime Fading/Sleep Restriction Therapy

The idea behind bedtime fading is to increase the homeostatic pressure to sleep by delaying the child's usual bedtime. Like the underlying rationale of sleep restriction therapy applied in adults with insomnia (Maurer et al., 2021), the child is supposed to enter bed while feeling tired enough to ensure that they would fall asleep rapidly (Piazza & Fisher, 1991). Parents are usually asked to devote the time before bed to a calming bedtime routine, and so the combination of bedtime fading and a bedtime routine is aimed at increasing sleepiness, reconditioning sleep cues, and promoting physiological and emotional down-regulation. When the child falls asleep easily, bedtime can be gradually advanced. Bedtime fading has rarely been studied as a standalone intervention, but a few studies show that it leads not only to shorter sleep latency but also to better nighttime sleep (Cooney et al., 2018; Gradisar et al., 2016).

TREATMENT OF INSOMNIA IN PRESCHOOL-AGED CHILDREN

Most of the interventions described above could also be employed with preschool and kindergarten children who present with insomnia, except for standard checking which might be more difficult to implement when the child can climb out of bed. At this age many children with insomnia mainly exhibit bedtime struggles and come out of the bedroom after lights-out. Bedtime refusal is usually treated by strengthening parental limit-setting skills and developing realistic and consistent bedtime rules (Tikotzky & Sadeh, 2010). Moreover, in light of the children's growing cognitive, verbal, and regulatory capacities, it is also possible to directly involve them in a positive reward system plan such as a token economy program. For instance, the child is rewarded each morning with a sticker for not getting out of bed, and when a certain number of stickers has been collected the child may choose a bigger reward. A few small studies examined the use of a *bedtime pass* program. A bedtime pass is an object, such as a decorated card or stuffed animal, that the child may exchange for one chance to shortly leave the bedroom (e.g., for a drink of water) or call a parent into the bedroom for a short visit. Parents then collect the pass and remind the child that once the pass has been used, an additional trip or calling the parent is not allowed anymore that night. If the child leaves the bed again, parents are guided to use extinction-based methods for the rest of the time (Friman et al., 1999; Moore et al., 2007). One RCT of 19 children aged 3–6 years found this intervention to be effective at reducing bedtime struggles, with treatment gains maintained at a 3-month follow-up (Moore et al., 2007).

Treatment of Nighttime Fears

In preschoolers, nighttime fears are often part and parcel of insomnia symptomology (Kushnir & Sadeh, 2011). Such fears have thus been addressed in several investigations of interventions for insomnia in this age group. For example, bibliotherapy was found to be superior to a wait-list control group at reducing nighttime fears and co-sleeping frequency, with gains maintained 3 months following the intervention (El Rafihi-Ferreira et al., 2018; Lewis et al., 2015). Kushnir and Sadeh (2012) used the *huggy puppy* intervention, in which children are asked to adopt and care for a puppy dog–shaped doll that is described as frightened at nighttime. Significant reductions in nighttime fears and improvements in sleep were indexed following the intervention, yet similar improvements were also observed in the comparison group, which was instructed to use the doll as a protector. Play therapy techniques were used in a multicomponent cognitive behavioral therapy (CBT) intervention, which included psychoeducation, problem-solving, in vivo exposure, reinforcement management, and parent-involved play (Kahn et al., 2017). In an RCT of 90 children aged 4–6 years, this intervention led to greater reductions in sleep problems and co-sleeping compared to non-directive play therapy, although reductions in nighttime fears were equivalent in both groups. Importantly, CBT interventions are usually very brief (two to six sessions, depending on the specific approach), and some can be delivered at home by parents (Kopcsó et al., 2022). A recent systematic review attested to the efficacy of these interventions at reducing nighttime fears in young children and called for further investigations into their long-term effects and mechanism of action (Lewis et al., 2021).

Insomnia in School-Age Children

Many young school-age children still rely on their parents to fall asleep or demonstrate bedtime resistance and refusal to sleep alone. As children mature, the presentation of insomnia begins to change, and they are likely to develop insomnia symptoms that more closely resemble the presentation seen in adolescents and adults, such as "racing thoughts" or catastrophizing (Dewald-Kaufmann et al., 2019; Paine & Gradisar, 2011; Tikotzky & Sadeh, 2010).

Although the etiology of insomnia in school-age children is not well established, it is probably multifactorial and could be influenced by child-related physiological factors as well as socio-environmental factors (e.g., sleeping environment and habits, family stress, socioeconomic status; Dewald-Kaufmann et al., 2019; El-Sheikh et al., 2014; Kelly & El-Sheikh, 2011). Importantly, most school-age children experience sleep problems over a long period, and thus the roots of their insomnia may lie in the first years of life and the difficulties they experienced then in developing nighttime self-regulatory capacities (Paine & Gradisar, 2011; Stein et al., 2001). In addition, insomnia in school-age children may be comorbid with other medical, neurodevelopmental, and mental health problems such as attention-deficit hyperactivity disorder (ADHD) and anxiety disorders (Gregory & Sadeh, 2012). Etiological and maintaining factors that could be specifically relevant to this age group are the growing ability of children to worry about their sleep and about the impact of poor sleep on their daytime functioning (school performance, social activities). Spending increased time in bed while worrying may lead to conditioned cognitive and physiological arousal (i.e., the bed becomes associated with arousal instead of sleep), thereby delaying sleep onset and perpetuating the sleeping difficulties. Moreover, as children mature, their sleep needs change, and they may become tired at later times. When parents send the child to bed too early, conditioned arousal may develop, leading to difficulties falling asleep (Meltzer & Mindell, 2006; Paine & Gradisar, 2011). Another factor which becomes prominent at this age and may exacerbate sleep initiation difficulties is prolonged screen media use before bedtime (Cain & Gradisar, 2010; Hale & Guan, 2015).

TREATMENT OF INSOMNIA IN SCHOOL-AGE CHILDREN

Given the complexity of factors that might be involved in the development of insomnia in this age group, the proper intervention should be chosen based on a comprehensive assessment that will consider specific behavioral, emotional, and environmental factors that underlie the problem in the individual child. Generally, in young school-aged children who still rely on their parents to facilitate sleep, parents should continue to actively participate in the treatment plan. Interventions in such cases closely resemble those used with younger children (e.g., checking, positive routines, bedtime fading), although direct behavioral work with children is also recommended. The involvement of parents in treatment is essential for cases in which parents continue to reinforce undesirable behaviors (e.g., co-sleeping, allowing the child to fall asleep while watching TV). Reinforcement of positive efforts and achievements (e.g., the child tries to go to sleep independently) is also warranted (Dewald-Kaufmann et al., 2019). As children mature, interventions usually focus more on direct work with the child, building on CBT for insomnia (CBT-I) for adults. Because CBT-I in adults is described comprehensively in other chapters of this book, we will not describe it in detail here. However, specific components of adult CBT-I that can be used with most school-age children include psychoeducation (e.g., regarding the circadian clock, sleep homeostatic pressure, recommended sleep duration), sleep hygiene (e.g., avoidance of screen exposure before sleep, avoidance of caffeine), stimulus control (e.g., go to bed only when sleepy, avoid daytime naps), sleep restriction (bedtime fading), relaxation techniques (e.g., guided imagery, mindfulness), and cognitive work (e.g., thought challenging; Aslund et al., 2018; Lunsford-Avery et al., 2021). With young school-age children, an adapted version, using a therapy puppet, for example, can be used to explain and model the different elements and increase cooperation (Schlarb et al., 2018).

Research on the effects of interventions for insomnia in school-age children has been very limited, although a few RCTs attest to their effectiveness (Aslund et al., 2018; Dewald-Kaufmann et al., 2019; Quach et al., 2011). In the first RCT conducted in school-age children, Paine and Gradisar (2011) randomly assigned 42 children aged between 7 and 13 years to a six-session CBT-I intervention or a waiting-list control group. Treatment included behavioral components such as sleep education, sleep hygiene, and bedtime fading, as well as somatic and cognitive arousal reduction techniques. Parents were asked to provide encouragement and reinforcement of successful coping with independent sleeping. Improvements were found in the CBT-I group for both sleep diary and actigraphic sleep latency and sleep efficiency, as well as with problematic sleep associations and child-reported anxiety. All gains were maintained at the 6-month follow-up. Schlarb and colleagues (2018) conducted an RCT to examine the effectiveness of CBT-I in a group of 112 children with insomnia (age range 5–11.5 years). The intervention consisted of three group sessions for parents and three for children and included most CBT-I components. Findings demonstrated improvement in both actigraphic and reported sleep quality measures in comparison to the wait-list control group, and improvement remained stable at follow-ups. A recent RCT (Cain et al., 2022) examined the effectiveness of two "doses" of sleep restriction therapy (bedtime only and nighttime) compared to control in 61 school-age children (ages 6–14). Both intervention groups showed improvement in insomnia symptoms relative to control. Gains were maintained at 1-month follow-up, suggesting that sleep restriction may be an effective standalone intervention for insomnia in school-age children.

These studies provide evidence for the effectiveness of CBT-I with school-age children diagnosed with insomnia. However, more RCTs are needed to further support these findings, to systematically assess which CBT-I components are especially effective at treating school-age children, and to adjust the role of parents in these interventions to the changing developmental needs of children during the school-age years.

Insomnia in Adolescence

Despite it being the most prevalent sleep disorder in adolescence, the incidence of insomnia diminishes somewhat with the transition into the teenage years and is estimated to be 9%–18% in this age group (Hysing et al., 2013; E. O. Johnson et al., 2006). Furthermore, a female predominance emerges in adolescence, with girls being twice as likely to be diagnosed as boys (Hysing et al., 2013). This gender difference suggests that hormonal changes may be implicated in the pathogenesis of adolescent insomnia. As in younger children, insomnia in adolescents emanates from an interplay between intrinsic and extrinsic factors. Intrinsic factors include genetic vulnerability, changes related to bioregulatory processes governing sleep (i.e., the sleep homeostat and circadian rhythm), and medical or neurodevelopmental conditions (de Zambotti et al., 2018). Hyperarousal is seen as a key contributor, given that adolescents with insomnia tend to have increased cortical arousal during sleep, as well as elevated inflammation and hyperaroused cardiac autonomic modulation (Fernandez-Mendoza et al., 2016, 2017; Rodríguez-Colón et al., 2015). Extrinsic factors include parental divorce, adverse parenting styles, and family stress, as well as lower socioeconomic background and ethnicity/minority status (Blake et al., 2018; Guglielmo et al., 2018). Increased media screen exposure, caffeine and alcohol intake, and social and academic responsibilities have also been proposed as precipitating and perpetuating factors (Bartel et al., 2015; Hale et al., 2019; Marmorstein, 2017; Owens et al., 2014).

The manifestation of insomnia in adolescents bears resemblance to that of adults, with increased cognitive hyperarousal (e.g., "racing thoughts"), sleep dissatisfaction, and maladaptive beliefs about sleep (e.g., "If I don't get 8 hours of sleep, I am sure to fail my exam tomorrow"). Clinical interviews begin to focus more on the young person's experience and perspective, yet parent reports may still be beneficial. As part of the assessment process in this age group, it is particularly important to inspect the adolescent's circadian rhythms and consider the possibility of a delayed sleep–wake phase disorder (DSWPD; see section "Circadian Rhythm Problems"). Assessment of the young person's sleep–wake patterns on weekends versus weekdays, and sometimes documenting a non-restricted sleep schedule for a few days, may help determine the presence of DSWPD, insomnia, or both.

Multiple studies have documented the maladaptive consequences of insomnia on adolescents' physical and mental health. Chronic insomnia has been associated with a two- to fourfold increase in risk for adolescent somatic health problems (Hedin et al., 2020; Roberts et al., 2008). Insomnia has also been linked with poorer executive functioning, which may underlie the greater likelihood of adolescents with insomnia engaging in risk-taking behaviors and substance abuse (Catrett & Gaultney, 2009; Mike et al., 2016; Thomas et al., 2015). Several mental disorders have additionally been linked with insomnia in adolescence, including mood disorders, suicidality, anxiety disorders, and anorexia nervosa (Allison et al., 2016; Blake et al., 2018). While sleep problems have traditionally been conceived of as symptoms of depression, recent evidence suggests that insomnia symptoms tend to precede the development of depression, rather than the other way around, albeit links are likely bidirectional (de Zambotti et al., 2018; Gradisar et al., 2022).

TREATMENT OF INSOMNIA IN ADOLESCENCE

As in the case of younger children, CBT-I is considered the first-line treatment of insomnia in adolescence (Blake et al., 2017; Medalie et al., 2021). Many of the treatment modalities described previously in this chapter are implemented in this age group as well, including psychoeducation, sleep hygiene, stimulus control, sleep restriction, graduated exposure, reinforcement management, cognitive restructuring, relaxation techniques, and mindfulness. Combinations of these interventions have been shown to alleviate insomnia symptoms when delivered face to face, both individually and in group formats, and digitally via telehealth or using a phone application (Blake et al., 2017; de Bruin et al., 2015; Werner-Seidler et al., 2019). Digital delivery methods may be particularly beneficial for adolescents, who are typically more concerned about stigmatization than younger children. Importantly, evidence has been documented for the efficacy of CBT-I in improving not only insomnia but also depression, anxiety, and ADHD symptoms (Blake et al., 2016; de Bruin et al., 2018; Orchard et al., 2020). Moreover, de Bruin and colleagues' RCT (2018) demonstrated that improvements in sleep mediated the positive effects of CBT-I on psychopathology. Targeting insomnia may thus be a promising first-step intervention for adolescents with comorbid mental disorders, given that acceptability and adherence may be higher when sleep—rather than emotions—is the initial focus of treatment (Gradisar et al., 2022).

Pharmacological interventions are also used to treat adolescent insomnia, either as stand-alone treatments or in combination with CBT-I. Exogenous melatonin is the most commonly used medication for pediatric insomnia. This synthetic hormone can advance circadian timing, reduce sleep-onset latency (when delivered in immediate-release form), and increase sleep consolidation (when delivered in prolonged-release form). A recent meta-analysis found that, compared to placebo, exogenous melatonin led to significantly greater reductions in sleep-onset latency and increases in total sleep time in children and adolescents with insomnia (Wei et al., 2020). Notably, despite concerns regarding the safety of exogenous melatonin use in pediatric populations, this meta-analysis yielded little to no difference in short-term side effects of melatonin compared to placebo. Still, the long-term side effects of this treatment should be further examined. Other pharmacological options, such as sedating antihistamines, benzodiazepines, and antidepressants, are also used to treat adolescent insomnia, particularly when there is a coexisting medical, psychiatric, and/or neurodevelopmental condition (Barrett et al., 2013; Bruni et al., 2019). Yet, neither melatonin nor any of these medications have been approved by the US Food and Drug Administration (FDA), and prolonged-release exogenous melatonin alone has been approved by the European Medicines Agency for treating insomnia in youth.

More research work is thus warranted to inform guidelines for the safe and effective use of pharmacotherapy in children and adolescents with insomnia.

Circadian Rhythm Problems

As previously mentioned, sleep undergoes dynamic changes in its underlying biology as the child develops into an adolescent. Comparisons between younger (age ~11 years) and older adolescents (age ~14 years) have demonstrated a reduction in sleep homeostatic pressure, such that older adolescents are more alert in the late evening (Taylor et al., 2005). However, it is not precisely known at what age the change in adolescents' sleep homeostat occurs, with one longitudinal study suggesting it likely occurs between 12 and 14 years (Gradisar et al., 2020). To compound this evening alertness, adolescents' timing of their circadian rhythm gradually delays across development (Crowley et al., 2018). At a population level, this can be observed from ages 10 to 20 years via the measurement of chronotype (i.e., the mid-point of sleep-on free days; Roenneberg et al., 2004). Indeed, a delay in sleep timing is the norm during adolescence, with analyses showing that such a sleep pattern occurs across many countries and continents (Gariepy et al., 2020; Gradisar, Gardner, & Dohnt, 2011). If delayed sleep timing is so prevalent among adolescents, this suggests it is not abnormal, and thus does not require intervention. Thus, the next logical question is, when does one intervene?

Clinical interventions are usually recommended when the individual, or someone close to them (e.g., family member), experiences a negative consequence. While there are a plethora of negative consequences stemming from a departure from healthy adolescent sleep—which is beyond the scope of this chapter (Shochat et al., 2014)—there are nevertheless two key consequences that are particularly relevant during adolescence.

First, academic achievement during the adolescent years dictates future academic study and/or career options, and academic achievement can be influenced by circadian timing (Phillips et al., 2017). Furthermore, due to the restriction of sleep that occurs for adolescents across the school week as they rise early to attend school (Crowley et al., 2018), there is an added influence of this sleep restriction on their academic performance (Dewald et al., 2010). Yet, it is the resultant daytime sleepiness that has shown more of an effect on adolescents' school performance than sleep duration and sleep quality (Dewald et al., 2010). Taken together, this suggests many adolescents may be trying to learn through the "fog" of daytime sleepiness and during times of the day (e.g., morning) that are not conducive to any waking behavior (as they should be sleeping).

A second common occurrence from delayed circadian timing in adolescents is depression (Bauducco et al., 2020; Gradisar et al., 2022). Delayed circadian timing independently relates to levels of depression (Bauducco et al., 2020). Compared to good-sleeping adolescents, those diagnosed with DSWPD self-report higher levels of depression (Richardson & Gradisar, 2022). Of note is that adolescents with DSWPD also report higher levels of ruminative thinking (i.e., worry and rumination; Richardson & Gradisar, 2022), which presents as another pathway linking poor sleep and depression (Gradisar et al., 2022). However, one does not observe this pattern only in adolescents with a diagnosed circadian disorder but also in those with a late chronotype (Bauducco et al., 2020). Regardless, higher levels of depression during adolescence are troublesome for them when entering adulthood (D. Johnson et al., 2018). Finally, a complex interaction exists whereby a higher proportion of evening-type adolescents experience greater daytime sleepiness and depression, which in turn may result in lower grades (Short et al., 2013). Given that the negative sleep outcomes resulting from a circadian delay may impact an adolescent's mental health and academic achievement, adolescence may be considered a sensitive period of development. As such, this suggests intervention need not be reserved just for those diagnosed with a circadian rhythm disorder like DSWPD but can also be used if there are significant consequences due to a late chronotype.

Treatment of Circadian Rhythm Problems

Recent years have seen the emergence of a new, more holistic sleep intervention intended to target a range of different sleep problems experienced by adolescents—with the weight of the evidence indicating benefits for late chronotypes (Harvey et al., 2018). The transdiagnostic sleep intervention (TranS-C-Youth) is modular therapy (Harvey, 2016) including four core modules, four "cross-cutting" modules that are taught in every session, and four optional modules (Harvey et al. 2018). The intention is that the TranS-C intervention is flexible enough that it can target various psychophysiological sleep issues experienced by adolescents, including insomnia, delayed sleep phase disorder, nightmares, and adherence to continuous positive airway pressure (CPAP) therapy for sleep apnea (Harvey, 2016). In the first RCT, TranS-C was designed to teach late chronotype adolescents techniques based on CBT-I, interpersonal and social rhythm therapy, chronotherapy, and motivational interviewing over six sessions (Harvey et al., 2018). Compared to a control group receiving psychoeducation, adolescents who received TranS-C showed improvements in phase-advancing their chronotype, as well as the sequalae of benefits that flow from an earlier sleep timing (i.e., reduced *social jetlag*, significant discrepancy in sleep timing between weekdays and weekends [Roenneberg et al., 2019]; increased sleep duration; decreased daytime sleepiness [Harvey et al., 2018]). The earlier sleep timing was the key outcome that was maintained, both at the 6-month follow-up (Dong et al., 2020) and 1 year after treatment cessation (Dolsen et al., 2023). While meaningful changes in various health domains were not observed (e.g., physical, behavioral, social, emotional; Harvey et al., 2018), it could be argued that maintaining a stable and earlier chronotype across a 12-month period may have prevented complications in these areas of functioning. Nevertheless, this data suggests that sleep interventions can be performed for subclinical circadian rhythm issues in adolescents.

But what happens when an adolescent crosses the line from a typical evening type to DSWPD? Recent research has shown that compared to their good-sleeping peers, those with DSWPD perform just as well on objective assessments of cognitive abilities (i.e., short-term memory, processing speed) despite reporting lower school grades (Richardson, Micic, et al., 2018). Adolescents with DSWPD report significantly higher levels of fatigue, daytime sleepiness, repetitive negative thinking, depressed mood, and overall impairment (Richardson, Cain, et al., 2018). While most adolescents with DSWPD appear to maintain their schooling, many have been at risk for school non-attendance (Gradisar, Dohnt, et al., 2011). Any of these above-mentioned self-reports flags that there is a "problem," and thus intervention is crucial. The sleep profile of adolescents with DSWPD may vary and could be argued to be age-dependent—with a more severe sleep profile as they age (e.g., later sleep-onset time, insufficient school night sleep). Due to the chronicity of a late sleep onset, many adolescents with DSWPD present with insomnia symptoms. Besides the classic long sleep-onset latency, sleep-related monitoring and sleep misperception have been observed (Richardson et al., 2019). Fortunately, chronotherapies are demonstrating that they can improve not only sleep but also a host of negative outcomes resulting from the DSWPD experience. At present, bright light therapy—timed at the end of the adolescent's sleep period—has the greatest amount of research evidence. Clinical trials have shown that bright light, in the form of natural outdoor light and/or indoor artificial light, can reduce sleep-onset latency, produce an earlier sleep-onset time, and increase sleep duration on school nights (Gradisar, Dohnt, et al., 2011; Kaplan et al., 2019; Richardson, Cain, et al., 2018; Saxvig et al., 2014; Wilhelmsen-Langeland et al., 2013).[1] Possibly the second-ranked chronobiologic agent to phase-advance sleep timing in adolescents is melatonin. As mentioned earlier in this chapter, a recent meta-analysis found that exogenous melatonin administered in the evening decreased sleep-onset latency (Wei et al., 2020). However, this meta-analysis also included children who typically do not display significantly delayed sleep timing. It is evident more clinical trials on oral melatonin are required to establish whether or not administration advances sleep and circadian timing in adolescents with DSWPD. Finally, scheduled morning exercise has recently been shown to phase-advance circadian timing in adolescents, relative to being sedentary in the morning (Lang et al., 2022). Worth noting is that this latter study was performed on adolescents with a late chronotype; therefore, replication is needed on adolescents with DSWPD.

Parasomnias

The term *parasomnia* is derived from the Greek prefix *para*, which means "alongside," and the Latin word *somnus*, which means sleep. Correspondingly, parasomnias are unwanted motor, verbal, emotional, or behavioral events occurring either during sleep or during the process of sleep onset or offset. These disorders are separately classified into non-rapid-eye-movement (NREM) parasomnias (e.g., sleep terrors), rapid-eye-movement (REM) parasomnias (e.g., nightmares), and other parasomnias (e.g., sleep enuresis), based on the typical stage of sleep in which the events occur (see Table 38.1; American Academy of Sleep Medicine, 2014).

Table 38.1 Classification of parasomnias based on the *International Classification of Sleep Disorders*, third edition

NREM-related parasomnias	REM-related parasomnias	Other
Confusional arousals[a]	REM sleep behavior disorder	Exploding head syndrome
Sleepwalking[a]	Recurrent isolated sleep paralysis	Sleep-related hallucinations
Sleep terrors[a]	Nightmare disorder[a]	Sleep enuresis[a]
Sleep-related eating disorder		Parasomnia due to medical disorder
		Parasomnia due to medication or substance
		Parasomnia, unspecified

[a]Parasomnias commonly occurring in childhood.

Note. NREM = non-rapid eye movement; REM = rapid eye movement.

While largely considered benign phenomena, parasomnias can be substantially disruptive for some children and families, and such cases require adequate assessment and intervention (Oliviero et al., 2007; Owens & Mohan, 2016). In the following sections, we review the main clinical features of the types of parasomnias commonly diagnosed in children and young people, as well as their pathophysiology, assessment, and treatment.

NREM-Related Parasomnias Common in Youth

NREM parasomnias, also referred to as *disorders of arousal* or *partial arousal parasomnias*, are dissociated states between NREM sleep and full awakenings. Criteria for these disorders include the following: (a) recurrent episodes of incomplete awakening, (b) absent or inappropriate responsiveness, (c) limited or no cognition of dream report, and (d) partial or complete amnesia for the episode (American Academy of Sleep Medicine, 2014). Arousal episodes occur predominantly during slow-wave sleep, usually within a few hours of sleep onset. These disorders occur in 1%–4% of adults (Maski & Owens, 2016) but are much more common in pediatric populations, with prevalence ranging from 7% to 34% (Bruni & Miano, 2021; Singh et al., 2018). Prevalence rates are even higher in children diagnosed with neurological or psychological disorders (e.g., epilepsy, ADHD; Maski & Owens, 2016). NREM parasomnias tend to be underdiagnosed in children. This may be because some awakenings may not come to parents' attention, and even when they do, they are often mistaken for nightmares or full arousals (Bruni & Miano, 2021). Often, different types of NREM parasomnias overlap; they exist on a continuum, with most cases exhibiting features of multiple subtypes. Yet, for classification purposes, NREM parasomnias have been categorized into confusional arousals, sleepwalking, sleep terrors, and sleep-related eating disorder. The latter is seldom reported in children and is thus beyond the scope of this chapter. The former three are hereby described.

CONFUSIONAL AROUSALS

Confusional arousals are characterized by disorientation to time and space, slow mentation, grogginess, and disorganized behavior upon arousal from NREM sleep. The child typically sits up in bed, looks confused, and often speaks slowly and incoherently, cries, or moans. Attempts to intervene may trigger agitation, whereas when left to themselves, children often return to sleep spontaneously after a few minutes (Bruni & Miano, 2021; Maski & Owens, 2016). Confusional arousals are prevalent in 17.3% of children and are most common from infancy to the preschool age (Kotagal, 2009).

SLEEP TERRORS

Sleep terrors (also known as *night terrors*) are abrupt dramatic arousals from slow-wave sleep, during which the child appears extremely distressed, fearful, or agitated. Crying and screaming are common, with marked autonomic discharges, such as increased heart rate, hyperventilation, and sweating (Gigliotti et al., 2021). These episodes tend to last 3–5 minutes, during which the child is unresponsive and cannot be consoled or woken. As with other NREM parasomnias, there is usually no recollection of the episode. Despite their alarming manifestation, sleep terrors have not been shown to cause harm. They are highly prevalent in the preschool years, particularly in boys, with estimates of up to 40%, yet prevalence dramatically declines in the school-age years and is approximately 2% in adulthood (Petit et al., 2007, 2015).

Differentiation between sleep terrors and nightmares is relatively straightforward and based mainly on the timing of occurrence as sleep terrors typically occur in the first third of the night, during NREM sleep, whereas nightmares generally occur in the last third, during REM sleep. The level of consciousness is also markedly different, with disorientation during sleep terrors compared to alertness and responsiveness following a nightmare and recall being absent following sleep terrors and partial or full following a nightmare. Differential diagnosis from sleep-related hypermotor epilepsy is also sometimes required, albeit these conditions can coexist (Tinuper et al., 2016).

SLEEPWALKING

Episodes of sleepwalking, or *somnambulism*, involve getting out of bed and moving around upon partial arousal from slow-wave sleep. Children may walk aimlessly, occasionally bumping into things, and sometimes engage in bizarre behaviors (Owens & Mohan, 2016). As in other NREM parasomnias, the child may seem dazed and unaware of their environment, vocalizations are often incomprehensible, and attempts to communicate are met with inappropriate responses or agitation (Bruni & Miano, 2021). In some cases, injuries can occur (e.g., falling, bumping into objects; Maski & Owens, 2016). Episode duration is usually 5–15 minutes. Onset is typically at age 4–8 years. Childhood prevalence has been estimated at 10%–17% (Petit et al., 2015; Singh et al., 2018), and compared to other NREM parasomnias, sleepwalking is more likely to persist into adolescence and beyond (Plazzi et al., 2005).

Pathophysiology

The underlying pathophysiology of NREM parasomnias is not yet clear. Immediate triggers in children include conditions that increase sleep homeostatic pressure, creating a compensatory increase in the depth of NREM sleep (e.g., sleep loss, hypnotic medication), as well as conditions that increase the likelihood of cortical arousals from sleep (e.g., environmental stimuli such as sudden loud noises, presence of OSA or RLS, fevered illness, and emotional stress; Irfan et al., 2021). Recent evidence indicates a greater likelihood of behavioral and emotional problems among children and adolescents diagnosed with NREM parasomnias compared to controls, although the causal relationships between these disorders are still unclear (Castelnovo et al., 2021). Genetic background is a considerable predisposing factor, and genetic anomalies have been associated with NREM parasomnias (Lecendreux et al., 2003; Licis et al., 2011). Moreover, roughly 80% of children who sleepwalk have at least one family member with a similar history (Hublin & Kaprio, 2003). Several anomalies in sleep microarchitecture have been associated with NREM parasomnias. Studies in adult patients demonstrated increased arousals and decreased slow-wave activity density during the early sleep cycles compared to controls (Gaudreau et al., 2000; Guilleminault et al., 2006). NREM instability, expressed via increased cyclic alternating pattern, referring to the intrinsic oscillation between cortical arousal and quiescence throughout NREM sleep, has also been found in NREM parasomnia patients, even on nights with no episodes (Bruni et al., 2008; Guilleminault et al., 2006). NREM parasomnias have also been suggested to result from activation of "central pattern generators," which are located in subcortical regions and regulate innate behavioral automatisms (e.g., violent gestures; Tassinari et al., 2009). During NREM sleep, these neural networks may be instigated in isolation from other neural structures that regulate normal wakeful behavior, thus generating stereotypical motor activity along with poor executive function and amnesia (Irfan et al., 2021). Future research is needed to elucidate the underlying mechanisms of these dissociated sleep–wake states.

Treatment

NREM parasomnias are usually infrequent and have no maladaptive consequences. In such cases, management could consist of psychoeducation and reassurance of the family that these are benign phenomena, which usually resolve spontaneously. Safety measures should be discussed (e.g., locking doors and windows), particularly in sleepwalking children. Parents should be advised against intervening or trying to wake the child up during an episode, given the potential for increased confusion or agitation (Attarian, 2010; Gigliotti et al., 2021). Precipitating factors should also be addressed, including sleep deprivation, stress, medications increasing slow-wave sleep, and external disturbances to sleep (e.g., noise). Practicing sleep hygiene and prescribing consistent, slightly extended (by 30–60 minutes) sleep opportunities may be sufficient for most cases (Owens & Mohan, 2016).

For children who experience frequent episodes, as well as comorbid sleep or psychological disorders, more intensive intervention is warranted. However, evidence for the efficacy of NREM parasomnia interventions is currently limited. Scheduled awakenings, in which parents wake the child 15–30 minutes prior to the typical time of episodes for a period of approximately 4 weeks, can be effective for children who experience very frequent episodes, occurring at roughly the same time of night (Tobin, 1993). While this technique has been shown to be effective in some case series (Lask, 1988), further research is needed to establish its efficacy and underlying mechanisms. Additionally, anecdotal evidence supports the use of psychological treatment, including behavioral therapy, relaxation, and hypnosis (Attarian, 2010; Hauri et al., 2007). In rare cases where episodes are extremely disruptive or perilous, pharmacological treatment may be considered. Prescribed medications may include slow-wave sleep suppressants (e.g., benzodiazepines), tricyclic antidepressants, or melatonin (Irfan et al., 2021; Jan et al., 2004). Families should be advised that use of each of these drugs to treat NREM parasomnias is considered "off-label" (Bruni & Miano, 2021).

REM-Related Parasomnias Common in Youth

REM-related sleep parasomnias are unpleasant experiences or behaviors occurring during or following REM sleep. These parasomnias include REM sleep behavior disorder, recurrent isolated sleep paralysis, and nightmare disorder (American Academy of Sleep Medicine, 2014). The former two are uncommon in youth, whereas nightmare disorder is highly prevalent in children and is thus the focus of the following section.

NIGHTMARE DISORDER

Nightmares are upsetting dreams usually occurring during REM sleep (thus often in the last third of the night), which usually result in awakening. The content of dreams is typically scary and vivid, eliciting intense fear or other negative emotions, such as rage or disgust. Following nightmares, individuals usually become fully alert, can recount the nightmare scenario, respond positively to comforting, and often find it difficult to resume sleep. To be classified as nightmare disorder, nightmares need to be frequent, extremely dysphoric, and associated with considerable distress or impairment (American Academy of Sleep Medicine, 2014; American Psychiatric Association, 2013). Occasional nightmares are very common in children, with prevalence rates of 60%–75% (Reynolds & Alfano, 2016; Zadra & Donderi, 2000). Yet, recurrent nightmares (>1 per week) are less common and affect approximately 3%–6% of youth (Gauchat et al., 2014; Schredl, 2020). These have been associated with a myriad of nighttime and daytime maladaptive consequences, including insomnia symptoms, severe nighttime fears, and social, emotional, and academic difficulties (Kushnir & Sadeh, 2011; Mindell & Barrett, 2002; Schredl et al., 2009).

The etiology of nightmare disorder is thought to include several intrinsic and environmental factors. Nighttime hyperarousal, as demonstrated in individuals diagnosed with insomnia (Riemann et al., 2010) and post-traumatic stress disorder (Woodward et al., 2000), may increase the likelihood of sleep fragmentation, with some evidence for increased REM fragmentation in particular (Habukawa et al., 2018; Riemann et al., 2012). Sleep disorders which induce arousals (e.g., OSA) have also been linked with elevated nightmare frequency, and treating sleep respiratory problems has been shown to reduce the incidence of nightmares (BaHammam & Almeneessier, 2019). Impairments in fear extinction have also been proposed as underlying mechanisms for nightmare phenomenology as previous fearful memories fail to be associated with novel neutral–positive dream contexts, and thus extinction learning is not acquired (Nielsen & Levin, 2007). Traumatic experiences and childhood adversity may predispose nightmare occurrence, disrupting the development of adaptive emotion regulation and neurological affect networks (Nielsen, 2017). Indeed, nightmares are a hallmark of post-traumatic stress disorder, although they often occur in individuals diagnosed with other psychological disorders (e.g., depression) as well.

Assessment of nightmare disorder is often straightforward, given the distinct dream recall and typical occurrence in the latter parts of the night (see above, differential diagnosis from sleep terrors). The most established treatment for nightmare disorder is imagery rehearsal therapy, in which children rehearse alternative dream storylines while awake, in an aim to reduce the likelihood of recurrence of negative dream scenarios (Krakow & Zadra, 2010). Other types of psychotherapy have also been used to treat nightmares, such as CBT with exposure, relaxation, and rescripting modules (Fernandez et al., 2013), as well as lucid dreaming (de Macêdo et al., 2019). A recent trial used a remote control–like device called the "Dream Changer" as a low-intensity intervention for childhood nightmares, showing reductions in nightmare frequency and related anxiety at post-treatment (Bourboulis et al., 2022). Finally, pharmacotherapy (e.g., prazosin, risperidone, or trazodone) is used in severe cases. However, evidence for the efficacy of interventions for nighttime disorder in youth is based mostly on small, uncontrolled studies; and more work is needed to understand the efficacy, predictors, and mechanistic pathways of intervention approaches.

Other Parasomnias Common in Youth

SLEEP ENURESIS

Of the "other parasomnias," which do not necessarily occur during a specific stage of sleep, nocturnal enuresis is the only disorder typically seen in youth. Sleep enuresis is diagnosed when involuntary passing of urine during sleep occurs at least twice a week for a period of at least 3 months (American Academy of Sleep Medicine, 2014). It is only considered a disorder after the age of 5, and prevalence rates dramatically decrease with age, from 5%–10% at age 7 years to 1%–2% in adolescence and beyond (Mota et al., 2015; Yeung et al., 2004). Boys are more likely to experience sleep enuresis than girls, yet gender differences are no longer apparent after puberty. Secondary enuresis is diagnosed when recurrent bedwetting occurs after a period of >6 months of being dry. Compared to primary enuresis (in which such remission never occurred), secondary enuresis is considerably less prevalent and tends to be associated with organic (e.g., diabetes, seizures) or psychological (e.g., parental neglect or abuse) factors.

While sleep structure is similar between nights in which enuresis does and does not occur for the same child, children with enuresis sleep differently than controls. Enuresis has been associated with more sleep fragmentation and daytime sleepiness (Dhondt et al., 2009; Soster et al., 2017). Elevated sleep pressure caused by this fragmentation may be responsible for the higher arousal threshold, potentially impairing the child's ability to awaken in response to bladder activity (Bruni & Miano, 2021). Other physiological pathways, such as abnormal bladder reservoir function during sleep and excess nighttime urine production, may also play a role in the development of this disorder (Pedersen et al., 2020). Genetics are another predisposing factor as the likelihood of a child experiencing enuresis is 77% when both parents have a history of enuresis, and twin-based heritability is estimated at approximately 70% (Hublin & Kaprio, 2003).

Assessment of enuresis may be based on sleep diary data, as well as detailed descriptions of urination and fluid intake. Physical examinations (e.g., observing bladder distention) may be useful, and in some cases additional testing is required to rule out other conditions (e.g., urine culture to exclude urinary tract infections). The first-line treatment of primary enuresis is conditioning using an alarm device (Neveus et al., 2010). Other approaches may include scheduled awakenings, continence reinforcement, and restriction of fluids at night. Pharmacological options include desmopressin—a synthetic analogue of arginine vasopressin which decreases urine production. Alternatively, bladder capacity may be increased using antimuscarinic drugs (Arda et al., 2016). Despite some success, up to a third of children do not benefit from these treatments, and thus improving treatment and developing novel interventions are still warranted.

Sleep-Related Movement Disorders

Sleep-related movement disorder refers to simple stereotyped movements, occurring predominantly around the sleep period, that interfere with sleep onset or continuity. They include RLS, periodic limb movement disorders (PLMDs), growing pains, restless sleep disorder (RSD), nocturnal leg cramps, rhythmic movement disorder, bruxism, benign sleep myoclonus in infancy, and propriospinal myoclonus at sleep onset. The diagnosis of a sleep-related movement disorder requires the presence of disturbed sleep with complaints of daytime fatigue or sleepiness.

RLS

RLS, or Willis-Ekbom disease, is a neurologic disorder initially described by Sir Thomas Willis in 1685. Diagnostic criteria for pediatric-onset RLS were introduced in 2003 and updated in 2013 (Picchietti et al., 2013). RLS is relatively common in pediatrics, with a prevalence ranging from 2% to 4% in school-aged children and adolescents (Picchietti et al., 2007). Early-onset RLS is highly familial, with a 71% presence of positive family history in children and 80% in adolescents, with mothers three times more likely to be affected than fathers (Picchietti et al., 2013).

The diagnosis of RLS in pediatrics is generally overlooked since children mainly complain about difficulty falling or staying asleep, rather than describe the typical symptoms of RLS like leg discomfort, paresthesia, and urge to move. RLS may also be misdiagnosed because of the mild and intermittent nature of the symptoms at younger ages or the inability of young children to describe the sensations or discomfort in the legs. Therefore, language and cognitive abilities will determine the applicability of the RLS diagnostic criteria (DelRosso, Mogavero, et al., 2021). Unlike adults, children do not report the typical escalation of symptoms during the evening or at night but report daytime leg discomfort that is often misdiagnosed as growing pains (GPs). GPs represent one of the common RLS mimics, have a peak prevalence at 4–6 years of age, and can occur in the evening. It is not easy to differentiate RLS and GPs: In RLS there is an urge to move the legs and a relief by movement that is not the case with GPs. Moreover, GPs are commonly described as painful, whereas only 45% of children with RLS report associated pain (Hamilton-Stubbs & Walters, 2017).

Periodic limb movements (PLMs) during sleep (PLMS) are often associated with RLS in adults, and PLMD may sometimes precede the diagnosis of RLS. Furthermore, the presence of more than five PLMs per hour and a positive family history of either RLS or more than five PLMs per hour among first-degree relatives are supportive criteria for the diagnosis of pediatric RLS (Picchietti et al., 2013).

RLS is associated with insomnia, poor sleep quality, cognitive dysfunction, and psychiatric disorders (e.g., depression, anxiety, and conduct disorder) but also with GPs, kidney disease, migraine, diabetes, epilepsy, rheumatologic disorders, cardiovascular disease, and liver and gastrointestinal disorders (Angriman et al., 2017). Pediatric RLS is highly comorbid with ADHD, especially the combined and hyperactive type; this comorbidity might be related to a common genetic substrate or a common dopaminergic dysfunction linked to iron deficiency. In fact, low iron stores and decreased vitamin D are predisposing factors, and RLS severity is correlated with both low serum ferritin level and vitamin D deficiency. Improvement in symptoms with iron and dopaminergic agents suggests an involvement of the dopaminergic pathways and basal nuclei, especially at the level of the substantia nigra and thalamus, with reduced iron uptake in these areas. However, the data is still conflicting, and there are no studies in children (DelRosso et al., 2022).

TREATMENT OF RLS

Treatment of RLS in children should include non-pharmacological management including sleep hygiene rules and bedtime routines, dietary modification with elimination of caffeine, and physical activity with stretching leg exercises and sensory stimulation with rubbing, massaging, cool pads, or heating pads that decrease symptoms of RLS. Some medications known to exacerbate RLS should be avoided; in particular, selective serotonin reuptake inhibitors, tricyclic antidepressants, metoclopramide, diphenhydramine, nicotine, and alcohol worsen leg movements at night (DelRosso & Bruni, 2019). There are currently no FDA-approved medications for RLS in children, and therapeutic protocols for pediatric RLS are lacking. The treatment of RLS due to iron deficiency in children requires fasting blood iron profile and ferritin levels to be checked before beginning oral iron supplementation. Iron supplementation is usually given to patients with ferritin levels <50 ng/ml, at a daily dose of 1–6 mg/kg of ferrous sulfate or 50–65 mg of elemental iron. Iron levels usually take some time to improve (i.e., 3 months or more). The most frequent adverse effects reported with oral iron administration are constipation, nausea, and unpleasant taste (Bruni & Angriman, 2017). When symptoms persist following iron supplementation, combination therapy with a second medication like clonazepam or pramipexole or clonidine may be needed. Gabapentin can be combined with iron supplementation in refractory cases. Dopaminergic medications have proven successful in case reports and small open-label studies of children with RLS with and without ADHD, but there is scarce data supporting their use (DelRosso & Bruni, 2019).

PLMD

The ICSD-3 (American Academy of Sleep Medicine, 2014) defines PLMD as episodes of repetitive, highly stereotyped limb movements that occur during sleep, with a frequency of more than five per hour in children associated with a clinical sleep disturbance or a complaint of daytime fatigue that cannot be better explained by another cause. The World Association of Sleep Medicine, in collaboration with the International Restless Legs Syndrome Group Study, defines PLMS as four or more consecutive limb movements with a duration of 0.5–10 seconds, with an electromyographic increase of >8 mV above the resting baseline and a minimum interval of 10 seconds and a maximum of 90 seconds between two consecutive leg movements (Ferri et al., 2016). PLMs occur at the lower extremities, most typically every 20–40 seconds during sleep, with the dorsiflexion of the big toe and ankle. PLMD is additionally defined as causing significant sleep disruption and/or daytime consequences in terms of mental, physical, educational, and behavioral functioning. Both PLMs and related symptoms should not be better explained by other medical, mental, neurological, or sleep disorders, such as PLMs in the context of sleep apnea, narcolepsy, or RLS (American Academy of Sleep Medicine, 2014).

Pediatric PLMD is thought to be a rare disorder, and the prevalence of PLMD in children ranges from 0.3% to 14%. Differences in estimated prevalence may be due to the methods and definition of PLMD used by researchers. The cause of PLMD is probably linked to a central dopamine dysfunction, and the pathophysiologic mechanisms largely overlap with those of RLS (Ferri et al., 2023).

In the PSG recording, PLMs appear with the onset of sleep Stage 1 (N1), are frequent during sleep Stage 2 (N2), and decrease in frequency in slow-wave sleep (N3). Each PLM is accompanied by a cortical excitation visible in the sleep electroencephalogram (EEG) and by a short autonomic activation (Ferri et al., 2023).

Children with an elevated PLM index have shown increased behavioral problems, mood disturbances, and morning headaches (Delrosso, Lockhart, et al., 2020). PLMD is often comorbid with ADHD: 26%–64% of children with ADHD met the criteria for PLMD, and reciprocally, 91% of another group of children with PLMD met the criteria for ADHD. Children with PLMD/ADHD are significantly more likely to have enuresis, nightmares, and difficulty initiating sleep than children with PLMD only. Furthermore, children with PLMD/ADHD have significantly more PLMs associated with EEG arousals with respect to children with PLMD but without ADHD (Ferri et al., 2023).

TREATMENT OF PLMD

Treatment of PLMD is similar to that of RLS. Asymptomatic PLMs do not warrant treatment. As for RLS, the use of antidopaminergic or antidepressant agents that increase PLMS should be excluded, and iron supplementation is recommended if serum ferritin level is <50 mg/l, with doses ranging 1–6 mg/kg/day (DelRosso & Bruni, 2019). Sleep hygiene rules should be applied, and caffeine, alcohol, and nicotine need to be avoided. Pharmacologic options for PLMD include oral or intravenous iron supplementation, dopamine agonists, gabapentin, opioids, and, to a lesser extent, benzodiazepines; but very few studies have assessed the efficacy in children (Aurora et al., 2012).

Sleep-Related Rhythmic Movement Disorder

Sleep-related rhythmic movement disorder (SRRMD) is characterized by repetitive, stereotyped, and rhythmic motor behaviors involving large muscle groups that occur predominantly during drowsiness or sleep. Sleep-related rhythmic movements are common in normal infants and children and are a part of normal childhood development. They should be regarded as a disorder only if the behaviors significantly interfere with normal sleep, cause significant impairment in daytime function, or result in self-inflicted bodily injury (American Academy of Sleep Medicine, 2014).

The ICSD-3 (American Academy of Sleep Medicine, 2014) defines four criteria for the diagnosis of SRRMD: (a) The patient exhibits repetitive, stereotyped, and rhythmic motor behaviors involving large muscle groups; (b) the movements are predominantly sleep-related, occurring near nap or bedtime or when the individual appears drowsy or asleep; (c) the behaviors result in a significant complaint as manifest by at least one of the following: interference with normal sleep, significant impairment in daytime function, and self-inflicted bodily injury or likelihood of injury if preventive measures are not used; and (d) the rhythmic movements are not better explained by another movement disorder or epilepsy.

Vestibular stimulation and/or learned behaviors, which soothe the child at sleep onset and following night awakenings, have been proposed as the initiating factors in infants and toddlers (Gwyther et al., 2017). Environmental stress and lack of external stimulation have been proposed as factors in children who are hospitalized for extended periods, similarly to children with cognitive deficits and psychopathologies. SRRMD is particularly frequent in children with developmental disabilities, intellectual disorders, ASD, and anxiety (Arnulf, 2014; Prihodova et al., 2019).

The clinical manifestations are various and include body rocking, body rolling, head banging, head rolling, and other variants. Typically, these appear at sleep onset, but they may occur during any time of the night and even during quiet wakeful activities. A combination of two or more rhythmic movement subtypes may be observed, which may be accompanied by inarticulate sounds that may be quite loud (Arnulf, 2014). The frequency of rhythmic movements is usually 0.5–2 movements per second, they occur in clusters, and the duration of individual clusters typically varies from several seconds to 15 minutes. PSG recordings show that rhythmic movements can present in any sleep stage but mostly during drowsiness and NREM sleep (American Academy of Sleep Medicine, 2014; Gwyther et al., 2017). Rhythmic movements generally resolve in healthy children before preschool age and only rarely persist until adolescence or adulthood (Prihodova et al., 2019).

TREATMENT OF RHYTHMIC MOVEMENT DISORDER

Treatment is not necessary unless rhythmic movements are associated with sleep disturbance or bodily harm or could result in injury. Cessation of movements may occur following environmental disturbance or verbal intervention. The main preventive measure is maintaining a safe sleeping environment to prevent injury. Behavioral therapy, wearing helmets, and treatment with benzodiazepines, citalopram, and imipramine may be helpful in violent forms (Hamilton-Stubs & Walters, 2017).

RSD

RSD represents a new diagnostic category, recently proposed by DelRosso et al. (2018). This disorder is found in children who are described by their parents as restless sleepers with excessive nocturnal motor activity consisting of large, often repositioning, movements involving all limbs, sometimes to the point of falling out of bed. These sleep patterns are consistent throughout the night and occur almost nightly. Excessive daytime sleepiness, irritability, and hyperactivity are usually noticed as consequences and impair academic performance and social functioning. Differently from children with RLS, children with RSD do not have difficulty falling asleep, symptoms of RLS, or nocturnal awakenings (DelRosso et al., 2018).

A task force appointed by the International RLS Study Group established eight essential criteria for the diagnosis of RSD (DelRosso, Ferri, et al., 2020). The main criteria to be met are (a) a complaint of "restless sleep" reported by the parents or caregivers; (b) movements during sleep involve large muscle groups of the whole body, all four limbs, arms, legs, or head; (c) a total movement index (by video analysis) of five or more per hour of sleep is present during video-PSG; (d) a complaint of restless sleep at least three times per week present for at least 3 months. RSD should also be associated with a clinically significant impairment in behavioral, educational, academic, social, occupational, or other important areas of functioning; and the condition should not be better explained by another disorder or factor or the physiological effects of a substance (DelRosso, Ferri, et al., 2020). The current diagnostic criteria apply to children aged 6–18 years. While the prevalence of RSD in the general population is unknown, its prevalence in a sleep center–referred pediatric population has been estimated to be 7.7% (DelRosso & Ferri, 2019).

Three potential pathophysiological mechanisms underlying RSD include iron deficiency, sleep instability, and sympathetic activation. In a recent study, all children with RSD had lower mean ferritin levels of around 20 ng/dl (DelRosso et al., 2022). RSD shares low ferritin and decreased sleep efficiency with pediatric RLS but no increase in sleep latency.

There are currently no FDA-approved medications or consensus recommendations for the treatment of RSD in children. Clinical symptoms improved in children with RSD after iron supplementation: Parents reported improved sleep, manifested as fewer movements per night, fewer nocturnal awakenings, and improvement in daytime symptoms (DelRosso, Picchietti, & Ferri, 2021). Still, more research is needed to establish a prognosis, confirm pathophysiology, and identify RSD in younger children and adults.

Pediatric OSA

In recent years, numerous studies have delineated the different features of pediatric OSA. OSA is part of the family of sleep disordered breathing (SDB) disorders that includes diseases with different levels of severity starting from primary snoring, upper airway resistance syndrome (UARS), obstructive hypoventilation, and ending with OSA syndrome (OSAS) (Kaditis et al., 2016).

Primary snoring comprises habitual snoring (>3 nights a week) without apneas, hypopneas, frequent arousals, or gas exchange abnormalities. UARS includes habitual snoring, increased work of breathing, and frequent arousals but with no recognizable obstructive events or gas exchange abnormalities. Obstructive hypoventilation is characterized by the presence of snoring and hypoventilation without recognizable obstructive events. OSA is defined as the recurrent intermittent complete or partial obstruction (obstructive apnea or hypopnea), prolonged partial upper airway obstruction, or both prolonged and intermittent obstructions that disrupt normal ventilation during sleep or normal sleep patterns (Kaditis et al., 2016). The ICSD-3 defined specific criteria for the diagnosis of OSA (Table 38.2).

Table 38.2 Diagnostic criteria pediatric obstructive sleep apnea

Criteria A and B must be met
A. The presence of one or more of the following: 1. Snoring. 2. Labored, paradoxical, or obstructed breathing during the child's sleep. 3. Sleepiness, hyperactivity, behavioral problems, or learning and other cognitive problems.
B. Polysomnography demonstrates one of the following: 1. One or more obstructive apneas, mixed apneas, or hypopneas per hour of sleep. 2. A pattern of obstructive hypoventilation, defined as at least 25% of total sleep time with hypercapnia ($PaCO_2$ > 50 mm Hg) in association with one or more of the following: a. Snoring. b. Flattening of the inspiratory nasal pressure waveform. c. Paradoxical thoracoabdominal motion.

Note. $PaCO_2$ = partial pressure of carbon dioxide. The *International Classification of Sleep Disorders*, third edition, text revision. Reproduced with permission of the American Academy of Sleep Medicine.

To define the level of severity of SDB, three specific PSG parameters have been developed: (a) apnea–hypopnea index (AHI): number of obstructive, mixed, and central apneas and hypopneas per hour of total sleep time; (b) obstructive AHI: number of obstructive and mixed apneas and hypopneas per hour of total sleep time; (c) oxyhemoglobin desaturation (≥3%) index: number of desaturations of at least 3% compared to the pre-event baseline per hour of total sleep time.

In 2016 the European Respiratory Society proposed two definitions of OSAS (Kaditis et al., 2016):

1. Obstructive AHI (obstructive and mixed apneas and hypopneas per hour of total sleep time) ≥2 episodes/hour or an obstructive apnea index (obstructive apneas per hour of total sleep time) ≥1 episode/hour in the presence of SDB symptoms and adenotonsillar hypertrophy with or without obesity.
2. Presence of SDB symptoms in combination with an AHI ≥1 episode/hour.

Based on the above definitions, OSAS is defined as mild (AHI = 1–5) and moderate to severe (AHI >5).

The first scientific report of pediatric OSA by Guilleminault et al. (1976) documented eight children with symptoms of excessive daytime sleepiness, nighttime snoring, nocturnal enuresis, decreased school performance, morning headaches, mood and personality changes, weight problems, and pulmonary hypertension. This first report highlighted the presence of nocturnal symptoms like snoring, excessive sweating, restless sleep, mouth breathing, apneas, gasping, labored or paradoxical breathing, and hyperextension of the neck during sleep, along with night terrors or nightmares but also daytime symptoms including hyperactivity, inattention, learning and conduct problems, morning headaches, excessive daytime sleepiness, and failure to thrive.

The peak prevalence of pediatric OSA occurs between 2 and 8 years of age and ranges between 1% and 5% in the general pediatric population, but the prevalence may be higher due to the pediatric obesity epidemic (Bixler et al., 2009; Marcus et al., 2012). Some studies suggest a bimodal peak in preschool children associated with adenotonsillar hypertrophy and obesity and, in adolescents, primarily associated with obesity (Gozal & Kheirandish-Gozal, 2012).

From a pathophysiological point of view pediatric OSAS may be related to anatomical factors (i.e., adenotonsillar hypertrophy) and factors that increase upper airway collapsibility, such as alterations in the neurological reflexes coordinating the upper airway musculature (Tan & Kaditis, 2021). Adenotonsillar hypertrophy alone does not lead to OSA but may be associated with midface hypoplasia or micrognathia/retrognathia or orthodontic dysfunction. Furthermore, there is no direct relationship between tonsil size and OSA severity. Obesity, muscular dystrophy, and cerebral palsy are other risk factors for childhood OSA (Tan et al., 2017). However, genetic and environmental factors determine the susceptibility to and severity of OSAS morbidity.

Clinically, children with OSA exhibit different forms of breathing patterns during sleep. More frequently, younger children have a pattern of obstructive hypoventilation, consisting of long periods of persistent partial upper airway obstruction associated with continuous snoring, hypercapnia, and arterial oxygen desaturation that occurs predominantly during REM sleep. Older children, similar to adults, have cyclic episodes of OSA (Tan & Kaditis, 2021).

The daytime consequences of pediatric OSAS may vary greatly from child to child. Excessive daytime sleepiness is a less common daytime symptom in young children with OSA than in adults, although it may be present in obese adolescents. Hyperactivity, inattention, learning, and cognitive behavioral dysfunction may be present. A study of 1,010 children showed significant effects of OSAS on cognitive and executive functioning related to a dose–response effect of OSA, with performance of the children in the moderate to severe OSA group being significantly more impaired (Hunter et al., 2016). The most prominent recent study to examine neurobehavioral outcomes as the primary outcome of interest was the Childhood Adenotonsillectomy study, based on children aged 5–9 years with mild OSA (median AHI = 4.7/hour of total sleep time). Adenotonsillectomy resulted in significant improvements in symptoms, behavior, PSG parameters, as well as parent-rated generic and OSA-specific quality-of-life measures (Garetz et al., 2015). However, not all children with OSA exhibit cognitive or behavioral deficits, and genetic and environmental factors likely play a role in modifying the phenotypic expression of this morbidity (e.g., differences in systemic inflammatory responses as reflected by plasma C-reactive protein levels; Kheirandish-Gozal & Gozal, 2013). The adverse consequences of OSAS also include decreased quality of life; morbidity of the cardiovascular, metabolic, and central nervous systems; as well as increased frequency of nocturnal enuresis and somatic growth delay (Kaditis et al., 2016). There is emerging evidence of cardiovascular and metabolic consequences of OSA in children, including abnormal cardiac function, elevated blood pressure, insulin resistance, and inflammation. OSA can impose subclinical effects on the autonomic and cardiovascular systems, promoting disturbances in blood pressure regulation, left ventricular remodeling, and endothelial dysfunction. Higher systolic and diastolic blood pressure during wakefulness have been identified in otherwise healthy children with moderate to severe OSAS compared to subjects with mild OSAS or control subjects without OSAS (Marcus et al., 1998). Children with OSAS also showed a significant risk for impairments in endothelial function, with greater severity in obese children who have OSA (Kheirandish-Gozal & Farre, 2013).

Children with neurodevelopmental disabilities like ASD, ADHD, Down syndrome, Prader-Willi syndrome, myelomeningocele, Chiari malformation, and 22q deletion syndrome have increased risk of SDB (Imran et al., 2021). Therefore, in the presence of symptoms of SDB in children with neurodevelopmental disabilities it is imperative to include the screening for OSAS. The management of SDB in these patients should consider syndrome-specific features of SDB, which is the subject of a dedicated chapter in the handbook (Chapter 45).

Treatment of OSA

Adenotonsillectomy (AT) represents the mainstay of treatment for pediatric OSA, but therapeutic approaches include pharmaceuticals and other medical or surgical interventions. Montelukast and intranasal steroids are indicated for reduction of mild to moderate OSA severity (Liming et al., 2019). CPAP is considered when AT is not indicated; however, CPAP adherence in children is low at best (Bhattacharjee et al., 2020). A recent alternative to CPAP is the use of high-flow nasal cannula support in the home setting (Amaddeo et al., 2019).

Orthodontic treatment with rapid maxillary expansion is greatly effective in patients with high-arched/narrow palates (Camacho et al., 2017). Myofunctional therapy, which involves re-entrainment of oral, tongue, and facial muscles to improve airway positioning and neuromuscular patency, may be associated with the different other treatments. Recently, drug-induced sleep endoscopy that involves direct visualization of a dynamic airway under light anesthesia (spontaneous breathing) might better identify the site of obstruction and allow a direct surgical intervention like lingual tonsillectomy, tongue-base reduction, revision adenoidectomy, turbinate reduction, and supraglottoplasty (Wilcox et al., 2017). Finally, bariatric surgery, used in adults, might be an option in obese adolescents (Amin et al., 2017).

There is a need for further research on pediatric OSA to identify the natural course of the disease, to evaluate new simplified diagnostic methods, and to develop potential biomarkers of susceptibility to and severity of OSA to individualize the treatment dependent on patient-specific requirements.

Hypersomnia and Narcolepsy

It should be noted before concluding this chapter that symptoms of the sleep–wake disorders of neurological origin, hypersomnia and narcolepsy, often start in early life with a first peak in clinical presentation of narcolepsy with cataplexy (Type 1 narcolepsy) occurring around the age of 14 years (Dauvilliers et al., 2001). These disorders characterized by REM sleep abnormalities and excessive daytime sleepiness are very relevant to pediatric sleep medicine and are the subject of a dedicated chapter in the handbook (Chapter 36).

Conclusions

Sleep problems in children are prevalent and are associated with various negative consequences for child and family functioning. Hence, early identification and routine assessment of children in mental health and medical settings are very important. Fortunately, there are many effective and empirically validated interventions (both psychological and medical) for the various sleep problems described in this chapter. As children live within families, most of these treatments should involve the caregivers, either directly as agents of change when, for instance, early childhood insomnia is the main complaint, or indirectly, when parental supervision or support is needed to facilitate the child's adherence to treatment.

Future Directions

Although the effectiveness of sleep interventions in improving children's sleep has been demonstrated repeatedly, there are still many open questions and research gaps that should be addressed in the future. For example, in the area of insomnia, most intervention studies on CBT-I have focused on early childhood insomnia, and more research is needed to establish the efficacy of CBT-I for older children. Another issue that has received only limited attention is the long-term consequences of extinction-based behavioral interventions on children's emotional functioning and parent–child relationship. Relevant to all sleep disorders is the need to identify predictors and moderators of intervention outcomes so that sleep interventions could be adjusted and tailored to the specific characteristics of the child and the family. Personalized treatments are expected to lead to better adherence and improved outcomes. Another area of concern is that sleep interventions have been mostly examined in typically developing children from middle to high socioeconomic status, and thus there is a clear need to assess their effectiveness in diverse populations and expand their availability to these populations. Finally, there is a need to increase the awareness of the importance of sleep health and of the consequences of pediatric sleep problems among parents, children, teachers, and healthcare providers. Training primary care providers in screening for sleep problems and increasing the availability and skills of sleep specialists are crucial for delivering optimal treatment for these problems and for curtailing their adverse effects on children and their families.

Note

1. Note: both Gradisar et al. and Kaplan et al. combined light therapy with CBT-I.

References

Allison, K. C., Spaeth, A., & Hopkins, C. M. (2016). Sleep and eating disorders. *Current Psychiatry Reports, 18*(10), 1–8.

Amaddeo, A., Khirani, S., Frapin, A., Teng, T., Griffon, L., & Fauroux, B. (2019). High-flow nasal cannula for children not compliant with continuous positive airway pressure. *Sleep Medicine, 63*, 24–28. https://doi.org/10.1016/j.sleep.2019.05.012

American Academy of Sleep Medicine. (2005). *International classification of sleep disorders: diagnostic and coding manual* (2nd ed.).

American Academy of Sleep Medicine. (2014). *The international classification of sleep disorders* (3rd ed.).

American Psychiatric Association. (2013). *Diagnostic and statistical manual of mental disorders* (5th ed.). https://doi.org/10.1176/appi.books.9780890425596

Amin, R., Simakajornboon, N., Szczesniak, R., & Inge, T. (2017). Early improvement in obstructive sleep apnea and increase in orexin levels after bariatric surgery in adolescents and young adults. *Surgery for Obesity and Related Diseases, 13*(1), 95–100. https://doi.org/10.1016/j.soard.2016.05.023

Anders, T. F. (1994). Infant sleep, nighttime relationships, and attachment. *Psychiatry, 57*(1), 11–21. https://doi.org/10.1080/00332747.1994.11024664

Anders, T. F., Halpern, L. F., & Hua, J. (1992). Sleeping through the night: A developmental perspective. *Pediatrics, 90*(4), 554–560.

Angriman, M., Cortese, S., & Bruni, O. (2017). Somatic and neuropsychiatric comorbidities in pediatric restless legs syndrome: A systematic review of the literature. *Sleep Medicine Reviews, 34*, 34–45. https://doi.org/10.1016/j.smrv.2016.06.008

Arda, E., Cakiroglu, B., & Thomas, D. T. (2016). Primary nocturnal enuresis: A review. *Nephro-urology Monthly, 8*(4), Article e35809. https://doi.org/10.5812%2Fnumonthly.35809

Armstrong, J. M., Ruttle, P. L., Klein, M. H., Essex, M. J., & Benca, R. M. (2014). Associations of child insomnia, sleep movement, and their persistence with mental health symptoms in childhood and adolescence. *Sleep, 37*(5), 901–909. https://doi.org/10.5665/sleep.3656

Arnulf, I. (2014). Sleep-related movement disorders. Clinical picture and diagnosis. In C. Bassetti, Z. Dogas, & P. Peigneux (Eds.), *Sleep medicine textbook* (pp. 433–446). European Sleep Research Society.

Aslund, L., Arnberg, F., Kanstrup, M., & Lekander, M. (2018). Cognitive and behavioral interventions to improve sleep in school-age children and adolescents: A systematic review and meta-analysis. *Journal of Clinical Sleep Medicine, 14*(11), 1937–1947. https://doi.org/10.5664/jcsm.7498

Attarian, H. (2010). Treatment options for parasomnias. *Neurologic Clinics, 28*(4), 1089–1106. https://doi.org/10.1016/j.ncl.2010.03.025

Aurora, R. N., Kristo, D. A., Bista, S. R., Rowley, J. A., Zak, R. S., Casey, K. R., Lamm, C. I., Tracy, S. L., Rosenberg, R. S., & American Academy of Sleep Medicine. (2012). The treatment of restless legs syndrome and periodic limb movement disorder in adults—An update for 2012: Practice parameters with an evidence-based systematic review and meta-analyses: An American Academy of Sleep Medicine clinical practice guideline. *Sleep, 35*(8), 1039–1062. https://doi.org/10.5665/sleep.1988

BaHammam, A. S., & Almeneessier, A. S. (2019). Dreams and nightmares in patients with obstructive sleep apnea: A review. *Frontiers in Neurology, 10*, Article 1127. https://doi.org/10.3389/fneur.2019.01127

Barrett, J. R., Tracy, D. K., & Giaroli, G. (2013). To sleep or not to sleep: A systematic review of the literature of pharmacological treatments of insomnia in children and adolescents with attention-deficit/hyperactivity disorder. *Journal of Child and Adolescent Psychopharmacology, 23*(10), 640–647. https://doi.org/10.1089/cap.2013.0059

Bartel, K. A., Gradisar, M., & Williamson, P. (2015). Protective and risk factors for adolescent sleep: A meta-analytic review. *Sleep Medicine Reviews, 21*, 72–85. https://doi.org/10.1016/j.smrv.2014.08.002

Bauducco, S., Richardson, C., & Gradisar, M. (2020). Chronotype, circadian rhythms and mood. *Current Opinion in Psychology, 34*, 77–83. https://doi.org/10.1016/j.copsyc.2019.09.002

Bayer, J. K., Hiscock, H., Hampton, A., & Wake, M. (2007). Sleep problems in young infants and maternal mental and physical health. *Journal of Paediatrics and Child Health, 43*(1–2), 66–73. http://www.ncbi.nlm.nih.gov/entrez/query.fcgi?cmd=Retrieve&db=PubMed&dopt=Citation&list_uids=17207059

Belanger, M. E., Simard, V., Bernier, A., & Carrier, J. (2014). Investigating the convergence between actigraphy, maternal sleep diaries, and the Child Behavior Checklist as measures of sleep in toddlers. *Frontiers in Psychiatry, 5*, Article 158. https://doi.org/10.3389/fpsyt.2014.00158

Bhattacharjee, R., Benjafield, A. V., Armitstead, J., Cistulli, P. A., Nunez, C. M., Pepin, J. L. D., Woehrle, H., Yan, Y., Malhotra, A., & Grp, M. (2020). Adherence in children using positive airway pressure therapy: A big-data analysis. *Lancet Digital Health, 2*(2), E94–E101. https://doi.org/10.1016/S2589-7500(19)30214-6

Bixler, E. O., Vgontzas, A. N., Lin, H. M., Liao, D., Calhoun, S., Vela-Bueno, A., Fedok, F., Vlasic, V., & Graff, G. (2009). Sleep disordered breathing in children in a general population sample: prevalence and risk factors. *Sleep, 32*(6), 731–736. https://doi.org/10.1093/sleep/32.6.731

Blader, J. C., Koplewicz, H. S., Abikoff, H., & Foley, C. (1997). Sleep problems of elementary school children. A community survey. *Archives of Pediatrics and Adolescent Medicine, 151*(5), 473–480. https://doi.org/10.1001/archpedi.1997.02170420043007

Blake, M., Schwartz, O., Waloszek, J. M., Raniti, M., Simmons, J. G., Murray, G., Blake, L., Dahl, R. E., Bootzin, R., & McMakin, D. L. (2017). The SENSE study: Treatment mechanisms of a cognitive behavioral and mindfulness-based group sleep improvement intervention for at-risk adolescents. *Sleep, 40*(6), Article zsx061. https://doi.org/10.1093/sleep/zsx061

Blake, M., Waloszek, J. M., Schwartz, O., Raniti, M., Simmons, J. G., Blake, L., Murray, G., Dahl, R. E., Bootzin, R., & Dudgeon, P. (2016). The SENSE study: Post intervention effects of a randomized controlled trial of a cognitive-behavioral and mindfulness-based group sleep improvement intervention among at-risk adolescents. *Journal of Consulting and Clinical Psychology, 84*(12), 1039–1051. https://doi.org/10.1037/ccp0000142

Blake, M. J., Sheeber, L. B., Youssef, G. J., Raniti, M. B., & Allen, N. B. (2017). Systematic review and meta-analysis of adolescent cognitive-behavioral sleep interventions. *Clinical Child and Family Psychology Review, 20*(3), 227–249. https://doi.org/10.1007/s10567-017-0234-5

Blake, M. J., Trinder, J. A., & Allen, N. B. (2018). Mechanisms underlying the association between insomnia, anxiety, and depression in adolescence: Implications for behavioral sleep interventions. *Clinical Psychology Review, 63*, 25–40. https://doi.org/10.1016/j.cpr.2018.05.006

Blunden, S., Etherton, H., & Hauck, Y. (2016). Resistance to cry intensive sleep intervention in young children: Are we ignoring children's cries or parental concerns? *Children (Basel), 3*(2), Article 8. https://doi.org/10.3390/children3020008

Bourboulis, S., Gradisar, M., & Kahn, M. (2022). The "Dream Changer": A randomized controlled trial evaluating the efficacy of a parent-based intervention for childhood nightmares. *Sleep, 45*(4), Article zsac004. https://doi.org/10.1093/sleep/zsac004

Bruni, O., & Angriman, M. (2017). Management of RLS in children (unique features). In M. Manconi & D. Garcia-Borreguero (Eds.), *Restless legs syndrome/Willis Ekbom disease* (pp. 261–278). Springer.

Bruni, O., Angriman, M., Melegari, M. G., & Ferri, R. (2019). Pharmacotherapeutic management of sleep disorders in children with neurodevelopmental disorders. *Expert Opinion on Pharmacotherapy, 20*(18), 2257–2271. https://doi.org/10.1080/14656566.2019.1674283

Bruni, O., Ferri, R., Novelli, L., Finotti, E., Miano, S., & Guilleminault, C. (2008). NREM sleep instability in children with sleep terrors: The role of slow wave activity interruptions. *Clinical Neurophysiology, 119*(5), 985–992. https://doi.org/10.1016/j.clinph.2008.01.015

Bruni, O., & Miano, S. (2021). Parasomnias. In D. Gozal & L. Kheirandish-Gozal (Eds.), *Pediatric sleep medicine: Mechanisms and comprehensive guide to clinical evaluation and management* (pp. 415–429). Springer.

Bruni, O., Ottaviano, S., Guidetti, V., Romoli, M., Innocenzi, M., Cortesi, F., & Giannotti, F. (1996). The Sleep Disturbance Scale for Children (SDSC): Construction and validation of an instrument to evaluate sleep disturbances in childhood and adolescence. *Journal of Sleep Research, 5*(4), 251–261. https://doi.org/10.1111/j.1365-2869.1996.00251.x

Burnham, M. M., Goodlin-Jones, B. L., Gaylor, E. E., & Anders, T. F. (2002). Nighttime sleep–wake patterns and self-soothing from birth to one year of age: A longitudinal intervention study. *Journal of Child Psychology and Psychiatry and Allied Disciplines, 43*(6), 713–725.

Cain, N., & Gradisar, M. (2010). Electronic media use and sleep in school-aged children and adolescents: A review. *Sleep Medicine, 11*(8), 735–742. https://doi.org/10.1016/j.sleep.2010.02.006

Cain, N., Richardson, C., Bartel, K., Whittall, H., Reeks, J., & Gradisar, M. (2022). A randomised controlled dismantling trial of sleep restriction therapies for chronic insomnia disorder in middle childhood: Effects on sleep and anxiety, and possible contraindications. *Journal of Sleep Research, 31*(6), Article e13658. https://doi.org/10.1111/jsr.13658

Camacho, M., Chang, E. T., Song, S. J. A., Abdullatif, J., Zaghi, S., Pirelli, P., Certal, V., & Guilleminault, C. (2017). Rapid maxillary expansion for pediatric obstructive sleep apnea: A systematic review and meta-analysis. *Laryngoscope, 127*(7), 1712–1719. https://doi.org/10.1002/lary.26352

Camerota, M., Propper, C. B., & Teti, D. M. (2019). Intrinsic and extrinsic factors predicting infant sleep: Moving beyond main effects. *Developmental Review, 53*, Article 100871. https://doi.org/10.1016/j.dr.2019.100871

Carter, K. A., Hathaway, N. E., & Lettieri, C. F. (2014). Common sleep disorders in children. *American Family Physician, 89*(5), 368–377.

Castelnovo, A., Turner, K., Rossi, A., Galbiati, A., Gagliardi, A., Proserpio, P., Nobili, L., Terzaghi, M., Manni, R., & Ferini Strambi, L. (2021). Behavioural and emotional profiles of children and adolescents with disorders of arousal. *Journal of Sleep Research, 30*(1), Article e13188. https://doi.org/10.1111/jsr.13188

Catrett, C. D., & Gaultney, J. F. (2009). Possible insomnia predicts some risky behaviors among adolescents when controlling for depressive symptoms. *The Journal of Genetic Psychology, 170*(4), 287–309.

Chervin, R. D., Hedger, K., Dillon, J. E., & Pituch, K. J. (2000). Pediatric Sleep Questionnaire (PSQ): Validity and reliability of scales for sleep-disordered breathing, snoring, sleepiness, and behavioral problems. *Sleep Medicine, 1*(1), 21–32. https://doi.org/10.1016/s1389-9457(99)00009-x

Cook, F., Giallo, R., Petrovic, Z., Coe, A., Seymour, M., Cann, W., & Hiscock, H. (2017). Depression and anger in fathers of unsettled infants: A community cohort study. *Journal of Paediatrics and Child Health, 53*(2), 131–135. https://doi.org/10.1111/jpc.13311

Cooney, M.R., Short, M. A., & Gradisar, M. (2018). An open trial of bedtime fading for sleep disturbances in preschool children: A parent group education approach. *Sleep Medicne, 46*, 98–106. https://doi.org/10.1016/j.sleep.2018.03.003

Crowley, S. J., Wolfson, A. R., Tarokh, L., & Carskadon, M. A. (2018). An update on adolescent sleep: New evidence informing the perfect storm model. *Journal of Adolescence, 67*, 55–65. https://doi.org/10.1016/j.adolescence.2018.06.001

Dauvilliers, Y., Montplaisir, J., Molinari, N., Carlander, B., Ondze, B., Besset, A., & Billiard, M. (2001). Age at onset of narcolepsy in two large populations of patients in France and Quebec. *Neurology, 57*(11), 2029–2033. https://doi.org/10.1212/wnl.57.11.2029

Daws, D., & Sutton, S. (2020). *Parent–infant psychotherpay for sleep problems through the night*. Routledge.

de Bruin, E. J., Bögels, S. M., Oort, F. J., & Meijer, A. M. (2015). Efficacy of cognitive behavioral therapy for insomnia in adolescents: A randomized controlled trial with internet therapy, group therapy and a waiting list condition. *Sleep, 38*(12), 1913–1926. https://doi.org/10.5665/sleep.5240

de Bruin, E. J., Bögels, S. M., Oort, F. J., & Meijer, A. M. (2018). Improvements of adolescent psychopathology after insomnia treatment: Results from a randomized controlled trial over 1 year. *Journal of Child Psychology and Psychiatry, 59*(5), 509–522. https://doi.org/10.1111/jcpp.12834

DeLeon, C. W., & Karraker, K. H. (2007). Intrinsic and extrinsic factors associated with night waking in 9-month-old infants. *Infant Behavior & Development, 30*(4), 596–605. https://doi.org/10.1016/j.infbeh.2007.03.009

DelRosso, L. M., & Bruni, O. (2019). Treatment of pediatric restless legs syndrome. *Advances in Pharmacology, 84*, 237–253. https://doi.org/10.1016/bs.apha.2018.11.001

DelRosso, L. M., Bruni, O., & Ferri, R. (2018). Restless sleep disorder in children: A pilot study on a tentative new diagnostic category. *Sleep, 41*(8), Article zsy102. https://doi.org/10.1093/sleep/zsy102

DelRosso, L. M., & Ferri, R. (2019). The prevalence of restless sleep disorder among a clinical sample of children and adolescents referred to a sleep centre. *Journal of Sleep Research, 28*(6), Article e12870. https://doi.org/10.1111/jsr.12870

DelRosso, L. M., Ferri, R., Allen, R. P., Bruni, O., Garcia-Borreguero, D., Kotagal, S., Owens, J. A., Peirano, P., Simakajornboon, N., Picchietti, D. L., & International Restless Legs Syndrome Study Group. (2020). Consensus diagnostic criteria for a newly defined pediatric sleep disorder: Restless sleep disorder (RSD). *Sleep Medicine, 75*, 335–340. https://doi.org/10.1016/j.sleep.2020.08.011

Delrosso, L. M., Lockhart, C., Wrede, J. E., Chen, M. L., Samson, M., Reed, J., Martin-Washo, S., Arp, M., & Ferri, R. (2020). Comorbidities in children with elevated periodic limb movement index during sleep. *Sleep*, *43*(2), Article zsz221. https://doi.org/10.1093/sleep/zsz221

DelRosso, L. M., Mogavero, M. P., Baroni, A., Bruni, O., & Ferri, R. (2021). Restless legs syndrome in children and adolescents. *Child and Adolescent Psychiatric Clinics of North America*, *30*(1), 143–157. https://doi.org/10.1016/j.chc.2020.08.010

DelRosso, L. M., Mogavero, M. P., & Ferri, R. (2022). Restless sleep disorder, restless legs syndrome, and periodic limb movement disorder—Sleep in motion! *Pediatric Pulmonologiststs*, *57*(8), 1879–1886. https://doi.org/10.1002/ppul.25305

DelRosso, L. M., Picchietti, D. L., & Ferri, R. (2021). Comparison between oral ferrous sulfate and intravenous ferric carboxymaltose in children with restless sleep disorder. *Sleep*, *44*(2), Article zsaa155. https://doi.org/10.1093/sleep/zsaa155

de Macêdo, T. C. F., Ferreira, G. H., de Almondes, K. M., Kirov, R., & Mota-Rolim, S. A. (2019). My dream, my rules: Can lucid dreaming treat nightmares? *Frontiers in Psychology*, *10*, Article 2618. https://doi.org/10.3389/fpsyg.2019.02618

Dewald, J. F., Meijer, A. M., Oort, F. J., Kerkhof, G. A., & Bogels, S. M. (2010). The influence of sleep quality, sleep duration and sleepiness on school performance in children and adolescents: A meta-analytic review. *Sleep Medicine Reviews*, *14*(3), 179–189. https://doi.org/10.1016/j.smrv.2009.10.004

Dewald-Kaufmann, J., de Bruin, E., & Michael, G. (2019). Cognitive behavioral therapy for insomnia (CBT-i) in school-aged children and adolescents. *Sleep Medicine Clinics*, *14*(2), 155–165. https://doi.org/10.1016/j.jsmc.2019.02.002

de Zambotti, M., Goldstone, A., Colrain, I. M., & Baker, F. C. (2018). Insomnia disorder in adolescence: Diagnosis, impact, and treatment. *Sleep Medicine Reviews*, *39*, 12–24. https://doi.org/10.1016/j.smrv.2017.06.009

Dhondt, K., Raes, A., Hoebeke, P., Van Laecke, E., Van Herzeele, C., & Walle, J. V. (2009). Abnormal sleep architecture and refractory nocturnal enuresis. *The Journal of Urology*, *182*(4), 1961–1966. https://doi.org/10.1016/j.juro.2009.05.103

Dolsen, E. A., Dong, L., & Harvey, A. G. (2023). Transdiagnostic sleep and circadian intervention for adolescents plus text messaging: Randomized controlled trial 12-month follow-up. *Journal of Clinical Child and Adolescent Psychology*, *52*(6), 750–762. https://doi.org/10.1080/15374416.2021.1978295

Dong, L., Dolsen, M. R., Martinez, A. J., Notsu, H., & Harvey, A. G. (2020). A transdiagnostic sleep and circadian intervention for adolescents: Six-month follow-up of a randomized controlled trial. *Journal of Child Psychology and Psychiatry*, *61*(6), 653–661. https://doi.org/10.1111/jcpp.13154

El Rafihi-Ferreira, R., Silvares, E. F., Asbahr, F. R., & Ollendick, T. H. (2018). Brief treatment for nighttime fears and co-sleeping problems: A randomized clinical trial. *Journal of Anxiety Disorders*, *58*, 51–60. https://doi.org/10.1016/j.janxdis.2018.06.008

El-Sheikh, M., & Kelly, R. J. (2017). Family functioning and children's sleep. *Child Development Perspectives*, *11*(4), 264–269. https://doi.org/10.1111/cdep.12243

El-Sheikh, M., Kelly, R. J., Sadeh, A., & Buckhalt, J. A. (2014). Income, ethnicity, and sleep: Coping as a moderator. *Cultural Diversity and Ethnic Minority Psychology*, *20*(3), 441–448. https://doi.org/10.1037/a0036699

Etherton, H., Blunden, S., & Hauck, Y. (2016). Discussion of extinction-based behavioral sleep interventions for young children and reasons why parents may find them difficult. *Journal of Clinical Sleep Medicine*, *12*(11), 1535–1543. https://doi.org/10.5664/jcsm.6284

Ferber, R. (1985). *Solve your child's sleep problems*. Simon & Schuster.

Fernandez, S., DeMarni Cromer, L., Borntrager, C., Swopes, R., Hanson, R. F., & Davis, J. L. (2013). A case series: Cognitive-behavioral treatment (exposure, relaxation, and rescripting therapy) of trauma-related nightmares experienced by children. *Clinical Case Studies*, *12*(1), 39–59. https://doi.org/10.1177%2F1534650112462623

Fernandez-Mendoza, J., Baker, J. H., Vgontzas, A. N., Gaines, J., Liao, D., & Bixler, E. O. (2017). Insomnia symptoms with objective short sleep duration are associated with systemic inflammation in adolescents. *Brain, Behavior, and Immunity*, *61*, 110–116. https://doi.org/10.1016/j.bbi.2016.12.026

Fernandez-Mendoza, J., Lenker, K. P., Calhoun, S. L., Qureshi, M., Ricci, A., Bourchtein, E., He, F., Vgontzas, A. N., Liao, J., Liao, D., & Bixler, E. O. (2022). Trajectories of insomnia symptoms from childhood through young adulthood. *Pediatrics*, *149*(3), Article e2021053616. https://doi.org/10.1542/peds.2021-053616

Fernandez-Mendoza, J., Li, Y., Vgontzas, A. N., Fang, J., Gaines, J., Calhoun, S. L., Liao, D., & Bixler, E. O. (2016). Insomnia is associated with cortical hyperarousal as early as adolescence. *Sleep, 39*(5), 1029–1036. https://doi.org/10.5665/sleep.5746

Ferri, R., DelRosso, L. M., Mogavero, M. P., & Bruni, O. (2023). Periodic limb movement disorder. In C. A. Kushida (Ed.), Encyclopedia of sleep and circadian rhythms (2nd ed., pp. 620–627). Academic Press. https://doi.org/10.1016/B978-0-12-822963-7.00121-3

Ferri, R., Fulda, S., Allen, R. P., Zucconi, M., Bruni, O., Chokroverty, S., Ferini-Strambi, L., Frauscher, B., Garcia-Borreguero, D., Hirshkowitz, M., Hogl, B., Inoue, Y., Jahangir, A., Manconi, M., Marcus, C. L., Picchietti, D. L., Plazzi, G., Winkelman, J. W., & Zak, R. S.; International and European Restless Legs Syndrome Study Groups. (2016). World Association of Sleep Medicine (WASM) 2016 standards for recording and scoring leg movements in polysomnograms developed by a joint task force from the International and the European Restless Legs Syndrome Study Groups (IRLSSG and EURLSSG). *Sleep Medicine, 26*, 86–95. https://doi.org/10.1016/j.sleep.2016.10.010

Fiese, B. H., Cai, T. Y., Sutter, C., & Bost, K. K. (2021). Bedtimes, bedtime routines, and children's sleep across the first 2 years of life. *Sleep, 44*(8), Article zsab045. https://doi.org/10.1093/sleep/zsab045

France, K. G., & Hudson, S. M. (1990). Behavior management of infant sleep disturbance. *Journal of Applied Behavior Analysis, 23*, 91–8. https://doi.org/10.1901/jaba.1990.23-91

Friman, P. C., Hoff, K. E., Schnoes, C., Freeman, K. A., Woods, D. W., & Blum, N. (1999). The bedtime pass—An approach to bedtime crying and leaving the room. *Archives of Pediatrics & Adolescent Medicine, 153*(10), 1027–1029. https://doi.org/10.1001/archpedi.153.10.1027

Gaina, A., Sekine, M., Chen, X., Hamanishi, S., & Kagamimori, S. (2004). Validity of child sleep diary questionnaire among junior high school children. *Journal of Epidemiology, 14*(1), 1–4. https://doi.org/10.2188/jea.14.1

Galland, B. C., Sayers, R. M., Cameron, S. L., Gray, A. R., Heath, A. M., Lawrence, J. A., Newlands, A., Taylor, B. J., & Taylor, R. W. (2017). Anticipatory guidance to prevent infant sleep problems within a randomised controlled trial: Infant, maternal and partner outcomes at 6 months of age. *BMJ Open, 7*(5), Article e014908. https://doi.org/10.1136/bmjopen-2016-014908

Garetz, S. L., Mitchell, R. B., Parker, P. D., Moore, R. H., Rosen, C. L., Giordani, B., Muzumdar, H., Paruthi, S., Elden, L., Willging, P., Beebe, D. W., Marcus, C. L., Chervin, R. D., & Redline, S. (2015). Quality of life and obstructive sleep apnea symptoms after pediatric adenotonsillectomy. *Pediatrics, 135*(2), E477–E486. https://doi.org/10.1542/peds.2014-0620

Gariepy, G., Danna, S., Gobina, I., Rasmussen, M., de Matos, M. G., Tynjala, J., Janssen, I., Kalman, M., Villerusa, A., Husarova, D., Brooks, F., Elgar, F. J., Klavina-Makrecka, S., Smigelskas, K., Gaspar, T., & Schnohr, C. (2020). How are adolescents sleeping? Adolescent sleep patterns and sociodemographic differences in 24 European and North American countries. *Journal of Adolescent Health, 66*(6), S81–S88. https://doi.org/10.1016/j.jadohealth.2020.03.013

Gauchat, A., Séguin, J., & Zadra, A. (2014). Prevalence and correlates of disturbed dreaming in children. *Pathologie Biologie, 62*(5), 311–318. https://doi.org/10.1016/j.patbio.2014.05.016

Gaudreau, H., Joncas, S., Zadra, A., & Montplaisir, J. (2000). Dynamics of slow-wave activity during the NREM sleep of sleepwalkers and control subjects. *Sleep, 23*(6), 755–760.

Gigliotti, F., Esposito, D., Basile, C., Cesario, S., & Bruni, O. (2021). Sleep terrors—A parental nightmare. *Pediatric Pulmonology, 57*(8), 1869–1878. https://doi.org/10.1002/ppul.25304

Golik, T., Avni, H., Nehama, H., Greenfeld, M., Sivan, Y., & Tauman, R. (2013). Maternal cognitions and depression in childhood behavioral insomnia and feeding disturbances. *Sleep Medicine, 14*(3), 261–265. https://doi.org/10.1016/j.sleep.2012.10.025

Goodlin-Jones, B. L., Burnham, M. M., Gaylor, E. E., & Anders, T. F. (2001). Night waking, sleep–wake organization, and self-soothing in the first year of life. *Journal of Developmental and Behavioral Pediatrics, 22*(4), 226–233.

Gozal, D., & Kheirandish-Gozal, L. (2012). Childhood obesity and sleep: Relatives, partners, or both?—A critical perspective on the evidence. *Annals of the New York Academy of Sciences, 1264*, 135–141. https://doi.org/10.1111/j.1749-6632.2012.06723.x

Gradisar, M., Dohnt, H., Gardner, G., Paine, S., Starkey, K., Menne, A., Slater, A., Wright, H., Hudson, J. L., Weaver, E., & Trenowden, S. (2011). A randomized controlled trial of cognitive-behavior therapy plus bright light therapy for adolescent delayed sleep phase disorder. *Sleep, 34*(12), 1671–1680. https://doi.org/10.5665/sleep.1432

Gradisar, M., Gardner, G., & Dohnt, H. (2011). Recent worldwide sleep patterns and problems during adolescence: A review and meta-analysis of age, region, and sleep. *Sleep Medicine, 12*(2), 110–118. https://doi.org/10.1016/j.sleep.2010.11.008

Gradisar, M., Jackson, K., Spurrier, N. J., Gibson, J., Whitham, J., Williams, A. S., Dolby, R., & Kennaway, D. J. (2016). Behavioral interventions for infant sleep problems: A randomized controlled trial. *Pediatrics, 137*(6), Article e20151486. https://doi.org/10.1542/peds.2015-1486

Gradisar, M., Kahn, M., Micic, G., Short, M., Reynolds, C., Orchard, F., Bauducco, S., Bartel, K., & Richardson, C. (2022). Sleep's role in the development and resolution of adolescent depression. *Nature Reviews Psychology, 1,* 512–523. https://doi.org/10.1038/s44159-022-00074-8

Gradisar, M., Short, M., Reynolds, C., Richardson, C., Heath, M., Kahn, M., Lack, L., & Carskadon, M. (2020). Development of evening waking homeostatic pressure during early adolescence. *Journal of Sleep Research, 29,* 181–181.

Gregory, A. M., & Sadeh, A. (2012). Sleep, emotional and behavioral difficulties in children and adolescents. *Sleep Medicine Re*views, *16*(2), 129–136. https://doi.org/10.1016/j.smrv.2011.03.007

Guglielmo, D., Gazmararian, J. A., Chung, J., Rogers, A. E., & Hale, L. (2018). Racial/ethnic sleep disparities in US school-aged children and adolescents: A review of the literature. *Sleep Health, 4*(1), 68–80. https://doi.org/10.1016/j.sleh.2017.09.005

Guilleminault, C., Eldridge, F. L., Simmons, F. B., & Dement, W. C. (1976). Sleep apnea in eight children. *Pediatrics, 58*(1), 23–30. https://www.ncbi.nlm.nih.gov/pubmed/934781

Guilleminault, C., Kirisoglu, C., da Rosa, A. C., Lopes, C., & Chan, A. (2006). Sleepwalking, a disorder of NREM sleep instability. *Sleep Medicine, 7*(2), 163–170. https://doi.org/10.1016/j.sleep.2005.12.006

Gwyther, A. R. M., Walters, A. S., & Hill, C. M. (2017). Rhythmic movement disorder in childhood: An integrative review. *Sleep Medicine Reviews, 35,* 62–75. https://doi.org/10.1016/j.smrv.2016.08.003

Habukawa, M., Uchimura, N., Maeda, M., Ogi, K., Hiejima, H., & Kakuma, T. (2018). Differences in rapid eye movement (REM) sleep abnormalities between posttraumatic stress disorder (PTSD) and major depressive disorder patients: REM interruption correlated with nightmare complaints in PTSD. *Sleep Medicine, 43,* 34–39. https://doi.org/10.1016/j.sleep.2017.10.012

Hale, L., & Guan, S. (2015). Screen time and sleep among school-aged children and adolescents: A systematic literature review. *Sleep Medicine Reviews, 21,* 50–58. https://doi.org/10.1016/j.smrv.2014.07.007

Hale, L., Li, X., Hartstein, L. E., & LeBourgeois, M. K. (2019). Media use and sleep in teenagers: What do we know? *Current Sleep Medicine Reports, 5*(3), 128–134. https://doi.org/10.1007/s40675-019-00146-x

Hall, W. A., Hutton, E., Brant, R. F., Collet, J. P., Gregg, K., Saunders, R., Ipsiroglu, O., Gafni, A., Triolet, K., Tse, L., Bhagat, R., & Wooldridge, J. (2015). A randomized controlled trial of an intervention for infants' behavioral sleep problems. *BMC Pediatrics, 15,* Article 181. https://doi.org/10.1186/s12887-015-0492-7

Hall, W. A., Liva, S., Moynihan, M., & Saunders, R. (2015). A comparison of actigraphy and sleep diaries for infants' sleep behavior. *Frontiers in Psychiatry, 6,* Article 19. https://doi.org/10.3389/fpsyt.2015.00019

Hamilton-Stubbs, P., & Walters, A. (2017). Sleep disorders in children: Simple sleep-related movement disorders. In S. Nevšímalová & O. Bruni (Eds.), Sleep disorders in children (pp. 227–251). Springer.

Harvey, A. G. (2016). A transdiagnostic intervention for youth sleep and circadian problems. *Cognitive and Behavioral Practice, 23*(3), 341–355. https://doi.org/10.1016/j.cbpra.2015.06.001

Harvey, A. G., Hein, K., Dolsen, M. R., Dong, L., Rabe-Hesketh, S., Gumport, N. B., Kanady, J., Wyatt, J. K., Hinshaw, S. P., Silk, J. S., Smith, R. L., Thompson, M. A., Zannone, N., & Blum, D. J. (2018). Modifying the impact of eveningness chronotype ("night-owls") in youth: A randomized controlled trial. *Journal of the American Academy of Child and Adolescent Psychiatry, 57*(10), 742–754. https://doi.org/10.1016/j.jaac.2018.04.020

Hauri, P. J., Silber, M. H., & Boeve, B. F. (2007). The treatment of parasomnias with hypnosis: A 5-year follow-up study. *Journal of Clinical Sleep Medicine, 3*(4), 369–373. https://doi.org/10.5664/jcsm.26858

Hedin, G., Norell-Clarke, A., Hagell, P., Tønnesen, H., Westergren, A., & Garmy, P. (2020). Insomnia in relation to academic performance, self-reported health, physical activity, and substance use among adolescents. *International Journal of Environmental Research and Public Health, 17*(17), Article 6433.

Henderson, J. M., France, K. G., & Blampied, N. M. (2011). The consolidation of infants' nocturnal sleep across the first year of life. *Sleep Medicine Reviews, 15*(4), 211–220. https://doi.org/10.1016/j.smrv.2010.08.003

Henderson, J. M., France, K. G., Owens, J. L., & Blampied, N. M. (2010). Sleeping through the night: The consolidation of self-regulated sleep across the first year of life. *Pediatrics, 126*(5), e1081–e1087. https://doi.org/10.1542/peds.2010-0976

Henderson, J. M. T., Blampied, N. M., & France, K. G. (2020). Longitudinal study of infant sleep development: Early predictors of sleep regulation across the first year. *Nature and Science of Sleep, 12*, 949–957. https://doi.org/10.2147/NSS.S240075

Hiscock, H., Bayer, J., Gold, L., Hampton, A., Ukoumunne, O. C., & Wake, M. (2007). Improving infant sleep and maternal mental health: A cluster randomised trial. *Archives of Disease in Childhood, 92*(11), 952–958. https://doi.org/10.1136/adc.2006.099812

Hiscock, H., Bayer, J. K., Hampton, A., Ukoumunne, O. C., & Wake, M. (2008). Long-term mother and child mental health effects of a population-based infant sleep intervention: Cluster-randomized, controlled trial. *Pediatrics, 122*(3), E621–E627. https://doi.org/10.1542/peds.2007-3783

Honaker, S. M., & Meltzer, L. J. (2016). Sleep in pediatric primary care: A review of the literature. *Sleep Medicine Reviews, 25*, 31–39. https://doi.org/10.1016/j.smrv.2015.01.004

Hublin, C., & Kaprio, J. (2003). Genetic aspects and genetic epidemiology of parasomnias. *Sleep Medicine Reviews, 7*(5), 413–421. https://doi.org/10.1053/smrv.2001.0247

Hunter, S. J., Gozal, D., Smith, D. L., Philby, M. F., Kaylegian, J., & Kheirandish-Gozal, L. (2016). Effect of sleep-disordered breathing severity on cognitive performance measures in a large community cohort of young school-aged children. *American Journal of Respiratory and Critical Care Medicine, 194*(6), 739–747. https://doi.org/10.1164/rccm.201510-2099OC

Hysing, M., Pallesen, S., Stormark, K. M., Lundervold, A. J., & Sivertsen, B. (2013). Sleep patterns and insomnia among adolescents: A population-based study. *Journal of Sleep Research, 22*(5), 549–556. https://doi.org/10.1111/jsr.12055

Imran, S., Arganbright, J. M., & Ingram, D. G. (2021). Sleep disordered breathing in neurodevelopmental disorders. *Current Sleep Medicine Reports, 7*, 48–56. https://doi.org/10.1007/s40675-021-00203-4

Insana, S. P., Williams, K. B., & Montgomery-Downs, H. E. (2013). Sleep disturbance and neurobehavioral performance among postpartum women. *Sleep, 36*(1), 73–81. https://doi.org/10.5665/Sleep.2304

Irfan, M., Schenck, C. H., & Howell, M. J. (2021). NonREM disorders of arousal and related parasomnias: An updated review. *Neurotherapeutics, 18*(1), 124–139. https://doi.org/10.1007/s13311-021-01011-y

Jan, J., Freeman, R., Wasdell, M., & Bomben, M. (2004). A child with severe night terrors and sleep-walking responds to melatonin therapy. *Developmental Medicine and Child Neurology, 46*(11), 789–789. https://doi.org/10.1017/s0012162204231358

Johnson, C. M., & Lerner, M. (1985). Amelioration of infant sleep disturbances: II. Effects of scheduled awakenings by compliant parents. *Infant Mental Health Journal, 6*(1), 21–30. https://doi.org/10.1002/1097-0355(198521)6:1%3C21::AID-IMHJ2280060105%3E3.0.CO;2-Q

Johnson, D., Dupuis, G., Piche, J., Clayborne, Z., & Colman, I. (2018). Adult mental health outcomes of adolescent depression: A systematic review. *Depression and Anxiety, 35*(8), 700–716. https://doi.org/10.1002/da.22777

Johnson, E. O., Roth, T., Schultz, L., & Breslau, N. (2006). Epidemiology of DSM-IV insomnia in adolescence: Lifetime prevalence, chronicity, and an emergent gender difference. *Pediatrics, 117*(2), e247–e256. https://doi.org/10.1542/peds.2004-2629

Johnson, N., & McMahon, C. (2008). Preschoolers' sleep behaviour: Associations with parental hardiness, sleep-related cognitions and bedtime interactions. *Journal of Child Psychology and Psychiatry, 49*(7), 765–773. https://doi.org/10.1111/j.1469-7610.2007.01871.x

Jones, C. H., & Ball, H. (2014). Exploring socioeconomic differences in bedtime behaviours and sleep duration in English preschool children. *Infant and Child Development, 23*(5), 518–531. https://doi.org/10.1002/icd.1848

Kaditis, A. G., Alonso Alvarez, M. L., Boudewyns, A., Alexopoulos, E. I., Ersu, R., Joosten, K., Larramona, H., Miano, S., Narang, I., Trang, H., Tsaoussoglou, M., Vandenbussche, N., Villa, M. P., Van Waardenburg, D., Weber, S., & Verhulst, S. (2016). Obstructive sleep disordered breathing in 2- to 18-year-old children: Diagnosis and management. *European Respiratory Journal, 47*(1), 69–94. https://doi.org/10.1183/13993003.00385-2015

Kahn, M., Barnett, N., Glazer, A., & Gradisar, M. (2021). Infant sleep during COVID-19: Longitudinal analysis of infants of US mothers in home confinement versus working as usual. *Sleep Health, 7*(1), 19–23. https://doi.org/10.1016/j.sleh.2020.11.004

Kahn, M., Bauminger, Y., Volkovich, E., Meiri, G., Sadeh, A., & Tikotzky, L. (2018). Links between infant sleep and parental tolerance for infant crying: Longitudinal assessment from pregnancy through six months postpartum. *Sleep Medicine, 50*, 72–78. https://doi.org/10.1016/j.sleep.2018.05.014

Kahn, M., & Gradisar, M. (2022). Sleeping through COVID-19: A longitudinal comparison of 2019 and 2020 infant auto-videosomnography metrics. *Journal of Child Psychology and Psychiatry, 63*(6), 693–700. https://doi.org/10.1111/jcpp.13509

Kahn, M., Juda-Hanael, M., Livne-Karp, E., Tikotzky, L., Anders, T. F., & Sadeh, A. (2020). Behavioral interventions for pediatric insomnia: One treatment may not fit all. *Sleep, 43*(4), Article zsz268. https://doi.org/10.1093/sleep/zsz268

Kahn, M., Livne-Karp, E., Juda-Hanael, M., Omer, H., Tikotzky, L., Anders, T. F., & Sadeh, A. (2020). Behavioral interventions for infant sleep problems: The role of parental cry tolerance and sleep-related cognitions. *Journal of Clinical Sleep Medicine, 16*(8), 1275–1283. https://doi.org/10.5664/jcsm.8488

Kahn, M., Ronen, A., Apter, A., & Sadeh, A. (2017). Cognitive-behavioral versus non-directive therapy for preschoolers with severe nighttime fears and sleep-related problems. *Sleep Medicine, 32*, 40–47. https://doi.org/10.1016/j.sleep.2016.12.011

Kaplan, K. A., Mashash, M., Williams, R., Batchelder, H., Starr-Glass, L., & Zeitzer, J. M. (2019). Effect of light flashes vs sham therapy during sleep with adjunct cognitive behavioral therapy on sleep quality among adolescents: A randomized clinical trial. *JAMA Network Open, 2*(9), Article e1911944. https://doi.org/10.1001/jamanetworkopen.2019.11944

Kelly, R. J., & El-Sheikh, M. (2011). Marital conflict and children's sleep: Reciprocal relations and socioeconomic effects. *Journal of Family Psychology, 25*(3), 412–422. https://doi.org/10.1037/a0023789

Kerr, S. M., Jowett, S. A., & Smith, L. N. (1996). Preventing sleep problems in infants: A randomized controlled trial. *Journal of Advanced Nursing, 24*(5), 938–942. https://doi.org/10.1111/j.1365-2648.1996.tb02929.x

Kheirandish-Gozal, L., & Farre, R. (2013). The injury theory, endothelial progenitors, and sleep apnea. *American Journal of Respiratory and Critical Care Medicine, 187*(1), 5–7. https://doi.org/10.1164/rccm.201210-1950ED

Kheirandish-Gozal, L., & Gozal, D. (2013). Genotype–phenotype interactions in pediatric obstructive sleep apnea. *Respiratory Physiology & Neurobiology, 189*(2), 338–343. https://doi.org/10.1016/j.resp.2013.03.016

Kopcsó, K., Láng, A., & Coffman, M. F. (2022). Reducing the nighttime fears of young children through a brief parent-delivered treatment—Effectiveness of the Hungarian version of Uncle Lightfoot. *Child Psychiatry & Human Development, 53*, 256–267. https://doi.org/10.1007/s10578-020-01103-4

Kotagal, S. (2009). Parasomnias in childhood. *Sleep Medicine Reviews, 13*(2), 157–168. https://doi.org/10.1016/j.smrv.2008.09.005

Koulouglioti, C., Cole, R., Moskow, M., McQuillan, B., Carno, M. A., & Grape, A. (2014). The longitudinal association of young children's everyday routines to sleep duration. *Journal of Pediatrics Health Care, 28*(1), 80–87. https://doi.org/10.1016/j.pedhc.2012.12.006

Krakow, B., & Zadra, A. (2010). Imagery rehearsal therapy: Principles and practice. *Sleep Medicine Clinics, 5*(2), 289–298. https://doi.org/10.1016/J.JSMC.2010.01.004

Kushnir, J., & Sadeh, A. (2011). Sleep of preschool children with night-time fears. *Sleep Medicine, 12*(9), 870–874. https://doi.org/10.1016/j.sleep.2011.03.022

Kushnir, J., & Sadeh, A. (2012). Assessment of brief interventions for nighttime fears in preschool children. *European Journal of Pediatrics, 171*(1), 67–75. https://doi.org/10.1007/s00431-011-1488-4

Lang, C., Richardson, C., Short, M. A., & Gradisar, M. (2022). Low-intensity scheduled morning exercise for adolescents with a late chronotype: A novel treatment to advance circadian phase. *Sleep Advances, 3*, Article zpac021.

Lask, B. (1988). Novel and non-toxic treatment for night terrors. *British Medical Journal, 297*(6648), 592. https://doi.org/10.1136%2Fbmj.297.6648.592

Lecendreux, M., Bassetti, C., Dauvilliers, Y., Mayer, G., Neidhart, E., & Tafti, M. (2003). HLA and genetic susceptibility to sleepwalking. *Molecular Psychiatry, 8*(1), 114–117. https://doi.org/10.1038/sj.mp.4001203

Lewis, K. M., Amatya, K., Coffman, M. F., & Ollendick, T. H. (2015). Treating nighttime fears in young children with bibliotherapy: Evaluating anxiety symptoms and monitoring behavior change. *Journal of Anxiety Disorders, 30*, 103–112. https://doi.org/10.1016/j.janxdis.2014.12.004

Lewis, K. M., El Rafihi-Ferreira, R., Freitag, G. F., Coffman, M., & Ollendick, T. H. (2021). A 25-year review of nighttime fears in children: Past, present, and future. *Clinical Child and Family Psychology Review, 24*, 391–413. https://doi.org/10.1007/s10567-021-00354-4

Licis, A., Desruisseau, D., Yamada, K., Duntley, S., & Gurnett, C. (2011). Novel genetic findings in an extended family pedigree with sleepwalking. *Neurology, 76*(1), 49–52. https://doi.org/10.1212/WNL.0b013e318203e964

Liming, B. J., Ryan, M., Mack, D., Ahmad, I., & Camacho, M. (2019). Montelukast and nasal corticosteroids to treat pediatric obstructive sleep apnea: A systematic review and meta-analysis. *Otolaryngology–Head and Neck Surgery, 160*(4), 594–602. https://doi.org/10.1177/0194599818815683

Lunsford-Avery, J. R., Bidopia, T., Jackson, L., & Sloan, J. S. (2021). Behavioral treatment of insomnia and sleep disturbances in school-aged children and adolescents. *Child and Adolescent Psychiatric Clinics of North America, 30*(1), 101–116. https://doi.org/10.1016/j.chc.2020.08.006

MacDuffie, K. E., Shen, M. D., Dager, S. R., Styner, M. A., Kim, S. H., Paterson, S., Pandey, J., St John, T., Elison, J. T., Wolff, J. J., Swanson, M. R., Botteron, K. N., Zwaigenbaum, L., Piven, J., & Estes, A. M. (2020). Sleep onset problems and subcortical development in infants later diagnosed with autism spectrum disorder. *American Journal of Psychiatry, 177*(6), 518–525. https://doi.org/10.1176/appi.ajp.2019.19060666

Marcus, C. L., Brooks, L. J., Draper, K. A., Gozal, D., Halbower, A. C., Jones, J., Schechter, M. S., Ward, S. D., Sheldon, S. H., Shiffman, R. N., Lehmann, C., & Spruyt, K. (2012). Diagnosis and management of childhood obstructive sleep apnea syndrome. *Pediatrics, 130*(3), e714–e755. https://doi.org/10.1542/peds.2012-1672

Marcus, C. L., Greene, M. G., & Carroll, J. L. (1998). Blood pressure in children with obstructive sleep apnea. *American Journal of Respiratory and Critical Care Medicine, 157*(4), 1098–1103. https://doi.org/10.1164/ajrccm.157.4.9704080

Marmorstein, N. R. (2017). Sleep patterns and problems among early adolescents: Associations with alcohol use. *Addictive Behaviors, 66*, 13–16. https://doi.org/10.1016/j.addbeh.2016.11.002

Maski, K., & Owens, J. A. (2016). Insomnia, parasomnias, and narcolepsy in children: Clinical features, diagnosis, and management. *Lancet Neurology, 15*(11), 1170–1181. https://doi.org/10.1016/S1474-4422(16)30204-6

Matthey, S., & Črnčec, R. (2012). Comparison of two strategies to improve infant sleep problems, and associated impacts on maternal experience, mood and infant emotional health: A single case replication design study. *Early Human Development, 88*(6), 437–442. https://doi.org/10.1016/j.earlhumdev.2011.10.010

Maurer, L. F., Schneider, J., Miller, C. B., Espie, C. A., & Kyle, S. D. (2021). The clinical effects of sleep restriction therapy for insomnia: A meta-analysis of randomised controlled trials. *Sleep Medicine Reviews, 58*, Article 101493. https://doi.org/10.1016/j.smrv.2021.101493

McKenna, J. J., Ball, H. L., & Gettler, L. T. (2007). Mother–infant cosleeping, breastfeeding and sudden infant death syndrome: What biological anthropology has discovered about normal infant sleep and pediatric sleep medicine. *American Journal of Physical Anthropology, 134*(S45), 133–161. https://doi.org/10.1002/ajpa.20736

Medalie, L., Dang, T., & Casnar, C. L. (2021). Pediatric insomnia: Etiology, impact, assessment, and treatment. In D. Gozal & L. Kheirandish-Gozal (Eds.), *Pediatric sleep medicine: Mechanisms and comprehensive guide to clinical evaluation and management* (pp. 333–339). Springer. https://doi.org/10.1007/978-3-030-65574-7_26

Meltzer, L. J., & Mindell, J. A. (2006). Sleep and sleep disorders in children and adolescents. *Psychiatric Clinics of North America, 29*(4), 1059–1076. https://doi.org/10.1016/j.psc.2006.08.004

Meltzer, L. J., & Mindell, J. A. (2014). Systematic review and meta-analysis of behavioral interventions for pediatric insomnia. *Journal of Pediatric Psychology, 39*(8), 932–948. https://doi.org/10.1093/jpepsy/jsu041

Meltzer, L. J., Williamson, A. A., & Mindell, J. A. (2021). Pediatric sleep health: It matters, and so does how we define it. *Sleep Medicine Reviews, 57*, Article 101425. https://doi.org/10.1016/j.smrv.2021.101425

Messayke, S., Franco, P., Forhan, A., Dufourg, M. N., Charles, M. A., & Plancoulaine, S. (2020). Sleep habits and sleep characteristics at age one year in the ELFE birth cohort study. *Sleep Medicine, 67*, 200–206. https://doi.org/10.1016/j.sleep.2019.11.1255

Mike, T. B., Shaw, D. S., Forbes, E. E., Sitnick, S. L., & Hasler, B. P. (2016). The hazards of bad sleep—Sleep duration and quality as predictors of adolescent alcohol and cannabis use. *Drug and Alcohol Dependence, 168*, 335–339. https://doi.org/10.1016/j.drugalcdep.2016.08.009

Mindell, J., & Barrett, K. (2002). Nightmares and anxiety in elementary-aged children: Is there a relationship? *Child: Care, Health and Development, 28*(4), 317–322. https://doi.org/10.1046/j.1365-2214.2002.00274.x

Mindell, J. A., Gould, R. A., Tikotzy, L., Leichman, E. S., & Walters, R. M. (2019). Norm-referenced scoring system for the Brief Infant Sleep Questionnairee–Revised (BISQ-R). *Sleep Medicine, 63*, 106–114. https://doi.org/10.1016/j.sleep.2019.05.010

Mindell, J. A., Kuhn, B., Lewin, D. S., Meltzer, L. J., & Sadeh, A. (2006). Behavioral treatment of bedtime problems and night wakings in infants and young children—An American Academy of Sleep Medicine review. *Sleep, 29*(10), 1263–1276.

Mindell, J. A., Li, A. M., Sadeh, A., Kwon, R., & Goh, D. Y. (2015). Bedtime routines for young children: A dose-dependent association with sleep outcomes. *Sleep, 38*(5), 717–722. https://doi.org/10.5665/sleep.4662

Mindell, J. A., & Owens, A. O. (2015). *A clinical guide to pediatric sleep: Diagnosis and management of sleep problems* (3rd ed.). Wolters Kluwer.

Mindell, J. A., Sadeh, A., Kohyama, J., & How, T. H. (2010). Parental behaviors and sleep outcomes in infants and toddlers: A cross-cultural comparison. *Sleep Medicine, 11*(4), 393–399. https://doi.org/10.1016/j.sleep.2009.11.011

Mindell, J. A., Telofski, L. S., Wiegand, B., & Kurtz, E. S. (2009). A nightly bedtime routine: Impact on sleep in young children and maternal mood. *Sleep, 32*(5), 599–606. https://doi.org/10.1093/sleep/32.5.599

Mindell, J. A., & Williamson, A. A. (2018). Benefits of a bedtime routine in young children: Sleep, development, and beyond. *Sleep Medicne Reviews, 40*, 93–108. https://doi.org/10.1016/j.smrv.2017.10.007

Moore, B. A., Friman, P. C., Fruzzetti, A. E., & MacAleese, K. (2007). Brief report: Evaluating the bedtime pass program for child resistance to bedtime—A randomized, controlled trial. *Journal of Pediatric Psychology, 32*(3), 283–287. https://doi.org/10.1093/jpepsy/jsl025

Morales-Munoz, I., Nolvi, S., Virta, M., Karlsson, H., Paavonen, E. J., & Karlsson, L. (2020). The longitudinal associations between temperament and sleep during the first year of life. *Infant Behavior & Development, 61*, Article 101485. https://doi.org/10.1016/j.infbeh.2020.101485

Morrell, J., & Cortina-Borja, M. (2002). The developmental change in strategies parents employ to settle young children to sleep, and their relationship to infant sleeping problems, as assessed by a new questionnaire: The Parental Interactive Bedtime Behaviour Scale. *Infant and Child Development, 11*(1), 17–41.

Morrell, J., & Steele, H. (2003). The role of attachment security, temperament, maternal perception, and care-giving behavior in persistent infant sleeping problems. *Infant Mental Health Journal, 24*(5), 447–468.

Mota, D. M., Barros, A. J., Matijasevich, A., & Santos, I. S. (2015). Prevalence of enuresis and urinary symptoms at age 7 years in the 2004 birth cohort from Pelotas, Brazil. *Jornal de Pediatría, 91*, 52–58. https://doi.org/10.1016/j.jped.2014.04.011

Neveus, T., Eggert, P., Evans, J., Macedo, A., Rittig, S., Tekgül, S., Vande Walle, J., Yeung, C., & Robson, L. (2010). Evaluation of and treatment for monosymptomatic enuresis: A standardization document from the International Children's Continence Society. *Journal of Urology, 183*(2), 441–447. https://doi.org/10.1016/j.juro.2009.10.043

Newton, A. T., Honaker, S. M., & Reid, G. J. (2020). Risk and protective factors and processes for behavioral sleep problems among preschool and early school-aged children: A systematic review. *Sleep Medicine Reviews, 52*, Article 101303. https://doi.org/10.1016/j.smrv.2020.101303

Nielsen, T. (2017). The stress acceleration hypothesis of nightmares. *Frontiers in Neurology, 8*, Article 201. https://doi.org/10.3389/fneur.2017.00201

Nielsen, T., & Levin, R. (2007). Nightmares: A new neurocognitive model. *Sleep Medicine Reviews, 11*(4), 295–310. https://doi.org/10.1016/j.smrv.2007.03.004

Oliviero, A., Della Marca, G., Tonali, P., Pilato, F., Saturno, E., Dileone, M., Rubino, M., & Di Lazzaro, V. (2007). Functional involvement of cerebral cortex in adult sleepwalking. *Journal of Neurology, 254*(8), 1066–1072. https://doi.org/10.1007/s00415-006-0489-0

Orchard, F., Pass, L., Chessell, C., Moody, A., Ellis, J., & Reynolds, S. (2020). Adapting brief CBT-I for depressed adolescents: A case illustration of the sleeping better program. *Cognitive and Behavioral Practice, 27*(3), 336–346. https://doi.org/10.1016/j.cbpra.2019.07.010

Owens, J. (2008). Classification and epidemiology of childhood sleep disorders. *Primary Care, 35*(3), 533–546. https://doi.org/10.1016/j.pop.2008.06.003

Owens, J., & Mohan, M. (2016). Behavioral interventions for parasomnias. *Current Sleep Medicine Reports, 2*(2), 81–86. https://doi.org/10.1007/s40675-016-0046-z

Owens, J. A., & Mindell, J. A. (2011). Pediatric insomnia. *Pediatric Clinics of North America, 58*(3), 555–569. https://doi.org/10.1016/j.pcl.2011.03.011

Owens, J. A., Mindell, J., & Baylor, A. (2014). Effect of energy drink and caffeinated beverage consumption on sleep, mood, and performance in children and adolescents. *Nutrition Reviews, 72*(S1), 65–71. https://doi.org/10.1111/nure.12150

Owens, J. A., Spirito, A., & McGuinn, M. (2000). The Children's Sleep Habits Questionnaire (CSHQ): Psychometric properties of a survey instrument for school-aged children. *Sleep, 23*(8), 1043–1051.

Paine, S., & Gradisar, M. (2011). A randomised controlled trial of cognitive-behaviour therapy for behavioural insomnia of childhood in school-aged children. *Behavior Research and Theraphy, 49*(6–7), 379–388. https://doi.org/10.1016/j.brat.2011.03.008

Pedersen, M. J., Rittig, S., Jennum, P. J., & Kamperis, K. (2020). The role of sleep in the pathophysiology of nocturnal enuresis. *Sleep Medicine Reviews, 49*, Article 101228. https://doi.org/10.1016/j.smrv.2019.101228

Petit, D., Pennestri, M.-H., Paquet, J., Desautels, A., Zadra, A., Vitaro, F., Tremblay, R. E., Boivin, M., & Montplaisir, J. (2015). Childhood sleepwalking and sleep terrors: A longitudinal study of prevalence and familial aggregation. *JAMA Pediatrics, 169*(7), 653–658. https://doi.org/10.1001/jamapediatrics.2015.127

Petit, D., Touchette, E., Tremblay, R. E., Boivin, M., & Montplaisir, J. (2007). Dyssomnias and parasomnias in early childhood. *Pediatrics, 119*(5), e1016–e1025. https://doi.org/10.1542/peds.2006-2132

Philbrook, L. E., & Teti, D. M. (2016). Bidirectional associations between bedtime parenting and infant sleep: Parenting quality, parenting practices, and their interaction. *Journal of Family Psychology, 30*(4), 431–441. https://doi.org/10.1037/fam0000198

Phillips, A. J. K., Clerx, W. M., O'Brien, C. S., Sano, A., Barger, L. K., Picard, R. W., Lockley, S. W., Klerman, E. B., & Czeisler, C. A. (2017). Irregular sleep/wake patterns are associated with poorer academic performance and delayed circadian and sleep/wake timing. *Scientific Reports, 7*, Article 3216. https://doi.org/10.1038/s41598-017-03171-4

Piazza, C. C., & Fisher, W. W. (1991). Bedtime fading in the treatment of pediatric insomnia. *Journal of Behavior Therapy and Experimental Psychiatry, 22*(1), 53–56. https://doi.org/10.1016/0005-7916(91)90034-3

Picchietti, D., Allen, R. P., Walters, A. S., Davidson, J. E., Myers, A., & Ferini-Strambi, L. (2007). Restless legs syndrome: Prevalence and impact in children and adolescents—The Peds REST study. *Pediatrics, 120*(2), 253–266. https://doi.org/10.1542/peds.2006-2767

Picchietti, D. L., Bruni, O., de Weerd, A., Durmer, J. S., Kotagal, S., Owens, J. A., Simakajornboon, N., & International Restless Legs Syndrome Study Group. (2013). Pediatric restless legs syndrome diagnostic criteria: An update by the International Restless Legs Syndrome Study Group. *Sleep Medicine, 14*(12), 1253–1259. https://doi.org/10.1016/j.sleep.2013.08.778

Plazzi, G., Vetrugno, R., Provini, F., & Montagna, P. (2005). Sleepwalking and other ambulatory behaviours during sleep. *Neurological Sciences, 26*, Article s193. https://doi.org/10.1007/s10072-005-0486-6

Price, A. M. H., Wake, M., Ukoumunne, O. C., & Hiscock, H. (2012). Five-year follow-up of harms and benefits of behavioral infant sleep intervention: Randomized trial. *Pediatrics, 130*(4), 643–651. https://doi.org/10.1542/peds.2011-3467

Prihodova, I., Skibova, J., & Nevsimalova, S. (2019). Sleep-related rhythmic movements and rhythmic movement disorder beyond early childhood. *Sleep Medicine, 64*, 112–115. https://doi.org/10.1016/j.sleep.2019.05.021

Quach, J., Hiscock, H., Ukoumunne, O. C., & Wake, M. (2011). A brief sleep intervention improves outcomes in the school entry year: A randomized controlled trial. *Pediatrics, 128*(4), 692–701. https://doi.org/10.1542/peds.2011-0409

Reynolds, K. C., & Alfano, C. A. (2016). Things that go bump in the night: Frequency and predictors of nightmares in anxious and nonanxious children. *Behavioral Sleep Medicine, 14*(4), 442–456. https://doi.org/10.1080/15402002.2015.1017099

Richardson, C., Cain, N., Bartel, K., Micic, G., Maddock, B., & Gradisar, M. (2018). A randomised controlled trial of bright light therapy and morning activity for adolescents and young adults with delayed sleep-wake phase disorder. *Sleep Medicine, 45*, 114–123. https://doi.org/10.1016/j.sleep.2018.02.001

Richardson, C., & Gradisar, M. (2022). Depressed mood and repetitive negative thinking in delayed sleep–wake phase disorder: Treatment effects and a comparison with good sleepers. *Journal of Sleep Research, 31*(1), Article e13452. https://doi.org/10.1111/jsr.13452

Richardson, C., Micic, G., Cain, N., Bartel, K., Maddock, B., & Gradisar, M. (2018). Cognitive performance in adolescents with delayed sleep-wake phase disorder: Treatment effects and a comparison with good sleepers. *Journal of Adolescence, 65*, 72–84. https://doi.org/10.1016/j.adolescence.2018.03.002

Richardson, C., Micic, G., Cain, N., Bartel, K., Maddock, B., & Gradisar, M. (2019). Cognitive "insomnia" processes in delayed sleep–wake phase disorder: Do they exist and are they responsive to chronobiological treatment? *Journal of Consulting and Clinical Psychology, 87*(1), 16–32. https://doi.org/10.1037/ccp0000357

Rickert, V. I., & Johnson, C. M. (1988). Reducing nocturnal awakening and crying episodes in infants and young children: A comparison between scheduled awakenings and systematic ignoring. *Pediatrics, 81*(2), 203–212.

Riemann, D., Spiegelhalder, K., Feige, B., Voderholzer, U., Berger, M., Perlis, M., & Nissen, C. (2010). The hyperarousal model of insomnia: A review of the concept and its evidence. *Sleep Medicine Reviews, 14*(1), 19–31. https://doi.org/10.1016/j.smrv.2009.04.002

Riemann, D., Spiegelhalder, K., Nissen, C., Hirscher, V., Baglioni, C., & Feige, B. (2012). REM sleep instability—A new pathway for insomnia? *Pharmacopsychiatry, 45*(5), 167–176. https://doi.org/10.1055/s-0031-1299721

Roberts, R. E., Roberts, C. R., & Duong, H. T. (2008). Chronic insomnia and its negative consequences for health and functioning of adolescents: A 12-month prospective study. *Journal of Adolescent Health, 42*(3), 294–302. https://doi.org/10.1016/j.jadohealth.2007.09.016

Rodríguez-Colón, S. M., He, F., Bixler, E. O., Fernandez-Mendoza, J., Vgontzas, A. N., Calhoun, S., Zheng, Z.-J., & Liao, D. (2015). Sleep variability and cardiac autonomic modulation in adolescents—Penn State Child Cohort (PSCC) study. *Sleep Medicine, 16*(1), 67–72. https://doi.org/10.1016/j.sleep.2014.10.007

Roenneberg, T., Kuehnle, T., Pramstaller, P. P., Ricken, J., Havel, M., Guth, A., & Merrow, M. (2004). A marker for the end of adolescence. *Current Biology, 14*(24), R1038–R1039. https://doi.org/10.1016/j.cub.2004.11.039

Roenneberg, T., Pilz, L. K., Zerbini, G., & Winnebeck, E. C. (2019). Chronotype and social jetlag: A (self-) critical review. *Biology, 54,* 1–19. https://doi.org/10.3390/biology8030054

Sadeh, A. (1994). Assessment of intervention for infant night waking: Parental reports and activity-based home monitoring. *Journal of Consulting and Clinical Psychology, 62*(1), 63–68. https://doi.org/10.1037//0022-006x.62.1.63

Sadeh, A. (1996). Evaluating night wakings in sleep-disturbed infants: A methodological study of parental reports and actigraphy. *Sleep, 19*(10), 757–762. http://www.ncbi.nlm.nih.gov/pubmed/9085482

Sadeh, A. (2004). A brief screening questionnaire for infant sleep problems: Validation and findings for an Internet sample. *Pediatrics, 113*(6), E570–E577. https://doi.org/10.1542/peds.113.6.e570

Sadeh, A. (2005). Cognitive-behavioral treatment for childhood sleep disorders. *Clinical Psychology Review, 25*(5), 612–628. http://www.ncbi.nlm.nih.gov/entrez/query.fcgi?cmd=Retrieve&db=PubMed&dopt=Citation&list_uids=15979219

Sadeh, A. (2011). The role and validity of actigraphy in sleep medicine: An update. *Sleep Medicine Reviews, 15*(4), 259–267. https://doi.org/10.1016/j.smrv.2010.10.001

Sadeh, A. (2015). Sleep assessment methods. *Monographs of the Society for Research in Child Development, 80*(1), 33–48. https://doi.org/10.1111/mono.12143

Sadeh, A., & Anders, T. F. (1993). Infant sleep problems: Origins, assessment, interventions. *Infant Mental Health Journal, 14*(1), 17–34.

Sadeh, A., Flint-Ofir, E., Tirosh, T., & Tikotzky, L. (2007). Infant sleep and parental sleep-related cognitions. *Journal of Family Psychology, 21*(1), 74–87. http://www.ncbi.nlm.nih.gov/entrez/query.fcgi?cmd=Retrieve&db=PubMed&dopt=Citation&list_uids=17371112

Sadeh, A., Juda-Hanael, M., Livne-Karp, E., Kahn, M., Tikotzky, L., Anders, T. F., Calkins, S., & Sivan, Y. (2016). Low parental tolerance for infant crying: An underlying factor in infant sleep problems? *Journal of Sleep Research, 25*(5), 501–507. https://doi.org/10.1111/jsr.12401

Sadeh, A., Mindell, J. A., Luedtke, K., & Wiegand, B. (2009). Sleep and sleep ecology in the first 3 years: A web-based study. *Journal of Sleep Research, 18*(1), 60–73. https://doi.org/10.1111/j.1365-2869.2008.00699.x

Sadeh, A., Tikotzky, L., & Kahn, M. (2014). Sleep in infancy and childhood: Implications for emotional and behavioral difficulties in adolescence and beyond. *Current Opinion in Psychiatry, 27*(6), 453–459. https://doi.org/10.1097/Yco.0000000000000109

Sadeh, A., Tikotzky, L., & Scher, A. (2010). Parenting and infant sleep. *Sleep Medicine Reviews, 14*(2), 89–96. https://doi.org/10.1016/j.smrv.2009.05.003

Santos, I. S., Del-Ponte, B., Tovo-Rodrigues, L., Halal, C. S., Matijasevich, A., Cruz, S., Anselmi, L., Silveira, M. F., Hallal, P. R. C., & Bassani, D. G. (2019). Effect of parental counseling on infants' healthy sleep habits in Brazil: A randomized clinical trial. *JAMA Network Open, 2*(12), Article e1918062. https://doi.org/10.1001/jamanetworkopen.2019.18062

Saxvig, I. W., Wilhelmsen-Langeland, A., Pallesen, S., Vedaa, O., Nordhus, I. H., & Bjorvatn, B. (2014). A randomized controlled trial with bright light and melatonin for delayed sleep phase disorder: Effects on subjective and objective sleep. *Chronobiology International, 31*(1), 72–86. https://doi.org/10.3109/07420528.2013.823200

Scher, A. (2008). Maternal separation anxiety as a regulator of infants' sleep. *Journal of Child Psychology and Psychiatry, 49*(6), 618–625. https://doi.org/10.1111/j.1469-7610.2007.01872.x

Scher, A., & Blumberg, O. (1999). Night waking among 1-year olds: A study of maternal separation anxiety. *Child: Care, Health and Development, 25*(5), 323–334. https://doi.org/10.1046/j.1365-2214.1999.00099.x

Schlarb, A. A., Bihlmaier, I., Velten-Schurian, K., Poets, C. F., & Hautzinger, M. (2018). Short- and long-term effects of CBT-I in groups for school-age children suffering from chronic insomnia: The KiSS-Program. *Behavioral Sleep Medicine, 16*(4), 380–397. https://doi.org/10.1080/15402002.2016.1228642

Schlarb, A. A., Seiler, D., Werner, A., & Kater, M. J. (2020). Modern strategies for settling infants to sleep: A comparison between sleep-disturbed and non-sleep-disturbed infants. *Somnologie, 24*(4), 237–244. https://doi.org/10.1007/s11818-020-00279-0

Schredl, M. (2020). Bad dreams, bedtime anxiety, and trait anxiety in school-aged children. *Somnologie, 24*(4), 267–273. https://doi.org/10.1007/s11818-020-00268-3

Schredl, M., Fricke-Oerkermann, L., Mitschke, A., Wiater, A., & Lehmkuhl, G. (2009). Longitudinal study of nightmares in children: Stability and effect of emotional symptoms. *Child Psychiatry and Human Development, 40*(3), 439–449. https://doi.org/10.1007/s10578-009-0136-y

Sen, T., & Spruyt, K. (2020). Pediatric sleep tools: An updated literature review. *Frontiers in Psychiatry, 11*, Article 317. https://doi.org/10.3389/fpsyt.2020.00317

Shochat, T., Cohen-Zion, M., & Tzischinsky, O. (2014). Functional consequences of inadequate sleep in adolescents: A systematic review. *Sleep Medicine Reviews, 18*(1), 75–87. https://doi.org/10.1016/j.smrv.2013.03.005

Short, M. A., Arora, T., Gradisar, M., Taheri, S., & Carskadon, M. A. (2017). How many sleep diary entries are needed to reliably estimate adolescent sleep? *Sleep, 40*(3), Article zsx006. https://doi.org/10.1093/sleep/zsx006

Short, M. A., Gradisar, M., Lack, L. C., & Wright, H. R. (2013). The impact of sleep on adolescent depressed mood, alertness and academic performance. *Journal of Adolescence, 36*(6), 1025–1033. https://doi.org/10.1016/j.adolescence.2013.08.007

Singh, S., Kaur, H., Singh, S., & Khawaja, I. (2018). Parasomnias: A comprehensive review. *Cureus, 10*(12), Article e3807. https://doi.org/https://org.doi/10.7759/cureus.3807

Sivertsen, B., Harvey, A. G., Pallesen, S., & Hysing, M. (2017). Trajectories of sleep problems from childhood to adolescence: A population-based longitudinal study from Norway. *Journal of Sleep Research, 26*(1), 55–63. https://doi.org/10.1111/jsr.12443

Soster, L. A., Alves, R. C., Fagundes, S. N., Lebl, A., Garzon, E., Koch, V. H., Ferri, R., & Bruni, O. (2017). Non-REM sleep instability in children with primary monosymptomatic sleep enuresis. *Journal of Clinical Sleep Medicine, 13*(10), 1163–1170. https://doi.org/10.5664/jcsm.6762

Spruyt, K. (2019). A review of developmental consequences of poor sleep in childhood. *Sleep Medicine, 60*, 3–12. https://doi.org/10.1016/j.sleep.2018.11.021

Spruyt, K., & Gozal, D. (2011). Pediatric sleep questionnaires as diagnostic or epidemiological tools: A review of currently available instruments. *Sleep Medicine Reviews, 15*(1), 19–32. https://doi.org/10.1016/j.smrv.2010.07.005

Staples, A. D., Bates, J. E., & Petersen, I. T. (2015). Bedtime routines in early childhood: Prevalence, consistency, and associations with nighttime sleep. *Monographs of the Society for Research in Child Development, 80*(1), 141–159. https://doi.org/10.1111/mono.12149

Stein, M. A., Mendelsohn, J., Obermeyer, W. H., Amromin, J., & Benca, R. (2001). Sleep and behavior problems in school-aged children. *Pediatrics, 107*(4), Article e60. https://doi.org/10.1542/peds.107.4.e60

Stremler, R., Hodnett, E., Lee, K., MacMillan, S., Mill, C., Ongcangco, L., & Willan, A. (2006). A behavioral–educational intervention to promote maternal and infant sleep: A pilot randomized, controlled trial. *Sleep, 29*(12), 1609–1615.

Tan, H. L., Gozal, D., & Kheirandish-Gozal, L. (2017). Obstructive sleep apnea in children: A short primer. In S. Nevšímalová & O. Bruni (Eds.), *Sleep disorders in children* (pp. 185–226). Springer. https://doi.org/10.1007/978-3-319-28640-2_10

Tan, H. L., & Kaditis, A. G. (2021). Phenotypic variance in pediatric obstructive sleep apnea. *Pediatric Pulmonology, 56*(6), 1754–1762. https://doi.org/10.1002/ppul.25309

Tassinari, C., Cantalupo, G., Högl, B., Cortelli, P., Tassi, L., Francione, S., Nobili, L., Meletti, S., Rubboli, G., & Gardella, E. (2009). Neuroethological approach to frontolimbic epileptic seizures and parasomnias: The same central pattern generators for the same behaviours. *Revue Neurologique, 165*(10), 762–768. https://doi.org/10.1016/j.neurol.2009.08.002

Taylor, D. J., Jenni, O. G., Acebo, C., & Carskadon, M. A. (2005). Sleep tendency during extended wakefulness: Insights into adolescent sleep regulation and behavior. *Journal of Sleep Research, 14*(3), 239–244.

Thomas, A. G., Monahan, K. C., Lukowski, A. F., & Cauffman, E. (2015). Sleep problems across development: A pathway to adolescent risk taking through working memory. *Journal of Youth and Adolescence, 44*(2), 447–464. https://doi.org/10.1007/s10964-014-0179-7

Tikotzky, L. (2017). Parenting and sleep in early childhood. *Current Opinion in Psychology, 15*, 118–124. https://doi.org/10.1016/j.copsyc.2017.02.016

Tikotzky, L., & Sadeh, A. (2001). Sleep patterns and sleep disruptions in kindergarten children. *Journal of Clinical Child Psychology, 30*(4), 579–589.

Tikotzky, L., & Sadeh, A. (2009). Maternal sleep-related cognitions and infant sleep: A longitudinal study from pregnancy through the first year. *Child Development, 80*(3), 860–874.

Tikotzky, L., & Sadeh, A. (2010). The role of cognitive-behavioral therapy in behavioral childhood insomnia. *Sleep Medicine, 11*(7), 686–691. https://doi.org/10.1016/j.sleep.2009.11.017

Tikotzky, L., Sadeh, A., Volkovich, E., Manber, R., Meiri, G., & Shahar, G. (2015). Infant sleep development from 3 to 6 months postpartum: Links with maternal sleep and paternal involvement. *Monographs of the Society for Research in Child Development, 80*(1), 107–124. https://doi.org/10.1111/mono.12147

Tikotzky, L., & Volkovich, E. (2019). Infant nocturnal wakefulness: A longitudinal study comparing three sleep assessment methods. *Sleep, 42*(1), Article zsy191. https://doi.org/10.1093/sleep/zsy191

Tinuper, P., Bisulli, F., Cross, J., Hesdorffer, D., Kahane, P., Nobili, L., Provini, F., Scheffer, I. E., Tassi, L., & Vignatelli, L. (2016). Definition and diagnostic criteria of sleep-related hypermotor epilepsy. *Neurology, 86*(19), 1834–1842. https://doi.org/10.1212/WNL.0000000000002666

Tobin, J. D. (1993). Treatment of somnambulism with anticipatory awakening. *Journal of Pediatrics, 122*(3), 426–427. https://doi.org/10.1016/s0022-3476(05)83433-x

Voltaire, S. T., & Teti, D. M. (2018). Early nighttime parental interventions and infant sleep regulation across the first year. *Sleep Medicine, 52*, 107–115. https://doi.org/10.1016/j.sleep.2018.07.013

Wei, S., Smits, M. G., Tang, X., Kuang, L., Meng, H., Ni, S., Xiao, M., & Zhou, X. (2020). Efficacy and safety of melatonin for sleep onset insomnia in children and adolescents: A meta-analysis of randomized controlled trials. *Sleep Medicine, 68*, 1–8. https://doi.org/10.1016/j.sleep.2019.02.017

Werner-Seidler, A., Wong, Q., Johnston, L., O'Dea, B., Torok, M., & Christensen, H. (2019). Pilot evaluation of the Sleep Ninja: A smartphone application for adolescent insomnia symptoms. *BMJ Open, 9*(5), Article e026502. https://doi.org/10.1136/bmjopen-2018-026502

Whittall, H., Kahn, M., Pillion, M., & Gradisar, M. (2021). Parents matter: Barriers and solutions when implementing behavioural sleep interventions for infant sleep problems. *Sleep Medicine, 84*, 244–252. https://doi.org/10.1016/j.sleep.2021.05.042

Wilcox, L. J., Bergeron, M., Reghunathan, S., & Ishman, S. L. (2017). An updated review of pediatric drug-induced sleep endoscopy. *Laryngoscope Investigative Otolaryngology, 2*(6), 423–431. https://doi.org/10.1002/lio2.118

Wilhelmsen-Langeland, A., Saxvig, I. W., Pallesen, S., Nordhus, I. H., Vedaa, O., Lundervold, A. J., & Bjorvatn, B. (2013). A randomized controlled trial with bright light and melatonin for the treatment of delayed sleep phase disorder: Effects on subjective and objective sleepiness and cognitive function. *Journal of Biological Rhythms, 28*(5), 306–321. https://doi.org/10.1177/0748730413500126

Williamson, A. A., Mindell, J. A., Hiscock, H., & Quach, J. (2020). Longitudinal sleep problem trajectories are associated with multiple impairments in child well-being. *Journal of Child Psychology and Psychiatry, 61*(10), 1092–1103. https://doi.org/10.1111/jcpp.13303

Wilson, K. E., Lumeng, J. C., Kaciroti, N., Chen, S. Y., LeBourgeois, M. K., Chervin, R. D., & Miller, A. L. (2015). Sleep hygiene practices and bedtime resistance in low-income preschoolers: Does temperament matter? *Behavioral Sleep Medicine, 13*(5), 412–423. https://doi.org/10.1080/15402002.2014.940104

Wolfson, A., Lacks, P., & Futterman, A. (1992). Effects of parent training on infant sleeping patterns, parents' stress, and perceived parental competence. *Journal of Consulting and Clinical Psychology, 60*(1), 41–48. https://doi.org/10.1037/0022-006X.60.1.41

Wolfson, A. R., Carskadon, M. A., Acebo, C., Seifer, R., Fallone, G., Labyak, S. E., & Martin, J. L. (2003). Evidence for the validity of a sleep habits survey for adolescents. *Sleep, 26*(2), 213–216. https://doi.org/10.1093/sleep/26.2.213

Woodward, S. H., Murburg, M. M., & Bliwise, D. L. (2000). PTSD-related hyperarousal assessed during sleep. *Physiology and Behavior, 70*(1–2), 197–203. https://doi.org/10.1016/S0031-9384(00)00271-7

Yau, S., Pickering, R. M., Gringras, P., Elphick, H., Evans, H. J., Farquhar, M., Martin, J., Joyce, A., Reynolds, J., Kingshott, R. N., Mindell, J. A., & Hill, C. M. (2019). Sleep in infants and toddlers with Down syndrome compared to typically developing peers: Looking beyond snoring. *Sleep Medicine, 63*, 88–97. https://doi.org/10.1016/j.sleep.2019.05.005

Yeung, C. K., Sihoe, J., Sit, F., Bower, W., Sreedhar, B., & Lau, J. (2004). Characteristics of primary nocturnal enuresis in adults: An epidemiological study. *BJU International, 93*(3), 341–345. https://doi.org/10.1111/j.1464-410X.2003.04612.x

Yu, X. T., Sadeh, A., Lam, H. S., Mindell, J. A., & Li, A. M. (2017). Parental behaviors and sleep/wake patterns of infants and toddlers in Hong Kong, China. *World Journal of Pediatrics, 13*(5), 496–502. https://doi.org/10.1007/s12519-017-0025-6

Zadra, A., & Donderi, D. C. (2000). Nightmares and bad dreams: Their prevalence and relationship to well-being. *Journal of Abnormal Psychology, 109*(2), 273–281. https://doi.org/10.1037//0021-843X.109.2.273

Zreik, G., Asraf, K., Tikotzky, L., & Haimov, I. (2020). Sleep ecology and sleep patterns among infants and toddlers: A cross-cultural comparison between the Arab and Jewish societies in Israel. *Sleep Medicine, 75*, 117–127. https://doi.org/10.1016/j.sleep.2020.07.017

CHAPTER

39 Sleep Disorders in the Elderly

Ali Amidi, Sonia Ancoli-Israel, Jeanne E. Maglione, *and* Lisa M. Wu

Abstract

Complaints about sleep are common in elderly adults. While changes in sleep architecture occur with normal aging, complaints about sleep are often related to pathological and treatable sleep disturbances. Primary sleep disturbances occurring in older adults include circadian rhythm disturbances, insomnia, sleep disordered breathing, rapid-eye-movement sleep behavior disorder, restless legs syndrome, and periodic limb movements in sleep. Particularly in older adults, sleep disturbances are likely to represent a multifactorial syndrome in which medical illness, psychiatric illness, and medications play a role. Sleep complaints necessitate the attention of the clinician as they are associated with poor outcomes. Because treatment strategies differ depending on the etiology of the sleep disturbance, a careful and systematic approach to diagnosis is crucial. This chapter reviews the normal changes in sleep that occur with age and sleep disorders frequently seen in older adults including in those with major neurocognitive disorders/ dementia. Diagnosis and treatment strategies are discussed.

Key Words: sleep, insomnia, elderly, aging, major neurocognitive disorder, dementia, sleep disordered breathing, RBD, PLMS, restless legs syndrome

Introduction

It has been projected that by 2050, 16% of the global population will be >65 years of age compared with 10% in 2022 (United Nations Department of Economic and Social Affairs, 2022). As the global population of older adults increases, societies will need to adapt public programs to meet specific challenges associated with increased age. In this regard, sleep is a vital focus area. Age-related changes in both objectively and subjectively measured sleep outcomes have been firmly established in older adults (Boulos et al., 2019; Kocevska et al., 2021) and include decreased total sleep time, sleep efficiency, slow-wave sleep, and rapid-eye-movement (REM) sleep, and increased time awake after sleep onset (WASO), nighttime arousals, and sleep latency (Miner & Kryger, 2020). Sleep complaints are common in older adults in both high- and middle-income countries (Foley et al., 2004; Mazzotti et al., 2012), with a majority of older adults endorsing at least one chronic complaint about their sleep (Foley et al., 1995). However, it is important to underscore that most sleep disturbances that occur in elderly adults are not a normal, inevitable part of aging. Evidence from prospective studies indicates that risk factors associated with sleep disturbances in older adults include female gender, depressed mood, and physical illness (Smagula et al., 2016). Sleep complaints are generally related to circadian rhythm disturbances, primary sleep disorders, and sleep disturbances related to medical and psychiatric illness or medications. Although common, sleep complaints in elderly patients warrant attention as they are associated with a number of poor outcomes such as decreased quality of life, increased depression and anxiety (Bao et al., 2017; Fang et al., 2019), suicidal ideation (Gallo et al., 2020), impaired cognition and risk of dementia (Bubu et al., 2020; Shi et al., 2018; Yaffe et al., 2014), risk of falls (Min & Slattum, 2018), and mortality (Dew et al., 2003; Guida et al., 2021; Svensson et al., 2021). Because treatment strategies differ depending on the etiology of the sleep disturbance, a careful and systematic approach to diagnosis is indicated. This chapter will review both the normal changes in sleep that occur with age and sleep disorders frequently seen in older adults.

Sleep and Consequences of Sleep Disturbances in Older Adults

Changes in Sleep in Older Adults

Older adults report a variety of subjective complaints about their sleep including difficulties falling asleep, increased nocturnal awakenings, early awakenings, daytime sleepiness, needing more naps, and not feeling rested. In one survey of 9,000 adults aged 65 or older from three US communities, over 80% of those surveyed reported at least one problem with sleep, and more than half reported that at least one sleep complaint occurred nearly all the time (Foley et al., 1995). Age-related changes in sleep and sleep quality are most likely multifactorial, arising from a myriad of factors including age-related changes in circadian and sleep regulatory mechanisms, lifestyle and behavioral factors, comorbidities, and the use of medication.

Studies and meta-analyses of polysomnographic (PSG) assessments of sleep have confirmed that a number of changes in sleep architecture occur with advanced age. The most reliable findings indicate that in later life, sleep becomes more fragmented with increased nighttime arousals and awakenings (Boulos et al., 2019; Luca et al., 2015; Mitterling et al., 2015; Ohayon et al., 2004). Furthermore, the proportion of time spent in the lighter stages of sleep (Stages 1 and 2) increases with age (Boulos et al., 2019; Luca et al., 2015; Ohayon et al., 2004), although some studies have not observed this (Mitterling et al., 2015). Conversely, there is a reduction in the amount of slow-wave sleep (deep sleep) and a decrease in REM sleep (Luca et al., 2015; Mitterling et al., 2015; Ohayon et al., 2004). A shift toward morning "preference" is also observed with advanced age (Fischer et al., 2017; Luca et al., 2015), as well as an increase in diurnal naps (Foley et al., 2007). Sleep efficiency and total sleep time also decrease with advanced age (Boulos et al., 2019; Luca et al., 2015). Boulos and colleagues (2019) found that in the adult population aged 18–80+ years, total sleep time decreased on average by 10.1 minutes per decade across this age span. Sleep efficiency declined 2.1% per decade, while the most substantial changes occurred in WASO, which was estimated to increase approximately 10 minutes per decade, amounting to an average of approximately 77 minutes in older adults aged 65–79 years. A study of more than 1,000 French adults over the age of 60 reported that the mean amount of nightly sleep was approximately 7 hours, with men sleeping slightly more than women, while the amount of sleep did not differ between age groups (Ohayon & Vecchierini, 2005). A recent meta-analysis of actigraphy-assessed sleep using data from 21,242 healthy participants across the life span from 78 published articles estimated sleep duration in older adults aged 60–89 years to be approximately 6.5 hours (Evans et al., 2021).

While the underlying mechanisms driving age-related changes in sleep macro- and micro-architecture in older adults are still being explored, emerging evidence points to several potential neurobiological mechanisms of importance, including changes in sleep–wake regulatory brain structures, general gray matter atrophy, and impaired homeostatic sleep drive and circadian regulation (Mander et al., 2017). It is important to note, however, that changes in sleep parameters do not easily explain the majority of sleep complaints in older adults. A number of primary sleep disorders occur in the elderly, including sleep disordered breathing (SDB), insomnia, periodic limb movements in sleep (PLMS), restless legs syndrome (RLS), and REM sleep behavior disorder (RBD; Table 39.1). Medical conditions, psychiatric illness, chronic pain, obesity, neurodegeneration, and medications are also often related to sleep disturbances, making diagnosis and treatment of sleep disorders in this complex patient population challenging.

Consequences of Poor Sleep in Older Adults

Sleep disorders are highly prevalent among older adults yet are often undiagnosed and therefore untreated (e.g., Braley et al., 2018; Grandner & Chakravorty, 2017). There is evidence that sleep problems are highly associated with coexisting chronic conditions and the number of chronic conditions (Koyanagi et al., 2014), and it is likely that these comorbid health conditions become the more immediate focus of the clinician's attention. Furthermore, there is evidence that older adults are likely to adapt their perceptions of sleep satisfaction as they get older, despite more impaired quantitative nighttime sleep features (Vitiello et al., 2004; Zilli et al., 2009). Although there is evidence that community-dwelling older adults may underreport sleep duration when compared with actigraphy-based assessments (Scarlett et al., 2021), individuals with insomnia may nevertheless be experiencing poor sleep quality during their sleep period (Van Den Berg et al., 2008). Due to the high co-occurrence of sleep problems with physical, psychiatric, and neurological conditions, sleep disorders must be addressed as part of a comprehensive treatment plan among older adults (McCarthy, 2021), especially since poor sleep is associated with numerous detrimental outcomes, including poorer physical and psychological

Table 39.1 Symptoms and clinical features of sleep disorders commonly encountered in the older adult

Risk factors and clinical features of sleep disorders amplified in older adults	
Obstructive sleep apnea	• Prevalence rates significantly increase with age. • Prevalence in males > females. • Commonly under-reported. • May be associated with age-related changes in airway anatomy. • With age, moderate or severe OSA is predominant in men, but mild OSA is predominant in women. • Dementia is a common comorbidity. • Obesity may or may not be a specific risk factor. • Other risk factors include hypertension and higher medication use. • Excessive daytime sleepiness associated with SDB may be due to increased nighttime arousals, sleep fragmentation, unintentional napping, phase-advanced circadian rhythms, and reduced circadian amplitude. • Dry mouth, nocturia, falls. • Cognitive difficulties and/or nocturnal confusion. • May report symptoms similar to insomnia. • Alzheimer's patients with depressive symptoms are less likely to comply with CPAP treatment than non-depressed patients.
Sleep-related movement disorders	• Prevalence of PLMS may increase with age, but severity does not. • Prevalence of RLS may increase with age but drops again over age 80. • Diagnosis complicated by cognitive and communication problems. • May report symptoms similar to insomnia. • Other conditions may be mistaken for RLS (including neuropathy, arthritic conditions, akathisia, dementia-related nonspecific pacing, pruritus, vascular insufficiency, anxiety, and depression). • May be secondary to a range of conditions and illnesses that ought to be treated first (including anemia, end-stage renal disease, rheumatoid arthritis, chronic obstructive pulmonary disease, asthma, fibromyalgia, diabetes mellitus, Parkinson's disease, medication use, and multiple sclerosis). • Treatment requires consideration of medication interactions and side effects. • Studies supporting use of pharmacologic agents for RLS have not typically been done in elderly patients.
REM sleep behavior disorder	• Detected more often in males, even though it may occur equally in the population. • May be early manifestation of neurodegenerative disease, typically Parkinson's disease. • Clonazepam has been used by clinicians to treat RBD but may increase risk of confusion in older adults and is contraindicated with OSAS.
Advanced sleep phase disorder	• Prevalence not established in older adults, but age is a likely risk factor. • May report symptoms similar to insomnia.
Insomnia	• Prevalence rates significantly increase with age. • Sleep maintenance difficulties represent the most common subtype in older adults. • Comorbid conditions are common (including heart disease, stroke, cancer, diabetes, hip fracture, self-reported physical disability or health status, depressive symptoms, and use of medications).

Note. CPAP = continuous positive airway pressure; OSA = obstructive sleep apnea; OSAS = OSA syndrome; PLMS = periodic limb movements in sleep; REM = rapid eye movement; RLS = restless legs syndrome; SDB = sleep disordered breathing.

well-being, cognitive decline, a greater risk of falls, and a greater risk of being placed in long-term care facilities; and it may even predict mortality.

The benefits of better sleep on physical and psychological well-being are evident in a number of studies of older adults. In a relatively large study of 1,503 older adults in primary care settings, the number and type of sleep complaints predicted poorer general physical and mental health-related quality of life status (Reid et al., 2006). Hanson and Ruthig (2012) also found associations between sleep quality and psychological well-being. Similarly, in a large European study of 8,934 older adults, sleep complaints were associated with an increased risk of future health and functional problems (Grossman et al., 2017). Poorer subjective sleep quality has also been found to be strongly associated with frailty status (Balomenos et al., 2021) and may even be associated with an increased risk of developing disability (Park et al., 2014).

Cognitive function is a common area of concern for older patients. There are numerous cross-sectional studies indicating associations between poor sleep and impaired cognition. In a prospective study of 740 older adults (Johar et al., 2016), difficulties maintaining sleep and long sleep duration were related to cognitive decline over 3 years of follow-up in normal and cognitively impaired older adults, respectively. The Study of Osteoporotic Fractures (SOF) estimated sleep objectively with actigraphy in more than 2,800 community-dwelling women over the age of 70 and found that lower sleep efficiency, more WASO, and longer sleep latency were associated with poorer cognition in this population (Blackwell et al., 2006).

Also of particular concern in older adults is the association between poor sleep and falls as falls are a major cause of morbidity and mortality in this age group. Numerous studies among older adults have found associations between sleep characteristics and falls. Studies of community-dwelling older adults have found associations between nighttime sleep complaints, long sleep duration, and history of falls (Brassington et al., 2000; Mesas et al., 2011). Prospective studies have also shown sleep to be predictive of future falls. In the SOF, those with sleep duration less than 5 hours per night had 1.5 times the risk of having two or more subsequent falls compared with those who had a normal sleep duration (defined as 7–8 hours of sleep per night), even after controlling for multiple factors, including benzodiazepine use (Stone et al., 2008). Poor sleep efficiency (<70% of time in bed spent sleeping) was also associated with an increased risk for falls (Stone et al., 2008). Poor subjective sleep quality has also been found to be associated with increased odds of experiencing falls (Takada et al., 2018). A large prospective study of 6,882 community-dwelling older adults also found that the number of insomnia symptoms and taking sleep medications (irrespective of insomnia symptoms) predicted 2-year fall risk (Chen et al., 2017).

Given the effects of sleep disturbance on cognition and falls, it is not surprising that sleep disturbance is an important risk factor for long-term care placement. Pollak and colleagues (1990) studied over 1,800 community-dwelling older adults and found that, in men, a complaint of insomnia was the strongest predictor for nursing home placement 3.5 years later, even when compared with cognitive impairment. In a study focused on 1,664 community-dwelling women, greater WASO and lower sleep efficiency were risk factors for nursing home or personal care home placement (Spira et al., 2012).

Sleep may also be important for predicting mortality in general. Indeed, a systematic review comprised of over 70,000 older adults found that long or short sleep duration is associated with an increased risk of all-cause mortality in older adults (Da Silva et al., 2016).

Daytime Napping in Older Adults

Daytime napping is common in older adults, with an estimated prevalence rate between 20% and 60% (Furihata et al., 2016; Ohayon & Zulley, 1999; Xin et al., 2020; Zhang et al., 2020). Studies suggest that the tendency to nap, frequency of napping, and duration of naps all increase with age and may be the result of various causes including disturbed nighttime sleep, psychiatric and medical comorbidities, phase-advanced circadian rhythms, decreased circadian amplitude, or lifestyle factors (Zhang et al., 2020). In the 2003 National Sleep Foundation "Sleep and Aging" survey, 25% of respondents 74–84 years of age reported taking regular naps compared with 10% of those who were 55–64 years old (Foley et al., 2007). Metz and Bunnell (1990) found that "older old" subjects (mean age 80 years) took an average of five naps per week compared to four naps per week in the "younger old" group (mean age 75 years) and took longer naps ("older old" naps averaged 67 minutes vs. 51 minutes in the "younger old" group).

Despite widely held cultural beliefs about the benefits of daytime napping, the research literature on the health-related impact of napping is conflicting; and while daytime napping has been associated with both positive and negative health outcomes, much remains to be determined (Vitiello, 2008).

Given the changes in nighttime sleep with age, one would expect that daytime napping might benefit older adults by compensating somewhat for the increased fragmentation of sleep. However, the relationship between nighttime sleep disruption and daytime napping in the older adult is not clear. Although some studies have found associations between napping and disrupted sleep at night in older adults (Goldman et al., 2008), other studies failed to observe a statistically significant association (Campbell et al., 2005; Mallon & Hetta, 1997).

Other detrimental correlates to daytime napping in older adults that have been reported include depression, pain, nocturia (Foley et al., 2007), risk of dementia (Li et al., 2023), burden of medical comorbidities (Martin et al., 2006), and risk of cardiovascular disease and all-cause mortality (Cheng et al., 2018; Pan et al., 2020; Wang et al., 2019; Yamada et al., 2015). A large prospective, observational cohort study of 1,140 community-dwelling older adults revealed that frequent and longer naps (exceeding 44 minutes) were associated with a 1.7-fold increase in risk of heart failure In a longitudinal study of a large representative sample of older adults in Singapore (N = 2,448), Cheng and colleagues (2018) found that compared to non-nappers, an increase or change in nap duration was associated with a significant increase in all-cause mortality risk. Similarly, Bursztyn and colleagues reported lower 6-year and 12-year survival rates among nappers compared with non-nappers (Bursztyn et al., 2002; Bursztyn & Stressman, 2005) independent of history of cancer, ischemic heart disease, hypertension, diabetes, smoking, renal disease, lipid levels, activities of daily living, and quality of life. Furthermore, increased daytime napping has been associated with a greater risk of falls and hip fracture (Stone et al., 2008).

Potential beneficial impacts of daytime napping in older adults have also been investigated, most notably in relation to cognitive functioning. While there is evidence to suggest that short daytime naps may result in improved cognitive performance in adult populations (Dutheil et al., 2021; Ficca et al., 2010), the role of napping for optimal cognitive health in older adults remains unclear. For example, in a small study of 50 participants, Scullin and colleagues (2017) found that while an afternoon nap had beneficial effects on episodic memory, such benefits decreased with advanced age. Yet in a cross-sectional cohort study of 2,974 Chinese older adults aged 65 and older, participants who were moderate nappers (30–90 minutes) evidenced improved overall cognition compared with non-nappers and extended nappers (Li et al., 2017). Similarly, Keage and colleagues (2012) reported that daytime napping in older adults above 65 years of age was associated with a lower risk of cognitive decline, as indicated by the Mini-Mental State Examination, 2 and 10 years later. It has, however, been argued that research on the effects of napping on health-related outcomes should avoid simplistic conceptualizations and assessment of naps (Vitiello, 2008). For example, one study found that specific nap characteristics such as nap "intention" may be of specific importance. In a study of 2,549 community-dwelling older adults, Owusu and colleagues (2019) reported that unintentional nappers evidenced poorer verbal memory performance and worse self-rated memory compared with intentional nappers.

Primary Sleep Disorders in Older Adults

SDB

A variety of breathing abnormalities may occur during sleep, ranging from benign snoring to partial (hypopnea) or complete (apnea) cessation of airflow. These events may be caused by airway collapse during sleep or alternatively may be due to impaired central nervous system signaling, both of which can lead to hypoxemia and repeated arousals throughout the night (Foldvary-Schaefer & Waters, 2017). The total number of apneas plus hypopneas per hour of sleep is called the *apnea-hypopnea index* (AHI), and a diagnosis of SDB is usually made when the AHI is greater than 5, 10, or even 15 (respiratory disturbances per hour; Ahmadi et al., 2009).

The prevalence of obstructive sleep apnea (OSA; defined as AHI ≥5) varies widely across studies, largely due to methodological heterogeneity. In a large Swiss population-based study of over 2,000 people, the prevalence among middle-aged adults (30–60 years) was around 80% for men and 47% for women but as high as 90% among men and 78% among women aged between 60 and 85 years (Heinzer et al., 2015). Furthermore, AHI scores among men over the age of 60 were approximately double those of women. Using the *International Classification of Sleep Disorders*, second edition, criteria (American Academy of Sleep Medicine, 2005), the prevalence of OSA syndrome was measured in a sample of over 1,000 São Paulo inhabitants in different age groups (Tufik et al., 2010). Prevalence rates steadily rose from 24% in the 30–39 year age group to 87% in the 70–80 year age group, with obesity being an important risk factor for moderate to severe OSA. In addition, with age, moderate or severe OSA tends to predominate in men and mild OSA in women (Senaratna et al., 2017).

SDB is also common in elderly nursing home residents, where a prevalence of 40%–70% has been reported (Ancoli-Israel, Klauber, et al., 1991; Martin et al., 2005). Several studies have suggested that SDB is particularly common in patients with dementia, and its severity has been shown to correlate with the severity of dementia in the nursing home setting (Ancoli-Israel, Klauber, et al., 1991). Another study reported the prevalence of SDB with AHI ≥5 to be as high as 89.5% in nursing home residents with a diagnosis of Alzheimer's disease (AD). In institutionalized AD patients with SDB, the frequency of oxygen desaturations has been shown to correlate with the severity of daytime aggressive agitation (Gehrman et al., 2003). Unfortunately, SDB is associated with poor cognitive and health outcomes (Aloia et al., 2003; Ancoli-Israel, Kripke, et al., 1991b; Newman et al., 2001; Nieto et al., 2000) and, in the presence of excessive daytime sleepiness (EDS), with an increase in all-cause mortality risk (Gooneratne et al., 2011). Given how severely underreported sleep apnea is among US nursing home residents (Resnick & Phillips, 2008), this raises the question of whether better diagnosis and treatment of SDB would be beneficial for this population.

Changes in airway anatomy with age that may play a role in the development of SDB in older individuals include an increased fat deposition in the pharyngeal fat pads, a decrease in the genioglossus muscle response to negative pressure in men, an increase in the length of the soft palate in women, and changes in the shape of the bony structures surrounding the pharyngeal airway (Malhotra et al., 2006). Other studies have shown that pharyngeal airway collapsibility may be worse in the elderly (Eikermann et al., 2007), particularly in the upper airway (McMillan & Morrell, 2016), as well as a greater frequency of spontaneous arousals (Redline et al., 2004). In a large study of 27,210 middle-aged and older adults from the Canadian Longitudinal Study of Aging (Thompson et al., 2022), risk factors for OSA included age 55 or older, being male or a postmenopausal woman, being overweight or obese, and having cardiovascular diseases, diabetes mellitus, cerebrovascular disease, anxio-depressive symptoms, and higher systemic inflammation. Additional risk factors include being on sedating medications, family history, and African American race (reviewed in Phillips & Ancoli-Israel, 2001). However, there is conflicting evidence regarding whether alcohol consumption and smoking (Hua-Huy et al., 2015; Kashyap et al., 2001; Peppard et al., 2013; Scanlan et al., 2000; Wetter et al., 1994) are risk factors.

Older adults with SDB may present with symptoms similar to younger adults such as loud snoring, EDS, night sweats, non-restorative sleep, gasping arousals from sleep, witnessed apneas, dry mouth, or headaches upon awakening (Norman & Loredo, 2008). However, EDS in older adults tends to occur due to recurrent nighttime arousals and sleep fragmentation, as well as unintentional napping during the day (J. Martin et al., 2002). SDB symptoms may also present quite differently. While the two most common symptoms of SDB are snoring and EDS, they may also present with complaints of insomnia, nocturnal confusion, cognitive difficulties, enuresis and nocturia, or falls (Launois et al., 2007; Table 39.1). Further, although body mass index is a risk factor for OSA in older adults, the older adult with OSA may not be obese. Indeed, as age advances, OSA is more likely to be associated with hypertension and higher medication use rather than anthropometric indicators (Silva et al., 2022). Together, these differences have led investigators to question whether OSA in older adults represents a different disease compared with OSA in younger adults and to raise the question of whether treatment criteria should be the same in the older adult as in the younger adult. However, most studies do suggest that older adults with SDB are excessively sleepy and that the SDB may contribute to decreased quality of life, increased cognitive impairment, and greater risk of nocturia, hypertension, cardiovascular disease, and cerebrovascular disease (Launois et al., 2007). Elderly individuals with both insomnia and OSA have more functional impairment than those with just insomnia, particularly significantly lower daytime functioning and longer psychomotor reaction times (Gooneratne et al., 2006).

Treatment of SDB in older patients does result in reduced apnea events with improved O_2 saturation, deeper sleep, reduced daytime sleepiness, improved sleep architecture, reduced self-reported symptoms such as snoring or gasping, improved or stable cognition and mood, vascular resistance, platelet coagulability, and other factors affecting cardiac function and has a positive effect on nocturia, reducing the number of voids per night (Netzer et al., 2016; Weaver & Chasens, 2007). Therefore, any older patient who presents with symptoms of impairment or with a history of traffic accidents or repeated falls should be evaluated for a sleep disturbance. Older adults and the frail elderly, particularly those with stroke, overlapping chronic obstructive pulmonary disease (COPD), and even AD or Parkinson's disease, may benefit from having their SDB treated (Netzer et al., 2016). Treatment of a symptomatic elderly patient should not be withheld on the basis of age as the consequence of SDB can be just as serious in older as in younger patients (Ancoli-Israel, 2007; Launois et al., 2007).

Assessment for SDB in the older adult should begin with a complete sleep history, including probing for the symptoms of SDB. It is particularly helpful to have input from a caregiver or spouse who may witness SDB symptoms that the patient is unaware of (such as snoring or gasping for air). A medical history may reveal comorbid medical conditions. If there is suspicion for SDB based on the initial evaluation, an overnight, attended sleep study is indicated.

Treatment should begin with education and encouragement of weight loss if appropriate. A prospective study of 690 randomly selected people in Wisconsin showed that a weight gain of 10% predicted a 32% increase in AHI, while a 10% weight loss predicted a 26% decrease in AHI (Peppard et al., 2000). The medication list should be reviewed, and medications that act as respiratory depressants, and therefore can increase the duration of apneas, should be avoided. Continuous positive airway pressure (CPAP) remains the gold-standard treatment for SDB. The efficacy of this treatment is well established, and there are few associated side effects. Compliance can be an issue with adults of any age. An effort must therefore be made to work with the patient to determine and address any obstacles to compliance. A study of 33 patients over the age of 65 found that noncompliance was associated with nocturia, smoking, and benign prostatic hypertrophy, whereas resolution of symptoms was associated with compliance (Russo-Magno et al., 2001). Interestingly, in older adults with AD and SDB, patients with depressive symptoms were less likely to comply with CPAP compared to those who were not depressed (Ayalon et al., 2006). It is therefore imperative to assess for psychiatric disorders and adequately address depression.

PLMS and RLS

PLMS are repetitive movements that can disrupt sleep (Vetrugno et al., 2007). When PLMS occur during drowsiness prior to sleep initiation, they can prevent the patient from falling asleep. Patients may not be aware of the movements and therefore may present with other symptoms including subjective poor sleep, difficulty falling asleep, difficulty staying asleep, or EDS. It can be helpful therefore to talk to the patient's bed partner when possible as they are likely to be aware of the kicks and jerks. The diagnosis of PLMS requires an overnight PSG. A periodic leg movement index (PLMI; number of PLMs per hour) >5 is considered pathologic. PLM disorder is defined as a PLMI >15 in the setting of an otherwise unexplained sleep complaint (American Academy of Sleep Medicine, 2005). Leg movements without arousals are unlikely to be pathological.

PLMS are common in elderly populations. Prevalence rates vary across studies. Notably, in one of the largest epidemiological studies to date in which 18,980 participants aged 15 to 100 years from five European countries were assessed through a diagnostic phone interview, prevalence rates ranged between 2.8% and 3.7% in adults aged 60 and over (Ohayon & Roth, 2002). Rates were actually highest in the 20–29 year age group at around 5%. However, studies of older adults that have used home- or laboratory-based PSG have tended to find much higher rates. In an early study of 422 community-dwelling elderly adults greater than 65 years of age, sleep was assessed with electromyogram (EMG) at home. Forty-five percent were found to have a PLMI >5 (Ancoli-Israel, Kripke, et al., 1991a). Richards and colleagues (2008) studied 102 adults over the age of 60 with cognitive impairment and found 33% to have a PLMI >15. In a cohort of 455 community-dwelling older women (mean age 82.9 years), 62% had a PLMI >5, 52% had a PLMI >15, and increased PLMI was associated with a higher arousal index (Claman et al., 2006). Despite the increase in prevalence of pathologic PLMS with age, longitudinal analysis suggests that the severity does not increase over time (Gehrman et al., 2002).

RLS is a neurologic condition in which patients experience an urge to move the legs or arms, usually accompanied by a dysesthesia that is relieved or partially relieved by movement (Table 39.1). The symptoms, which may be described as "creepy-crawly" feelings or "internal itching" sensations, usually occur at rest or are worse during periods of rest. The symptoms also tend to be worse during the evening and therefore can considerably disrupt sleep (Hornyak et al., 2007). A large general population study of 15,391 adults determined that the prevalence of RLS sufferers tends to increase with age, reaching approximately 4.3% to 5.0% for those over age 60 but dropping again to about 3% among those age 80 and above (Allen et al., 2005).

The diagnosis of RLS does not require a sleep study and can be made on the basis of history alone. A key diagnostic question is, "When you try to relax in the evening or sleep at night, do you ever have unpleasant, restless feelings in your legs that can be relieved by walking or movement?" In the cognitively impaired elderly patient, however, diagnosis is more challenging. Allen and colleagues (2003) developed a modified set of essential (left panel) and suggestive (right panel) criteria (Table 39.2) for diagnosis of RLS in cognitively impaired elderly patients. In this population, the presentation may include signs of discomfort in the legs such as rubbing or kneading the legs and increased motor activity that are present or worse during inactivity and are lessened by activity (Allen et al., 2003). In all cases a bed partner may again be helpful to elucidate a history of leg movements at night.

Careful exclusion of other conditions that may be mistaken for RLS in this setting is also required. These include painful neuropathy, arthritic conditions, akathisia, nonspecific pacing associated with dementia, pruritus, vascular insufficiency, anxiety disorder, and agitated depression (Allen et al., 2003). Diagnosis can be further complicated by cognitive and communication problems (Allen et al., 2014), as well as a tendency for PLMS and PLMs during wakefulness at night to increase with age (Pennestri et al., 2006). RLS may also be secondary to anemia and end-stage renal disease, and there is a growing body of evidence associating other chronic illnesses with RLS, including rheumatoid arthritis, COPD, asthma, fibromyalgia, diabetes mellitus, Parkinson's disease (possibly even associated with dopaminergic therapy for Parkinson's disease itself; Lee et al., 2009), and multiple sclerosis (Spiegelhalder & Hornyak, 2008). Therefore, some consideration should be given to assessment of these illnesses when a diagnosis of RLS is made (see Table 39.1).

Table 39.2 The International Restless Legs Syndrome (RLS) study group essential criteria for diagnosis of probable RLS in cognitively impaired older adults

Essential criteria	Suggested criteria
• Signs of leg discomfort such as rubbing or kneading the legs and groaning while holding the lower extremities are present. • Excessive motor activity in the lower extremities such as pacing, fidgeting, repetitive kicking, tossing and turning in bed, slapping the legs on the mattress, cycling movements of the lower limbs, repetitive foot tapping, rubbing the feet together, and inability to remain seated are present. • Signs of leg discomfort are exclusively present or worsen during periods of rest or inactivity. • Signs of leg discomfort are diminished with activity. • Criteria 1 and 2 occur only in the evening or at night or are worse at those times than during the day.	• Dopaminergic responsiveness. • Patient's past history—as reported by a family member, caregiver, or friend—is suggestive of RLS. • A first-degree, biological relative (sibling, child, or parent) has RLS. • Observed periodic limb movements while awake or during sleep. • Periodic limb movements in sleep recorded by polysomnography or actigraphy. • Significant sleep-onset problems. • Better-quality sleep in the day than at night. • The use of restraints at night (for institutionalized patients). • Low serum ferritin level. • End-stage renal disease. • Diabetes. • Clinical, electromyographic, or nerve conduction evidence of peripheral neuropathy or radiculopathy.

Note. RLS = restless legs syndrome. Reprinted from Allen et al. (2003) with permission from Elsevier.

The treatment of secondary RLS necessitates treatment of the underlying disease (e.g., iron deficiency; Allen et al., 2013). Otherwise, treatment of primary RLS/PLMS in the elderly involves the careful use of pharmacologic agents. In elderly patients, close attention must be paid to medication interactions and side effects, particularly orthostatic hypotension, nausea, and dizziness. Agents that may present a favorable risk–benefit profile include α-2-δ drugs or dopaminergic agents, so long as the risk of RLS augmentation associated with dopaminergic agents is carefully considered. Low-dose opioids may also be considered in the case of RLS augmentation (i.e., medication-related increase in symptoms after initial improvement; During & Winkelman, 2019). Currently, nonergot dopaminergic agonists including oral pramipexole, ropinirole, and transdermal rotigotine are approved by the US Food and Drug Administration for moderate to severe primary RLS and have been shown to reduce RLS symptoms, subjective (and possibly objective) sleep parameters, PLMS, quality of life, and possibly depression (Winkelman et al., 2016). Several studies have also found ergot agents such as cabergoline to be effective. However, they are also associated with an increased risk for valvulopathy and augmentation and are not considered to be first-line agents (reviewed in During & Winkelman, 2019, and Spiegelhalder & Hornyak, 2008). It should also be noted that none of the studies supporting the use of pharmacologic agents for RLS have been done in elderly patients. Carbidopa/levodopa is also effective but may cause augmentation at a higher rate than other drugs or a rebound (increase in symptoms after the medication wears off) phenomenon (Hening et al., 2004).

RBD

During REM sleep, atonia of voluntary skeletal muscles prevents us from physically acting out our dreams. RBD is a parasomnia in which the skeletal muscle atonia normally present in REM sleep is intermittently absent, resulting in movements such as punching, leaping from the bed, kicking, laughing, crying, or gesturing during REM sleep. Thus, the movements typically occur during the second half of the night when REM sleep is more prevalent (Dauvilliers et al., 2018; Table 39.1).

RBD is a rare sleep disorder that affects ~0.7%–2% of the elderly population as estimated by PSG studies (Kang et al., 2013; Pujol et al., 2017; Sasai-Sakuma et al., 2020). It typically affects older adults and is detected more often in elderly men in clinical cohorts, even though it may occur equally among men and women in population studies (Haba-Rubio et al., 2018; Roguski et al., 2020). The etiology of RBD is not known but likely involves the dysfunction of one or several pathways in the brainstem (Boeve, 2010; Gagnon, Postuma, Mazza, et al., 2006; Roguski et al., 2020). RBD can be either symptomatic when primarily associated with α-synucleinopathy neurodegenerative diseases such as Parkinson's disease, dementia with Lewy bodies, and multiple-system atrophy, or idiopathic (iRBD), ostensibly occurring in the absence of neurological disease (Dauvilliers et al., 2018). However, some studies suggest that RBD may be an early manifestation of neurodegenerative disease that precedes the onset of the clinical neurologic symptoms by years. In a lengthy follow-up study of men diagnosed with iRBD aged 50 years or older, Schenck and colleagues (2013) found that 80.8% of the 26 patients they were able to follow up with eventually developed parkinsonism/dementia, with mean time to onset being around 14 years.

The diagnosis of RBD requires a thorough sleep history including information from the patient's bed partner if possible. A number of screening tools have been used to assist in the diagnosis of RBD (Dauvilliers et al., 2018), with the most common being the REM Sleep Behavior Disorder Screening Questionnaire, which is a 10-item instrument that has been validated as a diagnostic tool and can be helpful in the assessment (Stiasny-Kolster et al., 2007). The questionnaire asks some questions about dreaming and about movements during sleep. However, it has a number of limitations. For example, its diagnostic value may depend on the clinical context (Stiasny-Kolster et al., 2015), and it may not be valid in de novo Parkinson's patients (Halsband et al., 2018). No matter the screening tool used, the relationship between REM sleep and reported complex motor behaviors should be confirmed with overnight PSG that includes video recording. Intermittent elevations in muscle tone or limb movements on the EMG channel during REM sleep are highly suggestive of RBD (Dauvilliers et al., 2018).

Treatment of RBD should begin with education of the patient and the bed partner, who may have been the target of the nighttime punches and kicks. Patients should take measures to increase the safety of their bedroom environment in order to reduce the risk of injury to themselves or their bed partners. Primary pharmacotherapy agents have not been tested in rigorous randomized controlled trials. However, clonazepam and melatonin have been used by clinicians. The long-acting benzodiazepine clonazepam may be effective and well tolerated in many patients, though not all patients respond to clonazepam; some patients may complain of daytime sedation due to the long half-life, and it has been shown in some studies to increase risk of confusion in the elderly. Further, clonazepam is contraindicated in patients with OSA. There have been several studies investigating the efficacy and tolerability of alternative treatments including melatonin, dopaminergic agents, and acetylcholinesterase inhibitors. However, more research is required (reviewed in Dauvilliers et al., 2018, and Gagnon, Postuma, & Montplaisir, 2006).

Circadian Rhythm Disturbances

Circadian rhythms are endogenously generated physiologic and behavioral cycles of approximately 24 hours. Examples of these rhythms include the melatonin secretion pattern, corticosteroid production, the sleep–wake cycle, and core body temperature. In humans, the circadian pacemaker is located in the suprachiasmatic nucleus (SCN) of the anterior hypothalamus (Hastings et al., 2018) and generates near 24-hour rhythmicity through a transcription–translation feedback loop (Patke et al., 2020). Circadian rhythms, including the sleep–wake cycle, are synchronized to environmental time by a number of external cues (called *zeitgebers*) of which light exerts the strongest influence (Hastings et al., 2018). Light, in particular light that includes short-wavelength frequencies (i.e., blue light), synchronizes the SCN through specialized and photosensitive retinal ganglion cells (Hattar et al., 2002). Other zeitgebers include food intake (Challet, 2019) and physical activity (Tahara et al., 2017). Circadian rhythm disturbances occur when there is desynchrony between the internal circadian system and the external environmental time. Such disturbances often have a detrimental impact on sleep.

Aging is associated with changes that can contribute to the development of circadian rhythm disturbances. There is evidence to suggest that circadian rhythms become less robust with age, resulting in weaker sleep rhythms (Munch et al., 2005). Most notably, shifts in circadian activity/rest rhythms have been observed in both cross-sectional and longitudinal studies, indicating a shift in older adults toward morning preference and earlier chronotype (Fischer et al., 2017; Hood & Amir, 2017). Evidence of gender differences indicates that female adults over 40 tend to be later chronotypes than men (Fischer et al., 2017). Other changes include increased activity rhythm fragmentation (Luik et al., 2013) and decreased rhythm amplitude (Musiek et al., 2018). The nocturnal endogenous secretion of melatonin also decreases with age (Touitou, 2001). Experimental studies with rodents have generally confirmed these observations (Nakamura et al., 2016).

Furthermore, exposure to synchronizing cues (i.e., zeitgebers) as well as the response to these cues may also change with age. Several studies have shown that, in general, older adults are exposed to less bright light (Campbell et al., 1988; Savides et al., 1986), although other studies report a higher level of light exposure in older adults (Scheuermaier et al., 2010). Specifically, older adults with dementia have been shown to be exposed to little light (Figueiro et al., 2012), with an average bright light exposure of 30 minutes per day for AD patients living at home (Campbell et al., 1988) and less than 10 minutes of exposure for those living in nursing homes (Ancoli-Israel et al., 1997). Less light exposure in these patients is associated with more awakenings (Shochat et al., 2000). In contrast, increased light exposure at nighttime has been associated with multiple adverse outcomes in older adults. For example, in a sample of 552 community-dwelling older adults, Kim and colleagues (2022) found associations between nighttime light exposure and obesity, diabetes, and hypertension.

Age-related changes in the responsiveness to light stimuli are also evident in older age. Reduced light responsiveness may be due to changes in ocular physiology such as reduced pupil diameter (Turner & Mainster, 2008), lens yellowing (Kessel et al., 2011), and increased density (Revell & Skene, 2010), resulting in reduced light transmission. Interventions to ameliorate these impairments may be one option to increase circadian health in older adults. For example, a recent randomized trial by Nishi et al. (2020) found that cataract surgery resulted in increased nocturnal melatonin production.

It should be mentioned that some experimental studies, however, do not find significant differences in the amount of phase delays in relation to bright light exposure between older and younger adults (Benloucif et al., 2006), whereas such differences have been reported for lower to moderate light intensity levels (Duffy et al., 2007). Given that the level of light exposure in older adults may be lower due to reduced mobility and changed retinal physiology, ensuring optimal lighting conditions in the indoor environment is of great importance.

Advanced Sleep Phase Disorder

As described above, the timing of the sleep/wake rhythm in the elderly advances such that sleep and wake times are routinely several hours earlier than the conventional sleep and wake times. Circadian rhythms of melatonin, cortisol, and core body temperature are similarly advanced (Duffy et al., 2015). A person with advanced rhythms, for example, may fall asleep between 6:00 p.m. and 9:00 p.m. and wake up 7–8 hours later between 2:00 a.m. and 5:00 a.m., with normal sleep during that time period. The phase shift typically becomes pathological when sleepiness in the afternoon or early evening prevents individuals from engaging in normal life activities. Attempts to stay awake despite the phase advance can result in insufficient sleep as the wake time remains advanced. Alternatively, some adults with advanced rhythms fall asleep while reading or watching television in the early evening and then, having napped, cannot fall asleep at bedtime. In these cases, advanced sleep phase disorder (ASPD) is diagnosed.

ASPD is characterized by a sleep schedule that is significantly advanced (usually 2–3 hours) compared with societal norms and is bothersome to the patient. The prevalence of ASPD in elderly adults has not been established, but it is more common in older adults compared with younger adults; and several studies suggest that age is a risk factor (Carrier et al., 1997; Sack et al., 2007). Furthermore, the prevalence is higher among men (Paine et al., 2014). In the general population, the prevalence is estimated to lie between 0.25% and 7% depending on the criteria used (Paine et al., 2014). The diagnosis of ASPD is largely based on clinical information. A careful sleep history, including a sleep diary, should be obtained and examined for the presence of a stable pattern of early sleep and wake times (Table 39.1). Collateral information from a caretaker or family member can also be helpful, as can actigraphy (Sack et al., 2007). PSG is not required to make the diagnosis, although it may be useful to rule out other sleep disorders, such as sleep apnea (Morgenthaler et al., 2007; Sack et al., 2007). Sleep-maintenance insomnia, as well as depression, which can also cause problems with sleep maintenance, should be assessed for and ruled out before a diagnosis of ASPD is made.

The American Academy of Sleep Medicine Clinical Practice Guideline reviewed the evidence regarding available treatments for ASPD and recommended evening light exposure (Auger et al., 2015). It was noted that the evidence for evening bright light therapy was "weak"; however, associated risks were assessed to be minimal, and patients reported reasonable compliance with high satisfaction (Auger et al., 2015). Prescribed sleep–wake scheduling was not recommended due to insufficient evidence.

Although little research has specifically investigated the use of evening light exposure in older adults with ASPD, it is often recommended and used in practice. This treatment relies on the ability of circadian stimulating light to act as a cue to synchronize circadian rhythms. Specifically, evening light exposure has been found to delay circadian rhythms in older adults and nursing home patients (Campbell et al., 1993, 1995; Lack et al., 2005; Suhner et al., 2002). While some studies have shown improvements in objective sleep measures with evening bright light treatment (Campbell et al., 1993; Lack et al., 2005), others have not (Friedman et al., 2009; Suhner et al., 2002). A study of older adults in the home setting also reported disruptive effects of evening light on sleep as indicated by prolonged sleep-onset latency (Obayashi et al., 2014). Most of the above studies, however, did not specifically target patients with ASPD. One study that included 47 patients with self-reported ASP, however, found no effect of evening light treatment (265 lux) on actigraphy-recorded sleep or urinary melatonin excretion patterns when compared with a placebo dim light (2 lux; Palmer et al., 2010). However, the lack of an effect could potentially be due to the relatively low light intensity level (256 lux) of the intervention. Despite these mixed results, the best time for bright light exposure is generally considered to be between 7:00 p.m. and 9:00 p.m. Depending on season and geographical location, the sun is rarely out at that time. Most commercial bright light boxes may be used as long as light intensity is adequately high (>1500 lux). Other types of wearable devices can also be used (e.g., light therapy glasses), which tend to emit lower light intensity due to a shorter distance to the retina. Here, choosing a tested device is important as efficacy will depend on the applied light specifications. Although there is no general consensus about the exact duration of light required, in practice, a minimum of 30 minutes is usually advised and longer if no effect is reported. In addition, bright light should be avoided in the morning hours as this may phase-advance the patient. One option is for patients to wear sunglasses when going for morning walks or using blue light–blocking glasses. If a light device is not available, it is recommended that patients spend time outdoors in the late afternoon and early evening before the sun has set.

Insomnia in Older Adults

A Multifactorial Syndrome

Insomnia is defined by difficulty initiating or maintaining sleep or non-restorative sleep resulting in clinically significant distress or functional impairment (American Psychiatric Association, 2013). Historically, insomnia was classified as primary (implying that there is no other cause of the sleep disturbance) or comorbid. However, contemporary guidance is that insomnia is actively treated whenever it presents without presumption of etiology or concurrent comorbid conditions. Overall, the estimated prevalence of insomnia disorder in the older population ranges between 12% and 20%, with sleep-maintenance difficulties being the most common insomnia subtype (Patel et al., 2018). Insomnia disorder is more common in middle-aged and older adults than it is in earlier adulthood, but this does not mean that insomnia is simply a normal part of aging (Brewster et al., 2018; Ohayon, 2002). Rather, comorbidity is the norm. In a survey of over 6,800 adults ages 65 years and older, only 7% of complaints of insomnia occurred in the absence of a risk factor including medical conditions (heart disease, stroke, cancer, diabetes, hip fracture), self-report of physical disability, depressive symptoms, perceived poor health status, or use of medications (Foley et al., 1999). It is therefore important not only to assess for the common primary sleep disturbances mentioned above but also to recognize that sleep complaints are often comorbid with medical and psychiatric conditions or related to medication use. Hence, the cause of disrupted sleep in older adults is often multifactorial in nature, and a careful assessment must be done to identify all contributing factors (Patel et al., 2018).

Medical Conditions and Pain

At any age, conditions that cause pain or discomfort during the night can disturb sleep. This is particularly important to keep in mind when evaluating sleep complaints in older adults, who are likely to have one or more chronic medical conditions that either cause or contribute to their sleep problems (Foley et al., 2004). There have been numerous studies showing that sleep complaints in the elderly are strongly associated with complaints about health (Foley et al., 2004; Foley et al., 1995; Quan et al., 2005). In the 2003

National Sleep Foundation Sleep in America Survey (Foley et al., 2004), more than 80% of those over the age of 65 reported at least one chronic medical condition, and 23.3% reported more than four conditions. The prevalence of disturbed sleep was increased in those with more reported medical conditions (Foley et al., 2004). In the general population, multi-comorbidity (i.e., having more than two coexisting chronic conditions) is found to be 62% in adults aged over 65 years (Salive, 2013). Chronic pain is particularly prevalent and troublesome in older adults (Larsson et al., 2017), with a recent meta-analysis reporting sleep difficulties in approximately 75% of chronic pain patients (Sun et al., 2021). Evidence also suggests a bidirectional link between sleep disturbance and pain in older adults (Griffin et al., 2021). Osteoarthritis, which is estimated to affect 27 million people in the United States (Lawrence et al., 2008), increases in frequency with age (Lawrence et al., 1998, 2008; Zhang & Jordan, 2008) and is associated with increased self-reported sleep problems including problems with sleep onset, sleep maintenance, and early-morning awakenings (Allen et al., 2008; Wilcox et al., 2000).

Symptoms of other illnesses may also be disruptive to sleep. Respiratory conditions that cause shortness of breath and hypoxemia such as COPD, congestive heart failure, and asthma are disruptive to sleep. In patients with COPD, the hypoxemia and hypercapnia that occur are amplified during REM sleep due to respiratory muscle atonia, leading to increased arousals and sleep disruption (Garcia, 2008; Gay, 2004; Lewis, 2001). If SDB is also present, the symptoms may be even more pronounced (Gay, 2004). Nocturia, which may be caused by a number of conditions including medication side effects, kidney or bladder stone, diabetes, prostatic disease, and overactive bladder, is common in older adults and can significantly impact sleep (Bliwise et al., 2009; Vaughan & Bliwise, 2018). In the National Sleep Foundation survey, nocturia was the most common self-perceived cause of sleep disturbance, with 53% of respondents aged 55 years and older reporting interrupted sleep related to nocturia "every night or almost every night." Gastroesophageal reflux disease and cancer are associated with high rates of sleep disturbance as well. While the prevalence of insomnia in cancer populations varies according to the specific cancer disease, insomnia and sleep disturbances are reported in 30%–50% of all cancer patients (Harrold et al., 2020; Strollo et al., 2020). With a global increase in the number of cancer survivors (Miller et al., 2022), these challenges need to be addressed. Furthermore, evidence suggests that poorer sleep in cancer patients is associated with clinical outcomes including overall survival and shorter time to progression (Strøm et al., 2022).

Psychiatric Illness

Psychiatric illnesses are also common in the elderly and can contribute to sleep disturbances, as well as vice versa. Older adults are more likely to experience certain stressors such as the death of a spouse, medical illness and injury, disability and functional decline, and lack of social contact, all of which can increase their risk for developing depression (Burke & Wengel, 2003). The prevalence of significant depressive symptomology in community-dwelling older adults ranges from 3% to 26% and increases to 15%–30% in the nursing home setting (reviewed in Hybels & Blazer, 2003). The association between depression and insomnia has been well established (Fang et al., 2019; Ford & Kamerow, 1989), and it is therefore important to screen for depression in all older patients presenting with sleep complaints. In addition, several meta-analyses have shown that insomnia is a significant predictive factor for the subsequent development of depression in adults of all ages (Baglioni et al., 2011; Hertenstein et al., 2019; L. Li et al., 2016). The association between insomnia and anxiety disorders, which affect up to 10.2% of adults aged 55–85, has also been well established (Chellappa & Aeschbach, 2022; Magee & Carmin, 2010; Spira et al., 2005).

Medications

Medications can cause or contribute to sleep problems in adults of all ages. Many drugs can disrupt sleep by impacting central sleep–wake regulatory mechanisms including important neurotransmitters and receptors (Van Gastel, 2018). It is particularly important to consider the effects of medications in older adults who are often taking multiple prescription and over-the-counter medications. Some examples of medications that may cause insomnia are central nervous system stimulants, antihypertensives, bronchodilators, corticosteroids, decongestants, diuretics, and many antidepressants. In contrast, sedating medications can lead to daytime sleepiness and napping, thereby disrupting nighttime sleep. Some examples of medications that can contribute to daytime sleepiness are sedative–hypnotic medications, antihistamines, some antidepressants (tricyclic antidepressants, trazodone, and mirtazapine), and dopamine agonists. All medications and administration times should be reviewed carefully. In some cases, the adverse effects of these medications on sleep may be avoided or minimized by scheduling sedating medications at night and stimulating medications in the morning.

Treatment of Insomnia in Older Adults

NON-PHARMACOLOGIC TREATMENT

Because older adults are often on multiple medications and may be more sensitive to the side effects of medications, non-pharmacologic interventions, which have been shown to be very effective, are often preferred as front-line treatments (Morin et al., 1999). Non-pharmacologic treatment typically includes a multicomponent cognitive behavioral therapy for insomnia (CBT-I), which combines behavioral interventions such as stimulus control, sleep restriction, cognitive therapy, relaxation techniques, and sleep hygiene (please refer to Chapter 28 for additional detail). CBT-I has been shown to be an efficacious treatment of insomnia in both younger and older adults (Nau et al., 2005) and in medical and psychiatric populations with comorbid insomnia (Geiger-Brown et al., 2015; Hertenstein et al., 2022; Johnson et al., 2016) with evidence of lasting effects (van der Zweerde et al., 2019). It has been shown to be as effective as medications, with the effects being more durable (Mitchell et al., 2012); and unlike medications, CBT-I has a lasting beneficial effect well beyond the termination of treatment (Amidi et al., 2022; Morin et al., 1999). However, evidence also suggests that a combination of CBT-I and medication can be especially effective (Kwon et al., 2021). Furthermore, digitally delivered CBT-I has been shown to be efficacious and comparable to face-to-face CBT-I (Zachariae et al., 2016), including in different clinical populations (Zachariae et al., 2018) and with evidence of sustained improvements (Amidi et al., 2022).

Descriptions of CBT component techniques can be found in Chapter 28 and elsewhere in this textbook. It should be noted that although there are no conceptual differences in the implementation of CBT-I between younger and older adults (Bélanger et al., 2012), depending on the specific challenges of the older individual, adaptations should be considered (Hughes & Martin, 2022). Considerations about adapting CBT-I to work with older adults are summarized in Table 39.3.

Stimulus control aims to strengthen the bed and bedroom as a cue for sleep and, as such, requires the elimination of all in-bed activities other than sleep (Bootzin & Epstein, 2000). Patients are not allowed to read, use smartphones, watch television, or do any other non-sleep-related activities in bed. Further, if they are unable to sleep within 20 minutes, they are not to stay in bed. In this way, the association between bed and sleep is

Table 39.3 Considerations in working with older adults with insomnia
General considerations • Consider patient's cognitive level, and adapt information and study materials accordingly. • When possible, involve caregivers in therapy.
Stimulus control and sleep restriction • Careful consideration of safety concerns before initiating sleep restriction and stimulus control. • Allow for greater flexibility depending on patient characteristics and conditions, for example, a lower cutoff for satisfactory sleep efficiency (e.g. 80%) can be applied for sleep restriction. • Consider pain, mobility difficulties, and general safety risks (e.g., falls from getting in and out of bed). • Consider stimulus control adaptations, such as sitting up in bed during periods of wakefulness instead of leaving bed.
Cognitive strategies • Psychoeducation regarding normal age-related changes in sleep may be helpful to change unrealistic expectations about sleep. • Psychoeducation regarding how planned daytime activities such as walks, social interactions, and other leisure activities may increase energy levels, improve nighttime sleep quality, and add to the patient's general quality of life. • Consider treating any comorbid depressive symptoms alongside sleep symptoms.
Sleep hygiene • Although naps should be avoided to enable adequate buildup of sleep pressure, scheduled naps may be beneficial for daytime vigilance and functioning. • Restrict naps to 20 minutes in the late morning or early afternoon. • Increase overall light exposure. • Maintain consistent sleep and wake times, as well as meal and activity schedules.

strengthened, while the association between bed and wakefulness is weakened. It may not always be feasible or safe for an older adult to leave the bed or bedroom. In this situation a patient might be encouraged to sit up in bed when unable to sleep and to return to the prone position when feeling sleepy again.

Sleep restriction therapy limits the time spent in bed to 15 minutes beyond the duration of time spent asleep at night (Spielman et al., 1987) to consolidate sleep by allowing for the buildup of a high sleep pressure. For example, a person who is spending 9 hours in bed but sleeps only 5 hours per night would be advised to limit time in bed to 5 hours and 15 minutes. As sleep efficiency improves, the amount of time spent in bed is also gradually increased in 15–20-minute intervals. Sleep restriction therapy is often modified in older adults whose baseline sleep efficiency is often lower (<80%) even among good sleepers. Sleep compression also offers an alternative to restriction.

A cognitive restructuring component employs standard CBT principals to help patients to identify maladaptive thoughts and beliefs about sleep, to challenge them, and finally to reframe them into more adaptive thoughts and beliefs (Belanger et al., 2006). The therapy is often structured and includes homework designed to help the patient gather evidence that challenges the maladaptive thought patterns and supports the adaptive ones. Some common maladaptive thought patterns targeted include unrealistic expectations about sleep, misconceptions about the causes of insomnia, distorted beliefs about the consequences of insomnia, and faulty beliefs about what promotes good sleep (Belanger et al., 2006). Recent research points to dysfunctional beliefs about sleep as an important mediator of CBT-I (Parsons et al., 2021). A considerable proportion of funded research on CBT has been on older adults, including the use of cognitive aspects of intervention. Similar interventions therefore may be used regardless of age.

Patients who have trouble getting to sleep often report becoming anxious about their sleep once they try to go to bed. Relaxation therapy is used to help people achieve a calm and relaxed state when they are trying to go to sleep. Some common relaxation techniques employed include progressive muscle relaxation (tensing and then relaxing muscle groups in a certain order), guided imagery, deep breathing, meditation, and biofeedback. For patients who have mobility/joint problems, relaxation methods can focus on breathing techniques and autogenic training rather than muscle tension–release cycles.

Sleep hygiene, which consists of a set of guidelines for the maintenance of healthy sleep and wake habits, should also be emphasized (see Table 39.3) with all patients, although correcting sleep hygiene alone is often not enough. Patients should be encouraged to maintain a regular bedtime and wake-time schedule. Alcohol, which is commonly considered by patients to be a sleep aid due to its ability to shorten sleep latency, should be discouraged as it has been shown to induce sleep fragmentation and early-morning awakenings (Roehrs & Roth, 2001). Caffeine and nicotine should also be minimized and avoided after lunchtime.

Sleep hygiene considerations are similar in older adults, but age-related challenges may affect expectations (e.g., concerning timing of sleep). The five principles of good sleep health continue to be relevant at all ages and offer a broader perspective (Espie, 2022).

The American Academy of Sleep Medicine recently published clinical practice guidelines with strong recommendations for a multicomponent CBT-I in adults with chronic insomnia (Edinger et al., 2021). Conditional recommendation was given to single-component treatments including stimulus control, sleep restriction therapy, and relaxation therapy, while there was insufficient evidence to recommend cognitive therapy as a stand-alone treatment. However, the use of sleep hygiene as a stand-alone treatment was not recommended.

Whether behavioral treatment of insomnia should include all or perhaps only some of the above components remains unclear. Furthermore, it remains to be elucidated whether certain components or component combinations are better suited to certain subgroups or subtypes of insomnia.

PHARMACOLOGIC TREATMENT

Pharmacological treatment of insomnia in the older adult population is generally not recommended. In the clinical practice guideline of chronic insomnia, the American Academy of Sleep Medicine finds that the evidence base for many individual drugs commonly used to treat insomnia is weak (Sateia et al., 2017). Studies have also shown that the use of sleep medication is more successful when combined with a behavioral intervention (Kwon et al., 2021). In older adults, it is particularly important to consider potential side effects and medication interactions prior to initiating treatment. Long-acting hypnotics can cause EDS and decrease motor coordination, which may lead to an increased risk of falls (Andrade, 2018). Cognitive impairment and respiratory depression are also potential side effects (Picton et al., 2018). While benzodiazepines have been shown to be effective in the treatment of acute insomnia (De Crescenzo et al., 2022), tolerability and safety profiles are not favorable. Furthermore, chronic use of long-acting benzodiazepines can lead to several negative outcomes, including tolerance, dependency, and insomnia rebound when discontinued (Markota et al., 2016), and the benefits of these agents for long-term use have not been sufficiently studied (De Crescenzo et al., 2022).

Non-benzodiazepine receptor agonists, or so-called Z-drugs, which include zolpidem, zopiclone, zaleplon, and eszopiclone, are more selective molecules and therefore are associated with less tolerance and a more benign side effect profile compared with the older benzodiazepines (Becker & Somiah, 2015; Dolder et al., 2007). These agents have been found to be effective in the short-term management of insomnia in the elderly (Scharner et al., 2021), and eszopiclone and zolpidem modified-release are approved for long-term use. Despite the improved side effect profile, safety concerns remain, which include increased risk of falls and fractures (Becker & Somiah, 2015). In one case–control study (n = 1,222 cases) of patients who had undergone surgical repair of a hip fracture, use of zolpidem in the past 180 days was associated with a significantly increased risk of hip fracture (adjusted odds ratio = 1.95, confidence interval [1.09, 3.51]; P. S. Wang et al., 2001). Finally, cases of psychiatric disturbances including delusions, hallucinations, and delirium have also been reported in older patients (Dolder et al., 2007; Scharner et al., 2021). Ramelteon, a melatonin receptor agonist, is another consideration. Several studies suggest that it is effective and tolerable in older adults with insomnia (Mini et al., 2008; Zammit et al., 2007). Of note, ramelteon is not extensively metabolized by the cytochrome P450 CYP3A4 isoenzyme, reducing the potential for drug–drug interactions with many other medications metabolized through this pathway (Dolder et al., 2007; Sateia et al., 2008). It is, however, extensively metabolized by first-pass metabolism, which should be taken into account when considering treatment for patients with hepatic impairment (Dolder et al., 2007; Sateia et al., 2008).

In practice, it is not uncommon to see medications from multiple other classes prescribed for insomnia in the elderly. There is no systematic evidence for the effectiveness of the antihistamines, antidepressants, antipsychotics, or anticonvulsants in the treatment of insomnia; and these are associated with risks, particularly in older adults (Ancoli-Israel et al., 2005). A newer class of drugs is the dual orexin receptor antagonist (DORA). This class of drugs works by antagonizing the two orexin receptors. Orexin is a known neuropeptide with an important role in the regulation and stability of arousal and wakefulness. Thus, DORAs constitute an alternative mechanism compared with commonly used hypnotics that target gamma-aminobutyric acid receptors. To date, several DORAs have been approved for the treatment of insomnia (Wu et al., 2022), and evidence has shown dose-dependent association with sleep outcomes in older participants aged >65 years (Zammit et al., 2020). In a recent comprehensive review of the pharmacological treatments for acute and long-term insomnia in adults, DORAs were shown to have the best efficacy and tolerability profile, but safety was variable (De Crescenzo et al., 2022). The efficacy and safety of DORAs in the older adults have also been highlighted recently (Wang et al., 2021). Finally, a rise in the use of melatonin for the treatment of insomnia has also been noted, as have associated safety concerns (Kuehn, 2022).

Sleep Disturbances in Older Adults With Major Neurocognitive Disorder/Dementia

While accumulating evidence points to poor (and short) sleep as an independent risk factor for neurodegenerative disorders including dementias (Sabia et al., 2021; Shi et al., 2018), this section will mainly focus on the nature and extent of sleep disturbances in populations already diagnosed with dementia or AD. Please note that our frequent use of the term *dementia* is largely synonymous with the more contemporary term *major neurocognitive disorder* (as per the *Diagnostic and Statistical Manual of Mental Disorders*, fifth edition; American Psychiatric Association, 2013).

Patients with dementia experience more fragmentation of sleep, as well as decreased sleep efficiency, total sleep time, and slow-wave sleep (Peter-Derex et al., 2015; Vitiello & Borson, 2001) compared with other older adults; and the severity of the dementia correlates with the severity of the sleep disruption (Pat-Horenczyk et al., 1998). Confirming these findings, a recent meta-analysis on PSG-assessed sleep in AD patients reported worse sleep across a range of outcomes compared with controls including decreased total sleep time, slow-wave sleep, REM, sleep efficiency, and increased number of awakenings, WASO, sleep-onset latency, and percentage of N1 sleep (Zhang et al., 2022). Accordingly, patients with dementia may also have EDS, nighttime wandering, confusion, and agitation (sundowning). All of these symptoms, in turn, increase the risk for long-term care placement (Ye & Richards, 2018), making it especially important to screen for and treat them. Furthermore, an increasing focus on the quality of life of dementia caregivers has revealed that many caregivers experience impaired sleep quality and shorter sleep compared with non-caregivers (Gao et al., 2019).

Sleep disturbances in dementia and AD may arise from a complex interplay between both environmental and pathophysiological factors, and there is increasing bidirectional evidence that, on the one hand, neurodegenerative processes occurring in dementia contribute to disturbances in sleep (Deschenes & McCurry, 2009; Wu & Swaab, 2007) and, on the other hand, sleep disturbances may contribute to the course of AD (Irwin & Vitiello, 2019). For example, there is evidence that neuropathological changes associated with AD have a deleterious effect on the circadian timing system. Early in the disease process, changes have been found to occur in the SCN, including alterations in the expression of key neuropeptides involved in the maintenance of the circadian rhythm (Van Erum et al., 2018; Wu & Swaab, 2007). Reduced nocturnal melatonin levels are also found in AD patients (Nous et al., 2021), as well as reduced melatonin levels in the cerebrospinal fluid and in the pineal glands of postmortem AD specimens (Liu et al., 1999; Zhou et al., 2003). These neuropathological changes are further exacerbated by reduced input of cues from environmental entrainers such as light. In particular, as mentioned above, older adults with dementia are exposed to less light (Figueiro et al., 2012), with an average bright light exposure of 30 minutes per day for AD patients living in the community (Campbell et al., 1988) and less than 10 minutes for those in nursing homes (Ancoli-Israel et al., 1997).

Hence, dementia adds an extra level of complexity to the diagnosis and treatment of sleep problems in this population. The same primary sleep disorders considered in the evaluation of all older adults should be considered when evaluating patients with dementia, including SDB, RLS, RBD, and circadian rhythm sleep disorders. Likewise, the possible contribution of secondary factors such as comorbid medical conditions, pain, psychiatric illnesses, and medications must be assessed. In this population it is particularly important to get input from the caregiver or bed partner as part of the evaluation process. Depending on the severity of the dementia, overnight sleep studies may not be feasible, and therefore actigraphy may serve as a useful method to assess sleep and circadian rhythms in these patients (Ancoli-Israel et al., 2003).

Although the evidence of efficacious treatments for sleep disturbance in populations with dementia is scarce (Blackman et al., 2021), treatment of specific sleep disturbances in this population should be guided by that specific sleep disorder. Maintenance of regular physical activity and social interaction can also promote a more robust sleep/wake cycle. Although sedating medications are frequently prescribed for the nighttime restlessness associated with dementia, they may paradoxically result in increased sleep disturbance, daytime sleepiness, impaired motor functioning, and impaired cognitive functioning. A recent Cochrane review on pharmacotherapies for sleep disturbances in dementia failed to find randomized controlled trials of any of the most commonly prescribed sleep medications (McCleery & Sharpley, 2020). Furthermore, no beneficial effects of melatonin were observed. In a recent randomized trial, administration of DORAs for insomnia in patients with probable AD led to significant improvements in total sleep time, sleep efficiency, and WASO. However, increased rates of daytime somnolence and other adverse effects were noted (Herring et al., 2020). Therefore, non-pharmacologic treatments are preferred in this population. For example, light therapy has been shown to have beneficial effects on a range of sleep disturbances in AD and dementia populations (van Maanen et al., 2016), although recent reviews conclude that larger and more rigorous trials are needed (Hjetland et al., 2020; Tan et al., 2022). CBT-I also may be successfully adapted to support older adults with dementia living at home (Livingston et al., 2019; Rapaport et al., 2024).

Sleep Disturbances in the Nursing Home Setting

Sleep disturbances are very common in nursing home settings (Morley, 2015), where elderly patients tend to have multiple risk factors including medical illnesses, use of multiple medications, psychiatric illnesses, and dementia (Neikrug & Ancoli-Israel, 2010). Nursing home residents tend to have disturbed nighttime sleep and disrupted circadian rhythms (J. L. Martin et al., 2006). Studies have shown that sleep in nursing home settings tends to be very fragmented (Ancoli-Israel, Parker, et al., 1989). Nursing home patients also tend to be excessively sleepy and fall asleep often during the daytime. One early study showed that patients fell asleep an average of 22 times and slept for an average of 2 hours, 10 minutes per day between 7:00 a.m. and 7:00 p.m. (Jacobs et al., 1989).

In the nursing home environment there is also a variety of environmental factors that contribute to problems with sleep (Morley, 2015). Most nursing homes are not set up in an ideal fashion to promote good sleep. Patients often share rooms, disruptive noises and exposure to light during the nighttime hours are common, and light exposure during the day tends to be inadequate. Both nighttime ambient light and nighttime noise have been shown to contribute significantly to sleep disruption in nursing home patients (Janus et al., 2021). Lack of bright light during the daytime is also a problem in nursing homes, where residents may be exposed to less than 10 minutes of bright light per day

(Ancoli-Israel et al., 1997). More light exposure is associated with fewer sleep disruptions in this population (Gammack & Burke, 2009; Shochat et al., 2000). As mentioned previously, light is the most important synchronizer and stabilizer of circadian rhythms in humans, and these environments therefore may cause or exacerbate circadian rhythm disruptions.

Because sleep disturbances and daytime sleepiness are so common in the nursing home setting, they may often be disregarded or thought of as "normal." Further, if they do not cause difficulties for the nursing home staff (e.g., napping during the day), they may not be brought to the attention of the clinician. However, as in other settings, sleep difficulties in the nursing home environment are associated with increased morbidity and mortality (Ancoli-Israel, Klauber, et al., 1989), and it is important that any problems be addressed.

As in all older adults, patients should be assessed for the presence of primary sleep disorders such as SDB, RLS/PLMS, RBD, and circadian rhythm disorders that, if present, should be treated accordingly. The contribution of medications, medical illnesses, and psychiatric illnesses must also be considered and addressed appropriately. Where possible, environmental factors contributing to the sleep problem should be addressed. We recommend keeping the environment dark at night and light during the day. When possible, dynamic lighting should be installed to strengthen the circadian rhythms (Baandrup & Jennum, 2021; Juda et al., 2020). Also, noise should be minimized during the night (Janus et al., 2021). Matching roommates with respect to sleeping patterns may be helpful in this regard. J. L. Martin and colleagues (2007) showed that a multicomponent non-pharmacological intervention including increased exposure to outdoor light, efforts to keep patients out of bed during the daytime, structured physical activity, institution of a bedtime routine, and efforts to reduce noise and light in patients' rooms resulted in improved robustness of circadian rest/activity rhythms in nursing home patients. Despite methodological issues, a recently published systematic review found promising support for the use of multicomponent non-pharmacological treatment to improve sleep in nursing homes (Wilfling et al., 2021).

While the use of sleep-promoting medication including hypnotics in the nursing home is very high (Conn & Madan, 2006), the general use of medications specifically for sleep is discouraged. Patients should have a full evaluation for primary sleep disorders and other contributing factors, as described above; and these should be treated before consideration is given to prescribing a sleep aid. If medications are employed, we recommend they be used sparingly, cautiously, and only in the short term. Special attention must be given to medication interactions and to the possibility of daytime sedation that may be a side effect of the medication use.

Summary

As the population proportion of older adults continues to grow globally, it is of increasing importance to adapt public programs to meet specific challenges associated with increased age. Sleep complaints and disorders are common in elderly adults. Primary sleep disturbances occurring in older adults include insomnia, circadian rhythm disturbances, SDB, RBD, PLMS, and RLS. Sleep disturbances in older adults often represent a multifactorial syndrome in which medical illness, psychiatric illness, and medications may play a role. Sleep complaints are associated with poor outcomes and must therefore be addressed as part of any complete treatment plan. Treatment strategies differ depending on the etiology of the sleep disturbance, and a careful and systematic approach to diagnosis is indicated.

Acknowledgment

Lisa M. Wu's effort on this chapter was supported by the European Union Horizon 2020 Research and Innovation Programme under Marie Sklodowska-Curie grant agreement no. 754513 and the Aarhus University Research Foundation.

References

Ahmadi, N., Shapiro, G. K., Chung, S. A., & Shapiro, C. M. (2009). Clinical diagnosis of sleep apnea based on single night of polysomnography vs. two nights of polysomnography. *Sleep and Breathing*, *13*(3), 221–226. https://doi.org/10.1007/s11325-008-0234-2

Allen, K. D., Renner, J. B., Devellis, B., Helmick, C. G., & Jordan, J. M. (2008). Osteoarthritis and sleep: The Johnston County Osteoarthritis Project. *The Journal of Rheumatology*, 35(6), 1102–1107.

Allen, R. P., Auerbach, S., Bahrain, H., Auerbach, M., & Earley, C. J. (2013). The prevalence and impact of restless legs syndrome on patients with iron deficiency anemia. *American Journal of Hematology*, *88*(4), 261–264. https://doi.org/10.1002/AJH.23397

Allen, R. P., Picchietti, D. L., Garcia-Borreguero, D., Ondo, W. G., Walters, A. S., Winkelman, J. W., Zucconi, M., Ferri, R., Trenkwalder, C., & Lee, H. B. (2014). Restless legs syndrome/Willis–Ekbom disease diagnostic criteria: Updated International Restless Legs Syndrome Study Group (IRLSSG) consensus criteria—History, rationale, description, and significance. *Sleep Medicine*, *15*(8), 860–873. https://doi.org/10.1016/J.SLEEP.2014.03.025

Allen, R. P., Picchietti, D., Hening, W. A., Trenkwalder, C., Walters, A. S., Montplaisi, J., Bara-Jimenez, W., Becker, P., Bell, G., Berger, K., Bliwise, D. L., Brooks, D., Consens, F., Earley, C. J., Ehrenberg, B. L., Foley, D., Murray, C. F., Garcia-Borreguero, D., Hallett, M., . . . Zucconi, M. (2003). Restless legs syndrome: Diagnostic criteria, special considerations, and epidemiology. A report from the restless legs syndrome diagnosis and epidemiology workshop at the National Institutes of Health. *Sleep Medicine*, *4*(2), 101–119. https://doi.org/10.1016/S1389-9457(03)00010-8

Allen, R. P., Walters, A. S., Montplaisir, J., Hening, W., Myers, A., Bell, T. J., & Ferini-Strambi, L. (2005). Restless legs syndrome prevalence and impact: REST general population study. *Archives of Internal Medicine*, *165*(11), 1286–1292. https://doi.org/10.1001/ARCHINTE.165.11.1286

Aloia, M. S., Ilniczky, N., Di Dio, P., Perlis, M. L., Greenblatt, D. W., & Giles, D. E. (2003). Neuropsychological changes and treatment compliance in older adults with sleep apnea. *Journal of Psychosomatic Research*, *54*(1), 71–76. https://doi.org/10.1016/S0022-3999(02)00548-2

American Academy of Sleep Medicine. (2005). *International classification of sleep disorders: Diagnostic and Coding Manual* (2nd ed.).

American Psychiatric Association. (2013). *Diagnostic and statistical manual of mental disorders*. (5th ed.).

Amidi, A., Buskbjerg, C. D. R., Damholdt1, M. F., Dahlgaard, J., Thorndike, F. P., Ritterband, L., & Zachariae, R. (2022). Changes in sleep following internet-delivered cognitive-behavioral therapy for insomnia in women treated for breast cancer: A 3-year follow-up assessment. *Sleep Medicine*, *96*, 35–41.

Ancoli-Israel, S. (2007). Sleep apnea in older adults – Is it real and should age be the determining factor in the treatment decision matrix? *Sleep Medicine Reviews*, *11*(2), 83–85. https://doi.org/10.1016/j.smrv.2006.11.002

Ancoli-Israel, S., Cole, R., Alessi, C., Chambers, M., Moorcroft, W., & Pollak, C. P. (2003). The role of actigraphy in the study of sleep and circadian rhythms. *Sleep*, *26*(3), 342–392. http://www.ncbi.nlm.nih.gov/pubmed/12749557

Ancoli-Israel, S., Klauber, M. R., Butters, N., Parker, L., & Kripke, D. F. (1991). Dementia in institutionalized elderly: Relation to sleep apnea. *Journal of the American Geriatrics Society*, *39*(3), 258–263. https://doi.org/10.1111/j.1532-5415.1991.tb01647.x

Ancoli-Israel, S., Klauber, M. R., Jones, D. W., Kripke, D. F., Martin, J., Mason, W., Pat-Horenczyk, R., & Fell, R. (1997). Variations in circadian rhythms of activity, sleep, and light exposure related to dementia in nursing-home patients. *Sleep*, *20*(1), 18–23. https://doi.org/10.1093/sleep/20.1.18

Ancoli-Israel, S., Klauber, M. R., Kripke, D. F., Parker, L., & Cobarrubias, M. (1989). Sleep apnea in female patients in a nursing home: Increased risk of mortality. *Chest*, *96*(5), 1054–1058. https://doi.org/10.1378/CHEST.96.5.1054

Ancoli-Israel, S., Kripke, D. F., Klauber, M. R., Mason, W. J., Fell, R., & Kaplan, O. (1991a). Periodic limb movements in sleep in community-dwelling elderly. *Sleep*, *14*(6), 496–500. https://doi.org/10.1093/sleep/14.6.496

Ancoli-Israel, S., Kripke, D. F., Klauber, M. R., Mason, W. J., Fell, R., & Kaplan, O. (1991b). Sleep-disordered breathing in community-dwelling elderly. *Sleep*, *14*(6), 486–495. https://doi.org/10.1093/SLEEP/14.6.486

Ancoli-Israel, S., Parker, L., Sinaee, R., Fell, R. L., & Kripke, D. F. (1989). Sleep fragmentation in patients from a nursing home. *Journal of Gerontology*, *44*(1), M18–M21. https://doi.org/10.1093/GERONJ/44.1.M18

Ancoli-Israel, S., Richardson, G. S., Mangano, R. M., Jenkins, L., Hall, P., & Jones, W. S. (2005). Long-term use of sedative hypnotics in older patients with insomnia. *Sleep Medicine*, *6*(2), 107–113. https://doi.org/10.1016/j.sleep.2004.10.015

Andrade, C. (2018). Sedative hypnotics and the risk of falls and fractures in the elderly. *Journal of Clinical Psychiatry*, *79*(3), Article 18f12340. https://doi.org/10.4088/JCP.18F12340

Auger, R. R., Burgess, H. J., Emens, J. S., Deriy, L. V., Thomas, S. M., & Sharkey, K. M. (2015). Clinical practice guideline for the treatment of intrinsic circadian rhythm sleep–wake disorders: Advanced sleep–wake phase disorder (ASWPD), delayed sleep–wake phase disorder (DSWPD), non-24-hour sleep–wake rhythm disorder (N24SWD), and irregular sleep–wake rhythm disorder (ISWRD). An update for 2015. *Journal of Clinical Sleep Medicine*, *11*(10), 1199–1236. https://doi.org/10.5664/JCSM.5100

Ayalon, L., Ancoli-Israel, S., Stepnowsky, C., Marler, M., Palmer, B. W., Liu, L., Loredo, J. S., Corey-Bloom, J., Greenfield, D., & Cooke, J. (2006). Adherence to continuous positive airway pressure treatment in patients with Alzheimer's disease and obstructive sleep apnea. *The American Journal of Geriatric Psychiatry : Official Journal of the American Association for Geriatric Psychiatry*, *14*(2), 176–180. https://doi.org/10.1097/01.JGP.0000192484.12684.cd

Baandrup, L., & Jennum, P. J. (2021). Effect of a dynamic lighting intervention on circadian rest–activity disturbances in cognitively impaired, older adults living in a nursing home: A proof-of-concept study. *Neurobiology of Sleep and Circadian Rhythms*, *11*, Article 100067. https://doi.org/10.1016/J.NBSCR.2021.100067

Baglioni, C., Battagliese, G., Feige, B., Spiegelhalder, K., Nissen, C., Voderholzer, U., Lombardo, C., & Riemann, D. (2011). Insomnia as a predictor of depression: A meta-analytic evaluation of longitudinal epidemiological studies. *Journal of Affective Disorders*, *135*(1–3), 10–19. https://doi.org/10.1016/J.JAD.2011.01.011

Balomenos, V., Ntanasi, E., Anastasiou, C. A., Charisis, S., Velonakis, G., Karavasilis, E., Tsapanou, A., Yannakoulia, M., Kosmidis, M. H., Dardiotis, E., Hadjigeorgiou, G., Sakka, P., & Scarmeas, N. (2021). Association between sleep disturbances and frailty: Evidence from a population-based study. *Journal of the American Medical Directors Association*, *22*(3), 551–558.e1. https://doi.org/10.1016/J.JAMDA.2020.08.012

Bao, Y. P., Han, Y., Ma, J., Wang, R. J., Shi, L., Wang, T. Y., He, J., Yue, J. L., Shi, J., Tang, X. D., & Lu, L. (2017). Cooccurrence and bidirectional prediction of sleep disturbances and depression in older adults: Meta-analysis and systematic review. *Neuroscience & Biobehavioral Reviews*, *75*, 257–273. https://doi.org/10.1016/J.NEUBIOREV.2017.01.032

Becker, P. M., & Somiah, M. (2015). Non–benzodiazepine receptor agonists for insomnia. *Sleep Medicine Clinics*, *10*(1), 57–76. https://doi.org/10.1016/J.JSMC.2014.11.002

Bélanger, L., LeBlanc, M., & Morin, C. M. (2012). Cognitive behavioral therapy for insomnia in older adults. *Cognitive and Behavioral Practice*, *19*(1), 101–115. https://doi.org/10.1016/J.CBPRA.2010.10.003

Belanger, L., Savard, J., & Morin, C. M. (2006). Clinical management of insomnia using cognitive therapy. *Behavioral Sleep Medicine, 4*(3), 179–198. https://doi.org/10.1207/s15402010bsm0403_4

Benloucif, S., Green, K., L'Hermite-Balériaux, M., Weintraub, S., Wolfe, L. F., & Zee, P. C. (2006). Responsiveness of the aging circadian clock to light. *Neurobiology of Aging, 27*(12), 1870–1879. https://doi.org/10.1016/J.NEUROBIOLAGING.2005.10.011

Blackman, J., Swirski, M., Clynes, J., Harding, S., Leng, Y., & Coulthard, E. (2021). Pharmacological and non-pharmacological interventions to enhance sleep in mild cognitive impairment and mild Alzheimer's disease: A systematic review. *Journal of Sleep Research, 30*(4), Article e13229. https://doi.org/10.1111/JSR.13229

Blackwell, T., Yaffe, K., Ancoli-Israel, S., Schneider, J. L., Cauley, J. A., Hillier, T. A., Fink, H. A., & Stone, K. L.; Study of Osteoporotic Fractures Group. (2006). Poor sleep is associated with impaired cognitive function in older women: The Study of Osteoporotic Fractures. *Journals of Gerontology: Series A, 61*(4), 405–410. https://doi.org/10.1093/GERONA/61.4.405

Bliwise, D. L., Foley, D. J., Vitiello, M. V., Ansari, F. P., Ancoli-Israel, S., & Walsh, J. K. (2009). Nocturia and disturbed sleep in the elderly. *Sleep Medicine, 10*(5), 540–548. https://doi.org/10.1016/J.SLEEP.2008.04.002

Boeve, B. F. (2010). REM sleep behavior disorder: Updated review of the core features, the REM sleep behavior disorder–neurodegenerative disease association, evolving concepts, controversies, and future directions. *Annals of the New York Academy of Sciences, 1184*, 15–54. https://doi.org/10.1111/J.1749-6632.2009.05115.X

Bootzin, R. R., & Epstein, D. (2000). Stimulus control. In K. L. Lichstein & C. M. Morin (Eds.), *Treatment of late-life insomnia* (pp. 167–184). Sage Publications.

Boulos, M. I., Jairam, T., Kendzerska, T., Im, J., Mekhael, A., & Murray, B. J. (2019). Normal polysomnography parameters in healthy adults: A systematic review and meta-analysis. *Lancet Respiratory Medicine, 7*(6), 533–543. https://doi.org/10.1016/S2213-2600(19)30057-8

Braley, T. J., Dunietz, G. L., Chervin, R. D., Lisabeth, L. D., Skolarus, L. E., & Burke, J. F. (2018). Recognition and diagnosis of obstructive sleep apnea in older Americans. *Journal of the American Geriatrics Society, 66*(7), 1296–1302. https://doi.org/10.1111/JGS.15372

Brassington, G. S., King, A. C., & Bliwise, D. L. (2000). Sleep problems as a risk factor for falls in a sample of community-dwelling adults aged 64–99 years. *Journal of the American Geriatrics Society, 48*(10), 1234–1240. https://doi.org/10.1111/J.1532-5415.2000.TB02596.X

Brewster, G. S., Riegel, B., & Gehrman, P. R. (2018). Insomnia in the older adult. *Sleep Medicine Clinics, 13*(1), 13–19. https://doi.org/10.1016/j.jsmc.2017.09.002

Bubu, O. M., Andrade, A. G., Umasabor-Bubu, O. Q., Hogan, M. M., Turner, A. D., de Leon, M. J., Ogedegbe, G., Ayappa, I., Jean-Louis G, G., Jackson, M. L., Varga, A. W., & Osorio, R. S. (2020). Obstructive sleep apnea, cognition and Alzheimer's disease: A systematic review integrating three decades of multidisciplinary research. *Sleep Medicine Reviews, 50*, Article 101250. https://doi.org/10.1016/J.SMRV.2019.101250

Burke, W. J., & Wengel, S. P. (2003). Late-life mood disorders. *Clinics in Geriatric Medicine, 19*(4), 777–797. https://doi.org/10.1016/s0749-0690(03)00041-7

Bursztyn, M., & Stessman, J. (2005). The siesta and mortality: twelve years of prospective observations in 70-year-olds. *Sleep, 28*(3), 345–347.

Bursztyn, M., Ginsberg, G., & Stessman, J. (2002). The siesta and mortality in the elderly: effect of rest without sleep and daytime sleep duration. *Sleep, 25*(2), 187–191. https://doi.org/10.1093/sleep/25.2.187

Campbell, S. S., Dawson, D., & Anderson, M. W. (1993). Alleviation of sleep maintenance insomnia with timed exposure to bright light. *Journal of the American Geriatrics Society, 41*(8), 829–836. https://doi.org/10.1111/J.1532-5415.1993.TB06179.X

Campbell, S. S., Kripke, D. F., Gillin, J. C., & Hrubovcak, J. C. (1988). Exposure to light in healthy elderly subjects and Alzheimer's patients. *Physiology & Behavior, 42*(2), 141–144. http://www.ncbi.nlm.nih.gov/pubmed/3368532

Campbell, S. S., Murphy, P. J., & Stauble, T. N. (2005). Effects of a nap on nighttime sleep and waking function in older subjects. *Journal of the American Geriatrics Society, 53*(1), 48–53. https://doi.org/10.1111/J.1532-5415.2005.53009.X

Campbell, S. S., Terman, M., Lewy, A. J., Dijk, D.-J., Eastman, C. I., & Boulos, Z. (1995). Light treatment for sleep disorders: Consensus report. *Journal of Biological Rhythms, 10*(2), 151–154. https://doi.org/10.1177/074873049501000207

Carrier, J., Monk, T. H., Buysse, D. J., & Kupfer, D. J. (1997). Sleep and morningness–eveningness in the "middle" years of life (20–59y). *Journal of Sleep Research, 6*(4), 230–237. https://doi.org/10.1111/J.1365-2869.1997.00230.X

Challet, E. (2019). The circadian regulation of food intake. *Nature Reviews Endocrinology, 15*(7), 393–405. https://doi.org/10.1038/S41574-019-0210-X

Chellappa, S. L., & Aeschbach, D. (2022). Sleep and anxiety: From mechanisms to interventions. *Sleep Medicine Reviews, 61*, Article 101583. https://doi.org/10.1016/J.SMRV.2021.101583

Chen, T. Y., Lee, S., & Buxton, O. M. (2017). A greater extent of insomnia symptoms and physician-recommended sleep medication use predict fall risk in community-dwelling older adults. *Sleep, 40*(11), Article zsx142. https://doi.org/10.1093/SLEEP/ZSX142

Cheng, G. H. L., Malhotra, R., Østbye, T., Chan, A., Ma, S., & Lo, J. C. (2018). Changes in nocturnal sleep and daytime nap durations predict all-cause mortality among older adults: The Panel on Health and Ageing of Singaporean Elderly. *Sleep, 41*(7), Article zsy087. https://doi.org/10.1093/sleep/zsy087

Claman, D. M., Redline, S., Blackwell, T., Ancoli-Israel, S., Surovec, S., Scott, N., Cauley, J. A., Ensrud, K. E., & Stone, K. L.; Study of Osteoporotic Fratures Research Group. (2006). Prevalence and correlates of periodic limb movements in older women. *Journal of Clinical Sleep Medicine : JCSM : Official Publication of the American Academy of Sleep Medicine, 2*(4), 438–445.

Conn, D. K., & Madan, R. (2006). Use of sleep-promoting medications in nursing home residents: Risks versus benefits. *Drugs and Aging, 23*(4), 271–287. https://doi.org/10.2165/00002512-200623040-00001

Da Silva, A. A., De Mello, R. G. B., Schaan, C. W., Fuchs, F. D., Redline, S., & Fuchs, S. C. (2016). Sleep duration and mortality in the elderly: A systematic review with meta-analysis. *BMJ Open, 6*(2), Article e00819. https://doi.org/10.1136/BMJOPEN-2015-008119

Dauvilliers, Y., Schenck, C. H., Postuma, R. B., Iranzo, A., Luppi, P. H., Plazzi, G., Montplaisir, J., & Boeve, B. (2018). REM sleep behaviour disorder. *Nature Reviews Disease Primers, 4*(1), Article 19. https://doi.org/10.1038/s41572-018-0016-5

De Crescenzo, F., D'Alò, G. L., Ostinelli, E. G., Ciabattini, M., Franco, V. Di, Watanabe, N., Kurtulmus, A., Tomlinson, A., Mitrova, Z., Foti, F., Del Giovane, C., Quested, D. J., Cowen, P. J., Barbui, C., Amato, L., Efthimiou, O., & Cipriani, A. (2022). Comparative effects of pharmacological interventions for the acute and long-term management of insomnia disorder in adults: A systematic review and network meta-analysis. *Lancet, 400*(10347), 170–184. https://doi.org/10.1016/S0140-6736(22)00878-9

Deschenes, C. L., & McCurry, S. M. (2009). Current treatments for sleep disturbances in individuals with dementia. *Current Psychiatry Reports, 11*(1), 20–26. https://doi.org/10.1007/s11920-009-0004-2

Dew, M. A., Hoch, C. C., Buysse, D. J., Monk, T. H., Begley, A. E., Houck, P. R., Hall, M., Kupfer, D. J., & Reynolds, C. F., 3rd. (2003). Healthy older adults' sleep predicts all-cause mortality at 4 to 19 years of follow-up. *Psychosomatic Medicine, 65*(1), 63–73.

Dolder, C., Nelson, M., & McKinsey, J. (2007). Use of non-benzodiazepine hypnotics in the elderly: Are all agents the same? *CNS Drugs, 21*(5), 389–405. https://doi.org/10.2165/00023210-200721050-00003

Duffy, J. F., Zeitzer, J. M., & Czeisler, C. A. (2007). Decreased sensitivity to phase-delaying effects of moderate intensity light in older subjects. *Neurobiology of Aging, 28*(5), 799–807. https://doi.org/10.1016/J.NEUROBIOLAGING.2006.03.005

Duffy, J. F., Zitting, K. M., & Chinoy, E. D. (2015). Aging and circadian rhythms. *Sleep Medicine Clinics, 10*(4), 423–434. https://doi.org/10.1016/J.JSMC.2015.08.002

During, E. H., & Winkelman, J. W. (2019). Drug treatment of restless legs syndrome in older adults. *Drugs & Aging, 36*, 939–946. https://doi.org/10.1007/s40266-019-00698-1

Dutheil, F., Danini, B., Bagheri, R., Fantini, M. L., Pereira, B., Moustafa, F., Trousselard, M., & Navel, V. (2021). Effects of a short daytime nap on the cognitive performance: A systematic review and meta-analysis. *International Journal of Environmental Research and Public Health, 18*(19), Article 10212. https://doi.org/10.3390/IJERPH181910212

Edinger, J. D., Arnedt, J. T., Bertisch, S. M., Carney, C. E., Harrington, J. J., Lichstein, K. L., Sateia, M. J., Troxel, W. M., Zhou, E. S., Kazmi, U., Heald, J. L., & Martin, J. L. (2021). Behavioral and psychological treatments for chronic insomnia disorder in adults: An American Academy of Sleep Medicine clinical practice guideline. *Journal of Clinical Sleep Medicine, 17*(2), 255–262. https://doi.org/10.5664/JCSM.8986

Eikermann, M., Jordan, A. S., Chamberlin, N. L., Gautam, S., Wellman, A., Lo, Y. L., White, D. P., & Malhotra, A. (2007). The influence of aging on pharyngeal collapsibility during sleep. *Chest, 131*(6), 1702–1709. https://doi.org/10.1378/CHEST.06-2653

Espie, C. A. (2022). The "5 principles" of good sleep health. *Journal of Sleep Research, 31*(3), e13502. https://doi.org/10.1111/jsr.13502
Evans, M. A., Buysse, D. J., Marsland, A. L., Wright, A. G. C., Foust, J., Carroll, L. W., Kohli, N., Mehra, R., Jasper, A., Srinivasan, S., & Hall, M. H. (2021). Meta-analysis of age and actigraphy-assessed sleep characteristics across the lifespan. *Sleep, 44*(9), Article zsab088. https://doi.org/10.1093/SLEEP/ZSAB088
Fang, H., Tu, S., Sheng, J., & Shao, A. (2019). Depression in sleep disturbance: A review on a bidirectional relationship, mechanisms and treatment. *Journal of Cellular and Molecular Medicine, 23*(4), 2324–2332. https://doi.org/10.1111/JCMM.14170
Ficca, G., Axelsson, J., Mollicone, D. J., Muto, V., & Vitiello, M. V. (2010). Naps, cognition and performance. *Sleep Medicine Reviews, 14*(4), 249–258. https://doi.org/10.1016/j.smrv.2009.09.005
Figueiro, M. G., Hamner, R., Higgins, P., Hornick, T., & Rea, M. S. (2012). Field measurements of light exposures and circadian disruption in two populations of older adults. *Journal of Alzheimer's Disease, 31*(4), 711–715. https://doi.org/10.3233/JAD-2012-120484
Fischer, D., Lombardi, D. A., Marucci-Wellman, H., & Roenneberg, T. (2017). Chronotypes in the US—Influence of age and sex. *PLOS ONE, 12*(6), Article e0178782. https://doi.org/10.1371/journal.pone.0178782
Foldvary-Schaefer, N. R., & Waters, T. E. (2017). Sleep-disordered breathing. *Continuum, 23*(4), 1093–1116. https://doi.org/10.1212/01.CON.0000522245.13784.F6
Foley, D., Ancoli-Israel, S., Britz, P., & Walsh, J. (2004). Sleep disturbances and chronic disease in older adults: Results of the 2003 National Sleep Foundation Sleep in America survey. *Journal of Psychosomatic Research, 56*(5), 497–502. https://doi.org/10.1016/J.JPSYCHORES.2004.02.010
Foley, D. J., Monjan, A. A., Brown, S. L., Simonsick, E. M., Wallace, R. B., & Blazer, D. G. (1995). Sleep complaints among elderly persons: An epidemiologic study of three communities. *Sleep, 18*(6), 425–432. https://doi.org/10.1093/SLEEP/18.6.425
Foley, D. J, Monjan, A. A., Izmirlian, G., Hays, J. C., & Blazer, D. G. (1999). Incidence and remission of insomnia among elderly adults in a biracial cohort. *Sleep, 22*(S2), S373–S378.
Foley, D. J., Vitiello, M. V., Bliwise, D. L., Ancoli-Israel, S., Monjan, A. A., & Walsh, J. K. (2007). Frequent napping is associated with excessive daytime sleepiness, depression, pain, and nocturia in older adults: Findings from the National Sleep Foundation "2003 Sleep in America" Poll. *American Journal of Geriatric Psychiatry, 15*(4), 344–350. https://doi.org/10.1097/01.JGP.0000249385.50101.67
Ford, D. E., & Kamerow, D. B. (1989). Epidemiologic study of sleep disturbances and psychiatric disorders. An opportunity for prevention? *JAMA, 262*(11), 1479–1484. https://doi.org/10.1001/jama.262.11.1479
Friedman, L., Zeitzer, J. M., Kushida, C., Zhdanova, I., Noda, A., Lee, T., Schneider, B., Guilleminault, C., Sheikh, J., & Yesavage, J. A. (2009). Scheduled bright light for treatment of insomnia in older adults. *Journal of the American Geriatrics Society, 57*(3), 441–452. https://doi.org/10.1111/j.1532-5415.2008.02164.x
Furihata, R., Kaneita, Y., Jike, M., Ohida, T., & Uchiyama, M. (2016). Napping and associated factors: A Japanese nationwide general population survey. *Sleep Medicine, 20*, 72–79. https://doi.org/10.1016/J.SLEEP.2015.12.006
Garcia, A. D. (2008). The effect of chronic disorders on sleep in the elderly. *Clinics in Geriatric Medicine, 24*, 27–38, vi. https://doi.org/10.1016/j.cger.2007.08.008
Gagnon, J. F., Postuma, R. B., Mazza, S., Doyon, J., & Montplaisir, J. (2006). Rapid-eye-movement sleep behaviour disorder and neurodegenerative diseases. *Lancet Neurology, 5*(5), 424–432. https://doi.org/10.1016/S1474-4422(06)70441-0
Gagnon, J. F., Postuma, R. B., & Montplaisir, J. (2006). Update on the pharmacology of REM sleep behavior disorder. *Neurology, 67*(5), 742–747. https://doi.org/10.1212/01.WNL.0000233926.47469.73
Gallo, J. J., Hwang, S., Truong, C., Reynolds, C. F., & Spira, A. P. (2020). Role of persistent and worsening sleep disturbance in depression remission and suicidal ideation among older primary care patients: The PROSPECT study. *Sleep, 43*(10), Article zsaa063. https://doi.org/10.1093/SLEEP/ZSAA063
Gammack, J. K., & Burke, J. M. (2009). Natural light exposure improves subjective sleep quality in nursing home residents. *Journal of the American Medical Directors Association, 10*(6), 440–441. https://doi.org/10.1016/J.JAMDA.2009.03.012
Gao, C., Chapagain, N. Y., & Scullin, M. K. (2019). Sleep duration and sleep quality in caregivers of patients with dementia: A systematic review and meta-analysis. *JAMA Network Open, 2*(8), Article e199891. https://doi.org/10.1001/JAMANETWORKOPEN.2019.9891
Gay, P. C. (2004). Chronic obstructive pulmonary disease and sleep. *Respiratory Care, 49*(1), 39–52.

Gehrman, P. R., Martin, J. L., Shochat, T., Nolan, S., Corey-Bloom, J., & Ancoli-Israel, S. (2003). Sleep-disordered breathing and agitation in institutionalized adults with Alzheimer disease. *American Journal of Geriatric Psychiatry, 11*(4), 426–433. https://doi.org/10.1097/00019442-200307000-00005

Gehrman, P., Stepnowsky, C., Cohen-Zion, M., Marler, M., Kripke, D. F., & Ancoli-Israel, S. (2002). Long-term follow-up of periodic limb movements in sleep in older adults. *Sleep, 25*(3), 340–343. https://doi.org/10.1093/sleep/25.3.340

Geiger-Brown, J. M., Rogers, V. E., Liu, W., Ludeman, E. M., Downton, K. D., & Diaz-Abad, M. (2015). Cognitive behavioral therapy in persons with comorbid insomnia: A meta-analysis. *Sleep Medicine Reviews, 23*, 54–67. https://doi.org/10.1016/J.SMRV.2014.11.007

Goldman, S. E., Hall, M., Boudreau, R., Matthews, K. A., Cauley, J. A., Ancoli-Israel, S., Stone, K. L., Rubin, S. M., Satterfield, S., Simonsick, E. M., & Newman, A. B. (2008). Association between nighttime sleep and napping in older adults. *Sleep, 31*(5), 733–740. https://doi.org/10.1093/SLEEP/31.5.733

Gooneratne, N. S., Gehrman, P. R., Nkwuo, J. E., Bellamy, S. L., Schutte-Rodin, S., Dinges, D. F., & Pack, A. I. (2006). Consequences of comorbid insomnia symptoms and sleep-related breathing disorder in elderly subjects. *Archives of Internal Medicine, 166*(16), 1732–1738. https://doi.org/10.1001/ARCHINTE.166.16.1732

Gooneratne, N. S., Richards, K. C., Joffe, M., Lam, R. W., Pack, F., Staley, B., Dinges, D. F., & Pack, A. I. (2011). Sleep disordered breathing with excessive daytime sleepiness is a risk factor for mortality in older adults. *Sleep, 34*(4), 435–442. https://doi.org/10.1093/SLEEP/34.4.435

Grandner, M. A., & Chakravorty, S. (2017). Insomnia in primary care: Misreported, mishandled, and just plain missed. *Journal of Clinical Sleep Medicine, 13*(8), 937–939. https://doi.org/10.5664/JCSM.6688

Griffin, S. C., Ravyts, S. G., Bourchtein, E., Ulmer, C. S., Leggett, M. K., Dzierzewski, J. M., & Calhoun, P. S. (2021). Sleep disturbance and pain in U.S. adults over 50: Evidence for reciprocal, longitudinal effects. *Sleep Medicine, 86*, 32–39. https://doi.org/10.1016/J.SLEEP.2021.08.006

Grossman, E. S. (2017). Enduring sleep complaints predict health problems: A six-year follow-up of the survey of health and retirement in Europe. *Aging & Mental Health, 21*(11), 1155–1163. https://doi.org/10.1080/13607863.2016.1209735

Guida, J. L., Alfini, A. J., Gallicchio, L., Spira, A. P., Caporaso, N. E., & Green, P. A. (2021). Association of objectively measured sleep with frailty and 5-year mortality in community-dwelling older adults. *Sleep, 44*(7), Article zsab003. https://doi.org/10.1093/SLEEP/ZSAB003

Haba-Rubio, J., Frauscher, B., Marques-Vidal, P., Toriel, J., Tobback, N., Andries, D., Preisig, M., Vollenweider, P., Postuma, R., & Heinzer, R. (2018). Prevalence and determinants of rapid eye movement sleep behavior disorder in the general population. *Sleep, 41*(2), Article zsx197. https://doi.org/10.1093/SLEEP/ZSX197

Halsband, C., Zapf, A., Sixel-Döring, F., Trenkwalder, C., & Mollenhauer, B. (2018). The REM Sleep Behavior Disorder Screening Questionnaire is not valid in de novo Parkinson's disease. Movement Disorders Clinical Practice, 5(2), 171–176. https://doi.org/10.1002/MDC3.12591

Hanson, B. L., & Ruthig, J. C. (2012). The unique role of sleep quality in older adults' psychological well-being. *Journal of Applied Gerontology, 31*(5), 587–607. https://doi.org/10.1177/0733464810392226

Harrold, E. C., Idris, A. F., Keegan, N. M., Corrigan, L., Teo, M. Y., O'Donnell, M., Tee Lim, S., Duff, E., O'Donnell, D. M., Kennedy, M. J., Sukor, S., Grant, C., Gallagher, D. G., Collier, S., Kingston, T., O'Dwyer, A. M., & Cuffe, S. (2020). Prevalence of insomnia in an oncology patient population: An Irish tertiary referral center experience. *Journal of the National Comprehensive Cancer Network, 18*(12), 1623–1630. https://doi.org/10.6004/JNCCN.2020.7611

Hastings, M. H., Maywood, E. S., & Brancaccio, M. (2018). Generation of circadian rhythms in the suprachiasmatic nucleus. *Nature Reviews Neuroscience, 19*(8), 453–469. https://doi.org/10.1038/s41583-018-0026-z

Hattar, S., Liao, H. W., Takao, M., Berson, D. M., & Yau, K. W. (2002). Melanopsin-containing retinal ganglion cells: Architecture, projections, and intrinsic photosensitivity. *Science, 295*(5557), 1065–1070. https://doi.org/10.1126/SCIENCE.1069609

Heinzer, R., Vat, S., Marques-Vidal, P., Marti-Soler, H., Andries, D., Tobback, N., Mooser, V., Preisig, M., Malhotra, A., Waeber, G., Vollenweider, P., Tafti, M., & Haba-Rubio, J. (2015). Prevalence of sleep-disordered breathing in the general population: The HypnoLaus study. *Lancet Respiratory Medicine, 3*(4), 310–318. https://doi.org/10.1016/S2213-2600(15)00043-0

Hening, W. A., Allen, R. P., Earley, C. J., Picchietti, D. L., & Silber, M. H. (2004). An update on the dopaminergic treatment of restless legs syndrome and periodic limb movement disorder. *Sleep, 27*(3), 560–583. https://doi.org/10.1093/SLEEP/27.3.560

Herring, W. J., Ceesay, P., Snyder, E., Bliwise, D., Budd, K., Hutzelmann, J., Stevens, J., Lines, C., & Michelson, D. (2020). Polysomnographic assessment of suvorexant in patients with probable Alzheimer's disease dementia and insomnia: A randomized trial. *Alzheimer's & Dementia, 16*(3), 541–551. https://doi.org/10.1002/ALZ.12035

Hertenstein, E., Feige, B., Gmeiner, T., Kienzler, C., Spiegelhalder, K., Johann, A., Jansson-Fröjmark, M., Palagini, L., Rücker, G., Riemann, D., & Baglioni, C. (2019). Insomnia as a predictor of mental disorders: A systematic review and meta-analysis. *Sleep Medicine Reviews, 43*, 96–105. https://doi.org/10.1016/j.smrv.2018.10.006

Hertenstein, E., Trinca, E., Wunderlin, M., Schneider, C. L., Züst, M. A., Fehér, K. D., Su, T., Straten, A. v., Berger, T., Baglioni, C., Johann, A., Spiegelhalder, K., Riemann, D., Feige, B., & Nissen, C. (2022). Cognitive behavioral therapy for insomnia in patients with mental disorders and comorbid insomnia: A systematic review and meta-analysis. *Sleep Medicine Reviews, 62*, Article 101597. https://doi.org/10.1016/J.SMRV.2022.101597

Hjetland, G. J., Pallesen, S., Thun, E., Kolberg, E., Nordhus, I. H., & Flo, E. (2020). Light interventions and sleep, circadian, behavioral, and psychological disturbances in dementia: A systematic review of methods and outcomes. *Sleep Medicine Reviews, 52*, Article 101310. https://doi.org/10.1016/J.SMRV.2020.101310

Hood, S., & Amir, S. (2017). The aging clock: circadian rhythms and later life. *Journal of Clinical Investigation, 127*(2), 437–446. https://doi.org/10.1172/JCI90328

Hornyak, M., Feige, B., Voderholzer, U., Philipsen, A., & Riemann, D. (2007). Polysomnography findings in patients with restless legs syndrome and in healthy controls: A comparative observational study. *Sleep, 30*(7), 861–865. https://doi.org/10.1093/sleep/30.7.861

Hua-Huy, T., Rouhani, S., Nguyen, X. Y., Luchon, L., Meurice, J. C., & Dinh-Xuan, A. T. (2015). Cardiovascular comorbidities in obstructive sleep apnoea according to age: A sleep clinic population study. *Aging Clinical and Experimental Research, 27*(5), 611–619. https://doi.org/10.1007/S40520-015-0318-3

Hughes, J. M., & Martin, J. L. (2022). CBT-I for older adults. In S. Nowakowski, S. N. Garland, M. A. Grandner, & L. J. Cuddihy (Eds.), *Adapting Cognitive Behavioral Therapy for Insomnia* (pp. 347–366). Elsevier. https://doi.org/10.1016/B978-0-12-822872-2.00005-0

Hybels, C. F., & Blazer, D. G. (2003). Epidemiology of late-life mental disorders. *Clinics in Geriatric Medicine, 19*(4), 663–696, v. https://doi.org/10.1016/s0749-0690(03)00042-9

Irwin, M. R., & Vitiello, M. V. (2019). Implications of sleep disturbance and inflammation for Alzheimer's disease dementia. *Lancet Neurology, 18*(3), 296–306. https://doi.org/10.1016/S1474-4422(18)30450-2

Jacobs, D., Ancoli-Israel, S., Parker, L., & Kripke, D. F. (1989). Twenty-four-hour sleep–wake patterns in a nursing home population. *Psychology and Aging, 4*(3), 352–356. https://doi.org/10.1037/0882-7974.4.3.352

Janus, S. I. M., Kosters, J., Van Den Bosch, K. A., Andringa, T. C., Zuidema, S. U., & Luijendijk, H. J. (2021). Sounds in nursing homes and their effect on health in dementia: A systematic review. *International Psychogeriatrics, 33*(6), 627–644. https://doi.org/10.1017/S1041610220000952

Johar, H., Kawan, R., Emeny, R. T., & Ladwig, K. H. (2016). Impaired sleep predicts cognitive decline in old people: Findings from the prospective KORA age study. *Sleep, 39*(1), 217–226. https://doi.org/10.5665/SLEEP.5352

Johnson, J. A., Rash, J. A., Campbell, T. S., Savard, J., Gehrman, P. R., Perlis, M., Carlson, L. E., & Garland, S. N. (2016). A systematic review and meta-analysis of randomized controlled trials of cognitive behavior therapy for insomnia (CBT-I) in cancer survivors. *Sleep Medicine Reviews, 27*, 20–28. https://doi.org/10.1016/j.smrv.2015.07.001

Juda, M., Liu-Ambrose, T., Feldman, F., Suvagau, C., & Mistlberger, R. E. (2020). Light in the senior home: Effects of dynamic and individual light exposure on sleep, cognition, and well-being. *Clocks & Sleep, 2*(4), 557–576. https://doi.org/10.3390/CLOCKSSLEEP2040040

Kang, S. H., Yoon, I. Y., Lee, S. D., Han, J. W., Kim, T. H., & Kim, K. W. (2013). REM sleep behavior disorder in the Korean elderly population: Prevalence and clinical characteristics. *Sleep, 36*(8), 1147–1152. https://doi.org/10.5665/SLEEP.2874

Kashyap, R., Hock, L. M., & Bowman, T. J. (2001). Higher prevalence of smoking in patients diagnosed as having obstructive sleep apnea. *Sleep & Breathing, 5*(4), 167–172. https://doi.org/10.1007/S11325-001-0167-5

Keage, H. A. D., Banks, S., Yang, K. L., Morgan, K., Brayne, C., & Matthews, F. E. (2012). What sleep characteristics predict cognitive decline in the elderly? *Sleep Medicine, 13*(7), 886–892. https://doi.org/10.1016/J.SLEEP.2012.02.003

Kessel, L., Siganos, G., Jørgensen, T., & Larsen, M. (2011). Sleep disturbances are related to decreased transmission of blue light to the retina caused by lens yellowing. *Sleep, 34*(9), 1215–1219. https://doi.org/10.5665/SLEEP.1242

Kim, M., Vu, T.-H., Maas, M. B., Braun, R. I., Wolf, M. S., Roenneberg, T., Daviglus, M. L., Reid, K. J., & Zee, P. C. (2022). Light at night in older age is associated with obesity, diabetes, and hypertension. *Sleep*, Article zsac130. https://doi.org/10.1093/SLEEP/ZSAC130

Kocevska, D., Lysen, T. S., Dotinga, A., Koopman-Verhoeff, M. E., Luijk, M. P. C. M., Antypa, N., Biermasz, N. R., Blokstra, A., Brug, J., Burk, W. J., Comijs, H. C., Corpeleijn, E., Dashti, H. S., de Bruin, E. J., de Graaf, R., Derks, I. P. M., Dewald-Kaufmann, J. F., Elders, P. J. M., Gemke, R. J. B. J., . . . Tiemeier, H. (2021). Sleep characteristics across the lifespan in 1.1 million people from the Netherlands, United Kingdom and United States: A systematic review and meta-analysis. *Nature Human Behaviour, 5*(1), 113–122. https://doi.org/10.1038/S41562-020-00965-X

Koyanagi, A., Garin, N., Olaya, B., Ayuso-Mateos, J. L., Chatterji, S., Leonardi, M., Koskinen, S., Tobiasz-Adamczyk, B., & Haro, J. M. (2014). Chronic conditions and sleep problems among adults aged 50 years or over in nine countries: A multi-country study. *PLOS ONE, 9*(12), Article e114742. https://doi.org/10.1371/JOURNAL.PONE.0114742

Kuehn, B. M. (2022). Climbing melatonin use for insomnia raises safety concerns. *JAMA, 328*(7), 605–607. https://doi.org/10.1001/JAMA.2022.11506

Kwon, C. Y., Lee, B., Cheong, M. J., Kim, T. H., Jang, B. H., Chung, S. Y., & Kim, J. W. (2021). Non-pharmacological treatment for elderly individuals with insomnia: A systematic review and network meta-analysis. *Frontiers in Psychiatry, 11*, Article 608896. https://doi.org/10.3389/FPSYT.2020.608896

Lack, L., Wright, H., Kemp, K., & Gibbon, S. (2005). The treatment of early-morning awakening insomnia with 2 evenings of bright light. *Sleep, 28*(5), 616–623. https://doi.org/10.1093/SLEEP/28.5.616

Larsson, C., Hansson, E. E., Sundquist, K., & Jakobsson, U. (2017). Chronic pain in older adults: prevalence, incidence, and risk factors. *Scandinavian Journal of Rheumatology, 46*(4), 317–325. https://doi.org/10.1080/03009742.2016.1218543

Launois, S. H., Pépin, J. L., & Lévy, P. (2007). Sleep apnea in the elderly: A specific entity? *Sleep Medicine Reviews, 11*(2), 87–97. https://doi.org/10.1016/J.SMRV.2006.08.005

Lawrence, R. C., Felson, D. T., Helmick, C. G., Arnold, L. M., Choi, H., Deyo, R. A., & Wolfe, F. (2008). Estimates of the prevalence of arthritis and other rheumatic conditions in the United States. Part II. *Arthritis and Rheumatism, 58*, 26–35.

Lawrence, R. C., Helmick, C. G., Arnett, F. C., Deyo, R. A., Felson, D. T., Giannini, E. H., & Wolfe, F. (1998). Estimates of the prevalence of arthritis and selected musculoskeletal disorders in the United States. *Arthritis and Rheumatism, 41*, 778–799.

Lee, J. E., Shin, H. W., Kim, K. S., & Sohn, Y. H. (2009). Factors contributing to the development of restless legs syndrome in patients with Parkinson disease. *Movement Disorders, 24*(4), 579–582. https://doi.org/10.1002/MDS.22410

Li, J., Cacchione, P. Z., Hodgson, N., Riegel, B., Keenan, B. T., Scharf, M. T., Richards, K. C., & Gooneratne, N. S. (2017). Afternoon napping and cognition in Chinese older adults: Findings from the China Health and Retirement Longitudinal Study baseline assessment. *Journal of the American Geriatrics Society, 65*(2), 373–380. https://doi.org/10.1111/jgs.14368

Li, L., Wu, C., Gan, Y., Qu, X., & Lu, Z. (2016). Insomnia and the risk of depression: A meta-analysis of prospective cohort studies. *BMC Psychiatry, 16*(1), Article 375. https://doi.org/10.1186/s12888-016-1075-3

Li, P., Gao, L., Yu, L., Zheng, X., Ulsa, M. C., Yang, H. W., Gaba, A., Yaffe, K., Bennett, D. A., Buchman, A. S., Hu, K., & Leng, Y. (2023). Daytime napping and Alzheimer's dementia: A potential bidirectional relationship. *Alzheimer's & Dementia, 19*(1), 158–168. https://doi.org/10.1002/ALZ.12636

Liu, R. Y., Zhou, J. N., van, H. J., Hofman, M. A., & Swaab, D. F. (1999). Decreased melatonin levels in postmortem cerebrospinal fluid in relation to aging, Alzheimer's disease, and apolipoprotein E-epsilon4/4 genotype. *Journal of Clinical Endocrinology & Metabolism, 84*, 323–327.

Livingston, G., Barber, J. A., Kinnunen, K. M., Webster, L., Kyle, S. D., Cooper, C., Espie, C. A., Hallam, B., Horsley, R., Pickett, J., & Rapaport, P. (2019). DREAMS-START (Dementia RElAted Manual for Sleep; STrAtegies for RelaTives) for people with dementia and sleep disturbances: A single-blind feasibility and acceptability randomized controlled trial. *International Psychogeriatrics, 31*(2), 251–265. https://doi.org/10.1017/S1041610218000753

Luca, G., Haba Rubio, J., Andries, D., Tobback, N., Vollenweider, P., Waeber, G., Marques Vidal, P., Preisig, M., Heinzer, R., & Tafti, M. (2015). Age and gender variations of sleep in subjects without sleep disorders. *Annals of Medicine, 47*(6), 482–491. https://doi.org/10.3109/07853890.2015.1074271

Luik, A. I., Zuurbier, L. A., Hofman, A., Van Someren, E. J. W., & Tiemeier, H. (2013). Stability and fragmentation of the activity rhythm across the sleep–wake cycle: The importance of age, lifestyle, and mental health. *Chronobiology International, 30*(10), 1223–1230. https://doi.org/10.3109/07420528.2013.813528

Magee, J. C., & Carmin, C. N. (2010). The relationship between sleep and anxiety in older adults. *Current Psychiatry Reports, 12*(1), 13–19. https://doi.org/10.1007/S11920-009-0087-9

Malhotra, A., Huang, Y., Fogel, R., Lazic, S., Pillar, G., Jakab, M., Kikinis, R., & White, D. P. (2006). Aging influences on pharyngeal anatomy and physiology: The predisposition to pharyngeal collapse. *American Journal of Medicine, 119*(1), 72.e9–72.e14. https://doi.org/10.1016/J.AMJMED.2005.01.077

Mallon, L., & Hetta, J. (1997). A survey of sleep habits and sleeping difficulties in an elderly Swedish population. *Upsala Journal of Medical Sciences, 102*(3), 185–197. https://doi.org/10.3109/03009739709178940

Mander, B. A., Winer, J. R., & Walker, M. P. (2017). Sleep and human aging. *Neuron, 94*(1), 19–36. https://doi.org/10.1016/J.NEURON.2017.02.004

Markota, M., Rummans, T. A., Bostwick, J. M., & Lapid, M. I. (2016). Benzodiazepine use in older adults: Dangers, management, and alternative therapies. *Mayo Clinic Proceedings, 91*(11), 1632–1639. https://doi.org/10.1016/J.MAYOCP.2016.07.024

Martin, J., Stepnowsky, C., & Ancoli-Israel, S. (2002). Sleep apnea in the elderly. In W. McNicholas & E. Phillipson (Eds.), *Breathing disorders during sleep* (pp. 278–387). W. B. Saunders Company.

Martin, J. L., Marler, M. R., Harker, J. O., Josephson, K. R., & Alessi, C. A. (2007). A multicomponent nonpharmacological intervention improves activity rhythms among nursing home residents with disrupted sleep/wake patterns. *Journals of Gerontology. Series A, 62*(1), 67–72. https://doi.org/10.1093/GERONA/62.1.67

Martin, J. L., Mory, A. K., & Alessi, C. A. (2005). Nighttime oxygen desaturation and symptoms of sleep-disordered breathing in long-stay nursing home residents. *Journals of Gerontology. Series A, 60*(1), 104–108. https://doi.org/10.1093/GERONA/60.1.104

Martin, J. L., Webber, A. P., Alam, T., Harker, J. O., Josephson, K. R., & Alessi, C. A. (2006). Daytime sleeping, sleep disturbance, and circadian rhythms in the nursing home. *American Journal of Geriatric Psychiatry, 14*(2), 121–129. https://doi.org/10.1097/01.JGP.0000192483.35555.A3

Mazzotti, D. R., Guindalini, C., Sosa, A. L., Ferri, C. P., & Tufik, S. (2012). Prevalence and correlates for sleep complaints in older adults in low and middle income countries: A 10/66 Dementia Research Group study. *Sleep Medicine, 13*(6), 697–702. https://doi.org/10.1016/J.SLEEP.2012.02.009

McCarthy, C. E. M. (2021). Sleep disturbance, sleep disorders and co-morbidities in the care of the older person. *Medical Sciences, 9*(2), Article 31. https://doi.org/10.3390/MEDSCI9020031

McCleery, J., & Sharpley, A. L. (2020). Pharmacotherapies for sleep disturbances in dementia. *Cochrane Database of Systematic Reviews, 2020*(11), Article CD009178. https://doi.org/10.1002/14651858.CD009178

McMillan, A., & Morrell, M. J. (2016). Sleep disordered breathing at the extremes of age: The elderly. *Breathe, 12*(1), 50–60. https://doi.org/10.1183/20734735.003216

Mesas, A. E., López-García, E., & Rodríguez-Artalejo, F. (2011). Self-reported sleep duration and falls in older adults. *Journal of Sleep Research, 20*(1, Pt. 1), 21–27. https://doi.org/10.1111/J.1365-2869.2010.00867.X

Metz, M. E., & Bunnell, D. E. (1990). Napping and sleep disturbances in the elderly. *The Family Practice Research Journal, 10*(1), 47–56. https://pubmed.ncbi.nlm.nih.gov/2382580/

Miller, K. D., Nogueira, L., Devasia, T., Mariotto, A. B., Yabroff, K. R., Jemal, A., Kramer, J., & Siegel, R. L. (2022). Cancer treatment and survivorship statistics, 2022. *CA: A Cancer Journal for Clinicians, 75*(5), 409–436. https://doi.org/10.3322/CAAC.21731

Min, Y., & Slattum, P. W. (2018). Poor sleep and risk of falls in community-dwelling older adults: A systematic review. *Journal of Applied Gerontology, 37*(9), 1059–1084. https://doi.org/10.1177/0733464816681149

Miner, B., & Kryger, M. H. (2020). Sleep in the aging population. *Sleep Medicine Clinics, 15*(2), 311–318. https://doi.org/10.1016/j.jsmc.2020.02.016

Mini, L., Wang-Weigand, S., & Zhang, J. (2008). Ramelteon 8 mg/d versus placebo in patients with chronic insomnia: Post hoc analysis of a 5-week trial using 50% or greater reduction in latency to persistent sleep as a measure of treatment effect. *Clinical Therapeutics, 30*(7), 1316–1323. https://doi.org/10.1016/S0149-2918(08)80056-2

Mitchell, M. D., Gehrman, P., Perlis, M., & Umscheid, C. A. (2012). Comparative effectiveness of cognitive behavioral therapy for insomnia: A systematic review. *BMC Family Practice, 13*(1), Article 40. https://doi.org/10.1186/1471-2296-13-40

Mitterling, T., Högl, B., Schönwald, S. V., Hackner, H., Gabelia, D., Biermayr, M., & Frauscher, B. (2015). Sleep and respiration in 100 healthy Caucasian sleepers—A polysomnographic study according to American Academy of Sleep Medicine standards. *Sleep, 38*(6), 867–875. https://doi.org/10.5665/SLEEP.4730

Morgenthaler, T., Alessi, C., Friedman, L., Owens, J., Kapur, V., Boehlecke, B., Brown, T., Chesson, A., Coleman, J., Lee-Chiong, T., Pancer, J., & Swick, T. J. (2007). Practice parameters for the use of actigraphy in the assessment of sleep and sleep disorders: An update for 2007. *Sleep, 30*(4), 519–529. https://doi.org/10.1093/SLEEP/30.4.519

Morin, C. M., Colecchi, C., Stone, J., Sood, R., & Brink, D. (1999). Behavioral and pharmacological therapies for late-life insomnia: A randomized controlled trial. *JAMA, 281*(11), 991–999. https://doi.org/10.1001/JAMA.281.11.991

Morley, J. E. (2015). Sleep and the nursing home. *Journal of the American Medical Directors Association, 16*(7), 539–543. https://doi.org/10.1016/J.JAMDA.2015.05.001

Münch, M., Knoblauch, V., Blatter, K., Schröder, C., Schnitzler, C., Kräuchi, K., Wirz-Justice, A., & Cajochen, C. (2005). Age-related attenuation of the evening circadian arousal signal in humans. *Neurobiology of Aging, 26*(9), 1307–1319. https://doi.org/10.1016/j.neurobiolaging.2005.03.004

Musiek, E. S., Bhimasani, M., Zangrilli, M. A., Morris, J. C., Holtzman, D. M., & Ju, Y. E. S. (2018). Circadian rest–activity pattern changes in aging and preclinical Alzheimer disease. *JAMA Neurology, 75*(5), 582–590. https://doi.org/10.1001/jamaneurol.2017.4719

Nakamura, T. J., Takasu, N. N., & Nakamura, W. (2016). The suprachiasmatic nucleus: Age-related decline in biological rhythms. *Journal of Physiological Sciences, 66*(5), 367–374. https://doi.org/10.1007/S12576-016-0439-2

Nau, S. D., McCrae, C. S., Cook, K. G., & Lichstein, K. L. (2005). Treatment of insomnia in older adults. *Clinical Psychology Review, 25*(5), 645–672. https://doi.org/10.1016/J.CPR.2005.04.008

Neikrug, A. B., & Ancoli-Israel, S. (2010). Sleep disturbances in nursing homes. *Journal of Nutrition, Health & Aging, 14*(3), 207–211. https://doi.org/10.1007/S12603-010-0051-8

Netzer, N. C., Ancoli-Israel, S., Bliwise, D. L., Fulda, S., Roffe, C., Almeida, F., Onen, H., Onen, F., Raschke, F., Garcia, M. A. M., & Frohnhofen, H. (2016). Principles of practice parameters for the treatment of sleep disordered breathing in the elderly and frail elderly: The consensus of the International Geriatric Sleep Medicine Task Force. *European Respiratory Journal, 48*(4), 992–1018. https://doi.org/10.1183/13993003.01975-2015

Newman, A. B., Nieto, F. J., Guidry, U., Lind, B. K., Redline, S., Shahar, E., Pickering, T. G., & Quan, S. F. (2001). Relation of sleep-disordered breathing to cardiovascular disease risk factors: The Sleep Heart Health Study. *American Journal of Epidemiology, 154*(1), 50–59. https://doi.org/10.1093/AJE/154.1.50

Nieto, F. J., Young, T. B., Lind, B. K., Shahar, E., Samet, J. M., Redline, S., D'Agostino, R. B., Newman, A. B., Lebowitz, M. D., & Pickering, T. G. (2000). Association of sleep-disordered breathing, sleep apnea, and hypertension in a large community-based study. Sleep Heart Health Study. *JAMA, 283*(14), 1829–1836. https://doi.org/10.1001/JAMA.283.14.1829

Nishi, T., Saeki, K., Miyata, K., Yoshikawa, T., Ueda, T., Kurumatani, N., Obayashi, K., & Ogata, N. (2020). Effects of cataract surgery on melatonin secretion in adults 60 years and older: A randomized clinical trial. *JAMA Ophthalmology, 138*(4), 405–411. https://doi.org/10.1001/JAMAOPHTHALMOL.2020.0206

Norman, D., & Loredo, J. S. (2008). Obstructive sleep apnea in older adults. *Clinics in Geriatric Medicine, 24*(1), 151–165, ix. https://doi.org/10.1016/j.cger.2007.08.006

Nous, A., Engelborghs, S., & Smolders, I. (2021). Melatonin levels in the Alzheimer's disease continuum: A systematic review. *Alzheimer's Research & Therapy, 13*(1), Article 52. https://doi.org/10.1186/S13195-021-00788-6

Obayashi, K., Saeki, K., Iwamoto, J., Okamoto, N., Tomioka, K., Nezu, S., Ikada, Y., & Kurumatani, N. (2014). Effect of exposure to evening light on sleep initiation in the elderly: A longitudinal analysis for repeated measurements in home settings. *Chronobiology International, 31*(4), 461–467. https://doi.org/10.3109/07420528.2013.840647

Ohayon, M. M. (2002). Epidemiology of insomnia: What we know and what we still need to learn. *Sleep Medicine Reviews, 6*(2), 97–111. https://doi.org/10.1053/smrv.2002.0186

Ohayon, M. M., Carskadon, M. A., Guilleminault, C., & Vitiello, M. V. (2004). Meta-analysis of quantitative sleep parameters from childhood to old age in healthy individuals: Developing normative sleep values across the human lifespan. *Sleep, 27*(7), 1255–1273. https://doi.org/10.1093/SLEEP/27.7.1255

Ohayon, M. M., & Roth, T. (2002). Prevalence of restless legs syndrome and periodic limb movement disorder in the general population. *Journal of Psychosomatic Research, 53*(1), 547–554. https://doi.org/10.1016/S0022-3999(02)00443-9

Ohayon, M. M., & Vecchierini, M. F. (2005). Normative sleep data, cognitive function and daily living activities in older adults in the community. *Sleep, 28*(8), 981–989. https://doi.org/10.1093/sleep/28.8.981

Ohayon, M. M., & Zulley, J. (1999). Prevalence of naps in the general population. *Sleep and Hypnosis, 1*(2), 88–97.

Owusu, J. T., Wennberg, A. M. V., Holingue, C. B., Tzuang, M., Abeson, K. D., & Spira, A. P. (2019). Napping characteristics and cognitive performance in older adults. *International Journal of Geriatric Psychiatry, 34*(1), 87–96. https://doi.org/10.1002/gps.4991

Paine, S. J., Fink, J., Gander, P. H., & Warman, G. R. (2014). Identifying advanced and delayed sleep phase disorders in the general population: A national survey of New Zealand adults. *Chronobiology International, 31*(5), 627–636. https://doi.org/10.3109/07420528.2014.885036

Palmer, C. R., Kripke, D. F., Savage, H. C., Cindrich, L. A., Loving, R. T., & Elliott, J. A. (2010). Efficacy of enhanced evening light for advanced sleep phase syndrome. *Behavioral Sleep Medicine, 1*(4), 213–226. https://doi.org/10.1207/S15402010BSM0104_4

Pan, Z., Huang, M., Huang, J., Yao, Z., & Lin, Z. (2020). Association of napping and all-cause mortality and incident cardiovascular diseases: A dose–response meta analysis of cohort studies. *Sleep Medicine, 74*, 165–172. https://doi.org/10.1016/j.sleep.2020.08.009

Park, M., Buchman, A. S., Lim, A. S. P., Leurgans, S. E., & Bennett, D. A. (2014). Sleep complaints and incident disability in a community-based cohort study of older persons. *American Journal of Geriatric Psychiatry, 22*(7), 718–726. https://doi.org/10.1016/j.jagp.2012.12.023

Parsons, C. E., Zachariae, R., Landberger, C., & Young, K. S. (2021). How does cognitive behavioural therapy for insomnia work? A systematic review and meta-analysis of mediators of change. *Clinical Psychology Review, 86*, Article 102027. https://doi.org/10.1016/J.CPR.2021.102027

Pat-Horenczyk, R., Klauber, M. R., Shochat, T., & Ancoli-Israel, S. (1998). Hourly profiles of sleep and wakefulness in severely versus mild-moderately demented nursing home patients. *Aging: Clinical and Experimental Research, 10*(4), 308–315. https://doi.org/10.1007/BF03339793

Patel, D., Steinberg, J., & Patel, P. (2018). Insomnia in the elderly: A review. *Journal of Clinical Sleep Medicine, 14*(6), 1017–1024. https://doi.org/10.5664/JCSM.7172

Patke, A., Young, M. W., & Axelrod, S. (2020). Molecular mechanisms and physiological importance of circadian rhythms. *Nature Reviews Molecular Cell Biology, 21*(2), 67–84. https://doi.org/10.1038/s41580-019-0179-2

Pennestri, M. H., Whittom, S., Adam, B., Petit, D., Carrier, J., & Montplaisir, J. (2006). PLMS and PLMW in healthy subjects as a function of age: Prevalence and interval distribution. *Sleep, 29*(9), 1183–1187. https://doi.org/10.1093/SLEEP/29.9.1183

Peppard, P. E., Young, T., Palta, M., Dempsey, J., & Skatrud, J. (2000). Longitudinal study of moderate weight change and sleep-disordered breathing. *JAMA, 284*(23), 3015–3021. https://doi.org/10.1001/jama.284.23.3015

Peppard, P. E., Young, T., Barnet, J. H., Palta, M., Hagen, E. W., & Hla, K. M. (2013). Increased prevalence of sleep-disordered breathing in adults. *American Journal of Epidemiology, 177*(9), 1006–1014. https://doi.org/10.1093/AJE/KWS342

Peter-Derex, L., Yammine, P., Bastuji, H., & Croisile, B. (2015). Sleep and Alzheimer's disease. *Sleep Medicine Reviews, 19*, 29–38. https://doi.org/10.1016/J.SMRV.2014.03.007

Phillips, B., & Ancoli-Israel, S. (2001). Sleep disorders in the elderly. *Sleep Medicine, 2*(2), 99–114. https://doi.org/10.1016/S1389-9457(00)00083-6

Picton, J. D., Brackett Marino, A., & Lovin Nealy, K. (2018). Benzodiazepine use and cognitive decline in the elderly. *American Journal of Health-System Pharmacy, 75*(1), e6–e12. https://doi.org/10.2146/AJHP160381

Pollak, C. P., Perlick, D., Linsner, J. P., Wenston, J., & Hsieh, F. (1990). Sleep problems in the community elderly as predictors of death and nursing home placement. *Journal of Community Health, 15*(2), 123–135. https://doi.org/10.1007/BF01321316

Pujol, M., Pujol, J., Alonso, T., Fuentes, A., Pallerola, M., Freixenet, J., Barbé, F., Salamero, M., Santamaría, J., & Iranzo, A. (2017). Idiopathic REM sleep behavior disorder in the elderly Spanish community: A primary care center study with a two-stage design using video-polysomnography. *Sleep Medicine, 40,* 116–121. https://doi.org/10.1016/J.SLEEP.2017.07.021

Quan, S. F., Katz, R., Olson, J., Bonekat, W., Enright, P. L., Young, T., & Newman, A. (2005). Factors associated with incidence and persistence of symptoms of disturbed sleep in an elderly cohort: The Cardiovascular Health Study. *American Journal of the Medical Sciences, 329*(4), 163–172. https://doi.org/10.1097/00000441-200504000-00001

Rapaport, P., Amador, S., Adeleke, M., Banerjee, S., Barber, J., Charlesworth, G., Clarke, C., Connell, C., Espie, C., Gonzalez, L., Horsley, R., Hunter, R., Kyle, S. D., Manela, M., Morris, S., Pikett, L., Raczek, M., Thornton, E., Walker, Z., . . . Livingston, G. (2024). Clinical and cost-effectiveness of DREAMS START (Dementia RElAted Manual for Sleep; STrAtegies for RelaTives) for people living with dementia and their carers: A study protocol for a parallel multicentre randomised controlled trial. *BMJ Open, 14*(2), e075273. https://doi.org/10.1136/bmjopen-2023-075273

Redline, S., Kirchner, H. L., Quan, S. F., Gottlieb, D. J., Kapur, V., & Newman, A. (2004). The effects of age, sex, ethnicity, and sleep-disordered breathing on sleep architecture. *Archives of Internal Medicine, 164*(4), 406–418. https://doi.org/10.1001/ARCHINTE.164.4.406

Reid, K. J., Martinovich, Z., Finkel, S., Statsinger, J., Golden, R., Harter, K., & Zee, P. C. (2006). Sleep: A marker of physical and mental health in the elderly. *American Journal of Geriatric Psychiatry, 14*(10), 860–866. https://doi.org/10.1097/01.JGP.0000206164.56404.BA

Resnick, H. E., & Phillips, B. (2008). Documentation of sleep apnea in nursing homes: United States 2004. *Journal of the American Medical Directors Association, 9*(4), 260–264. https://doi.org/10.1016/J.JAMDA.2008.01.001

Revell, V. L., & Skene, D. J. (2010). Impact of age on human non-visual responses to light. *Sleep and Biological Rhythms, 8*(2), 84–94. https://doi.org/10.1111/J.1479-8425.2009.00418.X

Richards, K. C., Roberson, P. K., Simpson, K., Lambert, C. W., Bliwise, D. L., Cole, C. S., Enderlin, C., Shue, V. M., Siddiqui, N., & Williams, J. S. (2008). Periodic leg movements predict total sleep time in persons with cognitive impairment and sleep disturbance. *Sleep, 31*(2), 224–230. https://doi.org/10.1093/sleep/31.2.224

Roehrs, T., & Roth, T. (2001). Sleep, sleepiness, and alcohol use. *Alcohol Research & Health : The Journal of the National Institute on Alcohol Abuse and Alcoholism, 25*(2), 101–109.

Roguski, A., Rayment, D., Whone, A. L., Jones, M. W., & Rolinski, M. (2020). A neurologist's guide to REM sleep behavior disorder. *Frontiers in Neurology, 11,* Article 610. https://doi.org/10.3389/FNEUR.2020.00610

Russo-Magno, P., O'Brien, A., Panciera, T., & Rounds, S. (2001). Compliance with CPAP therapy in older men with obstructive sleep apnea. *Journal of the American Geriatrics Society, 49*(9), 1205–1211. https://doi.org/10.1046/j.1532-5415.2001.49238.x

Sabia, S., Fayosse, A., Dumurgier, J., van Hees, V. T., Paquet, C., Sommerlad, A., Kivimäki, M., Dugravot, A., & Singh-Manoux, A. (2021). Association of sleep duration in middle and old age with incidence of dementia. *Nature Communications, 12*(1), Article 2289. https://doi.org/10.1038/S41467-021-22354-2

Sack, R. L., Auckley, D., Auger, R. R., Carskadon, M. A., Wright, K. P., Vitiello, M. V., & Zhdanova, I. V. (2007). Circadian rhythm sleep disorders: Part II, Advanced sleep phase disorder, delayed sleep phase disorder, free-running disorder, and irregular sleep–wake rhythm. An American Academy of Sleep Medicine review. *Sleep, 30*(11), 1484–1501. https://doi.org/10.1093/SLEEP/30.11.1484

Salive, M. E. (2013). Multimorbidity in older adults. *Epidemiologic Reviews, 35*(1), 75–83. https://doi.org/10.1093/EPIREV/MXS009

Sasai-Sakuma, T., Takeuchi, N., Asai, Y., Inoue, Y., & Inoue, Y. (2020). Prevalence and clinical characteristics of REM sleep behavior disorder in Japanese elderly people. *Sleep, 43*(8), Article zsaa024. https://doi.org/10.1093/SLEEP/ZSAA024

Sateia, M. J., Buysse, D. J., Krystal, A. D., Neubauer, D. N., & Heald, J. L. (2017). Clinical practice guideline for the pharmacologic treatment of chronic insomnia in adults: An American Academy of Sleep Medicine clinical practice guideline. *Journal of Clinical Sleep Medicine, 13*(2), 307–349. https://doi.org/10.5664/jcsm.6470

Sateia, M. J., Kirby-Long, P., & Taylor, J. L. (2008). Efficacy and clinical safety of ramelteon: An evidence-based review. *Sleep Medicine Reviews, 12*(4), 319–332. https://doi.org/10.1016/J.SMRV.2007.12.005

Savides, T. J., Messin, S., Senger, C., & Kripke, D. F. (1986). Natural light exposure of young adults. *Physiology and Behavior, 38,* 571–574.

Scanlan, M. F., Roebuck, T., Little, P. J., Redman, J. R., & Naughton, M. T. (2000). Effect of moderate alcohol upon obstructive sleep apnoea. *European Respiratory Journal, 16*(5), 909–913. https://doi.org/10.1183/09031936.00.16590900

Scarlett, S., Nolan, H. N., Kenny, R. A., & O'Connell, M. D. L. (2021). Discrepancies in self-reported and actigraphy-based sleep duration are associated with self-reported insomnia symptoms in community-dwelling older adults. *Sleep Health, 7*(1), 83–92. https://doi.org/10.1016/J.SLEH.2020.06.003

Scharner, V., Hasieber, L., Sönnichsen, A., & Mann, E. (2021). Efficacy and safety of Z-substances in the management of insomnia in older adults: A systematic review for the development of recommendations to reduce potentially inappropriate prescribing. *BMC Geriatrics, 22,* Article 87. https://doi.org/10.1186/s12877-022-02757-6

Schenck, C. H., Boeve, B. F., & Mahowald, M. W. (2013). Delayed emergence of a parkinsonian disorder or dementia in 81% of older men initially diagnosed with idiopathic rapid eye movement sleep behavior disorder: A 16-year update on a previously reported series. *Sleep Medicine, 14*(8), 744–748. https://doi.org/10.1016/J.SLEEP.2012.10.009

Scheuermaier, K., Laffan, A. M., & Duffy, J. F. (2010). Light exposure patterns in healthy older and young adults. *Journal of Biological Rhythms, 25*(2), 113–122. https://doi.org/10.1177/0748730410361916

Scullin, M. K., Fairley, J., Decker, M. J., & Bliwise, D. L. (2017). The effects of an afternoon nap on episodic memory in young and older adults. *Sleep, 40*(5), Article zsx035. https://doi.org/10.1093/SLEEP/ZSX035

Senaratna, C. V., Perret, J. L., Lodge, C. J., Lowe, A. J., Campbell, B. E., Matheson, M. C., Hamilton, G. S., & Dharmage, S. C. (2017). Prevalence of obstructive sleep apnea in the general population: A systematic review. *Sleep Medicine Reviews, 34,* 70–81. https://doi.org/10.1016/J.SMRV.2016.07.002

Shi, L., Chen, S. J., Ma, M. Y., Bao, Y. P., Han, Y., Wang, Y. M., Shi, J., Vitiello, M. V., & Lu, L. (2018). Sleep disturbances increase the risk of dementia: A systematic review and meta-analysis. *Sleep Medicine Reviews, 40,* 4–16. https://doi.org/10.1016/J.SMRV.2017.06.010

Shochat, T., Martin, J., Marler, M., & Ancoli-Israel, S. (2000). Illumination levels in nursing home patients: Effects on sleep and activity rhythms. *Journal of Sleep Research, 9*(4), 373–379. https://doi.org/10.1046/J.1365-2869.2000.00221.X

Silva, M. dos S., Poyares, D., Silva, L. O., Souza, K. M., Andersen, M. L., Ohayon, M. M., Tufik, S., & Piovezan, R. D. (2022). Associations of the severity of obstructive sleep apnea with age-related comorbidities: A population-based study. *Frontiers in Neurology, 13,* Article 802554. https://doi.org/10.3389/fneur.2022.802554

Smagula, S. F., Stone, K. L., Fabio, A., & Cauley, J. A. (2016). Risk factors for sleep disturbances in older adults: Evidence from prospective studies. *Sleep Medicine Reviews, 25,* 21–30. https://doi.org/10.1016/J.SMRV.2015.01.003

Spiegelhalder, K., & Hornyak, M. (2008). Restless legs syndrome in older adults. *Clinics in Geriatric Medicine, 24*(1), 167–180. https://doi.org/10.1016/J.CGER.2007.08.004

Spielman, A. J., Saskin, P., & Thorpy, M. J. (1987). Treatment of chronic insomnia by restriction of time in bed. *Sleep, 10,* 45–56.

Spira, A. P., Covinsky, K., Rebok, G. W., Stone, K. L., Redline, S., & Yaffe, K. (2012). Objectively measured sleep quality and nursing home placement in older women. *Journal of the American Geriatrics Society, 60*(7), 1237–1243. https://doi.org/10.1111/J.1532-5415.2012.04044.X

Spira, A. P., Friedman, L., Flint, A., & Sheikh, J. I. (2005). Interaction of sleep disturbances and anxiety in later life: Perspectives and recommendations for future research. *Journal of Geriatric Psychiatry and Neurology, 18*(2), 109–115. https://doi.org/10.1177/0891988705276062

Stiasny-Kolster, K., Mayer, G., Schäfer, S., Möller, J. C., Heinzel-Gutenbrunner, M., & Oertel, W. H. (2007). The REM sleep behavior disorder screening questionnaire—A new diagnostic instrument. *Movement Disorders, 22*(16), 2386–2393. https://doi.org/10.1002/MDS.21740

Stiasny-Kolster, K., Sixel-Döring, F., Trenkwalder, C., Heinzel-Gutenbrunner, M., Seppi, K., Poewe, W., Högl, B., & Frauscher, B. (2015). Diagnostic value of the REM sleep behavior disorder screening questionnaire in Parkinson's disease. *Sleep Medicine, 16*(1), 186–189. https://doi.org/10.1016/J.SLEEP.2014.08.014

Stone, K. L., Ancoli-Israel, S., Blackwell, T., Ensrud, K. E., Cauley, J. A., Redline, S., Hillier, T. A., Schneider, J., Claman, D., & Cummings, S. R. (2008). Actigraphy-measured sleep characteristics and risk of falls in older women. *Archives of Internal Medicine, 168*(16), 1768–1775. https://doi.org/10.1001/ARCHINTE.168.16.1768

Strollo, S. E., Fallon, E. A., Gapstur, S. M., & Smith, T. G. (2020). Cancer-related problems, sleep quality, and sleep disturbance among long-term cancer survivors at 9-years post diagnosis. *Sleep Medicine, 65*, 177–185. https://doi.org/10.1016/j.sleep.2019.10.008

Strøm, L., Danielsen, J. T., Amidi, A., Cardenas Egusquiza, A. L., Wu, L. M., & Zachariae, R. (2022). Sleep during oncological treatment—A systematic review and meta-analysis of associations with treatment response, time to progression and survival. *Frontiers in Neuroscience, 16*, Article 817837. https://doi.org/10.3389/fnins.2022.817837

Suhner, A. G., Murphy, P. J., & Campbell, S. S. (2002). Failure of timed bright light exposure to alleviate age-related sleep maintenance insomnia. *Journal of the American Geriatrics Society, 50*(4), 617–623. https://doi.org/10.1046/J.1532-5415.2002.50154.X

Sun, Y., Laksono, I., Selvanathan, J., Saripella, A., Nagappa, M., Pham, C., Englesakis, M., Peng, P., Morin, C. M., & Chung, F. (2021). Prevalence of sleep disturbances in patients with chronic non-cancer pain: A systematic review and meta-analysis. *Sleep Medicine Reviews, 57*, Article 101467. https://doi.org/10.1016/J.SMRV.2021.101467

Svensson, T., Saito, E., Svensson, A. K., Melander, O., Orho-Melander, M., Mimura, M., Rahman, S., Sawada, N., Koh, W. P., Shu, X. O., Tsuji, I., Kanemura, S., Park, S. K., Nagata, C., Tsugane, S., Cai, H., Yuan, J. M., Matsuyama, S., Sugawara, Y., . . . Inoue, M. (2021). Association of sleep duration with all- and major-cause mortality among adults in Japan, China, Singapore, and Korea. *JAMA Network Open, 4*(9), Article e2122837. https://doi.org/10.1001/JAMANETWORKOPEN.2021.22837

Tahara, Y., Aoyama, S., & Shibata, S. (2017). The mammalian circadian clock and its entrainment by stress and exercise. *Journal of Physiological Sciences*, 67(1), 1–10. https://doi.org/10.1007/s12576-016-0450-7

Takada, S., Yamamoto, Y., Shimizu, S., Kimachi, M., Ikenoue, T., Fukuma, S., Onishi, Y., Takegami, M., Yamazaki, S., Ono, R., Sekiguchi, M., Otani, K., Kikuchi, S. I., Konno, S. I., & Fukuhara, S. (2018). Association between subjective sleep quality and future risk of falls in older people: Results from LOHAS. *Journals of Gerontology: Series A, 73*(9), 1205–1211. https://doi.org/10.1093/GERONA/GLX123

Tan, J. S. I., Cheng, L. J., Chan, E. Y., Lau, Y., & Lau, S. T. (2022). Light therapy for sleep disturbances in older adults with dementia: A systematic review, meta-analysis and meta-regression. *Sleep Medicine, 90*, 153–166. https://doi.org/10.1016/J.SLEEP.2022.01.013

Thompson, C., Legault, J., Moullec, G., Baltzan, M., Cross, N., Dang-Vu, T. T., Martineau-Dussault, M. È., Hanly, P., Ayas, N., Lorrain, D., Einstein, G., Carrier, J., & Gosselin, N. (2022). A portrait of obstructive sleep apnea risk factors in 27,210 middle-aged and older adults in the Canadian Longitudinal Study on Aging. *Scientific Reports, 12*(1), Article 5127. https://doi.org/10.1038/S41598-022-08164-6

Touitou, Y. (2001). Human aging and melatonin. Clinical relevance. *Experimental Gerontology, 36*(7), 1083–1100. https://doi.org/10.1016/S0531-5565(01)00120-6

Tufik, S., Santos-Silva, R., Taddei, J. A., & Bittencourt, L. R. A. (2010). Obstructive sleep apnea syndrome in the Sao Paulo Epidemiologic Sleep Study. *Sleep Medicine, 11*(5), 441–446. https://doi.org/10.1016/J.SLEEP.2009.10.005

Turner, P. L., & Mainster, M. A. (2008). Circadian photoreception: Ageing and the eye's important role in systemic health. *British Journal of Ophthalmology, 92*(11), 1439–1444. https://doi.org/10.1136/BJO.2008.141747

United Nations Department of Economic and Social Affairs. (2022). *World population prospects 2022: Summary of results*.

Van Den Berg, J. F., Van Rooij, F. J. A., Vos, H., Tulen, J. H. M., Hofman, A., Miedema, H. M. E., Neven, A. K., & Tiemeier, H. (2008). Disagreement between subjective and actigraphic measures of sleep duration in a population-based study of elderly persons. *Journal of Sleep Research, 17*(3), 295–302. https://doi.org/10.1111/J.1365-2869.2008.00638.X

van der Zweerde, T., Bisdounis, L., Kyle, S. D., Lancee, J., & van Straten, A. (2019). Cognitive behavioral therapy for insomnia: A meta-analysis of long-term effects in controlled studies. *Sleep Medicine Reviews*, 48, Article 101208. https://doi.org/10.1016/j.smrv.2019.08.002

Van Erum, J., Van Dam, D., & De Deyn, P. P. (2018). Sleep and Alzheimer's disease: A pivotal role for the suprachiasmatic nucleus. *Sleep Medicine Reviews, 40*, 17–27. https://doi.org/10.1016/J.SMRV.2017.07.005

Van Gastel, A. (2018). Drug-induced insomnia and excessive sleepiness. *Sleep Medicine Clinics, 13*(2), 147–159. https://doi.org/10.1016/j.jsmc.2018.02.001

van Maanen, A., Meijer, A. M., van der Heijden, K. B., & Oort, F. J. (2016). The effects of light therapy on sleep problems: A systematic review and meta-analysis. *Sleep Medicine Reviews*, *29*, 52–62. https://doi.org/10.1016/J.SMRV.2015.08.009

Vaughan, C. P., & Bliwise, D. L. (2018). Sleep and nocturia in older adults. *Sleep Medicine Clinics*, *13*(1), 107–116. https://doi.org/10.1016/J.JSMC.2017.09.010

Vetrugno, R., D'Angelo, R., & Montagna, P. (2007). Periodic limb movements in sleep and periodic limb movement disorder. *Neurological Sciences : Official Journal of the Italian Neurological Society and of the Italian Society of Clinical Neurophysiology*, *28*(Suppl 1), S9–S14. https://doi.org/10.1007/s10072-007-0733-0

Vitiello, M. V. (2008). We have much more to learn about the relationships between napping and health in older adults. *Journal of the American Geriatrics Society*, *56*(9), 1753–1755. https://doi.org/10.1111/J.1532-5415.2008.01837.X

Vitiello, M. V., & Borson, S. (2001). Sleep disturbances in patients with Alzheimer's disease: Epidemiology, pathophysiology and treatment. *CNS Drugs*, *15*(10), 777–796. https://doi.org/10.2165/00023210-200115100-00004

Vitiello, M. V., Larsen, L. H., & Moe, K. E. (2004). Age-related sleep change: Gender and estrogen effects on the subjective–objective sleep quality relationships of healthy, noncomplaining older men and women. *Journal of Psychosomatic Research*, *56*(5), 503–510. https://doi.org/10.1016/S0022-3999(04)00023-6

Wang, C., Bangdiwala, S. I., Rangarajan, S., Lear, S. A., AlHabib, K. F., Mohan, V., Teo, K., Poirier, P., Tse, L. A., Liu, Z., Rosengren, A., Kumar, R., Lopez-Jaramillo, P., Yusoff, K., Monsef, N., Krishnapillai, V., Ismail, N., Seron, P., Dans, A. L., . . . Yusuf, S. (2019). Association of estimated sleep duration and naps with mortality and cardiovascular events: A study of 116 632 people from 21 countries. *European Heart Journal*, *40*(20), 1620–1629. https://doi.org/10.1093/EURHEARTJ/EHY695

Wang, L., Pan, Y., Ye, C., Guo, L., Luo, S., Dai, S., Chen, N., & Wang, E. (2021). A network meta-analysis of the long- and short-term efficacy of sleep medicines in adults and older adults. *Neuroscience & Biobehavioral Reviews*, *131*, 489–496. https://doi.org/10.1016/J.NEUBIOREV.2021.09.035

Wang, P. S., Bohn, R. L., Glynn, R. J., Mogun, H., & Avorn, J. (2001). Zolpidem use and hip fractures in older people. *Journal of the American Geriatrics Society*, *49*(12), 1685–1690. https://doi.org/10.1111/J.1532-5415.2001.49280.X

Weaver, T. E., & Chasens, E. R. (2007). Continuous positive airway pressure treatment for sleep apnea in older adults. *Sleep Medicine Reviews*, *11*(2), 99–111. https://doi.org/10.1016/J.SMRV.2006.08.001

Wetter, D. W., Young, T. B., Bidwell, T. R., Badr, M. S., & Palta, M. (1994). Smoking as a risk factor for sleep-disordered breathing. *Archives of Internal Medicine*, *154*(19), 2219–2224. https://doi.org/10.1001/archinte.1994.00420190121014

Wilcox, S., Brenes, G. A., Levine, D., Sevick, M. A., Shumaker, S. A., & Craven, T. (2000). Factors related to sleep disturbance in older adults experiencing knee pain or knee pain with radiographic evidence of knee osteoarthritis. *Journal of the American Geriatrics Society*, *48*(10), 1241–1251. https://doi.org/10.1111/j.1532-5415.2000.tb02597.x

Wilfling, D., Hylla, J., Berg, A., Meyer, G., Köpke, S., Halek, M., Möhler, R., & Dichter, M. N. (2021). Characteristics of multicomponent, nonpharmacological interventions to reduce or avoid sleep disturbances in nursing home residents: A systematic review. *International Psychogeriatrics*, *33*(3), 245–273. https://doi.org/10.1017/S1041610220000733

Winkelman, J. W., Armstrong, M. J., Allen, R. P., Chaudhuri, K. R., Ondo, W., Trenkwalder, C., Zee, P. C., Gronseth, G. S., Gloss, D., & Zesiewicz, T. (2016). Practice guideline summary: Treatment of restless legs syndrome in adults: Report of the Guideline Development, Dissemination, and Implementation Subcommittee of the American Academy of Neurology. *Neurology*, *87*(24), 2585–2593. https://doi.org/10.1212/WNL.0000000000003388

Wu, X., Xue, T., Chen, Z., Wang, Z., & Chen, G. (2022). Orexin receptor antagonists and insomnia. *Current Psychiatry Reports*, *24*, 509–521. https://doi.org/10.1007/S11920-022-01357-W

Wu, Y. H., & Swaab, D. F. (2007). Disturbance and strategies for reactivation of the circadian rhythm system in aging and Alzheimer's disease. *Sleep Medicine*, *8*(6), 623–636. https://doi.org/10.1016/J.SLEEP.2006.11.010

Xin, C., Zhang, B., Fang, S., & Zhou, J. (2020). Daytime napping and successful aging among older adults in China: A cross-sectional study. *BMC Geriatrics*, *20*(1), Article 2. https://doi.org/10.1186/s12877-019-1408-4

Yaffe, K., Falvey, C. M., & Hoang, T. (2014). Connections between sleep and cognition in older adults. *Lancet Neurology*, *13*(10), 1017–1028. https://doi.org/10.1016/S1474-4422(14)70172-3
Yamada, T., Hara, K., Shojima, N., Yamauchi, T., & Kadowaki, T. (2015). Daytime napping and the risk of cardiovascular disease and all-cause mortality: A prospective study and dose–response meta-analysis. *Sleep*, *38*(12), 1945–1953. https://doi.org/10.5665/sleep.5246
Ye, L., & Richards, K. C. (2018). Sleep and long-term care. *Sleep Medicine Clinics*, *13*(1), 117–125. https://doi.org/10.1016/J.JSMC.2017.09.011
Zachariae, R., Amidi, A., Damholdt, M. F., Clausen, C. D. R., Dahlgaard, J., Lord, H., Thorndike, F. P., & Ritterband, L. M. (2018). Internet-delivered cognitive-behavioral therapy for insomnia in breast cancer survivors: A randomized controlled trial. *Journal of the National Cancer Institute*, *110*(8), 880–887. https://doi.org/10.1093/jnci/djx293
Zachariae, R., Lyby, M. S., Ritterband, L. M., & O'Toole, M. S. (2016). Efficacy of internet-delivered cognitive-behavioral therapy for insomnia—A systematic review and meta-analysis of randomized controlled trials. *Sleep Medicine Reviews*, *30*, 1–10. https://doi.org/10.1016/j.smrv.2015.10.004
Zammit, G., Dauvilliers, Y., Pain, S., Sebök Kinter, D., Mansour, Y., & Kunz, D. (2020). Daridorexant, a new dual orexin receptor antagonist, in elderly subjects with insomnia disorder. *Neurology*, *94*(21), e2222–e2232. https://doi.org/10.1212/WNL.0000000000009475
Zammit, G., Erman, M., Wang-Weigand, S., Sainati, S., Zhang, J., & Roth, T. (2007). Evaluation of the efficacy and safety of ramelteon in subjects with chronic insomnia. *Journal of Clinical Sleep Medicine*, *3*(5), 495–504. https://doi.org/10.5664/jcsm.26914
Zhang, Y., & Jordan, J. M. (2008). Epidemiology of osteoarthritis. *Rheumatic Disease Clinics of North America*, *34*, 515–529.
Zhang, Y., Ren, R., Yang, L., Zhang, H., Shi, Y., Okhravi, H. R., Vitiello, M. V., Sanford, L. D., & Tang, X. (2022). Sleep in Alzheimer's disease: A systematic review and meta-analysis of polysomnographic findings. *Translational Psychiatry*, *12*(1), Article 136. https://doi.org/10.1038/s41398-022-01897-y
Zhang, Z., Xiao, X., Ma, W., & Li, J. (2020). Napping in older adults: A review of current literature. *Current Sleep Medicine Reports*, *6*(3), 129–135. https://doi.org/10.1007/S40675-020-00183-X
Zhang, Y., & Jordan, J. M. (2008). Epidemiology of osteoarthritis. *Rheumatic Diseases Clinics of North America*, *34*(3), 515–529. https://doi.org/10.1016/j.rdc.2008.05.007
Zhou, J. N., Liu, R. Y., Kamphorst, W., Hofman, M. A., & Swaab, D. F. (2003). Early neuropathological Alzheimer's changes in aged individuals are accompanied by decreased cerebrospinal fluid melatonin levels. *Journal of Pineal Research*, *35*(2), 125–130. https://doi.org/10.1034/j.1600-079x.2003.00065.x
Zilli, I., Ficca, G., & Salzarulo, P. (2009). Factors involved in sleep satisfaction in the elderly. *Sleep Medicine*, *10*(2), 233–239. https://doi.org/10.1016/J.SLEEP.2008.01.004

CHAPTER

40 Sleep and Psychiatric Disorders

Rachel Manber, Jessica R. Dietch, Nicole B. Gumport, *and* Norah Simpson

Abstract

Disturbed sleep is common in many psychiatric disorders and is a diagnostic symptom of mood and several anxiety disorders, including post-traumatic stress disorder and generalized anxiety disorder. This chapter discusses sleep in psychiatric disorders, including mood, anxiety, schizophrenia, eating, and personality disorders. For each psychiatric disorder, the authors describe what is known about associated sleep symptoms, polysomnographic findings pertaining to abnormal sleep architecture, comorbid sleep disorders and other sleep abnormalities, and the clinical significance of the sleep symptoms. They also discuss gaps in knowledge and future directions for research. They conclude with highlighting three sets of clinically relevant questions that will be important to address in the future.

Key Words: depression, bipolar, anxiety disorder, panic disorder, post-traumatic stress disorder, generalized anxiety disorder, social phobia, eating disorder, schizophrenia, personality disorder

Introduction

Disturbed sleep is common in many psychiatric disorders and is a diagnostic symptom of mood and several anxiety disorders, including post-traumatic stress disorder (PTSD) and generalized anxiety disorder (GAD). Individuals with multiple psychiatric disorders appear to experience greater levels of more disturbed sleep than those with a single diagnosis. For example, Leskin and colleagues (2002) examined data from the National Comorbidity Survey and found that patients with both PTSD and panic disorder (PD) reported higher rates of sleep symptoms (nightmares, difficulties initiating and maintaining sleep) than patients with PTSD alone. A similar interactive severity pattern is seen between PD and depression. Patients with PD who experience nocturnal panic and have a history of depression report having worse sleep and significantly reduced total sleep time than patients without nocturnal panic or depression (Singareddy & Uhde, 2009).

Disturbed sleep can predate a psychiatric disorder or emerge as one of its symptoms, as documented in a large study of 14,915 participants in four European countries that examined the relationship between the onset of insomnia symptoms and the onset of mood and anxiety disorders. Among participants with a first depressive episode and insomnia, insomnia symptoms emerged before major depressive disorder (MDD) in 41%, concurrently in 29%, and after the depressive episode in 30% (Ohayon & Roth, 2003). In contrast, when anxiety disorders were examined, insomnia appeared at the same time as or after the onset of an anxiety disorder in most cases. This data suggests that disturbed sleep might play different roles in different psychiatric disorders. Disturbed sleep can also emerge as a side effect of psychoactive medications used for treating psychiatric disorders. For example, selective serotonin reuptake inhibitors (SSRIs), which are the first-line pharmaceutical approach for depression and anxiety disorders, may cause restless legs syndrome (RLS) and lead to sleep continuity disturbances.

Historically, it was assumed that sleep continuity disturbances are caused by the psychiatric disorder and will resolve when the disorder is adequately treated. A large body of data, reviewed in this chapter, provides evidence that the relationship between sleep disturbance and psychiatric disorders is more complex. Specifically, there is increasing evidence that the disturbed sleep often does not fully resolve with effective psychiatric and psychological treatments of the psychiatric disorder (Carney et al., 2007). Even when sleep difficulties emerge as a symptom of a psychiatric disorder or its treatment, over time they may develop into a comorbid insomnia disorder. For example, persistent disturbed sleep may intensify distress about poor or insufficient sleep, leading to increased efforts to initiate sleep, anxiety about being unable to sleep, and conditioned arousal that in turn exacerbate the initial sleep disturbance. The original sleep symptoms then become a comorbid insomnia disorder. Consequently, current sleep disorder nosologies, such as the *Diagnostic and Statistical Manual of Mental Disorders*, fifth edition (DSM-5), replaced the category of *primary insomnia* with a new category, *insomnia disorder*, which can be comorbid with other psychiatric disorders, as long as comorbid mental disorders "do not adequately explain" the sleep symptoms (American Psychiatric Association, 2013). This change reflects current understanding that sleep disturbances can occur independently of other psychiatric disorders and may be an important therapeutic target.

This chapter aims to describe the current knowledge about sleep in psychiatric disorders. It covers mood, anxiety, psychotic, eating, and personality disorders, as well as obsessive–compulsive disorder (OCD) and PTSD. As we discuss each disorder, we describe what is known about sleep symptoms associated with the psychiatric disorder, polysomnographic (PSG) findings pertaining to abnormal sleep architecture, comorbid sleep disorders and other sleep abnormalities, and the clinical significance of the sleep symptoms. We note that older literature on sleep in psychiatric disorders used the term *insomnia* in reference to difficulties initiating and maintaining sleep rather than to a diagnostic entity. In this chapter, we use the term *insomnia symptoms* when referring to disturbed sleep (a nocturnal symptom of insomnia disorder).

Mood Disorders

We focus here on two mood disorders: MDD and bipolar disorder (BD). Historically, research on sleep in MDD has been more extensive than in BD; however, recently there has been an increase in research of sleep in BD.

MDD

Most individuals with MDD experience disturbed sleep or hypersomnia (Thase, 1999). Disturbed sleep includes difficulties initiating sleep, middle of the night awakenings, and early-morning awakenings. Hypersomnia, a sleep-related symptom in MDD, is much less common than poor sleep. It is defined as increased sleep duration and considered an "atypical" depression symptom, along with increased appetite, carbohydrate craving, and diurnal variations in mood. It has been suggested that hypersomnia may be more common among individuals with MDD who later experience hypomanic or manic episodes than among those whose disease course does not include manic features (Mitchell et al., 2008), although this was not replicated in a recent large cohort study of adolescents and young adults (Pfennig et al., 2016).

PSG FINDINGS IN DEPRESSION

Many studies document that the distribution of sleep stages is altered in MDD when compared with non-psychiatric controls (Baglioni et al., 2016; Krystal et al., 2008). The most robust findings pertain to alterations in rapid-eye-movement (REM) sleep, slow-wave sleep (SWS), and percent time spent awake. Alterations in REM sleep include shortened latency to the first REM episode, longer duration of the first REM episode, and greater density of eye movements during REM sleep, all reflecting disinhibition of REM sleep. *REM density* is the frequency of rapid eye movements during REM sleep. Though shortened REM latency was previously viewed as a specific marker of depression (Kupfer & Foster, 1972), it is no longer viewed as such. Indeed, there is evidence that it is present in other psychiatric disorders, such as schizophrenia (Zarcone et al., 1987), OCD (Insel et al., 1982), and eating disorders (Katz et al., 1984), among others. REM sleep abnormalities in depression and other psychiatric disorders might be a marker of emotion deregulation as REM sleep is involved in emotional processing (Baglioni et al., 2016; Fosse et al., 2001). Reduction in SWS has also been documented in depression (Kupfer et al., 1985), although there is some evidence that this may occur mostly in men (Armitage et al., 2000). For a review of sleep architecture findings in MDD and the effects of antidepressant treatment on sleep architecture, see Hutka et al. (2021).

COMORBID SLEEP DISORDERS

A 2016 meta-analysis reported that among 358,853 individuals with MDD, 19.8% had obstructive sleep apnea (OSA; Stubbs et al., 2016). This figure is remarkably similar to results from a large epidemiological study that did not include PSG, the standard diagnostic assessment for OSA, where the prevalence was estimated at 18% (Ohayon, 2003). It is possible that the prevalence of OSA is even higher in individuals with comorbid MDD and insomnia. In a separate study, we found that 39% of individuals with MDD and comorbid insomnia disorder had PSG-defined OSA (Ong et al., 2009). Older age, higher body mass index (BMI), and male gender, all common predictors of OSA in the general population, have also been reported to be the primary predictors of higher OSA severity among individuals with MDD (Ong et al., 2009; Reynolds et al., 1982). Several important clinical questions pertaining to OSA in MDD remain open. These include the impact of OSA on the presentation, natural course, and response to treatment of MDD and the effects of treating OSA on the depressive illness and response to its treatment. It is also not known whether the relationship between OSA and MDD is mediated by daytime sleepiness or sleep fragmentation rather than by levels of hypoxia (O'Hara & Schroder, 2006).

Compared to a population without depression, individuals with depressive disorders have higher rates of RLS and periodic limb movement disorder (PLMD; Lee et al., 2019), which may be related to use of antidepressant medications. Indeed, a large population study found that use of SSRIs increases threefold the risk for having RLS (Ohayon & Roth, 2002). A recent study reported that among individuals with depressive disorders receiving antidepressant medication, 13.5% had RLS and that those receiving an SSRI or a serotonin–norepinephrine reuptake inhibitor (SNRI) medication were at increased risk for experiencing RLS (Ocak et al., 2019); however, the study did not estimate whether the symptoms were treatment=emergent or preexisting, and the prevalence of RLS among unmedicated individuals with MDD is unknown.

CLINICAL RELEVANCE

Impact of Depression Treatment

The clinical relevance of PSG findings in MDD is not clear. It is also not yet clear which aspects of sleep REM and SWS abnormalities, if any, are truly state-dependent (i.e., specific to the depressive episode itself) because the extant literature is not consistent. It is possible that the extent of normalization in sleep electroencephalography (EEG) depends on the level of remission and/or time in remission, with greater normalization following full recovery (usually defined by at least 4 months of absence in core depressive symptoms) but not immediately following remission (Riemann et al., 2001). Evidence for sleep EEG predicting response to treatment is also not consistent and may depend on the type of treatment. For example, a 2021 review concluded that sleep EEG does not correlate strongly with remission after electroconvulsive therapy (Simon et al., 2021).

In contrast, the severity of subjectively reported sleep disturbance does correlate with overall depression severity and poorer quality of life (McCall et al., 2000). Moreover, subjective poor sleep incurs risk of suicide ideation and specific plans for suicide, and those reporting poor sleep are more likely to have had previous suicide attempts (Agargun et al., 1997; Chellappa & Araujo, 2007; Fawcett et al., 1990; Turvey et al., 2002). Further, abnormal sleep profiles, both physiological and self-reported, have been associated with poor response to pharmacological and psychotherapeutic treatments for depression (Boland et al., 2020).

Further, even successful treatment of depression leaves a substantial proportion of individuals with insomnia symptoms (Boland et al., 2020; Carney et al., 2011; Pigeon et al., 2009), and it does not appear to be improved with maintenance treatment for depression (Boland et al., 2020). Among individuals whose depression remitted, disturbed sleep is one of the most common residual symptoms following pharmacotherapy and cognitive therapy for depression (Carney et al., 2007; Nierenberg et al., 1999). In the study by Carney and colleagues, of the participants whose depression remitted 22% continue to experience difficulty falling asleep, 26% experienced difficulty with wakefulness after sleep onset, and 17% experienced early-morning awakenings.

It is likely that specific depression treatments produce differing levels of improvement in sleep disturbances. Consistent with this assertion, a large multicenter study of chronic depression found that the antidepressant nefazodone produced significantly greater improvements in subjective sleep than the cognitive analysis system of psychotherapy (Manber et al., 2003; Thase et al., 2002). Differential effects on sleep difficulties are evident even among individuals whose depression improves following different depression treatments. For example, a study comparing residual symptoms following response to reboxetine and fluoxetine found similar rates of overall residual insomnia symptoms (54% for fluoxetine vs. 56% for reboxetine); however, fluoxetine was associated with almost twice the rate of residual middle insomnia compared to reboxetine (Nelson et al., 2005). When insomnia symptoms persist following successful remission of depression, it may be that an insomnia disorder has developed and become comorbid with (now remitted) MDD.

Impact of Insomnia Treatment

Several studies have shown that an insomnia disorder that coexists with a depressive disorder can be successfully treated with cognitive behavioral therapy for insomnia (CBT-I; Carney et al., 2017; Manber et al., 2016), as well as with hypnotics (Fava et al., 2006). However, the effects of these sleep-focused treatments on depression outcomes are small. In a network meta-analysis, Ballesio and colleagues (2018) reported a small effect size ($d = 0.34$) of individual CBT-I on depression outcome among individuals with MDD who were not receiving concomitant depression treatment. In a study not included in this meta-analysis, where 107 participants with comorbid insomnia and MDD received antidepressant medications alone, CBT-I alone (CBT-I + pill placebo), or their combination, Carney and colleagues (2017) reported a significant reduction in depression symptom severity in each group, although with no difference between the three treatment types. The additive effects of CBT-I on depression outcomes, when provided along with a depression treatment, are more modest. Whereas a pilot study of CBT-I as an augmentation to an antidepressant medication found enhanced depression outcome in a sample of individuals with insomnia disorder and MDD, a more recent adequately powered study of CBT-I augmentation did not replicate this finding (Manber et al., 2016). Nonetheless, this study found that improvements in insomnia at treatment midpoint mediated eventual remission from depression; specifically, early change in insomnia severity predicted depression remission among those receiving CBT-I but not among those receiving the control insomnia intervention (Manber et al., 2016). Collectively, these findings suggest that treating insomnia disorder is a feasible and important therapeutic target in the overall management of MDD.

Insomnia as a Risk Factor for Future Depressive Episodes

Disturbed sleep and insomnia disorder predict subsequent depression (Riemann & Voderholzer, 2003). This conclusion has been reached by epidemiological studies with differing methodologies using varying definitions of insomnia symptoms and many examining depression and insomnia symptom severity, rather than diagnostic categories. Nonetheless, the picture that emerges is consistent; insomnia/disturbed sleep at Time 1 predicts depressive disorder/symptoms 1 to 3 years later. Two meta-analyses of longitudinal studies concluded that individuals with insomnia, compared to those without, are about twice as likely to develop depression (Baglioni et al., 2011; Li et al., 2016). Poor sleep predicts depression in various age groups, including adolescents (Johnson et al., 2006), young adults (Breslau et al., 1996; Buysse et al., 2008), and older adults (Cole & Dendukuri, 2003; Livingston et al., 1993; Perlis et al., 2006; Roberts et al., 2000). Disturbed sleep appears to also emerge as one of the first symptoms of recurrence among individuals whose depression previously remitted (Perlis et al., 1997).

KEY POINTS

- MDD is associated with difficulty initiating and maintaining sleep, as well as with REM and SWS abnormalities.
- Worse sleep quality and abnormal sleep profiles are associated with greater severity of depression, higher suicide risk, and worse response to depression treatment.
- Sleep difficulties among those with no current MDD predict future depressive episodes and, when present as residual symptoms following depression treatment, are associated with greater likelihood of relapse.
- CBT-I is effective for insomnia comorbid with MDD but has only small effects on depression symptoms.

BD

Sleep alterations are present in all three phases of BD, including the manic and the depressive states. For the majority (70%) of people with BD, insomnia symptoms persist into the inter-episodic period, and for a small proportion (25%), hypersomnia symptoms persist (Kaplan et al., 2011). Some of these alterations are phase-specific. In this section we discuss sleep in each of the three phases. Although beyond the scope of this chapter, we note that there has also been research in recent years on circadian factors in BD, including modest association with genes involved in circadian regulation and the possibility of increased prevalence eveningness tendency and blunted social rhythm (for a review, see Alloy et al., 2017).

SLEEP DURING A MANIC EPISODE

Decreased sleep need is one of seven diagnostic criteria for both manic and hypomanic episodes. It is defined by a reduction of time spent asleep that does not impact daytime energy levels or productivity. Disturbed or shorter-than-usual sleep is present in the vast majority of individuals during a manic state (Robillard et al., 2013). PSG of unmedicated individuals with BD during a manic state reveals abnormalities in REM and SWS that are similar to those reported in MDD (Hudson et al., 1988, 1992; Linkowski et al., 1986).

SLEEP DURING A DEPRESSIVE EPISODE

During depressive episodes, the sleep profiles of individuals with BD are largely similar to profiles of individuals with MDD, with higher prevalence of early-morning awakenings and greater REM fragmentation and density among those in a bipolar depressive episode (for reviews, see Harvey, 2008; Riemann et al., 2002). Experimentally induced sleep deprivation leads to improved mood during bipolar depressive episodes (Wu & Bunney, 1990), which is more pronounced than improvement in mood of individuals with unipolar depression (Barbini et al., 1998). The potential therapeutic use of sleep deprivation has been considered, but the procedure has not been adapted for clinical use because the benefit of forced sleep deprivation is lost after recovery sleep and because of concern that sleep deprivation incurs risk for a manic/hypomanic episode (Colombo et al., 1999). In considering ways to increase the clinical utility and efficacy of sleep deprivation among individuals with BD, researchers have reported that augmenting sleep deprivation with morning bright light exposure prolonged the benefits of sleep deprivation (Vai et al., 2015).

Hypersomnia, typically operationalized as increased sleep over 24 hours relative to euthymic states, is reported by many more individuals with bipolar than unipolar depression (Bowden, 2005; Frankland et al., 2015; Kaplan et al., 2015). A meta-analysis of 10 studies encompassing 1,824 individuals with BD estimated that approximately 30% of individuals with BD reported hypersomnia that was independent of the polarity of mood state or BD type (Grigolon et al., 2019). However, although hypersomnia is sometimes also construed as a high level of daytime sleepiness, Multiple Sleep Latency Tests, used as objective measures of daytime sleepiness, have not found clinically significant excessive daytime sleepiness (Nofzinger et al., 1991). This suggests that self-reported hypersomnia during a depressive episode might not index sleepiness per se but rather reflects related constructs such as low energy level, fatigue, anhedonia, or avoidance strategies.

SLEEP DURING INTER-EPISODIC PERIODS

Two meta-analyses published in recent years highlight that, as determined by actigraphy, sleep in the inter-episode phase of BD is characterized by both insomnia and hypersomnia symptoms, including long sleep-onset latency, long wake after sleep onset, and longer sleep durations (Geoffroy et al., 2015; Ng et al., 2015). (An actigraph is a sensitive motion sensor typically worn on the non-dominant wrist that provides estimates of sleep and wake states.) Ng and colleagues (2015) also found that, compared to healthy controls, adults with BD who were studied during inter-episodic periods report more severe daytime sleepiness, larger night-to-night variability in sleep duration, and more unstable rest–activity cycles based on actigraphy data. Findings regarding EEG differences between individuals with BD and healthy controls were sparse and inconsistent and hence do not support meaningful conclusions. It is estimated that 70% of individuals with BD experience sleep disruptions during the inter-episodic period and that 55% meet criteria for insomnia disorder (Harvey et al., 2005).

COMORBID SLEEP DISORDERS AND OTHER SLEEP ABNORMALITIES IN BD

Despite documentation of high prevalence of sleep continuity disturbances among individuals with BD during all phases of the disorder, the prevalence of an insomnia disorder (disturbed sleep associated with daytime impairment or distress) has not been documented. Circadian rhythm sleep–wake disorders, particularly delayed type, are also common in BD (e.g., Talih et al., 2018) and may predict shorter inter-episodic periods (Takaesu et al., 2017). The prevalence of OSA is estimated at 25% (Stubbs et al., 2016).

CLINICAL RELEVANCE

In their 2019 review of the literature on sleep alterations as prodromal symptoms of mood episodes in BD, Pancheri and colleagues (2019) concluded that decreased sleep need tends to precede the onset of a manic episode and that hypersomnia tends to precede depressive episodes; in contrast, insomnia symptoms were considered a non-specific prodrome, predicting both manic and depressive episodes. Wehr and colleagues (1987) proposed that the mood elevation caused by reduced sleep reinforces further curtailment of sleep and therefore progressively heightens mood to the level of a manic or hypomanic phase. It is estimated that 77% of individuals with BD report reduced sleep duration as a prodromal symptom to a manic episode (Jackson et al., 2003). Estimates are lower (44%) when sleep loss is measured objectively using actigraphy (Wehr et al., 1982) and even lower (5% and 12%) in studies that induce experimental sleep deprivation as a therapy for bipolar depression (Colombo et al., 1999; Kasper & Wehr, 1992). Individuals with rapid cycling between manic and depressive states might be particularly vulnerable to the effects of insufficient sleep.

Both light therapy and dark therapy have been studied among individuals with BD, the former for the treatment of depressive episodes and the latter for the treatment of manic episodes (Henriksen et al., 2016). Despite case reports cautioning about bright light exposure as contributing to poor sleep and a trigger for manic episodes among individuals with BD (Benedetti, 2018), a review of the literature and recent data suggest that bright light therapy for depression among adults with BP is safe (Benedetti, 2018; Sit et al., 2018; Zhou et al., 2018). There is some evidence that forced rest/darkness and use of blue light–blocking glasses during a window of time that overlaps with the goal sleep period could stabilize mood during the manic phase of BD, even when it does not result in lengthening of sleep duration (Barbini et al., 2005).

As in the case of unipolar depression, the moderating effects of insomnia symptoms could negatively impact response to treatment of BD, and this effect may depend on the intervention. For example, within the Systematic Treatment Enhancement Program for BD trial, individuals with BD who had sleep disturbances at baseline had a lower probability of sustained response to pharmacological treatment with quetiapine versus lithium compared to those without sleep disturbance; this was not the case for psychosocial interventions (Sylvia et al., 2018). A pilot randomized controlled trial provides initial evidence that treatment with CBT-I during an inter-episodic period is effective and has the potential to improve some bipolar outcomes (Harvey et al., 2015). Specifically, during the 6-month follow-up, CBT-I led to fewer days in a bipolar episode (mania, hypomania, depression) than an education control intervention (3 vs. 25 days). Moreover, individuals with bipolar I disorder who received CBT-I had a significantly lower rate of relapse into hypomania/mania (4.6% vs. 31.6%) than those receiving the control intervention. To promote safety, the CBT-I intervention introduced time in bed restriction later in the course of treatment than traditionally used when treating individuals without BD and only if needed. The intervention also included the RISE-UP routine (Kaplan et al., 2018), which consists of a set of behaviors and environmental cues to promote alertness upon waking up. This component of the intervention, introduced at the first session, led to reduced morning sleep inertia during the following week.

KEY POINTS

- Sleep abnormalities are present in all three phases of BD.
- During a depressive episode, sleep difficulties are similar to those experienced by individuals with MDD; however, early-morning awakenings and hypersomnia are experienced more often.
- During a manic episode, patients report more disturbed sleep and lower sleep need, and three-quarters of patients report sleep loss as a prodromal symptom.

- During a euthymic inter-episode phase, poor sleep quality is reported, but evidence for abnormal objective sleep profiles is mixed.
- Preliminary data suggests that CBT-I provided during an inter-episode phase is effective for insomnia and is associated with reduced risk for hypomania/mania relapse, and that the added RISE-UP component promotes alertness after waking.

Anxiety Disorders

PD

Sleep symptoms in PD are generally characterized by difficulties falling asleep, difficulties staying asleep, and nocturnal panic attacks. Some have attributed difficulties falling asleep to pre-sleep misappraisals of physiological events that may occur during sleep (Craske, Lang, Mystkowski, et al., 2002) or fears about a loss of vigilance to body-focused cues (Tsao & Craske, 2003). A recent study utilizing national claim data in South Korea estimates that 33% of individuals with PD also had insomnia (i.e., received an *International Classification of Diseases* code of insomnia; Park et al., 2018). This study also found that individuals with sleep disorders had a higher incidence of PD than those without, with the strongest association existing among those with an insomnia diagnosis; this association persisted even after adjusting for multiple variables, including comorbidities.

NOCTURNAL PANIC

People who experience nocturnal panic attacks describe awakening spontaneously, without a trigger, in sudden fear and with a number of associated physiological symptoms, such as heart palpitations, increased breathing rate, and a sensation of choking. Nocturnal panic (NP) attacks are frequent in individuals with PD, with 30%–45% reporting having experienced repeated NP (Craske & Tsao, 2005). PSG studies found that NP attacks tend to arise in the transition from Stage 2 to Stage 3 sleep as respiration slows and becomes more regular (Mellman & Uhde, 1989). As compared to healthy individuals, those with PD have increased micro-apneas and micro-hypopneas and more air inhaled and exhaled at each breath during REM sleep (e.g., Stein et al., 1995). These authors hypothesized that these micro-apnea and micro-hypopnea events increase sensitivity to carbon dioxide levels and that this hypersensitivity may trigger a panic attack.

Studies comparing levels of sleep disturbances in PD between individuals with and without NP have mixed findings. One study reports little evidence for greater levels of sleep disturbances in PD individuals with NP outside of sleep disruptions directly associated with NP; the only significant finding was increased difficulty with sleep onset (Craske, Lang, Mystkowski, et al., 2002). This observation of longer sleep-onset latency in the context of NP has been reported in one other previous study (Mellman & Uhde, 1989). The largest study (n = 773) of individuals with diagnosed PD with and without

NP, as well as with and without lifetime depression, reported high rates of self-reported sleep disturbances in all four groups, ranging between 67% and 91% (Singareddy & Uhde, 2009). Participants in the NP plus depression group endorsed the highest levels of sleep disturbances (91%) compared to the other groups (NP without lifetime depression: 78.5%, PD without depression or NP: 66.7%). The authors conclude that the presence of NP attacks and depression is independently and interactively associated with rates of sleep disturbance PD (Singareddy & Uhde, 2009).

Craske and colleagues propose an interoceptive conditioning model to explain NP attacks (Craske et al., 2005; Craske, Lang, Rowe, et al., 2002). They suggest that individuals with PD preferentially attend to somatic stimuli during sleep and that aberrations in internal stimuli trigger a panic attack. They further suggest that a person awakens from NP and then assigns catastrophic attributions to their body sensations. Consistent with this model, they have found that among people with PD, those with NP endorsed more panic symptoms when exposed to imagery of hypnosis than neutral scenes compared to those without NP. This has been interpreted as evidence that NP is related to fear of loss of vigilance (Tsao & Craske, 2003). Individuals with NP attacks who were led to believe that signals of physiological state during sleep were unexpected (vs. expected) had more NP attacks (Craske, Lang, Rowe, et al., 2002). Also consistent with this theory is the efficacy of CBT for NP attacks, which helps people learn how to restructure catastrophic beliefs about bodily sensations (Craske et al., 2005). Other theoretical models have postulated a biological diathesis for NP attacks. In support of these models, sleep deprivation (Mellman & Uhde, 1989; Roy-Byrne et al., 1986) and administration of caffeine and cholecystokinin-4 challenges during SWS appear to elicit NP (Craske & Tsao, 2005).

PSG FINDINGS IN PD

In general, objective sleep findings in PD are mixed. Multiple studies comparing individuals with PD to healthy controls have reported increased sleep-onset latency, decreased sleep efficiency, and decreased total sleep time compared to healthy adults, although some studies report no differences (for a review, see Cox & Olatunji, 2016). Individuals with PD and comorbid depression have PSG sleep profiles that are a mixture of both disorders but without shortened REM latency, which is present in MDD (Dube et al., 1986; Grunhaus et al., 1986). It is not known if and how the presence of NP contributes to EEG alterations among individuals with PD. One exception is the finding of modest reductions in SWS and some disruptions to sleep continuity (Arriaga et al., 1996; Stein, Enns, & Kryger, 1993) among individuals with NP without comorbid depression.

COMORBID SLEEP DISORDERS AND OTHER SLEEP ABNORMALITIES

Sleep paralysis is common among individuals with PD, with one study of 133 consecutive individuals presenting for treatment of panic symptoms (95% of whom met diagnostic criteria for PD) reporting that 29.3% experienced isolated sleep paralysis (Sharpless et al., 2010). However, the increased prevalence may not be unique to PD as Otto and colleagues (2006) did not find differences in the rates of sleep paralysis in PD compared with other anxiety disorders (GAD, social anxiety) in a primarily Caucasian sample with high levels of psychiatric comorbidity. There is evidence that African Americans with PD have higher rates of recurrent sleep paralysis than Caucasians with PD (59% vs. 7%; Paradis & Friedman, 2005). This is consistent with findings that African Americans are more likely to experience sleep paralysis in general (23% compared to 6% of Caucasians), which might be related to differential levels of stress and cultural/spiritual factors (Ohayon & Pakpour, 2022). Together, these results suggest that the experience of sleep paralysis is relatively common in PD, particularly among African Americans, and that this association may be a result of their experience of stress and/or anxious mood in general.

It has also been reported that individuals with PD have increased nocturnal movements (Hauri et al., 1989), especially on nights when NP attacks do not occur (Brown & Uhde, 2003). Moreover, among individuals with PD, those with no NP have the highest rate of nocturnal movement (Brown & Uhde, 2003). From these findings, Brown and Uhde suggest that increased nocturnal movement may be a protective factor against NP attacks. Specifically, they propose that movement may delay progression into SWS, which may allow chemoreceptors more time to accommodate to the hypercapnia associated with the transition to sleep onset, which might be the trigger for NP attacks.

CLINICAL RELEVANCE

Whereas sleep deprivation has been identified as a trigger for panic attacks (Mellman & Uhde, 1989; Roy-Byrne et al., 1986), the relationship between disturbed sleep and the severity of PD is not clear. More is known about the clinical relevance of experiencing NP attacks. Some, but not all (Craske, Lang, Mystkowski, et al., 2002; Norton et al., 1999), studies find greater disease severity among individuals with PD who experience NP attacks, as indexed by more somatic symptoms (Craske & Barlow, 1989), more severe fears of panic symptoms (Craske & Kreuger 1990), and higher rates of comorbid depression and anxiety disorders (Labbate et al., 1994). While one study found higher rates of suicidality among individuals with PD and NP compared to those without NP (Agargun & Kara, 1998), another found similar rates of suicidality in these two groups but reported that those with NP reported more past suicide attempts than individuals with daytime panic symptoms and rated themselves as more likely to make an attempt in the future (Smith et al., 2020). Individuals with PD and NP also report higher rates of trauma (Freed et al., 1999) and less agoraphobic avoidance (Craske, Lang, Mystkowski, et al., 2002).

Two studies have shed light on considerations for treatment of sleep disturbances in individuals with PD. The first of these two studies suggests that CBT of PD leaves a significant proportion of individuals with clinically meaningful problems with sleep at post-treatment (Cousineau et al., 2016). While it has not been replicated in other studies, this preliminary finding suggests that an insomnia-focused treatment is needed for addressing sleep difficulties among individuals with PD. The second study found that nicotine dependence partially mediated the relationship between insomnia and PD (as well as with insomnia and PTSD) even after adjusting for major depressive episodes, drug and alcohol dependence, and gender (Babson et al., 2008). This finding suggests that nicotine use is an important health behavior to assess and address when treating insomnia among people with PD.

KEY POINTS

- Individuals with PD report difficulties falling and staying asleep that continue even after successful treatment of PD.
- Individuals with PD also report NP attacks, which seem to emerge primarily in the transition between non-REM (NREM) Stages 2 and 3, and can be triggered by insufficient sleep.
- Individuals with PD are more likely to experience sleep paralysis than healthy controls.

GAD

In the DSM-5, disturbed sleep is characterized as a symptom of GAD within the vigilance and scanning symptom cluster. Insomnia symptoms in GAD are characterized by excessive worry and rumination. The vast majority (75%–90%) of individuals with GAD report insomnia symptoms (Arriaga et al., 1995; Belanger et al., 2004; Brenes et al., 2009; Monti & Monti, 2000). Belanger and colleagues (2004) studied a sample of 44 individuals with GAD and found that approximately 48% reported difficulties falling asleep, 64% reported difficulties staying asleep, and 57% reported difficulties awakening too early. Among older adults, those with GAD are more likely to report disturbed sleep than those classified as "worried well," suggesting that the intensity or excessiveness of worry and rumination may contribute to elevated rates of sleep disturbances in GAD (Brenes et al., 2009).

PSG FINDINGS IN GAD

Results from objective sleep assessments in GAD align with subjective reports of sleep disturbances. Monti and Monti (2000) conducted a systematic review of six PSG-based studies in GAD and found that the majority of studies documented longer sleep-onset latency and wake time after sleep onset and shorter total sleep time compared to controls. There is also evidence for increased percent of Stage 2 and Stage 4 (Arriaga & Paiva, 1990); one small study also reported increased REM latency among adults with GAD (Lund et al., 1991). This study additionally compared patients with GAD and MDD and found increased REM latency in GAD, a result consistent with two earlier studies (Papadimitriou, Kerkhofs, et al., 1988; Reynolds et al., 1983). Adults with both

GAD and MDD appear to have REM latency indices more similar to GAD than MDD (Papadimitriou, Linkowski, et al., 1988).

CLINICAL RELEVANCE

Generally, research has shown that sleep problems in GAD are of clinical concern but not as severe as they are in MDD (Papadimitriou, Linkowski, et al., 1988; Reynolds et al., 1983). Interestingly, insomnia symptom severity does not appear to correlate with GAD severity (Belanger et al., 2004). Findings regarding the effects of CBT for GAD on insomnia are mixed. In one study, individuals with GAD did not experience residual sleep problems after effective treatment with CBT for anxiety (Belanger et al., 2004); however, another study found that although CBT for GAD improved insomnia symptoms, one-third of those who met criteria for insomnia pre-treatment still met criteria post-treatment (Cousineau et al., 2016).

Several studies have examined the effectiveness of an insomnia-focused treatment, behavioral or pharmacological, among individuals with GAD. One open-label trial of CBT-I for individuals with comorbid insomnia and GAD reported moderate to large effect sizes for sleep and anxiety outcomes (Jansson-Frojmark & Jacobson, 2021). Two additional studies have examined the effects of sleep medications on insomnia and GAD outcomes. In one of these two studies, individuals with GAD and insomnia symptoms who had a partial response to GAD treatment with an SSRI or an SNRI were prescribed 8 mg ramelteon (open label). The study found that ramelteon was associated with pre- to post-treatment improvement in both sleep and anxiety symptoms (Gross et al., 2009). Another study found that the addition of a sleep medication to an anxiety-focused treatment led to greater improvements in anxiety than treatment for anxiety alone (Pollack et al., 2008).

Two additional studies have examined sequencing or relative efficacy of CBT for anxiety and CBT-I. One study addressed the question of sequencing. It compared two sequential orders of CBT for GAD and CBT-I in a sample with comorbid insomnia and GAD. It found that providing CBT-GAD first produced "superior clinical benefits in anxiety and sleep" compared to beginning treatment with CBT-I (Belleville et al., 2016). However, a study of the differential efficacy of CBT-I versus CBT for anxiety among individuals with both clinically significant insomnia and anxiety symptoms found that CBT-I was more effective at reducing insomnia symptoms and equally effective at reducing anxiety symptoms; at 3-month follow-up, however, gains in both treatment groups were equivalent (Mason et al., 2023). Together, these results suggest that treating insomnia in patients with clinically significant insomnia and anxiety symptoms is beneficial, although the presence of high levels of general anxiety, as seen in GAD, may interfere with maximum benefit of CBTI. In the latter case concomitant treatment of both symptoms might be the best strategy, but this assertion needs to be tested.

Interestingly, unlike depressive disorders, in which one night of sleep deprivation results in mood elevation on the following day, a night of sleep deprivation has little therapeutic benefit in GAD (Labbate et al., 1998). Transcranial magnetic stimulation (TMS) is a promising novel intervention for individuals with GAD and insomnia, with some evidence of significant improvements in both anxiety and insomnia symptoms (Huang et al., 2018). While anxiety and insomnia severity were not correlated at baseline in this study, improvement in anxiety and sleep (as measured by the Pittsburgh Sleep Quality Index) were, potentially suggesting a global positive impact of TMS on functioning. Another clinically relevant study of older adults with GAD concluded that a modest amount of alcohol may minimize the association between anxiety/worry and insomnia (Ivan et al., 2014). In this study, modest alcohol use was helpful for reducing anxiety without interfering with sleep; in fact, alcohol use was associated with less severe insomnia. This finding indicates that nuance is needed in providing psychoeducation about the impact of alcohol on sleep when working with older adults with GAD.

KEY POINTS

- Individuals with GAD report prolonged latency to sleep onset and difficulties staying asleep that are also detected in overnight sleep studies; however, the severity of these symptoms does not appear to correlate with the severity of GAD.
- Augmenting treatment for GAD with medications or with CBT-I enhances anxiety symptom reduction. In the case of non-pharmacological combination of treatments, sequencing matters: CBT for GAD followed by CBT-I produces better anxiety and insomnia outcomes than the reverse order.
- TMS is emerging as a novel intervention for patients with GAD and insomnia that improves both anxiety and insomnia symptoms.

OCD

Sleep-onset and sleep-maintenance difficulties in OCD are often associated with obsessional worries accompanied by checking behaviors (Insel et al., 1982). Approximately 0.2% of the general population qualifies for a diagnosis of insomnia related to OCD (Ohayon, 1997), and 5% of young adults with an insomnia diagnosis have OCD (Breslau et al., 1996). A nationally representative study sample from the United States (n = 2,073) found that individuals with sleep disturbance reported increased obsessive–compulsive (OC) symptom severity compared to those without sleep disturbances and, further, that sleep disturbance severity was associated with OC symptoms, even adjusting for depression and other anxiety-related disorders (Cox & Olatunji, 2016). A population study conducted in Sweden identified 31,856 individuals diagnosed with OCD in a cohort of over 13 million individuals living in Sweden (Sevilla-Cermeno et al., 2020). In this study, individuals with OCD had nearly sevenfold odds of receiving an insomnia diagnosis or receiving a drug with a specific indication for insomnia, compared to individuals without an OCD diagnosis. The strength of this relationship weakened when individuals with comorbid depression and anxiety disorder were excluded (odds ratio = 4.97 and 4.51, respectively).

Two large studies have examined the relationships between OCD symptomatology and sleep disturbances. One study found a significant relationship between insomnia and obsessions but not compulsions (Timpano et al., 2014), which was maintained when adjusting for depression symptoms. A second, more recent, study conducted a network analysis using data from 773 patients with a primary OCD diagnosis in residential and outpatient settings. It found only a "very weak" correlation between OCD symptoms and insomnia and hypersomnia symptoms, with low bridge and strength centrality (Litvin et al., 2022). It is possible that an association between sleep and OCD symptoms may vary by the extent to which the OCD symptoms occur during the time in bed or the time leading to it, but this possibility will need to be tested empirically.

There is also increasing evidence for a positive relationship between a delayed or eveningness tendency and OCD or OC symptoms. One publication examining both cross-sectional (n = 341) and prospective (n = 382) data found that while depression better accounted for cross-sectional associations between eveningness and OC symptoms, prospectively, eveningness was a stronger predictor of change in OC symptoms (Cox & Olatunji, 2016). In this prospective study, sleep disturbance, but not total sleep time, partially mediated the relationship between eveningness and OC symptoms. Another study of 74 participants categorized the sample into adults with OCD, adults without OCD (with another psychiatric disorder), and adults with no psychiatric disorders. It found that, compared to adults without any psychiatric disorder, adults with OCD had more symptoms suggestive of delayed circadian phase (higher eveningness tendency scores, later mid-sleep timing, higher rates of circadian rhythm sleep wake disorder [delayed sleep phase type]) and higher insomnia symptoms (Cox & Olatunji, 2022). Additionally, in the total sample, OCD severity was associated with insomna and delayed sleep phase, and insomnia symptoms mediated the relationship between OCD severity and delayed sleep phase symptoms. These findings suggest strong relationships between delayed circadian timing and OCD symptomatology as well as a potential mediating role for insomnia. Complementary support for this hypothesized relationship comes from one small study of adults consecutively hospitalized for inpatient treatment of severe OCD, which found that 41.9% met diagnostic criteria for delayed sleep phase syndrome, currently known as *circadian rhythm sleep–wake disorder, delayed sleep phase type* (Turner et al., 2007). Notably, this study excluded individuals who had comorbid major depression (or schizophrenia or other major medical comorbidities), removing the potential that depression was driving the relationship with delayed sleep phase.

PSG FINDINGS IN OCD

Two systematic reviews and meta-analyses of sleep and OCD have been completed (Cox et al., 2020; Diaz-Roman et al., 2015). The meta-analysis conducted by Diaz-Roman and colleagues, which included four studies, reported that total sleep time, time awake, sleep efficiency, and Stage 2 sleep differed between individuals with OCD and healthy controls. However, in a subgoup analysis, where individuals with comorbid major depression were excluded, as well as in the Cox and colleagues meta-analysis of two studies, only the sleep-latency variable was significant, suggesting that the presence of depression likely accounts for much of the abnormal PSG findings in this population. The Cox and colleagues (2020) review and meta-analysis of sleep and anxiety disorders identified 11 studies examining sleep patterns in OCD. Subsequent analyses found a large effect size for decreased total sleep time compared to healthy controls (average of 35.96 minutes less) and a trend-level medium effect for increased REM sleep. No differences were found in sleep continuity and sleep depth, and the authors state that they identified insufficient studies to examine subjective sleep disturbance. The (null) main effect of sleep continuity was significantly moderated by inclusion of comorbid MDD; individuals with comorbid MDD had a trend-level decrease in sleep continuity compared to controls, whereas this effect was not significant in those with OCD alone. Findings from these meta-analyses suggest that depression accounts for at least some of the relationship between OCD and sleep disturbances.

CLINICAL RELEVANCE

To our knowledge, no studies to date have examined the impact of sleep-specific treatments on OCD symptoms. One study deprived individuals with OCD of sleep for 3 days and found large individual differences in OC behaviors in response to sleep deprivation that were not related to changes in mood (Joffe & Swinson, 1988). Two studies have examined the impact of concentrated exposure treatment of OCD on sleep-related outcomes. The first study assessed 36 individuals before undergoing 4 days of concentrated exposure treatment for OCD and found that 70% had sleep difficulties indicative of insomnia disorder (Nordahl et al., 2018). Post-treatment (immediate and at 6-month follow-up), both OCD and insomnia symptoms improved, although a number of individuals still experienced subthreshold insomnia symptoms. The second study examined the effects of a concentrated exposure treatment (4 days) for OCD on insomnia symptoms (Hagen et al., 2021). In this study, 16 individuals received the concentrated exposure treatment and 16 received self-help treatment; an additional group of 16 individuals was assigned to a wait-list condition. This study found that insomnia symptoms did not improve with OCD treatment, but at the 3-month follow-up, there was improvement in insomnia symptoms for individuals receiving the concentrated exposure treatment. This change was largely related to change in depressive symptoms, suggesting that improving OCD symptoms may not directly impact insomnia symptoms.

Two studies have examined whether insomnia or circadian rhythm disturbances predicted response to OCD treatment with repetitive TMS (rTMS) combined with psychotherapy. In one small study of 22 adults with OCD, measures of circadian rhythm sleep disorders accurately predicted non-response to rTMS (combined with psychotherapy) with 83% sensitivity and 63% specificity, while models using insomnia symptoms did not accurately predict non-response (Donse et al., 2017). The authors hypothesize that circadian rhythm disturbances may represent a marker for different subtypes of OCD or for treatment response and highlight the need to consider the contribution of circadian factors when treating individuals with OCD and disturbed sleep. In a follow-up study of 61 adults with OCD treated with combined rTMS and CBT, several insomnia/sleep variables were found to predict treatment response; these variables included subjective sleep quality, sleep latency, daytime dysfunction, as well as insomnia severity (Gajadien et al., 2023). Additional research is needed to gain insight into the role of circadian factors versus more general sleep disruptions in predicting response to rTMS plus psychotherapy.

KEY POINTS

- Individuals with OCD report sleep initiation and maintenance difficulties that tend to be associated with their obsessions and, to a lesser degree, with their compulsions.
- To the extent that abnormal PSG-measured sleep abnormalities are present among people with OCD, they are believed to be related to comorbid depression, which is common among those with OCD.
- Increasing evidence suggests a relationship between OCD and circadian rhythm sleep–wake disorder, delayed sleep phase type, and a potential mediating role of insomnia symptoms in this relationship.

Social Anxiety Disorder

Among the anxiety disorders, the relationship between sleep and social anxiety has been studied the least. Ohayon (1997) found that 0.1% of the general population qualifies for a diagnosis of insomnia related to social phobia. In this large French epidemiological study, social phobia was one of the least prevalent among insomnia-related-to-anxiety disorders. In one study of college students with clinical levels of social anxiety, approximately 18% reported significant levels of insomnia symptoms (Buckner et al., 2008). In another study of 191 individuals with social anxiety disorders, a third of the sample were classified as likely having an insomnia disorder as measured with the Insomnia Severity Index (28.5% severe, 5% moderate), and an additional third were classified as having subthreshold insomnia (Raffray et al., 2011). In this study, where participants were recruited from a treatment clinic, approximately 40% of participants were taking psychotropic medications; further research is needed to assess rates of insomnia disorder among individuals with social anxiety disorder without this potential confounding effect. As is the case in other classes of anxiety disorders, depression may contribute to sleep disturbances in social anxiety disorders. One study found that depression symptoms may partially mediate the relationship between social anxiety and insomnia symptoms (Buckner et al., 2008), although others did not (Stein, Kroft, & Walker, 1993). One night of sleep deprivation does not increase social phobia behaviors in individuals with social anxiety disorder (Labbate et al., 1998).

No differences in objectively assessed sleep indices were found between normal controls and individuals with social anxiety disorder (e.g., Brown & Uhde, 2003; Papadimitriou & Linkowski, 2005). There were also no differences when comparing objective sleep parameters between individuals with social anxiety disorder and those with NP (Brown & Uhde, 2003).

KEY POINTS

- Individuals with social anxiety report difficulties initiating and maintaining sleep that are partially mediated by the presence of depression.
- PSG studies did not find differences in sleep of individuals with social anxiety and health controls.

PTSD

Disturbed sleep is a hallmark feature of PTSD (Germain, 2013). An estimated 70%–92% of individuals with PTSD report sleep disturbances including insomnia symptoms, nightmares, sleep disordered breathing (SDB), and parasomnias (Maher et al., 2006; Milanak et al., 2019; Ohayon & Shapiro, 2000). Sleep continuity difficulties and nightmares are the most commonly reported sleep symptoms in PTSD, and both are considered symptoms of PTSD within the DSM-5 nosology (American Psychiatric Association, 2013). Insomnia symptoms are characterized within the PTSD Criterion E ("alterations in arousal and reactivity") symptom cluster. Approximately 27%–60% of individuals with PTSD demonstrate clinically significant insomnia symptoms (Byrne et al., 2021; M. M. Jenkins et al., 2015; Ohayon & Shapiro, 2000). Nightmares are categorized within the PTSD Criterion B ("intrusion") symptom cluster. Approximately 52%–96% of individuals with PTSD experience nightmares (Leskin et al., 2002; Neylan et al., 2002). True prevalence estimates of sleep symptoms and disorders in the context of PTSD are highly limited by measurement approach and representativeness of samples.

In addition to insomnia symptoms and nightmares, individuals with PTSD demonstrate a range of other sleep disturbances. Individuals with PTSD report fear of sleep, which may be associated with avoidant bedtime behaviors and nocturnal self-reports of hypervigilance, two factors that could contribute to the development and maintenance of both insomnia and nightmare disorders (Werner et al., 2021). PTSD is also associated with elevated rates of OSA (Zhang et al., 2017), REM sleep behavior (Elliott et al., 2020), and periodic limb movements (Brown & Boudewyns, 1996) compared to the general population, though most of this work is focused exclusively on veteran samples. Recently, some have proposed the existence of a trauma-associated sleep disorder, which manifests as a combination of nightmares, REM without atonia, dream enactment, and disruptive nighttime behaviors including somnambulism, vocalizations, and combative behavior toward bed partners (Brock et al., 2019). Trauma-related sleep disorder has not yet been included in any diagnostic nosology, nor are prevalence estimates available.

PSG FINDINGS IN PTSD

There is little agreement between objective sleep assessments and subjective reports by individuals with PTSD (Breslau et al., 2004).

A meta-analysis of 20 studies (722 participants) found no consistent differences between participants with and without PTSD on PSG-defined sleep-onset or sleep-maintenance difficulties (Kobayashi et al., 2007). Nevertheless, a number of abnormalities in sleep architecture have been observed among individuals with PTSD. A meta-analysis concluded that individuals with PTSD have more Stage 1 sleep (light sleep), less SWS (deep sleep), and greater REM density than individuals without PTSD (Kobayashi et al., 2007). It has been suggested that the abnormalities in REM sleep may reflect increased REM pressure, likely a result of an overall fragmented and shorter REM sleep (Mellman et al., 2002).

Duration of continuous REM correlates inversely with subjective reports of insomnia symptoms (Mellman et al., 2002). As REM sleep is involved in emotional processing, interruption of REM may contribute to difficulties in emotional adaptation after a traumatic event (Levin & Nielsen, 2007). Supporting this notion is the fact that successful treatment of nightmares (e.g., imagery rehearsal therapy; exposure, relaxation, and rescripting therapy; and prazosin) leads to reduction in PTSD symptoms (Yucel et al., 2020). The therapeutic effects of these treatments are thought to be related to them leading to an increase in uninterrupted REM sleep; this mechanism of action has been preliminarily demonstrated for both prazosin (F. B. Taylor et al., 2008) and imagery rehearsal therapy (Germain et al., 2012).

One reason for mixed findings concerning sleep in PTSD may stem from unassessed comorbid depression (Kobayashi et al., 2007). Preliminary research suggests greater sleep disturbance when both disorders are present, as compared to PTSD alone (Leskin et al., 2002). Two studies have used PSG to assess sleep in a PTSD/MDD sample. One study suggested more similarities than differences between the MDD only and the PTSD/MDD groups (Dow et al., 1996). The study found that both PTSD/MDD and MDD had decreased REM latency, increased REM density, reduced total sleep time, and reduced sleep efficiency. The only detected difference was longer sleep-onset latency among individuals with MDD than among those with PTSD/MDD or PTSD only. The second study found shortened REM latency among individuals with PTSD/MDD as well as among those with only PTSD (Woodward et al., 1996). Also, the PTSD/MDD group had greater REM density and less SWS (common sleep abnormalities in MDD) than individuals with PTSD only (Woodward et al., 1996). These findings are consistent with results reported by Ohayon and Shapiro (2000), indicating that depression may explain a significant portion of insomnia symptoms in anxiety disorders.

COMORBID SLEEP DISORDERS AND OTHER SLEEP ABNORMALITIES

Several reports have found that individuals with PTSD have higher levels of automatic motor behavior (e.g., more periodic movements) during both REM and NREM sleep (Brown & Boudewyns, 1996), although they may have overall less body movement time (Leskin et al., 2002). There is higher prevalence of both PLMD and REM behavior disorder among individuals with PTSD than in the population at large (de Boer et al., 2020). There is also a high rate of SDB among individuals with PTSD (B. J. Krakow et al., 2015; Zhang et al., 2017), which may be due to indirect factors, such as increased obesity and use of sedatives. B. Krakow and colleagues (2002) noted that among individuals with PTSD, difficulties initiating or maintaining sleep were more frequently reported by those with SDB than excessive daytime sleepiness. These authors suggested that SDB and PTSD symptoms interact so that arousals and awakenings caused by SDB are prolonged by the PTSD symptom hypervigilance. This interaction might also contribute to increased nightmare frequency because a significant number of respiratory arousals tend to occur in REM sleep, leading to increased awakenings from dreams.

CLINICAL RELEVANCE

In general, few studies have examined the temporal relationships between sleep problems and PTSD. Emerging data suggests that individuals who report sleep disturbance within 1 month after trauma exposure may be more likely to develop PTSD (Babson & Feldner, 2010). However, PSG data collected shortly after the trauma in one of these studies indicated that individuals who develop PTSD after a trauma have faster sleep initiation, a shorter duration of continuous REM, and no differences in wakefulness after sleep onset compared to those who do not (Mellman et al., 2007).

As is the case in MDD, disturbed sleep often does not fully resolve following successful treatment of PTSD (Zayfert & DeViva, 2004). Zayfert and DeViva (2004) found that 48% of individuals with PTSD successfully treated with CBT for PTSD continued to experience insomnia symptoms even after their nightmares remitted. This is a remarkably similar figure to the estimated prevalence of residual sleep disturbance in those who remitted from MDD (Nierenberg et al., 2010). This suggests that disturbed sleep in PTSD merits separate targeted sleep intervention (Miller et al., 2020). Whereas the severity of subjectively reported disturbed sleep did not differ according to the type of trauma (Germain et al., 2004), individuals with PTSD whose trauma was experienced in a sleep-related context might be at higher risk for residual insomnia symptoms than those with childhood abuse history (Zayfert & DeViva, 2004).

Increasing evidence suggests sleep disturbances may be a risk factor for PTSD, not merely a symptom of the disorder (Koffel et al., 2016; Pruiksma et al., 2016; D. J. Taylor et al., 2016). Individuals with both preexisting and post-trauma sleep disturbances are at elevated risk for the development of PTSD (Bryant et al., 2010; Mellman et al., 2007). For example, pre-trauma insomnia symptoms prospectively predicted PTSD among injured and combat veterans (Bryant et al., 2010; Gehrman et al., 2013; Koffel et al., 2013). Also, one longitudinal study of victims of motor vehicle accidents (N = 102) found that the presence of insomnia symptoms at 1 month post-trauma was associated with the development of a PTSD diagnosis at the 12-month follow-up (Klein et al., 2003).

Sleep disturbances like insomnia and nightmares that develop during the course of PTSD are unlikely to remit without targeted treatment. A study of 108 active-duty Army soldiers successfully treated for PTSD found that insomnia complaints remained in 77% and nightmares remained in 52% of the sample (Pruiksma et al., 2016). Though PTSD may precipitate the development of sleep disturbances, these disturbances can and often do develop into co-occurring disorders which merit independent attention. There is emerging evidence that CBT-I is effective for improving sleep among individuals with PTSD (Talbot et al., 2014), as well as initial evidence that integrating CBT-I into psychotherapy for PTSD could increase sleep duration (Colvonen et al., 2019).

KEY POINTS

- Sleep symptoms experienced by individuals with PTSD include difficulties initiating and maintaining sleep, nightmares, and fear of going to sleep.
- Compared to healthy controls, those with PTSD are more likely to experience SDB, periodic limb movements, and parasomnias, including nightmare disorder.
- Whereas disturbed sleep does not fully resolve following successful treatment of PTSD, emerging evidence suggests that CBT-I is effective and may result in decreases in PTSD symptoms.
- The unique sleep symptoms experienced by individuals with PTSD have led to a proposal for a new disorder, *trauma-associated sleep disorder*, characterized by nightmares, REM without atonia, dream enactment, and disruptive nighttime behaviors.

Schizophrenia

Individuals with schizophrenia often report difficulty initiating and maintaining sleep and poor sleep quality (Hofstetter et al., 2005). Estimates of the prevalence of insomnia symptoms among individuals with schizophrenia range from 30% to 80% (Chan et al., 2017; Korenic et al., 2020). The wide range is likely due to differences in definitions of insomnia symptoms and differences in sample characteristics, including use of medications, types of medication used, and presence of current psychotic symptoms. When psychotic symptoms worsen, so do sleep quality and fatigue; there is also a reduction in sleep duration, an increase in occurrence of upsetting dreams and nightmares, and an increase in circadian rhythm disturbances such as delayed phase (Chung et al., 2018; Korenic et al., 2020; Lemyre et al., 2019; Wulff et al., 2012).

PSG FINDINGS IN SCHIZOPHRENIA

A meta-analysis of 31 studies that collected PSG data from 574 individuals with schizophrenia (both medicated and unmedicated) and 515 healthy controls found that individuals with schizophrenia had longer sleep-onset latency, shorter total sleep time, and lower sleep efficiency (Chan et al., 2017). This meta-analysis also found that the medication-naive individuals had more wakefulness after sleep onset and that the observed sleep disturbances were more severe among individuals who discontinued antipsychotic medications prior to study participation compared to those who were medication-naive. When looking across multiple systematic reviews, results on SWS and sleep spindles were inconclusive (Carruthers et al., 2021; Chan et al., 2017); however these studies suggest compared to healthy controls, individuals with schizophrenia have longer time in bed, shorter sleep duration, faster latency to REM sleep, and greater REM density (Carruthers et al., 2021; Chan et al., 2017).

COMORBID SLEEP DISORDERS

A population-based study found a low prevalence rate of OSA in schizophrenia and other psychotic disorders, estimating the rate to be 4.5% (Sharafkhaneh et al., 2005). However, it appears that for inpatient populations with schizophrenia the rate of comorbid OSA is much higher at 48% (Takahashi et al., 1998). Several reasons may account for the high prevalence of OSA among individuals with more severe schizophrenia. These include weight gain due to antipsychotic medication use, pre-medication use obesity, and the high prevalence of smoking in this population.

The presence of narcolepsy among individuals with schizophrenia was evaluated among 366 consecutive individuals with the diagnosis of schizophrenia or schizoaffective disorder (Sansa et al., 2016). The study initially found elevated rates of symptoms suggestive of narcolepsy, such as excessive daytime sleepiness, cataplexy-like experiences, sleep paralysis, and sleep-related hallucinations that occur during the transition between sleep and wakefulness. However, upon closer clinical evaluation, the authors estimate that the prevalence of narcolepsy in this group is at most 1% and that in the majority of people with schizophrenia, the excessive daytime sleepiness was temporally related to initiating an antipsychotic treatment.

CLINICAL RELEVANCE

Poor self-reported sleep quality has been associated with lower quality of life in individuals with schizophrenia (Kaskie et al., 2017; Reeve et al., 2015, 2019; Wulff et al., 2012). The presence of sleep disturbance has also been associated with more severe symptoms, including more severe paranoia and hallucinations (Reeve et al., 2019). Sleep disruption appear to predate and predict a psychosis relapse (Reeve et al., 2015). Sleep disturbance has been documented as an early prodromal feature of psychosis and one of the first features to reappear prior to a psychosis relapse (e.g., Freeman et al., 2012). These findings highlight the possible importance of early intervention on the sleep symptoms to improve functioning and prolong the duration of psychosis-free periods. Indeed, there is emerging evidence that CBT-I is effective at improving both sleep and psychosis symptoms among individuals with psychotic symptoms, including schizophrenia spectrum disorders (Freeman et al., 2017; Harvey et al., 2021).

Atypical antipsychotic medications help improve sleep by shortening sleep-onset latency, improving sleep continuity, and normalizing sleep stage distribution (Monti et al., 2017). However, daytime sedation is a common side effect that may contribute to extended time in bed and worsening of sleep. Indeed, a worldwide survey of 435 individuals with schizophrenia treated with antipsychotic medications found that 83% reported an increase in feeling sleepy during the day and that 74% reported an increase in difficulty sleeping (Tandon et al., 1992).

KEY POINTS

- Difficulties initiating and maintaining sleep reported by individuals with schizophrenia are also observed in PSG and are associated with poorer quality of life.
- Sleep worsens when psychosis symptoms are present.
- Disturbed sleep may be prodromal to psychosis relapse.
- There is preliminary evidence that CBT-I improves both sleep and psychosis symptoms.

Eating Disorders

Sleep disturbances are estimated to be reported by approximately 50% of individuals with eating disorders (Kim et al., 2010). In their study of 400 individuals with anorexia nervosa (AN) and bulimia nervosa (BN), the two most common eating disorders, Kim and colleagues (2010) reported that the most common symptoms were difficulty falling asleep (33%) and difficulty with middle of the night awakenings (18%). Early-morning awakenings, hypersomnia, and parasomnia were each present in 7%–8% of those interviewed (Kim et al., 2010). These authors report that those with disturbed sleep had higher binge and vomiting frequencies. Research has also documented a relationship between sleep duration and endogenous peptides involved in the regulation of eating behaviors, such as ghrelin and leptin (Ohno & Sakurai, 2008; Willie et al., 2001). Ghrelin, secreted by the stomach, stimulates hunger and promotes food ingestion. Leptin, a hormone released by the fat cells, signals satiety to the brain and thus suppresses appetite.

A recent meta-analysis suggests that complex associations between sleep duration and levels of leptin and ghrelin depend in part on whether sleep duration was experimentally manipulated or habitual (Lin et al., 2020). It found a significant elevation in ghrelin level among both those with habitual short sleep and those with experimentally induced sleep deprivation. For leptin, it found no association between short sleep duration and leptin levels in cross-sectional studies; however, higher levels were observed following experimentally induced sleep deprivation compared to those with normal sleep duration. These complex results suggest that insufficient sleep might alter the ability of leptin and ghrelin to signal caloric need and therefore raise the possibility that sleep behaviors might be more relevant to eating disorders, including obesity, than has been recognized historically. This highlights a need for more research on sleep and its potential impact on abnormal levels of leptin and ghrelin among individuals with eating disorders. For a review of alteration in these two hormones among individuals with AN and BN disorders, see Monteleone et al. (2000).

Here we focus on what is known about sleep in AN and BN. We note that, unfortunately, many studies of sleep of individuals with eating disorders include multiple eating disorders and did not report subgroup analyses within a specific eating disorder.

AN

AN is an eating disorder characterized by low body weight attributable to intentional energy intake restriction, intense fear of weight gain, and disturbances in self-perception surrounding weight (DSM-5; American Psychiatric Association, 2013). The scarce literature on sleep in AN that is discussed here is limited by inconsistent definitions of AN and sleep disorders, small samples, and use of non-validated sleep assessments. Additionally, most of this research was conducted mainly among young females, limiting generalizability.

A 1992 meta-analysis of sleep in psychiatric disorders concluded that the only aspect of sleep differentiating individuals with AN from healthy controls was shorter self-reported total sleep time (Benca et al., 1992). An actigraphy-based study also found no differences in any evidence for more disturbed sleep among those with and without AN (Latzer et al., 2001). In contrast, two more recent studies suggest that disturbed sleep is present among individuals with AN. In the first study, Sauchelli and colleagues (2016) found that individuals with AN reported poorer sleep quality and more disturbed sleep than healthy controls, with moderate effect sizes. In the second study, Kim and colleagues (2010) estimated that 58% of females with AN (N = 84) reported sleep disturbances, including symptoms of insomnia, parasomnias, and hypersomnia. Several studies have indicated that eating disorder symptomatology is more severe among AN individuals with sleep disturbances compared to those without (Bat-Pitault et al., 2021; Kim et al., 2010; Malcolm et al., 2022), but this association should not be interpreted as causal. Indeed, there may be a bidirectional relationship between AN and sleep, in which disturbed sleep may contribute to alternations in appetitive hormones, and symptoms of AN may have a disruptive effect on sleep.

Additionally, several psychiatric comorbidities that are associated with high rates of sleep disturbance (e.g., anxiety, depression, substance use disorders) are common among individuals with AN (O'Brien & Vincent, 2003; Woodside & Staab, 2006). In particular, lifetime prevalence of MDD ranges from 64% to 75% of individuals with AN (Godart et al., 2015). One recent cross-sectional study of college women found that symptoms of depression and anxiety mediated the relationship between insomnia and eating disorder symptomatology (Goel et al., 2021). However, research has yet to fully disentangle the relationship between sleep disturbances and psychiatric comorbidities in AN, and these relationships may be bidirectional (Christensen & Short, 2021). It has been suggested that low BMI and associated malnutrition may contribute to this association (Nobili et al., 2004). Partially consistent with this assertion is the observation that weight restoration among people with AN led to reduction in self-reported sleep disturbances (Delvenne et al., 1996; Pieters et al., 2004).

PSG FINDINGS IN AN

Most of the PSG-based work in AN was conducted during the 1980s and 1990s and had small sample sizes. Several studies report lower sleep efficiency, total sleep time, SWS stages, and slow-wave activity in people with AN compared to healthy controls (Asaad Abdou et al., 2018; Neil et al., 1980; Nobili et al., 2004). Most studies have found no significant differences in PSG-derived sleep-onset latency (Neil et al., 1980; Nobili et al., 2004). Elevations in Stage N1 percentage, number of awakenings, and wake after sleep onset have also been reported in multiple studies (Asaad Abdou et al., 2018; Levy et al., 1988; Neil et al., 1980). Some studies have found individuals with anorexia demonstrate elevated REM latency (Kupfer et al., 1976) and density (Katz et al., 1984; Neil et al., 1980), whereas others have found reduced or no difference in REM latency and density (Asaad Abdou et al., 2018) compared to controls.

CLINICAL RELEVANCE

There is some evidence that poor sleep is associated with poorer AN treatment outcome (Sauchelli et al., 2016). A few studies reported that treatments for AN, particularly those which result in weight gain, appear to have slight positive impacts on sleep disturbances. In particular, studies have shown increases in PSG-derived total sleep time (Crisp et al., 1971; Lacey et al., 1976), SWS (Lacey et al., 1975), and REM sleep (Lacey et al., 1976) and decreases in wake after sleep onset (Lauer & Krieg, 1992) and number of awakenings (Crisp et al., 1971). One study found no changes in PSG-derived sleep parameters following weight restoration but did observe increases in self-reported sleep quality, total sleep time, and sleep efficiency and decreases in self-reported sleep-onset latency and sleep disturbances (Pieters et al., 2004). Although it is posited that weight restoration is a primary pathway for improvements in sleep disturbances, there is evidence that sleep can also be improved without an increase in weight, as observed in a pilot study of adolescents with AN undergoing a Pilates-based treatment (Martinez-Sanchez et al., 2020).

KEY POINTS

- Insomnia symptoms and short sleep duration are common and are detected by PSG.
- Sleep disturbances are associated with greater severity of AN.
- Weight gain leads to improved sleep quality, fewer awakenings, and longer sleep duration.

BN

Compared to AN, there is less available research on the relationship between BN and sleep/sleep disturbances. In one study, individuals with BN reported difficulties with sleep initiation and maintenance, including early-morning awakenings (Latzer et al., 1999). Kim and colleagues (2010) documented that 49% of individuals with BN reported disturbed sleep. Additionally, one study found undergraduate students with bulimic behaviors who also report social pressure to eat were more likely to report difficulty falling and staying asleep 1 and 2 years later compared to those without such pressure (Bos et al., 2013). One study found that individuals with BN also have a delayed bedtime, possibly resulting from late-evening binges or irregular sleep schedules (Linnaranta et al., 2020).

PSG FINDINGS

Similar to findings in AN, objective measures of sleep do not always support self-reports in BN (Lauer et al., 1988). One study found no differences in sleep architecture between individuals with BN compared to healthy controls (Levy et al., 1988). A few other studies have similarly found no differences in REM latency and density between depression free individuals with BN and controls (Katz et al., 1984; Neil et al., 1980). In contrast, a recent small study reported increased sleep-onset latency and arousal index and decreased sleep efficiency, SWS, and REM percentage and density among individuals with AN and BN compared to controls; however, the two patient groups exhibited no difference in PSG-defined sleep parameter (Asaad Abdou et al., 2018).

CLINICAL RELEVANCE

Little is known about the clinical relevance of sleep difficulties in BN. There are reasons to believe that poor and irregular sleep could hinder response to psychological treatments of BN because these sleep issues can negatively impact some of the targets of these interventions, including emotion regulation (Cerolini et al., 2015), distress tolerance (Short et al., 2016), and cognitive functioning (Wardle-Pinkston et al., 2019). As is the case with AN, it is not known how common residual insomnia symptoms are following successful treatment of BN and whether they confer risk for relapse. It is also not known whether CBT-I is effective in BN.

KEY POINTS

- Insomnia symptoms are reported by patients with BN but data on PSG indices of sleep initiation and continuity are not conclusive.
- Individuals with BN have a delay in bedtime, possibly attributable to late-evening binges or irregular sleep schedules.

Personality Disorders

Only a handful of studies have examined sleep in personality disorders, most focused on borderline personality disorder (BPD) and several focused on antisocial personality disorder (ASPD).

BPD

A few studies suggest that BPD is associated with poor sleep quality compared to healthy control participants (Bromundt et al., 2013; C. A. Jenkins et al., 2022; Weibel et al., 2017). Data from the National Comorbidity Survey-Replication found that BPD is associated with self-reported complaints of trouble falling asleep and maintaining sleep, even when accounting for diagnoses of other mental health problems such as depression and anxiety (Selby, 2013). A recent review revealed a wide range of estimates of the prevalence of insomnia among individuals with BPD (5%–45%), which is likely because some of the samples were quite unique, such as prisoners (70% male), or had high rates of comorbidities, such as depression.

PSG FINDINGS IN BPD

A meta-analysis of 32 studies revealed that individuals with BPD compared to healthy controls had longer sleep latency, disturbances in sleep continuity, shorter sleep duration, decreased REM latency, increased REM density, and reduced delta power or SWS (Winsper et al., 2017). These authors found that among these sleep variables, only short REM latency was present regardless of past or current MDD.

COMORBID SLEEP DISORDERS IN BPD

We found no estimates of prevalence of comorbid sleep disorders in BPD, but some reported comorbid sleep symptoms. For example, although the prevalence of circadian sleep–wake disorders in BPD is not known, circadian symptoms, including delayed and irregular sleep–wake schedules, are common in BPD (C. A. Jenkins et al., 2022; Winsper et al., 2017). Similarly, whereas the prevalence of nightmare disorder in BPD is not known, a meta-analysis concluded that nightmare frequency is high among individuals with BPD symptoms (Winsper et al., 2017). However, some studies reported that comorbid PTSD accounts for at least some proportion of nightmares observed in BPD (Semiz et al., 2008), while others do not (Schredl et al., 2012).

CLINICAL RELEVANCE

To date, there is little research examining the clinical relevance of sleep disturbance in BPD. One study of 481 young adults found that emotion dysregulation predicted worse sleep quality in BPD and that sleep disturbance predicted worse emotion dysregulation (Grove et al., 2017). Given the association between emotion dysregulation and risk of self-harm and suicide in this population, it will be important to evaluate the impact of sleep interventions on improving emotion regulation skills.

There is some evidence that improving symptoms of BPD also improves sleep. A study of 105 individuals who had recovered from BPD versus 228 non-recovered individuals with BPD found that the individuals who had recovered had improved sleep quality (Plante et al., 2013).

ASPD

A few small studies suggest that ASPD is associated with poor self-reported sleep quality (Lindberg et al., 2003; Taherifard et al., 2015; Van Veen et al., 2017). In a study of 19 men with ASPD, Lindberg and colleagues (2003) reported more subjective problems with sleep onset and sleep maintenance than healthy controls and that these self-reported sleep continuity problems were confirmed by PSG. There is also some indication of more SWS among individuals with ASPD compared to healthy controls (Lindberg et al., 2003, 2006); however, further replication in larger samples is needed in order to determine if this observation is spurious and its clinical implications, if any. To the best of our knowledge, the clinical significance of sleep abnormalities in ASPD has yet to be investigated.

KEY POINTS

- Trouble falling and staying asleep are reported by individuals with BPD and ASPD and are detected in PSG.
- Individuals with BPD also report more nightmares than healthy controls.
- Among individuals with BPD, disturbed sleep is associated with emotion dysregulation.
- Improving symptoms of BPD appears to improve sleep.

Conclusions

In this chapter, we discussed subjective and physiological sleep symptoms in psychiatric disorders and their clinical relevance. These are summarized in Table 40.1. Historically, disturbed sleep has been conceptualized as a symptom of the psychiatric disease that is expected to resolve with its successful treatment. This conceptualization has been challenged by a wealth of research published in recent decades. The extant data indicates that

Table 40.1 Sleep Symptoms in Psychiatric Disorders

Psychiatric disorder	Subjective sleep symptoms	Polysomnography findings	Clinical relevance
Major depressive disorder (MDD)	• Difficulties with sleep initiation • Difficulties with sleep maintenance (very common) • Undesired early morning awakening • Hypersomnia (less common but increases the risk for manic or hypomanic episodes in the future • Sleep paralysis might be more prevalent in depression than in the general population	• Reduced latency to first REM episode • Longer duration of first REM episode • Greater REM density • Reduced SWS (mostly in men) • Sleep disordered breathing might be more prevalent in depression than the general population	• Poor sleep quality and disturbed sleep o correlate with depression severity and poorer quality of life o incur risk of suicide ideation, specific plans for suicide (those with poor sleep more likely to have had previous suicide attempts) o associated with poor response to depression treatment o do not always resolve with standard depression treatments o predict subsequent relapse (residual sleep symptoms) o emerge as one of the first symptoms of recurrence in previously remitted depressed patients • CBT-I is effective in insomnia with comorbid MDD. • Among patients with comorbid insomnia and depression receiving CBT-I, early improvement in insomnia severity predicts depression remission. • Experimentally induced sleep deprivation leads to transient mood elevation.
Bipolar disorder (BD)	• Manic episode o decrease in self-reported sleep need o short and disrupted sleep • Depressive episode o poor sleep and/or hypersomnia[a] o early-morning awakening and hypersomnia are more common in bipolar than unipolar depressive episodes • Euthymic state o poor sleep quality o night-to-night variability in sleep habit	• Manic episodes o REM and SWS abnormalities similar to those reported in MDD • Depressive episodes o higher prevalence of early-morning awakenings and greater REM density than MDD o longer REM latency in bipolar II than MDD • Inter-episode o results are mixed	• 77% of bipolar patients report sleep loss as a prodomal symptom to a manic episode. • Some evidence that forced rest or darkness, even when it does not result in lengthening of sleep, could stabilize mood. • Mood elevation following experimentally induced sleep deprivation is more pronounced in bipolar than unipolar depressive disorder, particularly for rapid cycling patients. • There is preliminary data that CBT-I provided during an inter-episode phase is effective for insomnia and is associated with reduced risk for hypomania/mania relapse. • A single-session intervention with the RISE-UP routine, provided during the inter-episode phase, promotes alertness upon waking up.

Continued

Table 40.1 *Continued*

Psychiatric disorder	Subjective sleep symptoms	Polysomnography findings	Clinical relevance
Panic disorder (PD)	• Difficulties with sleep initiation • Difficulties with sleep maintenance. • Nocturnal panic attacks • Sleep paralysis is more common compared with healthy control, particularly among African Americans	• Mixed result regarding o prolonged sleep latency o decreased sleep efficiency o decreased sleep duration • Nocturnal panic attacks arise mostly during the transition from Stage 2 to 3	• Sleep deprivation can trigger daytime panic attacks. • Nocturnal panic attacks are associated with o increased somatic symptoms o more daytime panic attacks o more severe fears of panic symptoms • A significant proportion of patients continue to experience sleep symptoms after treatment for panic disorder.
Generalized anxiety disorder (GAD)	• Difficulties with sleep initiation • Difficulties with sleep maintenance • Early-morning awakening	• Compared to healthy controls o longer sleep-onset latency o longer wake after sleep onset o more Stage 1 sleep o shorter total sleep time o shorter REM sleep duration • No difference in latency to first REM episode	• Insomnia symptoms do not correlate with GAD severity. • Effective anxiety treatment is not associated with significant residual sleep problems. • Sleep medications enhance pharmacological treatment of GAD. • Sequenced treatment with CBT for GAD followed by CBT-I produces better anxiety and insomnia outcomes than the reverse order. • TMS improves both anxiety and insomnia symptoms among has been tested as novel intervention for patients with GAD and insomnia.
Obsessive–compulsive disorder (OCD)	• Sleep onset or maintenance associated with obsessions and, to a lesser extent, with compulsions	• PSG findings in OCD might be largely explained by presence of a comorbid depression	• Individuals with OCD have nearly sevenfold odds of receiving an insomnia diagnosis or receiving sleep medications. • Increasing evidence suggests a relationship between OCD and circadian rhythm sleep wake disorder, delayed sleep phase type, and a potential mediating role of insomnia symptoms in this relationship. • Studies on the impact of OCD treatment on insomnia symptoms are too small to draw conclusions; however, sleep disturbances, including circadian rhythm factors, may predict response to combined repetitive TMS+psychotherapy treatment for OCD.

Social anxiety disorder	• Difficulties with sleep initiation • Difficulties with sleep maintenance	• No differences compared to controls	• Depression symptoms may partially mediate the relationship between social anxiety and insomnia symptoms.
Post-traumatic stress disorder (PTSD)	• Difficulties with sleep initiation • Difficulties with sleep maintenance • Nightmares • Fear of sleep	• Increase in Stage 1 sleep • Decrease in SWS • Greater REM density • Increased prevalence of o sleep-disordered breathing o parasomnias • Periodic limb movements	• Individuals who report sleep disturbances within 1 month after trauma exposure may be more likely to develop PTSD. • Disturbed sleep does not fully resolve following successful treatment of PTSD. • Treatment of disturbed sleep may result in decreases in PTSD symptoms. • Trauma-related sleep disorder is a new proposed diagnosis that includes a combination of nightmares, REM without atonia, dream enactment, and disruptive nighttime behaviors. • There is emerging evidence the CBT-I is effective for improving sleep among patients with PTSD.
Schizophrenia	• Difficulties with sleep initiation • Difficulties with sleep maintenance • Poor sleep quality	• Longer sleep latency • Less total sleep time • Lower sleep efficiency • Decreased REM latency	• Sleep quality worsens when psychotic symptoms are exacerbated. • Poor sleep quality has been associated with lower quality of life. • Disturbed sleep appears to precede a psychotic relapse. • There is preliminary evidence that CBT-I improves both sleep and psychosis symptoms.
Anorexia nervosa (AN)	• Insomnia symptoms • Poor sleep quality • Reduced total sleep time • Hypersomnia • Parasomonias	• Decreased total sleep time • Reduced sleep efficiency • Reduced SWS • Increased number of awakenings • Elevated percentage of Stage 1	• Eating disorder symptoms are more severe among those with sleep disturbances compared to those without. • Self-reported sleep quality improves after weight gain. • PSG-derived total sleep time, SWS, and REM sleep increase after treatment. • Number of awakenings may decrease after successful treatment.

Continued

Table 40.1 *Continued*

Psychiatric disorder	Subjective sleep symptoms	Polysomnography findings	Clinical relevance
Bulimia nervosa (BN)	• Difficulties with sleep initiation • Difficulties with sleep maintenance • Early-morning awakenings • Possible delayed bedtime	• Inconclusive findings	• Individuals with BN have a delay in bedtime, possibly attributable to late-evening binges or irregular sleep schedules.
Borderline personality disorder (BPD)	• Trouble falling and staying asleep	• Increased sleep latency • Less SWS and more delta power • Shortened REM latency • Less Stage 2 sleep	• More nightmares. • Disturbed sleep associated with emotion dysregulation. • Improving symptoms of BPD appears to improve sleep.
Antisocial personality disorder (ASPD)	• Difficulties with sleep initiation • Difficulties with sleep maintenance • Poor sleep quality	• Sleep continuity problems • Increase in SWS	• Unknown

[a]Hypersomnia is distinct from sleepiness

Note. All comparisons are relative to controls, unless otherwise specified. CBT-I = cognitive behavioral therapy for insomnia; PSG = polysomnography; REM = rapid eye movement; SWS = slow-wave sleep; TMS = transcranial magnetic stimulation.

disturbed sleep does not resolve without targeted attention and that, in many cases, it contributes to the severity and course of the comorbid psychiatric disorder.

The most common sleep symptoms among individuals with psychiatric disorders are symptoms of insomnia, present in all the disorders we have discussed in this chapter. In that way, sleep difficulties constitute a transdiagnostic mental health symptom. CBT-I has been established as an effective therapy for insomnia disorder, including when it is comorbid with psychiatric disorders (e.g., Hertenstein et al., 2022). For each of the disorders discussed, under the heading of *clinical significance*, we included a discussion on what is known about the efficacy of CBT-I when insomnia is comorbid with the disorder. There is strong evidence that CBT-I improves insomnia symptoms in unipolar depression and preliminary data supporting its efficacy in GAD, PTSD, BD, and schizophrenia. Studies also have shown that CBT-I has small effects on psychiatric symptoms, such as depression and anxiety (Ballesio et al., 2018; Benz et al., 2020; Jansson-Frojmark & Jacobson, 2021).

Future Directions

There is large variability in what is known about sleep in the different psychiatric disorders covered in this chapter. Below we highlight three sets of questions that we believe will be important to answer in future research as applied separately to these psychiatric disorders.

1. How do sleep symptoms impact the severity or course of each psychiatric disorder? The following are a few examples of questions that fall in this domain: Do sleep symptoms correlate with the severity of the comorbid disorder? Do they hinder response to the treatment of the psychiatric disorder? Do sleep symptoms resolve with successful treatment of the psychiatric disorder? Do residual sleep problems increase the risk of relapse?
2. When is the best time to intervene? For example, is a combined approach (simultaneous treatment of the psychiatric and the sleep disorder) superior to a sequential approach (augmenting the treatment of the psychiatric disorder with a sleep-specific intervention of residual insomnia symptoms)? If a sequential approach is selected, what is the best order?
3. What is the impact of the psychiatric disorder and its treatments on sleep disorders, and what is the best way to address them? For example, what modifications, if any, are needed when implementing CBT-I in different psychiatric disorders? What is the best way to address safety issues when implementing time in bed restriction in the presence of a psychotropic medication that contributes to excessive daytime sleepiness?

References

Agargun, M. Y., & Kara, H. (1998). Recurrent sleep panic, insomnia, and suicidal behavior in patients with panic disorder. *Comprehensive Psychiatry, 39*(3), 149–151. https://doi.org/10.1016/s0010-440x(98)90074-8

Agargun, M. Y., Kara, H., & Solmaz, M. (1997). Sleep disturbances and suicidal behavior in patients with major depression. *Journal of Clinical Psychiatry, 58*(6), 249–251. https://doi.org/10.4088/jcp.v58n0602

Alloy, L. B., Ng, T. H., Titone, M. K., & Boland, E. M. (2017). Circadian rhythm dysregulation in bipolar spectrum disorders. *Current Psychiatry Reports, 19*(4), Article 21. https://doi.org/10.1007/s11920-017-0772-z

American Psychiatric Association. (2013). *Diagnostic and statistical manual of mental disorders* (5th ed.). Washington, DC. https://doi.org/10.1176/appi.books.9780890425596

Armitage, R., Hoffmann, R., Trivedi, M., & Rush, A. J. (2000). Slow-wave activity in NREM sleep: Sex and age effects in depressed outpatients and healthy controls. *Psychiatry Research, 95*(3), 201–213. https://doi.org/10.1016/s0165-1781(00)00178-5

Arriaga, F., Lara, E., Matos-Pires, A., Cavaglia, F., & Bastos, L. (1995). Diagnostic relevance of sleep complaints in anxiety and mood disorders. *European Psychiatry, 10*(8), 386–390. https://doi.org/10.1016/0924-9338(96)80343-9

Arriaga, F., & Paiva, T. (1990). Clinical and EEG sleep changes in primary dysthymia and generalized anxiety: A comparison with normal controls. *Neuropsychobiology, 24*(3), 109–114. https://doi.org/10.1159/000119471

Arriaga, F., Paiva, T., Matos-Pires, A., Cavaglia, F., Lara, E., & Bastos, L. (1996). The sleep of non-depressed patients with panic disorder: A comparison with normal controls. *Acta Psychiatrica Scandinavica, 93*(3), 191–194. https://doi.org/10.1111/j.1600-0447.1996.tb10630.x

Asaad Abdou, T., Esawy, H. I., Abdel Razek Mohamed, G., Hussein Ahmed, H., Elhabiby, M. M., Khalil, S. A., & El-Hawary, Y. A. (2018). Sleep profile in anorexia and bulimia nervosa female patients. *Sleep Medicine, 48*, 113–116. https://doi.org/10.1016/j.sleep.2018.03.032

Babson, K. A., & Feldner, M. T. (2010). Temporal relations between sleep problems and both traumatic event exposure and PTSD: A critical review of the empirical literature. *Journal of Anxiety Disorders, 24*(1), 1–15. https://doi.org/10.1016/j.janxdis.2009.08.002

Babson, K. A., Feldner, M. T., Sachs-Ericsson, N., Schmidt, N. B., & Zvolensky, M. J. (2008). Nicotine dependence mediates the relations between insomnia and both panic and posttraumatic stress disorder in the NCS-R sample. *Depression and Anxiety, 25*(8), 670–679. https://doi.org/10.1002/da.20374

Baglioni, C., Battagliese, G., Feige, B., Spiegelhalder, K., Nissen, C., Voderholzer, U., Lombardo, C., & Riemann, D. (2011). Insomnia as a predictor of depression: A meta-analytic evaluation of longitudinal epidemiological studies. *Journal of Affective Disorders, 135*(1–3), 10–19. https://doi.org/10.1016/j.jad.2011.01.011

Baglioni, C., Nanovska, S., Regen, W., Spiegelhalder, K., Feige, B., Nissen, C., Reynolds, C. F., & Riemann, D. (2016). Sleep and mental disorders: A meta-analysis of polysomnographic research. *Psychological Bulletin, 142*(9), 969–990. https://doi.org/10.1037/bul0000053

Ballesio, A., Aquino, M., Feige, B., Johann, A. F., Kyle, S. D., Spiegelhalder, K., Lombardo, C., Rucker, G., Riemann, D., & Baglioni, C. (2018). The effectiveness of behavioural and cognitive behavioural therapies for insomnia on depressive and fatigue symptoms: A systematic review and network meta-analysis. *Sleep Medicine Reviews, 37*, 114–129. https://doi.org/10.1016/j.smrv.2017.01.006

Barbini, B., Benedetti, F., Colombo, C., Dotoli, D., Bernasconi, A., Cigala-Fulgosi, M., Florita, M., & Smeraldi, E. (2005). Dark therapy for mania: A pilot study. *Bipolar Disorders, 7*(1), 98–101. https://doi.org/10.1111/j.1399-5618.2004.00166.x

Barbini, B., Colombo, C., Benedetti, F., Campori, E., Bellodi, L., & Smeraldi, E. (1998). The unipolar–bipolar dichotomy and the response to sleep deprivation. *Psychiatry Research, 79*(1), 43–50. https://doi.org/10.1016/s0165-1781(98)00020-1

Bat-Pitault, F., Da Silva, C., Charvin, I., & Da Fonseca, D. (2021). Sleep disturbances in anorexia nervosa subtypes in adolescence. *Eating and Weight Disorders, 26*(6), 1845–1852. https://doi.org/10.1007/s40519-020-01033-z

Belanger, L., Morin, C. M., Langlois, F., & Ladouceur, R. (2004). Insomnia and generalized anxiety disorder: Effects of cognitive behavior therapy for gad on insomnia symptoms. *Journal of Anxiety Disorders, 18*(4), 561–571. https://doi.org/10.1016/S0887-6185(03)00031-8

Belleville, G., Ivers, H., Belanger, L., Blais, F. C., & Morin, C. M. (2016). Sequential treatment of comorbid insomnia and generalized anxiety disorder. *Journal of Clinical Psychology, 72*(9), 880–896. https://doi.org/10.1002/jclp.22300

Benca, R. M., Obermeyer, W. H., Thisted, R. A., & Gillin, J. C. (1992). Sleep and psychiatric disorders. A meta-analysis. *Archives of General Psychiatry, 49*(8), 651–668; discussion 669-670. https://doi.org/10.1001/archpsyc.1992.01820080059010

Benedetti, F. (2018). Rate of switch from bipolar depression into mania after morning light therapy: A historical review. *Psychiatry Research, 261*, 351–356. https://doi.org/10.1016/j.psychres.2018.01.013

Benz, F., Knoop, T., Ballesio, A., Bacaro, V., Johann, A. F., Rucker, G., Feige, B., Riemann, D., & Baglioni, C. (2020). The efficacy of cognitive and behavior therapies for insomnia on daytime symptoms: A systematic review and network meta-analysis. *Clinical Psychology Review, 80*, Article 101873. https://doi.org/10.1016/j.cpr.2020.101873

Boland, E. M., Vittengl, J. R., Clark, L. A., Thase, M. E., & Jarrett, R. B. (2020). Is sleep disturbance linked to short- and long-term outcomes following treatments for recurrent depression? *Journal of Affective Disorders, 262*, 323–332. https://doi.org/10.1016/j.jad.2019.10.033

Bos, S. C., Soares, M. J., Marques, M., Maia, B., Pereira, A. T., Nogueira, V., Valente, J., & Macedo, A. (2013). Disordered eating behaviors and sleep disturbances. *Eating Behaviors, 14*(2), 192–198. https://doi.org/10.1016/j.eatbeh.2013.01.012

Bowden, C. L. (2005). A different depression: Clinical distinctions between bipolar and unipolar depression. *Journal of Affective Disorders, 84*(2–3), 117–125. https://doi.org/10.1016/S0165-0327(03)00194-0

Brenes, G. A., Miller, M. E., Stanley, M. A., Williamson, J. D., Knudson, M., & McCall, W. V. (2009). Insomnia in older adults with generalized anxiety disorder. *American Journal of Geriatric Psychiatry, 17*(6), 465–472. https://doi.org/10.1097/jgp.0b013e3181987747

Breslau, N., Roth, T., Burduvali, E., Kapke, A., Schultz, L., & Roehrs, T. (2004). Sleep in lifetime posttraumatic stress disorder: A community-based polysomnographic study. *Archives of General Psychiatry, 61*(5), 508–516. https://doi.org/10.1001/archpsyc.61.5.508

Breslau, N., Roth, T., Rosenthal, L., & Andreski, P. (1996). Sleep disturbance and psychiatric disorders: A longitudinal epidemiological study of young adults. *Biological Psychiatry, 39*(6), 411–418. https://doi.org/10.1016/0006-3223(95)00188-3

Brock, M. S., Powell, T. A., Creamer, J. L., Moore, B. A., & Mysliwiec, V. (2019). Trauma associated sleep disorder: Clinical developments 5 years after discovery. *Current Psychiatry Reports, 21*(9), Article 80. https://doi.org/10.1007/s11920-019-1066-4

Bromundt, V., Wirz-Justice, A., Kyburz, S., Opwis, K., Dammann, G., & Cajochen, C. (2013). Circadian sleep–wake cycles, well-being, and light therapy in borderline personality disorder. *Journal of Personality Disorders, 27*(5), 680–696. https://doi.org/10.1521/pedi_2012_26_057

Brown, T. M., & Boudewyns, P. A. (1996). Periodic limb movements of sleep in combat veterans with posttraumatic stress disorder. *Journal of Traumatic Stress, 9*(1), 129–136. https://doi.org/10.1007/BF02116838

Brown, T. M., & Uhde, T. W. (2003). Sleep panic attacks: A micromovement analysis. *Depression and Anxiety, 18*(4), 214–220. https://doi.org/10.1002/da.10152

Bryant, R. A., Creamer, M., O'Donnell, M., Silove, D., & McFarlane, A. C. (2010). Sleep disturbance immediately prior to trauma predicts subsequent psychiatric disorder. *Sleep, 33*(1), 69–74. https://doi.org/10.1093/sleep/33.1.69

Buckner, J. D., Bernert, R. A., Cromer, K. R., Joiner, T. E., & Schmidt, N. B. (2008). Social anxiety and insomnia: The mediating role of depressive symptoms. *Depression and Anxiety, 25*(2), 124–130. https://doi.org/10.1002/da.20282

Buysse, D. J., Angst, J., Gamma, A., Ajdacic, V., Eich, D., & Rossler, W. (2008). Prevalence, course, and comorbidity of insomnia and depression in young adults. *Sleep, 31*(4), 473–480. https://doi.org/10.1093/sleep/31.4.473

Byrne, S. P., McCarthy, E., DeViva, J. C., Southwick, S. M., & Pietrzak, R. H. (2021). Prevalence, risk correlates, and health comorbidities of insomnia in US military veterans: Results from the 2019–2020 National Health and Resilience in Veterans Study. *Journal of Clinical Sleep Medicine, 17*(6), 1267–1277. https://doi.org/10.5664/jcsm.9182

Carney, C. E., Edinger, J. D., Kuchibhatla, M., Lachowski, A. M., Bogouslavsky, O., Krystal, A. D., & Shapiro, C. M. (2017). Cognitive behavioral insomnia therapy for those with insomnia and depression: A randomized controlled clinical trial. *Sleep, 40*(4), Article zsx019. https://doi.org/10.1093/sleep/zsx019

Carney, C. E., Harris, A. L., Friedman, J., & Segal, Z. V. (2011). Residual sleep beliefs and sleep disturbance following cognitive behavioral therapy for major depression. *Depression and Anxiety, 28*(6), 464–470. https://doi.org/10.1002/da.20811

Carney, C. E., Segal, Z. V., Edinger, J. D., & Krystal, A. D. (2007). A comparison of rates of residual insomnia symptoms following pharmacotherapy or cognitive-behavioral therapy for major depressive disorder. *Journal of Clinical Psychiatry, 68*(2), 254–260. https://doi.org/10.4088/jcp.v68n0211

Carruthers, S. P., Brunetti, G., & Rossell, S. L. (2021). Sleep disturbances and cognitive impairment in schizophrenia spectrum disorders: A systematic review and narrative synthesis. *Sleep Medicine, 84*, 8–19. https://doi.org/10.1016/j.sleep.2021.05.011

Cerolini, S., Ballesio, A., & Lombardo, C. (2015). Insomnia and emotion regulation: Recent findings and suggestions for treatment. *Journal of Sleep Disorders and Management, 1*(1), ISSN: 2572-4053.

Chan, M. S., Chung, K. F., Yung, K. P., & Yeung, W. F. (2017). Sleep in schizophrenia: A systematic review and meta-analysis of polysomnographic findings in case-control studies. *Sleep Medicine Reviews, 32*, 69–84. https://doi.org/10.1016/j.smrv.2016.03.001

Chellappa, S. L., & Araujo, J. F. (2007). Sleep disorders and suicidal ideation in patients with depressive disorder. *Psychiatry Research, 153*(2), 131–136. https://doi.org/10.1016/j.psychres.2006.05.007

Christensen, K. A., & Short, N. A. (2021). The case for investigating a bidirectional association between insomnia symptoms and eating disorder pathology. *International Journal of Eating Disorders, 54*(5), 701–707. https://doi.org/10.1002/eat.23498

Chung, K. F., Poon, Y. P. Y., Ng, T. K., & Kan, C. K. (2018). Correlates of sleep irregularity in schizophrenia. *Psychiatry Research, 270*, 705–714. https://doi.org/10.1016/j.psychres.2018.10.064

Cole, M. G., & Dendukuri, N. (2003). Risk factors for depression among elderly community subjects: A systematic review and meta-analysis. *American Journal of Psychiatry, 160*(6), 1147–1156. https://doi.org/10.1176/appi.ajp.160.6.1147

Colombo, C., Benedetti, F., Barbini, B., Campori, E., & Smeraldi, E. (1999). Rate of switch from depression into mania after therapeutic sleep deprivation in bipolar depression. *Psychiatry Research, 86*(3), 267–270. https://doi.org/10.1016/s0165-1781(99)00036-0

Colvonen, P. J., Drummond, S. P. A., Angkaw, A. C., & Norman, S. B. (2019). Piloting cognitive-behavioral therapy for insomnia integrated with prolonged exposure. *Psychological Trauma, 11*(1), 107–113. https://doi.org/10.1037/tra0000402

Cousineau, H., Marchand, A., Bouchard, S., Belanger, C., Gosselin, P., Langlois, F., Labrecque, J., Dugas, M. J., & Belleville, G. (2016). Insomnia symptoms following treatment for comorbid panic disorder with agoraphobia and generalized anxiety disorder. *Journal of Nervous and Mental Disease, 204*(4), 267–273. https://doi.org/10.1097/NMD.0000000000000466

Cox, R. C., & Olatunji, B. O. (2016). A systematic review of sleep disturbance in anxiety and related disorders. *Journal of Anxiety Disorders, 37*, 104–129. https://doi.org/10.1016/j.janxdis.2015.12.001

Cox, R. C, & Olatunji, B. O. (2022). Delayed circadian rhythms and insomnia symptoms in obsessive-compulsive disorder. *Journal of Affective Disorders, 318*, 94–102. https://doi.org/10.1016/j.jad.2022.08.118

Cox, R. C., Parmar, A. M., & Olatunji, B. O. (2020). Sleep in obsessive–compulsive and related disorders: A selective review and synthesis. *Current Opinion in Psychology, 34*, 23–26. https://doi.org/10.1016/j.copsyc.2019.08.018

Craske, M. G., & Barlow, D. H. (1989). Nocturnal panic. *Journal of Nervous and Mental Disease, 177*(3), 160–167. https://doi.org/10.1097/00005053-198903000-00006

Craske, M. G., & Kreuger, M. (1990). The prevalence of nocturnal panic in a college population. *Journal of Anxiety Disorders, 4*, 125–139.

Craske, M. G., Lang, A. J., Aikins, D., & Mystkowski, J. L. (2005). Cognitive behavioral therapy for nocturnal panic. *Behavior Therapy, 36*(1), 43–54.

Craske, M. G., Lang, A. J., Mystkowski, J. L., Zucker, B. G., Bystritsky, A., & Yan-Go, F. (2002). Does nocturnal panic represent a more severe form of panic disorder? *Journal of Nervous and Mental Disease, 190*(9), 611–618. https://doi.org/10.1097/00005053-200209000-00006

Craske, M. G., Lang, A. J., Rowe, M., DeCola, J. P., Simmons, J., Mann, C., Yan-Go, F., & Bystritsky, A. (2002). Presleep attributions about arousal during sleep: Nocturnal panic. *Journal of Abnormal Psychology, 111*(1), 53–62. https://doi.org/10.1037//0021-843x.111.1.53

Craske, M. G., & Tsao, J. C. (2005). Assessment and treatment of nocturnal panic attacks. *Sleep Medicine Reviews, 9*(3), 173–184. https://doi.org/10.1016/j.smrv.2004.11.003

Crisp, A. H., Stonehill, E., & Fenton, G. W. (1971). The relationship between sleep, nutrition and mood: A study of patients with anorexia nervosa. *Postgraduate Medical Journal, 47*(546), 207–213. https://doi.org/10.1136/pgmj.47.546.207

de Boer, M., Nijdam, M. J., Jongedijk, R. A., Bangel, K. A., Olff, M., Hofman, W. F., & Talamini, L. M. (2020). The spectral fingerprint of sleep problems in post-traumatic stress disorder. *Sleep, 43*(4), Article zsz269. https://doi.org/10.1093/sleep/zsz269

Delvenne, V., Goldman, S., De Maertelaer, V., Simon, Y., Luxen, A., & Lotstra, F. (1996). Brain hypometabolism of glucose in anorexia nervosa: Normalization after weight gain. *Biological Psychiatry, 40*(8), 761–768. https://doi.org/10.1016/0006-3223(95)00522-6

Diaz-Roman, A., Perestelo-Perez, L., & Buela-Casal, G. (2015). Sleep in obsessive–compulsive disorder: A systematic review and meta-analysis. *Sleep Medicine, 16*(9), 1049–1055. https://doi.org/10.1016/j.sleep.2015.03.020

Donse, L., Sack, A. T., Fitzgerald, P. B., & Arns, M. (2017). Sleep disturbances in obsessive–compulsive disorder: Association with non-response to repetitive transcranial magnetic stimulation (rTMS). *Journal of Anxiety Disorders, 49*, 31–39. https://doi.org/10.1016/j.janxdis.2017.03.006

Dow, B. M., Kelsoe, J. R., Jr., & Gillin, J. C. (1996). Sleep and dreams in Vietnam PTSD and depression. *Biological Psychiatry, 39*(1), 42–50. https://doi.org/10.1016/0006-3223(95)00103-4

Dube, S., Jones, D. A., Bell, J., Davies, A., Ross, E., & Sitaram, N. (1986). Interface of panic and depression: Clinical and sleep EEG correlates. *Psychiatry Research, 19*(2), 119–133. https://doi.org/10.1016/0165-1781(86)90005-3

Elliott, J. E., Opel, R. A., Pleshakov, D., Rachakonda, T., Chau, A. Q., Weymann, K. B., & Lim, M. M. (2020). Posttraumatic stress disorder increases the odds of REM sleep behavior disorder and other parasomnias in veterans with and without comorbid traumatic brain injury. *Sleep, 43*(3), Article zsz237. https://doi.org/10.1093/sleep/zsz237

Fava, M., McCall, W. V., Krystal, A., Wessel, T., Rubens, R., Caron, J., Amato, D., & Roth, T. (2006). Eszopiclone co-administered with fluoxetine in patients with insomnia coexisting with major depressive disorder. *Biological Psychiatry, 59*(11), 1052–1060. https://doi.org/10.1016/j.biopsych.2006.01.016

Fawcett, J., Scheftner, W. A., Fogg, L., Clark, D. C., Young, M. A., Hedeker, D., & Gibbons, R. (1990). Time-related predictors of suicide in major affective disorder. *American Journal of Psychiatry, 147*(9), 1189–1194. http://www.ncbi.nlm.nih.gov/pubmed/2104515

Fosse, R., Stickgold, R., & Hobson, J. A. (2001). The mind in REM sleep: Reports of emotional experience. *Sleep, 24*(8), 947–955. https://www.ncbi.nlm.nih.gov/pubmed/11766165

Frankland, A., Cerrillo, E., Hadzi-Pavlovic, D., Roberts, G., Wright, A., Loo, C. K., Breakspear, M., & Mitchell, P. B. (2015). Comparing the phenomenology of depressive episodes in bipolar I and II disorder and major depressive disorder within bipolar disorder pedigrees. *Journal of Clinical Psychiatry, 76*(1), 32–38; quiz 39. https://doi.org/10.4088/JCP.14m09293

Freed, S., Craske, M. G., & Greher, M. R. (1999). Nocturnal panic and trauma. *Depression and Anxiety, 9*(3), 141–145. https://doi.org/10.1002/(sici)1520-6394(1999)9:3<141::aid-da8>3.0.co;2-5

Freeman, D., Sheaves, B., Goodwin, G. M., Yu, L. M., Nickless, A., Harrison, P. J., Emsley, R., Luik, A. I., Foster, R. G., Wadekar, V., Hinds, C., Gumley, A., Jones, R., Lightman, S., Jones, S., Bentall, R., Kinderman, P., Rowse, G., Brugha, T., . . . Espie, C. A. (2017). The effects of improving sleep on mental health (OASIS): A randomised controlled trial with mediation analysis. *Lancet Psychiatry, 4*(10), 749–758. https://doi.org/10.1016/s2215-0366(17)30328-0

Freeman, D., Stahl, D., McManus, S., Meltzer, H., Brugha, T., Wiles, N., & Bebbington, P. (2012). Insomnia, worry, anxiety and depression as predictors of the occurrence and persistence of paranoid thinking. *Social Psychiatry and Psychiatric Epidemiology, 47*(8), 1195–1203. https://doi.org/10.1007/s00127-011-0433-1

Gajadien, P. T., Postma, T. S., van Oostrom, I., Scheepstra, K. W. F., van Dijk, H., Sack, A. T., van den Heuvel, O. A., & Arns, M. (2023). Sleep predicts the response to rTMS and CBT in patients with OCD: An open label effectiveness study. *International Journal of Clinical and Health Psychology, 23*(2), Article 100353. https://doi.org/10.1016/j.ijchp.2022.100353

Gehrman, P., Seelig, A. D., Jacobson, I. G., Boyko, E. J., Hooper, T. I., Gackstetter, G. D., Ulmer, C. S., & Smith, T. C. (2013). Predeployment sleep duration and insomnia symptoms as risk factors for new-onset mental health disorders following military deployment. *Sleep, 36*(7), 1009–1018. https://doi.org/10.5665/sleep.2798

Geoffroy, P. A., Scott, J., Boudebesse, C., Lajnef, M., Henry, C., Leboyer, M., Bellivier, F., & Etain, B. (2015). Sleep in patients with remitted bipolar disorders: A meta-analysis of actigraphy studies. *Acta Psychiatrica Scandinavica, 131*(2), 89–99. https://doi.org/10.1111/acps.12367

Germain, A. (2013). Sleep disturbances as the hallmark of PTSD: Where are we now? *American Journal of Psychiatry, 170*(4), 372–382. https://doi.org/10.1176/appi.ajp.2012.12040432

Germain, A., Krakow, B., Faucher, B., Zadra, A., Nielsen, T., Hollifield, M., Warner, T. D., & Koss, M. (2004). Increased mastery elements associated with imagery rehearsal treatment for nightmares in sexual assault survivors with PTSD. *Dreaming, 14*(4), 195–206. https://doi.org/10.1037/1053-0797.14.4.195

Germain, A., Richardson, R., Moul, D. E., Mammen, O., Haas, G., Forman, S. D., Rode, N., Begley, A., & Nofzinger, E. A. (2012). Placebo-controlled comparison of prazosin and cognitive-behavioral treatments for sleep disturbances in US military veterans. *Journal of Psychosomatic Research, 72*(2), 89–96. https://doi.org/10.1016/j.jpsychores.2011.11.010

Godart, N., Radon, L., Curt, F., Duclos, J., Perdereau, F., Lang, F., Venisse, J. L., Halfon, O., Bizouard, P., Loas, G., Corcos, M., Jeammet, P., & Flament, M. F. (2015). Mood disorders in eating disorder patients: Prevalence and chronology of ONSET. *Journal of Affective Disorders, 185*, 115–122. https://doi.org/10.1016/j.jad.2015.06.039

Goel, N. J., Sadeh-Sharvit, S., Trockel, M., Flatt, R. E., Fitzsimmons-Craft, E. E., Balantekin, K. N., Monterubio, G. E., Firebaugh, M. L., Wilfley, D. E., & Taylor, C. B. (2021). Depression and anxiety mediate the relationship between insomnia and eating disorders in college women. *Journal of American College Health, 69*(8), 976–981. https://doi.org/10.1080/07448481.2019.1710152

Grigolon, R. B., Trevizol, A. P., Cerqueira, R. O., Lee, Y., Mansur, R. B., McIntyre, R. S., & Brietzke, E. (2019). Hypersomnia and bipolar disorder: A systematic review and meta-analysis of proportion. *Journal of Affective Disorders, 246*, 659–666. https://doi.org/10.1016/j.jad.2018.12.030

Gross, P. K., Nourse, R., & Wasser, T. E. (2009). Ramelteon for insomnia symptoms in a community sample of adults with generalized anxiety disorder: An open label study. *Journal of Clinical Sleep Medicine, 5*(1), 28–33. https://www.ncbi.nlm.nih.gov/pubmed/19317378

Grove, J. L., Smith, T. W., Crowell, S. E., & Ellis, J. H. (2017). Preliminary evidence for emotion dysregulation as a mechanism underlying poor sleep quality in borderline personality disorder. *Journal of Personality Disorders, 31*(4), 542–552. https://doi.org/10.1521/pedi_2016_30_261

Grunhaus, L., Rabin, D., Harel, Y., Greden, J. F., Feinberg, M., & Hermann, R. (1986). Simultaneous panic and depressive disorders: Clinical and sleep EEG correlates. *Psychiatry Research, 17*(4), 251–259. https://doi.org/10.1016/0165-1781(86)90072-7

Hagen, K., Nordahl, H., Launes, G., Kvale, G., Ost, L. G., Hystad, S., Hansen, B., & Solem, S. (2021). Does concentrated exposure treatment for obsessive–compulsive disorder improve insomnia symptoms? Results from a randomized controlled trial. *Frontiers in Psychiatry, 12*, Article 625631. https://doi.org/10.3389/fpsyt.2021.625631

Harvey, A. G. (2008). Sleep and circadian rhythms in bipolar disorder: Seeking synchrony, harmony, and regulation. *American Journal of Psychiatry, 165*(7), 820–829. https://doi.org/10.1176/appi.ajp.2008.08010098

Harvey, A. G., Dong, L., Hein, K., Yu, S. H., Martinez, A. J., Gumport, N. B., Smith, F. L., Chapman, A., Lisman, M., Mirzadegan, I. A., Mullin, A. C., Fine, E., Dolsen, M. R., Gasperetti, C. E., Bukosky, J., Alvarado-Martinez, C. G., Kilbourne, A. M., Rabe-Hesketh, S., & Buysse, D. J. (2021). A randomized controlled trial of the Transdiagnostic Intervention for Sleep and Circadian Dysfunction (TranS-C) to improve serious mental illness outcomes in a community setting. *Journal of Consulting and Clinical Psychology, 89*(6), 537–550. https://doi.org/10.1037/ccp0000650

Harvey, A. G., Schmidt, D. A., Scarna, A., Semler, C. N., & Goodwin, G. M. (2005). Sleep-related functioning in euthymic patients with bipolar disorder, patients with insomnia, and subjects without sleep problems. *American Journal of Psychiatry, 162*(1), 50–57. https://doi.org/10.1176/appi.ajp.162.1.50

Harvey, A. G., Soehner, A. M., Kaplan, K. A., Hein, K., Lee, J., Kanady, J., Li, D., Rabe-Hesketh, S., Ketter, T. A., Neylan, T. C., & Buysse, D. J. (2015). Treating insomnia improves mood state, sleep, and functioning in bipolar disorder: A pilot randomized controlled trial. *Journal of Consulting and Clinical Psychology, 83*(3), 564–577. https://doi.org/10.1037/a0038655

Hauri, P. J., Friedman, M., & Ravaris, C. L. (1989). Sleep in patients with spontaneous panic attacks. *Sleep, 12*(4), 323–337. https://doi.org/10.1093/sleep/12.4.323

Henriksen, T. E., Skrede, S., Fasmer, O. B., Schoeyen, H., Leskauskaite, I., Bjorke-Bertheussen, J., Assmus, J., Hamre, B., Gronli, J., & Lund, A. (2016). Blue-blocking glasses as additive treatment for mania: A randomized placebo-controlled trial. *Bipolar Disorders, 18*(3), 221–232. https://doi.org/10.1111/bdi.12390

Hertenstein, E., Trinca, E., Wunderlin, M., Schneider, C. L., Zust, M. A., Feher, K. D., Su, T., Straten, A. V., Berger, T., Baglioni, C., Johann, A., Spiegelhalder, K., Riemann, D., Feige, B., & Nissen, C. (2022). Cognitive behavioral therapy for insomnia in patients with mental disorders and comorbid insomnia: A systematic review and meta-analysis. *Sleep Medicine Reviews, 62*, Article 101597. https://doi.org/10.1016/j.smrv.2022.101597

Hofstetter, J. R., Lysaker, P. H., & Mayeda, A. R. (2005). Quality of sleep in patients with schizophrenia is associated with quality of life and coping. *BMC Psychiatry, 5*, Article 13. https://doi.org/10.1186/1471-244x-5-13

Huang, Z., Li, Y., Bianchi, M. T., Zhan, S., Jiang, F., Li, N., Ding, Y., Hou, Y., Wang, L., Ouyang, Q., & Wang, Y. (2018). Repetitive transcranial magnetic stimulation of the right parietal cortex for comorbid generalized anxiety disorder and insomnia: A randomized, double-blind, sham-controlled pilot study. *Brain Stimulation, 11*(5), 1103–1109. https://doi.org/10.1016/j.brs.2018.05.016

Hudson, J. I., Lipinski, J. F., Frankenburg, F. R., Grochocinski, V. J., & Kupfer, D. J. (1988). Electroencephalographic sleep in mania. *Archives of General Psychiatry, 45*(3), 267–273. https://doi.org/10.1001/archpsyc.1988.01800270085010

Hudson, J. I., Lipinski, J. F., Keck, P. E., Jr., Aizley, H. G., Lukas, S. E., Rothschild, A. J., Waternaux, C. M., & Kupfer, D. J. (1992). Polysomnographic characteristics of young manic patients. Comparison with unipolar depressed patients and normal control subjects. *Archives of General Psychiatry, 49*(5), 378–383. http://www.ncbi.nlm.nih.gov/pubmed/1586273

Hutka, P., Krivosova, M., Muchova, Z., Tonhajzerova, I., Hamrakova, A., Mlyncekova, Z., Mokry, J., & Ondrejka, I. (2021). Association of sleep architecture and physiology with depressive disorder and antidepressants treatment. *International Journal of Molecular Sciences, 22*(3), Article 1333. https://doi.org/10.3390/ijms22031333

Insel, T. R., Gillin, J. C., Moore, A., Mendelson, W. B., Loewenstein, R. J., & Murphy, D. L. (1982). The sleep of patients with obsessive–compulsive disorder. *Archives of General Psychiatry, 39*(12), 1372–1377. https://doi.org/10.1001/archpsyc.1982.04290120008002

Ivan, M. C., Amspoker, A. B., Nadorff, M. R., Kunik, M. E., Cully, J. A., Wilson, N., Calleo, J., Kraus-Schuman, C., & Stanley, M. A. (2014). Alcohol use, anxiety, and insomnia in older adults with generalized anxiety disorder. *American Journal of Geriatric Psychiatry, 22*(9), 875–883. https://doi.org/10.1016/j.jagp.2013.04.001

Jackson, A., Cavanagh, J., & Scott, J. (2003). A systematic review of manic and depressive prodromes. *Journal of Affective Disorders, 74*(3), 209–217. https://doi.org/10.1016/s0165-0327(02)00266-5

Jansson-Frojmark, M., & Jacobson, K. (2021). Cognitive behavioural therapy for insomnia for patients with co-morbid generalized anxiety disorder: An open trial on clinical outcomes and putative mechanisms. *Behavioural and Cognitive Psychotherapy, 49*(5), 540–555. https://doi.org/10.1017/S1352465821000023

Jenkins, C. A., Thompson, K. N., Nicholas, C. L., & Chanen, A. M. (2022). Sleep in young people with features of borderline personality disorder: A scoping review. *Journal of Personality Disorders, 36*(1), 19–39. https://doi.org/10.1521/pedi_2021_35_525

Jenkins, M. M., Colvonen, P. J., Norman, S. B., Afari, N., Allard, C. B., & Drummond, S. P. (2015). Prevalence and mental health correlates of insomnia in first-encounter veterans with and without military sexual trauma. *Sleep, 38*(10), 1547–1554. https://doi.org/10.5665/sleep.5044

Joffe, R. T., & Swinson, R. P. (1988). Total sleep deprivation in patients with obsessive–compulsive disorder. *Acta Psychiatrica Scandinavica, 77*(4), 483–487. https://doi.org/10.1111/j.1600-0447.1988.tb05155.x

Johnson, E. O., Roth, T., & Breslau, N. (2006). The association of insomnia with anxiety disorders and depression: Exploration of the direction of risk. *Journal of Psychiatric Research, 40*(8), 700–708. https://doi.org/10.1016/j.jpsychires.2006.07.008

Kaplan, K. A., Gruber, J., Eidelman, P., Talbot, L. S., & Harvey, A. G. (2011). Hypersomnia in inter-episode bipolar disorder: Does it have prognostic significance? *Journal of Affective Disorders, 132*(3), 438–444. https://doi.org/10.1016/j.jad.2011.03.013

Kaplan, K. A., McGlinchey, E. L., Soehner, A., Gershon, A., Talbot, L. S., Eidelman, P., Gruber, J., & Harvey, A. G. (2015). Hypersomnia subtypes, sleep and relapse in bipolar disorder. *Psychological Medicine, 45*(8), 1751–1763. https://doi.org/10.1017/S0033291714002918

Kaplan, K. A., Talavera, D. C., & Harvey, A. G. (2018). Rise and shine: A treatment experiment testing a morning routine to decrease subjective sleep inertia in insomnia and bipolar disorder. *Behaviour Research and Therapy, 111*, 106–112. https://doi.org/10.1016/j.brat.2018.10.009

Kaskie, R. E., Graziano, B., & Ferrarelli, F. (2017). Schizophrenia and sleep disorders: Links, risks, and management challenges. *Nature and Science of Sleep, 9*, 227–239. https://doi.org/10.2147/nss.S121076

Kasper, S., & Wehr, T. A. (1992). The role of sleep and wakefulness in the genesis of depression and mania [Special issue]. *Encephale, 18*, 45–50. https://www.ncbi.nlm.nih.gov/pubmed/1600904

Katz, J. L., Kuperberg, A., Pollack, C. P., Walsh, B. T., Zumoff, B., & Weiner, H. (1984). Is there a relationship between eating disorder and affective disorder? New evidence from sleep recordings. *American Journal of Psychiatry, 141*(6), 753–759. https://doi.org/10.1176/ajp.141.6.753

Kim, K. R., Jung, Y. C., Shin, M. Y., Namkoong, K., Kim, J. K., & Lee, J. H. (2010). Sleep disturbance in women with eating disorder: Prevalence and clinical characteristics. *Psychiatry Research, 176*(1), 88–90. https://doi.org/10.1016/j.psychres.2009.03.021

Klein, E., Caspi, Y., & Gil, S. (2003). The relation between memory of the traumatic event and PTSD: Evidence from studies of traumatic brain injury. *Canadian Journal of Psychiatry, 48*(1), 28–33. https://doi.org/10.1177/070674370304800106

Kobayashi, I., Boarts, J. M., & Delahanty, D. L. (2007). Polysomnographically measured sleep abnormalities in PTSD: A meta-analytic review. *Psychophysiology, 44*(4), 660–669. https://doi.org/10.1111/j.1469-8986.2007.537.x

Koffel, E., Khawaja, I. S., & Germain, A. (2016). Sleep disturbances in posttraumatic stress disorder: Updated review and implications for treatment. *Psychiatric Annals, 46*(3), 173–176. https://doi.org/10.3928/00485713-20160125-01

Koffel, E., Polusny, M. A., Arbisi, P. A., & Erbes, C. R. (2013). Pre-deployment daytime and nighttime sleep complaints as predictors of post-deployment PTSD and depression in National Guard troops. *Journal of Anxiety Disorders, 27*(5), 512–519. https://doi.org/10.1016/j.janxdis.2013.07.003

Korenic, S. A., Klingaman, E. A., Wickwire, E. M., Gaston, F. E., Chen, H., Wijtenburg, S. A., & Rowland, L. M. (2020). Sleep quality is related to brain glutamate and symptom severity in schizophrenia. *Journal of Psychiatric Research, 120*, 14–20. https://doi.org/10.1016/j.jpsychires.2019.10.006

Krakow, B., Melendrez, D., Johnston, L., Warner, T. D., Clark, J. O., Pacheco, M., Pedersen, B., Koss, M., Hollifield, M., & Schrader, R. (2002). Sleep-disordered breathing, psychiatric distress, and quality of life impairment in sexual assault survivors. *Journal of Nervous and Mental Disease, 190*(7), 442–452. https://doi.org/10.1097/00005053-200207000-00004

Krakow, B. J., Ulibarri, V. A., Moore, B. A., & McIver, N. D. (2015). Posttraumatic stress disorder and sleep-disordered breathing: A review of comorbidity research. *Sleep Medicine Reviews, 24*, 37–45. https://doi.org/10.1016/j.smrv.2014.11.001

Krystal, A. D., Thakur, M., & Roth, T. (2008). Sleep disturbance in psychiatric disorders: Effects on function and quality of life in mood disorders, alcoholism, and schizophrenia. *Annals of Clinical Psychiatry, 20*(1), 39–46. https://doi.org/10.1080/10401230701844661

Kupfer, D. J., & Foster, F. G. (1972). Interval between onset of sleep and rapid-eye-movement sleep as an indicator of depression. *Lancet, 2*(7779), 684–686. https://doi.org/10.1016/s0140-6736(72)92090-9

Kupfer, D. J., Foster, F. G., Reich, L., Thompson, S. K., & Weiss, B. (1976). EEG sleep changes as predictors in depression. *American Journal of Psychiatry, 133*(6), 622–626. https://doi.org/10.1176/ajp.133.6.622

Kupfer, D. J., Ulrich, R. F., Coble, P. A., Jarrett, D. B., Grochocinski, V. J., Doman, J., Matthews, G., & Borbely, A. A. (1985). Electroencephalographic sleep of younger depressives. Comparison with normals. *Archives of General Psychiatry, 42*(8), 806–810. http://www.ncbi.nlm.nih.gov/pubmed/4015325

Labbate, L. A., Johnson, M. R., Lydiard, R. B., Brawman-Mintzer, O., Emmanuel, N., Crawford, M., Kapp, R., & Ballenger, J. C. (1998). Sleep deprivation in social phobia and generalized anxiety disorder. *Biological Psychiatry, 43*(11), 840–842. https://doi.org/10.1016/s0006-3223(97)00319-3

Labbate, L. A., Pollack, M. H., Otto, M. W., Langenauer, S., & Rosenbaum, J. F. (1994). Sleep panic attacks: An association with childhood anxiety and adult psychopathology. *Biological Psychiatry, 36*(1), 57–60. https://doi.org/10.1016/0006-3223(94)90063-9

Lacey, J. H., Crisp, A. H., Kalucy, R. S., Hartmann, M. K., & Chien, C. N. (1975). Weight gain and the sleeping electroencephalogram: Study of 10 patients with anorexia nervosa. *British Medical Journal, 4*(5996), 556–558. https://doi.org/10.1136/bmj.4.5996.556

Lacey, J. H., Crisp, A. H., Kalucy, R. S., Hartmann, M., & Chien, C. (1976). Study of EEG sleep characteristics in patients with anorexia nervosa before and after restoration of matched population mean weight consequent on ingestion of a "normal" diet. *Postgraduate Medical Journal, 52*(603), 45–49. https://doi.org/10.1136/pgmj.52.603.45

Latzer, Y., Tzischinsky, O., & Epstein, R. (2001). Sleep–wake monitoring in women suffering from anorexia nervosa. *Eating Disorders, 9*(2), 159–166. https://doi.org/10.1080/10640260127713

Latzer, Y., Tzischinsky, O., Epstein, R., Klein, E., & Peretz, L. (1999). Naturalistic sleep monitoring in women suffering from bulimia nervosa. *International Journal of Eating Disorders, 26*(3), 315–321. https://doi.org/10.1002/(sici)1098-108x(199911)26:3<315::aid-eat9>3.0.co;2-6

Nierenberg, A. A., Keefe, B. R., Leslie, V. C., Alpert, J. E., Pava, J. A., Worthington, J. J., 3rd, Rosenbaum, J. F., & Fava, M. (1999). Residual symptoms in depressed patients who respond acutely to fluoxetine. *Journal of Clinical Psychiatry*, *60*(4), 221–225. http://www.ncbi.nlm.nih.gov/pubmed/10221281

Nobili, L., Baglietto, M. G., Beelke, M., De Carli, F., Di Comite, R., Fiocchi, I., Rizzo, P., Veneselli, E., Savoini, M., Zanotto, E., & Ferrillo, F. (2004). Impairment of the production of delta sleep in anorectic adolescents. *Sleep*, *27*(8), 1553–1559. https://doi.org/10.1093/sleep/27.8.1553

Nofzinger, E. A., Thase, M. E., Reynolds, C. F., 3rd, Himmelhoch, J. M., Mallinger, A., Houck, P., & Kupfer, D. J. (1991). Hypersomnia in bipolar depression: A comparison with narcolepsy using the Multiple Sleep Latency Test. *American Journal of Psychiatry*, *148*(9), 1177–1181. http://www.ncbi.nlm.nih.gov/pubmed/1882995

Nordahl, H., Havnen, A., Hansen, B., Ost, L. G., & Kvale, G. (2018). Sleep disturbances in treatment-seeking OCD-patients: Changes after concentrated exposure treatment. *Scandinavian Journal of Psychology*, *59*(2), 186–191. https://doi.org/10.1111/sjop.12417

Norton, G. R., Norton, P. J., Walker, J. R., Cox, B. J., & Stein, M. B. (1999). A comparison of people with and without nocturnal panic attacks. *Journal of Behavior Therapy and Experimental Psychiatry*, *30*(1), 37–44. https://doi.org/10.1016/s0005-7916(98)00037-8

O'Brien, K. M., & Vincent, N. K. (2003). Psychiatric comorbidity in anorexia and bulimia nervosa: Nature, prevalence, and causal relationships. *Clinical Psychology Review*, *23*(1), 57–74. https://doi.org/10.1016/s0272-7358(02)00201-5

Ocak, D., Kotan, V. O., Paltun, S. C., & Aydemir, M. Ç. (2019). Is restless legs syndrome related with depression/anxiety disorders or medications used in these disorders? A cross-sectional, clinic-based study. *Psychiatry and Clinical Psychopharmacology*, *29*(4), 832–839. https://doi.org/10.1080/24750573.2019.1673943

O'Hara, R., & Schroder, C. (2006). Unraveling the relationship of obstructive sleep-disordered breathing to major depressive disorder. *Sleep Medicine*, *7*(2), 101–103. https://doi.org/10.1016/j.sleep.2005.11.011

Ohayon, M. M. (1997). Prevalence of DSM-IV diagnostic criteria of insomnia: Distinguishing insomnia related to mental disorders from sleep disorders. *Journal of Psychiatric Research*, *31*(3), 333–346. https://doi.org/10.1016/s0022-3956(97)00002-2

Ohayon, M. M. (2003). The effects of breathing-related sleep disorders on mood disturbances in the general population. *Journal of Clinical Psychiatry*, *64*(10), 1195–1200; quiz, 1274–1196. https://doi.org/10.4088/jcp.v64n1009

Ohayon, M. M., & Pakpour, A. H. (2022). Prevalence, incidence, evolution and associated factors of sleep paralysis in a longitudinal study of the US general population. *Sleep Medicine*, *98*, 62–67. https://doi.org/10.1016/j.sleep.2022.06.003

Ohayon, M. M., & Roth, T. (2002). Prevalence of restless legs syndrome and periodic limb movement disorder in the general population. *Journal of Psychosomatic Research*, *53*(1), 547–554. https://doi.org/10.1016/s0022-3999(02)00443-9

Ohayon, M. M., & Roth, T. (2003). Place of chronic insomnia in the course of depressive and anxiety disorders. *Journal of Psychiatric Research*, *37*(1), 9–15. https://doi.org/10.1016/s0022-3956(02)00052-3

Ohayon, M. M., & Shapiro, C. M. (2000). Sleep disturbances and psychiatric disorders associated with post-traumatic stress disorder in the general population. *Comprehensive Psychiatry*, *41*(6), 469–478. https://doi.org/10.1053/comp.2000.16568

Ohno, K., & Sakurai, T. (2008). Orexin neuronal circuitry: Role in the regulation of sleep and wakefulness. *Frontiers in Neuroendocrinology*, *29*(1), 70–87. https://doi.org/10.1016/j.yfrne.2007.08.001

Ong, J. C., Gress, J. L., San Pedro-Salcedo, M. G., & Manber, R. (2009). Frequency and predictors of obstructive sleep apnea among individuals with major depressive disorder and insomnia. *Journal of Psychosomatic Research*, *67*(2), 135–141. https://doi.org/10.1016/j.jpsychores.2009.03.011

Otto, M. W., Simon, N. M., Powers, M., Hinton, D., Zalta, A. K., & Pollack, M. H. (2006). Rates of isolated sleep paralysis in outpatients with anxiety disorders. *Journal of Anxiety Disorders*, *20*(5), 687–693. https://doi.org/10.1016/j.janxdis.2005.07.002

Pancheri, C., Verdolini, N., Pacchiarotti, I., Samalin, L., Delle Chiaie, R., Biondi, M., Carvalho, A. F., Valdes, M., Ritter, P., Vieta, E., & Murru, A. (2019). A systematic review on sleep alterations anticipating the onset of bipolar disorder. *European Psychiatry*, *58*, 45–53. https://doi.org/10.1016/j.eurpsy.2019.02.003

Papadimitriou, G. N., Kerkhofs, M., Kempenaers, C., & Mendlewicz, J. (1988). EEG sleep studies in patients with generalized anxiety disorder. *Psychiatry Research*, *26*(2), 183–190. https://doi.org/10.1016/0165-1781(88)90073-x

Papadimitriou, G. N., & Linkowski, P. (2005). Sleep disturbance in anxiety disorders. *International Review of Psychiatry, 17*(4), 229–236. https://doi.org/10.1080/09540260500104524

Papadimitriou, G. N., Linkowski, P., Kerkhofs, M., Kempenaers, C., & Mendlewicz, J. (1988). Sleep EEG recordings in generalized anxiety disorder with significant depression. *Journal of Affective Disorders, 15*(2), 113–118. https://doi.org/10.1016/0165-0327(88)90078-x

Paradis, C. M., & Friedman, S. (2005). Sleep paralysis in African Americans with panic disorder. *Transcultural Psychiatry, 42*(1), 123–134. https://doi.org/10.1177/1363461505050720

Park, H. J., Kim, M. S., Park, E. C., Jang, S. Y., Kim, W., & Han, K. T. (2018). Association between sleep disorder and panic disorder in South Korea: Nationwide nested case–control study of data from 2004 to 2013. *Psychiatry Research, 260*, 286–291. https://doi.org/10.1016/j.psychres.2017.11.076

Perlis, M. L., Giles, D. E., Buysse, D. J., Tu, X., & Kupfer, D. J. (1997). Self-reported sleep disturbance as a prodromal symptom in recurrent depression. *Journal of Affective Disorders, 42*(2–3), 209–212. https://doi.org/10.1016/s0165-0327(96)01411-5

Perlis, M. L., Smith, L. J., Lyness, J. M., Matteson, S. R., Pigeon, W. R., Jungquist, C. R., & Tu, X. (2006). Insomnia as a risk factor for onset of depression in the elderly. *Behavioral Sleep Medicine, 4*(2), 104–113. https://doi.org/10.1207/s15402010bsm0402_3

Pfennig, A., Ritter, P. S., Hofler, M., Lieb, R., Bauer, M., Wittchen, H. U., & Beesdo-Baum, K. (2016). Symptom characteristics of depressive episodes prior to the onset of mania or hypomania. *Acta Psychiatrica Scandinavica, 133*(3), 196–204. https://doi.org/10.1111/acps.12469

Pieters, G., Theys, P., Vandereycken, W., Leroy, B., & Peuskens, J. (2004). Sleep variables in anorexia nervosa: Evolution with weight restoration. *International Journal of Eating Disorders, 35*(3), 342–347. https://doi.org/10.1002/eat.10256

Pigeon, W. R., May, P. E., Perlis, M. L., Ward, E. A., Lu, N., & Talbot, N. L. (2009). The effect of interpersonal psychotherapy for depression on insomnia symptoms in a cohort of women with sexual abuse histories. *Journal of Traumatic Stress, 22*(6), 634–638. https://doi.org/10.1002/jts.20456

Plante, D. T., Frankenburg, F. R., Fitzmaurice, G. M., & Zanarini, M. C. (2013). Relationship between sleep disturbance and recovery in patients with borderline personality disorder. *Journal of Psychosomatic Research, 74*(4), 278–282. https://doi.org/10.1016/j.jpsychores.2013.01.006

Pollack, M., Kinrys, G., Krystal, A., McCall, W. V., Roth, T., Schaefer, K., Rubens, R., Roach, J., Huang, H., & Krishnan, R. (2008). Eszopiclone coadministered with escitalopram in patients with insomnia and comorbid generalized anxiety disorder. *Archives of General Psychiatry, 65*(5), 551–562. https://doi.org/10.1001/archpsyc.65.5.551

Pruiksma, K. E., Taylor, D. J., Wachen, J. S., Mintz, J., Young-McCaughan, S., Peterson, A. L., Yarvis, J. S., Borah, E. V., Dondanville, K. A., Litz, B. T., Hembree, E. A., & Resick, P. A. (2016). Residual sleep disturbances following PTSD treatment in active duty military personnel. *Psychological Trauma, 8*(6), 697–701. https://doi.org/10.1037/tra0000150

Raffray, T., Bond, T. L., & Pelissolo, A. (2011). Correlates of insomnia in patients with social phobia: role of depression and anxiety. *Psychiatry Research, 189*(2), 315–317. https://doi.org/10.1016/j.psychres.2011.03.004

Reeve, S., Sheaves, B., & Freeman, D. (2015). The role of sleep dysfunction in the occurrence of delusions and hallucinations: A systematic review. *Clinical Psychology Review, 42*, 96–115. https://doi.org/10.1016/j.cpr.2015.09.001

Reeve, S., Sheaves, B., & Freeman, D. (2019). Sleep disorders in early psychosis: Incidence, severity, and association with clinical symptoms. *Schizophrenia Bulletin, 45*(2), 287–295. https://doi.org/10.1093/schbul/sby129

Reynolds, C. F., 3rd, Coble, P. A., Spiker, D. G., Neil, J. F., Holzer, B. C., & Kupfer, D. J. (1982). Prevalence of sleep apnea and nocturnal myoclonus in major affective disorders: Clinical and polysomnographic findings. *Journal of Nervous and Mental Disease, 170*(9), 565–567. https://doi.org/10.1097/00005053-198209000-00008

Reynolds, C. F., 3rd, Shaw, D. H., Newton, T. F., Coble, P. A., & Kupfer, D. J. (1983). EEG sleep in outpatients with generalized anxiety: A preliminary comparison with depressed outpatients. *Psychiatry Research, 8*(2), 81–89. https://doi.org/10.1016/0165-1781(83)90094-x

Riemann, D., Berger, M., & Voderholzer, U. (2001). Sleep and depression—Results from psychobiological studies: An overview. *Biological Psychology, 57*(1–3), 67–103.

Riemann, D., & Voderholzer, U. (2003). Primary insomnia: A risk factor to develop depression? *Journal of Affective Disorders, 76*(1–3), 255–259. https://doi.org/10.1016/s0165-0327(02)00072-1

Riemann, D., Voderholzer, U., & Berger, M. (2002). Sleep and sleep–wake manipulations in bipolar depression. *Neuropsychobiology*, *45*(S1), 7–12. https://doi.org/10.1159/000049255

Roberts, R. E., Shema, S. J., Kaplan, G. A., & Strawbridge, W. J. (2000). Sleep complaints and depression in an aging cohort: A prospective perspective. *American Journal of Psychiatry*, *157*(1), 81–88. https://doi.org/10.1176/ajp.157.1.81

Robillard, R., Naismith, S. L., & Hickie, I. B. (2013). Recent advances in sleep–wake cycle and biological rhythms in bipolar disorder. *Current Psychiatry Reports*, *15*(10), 402. https://doi.org/10.1007/s11920-013-0402-3

Roy-Byrne, P. P., Uhde, T. W., & Post, R. M. (1986). Effects of one night's sleep deprivation on mood and behavior in panic disorder. Patients with panic disorder compared with depressed patients and normal controls. *Archives of General Psychiatry*, *43*(9), 895–899. https://doi.org/10.1001/archpsyc.1986.01800090085011

Sansa, G., Gavalda, A., Gaig, C., Monreal, J., Ercilla, G., Casamitjana, R., Ribera, G., Iranzo, A., & Santamaria, J. (2016). Exploring the presence of narcolepsy in patients with schizophrenia. *BMC Psychiatry*, *16*, Article 177. https://doi.org/10.1186/s12888-016-0859-9

Sauchelli, S., Jimenez-Murcia, S., Sanchez, I., Riesco, N., Custal, N., Fernandez-Garcia, J. C., Garrido-Sanchez, L., Tinahones, F. J., Steiger, H., Israel, M., Banos, R. M., Botella, C., de la Torre, R., Fernandez-Real, J. M., Ortega, F. J., Fruhbeck, G., Granero, R., Tarrega, S., Crujeiras, A. B., . . . Fernandez-Aranda, F. (2016). Orexin and sleep quality in anorexia nervosa: Clinical relevance and influence on treatment outcome. *Psychoneuroendocrinology*, *65*, 102–108. https://doi.org/10.1016/j.psyneuen.2015.12.014

Schredl, M., Paul, F., Reinhard, I., Ebner-Priemer, U. W., Schmahl, C., & Bohus, M., (2012). Sleep and dreaming in patients with borderline personality disorder: A polysomnography study. *Psychiatry Research*, *200*(2–3), 430–436. https://doi.org/10.1016/j.psychres.2012.04.036

Selby, E. A. (2013). Chronic sleep disturbances and borderline personality disorder symptoms. *Journal of Consulting and Clinical Psychology*, *81*(5), 941–947. https://doi.org/10.1037/a0033201

Semiz, U. B., Basoglu, C., Ebrinc, S., & Cetin, M. (2008). Nightmare disorder, dream anxiety, and subjective sleep quality in patients with borderline personality disorder. *Psychiatry and Clinical Neurosciences*, *62*(1), 48–55. https://doi.org/10.1111/j.1440-1819.2007.01789.x

Sevilla-Cermeno, L., Isomura, K., Larsson, H., Akerstedt, T., Vilaplana-Perez, A., Lahera, G., Mataix-Cols, D., & Fernandez de la Cruz, L. (2020). Insomnia in obsessive–compulsive disorder: A Swedish population-based cohort study. *Journal of Affective Disorders*, *266*, 413–416. https://doi.org/10.1016/j.jad.2020.01.122

Sharafkhaneh, A., Giray, N., Richardson, P., Young, T., & Hirshkowitz, M. (2005). Association of psychiatric disorders and sleep apnea in a large cohort. *Sleep*, *28*(11), 1405–1411. https://doi.org/10.1093/sleep/28.11.1405

Sharpless, B. A., McCarthy, K. S., Chambless, D. L., Milrod, B. L., Khalsa, S. R., & Barber, J. P. (2010). Isolated sleep paralysis and fearful isolated sleep paralysis in outpatients with panic attacks. *Journal of Clinical Psychology*, *66*(12), 1292–1306. https://doi.org/10.1002/jclp.20724

Short, N. A., Babson, K. A., Schmidt, N. B., Knight, C. B., Johnson, J., & Bonn-Miller, M. O. (2016). Sleep and affective functioning: Examining the association between sleep quality and distress tolerance among veterans. *Personality and Individual Differences*, 90, 247–253. https://doi.org/10.1016/j.paid.2015.10.054

Simon, L., Blay, M., Galvao, F., & Brunelin, J. (2021). Using EEG to predict clinical response to electroconvulsive therapy in patients with major depression: A comprehensive review. *Frontiers in Psychiatry*, *12*, Article 643710. https://doi.org/10.3389/fpsyt.2021.643710

Singareddy, R., & Uhde, T. W. (2009). Nocturnal sleep panic and depression: Relationship to subjective sleep in panic disorder. *Journal of Affective Disorders*, *112*(1–3), 262–266. https://doi.org/10.1016/j.jad.2008.04.026

Sit, D. K., McGowan, J., Wiltrout, C., Diler, R. S., Dills, J. J., Luther, J., Yang, A., Ciolino, J. D., Seltman, H., Wisniewski, S. R., Terman, M., & Wisner, K. L. (2018). Adjunctive bright light therapy for bipolar depression: A randomized double-blind placebo-controlled trial. *American Journal of Psychiatry*, *175*(2), 131–139. https://doi.org/10.1176/appi.ajp.2017.16101200

Smith, N. S., Martin, R. L., Bauer, B. W., Bandel, S. L., & Capron, D. W. (2020). The association between nocturnal panic attacks and suicidal ideation, plans, and attempts. *Psychiatry Research*, *291*, Article 113280. https://doi.org/10.1016/j.psychres.2020.113280

Stein, M. B., Enns, M. W., & Kryger, M. H. (1993). Sleep in nondepressed patients with panic disorder: II. Polysomnographic assessment of sleep architecture and sleep continuity. *Journal of Affective Disorders*, *28*(1), 1–6. https://doi.org/10.1016/0165-0327(93)90071-q

Stein, M. B., Kroft, C. D., & Walker, J. R. (1993). Sleep impairment in patients with social phobia. *Psychiatry Research, 49*(3), 251–256. https://doi.org/10.1016/0165-1781(93)90065-o
Stein, M. B., Millar, T. W., Larsen, D. K., & Kryger, M. H. (1995). Irregular breathing during sleep in patients with panic disorder. *American Journal of Psychiatry, 152*(8), 1168–1173. https://doi.org/10.1176/ajp.152.8.1168
Stubbs, B., Vancampfort, D., Veronese, N., Solmi, M., Gaughran, F., Manu, P., Rosenbaum, S., De Hert, M., & Fornaro, M. (2016). The prevalence and predictors of obstructive sleep apnea in major depressive disorder, bipolar disorder and schizophrenia: A systematic review and meta-analysis. *Journal of Affective Disorders, 197*, 259–267. https://doi.org/10.1016/j.jad.2016.02.060
Sylvia, L. G., Chang, W. C., Kamali, M., Tohen, M., Kinrys, G., Deckersbach, T., Calabrese, J. R., Thase, M. E., Reilly-Harrington, N., Bobo, W. V., Kocsis, J. H., McInnis, M. G., Bowden, C. L., Ketter, T. A., Friedman, E. S., Shelton, R. C., McElroy, S. L., Gao, K., Rabideau, D. J., & Nierenberg, A. A. (2018). Sleep disturbance may impact treatment outcome in bipolar disorder: A preliminary investigation in the context of a large comparative effectiveness trial. *Journal of Affective Disorders, 225*, 563–568. https://doi.org/10.1016/j.jad.2017.08.056
Taherifard, M., Abolghasemi, A., & Hajloo, N. (2015). Positive and negative urgency and sleep quality among patients with borderline and antisocial personality disorder. *Archives of Psychiatry and Psychotherapy, 17*, 105–112. https://doi.org/10.12740/APP/61255
Takaesu, Y., Inoue, Y., Ono, K., Murakoshi, A., Futenma, K., Komada, Y., & Inoue, T. (2017). Circadian rhythm sleep–wake disorders as predictors for bipolar disorder in patients with remitted mood disorders. *Journal of Affective Disorders, 220*, 57–61. https://doi.org/10.1016/j.jad.2017.05.041
Takahashi, K. I., Shimizu, T., Sugita, T., Saito, Y., Takahashi, Y., & Hishikawa, Y. (1998). Prevalence of sleep-related respiratory disorders in 101 schizophrenic inpatients. *Psychiatry and Clinical Neurosciences, 52*(2), 229–231. https://doi.org/10.1111/j.1440-1819.1998.tb01046.x
Talbot, L. S., Maguen, S., Metzler, T. J., Schmitz, M., McCaslin, S. E., Richards, A., Perlis, M. L., Posner, D. A., Weiss, B., Ruoff, L., Varbel, J., & Neylan, T. C. (2014). Cognitive behavioral therapy for insomnia in posttraumatic stress disorder: A randomized controlled trial. *Sleep, 37*(2), 327–341. https://doi.org/10.5665/sleep.3408
Talih, F., Gebara, N. Y., Andary, F. S., Mondello, S., Kobeissy, F., & Ferri, R. (2018). Delayed sleep phase syndrome and bipolar disorder: Pathogenesis and available common biomarkers. *Sleep Medicine Reviews, 41*, 133–140. https://doi.org/10.1016/j.smrv.2018.02.002
Tandon, R., Shipley, J. E., Taylor, S., Greden, J. F., Eiser, A., DeQuardo, J., & Goodson, J. (1992). Electroencephalographic sleep abnormalities in schizophrenia. Relationship to positive/negative symptoms and prior neuroleptic treatment. *Archives of General Psychiatry, 49*(3), 185–194. http://www.ncbi.nlm.nih.gov/pubmed/1348923
Taylor, D. J., Pruiksma, K. E., Hale, W. J., Kelly, K., Maurer, D., Peterson, A. L., Mintz, J., Litz, B. T., Williamson, D. E., & Consortium, S. S. (2016). Prevalence, correlates, and predictors of insomnia in the US Army prior to deployment. *Sleep, 39*(10), 1795–1806. https://doi.org/10.5665/sleep.6156
Taylor, F. B., Martin, P., Thompson, C., Williams, J., Mellman, T. A., Gross, C., Peskind, E. R., & Raskind, M. A. (2008). Prazosin effects on objective sleep measures and clinical symptoms in civilian trauma post-traumatic stress disorder: A placebo-controlled study. *Biological Psychiatry, 63*(6), 629–632. https://doi.org/10.1016/j.biopsych.2007.07.001
Thase, M. E. (1999). Antidepressant treatment of the depressed patient with insomnia. *Journal of Clinical Psychiatry, 60*(S17), 28–31; discussion 46–28. https://www.ncbi.nlm.nih.gov/pubmed/10446739
Thase, M. E., Rush, A. J., Manber, R., Kornstein, S. G., Klein, D. N., Markowitz, J. C., Ninan, P. T., Friedman, E. S., Dunner, D. L., Schatzberg, A. F., Borian, F. E., Trivedi, M. H., & Keller, M. B. (2002). Differential effects of nefazodone and cognitive behavioral analysis system of psychotherapy on insomnia associated with chronic forms of major depression. *Journal of Clinical Psychiatry, 63*(6), 493–500. http://www.ncbi.nlm.nih.gov/pubmed/12088160
Timpano, K. R., Carbonella, J. Y., Bernert, R. A., & Schmidt, N. B. (2014). Obsessive compulsive symptoms and sleep difficulties: Exploring the unique relationship between insomnia and obsessions. *Journal of Psychiatric Research, 57*, 101–107. https://doi.org/10.1016/j.jpsychires.2014.06.021
Tsao, J. C., & Craske, M. G. (2003). Reactivity to imagery and nocturnal panic attacks. *Depression and Anxiety, 18*(4), 205–213. https://doi.org/10.1002/da.10091
Turner, J., Drummond, L. M., Mukhopadhyay, S., Ghodse, H., White, S., Pillay, A., & Fineberg, N. A. (2007). A prospective study of delayed sleep phase syndrome in patients with severe resistant obsessive–compulsive disorder. *World Psychiatry, 6*(2), 108–111. https://www.ncbi.nlm.nih.gov/pubmed/18235868

Turvey, C. L., Conwell, Y., Jones, M. P., Phillips, C., Simonsick, E., Pearson, J. L., & Wallace, R. (2002). Risk factors for late-life suicide: A prospective, community-based study. *American Journal of Geriatric Psychiatry, 10*(4), 398–406. http://www.ncbi.nlm.nih.gov/pubmed/12095899

Vai, B., Poletti, S., Radaelli, D., Dallaspezia, S., Bulgarelli, C., Locatelli, C., Bollettini, I., Falini, A., Colombo, C., Smeraldi, E., & Benedetti, F. (2015). Successful antidepressant chronotherapeutics enhance fronto-limbic neural responses and connectivity in bipolar depression. *Psychiatry Research, 233*(2), 243–253. https://doi.org/10.1016/j.pscychresns.2015.07.015

Van Veen, M. M., Karsten, J., & Lancel, M. (2017). Poor sleep and its relation to impulsivity in patients with antisocial or borderline personality disorders. *Behavioral Medicine, 43*(3), 218–226. https://doi.org/10.1080/08964289.2017.1313719

Wardle-Pinkston, S., Slavish, D. C., & Taylor, D. J. (2019). Insomnia and cognitive performance: A systematic review and meta-analysis. *Sleep Medicine Reviews, 48*, 01205. https://doi.org/10.1016/j.smrv.2019.07.008

Wehr, T. A., Goodwin, F. K., Wirz-Justice, A., Breitmaier, J., & Craig, C. (1982). 48-Hour sleep–wake cycles in manic-depressive illness: Naturalistic observations and sleep deprivation experiments. *Archives of General Psychiatry, 39*(5), 559–565. https://doi.org/10.1001/archpsyc.1982.04290050037008

Wehr, T. A., Sack, D. A., & Rosenthal, N. E. (1987). Sleep reduction as a final common pathway in the genesis of mania. *American Journal of Psychiatry, 144*(2), 201–204. https://doi.org/10.1176/ajp.144.2.201

Weibel, S., Jermann, F., Weiner, L., Nicastro, R., Ardu, S., Pham, E., Hasler, R., Dayer, A., Prada, P., & Perroud, N. (2017). Insomnia in adult attention-deficit/hyperactivity disorder: A comparison with borderline personality disorder population in a clinical setting and control participants. *Comprehensive Psychiatry, 76*, 119–128. https://doi.org/10.1016/j.comppsych.2017.04.009

Werner, G. G., Riemann, D., & Ehring, T. (2021). Fear of sleep and trauma-induced insomnia: A review and conceptual model. *Sleep Medicine Reviews, 55*, Article 101383. https://doi.org/10.1016/j.smrv.2020.101383

Willie, J. T., Chemelli, R. M., Sinton, C. M., & Yanagisawa, M. (2001). To eat or to sleep? Orexin in the regulation of feeding and wakefulness. *Annual Review of Neuroscience, 24*, 429–458. https://doi.org/10.1146/annurev.neuro.24.1.429

Winsper, C., Tang, N. K., Marwaha, S., Lereya, S. T., Gibbs, M., Thompson, A., & Singh, S. P. (2017). The sleep phenotype of borderline personality disorder: A systematic review and meta-analysis. *Neuroscience & Biobehavioral Reviews, 73*, 48–67. https://doi.org/10.1016/j.neubiorev.2016.12.008

Woodside, B. D., & Staab, R. (2006). Management of psychiatric comorbidity in anorexia nervosa and bulimia nervosa. *CNS Drugs, 20*(8), 655–663. https://doi.org/10.2165/00023210-200620080-00004

Woodward, S. H., Bliwise, D. L., Friedman, M. J., & Gusman, D. F. (1996). Subjective versus objective sleep in Vietnam combat veterans hospitalized for PTSD. *Journal of Traumatic Stress, 9*(1), 137–143. https://doi.org/10.1007/BF02116839

Wu, J. C., & Bunney, W. E. (1990). The biological basis of an antidepressant response to sleep deprivation and relapse: Review and hypothesis. *American Journal of Psychiatry, 147*(1), 14–21. https://doi.org/10.1176/ajp.147.1.14

Wulff, K., Dijk, D. J., Middleton, B., Foster, R. G., & Joyce, E. M. (2012). Sleep and circadian rhythm disruption in schizophrenia. *British Journal of Psychiatry, 200*(4), 308–316. https://doi.org/10.1192/bjp.bp.111.096321

Yucel, D. E., van Emmerik, A. A. P., Souama, C., & Lancee, J. (2020). Comparative efficacy of imagery rehearsal therapy and prazosin in the treatment of trauma-related nightmares in adults: A meta-analysis of randomized controlled trials. *Sleep Medicine Reviews, 50*, Article 101248. https://doi.org/10.1016/j.smrv.2019.101248

Zarcone, V. P., Jr., Benson, K. L., & Berger, P. A. (1987). Abnormal rapid eye movement latencies in schizophrenia. *Archives of General Psychiatry, 44*(1), 45–48. https://doi.org/10.1001/archpsyc.1987.01800130047007

Zayfert, C., & DeViva, J. C. (2004). Residual insomnia following cognitive behavioral therapy for PTSD. *Journal of Traumatic Stress, 17*(1), 69–73. https://doi.org/10.1023/B:JOTS.0000014679.31799.e7

Zhang, Y., Weed, J. G., Ren, R., Tang, X., & Zhang, W. (2017). Prevalence of obstructive sleep apnea in patients with posttraumatic stress disorder and its impact on adherence to continuous positive airway pressure therapy: A meta-analysis. *Sleep Medicine, 36*, 125–132. https://doi.org/10.1016/j.sleep.2017.04.020

Zhou, T. H., Dang, W. M., Ma, Y. T., Hu, C. Q., Wang, N., Zhang, G. Y., Wang, G., Shi, C., Zhang, H., Guo, B., Zhou, S. Z., Feng, L., Geng, S. X., Tong, Y. Z., Tang, G. W., He, Z. K., Zhen, L., & Yu, X. (2018). Clinical efficacy, onset time and safety of bright light therapy in acute bipolar depression as an adjunctive therapy: A randomized controlled trial. *Journal of Affective Disorders, 227*, 90–96. https://doi.org/10.1016/j.jad.2017.09.038

CHAPTER

41 Women's Sleep and Circadian Rhythms From Puberty to Menopausal Transition

Bilgay Izci Balserak *and* Kathryn Aldrich Lee

Abstract

This chapter focuses on women's sleep and circadian rhythms from puberty to menopause. Sleep and circadian misalignment can influence menstrual cycle regularity and ovulation. Fluctuations in menstrual hormones are associated with menstrual symptoms like breast tenderness and uterine cramping that affect sleep and mood. Hormones, discomfort, and mood are also associated with gradual changes in sleep quality during pregnancy. Childbirth and lactation affect maternal sleep and circadian rhythms, primarily because of the newborn's unpredictable sleeping and feeding patterns. As women cycle through these reproductive phases, sleep may improve with more motherhood experience. However, during menopausal transition, sleep and circadian rhythms are impacted by irregular menstrual cycles, hormonal fluctuations, and nocturnal hot flashes in addition to the discomfort associated with aging or chronic health conditions. This chapter ends with suggestions for future research on these key reproductive stages.

Key Words: premenstrual syndrome, polycystic ovary syndrome, gestational diabetes, gestational hypertension, restless leg, co-sleeping, breastfeeding, postpartum depression, surgical menopause, breast cancer

Introduction

The purpose of this chapter is to describe sleep and circadian rhythms at key times in women's reproductive phase from menarche to menopause (Tables 41.1 and 41.2). These key times include regular monthly menstrual cycles, pregnancy and labor onset, early postpartum recovery and lactation, and the transition from regular menstrual cycles to menopause. Reproductive health issues affected by circadian misalignment or shift work, such as fertility, pregnancy loss, and breast cancer, are also included. The chapter concludes with specific questions to consider for future directions in potential research for these special populations of women.

Table 41.1 A summary of circadian rhythm changes at key reproductive stages

Circadian rhythms	Menstrual cycle
Menstrual cycle	
Melatonin	No evidence of luteal-phase difference in acrophase ↑ level in follicular phase, ↓ in luteal phase (dampened amplitude) Phase delay in morning offset time for women with PCOS ↓ melatonin amplitude in PMDD ↓ level across all phases in women with PMDD ↑ FSH responsiveness during follicular phase associated with progesterone production and risk of infertility ↑ oocytes in infertile women with sleep disturbance but does not improve their sleep No evidence for effects from low-dose oral contraceptives
Body temperature	No evidence of luteal-phase difference in acrophase ↑ in luteal phase (dampened amplitude) ↑ in luteal phase for women with PMDD compared to asymptomatic controls Low-dose oral contraceptives cause slight ↑ without phase changes
Circadian misalignment or shift work	↑ risk of irregular cycles ↑ risk of infertility
Pregnancy	
Melatonin	Continues to synchronize with estrogen and progesterone circadian rhythms ↑ level because also produced by the placenta Peak level in third trimester with abrupt reduction after birth Has role in entraining fetal circadian rhythms and maturation ↓ level or altered rhythm associated with preeclampsia Synergistic with oxytocin nocturnal peaks during labor
Body temperature	↑ slightly during pregnancy associated with ↑ progesterone
Circadian misalignment or shift work	Linked to risk of miscarriage, preeclampsia, and premature birth May be linked to glucose dysregulation May be linked to depression
Postpartum	
Melatonin	Secreted in breast milk
Body temperature	
Circadian misalignment or shift work	↑ risk of weight retention ↑ risk of postpartum depression ↑ risk of poor lactation ↑ risk of poor maternal-infant bonding and interactions
Menopausal transition (perimenopause)	
Melatonin	No evidence of change in amplitude Begins shifting to earlier peak seen with aging Begins shift to lower level seen with aging Associations with surgical menopause unclear

Continued

Table 41.1 *Continued*	
Circadian rhythms	**Menstrual cycle**
Body temperature	Loss of estrogen may narrow thermoneutral zone → hot flashes ↑ frequency of hot flashes in early evening Begins shift to earlier peak ↓ mean across the 24 hours
Circadian misalignment or shift work	Potential ↑ risk for breast cancer

Note. FSH = follicle-stimulating hormone; PCOS = polycystic ovary syndrome; PMDD = premenstrual dysphoric disorder.

Table 41.2 A summary of sleep changes at key reproductive stages	
Menstrual cycle	
PSG	No difference in Stage N2 (%) by phase Fragmented PSG associated with luteal rise in progesterone but not estrogen
Sleep-onset latency	No difference between follicular and luteal Latency may be associated with progesterone ↑ in women with polycystic ovaries
Sleep efficiency	No difference between follicular and luteal ↓ late luteal phase with menstrual cramping
Wakefulness and awakenings	No difference between follicular and luteal ↑ late luteal phase with menstrual cramping associated with irregular cycles
Duration	Shortest at ovulation; longest at luteal phase Short duration associated with infertility alters secretion of gonadal hormones Short duration may be associated with PMDD
Pregnancy	
PSG	↑ light sleep stages
Sleep-onset latency	Phase advance in first and second trimesters, returns to pre-pregnancy latency in third trimester
Sleep efficiency	↓ gradually across gestation Shortest on the night prior to onset of labor
Wakefulness and awakenings	More light sleep stages during pregnancy ↑ awakenings first and third trimesters ↑ awakenings from vivid dreams and nightmares ↑ wake due to bladder and other discomforts
Duration	↓ gradually across gestation; influenced by age, race, and parity Short-duration ↑ risk for longer labor Short-duration ↑ risk for cesarean birth Short-duration ↑ risk for depression Association with miscarriage or stillbirth unknown

Table 41.2 *Continued*

Postpartum	
PSG	Lactation and prolactin may ↑ slow-wave N3 sleep
Sleep-onset latency	Difficult to evaluate due to newborn
Sleep efficiency	↑ for breastfeeding mothers ↓ for bed-sharing mothers Low until infant skips nocturnal mid-sleep feeding
Wakefulness and awakenings	↑ awakenings for formula-feeding mothers High until infant skips nocturnal mid-sleep feeding
Duration	Short-duration ↑ risk for depression
Menopausal transition (perimenopause)	
PSG	↓ slow-wave N3 sleep in African Americans No changes in REM or non-REM stages ↓ duration about 30 minutes pre- to perimenopause
Sleep-onset latency	
Sleep efficiency	↓ late luteal premenstrual phase ↓ with hot flash events ↓ with abrupt onset surgical menopause ↓ with onset of age-related chronic pain
Wakefulness and awakenings	↑ associated with ↓ estrogen and steep ↑ FSH ↑ with hot flash events ↑ with chronic pain ↑ with abrupt onset surgical menopause
Duration	Short-duration prevalence ↑ in African Americans Association with breast cancer unclear

Note. FSH = follicle-stimulating hormone; PMDD = premenstrual dysphoric disorder; PSG = polysomnography; REM = rapid eye movement.

Menstrual Cycle

Overview

During the reproductive years, most women experience menstrual cycles that repeat every 25–35 days. The first day of menstrual bleeding marks the onset of a new cycle. There may be discomfort due to uterine cramping as the endometrial lining of the uterus is shed. Only basal levels of gonadal hormones are present during the first few days, but as the anterior pituitary signals the ovary to start developing follicles by secreting follicle-stimulating hormone (FSH) and luteinizing hormone (LH), a follicle begins to mature (follicular phase of the menstrual cycle), and ovarian secretion of estrogen increases and peaks, triggering ovulation around Day 14 with a peak in core temperature and a subsequent peak in estrogen and progesterone 5–7 days after ovulation. In the absence of fertilization, the corpus luteum degenerates (luteal phase of the menstrual cycle) and estrogen and progesterone sharply decline in preparation for a new menstrual cycle (Baker & Lee, 2018; Mihm et al., 2011). If the cycle is irregular, either too short or too long, it is likely that an ovarian follicle was not sufficiently stimulated, and there will be no rise in estrogen or progesterone and no rise in body temperature.

In addition to hormonal fluctuations associated with mood state, a higher nocturnal body temperature in the luteal phase dampens the circadian temperature rhythm (K. A. Lee, 1988; Shechter et al., 2010); and this dampening, an overall higher temperature, and no change in temperature have all been hypothesized to contribute to mood lability and premenstrual dysphoric disorder (PMDD; Baker et al., 2012; K. A. Lee, 1988; K. A. Lee et al., 1990; Parry, LeVeau, et al., 1997). Low-dose oral contraceptive hormones prescribed to treat PMDD not only prevent ovulation by inhibiting progesterone and estrogen production but maintain a consistent and slightly higher core temperature across the menstrual cycle (Baker et al., 2001; K. A. Lee, 1988). If fertilization occurs after ovulation and the pregnancy is viable, estrogen and progesterone levels continue to increase, shifting from ovarian production to placental production, and core temperature remains higher over the course of the pregnancy (see next section on pregnancy).

Circadian Factors

The complex monthly menstrual cycle is influenced by many factors orchestrated along the hypothalamic–pituitary–ovarian (HPO) axis. Any environmental or physiological stressor can alter ovarian function, sleep architecture, and mood state through the HPO axis (Tables 41.1 and 41.2). These stressors include intense physical exertion (Hrozanova et al., 2021), acute sleep deprivation or chronic short sleep duration, and 24-hour circadian rhythm misalignment from working night-shift schedules (Kervezee et al., 2018). Not only are there receptor sites for estrogen and progesterone in areas of the brain that control circadian rhythms, sleep, and mood (Buckley & Schatzberg, 2005), but LH and FSH also have a circadian rhythm during the follicular phase (Beroukhim et al., 2022); and there is evidence of melatonin action in the ovary itself (Tamura et al., 2009). Circadian rhythms altered by light exposure and melatonin production at night can affect the HPO axis and thus menstrual cycle regularity, ovulation, and fertility (Kloss et al., 2015).

Melatonin is primarily a circadian rhythm hormone produced in the pineal gland in response to darkness and is known to affect sleep patterns and mood state. Melatonin is also found in the ovary and exerts some control over ovarian function by enhancing FSH prior to ovulation and influencing estrogen and progesterone production (Cagnacci et al., 1995; Reiter et al., 2014; Woo et al., 2001). Higher melatonin levels are associated with delayed onset of puberty and menarche, while lower levels of melatonin have been associated with precocious puberty (Waldhauser et al., 1991). Melatonin's effect on ovarian function suggests that it may play a role in infertility (M. Zheng et al., 2018), with melatonin supplementation showing promising effects in treating infertility (Espino et al., 2019).

There is convincing evidence that circadian rhythms for core body temperature and melatonin levels in saliva and plasma have a lower amplitude after ovulation, but there is no evidence of a phase-delay or phase-advance in healthy asymptomatic menstruating women (Kervezee et al., 2018; K. A. Lee, 1988; Shechter et al., 2010). In women who experience PMDD, alterations in temperature and melatonin rhythms are seen (Parry, Berga, et al., 1997; Parry, LeVeau, et al., 1997), and temperature is even higher in women with PMDD (Baker et al., 1999). Despite the complex interaction between melatonin and core body temperature, more recent research points to melatonin rhythms as the culprit. Melatonin rhythm is dampened before and after ovulation in women with PMDD, but there is no evidence of a phase shift (Shechter et al., 2012). These findings in very small samples of women with PMDD are intriguing (Kervezee et al., 2018) and are further supported by recent results from a rigorous study of exogenous melatonin administration (Moderie et al., 2021).

Other risk factors for PMDD must be considered, however, to explain why all women who work night shift and have misaligned melatonin rhythms do not experience PMDD. Although there is a higher risk for mental health problems in women who work night shift (Shi et al., 2022), there is very little research on shift work and incidence of PMDD, likely due to exclusion of shift workers from studies of sleep and circadian rhythms, difficulty distinguishing premenstrual symptoms from irregular sleep schedules imposed by shift work during the premenstrual phase, and a higher prevalence of irregular menstrual cycles in women who work night shifts (Baker & Driver, 2007). Simulated night-shift schedules in controlled laboratory settings (M. R. Smith et al., 2009) may be a useful design for research on PMDD. Chellappa and colleagues (2020) used a simulated shift-work protocol to study mood; but their small sample included men and women, and the only mood rating was for happy/sad.

Sleep Factors

Although polysomnographic (PSG) studies in small samples of women may show subtle or inconclusive changes in sleep stages across the menstrual cycle, it is most likely the perception of poor sleep quality, whether associated with the menstrual cycle or not, that motivates women to seek clinical intervention.

Sleep Quality

Sleep quality may be affected by age as well as menstrual cycle as demonstrated in a sample of older premenopausal women in an actigraphy study who had lower sleep efficiency the week before menses (H. Zheng et al., 2015). Longitudinal self-report studies that include daily ratings for menstrual cycles, symptoms, and sleep quality and duration can be very informative, are more likely replicated by other researchers, and are more generalizable to the population. Most of these longitudinal studies describe sleep complaints just prior to onset of menses or during menstrual bleeding days (Baker & Driver, 2004; Kravitz et al.,

2005). In a study of 213 relatively healthy young women there were significant individual differences across the menstrual cycle in patterns of self-reported difficulty sleeping in daily logs (Van Reen & Kiesner, 2016). In a clinic sample of over 900 women complaining of sleep difficulty, women with irregular menstrual cycles were two times more likely to report sleep difficulties than women with regular cycles, even when controlling for age, body mass index (BMI), and premenstrual complaints (Hachul et al., 2010). These findings were supported in a meta-analysis of 10 studies on ovarian function which concluded that women with poor sleep had a 46% increased risk of irregular menstrual cycles (Caetano et al., 2021).

Sleep quality from the person's perception should be the valid gold-standard measure. However, objective PSG or actigraphy measures of sleep efficiency or wake time can offer accurate estimates of sleep quality if the invasive nature of the measure is considered. Wrist actigraphy results from 19 women indicated a weak association between sleep efficiency and estrogen and progesterone (Li et al., 2015), and results from a wearable sensor device (the Oura Ring) suggested a small decline in sleep efficiency in the mid-luteal phase (Alzueta et al., 2022), yet there were no significant differences in either self-reported sleep or sensor measures of sleep duration or sleep stages at four discrete time points across the menstrual cycle (menses, ovulation, mid- and late luteal).

Even results about sleep quality from well-designed studies of healthy research participants can conflict, with sleep quality deemed worse using wrist actigraphy measures (Li et al., 2015) compared to daily self-report (Romans et al., 2015). Results may also differ because of participants who are stressed in different ways, such as shift workers or endurance athletes (Hrozanova et al., 2021). In a sample of women with PMDD who did ovulate, Baker and colleagues (2007) found differences in self-reported sleep but not in PSG measures in the luteal phase compared to asymptomatic controls (Baker et al., 2007), a finding replicated in a follow-up study (Baker et al., 2012).

Conflicting results on sleep quality should not be discouraging, however, as they often create new avenues for research when attempting to understand why findings from various studies differ. For example, Sharkey and colleagues (2014) reported that more fragmented sleep during a one-night home PSG recording was associated with a sharper rise in progesterone levels from the follicular to the luteal phase but no effect from the rise in estrogen. For every 0.1 ng/dl increase in progesterone, wake after sleep onset (WASO) was 8.9% higher, with four additional wake episodes per hour of sleep. These were likely a sample of good sleepers, averaging only 3.5% WASO with PSG recordings in the home setting. It is critically important to note that WASO was reported as a percentage of each woman's sleep period, particularly given differences in total sleep time (TST). Although the difference in TST was not statistically significant in this small sample, the effect size difference was large and clinically meaningful (Cohen's $d = 0.87$) as the 16 women with high progesterone averaged <7 hours sleep and the 11 women with low progesterone averaged 8 hours (Sharkey et al., 2014). However, WASO does not include time to fall asleep, which varied greatly in the luteal phase (18 ± 21 minutes) and depended on whether ovulation occurred (22 ± 26 minutes for the high-progesterone group) or not (14 ± 10 minutes for the low-progesterone group).

Sharkey and colleagues (2014) were unable to measure the downslope of progesterone from its peak in the luteal phase to menses onset, but it could be hypothesized that the rate of fall in hormone levels prior to onset of menses (or precipitous fall at postpartum) may have more impact on sleep, circadian rhythms, and mood than the peak level or a measure taken on any given day. With long-standing evidence that progesterone administered to animals or humans has side effects that include sleepiness and elevated core body temperature, the precipitous withdrawal of a high level of endogenous progesterone prior to onset of menses could hypothetically result in prolonged sleep-onset latency in some women who may be more sensitive to progesterone. Very little research exists on how sleep or circadian rhythm is altered when hormonal interventions for long-term contraception or for infertility are used. These interventions are known to have adverse effects on psychological mood, yet how they alter sleep and circadian rhythms remains poorly understood.

Sleep Duration

In a carefully controlled laboratory study of 10 women, Baumgartner and colleagues (1993) showed that short sleep duration as a result of experimentally-induced awakening at 01:30 altered LH but not FSH (Baumgartner et al., 1993). Other researchers have also shown that brief wake episodes and sleep deprivation can alter LH secretion in the follicular phase (J. E. Hall et al., 2005). These types of studies with intense monitoring over a few days are costly, and while findings may not generalize to the home environment, they increase knowledge about potential mechanisms involved in ovulation and infertility.

There is also value in daily self-report measures addressing research questions about how sleep disturbance and circadian misalignment affect menstrual cycles and ovulation. Michels and colleagues (2020) collected daily sleep logs and salivary samples over two menstrual cycles and found no differences by night shift or chronotype. Controlling for shift work, BMI, age, and other factors, however, they found that the shortest sleep duration occurred at ovulation and the longest duration was associated with the luteal phase. Furthermore, for every additional hour of sleep during a 24-hour day, estrogen was 3.9% higher and progesterone was 9.4% higher; women reporting <7 hours sleep had 7% lower estrogen levels and 9.5% lower progesterone levels in the luteal phase (Michels et al., 2020).

There is growing evidence that short sleep duration is associated with lower FSH levels and thus is a potential risk factor for infertility (Beroukhim et al., 2022). Touzet and colleagues (2002) studied 106 French women 19–44 years old who provided daily urine samples for hormonal analyses to describe fertility in relation to sleep duration. FSH levels, but not estrogen or progesterone, were consistently lower across the menstrual cycle for the 42 women who reported sleeping <8 hours compared to the 64 women sleeping ≥8 hours (Touzet et al., 2002). Although <8 hours would not be typically regarded as short sleep duration, results are supported by other researchers. In a study of over 800 Korean adolescents up to 18 years old, 15% had irregular menstrual cycles, but those who reported sleeping ≤5 hours were twice as likely to have irregular cycles compared to the reference group sleeping ≥8 hours (Nam et al., 2017). The reasons for short sleep duration and cultural differences are difficult to discern in self-report studies. Some conflicting findings may be explained by short sleep duration or variable sleep durations across the week. Rather than sleep duration itself, other researchers have found that irregular sleep duration reported daily across one menstrual cycle was associated with levels of salivary estrogen levels (Merklinger-Gruchala et al., 2008).

Menstrual Cycle Disorders—Polycystic Ovary Syndrome

Polycystic ovary syndrome (PCOS) is the most common endocrine disorder, impacting over 5 million women of reproductive age in the United States; in PCOS, the ovaries fail to produce estrogen and progesterone (National Institutes of Health, 2012). A diagnosis of PCOS is made when women experience at least two of the following conditions: irregular menstrual cycles, high serum testosterone, and polycystic ovaries identified by ultrasound (Legro et al., 2013). Adverse health outcomes include obesity-related issues such as sleep disordered breathing (SDB), particularly in older menstruating women (Helvaci et al., 2017; Lin et al., 2017).

Accumulating evidence suggests that women with PCOS may have poorer sleep than their healthy peers. Among a clinical sample of Polish women (17–43 years) with PCOS (n = 95), over 70% reported difficulty falling asleep, 58% had poor sleep quality with Pittsburgh Sleep Quality Index (PSQI) scores >5, and about 25% had short sleep duration of <6 hours (Franik et al., 2016). In a one-night PSG study of 53 women with PCOS (16–45 years old), Vgontzas and colleagues (2001) did not find differences in sleep stages after controlling for BMI, but women with PCOS had a significantly longer sleep-onset latency (44 minutes) compared to over 400 controls randomly selected from their database of premenopausal patients (30 minutes). The prevalence of daytime sleepiness was also higher in women with PCOS (80.4%) compared to controls (27%), suggesting that BMI and daytime sleepiness with associated SDB may be confounding issues (Vgontzas et al., 2001).

Circadian rhythm studies in women with PCOS are rare. Simon and colleagues (2019) obtained hourly salivary melatonin samples to compare obese (BMI at 97th percentile) young women 12–21 years old with and without PCOS. Although adolescents may have a delayed circadian phase, the two groups did not differ on melatonin onset, but the PCOS group had an even later morning melatonin offset time relative to clock time and sleep timing, higher testosterone levels and apnea index, and a longer sleep-onset latency on school nights (Simon et al., 2019).

Design Issues in Menstrual Cycle Research

The effects of environmental and physiological stress on menstrual cycle regularity, sleep, circadian rhythms, and psychological mood state cannot be overemphasized. Although this section focuses on the menstrual cycle, research design issues are applicable to all reproductive stages including menstrual cycle, pregnancy, postpartum, and menopausal transition stages. Exposure to a strange environment, sleep deprivation, a venipuncture or other invasive procedure, and simply completing questionnaires are examples of stressors. Moreover, just paying attention to the cycle can change its characteristics. A woman who consistently reports regular cycles can suddenly experience an anovulatory cycle lasting 35 days or longer when attention is focused on it. This has prompted researchers to conduct a month or two of tracking cycles as part of a wait-list group prior to data collection for a study or to over-enroll participants to allow for substantial attrition due to anovulatory cycles. For example, Sharkey and colleagues (2014) enrolled 27 women with regular cycles over the preceding 6 months, yet during the home PSG monitoring, 11 (41%) had not ovulated according to their progesterone level. Driver and colleagues (1996) enrolled 18 women, and only 9 (50%) met phase criteria for analyses of PSG recordings across one menstrual cycle; and in a study with 259 women, 42 (16%) had anovulatory menstrual cycles (Michels et al., 2020).

To better understand how the reproductive stages (e.g., menstrual cycle, pregnancy) influence, or are influenced by, sleep and circadian rhythms, researchers need to consider design and methodology very carefully. For example, the characteristics of women motivated to participate in intensive laboratory studies may differ from characteristics of women who participate in larger epidemiological studies. Participating in laboratory studies away from home may not be feasible for most women, prompting a variety of research protocols. One design may involve PSG sleep recordings during a few consecutive nights in the follicular phase and a few consecutive nights in the luteal phase, using the first night at each time point as a night of adaptation and randomly starting at different phases (K. A. Lee et al., 1990). Another approach for PSG studies may involve sleeping in the laboratory every second or third night for an entire menstrual cycle (Driver et al., 1996; Shechter et al., 2012). Some very rigorous studies collect data daily at home from smaller cohorts of women for at least two (Hrozanova et al., 2021) to four (Romans et al., 2015) consecutive menstrual cycles, with statistical power derived from the large number of data points rather than the sample size.

There are strengths and limitations to each design, but results can build knowledge about the associations between hormone levels, sleep architecture, circadian rhythms, and psychological mood over the course of a menstrual cycle. A more acceptable approach for women may be ambulatory monitoring in the home (Sharkey et al., 2014), particularly if environmental issues of sleep disturbances from a bed partner, light, noise, and pets can be minimized. Ideally, however, each participant should be studied over two to three menstrual cycles to replicate the patterns and assess the stability of the findings.

Regardless of the study design, scientific rigor requires an objective measure of either hormone levels or a change in body temperature indicating that the salient point in the menstrual cycle is correctly identified. Yet enrollment in a laboratory study may be sufficiently stressful to alter ovulation and menstrual cycle regularity such that labeling the luteal phase according to day of the menstrual cycle may misrepresent actual luteal-phase associations with a change in circadian rhythms, sleep architecture, or psychological mood.

The need for rigor in accurately labeling phases of the menstrual cycle with an objective measure makes large cross-sectional studies less desirable. Nevertheless, knowledge can be gained by comparing large normative samples of healthy menstruating women to large samples of women in the population of interest, such as shift workers or clinical patients with infertility, polycystic ovaries and androgen excess, stress disorders, or PMDD. Sleep and menstrual cycle daily logs repeated over 2–3 months can be particularly informative in this regard, although statistical analyses can be quite complex.

Intense PSG studies are costly and typically consist of small samples, with results that may be replicated in subsequent studies or may conflict with other studies because of methodology or sampling bias. Researchers face the dilemma of recruiting from heterogeneous populations of women who may be "healthy" and consent to participate because they have a sleep problem and want answers, consent because they do not have a sleep problem but are at liberty to sleep anywhere without concern, or consent because of a primary interest in contributing to science and helping others.

Laboratory studies of potential mechanisms are critical to understanding women's physical and mental health, particularly if health can be improved by normalizing sleep and circadian rhythms. However, alternative approaches using self-report measures outside the laboratory are also useful in identifying potential mechanisms to explore. To study how the menstrual cycle affects sleep, or alternatively how sleep affects the menstrual cycle, researchers can use longitudinal data from women's daily sleep and menstrual cycle logs over 2–3 months. Because of the potential for response bias in self-report questionnaires, researchers should be cautious about using questionnaires for both sleep perception and menstrual cycle symptoms or psychological mood symptoms. Not only do some measures of sleep have items that overlap with anxiety and depression measures, but the participant's emotional state while completing the questionnaire can bias how they respond.

Pregnancy

Overview

Changes in anatomy and physiology during pregnancy can alter circadian rhythms and sleep patterns (Tables 41.1 and 41.2). These changes are often gestation-dependent and can affect physical and mental health (Beebe et al., 2017; Facco et al., 2010; Izci-Balserak et al., 2018; Tsai et al., 2012, 2017) as well as exacerbate an existing sleep disorder or create a new and persistent sleep disorder (Pien et al., 2014; Reid et al., 2017; Wilson et al., 2011). While there are many other hormonal changes occurring during pregnancy, this section focuses on estrogen, progesterone, and melatonin. Sleep and circadian rhythm disruption not only can affect maternal health but in turn can adversely influence fetal and pregnancy outcomes (Cunningham et al., 2022; Izci-Balserak, O'Brien, & Bei, 2022).

Once a fertilized ovum implants in the uterus, estrogen and progesterone production shifts from the corpus luteum to the placenta, and the markedly increasing levels during pregnancy peak in third trimester and decline after birth and delivery of the placenta (Cunningham et al., 2022; Póvoa et al., 2018). The rising estrogen (in this case estriol, a weaker form produced in the placenta) causes vasodilation and fluid accumulation that manifests as nasal congestion and ankle edema (Cunningham et al., 2022). Estrogen also stimulates prolactin production and suppresses dopamine release, which may contribute to restless legs syndrome (RLS) symptoms as pregnancy progresses (Srivanitchapoom et al., 2014).

FIRST TRIMESTER (1–12 WEEKS)

Dramatic hormonal changes begin in this trimester and contribute to sleep disturbances because of associated fatigue, daytime sleepiness, nausea in the morning or evening, increased urinary frequency, other physical discomforts like breast tenderness or nasal congestion, and mood changes (Hedman et al., 2002; K. A. Lee & Zaffke, 1999; Martin-Fairey et al., 2019; Mindell et al., 2015; Tsai et al., 2017).

SECOND TRIMESTER (13–26 WEEKS)

As the uterus continues enlarging, internal organs and the diaphragm begin to shift to make way for the growing fetus. The fatigue and nausea symptoms that are often the first signs of pregnancy attenuate, and sleep is often less disturbed in this trimester as women are now adjusting to their new hormonal milieu, particularly if this is not their first experience with motherhood (K. A. Lee et al., 2000).

THIRD TRIMESTER (27–42 WEEKS)

More pressure is exerted on the bladder and on the diaphragm as the fetus continues to develop. Most women experience urinary frequency, shortness of breath, heartburn, leg cramps, fetal movements and intermittent uterine contractions, fatigue, and physical discomforts such as breast tenderness, joint pain, backache, and itching (Beebe et al., 2017; Mindell et al., 2015; Tsai et al., 2012; Wilson et al., 2011). These physical symptoms can disrupt sleep, but many women also experience vivid dreams or nightmares (Schredl et al., 2016; Van et al., 2004), difficulty concentrating, or anxiety about potential birth complications, while also contending with external factors such as an adult bed partner or older children who may awaken during the night (Mindell et al., 2015; Palagini et al., 2014). Employment schedules can also contribute to sleep loss by minimizing nap opportunities (Facco et al., 2010; Gay et al., 2004; Manconi et al., 2012; Tsai et al., 2017).

Circadian Factors

Both estrogen and progesterone have circadian rhythms during pregnancy (Seron-Ferre et al., 1993), but it is melatonin that continues to play a key role in synchronizing all of these circadian rhythms to the 24-hour day (Reiter et al., 2014), while also entraining fetal circadian rhythms (McCarthy et al., 2019). Maternal melatonin production is higher during pregnancy due to the additional placental source of melatonin that reaches its highest levels in the third trimester and decreases abruptly after delivery, especially after cesarean delivery (Ejaz et al., 2020). Evening melatonin levels have been found to be significantly higher in multiple gestations (twins) after 28 weeks' gestation compared to a singleton pregnancy (Reiter et al., 2014).

In a recent study on chronotype changes during pregnancy, Martin-Fairey and colleagues (2019) collected wrist actigraphy data on 39 women living in St. Louis, Missouri, before conception and throughout the pregnancy. Even after controlling for seasons, weekends, and daylight savings time changes, women had a phase-advance in sleep-onset latency during the first two trimesters that returned to pre-pregnancy baseline values during the third trimester (Martin-Fairey et al., 2019).

Labor Onset and Birth

Evidence from several animal studies indicates that melatonin has a strong influence on birth timing (McCarthy et al., 2019; Takayama et al., 2003). Altered melatonin rhythm or low levels of melatonin secretion may be associated with pregnancy complications such as preeclampsia (Dou et al., 2019) because of its role in fetal maturation and placenta/uterine homeostasis (Reiter et al., 2014).

Oxytocin, a hormone released by the posterior pituitary, also has a circadian rhythm and has a major role in promoting uterine contractions. In late pregnancy, oxytocin reaches its highest level at night (Hirst et al., 1993) when the uterus is more sensitive to oxytocin. Melatonin and oxytocin act synergistically during labor, which could explain the higher incidence of nocturnal births (Hirst et al., 1993; Pires et al., 2010; Reiter et al., 2014). After a vaginal birth, prolactin peaks for 4–6 hours and then returns to a normal circadian pattern; however, concentrations are significantly lower after an elective cesarean birth if no labor is experienced (Izci-Balserak, O'Brien, & Bei, 2022).

Intravenous oxytocin for labor induction is commonly administered in developed countries, particularly for prolonged ruptured membranes or complications such as preeclampsia or hemorrhage. However, inductions are typically scheduled for the morning at the convenience of both clinician and hospitals. From a Cochrane review on the topic, no morning versus evening differences in length of labor or birth complications are apparent for nulliparas or multiparas with any form of pharmacologically induced labor, but women induced in the morning may have a better night's sleep prior to induction (Bakker et al., 2013).

Cortisol levels during pregnancy are affected by age, parity, and body weight in addition to the known effects of lifestyle stress (Bleker et al., 2017). Cortisol levels increase twofold by late pregnancy and quickly return to normal following birth (Seron-Ferre et al., 1993), but higher evening cortisol has been linked to worse self-reported (PSQI) sleep quality and shorter gestation in a secondary analysis of a sample of women with a history of depression (Bublitz et al., 2018).

Circadian Rhythm Misalignment

Pregnancy-related changes in melatonin, body temperature, physical activities, and eating patterns may lead to circadian misalignment (Balieiro et al., 2021; Izci-Balserak, O'Brien, & Bei, 2022; Logan & McClung, 2019; Silver et al., 2019). In the first trimester, 55% of women were found to experience misalignment (mismatch between circadian and social clocks) of >1 hour, and 77% experienced misalignment during at least one trimester that was influenced by excessive weight gain (Balieiro et al., 2021). Key zeitgebers, such as artificial light exposure due to frequent bathroom visits during pregnancy and changes in meal schedules due to heartburn, may also lead to circadian misalignment (Izci Balserak, Hermann, et al., 2022; van der Meijden et al., 2016).

Artificial lighting at night suppresses melatonin release, increases alertness, and shifts the timing of the circadian clock in such a way as to alter the brain's restorative slow waves during deep sleep (Izci Balserak, Hermann, et al., 2022; Opperhuizen et al., 2017; Park et al., 2019). Altered melatonin rhythm may be a risk factor for pregnancy complications given its role in fetal maturation and placenta homeostasis (Dou et al., 2019; Reiter et al., 2014). Circadian rhythm misalignment can also result in adverse health outcomes such as mood disorders, impaired glucose metabolism, and obesity (Izci Balserak, Hermann, et al., 2022; Liset et al., 2021; Qian & Scheer, 2020).

Circadian misalignment associated with shift work has been linked to risk of low birth weight, premature birth, miscarriage, preeclampsia, and gestational diabetes (Balieiro et al., 2021; Cai et al., 2019; Facco, Grobman, et al., 2017). Halabi and colleagues (2021) found that chronic circadian misalignment in pregnant rats had long-term detrimental effects on glucose homeostasis in male offspring, even into adulthood. Emerging evidence also suggests strong relationships between altered circadian rhythms in pregnancy and mood disorders, particularly depression (Logan & McClung, 2019; Sharkey et al., 2013). Light therapies and dosages that improve circadian rhythms in most adults need further study for potential safety issues regarding maternal–fetal dynamics and implications for the fetus (Faulkner et al., 2019).

Sleep Factors

The inhibitory effects of progesterone and its metabolites act on brain gamma-aminobutyric acid receptors to create a relaxing and soporific effect. Exogenous progesterone administration has been shown to shorten sleep-onset latency, lengthen rapid-eye-movement

(REM)–onset latency, and reduce total REM sleep (Pires et al., 2010). Progesterone also appears to raise body temperature and relaxes smooth muscle of the gastrointestinal tract, ureters, and bladder, which can indirectly disrupt sleep (Cunningham et al., 2022; Izci-Balserak & Pien, 2014). In contrast, the excitatory effects of estrogen on the nervous system are known to selectively decrease REM sleep activation in the ventrolateral pre-optic area (Hadjimarkou et al., 2008), but the less potent form (estriol) produced by the placenta may have less impact on sleep compared to progesterone.

Most PSG studies show less REM sleep, less N3 slow-wave delta power, and more light sleep stages during pregnancy when compared to non-pregnant controls or pre-pregnancy values (Hertz et al., 1992; Izci-Balserak et al., 2018; K. A. Lee et al., 2000; Wilson et al., 2011). However, research findings regarding sleep characteristics during pregnancy are not always consistent. Although night-to-night and individual variabilities exist (Signal et al., 2007), findings may differ due to study design, sleep location, objective or self-report measures, selection of comparison groups, and sample inclusion criteria considering age, parity, gestational week, mental health history, and employment schedule. In a recent meta-regression of seven cross-sectional studies the only significant predictor of prevalence of sleep problems among pregnant women was age (Alimoradi et al., 2022). Age can easily be confounded with parity, and in the case of pregnancy, age is not necessarily linear; younger women (< 21 years) may have as much risk as women of advanced maternal age (>35 years).

Sleep Quality

Sleep quality can be estimated by self-report measures that may be biased by mood state or attitudes toward sleep. Objective measures of sleep quality often refer to sleep efficiency (SE), known to progressively decrease across pregnancy, or amount of WASO, known to progressively increase due to more and longer nocturnal awakenings (Christian et al., 2019; Haney et al., 2014; K. A. Lee et al., 2000; Wilson et al., 2011). Psychosocial stressors can also lead to poor sleep quality (Ladyman & Signal, 2018). Most women (75%–100%) will report sleep disturbances with multiple nocturnal awakenings when approaching the final week of gestation (Kalmbach, Cheng, Roth, Roth, et al., 2022).

A woman expecting her first child (nullipara) is at higher risk for poor sleep quality compared to experienced (multipara) mothers (Ladyman & Signal, 2018). Although multiparas may self-report worse sleep quality during pregnancy compared to nulliparas, multiparas have better objectively measured SE (K. A. Lee & Zaffke, 1999; Signal et al., 2007). Tsai et al. (2017) found that nulliparas were significantly sleepier from the first trimester to delivery compared to experienced mothers. K. A. Lee and colleagues (2000) found that multiparas started to increase their sleep time as soon as they knew they were pregnant, likely compensating for normal nocturnal awakenings, but that nulliparas steadily lost sleep by continuing with their habitual pre-pregnancy bedtimes.

Most self-report and objective measures of sleep quality improve in the second trimester compared to the first and third trimesters (Facco et al., 2010; Haney et al., 2014; Hedman et al., 2002; Izci-Balserak & Pien, 2014; Ladyman & Signal, 2018; K. A. Lee et al., 2000; Mindell et al., 2015). However, Reid and colleagues (2017) found that women in a substudy of the Nulliparous Pregnancy Outcomes: Monitoring Mothers-to-Be (n = 782) spent a relatively long time in bed attempting to sleep, with WASO >42 minutes.

Sleep Duration and Napping

In addition to worse sleep quality, nulliparas are at higher risk for shorter sleep duration compared to multiparas (Ladyman & Signal, 2018), but this may be age-dependent. Women <30 years old have longer nocturnal sleep duration during the third trimester than women >30 years old (Hedman et al., 2002; Ladyman & Signal, 2018). Sleep duration also differs by race, with Black and Asian pregnant women having the shortest sleep durations (Izci-Balserak, O'Brien, & Bei, 2022; Kalmbach et al., 2019). Sleep duration may also differ between objective and self-reported measures, with self-report estimated durations being longer than PSG or actigraphy regardless of the trimester (Ladyman & Signal, 2018).

In an actigraphy study of nulliparas in the third trimester, there was a dose–response relationship between sleep duration and length of labor as well as incidence of cesarean births even after controlling for infant birth weight (K. A. Lee & Gay, 2004). Most (n = 74; 57%) of the nulliparas had ≥7 hours of sleep at night, and their labor averaged 17.7 hours, with only 11% cesarean births. In contrast, the 19 (15%) nulliparas with sleep duration <6 hours averaged 29 hours of labor and were 4.5 times more likely to have a cesarean birth (K. A. Lee & Gay, 2004). When controlling for parity, findings on nulliparas have been replicated in other countries where cesarean birth rates are typically lower (Naghi et al., 2011; Zafarghandi et al., 2012).

It is not known whether a daytime nap can counter the potential adverse effects of short nocturnal sleep duration. The 24-hour TST may approach pre-pregnancy values due to napping (Obeysekare et al., 2020). In fact, over 75% of women report at least one nap each week in the third trimester (Beebe et al., 2017; Hedman et al., 2002; Kalmbach, Cheng, Roth, Swanson, et al., 2022; Mindell et al., 2015; Palagini et al., 2014).

Labor and Birth

Both sleep quality and duration suffer once labor begins. Compared to multiparas, nulliparas tend to have longer labor and report being unable to sleep once contractions begin (Kennedy et al., 2007). Labor pains, anxiety, and medications all affect sleep quality (Beebe & Lee, 2007; Ladyman & Signal, 2018; Palagini et al., 2014). In an actigraphy study of 35 women, sleep quality and duration decreased during the last 5 days of pregnancy and were lowest the night before regular contractions prompted hospital admission for birth (Beebe & Lee, 2007).

Sleeping in the supine position has been implicated in risk of miscarriage or stillbirth (Gordon et al., 2015; Heazell et al., 2018). Supine position can compress the vena cava and impair placental circulation, but this is also confounded by maternal obesity and hypoxia associated with obstructive apnea. Women experiencing a stillbirth were significantly more likely to report sleeping supine the previous night and an absence of typically frequent bathroom visits at night (Stacey et al., 2011). Prospective data on sleep quality and duration associated with miscarriage or stillbirth are difficult to obtain as these participants typically become missing cases in longitudinal studies on birth outcomes.

Sleep Disorders During Pregnancy

SDB

SDB is common during pregnancy and worsens as the pregnancy progresses, particularly if weight gain is excessive or obesity is already present (Bourjeily et al., 2014, 2017; Facco, Parker, et al., 2017; Izci Balserak et al., 2020; O'Brien et al., 2012; Pien et al., 2014; Pien & Schwab, 2004). Pregnancy-related physical and hormonal changes may worsen preexisting obstructive sleep apnea (OSA) or lead to gestational OSA. Women with preexisting OSA need to continue treatment, but continuous positive airway pressure (CPAP) may need to be adjusted (Guilleminault et al., 2004) due to weight gain that can exacerbate OSA severity.

Most new-onset OSA cases are mild, but it affects 4%–8% in early pregnancy and 8%–20% in mid- to late pregnancy (Facco, Parker, et al., 2017; Pien et al., 2014). OSA likely causes repetitive hypoxemia, sympathetic overactivation, inflammation, and altered regulation of energy expenditure (Bouloukaki et al., 2017; Challis et al., 2009; Gozal & Kheirandish-Gozal, 2008; Javaheri et al., 2017). These changes can make women more vulnerable to pregnancy complications (Izci-Balserak & Pien, 2014). In fact, OSA is associated with increased risk of adverse pregnancy outcomes, including gestational diabetes mellitus (GDM), preeclampsia, and preterm birth (Bourjeily et al., 2017; Facco, Parker, et al., 2017; Izci Balserak et al., 2020; Louis et al., 2014).

Although CPAP is regarded as first-line therapy for pregnant women with OSA, data on effects of CPAP therapy are extremely limited, and gestational OSA likely improves after delivery (Edwards et al., 2005) due to abdominal weight reduction, although enlarged breast tissue in lactating women may continue to affect breathing. Treatment with CPAP might improve perinatal outcomes, but usefulness of CPAP therapy on these outcomes is not yet established (Migueis et al., 2022).

INSOMNIA

During pregnancy, women experience insomnia symptoms, but these symptoms need to be carefully differentiated from the sleep disruption seen in normal pregnancy (Facco et al., 2010; Pietikäinen et al., 2019; Quin et al., 2022). Recent meta-analytic studies conclude that prevalence of clinical insomnia is 25%–27% in the first and second trimesters, increasing to 40%–50% in the third trimester (Quin et al., 2022; Salari et al., 2021; Sedov et al., 2021; Sivertsen et al., 2015). Based on symptom scales, 50%–74% of women experience insomnia during pregnancy, and clinical follow-up is likely needed for as many as 30% (Quin et al., 2022; Sivertsen et al., 2015).

Risk factors for insomnia in pregnancy include age >30 years (Facco et al., 2010; Hedman et al., 2002); race/ethnicity, poverty, and obesity (Kalmbach et al., 2019); smoking (Fernandez-Alonso et al., 2012); single parenting (X. Xu et al., 2017); pre-pregnancy affective disorders or perinatal depression (Lewis et al., 2018; Palagini et al., 2014; Pietikäinen et al., 2019); negative body image (Hung et al., 2013); and environmental factors such as noise (Mindell et al., 2015). Women who experienced a prior pregnancy loss may have anxiety, insomnia, and bad dreams throughout the subsequent pregnancy or until after reaching the gestational week when the prior loss occurred (Schredl et al., 2016; Van et al., 2004).

During pregnancy, women may have insomnia comorbid with OSA or depression. As described in the 3P model (Spielman et al., 1987), the primary precipitating factors for prenatal insomnia are sleep-disrupting physical changes related to fetal growth, hormones, frequent urination, and short sleep duration due to role responsibilities at home or work (Facco et al., 2010; Gay et al., 2004). These sleep disruptions may lead to sleep-related worries, spending more time in bed, or higher caffeine intake (Fernandez-Alonso et al., 2012; Ladyman & Signal, 2018) that only perpetuate the problem and contribute to chronic insomnia.

Insomnia in pregnancy can significantly affect physical and cognitive function and has implications for pregnancy outcomes (Manber et al., 2019). Thus, timely assessment and appropriate management are essential. Various forms of cognitive behavioral therapy for insomnia (CBT-I) are recommended by sleep experts as primary options and preferred over medication by expecting couples (Manber et al., 2019; Miller et al., 2020; Sedov et al., 2019). These options include good sleep hygiene practices (e.g., establishing a bedtime routine, regular sleep–wake cycles, avoiding caffeine, and minimizing fluid intake in evenings to decrease nocturia) and CBT-I (Manber et al., 2019; Miller et al., 2020). A large randomized controlled trial of CBT-I for women diagnosed with prenatal insomnia significantly reduced insomnia severity with higher remission rates compared to an active control condition (K. A. Lee & Gay, 2017; Manber et al., 2019). Recent research focuses on making CBT-I more widely accessible and better integrated in perinatal care with telephone or group formats (Bei et al., 2019; Cain et al., 2019; Kalmbach, Cheng, Roth, Swanson, et al., 2022) as well as internet and digital (dCBT-I) formats (Felder et al., 2022; Kalmbach et al., 2020). Other interventions that address stress reduction to alleviate insomnia symptoms during pregnancy include mindful yoga, acupuncture, massage, and exercise (Beddoe et al., 2010; Xie et al., 2021) and decaffeinated herbal teas (K. A. Lee & Gay, 2017).

Histamine H1 receptor antagonists such as diphenhydramine and doxylamine are widely used as over-the-counter sleep aids during pregnancy and are considered unlikely to cause harm to the fetus, especially later in the third trimester (Chaudhry & Susser, 2018; Miller et al., 2020). Because higher pregnancy levels of progesterone can potentiate the dose of any hypnotic medication, clinicians should consider the risk/benefit ratio for benzodiazepines when treating insomnia during pregnancy and only consider medication if non-pharmacologic approaches are unavailable and potential benefits outweigh risks (Miller et al., 2020).

GESTATIONAL RLS (WILLIS-EKBOM DISEASE)

RLS follows a circadian pattern with intense symptoms at night before bedtime or while trying to fall asleep (see Chapter 37). Pregnancy is a risk factor in the onset or worsening of RLS. In a meta-analysis of 27 studies that involved about 50,000 women, the pooled prevalence of RLS during pregnancy was 21%, and the incidence of new-onset gestational RLS was 18% (Na et al., 2020). A meta-analysis of prospective and cross-sectional studies found that RLS increased from 8% in the first trimester to 22% in the third trimester, followed by a large decrease to only 4% after delivery (S. J. Chen et al., 2018; Srivanitchapoom et al., 2014)

RLS symptoms are associated with difficulty initiating sleep, shorter sleep duration, more daytime sleepiness, and depressive symptoms (K. A. Lee et al., 2001; Manconi et al., 2012; Srivanitchapoom et al., 2014; Wesstrom et al., 2014). RLS may coexist with periodic leg movements in sleep (PLMS), and risk factors are similar (multiple gestation with twins, older maternal age, obesity, multiparity) for both RLS and PLMS (Izci-Balserak, O'Brien, & Bei, 2022). Pre-pregnancy RLS was a risk factor for both antenatal and postnatal depression, while no added risk was seen in women with pregnancy-onset RLS (Lu et al., 2021; Wesstrom et al., 2014). PLMS, however, seem to have no adverse impact on objective sleep measures or sleepiness (Wilson et al., 2018).

The pathophysiology of gestational RLS is not firmly established. Potential factors include high estrogen level; iron, ferritin, and folate deficiencies; dopaminergic system dysfunction; genetic predisposition; or compressed nerves (K. A. Lee et al., 2001; Manconi et al., 2012; Minar et al., 2015; Srivanitchapoom et al., 2014; Telarovic & Condic, 2019). Medications such as selective serotonin reuptake inhibitors (SSRIs), antihistamines, and antiemetics may also increase the risk of RLS (P. H. Chen et al., 2012; Srivanitchapoom et al., 2014). In a meta-analysis of 16 studies, gestational RLS was associated with increased risk of gestational hypertension, preeclampsia, and perinatal depression (Steinweg et al., 2020).

Diagnosis of gestational RLS is based on symptoms after ruling out other possible causes (Izci-Balserak, O'Brien, & Bei, 2022). It is highly symptomatic, but given its short-term duration until onset of labor, the impact on the individual is central in the decision to treat. Consensus guidelines for treatment during pregnancy are published elsewhere

(Miller et al., 2020; Picchietti et al., 2015). Caffeine and alcohol should be avoided, and initial approaches should include non-pharmacologic comfort strategies like exercise, massage, pneumatic compression, or elastic stockings (Dunietz et al., 2017; Izci-Balserak, O'Brien, & Bei, 2022). In severe cases, iron therapy or the lowest dose of pharmacologic therapy for safe fetal development can be considered.

NARCOLEPSY

The prevalence of narcolepsy in pregnant women is similar to that in non-pregnant populations, but symptoms may be either exacerbated or attenuated. Differential diagnosis of narcolepsy during pregnancy may require consideration of gestational daytime sleepiness or vivid dreams. Narcolepsy in pregnancy is a risk factor for anemia, impaired glucose metabolism, obesity, and cesarean birth (Maurovich-Horvat et al., 2013).

Medication to treat narcolepsy should be used with caution during pregnancy as data are lacking on fetal risks (Thorpy et al., 2013). Risks may include prematurity, low birth weight, and withdrawal symptoms in infants of women taking amphetamines (Thorpy et al., 2013). Safety of armodafinil and sodium oxybate in pregnancy awaits comprehensive human studies. However, in a survey of 75 clinicians who treated narcolepsy during pregnancy, there was no evidence of teratogenicity with modafinil, sodium oxybate, methylphenidate, amphetamines, or SSRIs (Thorpy et al., 2013). Around 33% of women discontinue therapy during pregnancy (Pascoe et al., 2019). If medication is required, there is reassuring evidence that no considerable harm has been documented (Miller et al., 2020). Scheduled naps, stress management, and avoiding situations that trigger cataplexy can reduce risk of physical injury as well as unpredictable sleepiness.

Physical and Mental Health Consequences

Accumulating evidence indicates that circadian misalignment and late sleep timing during pregnancy, as well as poor sleep quality and short sleep duration, are risk factors for adverse outcomes such as GDM, pregnancy-induced hypertension (PIH), preterm labor, cesarean birth, and depression (Cai et al., 2016; Herring et al., 2014; K. A. Lee & Gay, 2004; Okun et al., 2011; Palagini et al., 2014; Reutrakul et al., 2017; Sedov et al., 2017; Warland et al., 2018).

PIH and Preeclampsia

PIH significantly increases the risk of maternal and fetal morbidity; thus, timely diagnosis and treatment are essential (Dunietz et al., 2014). In a large recent study using actigraphy, there was no association between sleep duration and PIH or preeclampsia (Facco, Grobman, et al., 2017). Accumulating evidence does link risk of PIH and preeclampsia to the sleep disruption seen with SDB (Facco, Parker, et al., 2017; Louis et al., 2014; O'Brien et al., 2012).

GDM

In a large study using actigraphy, short sleep (<7 hours per night) and late sleep midpoint were associated with a twofold increased risk of GDM (Facco, Grobman, et al., 2017). In a recent meta-analysis of 16 studies, researchers concluded that both short and long sleep duration, poor sleep quality, and OSA were associated with risk of GDM, with a U-shaped relationship between sleep duration and GDM (Zhang et al., 2020). Thus, sleep duration and poor sleep quality may modulate glucose regulation, and efforts to improve sleep early in pregnancy could be clinically important in lowering GDM risk.

Mental Health

Both self-reported poor sleep quality and short sleep duration during pregnancy concurrently and prospectively impact mental health. In a recent survey, insomnia in mid-pregnancy was associated with depression, suicidality, cognitive and somatic arousal, perinatal-focused rumination, and daytime sleepiness (Kalmbach, Cheng, Roth, Roth, et al., 2022). In a large population-based Norwegian survey, depressive symptoms during late pregnancy were associated with extremes in sleep duration (<5 or >10 hours), low SE (<75%), and prolonged sleep-onset latency (Dorheim et al., 2012; Pietikäinen et al., 2019), and poor self-reported sleep quality during early pregnancy also predicted depressive symptoms in late pregnancy in Finland (Pietikäinen et al., 2019). The same researchers also reported that prolonged sleep latency, anxiety in early pregnancy, and insufficient sleep during late pregnancy predicted the risk of postnatal depressive symptoms (Pietikainen et al., 2021). In an in-home study during early pregnancy, SDB predicted worse depressive symptoms later in pregnancy (Bublitz et al., 2021).

Postpartum Recovery (The First 3 Months)

Overview

There are abrupt changes in anatomy, physiology, and hormones after delivery (Cunningham et al., 2022; Izci-Balserak, O'Brien, & Bei, 2022); and sleep complaints are more prevalent after surgery for a cesarean birth than a vaginal birth (S. Y. Lee & Lee, 2007). Maternal sleep disturbance is prevalent during the first few weeks postpartum when recovering from labor and delivery and when the newborn has irregular feeding and sleep–wake cycles (Tables 41.1 and 41.2; Insana et al., 2013; Spaeth et al., 2021). In the first few weeks, however, novice mothers (primiparas) have lower SE compared to multiparas (K. A. Lee et al., 2000). After a few weeks, sleep begins to improve but does not necessarily return to pre-pregnancy quality or duration (Table 41.2; Badr & Zauszniewski, 2017; K. A. Lee et al., 2000; Sharkey et al., 2013).

Circadian Factors

Evidence suggests that consistent maternal circadian rhythms are important in shaping infant rhythms to synchronize with external light–dark cycles (Tsai et al., 2011). Circadian misalignment is associated with postpartum weight retention and adiposity (Stremler & Sharkey, 2022). Altered sleep timing during postpartum recovery may be in response to the infant's behaviors, mother's napping during the day, or juggling parental role responsibilities. Minimizing risk of circadian misalignment during postpartum recovery is crucial for mental and physical health as well as breastfeeding success and mother–infant interactions.

Sleep Factors

Breastfeeding and bed-sharing are critical postpartum issues with major implications for postpartum sleep and long-term health of the mother and infant. No one expects better sleep in the early postpartum phase of parenthood; but breastfeeding may help increase sleep duration for both parents, and bed-sharing practices may be planned or used as a coping strategy that can further worsen sleep quality for both parents.

Sleep Quality

There are postpartum sleep disparities among socioeconomically disadvantaged women of color who experience lower SE compared to socioeconomically advantaged women (K. A. Lee & Gay, 2011; Spaeth et al., 2021). The most common reason for lower SE is co-sleeping (Volkovich et al., 2015). Co-sleeping varies from room-sharing to bed-sharing, but survey data at 3 months postpartum indicate that most (85%) mothers room-share with the infant and that 34% bed-share (Hauck et al., 2008).

Bed-sharing may be controversial in some societies but is accepted in most cultures (Barry & McKenna, 2022), and the practice of bed-sharing in the first few months postpartum is linked more to breastfeeding practices (Buswell & Spatz, 2007) than socioeconomic resources or bed-partner preferences (Barry & McKenna, 2022). Results from cross-sectional studies make it difficult to ascertain whether frequent night awakenings occur before or after co-sleeping is initiated. Furthermore, what starts out as solitary sleeping at bedtime may become bed-sharing during the night. In a 4-night study of 44 mothers at 1 month postpartum, 14% reported bed-sharing at study enrollment, yet 50% indicated actual bed-sharing on some or all 4 nights, regardless of feeding type (Rosen, 2009).

Sleep Duration

While recommendations to breastfeed for at least 6 months are intended to improve the health of infants and maternal–infant interactions, milk production utilizes considerable calories and typically promotes postpartum weight loss. There is also an added benefit of longer sleep duration for parents. Using actigraphy measures at 3 months postpartum, TST was 45 minutes longer for both parents if the infant was exclusively breastfed compared to parents with formula-fed infants (Doan et al., 2007), and results were similar in a different sample of mothers as early as 1 month postpartum (Doan et al., 2014). In a recent systematic review and meta-analysis of seven studies, researchers concluded that breastfeeding is associated with a longer sleep duration, and co-sleeping with the infant was also associated with longer sleep duration in breastfeeding mothers (Srimoragot et al., 2022).

Physical and Mental Health Consequences

Co-sleeping or bed-sharing impacts overall sleep quality and duration and is confounded with infant feeding practices. In fact, Barry and McKenna (2022) have coined the term *breastsleeping* to describe this maternal–infant behavior. Breastsleeping is also confounded with postpartum depression, which affects up to 20% of women and worsens sleep quality (Stremler & Sharkey, 2022). Based on 72 hours of actigraphy data during hospitalization after birth, Japanese women who were rooming-in with their first baby slept as much as they breastfed, sleeping only 4.2 hours (±73 minutes) and breastfeeding 12 (±3.2) times or 4.1 hours (±102 minutes) per 24 hours; this amount of sleep deprivation was associated with postpartum depression scores during the first month (Kawashima et al., 2022). Kalmbach, O'Brien, and colleagues (2022) reported that maternal insomnia, nocturnal rumination, and daytime sleepiness were associated with poorer mother–infant bonding, independent of the effects of maternal depression and infant colic. This is especially the case for new mothers (Gallaher et al., 2018; Insana et al., 2013; Obeysekare et al., 2020; Sharkey et al., 2013).

Evidence suggests that women in the third trimester who report circadian dysregulation, substantial sleep loss, or later sleep timing are more likely to experience depressive symptoms in the first 3 months postpartum (Badr & Zauszniewski, 2017; Gallaher et al., 2018; Obeysekare et al., 2020; Sharkey et al., 2013; Stremler & Sharkey, 2022). In a prospective study with over 1,300 women, poor sleep quality and short sleep duration in the third trimester were associated with depressive symptoms 3 months postpartum (Pietikäinen et al., 2019). In particularly vulnerable women with bipolar disorder, postpartum recovery combined with acute sleep loss may trigger postpartum psychosis (Lewis et al., 2018). There is promising evidence from a recent randomized clinical trial that dCBT-I (Sleepio®) for insomnia symptoms during pregnancy has continuing efficacy for reducing postpartum depression and anxiety; at 3 months postpartum only 4% of the intervention group had depression compared to 18% of controls (Felder et al., 2022).

Menopausal Transition

Overview

The years spent in menopausal transition, or perimenopause stage, can vary greatly and unpredictably. Signs of ovarian aging and impact on the HPO axis begin about 5–7 years before the final menstrual cycle, as levels of ovarian estrogen fluctuate and diminish with each cycle. Without estrogen's negative feedback on pituitary FSH production, the level of FSH may be inconsistent each month, and irregular or occasionally missed cycles can

Menarche | FMP (0)

Stage	-5	-4	-3b	-3a	-2	-1	+1a	+1b	+1c	+2
Terminology	**REPRODUCTIVE**				**MENOPAUSAL TRANSITION**		**POSTMENOPAUSE**			
	Early	Peak	Late		Early	Late	Early			Late
					Perimenopause					
Duration	*variable*				*variable*	1-3 years	2 years (1+1)		3-6 years	*Remaining lifespan*
PRINCIPAL CRITERIA										
Menstrual Cycle	Variable to regular	Regular	Regular	Subtle changes in Flow/ Length	*variable Length* Persistent ≥7-day difference in length of consecutive cycles	Interval of amenorrhea of >=60 days				
SUPPORTIVE CRITERIA										
Endocrine										
FSH			Normal	Variable*	↑ Variable*	↑ >25 IU/L**	↑ Variable*		Stabilizes	
AMH			Low	Low	Low	Low	Low		Very Low	
Inhibin B			Low	Low	Low	Low	Low		Very Low	
Antral Follicle Count 2–10 mm			Low	Low	Low	Low	Very Low		Very Low	
DESCRIPTIVE CHARACTERISTICS										
Symptoms						Vasomotor symptoms *Likely*	Vasomotor symptoms *Most Likely*			*Increasing* symptoms of urogenital atrophy

* Blood draw on cycle days 2–5 = elevated
**Approximate expected level based on assays using current pituitary standard[67–69]

Figure 41.1 The Stages of Reproductive Aging Workshop (STRAW + 10) criteria for reproductive stage
Note. Criteria such as menstrual cycle length and regularity and FSH level (Harlow et al., 2012) are used to categorize women into late pre-, early peri-, and late perimenopause stages. AMH = anti-Mullerian hormone; FMP = final menstrual period; FSH = follicle-stimulating hormone. Reproduced from S. D. Harlow et al., (2012), "Executive summary of the stages of reproductive aging workshop + 10: Addressing the unfinished agenda of staging reproductive aging," *Journal of Clinical Endocrinology & Metabolism, 97*(4), 1159–116 by permission of The Endocrine Society.

occur in early and late perimenopausal stages. These stages have been differentiated in the Stages of Reproductive Aging Workshop (STRAW) criteria according to hormones and menstrual cycle characteristics (see Figure 41.1). Postmenopausal status becomes official once there has been no menstrual bleeding for 12 months (Harlow et al., 2012). Natural menopause occurs at about 50–51 years of age. However, younger women experiencing surgical removal of an ovary or surgical menopause have an abrupt loss of estrogen accompanied by elevated FSH.

Estrogen's role within the HPO axis includes thermoregulation and maintaining a wide thermoneutral zone controlled by the hypothalamus. In the absence of estrogen, it is thought that this zone narrows considerably (Freedman, 2014), prompting hypothalamic instability and vasomotor symptoms of hot flashes during the day and night sweats during sleep with just minor fluctuations in temperature. There is some evidence in a small sample of symptomatic women that hot flashes can occur as often as 30 times per day and follow a circadian rhythm, with peak frequency in the early evening around 6:30 p.m. (Freedman et al., 1995).

In most large cohort studies, the prevalence of sleep disturbance for women in menopausal transition varies between 30% and 40% depending on how sleep is measured, the stage of transition (see Figure 41.1), whether vasomotor symptoms are present, and what factors (such as age, BMI, and depression) are controlled in the analyses (Tables 41.1 and 41.2). For example, Woods and Mitchell (2010) asked specifically about nighttime awakenings in symptom diaries beginning at 41 years of age and observed increasing prevalence of moderate to severe awakenings over time from 18% initially to 22% and 30% during menopausal transition and 46% in early postmenopause. In contrast, women 40–55 years of age participating in the Study of Women's Health Across the Nation (SWAN) were asked about difficulty sleeping in the past 2 weeks, and the prevalence was 38% for the premenopause group, 45% for the late perimenopause group, and even higher (48%) in the group that experienced surgical menopause (Kravitz et al., 2003). The pattern was similar in a meta-analysis of cross-sectional data from 24 studies in which Q. Xu and Lang (2014) found increased risk for sleep disturbance among women in menopausal transition (odds ratio = 1.60) compared to premenopause, and women who experienced surgical menopause had twice the odds (odds ratio = 2.17) of sleep disturbance.

In annual surveys of women 45–54 years old in the United States, poor sleep was primarily associated with smoking, depression, and vasomotor symptoms; but premenopausal sleep complaints did not predict peri- or postmenopausal sleep (R. L. Smith et al., 2018). Another factor that may influence prevalence rates for sleep problems during menopausal transition is race/ethnicity. When age-adjusted percentages for sleep difficulty were examined in the SWAN cohort, sleep difficulty differed by race. For premenopausal women, sleep difficulty ranged from 21% in Japanese Americans to 26% in African Americans to 27% in Chinese Americans to 30% in Hispanic Americans to 37% in Caucasians, with significantly higher percentages in all five groups in early perimenopause (Kravitz et al., 2003). It should be noted, however, that racial groups were geocentric, with Chinese Americans in California and Hispanic Americans primarily from east coast Puerto Rican and Cuban heritage.

Circadian Factors

In addition to aging's effects on circadian rhythms, lower estrogen production in the ovaries and rising FSH levels from the pituitary influence the HPO axis and its control over circadian rhythms and melatonin production. Estrogen receptors are found throughout the circadian system, including the suprachiasmatic nucleus (Hatcher et al., 2020). Circadian rhythms are modulated in part by circulating estrogen in a bidirectional relationship, causing circadian misalignment with sudden or chronic shifts in estrogen signaling from the ovary as in the case of pregnancy or menopause, while light exposure at night due to shift work or jetlag can alter estrogen and reproductive functions that are critical for fertility and gestation (Hatcher et al., 2020). There is also preliminary research demonstrating melatonin's potential therapeutic use in inhibiting breast cancer metastasis (Lopes et al., 2016).

Age-related differences in melatonin rhythms exist between younger perimenopausal and older postmenopausal women (Cagnacci, 2017), but to our knowledge, no one has yet examined changes in circadian rhythms or specifically melatonin rhythm longitudinally during menopausal transition (Pines, 2016). In cross-sectional studies, postmenopausal women are more likely phase-advanced compared to premenopausal women, but this may be age-related rather than melatonin- or estrogen-mediated (Toffol et al., 2014, 2021). In a carefully controlled constant routine methodology comparing 10 premenopausal (mean age 42 years) and 10 postmenopausal (mean age 55 years) participants, melatonin amplitude did not differ; but melatonin acrophase was 1 hour earlier, and the time interval between melatonin onset and onset of sleepiness was significantly greater for the postmenopausal group compared to the premenopausal group (Walters et al., 2005). These findings were supported by findings from a larger study where wrist temperature monitoring for 8 days documented a 1-hour earlier acrophase as well as a lower mean temperature for 50 postmenopausal women compared to 120 premenopausal women (Gomez-Santos et al., 2016).

Sleep Factors

In comprehensive longitudinal and cross-sectional data collected on women in the United States as part of the large SWAN project, subsets of participants had more intense sleep measures over 7 years during menopausal transition (M. H. Hall et al., 2015; Kravitz et al., 2008). Demographics and health-related factors such as age, BMI, race, education, income, and chronic illness were controlled in all analyses. The prevalence of self-reported poor sleep quality and short sleep duration assessed with the PSQI were higher for African American women compared to other racial/ethnic groups, and the African American sample had less N3 slow-wave sleep on PSG (M. H. Hall et al., 2009; Kravitz & Joffe, 2011; Kravitz et al., 2008).

In a smaller SWAN sleep study, 9 years after baseline self-report sleep measures showed that 62% of the sleep cohort was still pre- or early perimenopausal (mean age 51 years), and M. H. Hall and colleagues (2015) reported on their chronic stress exposure using results from 3 nights of home PSG monitoring. PSG sleep duration averaged 380 ± 60 minutes, and SE was 84%; but there was no difference by stress level. For the 300 women in this cohort, the overall mean PSQI score was not only >5, indicating poor sleep quality, but varied from 5.6 for the low-stress group to 8.0 for the high-stress group. Similarly, prevalence of insomnia based on scores from the Insomnia Symptom Questionnaire was 15% overall but lowest (4%) in the low-stress group and highest (38%) in the high-stress group (M. H. Hall et al., 2015).

Sleep Quality

Fluctuating estrogen and FSH levels during menopausal transition are associated with poor sleep quality due to vasomotor symptoms that cause frequent awakenings. Sleep complaints are more prevalent when women self-report on their sleep than when they are studied in the laboratory, but the mechanisms associated with reports of poor sleep quality are complex and often difficult to isolate from the aging process itself, from the stress of family and social roles, or from the weight gain typically seen with aging. Furthermore, when women respond to a questionnaire about frequency or severity of "disturbed" sleep, the specific reason for the disturbance is seldom elucidated. For example, women prior to menopausal transition may have reasons for disturbed sleep associated with job stress, noise from children or pets, snoring bed partner, or nocturia (Baker, Wolfson, & Lee, 2009). In contrast, during menopausal transition children may no longer be in the home or the bed partner may be absent; but now hot flashes may occur, and age-related chronic pain or weight gain may predispose women to comorbid sleep disorders like chronic insomnia or OSA.

In one cross-sectional sleep laboratory study of women with no sleep complaints (43–52 years of age) in various stages of pre- and perimenopause, a higher FSH level was associated with more awakenings after adjusting for age and BMI (de Zambotti et al., 2015). Previous cross-sectional comparisons of PSG recordings for pre- and perimenopausal women did not measure FSH levels, but there was little difference in any sleep stages, SE was 84%–85%, and sleep duration was 370–380 minutes (Young et al., 2003).

Longitudinal studies that compare pre- and perimenopause sleep do show some differences. Lampio et al. (2017) conducted 1-night PSG laboratory studies in Finland on 60 women when they were premenopausal (mean age 46) and again 6 years later at various stages of perimenopausal transition. They found that TST decreased by about 30 minutes, SE did not change, WASO minutes increased, and awakenings per hour of sleep almost doubled. There was no difference in the amount of REM or non-REM sleep, but night sweats were occurring at least once per week in 12% at their premenopausal assessment, jumped to almost 36% at the follow-up assessment (Lampio et al., 2017), and remained at about 36% at their 10-year follow-up assessment (Kalleinen et al., 2021).

Sleep Duration

Sleep duration is likely shorter in perimenopausal transition due to frequent awakenings caused by symptoms such as pain or hot flashes. Baker et al. (2015) monitored PSG sleep and hot flashes in perimenopausal women (mean age 50 years) and compared 31 controls without insomnia to 36 women who met criteria for insomnia. Under the same laboratory conditions, the insomnia group averaged 40 minutes less sleep (mean 360 minutes) and had 12% WASO compared to only 8% WASO for controls. The insomnia group also self-reported shorter sleep duration in the sleep diary, reflecting their usual sleep at home; 47% slept <6 hours compared to 9% of controls (Baker et al., 2015). The insomnia group also had higher FSH and lower estrogen levels, and 56% had at least one nocturnal hot flash compared to only 16% of the control group.

Based on these laboratory data (Baker et al., 2015) and findings from the cohort of 60 women in Finland (Kalleinen et al., 2021; Lampio et al., 2017), shorter sleep duration seen with menopausal transition is more likely a result of aging. In contrast, poor sleep quality during menopausal transition is more likely a result of hormonal changes.

Sleep Quality and Surgical Menopause

Surgical menopause (removing the ovaries as part of a hysterectomy) is often an exclusion criterion for participation in menopausal transition research. There are surprisingly few studies on sleep before and after this surgery, but the impact on sleep during postoperative recovery would be in addition to the sudden onset of vasomotor symptoms from immediate loss of ovarian estrogen. Most researchers have assessed sleep during the immediate week after surgery when effects of anesthesia, vaginal or abdominal healing, and pain need to be considered. Nowakowski et al. (2020) reported on PSQI and actigraphy data for 7 days before and 7 days after hysterectomy. Only 7 of the 16 patients had ovaries removed; but notably their mean PSQI score was 9 (>5 indicates poor sleep quality), and mean actigraphy SE was only 75% (Nowakowski et al., 2020). In an earlier study of 25 women, mean preoperative actigraphy SE was 89%, and PSQI was 7.6. At 3 weeks after surgery, PSQI increased to 9.5 and returned to 7.6 at 6 weeks, with similar values for vaginal and abdominal hysterectomy (Kim & Lee, 2009).

In a population-based study of 962 women living in the United Kingdom, sleep was assessed annually from age 43 to 54 years. Trouble sleeping was initially present in 38%. By age 51, 20% had experienced a hysterectomy, and trouble sleeping was worse particularly for that group, for women who initiated hormone therapy in the prior year, and for those women who became postmenopausal. At 54 years of age, 48% had trouble sleeping (Tom et al., 2010).

The time since surgical menopause was not reported in SWAN's longitudinal data, but self-reported difficulty falling or staying asleep ≥3 nights per week was more common in the surgical menopause group compared to the natural menopause group and significantly worse for women not on hormone replacement compared to natural menopause or surgical menopause with hormone replacement (Kravitz et al., 2008). The frequency of self-reported awakenings was also associated with lower estrogen levels and a steeper rise in FSH (Cho et al., 2019).

Circadian Misalignment and Breast Cancer

Breast cancer is the most common type of cancer in women in the United States, and many researchers have hypothesized that surgery to remove the cancer is best done at either the follicular or luteal phase of the menstrual cycle to improve long-term survival. There are intriguing descriptive reports that support each phase, but most systematic reviews (Bernhardt et al., 2020) conclude that evidence is lacking from randomized clinical trials.

There are also many researchers hypothesizing that melatonin suppression due to light exposure at night can result in higher estrogen levels and proliferation of estrogen-sensitive cells in breast tissue (Razavi et al., 2019). While researchers have made a concerted effort to study risk of breast cancer from night-shift work, evidence to support this relationship is inconsistent. For example, in the Nurses' Health Study with over 114,500 women, there were 3,570 cases of breast cancer, but fewer than 30 nurses were in the highest-risk group of rotating on night shift for >20 years (Schernhammer et al., 2001; Wegrzyn et al., 2017). After adjusting for age and other factors such as parity and smoking history, there was twice the risk (hazard ratio = 2.15, 95% confidence interval [1.23, 3.73]) for the youngest of the premenopausal women who worked at least 20 years on rotating night shift (Schernhammer et al., 2001; Wegrzyn et al., 2017). In a meta-analysis of night-shift work and breast cancer, Megdal et al. (2005) reviewed 13 studies that included airline crews and other female shift workers and found overall risk of breast cancer to be 48% higher compared to the reference group of day-shift workers (hazard ratio = 1.48, 95% confidence interval [1.36, 1.61]). However, in a review of large epidemiological studies in the United Kingdom, Travis et al. (2016) concluded that night shift of any duration has no effect on risk of breast cancer regardless of occupation.

Sleep Duration and Breast Cancer Risk

The question of whether it is short sleep duration or light exposure at night that may increase the risk of breast cancer has not been adequately addressed. Risk of breast cancer is generally very weakly associated or not associated with short sleep or long sleep duration (McElroy et al., 2006; Merklinger-Gruchala et al., 2008). In a study of 95 women who recorded sleep duration across an entire menstrual cycle and provided daily morning salivary samples for estrogen, the group of women with the least variability in their sleep times (presumably day-shift workers) had the longest sleep duration (7.7 hours), and the group with more variability in sleep times (typical for night-shift workers) had the shortest duration (7.0–7.3 hours) and higher estrogen levels across the entire menstrual cycle even after controlling for sleep duration (Merklinger-Gruchala et al., 2008). These findings need to be replicated in other samples. While sleep duration itself was not significant, duration could affect the timing for morning saliva samples, and work schedules and melatonin levels were not assessed.

Conclusions

From menarche to menopause, each stage impacts sleep and circadian rhythms, mainly due to alterations in the HPO axis from hormonal changes and subsequent risks of adverse health outcomes. Poor sleep quality is seen in the late-luteal phase if PMDD is present, likely due to sudden hormonal changes. Younger women with polycystic ovaries or surgical menopause are at extreme risk of poor sleep, and women with hot flashes are also at risk.

During pregnancy, physiological changes contribute to poor sleep quality or short sleep duration even without onset of a sleep disorder or health problem. However, disorders like RLS, SDB, and insomnia should be re-evaluated postpartum after mother–infant dynamics are stabilized. Asking about sleep quality and duration should be a part of routine antepartum and postpartum care when assessing depression and breastsleeping.

Although sleep complaints are frequently attributed to hormonal changes during the menstrual cycle, during pregnancy and postpartum, and during menopausal transition, it is important to consider other factors like health problems, circadian misalignment from shift work, and stress associated with family and social relationships. Thus, it is imperative that clinicians evaluate sleep complaints within the context of these factors and that researchers consider these factors in their research.

Regardless of women's reproductive stage, clinicians faced with intervention options for sleep complaints need to evaluate whether the primary cause is circadian rhythm misalignment or a sleep issue as these two causes are often interrelated, but treatment approaches differ. Some women may want a quick pharmacological intervention such as melatonin or hypnotics for their acute time-limited complaint, and dosage (including amount of light therapy) needs to be considered when progesterone levels can potentiate the effects. Other women may prefer to remain vigilant during the night because of child- or elder-care responsibilities and would appreciate helpful behavioral strategies and ways to cope with stress. Evidence-based CBT-I programs address these issues, but motivation for behavioral change can be problematic. Because women planning to start a family are highly motivated to make any behavioral change that will result in a healthy infant, CBI-I as a component of childbirth preparation classes could improve the overall health of families for years to come.

Future Directions

Regardless of the woman's reproductive stage in life, sleep complaints are likely to have multifactorial origins. Fluctuations in ovarian hormones may play an important role, but contexts such as incident sleep disorder, comorbidity with a chronic health condition, or stressful relationships in the home may also be implicated. From a research perspective, laboratory environments may assist in evaluating some aspects of sleep–hormone interaction but may be unsuitable for other aspects where the more natural home environment is important or where longitudinal monitoring of physiology and behavior is indicated.

The success of many CBT-I programs is well documented regardless of number of sessions or mode of delivery, which can range from scheduled group sessions to individual appointments in person or by telephone. Promising findings from randomized clinical trials using dCBT-I (Sleepio®) for insomnia symptoms during pregnancy point to the high potential for success with populations of new mothers. Future research is needed with other populations of women, from puberty to menopause, who may differ in types or levels of motivation for behavior change.

Menstrual Cycle

The distinct phases of the menstrual cycle can affect sleep and circadian rhythms, and sleep (Tables 41.1 and 41.2) as well as circadian misalignment can affect ovulation and fertility. There is a need for research designed to answer questions about (1) how melatonin and estrogen interact with the HPO axis to impact fertility and sleep quality, (2) how short sleep duration can influence both melatonin and estrogen production from the brain and the ovary, and (3) how FSH levels are impacted by poor sleep quality or short sleep duration.

Pregnancy

Circadian and sleep issues can differ by week of gestation or onset of a sleep disorder (Tables 41.1 and 41.2). In addition to efficacy of short-term interventions that can be implemented early in pregnancy, there is a need for research designed to answer questions about (1) circadian and hormonal biomarkers that can best predict RLS, GDM, and OSA and (2) how circadian misalignment and sleep influence miscarriage, particularly in longitudinal studies where this population is usually a source of high attrition.

Postpartum

Infant feeding and sleeping patterns may lead to maternal poor sleep and altered circadian rhythms (Tables 41.1 and 41.2), particularly for the novice mother. There is a need for research designed to answer questions about (1) how parity and pregnancy mental health interact with sleep quality and duration to precipitate postpartum symptoms of anxiety and depression, (2) how sleep and circadian rhythms affect lactation, and (3) how poor sleep quality or short sleep duration influence breastsleeping.

Menopausal Transition

The perimenopausal transition typically begins at any time between 40 and 50 years of age, and physical and psychological symptoms fluctuate with the aging ovary's erratic ability to produce and respond to hormones within the HPO axis, like FSH, estrogen, and melatonin (Tables 41.1 and 41.2). Rather than recruiting women by age, STRAW (Figure 41.1) criteria should be used to characterize participants when designing research to answer questions about (1) how frequency and severity of hot flashes impact acrophase and amplitude for various circadian rhythms, (2) what factors account for differences between objective and self-report measures of sleep, and (3) how the rate of increase in FSH levels during the menopausal transition influences circadian rhythms and sleep.

References

Alimoradi, Z., Abdi, F., Gozal, D., & Pakpour, A. H. (2022). Estimation of sleep problems among pregnant women during COVID-19 pandemic: A systematic review and meta-analysis. *BMJ Open, 12*(4), Article e056044.

Alzueta, E., de Zambotti, M., Javitz, H., Dulai, T., Albinni, B., Simon, K. C., Sattari, N., Zhang, J., Shuster, A., Mednick, S. C., & Baker F. C. (2022). Tracking sleep, temperature, heart rate, and daily symptoms across the menstrual cycle with the Oura Ring in healthy women. *International Journal of Women's Health, 14*, 491–503.

Badr, H. A., & Zauszniewski, J. A. (2017). Meta-analysis of the predictive factors of postpartum fatigue. *Applied Nursing Research, 36*, 122–127.

Baker, F. C., & Driver, H. S. (2004). Self-reported sleep across the menstrual cycle in young, healthy women. *Journal of Psychosomatic Research, 56*(2), 239–243.

Baker, F. C., & Driver, H. S. (2007). Circadian rhythms, sleep, and the menstrual cycle. *Sleep Medicine, 8*(6), 613–622.

Baker, F. C., Driver, H. S., Rogers, G. G., Paiker, J., & Mitchell, D. (1999). High nocturnal body temperatures and disturbed sleep in women with primary dysmenorrhea. *American Journal of Physiology, 277*(6), E1013–E1021.

Baker, F. C., Kahan, T. L., Trinder, J., & Colrain, I. M. (2007). Sleep quality and the sleep electroencephalogram in women with severe premenstrual syndrome. *Sleep, 30*(10), 1283–1291.

Baker, F. C., & Lee, K. A. (2018). Menstrual cycle effects on sleep. *Sleep Medicine Clinics, 13*(3), 283–294.

Baker, F. C., Mitchell, D., & Driver, H. S. (2001). Oral contraceptives alter sleep and raise body temperature in young women. *Pflugers Archiv, 442*(5), 729–737.

Baker, F. C., Sassoon, S. A., Kahan, T., Palaniappan, L., Nicholas, C. L., Trinder, J., & Colrain I. M. (2012). Perceived poor sleep quality in the absence of polysomnographic sleep disturbance in women with severe premenstrual syndrome. *Journal of Sleep Research, 21*(5), 535–545.

Baker, F. C., Willoughby, A. R., Sassoon, S. A., Colrain, I. M., & de Zambotti, M. (2015). Insomnia in women approaching menopause: Beyond perception. *Psychoneuroendocrinology, 60*, 96–104.

Baker, F. C., Wolfson, A. R., & Lee, K. A. (2009). Association of sociodemographic, lifestyle, and health factors with sleep quality and daytime sleepiness in women: Findings from the 2007 National Sleep Foundation "Sleep in America Poll." *Journal of Women's Health (2002), 18*(6), 841–849.

Bakker, J. J., van der Goes, B. Y., Pel, M., Mol, B. W., & van der Post, J. A. (2013). Morning versus evening induction of labour for improving outcomes. *Cochrane Database of Systematic Reviews, 2*, Article CD007707.

Balieiro, L. C. T., Gontijo, C. A., Marot, L. P., Teixeira, G. P., Fahmy, W. M., Moreno, C. R. C., Maia, Y. C. P., & Crispim, C. A. (2021). Circadian misalignment measured by social jetlag from early to late pregnancy and its association with nutritional status: A longitudinal study. *Scientific Reports, 11*(1), Article 18678.

Barry, E. S., & McKenna, J. J. (2022). Reasons mothers bedshare: A review of its effects on infant behavior and development. *Infant Behavior & Development, 66*, Article 101684.

Baumgartner, A., Dietzel, M., Saletu, B., Wolf, R., Campos-Barros, A., Graf, K. J., Kürten, I., & Mannsmann, U. (1993). Influence of partial sleep deprivation on the secretion of thyrotropin, thyroid hormones, growth hormone, prolactin, luteinizing hormone, follicle stimulating hormone, and estradiol in healthy young women. *Psychiatry Research, 48*(2), 153–178.

Beddoe, A. E., Lee, K. A., Weiss, S. J., Kennedy, H. P., & Yang, C. P. (2010). Effects of mindful yoga on sleep in pregnant women: A pilot study. *Biological Research for Nursing, 11*(4), 363–370.

Beebe, K. R., Gay, C. L., Richoux, S. E., & Lee, K. A. (2017). Symptom experience in late pregnancy. *Journal of Obstetric, Gynecologic, and Neonatal Nursing, 46*(4), 508–520.

Beebe, K. R., & Lee, K. A. (2007). Sleep disturbance in late pregnancy and early labor. *Journal of Perinatal & Neonatal Nursing, 21*(2), 103–108.

Bei, B., Pinnington, D. M., Shen, L., Blumfield, M., Drummond, S. P. A., Newman, L. K., & Manber, R. (2019). A scalable cognitive behavioural program to promote healthy sleep during pregnancy and postpartum periods: Protocol of a randomised controlled trial (the SEED project). *BMC Pregnancy and Childbirth, 19*(1), Article 254.

Bernhardt, S. M., Dasari, P., Walsh, D., Townsend, A. R., Price, T. J., & Ingman, W. V. (2020). Timing of breast cancer surgery during the menstrual cycle—Is there an optimal time of the month? *Oncology Letters, 20*(3), 2045–2057.

Beroukhim, G., Esencan, E., & Seifer, D. B. (2022). Impact of sleep patterns upon female neuroendocrinology and reproductive outcomes: A comprehensive review. *Reproductive Biology and Endocrinology, 20*(1), Article 16.

Bleker, L. S., Roseboom, T. J., Vrijkotte, T. G., Reynolds, R. M., & de Rooij, S. R. (2017). Determinants of cortisol during pregnancy—The ABCD cohort. *Psychoneuroendocrinology, 83*, 172–181.

Bouloukaki, I., Mermigkis, C., Tzanakis, N., Kallergis, E., Moniaki, V., Mauroudi, E., & Schiza, S. E. (2017). Evaluation of inflammatory markers in a large sample of obstructive sleep apnea patients without comorbidities. *Mediators of Inflammation, 2017,* Article 4573756.

Bourjeily, G., Butterfield, K., Curran, P., & Messerlian, G. (2014). Obstructive sleep apnea is associated with alterations in markers of fetoplacental wellbeing. *Journal of Maternal–Fetal & Neonatal Medicine, 28*(3), 262–266.

Bourjeily, G., Danilack, V. A., Bublitz, M. H., Lipkind, H., Muri, J., Caldwell, D., Tong, I., & Rosene-Montella, K. (2017). Obstructive sleep apnea in pregnancy is associated with adverse maternal outcomes: A national cohort. *Sleep Medicine, 38,* 50–57.

Bublitz, M. H., Bourjeily, G., D'Angelo, C., & Stroud, L. R. (2018). Maternal sleep quality and diurnal cortisol regulation over pregnancy. *Behavioral Sleep Medicine, 16*(3), 282–293.

Bublitz, M. H., Sharp, M., Freeburg, T., Sanapo, L., Nugent, N. R., Sharkey, K., & Bourjeily, G. (2021). Sleep disordered breathing measures in early pregnancy are associated with depressive symptoms in late pregnancy. *Diagnostics (Basel), 11*(5), Article 858.

Buckley, T. M., & Schatzberg, A. F. (2005). On the interactions of the hypothalamic–pituitary–adrenal (HPA) axis and sleep: Normal HPA axis activity and circadian rhythm, exemplary sleep disorders. *Journal of Clinical Endocrinology & Metabolism, 90*(5), 3106–3114.

Buswell, S. D., & Spatz, D. L. (2007). Parent–infant co-sleeping and its relationship to breastfeeding. *Journal of Pediatric Health Care, 21*(1), 22–28.

Caetano, G., Bozinovic, I., Dupont, C., Leger, D., Levy, R., & Sermondade, N. (2021). Impact of sleep on female and male reproductive functions: A systematic review. *Fertility and Sterility, 115*(3), 715–731.

Cagnacci, A. (2017). Role of melatonin in circadian rhythm at menopause. *Climacteric, 20*(2), Article 183.

Cagnacci, A., Paoletti, A. M., Soldani, R., Orru, M., Maschio, E., & Melis, G. B. (1995). Melatonin enhances the luteinizing hormone and follicle-stimulating hormone responses to gonadotropin-releasing hormone in the follicular, but not in the luteal, menstrual phase. *Journal of Clinical Endocrinology & Metabolism, 80*(4), 1095–1099.

Cai, C., Vandermeer, B., Khurana, R., Nerenberg, K., Featherstone, R., Sebastianski, M., & Davenport, M. H. (2019). The impact of occupational shift work and working hours during pregnancy on health outcomes: A systematic review and meta-analysis. *American Journal of Obstetrics and Gynecology, 221*(6), 563–576.

Cai, S., Tan, S., Gluckman, P. D., Godfrey, K. M., Saw, S., Teoh, O. H., Chong, Y. S., Meaney, M. J., Kramer, M. S., & Gooley, J. J.; GUSTO Study Group. (2016). Sleep quality and nocturnal sleep duration in pregnancy and risk of gestational diabetes mellitus. *Sleep, 40*(2), Article zsw058.

Cain, M. A., Brumley, J., Louis-Jacques, A., Drerup, M., Stern, M., & Louis, J. M. (2019). A pilot study of a sleep intervention delivered through group prenatal care to overweight and obese women. *Behavioral Sleep Medicine, 18*(4), 477–487.

Challis, J. R., Lockwood, C. J., Myatt, L., Norman, J. E., Strauss, J. F., 3rd, & Petraglia, F. (2009). Inflammation and pregnancy. *Reproductive Sciences, 16*(2), 206–215.

Chaudhry, S. K., & Susser, L. C. (2018). Considerations in treating insomnia during pregnancy: A literature review. *Psychosomatics, 59*(4), 341–348.

Chellappa, S. L., Morris, C. J., & Scheer, F. (2020). Circadian misalignment increases mood vulnerability in simulated shift work. *Scientific Reports, 10*(1), Article 18614.

Chen, P. H., Liou, K. C., Chen, C. P., & Cheng, S. J. (2012). Risk factors and prevalence rate of restless legs syndrome among pregnant women in Taiwan. *Sleep Medicine, 13*(9), 1153–1157.

Chen, S. J., Shi, L., Bao, Y. P., Sun, Y. K., Lin, X., Que, J. Y., Vitiello, M. V., Zhou, Y. X., Wang, Y. Q., & Lu, L. (2018). Prevalence of restless legs syndrome during pregnancy: A systematic review and meta-analysis. *Sleep Medicine Reviews, 40,* 43–54.

Cho, N. Y., Kim, S., Nowakowski, S., Shin, C., & Suh, S. (2019). Sleep disturbance in women who undergo surgical menopause compared with women who experience natural menopause. *Menopause, 26*(4), 357–364.

Christian, L. M., Carroll, J. E., Porter, K., & Hall, M. H. (2019). Sleep quality across pregnancy and postpartum: Effects of parity and race. *Sleep Health, 5*(4), 327–334.

Cunningham, F. G., Leveno, K. J., Dashe, J. S., Hoffman, B. L., Spong, C. Y., & Casey, B. M. (Eds.). (2022). Implantation and placental development; maternal physiology; pulmonary disorders. In *Williams obstetrics* (26th ed.). McGraw Hill. https://accessmedicine-mhmedical-com.proxy.cc.uic.edu/content.aspx?bookid=2977&sectionid=252902560

de Zambotti, M., Colrain, I. M., & Baker, F. C. (2015). Interaction between reproductive hormones and physiological sleep in women. *Journal of Clinical Endocrinology & Metabolism, 100*(4), 1426–1433.

Doan, T., Gardiner, A., Gay, C. L., & Lee, K. A. (2007). Breast-feeding increases sleep duration of new parents. *Journal of Perinatal and Neonatal Nursing, 21*(3), 200–206.

Doan, T., Gay, C. L., Kennedy, H. P., Newman, J., & Lee, K. A. (2014). Nighttime breastfeeding behavior is associated with more nocturnal sleep among first-time mothers at one month postpartum. *Journal of Clinical Sleep Medicine, 10*(3), 313–319.

Dorheim, S. K., Bjorvatn, B., & Eberhard-Gran, M. (2012). Insomnia and depressive symptoms in late pregnancy: A population-based study. *Behavioral Sleep Medicine, 10*(3), 152–166.

Dou, Y., Lin, B., Cheng, H., Wang, C., Zhao, M., Zhang, J., & Wu, J. (2019). The reduction of melatonin levels is associated with the development of preeclampsia: A meta-analysis. *Hypertension in Pregnancy, 38*(2), 65–72.

Driver, H. S., Dijk, D. J., Werth, E., Biedermann, K., & Borbely, A. A. (1996). Sleep and the sleep electroencephalogram across the menstrual cycle in young healthy women. *Journal of Clinical Endocrinology & Metabolism, 81*(2), 728–735.

Dunietz, G. L., Chervin, R. D., & O'Brien, L. M. (2014). Sleep-disordered breathing during pregnancy: Future implications for cardiovascular health. *Obstetrical & Gynecological Survey, 69*(3), 164–176.

Dunietz, G. L., Lisabeth, L. D., Shedden, K., Shamim-Uzzaman, Q. A., Bullough, A. S., Chames, M. C., Bowden, M. F., & O'Brien, L. M. (2017). Restless legs syndrome and sleep–wake disturbances in pregnancy. *Journal of Clinical Sleep Medicine, 13*(7), 863–870.

Edwards, N., Blyton, D. M., Hennessy, A., & Sullivan, C. E. (2005). Severity of sleep-disordered breathing improves following parturition. *Sleep, 28*(6), 737–741.

Ejaz, H., Figaro, J. K., Woolner, A. M. F., Thottakam, B. M. V., & Galley, H. F. (2020). Maternal serum melatonin increases during pregnancy and falls immediately after delivery implicating the placenta as a major source of melatonin. *Frontiers in Endocrinology, 11*, Article 623038.

Espino, J., Macedo, M., Lozano, G., Ortiz, Á., Rodríguez, C., Rodríguez, A. B., & Bejarano, I. (2019). Impact of melatonin supplementation in women with unexplained infertility undergoing fertility treatment. *Antioxidants (Basel), 8*(9), Article 338.

Facco, F. L., Grobman, W. A., Reid, K. J., Parker, C. B., Hunter, S. M., Silver, R. M., Basner, R. C., Saade, G. R., Pien, G. W., Manchanda, S., Louis, J. M., Nhan-Chang, C. L., Chung, J. H., Wing, D. A., Simhan, H. N., Haas, D. M., Iams, J., Parry, S., & Zee, P. C. (2017). Objectively measured short sleep duration and later sleep midpoint in pregnancy are associated with a higher risk of gestational diabetes. *American Journal of Obstetrics and Gynecology*, 217(4), 447.e1–447.e13.

Facco, F. L., Kramer, J., Ho, K. H., Zee, P. C., & Grobman, W. A. (2010). Sleep disturbances in pregnancy. *Obstetrics and Gynecology, 115*(1), 77–83.

Facco, F. L., Parker, C. B., Reddy, U. M., Silver, R. M., Koch, M. A., Louis, J. M., Basner, R. C., Chung, J. H., Nhan-Chang, C. L., Pien, G. W., Redline, S., Grobman, W. A., Wing, D. A., Simhan, H. N., Haas, D. M., Mercer, B. M., Parry, S., Mobley, D., Hunter, S., Saade, G. R., Schubert, F. P., & Zee P. C. (2017). Association between sleep-disordered breathing and hypertensive disorders of pregnancy and gestational diabetes mellitus. *Obstetrics and Gynecology, 129*(1), 31–41.

Faulkner, S. M., Bee, P. E., Meyer, N., Dijk, D. J., & Drake, R. J. (2019). Light therapies to improve sleep in intrinsic circadian rhythm sleep disorders and neuro-psychiatric illness: A systematic review and meta-analysis. *Sleep Medicine Reviews, 46*, 108–123.

Felder, J. N., Epel, E. S., Neuhaus, J., Krystal, A. D., & Prather, A. A. (2022). Randomized controlled trial of digital cognitive behavior therapy for prenatal insomnia symptoms: Effects on postpartum insomnia and mental health. *Sleep, 45*(2), Article zsab280.

Fernandez-Alonso, A. M., Trabalon-Pastor, M., Chedraui, P., & Perez-Lopez, F. R. (2012). Factors related to insomnia and sleepiness in the late third trimester of pregnancy. *Archives of Gynecology and Obstetrics, 286*(1), 55–61.

Franik, G., Krysta, K., Madej, P., Gimlewicz-Pięta, B., Oślizło, B., Trukawka, J., & Olszanecka-Glinianowicz, M. (2016). Sleep disturbances in women with polycystic ovary syndrome. *Gynecological Endocrinology, 32*(12), 1014–1017.

Freedman, R. R. (2014). Menopausal hot flashes: Mechanisms, endocrinology, treatment. *Journal of Steroid Biochemistry and Molecular Biology, 142*, 115–120.

Freedman, R. R., Norton, D., Woodward, S., & Cornélissen, G. (1995). Core body temperature and circadian rhythm of hot flashes in menopausal women. *Journal of Clinical Endocrinology & Metabolism, 80*(8), 2354–2358.

Gallaher, K. G. H., Slyepchenko, A., Frey, B. N., Urstad, K., & Dorheim, S. K. (2018). The role of circadian rhythms in postpartum sleep and mood. *Sleep Medicine Clinics, 13*(3), 359–374.

Gay, C. L., Lee, K. A., & Lee, S. Y. (2004). Sleep patterns and fatigue in new mothers and fathers. *Biological Research for Nursing, 5*(4), 311–318.

Gomez-Santos, C., Saura, C. B., Lucas, J. A., Castell, P., Madrid, J. A., & Garaulet, M. (2016). Menopause status is associated with circadian- and sleep-related alterations. *Menopause, 23*(6), 682–690.

Gordon, A., Raynes-Greenow, C., Bond, D., Morris, J., Rawlinson, W., & Jeffery, H. (2015). Sleep position, fetal growth restriction, and late-pregnancy stillbirth: The Sydney stillbirth study. *Obstetrics and Gynecology, 125*(2), 347–355.

Gozal, D., & Kheirandish-Gozal, L. (2008). Cardiovascular morbidity in obstructive sleep apnea: Oxidative stress, inflammation, and much more. *American Journal of Respiratory and Critical Care Medicine, 177*(4), 369–375.

Guilleminault, C., Kreutzer, M., & Chang, J. L. (2004). Pregnancy, sleep disordered breathing and treatment with nasal continuous positive airway pressure. *Sleep Medicine, 5*(1), 43–51.

Hachul, H., Andersen, M. L., Bittencourt, L. R., Santos-Silva, R., Conway, S. G., & Tufik, S. (2010). Does the reproductive cycle influence sleep patterns in women with sleep complaints? *Climacteric, 13*(6), 594–603.

Hadjimarkou, M. M., Benham, R., Schwarz, J. M., Holder, M. K., & Mong, J. A. (2008). Estradiol suppresses rapid eye movement sleep and activation of sleep-active neurons in the ventrolateral preoptic area. *European Journal of Neuroscience, 27*(7), 1780–1792.

Halabi, D., Richter, H. G., Mendez, N., Kähne, T., Spichiger, C., Salazar, E., Torres, F., Vergara, K., Seron-Ferre, M., & Torres-Farfan, C. (2021). Maternal chronodisruption throughout pregnancy impairs glucose homeostasis and adipose tissue physiology in the male rat offspring. *Frontiers in Endocrinology (Lausanne), 12*, Article 678468.

Hall, J. E., Sullivan, J. P., & Richardson, G. S. (2005). Brief wake episodes modulate sleep-inhibited luteinizing hormone secretion in the early follicular phase. *Journal of Clinical Endocrinology & Metabolism, 90*(4), 2050–2055.

Hall, M. H., Casement, M. D., Troxel, W. M., Matthews, K. A., Bromberger, J. T., Kravitz, H. M., Krafty, R. T., & Buysse, D. J. (2015). Chronic stress is prospectively associated with sleep in midlife women: The SWAN sleep study. *Sleep, 38*(10), 1645–1654.

Hall, M. H., Matthews, K. A., Kravitz, H. M., Gold, E. B., Buysse, D. J., Bromberger, J. T., Owens, J. F., & Sowers, M. (2009). Race and financial strain are independent correlates of sleep in midlife women: The SWAN sleep study. *Sleep, 32*(1), 73–82.

Haney, A., Buysse, D. J., Rosario, B. L., Chen, Y. F., & Okun, M. L. (2014). Sleep disturbance and cardiometabolic risk factors in early pregnancy: A preliminary study. *Sleep Medicine, 15*(4), 444–450.

Harlow, S. D., Gass, M., Hall, J. E., Lobo, R., Maki, P., Rebar, R. W., Sherman, S., Sluss, P. M., & de Villiers, T. J.; STRAW + 10 Collaborative Group. (2012). Executive summary of the Stages of Reproductive Aging Workshop + 10: Addressing the unfinished agenda of staging reproductive aging. *Journal of Clinical Endocrinology & Metabolism, 97*(4), 1159–1168.

Hatcher, K. M., Royston, S. E., & Mahoney, M. M. (2020). Modulation of circadian rhythms through estrogen receptor signaling. *European Journal of Neuroscience, 51*(1), 217–228.

Hauck, F. R., Signore, C., Fein, S. B., & Raju, T. N. (2008). Infant sleeping arrangements and practices during the first year of life. *Pediatrics, 122*(S2), S113–S120.

Heazell, A., Li, M., Budd, J., Thompson, J., Stacey, T., Cronin, R. S., Martin, B., Roberts, D., Mitchell, E. A., & McCowan, L. (2018). Association between maternal sleep practices and late stillbirth—Findings from a stillbirth case–control study. *BJOG, 125*(2), 254–262.

Hedman, C., Pohjasvaara, T., Tolonen, U., Suhonen-Malm, A. S., & Myllyla, V. V. (2002). Effects of pregnancy on mothers' sleep. *Sleep Medicine, 3*(1), 37–42.

Helvaci, N., Karabulut, E., Demir, A. U., & Yildiz, B. O. (2017). Polycystic ovary syndrome and the risk of obstructive sleep apnea: A meta-analysis and review of the literature. *Endocrine Connections, 6*(7), 437–445.

Herring, S. J., Nelson, D. B., Pien, G. W., Homko, C., Goetzl, L. M., Davey, A., Foster, G. D. (2014). Objectively measured sleep duration and hyperglycemia in pregnancy. *Sleep Medicine, 15*(1), 51–55.

Hertz, G., Fast, A., Feinsilver, S. H., Albertario, C. L., Schulman, H., & Fein, A. M. (1992). Sleep in normal late pregnancy. *Sleep, 15*(3), 246–251.

Hirst, J. J., Haluska, G. J., Cook, M. J., & Novy, M. J. (1993). Plasma oxytocin and nocturnal uterine activity: Maternal but not fetal concentrations increase progressively during late pregnancy and delivery in rhesus monkeys. *American Journal of Obstetrics and Gynecology, 169*(2, Pt. 1), 415–422.

Hrozanova, M., Klockner, C. A., Sandbakk, O., Pallesen, S., & Moen, F. (2021). Sex differences in sleep and influence of the menstrual cycle on women's sleep in junior endurance athletes. *PLOS ONE, 16*(6), Article e0253376.

Hung, H. M., Tsai, P. S., Ko, S. H., & Chen, C. H. (2013). Patterns and predictors of sleep quality in Taiwanese pregnant women. *American Journal of Maternal Child Nursing, 38*(2), 95–101.

Insana, S. P., Williams, K. B., & Montgomery-Downs, H. E. (2013). Sleep disturbance and neurobehavioral performance among postpartum women. *Sleep, 36*(1), 73–81.

Izci Balserak, B., Hermann, R., Hernandez, T. L., Buhimschi, C., & Park, C. (2022). Evening blue-light exposure, maternal glucose, and infant birthweight. *Annals of the New York Academy of Sciences, 1515*(1), 276–284.

Izci-Balserak, B., Keenan, B. T., Corbitt, C., Staley, B., Perlis, M., & Pien, G. W. (2018). Changes in sleep characteristics and breathing parameters during sleep in early and late pregnancy. *Journal of Clinical Sleep Medicine, 14*(7), 1161–1168.

Izci-Balserak, B., O'Brien, L. M., & Bei, B. (2022). Sleep and sleep disorders associated with pregnancy. In M. Kryger, T. Roth, C. Goldstein, & W. Dement (Eds.), *Principles and practice of sleep medicine* (7th ed., pp. 1751–1763). Elsevier.

Izci-Balserak, B., & Pien, G. W. (2014). The relationship and potential mechanistic pathways between sleep disturbances and maternal hyperglycemia. *Current Diabetes Reports, 14*(2), Article 459.

Izci Balserak, B., Pien, G. W., Prasad, B., Mastrogiannis, D., Park, C., Quinn, L. T., Herdegen, J., & Carley, D. W. (2020). Obstructive sleep apnea is associated with newly diagnosed gestational diabetes mellitus. *Annals of the American Thoracic Society, 17*(6), 754–761.

Javaheri, S., Barbe, F., Campos-Rodriguez, F., Dempsey, J. A., Khayat, R., Javaheri, S., Malhotra, A., Martinez-Garcia, M. A., Mehra, R., Pack, A. I., Polotsky, V. Y., Redline, S., & Somers, V. K. (2017). Sleep apnea: Types, mechanisms, and clinical cardiovascular consequences. *Journal of the American College of Cardiology, 69*(7), 841–858.

Kalleinen, N., Aittokallio, J., Lampio, L., Kaisti, M., Polo-Kantola, P., Polo, O., Heinonen, O. J., & Saaresranta, T. (2021). Sleep during menopausal transition: A 10-year follow-up. *Sleep, 44*(6), Article zsaa283.

Kalmbach, D. A., Cheng, P., O'Brien, L. M., Swanson, L. M., Sangha, R., Sen, S., Guille, C., Cuamatzi-Castelan, A., Henry, A. L., Roth, T., & Drake, C. L. (2020). A randomized controlled trial of digital cognitive behavioral therapy for insomnia in pregnant women. *Sleep Medicine, 72*, 82–92.

Kalmbach, D. A., Cheng, P., Roth, A., Roth, T., Swanson, L. M., O'Brien, L. M., Fresco, D. M., Harb, N. C., Cuamatzi-Castelan, A. S., Reffi, A. N., & Drake, C. L. (2022). DSM-5 insomnia disorder in pregnancy: Associations with depression, suicidal ideation, and cognitive and somatic arousal, and identifying clinical cutoffs for detection. *Sleep Advances, 3*(1), Article zpac006.

Kalmbach, D. A., Cheng, P., Roth, T., Swanson, L. M., Cuamatzi-Castelan, A., Roth, A., Drake, C. L. (2022). Examining patient feedback and the role of cognitive arousal in treatment non-response to digital cognitive-behavioral therapy for insomnia during pregnancy. *Behavioral Sleep Medicine, 20*(2), 143–163.

Kalmbach, D. A., Cheng, P., Sangha, R., O'Brien, L. M., Swanson, L. M., Palagini, L., Bazan, L. F., Roth, T., & Drake, C. L. (2019). Insomnia, short sleep, and snoring in mid-to-late pregnancy: Disparities related to poverty, race, and obesity. *Nature and Science of Sleep, 11*, 301–315.

Kalmbach, D. A., O'Brien, L. M., Pitts, D. S., Sagong, C., Arnett, L. K., Harb, N. C., Cheng, P., & Drake, C. L. (2022). Mother-to-infant bonding is associated with maternal insomnia, snoring, cognitive arousal, and infant sleep problems and colic. *Behavioral Sleep Medicine, 20*(4), 393–409.

Kawashima, A., Detsuka, N., & Yano, R. (2022). Sleep deprivation and fatigue in early postpartum and their association with postpartum depression in primiparas intending to establish breastfeeding. *Journal of Rural Medicine, 17*(1), 40–49.

Kennedy, H. P., Gardiner, A., Gay, C., & Lee, K. A. (2007). Negotiating sleep: A qualitative study of new mothers. *Journal of Perinatal & Neonatal Nursing, 21*(2), 114–122.

Kervezee, L., Shechter, A., & Boivin, D. B. (2018). Impact of shift work on the circadian timing system and health in women. *Sleep Medicine Clinics, 13*(3), 295–306.

Kim, K. H., & Lee, K. A. (2009). Sleep and fatigue symptoms in women before and 6 weeks after hysterectomy. *Journal of Obstetric, Gynecologic, and Neonatal Nursing, 38*(3), 344–352.

Kloss, J. D., Perlis, M. L., Zamzow, J. A., Culnan, E. J., & Gracia, C. R. (2015). Sleep, sleep disturbance, and fertility in women. *Sleep Medicine Reviews, 22*, 78–87.

Kravitz, H. M., Ganz, P. A., Bromberger, J., Powell, L. H., Sutton-Tyrrell, K., & Meyer, P. M. (2003). Sleep difficulty in women at midlife: A community survey of sleep and the menopausal transition. *Menopause, 10*(1), 19–28.

Kravitz, H. M., Janssen, I., Santoro, N., Bromberger, J. T., Schocken, M., Everson-Rose, S. A., Karavolos, K., & Powell, L. H. (2005). Relationship of day-to-day reproductive hormone levels to sleep in midlife women. *Archives of Internal Medicine, 165*(20), 2370–2376.

Kravitz, H. M., & Joffe, H. (2011). Sleep during the perimenopause: A SWAN story. *Obstetrics and Gynecology Clinics of North America, 38*(3), 567–586.

Kravitz, H. M., Zhao, X., Bromberger, J. T., Gold, E. B., Hall, M. H., Matthews, K. A., Sowers, M. R. (2008). Sleep disturbance during the menopausal transition in a multi-ethnic community sample of women. *Sleep, 31*(7), 979–990.

Ladyman, C., & Signal, T. L. (2018). Sleep health in pregnancy: A scoping review. *Sleep Medicine Clinics, 13*(3), 307–333.

Lampio, L., Polo-Kantola, P., Himanen, S. L., Kurki, S., Huupponen, E., Engblom, J., Heinonen, O. J., Polo, O., & Saaresranta, T. (2017). Sleep during menopausal transition: A 6-year follow-up. *Sleep, 40*(7), Article zsx090.

Lee, K. A. (1988). Circadian temperature rhythms in relation to menstrual cycle phase. *Journal of Biological Rhythms, 3*(3), 255–263.

Lee, K. A., & Gay, C. L. (2004). Sleep in late pregnancy predicts length of labor and type of delivery. *American Journal of Obstetrics and Gynecology, 191*(6), 2041–2046.

Lee, K. A., & Gay, C. L. (2011). Can modifications to the bedroom environment improve the sleep of new parents? Two randomized controlled trials. *Research in Nursing & Health, 34*(1), 7–19.

Lee, K. A., & Gay, C. L. (2017). Improving sleep for hospitalized antepartum patients: A non-randomized controlled pilot study. *Journal of Clinical Sleep Medicine, 13*(12), 1445–1453.

Lee, K. A., Shaver, J. F., Giblin, E. C., & Woods, N. F. (1990). Sleep patterns related to menstrual cycle phase and premenstrual affective symptoms. *Sleep, 13*(5), 403–409.

Lee, K. A., & Zaffke, M. E. (1999). Longitudinal changes in fatigue and energy during pregnancy and the postpartum period. *Journal of Obstetric, Gynecologic, and Neonatal Nursing, 28*(2), 183–191.

Lee, K. A., Zaffke, M. E., & Baratte-Beebe, K. (2001). Restless legs syndrome and sleep disturbance during pregnancy: The role of folate and iron. *Journal of Women's Health & Gender-Based Medicine, 10*(4), 335–341.

Lee, K. A., Zaffke, M. E., & McEnany, G. (2000). Parity and sleep patterns during and after pregnancy. *Obstetrics and Gynecology, 95*(1), 14–18.

Lee, S. Y., & Lee, K. A. (2007). Early postpartum sleep and fatigue for mothers after cesarean delivery compared with vaginal delivery: An exploratory study. *Journal of Perinatal & Neonatal Nursing, 21*(2), 109–113.

Legro, R. S., Arslanian, S. A., Ehrmann, D. A., Hoeger, K. M., Murad, M. H., Pasquali, R., & Welt, C. K.; Endocrine Society. (2013). Diagnosis and treatment of polycystic ovary syndrome: An Endocrine Society clinical practice guideline. *Journal of Clinical Endocrinology & Metabolism, 98*(12), 4565–4592.

Lewis, K. J. S., Di Florio, A., Forty, L., Gordon-Smith, K., Perry, A., Craddock, N., Jones, L., & Jones, I. (2018). Mania triggered by sleep loss and risk of postpartum psychosis in women with bipolar disorder. *Journal of Affective Disorders, 225*, 624–629.

Li, D. X., Romans, S., De Souza, M. J., Murray, B., & Einstein, G. (2015). Actigraphic and self-reported sleep quality in women: Associations with ovarian hormones and mood. *Sleep Medicine, 16*(10), 1217–1224.

Lin, T. Y., Lin, P. Y., Su, T. P., Li, C. T., Lin, W. C., Chang, W. H., Chen, T. J., Bai, Y. M., & Chen, M. H. (2017). Risk of developing obstructive sleep apnea among women with polycystic ovarian syndrome: A nationwide longitudinal follow-up study. *Sleep Medicine, 36*, 165–169.

Liset, R., Gronli, J., Henriksen, R. E., Henriksen, T. E. G., Nilsen, R. M., & Pallesen, S. (2021). Sleep, evening light exposure and perceived stress in healthy nulliparous women in the third trimester of pregnancy. *PLOS ONE, 16*(6), Article e0252285.

Logan, R. W., & McClung, C. A. (2019). Rhythms of life: Circadian disruption and brain disorders across the lifespan. *Nature Reviews Neuroscience, 20*(1), 49–65.

Lopes, J., Arnosti, D., Trosko, J. E., Tai, M. H., & Zuccari, D. (2016). Melatonin decreases estrogen receptor binding to estrogen response elements sites on the OCT4 gene in human breast cancer stem cells. *Genes & Cancer, 7*(5–6), 209–217.

Louis, J. M., Mogos, M. F., Salemi, J. L., Redline, S., & Salihu, H. M. (2014). Obstructive sleep apnea and severe maternal-infant morbidity/mortality in the United States, 1998–2009. *Sleep, 37*(5), 843–849.

Lu, Q., Zhang, X., Wang, Y., Li, J., Xu, Y., Song, X., Su, S., Zhu, X., Vitiello, M. V., Shi, J., Bao, Y., & Lu, L. (2021). Sleep disturbances during pregnancy and adverse maternal and fetal outcomes: A systematic review and meta-analysis. *Sleep Medicine Reviews, 58*, Article 101436.

Manber, R., Bei, B., Simpson, N., Asarnow, L., Rangel, E., Sit, A., & Lyell, D. (2019). Cognitive behavioral therapy for prenatal insomnia: A randomized controlled trial. *Obstetrics and Gynecology, 133*(5), 911–919.

Manconi, M., Ulfberg, J., Berger, K., Ghorayeb, I., Wesstrom, J., Fulda, S., Allen, R. P., & Pollmächer, T. (2012). When gender matters: Restless legs syndrome. Report of the "RLS and Woman" workshop endorsed by the European RLS Study Group. *Sleep Medicine Reviews, 16*(4), 297–307.

Martin-Fairey, C. A., Zhao, P., Wan, L., Roenneberg, T., Fay, J., Ma, X., McCarthy, R., Jungheim, E. S., England, S. K., & Herzog, E. D. (2019). Pregnancy induces an earlier chronotype in both mice and women. *Journal of Biological Rhythms, 34*(3), 323–331.

Maurovich-Horvat, E., Kemlink, D., Hogl, B., Frauscher, B., Ehrmann, L., Geisler, P., Ettenhuber, K., Mayer, G., Peraita-Adrados, R., Calvo, E., Lammers, G. J., Van der Heide, A., Ferini-Strambi, L., Plazzi, G., Poli, F., Dauvilliers, Y., Jennum, P., Leonthin, H., Mathis, J., . . . Sonka, K.; European Narcolepsy Network. (2013). Narcolepsy and pregnancy: A retrospective European evaluation of 249 pregnancies. *Journal of Sleep Research, 22*(5), 496–512.

McCarthy, R., Jungheim, E. S., Fay, J. C., Bates, K., Herzog, E. D., & England, S. K. (2019). Riding the rhythm of melatonin through pregnancy to deliver on time. *Frontiers in Endocrinology (Lausanne), 10*, Article 616.

McElroy, J. A., Newcomb, P. A., Titus-Ernstoff, L., Trentham-Dietz, A., Hampton, J. M., & Egan, K. M. (2006). Duration of sleep and breast cancer risk in a large population-based case–control study. *Journal of Sleep Research, 15*(3), 241–249.

Megdal, S. P., Kroenke, C. H., Laden, F., Pukkala, E., & Schernhammer, E. S. (2005). Night work and breast cancer risk: A systematic review and meta-analysis. *European Journal of Cancer, 41*(13), 2023–2032.

Merklinger-Gruchala, A., Ellison, P. T., Lipson, S. F., Thune, I., & Jasienska, G. (2008). Low estradiol levels in women of reproductive age having low sleep variation. *European Journal of Cancer Prevention, 17*(5), 467–472.

Michels, K. A., Mendola, P., Schliep, K. C., Yeung, E. H., Ye, A., Dunietz, G. L., Wactawski-Wende, J., Kim, K., Freeman, J. R., Schisterman, E. F., & Mumford, S. L. (2020). The influences of sleep duration, chronotype, and nightwork on the ovarian cycle. *Chronobiology International, 37*(2), 260–271.

Migueis, D. P., Urel, A., Dos Santos, C. C., Accetta, A., & Burla, M. (2022). The cardiovascular, metabolic, fetal and neonatal effects of CPAP use in pregnant women: A systematic review [Special issue]. *Sleep Science, 15*, 264–277.

Mihm, M., Gangooly, S., & Muttukrishna, S. (2011). The normal menstrual cycle in women. *Animal Reproduction Science, 124*(3–4), 229–236.

Miller, M. A., Mehta, N., Clark-Bilodeau, C., & Bourjeily, G. (2020). Sleep pharmacotherapy for common sleep disorders in pregnancy and lactation. *Chest, 157*(1), 184–197.

Minar, M., Kosutzka, Z., Habanova, H., Rusnak, I., Planck, K., & Valkovic, P. (2015). Restless legs syndrome in pregnancy is connected with iron deficiency. *Sleep Medicine, 16*(5), 589–592.

Mindell, J. A., Cook, R. A., & Nikolovski, J. (2015). Sleep patterns and sleep disturbances across pregnancy. *Sleep Medicine, 16*(4), 483–488.

Moderie, C., Boudreau, P., Shechter, A., Lesperance, P., & Boivin, D. B. (2021). Effects of exogenous melatonin on sleep and circadian rhythms in women with premenstrual dysphoric disorder. *Sleep, 44*(12), Article zsab171.

Na, M., Wu, J., Li, M., Hinkle, S. N., Zhang, C., & Gao, X. (2020). New onset of restless legs syndrome in pregnancy in a prospective multiracial cohort: Incidence and risk factors. *Neurology, 95*(24), e3438–e3447.

Naghi, I., Keypour, F., Ahari, S. B., Tavalai, S. A., & Khak, M. (2011). Sleep disturbance in late pregnancy and type and duration of labour. *Journal of Obstetrics and Gynaecology, 31*(6), 489–491.

Nam, G. E., Han, K., & Lee, G. (2017). Association between sleep duration and menstrual cycle irregularity in Korean female adolescents. *Sleep Medicine, 35*, 62–66.

National Institutes of Health. (2012). *Final report: Evidence-based methodology workshop on polycystic ovary syndrome*. National Institutes of Health.
Nowakowski, S., Levy-Meeks, M. E., Dawson, D. B., Meers, J. M., Stout-Aguilar, J. S., Kilic, G. S., & Borahay, M. A. (2020). Association of preoperative sleep pattern with posthysterectomy pain: A pilot study. *Journal of Clinical Sleep Medicine, 16*(11), 1901–1908.
Obeysekare, J. L., Cohen, Z. L., Coles, M. E., Pearlstein, T. B., Monzon, C., Flynn, E. E., & Sharkey, K. M. (2020). Delayed sleep timing and circadian rhythms in pregnancy and transdiagnostic symptoms associated with postpartum depression. *Translational Psychiatry, 10*(1), Article 14.
O'Brien, L. M., Bullough, A. S., Owusu, J. T., Tremblay, K. A., Brincat, C. A., Chames, M. C., Kalbfleisch, J. D., & Chervin, R. D. (2012). Pregnancy-onset habitual snoring, gestational hypertension, and preeclampsia: prospective cohort study. *American Journal of Obstetrics and Gynecology, 207*(6), e481–e489.
Okun, M. L., Schetter, C. D., & Glynn, L. M. (2011). Poor sleep quality is associated with preterm birth. *Sleep, 34*(11), 1493–1498.
Opperhuizen, A. L., Stenvers, D. J., Jansen, R. D., Foppen, E., Fliers, E., & Kalsbeek, A. (2017). Light at night acutely impairs glucose tolerance in a time-, intensity- and wavelength-dependent manner in rats. *Diabetologia, 60*(7), 1333–1343.
Palagini, L., Gemignani, A., Banti, S., Manconi, M., Mauri, M., & Riemann, D. (2014). Chronic sleep loss during pregnancy as a determinant of stress: Impact on pregnancy outcome. *Sleep Medicine, 15*(8), 853–859.
Park, Y. M., White, A. J., Jackson, C. L., Weinberg, C. R., & Sandler, D. P. (2019). Association of exposure to artificial light at night while sleeping with risk of obesity in women. *JAMA Internal Medicine, 179*(8), 1061–1071.
Parry, B. L., Berga, S. L., Mostofi, N., Klauber, M. R., & Resnick, A. (1997). Plasma melatonin circadian rhythms during the menstrual cycle and after light therapy in premenstrual dysphoric disorder and normal control subjects. *Journal of Biological Rhythms, 12*(1), 47–64.
Parry, B. L., LeVeau, B., Mostofi, N., Naham, H. C., Loving, R., Clopton, P., & Gillin, J. C. (1997). Temperature circadian rhythms during the menstrual cycle and sleep deprivation in premenstrual dysphoric disorder and normal comparison subjects. *Journal of Biological Rhythms, 12*(1), 34–46.
Pascoe, M., Carter, L. P., Honig, E., Bena, J., & Foldvary-Schaefer, N. (2019). Pregnancy and contraception experiences in women with narcolepsy: A narcolepsy network survey. *Journal of Clinical Sleep Medicine, 15*(10), 1421–1426.
Picchietti, D. L., Hensley, J. G., Bainbridge, J. L., Lee, K. A., Manconi, M., McGregor, J. A., Silver, R. M., Trenkwalder, C., & Walters, A. S.; International Restless Legs Syndrome Study Group (IRLSSG). (2015). Consensus clinical practice guidelines for the diagnosis and treatment of restless legs syndrome/Willis-Ekbom disease during pregnancy and lactation. *Sleep Medicine Reviews, 22*, 64–77.
Pien, G. W., Pack, A. I., Jackson, N., Maislin, G., Macones, G. A., & Schwab, R. J. (2014). Risk factors for sleep-disordered breathing in pregnancy. *Thorax, 69*(4), 371–377.
Pien, G. W., & Schwab, R. J. (2004). Sleep disorders during pregnancy. *Sleep, 27*(7), 1405–1417.
Pietikainen, J. T., Harkanen, T., Polo-Kantola, P., Karlsson, H., Paunio, T., Karlsson, L., & Paavonen, E. J. (2021). Estimating the cumulative risk of postnatal depressive symptoms: The role of insomnia symptoms across pregnancy. *Social Psychiatry and Psychiatric Epidemiology, 56*(12), 2251–2261.
Pietikäinen, J. T., Polo-Kantola, P., Pölkki, P., Saarenpää-Heikkilä, O., Paunio, T., & Paavonen, E. J. (2019). Sleeping problems during pregnancy—A risk factor for postnatal depressiveness. *Archives of Women's Mental Health, 22*(3), 327–337.
Pines, A. (2016). Circadian rhythm and menopause. *Climacteric, 19*(6), 551–552.
Pires, G. N., Anderson, M. L., Giovenardi, M., & Tufik, S. (2010). Sleep impairment during pregnancy: Possible implications on mother–infant relationship. *Medical Hypotheses, 75*, 578–582.
Póvoa, A., Xavier, P., Matias, A., & Blickstein, I. (2018). First trimester β-hCG and estradiol levels in singleton and twin pregnancies after assisted reproduction. *Journal of Perinatal Medicine, 46*(8), 853–856.
Qian, J., & Scheer, F. (2020). Sex-dependent link between circadian misalignment and adiposity. *Nature Reviews Endocrinology, 16*(1), 13–15.
Quin, N., Lee, J. J., Pinnington, D. M., Newman, L., Manber, R., & Bei, B. (2022). Differentiating perinatal insomnia disorder and sleep disruption: A longitudinal study from pregnancy to 2 years postpartum. *Sleep, 45*(2), Article zsab293.

Razavi, P., Devore, E. E., Bajaj, A., Lockley, S. W., Figueiro, M. G., Ricchiuti, V., Gauderman, W. J., Hankinson, S. E., Willett, W. C., & Schernhammer, E. S. (2019). Shift work, chronotype, and melatonin rhythm in nurses. *Cancer Epidemiology, Biomarkers & Prevention, 28*(7), 1177–1186.

Reid, K. J., Facco, F. L., Grobman, W. A., Parker, C. B., Herbas, M., Hunter, S., Silver, R. M., Basner, R. C., Saade, G. R., Pien, G. W., Manchanda, S., Louis, J. M., Nhan-Chang, C. L., Chung, J. H., Wing, D. A., Simhan, H. N., Haas, D. M., Iams, J., Parry, S., & Zee, P. C. (2017). Sleep during pregnancy: The nuMoM2b pregnancy and sleep duration and continuity study. *Sleep, 40*(5), Article zsx045.

Reiter, R. J., Tan, D. X., Korkmaz, A., & Rosales-Corral, S. A. (2014). Melatonin and stable circadian rhythms optimize maternal, placental and fetal physiology. *Human Reproduction Update, 20*(2), 293–307.

Reutrakul, S., Anothaisintawee, T., Herring, S. J., Balserak, B. I., Marc, I., & Thakkinstian, A. (2017). Short sleep duration and hyperglycemia in pregnancy: Aggregate and individual patient data meta-analysis. *Sleep Medicine Reviews, 40*, 31–42.

Romans, S. E., Kreindler, D., Einstein, G., Laredo, S., Petrovic, M. J., & Stanley, J. (2015). Sleep quality and the menstrual cycle. *Sleep Medicine, 16*(4), 489–495.

Rosen, E. A. (2009). *Sleep characteristics in breastfeeding and formula-feeding mothers* [Unpublished doctoral dissertation]. University of Kansas.

Salari, N., Darvishi, N., Khaledi-Paveh, B., Vaisi-Raygani, A., Jalali, R., Daneshkhah, A., Bartina, Y., & Mohammadi, M. (2021). A systematic review and meta-analysis of prevalence of insomnia in the third trimester of pregnancy. *BMC Pregnancy and Childbirth, 21*(1), Article 284.

Schernhammer, E. S., Laden, F., Speizer, F. E., Willett, W. C., Hunter, D. J., Kawachi, I., & Colditz, G. A. (2001). Rotating night shifts and risk of breast cancer in women participating in the Nurses' Health Study. *Journal of the National Cancer Institute, 93*(20), 1563–1568.

Schredl, M., Gilles, M., Wolf, I., Peus, V., Scharnholz, B., Sutterlin, M., & Deuschle, M. (2016). Nightmare frequency in last trimester of pregnancy. *BMC Pregnancy and Childbirth, 16*(1), Article 346.

Sedov, I., Madsen, J. W., Goodman, S. H., & Tomfohr-Madsen, L. M. (2019). Couples' treatment preferences for insomnia experienced during pregnancy. *Families, Systems & Health, 37*(1), 46–55.

Sedov, I. D., Anderson, N. J., Dhillon, A. K., & Tomfohr-Madsen, L. M. (2021). Insomnia symptoms during pregnancy: A meta-analysis. *Journal of Sleep Research, 30*(1), Article e13207.

Sedov, I. D., Cameron, E. E., Madigan, S., & Tomfohr-Madsen, L. M. (2017). Sleep quality during pregnancy: A meta-analysis. *Sleep Medicine Reviews, 38*, 168–176.

Seron-Ferre, M., Ducsay, C. A., & Valenzuela, G. J. (1993). Circadian rhythms during pregnancy. *Endocrine Reviews, 14*(5), 594–609.

Sharkey, K. M., Crawford, S. L., Kim, S., & Joffe, H. (2014). Objective sleep interruption and reproductive hormone dynamics in the menstrual cycle. *Sleep Medicine, 15*(6), 688–693.

Sharkey, K. M., Pearlstein, T. B., & Carskadon, M. A. (2013). Circadian phase shifts and mood across the perinatal period in women with a history of major depressive disorder: A preliminary communication. *Journal of Affective Disorders, 150*(3), 1103–1108.

Shechter, A., Lesperance, P., Ng Ying Kin, N. M., & Boivin, D. B. (2012). Pilot investigation of the circadian plasma melatonin rhythm across the menstrual cycle in a small group of women with premenstrual dysphoric disorder. *PLOS ONE, 7*(12), Article e51929.

Shechter, A., Varin, F., & Boivin, D. B. (2010). Circadian variation of sleep during the follicular and luteal phases of the menstrual cycle. *Sleep, 33*(5), 647–656.

Shi, H., Huang, T., Schernhammer, E. S., Sun, Q., & Wang, M. (2022). Rotating night shift work and healthy aging after 24 years of follow-up in the Nurses' Health Study. *JAMA Network Open, 5*(5), Article e2210450.

Signal, T. L., Gander, P. H., Sangalli, M. R., Travier, N., Firestone, R. T., & Tuohy, J. F. (2007). Sleep duration and quality in healthy nulliparous and multiparous women across pregnancy and post-partum. *Australian & New Zealand Journal of Obstetrics & Gynaecology, 47*(1), 16–22.

Silver, R. M., Hunter, S., Reddy, U. M., Facco, F., Gibbins, K. J., Grobman, W. A., Mercer, B. M., Haas, D. M., Simhan, H. N., Parry, S., Wapner, R. J., Louis, J., Chung, J. M., Pien, G., Schubert, F. P., Saade, G. R., Zee, P., Redline, S., & Parker, C. B.; Nulliparous Pregnancy Outcomes Study: Monitoring Mothers-to-Be (NuMoM2b) Study. (2019). Prospective evaluation of maternal sleep position through 30 weeks of gestation and adverse pregnancy outcomes. *Obstetrics and Gynecology, 134*(4), 667–676.

Simon, S. L., McWhirter, L., Diniz Behn, C., Bubar, K. M., Kaar, J. L., Pyle, L., Rahat, H., Garcia-Reyes, Y., Carreau, A. M., Wright, K. P., Nadeau, K. J., & Cree-Green, M. (2019). Morning circadian misalignment is associated with insulin resistance in girls with obesity and polycystic ovarian syndrome. *Journal of Clinical Endocrinology & Metabolism, 104*(8), 3525–3534.

Sivertsen, B., Hysing, M., Dørheim, S. K., & Eberhard-Gran, M. (2015). Trajectories of maternal sleep problems before and after childbirth: A longitudinal population-based study. *BMC Pregnancy and Childbirth, 15*(1), Article 129.

Smith, M. R., Fogg, L. F., & Eastman, C. I. (2009). A compromise circadian phase position for permanent night work improves mood, fatigue, and performance. *Sleep, 32*(11), 1481–1489.

Smith, R. L., Flaws, J. A., & Mahoney, M. M. (2018). Factors associated with poor sleep during menopause: Results from the Midlife Women's Health Study. *Sleep Medicine, 45*, 98–105.

Spaeth, A. M., Khetarpal, R., Yu, D., Pien, G. W., & Herring, S. J. (2021). Determinants of postpartum sleep duration and sleep efficiency in minority women. *Sleep, 44*(4), Article zsaa246.

Spielman, A. J., Caruso, L. S., & Glovinsky, P. B. (1987). A behavioral perspective on insomnia treatment. *Psychiatric Clinics of North America, 10*(4), 541–553.

Srimoragot, M., Hershberger, P. E., Park, C., Hernandez, T. L., & Izci Balserak, B. (2022). Infant feeding type and maternal sleep during the postpartum period: A systematic review and meta-analysis. *Journal of Sleep Research, 32*(2), Article e13625.

Srivanitchapoom, P., Pandey, S., & Hallett, M. (2014). Restless legs syndrome and pregnancy: A review. *Parkinsonism & Related Disorders, 20*(7), 716–722.

Stacey, T., Thompson, J. M., Mitchell, E. A., Ekeroma, A. J., Zuccollo, J. M., & McCowan, L. M. (2011). Association between maternal sleep practices and risk of late stillbirth: a case-control study. *BMJ, 342*, Article d3403.

Steinweg, K., Nippita, T., Cistulli, P. A., & Bin, Y. S. (2020). Maternal and neonatal outcomes associated with restless legs syndrome in pregnancy: A systematic review. *Sleep Medicine Reviews, 54*, Article 101359.

Stremler, R., & Sharkey, K. (2022). Postpartum period and early parenthood. In M. Kryger, T. Roth, C. A. Goldstein, & W. Dement (Eds.), *Principle and practice of sleep medicine* (7th ed., pp. 1773–1780). Elsevier.

Takayama, H., Nakamura, Y., Tamura, H., Yamagata, Y., Harada, A., Nakata, M., Sugino, N., & Kato, H. (2003). Pineal gland (melatonin) affects the parturition time, but not luteal function and fetal growth, in pregnant rats. *Endocrine Journal, 50*(1), 37–43.

Tamura, H., Nakamura, Y., Korkmaz, A., Manchester, L. C., Tan, D. X., Sugino, N., & Reiter, R. J. (2009). Melatonin and the ovary: Physiological and pathophysiological implications. *Fertility and Sterility, 92*(1), 328–343.

Telarovic, S., & Condic, L. (2019). Frequency of iron deficiency anemia in pregnant and non-pregnant women suffering from restless legs syndrome. *Hematology, 24*(1), 263–267.

Thorpy, M., Zhao, C. G., & Dauvilliers, Y. (2013). Management of narcolepsy during pregnancy. *Sleep Medicine, 14*(4), 367–376.

Toffol, E., Kalleinen, N., Haukka, J., Vakkuri, O., Partonen, T., & Polo-Kantola, P. (2014). Melatonin in perimenopausal and postmenopausal women: Associations with mood, sleep, climacteric symptoms, and quality of life. *Menopause, 21*(5), 493–500.

Toffol, E., Kalleinen, N., Himanen, S. L., Partonen, T., Haukka, J., & Polo-Kantola, P. (2021). Nighttime melatonin secretion and sleep architecture: Different associations in perimenopausal and postmenopausal women. *Sleep Medicine, 81*, 52–61.

Tom, S. E., Kuh, D., Guralnik, J. M., & Mishra, G. D. (2010). Self-reported sleep difficulty during the menopausal transition: Results from a prospective cohort study. *Menopause, 17*(6), 1128–1135.

Touzet, S., Rabilloud, M., Boehringer, H., Barranco, E., & Ecochard, R. (2002). Relationship between sleep and secretion of gonadotropin and ovarian hormones in women with normal cycles. *Fertility and Sterility, 77*(4), 738–744.

Travis, R. C., Balkwill, A., Fensom, G. K., Appleby, P. N., Reeves, G. K., Wang, X. S., Roddam, A. W., Gathani, T., Peto, R., Green, J., Key, T. J., & Beral, V. (2016). Night shift work and breast cancer incidence: Three prospective studies and meta-analysis of published studies. *Journal of the National Cancer Institute, 108*(12), Article djw169.

Tsai, S. Y., Barnard, K. E., Lentz, M. J., & Thomas, K. A. (2011). Mother–infant activity synchrony as a correlate of the emergence of circadian rhythm. *Biological Research for Nursing, 13*(1), 80–88.

Tsai, S. Y., Lee, P. L., Lin, J. W., & Lee, C. N. (2017). Persistent and new-onset daytime sleepiness in pregnant women: A prospective observational cohort study. *International Journal of Nursing Studies, 66*, 1–6.

Tsai, S. Y., Lin, J. W., Kuo, L. T., & Thomas, K. A. (2012). Daily sleep and fatigue characteristics in nulliparous women during the third trimester of pregnancy. *Sleep, 35*(2), 257–262.

Van, P., Cage, T., & Shannon, M. (2004). Big dreams, little sleep: Dreams during pregnancy after prior pregnancy loss. *Holistic Nursing Practice, 18*(6), 284–292.

van der Meijden, W. P., Van Someren, J. L., Te Lindert, B. H., Bruijel, J., van Oosterhout, F., Coppens, J. E., Kalsbeek, A., Cajochen, C., Bourgin, P., & Van Someren, E. J. (2016). Individual differences in sleep timing relate to melanopsin-based phototransduction in healthy adolescents and young adults. *Sleep, 39*(6), 1305–1310.

Van Reen, E., & Kiesner, J. (2016). Individual differences in self-reported difficulty sleeping across the menstrual cycle. *Archives of Women's Mental Health, 19*(4), 599–608.

Vgontzas, A. N., Legro, R. S., Bixler, E. O., Grayev, A., Kales, A., & Chrousos, G. P. (2001). Polycystic ovary syndrome is associated with obstructive sleep apnea and daytime sleepiness: Role of insulin resistance. *Journal of Clinical Endocrinology & Metabolism, 86*(2), 517–520.

Volkovich, E., Ben-Zion, H., Karny, D., Meiri, G., & Tikotzky, L. (2015). Sleep patterns of co-sleeping and solitary sleeping infants and mothers: A longitudinal study. *Sleep Medicine, 16*(11), 1305–1312.

Waldhauser, F., Boepple, P. A., Schemper, M., Mansfield, M. J., & Crowley, W. F., Jr. (1991). Serum melatonin in central precocious puberty is lower than in age-matched prepubertal children. *Journal of Clinical Endocrinology & Metabolism, 73*(4), 793–796.

Walters, J. F., Hampton, S. M., Ferns, G. A., & Skene, D. J. (2005). Effect of menopause on melatonin and alertness rhythms investigated in constant routine conditions. *Chronobiology International, 22*(5), 859–872.

Warland, J., Dorrian, J., Morrison, J., & O'Brien, L. (2018). Maternal sleep during pregnancy and poor fetal outcomes: A scoping review of the literature with meta-analysis. *Sleep Medicine Reviews, 41*, 197–219.

Wegrzyn, L. R., Tamimi, R. M., Rosner, B. A., Brown, S. B., Stevens, R. G., Eliassen, A. H., Laden, F., Willett, W. C., Hankinson, S. E., & Schernhammer, E. S. (2017). Rotating night-shift work and the risk of breast cancer in the nurses' health studies. *American Journal of Epidemiology, 186*(5), 532–540.

Wesstrom, J., Skalkidou, A., Manconi, M., Fulda, S., & Sundstrom-Poromaa, I. (2014). Pre-pregnancy restless legs syndrome (Willis-Ekbom disease) is associated with perinatal depression. *Journal of Clinical Sleep Medicine, 10*(5), 527–533.

Wilson, D. L., Barnes, M., Ellett, L., Permezel, M., Jackson, M., & Crowe, S. F. (2011). Decreased sleep efficiency, increased wake after sleep onset and increased cortical arousals in late pregnancy. *Australian & New Zealand Journal of Obstetrics & Gynaecology, 51*(1), 38–46.

Wilson, D. L., Walker, S. P., Fung, A. M., O'Donoghue, F. J., Barnes, M., & Howard, M. E. (2018). Periodic limb movements in sleep during pregnancy: A common but benign disorder? *Sleep and Biological Rhythms, 16*(1), 11–20.

Woo, M. M., Tai, C. J., Kang, S. K., Nathwani, P. S., Pang, S. F., & Leung, P. C. (2001). Direct action of melatonin in human granulosa-luteal cells. *Journal of Clinical Endocrinology & Metabolism, 86*(10), 4789–4797.

Woods, N. F., & Mitchell, E. S. (2010). Sleep symptoms during the menopausal transition and early postmenopause: Observations from the Seattle Midlife Women's Health Study. *Sleep, 33*(4), 539–549.

Xie, Y., Liu, S., Chen, X. J., Yu, H. H., Yang, Y., & Wang, W. (2021). Effects of exercise on sleep quality and insomnia in adults: A systematic review and meta-analysis of randomized controlled trials. *Frontiers in Psychiatry, 12*, Article 664499.

Xu, Q., & Lang, C. P. (2014). Examining the relationship between subjective sleep disturbance and menopause: A systematic review and meta-analysis. *Menopause, 21*(12), 1301–1318.

Xu, X., Liu, D., Zhang, Z., Sharma, M., & Zhao, Y. (2017). Sleep duration and quality in pregnant women: A cross-sectional survey in China. *International Journal of Environmental Research and Public Health, 14*(7), Article 817.

Young, T., Rabago, D., Zgierska, A., Austin, D., & Laurel, F. (2003). Objective and subjective sleep quality in premenopausal, perimenopausal, and postmenopausal women in the Wisconsin Sleep Cohort Study. *Sleep, 26*(6), 667–672.

Zafarghandi, N., Hadavand, S., Davati, A., Mohseni, S. M., Kimiaiimoghadam, F., & Torkestani, F. (2012). The effects of sleep quality and duration in late pregnancy on labor and fetal outcome. *Journal of Maternal–Fetal & Neonatal Medicine, 25*(5), 535–537.

Zhang, X., Zhang, R., Cheng, L., Wang, Y., Ding, X., Fu, J., Dang, J., Moore, J., & Li, R. (2020). The effect of sleep impairment on gestational diabetes mellitus: A systematic review and meta-analysis of cohort studies. *Sleep Medicine, 74*, 267–277.

Zheng, H., Harlow, S. D., Kravitz, H. M., Bromberger, J., Buysse, D. J., Matthews, K. A., Gold, E. B., Owens, J. F., & Hall, M. (2015). Actigraphy-defined measures of sleep and movement across the menstrual cycle in midlife menstruating women: Study of Women's Health Across the Nation Sleep Study. *Menopause, 22*(1), 66–74.

Zheng, M., Tong, J., Li, W. P., Chen, Z. J., & Zhang, C. (2018). Melatonin concentration in follicular fluid is correlated with antral follicle count (AFC) and in vitro fertilization (IVF) outcomes in women undergoing assisted reproductive technology (ART) procedures. *Gynecological Endocrinology, 34*(5), 446–450.

CHAPTER

42 Sleep and Medical Disorders

Leanne Fleming, Megan Crawford, Bethany Martin, Mhairi Patience, *and* Samantha Fisher-Hicks

Abstract

Medical disorders are commonly associated with a high prevalence of sleep difficulties, which compound medical symptoms and can hinder treatment response. Sleep disturbance commonly follows diagnosis with a medical disorder, but in some cases, a sleep disorder may be a precursor to diagnosis with a medical disorder. Research of the complex and bidirectional relationship between sleep and illness can advance understanding of both medical and sleep disorders and advance the concept of patient-centered care for individuals with complex medical conditions. In this chapter, five common medical disorders that illustrate a diversity of relationships with sleep are outlined: cancer, obstructive sleep apnea, migraine, Type I diabetes, and traumatic brain injury. The chapter examines the prevalence, development, consequences, and treatment of sleep disturbance across these five conditions.

Key Words: medical disorder, sleep disorder, cancer, obstructive sleep apnea, migraine, Type I diabetes, traumatic brain injury, insomnia, comorbid

Introduction

Sleep health is increasingly recognized as fundamental to optimal mental and physical well-being, and studies have consistently reported a relationship between poor sleep and poor health (Chaput et al., 2020; Gadie et al., 2017; Sivertsen et al., 2021). Dimensions such as inappropriate sleep timing, poor sleep efficiency, insufficient sleep duration, poor sleep quality, and daytime sleepiness have all been associated with specific health outcomes such as diabetes, coronary heart disease, metabolic syndrome, and depression. Most is known about sleep continuity disturbance (e.g., insomnia), which has been identified as a precursor to and risk factor for mental illness and is strongly associated with the development of a range of physical health conditions.

Understanding and measuring key dimensions of sleep health and identifying and treating sleep disorders are important because of the associated risks, morbidities, and functional impairments. However, despite growing awareness of the importance of sleep as a central aspect of health, most is known about the relationship between insomnia and mental health, specifically anxiety and depression. Much less is known about the relationship between sleep (including sleep health and other sleep disorders) and physical health. This is the case despite the fact that sleep disturbance is a commonly reported problem across a range of somatic conditions (Ionescu et al., 2021).

Poor sleep is prevalent among patients with cancer (Strollo et al., 2020), obstructive sleep apnea (OSA; Sweetman, Melaku, et al., 2021), Type 1 diabetes (T1D; Ji et al., 2021), migraine (Tiseo et al., 2020), and traumatic brain injury (TBI; Mantua et al., 2018). The aim of this chapter is to explore interrelationships and proposed mechanisms between sleep health, sleep disturbance, and these five commonly reported medical disorders.

Sleep and Cancer

Cancer is not a single entity but a term for a multitude of diverse diseases in which abnormal cells divide without control and can invade nearby tissues. According to the World Health Organization, cancer is among the leading causes of death globally. In 2018, there were 18.1 million new cancer cases and 9.5 million cancer-related deaths worldwide. Lung cancer is the most common cancer worldwide in terms of incidence and mortality; breast cancer is the most common in women and is the leading cause of cancer death in women worldwide; colorectal cancer is the third most common cancer in both sexes worldwide; prostate cancer is the second most common in men worldwide. By 2040, the number of new cancer cases per year is expected to rise to 29.5 million and the number of cancer-related deaths to 16.4 million (International Agency for Research on Cancer, 2018).

Despite the anticipated global increase in cancer rates, recent developments in detection and treatment mean that cancer survival has doubled since the early 1980s (Hawkes, 2019). Such progress has resulted in an increasing number of cancer survivors living with persistent cancer-related side effects (e.g., sleep disturbance), with numbers expected to increase with an aging population (Zhou et al., 2020). However, cancer-related side effects are often poorly defined, inappropriately measured, and prone to bias (due to being assessed during active cancer treatment; Fleming et al., 2022), resulting in an absence of clear side effect–management protocols within oncology. This is especially true of sleep disturbance in cancer, which is reported as a common, persistent, and debilitating problem across various cancer groups yet is rarely addressed within cancer care (Mogavero et al., 2021).

The prevalence and nature of sleep disturbance vary by cancer type, which is unsurprising given its diversity. Lung cancer patients seem to experience a higher level of sleep disturbance compared to other cancer patients (Papadopoulos et al., 2018), particularly insomnia and OSA (Mogavero et al., 2021). Breast cancer and prostate cancer patients report a high prevalence of insomnia and circadian rhythm disorders, both before and after chemotherapy (Fleming et al., 2019; Leysen et al., 2019; Maguire et al., 2019), while OSA and insomnia are prevalent in patients with colorectal cancer (Lin et al., 2019).

Despite a growing interest in the field, less is known about sleep in patients with other cancer types (Mogavero et al., 2021). Across all cancer types, insomnia is the most commonly reported sleep disorder (López et al., 2016; Mogavero et al., 2021).

Prevalence and Etiology of Insomnia in Cancer

Insomnia is defined as difficulty falling or staying asleep or waking up earlier than intended, resulting in impairment to daytime functioning (American Psychiatric Association, 2013). It is recognized as a disabling, non-remitting condition and a causal factor in the evolution and maintenance of physical and mental ill-health, particularly depression and cardiometabolic disease (Vgontzas et al., 2013). People with cancer are disproportionately affected by insomnia relative to the general population. However, despite increasing awareness of the pervasiveness of insomnia within cancer groups, scientific reports of insomnia prevalence remain variable and wide-ranging. This is partly due to studies utilizing different insomnia definitions, measurements, and timing of assessments (Garland et al., 2014). Reported insomnia prevalence varies from 30% to 75% in newly diagnosed or recently treated cancer patients, with 18%–29% reporting sleep disturbance that meets diagnostic criteria for insomnia disorder (Ancoli-Israel, 2015; Harrold et al., 2020).

Insomnia prevalence also seems to vary by tumor type. The largest longitudinal studies (to date) of patients with heterogeneous cancer sites reported significant differences in insomnia prevalence across cancer groups (Palesh et al., 2010; Savard et al., 2011). The highest prevalence of insomnia was recorded in patients with breast cancer (Savard et al., 2011), gynecologic cancer (Savard et al., 2011), and lung cancer (Palesh et al., 2010). Patients with prostate cancer had the lowest prevalence of insomnia (Savard et al., 2011), and patients with breast cancer had the highest number of overall insomnia complaints (Palesh et al., 2010). Both studies controlled for sex in their analyses.

The development of persistent insomnia is complex and multifaceted, particularly in relation to cancer (Fleming et al., 2019; Schieber et al., 2019). Spielman's 3P model outlines the development and maintenance of insomnia and posits that predisposing (e.g., hyperreactivity), precipitating (e.g., diagnosis with serious illness), and perpetuating (e.g., time in bed extension) factors all contribute to the onset and persistence of insomnia (Spielman et al., 1987). An observational study by Fleming et al. (2019) explored the naturally occurring trajectory of insomnia in a sample of newly diagnosed breast cancer patients over a 12-month period. Prior to diagnosis, the point prevalence of insomnia (including clinical and subclinical complaints) was 25%, increasing to 46% at diagnosis and remaining stable thereafter at around 50%. In addition, most patients who met criteria for insomnia disorder retained that status throughout the 12-month study period. This data suggests that cancer diagnosis acts as a precipitating factor for persistent insomnia in cancer patients, which does not naturally remit over time without active intervention.

Cancer-Specific Risk Factors for Persistent Insomnia

In recent years, a bidirectional relationship between insomnia and cancer has been suggested. While research exploring cancer-induced insomnia is relatively well established, an increasing number of studies have attempted to evaluate whether insomnia increases cancer risk, with conflicting results. A recent review of these studies highlighted eight (those utilizing diagnostic criteria for insomnia) that demonstrated a 24% increased risk of cancer in individuals with an insomnia duration ≥10 years (Shi et al., 2020). This review suggests that long-term insomnia may be an early signal for cancer onset, emphasizing the importance of effective insomnia assessment and management. A full review of this literature is beyond the scope of this chapter, which will focus on cancer-specific risk factors for insomnia.

Disease-specific factors (e.g., direct effects of chemotherapy) and sleep-specific factors (e.g., daytime napping, time in bed extension) are known to contribute to the perpetuation of insomnia in cancer patients (Palesh, Scheiber, Kesler, Mustian, et al., 2018). Chemotherapy seems to pose a specific risk, with patients undergoing this treatment reporting more severe levels of insomnia than patients receiving other treatments such as surgery, radiation, or hormonal therapy (Palesh, Scheiber, Kesler, Mustian, et al., 2018). Fleming et al. (2019) reported that patients who received chemotherapy as part of their breast cancer treatment regimen were much more likely to develop persistent insomnia following the completion of active cancer treatment than those who did not receive chemotherapy.

Studies have attempted to explore the mechanisms by which chemotherapy exacerbates sleep disturbance, the most convincing of which relate to the impact of treatment side effects (Palesh, Scheiber, Kesler, Janelsins, et al., 2018). Chemotherapy-induced menopausal symptoms, such as nocturnal hot flashes and musculoskeletal pain, are known to impact sleep continuity and increase nighttime awakenings (Baker et al., 2018). Anticipatory anxiety and depression prior to chemotherapy onset have been identified as risk factors for later insomnia in prostate cancer survivors (Maguire et al., 2019). Cancer-related fatigue (CRF) is commonly reported by patients undergoing chemotherapy treatment, but unlike fatigue typically experienced by individuals without cancer, it is more severe, disabling, and challenging to relieve (Berger et al., 2015). For patients with CRF, non-restorative sleep is the most commonly reported symptom (Vethe et al., 2018), and daytime fatigue is known to predict nighttime sleep disruption (Ji et al., 2019).

In an attempt to compensate for nighttime sleep disruption during cancer treatment, patients often adopt strategies such as daytime napping or extending time in bed, leading to altered rest–activity rhythms (Van Dyk et al., 2021). While these strategies may occasionally yield more sleep, they often result in increased sleep fragmentation, wakefulness, and night-to-night variability in sleep timing, known to perpetuate persistent insomnia (Maurer et al., 2021). Exploring this association between rest–activity rhythms and persistent insomnia, Roh et al. (2022) reported that those with poorer rest–activity rhythms (low inter-day stability and high intra-daily variability) exhibited higher insomnia severity compared to those with better rest–activity rhythms (high inter-day stability and low intra-daily variability). Therefore, despite the disruption to sleep that commonly occurs during cancer treatment, maintenance of stable rest–activity rhythms during the active cancer treatment phase seems to be important for minimizing the development of insomnia disorder.

Treatment Approaches

Despite its pervasiveness in cancer patients, poor sleep remains a treatable yet neglected aspect of cancer care. This is due partly to a lack of understanding of the importance of good sleep health and poor access to effective treatments, such as cognitive behavioral therapy for insomnia (CBT-I; Reynolds-Cowie & Fleming, 2021). These factors contribute to patient underreporting of insomnia in oncology settings, leaving the majority to rely exclusively on pharmacological options and/or sleep hygiene education, neither of which are recommended for persistent insomnia (Zhou et al., 2020). Hypnotic drugs are commonly prescribed to cancer patients with insomnia, despite the fact that they have well-defined side effects, cause next-day functional impairment, and fail to increase sleep quantity (Kripke, 2018). In contrast, CBT-I is the recommended treatment for insomnia in the general population and in people with cancer (Johnson et al., 2016), demonstrating durable benefits for sleep and comorbid conditions in cancer patients (Fleming et al., 2014; Savard et al., 2021; Squires et al., 2022) and being safer than medication (Brasure et al., 2015).

CBT-I is a multicomponent intervention that targets the specific cognitive, physiological, and behavioral characteristics of persistent insomnia. Multicomponent CBT-I combines cognitive therapy with education about sleep regulation, stimulus control instructions, and sleep restriction therapy and often includes sleep hygiene education and relaxation training (Edinger et al., 2021). Traditionally, CBT-I is delivered in person by specialist behavioral sleep medicine therapists over four to eight sessions. However, trained therapists are limited in number, resulting in very long wait times or treatment inaccessibility for most patients. These barriers have led to the uptake of digital CBT-I as a translation pathway that offers a scalable solution, with promising results across a range of different populations. CBT-I can be delivered effectively to cancer patients as a self-help tool via the internet (Zachariae et al., 2018; Zhou et al., 2020), videos (Savard et al., 2021), and telemedicine (McCarthy et al., 2018). Crucially, treatment modality (in person vs. digital self-help) does not significantly impact CBT-I efficacy (Squires et al., 2022).

Despite the promise of scalable insomnia interventions in cancer populations, the majority of patients and clinicians remain unaware of their availability. Increasing awareness of the importance of sleep health within oncology services, and helping clinicians connect patients to evidence-based treatments, is a priority for supportive cancer care. In addition, a more sleep-focused approach is required within cancer care to identify those at high risk of insomnia, and further research is required to explore the implementation of CBT-I for acute, situational insomnia (e.g., upon diagnosis or during active cancer treatment). This is an important next step as offering insomnia prehabilitation may provide an opportunity to prevent, as well as treat, insomnia in cancer patients.

Insomnia and OSA

OSA is a condition that is characterized by a repeated reduction (hypopnea) or cessation (apnea) in airflow during sleep that is caused by an obstruction of the upper airway. Disease severity is dictated by the frequency of these obstructive events per hour of sleep. According to the *International Classification of Sleep Disorders*, third edition (ICSD-3; American Academy of Sleep Medicine, 2014), mild obstructive events on a polysomnogram (PSG) alone, without other presenting symptoms, is not sufficient for a diagnosis of OSA. Diagnosis is reserved for mild disease severity (apnea/hypopnea index [AHI] of 5–14) when other symptoms are also present.[1] While the cardinal symptoms are snoring, witnessed breathing interruptions during sleep, and sleepiness, one of the other symptoms listed is insomnia and, if present along with mild OSA, would suffice for a diagnosis of OSA. Thus, in compliance with the ICSD, it should be necessary to screen for insomnia in every potential OSA patient. This statement is reinforced by the high prevalence rates of comorbid insomnia and sleep apnea (COMISA). Depending on the diagnostic criteria used, approximately 40% of OSA patients experience insomnia symptoms (Zhang et al., 2019). Furthermore, COMISA has been linked to increased daytime impairment (Sweetman et al., 2017), cognitive impairment (Agudelo et al., 2022), and most recently increased risk of all-cause mortality (Lechat et al., 2022; Sweetman et al., 2022). Considering the significant overlap and impact, it is paramount to understand the pathophysiological mechanism in order to identify effective treatment targets.

OSA as a Risk Factor for Insomnia

Apneic events in OSA are often followed by cortical arousals. These arousals can lead to prolonged periods of wakefulness that can eventually lead to conditioned arousal, paving the way for chronic insomnia to develop (Robertson et al., 2007). Prevalence studies have demonstrated that difficulty maintaining sleep is the most prevalent insomnia symptom in COMISA patients (Bjornsdottir et al., 2013; Lundetrae et al., 2021). Repeated sleep fragmentation can lead to daytime sleepiness, which may result in increased napping during the day (Ye et al., 2014). This in turn may reduce the homeostatic drive for sleep, exacerbating the development of insomnia over time. Additionally, the frequent brief awakenings during the night can be misperceived as longer periods of wakefulness, a phenomenon associated with insomnia (Hermans et al., 2019).

Apneic events are typically more prevalent and more severe during rapid-eye-movement (REM) sleep (Findley et al., 1985) as a result of the muscle atonia during REM sleep. Thus, these frequent brief awakenings are particularly pronounced during REM sleep. REM sleep instability has been linked to disrupted processing of emotional events predating the sleep period (Riemann et al., 2012; M. P. Walker & van der Helm, 2009). If this is typical in OSA patients, there is a possibility that the emotional event of not being able to sleep is not processed appropriately (Wassing et al., 2019) and can bleed into the attribution of poor daytime performance to disrupted sleep at night. Many of these proposed mechanisms underlying the development of COMISA remain untested.

Some untreated OSA patients are fortunate enough not to develop insomnia. However, they may eventually struggle with their sleep once they start positive airway pressure (PAP), the treatment of choice for OSA. PAP, while effective at preventing the apneic events by creating a pneumatic split for the airway, can be intrusive (Berg et al., 2022; Luyster et al., 2016) and lead to side effects (Rotty et al., 2021), which may reduce the opportunity for a restful period of sleep onset. Insomnia then creates a barrier to optimal PAP adherence, with patients often using their machine less often than those without insomnia (El-Solh et al., 2021; Philip et al., 2018; Wallace et al., 2018) or giving up entirely (Eysteinsdottir et al., 2017). This leaves the OSA practically untreated (Kribbs et al., 1993), and a vicious pattern emerges. PAP can, however, reduce some of the insomnia symptoms, and there are now numerous prospective studies that have demonstrated moderate global improvement (Bjornsdottir et al., 2013; Bjorvatn et al., 2018; Krakow et al., 2019; Ong et al., 2020; Sweetman et al., 2019); and these improvements seem particularly pronounced for sleep maintenance insomnia (Bjornsdottir et al., 2013), especially following optimal PAP adherence.

Insomnia as a Risk Factor for OSA

While this global improvement in insomnia severity following OSA treatment has been reported, it is also important to acknowledge the symptom overlap between the disorders (Sweetman, Lack, et al., 2021), and improvements in symptoms associated with OSA would be captured in insomnia outcome measures such as the Insomnia Severity Index (Bastien et al., 2001). Other studies have demonstrated that insomnia does not completely resolve with PAP therapy, particularly onset insomnia (Bjornsdottir et al., 2013; Krakow et al., 2001), which indicates that comorbid insomnia is an independent condition with a unique pathophysiology and requires management, as opposed to simply a symptom of "underlying" OSA that would resolve with effective treatment of OSA. Supporting this statement are the possible pathways through which insomnia leads to or exacerbates the development of OSA. Sleep deprivation and sleep fragmentation associated with insomnia can reduce the airway patency (White, 2005) and thus increase the likelihood of airway collapse. Furthermore, sleep fragmentation and chronic deprivation and the concurrent daytime dysfunction associated with insomnia may lead to certain lifestyle changes such as a reduction in exercise, increased consumption of unhealthy foods, and sedentary behaviors, all of which can increase the risk of obesity, which has been linked to the development of OSA (Jehan et al., 2017). Lastly, the arousal profile characteristic for insomnia patients is consistent with a reduced arousal threshold. Such a reduced threshold can trigger apneic breathing events. During normal respiration at sleep onset, there is an increased risk of airway collapse as the pharyngeal muscles relax, and subsequent contraction of these muscles maintains airway patency if there is increased respiratory drive. A low arousal threshold (premature cortical arousal as a result of this change in respiration) will disrupt this process, meaning the pharyngeal muscles do not dilate and normal respiration does not immediately resume, leading to abnormal breathing patterns (apneas, hypopneas, and other respiratory events; Sands et al., 2018). Interestingly, providing CBT-I to untreated OSA patients has been associated with a reduced AHI, potentially as a result of increasing the arousal threshold (Sweetman et al., 2020). While CBT-I would not be recommended as a stand-alone treatment for COMISA, it has been evaluated in untreated OSA patients prior to PAP (Ong et al., 2020; Sweetman et al., 2019). This approach does not seem to be associated with increased adverse events and may be an effective treatment approach considering long waiting lists for PAP treatment in many countries.

A Bidirectional Relationship That Dictates a Combined Treatment Approach

While the above offers a snapshot of one-directional relationships and other authors have offered a more extensive overview of individual mechanisms (Meira et al., 2021; Sweetman, Lack, et al., 2021), it is clear that a bidirectional relationship exists, in which each condition exacerbates the other (Sweetman, Lack, et al., 2021). It may also be that a common pathway exists, mediated by the hypothalamic–pituitary–adrenal axis (HPA axis), where OSA and insomnia are both a consequence and a cause of alterations in HPA-axis activity, as outlined more extensively by Beneto and colleagues (2009). This dynamic relationship between OSA and insomnia, and the limitations of isolated therapeutic approaches, has led researchers to consider and evaluate combined treatment approaches.

To date there are only four clinical trials that have evaluated combined treatment of CBT-I and PAP (Alessi et al., 2021; Bjorvatn et al., 2018; Ong et al., 2020; Sweetman et al., 2019) using a randomized clinical trial design. Each trial contrasted some form of combined treatment with treatment as usual (PAP). CBT-I treatment was either in a self-help book (Bjorvatn et al., 2018) or face-to-face (Alessi et al., 2021; Ong et al., 2020; Sweetman et al., 2019) format, combined with a PAP adherence intervention (Alessi et al., 2021), and delivered either concurrently (Alessi et al., 2021; Bjorvatn et al., 2018; Ong et al., 2020) or prior to the start of PAP treatment (Ong et al., 2020; Sweetman et al., 2019). Two trials demonstrated that delivering CBT-I to untreated OSA patients and prior to PAP was an effective approach and resulted in large improvements in insomnia severity (Ong et al., 2020; Sweetman et al., 2019).A combined treatment approach led to significantly greater improvements in insomnia compared to PAP alone (Ong et al., 2020; Sweetman et al., 2019). Superior PAP adherence in the combined groups was also noted in some (Alessi et al., 2021; Sweetman et al., 2019) but not others (Bjorvatn et al., 2018; Ong et al., 2020). These results are encouraging for providers who are keen to implement CBT-I in COMISA patients (it is safe and effective); however, the impact on PAP adherence and the optimal treatment sequence are still unclear (Ong et al., 2020). A criticism of all of these approaches to treatment is the diagnostic approach to the care pathway, which dictates a specific pathway based on the diagnosis (i.e., COMISA). A more patient-centered approach would be to treat the presenting symptoms/symptom profile (Crawford et al., 2017; Keenan et al., 2018; Ye et al., 2014) and adapt treatment based on improvements. Such trials evaluating adaptive treatment strategies are currently ongoing (e.g., study by Edinger and Manber as registered on RePORTER, 2022) and will hopefully pave the way for more patient-tailored care for COMISA patients.

Sleep and Migraine

Migraine, characterized by severe head pain, is a headache condition ranked as the second leading medical condition for loss of labor globally (Stovner et al., 2018). In addition to head pain, migraines show varying neurological, gastrointestinal, and autonomic symptoms (Silberstein et al., 2018). Migraines, in contrast to tension-type headaches, are often accompanied by additional symptoms of nausea, vomiting, and sensitivity to movement, light, and sound. Chronic migraine, as defined by the International Classification of Headache Disorders, is persistent headaches for 15 or more days per month with eight of those meeting criteria for migraine (Headache Classification Committee of the International Headache Society, 2018). Migraine and tension-type headaches can be triggered by a wide variety of environmental (e.g., flickering lights, weather), psychological (e.g., emotional stressors), and physiological (e.g., hormones, fatigue) variables (Park et al., 2016; Peroutka, 2014). Pellegrino et al. (2018) determined that sleep was the second most frequently identified trigger across 85 studies in a meta-analysis. Further, insomnia has been linked to higher frequencies of headache attacks, providing a basis for the notion that sleep difficulties contribute to headaches (Bertisch et al., 2020; Fernández-de-Las-Peñas et al., 2018; Vgontzas et al., 2021).

It is widely recognized that there is an association between migraine and sleep (Petit et al., 2021; Vgontzas & Pavlović, 2018). For example, insomnia is reported as the most common sleep disorder in headache patients (Fernández-de-Las-Peñas et al., 2018; Rains, 2018; Uhlig et al., 2014). Further, migraine sufferers report poor sleep before and during migraine attacks, and around two-thirds of individuals with migraines experience headaches that awaken them (Engstrøm et al., 2014). The prevalence of insomnia increases in line with headache frequency; namely, individuals with chronic migraine experience more severe insomnia than those with episodic migraine (Buse et al., 2019). While the research strongly suggests an association between insomnia and headaches, the nuances of this complex relationship are poorly understood. As insomnia can be considered both a cause and an effect of headache attacks, further investigation into this interaction is required.

Biobehavioral Model of Chronic Headaches and Insomnia

Ong and Park (2012) proposed a biobehavioral model to explain the relationship between insomnia and migraines and the underlying mechanisms impacting this interaction. Based on the existing research evidence base, this theoretical model aims to describe the behaviors associated with migraine coping mechanisms, the effect of these behaviors on insomnia, and the increased predisposition for ongoing migraine attacks. The first tenet of the model posits that headache coping behaviors can cause and maintain insomnia. For example, individuals with migraine commonly utilize daytime naps or resting in a darkened room as a strategy to stop or cope with headache pain (Ong et al., 2023; Vgontzas & Pavlović, 2018). This coping mechanism of "sleeping it off" has been shown to have ongoing effects on sleep physiology (Rains, 2018). Specifically, Ong et al. (2023) report that in a sample of chronic migraine patients, increased headache severity was related to longer nap duration. Additionally, longer nap duration was significantly associated with decreased sleep efficiency, measured subjectively with diaries and objectively with actigraphy. As longer naps during the day have been shown to impact sleep pressure and lead to decreased sleep efficiency overnight, daytime napping behaviors in migraine patients may be instrumental in the development of insomnia. Combined with the tendency to utilize caffeine and sleep medication to support their ability to function, migraine sufferers can struggle with variable sleep patterns and inconsistent wake times (Ong et al., 2018, 2023). It could therefore be argued that continued use of these maladaptive coping behaviors may lead individuals into chronic insomnia (Ong & Park, 2012).

Secondly, Ong and Park (2012) argue that insomnia increases the likelihood of headache and migraine attacks. The research evidence base highlights that even slight sleep deprivation heightens the experience of pain and reduces pain-inhibitory functioning (Krause et al., 2019; Staffe et al., 2019). Individuals may then experience more severe headaches and migraine attacks due to increased sensitivity and a reduced pain threshold. Further, circadian system disruptions, and the resulting changes in melatonin levels, caused by insomnia may also affect the propensity for headaches. Melatonin, a hormone that regulates sleep–wake cycles, has been found to induce analgesic effects (Danilov & Kurganova, 2016), which may further lead to increased severity of migraine attacks. Research has identified that disruptions to sleep lead to an increased likelihood of future migraine attacks (Bertisch et al., 2020; Park et al., 2016; Sullivan & Martin, 2017). In particular, Vgontzas et al. (2021) found that in a sample of patients with episodic migraine, poor sleep was related to increased headache attacks over a 6-week period. Further, Houle and colleagues (2012) highlight that even 2 days of consecutive poor sleep increases headache risk. This evidence supports the tenet proposed by the biobehavioral model that disruptions to sleep increase the propensity for headaches.

Lastly, the third principle proposed by the biobehavioral model outlines that insomnia and the interaction of these mechanisms may lead to the chronification of migraines (Ong & Park, 2012). As migraine sufferers then further engage with these maladaptive coping mechanisms, a vicious cycle between chronic insomnia and migraine attacks can be created. The cycle of poor sleep and headaches may transform or perpetuate episodic headaches into chronic headache attacks. The two conditions of migraine and insomnia become entangled and may lead to the further perpetuation of both. Preliminary evidence suggests that insomnia plays a role in the chronification of migraine (Bigal & Lipton, 2011; Torres-Ferrús et al., 2020); however, further longitudinal studies to confirm this notion are required. While prospective research has indicated that insomnia can trigger and predict the onset of headaches by years (Harnod et al., 2015; Rains, 2018; Sivertsen et al., 2014), other research studies have also found migraine to precede insomnia (Lateef et al., 2011; Odegard et al., 2013). Therefore, further research is needed to continue exploring how insomnia and headaches interact and closely identify the preceding and perpetuating factors to inform clinical practice.

Treatment Approaches

Sleep is of particular interest as it can be considered a modifiable factor and offers an opportunity to intervene in the perpetuating cycle between chronic headaches and insomnia (Rains, 2018). Practitioners are recognizing that pain relief medication may not be the most effective approach as it does not target the underlying mechanisms of the identified bidirectional relationship and has limited efficacy at improving sleep quality and duration in migraine patients (Fernández-de-Las-Peñas et al., 2018). Moreover, sleep medications are not considered first-line treatment for insomnia (Ree et al., 2017), and individuals with chronic migraine typically have numerous acute or preventative medications prescribed and may be reluctant to consider an additional pharmacological option for sleep management. Contemporary research findings highlight that psychological treatments targeting better coping strategies and the mental and emotional burden of migraines are better placed. In particular, CBT-I has been shown to reduce the frequency and severity of headache (Calhoun & Ford, 2007; Crawford et al., 2020; Law et al., 2018; Smitherman et al., 2016). The results outline that approximately one-third of participants who completed the treatment reverted from chronic migraine to episodic (Calhoun & Ford, 2007; Crawford et al., 2020). Moreover, significant improvements in sleep efficiency as a result of the sleep intervention are concluded (Crawford et al., 2020; Smitherman et al., 2016). However, behavioral sleep treatments utilized in migraine patients represent a new approach, and the current limited studies suggest that the impact of CBT-I on headache, while statistically significant, is a small effect. For example, in a pilot study testing digital CBT-I, a 22% reduction in headache impairment was found (Crawford et al., 2020).

A hybrid cognitive behavioral intervention program targeting both insomnia and headache management has also been tested within an adolescent population (Law et al., 2018). The single-arm trial identified a significant reduction in headache frequency and improvements across all sleep measures (sleep quality, sleep hygiene, sleep latency, sleep efficiency, and insomnia symptoms) that were maintained at a 3-month follow-up

(Law et al., 2018). Specifically, the results highlight that the majority of participants achieved a 50% reduction or more in headache frequency and that pain-related disability due to migraine was significantly improved. This study on co-occurring insomnia and migraine in adolescents suggests that hybrid CBT is an effective avenue for treatment. The bidirectional relationship, as outlined by the biobehavioral model, supports the conclusion that addressing both migraine and insomnia simultaneously may be the most effective approach. While psychological sleep interventions show notable headache frequency and sleep improvements, the research provides contrasting results on headache intensity (Sullivan et al., 2019). Calhoun and Ford (2007) identified a significant reduction in headache intensity following CBT-I; however, Law et al. (2018) employing hybrid CBT did not achieve significant declines. A further study found that both the intervention and control groups experienced significant improvements on headache intensity (Smitherman et al., 2016). Overall, behavioral sleep treatments have been demonstrated to lead to significant changes in headache frequency, and the research so far shows promise for addressing both migraine attacks and insomnia with one non-invasive treatment.

Sleep and T1D in Adolescence

Diabetes mellitus, simply referred to as *diabetes*, describes a group of metabolic disorders (e.g., T1D, Type 2 diabetes [T2D]) in which there is a deficiency in the secretion and/or action of the hormone insulin. This results in chronic high blood glucose levels (hyperglycemia), which is the defining characteristic of diabetes (World Health Organization, 2019). Over an extended period, unregulated blood glucose levels can cause damage to vital organs, resulting in life-threatening and inhibiting health complications (e.g., cardiovascular disease, neuropathy, nephropathy, retinopathy, limb amputation). Appropriate management of the condition is required to minimize extreme blood glucose ranges and prevent any potential complications to health (Cole & Florez, 2020). Sleep research within the diabetes field has an increased focus on adults with T2D (Knutson et al., 2011; Ohkuma et al., 2013), which has resulted in an established recommendation to screen for T2D sleep behaviors (pattern and duration) and sleep disorders (particularly sleep apnea, insomnia, and restless legs syndrome; Schipper et al., 2021) as part of a comprehensive clinical care evaluation and assessment of comorbidities (American Diabetes Association, 2017). Sleep in T1D is also very pronounced yet not as researched.

Sleep in Adolescents With T1D

T1D is also referred to as *insulin-dependent diabetes mellitus* as daily insulin is crucial to the survival and management of the condition. T1D is often diagnosed during childhood or early adolescence (International Diabetes Federation, 2021). During this time, sleep curtailments are particularly problematic due to delayed sleep onset caused by bioregulatory (homeostatic sleep and circadian time systems) and psychosocial (bedtime autonomy, academic pressure, screen time, and social networking) pressures and early sleep offset caused by the societal pressure of school start times. The "perfect storm" of late sleep onset and earlier sleep offset results in short and ill-timed sleep for adolescents (Carskadon, 2011; Crowley et al., 2018). The perfect storm is even more problematic when it comes to adolescents with T1D as constant monitoring of blood glucose level, carbohydrate intake, and activity is required throughout the 24-hour period to ensure the correct level of insulin is administered and glycemic control is maintained. The perfect storm sleep curtailments already showcase the number of factors hampering sleep for adolescents without diabetes. Coupling this with the necessary 24-hour management required for T1D results in a hurricane of factors to consider if adolescents with T1D are to obtain a healthy sleep pattern.

Sleep Health

Sleep health has received recent traction within research, clinical, and regulatory environments and was originally defined by Buysse (2014, p. 12) as "a multidimensional pattern of sleep-wakefulness, adapted to individual, social and environmental demands, that promotes physical and mental well-being. Good sleep health is characterized by subjective satisfaction, appropriate timing, adequate duration, high efficiency, and sustained alertness during waking hours." The SATED (satisfaction, alertness, timing, efficiency, and duration) acronym was developed by Buysse to capture sleep health. This was later adapted to include sleep regularity (RU-SATED; Becker et al., 2018; Ravyts et al., 2021) and now, after review of the dimensions in the context of pediatrics, Peds B-SATED (Meltzer et al., 2021). The latter proposes that regularity should instead belong to a sleep-related "behavior" dimension, which is highly relevant for adolescents.

SLEEP DURATION

Sleep in adolescents with T1D has largely been investigated in relation to the duration dimension and refers to the total amount of sleep within the 24-hour day. The interest in duration likely stems from the increased utilization of the dimension as a public health outcome, and although there are currently no sleep duration guidelines developed specifically for adolescents with T1D, current recommendations for the general adolescent population advise 8–10 hours per 24-hour day (13–18 years; Paruthi et al., 2016; Watson et al., 2015). Several studies have highlighted adolescents with T1D not meeting these recommendations, reporting sleep duration ranges of 6.54 to 7.7 hours per day (Frye et al., 2019; Jaser & Ellis, 2016; Patel et al., 2018; Rechenberg et al., 2020; von Schnurbein et al., 2018). When adolescents do meet the sleep duration recommendations, they fall within the lower recommended limit (8 hours; McDonough et al., 2017; M. M. Perfect, 2014). This evidence suggests adolescents with T1D are consistently not achieving the sleep duration recommendations for health, and although this finding is not exclusive to T1D adolescents (Eaton et al., 2010; Gariepy et al., 2020), there is a strong degree of evidence suggesting adolescents with T1D obtain significantly less sleep than peers without T1D (de Lima et al., 2017; Reutrakul et al., 2016; Rose et al., 2021).

There is some contradictory evidence suggesting that T1D adolescents sleep longer than peers (Hazen et al., 2015; Yeshayahu & Mahmud, 2010) and another study reporting no significant differences between groups (Macaulay et al., 2020). The impact of sleep duration on glycated hemoglobin or HbA1c, the gold-standard measure of glycemic control (Nathan et al., 2005), has been investigated. However, the results of these studies yielded mixed findings, with longer sleep durations being associated with a worse HbA1c (Hazen et al., 2015) and improved HbA1c (Macaulay et al., 2020; M. M. Perfect, 2014; Silva et al., 2021) and no association between the variables (McDonough et al., 2017; Reutrakul et al., 2016). It is therefore important to scrutinize sleep further, to investigate other sleep health dimensions and better understand its complex interaction with important diabetes outcomes.

SLEEP TIMING AND REGULARITY

Research into timing and sleep-related behavior dimensions (specifically regularity) has gained traction over recent years within the T1D adolescent population. Timing refers to the placement of sleep within the 24-hour day and dictates obtainment of a sufficient sleep duration, which might explain why interest in this dimension has increased. Adolescents with T1D have a reported later sleep onset of ≥30 minutes compared to controls (Macaulay et al., 2020; Rose et al., 2021), and this later sleep onset has been associated with a worse HbA1c (Frye et al., 2019; Macaulay et al., 2020). The regularity (variability or consistency) definition has been subject to change in recent years and has been described as bedtime and wake time occurring at the same time, within 1 hour, every day. Now, it is considered a sleep behavior (e.g., consistent sleep schedule) and has been examined in the field using a variety of measurements, specifically the standard deviation of average total sleep time (SD TST) and social jetlag.

The social jetlag phenomenon is relevant to the adolescent population and describes an irregularity of sleep patterns in which adolescents compensate on weekend nights for insufficient sleep on weeknights and is also used as a measure of circadian misalignment (Roenneberg et al., 2004; Wittmann et al., 2006). Adolescents with T1D have a reported social jetlag of 0.7–2.5 hours, which has been associated with worse HbA1c (Frye et al., 2019; Silva et al., 2021; von Schnurbein et al., 2018). Studies investigating regularity using the SD TST measure have reported a range of 69–75 minutes (Frye et al., 2019; Patel et al., 2018; Rechenberg et al., 2020). One study conducted by Macaulay et al. (2020) used the daily variation in sleep and wake timing to investigate the difference between adolescents with T1D and controls, finding no difference between the groups. However, they did find that an increase in sleep timing variability resulted in worse HbA1c, which aligns with only one study using SD TST as a regulatory measure (Patel et al., 2018). The majority, however, showed no association with HbA1c (Frye et al., 2019; Rechenberg et al., 2020).

SLEEP QUALITY, EFFICIENCY, AND ALERTNESS

The quality dimension refers to an individual's subjective assessment of their own sleep. Most studies report adolescents with T1D having subjectively poor-quality sleep with no significant associations observed with HbA1c (Hamburger et al., 2020; Jaser & Ellis, 2016; Patel et al., 2018; M. M. Perfect et al., 2012; Rose et al., 2021). It is important to note that there are mixed findings in the literature between sleep quality and efficiency and HbA1c due to the heterogeneity of terms used to describe sleep dimensions as sleep efficiency derived via actigraphy has been used as a measure of sleep quality. However, the efficiency/continuity dimension in relation to sleep health refers to the ratio of time sleeping to time in bed trying to sleep and thus accounts for sleep-onset latency (time between lights-out and falling asleep) and wake after sleep onset (time awake after falling asleep; Meltzer et al., 2021). Studies have reported adolescents with T1D to have good *objective* sleep efficiency (Frye et al., 2019) but poorer *subjective* sleep efficiency (Rose et al., 2021). This finding was true for a variety of sleep patterns, which might suggest that adolescents with T1D perceive their sleep to be worse than that of their peers without diabetes (Bergner et al., 2018), thereby highlighting the necessity for both subjective and objective measures of sleep (Rose et al., 2021). Additionally, when T1D adolescents were compared to peers, there were no significant differences in actigraphy or PSG-measured sleep efficiency, and neither were significantly related to HbA1c (Macaulay et al., 2020).

The alertness/sleepiness dimension refers to the ability to maintain attentive wakefulness and is perhaps the least investigated dimension in adolescents with T1D, with no evidence suggesting excessive sleepiness in this population (Abdelmaksoud et al., 2021; M. M. Perfect et al., 2012; Silva et al., 2021). One study highlighted that adolescents with T1D with a higher HbA1c (≥7.5%) had significantly greater daytime sleepiness than those with a lower Hba1c (<7.5%; Silva et al., 2021).

Navigating the "Perfect Hurricane"

Examining each sleep dimension in relation to HbA1c reveals mixed results, and recently researchers have begun to scrutinize the complex relationship further. It is now broadly accepted that sleep impacts diabetes management activities, ultimately impacting HbA1c (Ji et al., 2021; Monzon et al., 2019). Diabetes management variables (e.g., blood glucose checks) could arguably be grouped into the sleep-related behavior dimension as it is known this activity can either promote or inhibit sleep. It is important to now consider all other specific T1D behaviors that may influence sleep obtainment, for example, necessary screen time behavior induced by diabetes technology (Cobry et al., 2022), physical activity timing and type (Colberg et al., 2016; Kredlow et al., 2015; Potter et al., 2022), diet (Campbell et al., 2015), and sedentary behavior pre-bed (Saunders et al., 2022). Research is beginning to examine all these sleep health dimensions in relation to HbA1c. Frye et al. (2019) investigated the associations of diabetes management and sleep duration with HbA1c in adolescents with T1D. While they found sleep duration was significantly associated to both management activities and Hba1c, the timing and regularity dimensions were significantly correlated with HbA1c and not with management activities, suggesting that perhaps the timing and regularity dimensions should be promoted alongside duration to optimize glycemic control (Frye et al., 2019). Sleep researchers should continue to examine all six of the sleep health dimensions, ensuring standardization across the domains utilizing both subjective and objective measures. Emphasis should be placed on identifying important sleep-related behaviors specific to T1D. These behaviors and the other sleep health dimensions should then be examined in relation to one another and how this might subsequently impact HbA1c. This will continue to unpick the complex sleep and glycemic control relationship and help inform clinicians and patients on how best to navigate the hurricane of factors influencing sleep health.

Sleep Health Interventions

Interventional research investigating the benefit of improving sleep health for glycemic control in T1D adolescents has recently gained traction. M. Perfect et al. (2018) conducted a randomized controlled trial to determine the impact of a 1-week sleep extension program in adolescents with T1D (n = 111; 10–16 years) and found that 80% of adolescents assigned to the intervention attained at least 15 minutes additional sleep and one-third of participants increased sleep duration by 1 hour (average increase 43 minutes). Additionally, an improvement of 7.4% in glucose levels for participants within the sleep extension intervention was reported, which translated into an additional 11 hours within the glucose control target range compared to participants within the control group. However, in a similar randomized pilot study of adolescents (n = 39; 13–17 years) with T1D no significant effects on glycemic control (HbA1c) were observed for participants in a sleep coach intervention despite significant improvements in sleep efficiency and sleep duration (average increase 48 minutes; Jaser et al., 2020).

Although there are currently available published protocols describing additional sleep interventions aiming to enhance glycemic control (M. M. Perfect et al., 2023; Rose et al., 2022), the interventional research within this field is still limited. Research should now place emphasis on building a solid base of experimental evidence to determine the impact of sleep interventions and how they can be utilized in clinical care to enhance glycemic control.

Sleep and TBI

Although there is no internationally accepted definition, TBI has been described as "an alteration in brain function, or other evidence of brain pathology, caused by an external force" (Menon et al., 2010, p. 1637). The consequences can include loss of consciousness, amnesia, and cognitive and/or neurological deficits. TBI can be categorized as mild, moderate, or severe, based on various markers of injury severity, including alteration in consciousness (typically assessed using the Glasgow Coma Scale; Teasdale & Jennett, 1974), loss of consciousness, post-traumatic amnesia, and evidence of neuroradiological abnormalities. Overall, 70%–90% of TBI cases are classified as mild (Skandsen et al., 2019). Common mild TBI symptoms include somatic complaints (e.g., headaches, tinnitus, dizziness, nausea, balance and coordination problems, and sleep difficulties), affective symptoms (depression, irritability, anxiety), and cognitive deficits (Prince & Bruhns, 2017) . Compared to moderate to severe TBI, most individuals with mild TBI recover from their symptoms within 3 months; however, approximately 10%–20% develop long-term post-concussive symptoms (Bergersen et al., 2017; Permenter et al., 2023). Moderate to severe TBI can result in long-term emotional, cognitive, and behavioral impairments (Carney et al., 1999; Dikmen et al., 2009), which can exert a negative, often devastating, impact on an individual's quality of life (Stocchetti & Zanier, 2016), interpersonal relationships, capacity for independence, and occupational, social (Cicerone et al., 2000; Decuypere & Klimo, 2012), and family functioning (Ponsford & Schönberger, 2010; Rasmussen et al., 2020).

Prevalence and Nature of Sleep Disturbances Following TBI

Sleep disturbances are among the most prevalent and persistent symptoms following TBI (Aoun et al., 2019; Duclos et al., 2014; Sandsmark et al., 2017), occurring at both the acute and chronic stages of recovery (Duclos et al., 2014; Fedele et al., 2020). However, the reported prevalence of sleep disturbances in the overall TBI population varies substantially, from 29% to 80% (e.g., Castriotta et al., 2007; Datta et al., 2009; Wickwire et al., 2016). This variation most likely reflects the heterogeneity of the populations studied (e.g., mild, moderate, or severe TBI), variations in sample size, and differences in criteria used to identify and measure sleep disturbances (e.g., subjective vs. objective, PSG or actigraphy, formal diagnostic criteria vs. informal diagnosis). Exploring some of these confounds, a meta-analysis of 21 studies, with 1,706 participants across the spectrum of TBI severity (Mathias & Alvaro, 2012), found a 50% prevalence of sleep–wake disturbances in individuals with TBI, which far exceeds that of the general population. In addition, approximately 30% were diagnosed with a clinical sleep disorder. When analysis was confined to individuals diagnosed as having a sleep disorder, a significantly higher prevalence of insomnia (29%), hypersomnia (28%), and sleep apnea (25%) was found for individuals with TBI relative to the general population (a prevalence of 10%, 10%, and 2%, respectively; Bixler et al., 2001; Breslau et al., 1996). Periodic limb movements and narcolepsy occurred less frequently (8% and 4%, respectively) but significantly more often than in the general population (4% and 0.047%, respectively). The influence of chronicity and severity could not be determined as few studies included this information (Mathias & Alvaro, 2012). A recent cohort study of 98,709 veterans with TBI and 98,709 age-matched veterans without TBI found that after an average follow-up of 5 (1–14) years, 23.4% of veterans with TBI developed sleep disorders compared with 15.8% of those without TBI. After adjusting for age, sex, race, education, and income, Leng et al. (2021) found that individuals with TBI were 50% more likely to develop any sleep disorder compared to those without TBI (hazard ratio = 1.50; 95% confidence interval [1.47, 1.53]). Additional adjustment for medical and psychiatric problems indicated that the likelihood of developing any sleep disorder was 41% higher in those with TBI (hazard ratio = 1.41; 95% confidence interval [1.37, 1.44]).

Objective measurements of sleep, including actigraphy and PSG, have generally corroborated subjective sleep complaints in the acute stage of recovery (Mantua et al., 2018). For instance, both subjective reports and objective measurement have frequently found nighttime awakenings and daytime sleepiness in individuals with TBI (Carrillo-Mora et al., 2022; Imbach et al., 2015; Mantua et al., 2018) as well as increased sleep need (hypersomnia; Imbach et al., 2015) and insomnia (Ouellet et al., 2006). Findings have been more variable in the chronic phase of recovery (e.g., Imbach et al., 2016; Kempf et al., 2010; Mantua et al., 2015). However, a meta-analysis (N. Grima et al., 2016), using pooled PSG data, revealed that individuals with TBI living in the community ($N = 637$) had poorer sleep efficiency, shorter total sleep duration, and greater wake after sleep onset time compared to controls ($N = 567$). Consistent with the PSG data, individuals with TBI reported greater subjective sleepiness and poorer perceived sleep quality. However, some studies have reported a weaker relationship between objective measures and subjective reports for individuals with TBI compared to non-injured controls (e.g., Lu et al., 2015).

Individuals with all severities of TBI are at increased risk of sleep disturbance, although the type of disturbance may vary; for example, some studies have found increased rates of insomnia in mild compared to severe TBI (Beetar et al., 1996; Clinchot et al., 1998; Ouellet et al., 2006), whereas hypersomnia has been associated with more severe TBI (Baumann et al., 2007; Wolfe et al., 2018).

Etiology of Sleep Disturbance Following TBI

The mechanisms underlying sleep disturbances in patients with TBI are complex, multifaceted, and not well understood. Damage or disruption to key brain areas involved in sleep such as the hypothalamus, brainstem reticular formation, and basal forebrain has been associated with sleep disturbances in individuals with TBI (Castriotta & Murthy, 2011; N. Grima et al., 2016). Other studies have found no structural abnormalities on cerebral imaging despite significant sleep disturbance (Boivin et al., 2003; Tobe et al., 1999). However, imaging techniques are not always sensitive to subtle pathology such as diffuse axonal injury or microhemorrhage. High cervical cord lesions have been known to cause sleepiness and OSA (Leduc et al., 2007). Disruption to neurotransmitter/hormonal systems involved in sleep has also been implicated; for example, reductions in hypocretin (Baumann et al., 2005, 2007, 2009), melatonin (Shekleton et al., 2010), and histamine (Sinclair et al., 2014) have been observed in the TBI population. Hypocretin and histamine are wake-promoting neurotransmitters, and low cerebrospinal fluid levels of these neurotransmitters have been associated with hypersomnia (N. A. Grima et al.,

2018; Mantua et al., 2018). Reduced melatonin has been associated with decreased REM sleep in TBI (N. Grima et al., 2016). In addition, genes involved in inflammation, glial function, immunity, neuronal plasticity, and circadian rhythm have been implicated in sleep disturbance following TBI (Imbach et al., 2015). Secondary psychological factors are also thought to play an important role in the development and/or maintenance of sleep disturbances. For example, anxiety, depression, and post-traumatic stress disorder are common sequelae of TBI (Ouellet et al., 2006; Ponsford et al., 2013; Rao et al., 2008), which have been associated with disrupted objective and subjective sleep in TBI (Ponsford et al., 2013; Shekleton et al., 2010). New-onset anxiety after TBI is a significant predictor of sleep disturbance, although the cause–effect relationship is unclear (Collen et al., 2012; Rao et al., 2008). Pain (Beetar et al., 1996), fatigue (Ouellet et al., 2006), hospitalization, headache, dizziness (Hou et al. 2013), higher use of medications such as antidepressants (N. Grima et al., 2016; Yasseen et al., 2008), and medical comorbidities (e.g., post-traumatic epilepsy) may also contribute to the development and exacerbation of sleep disturbances following TBI.

Sleep Disturbance as a Moderator of Outcomes Post-TBI

Sleep is critical for cognitive and behavioral functioning (Zielinski et al., 2016). Poor sleep is associated with disturbances of cognition, mood, and daily functioning (Cirelli, 2012; Orff et al., 2009; Rao et al., 2008; Van Dongen et al., 2003; Van Someren & Riemersma-Van Der Lek, 2007; Wickwire et al., 2018). Evidence is mounting that sleep disturbances can hamper recovery from TBI directly by inhibiting neural recovery and indirectly by increasing risk for cognitive, behavioral, and emotional difficulties (Wickwire et al., 2016, 2018). For example, in a prospective study of individuals with TBI (n = 87, at least 3 months post-injury), sleep disorders were associated with poorer cognitive performance, including slower reaction times and reduced vigilance (Castriotta et al., 2007). In individuals with TBI, the presence of OSA has been associated with greater impairment of sustained attention and memory than in patients with comparable severity TBI without OSA (Castriotta et al., 2007). Severity of sleep disturbances has also been associated with broad cognitive impairment (Kalmbach et al., 2018; Nakase-Richardson et al., 2013), post-traumatic amnesia (Kalmbach et al. 2018), post-concussive symptoms (Freeman et al., 2017), and global disability (Mollayeva et al., 2016). Individuals with TBI and sleep disturbances are more likely to suffer from headaches (Chaput et al., 2009), neurobehavioral deficits (Bloomfield et al., 2010; Dean & Sterr, 2013), and mood disturbances (Lew et al., 2009; Parcell et al., 2008). Importantly, evidence has suggested that sleep–wake disturbances impact clinical outcomes independent of associated mental health conditions (Sandsmark et al., 2017). Sleep disturbance has been shown to be predictive of prolonged recovery from concussion symptoms (Theadom et al., 2015). In addition, evidence has suggested that sleep and TBI have common neurological underpinnings that may impair glymphatic function (Bostock et al., 2016), reduce neurotoxin clearance, and accelerate neurodegeneration. Astroglial scars and inflammation caused by TBI may further damage the glymphatic system, increasing the buildup of neurotoxins (Sullan et al., 2018).

Treatment Approaches

Several treatment approaches relating to many of the commonly reported sleep disorders post-TBI (insomnia, circadian rhythm disorder, hypersomnia) have been evaluated; however, there are no well-controlled studies on treatment approaches for sleep apnea, periodic limb movement disorder, and parasomnia. A myriad of methodological limitations makes drawing valid conclusions from the extant literature difficult, including small sample sizes, inconsistencies in how sleep disturbances are defined and measured, and factors relating to injury severity, chronicity, premorbid factors, and comorbidity (Cheng et al., 2019).

In relation to insomnia, pharmacological studies have identified treatment effects associated with the use of melatonin (N. A. Grima et al., 2017; Kemp et al., 2004) and amitriptyline (Kemp et al., 2004). Non-pharmacological treatments have shown effects associated with CBT (Nguyen et al., 2017; Theadom et al., 2018), acupuncture (Zollman et al., 2012), and warm footbaths (Chiu et al., 2017). For hypersomnia post-TBI, pharmacological studies have shown support for the use of modafinil (Hershman et al., 2010; Jha et al., 2008) and armodafinil (Menn et al., 2014). A systematic review and network meta-analysis found moderate-quality evidence for blue-wavelength light therapy (BWLT; Srisurapanont et al., 2021). Some evidence has supported the use of pharmacological treatment for circadian rhythm disorder post-TBI using ramelteon (Lequerica et al., 2015), methylphenidate (Baumann et al., 2005), and sertraline (Baumann et al., 2005), as well as BWLT (Killgore et al., 2020). With regard to treatment of general sleep disturbance and fatigue post-TBI, amelioration of symptoms has been observed following the administration of *N*-acetyl cysteine (Hoffer et al., 2013), BWLT (Quera Salva et al., 2020; Raikes et al., 2020; Sinclair et al., 2014), and hyperbaric oxygen (J. M. Walker et al., 2018; Wolf et al., 2012).

Concerns have been raised about applying treatment approaches designed for the general population to individuals with TBI due to the potential risks of exacerbating common sequalae of TBI, including cognitive deficits, dizziness, motor problems, and fatigue. This includes concerns about side effects of commonly prescribed hypnotics (e.g., benzodiazepines, non-benzodiazepine receptor agonists) and medications which suppress slow-wave sleep (given the importance of this sleep stage for recovery after TBI; Morawska et al., 2016; Vermaelen et al., 2015). Moreover, there is now emerging evidence that long-term use of hypnotics may be associated with increased risk of dementia (Chen et al., 2012; Gallacher et al., 2012), particularly for individuals with TBI (Chiu et al., 2015). The use of sleep restriction (a component of CBT-I) also requires care because of the potential to exacerbate post-injury fatigue and cognitive deficits. Moreover, when applying generic treatment approaches to individuals with TBI, consideration also needs to be given to epileptic thresholds, potential for drug misuse, and deficits in self-awareness secondary to cognitive deficits (Ouellet et al., 2015; Stewart et al., 2022).

TBI is a heterogenous and complex disorder, and sleep disturbances, which are highly prevalent and underrecognized, can compromise recovery by initiating or exacerbating the psychological, cognitive, emotional, and physical (i.e., fatigue, pain) sequalae of TBI, thereby further impacting on quality of life (e.g. Gardani et al., 2015; Mollayeva et al., 2016; Zeitzer et al., 2009) and neurological recovery. Moreover, sleep disturbances can adversely affect rehabilitation, result in longer hospital stays, and increase health costs (Cheng et al., 2019; Fichtenberg et al., 2000; Ouellet et al., 2004).

Conclusion

Poor sleep health is common across a myriad of medical conditions. There is consensus that poor sleep is not merely a symptom of another medical condition but often a primary complaint that, if left unaddressed, can become persistent and costly for mental and physical health. This chapter has outlined a complex, bidirectional relationship between medical conditions and sleep disturbance, with significant symptom overlap, and offers hope in the form of evidence-based interventions to promote sleep health. The next steps are to make these interventions more available to patients, preferably through the healthcare system. The study of sleep and medical conditions furthers our knowledge not only of disease processes and of sleep processes but also of their reciprocal influences. As our understanding in this area progresses, the interaction of sleep with physiological and psychological aspects of medical conditions will become more integrated, paving the way for a transdiagnostic, patient-focused therapeutic approach that is not restricted by diagnostic categories and siloed treatments.

Future Directions

Insomnia is common across a range of chronic health conditions at all stages of the disease pathway (i.e., before treatment, during treatment, after completion of treatment). While disease-specific factors (e.g., pain, medications) are known to trigger the onset of sleep disturbance, less is known about the role of poor sleep in the development of chronic disease. More longitudinal and mechanistic studies are needed to increase our understanding of the influence of poor sleep on physical health and the disease pathway of chronic health conditions. Studies that characterize the natural course of sleep disturbance during the chronic illness trajectory would allow us to better understand the bidirectional relationship between sleep and health. Finally, we need to raise awareness among other healthcare providers of sleep disturbance as a transdiagnostic issue which, if addressed, may lead to improvements in the physical health condition and quality of life of these individuals. The efficacy of psychological interventions such as CBT-I is well established, yet most patients with sleep disturbance cannot access treatment. The integration of evidence-based interventions for sleep within standard healthcare systems would help raise the profile of sleep as a key public health concern and would facilitate patient access at the point of need.

Note

1. If the AHI≥15, then a diagnosis of OSA is made without the presence of symptoms.

References

Abdelmaksoud, A. A., Salah, N. Y., Ali, Z. M., Rashed, H. R., & Abido, A. Y. (2021). Disturbed sleep quality and architecture in adolescents with Type 1 diabetes mellitus: Relation to glycemic control, vascular complications and insulin sensitivity. *Diabetes Research and Clinical Practice, 174*, Article 108774.

Agudelo, C., Ramos, A. R., Sun, X., Kaur, S., Del Papa, D. F., Kather, J. M., Wallace, D. M., & Alzheimer's Disease Neuroimaging Initiative. (2022). Sleep-disordered breathing risk with comorbid insomnia is associated with mild cognitive impairment. *Applied Sciences, 12*(5), Article 2414. https://www.mdpi.com/2076-3417/12/5/2414

Alessi, C. A., Fung, C. H., Dzierzewski, J. M., Fiorentino, L., Stepnowsky, C., Rodriguez Tapia, J. C., Song, Y., Zeidler, M. R., Josephson, K., Mitchell, M. N., Jouldjian, S., & Martin, J. L. (2021). Randomized controlled trial of an integrated approach to treating insomnia and improving the use of positive airway pressure therapy in veterans with comorbid insomnia disorder and obstructive sleep apnea. *Sleep, 44*(4), Article zsaa235. https://doi.org/10.1093/sleep/zsaa235

American Academy of Sleep Medicine. (2014). *International classification of sleep disorders* (3rd ed.).

American Diabetes Association. (2017). 3. Comprehensive medical evaluation and assessment of comorbidities. *Diabetes Care, 40*(S1), S25–S32.

American Psychiatric Association. (2013). *Diagnostic and statistical manual of mental disorders* (5th ed.).

Ancoli-Israel, S. (2015). Sleep disturbances in cancer: A review. *Sleep Medicine Research, 6*(2), 45–49. https://doi.org/10.17241/smr.2015.6.2.45

Aoun, R., Rawal, H., Attarian, H., & Sahni, A. (2019). Impact of traumatic brain injury on sleep: An overview. *Nature and Science of Sleep, 11*, 131–140. https://doi.org/10.2147/NSS.S182158

Baker, F. C., Lampio, L., Saaresranta, T., & Polo-Kantola, P. (2018). Sleep and sleep disorders in the menopausal transition. *Sleep Medicine Clinics, 13*(3), 443–456. https://doi.org/10.1016/j.jsmc.2018.04.011

Bastien, C. H., Vallieres, A., & Morin, C. M. (2001). Validation of the Insomnia Severity Index as an outcome measure for insomnia research. *Sleep Medicine, 2*(4), 297–307. https://doi.org/10.1016/s1389-9457(00)00065-4

Baumann, C. R., Bassetti, C. L., Valko, P. O., Haybaeck, J., Keller, M., Clark, E., Stocker, R., Tolnay, M., & Scammell, T. E. (2009). Loss of hypocretin (orexin) neurons with traumatic brain injury. *Annals of Neurology, 66*(4), 555–559. https://doi.org/10.1002/ana.21836

Baumann, C. R., Stocker, R., Imhof, H. G., Trentz, O., Hersberger, M., Mignot, E., & Bassetti, C. L. (2005). Hypocretin-1 (orexin A) deficiency in acute traumatic brain injury. *Neurology, 65*(1), 147–149. https://doi.org/10.1212/01.wnl.0000167605.02541.f2

Baumann, C. R., Werth, E., Stocker, R., Ludwig, S., & Bassetti, C. L. (2007). Sleep–wake disturbances 6 months after traumatic brain injury: A prospective study. *Brain, 130*(Pt. 7), 1873–1883. https://doi.org/10.1093/brain/awm109

Becker, N. B., Martins, R. I. S., de Neves Jesus, S., Chiodelli, R., & Rieber, M. S. (2018). Sleep health assessment: A scale validation. *Psychiatry Research, 259*, 51–55.

Beetar, J. T., Guilmette, T. J., & Sparadeo, F. R. (1996). Sleep and pain complaints in symptomatic traumatic brain injury and neurologic populations. *Archives of Physical Medicine and Rehabilitation, 77*(12), 1298–1302. https://doi.org/10.1016/s0003-9993(96)90196-3

Beneto, A., Gomez-Siurana, E., & Rubio-Sanchez, P. (2009). Comorbidity between sleep apnea and insomnia. *Sleep Medicine Reviews, 13*(4), 287–293. https://doi.org/10.1016/j.smrv.2008.09.006

Berg, K. A., Marbury, M., Whaley, M. A., Perzynski, A. T., Patel, S. R., & Thornton, J. D. (2022). Experiences with continuous positive airway pressure among African American patients and their bed partners. *Behavioral Sleep Medicine, 21*(3), 242–253. https://doi.org/10.1080/15402002.2022.2075365

Berger, A. M., Mooney, K., Alvarez-Perez, A., Breitbart, W. S., Carpenter, K. M., Cella, D., Cleeland, C., Dotan, E., Eisenberger, M. A., Escalante, C. P., Jacobsen, P. B., Jankowski, C., LeBlanc, T., Ligibel, J. A., Loggers, E. T., Mandrell, B., Murphy, B. A., Palesh, O., Pirl, W. F., . . . Smith, C. (2015). Cancer-related fatigue, version 2.2015. *Journal of the National Comprehensive Cancer Network, 13*(8), 1012–1039. https://doi.org/10.6004/jnccn.2015.0122

Bergersen, K., Halvorsen, J., Tryti, E. A., Taylor, S. I., & Olsen, A. (2017). A systematic literature review of psychotherapeutic treatment of prolonged symptoms after mild traumatic brain injury. *Brain Injury, 31*(3), 279–289. https://doi.org/10.1080/02699052.2016.1255779

Bergner, E. M., Williams, R., Hamburger, E. R., Lyttle, M., Davis, A. C., Malow, B., Simmons, J. H., Lybarger, C., Capin, R., & Jaser, S. S. (2018). Sleep in teens with Type 1 diabetes: Perspectives from adolescents and their caregivers. *The Diabetes Educator, 44*(6), 541–548.

Bertisch, S. M., Li, W., Buettner, C., Mostofsky, E., Rueschman, M., Kaplan, E. R., Fung, J., Huntington, S., Murphy, T., Stead, C., Burstein, R., Redline, S., & Stead, C. (2020). Nightly sleep duration, fragmentation, and quality and daily risk of migraine. *Neurology, 94*(5), e489–e496.

Bigal, M. E., & Lipton, R. B. (2011). Migraine chronification. *Current Neurology and Neuroscience Reports, 11*(2), 139–148.

Bixler, E. O., Vgontzas, A. N., Lin, H. M., Ten Have, T., Rein, J., Vela-Bueno, A., & Kales, A. (2001). Prevalence of sleep-disordered breathing in women: Effects of gender. *American Journal of Respiratory and Critical Care Medicine, 163*(3, Pt. 1), 608–613. https://doi.org/10.1164/ajrccm.163.3.9911064

Bjornsdottir, E., Janson, C., Sigurdsson, J. F., Gehrman, P., Perlis, M., Juliusson, S., Arnardottir, E. S., Kuna, S. T., Pack, A. I., Gislason, T., & Benediktsdottir, B. (2013). Symptoms of insomnia among patients with obstructive sleep apnea before and after two years of positive airway pressure treatment. *Sleep, 36*(12), 1901–1909. https://doi.org/10.5665/sleep.3226

Bjorvatn, B., Berge, T., Lehmann, S., Pallesen, S., & Saxvig, I. W. (2018). No effect of a self-help book for insomnia in patients with obstructive sleep apnea and comorbid chronic insomnia—A randomized controlled trial. *Frontiers in Psychology, 9*, Article 2413. https://doi.org/10.3389/fpsyg.2018.02413

Bloomfield, I. L., Espie, C. A., & Evans, J. J. (2010). Do sleep difficulties exacerbate deficits in sustained attention following traumatic brain injury? *Journal of the International Neuropsychological Society, 16*(1), 17–25. https://doi.org/10.1017/s1355617709990798

Boivin, D. B., James, F. O., Santo, J. B., Caliyurt, O., & Chalk, C. (2003). Non-24-hour sleep–wake syndrome following a car accident. *Neurology, 60*(11), 1841–1843. https://doi.org/10.1212/01.wnl.0000061482.24750.7c

Bostock, S., Luik, A. I., & Espie, C. A. (2016). Sleep and productivity benefits of digital cognitive behavioral therapy for insomnia: A randomized controlled trial conducted in the workplace environment. *Journal of Occupational and Environmental Medicine, 58*(7), 683–689. https://doi.org/10.1097/jom.0000000000000778

Brasure, M., MacDonald, R., Fuchs, E., Olson, C. M., Carlyle, M., Diem, S., Koffel, E., Khawaja, I. S., Ouellete, J., Butler, M., Kane, R. L., & Wilt, T. J. (2015). *Management of insomnia disorder* (Comparative Effectiveness Reviews No. 159). Agency for Healthcare Research and Quality.

Bray, F., Ferlay, J., Soerjomataram, I., Siegel, R. L., Torre, L. A., & Jemal, A. (2018). Global cancer statistics 2018: GLOBOCAN estimates of incidence and mortality worldwide for 36 cancers in 185 countries. CA: A Cancer Journal for Clinicians, 68(6), 394–424. https://doi.org.10.3322/caac.21492

Breslau, N., Roth, T., Rosenthal, L., & Andreski, P. (1996). Sleep disturbance and psychiatric disorders: A longitudinal epidemiological study of young adults. *Biological Psychiatry, 39*(6), 411–418. https://doi.org/10.1016/0006-3223(95)00188-3

Buse, D. C., Rains, J. C., Pavlovic, J. M., Fanning, K. M., Reed, M. L., Manack Adams, A., & Lipton, R. B. (2019). Sleep disorders among people with migraine: Results from the chronic migraine epidemiology and outcomes (CaMEO) study. *Headache, 59*(1), 32–45.

Buysse, D. J. (2014). Sleep health: Can we define it? Does it matter? *Sleep, 37*(1), 9–17.

Calhoun, A. H., & Ford, S. (2007). Behavioral sleep modification may revert transformed migraine to episodic migraine. *Headache, 47*(8), 1178–1183.

Campbell, M. D., Walker, M., Bracken, R. M., Turner, D., Stevenson, E. J., Gonzalez, J. T., James, A. S., & West, D. J. (2015). Insulin therapy and dietary adjustments to normalize glycemia and prevent nocturnal hypoglycemia after evening exercise in Type 1 diabetes: A randomized controlled trial. *BMJ Open Diabetes Research and Care, 3*(1), Article e000085.

Carney, N., Chesnut, R. M., Maynard, H., Mann, N. C., Patterson, P., & Helfand, M. (1999). Effect of cognitive rehabilitation on outcomes for persons with traumatic brain injury: A systematic review. *Journal of Head Trauma Rehabilitation, 14*(3), 277–307. https://doi.org/10.1097/00001199-199906000-00008

Carrillo-Mora, P., Sidonio-Aguayo, B., Márquez-Vázquez, J. F., del Campo-Arias, S. M., Carrillo-Santos, M., Hernández-Arenas, C., Cervera-Delgadillo, N. G., & Samudio-Cruz, M. A. (2022). Sleep disorders in patients with acquired brain damage, associated factors and their impact on functionality. *Investigación en Discapacidad, 8*(1), 16–17.

Carskadon, M. A. (2011). Sleep in adolescents: The perfect storm. *Pediatric Clinics, 58*(3), 637–647.

Castriotta, R. J., & Murthy, J. N. (2011). Sleep disorders in patients with traumatic brain injury: A review. *CNS Drugs, 25*(3), 175–185. https://doi.org/10.2165/11584870-000000000-00000

Castriotta, R. J., Wilde, M. C., Lai, J. M., Atanasov, S., Masel, B. E., & Kuna, S. T. (2007). Prevalence and consequences of sleep disorders in traumatic brain injury. *Journal of Clinical Sleep Medicine, 3*(4), 349–356.

Chaput, G., Giguère, J. F., Chauny, J. M., Denis, R., & Lavigne, G. (2009). Relationship among subjective sleep complaints, headaches, and mood alterations following a mild traumatic brain injury. *Sleep Medicine, 10*(7), 713–716. https://doi.org/10.1016/j.sleep.2008.07.015

Chaput, J.-P., Dutil, C., Featherstone, R., Ross, R., Giangregorio, L., Saunders, T. J., Janssen, I., Poitras, V. J., Kho, M. E., Ross-White, A., & Carrier, J. (2020). Sleep duration and health in adults: An overview of systematic reviews. *Applied Physiology, Nutrition, and Metabolism, 45*(10, S2), S218–S231. https://doi.org/10.1139/apnm-2020-0034

Chen, P. L., Lee, W. J., Sun, W. Z., Oyang, Y. J., & Fuh, J. L. (2012). Risk of dementia in patients with insomnia and long-term use of hypnotics: A population-based retrospective cohort study. *PLOS ONE, 7*(11), Article e49113. https://doi.org/10.1371/journal.pone.0049113

Cheng, P., Luik, A. I., Fellman-Couture, C., Peterson, E., Joseph, C. L. M., Tallent, G., Tran, K. M., Ahmedani, B. K., Roehrs, T., Roth, T., & Drake, C. L. (2019). Efficacy of digital CBT for insomnia to reduce depression across demographic groups: A randomized trial. *Psychological Medicine, 49*(3), 491–500. https://doi.org/10.1017/S0033291718001113

Chiu, H. Y., Lin, E. Y., Chiu, H. T., & Chen, P. Y. (2017). A feasibility randomized controlled crossover trial of home-based warm footbath to improve sleep in the chronic phase of traumatic brain injury. *Journal of Neuroscience Nursing, 49*(6), 380–385. https://doi.org/10.1097/JNN.0000000000000325

Chiu, H. Y., Lin, E. Y., Wei, L., Lin, J. H., Lee, H. C., Fan, Y. C., & Tsai, P. S. (2015). Hypnotics use but not insomnia increased the risk of dementia in traumatic brain injury patients. *European Neuropsychopharmacology, 25*(12), 2271–2277. https://doi.org/10.1016/j.euroneuro.2015.09.011

Cicerone, K. D., Dahlberg, C., Kalmar, K., Langenbahn, D. M., Malec, J. F., Bergquist, T. F., Felicetti, T., Giacino, J. T., Harley, J. P., Harrington, D. E., Herzog, J., Kneipp, S., Laatsch, L., & Morse, P. A. (2000). Evidence-based cognitive rehabilitation: Recommendations for clinical practice. *Archives of Physical Medicine and Rehabilitation, 81*(12), 1596–1615. https://doi.org/10.1053/apmr.2000.19240

Cirelli, C. (2012). Brain plasticity, sleep and aging. *Gerontology, 58*(5), 441–445. https://doi.org/10.1159/000336149

Clinchot, D. M., Bogner, J., Mysiw, W. J., Fugate, L., & Corrigan, J. (1998). Defining sleep disturbance after brain injury. *American Journal of Physical and Medical Rehabilitation, 77*(4), 291–295. https://doi.org/10.1097/00002060-199807000-00006

Cobry, E. C., Karami, A. J., & Meltzer, L. J. (2022). Friend or foe: A narrative review of the impact of diabetes technology on sleep. *Current Diabetes Reports, 22*(7), 283–290.

Colberg, S. R., Sigal, R. J., Yardley, J. E., Riddell, M. C., Dunstan, D. W., Dempsey, P. C., Horton, E. S., Castorino, K., &Tate, D. F. (2016). Physical activity/exercise and diabetes: A position statement of the American Diabetes Association. *Diabetes Care, 39*(11), 2065–2079.

Cole, J. B., & Florez, J. C. (2020). Genetics of diabetes mellitus and diabetes complications. *Nature Reviews Nephrology, 16*(7), 377–390.

Collen, J., Orr, N., Lettieri, C. J., Carter, K., & Holley, A. B. (2012). Sleep disturbances among soldiers with combat-related traumatic brain injury. *Chest, 142*(3), 622–630. https://doi.org/10.1378/chest.11-1603

Crawford, M. R., Chirinos, D. A., Iurcotta, T., Edinger, J. D., Wyatt, J. K., Manber, R., & Ong, J. C. (2017). Characterization of patients who present with insomnia: Is there room for a symptom cluster-based approach? *Journal of Clinical Sleep Medicine, 13*(7), 911–921. https://doi.org/10.5664/jcsm.6666

Crawford, M. R., Luik, A. I., Espie, C. A., Taylor, H. L., Burgess, H. J., Jones, A. L., Rush University Sleep Research Team & Ong, J. C. (2020). Digital cognitive behavioral therapy for insomnia in women with chronic migraines. *Headache, 60*(5), 902–915.

Crowley, S. J., Wolfson, A. R., Tarokh, L., & Carskadon, M. A. (2018). An update on adolescent sleep: New evidence informing the perfect storm model. *Journal of Adolescence, 67*, 55–65.

Danilov, A., & Kurganova, J. (2016). Melatonin in chronic pain syndromes. *Pain and Therapy, 5*(1), 1–17.

Datta, S. G., Pillai, S. V., Rao, S. L., Kovoor, J. M., & Chandramouli, B. A. (2009). Post-concussion syndrome: Correlation of neuropsychological deficits, structural lesions on magnetic resonance imaging and symptoms. *Neurology India, 57*(5), 594–598. https://doi.org/10.4103/0028-3886.57810

Dean, P. J., & Sterr, A. (2013). Long-term effects of mild traumatic brain injury on cognitive performance. *Frontiers in Human Neuroscience, 7*, Article 30. https://doi.org/10.3389/fnhum.2013.00030

Decuypere, M., & Klimo, P., Jr. (2012). Spectrum of traumatic brain injury from mild to severe. *Surgical Clinics of North America, 92*(4), 939–957. https://doi.org/10.1016/j.suc.2012.04.005

de Lima, V. A., Mascarenhas, L. P. G., Decimo, J. P., de Souza, W. C., Monteiro, A. L. S., Lahard, I., Franca, S. N., & Leite, N. (2017). Physical activity levels of adolescents with Type 1 diabetes physical activity in T1D. *Pediatric Exercise Science, 29*(2), 213–219.

Dikmen, S. S., Corrigan, J. D., Levin, H. S., Machamer, J., Stiers, W., & Weisskopf, M. G. (2009). Cognitive outcome following traumatic brain injury. *Journal of Head Trauma Rehabilitation, 24*(6), 430–438. https://doi.org/10.1097/HTR.0b013e3181c133e9

Duclos, C., Dumont, M., Blais, H., Paquet, J., Laflamme, E., de Beaumont, L., Wiseman-Hakes, C., Menon, D. K., Bernard, F., & Gosselin, N. (2014). Rest–activity cycle disturbances in the acute phase of moderate to severe traumatic brain injury. *Neurorehabilitation and Neural Repair, 28*(5), 472–482. https://doi.org/10.1177/1545968313517756

Eaton, D. K., McKnight-Eily, L. R., Lowry, R., Perry, G. S., Presley-Cantrell, L., & Croft, J. B. (2010). Prevalence of insufficient, borderline, and optimal hours of sleep among high school students—United States, 2007. *Journal of Adolescent Health, 46*(4), 399–401.

Edinger, J. D., Arnedt, J. T., Bertisch, S. M., Carney, C. E., Harrington, J. J., Lichstein, K. L., Sateia, M. J., Troxel, W. M., Zhou, E. S., Kazmi, U., Heald, J. L., & Martin, J. L. (2021). Behavioral and psychological treatments for chronic insomnia disorder in adults: An American Academy of Sleep Medicine systematic review, meta-analysis, and GRADE assessment. *Journal of Clinical Sleep Medicine, 17*(2), 263–298. https://doi.org/10.5664/jcsm.8988

El-Solh, A. A., Lawson, Y., & Wilding, G. E. (2021). Impact of low arousal threshold on treatment of obstructive sleep apnea in patients with post-traumatic stress disorder. *Sleep and Breathing, 25*(2), 597–604. https://doi.org/10.1007/s11325-020-02106-0

Engstrøm, M., Hagen, K., Bjørk, M., Stovner, L., & Sand, T. (2014). Sleep quality and arousal in migraine and tension-type headache: The headache-sleep study. *Acta Neurologica Scandinavica, 129*, 47–54.

Eysteinsdottir, B., Gislason, T., Pack, A. I., Benediktsdottir, B., Arnardottir, E. S., Kuna, S. T., & Björnsdottir, E. (2017). Insomnia complaints in lean patients with obstructive sleep apnea negatively affect positive airway pressure treatment adherence. *Journal of Sleep Research, 26*(2), 159–165. https://doi.org/10.1111/jsr.12482

Fedele, B., Williams, G., McKenzie, D., Sutherland, E., & Olver, J. (2020). Subacute sleep disturbance in moderate to severe traumatic brain injury: A systematic review. *Brain Injury, 34*(3), 316–327. https://doi.org/10.1080/02699052.2019.1695288

Fernández-de-Las-Peñas, C., Fernández-Muñoz, J. J., Palacios-Ceña, M., Parás-Bravo, P., Cigarán-Méndez, M., & Navarro-Pardo, E. (2018). Sleep disturbances in tension-type headache and migraine. *Therapeutic Advances in Neurological Disorders, 11*, Article 1756285617745444.

Fichtenberg, N. L., Millis, S. R., Mann, N. R., Zafonte, R. D., & Millard, A. E. (2000). Factors associated with insomnia among post-acute traumatic brain injury survivors. *Brain Injury, 14*(7), 659–667. https://doi.org/10.1080/026990500500044015

Findley, L. J., Wilhoit, S. C., & Suratt, P. M. (1985). Apnea duration and hypoxemia during REM sleep in patients with obstructive sleep apnea. *Chest, 87*(4), 432–436. https://doi.org/10.1378/chest.87.4.432

Fleming, L., Agnew, S., Peddie, N., Crawford, M., Dixon, D., & MacPherson, I. (2022). The impact of medication side effects on adherence and persistence to hormone therapy in breast cancer survivors: A quantitative systematic review. *Breast, 64*, 63–84. https://doi.org/10.1016/j.breast.2022.04.010

Fleming, L., Randell, K., Harvey, C. J., & Espie, C. A. (2014). Does cognitive behaviour therapy for insomnia reduce clinical levels of fatigue, anxiety and depression in cancer patients? *Psycho-Oncology, 23*(6), 679–684. https://doi.org/10.1002/pon.3468

Fleming, L., Randell, K., Stewart, E., Espie, C. A., Morrison, D. S., Lawless, C., & Paul, J. (2019). Insomnia in breast cancer: A prospective observational study. *Sleep, 42*(3), Article zsy245. https://doi.org/10.1093/sleep/zsy245

Freeman, D., Sheaves, B., Goodwin, G. M., Yu, L.-M., Nickless, A., Harrison, P. J., Emsley, R., Luik, A. I., Foster, R. G., Wadekar, V., Hinds, C., Gumley, A., Jones, R., Lightman, S., Jones, S., Bentall, R., Kinderman, P., Rowse, G., Brugha, T., . . . Espie, C. A. (2017). The effects of improving sleep on mental health (OASIS): A randomised controlled trial with mediation analysis. *Lancet Psychiatry, 4*(10), 749–758. https://doi.org/10.1016/S2215-0366(17)30328-0

Frye, S. S., Perfect, M. M., & Silva, G. E. (2019). Diabetes management mediates the association between sleep duration and glycemic control in youth with Type 1 diabetes mellitus. *Sleep Medicine, 60*, 132–138.

Gadie, A., Shafto, M., Leng, Y., & Kievit, R. A. (2017). How are age-related differences in sleep quality associated with health outcomes? An epidemiological investigation in a UK cohort of 2406 adults. *BMJ Open, 7*(7), Article e014920. https://doi.org/10.1136/bmjopen-2016-014920

Gallacher, J., Elwood, P., Pickering, J., Bayer, A., Fish, M., & Ben-Shlomo, Y. (2012). Benzodiazepine use and risk of dementia: Evidence from the Caerphilly Prospective Study (CaPS). *Journal of Epidemiology & Community Health, 66*(10), 869–873. https://doi.org/10.1136/jech-2011-200314

Gardani, M., Morfiri, E., Thomson, A., O'Neill, B., & McMillan, T. M. (2015). Evaluation of sleep disorders in patients with severe traumatic brain injury during rehabilitation. *Archives of Physical Medicine and Rehabilitation, 96*(9), 1691–1697. https://doi.org/10.1016/j.apmr.2015.05.006

Gariepy, G., Danna, S., Gobiņa, I., Rasmussen, M., de Matos, M. G., Tynjälä, J., Janssen, I., Kalman, M., Villerusa, A., Husarova, D., Brooks, F., Elgar, F. J., Klavina-Makrecka, S., Smigelskas, K., Gaspar, T., & Schnohr, C. (2020). How are adolescents sleeping? Adolescent sleep patterns and sociodemographic differences in 24 European and North American countries. *Journal of Adolescent Health, 66*(6), S81–S88.

Garland, S. N., Johnson, J. A., Savard, J., Gehrman, P., Perlis, M., Carlson, L., & Campbell, T. (2014). Sleeping well with cancer: A systematic review of cognitive behavioral therapy for insomnia in cancer patients. *Neuropsychiatric Disease and Treatment, 10*, 1113–1124. https://doi.org/10.2147/NDT.S47790

Grima, N., Ponsford, J., Rajaratnam, S. M., Mansfield, D., & Pase, M. P. (2016). Sleep disturbances in traumatic brain injury: A meta-analysis. *Journal of Clinical Sleep Medicine, 12*(3), 419–428. https://doi.org/10.5664/jcsm.5598

Grima, N. A., Ponsford, J. L., & Pase, M. P. (2017). Sleep complications following traumatic brain injury. *Current Opinion in Pulmonary Medicine, 23*(6), 493–499. https://doi.org/10.1097/MCP.0000000000000429

Grima, N. A., Rajaratnam, S. M. W., Mansfield, D., Sletten, T. L., Spitz, G., & Ponsford, J. L. (2018). Efficacy of melatonin for sleep disturbance following traumatic brain injury: A randomised controlled trial. *BMC Medicine, 16*(1), Article 8. https://doi.org/10.1186/s12916-017-0995-1

Hamburger, E. R., Goethals, E. R., Choudhary, A., & Jaser, S. S. (2020). Sleep and depressive symptoms in adolescents with Type 1 diabetes not meeting glycemic targets. *Diabetes Research and Clinical Practice, 169*, Article 108442.

Harnod, T., Wang, Y.-C., & Kao, C.-H. (2015). Higher risk of developing a subsequent migraine in adults with nonapnea sleep disorders: A nationwide population-based cohort study. *European Journal of Internal Medicine, 26*(4), 232–236.

Harrold, E. C., Idris, A. F., Keegan, N. M., Corrigan, L., Teo, M. Y., O'Donnell, M., Kennedy, M. J., Sukor, S., Grant, C., Gallagher, D. G., Collier, S., Kingston, T., O'Dwyer, A. M., & Cuffe, S. (2020). Prevalence of insomnia in an oncology patient population: An Irish tertiary referral center experience. *Journal of the National Comprehensive Cancer Network, 18*(12), 1623–1630. https://doi.org/10.6004/jnccn.2020.7611

Hawkes, N. (2019). Cancer survival data emphasise importance of early diagnosis. *BMJ, 364*, Article l408. https://doi.org/10.1136/bmj.l408

Hazen, R. A., Fehr, K. K., Fidler, A., Cousino, M. K., MacLeish, S. A., & Gubitosi-Klug, R. (2015). Sleep disruption in adolescents with Type 1 diabetes mellitus: Relationships with adherence and diabetes control. *Diabetes Management, 5*(4), 257–265.

Headache Classification Committee of the International Headache Society. (2018). The International Classification of Headache Disorders, 3rd edition. *Cephalalgia, 38*(1), 1–211. https://doi.org/10.1177/0333102417738202

Hermans, L. W. A., Leufkens, T. R., van Gilst, M. M., Weysen, T., Ross, M., Anderer, P., Overeem, S., & Vermeeren, A. (2019). Sleep EEG characteristics associated with sleep onset misperception. *Sleep Medicine, 57*, 70–79. https://doi.org/10.1016/j.sleep.2019.01.031

Hershman, D. L., Kushi, L. H., Shao, T., Buono, D., Kershenbaum, A., Tsai, W. Y., Fehrenbacher, L., Gomez, S. L., Miles, S., & Neugut, A. I. (2010). Early discontinuation and nonadherence to adjuvant hormonal therapy in a cohort of 8,769 early-stage breast cancer patients. *Journal of Clinical Oncology, 28*(27), 4120–4128. https://doi.org/10.1200/jco.2009.25.9655

Hoffer, M. E., Balaban, C., Slade, M. D., Tsao, J. W., & Hoffer, B. (2013). Amelioration of acute sequelae of blast induced mild traumatic brain injury by *N*-acetyl cysteine: A double-blind, placebo controlled study. *PloS One, 8*(1), Article e54163. https://doi.org/10.1371/journal.pone.0054163

Houle, T. T., Butschek, R. A., Turner, D. P., Smitherman, T. A., Rains, J. C., & Penzien, D. B. (2012). Stress and sleep duration predict headache severity in chronic headache sufferers. *Pain, 153*(12), 2432–2440.

Hou, L., Han, X., Sheng, P., Tong, W., Li, Z., Xu, D., Yu, M., Huang, L., Zhao, Z., Lu, Y., & Dong, Y. (2013). Risk factors associated with sleep disturbance following traumatic brain injury: Clinical findings and questionnaire based study. *PloS One, 8*(10), e76087. https://doi.org/10.1371/journal.pone.0076087

Imbach, L. L., Buchele, F., Valko, P. O., Li, T., Maric, A., Stover, J. F., Bassetti, C. L., Mica, L., Werth, E., & Baumann, C. R. (2016). Sleep–wake disorders persist 18 months after traumatic brain injury but remain underrecognized. *Neurology, 86*(21), 1945–1949. https://doi.org/10.1212/WNL.0000000000002697

Imbach, L. L., Valko, P. O., Li, T., Maric, A., Symeonidou, E. R., Stover, J. F., Bassetti, C. L., Mica, L., Werth, E., &Baumann, C. R. (2015). Increased sleep need and daytime sleepiness 6 months after traumatic brain injury: A prospective controlled clinical trial. *Brain, 138*(Pt. 3), 726–735. https://doi.org/10.1093/brain/awu391

International Diabetes Federation. (2021). *The IDF diabetes atlas* (10th ed.).

Ionescu, C. G., Popa-Velea, O., Mihăilescu, A. I., Talaşman, A. A., & Bădărău, I. A. (2021). Somatic symptoms and sleep disorders: A literature review of their relationship, comorbidities and treatment. *Healthcare, 9*(9), Article 1128. https://doi.org/10.3390/healthcare9091128

Jaser, S. S., & Ellis, D. (2016). Sleep in adolescents and young adults with Type 1 diabetes: Associations with diabetes management and glycemic control. *Health Psychology and Behavioral Medicine, 4*(1), 49–55.

Jaser, S. S., Hamburger, E. R., Bergner, E. M., Williams, R., Slaughter, J. C., Simmons, J. H., & Malow, B. A. (2020). Sleep coach intervention for teens with Type 1 diabetes: Randomized pilot study. *Pediatric Diabetes, 21*(3), 473–478.

Jehan, S., Zizi, F., Pandi-Perumal, S. R., Wall, S., Auguste, E., Myers, A. K., Jean-Louis, G., & McFarlane, S. I. (2017). Obstructive sleep apnea and obesity: Implications for public health. *Sleep Medicine and Disorders, 1*(4), Article 00019. https://www.ncbi.nlm.nih.gov/pubmed/29517065

Jha, A., Weintraub, A., Allshouse, A., Morey, C., Cusick, C., Kittelson, J., Harrison-Felix, C., Whiteneck, G., & Gerber, D. (2008). A randomized trial of modafinil for the treatment of fatigue and excessive daytime sleepiness in individuals with chronic traumatic brain injury. *Journal of Head Trauma Rehabilitation, 23*(1), 52–63. https://doi.org/10.1097/01.HTR.0000308721.77911.ea

Ji, X., Ivers, H., Savard, J., Leblanc, M., & Morin, C. M. (2019). Residual symptoms after natural remission of insomnia: Associations with relapse over 4 years. *Sleep, 42*(8), Article zsz122. https://doi.org/10.1093/sleep/zsz122

Ji, X., Wang, Y., & Saylor, J. (2021). Sleep and Type 1 diabetes mellitus management among children, adolescents, and emerging young adults: A systematic review. *Journal of Pediatric Nursing, 61*, 245–253.

Johnson, J. A., Rash, J. A., Campbell, T. S., Savard, J., Gehrman, P. R., Perlis, M., Carlson, L. E., & Garland, S. N. (2016). A systematic review and meta-analysis of randomized controlled trials of cognitive behavior therapy for insomnia (CBT-I) in cancer survivors. *Sleep Medicine Reviews, 27*, 20–28. https://doi.org/10.1016/j.smrv.2015.07.001

Kalmbach, D. A., Cuamatzi-Castelan, A. S., Tonnu, C. V., Tran, K. M., Anderson, J. R., Roth, T., & Drake, C. L. (2018). Hyperarousal and sleep reactivity in insomnia: Current insights. *Nature and Science of Sleep, 10*, 193–201. https://doi.org/10.2147/nss.S138823

Keenan, B. T., Kim, J., Singh, B., Bittencourt, L., Chen, N. H., Cistulli, P. A., Magalang, U. J., McArdle, N., Mindel, J. W., Benediktsdottir, B., Arnardottir, E. S., Prochnow, L. K., Penzel, T., Sanner, B., Schwab, R. J., Shin, C., Sutherland, K., Tufik, S., Maislin, G., . . . Pack, A. I. (2018). Recognizable clinical subtypes of obstructive sleep apnea across international sleep centers: A cluster analysis. *Sleep, 41*(3), Article zsx214. https://doi.org/10.1093/sleep/zsx214

Kemp, S., Biswas, R., Neumann, V., & Coughlan, A. (2004). The value of melatonin for sleep disorders occurring post-head injury: A pilot RCT. *Brain Injury, 18*(9), 911–919. https://doi.org/10.1080/02699050410001671892

Kempf, J., Werth, E., Kaiser, P. R., Bassetti, C. L., & Baumann, C. R. (2010). Sleep–wake disturbances 3 years after traumatic brain injury. *Journal of Neurology, Neurosurgery & Psychiatry, 81*(12), 1402–1405. https://doi.org/10.1136/jnnp.2009.201913

Killgore, W. D. S., Vanuk, J. R., Shane, B. R., Weber, M., & Bajaj, S. (2020). A randomized, double-blind, placebo-controlled trial of blue wavelength light exposure on sleep and recovery of brain structure, function, and cognition following mild traumatic brain injury. *Neurobiology of Disease, 134*, Article 104679. https://doi.org/10.1016/j.nbd.2019.104679

Knutson, K. L., Van Cauter, E., Zee, P., Liu, K., & Lauderdale, D. S. (2011). Cross-sectional associations between measures of sleep and markers of glucose metabolism among subjects with and without diabetes: The Coronary Artery Risk Development in Young Adults (CARDIA) Sleep Study. *Diabetes Care, 34*(5), 1171–1176.

Krakow, B., McIver, N. D., Ulibarri, V. A., Krakow, J., & Schrader, R. M. (2019). Prospective randomized controlled trial on the efficacy of continuous positive airway pressure and adaptive servo-ventilation in the treatment of chronic complex insomnia. *EClinicalMedicine, 13*, 57–73. https://doi.org/10.1016/j.eclinm.2019.06.011

Krakow, B., Melendrez, D., Ferreira, E., Clark, J., Warner, T. D., Sisley, B., & Sklar, D. (2001). Prevalence of insomnia symptoms in patients with sleep-disordered breathing. *Chest, 120*(6), 1923–1929. https://doi.org/10.1378/chest.120.6.1923

Krause, A. J., Prather, A. A., Wager, T. D., Lindquist, M. A., & Walker, M. P. (2019). The pain of sleep loss: A brain characterization in humans. *Journal of Neuroscience, 39*(12), 2291–2300.

Kredlow, M. A., Capozzoli, M. C., Hearon, B. A., Calkins, A. W., & Otto, M. W. (2015). The effects of physical activity on sleep: A meta-analytic review. *Journal of Behavioral Medicine, 38*(3), 427–449.

Kribbs, N. B., Pack, A. I., Kline, L. R., Getsy, J. E., Schuett, J. S., Henry, J. N., & Dinges, D. F. (1993). Effects of one night without nasal CPAP treatment on sleep and sleepiness in patients with obstructive sleep apnea. *American Review of Respiratory Disease, 147*(5), 1162–1168.

Kripke, D. F. (2018). Hypnotic drug risks of mortality, infection, depression, and cancer: But lack of benefit. *F1000Research, 5*, Article 918. https://doi.org/10.12688/f1000research.8729.3

Lateef, T., Swanson, S., Cui, L., Nelson, K., Nakamura, E., & Merikangas, K. (2011). Headaches and sleep problems among adults in the United States: Findings from the National Comorbidity Survey–Replication Study. *Cephalalgia, 31*(6), 648–653.

Law, E. F., Wan Tham, S., Aaron, R. V., Dudeney, J., & Palermo, T. M. (2018). Hybrid cognitive-behavioral therapy intervention for adolescents with co-occurring migraine and insomnia: A single-arm pilot trial. *Headache, 58*(7), 1060–1073.

Lechat, B., Appleton, S., Melaku, Y. A., Hansen, K., McEvoy, R. D., Adams, R., Catcheside, P., Lack, L., Eckert, D. J., & Sweetman, A. (2022). Comorbid insomnia and sleep apnoea is associated with all-cause mortality. *European Respiratory Journal, 60*(1). https://doi.org/10.1183/13993003.01958-2021

Leduc, B. E., Dagher, J. H., Mayer, P., Bellemare, F., & Lepage, Y. (2007). Estimated prevalence of obstructive sleep apnea–hypopnea syndrome after cervical cord injury. *Archives of Physical Medicine and Rehabilitation, 88*(3), 333–337. https://doi.org/10.1016/j.apmr.2006.12.025

Leng, Y., Byers, A. L., Barnes, D. E., Peltz, C. B., Li, Y., & Yaffe, K. (2021). Traumatic brain injury and incidence risk of sleep disorders in nearly 200,000 US veterans. *Neurology, 96*(13), e1792–e1799. https://doi.org/10.1212/WNL.0000000000011656

Lequerica, A., Jasey, N., Portelli Tremont, J. N., & Chiaravalloti, N. D. (2015). Pilot study on the effect of ramelteon on sleep disturbance after traumatic brain injury: Preliminary evidence from a clinical trial. *Archives of Physical Medicine and Rehabilitation, 96*(10), 1802–1809. https://doi.org/10.1016/j.apmr.2015.05.011

Lew, H. L., Otis, J. D., Tun, C., Kerns, R. D., Clark, M. E., & Cifu, D. X. (2009). Prevalence of chronic pain, posttraumatic stress disorder, and persistent postconcussive symptoms in OIF/OEF veterans: Polytrauma clinical triad. *Journal of Rehabilitation Research & Development, 46*(6), 697–702. https://doi.org/10.1682/jrrd.2009.01.0006

Leysen, L., Lahousse, A., Nijs, J., Adriaenssens, N., Mairesse, O., Ivakhnov, S., Bilterys, T., Van Looveran, E., Pas, R., & Beckwée, D. (2019). Prevalence and risk factors of sleep disturbances in breast cancersurvivors:

Systematic review and meta-analyses. *Supportive Care in Cancer, 27*(12), 4401–4433. https://doi.org/10.1007/s00520-019-04936-5

Lin, C.-L., Liu, T.-C., Wang, Y.-N., Chung, C.-H., & Chien, W.-C. (2019). The association between sleep disorders and the risk of colorectal cancer in patients: A population-based nested case–control study. *In Vivo, 33*(2), 573–579. https://doi.org/10.21873/invivo.11513

López, E., de la Torre-Luque, A., Lazo, A., Álvarez, J., & Buela-Casal, G. (2016). Assessment of sleep disturbances in patients with cancer: Cross-sectional study in a radiotherapy department. *European Journal of Oncology Nursing, 20*, 71–76. https://doi.org/10.1016/j.ejon.2014.12.008

Lu, W., Cantor, J. B., Aurora, R. N., Gordon, W. A., Krellman, J. W., Nguyen, M., Ashman, T. A., Spielman, L., & Ambrose, A. F. (2015). The relationship between self-reported sleep disturbance and polysomnography in individuals with traumatic brain injury. *Brain Injury, 29*(11), 1342–1350. https://doi.org/10.3109/02699052.2015.1043947

Lundetrae, R. S., Saxvig, I. W., Aurlien, H., Lehmann, S., & Bjorvatn, B. (2021). Effect of continuous positive airway pressure on symptoms and prevalence of insomnia in patients with obstructive sleep apnea: A longitudinal study. *Frontiers in Psychology, 12*, Article 691495. https://doi.org/10.3389/fpsyg.2021.691495

Luyster, F. S., Dunbar-Jacob, J., Aloia, M. S., Martire, L. M., Buysse, D. J., & Strollo, P. J. (2016). Patient and partner experiences with obstructive sleep apnea and CPAP treatment: A qualitative analysis. *Behavioral Sleep Medicine, 14*(1), 67–84. https://doi.org/10.1080/15402002.2014.946597

Macaulay, G. C., Galland, B. C., Boucher, S. E., Wiltshire, E. J., Haszard, J. J., Campbell, A. J., Black, S. M., Smith, C., Elder, D., & Wheeler, B. J. (2020). Impact of Type 1 diabetes mellitus, glucose levels, and glycemic control on sleep in children and adolescents: A case–control study. *Sleep, 43*(2), Article zsz226.

Maguire, R., Drummond, F. J., Hanly, P., Gavin, A., & Sharp, L. (2019). Problems sleeping with prostate cancer: Exploring possible risk factors for sleep disturbance in a population-based sample of survivors. *Supportive Care in Cancer, 27*(9), 3365–3373. https://doi.org/10.1007/s00520-018-4633-z

Mantua, J., Grillakis, A., Mahfouz, S. H., Taylor, M. R., Brager, A. J., Yarnell, A. M., Balkin, T. J., Capaldi, V. F., & Simonelli, G. (2018). A systematic review and meta-analysis of sleep architecture and chronic traumatic brain injury. *Sleep Medicine Reviews, 41*, 61–77. https://doi.org/10.1016/j.smrv.2018.01.004

Mantua, J., Mahan, K. M., Henry, O. S., & Spencer, R. M. (2015). Altered sleep composition after traumatic brain injury does not affect declarative sleep-dependent memory consolidation. *Frontiers in Human Neuroscience, 9*, Article 328. https://doi.org/10.3389/fnhum.2015.00328

Mathias, J. L., & Alvaro, P. K. (2012). Prevalence of sleep disturbances, disorders, and problems following traumatic brain injury: A meta-analysis. *Sleep Medicine, 13*(7), 898–905. https://doi.org/10.1016/j.sleep.2012.04.006

Maurer, L. F., Schneider, J., Miller, C. B., Espie, C. A., & Kyle, S. D. (2021). The clinical effects of sleep restriction therapy for insomnia: A meta-analysis of randomised controlled trials. *Sleep Medicine Reviews, 58*, Article 101493. https://doi.org/10.1016/j.smrv.2021.101493

McCarthy, B., Trace, A., O'Donovan, M., O'Regan, P., Brady-Nevin, C., O'Shea, M., Martin, A. M., & Murphy, M. (2018). Coping with stressful events: A pre-post-test of a psycho-educational intervention for undergraduate nursing and midwifery students. *Nurse Education Today, 61*, 273–280.

McDonough, R. J., Clements, M. A., DeLurgio, S. A., & Patton, S. R. (2017). Sleep duration and its impact on adherence in adolescents with Type 1 diabetes mellitus. *Pediatric Diabetes, 18*(4), 262–270.

Meira, E. C. M., Kryger, M. H., Morin, C. M., Palombini, L., Salles, C., & Gozal, D. (2021). Comorbid insomnia and sleep apnea: Mechanisms and implications of an underrecognized and misinterpreted sleep disorder. *Sleep Medicine, 84*, 283–288. https://doi.org/10.1016/j.sleep.2021.05.043

Meltzer, L. J., Williamson, A. A., & Mindell, J. A. (2021). Pediatric sleep health: It matters, and so does how we define it. *Sleep Medicine Reviews, 57*, Article 101425.

Menn, S. J., Yang, R., & Lankford, A. (2014). Armodafinil for the treatment of excessive sleepiness associated with mild or moderate closed traumatic brain injury: A 12-week, randomized, double-blind study followed by a 12-month open-label extension. *Journal of Clinical Sleep Medicine, 10*(11), 1181–1191. https://doi.org/10.5664/jcsm.4196

Menon, D. K., Schwab, K., Wright, D. W., & Maas, A. I. (2010). Position statement: Definition of traumatic brain injury. *Archives of Physical Medicine and Rehabilitation, 91*(11), 1637–1640. https://doi.org/10.1016/j.apmr.2010.05.017

Mogavero, M. P., DelRosso, L. M., Fanfulla, F., Bruni, O., & Ferri, R. (2021). Sleep disorders and cancer: State of the art and future perspectives. *Sleep Medicine Reviews, 56*, Article 101409. https://doi.org/10.1016/j.smrv.2020.101409

Mollayeva, T., Pratt, B., Mollayeva, S., Shapiro, C. M., Cassidy, J. D., & Colantonio, A. (2016). The relationship between insomnia and disability in workers with mild traumatic brain injury/concussion: Insomnia and disability in chronic mild traumatic brain injury. *Sleep Medicine, 20*, 157–166. https://doi.org/10.1016/j.sleep.2015.09.008

Monzon, A., McDonough, R., Meltzer, L. J., & Patton, S. R. (2019). Sleep and Type 1 diabetes in children and adolescents: Proposed theoretical model and clinical implications. *Pediatric Diabetes, 20*(1), 78–85.

Morawska, M. M., Büchele, F., Moreira, C. G., Imbach, L. L., Noain, D., & Baumann, C. R. (2016). Sleep modulation alleviates axonal damage and cognitive decline after rodent traumatic brain injury. *Journal of Neuroscience, 36*(12), 3422–3429. https://doi.org/10.1523/jneurosci.3274-15.2016

Nakase-Richardson, R., Sherer, M., Barnett, S. D., Yablon, S. A., Evans, C. C., Kretzmer, T., Schwartz, D. J., & Modarres, M. (2013). Prospective evaluation of the nature, course, and impact of acute sleep abnormality after traumatic brain injury. *Archives of Physical Medicine and Rehabilitation, 94*(5), 875–882. https://doi.org/10.1016/j.apmr.2013.01.001

Nathan, D. M., Cleary, P. A., Backlund, J.-Y. C., Genuth, S. M., Lachin, J. M., Orchard, T. J., Raskin, P., & Zinman, B.; Diabetes Control and Complications Trial/Epidemiology of Diabetes and Complications Interventions Study Research Group. (2005). Intensive diabetes treatment and cardiovascular disease in patients with Type 1 diabetes. *New England Journal of Medicine, 353*(25), 2643–2653.

Nguyen, S., McKay, A., Wong, D., Rajaratnam, S. M., Spitz, G., Williams, G., Mansfield, D., & Ponsford, J. L. (2017). Cognitive behavior therapy to treat sleep disturbance and fatigue after traumatic brain injury: A pilot randomized controlled trial. *Archives of Physical Medicine and Rehabilitation, 98*(8), 1508–1517. https://doi.org/10.1016/j.apmr.2017.02.031

Odegard, S., Sand, T., Engstrom, M., Stovner, L., Zwart, J., & Hagen, K. (2013). The impact of headache and chronic musculoskeletal complaints on the risk of insomnia: Longitudinal data from the Nord-Trondelag Health Study. *The Journal of Headache and Pain, 14*, 1–10.

Ohkuma, T., Fujii, H., Iwase, M., Kikuchi, Y., Ogata, S., Idewaki, Y., Ide, H., Doi, Y., Hirakawa, Y., Nakamura, U., & Kitazono, T. (2013). Impact of sleep duration on obesity and the glycemic level in patients with Type 2 diabetes: The Fukuoka Diabetes Registry. *Diabetes Care, 36*(3), 611–617.

Ong, J. C., Crawford, M. R., Dawson, S. C., Fogg, L. F., Turner, A. D., Wyatt, J. K., Crisostomo, M. I., Chhangani, B. S., Kushida, C. A., Edinger, J. D., Abbott, S. A., Malkani, R. G., Attarian, H. P., & Zee, P. C. (2020). A randomized controlled trial of CBT-I and PAP for obstructive sleep apnea and comorbid insomnia: Main outcomes from the MATRICS study. *Sleep, 43*(9), Article zsaa041. https://doi.org/10.1093/sleep/zsaa041

Ong, J. C., Dawson, S. C., Taylor, H. L., Park, M., Burgess, H. J., Crawford, M. R., Rains, J. C., Smitherman, T. A., Espie, C. A., Jones, A. L., & Wyatt, J. K. (2023). A micro-longitudinal study of naps, sleep disturbance, and headache severity in women with chronic migraine. *Behavioral Sleep Medicine, 21*(2), 117–128.

Ong, J. C., & Park, M. (2012). Chronic headaches and insomnia: Working toward a biobehavioral model. *Cephalalgia, 32*(14), 1059–1070.

Ong, J. C., Taylor, H. L., Park, M., Burgess, H. J., Fox, R. S., Snyder, S., Rains, J. C., Espie, C. A., & Wyatt, J. K. (2018). Can circadian dysregulation exacerbate migraines? *Headache, 58*(7), 1040–1051.

Orff, H. J., Ayalon, L., & Drummond, S. P. (2009). Traumatic brain injury and sleep disturbance: A review of current research. *Journal of Head Trauma Rehabilitation, 24*(3), 155–165. https://doi.org/10.1097/HTR.0b013e3181a0b281

Ouellet, M. C., Beaulieu-Bonneau, S., & Morin, C. M. (2006). Insomnia in patients with traumatic brain injury: Frequency, characteristics, and risk factors. *Journal of Head Trauma Rehabilitation, 21*(3), 199–212. https://doi.org/10.1097/00001199-200605000-00001

Ouellet, M. C., Beaulieu-Bonneau, S., & Morin, C. M. (2015). Sleep–wake disturbances after traumatic brain injury. *Lancet Neurology, 14*(7), 746–757. https://doi.org/10.1016/s1474-4422(15)00068-x

Ouellet, M. C., Savard, J., & Morin, C. M. (2004). Insomnia following traumatic brain injury: A review. *Neurorehabilitation and Neural Repair, 18*(4), 187–198. https://doi.org/10.1177/1545968304271405

Palesh, O., Roscoe, J., & Mustian, K. (2010). Prevalence, demographics, and psychological associations of sleep disruption in patients with cancer: University of Rochester Cancer Center-Community Clinical Oncology Program. *Journal of Clinical Oncology, 28*, 292–298. https://doi.org/10.1200/jco.2009.22.5011

Palesh, O., Scheiber, C., Kesler, S., Janelsins, M. C., Guido, J. J., Heckler, C., Cases, M. G., Miller, J., Chrysson, N. G., & Mustian, K. M. (2018). Feasibility and acceptability of brief behavioral therapy for cancer-related insomnia: Effects on insomnia and circadian rhythm during chemotherapy: A Phase II randomised multicentre controlled trial. *British Journal of Cancer, 119*(3), 274–281. https://doi.org/10.1038/s41416-018-0154-2

Palesh, O., Scheiber, C., Kesler, S., Mustian, K., Koopman, C., & Schapira, L. (2018). Management of side effects during and post-treatment in breast cancer survivors. *Breast Journal, 24*(2), 167–175. https://doi.org/10.1111/tbj.12862

Papadopoulos, D., Papadoudis, A., Kiagia, M., & Syrigos, K. (2018). Nonpharmacologic interventions for improving sleep disturbances in patients with lung cancer: A systematic review and meta-analysis. *Journal of Pain and Symptom Management, 55*(5), 1364–1381. https://doi.org/10.1016/j.jpainsymman.2017.12.491

Parcell, D. L., Ponsford, J. L., Redman, J. R., & Rajaratnam, S. M. (2008). Poor sleep quality and changes in objectively recorded sleep after traumatic brain injury: A preliminary study. *Archives of Physical Medicine and Rehabilitation, 89*(5), 843–850. https://doi.org/10.1016/j.apmr.2007.09.057

Park, J.-W., Chu, M. K., Kim, J.-M., Park, S.-G., & Cho, S.-J. (2016). Analysis of trigger factors in episodic migraineurs using a smartphone headache diary applications. *PLOS ONE, 11*(2), Article e0149577.

Paruthi, S., Brooks, L. J., D'Ambrosio, C., Hall, W. A., Kotagal, S., Lloyd, R. M., Malow, B. A., Maski, K., Nichols, C., Quan, S. F., Rosen, C. L., Troester, M. M., & Wise, M. S. (2016). Recommended amount of sleep for pediatric populations: A consensus statement of the American Academy of Sleep Medicine. *Journal of Clinical Sleep Medicine, 12*(6), 785–786.

Patel, N. J., Savin, K. L., Kahanda, S. N., Malow, B. A., Williams, L. A., Lochbihler, G., & Jaser, S. S. (2018). Sleep habits in adolescents with Type 1 diabetes: Variability in sleep duration linked with glycemic control. *Pediatric Diabetes, 19*(6), 1100–1106.

Pellegrino, A. B. W., Davis-Martin, R. E., Houle, T. T., Turner, D. P., & Smitherman, T. A. (2018). Perceived triggers of primary headache disorders: A meta-analysis. *Cephalalgia, 38*(6), 1188–1198.

Perfect, M., Frye, S., & Bluez, G. P. (2018). The effects of a sleep extension intervention on glucose control in youth with Type 1 diabetes. *Diabetes, 67*(S1), 849-P.

Perfect, M. M. (2014). The relations of sleep and quality of life to school performance in youth with Type 1 diabetes. *Journal of Applied School Psychology, 30*(1), 7–28.

Perfect, M. M., Patel, P. G., Scott, R. E., Wheeler, M. D., Patel, C., Griffin, K., Sorensen, S. T., Goodwin, J. L., & Quan, S. F. (2012). Sleep, glucose, and daytime functioning in youth with Type 1 diabetes. *Sleep, 35*(1), 81–88.

Perfect, M. M., Silva, G. E., Chin, C. N., Wheeler, M. D., Frye, S. S., Mullins, V., & Quan, S. F. (2023). Extending sleep to improve glycemia: The Family Routines Enhancing Adolescent Diabetes by Optimizing Management (FREADOM) randomized clinical trial protocol. *Contemporary Clinical Trials, 124*, Article 106929.

Permenter, C. M., Fernández-de Thomas, R. J., & Sherman, A. L. (2023). Postconcussive syndrome. In *StatPearls*. StatPearls Publishing. PMID: 30521207.

Peroutka, S. J. (2014). What turns on a migraine? A systematic review of migraine precipitating factors. *Current Pain and Headache Reports, 18*(10), 1–6.

Petit, J., Eren-Koçak, E., Karatas, H., Magistretti, P., & Dalkara, T. (2021). Brain glycogen metabolism: A possible link between sleep disturbances, headache and depression. *Sleep Medicine Reviews, 59*, Article 101449.

Philip, P., Bioulac, S., Altena, E., Morin, C. M., Ghorayeb, I., Coste, O., Monteyrol, P. J., & Micoulaud-Franchi, J. A. (2018). Specific insomnia symptoms and self-efficacy explain CPAP compliance in a sample of OSAS patients. *PLOS ONE, 13*(4), Article e0195343. https://doi.org/10.1371/journal.pone.0195343

Ponsford, J., & Schönberger, M. (2010). Family functioning and emotional state two and five years after traumatic brain injury. *Journal of the International Neuropsychological Society, 16*(2), 306–317. https://doi.org/10.1017/s1355617709991342

Ponsford, J. L., Parcell, D. L., Sinclair, K. L., Roper, M., & Rajaratnam, S. M. (2013). Changes in sleep patterns following traumatic brain injury: A controlled study. *Neurorehabilitation and Neural Repair, 27*(7), 613–621. https://doi.org/10.1177/1545968313481283

Potter, R. L., Moore, E. M., & Lopez, R. M. (2022). Effects of physical activity timing and intensity on the occurrence and risk of nocturnal hypoglycemia in adolescents with Type 1 diabetes. *International Journal of Athletic Therapy and Training, 1*, 1–6.

Prince, C., & Bruhns, M. E. (2017). Evaluation and treatment of mild traumatic brain injury: The role of neuropsychology. *Brain Sciences*, *7*(8), Article 105. https://doi.org/10.3390/brainsci7080105

Quera Salva, M. A., Azabou, E., Hartley, S., Sauvagnac, R., Leotard, A., Vaugier, I., Pradat Diehl, P., Vallat-Azouvi, C., Barbot, F., & Azouvi, P. (2020). Blue-enriched white light therapy reduces fatigue in survivors of severe traumatic brain injury: A randomized controlled trial. *Journal of Head Trauma Rehabilitation*, *35*(2), E78–E85. https://doi.org/10.1097/htr.0000000000000500

Raikes, A. C., Dailey, N. S., Shane, B. R., Forbeck, B., Alkozei, A., & Killgore, W. D. S. (2020). Daily morning blue light therapy improves daytime sleepiness, sleep quality, and quality of life following a mild traumatic brain injury. *Journal of Head Trauma Rehabilitation*, *35*(5), E405–E421. https://doi.org/10.1097/htr.0000000000000579

Rains, J. C. (2018). Sleep and migraine: Assessment and treatment of comorbid sleep disorders. *Headache*, *58*(7), 1074–1091.

Rao, V., Spiro, J., Vaishnavi, S., Rastogi, P., Mielke, M., Noll, K., Cornwell, E., Schretlen, D., & Makley, M. (2008). Prevalence and types of sleep disturbances acutely after traumatic brain injury. *Brain Injury*, *22*(5), 381–386. https://doi.org/10.1080/02699050801935260

Rasmussen, M. S., Arango-Lasprilla, J. C., Andelic, N., Nordenmark, T. H., & Soberg, H. L. (2020). Mental health and family functioning in patients and their family members after traumatic brain injury: A cross-sectional study. *Brain Sciences*, *10*(10), Article 670. https://doi.org/10.3390/brainsci10100670

Ravyts, S. G., Dzierzewski, J. M., Perez, E., Donovan, E. K., & Dautovich, N. D. (2021). Sleep health as measured by RU SATED: A psychometric evaluation. *Behavioral Sleep Medicine*, *19*(1), 48–56.

Rechenberg, K., Griggs, S., Jeon, S., Redeker, N., Yaggi, H. K., & Grey, M. (2020). Sleep and glycemia in youth with Type 1 diabetes. *Journal of Pediatric Health Care*, *34*(4), 315–324.

Ree, M., Junge, M., & Cunnington, D. (2017). Australasian Sleep Association position statement regarding the use of psychological/behavioral treatments in the management of insomnia in adults. *Sleep Medicine*, *36*, S43–S47.

RePORTER. (2022). *Stepped-care management of insomnia co-occuring with sleep apnea*. Retrieved August 11, 2022, from https://reporter.nih.gov/search/KjF1M0W7e0y7XKqtBgQ9PQ/project-details/9969403

Reutrakul, S., Thakkinstian, A., Anothaisintawee, T., Chontong, S., Borel, A.-L., Perfect, M. M., Janovsky, C. C. P. S., Kessler, R., Schultes, B., Harsch, I. A., van Dijk, M., Bouhassira, D., Matejko, B., Lipton, R. B., Suwannalai, P., Chirakalwasan, N., Schober, A. K., & Knutson, K. L. (2016). Sleep characteristics in Type 1 diabetes and associations with glycemic control: Systematic review and meta-analysis. *Sleep Medicine*, *23*, 26–45.

Reynolds-Cowie, P., & Fleming, L. (2021). Living with persistent insomnia after cancer: A qualitative analysis of impact and management. *British Journal of Health Psychology*, *26*(1), 33–49. https://doi.org/10.1111/bjhp.12446

Riemann, D., Spiegelhalder, K., Nissen, C., Hirscher, V., Baglioni, C., & Feige, B. (2012). REM sleep instability—A new pathway for insomnia? *Pharmacopsychiatry*, *45*(5), 167–176. https://doi.org/10.1055/s-0031-1299721

Robertson, J. A., Broomfield, N. M., & Espie, C. A. (2007). Prospective comparison of subjective arousal during the pre-sleep period in primary sleep-onset insomnia and normal sleepers. *Journal of Sleep Research*, *16*(2), 230–238. https://doi.org/10.1111/j.1365-2869.2007.00579.x

Roenneberg, T., Kuehnle, T., Pramstaller, P. P., Ricken, J., Havel, M., Guth, A., & Merrow, M. (2004). A marker for the end of adolescence. *Current Biology*, *14*(24), R1038–R1039.

Roh, H. W., Choi, S. J., Jo, H., Kim, D., Choi, J.-g., Son, S. J., & Joo, E. Y. (2022). Associations of actigraphy derived rest activity patterns and circadian phase with clinical symptoms and polysomnographic parameters in chronic insomnia disorders. *Scientific Reports*, *12*(1), Article 4895. https://doi.org/10.1038/s41598-022-08899-2

Rose, S., Boucher, S. E., Galland, B. C., Wiltshire, E. J., Stanley, J., Smith, C., de Bock, M. I., Rayns, J. A., MacKenzie, K. E. & Wheeler, B. J. (2021). Impact of high-risk glycemic control on habitual sleep patterns and sleep quality among youth (13–20 years) with Type 1 diabetes mellitus compared to controls without diabetes. *Pediatric Diabetes*, *22*(5), 823–831.

Rose, S., Haszard, J. J., Galland, B. C., Wiltshire, E. J., de Bock, M. I., Smart, C. E., Ketu-McKenzie, M., Campbell, A., Thomson, R., Jefferies, C. A., Wheeler, B. J., & Jefferies, C. A. (2022). The OPTIMISE study protocol: A multicentre optimisation trial comparing continuous glucose monitoring, snacking habits, sleep extension and values-guided self-care interventions to improve glucose time-in-range in young people (13–20 years) with Type 1 diabetes. *Journal of Diabetes & Metabolic Disorders, 21*(2), 2023–2033.

Rotty, M. C., Suehs, C. M., Mallet, J. P., Martinez, C., Borel, J. C., Rabec, C., Bertelli, F., Bourdin, A., Molinari, N., & Jaffuel, D. (2021). Mask side-effects in long-term CPAP-patients impact adherence and sleepiness: The InterfaceVent real-life study. *Respiratory Research, 22*(1), 17. https://doi.org/10.1186/s12931-021-01618-x

Sands, S. A., Terrill, P. I., Edwards, B. A., Taranto Montemurro, L., Azarbarzin, A., Marques, M., de Melo, C. M., Loring, S. H., Butler, J. P., White, D. P., & Wellman, A. (2018). Quantifying the arousal threshold using polysomnography in obstructive sleep apnea. *Sleep, 41*(1), Article zsx183. https://doi.org/10.1093/sleep/zsx183

Sandsmark, D. K., Elliott, J. E., & Lim, M. M. (2017). Sleep–wake disturbances after traumatic brain injury: Synthesis of human and animal studies. *Sleep, 40*(5), Article zsx044. https://doi.org/10.1093/sleep/zsx044

Saunders, T. J., McIsaac, T., Campbell, J., Douillette, K., Janssen, I., Tomasone, J. R., Ross-White, A., Prince, S. A., & Chaput, J.-P. (2022). Timing of sedentary behaviour and access to sedentary activities in the bedroom and their association with sleep quality and duration in children and youth: A systematic review. *Health Promotion and Chronic Disease Prevention in Canada: Research, Policy and Practice, 42*(4), 139–149.

Savard, J., Ivers, H., Savard, M.-H., Morin, C. M., Caplette-Gingras, A., Bouchard, S., & Lacroix, G. (2021). Efficacy of a stepped care approach to deliver cognitive-behavioral therapy for insomnia in cancer patients: a noninferiority randomized controlled trial. *Sleep, 44*(11), Article zsab166. https://doi.org/10.1093/sleep/zsab166

Savard, J., Ivers, H., Villa, J., Caplette-Gingras, A., & Morin, C. M. (2011). Natural course of insomnia comorbid with cancer: An 18-month longitudinal study. *Journal of Clinical Oncology, 29*(26), 3580–3586. https://doi.org/10.1200/jco.2010.33.2247

Schieber, K., Niecke, A., Geiser, F., Erim, Y., Bergelt, C., Büttner-Teleaga, A., Maatouk, I., Stein, B., Teufel, M., Wickert, M., Wuensch, A., & Weis, J. (2019). The course of cancer-related insomnia: Don't expect it to disappear after cancer treatment. *Sleep Medicine, 58*, 107–113. https://doi.org/10.1016/j.sleep.2019.02.018

Schipper, S. B., Van Veen, M. M., Elders, P. J., van Straten, A., Van Der Werf, Y. D., Knutson, K. L., & Rutters, F. (2021). Sleep disorders in people with Type 2 diabetes and associated health outcomes: A review of the literature. *Diabetologia, 64*(11), 2367–2377.

Shekleton, J. A., Parcell, D. L., Redman, J. R., Phipps-Nelson, J., Ponsford, J. L., & Rajaratnam, S. M. (2010). Sleep disturbance and melatonin levels following traumatic brain injury. *Neurology, 74*(21), 1732–1738. https://doi.org/10.1212/WNL.0b013e3181e0438b

Shi, T., Min, M., Sun, C., Zhang, Y., Liang, M., & Sun, Y. (2020). Does insomnia predict a high risk of cancer? A systematic review and meta-analysis of cohort studies. *Journal of Sleep Research, 29*(1), Article e12876. https://doi.org/10.1111/jsr.12876

Silberstein, S. D., Upton, R. B., & Goadsby, P. J. (2018). *Headache in clinical practice.* Routledge.

Silva, R. A., Ganen, A. D. P., Fernandes, V. d. F. T., Evangelista, N. M. d. A., Figueiredo, C. C., Pacheco, L. d. A., & Colares Neto, G. d. P. (2021). Evaluation of sleep characteristics of children and adolescents with Type 1 diabetes mellitus. *Revista Paulista de Pediatria, 40*, Article e2020407.

Sinclair, K. L., Ponsford, J. L., Taffe, J., Lockley, S. W., & Rajaratnam, S. M. (2014). Randomized controlled trial of light therapy for fatigue following traumatic brain injury. *Neurorehabilitation and Neural Repair, 28*(4), 303–313. https://doi.org/10.1177/1545968313508472

Sivertsen, B., Hysing, M., Harvey, A. G., & Petrie, K. J. (2021). The epidemiology of insomnia and sleep duration across mental and physical health: The SHoT study. *Frontiers in Psychology, 12*, Article 662572. https://doi.org/10.3389/fpsyg.2021.662572

Sivertsen, B., Lallukka, T., Salo, P., Pallesen, S., Hysing, M., Krokstad, S., & Øverland, S. (2014). Insomnia as a risk factor for ill health: Results from the large population-based prospective HUNT study in Norway. *Journal of Sleep Research, 23*(2), 124–132.

Skandsen, T., Nilsen, T. L., Einarsen, C., Normann, I., McDonagh, D., Haberg, A. K., & Vik, A. (2019). Incidence of mild traumatic brain injury: A prospective hospital, emergency room and general practitioner–based study. *Frontiers in Neurology, 10*, Article 638. https://doi.org/10.3389/fneur.2019.00638

Smitherman, T. A., Walters, A. B., Davis, R. E., Ambrose, C. E., Roland, M., Houle, T. T., & Rains, J. C. (2016). Randomized controlled pilot trial of behavioral insomnia treatment for chronic migraine with comorbid insomnia. *Headache, 56*(2), 276–291.

Spielman, A. J., Caruso, L. S., & Glovinsky, P. B. (1987). A behavioral perspective on insomnia treatment. *Psychiatric Clinics of North America, 10*(4), 541–553.

Squires, L. R., Rash, J. A., Fawcett, J., & Garland, S. N. (2022). Systematic review and meta-analysis of cognitive-behavioural therapy for insomnia on subjective and actigraphy-measured sleep and comorbid symptoms in cancer survivors. *Sleep Medicine Reviews, 63,* Article 101615. https://doi.org/10.1016/j.smrv.2022.101615

Srisurapanont, K., Samakarn, Y., Kamklong, B., Siratrairat, P., Bumiputra, A., Jaikwang, M., & Srisurapanont, M. (2021). Blue-wavelength light therapy for post-traumatic brain injury sleepiness, sleep disturbance, depression, and fatigue: A systematic review and network meta-analysis. *PLOS ONE, 16*(2), Article e0246172. https://doi.org/10.1371/journal.pone.0246172

Staffe, A. T., Bech, M. W., Clemmensen, S. L. K., Nielsen, H. T., Larsen, D. B., & Petersen, K. K. (2019). Total sleep deprivation increases pain sensitivity, impairs conditioned pain modulation and facilitates temporal summation of pain in healthy participants. *PLOS ONE, 14*(12), Article e0225849.

Stewart, K., Shakarishvili, N., Michalak, A., Maschauer, E. L., Jenkins, N., & Riha, R. L. (2022). Treating sleep disorders following traumatic brain injury in adults: Time for renewed effort? *Sleep Medicine Reviews, 63,* Article 101631. https://doi.org/10.1016/j.smrv.2022.101631

Stocchetti, N., & Zanier, E. R. (2016). Chronic impact of traumatic brain injury on outcome and quality of life: A narrative review. *Critical Care, 20*(1), 148. https://doi.org/10.1186/s13054-016-1318-1

Stovner, L. J., Nichols, E., Steiner, T. J., Abd-Allah, F., Abdelalim, A., Al-Raddadi, R. M., Ansha, M. G., Barac, A., Bensenor, I. M. Doan, L. P., Edessa, D., Endres, M., Foreman, K. J., Gankpe, F. G., Gopalkrishna, G., Goulart, A. C., Gupta, R., Hankey, G. J., Hay, S. I. . . . Murray, C. J. L. (2018). Global, regional, and national burden of migraine and tension-type headache, 1990–2016: A systematic analysis for the Global Burden of Disease Study 2016. *Lancet Neurology, 17*(11), 954–976.

Strollo, S. E., Fallon, E. A., Gapstur, S. M., & Smith, T. G. (2020). Cancer-related problems, sleep quality, and sleep disturbance among long-term cancer survivors at 9-years post diagnosis. *Sleep Medicine, 65,* 177–185. https://doi.org/10.1016/j.sleep.2019.10.008

Sullan, M. J., Asken, B. M., Jaffee, M. S., DeKosky, S. T., & Bauer, R. M. (2018). Glymphatic system disruption as a mediator of brain trauma and chronic traumatic encephalopathy. *Neuroscience & Biobehavioral Reviews, 84,* 316–324. https://doi.org/10.1016/j.neubiorev.2017.08.016

Sullivan, D. P., & Martin, P. R. (2017). Sleep and headaches: Relationships between migraine and non-migraine headaches and sleep duration, sleep quality, chronotype, and obstructive sleep apnoea risk. *Australian Journal of Psychology, 69*(3), 210–217.

Sullivan, D. P., Martin, P. R., & Boschen, M. J. (2019). Psychological sleep interventions for migraine and tension-type headache: A systematic review and meta-analysis. *Scientific Reports, 9*(1), 1–8.

Sweetman, A., Lack, L., Catcheside, P. G., Antic, N. A., Smith, S., Chai-Coetzer, C. L., Douglas, J., O'Grady, A., Dunn, N., Robinson, J., Paul, D., Williamson, P., & McEvoy, R. D. (2019). Cognitive and behavioral therapy for insomnia increases the use of continuous positive airway pressure therapy in obstructive sleep apnea participants with comorbid insomnia: A randomized clinical trial. *Sleep, 42*(12), Article zsz178. https://doi.org/10.1093/sleep/zsz178

Sweetman, A., Lack, L., Lambert, S., Gradisar, M., & Harris, J. (2017). Does comorbid obstructive sleep apnea impair the effectiveness of cognitive and behavioral therapy for insomnia? *Sleep Medicine, 39,* 38–46. https://doi.org/10.1016/j.sleep.2017.09.003

Sweetman, A., Lack, L., McEvoy, R. D., Antic, N. A., Smith, S., Chai-Coetzer, C. L., Douglas, J., O'Grady, A., Dunn, N., Robinson, J., Paul, D., Eckert, D., & Catcheside, P. G. (2020). Cognitive behavioural therapy for insomnia reduces sleep apnoea severity: A randomised controlled trial. *ERJ Open Research, 6*(2), Article 00161-2020. https://doi.org/10.1183/23120541.00161-2020

Sweetman, A., Lack, L., McEvoy, R. D., Smith, S., Eckert, D. J., Osman, A., Carberry, J. C., Wallace, D., Nguyen, P. D., & Catcheside, P. (2021). Bi-directional relationships between co-morbid insomnia and sleep apnea (COMISA). *Sleep Medicine Reviews, 60,* Article 101519. https://doi.org/10.1016/j.smrv.2021.101519

Sweetman, A., Lechat, B., Appleton, S., Reynolds, A., Adams, R., & Melaku, Y. A. (2022). Association of co-morbid insomnia and sleep apnoea symptoms with all-cause mortality: Analysis of the NHANES 2005–2008 data. *Sleep Epidemiology, 2,* Article 100043. https://doi.org/10.1016/j.sleepe.2022.100043

Sweetman, A., Melaku, Y. A., Lack, L., Reynolds, A., Gill, T. K., Adams, R., & Appleton, S. (2021). Prevalence and associations of co-morbid insomnia and sleep apnoea in an Australian population-based sample. *Sleep Medicine, 82,* 9–17. https://doi.org/10.1016/j.sleep.2021.03.023

Teasdale, G., & Jennett, B. (1974). Assessment of coma and impaired consciousness. A practical scale. *Lancet, 2*(7872), 81–84. https://doi.org/10.1016/s0140-6736(74)91639-0

Theadom, A., Barker-Collo, S., Jones, K., Dudley, M., Vincent, N., & Feigin, V. (2018). A pilot randomized controlled trial of on-line interventions to improve sleep quality in adults after mild or moderate traumatic brain injury. *Clinical Rehabilitation, 32*(5), 619–629. https://doi.org/10.1177/0269215517736671

Theadom, A., Cropley, M., Parmar, P., Barker-Collo, S., Starkey, N., Jones, K., Feigin, V. L., & BIONIC Research Group. (2015). Sleep difficulties one year following mild traumatic brain injury in a population-based study. *Sleep Medicine, 16*(8), 926–932. https://doi.org/10.1016/j.sleep.2015.04.013

Tiseo, C., Vacca, A., Felbush, A., Filimonova, T., Gai, A., Glazyrina, T., Hubalek, I. A., Marchenko, Y., Overeem, L. H., Piroso, S., Tkachev, A., Martelleti, P., & Sacco, S. (2020). Migraine and sleep disorders: A systematic review. *Journal of Headache and Pain, 21*(1), Article 126. https://doi.org/10.1186/s10194-020-01192-5

Tobe, E. H., Schneider, J. S., Mrozik, T., & Lidsky, T. I. (1999). Persisting insomnia following traumatic brain injury. *Journal of Neuropsychiatry and Clinical Neurosciences, 11*(4), 504–506. https://doi.org/10.1176/jnp.11.4.504

Torres-Ferrús, M., Ursitti, F., Alpuente, A., Brunello, F., Chiappino, D., de Vries, T., Di Marco, S., Ferlisi, S., Guerritore, L., Gonzalez-Garcia, N., Gonzalez-Martinez, A., Khutorov, D., Kritsilis, M., Kyrou, M., Makeeva, T., Minguez-Olaondo, A., Pilati, L., Serrien, A., Tsurkalenko, O., . . . Lampl, C. (2020). From transformation to chronification of migraine: Pathophysiological and clinical aspects. *Journal of Headache and Pain, 21*(1), 1–12.

Uhlig, B., Engstrøm, M., Ødegård, S., Hagen, K., & Sand, T. (2014). Headache and insomnia in population-based epidemiological studies. *Cephalalgia, 34*(10), 745–751.

Van Dongen, H. P., Maislin, G., Mullington, J. M., & Dinges, D. F. (2003). The cumulative cost of additional wakefulness: Dose–response effects on neurobehavioral functions and sleep physiology from chronic sleep restriction and total sleep deprivation. *Sleep, 26*(2), 117–126. https://doi.org/10.1093/sleep/26.2.117

Van Dyk, K., Joffe, H., & Carroll, J. E. (2021). Sleep and endocrine therapy in breast cancer. *Current Opinion in Endocrine and Metabolic Research, 18*, 165–170. https://doi.org/10.1016/j.coemr.2021.03.007

Van Someren, E. J., & Riemersma-Van Der Lek, R. F. (2007). Live to the rhythm, slave to the rhythm. *Sleep Medicine Reviews, 11*(6), 465–484. https://doi.org/10.1016/j.smrv.2007.07.003

Vermaelen, J., Greiffenstein, P., & deBoisblanc, B. P. (2015). Sleep in traumatic brain injury. *Critical Care Clinics, 31*(3), 551–561. https://doi.org/10.1016/j.ccc.2015.03.012

Vethe, D., Kallestad, H., Jacobsen, H. B., Landrø, N. I., Borchgrevink, P. C., & Stiles, T. C. (2018). The relationship between improvement in insomnia severity and long-term outcomes in the treatment of chronic fatigue. *Frontiers in Psychology, 9*, Article 1764. https://doi.org/10.3389/fpsyg.2018.01764

Vgontzas, A., Li, W., Mostofsky, E., Mittleman, M. A., & Bertisch, S. M. (2021). Baseline sleep quality, stress, and depressive symptoms, and subsequent headache occurrence in a six-week prospective cohort study of patients with episodic migraine. *Headache, 61*(5), 727–733.

Vgontzas, A., & Pavlović, J. M. (2018). Sleep disorders and migraine: Review of literature and potential pathophysiology mechanisms. *Headache, 58*(7), 1030–1039.

Vgontzas, A. N., Fernandez-Mendoza, J., Liao, D., & Bixler, E. O. (2013). Insomnia with objective short sleep duration: The most biologically severe phenotype of the disorder. *Sleep Medicine Reviews, 17*(4), 241–254. https://doi.org/10.1016/j.smrv.2012.09.005

von Schnurbein, J., Boettcher, C., Brandt, S., Karges, B., Dunstheimer, D., Galler, A., Deller, A., Denzer, C., Denzer, F., Vollbach, H., Wabitsch, M., Roenneberg, T., & Vetter, C. (2018). Sleep and glycemic control in adolescents with Type 1 diabetes. *Pediatric Diabetes, 19*(1), 143–149.

Walker, J. M., Mulatya, C., Hebert, D., Wilson, S. H., Lindblad, A. S., & Weaver, L. K. (2018). Sleep assessment in a randomized trial of hyperbaric oxygen in U.S. service members with post concussive mild traumatic brain injury compared to normal controls. *Sleep Medicine, 51*, 66–79. https://doi.org/10.1016/j.sleep.2018.06.006

Walker, M. P., & van der Helm, E. (2009). Overnight therapy? The role of sleep in emotional brain processing. *Psychological Bulletin, 135*(5), 731–748. https://doi.org/10.1037/a0016570

Wallace, D. M., Sawyer, A. M., & Shafazand, S. (2018). Comorbid insomnia symptoms predict lower 6-month adherence to CPAP in US veterans with obstructive sleep apnea. *Sleep and Breathing, 22*(1), 5–15. https://doi.org/10.1007/s11325-017-1605-3

Wassing, R., Benjamins, J. S., Talamini, L. M., Schalkwijk, F., & Van Someren, E. J. W. (2019). Overnight worsening of emotional distress indicates maladaptive sleep in insomnia. *Sleep, 42*(4), Article zsy268. https://doi.org/10.1093/sleep/zsy268

Watson, N. F., Badr, M. S., Belenky, G., Bliwise, D. L., Buxton, O. M., Buysse, D., Dinges, D. F., Gangwisch, J., Grander, M. A., Kushida, C., Malhotra, R. K., Martin, J. L., Patel, S. R., Quan, S. F., & Tasali, E. (2015). Recommended amount of sleep for a healthy adult: A joint consensus statement of the American Academy of Sleep Medicine and Sleep Research Society. *Journal of Clinical Sleep Medicine, 11*(6), 591–592.

White, D. P. (2005). Pathogenesis of obstructive and central sleep apnea. *American Journal of Respiratory and Critical Care Medicine, 172*(11), 1363–1370. https://doi.org/10.1164/rccm.200412-1631SO

Wickwire, E. M., Schnyer, D. M., Germain, A., Williams, S. G., Lettieri, C. J., McKeon, A. B., Scharf, S. M., Stocker, R., Albrecht, J., Badjatia, N., Markowitz, A. J., & Manley, G. T. (2018). Sleep, sleep disorders, and circadian health following mild traumatic brain injury in adults: Review and research agenda. *Journal of Neurotrauma, 35*(22), 2615–2631. https://doi.org/10.1089/neu.2017.5243

Wickwire, E. M., Williams, S. G., Roth, T., Capaldi, V. F., Jaffe, M., Moline, M., Motamedi, G. K., Morgan, G. W., Mysliwiec, V., Germain, A., Pazdan, R. M., Ferziger, R., Balkin, T. J., MacDonald, M. E., Macek, T. A., Yochelson, M. R., Scharf, S. M., & Lettieri, C. J. (2016). Sleep, sleep disorders, and mild traumatic brain injury. What we know and what we need to know: Findings from a national working group. *Neurotherapeutics, 13*(2), 403–417. https://doi.org/10.1007/s13311-016-0429-3

Wittmann, M., Dinich, J., Merrow, M., & Roenneberg, T. (2006). Social jetlag: Misalignment of biological and social time. *Chronobiology International, 23*(1–2), 497–509.

Wolf, G., Cifu, D., Baugh, L., Carne, W., & Profenna, L. (2012). The effect of hyperbaric oxygen on symptoms after mild traumatic brain injury. *Journal of Neurotrauma, 29*(17), 2606–2612. https://doi.org/10.1089/neu.2012.2549

Wolfe, L. F., Sahni, A. S., & Attarian, H. (2018). Sleep disorders in traumatic brain injury. *NeuroRehabilitation, 43*(3), 257–266. https://doi.org/10.3233/NRE-182583

World Health Organization. (2019). *Classification of diabetes mellitus.*

World Health Organization. (2020). Cancer. Retrieved from https://www.who.int/news-room/factsheets/detail/cancer#:~:text=Key%20facts%201%20Cancer%20is%20a%20leading%20cause,and%20lack%20of%20physical%20activity.%20...%20More%20items

Yasseen, B., Colantonio, A., & Ratcliff, G. (2008). Prescription medication use in persons many years following traumatic brain injury. Brain Injury, 22(10), 752–757. https://doi.org/10.1080/02699050802320132

Ye, L., Pien, G. W., Ratcliffe, S. J., Bjornsdottir, E., Arnardottir, E. S., Pack, A. I., Benediktsdottir, B., & Gislason, T. (2014). The different clinical faces of obstructive sleep apnoea: A cluster analysis. *European Respiratory Journal, 44*(6), 1600–1607. https://doi.org/10.1183/09031936.00032314

Yeshayahu, Y., & Mahmud, F. H. (2010). Altered sleep patterns in adolescents with Type 1 diabetes: Implications for insulin regimen. *Diabetes Care, 33*(11), Article e142.

Zachariae, R., Amidi, A., Damholdt, M. F., Clausen, C. D., Dahlgaard, J., Lord, H., Thorndike, F. P., & Ritterband, L. M. (2018). Internet-delivered cognitive-behavioral therapy for insomnia in breast cancer survivors: A randomized controlled trial. *JNCI: Journal of the National Cancer Institute, 110*(8), 880–887. https://doi.org/10.1093/jnci/djx293

Zeitzer, J. M., Friedman, L., & O'Hara, R. (2009). Insomnia in the context of traumatic brain injury. *Journal of Rehabilitation Research & Development, 46*(6), 827–836. https://doi.org/10.1682/jrrd.2008.08.0099

Zhang, Y., Ren, R., Lei, F., Zhou, J., Zhang, J., Wing, Y. K., Sanford, L. D., & Tang, X. (2019). Worldwide and regional prevalence rates of co-occurrence of insomnia and insomnia symptoms with obstructive sleep apnea: A systematic review and meta-analysis. *Sleep Medicine Reviews, 45*, 1–17. https://doi.org/10.1016/j.smrv.2019.01.004

Zhou, E. S., Michaud, A. L., & Recklitis, C. J. (2020). Developing efficient and effective behavioral treatment for insomnia in cancer survivors: Results of a stepped care trial. *Cancer, 126*(1), 165–173. https://doi.org/10.1002/cncr.32509

Zielinski, M. R., McKenna, J. T., & McCarley, R. W. (2016). Functions and mechanisms of sleep. *AIMS Neuroscience, 3*(1), 67–104. https://doi.org/10.3934/Neuroscience.2016.1.67

Zollman, F. S., Larson, E. B., Wasek-Throm, L. K., Cyborski, C. M., & Bode, R. K. (2012). Acupuncture for treatment of insomnia in patients with traumatic brain injury: A pilot intervention study. *Journal of Head Trauma Rehabilitation, 27*(2), 135–142. https://doi.org/10.1097/HTR.0b013e3182051397

CHAPTER

43 Sleep in Patients With Substance Use Disorders

M. Elizabeth Cardoni, Bhanu Prakash Kolla, Mandilyn Graham,
Yosef Bronsteyn, *and* J. Todd Arnedt

Abstract

There is a bidirectional relationship between substance use disorders and sleep disturbances. Substance misuse, including chronic use of alcohol, cannabis, opioids, and cocaine, impacts both the subjective quality and objective measures of sleep. In turn, sleep disturbances, including insomnia, have been linked to the initiation, maintenance, and relapse of substance use disorder. This chapter summarizes recent research findings on the characteristics of sleep disturbances among individuals with substance use disorders. It then discusses available tools to aid sleep clinicians in diagnosing substance use disorders in their patients. Finally, it outlines key options and considerations for non-pharmacological and pharmacological treatments of sleep disorders in the substance use disorder population.

Key Words: substance use disorder, alcohol use disorder, alcohol, cannabis, opioid, cocaine, sleep disturbance, insomnia, nonpharmacological treatment

Introduction

In 2023, an estimated 17.1% of the US population aged 12 years and above met *Diagnostic and Statistical Manual of Mental Disorders*, fifth edition (DSM-5) criteria for substance use disorders (SUDs) (Substance Abuse and Mental Health Services Administration, 2024). Recent data indicates that the COVID-19 pandemic has contributed to an increase in overall substance use, with 13% of US adults reporting initiating or increasing substance use to help cope with the stress of the pandemic (Czeisler et al., 2020). In patients with SUD, sleep disturbances are common. One study found that nearly 70% of inpatients seeking detoxification from various substances reported sleep problems prior to their admission and that 80% of them attributed these sleep difficulties to their substance misuse (Roncero et al., 2011). The bidirectional relationship between SUD and sleep problems has been well established, with recent studies suggesting that sleep plays an important role in the initiation, maintenance, and relapse of SUD, most significantly with alcohol misuse, and that SUD, in turn, contributes to disturbances of sleep.

For these reasons, it is essential that sleep clinicians understand the sleep difficulties that are likely to present in patients with SUD during active substance use and with withdrawal and abstinence. This chapter aims to provide information of clinical relevance to the sleep specialist by (1) outlining the subjective and objective sleep disturbances present in adults with the most common SUDs (alcohol, cannabis, opioids, and cocaine), (2) presenting a brief description of screening tools that can be used to identify SUD in a clinical sleep population, and (3) outlining current findings on treatment options and considerations for sleep clinicians managing sleep disorders in people with SUD.

Prevalence of SUD

The rates of substance use and SUD in the general population have shifted in recent years. Most US adults (72%) endorsed alcohol use in the past year (Grant et al., 2017), and just over half of people aged 12 or above (50.8%) endorsed alcohol use in the past month (SAMHSA, 2020). The prevalence of alcohol use disorder (AUD) had decreased, with approximately 5.3% of the US population meeting criteria for AUD in 2019 (SAMHSA, 2020). However, there has been a COVID-19 pandemic–related increase in overall alcohol consumption and heavy drinking, which was more pronounced in women (Pollard et al., 2020).

Conversely, the increasing acceptance and legalization of recreational cannabis use has coincided with a substantial increase in its use in the general population, making it the most used illicit substance: Close to 17.5% of people aged 12 or above reported using cannabis in the previous year, and 1.8% met criteria for cannabis use disorder (SAMHSA, 2020). The United States is also currently amid the fourth wave of the opioid epidemic, resulting in an increased use of synthetic opioids and psychostimulants (Blanco et al., 2020). Roughly 0.3% of the US population endorsed heroin use in 2019, and close to two million people aged 12 or above meet criteria for an opioid use disorder (SAMHSA, 2020). The pandemic has also impacted opioid use patterns, with a significant increase in opioid use–related emergency department visits, which has exceeded the pre-pandemic baseline (Venkatesh et al., 2022). In 2019, approximately 5.5 million people aged 12 or above reported using cocaine in the last year (SAMHSA, 2020). Overall, the prevalence of SUD continues to remain quite high, and there has been a significant pandemic-related increase in the use of alcohol and other drugs, with a consequent significant increase in morbidity and mortality associated with these conditions.

Diagnostic Criteria for SUD

The DSM-5 made substantial changes to the way SUDs are classified, including that prior classifications were dropped in favor of severity indicators of diagnoses (mild, moderate, or severe; American Psychiatric Association, 2013). Among the criteria themselves, the DSM-5 classification system added *craving*, which is defined as a strong subjective desire to obtain/use the substance. These diagnostic criteria are consistent across all classes of

Box 43.1 Diagnostic criteria for substance use disorders

- Taken in larger quantities/longer periods
- Desire/unsuccessful efforts to cut down
- Time spent obtaining/using
- Failure to fulfill role obligations
- Use despite social/interpersonal problems
- Recurrent use in physically hazardous situations
- Important social, occupational/recreational activities given up
- Use despite physical/psychological problems
- Tolerance
- Withdrawal
- Craving

Mild: 2–3 Moderate: 4–5 Severe: ≥6

Note. Adapted from American Psychiatric Association (2013).

substances (see Box 43.1). In addition, the DSM-5 substance-related disorders are further divided into two groups: SUD and substance-induced disorders. The substance-induced disorders include intoxication, withdrawal, and other substance/medication-induced mental disorders. Of relevance to sleep specialists, patients with both SUD and substance-induced disorders can experience sleep disruption.

Screening for SUD

A thorough history and clinical exam continue to remain the foundation for making an SUD diagnosis. However, screening tools and targeted testing can significantly aid clinicians in identifying patients who might be at higher risk of SUD, allowing for appropriate counseling and referral.

Screening Tools

The Alcohol Use Disorder Identification Test (AUDIT) is a 10-item questionnaire that is considered the gold standard in screening for AUD. A shorter version, the AUDIT-C, a three-item questionnaire scored on a scale of 0–12 with cutoffs of 3, providing a sensitivity of 90%–98% and specificity of 60% in identifying AUD (Bush et al., 1998), is a more user-friendly option for busy clinical sleep practices. The Cannabis Use Disorder Identification Test is an eight-item questionnaire helpful in identifying potentially hazardous cannabis use (scores ≥8) or cannabis use disorder (scores ≥13) to guide future clinical follow-up (Adamson et al., 2010). The Drug Abuse Screening Test is a 10-item questionnaire that helps identify patients with risky/harmful/severe drug use and allows clinicians to detect patients who might require a referral to a specialized service. Identification of patients at high risk of drug abusive behaviors is critical when considering opioids as a rescue treatment option for patients with refractory restless legs syndrome. The opioid risk tool is a self-reported screening instrument that can identify these patients, and it is standard practice to administer this assessment prior to prescribing opioids (Webster, 2005).

Drug Testing in Sleep Practices

Current guidelines indicate that drug testing, such as a urine drug screen, should be considered in patients undergoing multiple sleep latency testing (Krahn et al., 2021). Studies have shown that up to 33% of patients undergoing this testing have positive urine drug screens, with about 80% of them not having reported the use of the drug prior to testing (Kosky et al., 2016). Drug testing is also an integral part of opioid prescribing contracts in patients on chronic opioid therapy, and sleep practices should partner with addiction services with expertise in conduct and interpretation of these tests (Kosky et al., 2016).

Characteristics of Sleep Disturbances in SUDs

Alcohol

SUBJECTIVE REPORTS

Insomnia symptoms are reported by 36%–91% of people who are actively drinking, and sleep complaints are positively associated with alcohol problem severity during all stages of AUD (Chakravorty et al., 2016; He et al., 2019). Among treatment-seeking patients with AUD, 32% report insomnia as a withdrawal symptom (Brower & Perron, 2010). During early recovery, 70% report persistent symptoms, and more than 50% continue to experience symptoms after several weeks of abstinence (Brower et al., 2001; Brower, Krentzman, & Robinson, 2011; Chaudhary et al., 2015; Kolla et al., 2014). In one study, more than half (53%, n = 267) of individuals with persistent insomnia at 6-month follow-up had significantly reduced or discontinued alcohol use (Brower, Krentzman, & Robinson, 2011).

Insomnia is experienced across all phases of the night in patients with AUD. One study demonstrated that 62% (n = 302) reported sleep-onset insomnia, 57% reported sleep-maintenance insomnia, and 41% complained of early-morning awakenings (Zhabenko et al., 2012). Risk factors for insomnia in this population include more severe addiction, earlier age of alcohol use onset, frequent use of alcohol as a sleep aid, concomitant drug use, and psychiatric comorbidities (Brower, 2015; Zhabenko et al., 2012).

OBJECTIVE FINDINGS

Most polysomnography studies have been conducted in treatment-seeking patients with AUD, rather than those actively drinking; and samples have been generally small and heterogeneous. Some early studies administered alcohol to small numbers of actively drinking male participants in inpatient settings and found that alcohol generally increased slow-wave sleep (SWS) and reduced rapid eye movement (REM), findings that were reversed during withdrawal (Gross & Best, 1975; Gross et al., 1973; Wagman & Allen, 1975). Cross-sectional, observational studies evaluating sleep among individuals recovering from AUD using polysomnography are consistent with complaints of insomnia. Compared to healthy controls, patients with AUD in early abstinence have less total sleep time, take longer to fall asleep, and experience more nighttime wakefulness (wake after sleep onset) in addition to disrupted sleep architecture, characterized by more light Stage 1 sleep, less deep SWS, and increased REM sleep (Gann et al., 2001, 2004; Gillin et al., 1990a; Le Bon et al., 1997). Objective sleep disturbances may be more pronounced in older individuals (Brower & Hall, 2001), African Americans (Irwin et al., 2000), and individuals with comorbid depression (Gillin et al., 1990b). Age-related changes in SWS and REM may additionally be accelerated in individuals with AUD (Irwin et al., 2016).

Cross-sectional and longitudinal studies have found that subjective and objective sleep-related disturbances persist for up to 3 years into abstinence. In general, studies during recovery from AUD demonstrate some recuperation of sleep continuity (e.g., sleep efficiency), but arousals from sleep, stage changes, and REM sleep disruptions remained after 2 years of continued abstinence (Drummond et al., 1998; Williams & Rundell, 1981).

In addition to changes in sleep continuity and architecture, AUD significantly impacts circadian and homeostatic sleep regulatory systems. For instance, during acute alcohol withdrawal and with abstinence, overall melatonin levels are reduced (Schmitz et al., 1996; Wetterberg et al., 1992), and peak melatonin production may be delayed (Kuhlwein et al., 2003). One study found that, compared to healthy controls, individuals with AUD in early abstinence (57.9 ± 19.3 days abstinent) demonstrated a slower rate of rise and a lower maximal amplitude of dim light melatonin onset (Conroy et al., 2012). Several studies have suggested that the homeostatic sleep drive is disrupted in individuals with AUD during abstinence (Armitage et al., 2012; Brower, Hoffmann, et al., 2011; Colrain, Crowley, et al., 2009; Colrain, Turlington, & Baker, 2009; Irwin et al., 2000, 2002). One study, utilizing a partial sleep deprivation challenge, found that subjects with AUD in the first month of abstinence did not show an increase in slow-wave activity power during the first non-REM period of recovery sleep that is typical of healthy controls (Irwin et al., 2002). Another experimental study found that subjects with AUD after 3–12 weeks of abstinence had a diminished response to a 3-hour sleep delay compared to healthy controls, demonstrated by lower slow-wave activity power during the first non-REM period and a slower dissipation of slow-wave activity across the night (Armitage et al., 2012). These findings, in the context of other objective studies, strongly suggest that sleep homeostasis is disrupted in subjects with AUD, both at baseline and when subjected to a sleep deprivation or sleep delay challenge.

OTHER SLEEP DISORDERS

AUD may contribute to or exacerbate other clinically relevant sleep disorders, including obstructive sleep apnea (OSA), nightmares, restless legs syndrome, and sleep-related movement disorders (Garcia & Salloum, 2015; He et al., 2019; Chakravorty et al., 2016). Alcohol use has been shown to worsen OSA symptoms, especially in patients with a prior diagnosis of OSA or a history of snoring (Kolla et al., 2018), including prolonging respiratory events and lowering minimum oxygen saturation levels (He et al., 2019). In one study, OSA prevalence in treatment-seeking patients with AUD compared to controls was 19% versus 7% (<55 years of age) and 67% versus 31% (≥55 years of age; Aldrich et al., 1999). Nightmares are more prevalent during acute alcohol withdrawal than during active alcohol use and, while most frequent in the first week of abstinence, may still occur for several weeks into abstinence (Nielsen & Zadra, 2005). Periodic limb movements in sleep have been found to be both higher than (Gann et al., 2002) and not different from (Le Bon et al., 1997) healthy controls. Finally, despite studies indicating circadian abnormalities among subjects with AUD (Conroy et al., 2012; Kühlwein et al., 2003), no studies have evaluated circadian rhythm sleep–wake disorders in this population.

Cannabis

SUBJECTIVE REPORTS

Cannabis is the most used Schedule I substance in the United States (SAMHSA, 2020). Of the many unique compounds in cannabis, tetrahydrocannabinol (THC) and cannabidiol (CBD) are of particular interest. THC is the primary psychoactive component in cannabis, leading to a feeling of euphoria as well as subjective sleepiness, which may make it beneficial as a sleep aid (Babson et al., 2015). However, tolerance to the effects of THC on sleep develops quickly (Babson et al., 2015). CBD has differential effects on sleep depending on dose; a stimulating effect has been found at low doses, while moderate to high doses are generally sedating (Babson et al., 2015). Additionally, CBD may counteract the effects of THC, and the ratio of THC:CBD is likely to impact the subjective experience of sleepiness and effects on sleep (Babson et al., 2015).

Findings of subjective sleep quality changes with cannabis have been mixed. Subjects in one study reported a 30-minute decrease in sleep latency following cannabis use (Tringale & Jensen, 2011), and in another, roughly 65% (n = 1513) reported reducing their use of sleep medications after initiating medical cannabis, suggesting that cannabis is perceived as an effective sleep aid by its users (Piper et al., 2017). Conversely, other studies have found that daily and treatment-seeking cannabis users report poor overall sleep quality (Conroy et al., 2016; Pacek et al., 2017). In a cohort study of more than 800 adults seeking medical cannabis, more than half reported difficulties falling asleep (53%) or staying asleep (54%) at least twice weekly despite using cannabis for sleep; 25% of these individuals had symptoms almost nightly. Additionally, nearly two-thirds of respondents reported a worsening of insomnia during the previous 2 weeks as a result of cannabis withdrawal (Cranford et al., 2017).

OBJECTIVE FINDINGS

Chronic cannabis use is associated with increased sleep latency and decreased SWS in addition to subjective reports of poor sleep quality (Babson et al., 2017; Garcia & Salloum, 2015; Kesner & Lovinger, 2020). One study of 87 treatment-seeking cannabis users using unattended polysomnography found that 31% took longer than 30 minutes to fall asleep, only 19.5% obtained 7 to 9 hours of sleep per night, and more than half the sample had abnormal sleep efficiencies (<85%; Pacek et al., 2017). A recent study of 187 adults found that higher doses of cannabis per day were associated with more nighttime awakenings as measured by actigraphy, despite improved ability to fall asleep (Bell et al., 2022). Overall, the data suggests that any potential benefits observed with short-term use of cannabis for sleep are offset by the tolerance that develops with more chronic use.

Insomnia symptoms during withdrawal from chronic cannabis use have been a consistent finding (Babson et al., 2017; Huhn & Finan, 2022; Kesner & Lovinger, 2020), lasting from 1 to several weeks and frequently severe (Bonnet & Preuss, 2017; Budney et al., 2003, 2010; Ek et al., 2021). A review of 15 studies, comprising 8,000 cannabis-dependent/treatment-seeking persons, found that during withdrawal 41.5% reported trouble sleeping, 33.2% reported waking up too early, and 34.4% reported strange dreams. Latency to REM sleep is also consistently reduced during cannabis withdrawal (Gates et al., 2016). A small polysomnography study (n = 18) found that quitting cannabis after heavy use was associated with reduced sleep efficiency, total sleep time, and REM sleep, as well as increased sleep latency and periodic limb movements and more interrupted sleep overall, especially during the first 2 weeks of abstinence (Bolla et al., 2010).

Opioids

Opioids have several therapeutic uses including management of chronic pain, treatment of refractory restless legs syndrome, and as an adjunct to anesthesia. Opioids are also among the most misused licit drugs, and misuse frequently starts with appropriate use of prescription or other opioids for pain management. In fact, according to the National Institute on Drug Abuse (2021), 4%–6% of people who misuse prescription opioids will eventually transition to using heroin, and 80% of heroin users report initially abusing a different opioid. Heroin, a derivative of morphine, is a rapidly acting and addictive illicit opioid. As with most clinically used opioid medications, heroin is fairly selective for μ-opioid receptors, and sleep effects of these agents are mediated in part by the ventrolateral preoptic nucleus (Reid-Varley et al., 2020; Teichtahl & Wang, 2007). Buprenorphine, on the other hand, is a partial μ-opioid receptor agonist and is commonly used to treat opioid use disorder.

Adverse sleep outcomes have been documented in populations reporting current opioid use, during withdrawal and post-withdrawal periods, and in those recently initiating medication-assisted treatments for opioid use disorder, utilizing methadone, buprenorphine (Huhn et al., 2022), or diacetylmorphine (Chrobok et al., 2020). Daytime effects associated with sleep dysfunction, including excessive daytime sleepiness, daytime fatigue, and symptoms of depression, have also been observed (Cao & Javaheri, 2018). Notably, much of the research on sleep in opioid use disorder has been conducted with treatment-seeking samples, rather than in individuals actively misusing heroin or other opioids; thus, sleep findings may not extend to non-treatment-seeking users of both licit and illicit opioids.

SUBJECTIVE REPORTS

Subjective sleep disturbances and related daytime sleepiness are common complaints among patients about to initiate or receiving medication-assisted treatment. Studies have found that as many as 76% of patients report poor sleep quality in the month prior to initiating methadone maintenance therapy (Chen et al., 2017) and that 70%–90% of patients in active methadone maintenance therapy report poor sleep quality (Baldassarri et al., 2020; Finan et al., 2020; Stein et al., 2004). Among the most common sleep complaints in methadone maintenance therapy patients are night sweats, nightmares, and difficulty falling asleep (Ellis et al., 2022). These complaints are not always resolved with the initiation of therapy, and, in fact, new-onset sleep disturbances may emerge during treatment. One study found that 19% of patients developed a new sleep disturbance warranting medical intervention within 2 years of initiating methadone maintenance therapy for heroin dependence (Li et al., 2018). Patients reporting sleep disturbances have more severe disease and worse psychosocial functioning than individuals without sleep disturbance during treatment (Chen et al., 2017).

Insomnia during withdrawal from opioids is significant as studies suggest that sleep disturbance is persistent throughout withdrawal, recovery, and abstinence and that persistent sleep disturbance is associated with increased drug cravings (Lydon-Staley et al., 2017) and serves as a motivator for continued opioid use (Huhn et al., 2022).

OBJECTIVE FINDINGS

Objective sleep monitoring in people with opioid use disorder consistently demonstrates many deviations from standard values in healthy populations: Sleep efficiency, SWS, REM, total sleep time, and time in Stage N2 are all consistently decreased relative to healthy sleeper controls, while sleep latency, wake after sleep onset, and periodic limb movements are all increased (Finan et al., 2020; Mehtry et al., 2014; Teichtahl et al., 2001). One marker of particular importance in patients with opioid use disorder is sleep disordered breathing. Chronic use of opioids contributes to various abnormal breathing patterns, which may present as hypoventilation, hypoxemia, central or obstructive apneas, periodic breathing, and/or ataxic or uncoordinated breathing (Cao & Javaheri, 2018). Central sleep apnea is common in opioid use disorder, with one recent review of eight studies, comprising 560 subjects with opioid use disorder, demonstrating central sleep apnea in 24% of subjects (Correa et al., 2015). Other studies have found OSA to be more prevalent than central sleep apnea, with prevalence rates for OSA and central sleep apnea at 35.2% and 14.1%, respectively, in one study of 71 patients receiving methadone maintenance therapy (Sharkey et al., 2010). Furthermore, longer-duration methadone maintenance therapy is associated with a higher prevalence of sleep disordered breathing, underscoring the importance of consistent monitoring of sleep in opioid use disorder patients receiving long-term methadone maintenance therapy (Sharkey et al., 2010). Finally, while buprenorphine has a different mechanism of action from methadone, its use is also associated with significant central sleep apnea (Farney et al., 2013); thus, patients in buprenorphine maintenance therapy may also require long-term sleep monitoring.

Studies examining both subjective and objective sleep measures in methadone or buprenorphine maintenance therapy patients frequently report conflicting results, suggesting that more research into the mechanisms and relationships among different sleep measures in patients with opioid use disorder is required. This discrepancy is illustrated by a few studies: Sharkey et al. (2011) found that polysomnography and subjective sleep findings largely matched for patients receiving methadone maintenance therapy. In contrast, Finan et al. (2020) and Baldassarri et al. (2020) found that patients receiving either methadone or buprenorphine maintenance therapy reported improvements in sleep quality over time, despite objective findings indicating worsening sleep.

The objective sleep disturbances found during active opioid use disorder remain consistent during medication-assisted treatment, even following a detoxification period (Finan et al., 2020; Mehtry et al., 2014), and do not significantly change when monitored 6 and 12 months after the initiation of treatment (Peles et al., 2011). Following withdrawal, patients may experience a pronounced and protracted REM withdrawal and altered sleep–wake patterns (Huhn et al., 2022). When comparing patients who are abstinent following detoxification to those in medication-assisted treatment, the abstinent patients displayed fewer sleep disturbances, with no significant differences found between medication types (Chrobok et al., 2020). These findings suggest that monitoring for sleep disturbances remains equally important for patients with opioid use disorder at all stages of treatment and regardless of medications used.

Cocaine

Cocaine, derived from the coca plant, is a highly addictive stimulant. Many symptoms of cocaine use disorder have a significant impact on sleep patterns, including psychomotor agitation, significant changes in blood pressure, euphoria, and hypervigilance. Available data on sleep in this population is limited, especially for subjects actively using cocaine.

SUBJECTIVE REPORTS

The subjective sleep experience of chronic cocaine users is not consistent with objective reports (Angarita et al., 2014; Toda et al., 2003). On subjective measures, chronic cocaine users have reported sleep disturbances, including hypersomnia and daytime sleepiness, vivid/unpleasant dreams, and depressed mood, in addition to physiological changes during the withdrawal period. With continued abstinence, the subjective reports of sleep-related symptoms improve (Angarita et al., 2014, 2016; Matuskey et al., 2011; Morgan et al., 2006; Pace-Schott et al., 2005).

OBJECTIVE FINDINGS

During the initial period of abstinence, individuals diagnosed with cocaine use disorder demonstrate occult insomnia, defined as an objective worsening of sleep with no corresponding subjective change or improved subjective sleep quality (Angarita et al., 2016; Hodges et al., 2017). This period of occult insomnia can continue for months or longer. Following sustained abstinence, chronic users of cocaine are likely to experience further objective symptoms, including impaired vigilance, which can be a consequence of chronic insomnia (Morgan et al., 2006).

Objective sleep quality is likely to continue to decline throughout periods of abstinence, particularly at Days 14–17, as evidenced by increased sleep latency (Morgan et al., 2006, 2010). Morgan et al. (2008) also found that REM sleep, which is suppressed during acute cocaine use, is typically increased during the initial phase of abstinence. SWS has also been shown to increase during periods of abstinence, though not to the level of healthy sleepers in comparable age groups (Angarita et al., 2014; Matuskey et al., 2011; Morgan et al., 2010). Additional studies have demonstrated a near complete absence of SWS or Stage N3 sleep in a substantial proportion of subjects in the early stages of abstinence (Irwin et al., 2016; Morgan et al., 2006).

Clinical Relevance of Sleep in Substance-Related Disorders

The relationship between sleep disturbances and the development and maintenance of SUD is bidirectional. Alcohol and all drugs of abuse disrupt sleep and have consequences for next-day functioning (e.g., impaired alertness, cognitive functioning). These daytime impacts of sleep disturbance, including increased stress, mood disturbance, and greater sensitivity to pain, in turn may contribute to the initiation, maintenance, and relapse of SUD (T. Roehrs et al., 2021; T. A. Roehrs & Roth, 2015). Research has demonstrated that insomnia frequently precedes alcohol misuse, suggesting alcohol use as a sleep aid. In one longitudinal population-based study, patients with insomnia had a 75% higher risk of AUD compared to healthy controls, even while controlling for confounding factors (Lin et al., 2020). Further illustrating the bidirectional relationship, one review observed that sleep disturbances are prominent symptoms of nearly all substance-related disorders and that substance-related sleep disorders could account for a substantial proportion of all sleep problems, while 10% of all alcohol-related costs could be attributed to insomnia and other sleep disorders (Garcia & Salloum, 2015).

Substance use is consistently associated with a pattern of preference for later timing of activity or sleep, or having an evening chronotype (Gulick & Gamsby, 2018; Hasler & Pedersen, 2020). Later sleep timing may in turn promote substance use to cope with and mitigate the effects of circadian misalignment, or a mismatch between an individual's internal sleep–wake cycle and environmental schedules and demands (Chellappa et al., 2019). Circadian misalignment often presents when later sleep time conflicts with next-day obligations, such as school start times or a variable shift-work schedule. This sleep–wake mismatch accumulates sleep debt over time, which may contribute to behaviors to help "catch up" on sleep, such as sleeping in on days off. Attempts to catch up on sleep help to satisfy the homeostatic sleep need but also reinforce a later sleep time the following night, maintaining both circadian misalignment and insomnia (Wittmann et al., 2006); and substances may be used to cope with these disturbances (Brown et al., 2020; Gulick & Gamsby, 2018).

Sleep disturbances may also motivate differential use of substances to cope with next-day effects of disturbed sleep, such as alcohol or cannabis to reduce anxiety, cocaine to avoid sleepiness, or opioids to regulate affect (Booker et al., 2020; Conroy et al., 2016; Dolsen & Harvey, 2017; Lydon-Staley et al., 2017; T. Roehrs & Roth, 2018). Additionally, cannabis and alcohol may become reinforcers and lead to substance misuse through their ability to induce sleep in individuals with insomnia (T. A. Roehrs & Roth, 2015). Taken together, this data suggests that substance use functions to temporarily alleviate some sleep disturbances and their consequences and that people more susceptible to circadian misalignment, including adolescents and shift workers, may be at increased risk of relying on substances for this purpose (Brown et al., 2020; Edwards et al., 2015; Gulick & Gamsby, 2018).

Sleep disturbances in individuals with SUD are complicated by the effects of tolerance, withdrawal, and abstinence. Alcohol may provide short-term relief of sleep disturbances, but tolerance to these effects develops quickly, which then motivates increased use (Koob & Colrain, 2020; T. Roehrs & Roth, 2001, 2018). A similar process is observed with other substances, including cannabis and opioids for sleep (Babson et al., 2017; Reid-Varley et al., 2020; Winiger et al., 2021). Sleep disturbances are additionally associated with withdrawal following chronic use of alcohol, cannabis, cocaine, and opioids (American Psychiatric Association, 2013). Abstinence from any of these substances leads to disturbed sleep, which has further negative downstream effects, including negative affect, and may drive craving and impulsivity contributing to relapse (Valentino & Volkow, 2020). Further, given that sleep disturbances frequently persist despite sustained abstinence, individuals who learned to use substances to relieve insomnia may be at increased risk for relapse following treatment (Brower et al., 2001; Cohen-Zion et al., 2009; Matuskey et al., 2011; Reid-Varley et al., 2020; Thompson et al., 1995).

Sleep is additionally important to memory consolidation and extinction, both of which are required for learning non-reinforced drug associations necessary to recovery, suggesting another way in which sleep dysfunction may impact recovery (Valentino & Volkow, 2020).

Recognizing and treating sleep disorders may be an important preventive measure against future drug misuse and SUD (Valentino & Volkow, 2020) in all stages of treatment. Higher insomnia symptoms at the start of an intensive outpatient SUD treatment program were found to be associated with lower likelihood of treatment completion, regardless of SUD diagnosis (Wilkerson et al., 2019). Upon discharge from SUD treatment, sleep quality remains critical to long-term recovery. In fact, sleep-related relapse risk to AUD is greater than risks associated with age, marital status, employment, duration/severity of alcoholism, hepatic enzymes, and depression ratings (T. A. Roehrs & Roth, 2015). One study of individuals receiving inpatient treatment for AUD demonstrated that poorer subjective sleep quality at discharge predicted self-reported relapse to drinking 4 weeks later (Brooks et al., 2021). Another large multisite study found that a lifetime history of insomnia and hypersomnia prospectively predicted cocaine use 12 months following substance use treatment (Dolsen & Harvey, 2017). Collectively, these studies highlight the importance of managing sleep within the context of SUD treatment and recovery.

Treatment of Sleep Disturbances in AUD and SUD

Treatment Considerations

Sleep disturbances often require treatment in individuals with SUD, but the timing and choice of sleep treatment are of particular importance. Abstinence frequently does not guarantee resolution of sleep problems; thus, an independent evaluation of any sleep complaint in a patient with SUD should be undertaken, with particular attention to the onset and course of sleep complaints in relation to the pattern of substance misuse. Independent sleep-focused intervention is likely necessary when there is evidence that the sleep disturbance predated the SUD or persisted during prior episodes of abstinence. Signs and symptoms consistent with a sleep-related breathing disorder or another intrinsic sleep disorder should be addressed immediately following recommended guidelines (Adult Obstructive Sleep Apnea Task Force of the American Academy of Sleep Medicine, 2009) as these will not ameliorate with improvement in SUD alone and could hinder recovery. Insomnia complaints that persist beyond 1 month of abstinence are associated with daytime symptoms and cause concern or distress that should also be the focus of appropriate assessment and treatment. Insomnia symptoms can be characterized early in SUD treatment with daily sleep/wake diaries, which provide a simple, cost-effective means of evaluating the sleep problem while engaging the patient in the treatment process. Ideally, treatment of sleep disturbances would complement SUD treatment and support abstinence efforts.

Individuals with SUD have historically been excluded from randomized controlled trials (RCTs) of insomnia, so limited information exists on the efficacy and safety of most pharmacological and non-pharmacological insomnia treatments in this population. When subjects with SUD are included, most trials have included subjects with AUD, and the majority fail to use rigorous assessment methods for selecting patients with clinically defined insomnia. The use of sleep medications among patients with SUD deserves careful consideration because of the potential for misuse and overdose when mixed with alcohol or other substances. Given these considerations, providers who work with patients with SUD are frequently reluctant to prescribe hypnotics; and, as a result, insomnia is frequently undertreated in this population (Friedmann et al., 2003).

Pharmacological Treatments

BENZODIAZEPINES AND OTHER BENZODIAZEPINE RECEPTOR AGONISTS

Benzodiazepines and other benzodiazepine receptor agonists (e.g., zolpidem) are used during acute and subacute alcohol withdrawal (Aubin et al., 1994), but no controlled studies of these medications have been conducted post-withdrawal in individuals with SUD and insomnia. Most addiction treatment specialists discourage benzodiazepine-related hypnotics for chronic use in patients with SUD because of their potential for misuse, rebound insomnia when discontinued, and overdose when mixed with alcohol (Griffiths & Johnson, 2005; B. Johnson & Longo, 1998). In a small study of 20 daily cannabis users, extended-release (XR) zolpidem was found to attenuate some of the adverse effects of short-term cannabis abstinence on sleep architecture and resulted in improvements in sleep efficiency (Vandrey et al., 2011). When considering benzodiazepine-related medications for insomnia, it is recommended that a shared decision-making approach be followed with the patient with SUD, including a discussion of the benefits, harms, and cost of short-term use of these medications. In addition, patients should be closely monitored, and additional precautions may be taken, such as obtaining written informed consent about their potential for misuse, conducting urine drug screens as a condition for refills, and limiting the number of refills to support short-term use only.

ANTICONVULSANTS

Anticonvulsant medications have low abuse potential, and their anti-kindling effect may reduce the likelihood of relapse (B. A. Johnson et al., 2004). Carbamazepine (Malcolm et al., 2002) and gabapentin (Malcolm et al., 2007) were both found to be superior to lorazepam for treating sleep disturbance and sleepiness associated with acute alcohol withdrawal. Gabapentin also reduced the likelihood of drinking during withdrawal and in the immediate post-withdrawal week compared to lorazepam (Myrick et al., 2009). Gabapentin is sedating (likely through gamma-aminobutyric acid enhancement and glutamate modulation), is not metabolized in the liver, does not interact with other medication, and does not require blood monitoring for therapeutic concentrations, hepatotoxicity, and hematological toxicity (LaRoche & Helmers, 2004). Initial open-label studies found that it improved the sleep of recovering patients with AUD over 4–6 weeks of treatment and that it was superior to trazodone with fewer side effects (Karam-Hage & Brower, 2000, 2003). In a small RCT of treatment-seeking subjects with AUD and insomnia, the onset to heavy drinking was delayed in gabapentin-treated patients (1,500 mg at bedtime), but no subjective or polysomnography-measured sleep differences between gabapentin and placebo were found (Brower et al., 2008). However, subsequent larger trials of gabapentin, alone and as a combination treatment (Anton et al., 2009, 2011; Mason et al., 2014) in adults with AUD, found that drinking and subjective sleep disturbances improved more for gabapentin-treated subjects. Interestingly, the positive findings for alcohol and sleep outcomes did not generalize to the XR formulation of gabapentin (gabapentin enacarbil XR, 600 mg twice a day; Falk et al., 2019). Given the relative advantages of these medications in this population, future controlled studies of anticonvulsants with larger samples of patients with SUD and comorbid insomnia are needed.

ANTIDEPRESSANTS

Some antidepressants may be of use for treating insomnia in patients with SUD because of their sedating side effects and because depression frequently co-occurs with SUD. Trazodone has been used safely and effectively in uncontrolled studies of patients with alcohol dependence (Karam-Hage & Brower, 2003). One randomized controlled study found that polysomnography measures of wake after sleep onset, sleep efficiency, and total sleep time were improved more after the first night of trazodone 50–200 mg compared to placebo, but only wake after sleep onset improvements were sustained after 4 weeks of treatment. Clinical global impression scales and depression scores were more improved in the trazodone group, however (Le Bon et al., 2003). A subsequent 12-week double-blind study in patients with AUD and insomnia recruited from detoxification found that trazodone 50–150 mg at bedtime improved sleep quality relative to placebo, but the trazodone group showed less improvement in the proportion of days abstinent during the treatment phase and consumed more drinks on drinking days following medication discontinuation (Friedmann et al., 2008). It was hypothesized that m-chlorophenylpiperazine, a trazodone metabolite that exerts ethanol-like effects, may have induced craving during treatment and impacted the drinking outcomes. Discontinuation of trazodone may have also triggered withdrawal symptoms, including sleep disturbances, and contributed to relapse. This association between trazodone and increased relapse risk was not replicated in a large retrospective study of 283 patients evaluated 6 months following discharge from a residential treatment program (Kolla et al., 2011). Nevertheless, trazodone should be used with caution in patients with AUD, with close monitoring advisable if prescribed. Its benefits and harms in patients with other SUDs have not been evaluated.

Limited evidence supports the use of mirtazapine, an antidepressant with sedative and anxiolytic properties, in patients with SUD and comorbid depression, although findings on sleep outcomes have been mixed. In a small open-label study of 12 adults with AUD and comorbid depression, patients were treated with mirtazapine 15 mg daily for the first 2 weeks and then 30 mg daily for 6 weeks (Cornelius et al., 2012). Insomnia symptoms were reduced at 8 weeks as measured by the Hamilton Rating Scale for Depression, improvements that were maintained at 2-year follow-up (Cornelius et al., 2013). Depression scores and alcohol use also improved at both time points (Afshar et al., 2012; Cornelius et al., 2012, 2013). A 12-week RCT of mirtazapine 45 mg versus placebo in 24 people with cocaine dependence and depression found reductions in sleep latency over the first month, but these did not persist (Afshar et al., 2012). No differences in depression or substance use were observed.

Use of other antidepressants, such as tricyclics, is complicated because alcohol-induced changes in liver metabolism can result in decreased blood levels of these medications at typical doses, reducing their efficacy. No studies have been conducted at higher than typical doses in patients with SUD, and there is an added concern of overdose potential in a population that is prone to suicide. Nevertheless, one small randomized trial in patients with opioid use disorder and insomnia during withdrawal ($N = 27$) found that amitriptyline and lorazepam were equally efficacious for sleep disturbances, but the former caused more daytime sedation (Srisurapanont & Jarusuraisin, 1998). Taken together, these findings highlight the need for larger and better-controlled studies of sedating antidepressants in diverse samples with SUD and insomnia to determine their efficacy and safety in this population.

ANTIPSYCHOTICS

Antipsychotics also have sedating properties and are not prone to misuse, making them potentially useful for managing insomnia among patients with SUD. Quetiapine, an atypical antipsychotic with sedating and anxiolytic effects (Cohrs et al., 2004), has been the most widely studied for treating insomnia in patients with AUD. Early retrospective studies found that patients with AUD treated with quetiapine 25–300 mg had more days of abstinence, fewer hospitalizations, and reduced craving; but neither used validated sleep measures to assess sleep effects (Monnelly et al., 2004; Sattar et al., 2004). In a placebo-controlled 8-week pilot study of 20 treatment-seeking veterans with AUD and sleep disturbance, 400 mg of quetiapine XR at bedtime improved objectively measured wake after sleep onset more and insomnia symptoms faster than placebo (Chakravorty et al., 2014). The subjective findings from this pilot study were replicated in a 12-week RCT of quetiapine XR 400 mg in heavy-drinking patients with AUD, although quetiapine did not reduce alcohol consumption (Litten et al., 2012). However, a reanalysis of another randomized trial of treatment-seeking patients with AUD found that quetiapine did improve craving symptoms more than placebo among participants with insomnia (He et al., 2019). Although quetiapine may benefit insomnia in patients with SUD and have particular utility for those with co-occurring mood or psychotic disorders, its potential benefits must be weighed against its many side effects, including the potential for akathisia, increased periodic limb movements when used to promote sleep (Cohrs et al., 2004), and adverse metabolic effects.

MELATONIN AGONISTS

Ramelteon is a US Food and Drug Administration (FDA)–approved melatonin receptor agonist with sedative effects and low abuse potential (M. W. Johnson et al., 2006) that may be appropriate for patients with AUD who exhibit abnormal melatonin profiles (Kühlwein et al., 2003). Consistent with this hypothesis, a 4-week trial of ramelteon 8 mg at bedtime improved scores on the Insomnia Severity Index from 17.6 ± 3.6 to 9.8 ± 7.6, increased subjective total sleep time from 5.0 ± 1.0 to 6.3 ± 1.6 hours, and reduced subjective sleep latency from 50.3 ± 20.9 to 23.5 ± 21.4 minutes in a case series of five individuals with AUD who had been abstinent for 2–13 weeks (Brower, Conroy, et al., 2011). Agomelatine 25–50 mg, an antidepressant that shares with ramelteon agonistic action of melatonin receptors 1 and 2, improved sleep disturbances in nine patients with AUD treated for 6 weeks (Grosshans et al., 2014), although concerns of hepatotoxicity exist. Conversely, the only placebo-controlled trial of melatonin (5 mg) in 60 treatment-seeking adults with AUD found improvements in sleep disturbances after 4 weeks of treatment in both groups, with no significant differences between conditions (Gendy et al., 2020). Given demonstrated abnormalities in melatonin profiles in individuals with SUD and the positive safety profile of melatonin agonists in this population, further controlled studies are needed.

OTHER MEDICATIONS

Acamprosate, one of three FDA-approved medications for AUD, has been evaluated in two RCTs for its effects on sleep disturbances among subjects with AUD. The first, which evaluated two tablets of 333 mg three times daily initiated 8 days before alcohol withdrawal and for 15 additional days, found that acamprosate reduced wake after sleep onset and increased Stage N3 and latency to REM sleep compared to placebo (Luc et al., 2006). A subsequent larger trial in 592 patients with AUD found that the proportion of subjects with sleep disturbances at baseline (40.2%) reduced to 19.5% after 24 weeks of acamprosate compared to 26.1% following placebo (Perney et al., 2012). Finally, an individual patient data meta-analysis found that acamprosate reduced insomnia (as measured by the Short Sleep Index, a four-item index of sleep quality derived from the insomnia items on the Hamilton Anxiety and Depression Scales) more than placebo among 3,508 patients with AUD (–45% for acamprosate vs. –26% for placebo, $p < .001$; Perney & Lehert, 2018; Perney et al., 2015). Although more studies are needed in samples of patients with SUD and well-characterized insomnia, acamprosate may be a good choice for subjects with AUD and sleep disturbances.

Modafinil, a wakefulness-promoting agent with effects on dopamine neurotransmission and apparent effects on glutamate and other neurotransmitters (Ballon & Feifel,

2006), has been shown to decrease sleep latency and increase SWS compared to placebo among individuals with cocaine use disorder (Morgan et al., 2010). In an RCT of 57 treatment-seeking subjects, morning-dosed modafinil 400 mg increased deep SWS and was associated with a higher percentage of cocaine-free urine drug screens (52% vs. 26%), more consecutive days abstinent, greater survival of abstinence, and higher daily rates of abstinence compared to placebo. The increase in SWS mediated the higher rate of cocaine-free urine drug screens (Morgan et al., 2016). Although further confirmatory controlled studies are needed, modafinil may be uniquely suited as both a sleep and a substance use treatment for patients with cocaine use disorder.

Dual orexin-receptor antagonists, such as suvorexant, lemborexant, and daridorexant, may have the potential to both improve sleep disturbances and reduce withdrawal and craving in SUD (Campbell, Marchant, & Lawrence, 2020). Evidence from preclinical studies indicates that orexin antagonism can alter drug-seeking behavior (Flores-Ramirez et al., 2022), but studies of the effects of dual orexin-receptor agonists in humans are still lacking. One small placebo-controlled preliminary study of non-treatment-seeking subjects with cocaine use disorder found that suvorexant improved actigraphy-measured sleep and reduced cocaine craving more than placebo (Suchting et al., 2020). Other studies of suvorexant are being conducted in individuals with insomnia comorbid with AUD (Campbell, Norman, et al., 2020). The preliminary findings for these agents are encouraging, but additional controlled studies in individuals with insomnia and comorbid SUD are needed.

NON-PHARMACOLOGICAL TREATMENTS

Few studies have evaluated the efficacy of non-pharmacological approaches to sleep disturbances in patients with SUD. One early study found that sleep quality ratings improved more in a group of male inpatients with AUD following 2 weeks of daily progressive muscle relaxation training than no treatment (Greeff & Conradie, 1998). More recent studies have evaluated cognitive behavioral treatment for insomnia (CBT-I) in subjects with AUD (Arnedt et al., 2011; Chakravorty et al., 2019; Currie et al., 2004) and cannabis use disorder (Babson et al., 2015). The findings from these RCTs are summarized in Table 43.1.

An 8-week RCT of 17 subjects with AUD and insomnia found greater improvements in self-reported wake after sleep onset, sleep efficiency, and daytime functioning in CBT-treated participants (Arnedt et al., 2011). A larger controlled study randomized 60 outpatients with AUD to individual CBT-I (five sessions over 7 weeks), self-help manual with five telephone support calls, or wait-list control (Currie et al., 2004). Participants in both active treatment groups had greater post-treatment improvements than controls on diary measures of sleep quality, sleep latency, sleep efficiency, and number of awakenings; and treatment gains were maintained at 3- and 6-month follow-up. More recently, Chakravorty and colleagues (2019) randomized 22 male veterans with AUD to CBT-I

Table 43.1 Non-pharmacological treatment for comorbid insomnia and substance misuse

Substance	Author, year	*N*	Sample	Conditions	Treatment dose/ duration	Treatment vs. control	
						Effect on insomnia	Effect on substance use
Alcohol	Greeff & Conradie (1998)	22	Institutionalized male subjects with AUD	Treatment: PMR Control: None	10 sessions/2 weeks	↓	Not studied
	Currie et al. (2004)	60	Subjects in outpatient treatment for AUD	Treatment: CBT, self-help with phone support Control: Wait list	5 sessions/7 weeks	↓	↔
	Arnedt et al. (2011)	17	Abstinent subjects with AUD	Treatment: CBT Control: Behavioral placebo therapy	8 sessions/8 weeks	↓	↔
	Chakravorty et al. (2019)	22	Veteran sample with AUD	Treatment: CBT Control: Monitoring only	8 sessions/8 weeks	↓	↔
Cannabis	Babson et al. (2015)	4	Male veterans with CUD	Treatment: Mobile application–delivered CBT-I Control: Mood tracking mobile application	Daily use/ 14 days	↓	↓
	Short et al. (2021)	56	Trauma-exposed sample with regular cannabis use	Treatment: Brief behavioral treatment for insomnia Control: Wait list	4 sessions/4 weeks	↓	↓

Note. AUD = alcohol use disorder; CBT = cognitive behavioral therapy; CBT-I = CBT for insomnia; CUD = cannabis use disorder; PMR = progressive muscle relaxation.

or a monitoring only control for 8 weeks. CBT-treated subjects showed greater improvements in both insomnia symptom severity and self-reported sleep latency. Despite consistently finding improvements in sleep and daytime outcomes with CBT, none of the three studies found CBT to differentially impact drinking outcomes relative to placebo. Importantly, none of these studies was sufficiently powered to properly evaluate drinking outcomes; thus, further studies are needed.

Bright light therapy is another non-pharmacological treatment commonly used in the treatment of circadian rhythm and mood disorders, but its efficacy and safety have undergone only preliminary evaluation in patients with SUD. Schmitz and colleagues (1997) administered bright light therapy (3,000 lux) to 10 patients with AUD on Day 3 of alcohol withdrawal from 7:00 to 9:00 a.m. and from 5:00 to 9:00 p.m. Subjective sleep quality and objectively measured sleep latency, sleep efficiency, latency to SWS, and percentage of REM improved on the night following treatment and persisted on the subsequent night. Bright light treatment was administered for only 1 day, and sleep was not evaluated beyond the first post-therapy night, however. Given the potential circadian abnormalities in this population, bright light therapy and other therapies targeting the circadian timing system are worthy of further evaluation.

One study has tested the benefits of combining CBT-I and light therapy in SUD. Fifty-five adolescents (13–19 years of age) with insomnia or sleepiness who had completed an outpatient addiction treatment program participated in a six-session group treatment that included components of CBT-I, bright light therapy, and mindfulness-based stress reduction. Compared to non-completers, treatment completers had greater improvements in subjective sleep parameters (sleep latency, number of awakenings, total sleep time, sleep efficiency) and reported fewer drug use problems at 12-month follow-up compared to non-completers (Bootzin & Stevens, 2005). Participants with greater increases in total sleep time during treatment were also less likely to report aggressive ideation and actions (Haynes et al., 2006).

Conclusions and Future Directions

SUD clearly has an impact on sleep health, and that relationship has been shown to be bidirectional. When evaluating and treating sleep disturbances in this population, it is critical to recognize that sleep effects differ among substances and among stages of SUD (active use, withdrawal, and abstinence) and that effective management of sleep disturbances can be beneficial in promoting SUD recovery. While there are several sleep treatment options in this population, data on long-term SUD outcomes are limited.

There are several areas where further research is needed in this population. The current literature is limited by inconsistent definitions of insomnia, minimal assessment of comorbid sleep and psychiatric disorders, and small and heterogeneous samples of individuals with SUD. Most studies have evaluated sleep treatments as monotherapies in this population; thus, further investigations to evaluate combinations of sleep (pharmacological and non-pharmacological) and SUD treatments are needed to maximize benefits and mitigate harms. Another important future direction will be to examine the effects of polysubstance use on sleep. Misuse of multiple substances is common in the SUD population, and, in fact, nearly 50% of drug overdose deaths in 2019 resulted from abuse of multiple drugs (O'Donnell et al., 2020). For sleep medicine, it will be important to identify the effects of polysubstance misuse on sleep, especially considering that some substances may exert differing or opposite effects on sleep when taken together. Finally, further research into improving sleep in users of licit substances is warranted, which, in many states, includes cannabis. Certainly, many licit substances, including routinely prescribed medications, may adversely impact sleep; and appropriate intervention to mitigate these consequences will be beneficial.

References

Adamson, S. J., Kay-Lambkin, F. J., Baker, A. L., Lewin, T. J., Thornton, L., Kelly, B. J., & Sellman, J. D. (2010). An improved brief measure of cannabis misuse: The Cannabis Use Disorders Identification Test-Revised (CUDIT-R). *Drug and Alcohol Dependence, 110*(1–2), 137–143.

Adult Obstructive Sleep Apnea Task Force of the American Academy of Sleep Medicine. (2009). Clinical guideline for the evaluation, management, and long-term care of obstructive sleep apnea in adults. *Journal of Clinical Sleep Medicine, 5*(3), 263–276.

Afshar, M., Knapp, C. M., Sarid-Segal, O., Devine, E., Colaneri, L. S., Tozier, L., & Ciraulo, D. A. (2012). The efficacy of mirtazapine in the treatment of cocaine dependence with comorbid depression. *The American Journal of Drug and Alcohol Abuse, 38*(2), 181–186.

Aldrich, M. S., Brower, K. J., & Hall, J. M. (1999). Sleep-disordered breathing in alcoholics. *Alcoholism: Clinical and Experimental Research, 23*(1), 134–140.

American Psychiatric Association. (2013). *Diagnostic and statistical manual of mental disorders* (5th ed.).

Angarita, G. A., Canavan, S. V., Forselius, E., Bessette, A., Pittman, B., & Morgan, P. T. (2014). Abstinence-related changes in sleep during treatment for cocaine dependence. *Drug and Alcohol Dependence, 134*, 343–347.

Angarita, G. A., Emadi, N., Hodges, S., & Morgan, P. T. (2016). Sleep abnormalities associated with alcohol, cannabis, cocaine, and opiate use: A comprehensive review. *Addiction Science & Clinical Practice, 11*(1), 1–17.

Anton, R. F., Myrick, H., Baros, A. M., Latham, P. K., Randall, P. K., Wright, T. M., & Malcolm, R. (2009). Efficacy of a combination of flumazenil and gabapentin in the treatment of alcohol dependence: relationship to alcohol withdrawal symptoms. *Journal of Clinical Psychopharmacology, 29*(4), 334–342.

Anton, R. F., Myrick, H., Wright, T. M., Latham, P. K., Baros, A. M., Waid, L. R., & Randall, P. K. (2011). Gabapentin combined with naltrexone for the treatment of alcohol dependence. *American Journal of Psychiatry, 168*(7), 709–717.

Armitage, R., Hoffmann, R., Conroy, D. A., Arnedt, J. T., & Brower, K. J. (2012). Effects of a 3-hour sleep delay on sleep homeostasis in alcohol dependent adults. *Sleep, 35*(2), 273–278.

Arnedt, J. T., Conroy, D. A., Armitage, R., & Brower, K. J. (2011). Cognitive-behavioral therapy for insomnia in alcohol dependent patients: A randomized controlled pilot trial. *Behaviour Research and Therapy, 49*(4), 227–233.

Aubin, H. J., Goldenberg, F., Benoit, O., Gillet, C., Roullet-Volmi, M. C., & Barrucand, D. (1994). Effects of tetrabamate and of diazepam on sleep polygraphy during subacute withdrawal in alcohol-dependent patients. *Human Psychopharmacology: Clinical and Experimental, 9*(3), 191–195.

Babson, K. A., Ramo, D. E., Baldini, L., Vandrey, R., & Bonn-Miller, M. O. (2015). Mobile app-delivered cognitive behavioral therapy for insomnia: Feasibility and initial efficacy among veterans with cannabis use disorders. *JMIR Research Protocols, 4*(3), Article e3852.

Babson, K. A., Sottile, J., & Morabito, D. (2017). Cannabis, cannabinoids, and sleep: A review of the literature. *Current Psychiatry Reports, 19*, 1–12.

Baldassarri, S. R., Beitel, M., Zinchuk, A., Redeker, N. S., Oberleitner, D. E., Oberleitner, L. M., & Barry, D. T. (2020). Correlates of sleep quality and excessive daytime sleepiness in people with opioid use disorder receiving methadone treatment. *Sleep and Breathing, 24*, 1729–1737.

Ballon, J. S., & Feifel, D. (2006). A systematic review of modafinil: Potential clinical uses and mechanisms of action. *Journal of Clinical Psychiatry, 67*(4), 554–566.

Bell, K. A., Coleman, E., Cooke, B. G., & Keen, L. D. (2022). Recreational cannabis use is associated with poorer sleep outcomes in young adult African Americans. *Addictive Behaviors, 134*, Article 107399.

Blanco, C., Wiley, T. R., Lloyd, J. J., Lopez, M. F., & Volkow, N. D. (2020). America's opioid crisis: The need for an integrated public health approach. *Translational Psychiatry, 10*(1), Article 167.

Bolla, K. I., Lesage, S. R., Gamaldo, C. E., Neubauer, D. N., Wang, N. Y., Funderburk, F. R., & Cadet, J. L. (2010). Polysomnogram changes in marijuana users who report sleep disturbances during prior abstinence. *Sleep Medicine, 11* (9), 882–889.

Bonnet, U., & Preuss, U. W. (2017). The cannabis withdrawal syndrome: Current insights. *Substance Abuse and Rehabilitation, 8*, 9–37.

Booker, L. A., Sletten, T. L., Alvaro, P. K., Barnes, M., Collins, A., Chai-Coetzer, C. L., & Howard, M. E. (2020). Exploring the associations between shift work disorder, depression, anxiety and sick leave taken amongst nurses. *Journal of Sleep Research, 29*(3), Article e12872.

Bootzin, R. R., & Stevens, S. J. (2005). Adolescents, substance abuse, and the treatment of insomnia and daytime sleepiness. *Clinical Psychology Review, 25*(5), 629–644.

Brooks, A. T., Kazmi, N., Yang, L., Tuason, R. T., Krumlauf, M. C., & Wallen, G. R. (2021). Sleep-related cognitive/behavioral predictors of sleep quality and relapse in individuals with alcohol use disorder. *International Journal of Behavioral Medicine, 28*, 73–82.

Brower, K. J. (2015). Assessment and treatment of insomnia in adult patients with alcohol use disorders. *Alcohol, 49*(4), 417–427.

Brower, K. J., Aldrich, M. S., Robinson, E. A., Zucker, R. A., & Greden, J. F. (2001). Insomnia, self-medication, and relapse to alcoholism. *American Journal of Psychiatry, 158*(3), 399–404.

Brower, K. J., Conroy, D. A., Kurth, M. E., Anderson, B. J., & Stein, M. D. (2011). Ramelteon and improved insomnia in alcohol-dependent patients: A case series. *Journal of Clinical Sleep Medicine, 7*(3), 274–275.

Brower, K. J., & Hall, J. M. (2001). Effects of age and alcoholism on sleep: A controlled study. *Journal of Studies on Alcohol, 62*(3), 335–343.

Brower, K. J., Hoffmann, R., Conroy, D. A., Arnedt, J. T., & Armitage, R. (2011). Sleep homeostasis in alcohol-dependent, depressed and healthy control men. *European Archives of Psychiatry and Clinical Neuroscience, 261*, 559–566.

Brower, K. J., Kim, H. M., Strobbe, S., Karam-Hage, M. A., Consens, F., & Zucker, R. A. (2008). A randomized double-blind pilot trial of gabapentin versus placebo to treat alcohol dependence and comorbid insomnia. *Alcoholism: Clinical and Experimental Research, 32*(8), 1429–1438.

Brower, K. J., Krentzman, A., & Robinson, E. A. (2011). Persistent insomnia, abstinence, and moderate drinking in alcohol-dependent individuals. *The American Journal on Addictions, 20*(5), 435–440.

Brower, K. J., & Perron, B. E. (2010). Sleep disturbance as a universal risk factor for relapse in addictions to psychoactive substances. *Medical Hypotheses, 74*(5), 928–933.

Brown, J. P., Martin, D., Nagaria, Z., Verceles, A. C., Jobe, S. L., & Wickwire, E. M. (2020). Mental health consequences of shift work: An updated review. *Current Psychiatry Reports, 22*, 1–7.

Budney, A. J., Moore, B. A., Vandrey, R. G., & Hughes, J. R. (2003). The time course and significance of cannabis withdrawal. *Journal of Abnormal Psychology, 112*(3), 393–402.

Budney, A. J., Vandrey, R. G., & Stanger, C. (2010). Pharmacological and psychosocial interventions for cannabis use disorders. *Brazilian Journal of Psychiatry, 32*, 546–555.

Bush, K., Kivlahan, D. R., McDonell, M. B., Fihn, S. D., Bradley, K. A., & Ambulatory Care Quality Improvement Project. (1998). The AUDIT alcohol consumption questions (AUDIT-C): An effective brief screening test for problem drinking. *Archives of Internal Medicine, 158*(16), 1789–1795.

Campbell, E. J., Marchant, N. J., & Lawrence, A. J. (2020). A sleeping giant: Suvorexant for the treatment of alcohol use disorder? *Brain Research, 1731*, Article 145902.

Campbell, E. J., Norman, A., Bonomo, Y., & Lawrence, A. J. (2020). Suvorexant to treat alcohol use disorder and comorbid insomnia: Plan for a Phase II trial. *Brain Research, 1728*, Article 146597.

Cao, M., & Javaheri, S. (2018). Effects of chronic opioid use on sleep and wake. *Sleep Medicine Clinics, 13*(2), 271–281.

Chakravorty, S., Chaudhary, N. S., & Brower, K. J. (2016). Alcohol dependence and its relationship with insomnia and other sleep disorders. *Alcoholism: Clinical and Experimental Research*, *40*(11), 2271–2282.

Chakravorty, S., Hanlon, A. L., Kuna, S. T., Ross, R. J., Kampman, K. M., Witte, L. M., & Oslin, D. W. (2014). The effects of quetiapine on sleep in recovering alcohol-dependent subjects: A pilot study. *Journal of Clinical Psychopharmacology*, *34*(3), 350–354.

Chakravorty, S., Morales, K. H., Arnedt, J. T., Perlis, M. L., Oslin, D. W., Findley, J. C., & Kranzler, H. R. (2019). Cognitive behavioral therapy for insomnia in alcohol-dependent veterans: A randomized, controlled pilot study. *Alcoholism: Clinical and Experimental Research*, *43*(6), 1244–1253.

Chaudhary, N. S., Kampman, K. M., Kranzler, H. R., Grandner, M. A., Debbarma, S., & Chakravorty, S. (2015). Insomnia in alcohol dependent subjects is associated with greater psychosocial problem severity. *Addictive Behaviors*, *50*, 165–172.

Chellappa, S. L., Morris, C. J., & Scheer, F. A. (2019). Effects of circadian misalignment on cognition in chronic shift workers. *Scientific Reports*, *9*(1), Article 699.

Chen, V. C. H., Ting, H., Wu, M. H., Lin, T. Y., & Gossop, M. (2017). Sleep disturbance and its associations with severity of dependence, depression and quality of life among heroin-dependent patients: A cross-sectional descriptive study. *Substance Abuse Treatment, Prevention, and Policy*, *12*(1), 1–8.

Chrobok, A. I., Krause, D., Winter, C., Plörer, D., Martin, G., Koller, G., & Pogarell, O. (2020). Sleeping patterns in patients with opioid use disorder: Effects of opioid maintenance treatment and detoxification. *Journal of Psychoactive Drugs*, *52*(3), 203–210.

Cohen-Zion, M., Drummond, S. P., Padula, C. B., Winward, J., Kanady, J., Medina, K. L., & Tapert, S. F. (2009). Sleep architecture in adolescent marijuana and alcohol users during acute and extended abstinence. *Addictive Behaviors*, *34*(11), 976–979.

Cohrs, S., Rodenbeck, A., Guan, Z., Pohlmann, K., Jordan, W., Meier, A., & Rüther, E. (2004). Sleep-promoting properties of quetiapine in healthy subjects. *Psychopharmacology*, *174*, 421–429.

Colrain, I. M., Crowley, K. E., Nicholas, C. L., Padilla, M., & Baker, F. C. (2009). The impact of alcoholism on sleep evoked Δ frequency responses. *Biological Psychiatry*, *66*(2), 177–184.

Colrain, I. M., Turlington, S., & Baker, F. C. (2009). Impact of alcoholism on sleep architecture and EEG power spectra in men and women. *Sleep*, *32*(10), 1341–1352.

Conroy, D. A., Hairston, I. S., Arnedt, J. T., Hoffmann, R. F., Armitage, R., & Brower, K. J. (2012). Dim light melatonin onset in alcohol-dependent men and women compared with healthy controls. *Chronobiology International*, *29*(1), 35–42.

Conroy, D. A., Kurth, M. E., Strong, D. R., Brower, K. J., & Stein, M. D. (2016). Marijuana use patterns and sleep among community-based young adults. *Journal of Addictive Diseases*, *35*(2), 135–143.

Cornelius, J. R., Douaihy, A. B., Clark, D. B., Chung, T., Wood, D. S., & Daley, D. (2012). Mirtazapine in comorbid major depression and alcohol dependence: An open-label trial. *Journal of Dual Diagnosis*, *8*(3), 200–204.

Cornelius, J. R., Douaihy, A. B., Clark, D. B., Daley, D. C., Chung, T. A., Wesesky, M. A., & Salloum, I. (2013). Mirtazapine in comorbid major depression and alcohol use disorder: A long-term follow-up study. *Journal of Addictive Behaviors, Therapy & Rehabilitation*, *3*(1), Article 1560.

Correa, D., Farney, R. J., Chung, F., Prasad, A., Lam, D., & Wong, J. (2015). Chronic opioid use and central sleep apnea: A review of the prevalence, mechanisms, and perioperative considerations. *Anesthesia & Analgesia*, *120*(6), 1273–1285.

Cranford, J. A., Arnedt, J. T., Conroy, D. A., Bohnert, K. M., Bourque, C., Blow, F. C., & Ilgen, M. (2017). Prevalence and correlates of sleep-related problems in adults receiving medical cannabis for chronic pain. *Drug and Alcohol Dependence*, *180*, 227–233.

Currie, S. R., Clark, S., Hodgins, D. C., & El-Guebaly, N. (2004). Randomized controlled trial of brief cognitive-behavioural interventions for insomnia in recovering alcoholics. *Addiction*, *99*(9), 1121–1132.

Czeisler, M. E., Lane, R. I., Petrosky, E., Wiley, J. F., Christensen, A., Njai, R., Weaver, M. D., Robbins, R., Facer-Childs, E. R., Barger, L. K., Czeisler, C. A., Howard, M. E., & Rajaratnam, S. M. W. (2020). Mental health, substance use, and suicidal ideation during the COVID-19 pandemic – United States, June 24–30, 2020. *MMWR Morbidity and Mortality Weekly Report*, 69(32), 1049–1057.

Dolsen, E. A., & Harvey, A. G. (2017). Life-time history of insomnia and hypersomnia symptoms as correlates of alcohol, cocaine and heroin use and relapse among adults seeking substance use treatment in the United States from 1991 to 1994. *Addiction*, *112*(6), 1104–1111.

Drummond, S. P., Gillin, J. C., Smith, T. L., & DeModena, A. (1998). The sleep of abstinent pure primary alcoholic patients: Natural course and relationship to relapse. *Alcoholism: Clinical and Experimental Research, 22*(8), 1796–1802.

Edwards, S., Reeves, G. M., & Fishbein, D. (2015). Integrative model of the relationship between sleep problems and risk for youth substance use. *Current Addiction Reports, 2*, 130–140.

Ek, J., Jacobs, W., Kaylor, B., & McCall, W. V. (2021). Addiction and sleep disorders. *Cannabinoids and Sleep: Molecular, Functional and Clinical Aspects, 1297*, 163–171.

Ellis, J. D., Mayo, J. L., Gamaldo, C. E., Finan, P. H., & Huhn, A. S. (2022). Worsening sleep quality across the lifespan and persistent sleep disturbances in persons with opioid use disorder. *Journal of Clinical Sleep Medicine, 18*(2), 587–595.

Falk, D. E., Ryan, M. L., Fertig, J. B., Devine, E. G., Cruz, R., Brown, E. S., & National Institute on Alcohol Abuse and Alcoholism Clinical Investigations Group Study Group. (2019). Gabapentin enacarbil extended-release for alcohol use disorder: A randomized, double-blind, placebo-controlled, multisite trial assessing efficacy and safety. *Alcoholism: Clinical and Experimental Research, 43*(1), 158–169.

Farney, R. J., McDonald, A. M., Boyle, K. M., Snow, G. L., Nuttall, R. T., Coudreaut, M. F., & Walker, J. M. (2013). Sleep disordered breathing in patients receiving therapy with buprenorphine/naloxone. *European Respiratory Journal, 42*(2), 394–403.

Finan, P. H., Mun, C. J., Epstein, D. H., Kowalczyk, W. J., Phillips, K. A., Agage, D., & Preston, K. L. (2020). Multimodal assessment of sleep in men and women during treatment for opioid use disorder. *Drug and Alcohol Dependence, 207*, Article 107698.

Flores-Ramirez, F. J., Illenberger, J. M., Pascasio, G. E., Matzeu, A., Mason, B. J., & Martin-Fardon, R. (2022). Alternative use of suvorexant (Belsomra®) for the prevention of alcohol drinking and seeking in rats with a history of alcohol dependence. *Frontiers in Behavioral Neuroscience, 16*, Article 1085882.

Friedmann, P. D., Herman, D. S., Freedman, S., Lemon, S. C., Ramsey, S., & Stein, M. D. (2003). Treatment of sleep disturbance in alcohol recovery: A national survey of addiction medicine physicians. *Journal of Addictive Diseases, 22*(2), 91–103.

Friedmann, P. D., Rose, J. S., Swift, R., Stout, R. L., Millman, R. P., & Stein, M. D. (2008). Trazodone for sleep disturbance after alcohol detoxification: A double-blind, placebo-controlled trial. *Alcoholism: Clinical and Experimental Research, 32*(9), 1652–1660.

Gann, H., Feige, B., Fasihi, S., van Calker, D., Voderholzer, U., & Riemann, D. (2002). Periodic limb movements during sleep in alcohol dependent patients. *European Archives of Psychiatry and Clinical Neuroscience, 252*, 124–129.

Gann, H., Feige, B., Hohagen, F., van Calker, D., Geiss, D., & Dieter, R. (2001). Sleep and the cholinergic rapid eye movement sleep induction test in patients with primary alcohol dependence. *Biological Psychiatry, 50*(5), 383–390.

Gann, H., Van Calker, D., Feige, B., Cloot, O., Brück, R., Berger, M., & Riemann, D. (2004). Polysomnographic comparison between patients with primary alcohol dependency during subacute withdrawal and patients with a major depression. *European Archives of Psychiatry and Clinical Neuroscience, 254*, 263–271.

Garcia, A. N., & Salloum, I. M. (2015). Polysomnographic sleep disturbances in nicotine, caffeine, alcohol, cocaine, opioid, and cannabis use: A focused review. *The American Journal on Addictions, 24*(7), 590–598.

Gates, P., Albertella, L., & Copeland, J. (2016). Cannabis withdrawal and sleep: A systematic review of human studies. *Substance Abuse, 37*(1), 255–269.

Gendy, M. N., Lagzdins, D., Schaman, J., & Le Foll, B. (2020). Melatonin for treatment-seeking alcohol use disorder patients with sleeping problems: A randomized clinical pilot trial. *Scientific Reports, 10*(1), 1–10.

Gillin, J. C., Smith, T. L., Irwin, M., Kripke, D. F., Brown, S., & Schuckit, M. (1990a). Short REM latency in primary alcoholic patients with secondary depression. *The American Journal of Psychiatry, 147*(1), 106–109.

Gillin, J. C., Smith, T. L., Irwin, M., Kripke, D. F., & Schuckit, M. (1990b). EEG sleep studies in "pure" primary alcoholism during subacute withdrawal: Relationships to normal controls, age, and other clinical variables. *Biological Psychiatry, 27*(5), 477–488.

Grant, B. F., Chou, S. P., Saha, T. D., Pickering, R. P., Kerridge, B. T., Ruan, W. J., & Hasin, D. S. (2017). Prevalence of 12-month alcohol use, high-risk drinking, and DSM-IV alcohol use disorder in the United States, 2001–2002 to 2012–2013: Results from the National Epidemiologic Survey on Alcohol and Related Conditions. *JAMA Psychiatry, 74*(9), 911–923.

Greeff, A. P., & Conradie, W. S. (1998). Use of progressive relaxation training for chronic alcoholics with insomnia. *Psychological Reports, 82*(2), 407–412.

Griffiths, R. R., & Johnson, M. W. (2005). Relative abuse liability of hypnotic drugs: A conceptual framework and algorithm for differentiating among compounds. *Journal of Clinical Psychiatry, 66*(S9), 31–41.

Gross, M. M., & Best, S. (1975). Behavioral concomitants of the relationship between baseline slow wave sleep and carry-over of tolerance and dependence in alcoholics. In M. M. Gross (Ed.), *Alcohol intoxication and withdrawal: Experimental studies II* (pp. 633–643). Springer.

Gross, M. M., Goodenough, D. R., Hastey, J., & Lewis, E. (1973). Experimental study of sleep in chronic alcoholics before, during, and after four days of heavy drinking, with a nondrinking comparison. *Annals of the New York Academy of Sciences, 215*(1), 254–265.

Grosshans, M., Mutschler, J., Luderer, M., Mann, K., & Kiefer, F. (2014). Agomelatine is effective in reducing insomnia in abstinent alcohol-dependent patients. *Clinical Neuropharmacology, 37*(1), 6–8.

Gulick, D., & Gamsby, J. J. (2018). Racing the clock: The role of circadian rhythmicity in addiction across the lifespan. *Pharmacology & Therapeutics, 188*, 124–139.

Hasler, B. P., & Pedersen, S. L. (2020). Sleep and circadian risk factors for alcohol problems: A brief overview and proposed mechanisms. *Current Opinion in Psychology, 34*, 57–62.

Haynes, P. L., Bootzin, R. R., Smith, L., Cousins, J., Cameron, M., & Stevens, S. (2006). Results from an integrative behavioral sleep-treatment pilot program. *Sleep, 29*(4), 512–520.

He, S., Hasler, B. P., & Chakravorty, S. (2019). Alcohol and sleep-related problems. *Current Opinion in Psychology, 30*, 117–122.

Hodges, S. E., Pittman, B., & Morgan, P. T. (2017). Sleep perception and misperception in chronic cocaine users during abstinence. *Sleep, 40*(3), Article zsw069.

Huhn, A. S., Dunn, K. E., Ellis, J. D., Sholler, D. J., Tabaschek, P., Burns, R., & Strain, E. C. (2022). Objective sleep outcomes in randomized-controlled trials in persons with substance use disorders: A systematic review. *Drug and Alcohol Dependence, 237*, Article 109509.

Huhn, A. S., & Finan, P. H. (2022). Sleep disturbance as a therapeutic target to improve opioid use disorder treatment. *Experimental and Clinical Psychopharmacology, 30*(6), Article 1024.

Irwin, M., Gillin, J. C., Dang, J., Weissman, J., Phillips, E., & Ehlers, C. L. (2002). Sleep deprivation as a probe of homeostatic sleep regulation in primary alcoholics. *Biological Psychiatry, 51*(8), 632–641.

Irwin, M., Miller, C., Gillin, J. C., Demodena, A., & Ehlers, C. L. (2000). Polysomnographic and spectral sleep EEG in primary alcoholics: An interaction between alcohol dependence and African-American ethnicity. *Alcoholism: Clinical and Experimental Research, 24*(9), 1376–1384.

Irwin, M. R., Bjurstrom, M. F., & Olmstead, R. (2016). Polysomnographic measures of sleep in cocaine dependence and alcohol dependence: Implications for age-related loss of slow wave, Stage 3 sleep. *Addiction, 111*(6), 1084–1092.

Johnson, B., & Longo, L. P. (1998). Considerations in the physician's decision to prescribe benzodiazepines to patients with addiction. *Psychiatric Annals, 28*(3), 160–165.

Johnson, B. A., Swift, R. M., Ait-Daoud, N., DiClemente, C. C., Javors, M. A., & Malcolm, R. J., Jr. (2004). Development of novel pharmacotherapies for the treatment of alcohol dependence: Focus on antiepileptics. *Alcoholism: Clinical and Experimental Research, 28*(2), 295–301.

Johnson, M. W., Suess, P. E., & Griffiths, R. R. (2006). Ramelteon: A novel hypnotic lacking abuse liability and sedative adverse effects. *Archives of General Psychiatry, 63*(10), 1149–1157.

Karam-Hage, M., & Brower, K. J. (2000). Gabapentin treatment for insomnia associated with alcohol dependence. *American Journal of Psychiatry, 157*(1), 151–151.

Karam-Hage, M., & Brower, K. J. (2003). Open pilot study of gabapentin versus trazodone to treat insomnia in alcoholic outpatients. *Psychiatry and Clinical Neurosciences, 57*(5), 542–544.

Kesner, A. J., & Lovinger, D. M. (2020). Cannabinoids, endocannabinoids and sleep. *Frontiers in Molecular Neuroscience, 13*, Article 125.

Kolla, B. P., Foroughi, M., Saeidifard, F., Chakravorty, S., Wang, Z., & Mansukhani, M. P. (2018). The impact of alcohol on breathing parameters during sleep: A systematic review and meta-analysis. *Sleep Medicine Reviews, 42*, 59–67.

Kolla, B. P., Schneekloth, T. D., Biernacka, J. M., Frye, M. A., Mansukhani, M. P., Hall-Flavin, D. K., & Mrazek, D. (2011). Trazodone and alcohol relapse: a retrospective study following residential treatment. *The American Journal on Addictions, 20*(6), 525–529.

Kolla, B. P., Schneekloth, T., Biernacka, J., Mansukhani, M., Geske, J., Karpyak, V., & Frye, M. A. (2014). The course of sleep disturbances in early alcohol recovery: An observational cohort study. *The American Journal on Addictions, 23*(1), 21–26.

Koob, G. F., & Colrain, I. M. (2020). Alcohol use disorder and sleep disturbances: A feed-forward allostatic framework. *Neuropsychopharmacology, 45*(1), 141–165.
Kosky, C. A., Bonakis, A., Yogendran, A., Hettiarachchi, G., Dargan, P. I., & Williams, A. J. (2016). Urine toxicology in adults evaluated for a central hypersomnia and how the results modify the physician's diagnosis. *Journal of Clinical Sleep Medicine, 12*(11), 1499–1505.
Krahn, L. E., Arand, D. L., Avidan, A. Y., Davila, D. G., DeBassio, W. A., Ruoff, C. M., & Harrod, C. G. (2021). Recommended protocols for the Multiple Sleep Latency Test and Maintenance of Wakefulness Test in adults: Guidance from the American Academy of Sleep Medicine. *Journal of Clinical Sleep Medicine, 17*(12), 2489–2498.
Kühlwein, E., Hauger, R. L., & Irwin, M. R. (2003). Abnormal nocturnal melatonin secretion and disordered sleep in abstinent alcoholics. *Biological Psychiatry, 54*(12), 1437–1443.
LaRoche, S. M., & Helmers, S. L. (2004). The new antiepileptic drugs: Scientific review. *JAMA, 291*(5), 605–614.
Le Bon, O., Murphy, J. R., Staner, L., Hoffmann, G., Kormoss, N., Kentos, M., & Verbanck, P. (2003). Double-blind, placebo-controlled study of the efficacy of trazodone in alcohol post-withdrawal syndrome: Polysomnographic and clinical evaluations. *Journal of Clinical Psychopharmacology, 23*(4), 377–383.
Le Bon, O., Verbanck, P., Hoffmann, G., Murphy, J. R., Staner, L., De Groote, D., & Pelc, I. (1997). Sleep in detoxified alcoholics: Impairment of most standard sleep parameters and increased risk for sleep apnea, but not for myoclonias—A controlled study. *Journal of Studies on Alcohol, 58*(1), 30–36.
Li, D. J., Chung, K. S., Wu, H. C., Hsu, C. Y., & Yen, C. F. (2018). Predictors of sleep disturbance in heroin users receiving methadone maintenance therapy: A naturalistic study in Taiwan. *Neuropsychiatric Disease and Treatment, 14*, 2853–2859.
Lin, C. L., Sun, J. C., Lin, C. P., Chung, C. H., & Chien, W. C. (2020). Risk of alcohol use disorders in patients with insomnia: A population-based retrospective cohort study. *Alcohol, 89*, 123–128.
Litten, R. Z., Fertig, J. B., Falk, D. E., Ryan, M. L., Mattson, M. E., Collins, J. F., & NCIG 001 Study Group. (2012). A double-blind, placebo-controlled trial to assess the efficacy of quetiapine fumarate XR in very heavy-drinking alcohol-dependent patients. *Alcoholism: Clinical and Experimental Research, 36*(3), 406–416.
Luc, S., Peter, B., Thierry, D., Isabelle, G., Muriel, M., Frédéric, L., & Rémy, L. (2006). Effects of acamprosate on sleep during alcohol withdrawal: A double-blind placebo-controlled polysomnographic study in alcohol-dependent subjects. *Alcoholism: Clinical and Experimental Research, 30*(9), 1492–1499.
Lydon-Staley, D. M., Cleveland, H. H., Huhn, A. S., Cleveland, M. J., Harris, J., Stankoski, D., & Bunce, S. C. (2017). Daily sleep quality affects drug craving, partially through indirect associations with positive affect, in patients in treatment for nonmedical use of prescription drugs. *Addictive Behaviors, 65*, 275–282.
Malcolm, R., Myrick, H., Roberts, J., Wang, W., & Anton, R. F. (2002). The differential effects of medication on mood, sleep disturbance, and work ability in outpatient alcohol detoxification. *American Journal on Addictions, 11*(2), 141–150.
Malcolm, R., Myrick, L. H., Veatch, L. M., Boyle, E., & Randall, P. K. (2007). Reported sleep, sleepiness, and repeated alcohol withdrawals: a randomized, double blind, controlled comparison of lorazepam vs gabapentin. *Journal of Clinical Sleep Medicine, 3*(1), 24–32.
Mason, B. J., Quello, S., Goodell, V., Shadan, F., Kyle, M., & Begovic, A. (2014). Gabapentin treatment for alcohol dependence: A randomized clinical trial. *JAMA Internal Medicine, 174*(1), 70–77.
Matuskey, D., Pittman, B., Forselius, E., Malison, R. T., & Morgan, P. T. (2011). A multistudy analysis of the effects of early cocaine abstinence on sleep. *Drug and Alcohol Dependence, 115*(1–2), 62–66.
Mehtry, V., Nizamie, S. H., Parvez, N., & Pradhan, N. (2014). Sleep profile in opioid dependence: A polysomnographic case–control study. *Journal of Clinical Neurophysiology, 31*(6), 517–522.
Monnelly, E. P., Ciraulo, D. A., Knapp, C., LoCastro, J., & Sepulveda, I. (2004). Quetiapine for treatment of alcohol dependence. *Journal of Clinical Psychopharmacology, 24*(5), 532–535.
Morgan, P. T., Angarita, G. A., Canavan, S., Pittman, B., Oberleitner, L., Malison, R. T., & Forselius, E. (2016). Modafinil and sleep architecture in an inpatient–outpatient treatment study of cocaine dependence. *Drug and Alcohol Dependence, 160*, 49–56.
Morgan, P. T., Pace-Schott, E., Pittman, B., Stickgold, R., & Malison, R. T. (2010). Normalizing effects of modafinil on sleep in chronic cocaine users. *American Journal of Psychiatry, 167*(3), 331–340.

Morgan, P. T., Pace-Schott, E. F., Sahul, Z. H., Coric, V., Stickgold, R., & Malison, R. T. (2006). Sleep, sleep-dependent procedural learning and vigilance in chronic cocaine users: Evidence for occult insomnia. *Drug and Alcohol Dependence, 82*(3), 238–249.

Morgan, P. T., Pace-Schott, E. F., Sahul, Z. H., Coric, V., Stickgold, R., & Malison, R. T. (2008). Sleep architecture, cocaine and visual learning. *Addiction, 103*(8), 1344–1352.

Myrick, H., Malcolm, R., Randall, P. K., Boyle, E., Anton, R. F., Becker, H. C., & Randall, C. L. (2009). A double-blind trial of gabapentin versus lorazepam in the treatment of alcohol withdrawal. *Alcoholism: Clinical and Experimental Research, 33*(9), 1582–1588.

National Institute on Drug Abuse. (2021, June 1). *Heroin drug facts*. Retrieved August 8, 2022, from https://nida.nih.gov/publications/drugfacts/heroin

Nielsen, T. A., & Zadra, A. (2005). Nightmares and other common dream disturbances. In M. H. Kryger, T. Roth, & W. C. Dement (Eds.), *Principles and practice of sleep medicine* (4th ed., pp. 926–935). W. B. Saunders.

O'Donnell, J., Gladden, R. M., Mattson, C. L., Hunter, C. T., & Davis, N. L. (2020). Vital signs: Characteristics of drug overdose deaths involving opioids and stimulants—24 states and the District of Columbia, January–June 2019. *Morbidity and Mortality Weekly Report, 69*(35), 1189–1197.

Pacek, L. R., Herrmann, E. S., Smith, M. T., & Vandrey, R. (2017). Sleep continuity, architecture and quality among treatment-seeking cannabis users: An in-home, unattended polysomnographic study. *Experimental and Clinical Psychopharmacology, 25*(4), 295–302.

Pace-Schott, E. F., Stickgold, R., Muzur, A., Wigren, P. E., Ward, A. S., Hart, C. L., & Hobson, J. A. (2005). Sleep quality deteriorates over a binge–abstinence cycle in chronic smoked cocaine users. *Psychopharmacology, 179*(4), 873–883.

Peles, E., Schreiber, S., Hamburger, R. B., & Adelson, M. (2011). No change of sleep after 6 and 12 months of methadone maintenance treatment. *Journal of Addiction Medicine, 5*(2), 141–147.

Perney, P., & Lehert, P. (2018). Insomnia in alcohol-dependent patients: prevalence, risk factors and acamprosate effect: An individual patient data meta-analysis. *Alcohol and Alcoholism, 53*(5), 611–618.

Perney, P., Lehert, P., & Mason, B. J. (2012). Sleep disturbance in alcoholism: Proposal of a simple measurement, and results from a 24-week randomized controlled study of alcohol-dependent patients assessing acamprosate efficacy. *Alcohol and Alcoholism, 47*(2), 133–139.

Perney, P., Rigole, H., Mason, B., Dematteis, M., & Lehert, P. (2015). Measuring sleep disturbances in patients with alcohol use disorders: A short questionnaire suitable for routine practice. *Journal of Addiction Medicine, 9*(1), 25–30.

Piper, B. J., DeKeuster, R. M., Beals, M. L., Cobb, C. M., Burchman, C. A., Perkinson, L., & Abess, A. T. (2017). Substitution of medical cannabis for pharmaceutical agents for pain, anxiety, and sleep. *Journal of Psychopharmacology, 31*(5), 569–575.

Pollard, M. S., Tucker, J. S., & Green, H. D. (2020). Changes in adult alcohol use and consequences during the COVID-19 pandemic in the US. *JAMA Network Open, 3*(9), Article e2022942.

Reid-Varley, W. B., Martinez, C. P., & Khurshid, K. A. (2020). Sleep disorders and disrupted sleep in addiction, withdrawal and abstinence with focus on alcohol and opioids. *Journal of the Neurological Sciences, 411*, Article 116713.

Roehrs, T., & Roth, T. (2001). Sleep, sleepiness, and alcohol use. *Alcohol Research & Health, 25*(2), 101–109.

Roehrs, T., & Roth, T. (2018). Insomnia as a path to alcoholism: Tolerance development and dose escalation. *Sleep, 41*(8), Article zsy091.

Roehrs, T., Sibai, M., & Roth, T. (2021). Sleep and alertness disturbance and substance use disorders: A bi-directional relation. *Pharmacology Biochemistry and Behavior, 203*, Article 173153.

Roehrs, T. A., & Roth, T. (2015). Sleep disturbance in substance use disorders. *Psychiatric Clinics, 38*(4), 793–803.

Roncero, C., Grau-López, L., Díaz-Morán, S., Miquel, L., Martínez-Luna, N., & Casas, M. (2011). Evaluation of sleep disorders in drug dependent inpatients. *Medicina Clinica, 138*(8), 332–335.

Sattar, S. P., Bhatia, S. C., & Petty, F. (2004). Potential benefits of quetiapine in the treatment of substance dependence disorders. *Journal of Psychiatry and Neuroscience, 29*(6), 452–457.

Schmitz, M., Frey, R., Pichler, P., Röpke, H., Anderer, P., Saletu, B., & Rudas, S. (1997). Sleep quality during alcohol withdrawal with bright light therapy. *Progress in Neuro-Psychopharmacology and Biological Psychiatry, 21*(6), 965–977.

Schmitz, M. M., Sepandj, A., Pichler, P. M., & Rudas, S. (1996). Disrupted melatonin-secretion during alcohol withdrawal. *Progress in Neuro-Psychopharmacology and Biological Psychiatry, 20*(6), 983–995.

Sharkey, K. M., Kurth, M. E., Anderson, B. J., Corso, R. P., Millman, R. P., & Stein, M. D. (2010). Obstructive sleep apnea is more common than central sleep apnea in methadone maintenance patients with subjective sleep complaints. *Drug and Alcohol Dependence, 108*(1–2), 77–83.

Sharkey, K. M., Kurth, M. E., Anderson, B. J., Corso, R. P., Millman, R. P., & Stein, M. D. (2011). Assessing sleep in opioid dependence: A of subjective ratings, sleep diaries, and home polysomnography in methadone maintenance patients. *Drug and Alcohol Dependence, 113*(2–3), 245–248.

Short, N. A., Zvolensky, M. J., & Schmidt, N. B. (2021). A pilot randomized clinical trial of brief behavioral treatment for insomnia to reduce problematic cannabis use among trauma-exposed young adults. *Journal of Substance Abuse Treatment, 131*, Article 108537.

Srisurapanont, M., & Jarusuraisin, N. (1998). Amitriptyline vs. lorazepam in the treatment of opiate-withdrawal insomnia: A randomized double-blind study. *Acta Psychiatrica Scandinavica, 97*(3), 233–235.

Stein, M. D., Herman, D. S., Bishop, S., Lassor, J. A., Weinstock, M., Anthony, J., & Anderson, B. J. (2004). Sleep disturbances among methadone maintained patients. *Journal of Substance Abuse Treatment, 26*(3), 175–180.

Substance Abuse and Mental Health Services Administration. (2024). Key substance use and mental health indicators in the United States: Results from the 2023 National Survey on Drug Use and Health (HHS Publication No. PEP24-07-021 2024).

Suchting, R., Yoon, J. H., San Miguel, G. G., Green, C. E., Weaver, M. F., Vincent, J. N., & Lane, S. D. (2020). Preliminary examination of the orexin system on relapse-related factors in cocaine use disorder. *Brain Research, 1731*, Article 146359.

Teichtahl, H., Prodromidis, A., Miller, B., Cherry, G., & Kronborg, I. (2001). Sleep-disordered breathing in stable methadone programme patients: A pilot study. *Addiction, 96*(3), 395–403.

Teichtahl, H., & Wang, D. (2007). Sleep-disordered breathing with chronic opioid use. *Expert Opinion on Drug Safety, 6*(6), 641–649.

Thompson, P. M., Gillin, J. C., Golshan, S., & Irwin, M. (1995). Polygraphic sleep measures differentiate alcoholics and stimulant abusers during short-term abstinence. *Biological Psychiatry, 38*(12), 831–836.

Toda, S., Alguacil, L. F., & Kalivas, P. W. (2003). Repeated cocaine administration changes the function and subcellular distribution of adenosine A1 receptor in the rat nucleus accumbens. *Journal of Neurochemistry, 87*(6), 1478–1484.

Valentino, R. J., & Volkow, N. D. (2020). Drugs, sleep, and the addicted brain. *Neuropsychopharmacology, 45*(1), 3–5.

Vandrey, R., Smith, M. T., McCann, U. D., Budney, A. J., & Curran, E. M. (2011). Sleep disturbance and the effects of extended-release zolpidem during cannabis withdrawal. *Drug and Alcohol Dependence, 117*(1), 38–44.

Venkatesh, A. K., Janke, A. T., Kinsman, J., Rothenberg, C., Goyal, P., Malicki, C., & Hawk, K. (2022). Emergency department utilization for substance use disorders and mental health conditions during COVID-19. *PLOS ONE, 17*(1), Article e0262136.

Wagman, A. M., & Allen, R. P. (1975). Effects of alcohol ingestion and abstinence on slow wave sleep of alcoholics. In M. M. Gross (Ed.), *Alcohol intoxication and withdrawal: Experimental studies II* (pp. 453–466). Springer.

Webster, L. (2005). Efficacy of intrathecal ziconotide for the treatment of severe chronic pain in adults. *Pain Medicine, 6*, 195–196.

Wetterberg, L., Aperia, B., Gorelick, D. A., Gwirtzman, H. E., McGuire, M. T., Serafetinides, E. A., & Yuwiler, A. (1992). Age, alcoholism and depression are associated with low levels of urinary melatonin. *Journal of Psychiatry and Neuroscience, 17*(5), 215–224.

Wilkerson, A. K., Sahlem, G. L., Bentzley, B. S., Lord, J., Smith, J. P., Simmons, R. O., & Book, S. W. (2019). Insomnia severity during early abstinence is related to substance use treatment completion in adults enrolled in an intensive outpatient program. *Journal of Substance Abuse Treatment, 104*, 97–103.

Williams, H. L., & Rundell, O. H., Jr. (1981). Altered sleep physiology in chronic alcoholics: Reversal with abstinence. *Alcoholism: Clinical and Experimental Research, 5*(2), 318–325.

Winiger, E. A., Hitchcock, L. N., Bryan, A. D., & Bidwell, L. C. (2021). Cannabis use and sleep: Expectations, outcomes, and the role of age. *Addictive Behaviors, 112*, Article 106642.

Wittmann, M., Dinich, J., Merrow, M., & Roenneberg, T. (2006). Social jetlag: Misalignment of biological and social time. *Chronobiology International, 23*(1-2), 497–509.

Zhabenko, N., Wojnar, M., & Brower, K. J. (2012). Prevalence and correlates of insomnia in a Polish sample of alcohol-dependent patients. *Alcoholism: Clinical and Experimental Research, 36*(9), 1600–1607.

CHAPTER

44 Sleep–Wake Disturbances in Individuals With Traumatic Brain Injury

Marie-Christine Ouellet, Simon Beaulieu-Bonneau, *and* Charles M. Morin

Abstract

Traumatic brain injury (TBI) is a prevalent and important public health issue which can lead to long-term consequences in various domains of functioning, especially for those sustaining moderate or severe injuries. Often overlooked, sleep disturbances are among the most prevalent and persistent negative consequences of TBI. Research on the etiology, evolution, and treatment of sleep–wake disturbances is still emerging, and rehabilitation professionals are giving increasing attention to these problems. This chapter starts with a general description of the clinical presentation of patients with TBI. It then discusses data on the prevalence, etiology, and nature of sleep disturbances in this patient population and presents considerations for assessment and treatment of insomnia, excessive daytime sleepiness, and circadian rhythm dysregulation in the context of TBI.

Key Words: traumatic brain injury, sleep, insomnia, sleepiness, fatigue, epidemiology, etiology, assessment, treatment

Introduction

Traumatic brain injury (TBI) represents a major source of disability and disease burden worldwide (Dewan et al., 2018; GBD 2016 Traumatic Brain Injury and Spinal Cord Injury Collaborators, 2019; Silver et al., 2005). TBI refers to any lesion to the brain caused by an external force, for example, in the context of a motor vehicle accident, a fall, or a sport-related collision. It can involve open (penetrating) lesions, where objects or parts of the skull directly damage cerebral tissue, or closed (blunt) lesions caused by forces such as acceleration, deceleration, or rotation, where the brain collides rapidly with the skull or is twisted around itself. It is estimated that about 1.7 million individuals sustain TBI each year in the United States, with a rate of about 500 to 600 per 100,000 inhabitants (Langlois et al., 2006; Rutland-Brown et al., 2006). In 2013, the US Centers for Disease Control recorded 2.8 million TBI-related visits to emergency departments, hospitalizations, or deaths (Taylor et al., 2017). The vast majority of TBIs are mild (about 80%), about 10% are moderate, and about 10% are severe (Kraus & Chu, 2005).

TBI can bring about a broad range of physical, cognitive, and emotional sequelae, thereby affecting several life habits as well as social participation. TBI can thus have considerable repercussions for the injured person as well as their families and larger social circles. Even in cases of mild TBI, individuals can suffer from a variety of difficulties which can seriously impede the return to satisfactory psychological, social, and professional functioning; and outcome and prognosis are extremely variable across individuals. Individuals having sustained mild TBI may feel various symptoms (e.g., dizziness, headaches, fatigue, inattentiveness, depressed mood) for several weeks or several months but are thought to usually recover within 3 to 12 months post-injury (Carroll et al., 2004). However, an important proportion of persons having sustained mild TBI experience persisting symptoms, functional impairments, or reduced quality of life, for example, in the form of work limitations (Carroll et al., 2020; Nelson et al., 2019; Theadom et al., 2017). Most persons with moderate or severe TBI often endure permanent deficits (of various degrees of severity) in cognition (e.g., attention, memory, executive function, social cognition), in physical function (e.g., pain, visual deficits, issues with balance or gait), in mental health (e.g., depression, anxiety), and in the social and occupational spheres (e.g., marital problems, problems returning to work).

Among the perduring consequences of TBI, sleep disturbances are quite prominent but have only received more scientific and clinical attention in recent decades. Self-reported problems with sleep are observed in proportions as high as 50% to 70% of TBI survivors and can appear during the acute phase after the injury, during hospitalization and inpatient rehabilitation care, or in the later and chronic phases following the accident when the individual is facing stressors linked to community reintegration (Montgomery et al., 2022; Ouellet et al., 2004; Rao et al., 2008; Verma et al., 2007). Common complaints include difficulties falling asleep or maintaining sleep, excessive daytime sleepiness (EDS) and fatigue, alterations in sleep–wake rhythms, and increased need for sleep. Sleep disorders such as insomnia, sleep-related breathing disorders, hypersomnia, and narcolepsy are in fact 3 to 10 times more prevalent in persons with TBI compared to the general population (Mathias & Alvaro, 2012). Several etiological factors are at play, including pathophysiological factors linked to the brain injury per se, effects of medications administered to treat the injury or its impacts, the presence of pain (e.g., headaches or pain to other parts of the body that have been injured), the presence of comorbid stress and psychopathology (e.g., depression, anxiety), and life habits affected by the injury (e.g., lack of routine because of being off work, naps to attempt to cope with fatigue). Because sleep–wake disturbances can exacerbate the functional consequences of TBI such as pain, physical problems, cognitive issues, or emotional disorders, they can potentially hamper the rehabilitation process as a whole (Lowe et al., 2020). Researchers and clinicians are thus stressing the importance of paying closer attention to post-TBI sleep–wake disturbances (Agrawal et al., 2008), and more systematic research on these issues is emerging.

Pathophysiology of Sleep–Wake Disturbances After TBI

A variety of pathophysiological factors can contribute to alterations in sleep after TBI. Structural changes induced by lesions may lead to changes in systems responsible for sleep–wake functions. Increased intracranial pressure, elevated levels of inflammatory cytokines, and abnormal neurotransmitter, protein, or hormonal secretion patterns may all play a potential role (Baumann et al., 2005, 2007; Frieboes et al., 1999; Gottshall et al., 2021; Mahowald, 2000).

Secretion and regulation of melatonin have been observed to be reduced in both the acute and chronic phases after TBI (Chen et al., 2015; N. A. Grima et al., 2016; Osier et al., 2017; Paparrigopoulos et al., 2006; Shekleton et al., 2010). A good body of evidence in both humans and animals links abnormal hypothalamic function to sleep–wake alterations early after TBI, particularly a decrease in secretion of hypocretin-I in the acute phase. This could explain, at least in part, an increased need for sleep (pleiosomnia), especially early after more severe injuries, and could also explain lingering issues with EDS (Baumann et al., 2005, 2007, 2009; Lim et al., 2013; Nardone et al., 2011; Sabir et al., 2015; Skopin et al., 2014; Valko et al., 2015; Willie et al., 2012). TBI may also cause damage to arousal-promoting neural circuiteries (Jang & Kwon, 2016; Valko et al., 2016).

Sleep–Wake Changes in the Acute Phase After TBI

In the first few days after a moderate or severe TBI, while patients are in the intensive care unit and often suffer from post-traumatic amnesia, sleep–wake patterns are likely to be disrupted, and hypersomnolence is frequent (Billiard & Podesta, 2013; Chiu et al., 2013; Friese et al., 2007; Gabor et al., 2001; Sanchez et al., 2022; Sommerauer et al., 2013). Several studies suggest that favorable evolutions in terms of return of consciousness and cognitive recovery (i.e., resolution of post-traumatic amnesia) are paralleled with a normalization of sleep quality during the acute phase after TBI (Chiu et al., 2014; Duclos et al., 2013, 2016, 2017; Makley et al., 2009; Nakase-Richardson et al., 2013; Sherer et al., 2009; Urakami, 2012). As such, if sleep is a marker or a stepping stone of recovery, this evidence underscores the importance of giving more attention to sleep quality early in the rehabilitation process, for example, by paying attention to environmental (frequent therapeutic or diagnostic procedures, noise, light, bed discomfort) and psychological (e.g., anxiety, loneliness, irregular routines) factors. In a prospective study of a large sample of patients with moderate to severe TBI, Nakase-Richardson and colleagues found that the proportion of persons with severely disorganized sleep decreased over the first month post-TBI during acute hospitalization, but 84% still had significant sleep–wake problems when admitted to the rehabilitation unit. Patients with moderate or severe sleep disturbances at 1 month post-TBI were found to have longer length of stay in acute care and rehabilitation and longer duration of post-traumatic amnesia (Nakase-Richardson et al., 2013).

Self-reported sleep problems in the subacute phase after mild TBI have been shown to be related to poorer life satisfaction and to an increased level of post-concussion symptoms including cognitive issues (concentration, memory) and irritability (Tang et al., 2022). In moderate to severe TBI, a higher quality of sleep during hospitalization (fewer awakenings, more slow–wave sleep, higher spindle density) has been associated with more favorable cognitive outcomes even several years after the accident (Sanchez et al., 2022). Similar results have been found in children (Williams et al., 2022), with sleep–wake disturbances being linked to worse executive function up to 3 months after hospital discharge. Taken together, the recent literature is clearly linking sleep quality early after TBI to long-term outcomes after TBI and should thus underscore the importance of monitoring and addressing sleep issues in this population.

Sleep Architecture in the Chronic Phase After TBI

Polysomnography (PSG) studies have yield mixed results regarding sleep architecture in the chronic phase after TBI (regardless of severity). In general, the frequent insomnia complaints seen up to several months and years post-injury are corroborated with PSG, which indicates reduced total sleep time, increased wake time after sleep onset, and longer sleep-onset latencies (Grima et al., 2016). Further examining the different sleep stages, several studies observed an increase in the proportion of slow-wave sleep (Shekleton et al., 2010; Sommerauer et al., 2013), decreased proportion of rapid-eye-movement (REM) sleep (Schreiber et al., 2008; Verma et al., 2007), decreased latencies to REM sleep (Stone et al., 2014; Verma et al., 2007; Williams et al., 2008), and increased proportion of N1 (Ouellet & Morin, 2006; Verma et al., 2007) and N2 (Schreiber et al., 2008; Verma et al., 2007). In mild TBI more specifically, Mollayeva and colleagues (2017) observed longer time spent awake compared to normative samples and less time spent in N2 and REM stages. In a meta-analysis of 14 studies conducted at least 6 months post-TBI, Mantua and colleagues (2018) concluded that, compared to control groups, the only clear result is that patients with TBI show an increased proportion of slow-wave sleep. The authors suggest that this difference may be linked to more severe injuries and could reflect ongoing neuroplasticity (synaptic remodeling, axonal sprouting) even several months post-injury.

Insomnia

Prevalence, Correlates, and Impacts of Insomnia Following TBI

Various studies conducted from a few weeks up to many years post-TBI have reported a prevalence of symptoms of insomnia ranging from about 30% to 70% (Mathias & Alvaro, 2012; Mosti et al., 2019; Ouellet et al., 2004; Wickwire et al., 2022). A recent meta-analysis of 20 studies indicates that following mild TBI, the prevalence of an insomnia disorder is 27% but that 71.7% suffer from insomnia symptoms (Montgomery et al., 2022). For a majority of patients, sleep disturbances are a new reality post-injury, with only 5%–10% reporting having had sleep problems before the injury, yet for many the condition remains untreated (Ouellet et al., 2006; Theadom et al., 2015).

Although insomnia is observed at all levels of severity of TBI (Farrell-Carnahan et al., 2015; Hou et al., 2013), several studies have shown that a milder TBI is associated with more insomnia complaints (Beetar et al., 1996; Farrell-Carnahan et al., 2015; Fichtenberg et al., 2000; Mahmood et al., 2004; Ouellet et al., 2006; Shekleton et al., 2010; Viola-Saltzman & Watson, 2012). This could be due to higher levels of self-awareness in milder injuries compared with moderate to severe TBI (which is known to cause anosognosia, a lack of self-awareness) which may in turn lead to more psychological distress (e.g., depression, anxiety, insomnia). Also, persons with mild TBI often return more rapidly to their pre-injury roles and activities, and thus may more readily perceive changes in their functioning and be distressed by these (Demakis et al., 2010). This could cause more worrying and tension and thus impact sleep quality. Pain and depressive symptoms also seem to emerge as risk factors for insomnia in some studies (Clinchot et al., 1998; Fichtenberg et al., 2000; Ouellet et al., 2006). Additional factors which have been suggested to be linked to insomnia following TBI include post-TBI fatigue and alcohol misuse (Clinchot et al., 1998; Ouellet et al., 2006).

In terms of impacts of insomnia after TBI, it has been shown to exacerbate psychological issues such as pain, psychological distress, depression, and post-traumatic stress symptoms (Chaput et al., 2009; Miller et al., 2022; Ouellet et al., 2006; Pattinson et al., 2021; Saksvik et al., 2021). Furthermore, in children (Chung et al., 2019), adolescents (Bramley et al., 2017; Brooks et al., 2019), and adults (Hoffman et al., 2020), sleep disturbances are associated with a significantly longer recovery time from concussion or mild TBI.

Evidence is accumulating that insomnia can exacerbate cognitive issues after TBI. Studies conducted with veterans have seen a link between higher insomnia severity and lower cognitive performance, for example, issues with memory (Waldron-Perrine et al., 2012), slower cognitive processing speed (Miller et al., 2022), sustained attention tasks (Bloomfield et al., 2010), and executive functioning (Shay et al., 2014). Even in cases of mild TBI with persistent symptoms, a correlation can be observed between poorer sleep quality and poorer cognitive performance, up to several years after the injury (Anderson & Jordan, 2021; Blaney et al., 2021; Dean & Sterr, 2013; Theadom, Starkey, et al., 2018). Interestingly, Wiseman-Hakes et al. (2013) observed that if they treated sleep disturbances in patients with TBI, they could measure significant improvements on tests of attention, memory, processing speed, and language.

Assessment of Insomnia in the Context of TBI

Recent clinical practice guidelines (Institut national d'excellence en santé et en services sociaux & Ontario Neurotrauma Foundation [INESSS-ONF], 2016; ONF, 2018) suggest systematically screening for sleep disturbances following TBI to identify persons in need of a more thorough assessment. We could add that this screening should probably be completed at different time points. Screening for insomnia or other sleep disturbances can be done effectively with simple questions or the sleep disturbance item of the Patient Health Questionnaire (Lequerica et al., 2022). A thorough evaluation of insomnia in patients with TBI ideally requires a comprehensive appraisal of all potential contributing factors. Clinicians should investigate both the individual's present and pre-accident sleep–wake patterns including questions on the nature, severity, duration, and evolution of insomnia, as well as typical sleep–wake cycles, daytime functioning, and levels of fatigue and alertness. In addition, clinicians must have a clear portrait of the physical condition of the patient, determining, for example, whether pain could explain the insomnia symptoms. Medications taken and interactions between medications should be examined closely because of frequent polypharmacy in this population. Moreover, a thorough assessment of potentially comorbid psychopathology is essential. In most cases of TBI, cognitive deficits are not severe enough to preclude the use of widely used self-reported instruments such as the Pittsburgh Sleep Quality Index (Buysse et al., 1989) or the Insomnia Severity Index (Morin, 1993). When severe cognitive deficits do exclude the possibility of using such instruments, the information provided by a significant other can complement the clinical interview with the patient.

If the presence of other sleep disorders is suspected (e.g., sleep-related breathing disorders, periodic limb movement disorder), a sleep laboratory evaluation is useful, although it may not always be readily accessible. Even when there are discrepancies between subjective reports and objective (PSG) measures of sleep—a frequent finding among individuals with insomnia—the diagnosis of insomnia should not be discarded (Ouellet & Morin, 2006). Our team has proposed an interview canvas adapted for insomnia in the TBI context (Ouellet et al., 2020).

Pharmacological Interventions

To date, there are very few studies informing clinicians about the safety and efficacy of medications for insomnia in persons with brain injury. Most clinicians probably thus rely on evidence obtained in non-rehabilitation patients and use the hypnotic medications which are presently known to have the best therapeutic efficacy and least side effects. When treating patients with TBI, however, several authors and clinicians urge caution because some medications have deleterious effects or may exacerbate brain injury–related problems, such as neuropsychological deficits, motor issues, or dizziness. When reviewing recent clinical practice guidelines for the rehabilitation and management of mild to severe brain injury, it is very clear that non-pharmacological interventions for insomnia are recommended over pharmacological interventions as a first-line treatment. Several authors advise complete avoidance of benzodiazepines in the TBI population or use of these as a last resort only and for only a few days, due to potential adverse effects such as memory impairment, impaired psychomotor skills, dizziness, potential for abuse and addiction, and impact on sleep architecture (Flanagan et al., 2007; INESSS-ONF, 2016). Flanagan and colleagues (2007) also do not recommend the use of drugs with anticholinergic effects (e.g., tricyclic antidepressants, diphenhydramine) because of their effects on memory and attention and because they have been shown to potentially lower the seizure threshold. Even with the "z-drugs" (i.e., zaleplon, zopiclone, zolpidem, eszopiclone), which are often prescribed for insomnia in the general population, some authors nonetheless recommend caution and only short-term use after TBI as these may also have deleterious effects on cognition in the short or long term (Larson & Zollman, 2010). Of note, Chiu and colleagues (2015) have presented data suggesting that in TBI patients suffering from insomnia, those using hypnotics were at increased risk of dementia compared to those not using any sleep medication. The latter group had a similar risk than persons who did not have insomnia after their TBI.

Other medications are also sometimes used off-label for insomnia (e.g., antidepressants such as trazodone or doxepin, antipsychotics such as gabapentin or tiagabine). Again, caution is advised to avoid deleterious or exacerbation effects on memory and attention or seizure activity. In the realm of natural products, there is some evidence that melatonin (2–5 mg) can be beneficial for post-TBI insomnia (Grima et al., 2018; INESSS-ONF, 2016; Kemp et al., 2004; Shekleton et al., 2010).

Cognitive Behavioral Therapy

There is now accumulating evidence that cognitive behavioral therapy (CBT) is an effective treatment for insomnia after TBI, which can also yield additional benefits for other related issues such as fatigue, depression, and anxiety (Ford et al., 2022; Lah et al., 2021; Lowe et al., 2022; Nguyen et al., 2017, 2018; Ouellet & Morin, 2004, 2007; Ymer et al., 2021, 2022). A recent systematic review (Pilon et al., 2021) that included patients with different types of brain injury concluded that CBT is recommended as the treatment of choice. The treatment protocols that have been used generally involve a combination of sleep hygiene education, stimulus control, restriction of time in bed, and cognitive therapy techniques. In addition, several teams have chosen to add fatigue management components, for example, activity pacing and graded physical activity.

After our team published preliminary data on the efficacy of CBT for insomnia in the context of TBI with a series of rigorous case studies (Ouellet & Morin, 2004, 2007), a first randomized controlled trial was published by another team in 2017 to further establish its efficacy. This study, however, involved patients with either TBI or stroke and targeted fatigue (Nguyen et al., 2017). The therapy consisted of psychoeducation, stimulus control, sleep restriction procedures, cognitive therapy, relaxation, and strategies for managing physical and mental fatigue (e.g., reorganization of daily schedules, graded physical activity). Compared to a treatment-as-usual control group, they found significant improvements in sleep quality and insomnia symptoms, with 70% of the CBT group improving compared to 27% of the control group. Fatigue improved in 55% of the CBT group, whereas 30% improved in the control group. A decrease in depressive symptoms was also observed. In terms of treatment response, this team found that better memory functioning was associated with better therapy outcomes, suggesting that clinicians should be attentive to patients with more important issues with memory after their TBI, for example, by planning shorter and more frequent treatment sessions, simplifying the content of therapy and monitoring patients more closely (Nguyen et al., 2018).

In a pilot randomized trial, the same research group recently compared CBT for sleep and fatigue to a health education control condition (Ymer et al., 2021). Again, CBT led to more improvements in sleep quality both during treatment and at a 2-month follow-up. These authors conclude that either CBT administered face to face or via videoconference is an effective treatment for sleep disturbance and fatigue following TBI or stroke (Ymer et al., 2021, 2022). Two other teams have also tested shorter (4 and 6 weeks) and online CBT protocols (Ford et al., 2022; Theadom, Barker-Collo, et al., 2018) and found them to be effective and feasible as well.

In a recent treatment manual published by our team (Ouellet et al., 2020), we have proposed simple adaptations made to the original treatment protocol developed by Morin (1993) in order to apply CBT to persons with TBI (see Box 44.1 and Table 44.1).

Box 44.1 Special Considerations for the Administration of Cognitive Behavioral Therapy for Insomnia Following Traumatic Brain Injury

Cognitive Deficits

Memory or attention problems may be present but in most cases do not preclude the use of cognitive behavioral therapy (CBT) or of self-reported questionnaires and sleep logs.

Shorter sessions are sometimes needed in some cases to compensate for fatigue or issues with sustained attention or vigilance. The latter may vary during sessions and from one session to another.

Simplified written material can be useful to enhance encoding and regular use of the information provided during therapy.

As needed, use simple sleep logs, and practice filling these out and interpreting them with the patients during sessions.

Repetition of therapeutic content may be useful to ensure retention.

Involvement of a significant other can be considered (explain the rationale and techniques to this person to promote collaboration and support during therapy).

Use concrete examples as needed.

For cognitive therapy, use the Dysfunctional Beliefs and Attitudes Scale (Morin, 1993) to elicit thoughts and beliefs. Suggest more appropriate or alternative interpretations as needed.

Behavioral Particularities

Particularly with patients with more severe injuries, adapt to occasional behavioral elements such as disinhibition, fluctuating adherence, missed appointments.

Discuss adherence issues with the patient, and encourage patients to adhere to treatment recommendations but stay flexible.

Discuss use of drugs (e.g., marijuana) and alcohol in interaction with sleep–wake issues.

As needed, discuss or remind patients of the parameters and structure of therapy. Consider that patients often receive a variety of healthcare services simultaneously and have several healthcare providers.

Fatigue

Persons with traumatic brain injury (TBI) often experience severe and persistent fatigue. Part of this fatigue may be due to insomnia, but another very important part is independent of sleep quality and quantity. Patients should be made aware of this before CBT starts so as to help them conserve realistic expectations.

Fatigue can lead to frequent nap- and rest-taking following TBI, habits that are known to influence the sleep–wake cycle. The efficacy of naps to relieve from fatigue should be carefully evaluated. The need for a nap must be evaluated depending on the time since the injury and the severity of daytime sleepiness (and not fatigue). The timing and length of naps should also be revised carefully.

A careful evaluation of behaviors and thoughts or beliefs relative to fatigue is warranted. Furthermore, fatigue management techniques should be added to CBT for insomnia.

Because stimulus control and sleep restriction are known to produce fatigue, at least in the first few weeks of treatment, patients should be made aware that their level of fatigue may be exacerbated. Particular attention should be given to the timing of the initiation of treatment so as to minimize the impacts related to fatigue or excessive daytime sleepiness.

Particular attention should be given to the timing of the intervention (does the patient have particularly cognitively or physically demanding or emotionally challenging events concurrent with treatment) and to inform the patient as to what to expect in the first weeks (normalize the increase in fatigue, encourage persistence).

Daily Routine

Pay attention to irregular sleep–wake schedules such as fluctuating bedtimes, excessive time spent in bed, frequent nap-taking or inactivity during the day. These elements could be more prominent in persons who have not yet returned to work following the injury.

One challenge of CBT for insomnia following TBI is to find, in collaboration with the patient, motivating activities to encourage the adherence to the sleep windows and stimulus control instructions. Indeed, because of cognitive or physical issues, the range of possible activities may be restricted.

Particular attention should be given to find activities that motivate the patient to arise in the morning. This may be a challenge for individuals who have not returned to work.

Depression and Anxiety Symptoms

Patients with depressive symptoms should be carefully evaluated. Sleep restriction should not be started before a major depressive episode is ruled out or controlled with appropriate treatment.

Address anxiety and depressive issues in therapy if they come up. Encourage the use of behavioral and cognitive techniques taught in the context of insomnia during therapy (i.e., behavioral activation and cognitive restructuring) but applied to depressive and anxious thoughts and behaviors. Explain the interconnections between sleep disturbance, fatigue, depression, anxiety, and other relevant factors (e.g., pain).

Encourage a balance in activities (physical, gratifying or useful, social, pleasurable).

Encourage the patient to seek and expand social support (an area which may have suffered after TBI).

Refer the patient to appropriate resources if the severity of psychiatric symptoms warrants treatment.

Physical Function

Some patients may be limited in their activities by physical issues. These patients may be more limited in their range of possible activities and more prone to maladaptive habits such as inactivity or nap-taking.

Evaluate the potential role of pain in insomnia. Keep informed about medications prescribed for pain or other problems.

Inform (i.e., explain the modalities and rationale of CBT for insomnia) and stay in contact with physicians and other key healthcare providers (e.g., neuropsychologist, rehabilitation counselor, occupational therapist) to ensure they know how the patient is evolving through the treatment.

Box 44.1 presents some general considerations for treatment planning or implementation with patients with TBI, and Table 44.1 summarizes the adaptations made to the original protocol. These include, for example, strategies to optimize encoding of information during therapy (to account for potential attentional and memory issues), simplification of cognitive therapy, involvement of a significant other, and addition of fatigue management skills (activity pacing, planning activities realistically into manageable steps, using rest periods efficiently, and exploring different ways to rest [not only by napping]).

Other Non-Pharmacological Interventions

Several other non-pharmacological interventions are worth noting, although research is very limited. Some research groups have studied the effects of exercise for alleviating insomnia symptoms with mixed results (Chin et al., 2015; Damiano et al., 2016; Hoffman et al., 2010). One study found that an 8-week program of five weekly sessions of 30 minutes of aerobic exercise produced significant improvement on the Pittsburgh Sleep Quality Index (Damiano et al., 2016). In a very different intervention focused on problem-solving skills for injury-related issues in military personnel with mild TBI, Vuletic and colleagues (2016) found that the intervention led to significant improvements in sleep quality, sleep-onset latency, sleep efficiency, and sleep duration. The intervention seemed to be particularly efficacious when sleep problems were associated with the presence of pain (Vuletic et al., 2016).

One group proposed a behavioral intervention to be implemented by nurses in the acute phase after the injury (De La Rue-Evans et al., 2013). The intervention included changes to the hospital environment, systematic routines, sleep hygiene education for both nurses and patients, and stimulus control strategies. Clinicians were trained to modify the environment to make it more conducive to sleep by reducing noise levels, dimming lights at night, opening blinds before dawn, and offering decaffeinated drinks when more

Table 44.1 Adaptations to the cognitive behavioral therapy protocol proposed by Morin (1993) for traumatic brain injury

CBT component	Brief description in the original protocol	Adaptation for the context of TBI
Introduction to the self-management approach	• Presentation of basic CBT principles.	• Keep expectations realistic, avoid comparisons to before the accident, keep focus on recent progress. • Explain that improving sleep quality will not necessarily eradicate TBI-related fatigue; these problems may be independent. • Aim for an increase in quality of life and social participation. • Use motivational interviewing techniques as needed.
Self-monitoring of sleep and fatigue	• Self-observation through a sleep diary to identify behaviors associated with insomnia, facilitate the application of therapy, and measure progress.	• Supervision of the sleep diary completion at the beginning of therapy, according to the client's needs. • Establishment of an effective self-monitoring routine (e.g., use reminders as needed). • Integrated self-monitoring of energy/fatigue. • Use a simplified version of the sleep diary if needed.
Psychoeducation about sleep and insomnia	• Conveying basic knowledge about sleep and the development of insomnia. • Normalize patient experiences, and validate subjective experiences.	• Communicate additional information about the impact of brain injury on sleep and the prevalence of insomnia and fatigue.
Sleep hygiene education	Basic recommendations: • Avoid stimulants. • Avoid late-night alcohol consumption. • Avoid electronic devices near bedtime and during the night. • Prefer regular physical activity (avoid near bedtime). • Keep the bedroom cool, dark, quiet, and comfortable.	• Gradual increase in physical activity to improve sleep and fatigue symptoms. • Pay particular attention to use of alcohol or soft drugs used in part to manage sleep issues.

Stimulus control	• Reinforce the association between sleep, and temporal and spatial stimuli associated with sleep. Recommendations: • Set aside at least 1 hour before bedtime to relax and unwind. • Go to bed only when drowsiness is felt. • If unable to fall asleep or to fall back asleep in 15–20 minutes, get out of bed, do a quiet activity, and return to bed when drowsiness returns. • Get up at the same time each morning, regardless of how much sleep you get. • Reserve the bed and bedroom for sleep and sexual activity only. • Avoid naps during the day.	• For clients with pain or mobility issues (risk of falling), accommodations can be made to the original protocol: using a comfortable chair or couch to alter the environment during nighttime awakenings (e.g., listening to music in a comfortable chair with a blanket while waiting for signs of drowsiness). • For clients with significant post-TBI fatigue, naps may be difficult to avoid, especially in the first few months post-accident. However, to limit the negative impact of naps and maximize their usefulness, encourage patients to keep naps short (e.g., 15–30 minutes) and to avoid naps after 3:00 p.m. When implementing restriction of time in bed (see next point), some flexibility about daytime naps may promote better adherence to the nighttime sleep window.
Restriction of time in bed	• Limit time in bed as close as possible to actual sleep time. • Consolidate sleep into a shorter period of time. • Define, in collaboration with the client, a sleep window based on the number of hours slept per night in the past week (on the sleep diary). • Adhere to the sleep window for at least 1 week, then adjust it based on the average sleep efficiency for the week.	• Some clients are off work for several weeks, months, or indefinitely as a result of brain injury, and therefore may not have a regular routine. Explore different types of activities adapted to the person's condition in order to establish a morning routine to help them get up and be active at a regular time (e.g., plan pleasant morning activities, explore appropriate activities for nighttime).
Cognitive therapy	• Identify and modify beliefs and attitudes that perpetuate insomnia (e.g., performance anxiety, worries about the possible consequences of insomnia, unrealistic expectations about sleep or energy level, etc.).	• A simplified cognitive therapy is suggested: identification of targets via the Sleep Belief and Attitude Scale followed by a more psychoeducational than Socratic approach. • For clients with less introspection, guide toward other interpretations if unable to do so spontaneously, and write down alternative thoughts (e.g., on a memory card, in the sleep diary, or in a personal diary/agenda). • Detect and modify TBI-related thoughts that may be contributing to insomnia (e.g., "If I don't sleep well, my brain will never recover from the injury," "If I can't sleep, I'll never be able to return to work.").

Continued

Table 44.1 *Continued*

CBT component	Brief description in the original protocol	Adaptation for the context of TBI

Having a significant other or caregiver involved in therapy	Not in the original protocol.	• Significant others can contribute to promote client motivation and compliance if they are well aware of the rationale of different treatment components: they can be invited to important sessions (e.g., second session).
		• Take into account changes in family roles due to TBI. Be mindful of potentially counterproductive habits. Examples:
		  • A loved one who takes on a large number of family tasks after the accident for fear of "tiring out" their injured loved one, which impedes reactivation.
		  • A loved one who cancels the client's medical, social, or work-related appointments because their loved one is too tired or had a bad night's sleep.
		  • A loved one who discourages the client from exercising for fear that the client will fall and suffer another injury.

Stress-management techniques	Not in the original protocol.	• Consider concerns related to health, brain recovery, and multiple psychosocial stressors that may arise from the accident (e.g. multiple medical constraints, absence from work litigation). • Include worry management techniques as needed ("worry chair," relaxation, mindfulness, or imagery techniques to manage thoughts or worries throughout the day).
Psychoeducation about fatigue and links between activities and energy levels	Not in the original protocol.	• Provide information on post-TBI fatigue, normalizing the person's experience. • Underscore the importance of taking time to adjust to this symptom. • Present the link between energy levels, mood, physical activity, and other types of activity. • Present the different types of fatigue (physical or mental) and their impact on motivation and mood. • Distinguish between fatigue and daytime sleepiness.

Recognition of signs of fatigue	Not in the original protocol.	• Since fatigue appears suddenly after the accident, offer training to self-observe one's energy level through activities (use of a fatigue barometer). • Provide training to enhance the perception of signs of fatigue. • Identify activities that are more or less tiring and those that restore energy.
Activity pacing	Not in the original protocol.	• Encourage clients to plan activities according to available energy and to manage energy during activities. • Plan behavioral experiments with these strategies. • Encourage clients to plan rest periods in advance. • Encourage clients to divide activities into shorter periods or more manageable units so as not to aggravate fatigue. • Encourage clients to alternate between different types of tasks (e.g., alternating between cognitive and physical tasks).
Attitudes regarding fatigue	Not in the original protocol.	• Identify fatigue-related factors that are controllable. • Discuss different strategies for resting, explore different ways to rest even while being somewhat active. • Discuss the balance between different types of activities (obligations, responsibilities, social, physical, mental, leisure, etc.) to contribute to self-esteem (e.g., productive tasks), social support and bonding, and overall mental and physical health. • Maintain realistic expectations about energy levels, and acknowledge when help is needed. • Reinforce what is accomplished despite fatigue rather than what is not done because of fatigue. • Explore with the patient how to resume or adapt certain activities that have been put aside because of fatigue. • Explore new leisure, productive, or satisfying activities if some are no longer possible because of the injury.

Note. Please see the treatment manual (Ouellet et al., 2020) for a more precise description of these adaptations. CBT = cognitive behavioral therapy; TBI = traumatic brain injury.

appropriate. Clinicians were encouraged to keep TBI patients active and awake during the day, to help them maintain a regular sleep–wake schedule, and to pay attention to naps. Although this was a pilot study, the intervention was found to be feasible and to produce some clinical benefits.

In veterans with TBI (Elliott et al., 2022), a 4-week exposure to bright light therapy showed promise for improving symptoms related to insomnia, mood, and pain. In one pilot study, patients receiving acupuncture after TBI were observed to take less hypnotics and had improved sleep quality and higher scores on cognitive tests (Zollman et al., 2012). There is, however, to our knowledge, no other research relative to the efficacy of acupuncture for post-TBI insomnia.

Disorders Causing EDS Following TBI

Prevalence, Correlates, and Impacts of EDS in TBI

SUBJECTIVE EDS

Following TBI, sleepiness can appear either alone or as a symptom of another condition. Indeed, EDS is a core feature of several sleep disorders that may develop after a TBI. EDS has often been described as a persistent symptom, lasting several years after the injury, some authors even reporting an increased prevalence of EDS with time (Cohen et al., 1992; Parcell et al., 2006). Several studies have estimated the frequency of occurrence of subjective sleepiness, and their results suggest that it affects between about 15% and 60% of individuals with TBI (Baumann et al., 2007; Beetar et al., 1996; Cohen et al., 1992; Kempf et al., 2010; Parcell et al., 2006; Verma et al., 2007; Watson et al., 2007). The variability of the results in the literature can be attributed to methodological discrepancies regarding sample characteristics (e.g., TBI severity range, time elapsed since injury, age), definitions of subjectively assessed EDS (e.g., increased napping, sleep propensity), and assessment methods (e.g., symptom checklist, self-reported sleepiness questionnaire). In their meta-analysis, Mathias and Alvaro (2012) found that 60% of patients complained of snoring, and 27% reported daytime sleepiness.

OBJECTIVE MEASURES OF EDS

In addition to evaluating subjective complaints of sleepiness after TBI with self-reported interviews or questionnaires, some studies have used the Multiple Sleep Latency Test (MSLT) to derive an objective (physiological) measure of EDS. Those studies have yielded rates of occurrence of 11% at least 3 months after the injury (Castriotta et al., 2007) and of 25% at least 6 months after the injury (Baumann et al., 2007). Overall, when using objective investigations of EDS with PSG measures, 10% to 28% meet criteria for objective EDS (Baumann et al., 2007; Castriotta et al., 2007; Hartvigsen et al., 2014). In the general population, the weak association between subjective and objective sleepiness is well documented, especially with regard to the most frequently used instruments, the

Epworth Sleepiness Scale, a self-reported questionnaire on subjective sleep propensity, and the MSLT. The fact that subjective and objective EDS are different constructs is perhaps even more noticeable in special populations such as individuals with TBI (Baumann et al., 2007; Castriotta et al., 2007; Verma et al., 2007). Another challenge in this population is to differentiate subjective EDS from fatigue. In a review, Castriotta and Murthy (2011) estimate that about 46% of all chronic TBI patients have sleep disorders, 23% have obstructive sleep apnea (OSA), 11% can be diagnosed with post-traumatic hypersomnia, 6% have narcolepsy, and 7% have periodic leg movement syndrome. In addition, 25% have objective EDS as measured by an MSLT score <10.

SLEEP APNEA

There is good evidence that sleep apnea is much more frequent after TBI compared to the general population, with estimates of prevalence ranging from 23% to 75% in different samples (Castriotta & Lai, 2001; Castriotta & Murthy, 2011; Castriotta et al., 2007; Holcomb et al., 2016; Mathias & Alvaro, 2012; Wilde et al., 2007). In a sample of 28 TBI patients studied on average 35 days after their injury, the apnea/hypopnea index (AHI) was above clinical threshold (≥5) in 30% and moderately severe (≥10) in 11% (Webster et al., 2001). In another study, with 60 patients complaining of poor sleep between 3 and 24 months after the injury, a severely abnormal AHI was found in 30% of the sample (Verma et al., 2007). The authors also noted that 74% of the respiratory events were obstructive. Another investigation reported that 32% of patients who were referred for a sleep evaluation because of complaints of EDS were diagnosed with sleep apnea following their TBI (Guilleminault et al., 2000). A more recent study prospectively examined the incidence of sleep apnea in 86 consecutive brain injury rehabilitation admissions and found half of the sample (49%) to be diagnosable with sleep apnea (Holcomb et al., 2016).

NARCOLEPSY

Narcolepsy is more rarely associated with TBI. Nonetheless, Ebrahim et al. (2005) published a review of the literature, reporting on 22 published cases of narcolepsy following TBI. According to their results, post-traumatic narcolepsy is highly variable across patients. In fact, symptom onset ranges from a few hours to 18 months post-TBI, and the presenting symptom can be EDS, cataplexy, or both. It appears that the development of narcolepsy is independent of various indices of TBI severity (e.g., presence of loss of consciousness, computed tomographic [CT] scan or magnetic resonance imaging findings). For most patients, the disorder worsens over time if left untreated.

POST-TRAUMATIC HYPERSOMNIA

When other sleep disorders and other medical or psychiatric conditions associated with sleepiness have been ruled out, a diagnosis of post-traumatic hypersomnia can be considered as part of the broader diagnostic category of hypersomnia due to a medical condition in the *International Classification of Sleep Disorders*, 3rd edition (American Academy of Sleep Medicine, 2014). A complaint of EDS has to be present almost daily following TBI in the absence of premorbid history of sleepiness or other sleep–wake problems. In four studies assessing the prevalence of sleep disorders with nocturnal and diurnal PSG, post-traumatic hypersomnia was diagnosed in 10% to 30% of participants (Baumann et al., 2007; Castriotta & Lai, 2001; Castriotta et al., 2007; Masel et al., 2001).

INCREASED NEED FOR SLEEP

The term *post-traumatic pleiosomnia* has been proposed to describe the increased need for sleep often observed after moderate or severe TBI (Imbach et al., 2015; Sommerauer et al., 2013). Using actigraphy 6 months after the injury, Imbach and colleagues (2015) found that patients with TBI slept 1.5 hours more per 24-hour period compared to a control group. They also observed that 57% of the TBI group had objective sleepiness on the MSLT compared to 19% in the control group. Another finding was more consolidated non-REM sleep in the TBI group. The authors hypothesized that pleiosomnia after TBI might reflect a heightened need for neuroplasticity. If assessed with a subjective measure, the Epworth Sleepiness Scale, patients were found to underestimate their EDS. Pleiosomnia was strongly linked with more severe injuries (lower Glasgow Coma Scale scores, presence of hemorrhage on CT scans), which is in line with previous research (Baumann et al., 2007; Chiu et al., 2014; Guilleminault et al., 2000; Hou et al., 2013).

IMPACTS OF EDS

In the general population, sleepiness has been associated with a number of negative outcomes, such as cognitive problems, mostly in the attentional domain; depressed mood; increased risk of road accidents; and disrupted family and social life (Roehrs et al., 2005). Few studies have documented the correlates and impacts of EDS specifically in the context of TBI. Parcell and colleagues (2006) found that a higher level of subjective EDS is associated with a higher level of anxiety symptoms and longer daytime naps. Patients suffering from EDS or patients with sleep apnea have been shown to perform significantly worse than patients without EDS on tests of attention and memory (Castriotta et al., 2007; Wilde et al., 2007). In adolescents, EDS was observed to be linked with more executive function deficits as reported by both parents and adolescent patients themselves (Osorio et al., 2013).

EDS may also affect participation in rehabilitation. Worthington and Melia (2006) asked rehabilitation clinicians to evaluate the impact of sleep and arousal disturbances during therapy in 135 patients with TBI: 47.4% of their sample had disturbances in sleep or arousal, and in 65.6% of cases, these sleep–wake disturbances interfered with rehabilitation therapy sessions and with patients' daily activities (e.g., patient unable to stay awake during an intervention or activity, patient missing appointments or opportunities due to late awakening time). Similarly, Silva and colleagues (2012) observed that hypersomnolence could predict post-traumatic confusion and impacted patient collaboration during inpatient rehabilitation interventions.

Assessment of EDS in the Context of TBI

In order to obtain a complete picture of the experience of sleepiness, clinicians ought to use various sources of information. Ideally, information obtained from the patient should be validated with a reliable informant, especially if the patient has important cognitive and/or self-awareness impairments. Patients and informants should be asked for the frequency, duration, severity, context, and physiological manifestations of daytime sleepiness. Other questions may target nighttime sleep pattern, quality and duration, napping, common symptoms of specific sleep disorders associated with EDS (e.g., presence of snoring, breathing interruptions, cataplexy), as well as the impact of comorbid psychiatric (e.g., mood disturbances, substance abuse) and medical (e.g., pain, epilepsy) conditions and of medications. It is also essential to document premorbid sleep history. In fact, it is possible that some patients had non-diagnosed sleep disorders involving EDS such as sleep apnea syndromes prior to their injury (Castriotta & Lai, 2001; Castriotta et al., 2007). Moreover, EDS associated with the presence of such a sleep disorder may even have contributed to the accident causing TBI.

Clinical interviews should be complemented with more systematic data obtained from subjective, behavioral, or physiological assessment tools. One commonly used self-reported instrument assessing EDS is the Epworth Sleepiness Scale (Johns, 1991), which evaluates the probability of falling asleep in eight situations, yet some patients may have difficult completing this measure. Other questionnaires, such as the Stanford Sleepiness Scale (Hoddes et al., 1973), aim at measuring sleepiness by asking the patient how sleepy they are at the present moment. As for clinical interviews, informants may be asked to complete subjective questionnaires when deemed relevant.

Despite its high costs and low availability, PSG recording remains the method of choice to evaluate more objectively daytime sleepiness and screen for disorders associated with such symptoms. Daytime PSG can thus be considered to evaluate EDS, using either the MSLT or the Maintenance of Wakefulness Test (MWT; Arand et al., 2005). The MWT is less useful for diagnostic purposes, mainly for narcolepsy, but may be more appropriate when the goal is to determine whether patients can remain awake during the day in the absence of external stimulations. This could be relevant when evaluating the capacity of TBI patients to perform tasks such as working or driving long distances, which are extremely important issues in rehabilitation.

When evaluating EDS, it is also essential to rule out the effects of medications used for other issues after TBI. Indeed, sleepiness is a potential side effect of numerous agents commonly used with the TBI population, specifically pain medication, hypnotics (including benzodiazepines and non-benzodiazepines), antidepressants, anticonvulsants, antipsychotics, and muscle relaxants (Pagel, 2005). To avoid a decrease in daytime alertness and other related undesirable consequences, a careful evaluation and monitoring of the potential side effects and medication interactions should be made before and during psychopharmacological treatment with TBI patients. Recently, Martin and colleagues (2021) observed that patients receiving opioid medications following moderate to severe TBI had increased markers of sleep-related breathing disorders including a higher frequency of central sleep apnea and OSA events as well as lower oxygen saturation nadir and higher oxygen desaturations across REM and non-REM sleep. Since the use of opioids is frequent following TBI, these authors underline that there is a need for more research to establish the potential link with sleep-disordered breathing.

Treatment of EDS Following TBI

As for insomnia, there are very few available data or recommendations regarding treatment of EDS and associated sleep disorders in TBI patients.

STIMULANTS

A handful of studies have documented the use of specific neurostimulants (i.e., modafinil, methylphenidate) as these agents have been found to be effective in other populations. In one study, daytime alertness was improved by methylphenidate but not by sertraline, an antidepressant, in a sample of 30 TBI patients (Lee et al., 2005). According to a retrospective study on 30 TBI patients, methylphenidate does not seem to significantly reduce the number of hours slept during the night or the day (Al-Adawi et al., 2006). Modafinil, another neurostimulant, is known to be effective at alleviating EDS in narcolepsy, OSA, and shift-work sleep disorder (Kumar, 2008). However, a randomized controlled trial with 51 mild to severe TBI patients revealed that modafinil did not provide any benefit compared to placebo on sleepiness and fatigue symptoms (Jha et al., 2008). Moreover, insomnia was more frequently reported as an adverse effect following modafinil treatment compared to placebo in this study.

CONTINUOUS POSITIVE AIRWAY PRESSURE FOR SLEEP APNEA

Treatment with continuous positive airway pressure (CPAP), which is the typical therapeutic device for OSA, has seldom been studied for sleepiness or apnea symptoms with the TBI population. Clearly, given the relatively high prevalence of sleep apnea in the TBI population, research on CPAP is warranted to document its efficacy and acceptability in these patients. In 13 patients with TBI, Castriotta and colleagues (2009) found significant improvements in the number of respiratory events during sleep (decreased AHI) after 3 months of CPAP use. It must be noted, however, that this result was not accompanied by improvements on the Epworth Sleepiness Scale or on an objective assessment of EDS with the MSLT. There is very little data on adherence to CPAP within the TBI population, which is surprising as behavioral issues might complicate adaptation and compliance with treatment. Recently, Silva and colleagues (2020) performed a retrospective chart study of 230 persons with acquired brain injury (traumatic and non-traumatic) treated with CPAP for moderate or severe OSA. Almost two-thirds of their sample were not adhering to CPAP.

LIGHT THERAPY

Some evidence is emerging concerning the efficacy of light therapy for EDS in the context of TBI. One randomized controlled trial of 30 patients with TBI with fatigue or sleep–wake disturbances compared blue light therapy (45 minutes per morning for 4 weeks) to placebo yellow light and to a no-treatment control group (Sinclair et al., 2014). Blue light therapy was found to reduce both fatigue and daytime sleepiness, results not found in the other two comparison groups. With a multimodal brain imaging battery, Raikes and colleagues (2021) recently documented effects of blue light therapy. They found that, compared to a placebo amber light, patients treated with blue light therapy had greater gray matter volume in 15 regions of the brain and an increase in functional connectivity between attention and cognitive control networks. These imaging findings were accompanied by improvements in daytime sleepiness.

Circadian Rhythm Sleep Disorders Following TBI

Prevalence and Correlates

Following TBI, a disruption of circadian rhythms may arise. For instance, in a study on changes in sleep schedules, three of 10 TBI patients reported an earlier bedtime and four reported a later bedtime compared to their pre-injury status (Steele et al., 2005). These patients were assessed from 74 to 1,194 days post-TBI. When the sleep–wake cycle disruption persists over time and is accompanied by significant functional impairments, a circadian rhythm sleep disorder (CRSD) can be diagnosed. CRSDs are characterized by a mismatch between the individual's sleep–wake rhythm and the 24-hour environment. Several 24-hour rhythms can be disturbed in CRSD, including the sleep–wake cycle, melatonin secretion, and body temperature. As CRSD is a less frequent problem following TBI compared to insomnia and EDS, epidemiological data is lacking. Most studies reporting post-TBI sleep–wake cycle disruptions are case studies. Cases of delayed sleep phase disorder (DSPD), characterized by a prolonged delay (usually more than 2 hours) in the sleep–wake episodes relative to conventional times, have been reported in the literature (Boivin et al., 2004; Nagtegaal et al., 1997; Patten & Lauderdale, 1992; Quinto et al., 2000). One of these cases also displayed a hypernycthemeral syndrome (i.e., non-24-hour sleep–wake cycle) in addition to DSPD (Boivin et al., 2004). A more recent investigation reported data on 15 mild TBI patients diagnosed with CRSD based on actigraphic recordings, eight of them having DSPD and seven having irregular sleep–wake rhythm disorder (i.e., high day-to-day variability in sleep onset and offset; Ayalon et al., 2007). In this study, melatonin and body temperature rhythms were also delayed in TBI compared to control participants. The differential diagnosis with insomnia must be considered. Recently, Zalai and colleagues (2020) found that 26% of their sample reporting chronic insomnia following mild TBI actually had a CRSD. Some overlap of those two conditions is often reported in clinical practice.

Even in the absence of a definite CRSD, there are some indications that the sleep–wake cycle is disturbed following TBI. In an investigation comparing 17 moderate to severe TBI patients to 12 healthy controls, Beaulieu-Bonneau and colleagues (2009) observed that TBI patients were more likely to report sleepiness and decreased alertness in the early afternoon hours and following a driving simulator task. Consequently, it may be hypothesized that individuals with TBI could be more vulnerable to circadian variations of alertness level.

Assessment of CRSD in the Context of TBI

As is the case for other sleep-related disturbances, a thorough assessment of sleep schedules should include information from both the individual with TBI and a significant other, ideally a spouse or a person able to document sleep patterns. Sleep diaries and actigraphy are obviously useful instruments to document habitual bedtime and arising time, night-to-night variability, as well as sleep quality. Moreover, a few questionnaires have been developed specifically to evaluate circadian issues. First, the Morningness–Eveningness Questionnaire (MEQ; Horne & Ostberg, 1976) can be used to determine preferences in sleep–wake schedules (e.g., morning type, evening type). Results from this instrument have to be interpreted with caution while taking into account the psychological and cognitive factors that may influence the answers of the patient. As the MEQ can be influenced by cognitive limitations, especially with severe TBI patients, some authors (Steele et al., 2005) have suggested that it may be preferable to use the Sleep Timing Questionnaire (Monk et al., 2003) as it relies to a lesser extent on hypothetical situations.

Treatment of CRSD in the Context of TBI

Data regarding pharmacological treatment options for post-TBI CRSD is very limited. While sedatives and hypnotics have been tried, melatonin remains a more likely effective candidate. Nagtegaal and colleagues (1997) successfully treated a 15-year-old girl with DSPD with 5 mg melatonin: her sleep schedule was initially delayed almost half a day and reverted to normal with treatment. Among non-pharmacological interventions for disturbed sleep patterns, chronotherapy (i.e., gradually and systematically shifting bedtime and arising time toward desired schedule) is probably the most promising alternative, although the only available study found that chronotherapy was unsuccessful with a 48-year-old man with DSPD (Quinto et al., 2000). Some elements of CBT for insomnia (e.g., restriction of time in bed, scheduled naps, regular arising time) can be adapted to assist in the management of CRSD in patients with TBI. Light therapy is another option. In a recent randomized controlled trial of daily morning blue-wavelength light exposure versus amber placebo light after a mild TBI (Killgore et al., 2020), blue light therapy was found to produce phase advancing. More research is needed to evaluate the efficacy of non-pharmacological treatments for sleep–wake cycle disruptions after TBI. Of note, special attention should be put on reinforcing compliance to recommendations as this is often the main reason for lack of success of chronotherapy and light therapy.

Future Research

Despite a recent surge in scientific interest with regard to sleep–wake disturbances following TBI, much work remains to be done in order to improve the clinical characterization and management of these problems. For example, it would help to better understand the specific etiology and neurophysiological bases of sleep disorders in TBI. This would further guide the development of safe and effective treatments truly adapted to these patients with complex clinical presentations where neurophysiological, psychological, and environmental factors interact closely. Future research should clarify how the severity of the injury and time since the injury impact sleep. For example, hypersomnia and increased need for sleep seem to be more frequently observed after severe TBI and in the acute phase after TBI, whereas insomnia seems to be more frequently observed in the longer term following the injury and is quite prevalent after mild TBI but also in the rest of the severity spectrum.

There is also much research needed to further evaluate the efficacy of different treatment avenues and to explore issues linked to compliance. It is essential that this research examine outcomes beyond sleep, integrating more distal outcomes that are also affected by TBI, such as daytime functioning (e.g., fatigue), cognition, mood, pain, and overall quality of life and social participation. It seems also essential to further our understanding of the scope and particularities of sleep-related issues in other age groups with TBI such as children, adolescents, and older adults. For example, it remains unclear how CBT or pharmacological treatments must be adapted for these specific groups.

Conclusion

Sleep and daytime sleepiness are becoming increasingly important issues in the rehabilitation of patients with TBI. Indeed, sleep–wake disturbances have until recently been often overlooked, probably because of the high predominance of physical, cognitive, and functional impairments which need rapid and massive attention following trauma. It is now clear that insomnia and sleepiness affect large proportions of patients, and this is unfortunately true up to several years post-injury. Given the now documented different impacts of sleep–wake disturbances on functioning and recovery after a brain injury, it is becoming increasingly clear that it is imperative to pay more clinical attention to sleep in both the acute and chronic phases after the injury. Indeed, improving sleep quality has the potential to promote neural and functional recovery and to facilitate rehabilitation interventions.

References

Agrawal, A., Cincu, R., & Joharapurkar, S. R. (2008). Traumatic brain injury and sleep disturbances. *Journal of Clinical Sleep Medicine, 4*(2), 177. http://www.ncbi.nlm.nih.gov/entrez/query.fcgi?cmd=Retrieve&db=PubMed&dopt=Citation&list_uids=18468317

Al-Adawi, S., Burke, D. T., & Dorvlo, A. S. (2006). The effect of methylphenidate on the sleep–wake cycle of brain-injured patients undergoing rehabilitation. *Sleep Medicine, 7*(3), 287–291. https://doi.org/10.1016/j.sleep.2005.11.008

American Academy of Sleep Medicine. (2014). *International classification of sleep disorders: Diagnostic and coding manual* (3rd ed.).

Anderson, J. F. I., & Jordan, A. S. (2021). An observational study of the association between sleep disturbance, fatigue and cognition in the post-acute period after mild traumatic brain injury in prospectively studied premorbidly healthy adults. *Neuropsychological Rehabilitation, 31*(9), 1444–1465. https://doi.org/10.1080/09602011.2020.1781665

Arand, D., Bonnet, M., Hurwitz, T., Mitler, M., Rosa, R., & Sangal, R. B. (2005). The clinical use of the MSLT and MWT. *Sleep, 28*(1), 123–144. http://www.ncbi.nlm.nih.gov/entrez/query.fcgi?cmd=Retrieve&db=PubMed&dopt=Citation&list_uids=15700728

Ayalon, L., Borodkin, K., Dishon, L., Kanety, H., & Dagan, Y. (2007). Circadian rhythm sleep disorders following mild traumatic brain injury. *Neurology, 68*(14), 1136–1140. https://doi.org/10.1212/01.wnl.0000258672.52836.30

Baumann, C. R., Bassetti, C. L., Valko, P. O., Haybaeck, J., Keller, M., Clark, E., Stocker, R., Tolnay, M., & Scammell, T. E. (2009). Loss of hypocretin (orexin) neurons with traumatic brain injury. *Annals of Neurology, 66*(4), 555–559. https://doi.org/10.1002/ana.21836

Baumann, C. R., Stocker, R., Imhof, H. G., Trentz, O., Hersberger, M., Mignot, E., & Bassetti, C. L. (2005). Hypocretin-1 (orexin A) deficiency in acute traumatic brain injury. *Neurology, 65*(1), 147–149. https://doi.org/10.1212/01.wnl.0000167605.02541.f2

Baumann, C. R., Werth, E., Stocker, R., Ludwig, S., & Bassetti, C. L. (2007). Sleep–wake disturbances 6 months after traumatic brain injury: A prospective study. *Brain, 130*(7), 1873–1883. https://doi.org/10.1093/brain/awm109

Beaulieu-Bonneau, S., Roy, M.-A., & Morin, C. M. (2009). Daytime sleepiness after moderate/severe traumatic brain injury: Preliminary findings. *Sleep, 32*(S1), Article A311.

Beetar, J. T., Guilmette, T. J., & Sparadeo, F. R. (1996). Sleep and pain complaints in symptomatic traumatic brain injury and neurologic populations. *Archives of Physical and Medical Rehabilitation, 77*(12), 1298–1302. https://doi.org/10.1016/S0003-9993(96)90196-3

Billiard, M., & Podesta, C. (2013). Recurrent hypersomnia following traumatic brain injury. *Sleep Medicine, 14*(5), 462–465. https://doi.org/10.1016/j.sleep.2013.01.009

Blaney, N. A., Trbovich, A., Ernst, N., Eagle, S. R., Collins, M. W., & Kontos, A. P. (2021). Influence of sleep dysfunction on concussion assessment outcomes among adolescent athletes after concussion and healthy controls. *Clinical Journal of Sport Medicine, 31*(6), 481–487. https://doi.org/10.1097/JSM.0000000000000860

Bloomfield, I. L., Espie, C. A., & Evans, J. J. (2010). Do sleep difficulties exacerbate deficits in sustained attention following traumatic brain injury? *Journal of the International Neuropsychological Society, 16*(1), 17–25. https://doi.org/10.1017/S1355617709990798

Boivin, D. B., Caliyurt, O., James, F. O., & Chalk, C. (2004). Association between delayed sleep phase and hypernyctohemeral syndromes: A case study. *Sleep, 27*(3), 417–421. http://www.ncbi.nlm.nih.gov/entrez/query.fcgi?cmd=Retrieve&db=PubMed&dopt=Citation&list_uids=15164893

Bramley, H., Henson, A., Lewis, M. M., Kong, L., Stetter, C., & Silvis, M. (2017). Sleep disturbance following concussion is a risk factor for a prolonged recovery. *Clinical Pediatrics, 56*(14), 1280–1285. https://doi.org/10.1177/0009922816681603

Brooks, B. L., Sayers, P. Q., Virani, S., Rajaram, A. A., & Tomfohr-Madsen, L. (2019). Insomnia in adolescents with slow recovery from concussion. *Journal of Neurotrauma, 36*(16), 2391–2399. https://doi.org/10.1089/neu.2018.6257

Buysse, D. J., Reynolds, C. F., 3rd, Monk, T. H., Berman, S. R., & Kupfer, D. J. (1989). The Pittsburgh Sleep Quality Index: A new instrument for psychiatric practice and research. *Psychiatry Research, 28*(2), 193–213. http://www.ncbi.nlm.nih.gov/entrez/query.fcgi?cmd=Retrieve&db=PubMed&dopt=Citation&list_uids=2748771

Carroll, E. L., Outtrim, J. G., Forsyth, F., Manktelow, A. E., Hutchinson, P. J. A., Tenovuo, O., Posti, J. P., Wilson, L., Sahakian, B. J., Menon, D. K., & Newcombe, V. F. J. (2020). Mild traumatic brain injury recovery: A growth curve modelling analysis over 2 years. *Journal of Neurology, 267*(11), 3223–3234. https://doi.org/10.1007/s00415-020-09979-x

Carroll, L. J., Cassidy, J. D., Peloso, P. M., Borg, J., von Holst, H., Holm, L., Paniak, C., & Pepin, M. (2004). Prognosis for mild traumatic brain injury: Results of the WHO Collaborating Centre Task Force on Mild Traumatic Brain Injury. *Journal of Rehabilitation Medicine, 43*, 84–105. http://www.ncbi.nlm.nih.gov/entrez/query.fcgi?cmd=Retrieve&db=PubMed&dopt=Citation&list_uids=15083873

Castriotta, R. J., Atanasov, S., Wilde, M. C., Masel, B. E., Lai, J. M., & Kuna, S. T. (2009). Treatment of sleep disorders after traumatic brain injury. *Journal of Clinical Sleep Medicine : JCSM : official publication of the American Academy of Sleep Medicine, 5*(2), 137–144.

Castriotta, R. J., & Lai, J. M. (2001). Sleep disorders associated with traumatic brain injury. *Archives of Physical Medicine and Rehabilitation, 82*(10), 1403–1406. https://doi.org/10.1053/apmr.2001.26081

Castriotta, R. J., & Murthy, J. N. (2011). Sleep disorders in patients with traumatic brain injury: A review. *CNS Drugs, 25*(3), 175–185. https://doi.org/10.2165/11584870-000000000-00000

Castriotta, R. J., Wilde, M. C., Lai, J. M., Atanasov, S., Masel, B. E., & Kuna, S. T. (2007). Prevalence and consequences of sleep disorders in traumatic brain injury. *Journal of Clinical Sleep Medicine, 3*(4), 349–356.

Chaput, G., Giguere, J. F., Chauny, J. M., Denis, R., & Lavigne, G. (2009). Relationship among subjective sleep complaints, headaches, and mood alterations following a mild traumatic brain injury. *Sleep Medicine, 10*(7), 713–716. https://doi.org/10.1016/j.sleep.2008.07.015

Chen, P. Y., Tsai, P. S., Chen, N. H., Chaung, L. P., Lee, C. C., Chen, C. C., Chiu, H. T., Lu, Y. J., Wei, K. C., Chiu, H. Y., Chiu, H. Y., Chen, P. Y., Chen, N. H., Chuang, L. P., & Tsai, P. S. (2015). Trajectories of sleep and its predictors in the first year following traumatic brain injury. *Journal of Head Trauma Rehabilitation, 30*(4), E50–E55. https://doi.org/10.1097/htr.0000000000000086

Chin, L. M., Keyser, R. E., Dsurney, J., & Chan, L. (2015). Improved cognitive performance following aerobic exercise training in people with traumatic brain injury. *Archives of Physical and Medical Rehabilitation, 96*(4), 754–759. https://doi.org/10.1016/j.apmr.2014.11.009

Chiu, H. Y., Chen, P. Y., Chen, N. H., Chuang, L. P., & Tsai, P. S. (2013). Trajectories of sleep changes during the acute phase of traumatic brain injury: A 7-day actigraphy study. *Journal of the Formosan Medical Association, 112*(9), 545–553. https://doi.org/10.1016/j.jfma.2013.06.007

Chiu, H. Y., Lin, E. Y., Wei, L., Lin, J. H., Lee, H. C., Fan, Y. C., & Tsai, P. S. (2015). Hypnotics use but not insomnia increased the risk of dementia in traumatic brain injury patients. *European Neuropsychopharmacology, 25*(12), 2271–2277. https://doi.org/10.1016/j.euroneuro.2015.09.011

Chiu, H. Y., Lo, W. C., Chiang, Y. H., & Tsai, P. S. (2014). The effects of sleep on the relationship between brain injury severity and recovery of cognitive function: A prospective study. *International Journal of Nursing Studies, 51*(6), 892–899. https://doi.org/10.1016/j.ijnurstu.2013.10.020

Chung, J. S., Zynda, A. J., Didehbani, N., Hicks, C., Hynan, L. S., Miller, S. M., Bell, K. R., & Cullum, C. M. (2019). Association between sleep quality and recovery following sport-related concussion in pediatrics. *Journal of Child Neurology, 34*(11), 639–645. https://doi.org/10.1177/0883073819849741

Clinchot, D. M., Bogner, J., Mysiw, W. J., Fugate, L., & Corrigan, J. (1998). Defining sleep disturbance after brain injury. *American Journal of Physical Medicine & Rehabilitation, 77*(4), 291–295. http://www.ncbi.nlm.nih.gov/entrez/query.fcgi?cmd=Retrieve&db=PubMed&dopt=Citation&list_uids=9715917

Cohen, M., Oksenberg, A., Snir, D., Stern, M. J., & Groswasser, Z. (1992). Temporally related changes of sleep complaints in traumatic brain injured patients. *Journal of Neurology, Neurosurgery, and Psychiatry, 55*(4), 313–315. http://www.ncbi.nlm.nih.gov/entrez/query.fcgi?cmd=Retrieve&db=PubMed&dopt=Citation&list_uids=1583518

Damiano, D. L., Zampieri, C., Ge, J., Acevedo, A., & Dsurney, J. (2016). Effects of a rapid-resisted elliptical training program on motor, cognitive and neurobehavioral functioning in adults with chronic traumatic brain injury. *Experimental Brain Research, 234*(8), 2245–2252. https://doi.org/10.1007/s00221-016-4630-8

Dean, P. J., & Sterr, A. (2013). Long-term effects of mild traumatic brain injury on cognitive performance. *Frontiers in Human Neuroscience, 7*, Article 30. https://doi.org/10.3389/fnhum.2013.00030

De La Rue-Evans, L., Nesbitt, K., & Oka, R. K. (2013). Sleep hygiene program implementation in patients with traumatic brain injury. *Rehabilitation Nursing, 38*(1), 2–10. https://doi.org/10.1002/rnj.66

Demakis, G. J., Hammond, F. M., & Knotts, A. (2010). Prediction of depression and anxiety 1 year after moderate–severe traumatic brain injury. *Applied Neuropsychology, 17*(3), 183–189. https://doi.org/10.1080/09084282.2010.499752

Dewan, M. C., Rattani, A., Gupta, S., Baticulon, R. E., Hung, Y. C., Punchak, M., Agrawal, A., Adeleye, A. O., Shrime, M. G., Rubiano, A. M., Rosenfeld, J. V., & Park, K. B. (2018). Estimating the global incidence of traumatic brain injury. *Journal of Neurosurgery, 130*(4), 1080–1097. https://doi.org/10.3171/2017.10.JNS17352

Duclos, C., Dumont, M., Arbour, C., Paquet, J., Blais, H., Menon, D. K., De Beaumont, L., Bernard, F., & Gosselin, N. (2017). Parallel recovery of consciousness and sleep in acute traumatic brain injury. *Neurology, 88*(3), 268–275.

Duclos, C., Dumont, M., Blais, H., Paquet, J., Laflamme, E., de Beaumont, L., Wiseman-Hakes, C., Menon, D. K., Bernard, F., & Gosselin, N. (2013). Rest–activity cycle disturbances in the acute phase of moderate to severe traumatic brain injury. *Neurorehabilitation and Neural Repair, 28*(5), 472–482. https://doi.org/10.1177/1545968313517756

Duclos, C., Dumont, M., Potvin, M. J., Desautels, A., Gilbert, D., Menon, D. K., Bernard, F., & Gosselin, N. (2016). Evolution of severe sleep–wake cycle disturbances following traumatic brain injury: A case study in both acute and subacute phases post-injury. *BMC Neurology, 16*(1), Article 186. https://doi.org/10.1186/s12883-016-0709-x

Ebrahim, I. O., Peacock, K. W., & Williams, A. J. (2005). Posttraumatic narcolepsy—Two case reports and a mini review. *Journal of Clinical Sleep Medicine, 1*(2), 153–156. http://www.ncbi.nlm.nih.gov/entrez/query.fcgi?cmd=Retrieve&db=PubMed&dopt=Citation&list_uids=17561629

Elliott, J. E., McBride, A. A., Balba, N. M., Thomas, S. V., Pattinson, C. L., Morasco, B. J., Wilkerson, A., Gill, J. M., & Lim, M. M. (2022). Feasibility and preliminary efficacy for morning bright light therapy to improve sleep and plasma biomarkers in US veterans with TBI. A prospective, open-label, single-arm trial. *PLOS ONE, 17*(4), Article e0262955. https://doi.org/10.1371/journal.pone.0262955

Farrell-Carnahan, L., Barnett, S., Lamberty, G., Hammond, F. M., Kretzmer, T. S., Franke, L. M., Geiss, M., Howe, L., & Nakase-Richardson, R. (2015). Insomnia symptoms and behavioural health symptoms in veterans 1 year after traumatic brain injury. *Brain Injury, 29*(12), 1400–1408. https://www.ncbi.nlm.nih.gov/pubmed/26274494

Fichtenberg, N. L., Millis, S. R., Mann, N. R., Zafonte, R. D., & Millard, A. E. (2000). Factors associated with insomnia among post-acute traumatic brain injury survivors. *Brain Injury, 14*(7), 659–667. http://www.ncbi.nlm.nih.gov/pubmed/10914647

Flanagan, S. R., Greenwald, B., & Wieber, S. (2007). Pharmacological treatment of insomnia for individuals with brain injury. *Journal of Head Trauma Rehabilitation, 22*(1), 67–70. https://doi.org/10.1097/00001199-200701000-00009

Ford, M. E., Geurtsen, G. J., Groet, E., Rambaran Mishre, R. D., Van Bennekom, C. A. M., & Van Someren, E. J. W. (2022). A blended eHealth intervention for insomnia following acquired brain injury: A randomised controlled trial. *Journal of Sleep Research*, Article e13629. https://doi.org/10.1111/jsr.13629

Frieboes, R. M., Muller, U., Murck, H., von Cramon, D. Y., Holsboer, F., & Steiger, A. (1999). Nocturnal hormone secretion and the sleep EEG in patients several months after traumatic brain injury. *Journal of Neuropsychiatry and Clinical Neurosciences, 11*(3), 354–360. http://www.ncbi.nlm.nih.gov/entrez/query.fcgi?cmd=Retrieve&db=PubMed&dopt=Citation&list_uids=10440012

Friese, R. S., Diaz-Arrastia, R., McBride, D., Frankel, H., & Gentilello, L. M. (2007). Quantity and quality of sleep in the surgical intensive care unit: Are our patients sleeping? *Journal of Trauma, 63*(6), 1210–1214. https://doi.org/10.1097/TA.0b013e31815b83d7

Gabor, J. Y., Cooper, A. B., & Hanly, P. J. (2001). Sleep disruption in the intensive care unit. *Current Opinion in Critical Care, 7*(1), 21–27. http://www.ncbi.nlm.nih.gov/entrez/query.fcgi?cmd=Retrieve&db=PubMed&dopt=Citation&list_uids=11373507

GBD 2016 Traumatic Brain Injury and Spinal Cord Injury Collaborators. (2019). Global, regional, and national burden of traumatic brain injury and spinal cord injury, 1990–2016: A systematic analysis for the Global Burden of Disease Study 2016. *Lancet Neurology, 18*(1), 56–87. https://doi.org/10.1016/S1474-4422(18)30415-0

Gottshall, J. L., Guedes, V. A., Pucci, J. U., Brooks, D., Watson, N., Sheth, P., Gabriel, A., Mithani, S., Leete, J. J., Lai, C., Qu, B. X., Devoto, C., Gill, J. M., Kenney, K., & Werner, J. K. (2021). Poor sleep quality is linked to elevated extracellular vesicle-associated inflammatory cytokines in warfighters with chronic mild traumatic brain injuries. *Frontiers in Pharmacology, 12*, Article 762077. https://doi.org/10.3389/fphar.2021.762077

Grima, N., Ponsford, J., Rajaratnam, S. M., Mansfield, D., & Pase, M. P. (2016). Sleep disturbances in traumatic brain injury: A meta-analysis. *Journal of Clinical Sleep Medicine, 12*(3), 419–428. https://doi.org/10.5664/jcsm.5598

Grima, N. A., Ponsford, J. L., St Hilaire, M. A., Mansfield, D., Rajaratnam, S. M., Grima, N., Ponsford, J., Rajaratnam, S. M., Mansfield, D., & Pase, M. P. (2016). Circadian melatonin rhythm following traumatic brain injury. *Neurorehabilitation and Neural Repair, 30*(10), 972–977. https://doi.org/10.1177/1545968316650279

Grima, N. A., Rajaratnam, S. M. W., Mansfield, D., Sletten, T. L., Spitz, G., & Ponsford, J. L. (2018). Efficacy of melatonin for sleep disturbance following traumatic brain injury: A randomised controlled trial. *BMC Medicine, 16*(1), Article 8.

Guilleminault, C., Yuen, K. M., Gulevich, M. G., Karadeniz, D., Leger, D., & Philip, P. (2000). Hypersomnia after head–neck trauma: A medicolegal dilemma. *Neurology, 54*(3), 653–659. http://www.ncbi.nlm.nih.gov/entrez/query.fcgi?cmd=Retrieve&db=PubMed&dopt=Citation&list_uids=10680799

Hartvigsen, J., Boyle, E., Cassidy, J. D., & Carroll, L. J. (2014). Mild traumatic brain injury after motor vehicle collisions: What are the symptoms and who treats them? A population-based 1-year inception cohort study. *Archives of Physical and Medical Rehabilitation, 95*(S3), S286–S294. https://doi.org/10.1016/j.apmr.2013.07.029

Hoddes, E., Zarcone, V., Smythe, H., Phillips, R., & Dement, W. C. (1973). Quantification of sleepiness: A new approach. *Psychophysiology, 10*(4), 431–436. http://www.ncbi.nlm.nih.gov/entrez/query.fcgi?cmd=Retrieve&db=PubMed&dopt=Citation&list_uids=4719486

Hoffman, J. M., Bell, K. R., Powell, J. M., Behr, J., Dunn, E. C., Dikmen, S., & Bombardier, C. H. (2010). A randomized controlled trial of exercise to improve mood after traumatic brain injury. *PM&R, 2*(10), 911–919. https://doi.org/10.1016/j.pmrj.2010.06.008

Hoffman, N. L., O'Connor, P. J., Schmidt, M. D., Lynall, R. C., & Schmidt, J. D. (2020). Relationships between post-concussion sleep and symptom recovery: A preliminary study. *Journal of Neurotrauma, 37*(8), 1029–1036. https://doi.org/10.1089/neu.2019.6761

Holcomb, E. M., Schwartz, D. J., McCarthy, M., Thomas, B., Barnett, S. D., & Nakase-Richardson, R. (2016). Incidence, characterization, and predictors of sleep apnea in consecutive brain injury rehabilitation admissions. *Journal of Head Trauma Rehabilitation, 31*(2), 82–100. https://doi.org/10.1097/HTR.0000000000000230

Horne, J. A., & Ostberg, O. (1976). A self-assessment questionnaire to determine morningness–eveningness in human circadian rhythms. *International Journal of Chronobiology, 4*(2), 97–110. http://www.ncbi.nlm.nih.gov/entrez/query.fcgi?cmd=Retrieve&db=PubMed&dopt=Citation&list_uids=1027738

Hou, L., Han, X., Sheng, P., Tong, W., Li, Z., Xu, D., Yu, M., Huang, L., Zhao, Z., Lu, Y., & Dong, Y. (2013). Risk factors associated with sleep disturbance following traumatic brain injury: Clinical findings and questionnaire based study. *PLOS ONE, 8*(10), Article e76087. https://doi.org/10.1371/journal.pone.0076087

Imbach, L. L., Valko, P. O., Li, T., Maric, A., Symeonidou, E. R., Stover, J. F., Bassetti, C. L., Mica, L., Werth, E., & Baumann, C. R. (2015). Increased sleep need and daytime sleepiness 6 months after traumatic brain injury: A prospective controlled clinical trial. *Brain, 138*(Pt. 3), 726–735.

Institut national d'excellence en santé et en services sociaux & Ontario Neurotrauma Foundation. (2016). *Clinical practice guideline for the rehabilitation of adults with moderate to severe traumatic brain injury.* http://www.braininjuryguidelines.org/

Jang, S. H., & Kwon, H. G. (2016). Injury of the ascending reticular activating system in patients with fatigue and hypersomnia following mild traumatic brain injury: Two case reports. *Medicine (Baltimore), 95*(6), Article e2628.

Jha, A., Weintraub, A., Allshouse, A., Morey, C., Cusick, C., Kittelson, J., Harrison-Felix, C., Whiteneck, G., & Gerber, D. (2008). A randomized trial of modafinil for the treatment of fatigue and excessive daytime sleepiness in individuals with chronic traumatic brain injury. *Journal of Head Trauma Rehabilitation, 23*(1), 52–63. https://doi.org/10.1097/01.HTR.0000308721.77911.ea

Johns, M. W. (1991). A new method for measuring daytime sleepiness: The Epworth Sleepiness Scale. *Sleep, 14*(6), 540–545. http://www.ncbi.nlm.nih.gov/entrez/query.fcgi?cmd=Retrieve&db=PubMed&dopt=Citation&list_uids=1798888

Kemp, S., Biswas, R., Neumann, V., & Coughlan, A. (2004). The value of melatonin for sleep disorders occurring post-head injury: A pilot RCT. *Brain Injury, 18*(9), 911–919. https://doi.org/10.1080/02699050410001671892

Kempf, J., Werth, E., Kaiser, P. R., Bassetti, C. L., & Baumann, C. R. (2010). Sleep–wake disturbances 3 years after traumatic brain injury. *Journal of Neurology, Neurosurgery, and Psychiatry, 81*(12), 1402–1405.

Killgore, W. D. S., Vanuk, J. R., Shane, B. R., Weber, M., & Bajaj, S. (2020). A randomized, double-blind, placebo-controlled trial of blue wavelength light exposure on sleep and recovery of brain structure, function, and cognition following mild traumatic brain injury. *Neurobiology of Disease, 134*, Article 104679. https://doi.org/10.1016/j.nbd.2019.104679

Kraus, J. F., & Chu, L. D. (2005). Epidemiology. In J. M. Silver, T. W. McAllister, & S. C. Yudofsky (Eds.), *Textbook of traumatic brain injury* (pp. 3–26). American Psychiatric Publishing.

Kumar, R. (2008). Approved and investigational uses of modafinil: An evidence-based review. *Drugs, 68*(13), 1803–1839. http://www.ncbi.nlm.nih.gov/pubmed/18729534

Lah, S., Phillips, N. L., Palermo, T. M., Bartlett, D., Epps, A., Teng, A., Brookes, N., Parry, L., & Naismith, S. L. (2021). A feasibility and acceptability study of cognitive behavioural treatment for insomnia in adolescents with traumatic brain injury: A–B with follow up design, randomized baseline, and replication across participants. *Neuropsychological Rehabilitation, 31*(3), 345–368. https://doi.org/10.1080/09602011.2019.1693404

Langlois, J. A., Rutland-Brown, W., & Wald, M. M. (2006). The epidemiology and impact of traumatic brain injury: A brief overview. *Journal of Head Trauma Rehabilitation, 21*(5), 375–378. https://doi.org/10.1097/00001199-200609000-00001

Larson, E. B., & Zollman, F. S. (2010). The effect of sleep medications on cognitive recovery from traumatic brain injury. *Journal of Head Trauma Rehabilitation, 25*(1), 61–67.

Lee, H., Kim, S. W., Kim, J. M., Shin, I. S., Yang, S. J., & Yoon, J. S. (2005). Comparing effects of methylphenidate, sertraline and placebo on neuropsychiatric sequelae in patients with traumatic brain injury. *Human Psychopharmacology, 20*(2), 97–104. https://doi.org/10.1002/hup.668

Lequerica, A. H., Watson, E., Dijkers, M. P., Goldin, Y., Hoffman, J. M., Niemeier, J. P., Silva, M. A., Rabinowitz, A., & Chiaravalloti, N. D. (2022). The utility of the Patient Health Questionnaire (PHQ-9) sleep disturbance item as a screener for insomnia in individuals with moderate to severe traumatic brain injury. *Journal of Head Trauma Rehabilitation, 37*(5), E383–E389. https://doi.org/10.1097/HTR.0000000000000746

Lim, M. M., Elkind, J., Xiong, G., Galante, R., Zhu, J., Zhang, L., Lian, J., Rodin, J., Kuzma, N. N., Pack, A. I., & Cohen, A. S. (2013). Dietary therapy mitigates persistent wake deficits caused by mild traumatic brain injury. *Science Translational Medicine, 5*(215), Article 215ra173. https://doi.org/10.1126/scitranslmed.3007092

Lowe, A., Bailey, M., O'Shaughnessy, T., & Macavei, V. (2022). Treatment of sleep disturbance following stroke and traumatic brain injury: A systematic review of conservative interventions. *Disability and Rehabilitation, 44*(13), 2975–2987. https://doi.org/10.1080/09638288.2020.1856948

Lowe, A., Neligan, A., & Greenwood, R. (2020). Sleep disturbance and recovery during rehabilitation after traumatic brain injury: A systematic review. *Disability and Rehabilitation, 42*(8), 1041–1054. https://doi.org/10.1080/09638288.2018.1516819

Mahmood, O., Rapport, L. J., Hanks, R. A., & Fichtenberg, N. L. (2004). Neuropsychological performance and sleep disturbance following traumatic brain injury. *Journal of Head Trauma Rehabilitation, 19*(5), 378–390. http://www.ncbi.nlm.nih.gov/entrez/query.fcgi?cmd=Retrieve&db=PubMed&dopt=Citation&list_uids=15597029

Mahowald, M. W. (2000). Sleep in traumatic brain injury and other acquired CNS conditions. In A. Culebras (Ed.), *Sleep disorders and neurological disease* (pp. 365–385). Dekker.

Makley, M. J., Johnson-Greene, L., Tarwater, P. M., Kreuz, A. J., Spiro, J., Rao, V., & Celnik, P. A. (2009). Return of memory and sleep efficiency following moderate to severe closed head injury. *Neurorehabilitation and Neural Repair, 23*(4), 320–326. http://www.ncbi.nlm.nih.gov/entrez/query.fcgi?cmd=Retrieve&db=PubMed&dopt=Citation&list_uids=19171947

Mantua, J., Grillakis, A., Mahfouz, S. H., Taylor, M. R., Brager, A. J., Yarnell, A. M., Balkin, T. J., Capaldi, V. F., Simonelli, G., Borniger, J. C., Ungerleider, K., Zhang, N., Karelina, K., Magalang, U. J., Weil, Z. M., Grima, N. A., Rajaratnam, S. M. W., Mansfield, D., Sletten, T. L., . . . & Ponsford, J. L. (2018). A systematic review and meta-analysis of sleep architecture and chronic traumatic brain injury. *Sleep Medicine Reviews, 375*(1), 74–83. https://doi.org/10.1016/j.smrv.2018.01.004

Martin, A. M., Almeida, E. J., Starosta, A. J., Hammond, F. M., Hoffman, J. M., Schwartz, D. J., Fann, J. R., Bell, K. R., & Nakase-Richardson, R. (2021). The impact of opioid medications on sleep architecture and nocturnal respiration during acute recovery from moderate to severe traumatic brain injury: A TBI model systems study. *Journal of Head Trauma Rehabilitation*, *36*(5), 374–387. https://doi.org/10.1097/HTR.0000000000000727

Masel, B. E., Scheibel, R. S., Kimbark, T., & Kuna, S. T. (2001). Excessive daytime sleepiness in adults with brain injuries. *Archives of Physical Medicine and Rehabilitation*, *82*(11), 1526–1532. http://www.ncbi.nlm.nih.gov/entrez/query.fcgi?cmd=Retrieve&db=PubMed&dopt=Citation&list_uids=11689971

Mathias, J. L., & Alvaro, P. K. (2012). Prevalence of sleep disturbances, disorders, and problems following traumatic brain injury: A meta-analysis. *Sleep Medicine*, *13*(7), 898–905. https://doi.org/10.1016/j.sleep.2012.04.006

Miller, M., Williams, R., Pagulayan, K., Barber, J., Ehde, D. M., & Hoffman, J. (2022). Correlates of sleep disturbance in veterans with traumatic brain injury and chronic pain: A cross-sectional study. *Disability and Health Journal*, *15*(1), Article 101203. https://doi.org/10.1016/j.dhjo.2021.101203

Mollayeva, T., Colantonio, A., Cassidy, J. D., Vernich, L., Moineddin, R., & Shapiro, C. M. (2017). Sleep stage distribution in persons with mild traumatic brain injury: A polysomnographic study according to American Academy of Sleep Medicine standards. *Sleep Medicine*, *34*, 179–192. https://doi.org/10.1016/j.sleep.2017.02.021

Monk, T. H., Buysse, D. J., Kennedy, K. S., Pods, J. M., DeGrazia, J. M., & Miewald, J. M. (2003). Measuring sleep habits without using a diary: The Sleep Timing Questionnaire. *Sleep*, *26*(2), 208–212.

Montgomery, M. C., Baylan, S., & Gardani, M. (2022). Prevalence of insomnia and insomnia symptoms following mild-traumatic brain injury: A systematic review and meta-analysis. *Sleep Medicine Reviews*, *61*, Article 101563. https://doi.org/10.1016/j.smrv.2021.101563

Morin, C. M. (1993). *Insomnia: Psychological assessment and management*. Guilford Press.

Mosti, C. B., Klingaman, E. A., Brownlow, J. A., & Gehrman, P. R. (2019). Insomnia prevalence among U.S. Army soldiers with history of TBI. *Rehabilitation Psychology*, *64*(4), 475–481. https://doi.org/10.1037/rep0000283

Nagtegaal, J. E., Kerkhof, G. A., Smits, M. G., Swart, A. C., & van der Meer, Y. G. (1997). Traumatic brain injury–associated delayed sleep phase syndrome. *Functional Neurology*, *12*(6), 345–348. http://www.ncbi.nlm.nih.gov/entrez/query.fcgi?cmd=Retrieve&db=PubMed&dopt=Citation&list_uids=9503198

Nakase-Richardson, R., Sherer, M., Barnett, S. D., Yablon, S. A., Evans, C. C., Kretzmer, T., Schwartz, D. J., & Modarres, M. (2013). Prospective evaluation of the nature, course, and impact of acute sleep abnormality after traumatic brain injury. *Archives of Physical and Medical Rehabilitation*, *94*(5), 875–882. https://doi.org/10.1016/j.apmr.2013.01.001

Nardone, R., Bergmann, J., Kunz, A., Caleri, F., Seidl, M., Tezzon, F., Gerstenbrand, F., Trinka, E., & Golaszewski, S. M. (2011). Cortical excitability changes in patients with sleep–wake disturbances after traumatic brain injury. *Journal of Neurotrauma*, *28*(7), 1165–1171.

Nelson, L. D., Temkin, N. R., Dikmen, S., Barber, J., Giacino, J. T., Yuh, E., Levin, H. S., McCrea, M. A., Stein, M. B., Mukherjee, P., Okonkwo, D. O., Robertson, C. S., Diaz-Arrastia, R., Manley, G. T., & TRACK-TBI Investigators. (2019). Recovery after mild traumatic brain injury in patients presenting to US Level I trauma centers: A transforming research and clinical knowledge in traumatic brain injury (TRACK-TBI) study. *JAMA Neurology*, *76*(9), 1049–1059. https://doi.org/10.1001/jamaneurol.2019.1313

Nguyen, S., McKay, A., Wong, D., Rajaratnam, S. M., Spitz, G., Williams, G., Mansfield, D., & Ponsford, J. L. (2017). Cognitive behavior therapy to treat sleep disturbance and fatigue after traumatic brain injury: A pilot randomized controlled trial. *Archives of Physical and Medical Rehabilitation*, *98*(8), 1508–1517. https://doi.org/10.1016/j.apmr.2017.02.031

Nguyen, S., McKenzie, D., McKay, A., Wong, D., Rajaratnam, S. M. W., Spitz, G., Williams, G., Mansfield, D., Ponsford, J., Nguyen, S., McKay, A., Wong, D., Rajaratnam, S. M., Spitz, G., Williams, G., Mansfield, D., & Ponsford, J. L. (2018). Exploring predictors of treatment outcome in cognitive behavior therapy for sleep disturbance following acquired brain injury. *Disability and Rehabilitation*, *40*(16), 1906–1913. https://doi.org/10.1080/09638288.2017.1315461

Ontario Neurotrauma Foundation. (2018). *Guideline for concussion/mild traumatic brain injury & persistent symptoms: Adults (18+ years of age)* (3rd ed.). https://concussionsontario.org/sites/default/files/2023-03/Third_Edition.pdf

Osier, N. D., Pham, L., Pugh, B. J., Puccio, A., Ren, D., Conley, Y. P., Alexander, S., & Dixon, C. E. (2017). Brain injury results in lower levels of melatonin receptors subtypes MT1 and MT2. *Neuroscience Letters*, *650*, 18–24.

Osorio, M. B., Kurowski, B. G., Beebe, D., Taylor, H. G., Brown, T. M., Kirkwood, M. W., & Wade, S. L. (2013). Association of daytime somnolence with executive functioning in the first 6 months after adolescent traumatic brain injury. *PM&R, 5*(7), 554–562. https://doi.org/10.1016/j.pmrj.2012.11.006

Ouellet, M.-C., Beaulieu-Bonneau, S., & Morin, C. M. (2006). Insomnia in patients with traumatic brain injury: Frequency, characteristics, and risk factors. *Journal of Head Trauma Rehabilitation, 21*, 199–212.

Ouellet, M.-C., Beaulieu-Bonneau, S., Savard, J., & Morin, C. (2020). *Insomnia and fatigue after traumatic brain injury: A CBT approach to assessment and treatment.* Elsevier.

Ouellet, M.-C., & Morin, C. M. (2006). Subjective and objective measures of insomnia in the context of traumatic brain injury: A preliminary study. *Sleep Medicine, 7*(6), 486–497. http://www.ncbi.nlm.nih.gov/entrez/query.fcgi?cmd=Retrieve&db=PubMed&dopt=Citation&list_uids=16934524

Ouellet, M. C., & Morin, C. M. (2004). Cognitive behavioral therapy for insomnia associated with traumatic brain injury: A single-case study. *Archives of Physical Medicine and Rehabilitation, 85*(8), 1298–1302. http://www.ncbi.nlm.nih.gov/entrez/query.fcgi?cmd=Retrieve&db=PubMed&dopt=Citation&list_uids=15295756

Ouellet, M.-C., & Morin, C. M. (2007). Efficacy of cognitive-behavioral therapy for insomnia associated with traumatic brain injury: A single-case experimental design. *Archives of Physical and Medical Rehabilitation, 88*(12), 1581–1592. https://doi.org/10.1016/j.apmr.2007.09.006

Ouellet, M. C., Savard, J., & Morin, C. M. (2004). Insomnia following traumatic brain injury: A review. *Neurorehabilitation and Neural Repair, 18*(4), 187–198. http://www.ncbi.nlm.nih.gov/entrez/query.fcgi?cmd=Retrieve&db=PubMed&dopt=Citation&list_uids=15669131

Pagel, J. F. (2005). Medications and their effects on sleep. *Primary Care, 32*(2), 491–509. http://www.ncbi.nlm.nih.gov/entrez/query.fcgi?cmd=Retrieve&db=PubMed&dopt=Citation&list_uids=15935197

Paparrigopoulos, T., Melissaki, A., Tsekou, H., Efthymiou, A., Kribeni, G., Baziotis, N., & Geronikola, X. (2006). Melatonin secretion after head injury: A pilot study. *Brain Injury, 20*(8), 873–878.

Parcell, D. L., Ponsford, J. L., Rajaratnam, S. M., & Redman, J. R. (2006). Self-reported changes to nighttime sleep after traumatic brain injury. *Archives of Physical Medicine and Rehabilitation, 87*(2), 278–285. http://www.ncbi.nlm.nih.gov/entrez/query.fcgi?cmd=Retrieve&db=PubMed&dopt=Citation&list_uids=16442985

Patten, S. B., & Lauderdale, W. M. (1992). Delayed sleep phase disorder after traumatic brain injury. *Journal of the American Academy of Child and Adolescent Psychiatry, 31*(1), 100–102. http://www.ncbi.nlm.nih.gov/entrez/query.fcgi?cmd=Retrieve&db=PubMed&dopt=Citation&list_uids=1537759

Pattinson, C. L., Brickell, T. A., Bailie, J., Hungerford, L., Lippa, S. M., French, L. M., & Lange, R. T. (2021). Sleep disturbances following traumatic brain injury are associated with poor neurobehavioral outcomes in US military service members and veterans. *Journal of Clinical Sleep Medicine, 17*(12), 2425–2438. https://doi.org/10.5664/jcsm.9454

Pilon, L., Frankenmolen, N., & Bertens, D. (2021). Treatments for sleep disturbances in individuals with acquired brain injury: A systematic review. *Clinical Rehabilitation, 35*(11), 1518–1529. https://doi.org/10.1177/02692155211014827

Quinto, C., Gellido, C., Chokroverty, S., & Masdeu, J. (2000). Posttraumatic delayed sleep phase syndrome. *Neurology, 54*(1), 250–252. http://www.ncbi.nlm.nih.gov/entrez/query.fcgi?cmd=Retrieve&db=PubMed&dopt=Citation&list_uids=10636163

Raikes, A. C., Dailey, N. S., Forbeck, B., Alkozei, A., & Killgore, W. D. S. (2021). Daily morning blue light therapy for post-mTBI sleep disruption: Effects on brain structure and function. *Frontiers in Neurology, 12*, Article 625431. https://doi.org/10.3389/fneur.2021.625431

Rao, V., Spiro, J., Vaishnavi, S., Rastogi, P., Mielke, M., Noll, K., Cornwell, E., Schretlen, D., & Makley, M. (2008). Prevalence and types of sleep disturbances acutely after traumatic brain injury. *Brain Injury, 22*(5), 381–386. https://doi.org/10.1080/02699050801935260

Roehrs, T., Carskadon, M. A., Dement, W. C., & Roth, T. (2005). Daytime sleepiness and alertness. In M. H. Kryger, T. Roth, & W. C. Dement (Eds.), *Principles and practice of sleep medicine* (4th ed., pp. 39–50). Elsevier Saunders.

Rutland-Brown, W., Langlois, J. A., Thomas, K. E., & Xi, Y. L. (2006). Incidence of traumatic brain injury in the United States, 2003. *Journal of Head Trauma Rehabilitation, 21*(6), 544–548. https://doi.org/10.1097/00001199-200611000-00009

Sabir, M., Gaudreault, P. O., Freyburger, M., Massart, R., Blanchet-Cohen, A., Jaber, M., Gosselin, N., & Mongrain, V. (2015). Impact of traumatic brain injury on sleep structure, electrocorticographic activity and transcriptome in mice. *Brain, Behavior, and Immunity, 47*, 118–130. https://doi.org/10.1016/j.bbi.2014.12.023

Saksvik, S. B., Smevik, H., Stenberg, J., Follestad, T., Vik, A., Haberg, A., Asarnow, R. F., Kallestad, H., Skandsen, T., & Olsen, A. (2021). Poor sleep quality is associated with greater negative consequences for cognitive control function and psychological health after mild traumatic brain injury than after orthopedic injury. *Neuropsychology, 35*(7), 706–717. https://doi.org/10.1037/neu0000751

Sanchez, E., Blais, H., Duclos, C., Arbour, C., Van Der Maren, S., El-Khatib, H., Baril, A. A., Bernard, F., Carrier, J., & Gosselin, N. (2022). Sleep from acute to chronic traumatic brain injury and cognitive outcomes. *Sleep, 45*(8), Article zsac123. https://doi.org/10.1093/sleep/zsac123

Schreiber, S., Barkai, G., Gur-Hartman, T., Peles, E., Tov, N., Dolberg, O. T., & Pick, C. G. (2008). Long-lasting sleep patterns of adult patients with minor traumatic brain injury (mTBI) and non-mTBI subjects. *Sleep Medicine, 9*(5), 481–487. https://doi.org/10.1016/j.sleep.2007.04.014

Shay, N., Yeates, K. O., Walz, N. C., Stancin, T., Taylor, H. G., Beebe, D., Caldwell, C., Krivitzky, L., Cassedy, A., & Wade, S. L. (2014). Sleep problems and their relationship to cognitive and behavioral outcomes in young children with traumatic brain injury. *Journal of Neurotrauma, 31*(14), 1305–1312. https://doi.org/10.1089/neu.2013.3275

Shekleton, J. A., Parcell, D. L., Redman, J. R., Phipps-Nelson, J., Ponsford, J. L., & Rajaratnam, S. M. (2010). Sleep disturbance and melatonin levels following traumatic brain injury. *Neurology, 74*(21), 1732–1738. https://doi.org/10.1212/WNL.0b013e3181e0438b

Sherer, M., Yablon, S. A., & Nakase-Richardson, R. (2009). Patterns of recovery of posttraumatic confusional state in neurorehabilitation admissions after traumatic brain injury. *Archives of Physical and Medical Rehabilitation, 90*(10), 1749–1754. https://doi.org/10.1016/j.apmr.2009.05.011

Silva, M. A., Calvo, D., Brennan, E. M., Reljic, T., Drasher-Phillips, L., Schwartz, D. J., Kumar, A., Cotner, B. A., Taylor, D. J., & Nakase-Richardson, R. (2020). Incidence and predictors of adherence to sleep apnea treatment in rehabilitation inpatients with acquired brain injury. *Sleep Medicine, 69*, 159–167. https://doi.org/10.1016/j.sleep.2020.01.016

Silva, M. A., Nakase-Richardson, R., Sherer, M., Barnett, S. D., Evans, C. C., & Yablon, S. A. (2012). Posttraumatic confusion predicts patient cooperation during traumatic brain injury rehabilitation. *American Journal of Physical Medicine & Rehabilitation, 91*(10), 890–893. https://doi.org/10.1097/PHM.0b013e31825a1648

Silver, J. M., McAllister, T. W., & Yudofsky, S. C. (Eds.). (2005). *Textbook of traumatic brain injury*. American Psychiatric Publishing.

Sinclair, K. L., Ponsford, J. L., Taffe, J., Lockley, S. W., & Rajaratnam, S. M. (2014). Randomized controlled trial of light therapy for fatigue following traumatic brain injury. *Neurorehabilitation and Neural Repair, 28*(4), 303–313. https://doi.org/10.1177/1545968313508472

Skopin, M. D., Kabadi, S. V., Viechweg, S. S., Mong, J. A., & Faden, A. I. (2014). Chronic decrease in wakefulness and disruption of sleep–wake behavior after experimental traumatic brain injury. *Journal of Neurotrauma, 32*(5), 289–296. https://doi.org/10.1089/neu.2014.3664

Sommerauer, M., Valko, P. O., Werth, E., & Baumann, C. R. (2013). Excessive sleep need following traumatic brain injury: A case–control study of 36 patients. *Journal of Sleep Research, 22*(6), 634–639. https://doi.org/10.1111/jsr.12068

Steele, D. L., Rajaratnam, S. M., Redman, J. R., & Ponsford, J. L. (2005). The effect of traumatic brain injury on the timing of sleep. *Chronobiology International, 22*(1), 89–105. https://doi.org/10.1081/CBI-200042428

Stone, J. J., Childs, S., Smith, L. E., Battin, M., Papadakos, P. J., & Huang, J. H. (2014). Hourly neurologic assessments for traumatic brain injury in the ICU. *Neurological Research, 36*(2), 164–169. https://doi.org/10.1179/1743132813y.0000000285

Tang, S., Sours Rhodes, C., Jiang, L., Chen, H., Roys, S., Badjatia, N., Raghavan, P., Zhuo, J., & Gullapalli, R. P. (2022). Association between sleep disturbances at subacute stage of mild traumatic brain injury and long-term outcomes. *Neurotrauma Reports, 3*(1), 276–285. https://doi.org/10.1089/neur.2022.0004

Taylor, C. A., Bell, J. M., Breiding, M. J., & Xu, L. (2017). Traumatic brain injury–related emergency department visits, hospitalizations, and deaths—United States, 2007 and 2013. *MMWR Surveillance Summaries, 66*(9), 1–16. https://doi.org/10.15585/mmwr.ss6609a1

Theadom, A., Barker-Collo, S., Jones, K., Dudley, M., Vincent, N., Feigin, V., Theadom, A., Rowland, V., Levack, W., Starkey, N., Wilkinson-Meyers, L., & McPherson, K. (2018). A pilot randomized controlled trial of on-line interventions to improve sleep quality in adults after mild or moderate traumatic brain injury. *Clinical Rehabilitation, 32*(5), 619–629. https://doi.org/10.1177/0269215517736671

Theadom, A., Barker-Collo, S., Jones, K., Kahan, M., Te Ao, B., McPherson, K., Starkey, N., & Feigin, V.; BIONIC4you Research Group. (2017). Work limitations 4 years after mild traumatic brain injury: A cohort study. *Archives of Physical and Medical Rehabilitation, 98*(8), 1560–1566. https://doi.org/10.1016/j.apmr.2017.01.010

Theadom, A., Cropley, M., Parmar, P., Barker-Collo, S., Starkey, N., Jones, K., & Feigin, V. L. (2015). Sleep difficulties one year following mild traumatic brain injury in a population-based study. *Sleep Medicine, 16*(8), 926–932. https://doi.org/10.1016/j.sleep.2015.04.013

Theadom, A., Starkey, N., Barker-Collo, S., Jones, K., Ameratunga, S., & Feigin, V. (2018). Population-based cohort study of the impacts of mild traumatic brain injury in adults four years post-injury. *PLOS ONE, 13*(1), Article e0191655.

Urakami, Y. (2012). Relationship between, sleep spindles and clinical recovery in patients with traumatic brain injury: A simultaneous EEG and MEG study. *Clinical EEG and Neuroscience, 43*(1), 39–47.

Valko, P. O., Gavrilov, Y. V., Yamamoto, M., Finn, K., Reddy, H., Haybaeck, J., Weis, S., Scammell, T. E., & Baumann, C. R. (2015). Damage to histaminergic tuberomammillary neurons and other hypothalamic neurons with traumatic brain injury. *Annals of Neurology, 77*(1), 177–182. https://doi.org/10.1002/ana.24298

Valko, P. O., Gavrilov, Y. V., Yamamoto, M., Noain, D., Reddy, H., Haybaeck, J., Weis, S., Baumann, C. R., & Scammell, T. E. (2016). Damage to arousal-promoting brainstem neurons with traumatic brain injury. *Sleep, 39*(6), 1249–1252.

Verma, A., Anand, V., & Verma, N. P. (2007). Sleep disorders in chronic traumatic brain injury. *Journal of Clinical Sleep Medicine, 3*(4), 357–362.

Viola-Saltzman, M., & Watson, N. F. (2012). Traumatic brain injury and sleep disorders. *Neurologic Clinics, 30*(4), 1299–1312. https://doi.org/10.1016/j.ncl.2012.08.008

Vuletic, S., Bell, K. R., Jain, S., Bush, N., Temkin, N., Fann, J. R., Stanfill, K. E., Dikmen, S., Brockway, J. A., He, F., Ernstrom, K., Raman, R., Grant, G., Stein, M. B., & Gahm, G. A. (2016). Telephone problem-solving treatment improves sleep quality in service members with combat-related mild traumatic brain injury: Results from a randomized clinical trial. *Journal of Head Trauma Rehabilitation, 31*(2), 147–157. https://doi.org/10.1097/htr.0000000000000221

Waldron-Perrine, B., McGuire, A. P., Spencer, R. J., Drag, L. L., Pangilinan, P. H., & Bieliauskas, L. A. (2012). The influence of sleep and mood on cognitive functioning among veterans being evaluated for mild traumatic brain injury. *Military Medicine, 177*(11), 1293–1301.

Watson, N. F., Dikmen, S., Machamer, J., Doherty, M., & Temkin, N. (2007). Hypersomnia following traumatic brain injury. *Journal of Clinical Sleep Medicine, 3*(4), 363–368.

Webster, J. B., Bell, K. R., Hussey, J. D., Natale, T. K., & Lakshminarayan, S. (2001). Sleep apnea in adults with traumatic brain injury: A preliminary investigation. *Archives of Physical Medicine and Rehabilitation, 82*(3), 316–321. http://www.ncbi.nlm.nih.gov/entrez/query.fcgi?cmd=Retrieve&db=PubMed&dopt=Citation&list_uids=11245752

Wickwire, E. M., Albrecht, J. S., Capaldi, V. F., 2nd, Jain, S. O., Gardner, R. C., Werner, J. K., Mukherjee, P., McKeon, A. B., Smith, M. T., Giacino, J. T., Nelson, L. D., Williams, S. G., Collen, J., Sun, X., Schnyer, D. M., Markowitz, A. J., Manley, G. T., & Krystal, A. D.; Transforming Research and Clinical Knowledge in Traumatic Brain Injury (TRACK-TBI) Investigators. (2022). Trajectories of insomnia in adults after traumatic brain injury. *JAMA Network Open, 5*(1), Article e2145310. https://doi.org/10.1001/jamanetworkopen.2021.45310

Wilde, M. C., Castriotta, R. J., Lai, J. M., Atanasov, S., Masel, B. E., & Kuna, S. T. (2007). Cognitive impairment in patients with traumatic brain injury and obstructive sleep apnea. *Archives of Physical and Medical Rehabilitation, 88*(10), 1284–1288. https://doi.org/10.1016/j.apmr.2007.07.012

Williams, B. R., Lazic, S. E., & Ogilvie, R. D. (2008). Polysomnographic and quantitative EEG analysis of subjects with long-term insomnia complaints associated with mild traumatic brain injury. *Clinical Neurophysiology, 119*(2), 429–438. https://doi.org/10.1016/j.clinph.2007.11.003

Williams, C. N., McEvoy, C. T., Lim, M. M., Shea, S. A., Kumar, V., Nagarajan, D., Drury, K., Rich-Wimmer, N., & Hall, T. A. (2022). Sleep and executive functioning in pediatric traumatic brain injury survivors after critical care. *Children, 9*(5), Article 748. https://doi.org/10.3390/children9050748

Willie, J. T., Lim, M. M., Bennett, R. E., Azarion, A. A., Schwetye, K. E., & Brody, D. L. (2012). Controlled cortical impact traumatic brain injury acutely disrupts wakefulness and extracellular orexin dynamics as determined by intracerebral microdialysis in mice. *Journal of Neurotrauma, 29*(10), 1908–1921. https://doi.org/10.1089/neu.2012.2404

Wiseman-Hakes, C., Murray, B., Moineddin, R., Rochon, E., Cullen, N., Gargaro, J., & Colantonio, A. (2013). Evaluating the impact of treatment for sleep/wake disorders on recovery of cognition and communication in adults with chronic TBI. *Brain Injury, 27*(12), 1364–1376. https://doi.org/10.3109/02699052.2013.823663

Worthington, A. D., & Melia, Y. (2006). Rehabilitation is compromised by arousal and sleep disorders: Results of a survey of rehabilitation centres. *Brain Injury, 20*(3), 327–332. https://doi.org/10.1080/02699050500488249

Ymer, L., McKay, A., Wong, D., Frencham, K., Grima, N., Tran, J., Nguyen, S., Junge, M., Murray, J., Spitz, G., & Ponsford, J. (2021). Cognitive behavioural therapy versus health education for sleep disturbance and fatigue after acquired brain injury: A pilot randomised trial. *Annals of Physical and Rehabilitation Medicine, 64*(5), Article 101560. https://doi.org/10.1016/j.rehab.2021.101560

Ymer, L., McKay, A., Wong, D., Frencham, K., Grima, N., Tran, J., Nguyen, S., & Ponsford, J. (2022). Cognitive behavioral therapy for sleep disturbance and fatigue following acquired brain injury: Predictors of treatment response. *Journal of Head Trauma Rehabilitation, 37*(3), E220–E230. https://doi.org/10.1097/HTR.0000000000000705

Zalai, D. M., Girard, T. A., Cusimano, M. D., & Shapiro, C. M. (2020). Circadian rhythm in the assessment of postconcussion insomnia: A cross-sectional observational study. *CMAJ Open, 8*(1), E142–E147. https://doi.org/10.9778/cmajo.20190137

Zollman, F. S., Larson, E. B., Wasek-Throm, L. K., Cyborski, C. M., & Bode, R. K. (2012). Acupuncture for treatment of insomnia in patients with traumatic brain injury: A pilot intervention study. *Journal of Head Trauma Rehabilitation, 27*(2), 135–142. https://doi.org/10.1097/HTR.0b013e3182051397

CHAPTER
45 Sleep in People With Intellectual Disabilities

Luci D. Wiggs

Abstract

Adequate amounts of good-quality sleep are vital for optimal functioning. Children and adults with intellectual disabilities (ID) appear to have increased risk for various forms of sleep disturbance, with implications for their daytime functioning, caregivers' stress, and the professionals involved in their care. Multiple biological and psychosocial factors likely interact to increase the risk for sleep disturbances and should be considered as part of assessment. Various forms of treatment for sleep difficulties have been used in people with ID (including sleep hygiene, behavioral therapy, chronotherapy, light therapy, and melatonin), but the evidence base is limited in quantity and quality, particularly for adults with ID. Given the scale of the problem in this population, there is an urgent need for studies which attempt to understand the mechanisms underlying different forms of sleep disturbance (including in association with discrete genetic disorders or syndromes) and permit the development of clear management guidelines.

Key Words: intellectual disability, adult, child, assessment, treatment, behavioral therapy, light therapy, melatonin, sleep hygiene, chronotherapy

Introduction

The importance of having sufficient amounts of good-quality sleep for optimal cognitive, emotional, behavioral, and physical functioning is now well documented, across all age groups. This is of note because sleep disturbance is widespread among the general population. However, there are certain subgroups for whom sleep disturbance seems to be particularly common. Individuals with intellectual disabilities (ID) are one of those groups. ID is characterized by co-occurring deficits in intellectual ability (often defined as an IQ <70) and deficits in day-to-day functioning (American Psychiatric Association, 2013). Many people with ID also have sensory and physical impairments. Many people with autism spectrum disorder (ASD) also have ID, although it should be noted that individuals with higher-functioning ASD may have average or even above-average IQs and so would not be considered to have an "intellectual disability" according to this definition. This definition of ID includes both IQ and functional aspects that make it distinct from the use of the term "learning difficulties," which has wider application in education settings.

Increased risk of sleep disturbance for individuals with ID is likely not only to increase their risk of suffering from the negative effects of sleep disturbance but also to impact upon their parents/caregivers, whose own sleep might be disturbed as a result of nocturnal caregiving demands.

Early identification and intervention are clearly important, perhaps especially so in young people, as some cognitive impairments associated with sleep disorders may be less easily reversed, if at all, if they occur at critical stages of development (Brouillette et al., 1982). Furthermore, sleep disturbance in childhood may even be predictive of poor psychiatric state in adulthood (Gregory et al., 2005; van Lang et al., 2007). For people with ID, who are already prone to cognitive, emotional, and behavioral difficulties, ensuring that sleep disruption is not playing a causal role in such problems is imperative as it may be one of the more easily treatable aspects of their condition. For caregivers of individuals with ID, improving sleep may be one way of reducing their burden of care and helping them to be able to cope optimally with other caregiving demands.

This chapter will discuss the nature, prevalence, and possible etiology of sleep disturbance in individuals with ID and special considerations of assessment for this population. Common approaches to treatment will be summarized and, where appropriate, the reader referred to other sources of relevant material for further details.

It is beyond the scope of this chapter to provide detailed information specific to individual etiologies underlying the presence of ID, although where possible readers will be directed to research concerning populations with discrete diagnoses, the availability of such literature being a growing trend at least for some of the most common etiologies.

In contrast to most sleep research with typically developing populations, most work with ID samples has addressed children, with the sleep of adults with ID being relatively neglected. In this chapter, the age groups of the participants in cited studies are indicated, and research concerning child and adult populations is integrated in the discussion of general points.

Sleep Abnormalities Associated With ID

Abnormalities of sleep and high rates of sleep problems and disorders have been consistently described in children and adults with ID. However, there are a number of challenges to both summarizing and interpreting the findings concerning sleep associated with ID due to methodological differences (e.g., in terms of the aspect of sleep being assessed and the type of measurement/assessment tool used) and the heterogeneity of (often small) samples in terms of their intellectual impairment being of mixed etiology and severity, their chronological age, and the presence of comorbid medical and psychological factors. This is particularly relevant since other conditions that can be associated with sleep disturbance, such as epilepsy, psychiatric disorders, sensory impairments, and discomfort due to muscle spasms, are generally present at elevated rates in ID samples.

Even basic definitions of the sleep area of enquiry can be ambiguous. For example, despite there being clear criteria for insomnia disorder (American Academy of Sleep Medicine [AASM], 2014), a literature review of the definitions used to characterize insomnia symptoms and disorder in adults and children with an ID found considerable variation in the definitions used, making synthesis of the results most challenging (van den Brok et al., 2022). With those limitations in mind, some general comments about areas of identified sleep abnormalities are presented.

Sleep Physiology and ID

Some of the earliest studies exploring sleep architecture of people with ID of mixed etiology documented associated rapid-eye-movement (REM) sleep abnormalities. This is of note given that the relationship between REM sleep and learning and memory appears to be strong (e.g., Maquet, 2001; Stickgold et al., 2001). Specific abnormalities associated with ID include a relative overall deficiency in amount, fewer and/or shorter REM sleep periods, and fewer eye movements ("low REM density"), which have been reported in adults and adolescents (Castaldo & Krynicki, 1973; Espie et al., 1998; Espie & Tweedie, 1991; Petre-Quadens & Jouvet, 1967), and a correlation between the amount of REM sleep and the degree of intellectual impairment (Grubar, 1983). Sleep spindle activity has also been an area of interest, not least because the mechanisms underlying spindle generation play a role in both plasticity and the stabilization of sleep. Sleep spindle activity in ID has also been noted to be abnormal, with spindles being absent or unusually frequent, high-voltage, and continuous ("extreme spindles"), with a pattern of development that may be abnormal (Shibagaki et al., 1982). Gruber and Wise (2016) provide a helpful review of sleep spindles in children with neurodevelopmental disorders, exploring possible associations between spindle characteristics and cognitive function, including in some discrete groups of neurodevelopmental disorders.

Studies comparing the polysomnographic (PSG) profiles of individuals with different syndromes suggest that there might be features of sleep physiology that are specific to different syndromes (e.g., Diomedi et al., 1999; Elia et al., 2000). For example, individuals with fragile X syndrome may have more REM sleep than individuals with ASD and Down syndrome, and individuals with ASD were reported to have more undifferentiated sleep than those with Down syndrome. The ASD group also had more electromyographic activity during sleep, especially during REM sleep. Such results suggest that there may be PSG characteristics associated with particular conditions and that greater knowledge of these may contribute to our understanding of normal and abnormal sleep processes.

Sleep Problems in ID

Problems with sleep, particularly sleeplessness, appear to be prominent in child (Richdale & Baker, 2014; Tietze et al., 2012) and, although less investigated, in adult (van de Wouw et al., 2012, 2013) populations with ID.

For example, Bartlett et al. (1985) found that up to 86% of children with ID aged less than 6 years were reported by parents to have "sleep problems," with similarly high rates (77%) even for adolescents aged 12–16 years. Problems of sleeplessness (i.e., difficulty getting to sleep, night waking, or early waking) appear to be the most commonly reported problems and frequently coexist. Quine's (1991) study of 200 children and adolescents aged 1–18 years with ID reported 51% to have night waking problems and 67% to have difficulties settling to sleep, and Wiggs and Stores' (1996a) sample of 209 young people with ID (aged 5–16 years) included 41% with severe sleeplessness problems and reported that 100% of the children had one type of sleep problem occurring more than three times a week.

Importantly, these problems are generally persistent. Quine (1991) conducted a 3-year follow-up study that indicated that over half of the children with settling and night waking difficulties still had such problems. In addition, about a quarter of children had developed sleep problems that had not been present 3 years previously (Pahl & Quine, 1984).

Studies of adult samples, although limited in number, concur with the idea that these problems are not all "outgrown": Espie and Tweedie (1991) suggested that around 15% of adults with ID have significant sleep disturbance, with similar rates reported by Gunning and Espie (2003) in their survey of 155 adults with ID attending adult training centers (17% difficulty getting to sleep, 11% difficulty remaining asleep). Brylewski and Wiggs's (1998) survey of 210 adults found higher rates of 27% for settling problems and 56% for night waking. M. T. Harvey et al.'s, (2003) survey of 237 adults living in community settings included reports of 36% being awake for more than 1 hour during the night and 60% taking more than 30 minutes to fall asleep. A systematic review conducted by van de Wouw et al. (2012) reported estimated overall prevalence rates of sleep problems in adults with ID ranging from 8.5% to 34.1%, based on the 50 studies included for review.

Consistent with these reports, recent meta-analyses (Brown et al., 2024; Surtees et al., 2018) found that people whose ID was associated with specific genetic syndromes or developmental disorders experienced significant deficits in both the duration and quality of their sleep; where ID was of mixed origin, only impairments in sleep quality, not duration, were noted, although there was considerable heterogeneity in the data for the analysis of sleep duration in those with ID of mixed origin and age might be an important moderator.

While true prevalence rates are difficult to assess and likely to vary as a function of age, underling etiology of ID, and the types of sleep disturbance being investigated, it seems warranted to conclude that perhaps the majority of children with ID and many adults with ID suffer from some form of sleep disturbance, commonly sleeplessness, that may well develop into long-standing problems without intervention; importantly, the presence of sleep disturbance is related to physical health, mental health, and quality of life of individuals with ID and their families/carers (see Harper et al., 2023).

Of note, the nature of behavioral disturbance during any wakeful periods can pose particular and variable challenges for caregivers of people with ID. For example, a recent survey and interview study of caregivers of children and adults with Smith-Magenis syndrome emphasized that challenging and self-injurious behavior during the night were common and that caregivers felt the need to be vigilant as they were highly concerned about the safety of the individual during nocturnal wake episodes (Agar et al., 2022); unusual "emotional" nighttime behavior (e.g., laughing, crying, screaming) in 50%–83% of girls with Rett syndrome (Coleman et al., 1988; Sansom et al., 1993) as well as in ASD (Wiggs & Stores, 2004) has been reported. Guidance to manage behavior during the episodes, as well as the sleep disturbance, is required by many families.

Sleep Disorders in ID

Much of the literature concerning sleep abnormalities of individuals with ID describes somewhat ill-defined "sleep problems" (i.e., a nonspecific description of presenting symptoms, e.g., "difficulty getting to sleep") and does not make the distinction between "sleep problems" and "sleep disorders" (i.e., disorders with discrete diagnostic criteria as defined in the *International Classification of Sleep Disorders*-3; AASM, 2014). This is a limitation both for characterizing any profiles of difficulties in particular groups of people with ID and for fully understanding the available prevalence data. Distinguishing between sleep problems and sleep disorders is also important clinically because management decisions need to be based upon correcting the underlying disorder, not treating symptoms, and different sleep disorders can present with similar symptoms. For example, sleeplessness, taking the form of difficulty getting to sleep at night, may, among other things, result from disorders of the body clock, failure to learn appropriate bedtime behavior, or restless legs syndrome. Treatment for each of these causes, or underlying disorders, would be very different.

Clinically, it is therefore important to remember that co-occurring sleep disorders may present in ID populations, just as they can in typically developing populations. Although whether etiology, presentation, course, and optimal intervention are the same for individuals with and without ID remains largely unexplored. For example, in addition to insomnia disorder (Boyle et al., 2010; van den Broek et al., 2022; van de Wouw et al., 2012, 2013) and sleep apnea (Gulotta et al., 2019; C. M. Hill et al., 2016; E. A. Hill, 2016; Stores, 2018), which are widely documented in a number of ID populations, sleep terrors (Durand, 2002), rhythmic movement disorders (De Leon et al., 2004), periodic limb movements (Arens et al., 1998; Gruber et al., 2022), nightmares (Willner, 2004), and REM sleep behavior disorder (Thirumalai et al., 2002) have all been described. Indeed, there are indications that a range of sleep disorders might be more prevalent in ID populations than in typically developing populations (Agar et al., 2021; Didden & Sigafoos, 2001).

Sleep Disorders Associated With Specific Syndromes and Conditions

The sleep patterns and disturbances associated with particular syndromes are increasingly being documented (e.g., Agar et al., 2021; Blackmer & Feinstein, 2016; Grigg-Damburger & Ralls, 2013; San José Cáceres et al., 2023). Documented links between particular syndromes and sleep disturbance profiles are limited in quantity for some syndromes (e.g., a single case report), but for other syndromes there is more plentiful/detailed information, allowing one to more confidently identify primary sleep disorders or particular patterns of sleep disturbance occurring in association with particular underlying conditions.

For example, both obstructive and, less commonly, central sleep apneas have been described in association with Down syndrome; but, importantly, insomnia disorder and sleep-related movement disorders may also feature prominently (Giménez et al., 2021); circadian rhythm sleep–wake disorders have been linked to an inverted endogenous melatonin secretion pattern in Smith-Magenis syndrome (De Leersnyder et al., 2001, 2006); in ASD, problems with insomnia and circadian rhythm sleep–wake disorders predominate, although parasomnias are also common (Cuomo et al., 2017) and Thirumalai et al. (2002) documented REM sleep behavior disorder in five of their series of 11 children with ASD who presented with disturbed sleep and nocturnal awakenings; in Williams syndrome, bedtime resistance, sleep anxiety, nighttime awakening, daytime sleepiness, and enuresis have all been highlighted as particularly common complaints (Annaz et al., 2011; Ashworth et al., 2013), with periodic limb movements also described (Arens et al., 1998); a disrupted maintenance of sleep (or wakefulness) state characterized by difficulties with initiating and maintaining sleep as well as excessive daytime sleepiness has been described in Rett syndrome (Spruyt, 2022); circadian rhythm sleep–wake disorders have been described in Sanfilippo syndrome (Hare et al., 2018); and sleep disordered breathing has been described in Prader-Willi syndrome, including central sleep apnea, obstructive sleep apnea (OSA), sleep-related hypoventilation disorder, and hypoxemia (Cataldi et al., 2021)—although the characteristic excessive daytime sleepiness can persist even once sleep disordered breathing is treated, and it is suggested that the excessive daytime sleepiness and REM sleep abnormalities reflect hypothalamic dysfunction, with generalized hypoarousal (Camfferman et al., 2008).

The potential insights to be gained from trying to document sleep disorders, and not just describe difficulties symptomatically, is exemplified by a recent meta-analysis of sleep in Angelman syndrome, which reported that disorders of arousal, such as nightmares and sleep terrors, were distinguishing (along with sleepiness; Spruyt et al., 2018). The authors make the point that while such sleep disorders are not incompatible with the widely reported sleep complaints of nighttime disruptive behaviors and fragmented sleep, they do contrast with the common interpretation of these sleep difficulties (e.g., see Egan et al., 2020) including in consensus guidelines (Williams et al., 2006), which propose that disorders related to the sleep–wake cycle underlie these sleep problems. The results of this meta-analysis illustrate the importance of trying to document sleep disorders, along with characterizing sleep difficulties at the symptomatic level. Such information is clinically valuable and has the potential to advance our understanding of both the mechanisms underlying sleep disorders and the relationships between sleep and other aspects of the individual's functioning.

Assessment of Sleep

An overview of sleep assessment methods is provided elsewhere in this handbook; hence, the current chapter confines itself to raising some key considerations for assessment of sleep in ID populations.

Taking a Sleep History in the Context of ID

Perhaps most fundamentally, given the elevated rates of difficulties with sleep in people with ID, it is important that screening for any problems forms a part of routine care; of note is that sleep has also been identified as an area of key concern (for individuals, parents/carers, and clinicians) which should be considered as an outcome in studies with children with ID (Morris et al., 2015). When making these preliminary enquiries, one needs to keep in mind the nature of the informant (usually not the individual themselves but often a parent or carer) and the precise phrasing of one's questioning; what is considered "problematic" will depend upon to whom one is speaking. For example, we know that sometimes sleepiness in children with ID may not be considered "problematic" by parents but perhaps rather be viewed as positive respite (Espie, 1992), although excessive sleepiness is likely to reflect a problem of some sort for the child.

As part of history taking, the timing of any nocturnal episodes can be helpful diagnostically when trying to clinically differentiate between parasomnias because, as outlined in Chapter 21, parasomnias are classified according to the stage of sleep from which they originate, and typically one has most deep non-REM (NREM) sleep in the first third of the night and most REM sleep in the last third of the night (although young children may also have a brief period of deep NREM shortly before waking in the morning). It is important to remember that for individuals with severe or profound ID whose basic sleep architecture may not be typical, these generalizations may not apply, and the timing of any nocturnal "episodes" may be less diagnostically informative. Appropriate further assessments may be required to identify and diagnose any episodes associated with sleep to avoid misdiagnosing one form of parasomnia for another or misdiagnosing parasomnias with other "episodic" conditions, notably epilepsy. Of course, if an individual has daytime seizures, it should not be assumed that nocturnal episodes are also epileptic in origin. Similarly, a lack of daytime seizures does not preclude the possibility of nocturnal episodes being epileptic. Moreover, because sleep disordered breathing is commonly associated with many underlying syndromes, one also needs to be particularly mindful of this possibility. Obtaining appropriate information to allow review of an individual's 24-hour sleep–wake pattern—not just the nighttime period—may be an especially important part of the clinical history as daytime sleep opportunities may be more plentiful for some individuals with ID (e.g., some special schools may allow naps, transport times to and from school/day centers may be of long duration).

Predisposing, Precipitating, and Maintaining Factors Relevant to History Taking in ID

The high rates of sleep disturbance in ID populations likely arise due to the interaction of physical and psychosocial factors. When taking a clinical history, special attention needs to be paid to potential predisposing, precipitating, and maintaining factors as well as to what is known about sleep disturbances associated with any syndrome and the fact that multiple sleep disorders can occur in the same individual (see Table 45.1 for a summary). Careful consideration of these factors, and their inter-relationships, may have helpful management implications.

Table 45.1 Factors relevant to history taking in intellectual disabilities

Factors to consider	Examples of factors linked with sleep disturbance
Syndrome-specific sleep phenotype	Down syndrome associated with increased risk for sleep-related breathing disorders, insomnia, and sleep-related movement disorders
Co-occurring sleep disorders	Impaired sleep quality/duration due to one sleep disorder (e.g., obstructive sleep apnea) may serve as a risk factor for other types of sleep disorders (e.g., arousal disorders, insomnia)
Neurodevelopmental factors	Neurodevelopmental problems and related brain abnormalities or damage associated with atypical functioning of the brain structures and processes involved in the control of sleep and wake states; sensory impairment
Medical conditions	Epilepsy, gastroesophageal reflux, neuromuscular disease
Psychiatric conditions	Anxiety, depression, attention-deficit hyperactivity disorder, autism spectrum disorder
Medication effects	Side effects of medications for medical and psychiatric conditions, drug interaction effects
Difficulties with learning	Difficulty with learning appropriate sleep behaviors or "unlearning" inappropriate behaviors as part of behavior change; exacerbated by communication difficulties
Challenging behavior	Challenging behavior associated with arousal (therefore sleep-incompatible), representing another underlying state (e.g., pain); safety concerns requiring caregiver involvement during the nighttime period
Environmental factors	Light levels, activity/stimulation patterns, 24-hourly routines
Caregiver factors	Caregiver/family stress, caregiver anxiety/concern, cultural/developmental expectations of sleep
Attributions	Normalization of sleep disturbance by parents and/or professionals can mean that appropriate help is not sought/implemented

Developmental, medical, and psychiatric factors that may play a causal or maintaining role in sleep disturbance are plentiful:

- Extensive neurodevelopmental problems and related brain abnormalities or damage may be associated with atypical functioning of the brain structures and processes involved in the control of sleep and wake states, resulting in a predisposition to various sleep difficulties. Circadian dysregulation, which is commonly seen in individuals with ID, is a good illustration of how underlying atypical physical functioning may, in isolation or by interaction with psychosocial factors, be causal of sleep disturbance. For example, an abnormal endogenous melatonin rhythm (in terms of production, secretion, distribution, or metabolism) that has been described in association with particular syndromes, likely with a genetic basis (e.g., an inverted rhythm in Smith-Magenis syndrome [De Leersnyder et al., 2001; Poisson et al., 2019], a "flattened" profile in ASD [Lorsung et al., 2021; Nir et al., 1995], and lower nocturnal levels in association with many rare genetic neurodevelopmental syndromes [Woodford et al., 2021]), in itself is likely to predispose to problems with sleep timing and/or continuity. However, the circadian clock is influenced by both endogenous and exogenous factors. Exogenous factors that may play a particular role in ID include reduced exposure to daytime light in some care environments when outdoor exposure is limited, reduced differentiation between "daytime" and "nighttime" in terms of extent and nature of activities and the environment in which they occur, reduced flexibility to link key zeitgebers (like bedtimes, mealtimes) to each individual's particular sleep–wake rhythm for people living in group residential settings, and impaired learning of the association between social zeitgebers and sleep. Addressing these exogenous factors in assessment and management may be of critical importance even when endogenous abnormalities exist.
- Sensory impairments are more common in ID populations and in themselves may be associated with sleep problems. With visual impairment, circadian rhythm sleep disorders are common (Lockley et al., 2007; Stores, 2001a) due to the effects of compromised light perception and possibly reduced social or environmental cues for sleeping and waking (Lockley et al., 1999). Fazzi et al. (2008) describe a wide range of sleep problems in their sample of visually impaired children, which were worse in association with developmental delay. Psychiatric aspects of associated conditions need to be considered too; for example, Moseley et al. (1996) found depression to be a strong predictor of sleep disturbance in blind adults, and Schakel et al. (2019) note the complex interplay between depression, sleep disturbance, and daytime fatigue in adults with a visual impairment. Sleep problems

associated with hearing impairment are less explored, but reduced social and environmental cues, in addition to the possible effects of tinnitus, and anxiety associated with hearing-aid removal at night have all been suggested (see Clarke et al., 2019; Stores, 2001b) as well as neuroplastic negative alterations to sleep through diminished auditory input (Velluti et al., 2010).

- Associated medical/neurological conditions may also play a role. For example, in cerebral palsy, sleep disordered breathing, circadian rhythm disorders, and sleeplessness have all been reported (Kotagal et al., 1994; Lélis et al., 2016; Newman et al., 2006; Palm et al., 1997), with possible causal factors including areas of brain insult, discomfort during sleep, and comorbid epilepsy. In neuromuscular disease, sleep disordered breathing, restless legs syndrome, sleeplessness, and excessive daytime sleepiness may occur, with discomfort/pain suggested to play a role in sleeplessness difficulties (see Fermin et al., 2016; Simakajornboon & Beckerman, 2001a; Tieleman et al., 2010). Craniofacial abnormalities are associated with sleep disordered breathing (see Samadi et al., 2003; Simakajornboon & Beckerman, 2001b; Zaffanello et al., 2018). Gastroesophageal reflux may be associated with a variety of sleep difficulties including OSA (Dimarino et al., 2005; Ghaem et al., 1998; Kurin et al., 2021).
- It should be particularly noted that epilepsy can be associated with sleep in a number of ways, depending on the type of epilepsy (Chan, 2020; Foldvary-Schaefer & Grigg-Damberger, 2009; Gibbon et al., 2019; Loddenkemper et al., 2011; St Louis, 2011). Sleep may induce (or suppress) seizure activity, sleep loss may lead to increased seizure frequency, and seizures can occur predominantly (or exclusively) during sleep. Seizures may hinder sleep onset, disrupt sleep during the night, impact sleep architecture, reduce sleep duration, and be associated with daytime sleepiness (as a result of impaired night sleep or daytime seizures or as a consequence of antiepileptic medication side effects). Furthermore, electrical status epilepticus during sleep (ESES), which in itself may be asymptomatic, is associated with neuropsychological impairment such as cognitive regression, behavioral disturbance, and motor impairment. Longer duration of ESES, abnormal development before the onset of ESES, and severity of initial regression are key risk factors for poorer neuropsychological outcome of cognitive impairment in the long term (Jansen et al., 2019), highlighting the importance of early recognition and effective treatment, especially for people with ID.
- When considering the relationship between sleep and epilepsy, an additional area of significance is that there can be diagnostic confusion between epilepsy and sleep disorders, perhaps particularly with complex partial seizures that may include vocalizations, motor behavior, and changes in affect along

with loss of consciousness, all of which might be expected in partial arousal disorders. OSA may also be mistaken, with choking sensations, motor disturbance, and daytime sleepiness being overlapping features (Oldani et al., 1998; Velluti et al., 2010).

- Psychiatric conditions may be associated with various types of sleep disturbance, perhaps most commonly insomnia and hypersomnia (see Cox & Olatunji, 2020; Gregory & Sadeh, 2016; Riemann et al., 2020). Psychiatric disorders are also common in ID populations (Mazza et al., 2020), although there can be challenges in identifying some psychiatric disorders in people with ID who may find it more difficult to report on their own internal state. However, Eaton et al. (2021) reported that adults with severe to profound ID presented with many classic symptoms, including sleep disturbance, as described in standardized diagnostic schemes (such as the *Diagnostic and Statistical Manual* and the *International Classification of Diseases*), although they highlight the possibility for additional, atypical behavioral presentations (such as challenging behavior and self-injurious behavior).
- Importantly, the bidirectional relationships between sleep and psychiatric disorders emphasize the need for difficulties with sleep to be identified and, where possible, managed to reduce any contribution that impaired sleep is making to psychiatric symptoms (Freeman et al., 2020). For example, sleep disordered breathing, motor restlessness during sleep, periodic limb movement disorder, and sleeplessness can occur in attention-deficit hyperactivity disorder (ADHD; van der Heijden et al., 2005), and ADHD is commonly comorbid with ID. It has been suggested that for some children with ADHD, their daytime symptoms of attentional difficulties and hyperactive behavior are caused by a primary sleep disorder (Fallone et al., 2002), with ADHD symptoms reversed by treatment of the sleep disorder (Dahl et al., 1991; Guilleminault et al., 1982; Hansen & Vandenberg, 1997; Konofal et al., 2001).
- A further consideration, of course, is that medications for coexisting physical and psychiatric conditions (to which people with ID may be prone) may have a disruptive effect on sleep in various ways (Schweitzer & Malhotra, 2021). Classic antiepileptic medications (e.g., phenobarbital, carbamazepine, valproate, and phenytoin) have been associated with reduced sleep latency, more slow-wave sleep (SWS), and more daytime sleepiness. Newer antiepileptic medications (e.g., gabapentin, lamotrigine, vigabatrin, zonisamide) tend to have less of a sedating effect after the medication is established, but effects on sleep architecture are variable (e.g., increased SWS with gabapentin and decreased SWS with lamotrigine). Antidepressant drugs may also have variable effects. For example, tricyclic

antidepressant drugs generally improve sleep; monoamine oxidase inhibitors may eliminate REM sleep, reduce total sleep time, and be associated with increased daytime sleepiness, with the effect related to dose and duration of treatment; selective serotonin reuptake inhibitors are frequently associated with insomnia, periodic limb movements, and REM sleep without atonia; and lithium may improve nocturnal sleep but increase daytime sleepiness. Older antipsychotic agents (e.g., chlorpromazine, thioridazine) are typically sedating, although newer options (e.g., clozapine, risperidone, olanzapine, sertindole) are more variable (e.g., clozapine most sedating, then olanzapine, risperidone, and sertindole least sedating). Methylphenidate for the treatment of ADHD appears to increase sleep latency, although sleep may be consolidated. Anxiolytics (especially benzodiazepines), antihistamines, and cardiovascular drugs may also be associated with sedation, although clonidine, an alpha2 agonist used in the treatment of tic disorder and Tourette syndrome, has been reported to be associated with insomnia and nightmares. Corticosteroids tend to be associated with increased wakefulness during sleep and increased alertness during the day. The action of analgesics depends on the compound used; non-steroidal anti-inflammatory drugs may well increase wakefulness, whereas opioids are associated with sedation and, importantly, respiratory depression during sleep. Other drugs known to be associated with increased insomnia include theophylline (a respiratory stimulant and bronchodilator), anorectic agents (used to treat obesity), pseudoephedrine, and phenylpropanolamine (used to treat nasal congestion and available in many over-the-counter preparations). The effect of medications on daytime functioning, drug interaction effects, and the possibility of paradoxical or atypical side effects for people with ID need to be recognized.

Relevant psychosocial factors also need to be considered as part of history taking, including the individual's cognitive/emotional/behavioral state, sleep environment, and matters related to parents'/caregivers' behavior and beliefs:

- There are aspects of sleep behavior that are learned, varying from family to family and culture to culture (Jenni & O'Connor, 2005; Wiggs, 2007, 2009). As such, for people with learning impairments, it may be more difficult for them to learn appropriate sleep behaviors in the first place or to "unlearn" inappropriate behaviors. Facilitating learning may be especially difficult for individuals with communication difficulties (Quine, 1991). Creative use of appropriate communication methods (e.g., picture exchange communication system, social stories, etc.; Moore, 2004) may help individuals to understand more clearly what is the expected and desired behavior.

- As noted above, emotional and behavioral disturbance and psychiatric problems are common in individuals with ID and may both in themselves be associated with various forms of sleep disturbance (Chawla et al., 2020) and impede the process of establishing good sleep habits. It should be emphasized that challenging daytime behavioral and emotional disturbance may well arise as a consequence of sleep disturbance (if sleep is compromised in terms of quality or quantity) and that successful treatment of sleep disturbance has been associated with improvements in daytime behavior. In addition to numerous positive anecdotal reports, assessments of daytime behavior, utilizing questionnaires and analog rating scales, have shown improvements following interventions for sleeplessness problems (Bramble, 1996; Espie, 1992; Quine, 1992; Schroder et al., 2019; Thackeray & Richdale, 2002). However, classroom behavior observations conducted by Thackery and Richdale (2002) failed to convincingly support their questionnaire data, and others too have failed to document associated improvements with either questionnaires (Esbensen et al., 2022; Gringras et al., 2012; Weiskop et al., 2001) or video analysis of mother/child interactions (Weiskop et al., 2005).
- While daytime behavior improvements associated with successful treatment of sleep difficulties appear to be a realistic possibility, the lack of consistency between different behavioral measures and the possible tendency for observational methods to be less likely to detect change than questionnaire measures raises the possibility of methodological inadequacy or that reported behavior change is small, is detected only by parents, or occurs secondary to improvements in parental functioning, affecting their reporting/perceptions of their children. Improvements in mother, father, and family functioning (e.g., increased ability to cope, less stress, improvements in their own subjective and objective sleep) have certainly been seen (Bramble, 1996; Quine, 1992; Schroder et al., 2019; Stuttard et al., 2015; Wiggs & Stores, 2001). The importance of these benefits for the parents should not be underestimated, and, of course, even improvements in family functioning (as opposed to direct improvements in the individual's behavior) are likely, in turn, to have indirect benefits for the person with ID.
- For individuals living at home, parent/caregiver factors may play a role; stress, psychological problems, and marital difficulties are elevated in the parents of children with ID and may make it more difficult for parents to manage the individual's sleep with consistency (Quine, 1992; A. Richdale et al., 2000; Wiggs & Stores, 2001). Parental anxieties about their child's safety and health during the nighttime period may also be present (Beresford et al., 2016; Cook et al., 2021). These may compromise parents'/caregivers'

ability to manage their child's sleep behavior in the way that is needed to avoid some sleep-related behavioral problems, especially those involving overdependence on parents/caregivers when settling to sleep or on waking during the night.

- For individuals in residential settings, other environmental factors may play a part (e.g., reduced day/night differentiation in activity level, environment and light level, increased caffeine consumption, or the inflexibility of routines).
- It is also perhaps worth highlighting that parents/caregivers of ID children and adults, and some professionals involved with their care, may hold the mistaken belief that sleep problems are an inevitable part of the individual's basic condition so that problems are not being presented or appropriately managed. As such, treatment and prevention opportunities may be being missed in ID populations (Brylewski & Wiggs, 1998; Chawla et al., 2023; Robinson & Richdale, 2004; Wiggs & Stores, 1996b), contributing to the maintenance of sleep problems.

Questionnaires and Rating Scales

Given the broad array of sleep difficulties that can present in people with ID, questionnaires offer an efficient way to screen for symptoms. Standardized scales that have been widely used to assess sleep in neurotypical populations have also been used with ID populations—for example, the Sleep Disturbance Scale for Children (Bruni et al., 1996), the Behavior Evaluation of Disorders of Sleep (Schreck et al., 2003), the Pediatric Sleep Questionnaire (Chervin et al., 2000), the Pittsburgh Sleep Quality Index (Buysse et al., 1989), and the Epworth Sleepiness Scale (Johns, 1991). The Children's Sleep Habits Questionnaire (CSHQ; Owens et al., 2000) and modified versions of the Simonds and Parraga Sleep Questionnaire (Simonds & Parraga, 1982) have perhaps been most widely used with child populations with ID. Good psychometric properties were reported for the modified Simonds and Parraga Sleep Questionnaire in a sample of adults and children with ID (Maas et al., 2011), and good correspondence between this and the CSHQ was reported by Johnson et al. (2012) for a sample of children with ASD.

However, whether the use/adaptation of scales designed for assessing sleep in neurotypical populations is really adequate was raised by Johnson et al. (2016), in relation to children with ASD. The SNAKE (Schlaffragebogen für Kinder mit Neurologischen und Anderen Komplexen Erkrankungen; Dreier et al., 2018) and the HOST (Holistic Assessment of Sleep and Daily Troubles in Parents; Tietze et al., 2014) questionnaires were designed with this in mind, to, respectively, assess the sleep of children with severe psychomotor impairment and the impact of child sleep disturbances on their parents/carers, taking into account the specific challenges they may face. Despite promising results from these development studies, use and further development of these scales unfortunately have been limited. Consequently, there remains an urgent need for valid and reliable screening questionnaires for use with people with ID, which are tailored to assess the aspects of sleep, and related factors, which are particularly pertinent for this group.

Actigraphy

Where individuals will not tolerate PSG, actigraphy may be the only way of obtaining some "objective" information about sleep. Actigraphy may also be particularly helpful where parents/caregivers are unable to provide information about sleep timing, either because they are unaware of the individual's sleep/wake times or because they are too exhausted themselves to be able to systematically record the information. Although some individuals will not tolerate actigraphy, many problems can be overcome by allowing adequate time for familiarization with the monitor and/or wearing the monitor over nightwear (so that it does not come into contact with the skin) or even on the ankle, where it can be less obtrusive than when worn on the wrist. Although actigraphy does not provide any information about sleep staging, it can be used to detect periodic limb movements (Kemlink et al., 2008), again offering a useful alternative for those who will not tolerate PSG. While actigraphy has been used widely with ID populations, one needs to be mindful of the fact that validation studies have not been performed in ID populations. As actigraphy is a movement-based assessment method, the validity of this approach with individuals with motor dysfunction remains to be adequately documented.

PSG

As noted, PSG may prove practically difficult with some individuals with ID. Nevertheless, many obstacles can be overcome by experienced technicians sensitive to the needs of the family and the individual (Zaremba et al., 2005). It should be acknowledged that PSG may not be particularly revealing for some individuals with profound ID, for whom it can be difficult to distinguish physiologically between waking and sleeping states ("undifferentiated sleep"). Further, as indicated earlier, features of PSG specific to particular conditions and syndromes may make the use of existing "normal" reference values less instructive (M. T. Harvey & Kennedy, 2002). The disrupting effect of the procedure itself upon sleep, with neurotypical individuals, can be overcome by disregarding the first night of recording and making greater use of a subsequent night. However, the rate of adaptation for individuals with ID has not been addressed. It is possible that it may not be as rapid, and therefore the generalizability of such information might be compromised.

Treatment

There is a wide variety of treatments from which to choose depending on the nature of the sleep disorder, and such interventions are described elsewhere in this handbook. These same types of treatments for sleep disorders that are used with children and adults from the general population are generally used with ID populations, although some adaptations might be required, taking into account the individual's environment, clinical condition, and the caregivers' resources. The reader is referred to Korb et al. (2021) for discussion of these issues, and Wiggs (2012) gives special consideration to the delivery of behavior therapy for sleep difficulties in ID populations.

Clinical management guidelines for sleep disorders are typically based mainly on evidence derived from typically developing populations given the paucity of good-quality research with specific ID populations, although there are increasing attempts to provide more population-specific advice (e.g., see Souders et al., 2017, for children with ASD). The need to document response to intervention for discrete groups is emphasized by the findings of Lee et al.'s (2020) meta-analysis, which reports, for example, that while adenotonsillectomy (AT) was associated with OSA improvement among children with Prader-Willi syndrome, residual OSA was frequently observed postoperatively; awareness of this clearly facilitates appropriate clinical monitoring and, if required, adjunct therapy.

Importantly, the complex and varied factors that may play a causal or maintaining role in sleep disturbance in ID populations need to be considered, and a holistic approach to assessment and management is usually required. For example, Böhmer et al. (2022) found that installation of carefully timed and lux level–controlled light in the communal living areas of a care home failed to result in changes to the sleep–wake patterns of elderly adults with ID, although mood and behavior were positively affected. These authors speculate that other elements of the individual's care (e.g., adhering to optimal sleep hygiene, having appropriate bedtimes, increasing daytime activities, etc.) would also need to be addressed for optimal benefits.

In this chapter, emphasis is placed on common management approaches for which there is some indication of efficacy or effectiveness in ID populations. Useful links to online resources for parents and young people, among other things, are helpfully provided by Ogundele and Yemula (2022).

Sleep Hygiene

An important precursor to most treatments is addressing sleep hygiene, that is, sleep-related behaviors that expose individuals to cues that prepare them for and promote appropriately timed and effective sleep (Meltzer & Mindell, 2004). These include environmental factors (temperature, light, noise), scheduling of sleep/wake times (including regularity of sleep times), sleep practices and behaviors (e.g., bedtime routine), and physiological factors (e.g., caffeine consumption, timing of meals, activity patterns). Identification and modification of any practices that may be contributing to the sleep disorder should be a priority before embarking upon other specific interventions to optimize the chances of their success and may sometimes be effective in isolation. Jan et al. (2008) provide a thoughtful review of the use of sleep hygiene with children with neurodevelopmental disabilities, drawing on the literature and clinical experience. They also stress the need to consider the sleep hygiene of caregivers and other family members living in the household. Although use of sleep hygiene is frequently suggested as a first-line treatment, the evidence base for people with ID is small; but results suggest it is likely to be useful (Spruyt & Curfs, 2015). Sutton et al. (2021) has worked with parents to co-produce a helpful framework for addressing sleep hygiene education with parents of children with ID, although its effectiveness has yet to be investigated.

Behavioral Therapy

Behavioral interventions aim to encourage behaviors that facilitate sleep and to decrease behaviors that are detrimental to sleep. Addressing the antecedents and consequences of a behavior, identified by functional assessment, may suggest the use of a range of behavioral techniques such as reinforcement of desirable behaviors, removing/reducing reinforcement for undesirable behavior, and stimulus control, including environmental changes. Cooper et al. (2007) provide helpful details of applied behavior analysis, Spruyt and Curfs (2015) describe techniques as applied to the management of insomnia, and functional analysis is also discussed in Chapters 26 and 27 of this textbook. Frequently, reports of behavioral intervention studies extend the strict definition to include addressing sleep hygiene and sleep timing/scheduling.

Behavior therapy is recommended as the first-line approach for insomnia in typically developing young children (Morgenthaler et al., 2006), and cognitive behavior therapy (CBT) is recommended for adults (Wilson et al., 2019), including when delivered digitally (National Institute for Health and Care Excellence, 2022). For children and adults with neurodevelopmental disorders, however, such a guideline is only formalized for children with ASD (Williams Buckley et al., 2020). Nevertheless, behavioral therapy for insomnia has been used successfully with adult and child ID populations. Readers are directed to reviews for details of the specific interventions and participants for child populations (Phillips et al., 2020; A. Richdale & Wiggs 2005; Rigney et al., 2018; Spruyt & Curfs, 2015; Wiggs & France, 2000), adult populations (Shanahan et al., 2019; van de Wouw et al., 2012), and mixed-age groups (Didden & Sigafoos, 2001; Harper et al., 2023; Lancioni et al., 1999; Priday et al., 2017; A. L. Richdale & Baker, 2014). It is noteworthy that while the majority of studies considered in the above reviews have used traditional, face-to-face delivery of behavior therapy, there is also work to suggest that delivery of behavior therapy in a booklet form to parents of children with ID can be effective (Montgomery et al., 2004). Taken together, results from group and single-case experimental designs with children with ID report moderate to large effect sizes, suggesting that behavioral therapy has the potential to offer relief for problems with both sleep initiation and sleep maintenance, although the duration of the effects may be highly variable. Whether post-intervention support would be a helpful addition for some families, to help encourage maintenance of any gains, remains an area for future study. Intervention studies with adults are more limited in number and quality, with most being case studies of young to middle-aged adults and utilizing subjective report sleep outcomes (see

Shanahan et al., 2019; van de Wouw et al., 2012). Results are generally encouraging and suggest that behavior therapy has the potential to be helpful for sleeplessness problems in adults with ID, although there is clearly a need for high-quality evidence (including in the elderly) to underpin clinical guidance.

There are increasing attempts to identify the effectiveness of behavior therapy for sleeplessness with discrete groups, for example, children and adults with Angelman syndrome (Egan et al., 2020), children with ASD (Cuomo et al., 2017; Kirkpatrick et al., 2019) and adults with Down syndrome (Giménez et al., 2021). Such an approach is helpful both for identifying groups who might be expected to respond favorably (e.g., children with ASD) and, unfortunately more commonly given the current paucity of information, for highlighting the lack of evidence base and suggesting areas in need of more research.

It is worth noting that behavioral intervention for insomnia frequently will include use of multiple elements (e.g., stimulus control to encourage sleep onset, reinforcement of positive behaviors, etc.), and few studies have explored the relative efficacy of different techniques. This makes it challenging to determine the contribution of the individual components of therapy, although, of course, such information would be useful to guide practice.

Although less commonly reported, behavioral interventions have been used successfully with young people with ID for sleep difficulties other than sleeplessness; for example, for sleep terrors (Durand, 2002), rhythmic movement disorders (DeLeon et al., 2004; Weiher & Harman, 1975), and daytime sleepiness (Friedman & Luiselli, 2008), although the very limited available empirical data does not meet the necessary criteria to allow one to make conclusions about likely efficacy. Behavior therapy may also have a role in accompanying other types of sleep intervention. For example, Koontz et al. (2003) describe the successful use of behavior therapy to facilitate continuous positive airway pressure (CPAP) compliance in children with ID who had OSA, and, as described below, behavioral intervention is often recommended as part of the management plan when using melatonin.

Cognitive Therapy

Cognitive therapy has a significant role to play in the treatment of some sleep disorders, notably insomnia and parasomnias, but, traditionally, has not been widely used with ID populations. Willner (2004) describes a case report of a 29-year-old man with ID and recurrent and persistent nightmares that were improved by "rescripting" (c.f. Wittman et al., 2006) the end of his nightmares, followed by rehearsal of this alternative ending morning and night for 1 week. Effects were maintained at 6- and 12-month follow-ups. Willner speculates that the nature of this intervention (essentially requiring the man to remember a new set of "facts") might be easier for individuals with ID rather than cognitive interventions that aim to change beliefs and attitudes. Adapted imagery rehearsal was also used successfully to ameliorate post-traumatic nightmares in two adults with ID (Stenfert-Kroese & Thomas, 2006). Gunning and Espie (2003) further describe the beneficial use of mental imagery with adults with ID who had difficulty initiating and maintaining sleep, along with cognitive work with their parents to address the parents' concerns and worries. Given the role that cognitions play in the maintenance of insomnia in typically developing adults (A. G. Harvey, 2002) and likely in typically developing children too (Gregory et al., 2008), therapeutic options addressing the cognitions of people with ID who have insomnia, and cognitive work with their parents/caregivers if appropriate, remains an important area for future research to address.

Chronotherapy

Chronotherapy refers to interventions designed to affect the circadian pattern of the sleep–wake cycle, used in the treatment of circadian rhythm sleep–wake disorders. They include behavioral chronotherapy, timed light exposure, and the use of chronobiotic medications, such as melatonin.

BEHAVIORAL CHRONOTHERAPY

Behavioral chronotherapy involves systematic and progressive altering of sleep and wake times along with other circadian cues (activities, mealtimes, etc.) to synchronize the endogenous circadian rhythm with the exogenous daily schedule. Many behavioral interventions involve altering the timing of sleep and wake, and the distinction between behavioral interventions and chronotherapeutic interventions (in this text) is somewhat opaque, especially since behavioral and circadian sleep disorders commonly co-occur. The studies referred to in this section are those that address the timing of sleep as their primary concern. Sleep scheduling has been used with children with ID, delivered in hospital settings. Okawa et al. (1987) described mixed results of strict sleep scheduling combined with hypnotic drugs in three blind school-aged girls with moderate to severe ID. Unfortunately, it is not possible to determine the contribution of the different treatment components. Piazza et al. (1998) had more success with an 8-year-old girl with severe ID and ASD who had a fragmented sleep–wake pattern and a reduced total sleep time. Systematically delaying bedtime and scheduling regular daytime activities improved sleep, with effects maintained at a 4-month follow-up.

There is clearly a need for considerably more research in this area with ID populations, to assess not only the effects of chronotherapy in isolation but also how its use can be facilitated by other agents (e.g., light therapy, melatonin) known to affect the circadian pacemaker.

LIGHT THERAPY

Exposure to bright light early in the biological night (i.e., close to sleep onset) delays the sleep phase, and exposure in the late biological night (i.e., close to waking time) promotes phase advances (Czeisler et al., 1989; Khalsa et al., 2003). Light therapy (i.e., appropriately timed exposure to bright light) is reported to have been helpful for dealing with cyclical sleeplessness problems in a child with Smith-Magenis syndrome (Smith et al., 1998) and for settling night waking problems in an adult with profound ID and visual impairment (Short & Carpenter, 1998). In both cases light was applied in the morning, and in the latter case light exposure was achieved by taking the man outside rather than using a commercially available light box. Because light was administered at a set time each morning, the interventions included a sleep-scheduling component, so discerning the precise mechanisms of treatment is difficult.

Light therapy may be combined with behavioral treatment. Guilleminault et al. (1993) found that five of 14 young children with moderate to severe ID responded to bright light treatment (with concurrent behavioral approaches) when other interventions (behavioral and pharmacological) had failed. Gunning and Espie (2003) also found light therapy, behavioral therapy, and the use of sleep hygiene to be effective at reducing sleep-onset latency in a 40-year-old female with moderate ID and delayed sleep phase syndrome. It is worth noting that light therapy has been shown to be effective for some blind patients, presumably because photosensitive retinal ganglion cells remain intact (Czeisler et al., 1995). However, Okawa et al.'s (1987) case series included a report of light therapy being unsuccessful for a 10-year-old girl with congenital blindness and moderate ID, serving as a reminder that this is not always the case. As discussed earlier, light therapy delivered in a residential setting for elderly with ID failed to also demonstrate benefits for sleep (Böhmer et al., 2022).

The AASM's guidelines for the treatment of circadian rhythm sleep–wake disorders suggests there is weak evidence to support the use of light therapy with or without accompanying behavioral interventions for adults with advanced sleep–wake phase disorder and for children and adolescents with delayed sleep wake phase disorder (Augur et al., 2015), but no specific recommendations are made for ID populations. It should be recognized that certain medications (including antipsychotics and some antidepressants) are photosensitizing, and the use of light therapy should be closely monitored in patients taking such medications (Terman & Terman, 1999).

Pharmacotherapy

Melatonin also may be considered a chronotherapeutic; however, as it is increasingly associated with pharmacotherapy in the ID population, it is given special attention in this section, followed by consideration of other pharmacological approaches.

MELATONIN

Endogenous melatonin is a hormone secreted by the pineal gland. Its production and release are suppressed by light and promoted in response to darkness. It is well documented that melatonin, acting via the suprachiasmatic nucleus, plays a role in the promotion of sleep (Wehr et al., 2001). Abnormalities of melatonin secretion may be associated with sleep disturbance in some groups, for example, an inverted rhythm in Smith-Magenis syndrome (De Leersnyder et al., 2001) and low levels in children with Williams syndrome (Sniecinska-Cooper et al., 2015) and Angelman syndrome (Paprocka et al., 2017). However, the profile of melatonin secretion and the relationships between this profile and sleep disturbance appear to vary considerably across and within discrete groups of individuals with neurodevelopmental disorders (see Woodford et al., 2021).

Synthetic exogenous melatonin is produced in tablet, capsule, and liquid forms; and both immediate and sustained-release formulations are available. Melatonin sustained-release tablets were approved by the European Medicines Agency in September 2018 and indicated for the treatment of insomnia in children and adolescents aged 2–18 with ASD and/or Smith-Magenis syndrome, where sleep hygiene measures have been insufficient, but are also used "off-label" with children with many neurodevelopmental disorders.

Results from the increasing number of randomized controlled trials (RCTs) with children with ID (see Blackmer & Feinstein, 2016; Braam et al., 2009; Cuomo et al., 2017; Rossignol & Frye 2011; Sajith & Clarke, 2007; Shanahan et al., 2019, for reviews) generally suggest a reduction in sleep latency (using immediate release; e.g., Gringras et al., 2012; Yuge et al., 2020) but that total sleep time is only increased by using sustained-release formulations (Gringras et al., 2017; Wasdell et al., 2008). The variability of findings from investigation of therapeutic use of melatonin in discrete groups of children raises important questions for further study; for example, melatonin has been generally associated with improvements in sleep in children with ASD (Cuomo et al., 2017), whereas results are more mixed for Angelman syndrome (Egan et al., 2020); and no objective changes in sleep were documented for children with Dravet syndrome compared to placebo, although there appeared to be individual children who showed response (Myers et al., 2018). Increased understanding of the individual factors which affect response will be helpful to inform therapeutic guidelines about the use of melatonin in ID populations.

It is of note that, appropriately, most intervention studies have used behavioral interventions in conjunction with melatonin treatment, so mechanisms underlying improvements are difficult to fully unravel, especially as sleep outcomes are better when melatonin is used alongside behavioral advice than when used alone (Cortesi et al., 2012). A further important consideration when evaluating this literature is that the administration of melatonin has varied considerably between studies, with doses of between 0.5 mg and 12 mg given at various times in relation to bedtime (e.g., at bedtime or several hours before bedtime).

For adults with an ID, studies evaluating the effects of melatonin (immediate- and sustained-release) are more limited (see Braam et al., 2009, and Shanahan et al., 2019, for reviews). Although there is some indication of benefits in reducing sleep-onset latency from a small RCT comparing 5 mg melatonin with placebo (Braam et al., 2008) and mixed results from case series studies (Dodd et al., 2008; Richings & Feroz-Nainar, 2010; Ward et al., 2015), associated agitation, aggression, and restlessness were also noted in some individuals in all studies. Relatedly, Ballester et al. (2019) conducted an RCT of agomelatine (a melatonin receptor agonist and a selective serotonin-receptor antagonist) with adults with ASD and ID. Compared to placebo they found agomelatine to be associated with significant increases in total sleep time, desirable circadian phase shifts, and increased stability of the sleep–wake rhythm.

Compared to other pharmacological preparations used in the treatment of sleeplessness, reported adverse effects associated with the use of melatonin are typically minimal (Foley & Steel, 2019), including with longer-term use over 26 weeks for children with ID (immediate-release melatonin; Yuge et al., 2020) and over 52 weeks with children with ASD and Smith-Magenis syndrome (sustained-release; Maras et al., 2018). Although there remain gaps in knowledge about the safety of the long-term use of melatonin and its effectiveness in adults, it may be used with caution, with awareness of the limitations in scientific and clinical knowledge. Since positive responses have been documented with low doses, it seems prudent to start with the smallest possible dose and to increase as needed. Benefits, if present, have typically been evident within a few days at most, allowing for a fairly rapid dose escalation if required.

OTHER PHARMACOTHERAPIES

Pharmacological approaches other than melatonin clearly have a role to play in the treatment of sleep disorders (see Chapter 18). While specific guiding information about the use of pharmacotherapy for management of sleep disorders in ID populations is lacking due to the absence of rigorous evidence, there are preliminary reports of medications being helpful for the sleep problems associated with psychiatric conditions common in ID populations, such as clonidine reported as useful in children with ADHD (Prince et al., 1996) and ASD (Ming et al., 2008) as well as for the sleep of children with ID of mixed etiology (Ingrassia & Turk, 2005); fluvoxamine in a child with Asperger's syndrome (Furusho et al., 2001); and possibly iron supplementation for children with ASD, although results are contradictory (Dosman et al., 2007; Lane et al., 2015); clonazepam was noted to be helpful for improving sleep continuity and reducing periodic limb movements in a small series of children with Williams syndrome (Arens et al., 1998); and CBD oil use was associated with improved parent-reported sleep of a small series of children and young people with severe ID (Efron et al., 2021).

Management of Sleep-Related Breathing Disorders

Treatment of sleep-related breathing disorders is discussed in detail in Chapter 35. Options for management are fundamentally the same for ID as for typically developing populations. These include lifestyle changes, such as weight loss, use of nasal decongestants or allergy medications and positional therapy for milder cases, and use of additional approaches, such as positive airway pressure (PAP) therapy, oral appliances, and surgery where this is required (e.g., for moderate/severe cases, where preliminary measures have been unsuccessful). As mentioned earlier in the present chapter, recognition needs to be given to both the elevated prevalence of OSA in people with ID and the additional management complexities and challenges that may present for children and adults with ID. Unfortunately, there are limited good-quality data assessing treatment outcome specifically in ID samples, but some important management considerations can be highlighted from the existing work.

For example, while AT is the most common first-line treatment for OSA in children, including those with ID, it may be less successful at treating OSA in ID populations compared with the general population. For example, between 50% and 75% of patients with OSA and Down syndrome will have clinically significant residual disease postoperatively (Ingram et al., 2017; Nation & Brigger, 2017), with similar rates of success reported for children with Prader-Willi syndrome (Lee et al., 2020). This is perhaps unsurprising as for many children with ID there can be multiple comorbidities that can affect airway obstruction and gas exchange, including various (and multiple) craniofacial/airway abnormalities, obesity, and hypotonia. As such, while AT might confer some important benefits, it might not be the only form of treatment required. Further, compared to use in typically developing samples it may also be associated with higher rates of postoperative problems including respiratory complications in Down syndrome (Goldstein et al., 1998) and velopharyngeal insufficiency in Prader-Willi syndrome (Lee et al., 2020). Awareness of elevated risks and treatment limitations is therefore important both to manage families' expectations and to alert clinicians to the need for ongoing postoperative monitoring (with additional treatment if required).

PAP has been shown to be effective at maintaining airway patency and improving neurobehavioral outcomes (including in ID samples; e.g., E. A. Hill et al., 2020; Marcus et al., 2006; van den Broek et al., 2021). Outcomes are, of course, at least somewhat related to treatment compliance and adherence, which raises questions for the use of such approaches with ID samples. It is therefore important to note that treatment using CPAP is possible both in adults (van den Broek et al., 2021) and in children with ID (Kang et al., 2019; Marcus et al., 2006), especially when appropriate guidance, support, and training are provided (see Luijks et al., 2017, for a suggested intensive training protocol). Some studies have suggested that, compared to the general population, adherence in adults with ID is comparable (Luijks et al., 2017) and in children with ID may be even greater (Kang et al., 2019). Reasons for this are difficult to fully delineate, but the authors speculate that the good adherence is related to the intensity of guidance from clinicians/input from carers (especially during the early stages of use) as well as the use of higher PAP pressures and perceived benefits of treatment. Awareness of potential barriers to CPAP implementation and compliance in individuals with ID, such as coexisting behavior problems, insomnia, anxiety, and nasal congestion, is particularly important so that these can be actively addressed. Indeed, as described in the earlier section on behavior therapy, this approach can be used to facilitate successful CPAP treatment through encouraging familiarity with the equipment, establishing routines, managing stress points, and addressing comorbid sleep difficulties such as insomnia.

Conclusions

Sleep disturbances are common in people with ID, posing a significant clinical challenge, increasing the burden of care, and potentially exposing the individual to the wide-reaching problems associated with impaired sleep quantity/quality. As such, sleep disturbance should be routinely screened for, to facilitate early identification and treatment, where possible. The increased risk for sleep disturbance is likely due to various biological and psychosocial factors which need to be considered to allow comprehensive case formulation and to facilitate appropriate management decisions.

For sleeplessness problems in children with ID, there is growing evidence to suggest that behavior therapy and melatonin may be helpful. Interventions for other forms of sleep disturbance in children are required, and more generally adult populations have been less studied. There is also an urgent need for information about the efficacy and relative efficacy of different interventions for particular sleep disorders within discrete ID populations (e.g., according to underlying etiology, age, etc.) to guide clinical practice. Given that sleep problems are so common in ID, exploration of ways to increase access to support and intervention and ongoing post-intervention support (e.g., using digital platforms) would likely be useful for both families and clinicians, as well as potentially proving cost-effective.

Future Directions

- Continued efforts are needed to document the sleep behaviors/disorders, PSG phenotypes, and response to treatment associated with a broader range of discrete syndromes to inform about potential mechanisms and to facilitate more personalized medicine.
- More work is needed investigating sleep disturbance in adults and older adults with ID, including identification of the key problems (in both home and residential settings) and intervention studies to provide guidance about how any problems might successfully be managed.
- The development and evaluation of digital tools to support parents and carers managing sleep in children and adults with ID (and parallel tools for the individuals themselves) would be valuable, affording the possibilities of increasing access and cost-effectiveness.
- The development of digital support could helpfully be informed by qualitative methods and patient and public involvement work to better understand the needs and preferences of the end users. For an example of this approach, see Wiggs et al. (2021) and Cook et al. (2021).

- The role of cognitions (of the individual and/or the parent/caregiver) in the onset and maintenance of some sleep disorders in individuals with ID is understudied, and increased understanding of this could feed into intervention development. Cognitive work may be synergistic with behavioral intervention, as it has proven to be when CBT is applied to sleep disorders in other populations.

References

Agar, G., Bissell, S., Wilde, L., Over, N., Williams, C., Richards, C., & Oliver, C. (2022). Caregivers' experience of sleep management in Smith-Magenis syndrome: A mixed-methods study. *Orphanet Journal of Rare Diseases*, 17, Article 35. https://doi.org/10.1186/s13023-021-02159-8

Agar, G., Brown, C., Sutherland, D., Coulborn, S., Oliver, C., & Richards, C. (2021). Sleep disorders in rare genetic syndromes: A meta-analysis of prevalence and profile. *Molecular Autism*, 12, Article 18. https://doi.org/10.1186/s13229-021-00426-w

American Academy of Sleep Medicine. (2014). *International classification of sleep disorders* (3rd ed.).

American Psychiatric Association. (2013). *Diagnostic and statistical manual of mental disorders* (5th ed.).

Annaz, D., Hill, C. M., Ashworth, A., Holley, S., & Karmiloff-Smith, A. (2011). Characterisation of sleep problems in children with Williams syndrome. *Research in Developmental Disabilities*, *32*(1), 164–169. https://doi.org/10.1016/j.ridd.2010.09.008

Arens, R., Wright, B., Elliott, J., Zhao, H., Wang, P. P., Brown, L. W., Namey, T., & Kaplan, P. (1998). Periodic limb movement in sleep in children with Williams syndrome. *The Journal of Pediatrics*, *133*, 670–674. https://doi.org/10.1016/s0022-3476(98)70110-6

Ashworth, A., Hill, C. M., Karmiloff-Smith, A., & Dimitriou, D. (2013). Cross syndrome comparison of sleep problems in children with Down syndrome and Williams syndrome. *Research in Developmental Disabilities*, *34*, 1572–1580. https://doi.org/10.1016/j.ridd.2013.01.031

Auger, R. R., Burgess, H. J., Emens, J. S., Deriy, L. V., Thomas, S. M., & Sharkey, K. M. (2015). Clinical practice guideline for the treatment of intrinsic circadian rhythm sleep–wake disorders: Advanced sleep–wake phase disorder (ASWPD), delayed sleep–wake phase disorder (DSWPD), non-24-hour sleep–wake rhythm disorder (N24SWD), and irregular sleep–wake rhythm disorder (ISWRD). An update for 2015: An American Academy of Sleep Medicine clinical practice guideline. *Journal of Clinical Sleep Medicine*, *11*(10), 1199–1236. https://doi.org/10.5664/jcsm.5100

Ballester, P., Martínez, M. J., Inda, M. D., Javaloyes, A., Richdale, A. L., Muriel, J., Belda, C., Toral, N., Morales, D., Fernández. E., & Peiró, A. M. (2019). Evaluation of agomelatine for the treatment of sleep problems in adults with autism spectrum disorder and co-morbid intellectual disability. *Journal of Psychopharmacology*, *33*(11), 1395–1406. https://doi.org/10.1177/0269881119864968

Bartlett, L. B., Rooney, V., & Spedding, S. (1985). Nocturnal difficulties in a population of mentally handicapped children. *British Journal of Mental Subnormality*, *31*, 54–59. https://doi.org/10.1179/bjms.1985.009

Beresford, B., Stuttard, L., Clarke, S., & Maddison, J. (2016). Parents' experiences of psychoeducational sleep management interventions: A qualitative study of parents of children with neurodevelopmental disabilities. *Clinical Practice in Pediatric Psychology*, *4*(2), 164–175. https://doi.org/10.1037/cpp0000144

Blackmer, A. B., & Feinstein, J. A. (2016). Management of sleep disorders in children with neurodevelopmental disorders: A review. *Pharmacotherapy*, *36*(1), 84–98. https://doi.org/10.1002/phar.1686

Böhmer, M. N., Oppewal, A., Valstar, M. J., Bindels, P. J. E., van Someren, E. J. W., & Maes-Festen, D. A. M. (2022). Light up: An intervention study of the effect of environmental dynamic lighting on sleep–wake rhythm, mood and behaviour in older adults with intellectual disabilities. *Journal of Intellectual Disability Research*, *66*, 756–781. https://doi.org/10.1111/jir.12969

Boyle, A., Melville, C. A., Morrison, J., Allan, L., Smiley, E., Espie, C. A., & Cooper, S. A. (2010). A cohort study of the prevalence of sleep problems in adults with intellectual disabilities. *Journal of Sleep Research*, *19*(1), 42–53. https://doi.org/10.1111/j.1365-2869.2009.00788.x

Braam, W., Didden, R., Smits, M., & Curfs, L. (2008). Melatonin treatment in individuals with intellectual disability and chronic insomnia: A randomized placebo-controlled study. *Journal of Intellectual Disability Research*, *52*, 256–264. https://doi.org/10.1111/j.1365-2788.2007.01016.x

Braam, W., Smits, M. G., Didden, R., Korzilius, H., Van Geijlswijk, I. M., & Curfs, L. M. (2009). Exogenous melatonin for sleep problems in individuals with intellectual disability: A meta-analysis. *Developmental Medicine and Child Neurology, 51*, 340–349. https://doi.org/10.1111/j.1469-8749.2008.03244.x

Bramble, D. (1996). Consumer opinion concerning the treatment of a common sleep problem. *Child: Care, Health and Development, 22*, 355–366.

Brouillette, R. T., Fernbach, S. K., & Hunt, C. E. (1982). Obstructive sleep apnea in infants and children. *Journal of Pediatrics, 100*, 31–40. https://doi.org/10.1016/s0022-3476(82)80231-x

Browne, E. G., King, J. R., & Surtees, A. D. R. (2024). Sleep in people with and without intellectual disabilities: A systematic review and meta-analysis. *Journal of Intellectual Disability Research, 68*, 1–22. https://doi.org/10.1111/jir.13093

Bruni, O., Ottaviano, S., Guidetti, V., Romoli, M., Innocenzi, M., Cortesi, F., & Giannotti, F. (1996). The Sleep Disturbance Scale for Children (SDSC). Construction and validation of an instrument to evaluate sleep disturbances in childhood and adolescence. *Journal of Sleep Research, 5*, 251–261. https://doi.org/10.1111/j.1365-2869.1996.00251.x

Brylewski, J., & Wiggs, L. (1998). A questionnaire survey of sleep and night-time behaviour in a community-based sample of adults with intellectual disability. *Journal of Intellectual Disability Research, 42*, 154–162. https://doi.org/10.1046/j.1365-2788.1998.00111.x

Buysse, D. J., Reynolds, C. F., 3rd, Monk, T. H., Berman, S. R., & Kupfer, D. J. (1989). The Pittsburgh Sleep Quality Index: A new instrument for psychiatric practice and research. *Psychiatry Research, 28*, 193–213. https://doi.org/10.1016/0165-1781(89)90047-4

Camfferman, D., McEvoy, R. D., O'Donoghue, F., & Lushington, K. (2008). Prader-Willi syndrome and excessive daytime sleepiness. *Sleep Medicine Reviews, 12*, 65–75. https://doi.org/10.1016/j.smrv.2007.08.005

Castaldo, V., & Krynicki, V. (1973). Sleep pattern and intelligence in functional mental retardation. *Journal of Mental Deficiency Research, 17*, 231–235. https://doi.org/10.1111/j.1365-2788.1973.tb01206.x

Cataldi, M., Arnaldi, D., Tucci, V., De Carli, F. Patti, G., Napoli, F., Pace, M., Maghnie, M., & Nobili, L. (2021). Sleep disorders in Prader-Willi syndrome, evidence from animal models and humans. *Sleep Medicine Reviews, 57*, Article 101432. https://doi.org/10.1016/j.smrv.2021.101432

Chan, S. Y.-S. (2020). Sleep architecture and homeostasis in children with epilepsy: A neurodevelopmental perspective. *Developmental Medicine and Child Neurology, 62*, 426–433. https://doi.org/10.1111/dmcn.14437

Chawla, J. K., Burgess, S., & Heussler, H. (2020). The impact of sleep problems on functional and cognitive outcomes in children with Down syndrome: A review of the literature. *Journal of Clinical Sleep Medicine, 16*(10), 1785–1795. https://doi.org/10.5664/jcsm.8630

Chawla, J. K., Cooke, E., Miguel, M. C., Burgess, S., & Staton, S. (2023). Parents' experiences of having a child with Down syndrome and sleep difficulties. *Behavioral Sleep Medicine, 3*, 21(5), 570–584. https://doi.org/ 10.1080/15402002.2022.2143359

Chervin, R. D., Hedger, K., Dillon, J. E., & Pituch, K. J. (2000). Pediatric Sleep Questionnaire (PSQ): Validity and reliability of scales for sleep-disordered breathing, snoring, sleepiness, and behavioral problems. *Sleep Medicine, 1*, 21–32. https://doi.org/10.1016/s1389-9457(99)00009-x

Clarke, N. A., Hoare, D. J., & Killan, E. C. (2019). Evidence for an association between hearing impairment and disrupted sleep: Scoping review. *American Journal of Audiology, 28*(4), 1015–1024. https://doi.org/10.1044/2019_AJA-19-0026

Coleman, M., Brubaker, J., Hunter, K., & Smith, G. (1988). Rett syndrome: A survey of North American patients. *Journal of Mental Deficiency Research, 32*, 117–124. https://doi.org/10.1111/j.1365-2788.1988.tb01397.x

Cook, G., Gringras, P., Hiscock, H., Pal, D. K., & Wiggs, L. (2021). A qualitative investigation into what parents want from an online behavioural sleep intervention for children with epilepsy. *Frontiers in Psychology*, 29(12), Article 628605. https://doi.org/10.3389/fpsyg.2021.628605

Cooper, J. O., Heron, T. E., & Heward, W. L. (2007). *Applied behaviour analysis* (2nd ed.). Pearson Prentice Hall.

Cortesi, F., Giannotti, F., Sebastiani, T., Panunzi, S., & Valente, D. (2012). Controlled-release melatonin, singly and combined with cognitive behavioural therapy, for persistent insomnia in children with autism spectrum disorders: A randomized placebo-controlled trial. *Journal of Sleep Research, 21*, 700–709. https://doi.org/10.1111/j.1365-2869.2012.01021.x

Cox, R. C., & Olatunji, B. O. (2020). Sleep in the anxiety-related disorders: A meta-analysis of subjective and objective research. *Sleep Medicine Reviews, 51*, Article 101282, https://doi.org/10.1016/j.smrv.2020.101282

Cuomo, B. M., Vaz, S., Lee, E. A. L., Thompson, C., Rogerson, J. M., & Falkmer, T. (2017). Effectiveness of sleep-based interventions for children with autism spectrum disorder: A meta-synthesis. *Pharmacotherapy, 37*(5), 555–578. https://doi.org/10.1002/phar.1920

Czeisler, C. A., Kronauer, R. E., Allan, J. S., Duffy, J. F., Jewett, M. E., Brown, E. N., & Ronda, J. M. (1989). Bright light induction of strong (Type 0) resetting of the human circadian pacemaker. *Science, 244*, 1328–1333. https://doi.org/10.1126/science.2734611

Czeisler, C. A., Shanahan, T. L., Klerman, E. B., Martens, H., Brotman, D. J., Emens, J. S., Klein, T., & Rizzo, J. F. (1995). Suppression of melatonin in some blind patients by exposure to bright light. *New England Journal of Medicine, 332*, 6–11. https://doi.org/10.1056/NEJM199501053320102

Dahl, R. E., Pelham, W. E., & Wierson, M. (1991). The role of sleep disturbance in attention deficit disorder symptoms: A case study. *Journal of Pediatric Psychology, 16*, 229–239. https://doi.org/10.1093/jpepsy/16.2.229

De Leersnyder, H., Claustrat, B., Munnich, A., & Verloes, A. (2006). Circadian rhythm disorder in a rare disease: Smith-Magenis syndrome. *Molecular and Cellular Endocrinology, 27*, 88–91. https://doi.org/10.1016/j.mce.2006.03.043

De Leersnyder, H., De Blois, M. C., Claustrat, B., Romana, S., Albrecht, U., Von Kleist-Retzow, J. C., Delobel, B., Viot, G., Lyonnet, S., Vekemans, M., & Munnich, A. (2001). Inversion of the circadian rhythm of melatonin in the Smith-Magenis syndrome. *Journal of Pediatrics, 139*, 111–116. https://doi.org/10.1067/mpd.2001.115018

DeLeon, I. G., Fisher, W. W., & Marhefka, J. M. (2004). Decreasing self-injurious behavior associated with awakening in a child with autism and developmental delays. *Behavioral Interventions, 19*, 111–119. https://doi.org/10.1002/bin.154

Didden, R., & Sigafoos, J. (2001). A review of the nature and treatment of sleep disorders in individuals with developmental disabilities. *Research in Developmental Disabilities, 22*, 255–272. https://doi.org/10.1016/s0891-4222(01)00071-3

Dimarino, A. J., Jr., Banwait, K. S., Eschinger, E., Greenberg, A., Dimarino, M., Doghramji, K., & Cohen, S. (2005). The effect of gastro-oesophageal reflux and omeprazole on key sleep parameters. *Alimentary Pharmacology and Therapeutics, 22*, 325–329. https://doi.org/10.1111/j.1365-2036.2005.02573.x

Diomedi, M., Curatolo, P., Scalise, A., Placidi, F., Caretto, F., & Gigli, G. L. (1999). Sleep abnormalities in mentally retarded autistic subjects: Down's syndrome with mental retardation and normal subjects. *Brain and Development, 21*, 548–553. https://doi.org/10.1016/s0387-7604(99)00077-7

Dodd, A., Hare, D. J., & Arshad, P. (2008). The use of melatonin to treat sleep disorder in adults with intellectual disabilities in community settings—The evaluation of three cases using actigraphy. *Journal of Intellectual Disability Research, 52*, 547–553. https://doi.org/10.1111/j.1365-2788.2008.01063.x

Dosman, C. F., Brian, J. A., Drmic, I. E., Senthilselvan, A., Harford, M. M., Smith, R. W., Sharieff, W., Zlotkin, S. H., Moldofsky, H., & Roberts, S. W. (2007). Children with autism: Effect of iron supplementation on sleep and ferritin. *Pediatric Neurology, 36*, 152–158. https://doi.org/10.1016/j.pediatrneurol.2006.11.004

Dreier, L. A., Zernikow, B., Blankenburg, M., & Wager, J. (2018). A sleep questionnaire for children with severe psychomotor impairment (SNAKE)—Concordance with a global rating of sleep quality. *Children, 5*(2), Article 20. https://doi.org/10.3390/children5020020

Durand, V. M. (2002). Treating sleep terrors in children with autism. *Journal of Positive Behavior Interventions, 4*, 66–72. https://doi.org/10.1177/109830070200400201

Eaton, C., Tarver, J., Shirazi, A., Pearson, E., Walker, L., Bird, M., Oliver, C., & Waite, J. A. (2021). A systematic review of the behaviours associated with depression in people with severe-profound intellectual disability. *Journal of Intellectual Disability* Research, *65*(3), 211–229. https://doi.org/10.1111/jir.12807

Efron, D., Freeman, J. L., Cranswick, N., Payne J. M., Mulraney, M., Prakash, C., Lee, K. J., Taylor, K., & Williams, K. (2021). A pilot randomised placebo-controlled trial of cannabidiol to reduce severe behavioural problems in children and adolescents with intellectual disability. *British Journal of Clinical Pharmacology, 87*, 436–446. https://doi.org/10.1111/bcp.14399

Egan, M., Farrell, K., Hoey, E., McGuire, B. E., & Lydon, H. K. (2020). Interventions to improve sleep for individuals with Angelman syndrome: A systematic review. *Research in Developmental Disabilities, 97*, Article 103554. https://doi.org/10.1016/j.ridd.2019.103554

Elia, M., Ferri, R., Musumeci, S. A., Del Gracco, S., Bottitta, M., Scuderi, C., Miano, G., Paneirai, S., Bertrand, T., & Grubar, J. C. (2000). Sleep in subjects with autistic disorder: A neuropsychological and psychological study. *Brain Development, 22*, 88–92. https://doi.org/10.1016/s0387-7604(99)00119-9

Esbensen, A. J., Hoffman, E. K., Beebe, D. W., Byars, K., Carle, A. C., Epstein, J. N., & Johnson, C. (2022). Randomized behavioral sleep clinical trial to improve outcomes in children with Down syndrome. *American Journal of Intellectual and Developmental Disabilities, 127*(2), 149–164. https://doi.org/10.1352/1944-7558-127.2.149

Espie, C. A. (1992). Optimal sleep–wake scheduling and profound mental handicap: Potential benefits. *Mental Handicap, 20*, 102–107. https://doi.org/10.1111/j.1468-3156.1992.tb00668.x

Espie, C. A., Paul, A., McFie, J., Amos, P., Hamilton, D., McColl, J. H., Tarassenko, L., & Pardey, J. (1998). Sleep studies in adults with severe or profound mental retardation and epilepsy. *American Journal on Mental Retardation, 103*, 47–59. https://doi.org/10.1352/0895-8017(1998)103<0047:SSOAWS>2.0.CO;2

Espie, C. A., & Tweedie, F. M. (1991). Sleep patterns and sleep problems amongst people with mental handicap. *Journal of Mental Deficiency Research, 35*, 25–36. https://doi.org/10.1111/j.1365-2788.1991.tb01028.x

Fallone, G., Owens, J. A., & Deane, J. (2002). Sleepiness in children and adolescents: Clinical implications. *Sleep Medicine Reviews, 6*, 287–306. https://doi.org/10.1053/smrv.2001.0192

Fazzi, E., Zaccagnino, M., Gahagan, S., Capsoni, C., Signorini, S., Ariaudo, G., Lanners, J., & Orcesi, S. (2008). Sleep disturbances in visually impaired toddlers. *Brain Development, 30*, 572–578. https://doi.org/10.1016/j.braindev.2008.01.008

Fermin, A. M., Afzal, U., & Culebras, A. (2016). Sleep in neuromuscular diseases. *Sleep Medicine Clinics, 11*(1), 53–64. https://doi.org/10.1016/j.jsmc.2015.10.005

Foldvary-Schaefer, N., & Grigg-Damberger, M. (2009). Sleep and epilepsy. *Seminars in Neurology, 29*, 419–428. https://doi.org/10.1055/s-0029-1237115

Foley, H. M., & Steel, A. E. (2019). Adverse events associated with oral administration of melatonin: A critical systematic review of clinical evidence. *Complementary Therapies in Medicine, 42*, 65–81. https://doi.org/10.1016/j.ctim.2018.11.003

Freeman, D., Sheaves, B., Waite, F., Harvey, A. G., & Harrison, P. J. (2020). Sleep disturbance and psychiatric disorders. *The Lancet Psychiatry, 7*(7), 628–637. https://doi.org/10.1016/S2215-0366(20)30136-X

Friedman, A., & Luiselli, J. K. (2008). Excessive daytime sleep: Behavioral assessment and intervention in a child with autism. *Behavior Modification, 32*, 548–555. https://doi.org/10.1177/0145445507312187

Furusho, J., Matsuzaki, K., Ichihashi, I., Satoh, H., Yamaguchi, K., & Kumagai, K. (2001). Alleviation of sleep disturbance and repetitive behavior by a selective serotonin re-uptake inhibitor in a boy with Asperger's syndrome. *Brain Development, 23*, 135–137. https://doi.org/10.1016/s0387-7604(01)00182-6

Ghaem, M., Armstrong, K., Trocki, O., Cleghorn, G., Patrick, M., & Shepherd, R. (1998). The sleep patterns of infants and young children with gastro-oesophageal reflux. *Journal of Paediatrics and Child Health, 34*, 160–163. https://doi.org/10.1046/j.1440-1754.1998.00191.x

Gibbon, F. M., Maccormac, E., & Gringras, P. (2019). Sleep and epilepsy: Unfortunate bedfellows. *Archives of Disease in Childhood, 104*(2), 189–192. https://doi.org/10.1136/archdischild-2017-313421

Giménez, S., Altuna, M., Blessing, E., Osorio, R. M., & Fortea, J. (2021). Sleep disorders in adults with Down syndrome. *Journal of Clinical Medicine, 10*, Article 3012. https://doi.org/10.3390/jcm10143012

Goldstein, N. A., Armfield, D. R., Kingsley, L. A., Borland, L. M., Allen, G. C., & Post, J. C. (1998). Postoperative complications after tonsillectomy and adenoidectomy in children with Down syndrome. *Archives of Otolaryngology–Head and Neck Surgery, 124*(2), 171–176. https://doi.org/10.1001/archotol.124.2.171

Gregory, A. M., Caspi, A., Eley, T. C., Moffitt, T. E., O'Connor, T. G., & Poulton, R. (2005). Prospective longitudinal associations between persistent sleep problems in childhood and anxiety and depression disorders in adulthood. *Journal of Abnormal Child Psychology, 33*, 157–163. https://doi.org/10.1007/s10802-005-1824-0

Gregory, A. M., & Sadeh, A. (2016). Annual research review: Sleep problems in childhood psychiatric disorders—A review of the latest science. *Journal of Child Psychology and Psychiatry, 57*(3), 296–317. https://doi.org/10.1111/jcpp.12469

Gregory, A. M., Willis, T. A., Wiggs, L. Harvey, A. G., & The STEPS Team. (2008). Pre-sleep arousal and sleep disturbances in children. *Sleep, 31*, 1745–1747. https://doi.org/10.1093/sleep/31.12.1745

Grigg-Damberger, M., & Ralls, F. (2013). Treatment strategies for complex behavioral insomnia in children with neurodevelopmental disorders. *Current Opinions in Pulmonary Medicine, 19*(6), 616–625. https://doi.org/10.1097/MCP.0b013e328365ab89

Gringras, P., Gamble, C., Jones, A. P., Wiggs, L., Williamson, P. R., Sutcliffe, A., Montgomery, P., Whitehouse, W. P., Choonara, I., Allport, T., Edmond, A., Appleton, R., & MENDS Study Group. (2012). Melatonin for sleep problems in children with neurodevelopmental disorders: Randomised double masked placebo controlled trial. *British Medical Journal, 345*, Article e6664. https://doi.org/10.1136/bmj.e6664

Gringras, P., Nir, T., Breddy, J., Frydman-Marom, A., & Findling, R. L. (2017). Efficacy and safety of pediatric prolonged-release melatonin for insomnia in children with autism spectrum disorder. *Journal of the American Academy of Child and Adolescent Psychiatry, 56*(11), 948–957.e4. https://doi.org/10.1016/j.jaac.2017.09.414

Grubar, J. C. (1983). Sleep and mental deficiency. *Review of Electroencephalography Neurophysiology Clinic, 13*, 107–114. https://doi.org/10.1016/s0370-4475(83)80068-9

Gruber, R., Scholes, S., Bertone, A., McKinney, R. A., Orlowski, J., & Wise, M. S. (2022). Sleep and daytime behavior in individuals with Christianson syndrome. *Sleep Medicine, 89*, 55–59. https://doi.org/10.1016/j.sleep.2021.11.007

Gruber, R., & Wise, M. S. (2016). Sleep spindle characteristics in children with neurodevelopmental disorders and their relation to cognition. *Neural Plasticity, 2016*, Article 4724792. https://doi.org/10.1155/2016/4724792

Guilleminault, C., McCann, C. C., Quera-Salva, M., & Cetel, M. (1993). Light therapy as treatment of dyschronosis in brain impaired children. *European Journal of Pediatrics, 152*, 754–759. https://doi.org/10.1007/BF01953995

Guilleminault, C., Winkle, R., Korobkin, R., & Simmons, B. (1982). Children and nocturnal snoring—Evaluation of the effects of sleep related respiratory resistive load and daytime functioning. *European Journal of Pediatrics, 139*, 165–171. https://doi.org/10.1007/BF01377349

Gulotta, G., Iannella, G., Vicini, C., Polimeni, A., Greco, A., de Vincentiis, M., Visconti, I. C., Meccariello, G., Cammaroto, G., De Vito, A., Gobbi, R., Bellini, C., Firinu, E., Pace, A., Colizza, A., Pelucchi, S., & Magliulo, G. (2019). Risk factors for obstructive sleep apnea syndrome in children: State of the art. *International Journal of Environmental Research and Public Health, 16*(18), Article 3235. https://doi.org/10.3390/ijerph16183235

Gunning, M. J., & Espie, C. A. (2003). Psychological treatment of reported sleep disorder in adults with intellectual disability using a multiple baseline design. *Journal of Intellectual Disability Research, 47*, 191–202. https://doi.org/10.1046/j.1365-2788.2003.00461.x

Hansen, D., & Vandenberg, B. (1997). Neuropsychological features and differential diagnosis of sleep apnea syndrome in children. *Journal of Clinical Child Psychology, 26*, 304–310. https://doi.org/10.1207/s15374424jccp2603_9

Hare, D., Mahon, L., & Rust, S. (2018). Assessment and management of over-activity and sleep disorder in mucopolysaccharidoses *Journal of Child Science, 8*(1), e124–e127. https://doi.org/10.1055/s-0038-1667348

Harper, L., McAnelly, S., Walshe, I., Ooms, A., & Tuffrey-Wijne, I. M. (2023). Behavioural sleep problems in children and adults with intellectual disabilities: An integrative literature review. *Journal of Applied Research in Intellectual Disabilities, 36*(5), 916–928. https://doi.org/10.1111/jar.13116

Harvey, A. G. (2002). A cognitive model of insomnia. *Behaviour Research and Therapy, 40*, 869–893. https://doi.org/10.1016/s0005-7967(01)00061-4

Harvey, M. T., Baker, D. J., Horner, R. H., & Blackford, J. U. (2003). A brief report on the prevalence of sleep problems in individuals with mental retardation living in the community. *Journal of Positive Behavior Interventions, 5*, 195–200. https://doi.org/10.1177/10983007030050040201

Harvey, M. T., & Kennedy, C. H. (2002). Polysomnographic phenotypes in developmental disabilities. *International Journal of Developmental Neuroscience, 20*, 443–448. https://doi.org/10.1016/s0736-5748(02)00008-4

Hill, C. M., Evans, H. J., Elphick, H., Farquhar, M., Pickering, R. M., Kingshott, R., Martin, J., Reynolds, J., Joyce, A., Rush, C., Gavlak, J. C., & Gringras, P. (2016). Prevalence and predictors of obstructive sleep apnoea in young children with Down syndrome. *Sleep Medicine, 27–28*, 99–106. https://doi.org/10.1016/j.sleep.2016.10.001

Hill, E. A. (2016). Obstructive sleep apnoea/hypopnoea syndrome in adults with Down syndrome. *Breathe (Sheff)*, *12*(4), 91–96. https://doi.org/10.1183/20734735.012116

Hill, E. A., Fairley, D. M., Williams, L. J., Spanò, G., Cooper, S. A., & Riha, R. L. (2020). Prospective trial of CPAP in community-dwelling adults with Down syndrome and obstructive sleep apnea syndrome. *Brain Sciences*, *10*(11), Article 844. https://doi.org/10.3390/brainsci10110844

Ingram, D. G., Ruiz, A. G., Gao, D., & Friedman, N. R. (2017). Success of tonsillectomy for obstructive sleep apnea in children with Down syndrome. *Journal of Clinical Sleep Medicine*, *13*(8), 975–980. https://doi.org/10.5664/jcsm.6698

Ingrassia, A., & Turk, J. (2005). The use of clonidine for severe and intractable sleep problems in children with neurodevelopmental disorders—A case series. *European Child and Adolescent Psychiatry*, *14*, 34–40. https://doi.org/10.1007/s00787-005-0424-4

Jan, J. E., Owens, J. A., Weiss, M. D., Johnson, K. P., Wasdell, M. B., Freeman, R. D., & Ipsiroglu, O. (2008). Sleep hygiene for children with neurodevelopmental disabilities. *Pediatrics*, *122*, 1343–1350. https://doi.org/10.1542/peds.2007-3308

Jansen, F. E., Nikanorova, M., & Peltola, M. (2019). Current treatment options for encephalopathy related to status epilepticus during slow sleep. *Epileptic Disorders*, *21*, 76–81. https://doi.org/10.1684/epd.2019.1061

Jenni, O. G., & O'Connor, B. (2005). Children's sleep: An interplay between culture and biology. *Pediatrics*, *115*, 204–216. https://doi.org/10.1542/peds.2004-0815B

Johns, M. W. (1991). A new method for measuring daytime sleepiness: The Epworth Sleepiness Scale. *Sleep*, *14*, 540–545. https://doi.org/10.1093/sleep/14.6.540

Johnson, C. R., DeMand, A., Lecavalier, L., Smith, T., Aman, M., Foldes, E., & Scahill, L. (2016). Psychometric properties of the children's sleep habits questionnaire in children with autism spectrum disorder. *Sleep Medicine*, *20*, 5–11. https://doi.org/10.1016/j.sleep.2015.12.005

Johnson, C. R., Turner, K. S., Foldes, E. L., Malow, B. A., & Wiggs, L. (2012). Comparison of sleep questionnaires in the assessment of sleep disturbances in children with autism spectrum disorders. *Sleep Medicine*, *13*(7), 795–801. https://doi.org/10.1016/j.sleep.2012.03.005

Kang, E. K., Xanthopoulos, M. S., Kim, J. Y., Arevalo, C., Shults, J., Beck, S. E., Marcus, C. L., & Tapia, I. E. (2019). Adherence to positive airway pressure for the treatment of obstructive sleep apnea in children with developmental disabilities. *Journal of Clinical Sleep Medicine*, *15*(6), 915–921. https://doi.org/10.5664/jcsm.7850

Kemlink, D., Pretl, M., Sonka, K., & Nevsimalova, S. (2008). A comparison of polysomnographic and actigraphic evaluation of periodic limb movements in sleep. *Neurology Research*, *30*, 234–238. https://doi.org/10.1179/016164107X229911

Khalsa, S. B. S., Jewett, M. E., Cajochen, C., & Czeisler, C. A. (2003). A phase response curve to single bright light pulses in human subjects. *Journal of Physiology*, *549*, 945–952. https://doi.org/10.1113/jphysiol.2003.040477

Kirkpatrick, B., Louw, J. S., & Leader, G. (2019). Efficacy of parent training incorporated in behavioral sleep interventions for children with autism spectrum disorder and/or intellectual disabilities: A systematic review. *Sleep Medicine*, *53*, 141–152. https://doi.org/10.1016/j.sleep.2018.08.034

Konofal, E., Lecendreux, M., Bouvard, M. P., & Mouren-Simeoni, M. C. (2001). High levels of nocturnal activity in children with attention-deficit hyperactivity disorder: A video analysis. *Psychiatry and Clinical Neurosciences*, *55*, 97–103. https://doi.org/10.1046/j.1440-1819.2001.00808.x

Koontz, K. L., Slifer, K. J., Cataldo, M. D., & Marcus, C. L. (2003). Improving pediatric compliance with positive airway pressure therapy: The impact of behavioral intervention. *Sleep*, *26*(8), 1010–1015. https://doi.org/10.1093/sleep/26.8.1010

Korb, L., O'Regan, D., Conley, J., Dillon, E., Briggs, R., Courtenay, K., & Perera, B. (2021). Sleep: The neglected life factor in adults with intellectual disabilities. *BJPsych Bulletin*, *47*(3), 139–145. https://doi.org/10.1192/bjb.2021.122

Kotagal, S., Gibbons, V. P., & Stith, J. A. (1994). Sleep abnormalities in patients with severe cerebral palsy. *Developmental Medicine and Child Neurology*, *36*, 304–311. https://doi.org/10.1111/j.1469-8749.1994.tb11850.x

Kurin, M., Shibli, F., Kitayama, Y., Kim, Y., & Fass, R. (2021). Sorting out the relationship between gastroesophageal reflux disease and sleep. *Current Gastroenterology Reports*, *23*(9), Article 15. https://doi.org/10.1007/s11894-021-00815-4

Lancioni, G. E., O'Reilly, M. F., & Basili, G. (1999). Review of strategies for treating sleep problems in persons with severe or profound mental retardation or multiple handicaps. *American Journal on Mental Retardation, 104*, 170–186. https://doi.org/10.1352/0895-8017(1999)104<0170:ROSFTS>2.0.CO;2

Lane, R., Kessler, R., Buckley, A. W., Rodriguez, A., Farmer, C., Thurm, A., Swedo, S., & Felt, B. (2015). Evaluation of periodic limb movements in sleep and iron status in children with autism. *Pediatric Neurology, 53*, 343–349. https://doi.org/10.1016/j.pediatrneurol.2015.06.014

Lee, C. H., Hsu, W. C., Ko, J. Y., Yeh, T. H., Lin, M. T., & Kang, K. T. (2020). Adenotonsillectomy for the treatment of obstructive sleep apnea in children with Prader-Willi syndrome: A meta-analysis. *Otolaryngology–Head and Neck Surgery, 162*(2), 168–176. https://doi.org/10.1177/0194599819893115

Lélis, A. L., Cardoso, M. V., & Hall, W. A. (2016). Sleep disorders in children with cerebral palsy: an integrative review. *Sleep Medicine Reviews, 30*, 63–71. https://doi.org/10.1016/j.smrv.2015.11.008

Lockley, S. W., Arendt, J., & Skene, D. J. (2007). Visual impairment and circadian rhythm disorders. *Dialogues in Clinical Neuroscience, 9*, 301–314. https://doi.org/10.31887/DCNS.2007.9.3/slockley

Lockley, S. W., Skene, D. J., Butler, L. J., & Arendt, J. (1999). Sleep and activity rhythms are related to circadian phase in the blind. *Sleep, 22*, 616–623. https://doi.org/10.1093/sleep/22.5.616

Loddenkemper, T., Vendrame, M., Zarowski, M., Gregas, M., Alexopoulos, A. V., Wyllie, E., & Kothare, S. V. (2011). Circadian patterns of pediatric seizures. *Neurology, 76*(2), 145–153. https://doi.org/10.1212/WNL.0b013e318206ca46

Lorsung, E., Karthikeyan, R., & Cao, R. (2021). Biological timing and neurodevelopmental disorders: A role for circadian dysfunction in autism spectrum disorders. *Frontiers in Neuroscience, 15*, Article 642745. https://doi.org/10.3389/fnins.2021.642745

Luijks, K. A., Vandenbussche, N. L., Pevernagie, D., Overeem, D., & Pillen, S. (2017). Adherence to continuous positive airway pressure in adults with an intellectual disability. *Sleep Medicine, 34*, 234–239. https://doi.org/10.1016/j.sleep.2017.02.029

Maas, A. P., Didden, R., Korzilius, H., Braam, W., Collin, P., Smits, M. G., & Curfs, L. M. (2011). Psychometric properties of a sleep questionnaire for use in individuals with intellectual disabilities. *Research in Developmental Disabilities, 32*(6), 2467–2479. https://doi.org/10.1016/j.ridd.2011.07.013

Maquet, P. (2001). The role of sleep in learning and memory. *Science, 294*, 1048–1052. https://doi.org/10.1126/science.1062856

Maras, A., Schroder, C. M., Malow, B. A., Findling, R. L., Breddy, J., Nir, T., Shahmoon, S., Zisapel, N., & Gringras, P. (2018). Long-term efficacy and safety of pediatric prolonged-release melatonin for insomnia in children with autism spectrum disorder. *Journal of Child and Adolescent Psychopharmacology, 28*(10), 699–710. https://doi.org/10.1089/cap.2018.0020

Marcus, C. L., Rosen, G., Ward, S. L., Halbower, A. C., Sterni, L., Lutz, J., Stading, P. J., Bolduc, D., & Gordon, N. (2006). Adherence to and effectiveness of positive airway pressure therapy in children with obstructive sleep apnea. *Pediatrics, 117*(3), e442–e451. https://doi.org/10.1542/peds.2005-1634

Mazza, M. G., Rossetti, A., Crespi, G., & Clerici, M. (2020). Prevalence of co-occurring psychiatric disorders in adults and adolescents with intellectual disability: A systematic review and meta-analysis. *Journal of Applied Research in Intellectual Disabilities, 33*, 126–138. https://doi.org/10.1111/jar.12654

Meltzer, L. J., & Mindell, J. A. (2004). Nonpharmacologic treatments for pediatric sleeplessness. *Pediatric Clinics of North America, 51*, 135–151. https://doi.org/10.1016/s0031-3955(03)00178-0

Ming, X., Gordon, E., Kang, N., & Wagner, G. C. (2008). Use of clonidine in children with autism spectrum disorders. *Brain Development, 30*, 454–460. https://doi.org/10.1016/j.braindev.2007.12.007

Montgomery, P., Stores, G., & Wiggs, L. (2004). The relative efficacy of two brief treatments for sleep problems in young learning disabled (mentally retarded) children: A randomised controlled trial. *Archives of Disease in Childhood, 89*, 125–130. https://doi.org/10.1136/adc.2002.017202

Moore, P. S. (2004). The use of social stories in a psychology service for children with learning disabilities: A case study of a sleep problem. *British Journal of Learning Disabilities, 32*, 133–138. https://doi.org/10.1111/j.1468-3156.2004.00278.x

Morgenthaler, T. I., Owens, J., Alessi, C., Boehlecke, B., Brown, T. M., Coleman, C., Friedman, L., Kapur, V. K., Lee-Chiong, T., Pancer, J., & Swick, T. J. (2006). Practice parameters for behavioral treatment of bedtime problems and night wakings in infants and young children. *Sleep, 29*, 1277–1281.

Morris, C., Janssens, A., Shilling, V., Allard, A., Fellowes, A., Tomlinson, R., Williams, J., Thompson Coon, J., Rogers, M., Beresford, B., Green, C., Jenkinson, C., Tennant, A., & Logan, S. (2015). Meaningful health outcomes for paediatric neurodisability: Stakeholder prioritisation and appropriateness of patient reported outcome measures. *Health and Quality of Life Outcomes, 13*, Article 87. https://doi.org/10.1186/s12955-015-0284-7

Moseley, M. J., Fouladi, M., Jones, H. S., & Tobin, M. J. (1996). Sleep disturbance and blindness. *Lancet, 348*, 1514–1515. https://doi.org/10.1016/S0140-6736(05)65928-4

Myers, K. A., Davey, M. J., Ching, M., Ellis, C., Grinton, B. E., Roten, A., Lightfoot, P. A., & Scheffer, I. E. (2018). Randomized controlled trial of melatonin for sleep disturbance in Dravet syndrome: The DREAMS study. *Journal of Clinical Sleep Medicine, 14*(10), 1697–1704. https://doi.org/10.5664/jcsm.7376

Nation, J., & Brigger, M. (2017). The efficacy of adenotonsillectomy for obstructive sleep apnea in children with Down syndrome: A systematic review. *Otolaryngology–Head and Neck Surgery, 157*(3), 401–408. https://doi.org/10.1177/0194599817703921

National Institute for Health and Care Excellence. (2022). *Sleepio to treat insomnia and insomnia symptoms* (Medical Technologies Guidance No. 70). www.nice.org.uk/guidance/mtg70

Newman, C. J., O'Regan, M., & Hensey, O. (2006). Sleep disorders in children with cerebral palsy. *Developmental Medicine and Child Neurology, 48*, 564–568. https://doi.org/10.1017/S0012162206001198

Nir, I., Meir, D., Zilber, N., Knobler, H., Hadjez, J., & Lerner, Y. (1995). Brief report: Circadian melatonin, thyroid-stimulating hormone, prolactin, and cortisol levels in serum of young adults with autism. *Journal of Autism and Developmental Disorders, 25*, 641–654. https://doi.org/10.1007/BF02178193

Ogundele, M. O., & Yemula, C. (2022). Management of sleep disorders among children and adolescents with neurodevelopmental disorders: A practical guide for clinicians. *World Journal of Clinical Pediatrics, 11*(3), 239–252. https://doi.org/10.5409/wjcp.v11.i3.239

Okawa, M., Nanami, T., Wada, S., Shimizu, T., Hishikawa, Y., Sasaki, H., Nagamine, H., & Takahashi, K. (1987). Four congenitally blind children with circadian sleep–wake rhythm disorder. *Sleep, 10*, 101–110. https://doi.org/10.1093/sleep/10.2.101

Oldani, A., Zucconi, M., Castronovo, C., & Ferini-Strambi, L. (1998). Nocturnal frontal lobe epilepsy misdiagnosed as sleep apnea syndrome. *Acta Neurologica Scandinavica, 98*, 67–91. https://doi.org/10.1111/j.1600-0404.1998.tb07381.x

Owens, J. A., Spirito, A., & McGuinn, M. (2000). The Children's Sleep Habits Questionnaire (CSHQ): Psychometric properties of a survey instrument for school-aged children. *Sleep, 23*, 1043–1051.

Pahl, J., & Quine, L. (1984). *Families with mentally handicapped children: A study of stress and service response.* University of Kent, Health Services Research Unit.

Palm, L., Blennow, G., & Wetterberg, L. (1997). Long-term melatonin treatment in blind children and young adults with circadian rhythm disorders. *Developmental Medicine and Child Neurology, 39*, 319–325. https://doi.org/10.1111/j.1469-8749.1997.tb07438.x

Paprocka, J., Kijonka, M., Wojcieszek, P., Pecka, M., Emich-Widera, E., & Sokol, M. (2017). Melatonin and Angelman syndrome: Implications and mathematical model of diurnal secretion. *International Journal of Endocrinology, 2017*, Article 5853167. https://doi.org/10.1155/2017/5853167

Petre-Quadens, O., & Jouvet, M. (1967). Sleep in the mentally retarded. *Journal of the Neurological Sciences, 4*, 354–357. https://doi.org/10.1016/0022-510x(67)90113-x

Phillips, N. L., Moore, T., Teng, A., Brookes, N., Palermo, T. M., & Lah, S. (2020). Behavioral interventions for sleep disturbances in children with neurological and neurodevelopmental disorders: A systematic review and meta-analysis of randomized controlled trials. *Sleep, 43*(9), zsaa040. https://doi.org/10.1093/sleep/zsaa040

Piazza, C. C., Hagopian, L. P., Hughes, C. R., & Fisher, W. W. (1998). Using chronotherapy to treat severe sleep problems: A case study. *American Journal on Mental Retardation, 102*, 358–366. https://doi.org/10.1352/0895-8017(1998)102<0358:ucttss>2.0.co;2

Poisson, A., Nicolas, A., Bousquet, I., Raverot, V., Gronfier, C., & Demily, C. (2019). Smith-Magenis syndrome: Molecular basis of a genetic-driven melatonin circadian secretion disorder. *International Journal of Molecular Science, 20*(14), Article 3533. https://doi.org/10.3390/ijms20143533

Priday, L. J., Byrne, C., & Totsika, V. (2017). Behavioural interventions for sleep problems in people with an intellectual disability: A systematic review and meta-analysis of single case and group studies. *Journal of Intellectual Disability Research, 61*(1), 1–15. https://doi.org/10.1111/jir.12265

Prince, J. B., Wilens, T. E., Biederman, J., Spencer, T. J., & Wozniak, J. R. (1996). Clonidine for sleep disturbances associated with attention-deficit hyperactivity disorder: A systematic chart review of 62 cases. *Journal of the American Academy of Child and Adolescent Psychiatry, 35*, 599–605. https://doi.org/10.1097/00004583-199605000-00014

Quine, L. (1991). Sleep problems in children with mental handicap. *Journal of Mental Deficiency Research, 35*, 269–290. https://doi.org/10.1111/j.1365-2788.1991.tb00402.x

Quine, L. (1992). Helping parents to manage children's sleep disturbance. An intervention trial using health professionals. In J. Gibbons (Ed.), *The Children Act 1989 and family support: Principles into practice* (pp. 101–141). HMSO.

Richdale, A., Gavidia-Payne, S., Francis, A., & Cotton, S. (2000). Stress, behaviour, and sleep problems in children with an intellectual disability. *Journal of Intellectual and Developmental Disability, 25*, 147–161. https://doi.org/10.1080/13269780050033562

Richdale, A., & Wiggs, L. (2005). Behavioral approaches to the treatment of sleep problems in children with developmental disorders. What is the state of the art? *International Journal of Behavioral and Consultation Therapy, 1*, 165–189. https://doi.org/10.1037/h0100743

Richdale, A. L., & Baker, E. K. (2014). Sleep in individuals with an intellectual or developmental disability: Recent research reports. *Current Developmental Disorders Reports, 1*, 74–85. https://doi.org/10.1007/s40474-014-0010-x

Richings, C., & Feroz-Nainar, C. (2010). Case series: Melatonin induced agitation in three patients with intellectual disability. *British Journal of Developmental Disabilities, 56*, 77–82. https://doi.org/10.1179/096979510799103032

Riemann, D., Krone, L. B., Wulff, K., & Nissen, C. (2020). Sleep, insomnia, and depression. *Neuropsychopharmacology, 45*(1), 74–89. https://doi.org/10.1038/s41386-019-0411-y

Rigney, G., Ali, N. S., Corkum, P. V., Brown, C. A., Constantin, E., Godbout, R., Hanlon-Dearman, A., Ipsiroglu, O., Reid, G. J., Shea, S., Smith, I. M., Van der Loos, H. F. M., & Weiss, S. K. (2018). A systematic review to explore the feasibility of a behavioural sleep intervention for insomnia in children with neurodevelopmental disorders: A transdiagnostic approach. *Sleep Medicine Reviews, 41*, 244–254. https://doi.org/10.1016/j.smrv.2018.03.008

Robinson, A. M., & Richdale, A. L. (2004). Sleep problems in children with an intellectual disability: Parental perceptions of sleep problems, and views of treatment effectiveness. *Child: Care, Health & Development, 30*, 139–150. https://doi.org/10.1111/j.1365-2214.2004.00395.x

Rossignol, D. A., & Frye, R. E. (2011). Melatonin in autism spectrum disorders: A systematic review and meta-analysis. *Developmental Medicine and Child Neurology, 53*(9), 783–792. https://doi.org/10.1111/j.1469-8749.2011.03980.x

Sajith, S. G., & Clarke, D. (2007). Melatonin and sleep disorders associated with intellectual disability: A clinical review. *Journal of International Disability Research, 51*, 2–13. https://doi.org/10.1111/j.1365-2788.2006.00893.x

Samadi, D. S., Shah, U. K., & Handler, S. D. (2003). Choanal atresia: A twenty-year review of medical comorbidities and surgical outcomes. *Laryngoscope, 113*, 254–258. https://doi.org/10.1097/00005537-200302000-00011

San José Cáceres, A., Landlust, A. M., Carbin, J. M., & Loth, E. (2023). Consensus recommendations on sleeping problems in Phelan-McDermid syndrome. *European Journal of Medical Genetics, 66*(6), 104750. https://doi.org/10.1016/j.ejmg.2023.104750

Sansom, D., Krishnan, V. H. R., Corbett, J., & Kerr, A. (1993). Emotional and behavioral aspects of Rett syndrome. *Developmental Medicine and Child Neurology, 35*, 340–345. https://doi.org/10.1111/j.1469-8749.1993.tb11646.x

Schakel, W., Bode, C., van de Ven, P. M., van der Aa, H. P. A., Hulshof, C. T. J., van Rens, G. H. M. B., & Nispen, R. M. A. (2019). Understanding fatigue in adults with visual impairment: A path analysis study of sociodemographic, psychological and health-related factors. *PLOS ONE, 14*(10), Article e0224340. https://doi.org/10.1371/journal.pone.0224340

Schreck, K. A., Mulick, J. A., & Rojahn, J. (2003). Development of the behavioral evaluation of disorders of sleep. *Journal of Child and Family Studies, 12*, 349–359. https://doi.org/10.1023/A:1023995912428

Schroder, C. M., Malow, B. A., Maras, A., Melmed, R. D., Findling, R. L., Breddy, J., Nir, T., Shahmoon, S., Zisapel, N., & Gringras, P. (2019). Pediatric prolonged-release melatonin for sleep in children with autism spectrum disorder: Impact on child behavior and caregiver's quality of life. *Journal of Autism and Developmental Disorders, 49*(8), 3218–3230. https://doi.org/10.1007/s10803-019-04046-5

Schweitzer, P. K., & Malhotra, R. K. (2021). Clinical pharmacology of drugs that disturb sleep and wakefulness. In M. Kryger, T. Roth, & C. A. Goldstein (Eds.), *Principles and practice of sleep medicine* (7th ed., pp. 519–546). Elsevier.

Shanahan, P. J., Palod, S., Smith, K. J., Fife-Schaw, C., & Mirza, N. (2019). Interventions for sleep difficulties in adults with an intellectual disability: A systematic review. *Journal of Intellectual Disability Research, 63*, 372–385. https://doi.org/10.1111/jir.12587

Shibagaki, M., Kiyonon, S., & Watanabe, K. (1982). Spindle evolution in normal and mentally retarded children: A review. *Sleep, 5*, 47–57. https://doi.org/10.1093/sleep/5.1.47

Short, C. A., & Carpenter, P. K. (1998). The treatment of sleep disorders in people with learning disabilities using light therapy. *International Journal of Psychiatry in Clinical Practice, 2*, 143–145. https://doi.org/10.3109/13651509809115347

Simakajornboon, N., & Beckerman, R. (2001a). Sleep disorders and neuromuscular disease. In G. Stores & L. Wiggs (Eds.), *Sleep disturbance in children and adolescents with disorders of development: Its significance and management* (pp. 111–119). Mac Keith Press.

Simakajornboon, N., & Beckerman, R. (2001b). Sleep disorders and craniofacial syndromes. In G. Stores & L. Wiggs (Eds.), *Sleep disturbance in children and adolescents with disorders of development: Its significance and management* (pp. 54–72). Mac Keith Press.

Simonds, J. F., & Parraga, H. (1982). Prevalence of sleep disorders and sleep behaviors in children and adolescents. *Journal of the American Academy of Child Psychiatry, 21*, 383–388. https://doi.org/10.1016/s0002-7138(09)60942-0

Smith, A. C., Dykens, E., & Greenberg, F. (1998). Sleep disturbance in Smith-Magenis syndrome (del17 p11.1). *American Journal of Medical Genetics, 81*, 186–191.

Sniecinska-Cooper, A. M., Iles, R. K., Butler, S. A., Jones, H., Bayford, R., & Dimitriou, D. (2015). Abnormal secretion of melatonin and cortisol in relation to sleep disturbances in children with Williams syndrome. *Sleep Medicine, 16*(1), Article 94e100. https://doi.org/10.1016/j.sleep.2014.09.003

Souders, M. C., Zavodny, S., Eriksen, W., Sinko, R., Connell, J., Kerns, C., Schaaf, R., & Pinto-Martin, J. (2017). Sleep in children with autism spectrum disorder. *Current Psychiatry Reports, 19*(6), Article 34. https://doi.org/10.1007/s11920-017-0782-x

Spruyt, K. (2022). Sleep problems in individuals with Rett syndrome: A systematic review and meta-analysis, *Sleep Epidemiology, 2*, Article 100027. https://doi.org/10.1016/j.sleepe.2022.100027

Spruyt, K., Braam, W., & Curfs, L. M. G. (2018). Sleep in Angelman syndrome: A review of evidence. *Sleep Medicine Reviews, 37*, 69–84. https://doi.org/10.1016/j.smrv.2017.01.002

Spruyt, K., & Curfs, L. M. G. (2015). Non-pharmacological management of problematic sleeping in children with developmental disabilities. *Developmental Medicine and Child Neurology, 57*, 120–136. https://doi.org/10.1111/dmcn.12623

Stenfert-Kroese, B., & Thomas, G. (2006). Treating chronic nightmares of sexual assault survivors with an intellectual disability—Two descriptive case studies. *Journal of Applied Research in Intellectual Disabilities, 19*, 75–80. https://doi.org/10.1111/j.1468-3148.2005.00275.x

Stickgold, R., Hobson, J. A., Fosse, R., & Fosse, M. (2001). Sleep, learning and dreams: Off-line memory processing. *Science, 294*, 1052–1057. https://doi.org/10.1126/science.1063530

St Louis, E. K. (2011). Sleep and epilepsy: Strange bedfellows no more. *Minerva Pneumologica, 50*(3), 159–176.

Stores, G. (2001a). Disordered sleep in other neurological conditions. In G. Stores & L. Wiggs (Eds.), *Sleep disturbance in children and adolescents with disorders of development: Its significance and management* (pp. 126–133). Mac Keith Press.

Stores, G. (2001b). Visual impairment and associated sleep abnormalities. In G. Stores & L. Wiggs (Eds.), *Sleep disturbance in children and adolescents with disorders of development: Its significance and management* (pp. 120–125). Mac Keith Press.

Stores, R. J. (2018). Sleep problems in adults with Down syndrome and their family carers. *Journal of Applied Research in Intellectual Disabilities, 32*(4), 831–840. https://doi.org/10.1111/jar.12572

Stuttard, L., Beresford, B., Clarke, S., Beecham, J., & Curtis, J. (2015). A preliminary investigation into the effectiveness of a group-delivered sleep management intervention for parents of children with intellectual disabilities. *Journal of Intellectual Disabilities, 19*(4), 342–355. https://doi.org/10.1177/1744629515576610

Surtees, A. D. R., Oliver, C., Jones, C. A., Evans, D. L., & Richards, C. (2018). Sleep duration and sleep quality in people with and without intellectual disability: A meta-analysis. *Sleep Medicine Reviews, 40*, 135–150. https://doi.org/10.1016/j.smrv.2017.11.003

Sutton, J., Huws, J. C., & Burton, C. (2021). A sleep intervention for children with developmental disabilities. *Nursing Times, 117*(1), 32–36.

Terman, M., & Terman, J. S. (1999). Bright light therapy: Side effects and benefits across the symptom spectrum. *Journal of Clinical Psychiatry, 60*, 799–808.

Thackeray, E., & Richdale, A. (2002). The behavioural treatment of sleep difficulties in children with an intellectual disability. *Behavioral Interventions, 17*, 211–231. https://doi.org/10.1002/bin.123

Thirumalai, S. S., Shubin, R. A., & Robinson, R. (2002). Rapid eye movement sleep behavior disorder in children with autism. *Journal of Child Neurology, 17*, 173–178. https://doi.org/10.1177/088307380201700304

Tieleman, A. A., Knoop, H., van de Logt, A.-E., Bleijenberg, G., van Engelen, B. G. M., & Overeem, S. (2010). Poor sleep quality and fatigue but no excessive daytime sleepiness in myotonic dystrophy type 2. *Journal of Neurology, Neurosurgery and Psychiatry, 81*, 963–967. https://doi.org/10.1136/jnnp.2009.192591

Tietze, A.-L., Blankenburg, M., Hechler, T., Michel, E., Koh, M., Schlüter, B., & Zernikow, B. (2012). Sleep disturbances in children with multiple disabilities. *Sleep Medicine Reviews, 16*(2), 117–127. https://doi.org/10.1016/j.smrv.2011.03.006

Tietze, A.-L., Zernikow, B., Otto, M., Hirschfeld, G., Michel, E., Koh, M., & Blankenburg, M. (2014). The development and psychometric assessment of a questionnaire to assess sleep and daily troubles in parents of children and young adults with severe psychomotor impairment. *Sleep Medicine, 15*(2), 219–227. https://doi.org/10.1016/j.sleep.2013.09.019

van den Broek, N., Broer, L., Vandenbussche, N., Tan, I., Overeeem, S., & Pillen, S. (2021). Obstructive sleep apnea in people with intellectual disabilities: Adherence to and effect of CPAP. *Sleep and Breathing, 25*, 1257–1265. https://doi.org/10.1007/s11325-020-02221-y

van den Broek, N., Festen, D., Tan, F., Overeem, S., & Pillen, S. (2022). What is in a name? Definitions of insomnia in people with intellectual disabilities. *Journal of Applied Research in Intellectual Disabilities, 35*(2), 506–518. https://doi.org/10.1111/jar.12960

van der Heijden, K. B., Smits, M. G., & Gunning, W. B. (2005). Sleep-related disorders in ADHD: A review. *Clinical Pediatrics, 44*, 201–210. https://doi.org/10.1177/000992280504400303

van de Wouw, E., Evenhuis, H. M., & Echteld, M. A. (2012). Prevalence, associated factors and treatment of sleep problems in adults with intellectual disability: A systematic review. *Research in Developmental Disabilities, 33*, 1310–32. https://doi.org/10.1016/j.ridd.2012.03.003

van de Wouw, E., Evenhuis, H. M., & Echteld, M. A. (2013). Objective assessment of sleep and sleep problems in older adults with intellectual disabilities. *Research in Developmental Disabilities, 34*(8), 2291–2303. https://doi.org/10.1016/j.ridd.2013.04.012

van Lang, N. D. J., Ferdinand, R. F., & Verhulst, F. C. (2007). Predictors of future depression in early and late adolescence. *Journal of Affective Disorders, 97*, 137–144. https://doi.org/10.1016/j.jad.2006.06.007

Velluti, R. A., Pedemonte, M., Suárez, H., Bentancor, C., & Rodríguez-Servetti, Z. (2010). Auditory input modulates sleep: An intra-cochlear-implanted human model. *Journal of Sleep Research, 19*(4), 585–590. https://doi.org/10.1111/j.1365-2869.2010.00829.x

Ward, F., Nanjappa, M., Hinder, S. A. J., & Roy, M. (2015). Use of melatonin for sleep disturbance in a large intellectual disability psychiatry service. *International Journal of Developmental Disabilities, 61*, 182–187. https://doi.org/10.1179/2047387714Y.0000000051

Wasdell, M. B., Jan, J. E., Bomben, M. M., Freeman, R. D., Rietveld, W. J., Tai, J., Hamilton, D., & Weiss, M. D. (2008). A randomized, placebo-controlled trial of controlled release melatonin treatment of delayed sleep phase syndrome and impaired sleep maintenance in children with neurodevelopmental disabilities. *Journal of Pineal Research, 44*, 57–64. https://doi.org/10.1111/j.1600-079X.2007.00528.x

Wehr, T. A., Aeschbach, D., & Duncan, W. C., Jr. (2001). Evidence for a biological dawn and dusk in the human circadian timing system. *Journal of Physiology, 535*(3), 937–951. https://doi.org/10.1111/j.1469-7793.2001.t01-1-00937.x

Weiher, R. G., & Harman, R. E. (1975). The use of omission training to reduce self-injurious behavior in a retarded child. *Behavior Therapy, 6*, 261–268. https://doi.org/10.1016/S0005-7894(75)80151-1

Weiskop, S., Matthews, J., & Richdale, A. (2001). Treatment of sleep problems in a 5-year-old boy with autism using behavioural principles. *Autism, 5*, 209–221. https://doi.org/10.1177/1362361301005002009

Weiskop, S., Richdale, A., & Matthews, J. (2005). Behavioural treatment to reduce sleep problems in children with autism or fragile X. *Developmental Medicine & Child Neurology, 47*, 94–104. https://doi.org/10.1017/s0012162205000186

Wiggs, L. (2007). Are children getting enough sleep? Implications for parents. *Sociological Research Online, 12*, 104–119. https://doi.org/10.5153/sro.1557

Wiggs, L. (2009). Behavioural aspects of children's sleep. *Archives of Disease in Childhood, 94*, 59–62. https://doi.org/10.1136/adc.2007.125278

Wiggs, L. (2012). Sleep disturbances and learning disability (mental retardation). In C. M. Morin & C. A. Espie (Eds.), *The Oxford handbook of sleep and sleep disorders* (pp. 788–819). Oxford University Press. https://doi.org/10.1093/oxfordhb/9780195376203.013.0038

Wiggs, L., Cook, G., Hiscock, H., Pal, D. K., & Gringras, P. (2021). Development and evaluation of the CASTLE trial online sleep intervention for parents of children with epilepsy. *Frontiers in Psychology, 12*, Article 679804. https://doi.org/10.3389/fpsyg.2021.679804

Wiggs, L., & France, K. (2000). Behavioural treatments for sleep problems in children and adolescents with physical illness, psychological problems or intellectual disabilities: A review. *Sleep Medicine Reviews, 4*, 299–314. https://doi.org/10.1053/smrv.1999.0094

Wiggs, L., & Stores, G. (1996a). Severe sleep disturbance and daytime challenging behaviour in children with severe learning disabilities. *Journal of Intellectual Disability Research, 40*, 518–528. https://doi.org/10.1046/j.1365-2788.1996.799799.x

Wiggs, L., & Stores, G. (1996b). Sleep problems in children with severe intellectual disabilities: What help is being provided? *Journal of Applied Research in Intellectual Disabilities, 9*, 159–164. https://doi.org/10.1111/j.1468-3148.1996.tb00105.x

Wiggs, L., & Stores, G. (2001). Behavioural treatment for sleep problems in children with severe intellectual disabilities and daytime challenging behaviour: Effect on mothers and fathers. *British Journal of Health Psychology, 6*, 257–269. https://doi.org/10.1348/135910701169197

Wiggs, L., & Stores, G. (2004). Sleep patterns and sleep disorders in children with autistic spectrum disorders. *Developmental Medicine and Child Neurology, 46*, 372–380. https://doi.org/10.1017/s0012162204000611

Williams, C. A., Beaudet, A. L., Clayton-Smith, J., Knoll, J. H., Kyllerman, M., Laan, L. A., Magenis, R. E., Moncla, A., Schinzel, A. A., Summers, J. A., & Wagstaff, J. (2006). Angelman syndrome 2005: Updated consensus for diagnostic criteria. *American Journal of Medical Genetics, 140*(5), 413–418. https://doi.org/10.1002/ajmg.a.31074

Williams Buckley, A., Hirtz, D., Oskoui, M., Armstrong, M. J., Batra, A., Bridgemohan, C., Coury, D., Dawson, G., Donley, D., Findling, R. L., Gaughan, T., Gloss, D., Gronseth, G., Kessler, R., Merillat, S., Michelson, D., Owens, J., Pringsheim, T., Sikich, L., . . . Ashwal, S. (2020). Practice guideline: Treatment for insomnia and disrupted sleep behavior in children and adolescents with autism spectrum disorder: Report of the guideline development, dissemination, and implementation subcommittee of the American Academy of Neurology. *Neurology, 94*, 392–404. https://doi.org/10.1212/WNL.0000000000009033

Willner, P. (2004). Brief cognitive therapy of nightmares and post-traumatic ruminations in a man with a learning disability. *British Journal of Clinical Psychology, 43*, 459–464. https://doi.org/10.1348/0144665042388919

Wilson, S., Anderson, K., Baldwin, D., Dijk, D. J., Espie, A., Espie, C., Gringras, P., Krystal, A., Nutt, D., Selsick, H., & Sharpley, A. (2019). British Association for Psychopharmacology consensus statement on evidence-based treatment of insomnia, parasomnias and circadian rhythm disorders: An update. *Journal of Psychopharmacology, 33*(8), 923–947. https://doi.org/10.1177/0269881119855343

Wittmann, L., Schredl, M., & Kramer, M. (2006). Dreaming in posttraumatic stress disorder: A critical review of phenomenology, psychophysiology and treatment. *Psychotherapy and Psychosomatics, 76*(1), 25–39. https://doi.org/10.1159/000096362

Woodford, E. C., McLay, L., France, K. G., Blampied, N. M., Gibbs, R., Swan, C. E., & Eggleston, M. (2021). Endogenous melatonin and sleep in individuals with rare genetic neurodevelopmental disorders (RGND): A systematic review. *Sleep Medicine Reviews, 57*, Article 101433. https://doi.org/10.1016/j.smrv.2021.101433

Yuge, K., Nagamitsu, S., Ishikawa, Y., Hamada, I., Takahashi, H., Sugioka, H., Yotsuya, O., Mishima, K., Hayashi, M., & Yamashita, Y. (2020). Long-term melatonin treatment for the sleep problems and aberrant behaviors of children with neurodevelopmental disorders. *BMC Psychiatry, 20*, Article 445. https://doi.org/10.1186/s12888-020-02847-y

Zaffanello, M., Antoniazzi, F., Tenero, L., Nosetti, L., Piazza, M., & Piacentini, G. (2018). Sleep-disordered breathing in paediatric setting: Existing and upcoming of the genetic disorders. *Annals of Translational Medicine, 6*(17), Article 343. https://doi.org/10.21037/atm.2018.07.13

Zaremba, E. K., Barkey, M. E., Mesa, C., Sannita, K., & Rosen, C. L. (2005). Making polysomnography more "child friendly": A family-centered care approach. *Journal of Clinical Sleep Medicine, 15*, 189–198.

CHAPTER

46 Sexsomnia and Sexual Assault: The Role of the Sleep Forensics Investigator in Court

Michel A. Cramer Bornemann *and* Carlos H. Schenck

Abstract

Parasomnias are undesirable physical events or experiences that occur during entry into sleep, within rapid-eye-movement (REM) or non-REM (NREM) sleep, or during arousals from sleep. Parasomnias encompass abnormal sleep-related movements, behaviors, emotions, perceptions, dreaming, and autonomic nervous system functioning. Also, instinctual behaviors can be involuntarily and pathologically released with the parasomnias, including sexual behaviors (sexsomnia), aggression, locomotion, and eating. The clinical consequences of a parasomnia can affect the patient, the bed partner, and any nearby individual. Sexsomnia is classified as a variant of confusional arousals (and sleepwalking), an NREM parasomnia, with amnesia for the sexual behaviors virtually always reported. The cumulative world published literature on sexsomnia consists of 220 cases, 84% males and predominant age in the 30s and 40s. Most cases were identified as NREM parasomnias, although obstructive sleep apnea was the identified trigger in 10.4% of cases. Various other triggers were identified. Forensic consequences were reported in 15 of the reported clinical cases. Sleep medicine physicians can expect inquiries from attorneys to solicit their involvement in criminal trials as forensic implications of parasomnias become increasingly more apparent. As courts generally have an implicit bias that is not favorable to the "sleepwalking defense," sleep medicine physicians who take on the mantle of an expert medical witness should define their role and understand that supporting justice in the courtroom can only be optimally done through a strong collaborative effort with the attorney throughout the legal process.

Key Words: parasomnia, sexsomnia, sexual behavior, sleep disorder, sleep violence, sexual assault, forensic medicine, law

Introduction

Parasomnias are defined as unpleasant or undesirable behavioral or experiential phenomena that occur predominately or exclusively during the sleep period. Though initially thought to be attributed to an underlying psychiatric condition, refined neuroimaging studies coupled with careful analysis of clinical and polysomnographic (PSG) studies have revealed that parasomnias are now best understood as resulting from the dynamic interplay of complex neurologic processes. Parasomnias represent a large number of completely different conditions which are more prevalent than generally appreciated. Despite their broad range of possible manifestations, most parasomnias are readily diagnosable and treatable. Once asleep, an individual transitions approximately every 90 minutes between non-rapid-eye-movement (NREM) sleep and rapid-eye-movement (REM) sleep four to six times in a typical 8-hour night. Parasomnias are generally classified according to the sleep state from which they arise, NREM sleep or REM sleep, and can be further categorized as either "primary" (instability within the sleep process) or "secondary" (disorders of other organ systems that destabilize the sleep process). There are 10 core categories of parasomnias in the *International Classification of Sleep Disorders*, third edition, Text Revision (ICSD-3TR): four from NREM sleep, involving the disorders of arousal (DOA; confusional arousals, sleepwalking [SW], sleep terrors [STs], and sleep-related eating disorder); three from REM sleep (REM sleep behavior disorder [RBD], recurrent isolated sleep paralysis, nightmare disorder); exploding head syndrome; sleep-related hallucinations; and sleep-related urologic dysfunction (formerly named *sleep enuresis*). Other categories include parasomnia due to a medical disorder; parasomnia due to a medication or substance; and parasomnia, unspecified. The final category of isolated symptoms and normal variants includes sleep talking (American Academy of Sleep Medicine, 2023). The clinical manifestations of primary parasomnias occur during transitions between NREM and REM sleep when brain processes are reorganizing toward a fully declared state. Interestingly, human brain electrical connectivity is astronomically vast, comprised of an estimated average of 86 billion neurons that is further supported by 85 billion non-neuronal cells (Azevedo et al., 2009). With such frequent state transitions in sleep coupled with the vast number of neural networks, neurotransmitters, and other state-determining substances that must be recruited synchronously for full state declaration, errors in state declaration likely occur more frequently than we are aware (Mahowald & Schenck, 2001).

In understanding parasomnias, it is first important to recognize that wakefulness and sleep are not strictly all-or-none propositions. This concept is likely to be problematic in the courtroom where the medical and legal paradigms in assessing an individual's mental state are often in conflict. Relatively recent advances in neuroscience fully support the concept that wakefulness and sleep are not dichotomous states and that elements often attributed to each are not invariably mutually exclusive. This concept along with an appreciation that the various state-determining variables of wakefulness, NREM sleep, and REM sleep may occur simultaneously or oscillate rapidly are the foundations to explain broad manifestations of parasomnias. In this regard, it is the admixture of wakefulness and NREM sleep which explains confusional arousals, automatic behaviors, and the inadvertent intrusion of episodes of microsleep (Mahowald & Schenck, 2001). Additionally, it is the admixture of wakefulness and REM sleep which explains cataplexy, sleep paralysis, hypnagogic hallucinations, and dream-enactment behaviors (Mahowald & Schenck, 1994).

Despite the public's perception, sleep is not necessarily a quiescent period. With parasomnias, these unstable admixed states may abruptly trigger outwardly violent behaviors which potentially pose an injurious threat to self and/or others. As a result and with increasing regularity, defense attorneys have been approaching sleep medicine physicians, especially those with focused expertise in parasomnias, to investigate and analyze a broad spectrum of criminal allegations. If the expert determines that the acts were committed in an altered state without conscious awareness, this expert medical opinion could support the defense attorney in seeking, if not a complete acquittal, at least a less severe charge or less severe sentence. Conversely, a sleep medicine physician may be approached by the prosecution to combat the defense counsel's largely improbable, if not entirely bogus, "sleepwalking defense."

Sleep medicine physicians considering stepping into the legal arena to investigate outwardly violent criminal allegations such as homicide, manslaughter, assault/battery, and rape need to be directly and consistently clinically active in the diagnosis and management of parasomnias. Their knowledge of parasomnias should remain current and consistent with accepted recognized community standards, such as those put forth by the American Academy of Sleep Medicine (AASM), and with reports published in recognized international peer-reviewed scientific publications. Though criminal allegations involving possible parasomnias indeed cover a broad spectrum, many of which have forensics implications, our extensive direct experience in sleep forensics investigations has consistently found an inordinately high case referral load related to inquiries into sexual assault (Cramer Bornemann et al., 2019). Consequently, this chapter will primarily focus on sleep-related abnormal sexual behavior, popularly and lasciviously referred to as *sexsomnia*, by providing an update on its characteristic features, prevalence, and conditions that increase its risk. A significant portion of this chapter will then review the legal process and discuss how to present clinical science in the courtroom.

The culmination of a comprehensive sleep forensics investigative process is expected to result in a formal medical opinion that ultimately may be presented in court or assist in pre-trial conflict resolution. However, physicians are often reluctant to consider involvement in the directly adversarial nature of courtroom dynamics in which science can be misapplied, misrepresented, or frustratingly mired in irrelevant disingenuous technicalities attempting to attain an advantage in securing a desired outcome. Physicians stepping into the legal arena should actually embrace this combative nature in the courtroom and acknowledge that convictions related to high-level felonies have very severe, often arguably unreasonable, punitive consequences. The stakes are indeed high. It is not the goal of the expert medical witness to win the case for their attorney's client. Instead, an essential role of the expert medical witness is to educate the court in scientifically valid and current information with which the jury may render a decision based upon sound scientific evidence. In most situations, simply providing a diagnosis, submitting a final case report, and testifying on the stand are not sufficient to facilitate a fair and informed legal resolution. The expert medical witness also has to be adept at clearly and succinctly distilling complex scientific concepts for those in the legal system as well as the laypersons chosen to serve on a jury.

Finally, in addition to providing a current salient update on those parasomnias associated with sleep-related violence (SRV), this chapter will concisely review the criminal justice process and the manner in which a sleep forensics expert medical witness may be involved. This chapter will also set the foundation for effective communication which can only be optimally done through a strong collaborative effort with the attorney. This should occur throughout the legal process from the initial investigative phase to the adjudication phase including extensive pre-trial as well as cross-examination preparations and up to post-trial motions, which might involve the sentencing phase, the development of safety disposition planning, or the filing of an appeal. With such involvement the expert medical witness needs to be prepared for the various actions which may be encountered during the legal process and to devise strategies to deal with those anticipated emotional, stressful, and unfamiliar situations.

Medico-Legal Sexsomnia Cases

The following is a summary of two actual US criminal cases accepted by our sleep forensics team. To maintain confidentiality, acronyms for individuals involved in these cases do not reflect actual names. In both cases, the sleep forensics expert was retained by the defense team.

LEGAL CASE 1

FT is a healthy 40-year-old Caucasian American male who on an early Sunday morning in the summer of 2021 was alleged to have willfully, unlawfully, and feloniously, for the purpose of gratifying his lust or indulging his depraved licentious sexual desires, handled, touched, or rubbed his hands or any part of his body on his biological daughter, DT, a child under 12 years. The incident is said to have occurred in the defendant's rural single-bedroom home. FT had been divorced from the victim's mother for over 2 years. According to FT, the couple had held joint custody of their two children, DT and her younger brother, ST. The children would alternate residences with their parents every other week, though during the summer months they would alternate 2 consecutive weeks with their father and 1 week with their mother.

Preceding the night of the criminal allegation, FT noted that he and his children, DT and ST, had a routine, easy, and uneventful Saturday. Citing significant fatigue due to his demanding work schedule, FT and his children all retired together to his bedroom at a reasonable time that evening. It was customary for his children to co-sleep with their father in his king-sized bed, with him always sleeping on the outside of his bed. As both children wanted to sleep close beside their father, FT would create and post a schedule to determine which would sleep in the middle of his bed right beside him. On this evening, his young daughter was elated to have been scheduled to sleep in the middle. FT characterized his father/daughter relationship as appropriately supportive, and she often openly exhibited affection toward him. On that early Sunday morning at approximately 4:30

a.m., FT abruptly woke up with an emotionally oppressive ominous feeling. He felt as though he was in the midst of a nonsexual dream but could not recall any specific imagery. His hands were not upon his daughter when he awoke, but he sensed that he had inadvertently touched the surface of his daughter's pubic and vaginal areas. Though his recollection of the event was sparse, he believed that the duration of the incident must have been very brief, likely less than 30 seconds. Upset, profusely tearful, and very confused as to what might have just occurred, FT immediately removed himself from his bedroom and made his way to the living room sofa to compose himself, where he eventually fell back to sleep. At breakfast, as FT was not certain about what had transpired between him and his daughter, he decided not to approach her concerning this uncomfortable topic. Later that morning, FT arranged for his teenage niece to babysit for his children as he had to leave to address pressing work-related responsibilities. DT reluctantly told her cousin, FT's niece, that something awkward had taken place with her father that had woken her up. The niece soon relayed what she had been told by her cousin to her mother, FT's sister, who brought it to his attention that evening. FT has never doubted his daughter's integrity, has never denied inappropriately touching his daughter, and has accepted her narrative of the incident.

The next Monday morning, FT contacted the local Child Protective Services (CPS) agency and requested that his daughter be urgently evaluated so that she could receive appropriate mental health support and counseling. In the course of the CPS evaluation, DT revealed that she woke up with her father rubbing her abdomen and vagina. She remembers that her panties had been pulled down a bit, that his hand was underneath her panties, and that she felt trapped with his legs on top of hers. DT believed that her father was asleep and must have had a "bad dream." Furthermore, DT confirmed that her father immediately became tearful after he "woke up" and removed himself from her by quickly going to the living room. Upon completion of their evaluation, the CPS agency contacted the police department to file a mandatory report of suspected sexual abuse and maltreatment. The police department conducted an investigation into this matter and found probable cause that FT had committed a crime; he then was arrested and charged with a single felony count of child molestation. If convicted, FT would face harsh penalties including fines, up to 15 years of imprisonment, and mandatory lifetime registration as a sex offender.

Consequently, FT posted bail, was released from custody, and quickly retained the services of a well-known and respected private criminal defense attorney. In addition, FT conducted his own exhaustive internet research and came across references to sexsomnia, which he brought to the attention of his sleep medicine physician who had been treating him for his recently diagnosed severe obstructive sleep apnea (OSA). The physician informed FT and his attorney that he was not qualified to become involved in criminal proceedings and strongly encouraged them to solicit the services of a seasoned sleep forensics expert, specifically recommending our medico-legal consulting group (Sleep Forensics Associates [SFA]). After a brief discussion concerning the merits of this case, SFA accepted FT's attorney's offer to become involved and was retained.

Upon the completion of an extensive sleep forensics investigation, the following facts were also found during discovery in this case:

1. FT had previously engaged in similar episodes of sleep-related events. Though FT did not have a childhood history of parasomnias, his fiancée, EV, estimated there were 5–10 episodes of sleep-related sexual behaviors since the time that they first began dating in the fall of 2017. Such behaviors were often expressed as intimate affectionate embraces (i.e., "spooning"), which might progress to touch involving her breasts and/or vaginal area. It is also important to note that EV also observed an association between such behaviors and the severity of FT's snoring.
2. DT noted that the allegation was an isolated incident that had never occurred to her before, though she often co-sleeps with her father.
3. FT was likely suffering from the effects of significant insufficient sleep. At the time of the allegation, FT was working long, unpredictable hours as an on-call industrial electrician. He estimated that he was working 70+ hours per week. He has estimated an average daily total sleep time of approximately 5 hours.
4. FT was suffering from untreated severe OSA. Just weeks prior to the allegations, FT underwent a clinical evaluation at an accredited sleep medicine facility. He underwent a home sleep test, which confirmed severe OSA with a reported estimated apnea/hypopnea index (AHI) of 58 events/hour and a hemoglobin oxygen desaturation nadir to 70%. Though treatment options had been discussed, including positive airway pressure, FT had yet to initiate any form of therapy at the time of the allegation.
5. FT's past medical history was also remarkable for a lumbar spine injury that was sustained in a work-related mishap. He was prescribed narcotics to control pain, and he eventually developed a chemical dependency. FT sought treatment for his addiction with his primary care physician and was prescribed Suboxone.
6. FT has denied any exposure to alcohol or illicit drugs during times when his children are under his care, though he admits that he was on a stable maintenance dose of Suboxone on the night of the allegation.
7. FT did not have a past criminal record.

LEGAL CASE 2

KD is a healthy 42-year-old African American male who on a Thursday mid-afternoon in the summer of 2020 was alleged, as in the previous case, to have willfully, unlawfully, and feloniously, for the purpose of gratifying his lust or indulging his depraved licentious sexual desires, handled, touched, or rubbed his hands or any part of his body on his biological daughter, HD, a child under 12 years. At the time, KD was the husband of LD and, in addition to the victim, was the biological father of their three sons, DD1, DD2, and DD3, with ages ranging from 13 to 18 years. The event is said to have occurred in their modest inner-city two-level home. Specifically, the second floor had three small separate bedrooms, which had been divided among their children. The first floor had a living room, kitchen/dining area, and the garage. As KD and his wife do not have a regular bedroom in which to sleep, the living room also served as their makeshift bedroom.

Though KD was often unemployed, in the summer of 2017, he was able with difficulty to pursue several part-time jobs including installing automobile tires, servicing returning automobiles at a large rental agency, and loading cargo for a long-haul freight company. On the day of the allegation, he drove his eldest son to his morning classes at a nearby community college despite being exhausted after finishing his overnight shift at the freight company. Upon his return home, he went upstairs to see if any of his other children were around and inquired whether any might be interested in watching a movie with him in the living room. Only KD's daughter, HD, was interested; and soon they both lay down close beside each other on the pullout living room sofa and began to watch the popular movie she had requested.

Shortly thereafter, HD recalled that her father's hand slid underneath her tank top to fondle her breasts underneath her bra, and on several occasions she urged her father to stop. She reported that the incident was rather brief, lasting not more than 2 minutes. KD's behavior was halted when HD finally decided to suddenly step away, making up an excuse that she needed to visit the upstairs bathroom. According to HD, her father also got up, followed her, grabbed her by the arm before she got to the stairs, and apologized for his behavior. KD noted that he was confused and not certain as to what had just occurred. He stated that he only offered an apology as he sensed that he had upset his daughter in some manner. KD's then-wife, LD, recalled that she received a text message from her daughter soon after the incident. She immediately left work to angrily confront her husband about the allegations. According to LD, her husband at first denied the allegations but, in her words, stated, "he said he didn't know why . . . it just happened." KD has consistently stated that he had no recollection of the incident, noting that he fell asleep on the sofa beside his daughter shortly after the movie started. KD continued to declare that if he did touch his daughter, it would have been an unintended mistake while still asleep. LD immediately ordered her husband leave their home and called the police department to report the incident. KD was charged with a single felony count of criminal sexual conduct in the fourth degree, which, if he were found guilty, could result in up to 10 years of imprisonment and/or $20,000 in fines as well as mandatory lifetime registration as a sex offender. An arrest warrant for KD was issued by the judge. He was found 2 days later camping out of his automobile in the parking lot of the long-haul freight company.

Unlike the previous case, KD was not able to secure funds to post his bail and remained in custody to await his trial. He also could not afford a private criminal defense attorney and was assigned to a county public defender. In attempting to formulate potential defenses for his client, the public defender likewise ordered their legal assistant to conduct a literature search hoping to link sleep with unconscious sexual behavior. The legal assistant found several manuscripts on sexsomnia, a condition for which the public defender's office was completely unaware, prompting their office to locate a sleep forensics expert.

Upon the completion of an extensive sleep forensics investigation, the following facts were also found during discovery in this case:

1. KD had previously experienced similar episodes of sleep-related events, which he characterized as rather benign sleepwalking. Unfortunately, this information could not be corroborated as his parents were deceased and he no longer had contact with his siblings.
2. KD and his daughter both noted that the allegation was an isolated incident that had never occurred with her or others before. Past hardships often compelled family members to share and sleep in the same space.
3. KD was likely suffering from the effects of significant insufficient sleep while shuttling between part-time employments and working long, unpredictable hours during both day and night. Just prior to the allegations, KD was loading cargo from midnight until 8:00 a.m.
4. KD was likely suffering from untreated severe OSA. A validated OSA screening tool, the STOP BANG questionnaire, revealed KD to have a high pretest probability for severe OSA. Unfortunately, due to constraints of the legal system and limitations related to the COVID pandemic, diagnostic testing could not be performed.
5. KD had an extensive past medical and mental health history documented as post-traumatic stress disorder, hospital admissions for major depressive disorder with suicidal ideation, escitalopram overdose, and homelessness.
6. KD has denied any exposure to alcohol or illicit drugs in the hours or days preceding the allegation.
7. KD's past criminal record included multiple arrests related to possession of marijuana with intent to distribute and possession of drug paraphernalia.

Both cases underwent Daubert hearings to qualify the sleep medicine physician to appear in court as a medical expert witness in parasomnias as well as to offer sexsomnia as evidence. Both cases eventually proceeded to a jury trial to render a final decision.

Parasomnia: Essential Pathophysiologic Mechanisms

The pathophysiologic mechanisms underlying parasomnias have been extensively discussed elsewhere but are firmly grounded on central pattern generators (CPGs) and fixed action patterns (FAPs) and rounded out by the unifying concept of state dissociation. CPGs are distinct, well-circumscribed neuronal aggregates found throughout the central nervous system (CNS). The CPGs involved with parasomnias are largely located in the brainstem in close proximity to and downstream from the sleep/wake generating centers in the hypothalamus. Factors which destabilize the sleep process can trigger a CPG, which then elicits a FAP, subserving programmed primitive behaviors. This activated CPG/FAP axis is then inappropriately overtly expressed as a parasomnia because the inhibitory control usually exerted by the prefrontal cortex has remained offline during sleep. Figure 46.1 provides a useful clinical-scientific framework for understanding parasomnia behavioral release and its triggers (Castelnovo et al., 2022, 2024; Mahowald et al., 2011). CPGs in the brainstem are the substrate for the release of parasomnia behaviors that can be

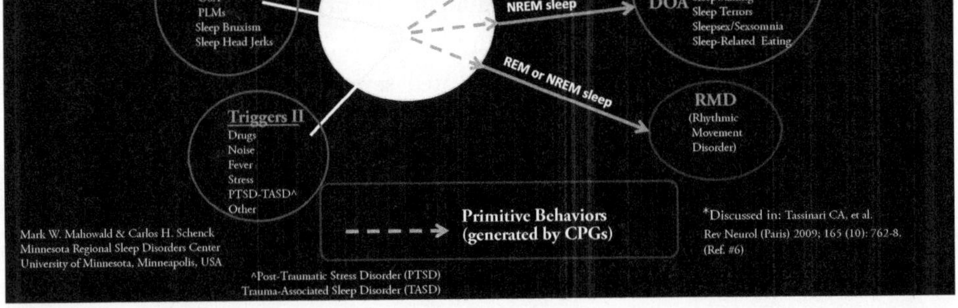

Figure 46.1 Parasomnia mechanisms

Note. Framework for understanding parasomnia behavioral release and its triggers. Reprinted (with slight modification), with permission from Schenck CH. RBD, sexsomnia, sleepwalking, and sleep paralysis comorbidities: relevance to pulmonary, dental, and behavioral sleep medicine. *Sleep Sci. 2021;14*(2):87–91. CPG = central pattern generator; DOA = disorders of arousal; NREM = non–rapid eye movement; OSA = obstructive sleep apnea; PLM = periodic limb movement; PLMD = periodic limb movement disorder; RBD = REM sleep behavior disorder; PTSD = post-traumatic stress disorder; REM = rapid eye movement; TASD = trauma-associated sleep disorder.

activated by a broad range of triggers, together with predisposing conditions. In regard to sexual behaviors that typically emerge during partial arousals from (deep) NREM sleep, triggers shown in Figure 46.1 that have been reported to promote release of sexual behaviors during sleep, as discussed below, include OSA, sleep bruxism, periodic limb movements (PLMs), sleep-related head jerks, drugs, and various types of stress (psychological, sleep deprivation, circadian disruption with shift work). Predisposing conditions include a history of NREM parasomnias, parasomnia overlap disorder, narcolepsy, and circadian rhythm disorders.

Sexsomnia: Clinical Features and Update

Sexsomnia is a chronic disorder that can cause relationship and marital strain (including accusations of sexual assault/rape within marriage) and can result in legal charges, which will be discussed in more detail in a subsequent section. Problems with sexsomnia include disrupting the sleep of the bed partner; physical injury to the bed partner or to oneself from aggressive sexual behaviors; and psychological disturbance of the bed partner from offensive sleep sex talking, the inappropriate time of sex, the inappropriate type of sex, and nonconsensual sexual behaviors (since the bed partner is asleep; Muza et al., 2016). Also, the bed partner often experiences shock, alarm, annoyance, bewilderment, and anger. Psychological disturbance to the sexsomniac can involve confusion, shame, guilt, and despair experienced within the context of amnesia for the event and being told about one's objectionable sleep behaviors by the bed partner after awakening in the morning (Schenck et al., 2007).

The full range of sexuality is expressed with sexsomnia, including spontaneous orgasms, masturbation, sexual fondling, sexual intercourse/attempted intercourse, and sexual vocalizations/verbalizations (*sleep sex talking*). The first classification of sleep-related abnormal sexual behaviors and experiences was published in 2007 (Schenck et al., 2007), with a subsequent update of the world literature published in 2015 (Schenck, 2015), followed by more recently published case series and case reports on sexsomnia (Muza et al., 2016). The total number of sexsomnia cases reported to date in the peer-reviewed world medical literature is 220 cases (Bušková et al., 2022; Contreras et al., 2019; Dubessy et al., 2017; Fernandez & Soca, 2021; Irfan & Schenck, 2018; Khawaja et al., 2017; Kim et al., 2021; Kumar et al., 2020; Martynowicz et al., 2018; Meira et al., 2016; Mioč et al., 2018; Muza et al., 2016; Pirzada et al., 2019; Riha et al., 2023; Rossi et al., 2023; Schenck, 2015; Schenck et al., 2007; Soca et al., 2016; Toscanini et al., 2021; Yeh & Schenck, 2016), 84.2% (n = 171) male and 15.8% (n = 32) female, with predominant age being in the 30s and 40s (n = 203; four cases excluded with no reported age or gender, involving pramipexole-induced sexsomnia [Schenck et al., 2007], and 13 other cases excluded due to lack of gender clarification among patients partially overlapping in two studies by the same group [Dubessy et al., 2017; Rossi et al., 2023]). OSA as the underlying diagnosis triggering the sexsomnia was identified in 14 (10.4%) of 135 cases (n = 85 cases excluded from two series that did not address the issue of OSA triggers [Riha et al., 2023; Rossi et al., 2023]), although this may be an underestimate. The cases were reported from 15 countries (United States, Canada, Brazil, France, England, Scotland, Italy, Spain, Portugal, Holland, Poland, Czech Republic, Taiwan, Turkey, Saudi Arabia) and five continents. The youngest cases were a 15-year-old male (Riha et al., 2023), a 16-year-old male (Contreras et al., 2019), and a 17-year-old (Dubessy et al., 2017; gender not reported). Two females were 76 and 77 years old, respectively. Triggers for sexsomnia were OSA, sleep bruxism, sleep-related head jerks, PLMs, shift work, sleep deprivation, stress, alcohol use (without intoxication), and medications (zolpidem, sodium oxybate, escitalopram, and pramipexole therapy of Parkinson's disease). Close contact with a bed partner is also a common trigger. In addition, predisposing conditions for sexsomnia include narcolepsy, circadian rhythm disorders, and parasomnia overlap disorder. Familial sexsomnia has been reported in two families, one involving a son and father in Australia with long-standing, high-frequency sleep intercourse with their respective partners and the other involving a daughter and mother in Turkey with spontaneous sleep orgasms (Irfan & Schenck, 2018; Schenck et al., 2007). Six cases of sexsomnia have been reported in military personnel, five cases in the United States and one case in Taiwan. These military cases involved concerns about continued suitability for remaining in the military because of the sexsomnia. Forensic consequences from the sexsomnia have been reported in 15 cases (Dubessy et al., 2017; Muza et al., 2016; Schenck et al., 2007). In addition, 9%–11% of patients in two series with SW/ST reported involuntary sexual behaviors during sleep (Carrillo-Solano et al., 2016; van Mierlo et al., 2022). Furthermore, the first assessment of sexsomnia frequency in a general sleep clinic population, involving 832 consecutive patients undergoing video PSG (vPSG) found a 7.6% prevalence of sexsomnia, with male predominance (11% male vs. 4% female; Chung et al. 2010). Finally, nocturnal sleep-related sexual seizures have also been reported (Muza et al., 2016; Schenck et al., 2007; Voges et al. 2019).

Sexsomnia is classified as a clinical subtype of confusional arousals in the ICSD-3TR but is also recognized to emerge from SW. Amnesia associated with sexsomnia has been reported in the vast majority of published cases. Sexsomnia is predominantly a young-adult male disorder, at least for cases that present to a sleep clinic. However, there may be a referral bias since it is the female bed partner who identifies the sexsomnia problem and then initiates the clinical referral. Perhaps just as many females have sexsomnia, but the male partners are not as frequently bothered or concerned about this behavior. (An analogous situation was identified for RBD, with a male-predominant sleep clinic referral bias resulting from males having more aggressive/violent RBD episodes; however, a community-based clinical and PSG study of RBD found an equal male-to-female ratio [Haba-Rubio et al., 2018].)

Sexsomnia usually emerges in the context of either (i) a long-standing, complex history of NREM sleep parasomnias, with sexsomnia being the latest NREM parasomnia to emerge, or (ii) OSA, with the onset of sexsomnia emerging in tandem with snoring, observed apneas, and the other hallmark symptoms of OSA. A first-time sexsomnia episode that results in legal charges, especially without a robust history of NREM parasomnia(s) observed by others and without any current documented moderately severe or severe OSA, should be regarded with extreme skepticism as being bona fide sexsomnia.

The number of reported cases of vPSG-documented sexual behaviors during sleep is currently nine, which involved sleep masturbation (with or without sexual pelvic movements and sexual moaning), n = 7; sexual pelvic movements (with dreaming), n = 1; and sexual intercourse, n = 1. The gender distribution was seven males (77.8%) and two females (22.2%). A 60-year-old married woman with parasomnia overlap disorder (American Academy of Sleep Medicine, 2023; RBD and four NREM parasomnias) had one episode of masturbation emerging from N3 sleep (Cicolin et al., 2011). A 42-year-old married woman had four episodes of masturbation with sexual movements and moaning emerging from N2 and N3 sleep (Toscanini et al., 2021). The seven males were 16–49 years old, including one male who had one episode of sexual intercourse, initiated by his wife's touch during his N1 sleep (Shapiro et al., 2003), and six males who had 38 documented episodes of sleep masturbation (range 1–16 episodes per patient; Contreras et al., 2019; Martynowicz et al., 2018; Mioč et al., 2018; Pirzada et al., 2019; Yeh & Schenck, 2016). There was no associated dreaming in eight of nine cases during these vPSG-documented sexual behaviors during sleep. Triggers for the sexsomnia episodes included spontaneous NREM sleep partial arousals (n = 6), OSA (n = 1), sleep bruxism (n = 1), combined OSA–sleep bruxism (n = 1), and being touched by his wife while asleep (N1). One patient had four episodes of sleep masturbation triggered by OSA in one vPSG study, and then after the OSA was fully treated with continuous positive airway pressure (CPAP), he had four more episodes of sleep masturbation triggered by NREM partial arousals in a second vPSG study (Contreras et al., 2019).

One striking sexsomnia scenario involved two married women, one in Paris (Dubessy et al., 2017) and the other in São Paulo (Toscanini et al., 2021), who repeatedly uttered the names of men not their husbands while sleeping and masturbating in bed alongside their husbands. This is an example of sleep state–dependent verbal–behavioral activation without any correlate during waking life.

The first case (Dubessy et al., 2017, Appendix Case 3) involved a 76-year-old happily married woman (for 50 years), without prior parasomnia history, who spontaneously developed a 3-year history of nightly amnestic sleep masturbation, observed by her husband. While masturbating in her sleep, she repeatedly uttered the name *Mike*, who was not her husband. She denied knowing any man named Mike and denied any extramarital affair. Her husband was suspicious but only because of her sleep masturbation, without any evidence of an affair. She felt shame from her sleep masturbation, became suicidal, left a suicide note, and departed the home—but returned home without any attempted suicide. She resumed sleeping with her husband. During vPSG, she had arousals from N3 sleep. The second case involved a 42-year-old married woman with 10-year history of amnestic sleep masturbation, observed by her husband (Toscanini et al., 2021). The episodes occurred up to twice monthly and involved "dirty talk" and sexual moaning during the sleep masturbation. Also, the woman uttered the names of men not her husband (and of inanimate objects) while masturbating during sleep. There was no evidence for an extramarital affair. However, there was major marital discord, with arguments over the recurrent sleep masturbation and the uttering of names of other men. vPSG documented confusional arousals during four episodes from N3 and five episodes from N2, accompanied by movements of hips and limbs and moaning. Also, quasi (incipient) sleep masturbation behaviors, with moaning, occurred during two of the N3 and two of the N2 arousals.

Finally, treatment of sexsomnia is highly effective in most of the reported cases, including both CPAP and mandibular advancement device therapy of OSA; but a discussion of this topic is beyond the scope of this chapter.

Other Parasomnias Associated With SRV

SRV is a common phenomenon spanning a wide spectrum of sleep disorders, particularly the parasomnias, with forensic consequences. The entire human life span, and all of sleep, carries a risk for SRV. The crucial role played by experienced sleep medicine clinicians in evaluating parasomnia cases at accredited sleep disorder centers with hospital-based extensive vPSG should be recognized for both clinical and forensic purposes. General discussions of parasomnias associated with SRV with possible forensic implications have been provided elsewhere (Ohayon et al., 1997; Ohayon & Schenck, 2010; Schenck et al., 1989). Specific parasomnia subtypes, in this regard, include NREM sleep parasomnias (DOA; Bhat et al., 2012; Castelnovo et al., 2021; Pillmann, 2009; Rocha & Arnulf, 2020; Szűcs et al., 2014), RBD (Schenck et al., 2009; Schenck & Mahowald, 2002), sleep-related dissociative disorder (Dumitrascu et al., 2013; Lopez et al., 2022; Schenck et al., 2021), nocturnal seizure disorder (Boursoulian et al., 2012), OSA/PLM disorder (Ingravallo et al., 2018; Schenck et al., 1989), and OSA/NREM sleep parasomnia (Baron & Auckley, 2005; Danish et al., 2018; Iranzo & Santamaria, 2005; Lateef et al., 2005; Nofzinger & Wettstein, 1995; Schenck, 2019).

Sleep Forensics

There is overwhelming evidence that very complex behaviors potentially resulting in violent or criminal acts may arise from the sleep period, often without conscious awareness and therefore without culpability (Siclari et al., 2010). Historical reviews of legal case reports involving SRV have been reported in the medical literature (Pressman, 2007, 2018). The legal implications of automatic behaviors, or automatisms, have been discussed and debated in both the medical and legal literature (Fitzgerald, 1961; Prevezer, 1958; Shroder & Mather, 1976). The landmark legal case successfully utilizing the "sleepwalking defense" remains the 1992 homicide case *Regina v. Parks*. In this bizarre criminal case, the then-23-year-old defendant, Kenneth Parks, was reported to have driven 14 miles in the early morning hours to the home of his wife's parents. His in-laws' response presumably triggered a violent response while Mr. Parks remained in the midst of a prolonged SW episode. Mr. Parks attacked both of them, killing the mother-in-law and grievously injuring the father-in-law. In a courtroom jury trial, the defendant was acquitted of all charges, a result eventually upheld in a landmark Supreme Court of Canada decision not to characterize SW as a mental health disorder (Broughton et al., 1994).

In 2006, we established the first formal sleep forensics consulting program within the Department of Sleep Medicine at a US academic institution, and named it Sleep Forensics Associates. At first, commensurate with the expertise of our group, the primary focus of this initiative was on parasomnias. However, we quickly found that the forensic implications of sleep disorders extended well beyond parasomnias. Attorney requests for investigative consultations also involved inquiries into a broad array of possible conditions including sleep deprivation, fatigue/hypersomnolence, insomnia, OSA, and unusual side effects of prescription sedative-hypnotic agents or stimulants. The goal of our sleep forensics program was not only to be an expert medical resource for the legal and law enforcement communities but also to facilitate clinical research by collecting case information to create a database for subsequent medical as well as legal analysis.

From our sleep forensics program's inception in 2006, we have been involved in over 400 legal cases from either the prosecution or the defense. The vast majority of these were criminal, though a few civil cases were also encountered. Our direct involvement in criminal cases typically ranged 1–2 years from the time of being formally assigned to the case to its legal resolution. The majority of our cases were settled out of court, and the time expended was chiefly attributed to case file analysis, interviews, and case report development. Our experience has been consistent with the current state of legal affairs in the United States: Plea bargaining is common, and a trial is the exception rather than the rule as less than 5% of federal criminal cases proceed to trial (Smith & MacQueen, 2017). Civil cases were rare but were especially remarkable for their sheer bulk of case files, some filling four banker's storage boxes. Subsequently, our involvement with these cases took the most time, often more than 5 years. In a case retained by the Office of the District Attorney Insurance Fraud Unit of a large US West Coast metropolitan city, the duration of our involvement was 12 years including case reviews, hearings, grand jury testimonies, and, finally, testimony leading to jury trial resolution.

In 2019, our group published the first report on the spectrum of legal complaints referred by the legal community to a single academic sleep medicine center. This report summarized the characteristics of 351 consecutive legal cases. We encountered 23 categories of criminal and civil complaints. Criminal allegations of homicide, manslaughter, assault/battery, and sexual assault were most prevalent. By far the most common criminal complaint was sexual assault, accounting for approximately 41% of all cases. As anticipated, of the possible sleep-related conditions implicated, parasomnias were most prevalent. Interestingly, our group found that forensic implications were closely associated with NREM parasomnias, specifically confusional arousals. Initial reviews of criminal allegations perhaps involving RBD were rare. This finding was surprising as one of the most frequent presenting clinical complaints with RBD involves violent dream-enactment behaviors (Cramer Bornemann et al., 2019).

Guidelines to Assess SRV

To assist in the determination of the role of a possible parasomnia in a criminal allegation, following is a summary of noteworthy features selected from the medical literature (Cramer Bornemann & Mahowald, 2021):

1. There should be reason (by history or formal sleep medicine center assessment) to suspect a bona fide sleep disorder. Similar episodes, with benign or morbid outcome, should have occurred previously.
2. The behavior is usually abrupt, immediate, impulsive, and senseless; often primal in nature; without apparent motivation; and in stark contrast to the individual's behavior and/or personality when fully awake.
3. Behaviors associated with NREM sleep typically occur in the first one-third of the sleep period, or within 2–3 hours after falling asleep. Under certain conditions, especially sleep deprivation, NREM behaviors may occur very shortly after falling asleep. In contrast, behaviors associated with REM sleep typically occur in the latter one-third of the sleep period, or within approximately 2–3 hours prior to waking up.
4. In the cases of ST, SW, or sleep inertia, the act may occur on awakening (rarely immediately upon falling asleep) and usually at least 1 hour after sleep onset. It may occur on attempts to awaken the subject.
5. The duration of the action is usually brief (seconds), although action of longer duration (minutes) does not necessarily exclude a sleep-related behavior.
6. Close proximity is a key feature, particularly in cases involving sexualized behaviors arising from sleep. The victim is someone who merely happened to be present and who may have been the stimulus for the arousal. Sleepwalkers rarely, if ever, seek out victims.
7. Immediately upon the return of consciousness there is no persistent attempt to conceal or cover up the action. There is generally a lack of awareness on the part of the individual during the event. At other times with abrupt awakenings from sleep, there may be strong emotionally dysphoric reactions such as horror, confusion, and heightened anxiety.
8. The individual is usually amnestic for the events, though the amnesia may not be complete. There is usually minimal, if any, dream imagery recalled, but notable exceptions have been reported with dream-enacting behaviors

during sleepwalking and sleep terrors in adults. Though possible to a much lesser degree, reported cases of sexsomnia are usually without any significant dream recall (Castelnovo et al., 2021; Pillmann, 2009; Rocha & Arnulf, 2020; Uguccioni et al., 2013).

9. Rule of Exclusion—The violent behavior cannot be better explained by another mental disorder, medical condition, medication, or substance use. Unlike that which may present in a clinical scenario, this rule is particularly important as longitudinal assessment of the afflicted individual is not practical, or possible, in legal cases. Thus, outright alcohol intoxication or significant exposure involving illicit substances precludes further consideration of the "sleepwalking defense."

The role of vPSG in sleep forensics cases is often debated. Whether a vPSG is indicated is based upon clinical judgment by experienced sleep medicine physicians in accordance with AASM standards and diagnostic guidelines. Certainly, vPSG would appear to be required if RBD is a consideration. However, NREM parasomnias, including sexsomnia, are clinical diagnoses whereby a vPSG is not an absolute requirement (American Academy of Sleep Medicine, 2023). Regardless of the type of parasomnia under consideration, vPSG performed after the fact is of absolutely no value in confirming whether the defendant was engaged in SRV at the time of the criminal allegation as the two are not temporally associated. Even complex SW captured during vPSG, however exceedingly rare, would only indicate that the person was a sleepwalker, not that SW was involved at the time of the crime. In criminal cases for which an NREM parasomnia may be involved, a vPSG may be considered to assess potential preexisting chronic conditions, such as OSA and PLMs, which are known to increase the defendant's propensity for abnormal arousals and SRV. Additionally, results from a vPSG may be helpful in developing a parasomnia safety plan for the defendant after the completion of the trial to ensure their safety and that of others. It should be emphasized that the undisciplined use of scientific technical data in court is a real concern, especially given the public's fascination with new technologies coupled with their misperception that science is a field that deals with absolute certainties when in actuality it is a field that reflects probabilities of occurrence. It is not uncommon to use irrelevant, disingenuous technicalities in an attempt to deceive so as to attain an advantage to secure the decision. It is important for the expert medical witness to appreciate and succinctly communicate the limitations of neuroscientific data in the courtroom.

Alcohol and Sedative-Hypnotic Drugs: Triggers for Parasomnias?

The recently approved (by the AASM) ICSD-3TR contains the following important statements about alcohol and SW with direct forensic implications that also apply to sexsomnia (italics provided by the authors):

Alcohol has been identified in previous reports as a potential sleepwalking trigger. However, the amnesia associated with disorders of arousal makes these reports unreliable. More recent evidence-based reviews have found no compelling relationship between alcohol and disorders of arousal. In addition, there is no evidence indicating that behavior resulting from alcohol intoxication can be distinguished from behavior resulting from a disorder of arousal. *Thus a disorder of arousal cannot be diagnosed in the context of alcohol intoxication. This assertion holds for any claim that an intoxicated person fell asleep and then engaged in an arousal disorder episode since "passing out" from alcohol intoxication cannot be distinguished from actual sleep by any observer.* Likewise, the association between therapeutic doses of sedative-hypnotic drugs and apparent parasomnias should be carefully distinguished from the expected effects of drug abuse or misuse that result in CNS depression. Investigations of drivers who had accidents attributed to drug-related sleep-driving are reported to show that: 1) blood levels of prescribed sedative-hypnotics exceeded therapeutic ranges; 2) the individuals failed to take the medication at the correct time or remain in bed for sufficient time following ingestion; or 3) the individuals combined sedative-hypnotics with other CNS depressants or alcohol. Driving with a high blood level of a sedative-hypnotic can result in significant cognitive and motor impairment. Serious accidents can result. Sleep driving and other complex behaviors in this population are more likely to have resulted from drug misuse and abuse rather than true parasomnias. *The ICSD-3TR advocates that disorders of arousal should not be diagnosed in the presence of alcohol intoxication or in the setting of sedative-hypnotic exposure resulting in elevated blood levels.* (American Academy of Sleep Medicine, 2023)

Common Scenarios of Sexsomnia Resulting in Allegations of Sexual Assault

With greater awareness in part influenced by the MeToo social media movement and stricter enforcement in US universities of Title IX of the US Civil Rights Act, referrals to evaluate sexual assault cases have become increasingly common, now approaching 75% of sleep forensics referrals to our group since 2020. However, in those cases where sexsomnia was determined to account for the sexual assault, the demographics have remained consistent over our experience and include the following characteristic features (Cramer Bornemann & Mahowald, 2021):

1. Gender of the perpetrator was predominantly male, with an age range of 18–55 years.
2 Gender of the victim was predominantly female, with an age range of 3–17 years.
3. A vast majority of the victims knew the perpetrator as a family member, significant other, or friend. Most often the perpetrator was a father.
4. Inappropriate touch of brief duration with hands upon breasts/genitals was the most common sexualized behavior eliciting a criminal charge.

5. The perpetrator often had a compelling history of symptoms suggestive of an NREM parasomnia, notably a DOA, some with sexualized attributes.
6. Close proximity was a key feature where the victim and perpetrator were either co-sleeping or at least sharing the same room.

At the annual meeting of the Associated Professional Sleep Societies held in Minneapolis in 2014 (SLEEP 2014), our group presented a summary of findings attributed to sexsomnia related to 103 consecutive cases of sexual assault. In the ensuing years these characteristic features have remained remarkably consistent (Cramer Bornemann et al., 2014). In situations supporting sexsomnia as a legal defense, the most common scenario involved the father of a young daughter, or step-daughter, who was under 14 years of age at the time of the allegations. The parents of the daughter were divorced or separated and continued to have a contentious relationship. Typically, the child would reside with the mother, with the father having contact on weekends. These families were most often of a low socioeconomic status and lived within confined quarters where co-sleeping or sleeping nearby one another was common. Allegations of sexual assault often involved the father and daughter either co-sleeping, sharing the same bedroom, or having inadvertently fallen asleep beside each other while watching a show on television or streaming on a laptop computer. The inappropriate sexualized touch by the father of the daughter usually occurred shortly after falling asleep and was of short duration (lasting seconds to a few minutes). The event was most often an isolated episode without any dream recall, and the father was unaware of it until a complaint by the daughter. In other instances, the father would first become aware of the episode only after being approached by law enforcement investigating the allegations. The legal process was typically initiated when the daughter confided in her mother, who then immediately contacted CPS or law enforcement. Such reports trigger mandatory preliminary criminal investigations. At other times, the legal process began with a daughter who shared her concerns with a trusted school counselor. Most US states have mandatory reporting laws which require certain professionals to report suspected child abuse to the proper authorities. In many states, the charge of aggravated sexual assault does not require sexual intercourse or penetration but only requires that a simple manual touch of the sexual organ (i.e., breast, vagina, buttocks, or any part which the complainant considers "private") or anus. If the defendant is found guilty, the outcome of the punitive phase of the legal proceedings is likely to be very severe. For example, in Texas under state criminal penal code §22.021, aggravated sexual assault of a victim under 14 years of age is a first-degree felony, and the minimum term for imprisonment is increased to 25 years. In Oregon, subjecting a person under 14 years to sexual contact is a Class B felony carrying a mandatory minimum penitentiary term of 75 months with no credit for good behavior. Our experience suggests that the vast majority of cases best explained by sexsomnia are situations where a father inadvertently fell asleep beside his prepubescent daughter. Whether such sleeping arrangements are appropriate is arguable when factoring in economic and/or cultural factors; likewise, one should consider whether such an event may have been anticipated by a father with a history suggestive of sleep-related behaviors.

The Expert Medical Witness in the Legal Process

The criminal justice system is like a funnel; the process starts wide with many cases but then diminishes as decision makers in the legal system remove cases from the process. Some of these cases are dismissed, while others are referred for counseling. In the US criminal justice system, the state (i.e., the prosecution) is required by law to support every deprivation of life, liberty, or property by establishing facts supporting its contentions. Thus, the greater the degree of deprivation, the more facts the state is required to produce. For instance, an arrest requires fewer facts than an indictment, and an indictment requires fewer facts than a criminal conviction. In Anglo-American law, the state has traditionally defined criminal offenses as requiring both an actus reus and a mens rea in order to secure a conviction. *Actus reus*, or "guilty act," essentially refers to the affirmative act that comprises the physical elements of the crime. *Mens rea*, or "guilty mind," refers to the state of mind required to be held accountable for the crime. The state, or prosecution, is required to prove the union, or joint operation, of act and wrongful intent. In a sexual assault case, the "wrongful intent" is for the purpose of sexual gratification. Sleep forensics investigations are largely concerned about addressing issues related to mens rea as opposed to those related to actus reus, which are usually not in doubt. An effective sleep forensics expert medical witness must be able to provide an opinion connecting violent sleep-related behaviors to the defendant's degree of consciousness and awareness at the time of the crime. Criminal intent is an important element in the state's argument against a defendant. Sleep forensics investigations do not provide an opinion on intent. The determination of the perpetrator's intent is a question for the trier of fact—either the jury or the judge (if a jury trial has been waived). Experts are not permitted to testify to the ultimate question of fact in connection with a perpetrator's ultimate intent.

Overview of the Legal Process

A wide variety of formal and informal processes are involved before the actual courtroom trial takes place. The major steps in the criminal justice process are as follows (American Bar Association, 2021):

1. Report of a possible crime.
2. Investigation of a possible crime by law enforcement. An investigation may require a search of the person or property. *Probable cause* means that there exists a reasonable basis that a crime may have been committed and that a specific person committed it. Probable cause is a requirement to execute a search.

3. Arrest of the suspect by law enforcement. Probable cause is a requirement for an arrest and placing the suspect in custody.
4. Prosecution of a defendant by the state. Once completed, the investigation is referred to the officers of the district attorney for filing considerations. Then, the prosecutor must determine which charges can be proven against the perpetrator beyond a reasonable doubt prior to submitting charges against them.
5. Indictment by a grand jury. All federal cases require a grand jury indictment for felony charges. Whether a grand jury indictment is required is variable from state to state. The grand jury proceeding is a closed hearing from the defendant in which the prosecution presents evidence. Probable cause alone is the standard for indicting an individual for a crime.
6. Arraignment by a judge. At this stage a defendant is informed of the formal charges. The judge ensures that the defendant understands the charges and their right to legal representation. The defendant is usually then asked to enter a plea. Sometimes entry of a plea is deferred so that both parties may engage in negotiations. Eventually, a defendant may plead guilty, not guilty, or not guilty by reason of insanity. On occasion, an Alford Plea may be offered whereby the defendant may plead no contest, thereby admitting the facts of the case but not guilt.
7. Pretrial detention and/or bail. The defendant is typically placed into custody at their arraignment, when the judge sets their bail. If bail cannot be posted or if conditions for their bail had been violated while awaiting trial, the defendant is remanded into custody of the local jail pending resolution of their case.
8. Plea bargaining between the defense attorney and the prosecutor. The defendant may consider pleading guilty in exchange for a reduction of the criminal charge and a lighter sentence. In our sleep forensics experience, we often encounter plea bargains in homicide cases. In contrast, with sexual assault cases defendants typically will not accept any plea bargain as they do not want to accept responsibility for their conduct given the stigma of their crime and the consequence of a lifetime registration as a sex offender. Prosecutors angle for a plea bargain in sexual assault cases to avoid having to force the victim to testify, which could incur additional trauma.
9. Adjudication phase. The case is resolved by a trial before a jury or, if the defendant so chooses, before the judge alone (referred to as a *bench trial*) after a waiver of the right to a jury. Prior to the trial, the judge reviews the evidence submitted by the prosecution and the defense to determine what is admissible in court. In cases involving a parasomnia, especially sexsomnia, the prosecution may request a Daubert (or Frye) hearing to determine

whether new or novel scientific evidence to be presented to the court should be allowed at trial. Such a hearing occurs outside the presence of the jury or before the jury trial has begun. Typically, the defense calls the sleep forensics expert to testify as an "offer of proof" in which they outline the areas of their testimony. The prosecutor will then cross-examine them, and the judge determines whether and to what extent their testimony will be allowed before the jury.

At trial, the burden is upon the prosecution to prove beyond a reasonable doubt that the defendant committed the crime. The defense attorney will have an opportunity to cross-examine the prosecution's witnesses. The defense attorney will also present evidence and witnesses to support their argument. The prosecution is then given an opportunity to cross-examine defense witnesses. After all the evidence and witnesses have been presented before the court, the prosecution and defense attorneys will offer their closing statements. The judge then instructs the jury about applying the law to the facts presented and then hands it to the jury for a final decision on the charges.

10. Sentencing by the judge if the defendant is found guilty. Possible sentences include a period of incarceration in a correctional facility, fines, or probation.
11. Appeals. The defense has a right to appeal the court's legal rulings as well as the sufficiency of the facts to support the jury's verdict. A lawyer files an appeal in formal proceedings before the appellate court, which is then ruled on by appellate judges. The appellate courts give great weight to the jury's findings on the facts and to the trial judge's rulings on the law. If the appellate court overturns a court decision, the case will return to the trial court for a new trial.
12. Punishment and/or rehabilitation as determined by sentencing guidelines for the criminal conviction. Often at sentencing where the defendant has no criminal history the judge has the discretion to grant the defendant probation. Especially in cases involving sexual assault, the defense will often employ experts to mitigate the defendant's guilt and encourage the judge to grant the defendant probation.

The sleep forensics investigator usually becomes involved once formal legal proceedings have begun. Only infrequently does the sleep forensics investigator first become involved at the investigatory stage or the stage beginning with grand jury hearings. In our experience, the entry point for the sleep forensics investigator most often begins at the adjudication phase (Figure 46.2). The degree to which a sleep forensics investigator is involved in a criminal case can increase or decrease the likelihood that it will go to trial

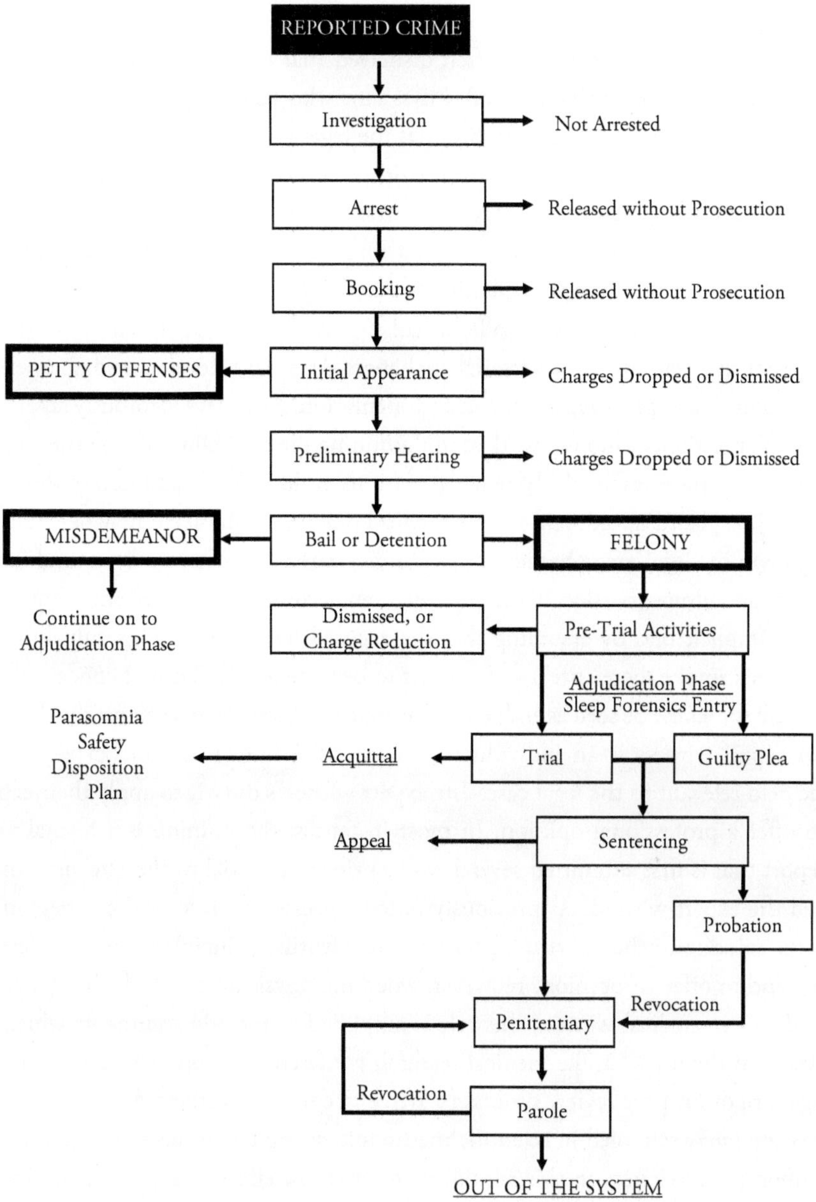

Figure 46.2 Sleep forensics entry into the legal process

long before such an expert is called to take the stand. Whether retained by the prosecution or the defense, our involvement as a sleep forensics expert medical witness is often completed with our testimony on the stand, usually on the last day of the trial before jury deliberations. On rare occasions, we have remained involved toward the end of the process as a resource for the defense team during sentencing and with appeals.

Roles of the Expert Medical Witness

Physicians who testify in court are often dismayed that the legal system does not share the same goals as the scientific method. Physicians who take on the privileged mantle of an expert medical witness need to realize that the legal process is not inherently scientific in nature nor is the endeavor simply to provide a clinical diagnosis. Science works with well-defined research questions, observations, testing/retesting hypotheses under carefully controlled conditions, peer review of results through open discussions, and advancing knowledge through publication. Scientific principles gain acceptance based on statistical relevance and a consensus-driven collegial collaborative approach. In contrast, attorneys receive extensive training in adversarial exchange. Attorneys develop and sharpen their skills through challenge, persuasion, and argumentation. Attorneys vigorously advocate for their client's position, arduously work at undermining the credibility of the other side, and often entertain strategies involving reinterpretations of the facts. In addition to the obvious inconvenience placed upon their routine medical practice, a physician may be reluctant to participate in the legal arena because of its conflict with scientific paradigms and its unfamiliar foreign culture (Barsky, 2012). Although an accused is presumed innocent, experts may have implicit bias by assuming that the accused has some level of culpability (i.e., "where there's smoke there's fire") and hesitate to become involved out of concern that this posture will somehow be seen as endorsing the abhorrent acts alleged against the defendant.

An expert witness is an individual with extensive knowledge and experience in a specific field relevant to the legal case. The expert witness's duty is to apply their expertise and to offer a professional opinion. In most instances, the opinion is a formal written case report that is first submitted several weeks prior to the trial to the attorney who had retained the expert witness. As previously noted, an essential role of the expert medical witness is to educate the courtroom on current scientific principles that are relevant to the case and to offer an opinion. However, when the physician enters the legal arena as a qualified expert medical witness, this role is amplified to include arguments which must resonate with the jury. Unlike medical research conferences where data and conclusions undergo a rigorous peer-review process to arrive at consensus-driven decisions, members of a jury are rarely schooled in scientific methodology and are unlikely to reach decisions solely upon good science. In this adjudicative phase, an effective expert medical witness is thereby one who can persuasively communicate facts and opinions about those facts in a succinct and credible manner. A jury is likely to believe an expert medical witness who is amiable, respectful, and nonconfrontational, all the while exhibiting qualities which convey credibility such as knowledge, confidence, honesty, openness, impartiality, and trustworthiness.

Qualifications of the Medical Expert Witness in Sleep Forensics

To ensure that the appropriate degree of expertise is provided in any given criminal case and to address the problem of pseudoscience in the courtroom, many professional societies have developed guidelines for medical expert witness qualifications. In general, the AASM's stance on medical expert witness testimony is to accept those views held by the American Medical Association (AMA). Influenced by position papers from both the AMA and the American Academy of Neurology, the following guidelines for expert medical witness qualifications in criminal cases involving a parasomnia should serve as a compass (Freeman & Nelson, 2004; Goldrich, 2004):

1. Must have a current, valid, unrestricted medical license
2. Must have successfully completed a formal sleep medicine fellowship training program
3. Must be a diplomat of the American Board of Sleep Medicine or have passed the American Board of Medical Specialties examination in sleep medicine
4. Must be clinically active as a physician in sleep medicine and involved in clinical practice in a manner relevant to the requirements of the criminal case at the time of the event
5. Must be a recognized resource within the sleep medicine community in the diagnosis and management of parasomnias
6. Membership in the Sleep Research Society is strongly encouraged.

As the stakes are indeed high in criminal felony cases involving homicide, manslaughter, or sexual assault, it would appear to be unethical for a physician to be involved as an expert medical witness without appropriate training and extensive clinical experience in parasomnias. Forensic psychiatrists (or forensic nurses) without formal sleep medicine training or sleep medicine physicians who have very limited knowledge and have rarely encountered parasomnias should not be qualified as an expert medical witness in these cases. Should opposing legal counsel also retain their own expert medical witness to provide an opinion on parasomnias, it is critical to review the credentials of this physician in light of these guidelines in order to maintain the integrity of the court and to steer clear of confusing, misleading statements. When the opposing counsel retains their own expert medical witness, the court may be inclined to permit their testimony, regardless of their qualifications, simply to "level the playing field."

Legal Cases 1 and 2 Redux

As previously described in this chapter, both Legal Cases 1 and 2 present fathers who allegedly sexually assaulted, to various degrees, their biological daughters. Assuming the integrity and honesty of those involved, the comprehensive sleep forensics investigative analysis did not uncover any substantive inconsistencies or contradictions. There were no findings to suggest malingering in either case. Both cases were consistent with the guidelines determining the role of a possible parasomnia in a criminal allegation and with the demographics which we reported on criminal cases where sexsomnia was supported. Each father also suffered from chronic insufficient sleep and likely struggled with troublesome OSA at the time of the allegations, thereby notably increasing their risk for a parasomnia. Furthermore, both fathers fulfilled ICSD-3TR diagnostic criteria for confusional arousal, an NREM parasomnia. In addition, the array of behaviors that are without awareness and memory attributed by such a condition can be scientifically explained through the lens of sleep/wake dissociative states founded upon currently accepted principles of neurophysiology. Though clinical science can never make determinations with absolute certainty, it was not only plausible but also highly likely that sexsomnia was at the core of both fathers' inappropriate sexual behaviors involving their daughters, resulting in criminal felony charges. In each case, the sleep forensics investigation concluded that sexsomnia was highly likely to have been the cause of the fathers' inappropriate sexual touch that ultimately prompted the criminal charges.

Despite their striking similarities and being comparable reflections of each other, very different court decisions were rendered by the juries in each case. In Legal Case 1, the jury found the father not guilty; he was acquitted of all charges. The sleep forensics team formulated a safety disposition plan for the father to ensure the safety and well-being of his daughter during times they spend evenings together. Consequently, this court's decision was pivotal in maintaining the integrity of this father's family, a decision that was also unequivocally supported by his daughter, the victim. In Legal Case 2, the jury found the father guilty of criminal sexual conduct. He was sentenced to 10 years' imprisonment with parole and must comply with a mandatory lifetime registration as a sex offender. As a result, his wife divorced him, and he lost contact not only with his daughter, the victim, but, sadly, with his three sons as well. Differences in trial outcomes between apparently similar cases can be attributed to many intangible factors including the makeup of the jury, the jury's implicit (possible racial) bias, the behavior of the judge, and the competence of the attorneys. It is imperative that the expert medical witness understand their role and not lose sight of it during the trial process.

Supporting Parasomnias Throughout the Legal Process

Even with a sleep forensics investigation that culminates in testimony firmly based upon sound science that adheres to widely accepted community standards and procedures, courtroom decisions can be unpredictable, inconsistent, and even diametrically opposed, as our experience with the recent court decisions above reflects. In our experience, submitting a final case report and providing testimony in support of a case at trial are not sufficient. The stakes in trials involving homicide and sexual assault, those criminal charges where a sleep forensics investigation are most often involved, are very high. Regardless of the trial's outcome, facilitating a fair and informed legal resolution can only be best supported by an expert medical witness working closely alongside their attorney throughout the legal process.

Criminal courtroom proceedings are not a scientific endeavor. A physician might find it difficult to understand how well-informed and intellectually honest individuals can argue the facts of the case and arrive at very divergent conclusions. The tenets of law are based upon legal text, the drafter's intent, judicial precedent, traditions, and sound policy. Some of these tenets may be outdated or conflict with currently held scientific principles. Whether from the prosecution or the defense, arguments in a courtroom will typically stem from these essential tenets. During the course of a courtroom trial, the main issue for the jury to decide is whose version of the facts is more likely to be believed. Accordingly, the persuasiveness of the argument is a key influence upon the jury's decision. An expert medical witness who provides support throughout the legal process is instrumental in contributing to the persuasiveness of their legal team's argument.

Once a sleep forensics investigation has been completed, an opinion, most often in the form of a written case report, is offered to the attorney for consideration to be submitted to the court as a form of evidence in support of their argument. Submitting a final case report should not be perceived to be analogous to a hospital discharge summary but should be considered as the next step in the collaborative process with the attorney in the ongoing support of the case's legal argument. Moreover, it does not necessarily follow that an expert medical witness will later appear in court to offer their testimony. The expert medical witness needs to be cognizant that the next step within the adjudication phase involves the court's rules of evidence. These rules determine what facts will be admissible in a jury trial. The rules of evidence not only may vary from state to state but also may differ among civil, criminal, and family court cases. Evidentiary rules in the United States have a reputation for being very complex, and any objections to a ruling on evidence must be made carefully to preserve the record for appeal (Friedman, 2019). Whether a physician will be qualified as an expert medical witness and whether their findings and opinions are ruled admissible in court depend upon these rules. In this regard, a physician can expect a vigorous unsettling confrontation from opposing counsel. Prosecutors may be particularly vigorous in objecting to evidence when a parasomnia is offered as the defense because most are either skeptical of or completely unwilling to believe the spectrum and complexity of behaviors possible with this condition. It should be emphasized that the judge determines the admissibility of evidence, but the actual trier of facts in a jury trial is the jury. In other words, it is the jury that determines the facts from the evidence which was allowed in court by the judge. Not to be overlooked, another type of trial is a bench trial, where the judge determines both the evidence and the facts in a case. Bench trials are rare in criminal cases involving serious charges. In our sleep forensics experience, we have only encountered bench trials in court martial cases within the US military judicial system.

To allow a physician to present their findings and opinion at trial, they first need to be qualified by the judge as an expert medical witness, and their testimony must satisfy legal standards (Barsky, 2012). The legal standard to qualify as an expert witness in any realm is surprisingly a minimal one and includes knowledge, skill, experience, training, and education. Most scientists would recognize that ill-defined standards or poorly controlled conditions create processes whose results are unpredictable and confusing to interpret. Accordingly, physicians should maintain their attitude of scientific rigor and hold themselves accountable to a much higher standard when supporting justice. In cases involving parasomnias, we strongly advocate for the aforementioned "Qualifications of the Medical Expert Witness in Sleep Forensics." The process of qualification to determine a physician's competence as an expert medical witness at trial can be performed through an offer of proof or a Daubert (or Frye) hearing, depending upon the state. An offer of proof occurs at trial before a witness is allowed to appear before the jury, but a Daubert (or Frye) hearing usually occurs before the scheduled start of the trial. In either situation, the process of qualification is straightforward. Each side questions the witness, who is called to testify under oath. Usually, the attorney presents the physician's curriculum vitae to the court and highlights important features relevant to their opinion. Both the judge and opposing counsel during these proceedings may ask for clarifications or challenge the physician's expertise, the work performed, and its relevance to the particular case. Though opposing counsel may object to admitting the physician as a qualified expert, the judge makes the final decision on whether the physician is to be qualified as an expert medical witness and upon the parameters of their opinion evidence at trial. In our sleep forensics experience during offers of proof, our qualifications as an expert medical witness have never been contested, and we have always been allowed to offer testimony. Our experience with Daubert hearings has been an altogether different matter.

Determining Admissibility of Scientific Evidence

A Daubert (or Frye) hearing refers to one of the two standards in the US legal system used to determine the admissibility of novel scientific expert witness testimony (Jensen, 2003). These hearings typically begin with the qualification process of the physician, similar to that of an offer of proof at trial and followed by the process of determining admissibility. The Frye standard dictates that the principle or methodology that is offered "be sufficiently established to have gained general acceptance within the relevant scientific community" (Frye v. United States, 1923). Curiously, the Frye standard was devised over 100 years ago as a response to an attempt at introducing the results of a lie detector test, specifically the systolic blood pressure deception test. It was eventually ruled inadmissible in trial. To aid the trial judge in determining whether novel evidence is scientifically valid and whether it aids the jury in evaluating a fact, the Daubert standard asks the following:

1. Can the scientific knowledge be tested, or has it been tested?
2. Has the theory or methodology been subjected to peer review and publication?
3. Does the methodology have a known or potential rate of error?
4. Is there general acceptance of the scientific technique? (Note: This fourth standard is a reiteration of the Frye standard.)

The Daubert standard came from the 1993 court case, *Daubert v. Merrell Dow Pharmaceuticals, Inc.* 43 F.3d 1311(9th Cir. 1995) and sets a higher standard for expert scientific testimony. It focuses on relevance, assumes that the expert witness opinion is founded upon a reliable basis, and attempts to make certain that the expert witness employs in the courtroom the same level of intellectual rigor that epitomizes their scientific practice in their specific field.

Challenges to Submitting Scientific Evidence

From our sleep forensics experience, motions for Daubert (or Frye) hearings appear to go beyond the determination of admissibility of novel scientific evidence and may be filed for several reasons. It may be a means to test the parasomnia argument, thereby providing the opposing counsel an opportunity to anticipate and be more prepared with opposing arguments at trial. Information elicited at such a hearing may prompt them to retain their own medical expert. Another reason may be an attempt to disqualify the physician as an expert medical witness based upon technical legal grounds. In a sexsomnia case for which we were retained by the defense, we were disqualified by a judge primarily because the judge found no legal decisions in that jurisdiction remotely related to admissibility of evidence of a parasomnia. In this case, the judge found a 40-year-old court ruling related to criminal involuntary behaviors associated with *psychomotor epilepsy*, a term first proposed in 1937 to describe seizures associated with mental, emotional, and motor phenomena (Bell, 2011). In this ruling, evidence about the "mental defect" attributed to the "psychomotor epilepsy" was admissible when given by a psychiatrist, or a specialist well-versed in mental disorders. Based upon this outdated precedent, the judge ruled that a specialist in sleep medicine was not qualified to provide opinions in court concerning the mental status of an individual with sexsomnia. Despite the defense attorney offering to the court that such parasomnias are not a psychiatric condition and opinions regarding altered mental status with this condition are within the domain of a sleep medicine specialist, not a psychiatrist, the judge stood steadfast with his ruling. This further accentuates the conflict between the law and medicine, reflecting how law may be founded upon tradition and precedent which may not be consistent with current science. It is the judge who is the gatekeeper of the evidence. Interestingly, *psychomotor epilepsy* is now considered a misleading, antiquated term, which has long been replaced by *temporal lobe epilepsy*, the most common form of focal epilepsy.

Regardless of whether the state jurisdiction utilizes the Daubert or Frye standard, the expert medical witness can expect much of the cross-examination from opposing counsel to stem directly from elements within these standards. These inquiries will certainly occur if the hearing on evidence admissibility occurs before trial. Should the case proceed to trial, the elements found within the Daubert standard will likely serve as the template for additional vigorous cross-examination.

For some time, sexsomnia was considered a novel clinical condition in the courts, and the question of whether it was generally accepted was always raised. Some courts ruled sexsomnia to be inadmissible because it had not been formally cited in medical professional society diagnostic manuals at the time, such as the ICSD-2 or *Diagnostic and Statistical Manual* (DSM)-IV. Other courts did admit the evidence solely on the extent of peer-reviewed medical literature. With the updated revisions found in the DSM-V in 2013, the ICSD-3 in 2014, and the ICSD-3-TR in 2023, sexsomnia is now formally recognized as sleep-related abnormal sexual behavior under confusional arousals, an NREM parasomnia subtype. As a diagnosable and treatable condition also recognized by health insurance providers as codable and billable, the admissibility of sexsomnia is no longer challenged in court—at least insofar as it pertains to fulfilling the standard of general acceptance. Infrequently, we have observed attempts by the prosecution to deny sexsomnia's admissibility by challenging its relevance in their case. Here, the prosecution will declare that sexsomnia is an extremely rare condition and cite the dearth of published case reports in the medical literature on this condition to support this claim. (However, as documented above, 220 cases of sexsomnia have now been published in the growing medical literature). This argument is unlikely to gain any traction in a pre-trial admissibility hearing at which the judge would probably say the evidence can be admitted, but the objection goes to its weight. In that situation, counsel should carefully prepare for this argument because it may have a significant impact on an already skeptical conservative jury. As we experienced in Legal Case 2, this might be of particular concern in cases where the defendant has a checkered past and a character as well as credibility that can be easily assailed.

During the closing statements to the jury in another trial, a prosecutor actually argued, "Do you believe that there are aliens from Mars on earth? I do not . . . but if they do exist they must be extremely rare. Do you see any aliens from Mars in this courtroom? I do not. . . . I also do not see anyone with sexsomnia in this courtroom." Counsel should be prepared to object to such claims as improper argument which reinforces a jury's bias against this evidence. These claims rest on the false impression that sexsomnia is such an exceedingly rare condition that even its consideration is unreasonable, and thereby the evidence is irrelevant. Though the number of published cases reports on sexsomnia is ever-increasing (as reported above), it is still apparently a rare condition—but certainly not as rare as finding an "alien from Mars on earth."

Maintaining Reliability and Credibility

Once the general acceptance of parasomnias, including sexsomnia, has been established, the medical expert witness can expect subsequent challenges to the submission of their evidence, attempting to create serious doubts and to undermine their credibility. Physicians lack knowledge on how to approach their evidence in a court of law. It is extremely important to maintain credibility as the jury is then more likely to consider the evidence and opinions presented by the expert medical witness as true. Again, these challenges largely arise from or are influenced by Daubert standards addressing testability, methodology, degree of certainty, and reliability. Not to be neglected, findings submitted as evidence also need to be relevant and helpful in the jury's understanding of the case. Specific questions we have often encountered include the following:

1. What methods did you rely upon to arrive at your conclusions?
2. What tests did you perform to confirm the conclusions or diagnosis?
3. How many patients with a parasomnia, or sexsomnia, have you taken care of? What is the rate of error in your diagnosis? What is your calculated degree of certainty?

Most questions of this nature confuse "hard" science with "soft" science and are misconstrued when directed toward many areas in clinical medicine, such as parasomnias. The hard sciences include fields such as particle physics, molecular biology, and organic chemistry. Studies involving hard sciences involve strict control of variables and use mathematical tools to exactly measure and calculate outcomes. From this, outcomes can be confirmed and error rates explicitly determined. Training in medical school certainly begins with an emphasis on learning the hard sciences that include anatomy, physiology, biochemistry, and microbiology, to name a few. However, the practice of clinical medicine, with diagnosing and managing patient conditions, is best understood as being at the intersection of these two types of science. The soft sciences, at times referred to as the *social sciences*, include psychiatry, psychology, sociology, and anthropology. Soft sciences in medicine apply scientific principles to deal with intangibles related to human behaviors and emotions whose complexities are difficult to measure with certainty. This softer side of clinical medicine is an inexact and bewildering process for which the hard sciences provide little help. For instance, when a psychiatrist evaluates a patient and determines that the diagnosis is schizophrenia, what was the rate of error? Did any test confirm the diagnosis? When a neurologist sees a patient for an event characterized as right-sided facial droop of brief duration that occurred several days ago but has since resolved and determines the cause to have been a transient ischemic attack, what was the rate of error? Did any test confirm the diagnosis? In both examples, there is no way to determine the clinician's rate of error with any mathematical exactitude nor would a test have confirmed either diagnosis. Parasomnias are akin to these two examples. Though diagnostic tests may be considered to support the diagnosis of parasomnia, especially for RBD, these do not confirm the cause for the criminal event as it is not directly temporally connected. In many instances in sleep forensics investigations, the alleged crime is often months to years removed before case files are even received. All this is not to imply that the soft sciences cannot generate reliable knowledge, but their methods of inquiry are qualitatively different from those associated with the hard sciences.

Presenting Clinical Medicine—Hard or Soft Science?

The hard sciences, such as pathophysiology, serve as the basis of medical research that focuses on the systematic collection of data about diseases in individual patients in order to gain verifiable knowledge and develop treatment strategies. The standard of proof in the hard sciences requires control of variables and strict regularity of outcomes in all cases to attain an objectively measured level of evidence that is irrefutable—a level that cannot be attained with most medical research. For clinical medicine, attaining such a standard is not only impossible but inappropriate and unnecessary (Miller & Miller, 2014). Published case studies and case series are a means of obtaining valuable information that can provide knowledge of potentially exceptionally high certainty. Consequently, this knowledge base can contribute to predicting various outcomes by establishing reliable general theories while falsifying others. Community- or consensus-driven standards of clinical practice of formally recognized medical conditions are routinely reviewed, updated, and published in authoritative medical professional society manuals, such as the ICSD-3TR (American Academy of Sleep Medicine, 2023). These manuals are the final product of several years of a rigorous international peer-review process reflective of the distillation of the most current, widely accepted scientific principles and comprehensive literature searches that included clinical case reports published in prominent medical journals. True expertise in any profession can only be acquired through accumulated experience. A physician becomes an expert on the basis of intimate knowledge of a tremendous number of clinical cases specific to their area of interest. It is with the cumulative number of these cases combined with knowledge of the paradigmatic and extremely unusual cases that transforms the physician from a knowledgeable, proficient clinician into a seasoned expert. Though a medical diagnosis is intrinsically probabilistic, physicians can attain high levels of reliability and certainty for their patients by their fund of specific medical knowledge and experience, maintaining community standards of clinical practice, and continuing to incorporate a standard systematic approach, or methodology, to patient assessment. In anticipation of inquiries concerning methodology in the courtroom, we have taken a standard systematic approach to patient assessment routinely used in our parasomnia specialty clinic and have adapted it into a flowsheet for use in the legal arena (Figure 46.3). As high-level criminal felony cases involving a parasomnia are exceedingly rare, this flowsheet emphasizes data collection in a measured, stepwise, as well as cost-effective manner that is heavily skewed toward meticulously uncovering much more common causes attributed to violent asocial behaviors. This bias is represented by variable degrees of thickness in the widths of each directional arrow in Figure 46.3. In cases specifically involving a possible parasomnia, we have offered this very helpful flowsheet to the attorney for consideration to be included as evidence in the formal case report. Alternatively, it could also be used as a source for discussion with the attorney during pre-trial preparations, especially when an aggressive cross-examination attacking the methodical reliability is expected.

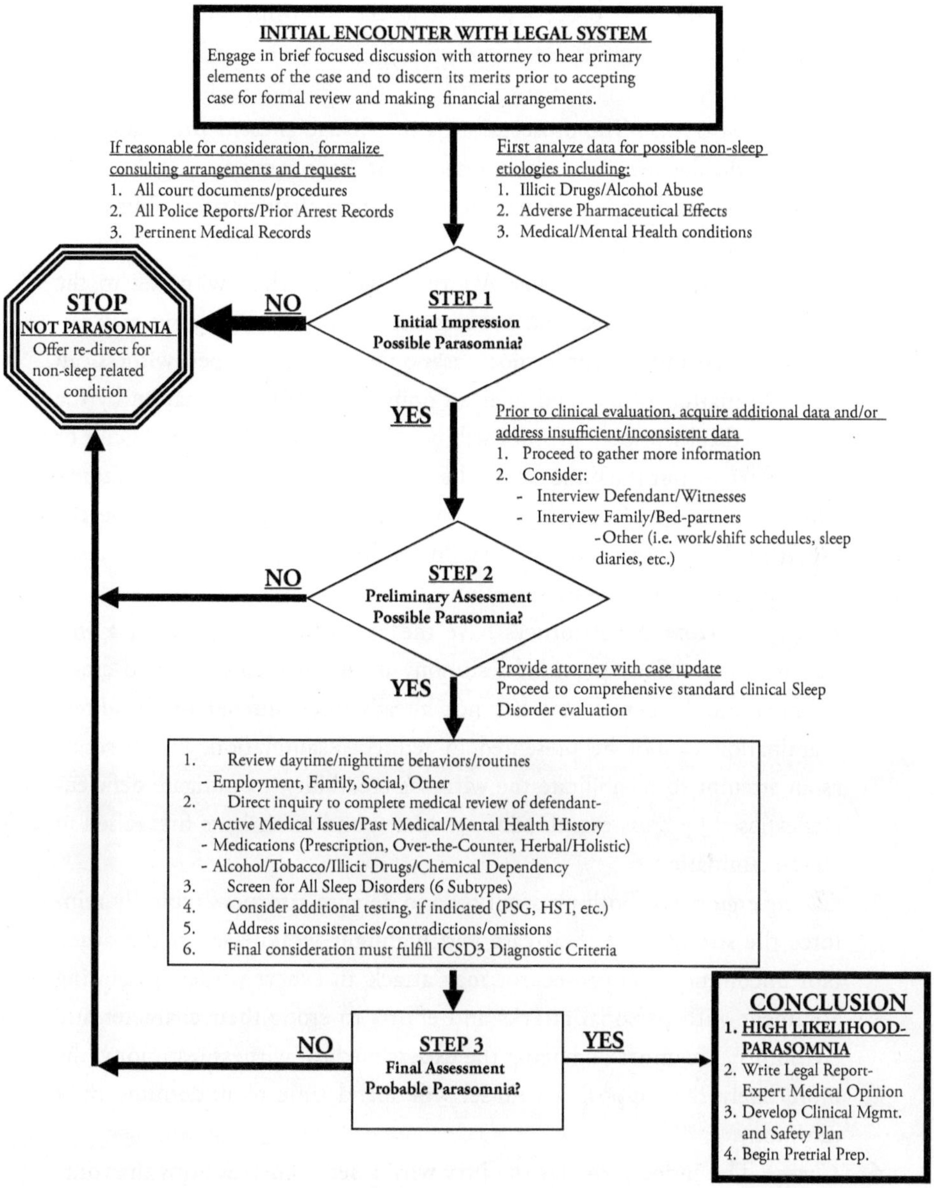

Figure 46.3 Parasomnia clinical methodology
Note. HST = home sleep test; ICSD3 = *International Classification of Sleep Disorders*, third edition; PSG = polysomnography.

On the Stand: The Courtroom Process

The most capable expert medical witnesses are those with significant legal experience or at least those who are well informed about the court proceedings and their role within the legal process as an effective communicator. Should the criminal case actually proceed to trial, elements of the trial process proceed in the following order (American Bar Association, 2019):

1. *Opening statements*: The prosecution is the first to present their case, followed by the defense. Here, they present their theories concerning the crime and provide an overview of evidence to support their position, but argument is not permitted.
2. *Direct examination of witnesses*: Attorneys will call their witnesses to the stand to elicit both direct and circumstantial evidence. Witnesses may testify to matters of fact, but in most cases only a qualified expert witness can testify to matters of fact and offer an opinion. Direct examination by the expert medical witness's attorney will not ask questions that are difficult or inappropriate, but the same cannot be expected during cross-examination.
3. *Cross-examination of witnesses*: The opposing attorney will challenge the expert medical witness to test reliability, accuracy, and credibility of testimony provided in direct examination.
4. *Redirect examination*: Attorneys have the opportunity to question a witness who has already provided testimony in response to direct and cross-examination. Evidence that has not already been offered in the direct examination cannot be presented in redirect examination, which serves as an attempt to rehabilitate the witness's credibility, to mitigate deficiencies exposed by cross-examination, or to respond to an issue first raised in cross-examination.
5. *Closing arguments*: Both prosecution and defense attorneys typically reinforce the strengths of their case and highlight weaknesses in the other. Not uncommonly, a prosecutor may attack an expert witness in closing argument with personal attacks and efforts to erode their character and credibility. The more damaging the expert medical witness testimony, the more likely that opposing counsel will spend time to undermine their testimony.
6. *Charge*: The judge provides the jury with a set of instructions that outline the legal principles and statutes, summarizes the evidence, and presents verdict forms that outline the factual questions for them to answer.
7. *Jury deliberations*: The jury deliberates in private, taking into account the applicable law as laid out by the court and the facts presented in court. To prevail, the prosecution must establish beyond a reasonable doubt that every element of the crime has been proven. If the jury is unclear about what occurred, they must render a verdict of not guilty.

For both the attorney and the expert medial witness, pre-trial preparations are very important but may be shortened or overlooked entirely because of limited financial resources, time constraints, and scheduling conflicts. Pre-trial preparation may also involve advising the attorney about the selection of jurors and how to determine which prospective jurors might be favorably sympathetic.

The expert medical witness needs to be very aware that educating the courtroom is not the same as giving a medical lecture. During direct examination, the medical expert witness can only answer questions in a very concise and exacting manner. Failure to do so might be perceived as "pontificating" and is likely to raise strong objections by the opposing counsel. In order to effectively and efficiently educate the courtroom on unfamiliar and complex medical conditions, such as those involving uncommon, bizarre SRV, our sleep forensics experience strongly recommends that the expert medical witness support their attorney by developing a point-summary of important questions that need to be presented. A list of questions for the attorney to consider in questioning the sleep forensics expert medical witness during testimony may start with those related to normal sleep processes, a review of the spectrum of sleep disorders, the definition of parasomnias, an explanation of how parasomnias arise and factors that increase their risk, prevalence of parasomnias, diagnostic criteria and treatment of parasomnias, and, finally, the degree of certainty in their opinion. As previously noted, degree of certainty cannot be mathematically calculated in many clinical conditions including parasomnias. This threshold for certainty would appear low compared to medical standards. If inquired about what evidence was relied upon to arrive at their opinion, we suggest that the sleep forensics expert medical witness specifically refer to Figure 46.3 of the parasomnia-based standard systematic approach to patient assessment. The sleep forensics expert medical witness should emphasize that the opinion is not based on one or a few pieces of evidence, as the prosecution may attempt to suggest in order to erode reliability, but rather that the opinion relied upon the entirety of the standard systematic approach. Conversely, if the prosecution relies on an expert witness whose opinion is that a result is "more likely than not"—the civil standard—the state has not met its burden to prove the case beyond a reasonable doubt, and the jury must acquit.

Preparing for Cross-Examination Challenges

Cross-examination is often an unsettling experience for any witness and may be particularly difficult for a physician serving as an expert medical witness. It cannot be overstated that the expert medical witness must set time aside to prepare for their testimony with the attorney prior to trial. As mentioned above, the expert medical witness can expect the elements found within the Daubert standard to be the template for a cross-examination. Cross-examination may also be viewed as a safety check to clarify and ensure that the expert medical witness's findings and opinions are correct. Common cross-examination tactics (Barsky, 2012) by opposing counsel we have encountered for which an expert medical witness should also be prepared include the following:

1. Leading questions—used to encourage the expert witness to agree with the attorney's false claims
2. Intentional ambiguity—employing double meanings or false assumptions meant to obfuscate the expert witness into admitting that which was not intended
3. Fog of war—creating uncertainty in the course of argumentative battle by rapidly raising questions, often ambiguous or tangential, to subvert the expert witness, thereby confusing the jury, clouding their judgment, and making it difficult for them to keep focus
4. Character assassination—use of insults or ridicule in an effort to make the expert witness appear weak and less credible
5. Raising doubt—getting the expert to acknowledge that they may not have been allowed to testify in a prior case and implying that, somehow, such a decision cast doubt on their credibility in this case
6. Financial consideration—the witness may be examined about the amount they are being paid with an implication that the fees are to assure a certain result
7. Friendship bias—the number of times the expert has worked with this attorney and if they have had a social relationship in an effort to impugn the witness's objectivity

The attorney and their expert witness should prepare carefully for all of these types of questions and many others which are routine efforts by a zealous opponent to undermine the expert witness's confidence and then make them appear uncertain before the jury about their conclusions.

After the trial, if the defendant has been found guilty, the expert medical witness may be asked to assist in the sentencing phase and/or the appeals process if they were retained by the defense. In our sleep forensics experience, this, however, has been extremely rare. More commonly, if we supported sexsomnia and the defendant was acquitted of sexual assault, we have been asked to develop a safety disposition plan for the defendant. Devised from characteristic features that have been recognized to increase the risk for sexsomnia, we offer the following standardized approach (which can also be easily modified for parasomnias in general).

Sexsomnia Post-Trial Safety Plan

The following safety plan is offered to ensure the safety and well-being of any children under 18 years of age when under the direct care of the parent or caregiver with a recognized vulnerability toward sexsomnia.

1. It is recommended that the caregiver's children, especially those children directly implicated with the legal proceedings, be referred to an appropriate adolescent psychologist.
   GOAL: To educate the children about their caregiver's vulnerability for NREM parasomnias and its potential impact on them and their family. Such therapy is indicated to proactively address anxieties and fears which children are likely to develop as a consequence of the court-mandated implementation of the caregiver's safety plan.

2. The caregiver with sexsomnia should not co-sleep with any children under 18 years of age.
   GOAL: Proximity is a key characteristic feature of all parasomnias where those sleeping close beside the affected individual could unknowingly have triggered the confusional arousal, or other sleep-related behaviors, by their movements and/or sounds.
   - 2.1.1. This caregiver should not sleep in the same room with any children under 18 years of age.
   - 2.1.2. When on vacation, this caregiver and any children under 18 years of age should have separate accommodations.
   - 2.1.3. This caregiver should inform any adult bed-partners of their condition and its potential impact. Those afflicted with NREM parasomnias are typically not aware of their behaviors. Informing such a bed-partner would allow them to relay this information to the afflicted individual for further consideration in the management of their condition. Additionally, this would allow the bed-partner to be directly involved in important decisions concerning risks to ensure their family's safety.

3. The caregiver with sexsomnia should sleep within their own bedroom with door closed and a loud alarm placed inside this caregiver's bedroom door.
   GOAL: In the very unlikely event that the caregiver's expression of an NREM parasomnia should progress beyond their bedroom, the triggered alarm would thereby awaken the caregiver and then likely abort their problematic behaviors from progressing any further.
   - 3.1.1. It is also very strongly recommended that a loud alarm be placed inside their children's bedroom door.
     - 3.1.1.1. *Note*: It is anticipated that children are likely to become anxious or fearful once they learn about the caregiver's propensity for bizarre sleep-related behaviors. In this regard, the children would gain some control and feel more secure knowing that a triggered alarm would warn them of their caregiver's unintended nighttime forays beyond the bedroom.

3.1.2. In cases involving parasomnias, locks on bedroom doors are not recommended as these could potentially compromise immediate access into the bedroom during emergencies of any type.

4. The caregiver with sexsomnia should remove any weapons, or any instruments that can potentially be used as such, from near the bed and bedroom. *GOAL*: Again, proximity is a key characteristic feature of all parasomnias. Individuals with a vulnerability for parasomnias may abruptly exhibit a defensive or predatory posture and haphazardly reach for anything nearby that could be used as an instrument of violence.

   4.1.1. The caregiver with sexsomnia should secure all firearms in the home. These firearms should be kept unloaded and secured in a locked gun safe, ideally situated separate from their bedroom.

      4.1.1.1. *Note*: It is appreciated that those with sexsomnia are also vulnerable to other sleep-related behaviors and not just to those with sexualized attributes alone.

5. In cases where the caregiver with sexsomnia also has OSA, the OSA should be effectively treated to an acceptable degree by a therapeutic modality as determined by their clinical sleep medicine physician.
GOAL: OSA is a well-recognized independent risk factor increasing the likelihood to trigger parasomnias, including sexsomnia, through sleep fragmentation induced by obstructive respiratory-related events.

   5.1. OSA treatment considerations:

      5.1.1. Weight reduction/maintenance of effective weight: It is recommended that their sleep medicine physician routinely perform, on intervals at their discretion, appropriate diagnostic studies (PSG or home sleep test) to objectively confirm ongoing resolution of OSA.

      5.1.2. CPAP (or similar such devices): The caregiver with sexsomnia should be made aware of and have access to laptop or cellphone applications which monitor device compliance and clinical effectiveness. This caregiver should be educated by their sleep medicine physician and made aware of effective CPAP outcome measures. This caregiver should remain actively and regularly involved in confirming the ongoing resolution of their OSA.

      5.1.3. The schedule of this caregiver's sleep medicine clinic follow-up appointments is to be made at the discretion of their sleep medicine physician but should occur no less than once per year.

5.1.4. This caregiver's CPAP monitoring data should also be made available to their partner, or former partner, on a monthly basis for them to review. This caregiver should agree to a medical release of information allowing their partner, or former partner, access to this CPAP monitoring data. Device compliance data can be easily acquired through wireless transmission at minimal inconvenience to this caregiver. Their partner, or former partner, should be educated on effective CPAP outcomes measures by this caregiver's sleep medicine physician. For average monthly CPAP outcome measures, it is advocated that the AHI should attain a goal of five or fewer events per hour, with a minimum device compliance of ≥70% of 4 hours of nightly use. If the minimum monthly compliance of 70% has not been met and/or the AHI reveals a trend that is consistently above 10 events/hour, it is recommended that this caregiver contact their sleep medicine provider to discuss possible device adjustments, equipment replacement, or other therapeutic considerations.

5.1.4.1. *Note*: Ex-spouses often harbor ongoing distrust toward each other. Allowing ex-spouses, or former partners, the option to regularly access this caregiver's monthly CPAP monitoring data gives them the opportunity to independently and objectively verify continued effective OSA resolution. Such access serves as another indicator reassuring the ex-spouse of this caregiver's commitment to ensuring the safety of their children.

6. Pharmaceutical management of the caregiver with sexsomnia with medications, such as clonazepam, is to be determined after a risk/benefit analysis by the patient and is considered *optional.*
7. The caregiver with sexsomnia is to completely refrain from all illicit drug use when caring for children and should only consume alcohol in an absolutely responsible manner guided by legal standards of intoxication.

Conclusion

It has been well established that parasomnias have been associated with asocial, violent, and sexual behaviors that may have forensic implications. When these do occur, they occur without consciousness or awareness, which has implications for culpability in a court of law. Parasomnias are not directly the result of an underlying psychiatric condition but can be explained through neurophysiologic processes that also involve CPGs, FAPs, and the unifying concept of state dissociation. The parasomnias that carry the strongest risk for medical–legal consequences are the DOA from NREM sleep, predominantly confusional arousals (with sexual behaviors and/or aggressive/violent behaviors) and SW (with aggression and at times with sexual behaviors and sleep-driving). ST comprise the third DOA but carry potential forensic consequences only when combined with SW. However, it is remotely possible that an ST episode in one person (with loud screaming) could trigger a violent involuntary reaction from sleep in the bed-partner, with forensic consequences. Also, RBD, the only parasomnia that requires PSG confirmation, carries a risk for forensic consequences because of the emergence of violent dream-enacting behaviors, with major risk of injury (including life-threatening injury, as described below) to self and bed-partner. Though both NREM-related and REM-related parasomnias have forensic implications, sexsomnia, a subtype of confusional arousal, has accounted for the majority of referrals to our sleep forensics practice. Those parasomnias with potential for violence have consistent characteristics which help to determine likelihood for any given event to relatively high degrees of certainty and reliability. With greater awareness of the forensic implications of parasomnias, in particular those of sexsomnia, sleep medicine physicians can expect a continued increase in inquiries from attorneys for their involvement in the legal arena. Both Legal Cases 1 and 2 involved criminal allegations of sexual assault for which sexsomnia was highly likely to have been the cause, at least to a level of certainty well beyond that of reasonable doubt. Civil attorneys often use 51% as their definition of a preponderance of the evidence—the standard of proof in such cases—or "more likely than not." In criminal law, the reasonable doubt standard is far higher. Despite their similarities and compelling medical evidence supporting each of these two cases, the separate courts arrived at contradictory final decisions. From our vantage point over the years as dedicated sleep forensics investigators, a sleep medicine physician's role as an expert medical witness involves more than presenting relevant, up-to-date clinical science to the legal process—more than just review the legal case files, formulate an opinion, draft a formal written report, and testify on the stand. Given the very high stakes for all involved in sleep forensics cases, supporting justice in the courtroom can only be optimally done through a strong collaborative effort with the attorney throughout the legal process. Given the foreign nature of science for most attorneys, such a collaborative approach would greatly aid the attorney to better utilize an expert medical witness to their fullest degree—a degree of support from which the legal system would also most certainly benefit.

Future Directions

1. For those convicted in criminal cases, the penalties are very severe and at times involve decades of incarceration. One essential goal of an expert medical witness is to ensure that the court is adequately educated and up to date on the current state of clinical science. Unfortunately, there are no published guidelines in sleep medicine which outline the minimum qualifications in formal training and experience required by physicians to serve as an expert

medical witness. Thus, professional medical societies, such as the AASM, are strongly encouraged to develop an international task force to address this deficiency. The task force's recommendations on expert medical witness qualifications should undergo further outside peer review to eventually be published in an appropriate medical journal. Such formal recommendations would provide both attorneys and physicians much needed clarity in identifying appropriate specialists to support fair decisions in court.

2. Just as the courtroom is foreign to physicians, most attorneys are unfamiliar with science and its methodology. This unfamiliarity contributes to less than optimal utilization of the expert medical witness as a valuable resource throughout the legal process and can contribute to inconsistent courtroom decisions. To bridge this divide, legal professional associations should inculcate a culture of closer collaboration between medicine and law. This goal can be attained by organizing conferences, such as those developed for continued legal education or continued medical education, focused on the effective use of clinical science and the expert medical witness in the courtroom.
3. The implications of sexsomnia encompass a broad spectrum involving both clinical and legal realms. Sexsomnia is likely more prevalent than currently appreciated. However, reliable estimates concerning the prevalence of sexsomnia, its demographics, and its various expressions are sorely lacking. To attain these goals, a multicenter research project that includes both academic and community-based sleep medicine programs should be undertaken to collect such important data using random selection methods of sample groups within the population to be described.
4. The practice in many courts is to treat "automatism" and behaviors attributed to a state of "unconsciousness" as virtually synonymous. Automatism is not a medical condition but a legal term that refers to an act committed without volition in which the critical issue concerns the absence of the defendant's will. The use of automatism to support the defense arises from a basic tenet embedded in criminal law whereby a defendant cannot be found guilty of an act which occurred independently of their will. Automatism is less a defense and more an assertion that the prosecution is unable to prove to the jury that the defendant acted on their own volition. In general, automatisms are divided into those that are insane and those that are sane (Mackay, 2015; Prevezer, 1958). Insane automatisms result from a preexisting "disease of the mind[brain]" or mental illness which may lead to disinhibited fear/aggression, delusions, or hallucinations. Conditions associated with an insane automatism include schizophrenia and a brain tumor.

The University of Texas Clock Tower shooting on August 1, 1966 is often cited as the premiere example of a possible insane automatism. It is also recognized as the first mass shooting that unfolded "live" on television (Lavergne, 1997). Charles Whitman, a former marine sharpshooter, began that day by first killing his wife and mother. Thereafter, with a footlocker filled with an assortment of weapons including an M-1 carbine rifle, he got access to the observation deck of the clock tower after fatally bludgeoning the receptionist. After barricading himself atop the clock tower, he opened fire at people below, killing 16 and wounding 32 before he was killed by Austin police officers. Whitman was literally a childhood choirboy and became one of the youngest Eagle Scouts in Boy Scout history. At the time of the shootings, he appeared to be a happily married engineering student with an IQ in the 99th percentile. In the prior year, he had seen physicians with complaints of severe headaches, feelings of rage and confusion, along with violent impulses. His typed suicide note proclaimed his love for his wife, puzzlement for his actions, and request that an autopsy be performed on his brain. Curiously, he also requested that any money left in his bank account be given to a mental health foundation. The autopsy supported Whitman's intuitions as it revealed a glioblastoma tumor pressing upon his amygdala. There is considerable evidence that links the amygdala with the axis of fear, anxiety, and aggression (LeDoux, 1998). An insane automatism could thereby possibly lead to a verdict of not guilty by reason of insanity, often leading to institutionalization. In contrast, sane automatisms are not an inherent "disease of the mind[brain]" and are caused by external stimuli. Common conditions associated with a sane automatism include head trauma and involuntary intoxication due to adverse medication reactions. An example of a sane automatism might be an individual who sustained a significant blow to the head, is dazed and confused but not rendered unconscious, and then engages in any number of behaviors for which they have no control, are unaware, and have no memory. A sane automatism could lead to a full acquittal. The distinction between an insane versus a sane automatism may be confusing to many physicians, as the result may indeed share a common neurophysiologic pathway despite the dissimilarity in the underpinnings of the event. The distinction between an insane versus a sane automatism is largely an arbitrary legal construct, not a medical one, which has been based upon legal precedent. Simply stated, an insane automatism refers to a primary cause within the actor to which their brain had already been predisposed whereas a sane automatism refers to a cause that is external first beginning outside of the actor. The SW defense is largely built upon the premise that the defendant committed an offense involuntarily. Thus, on occasion, SW may be referred to in the courts as a type of automatism. In criminal courts in the United States, automatism is rarely used as a defense and appears to be more often encountered in case law in Commonwealth countries such as the United Kingdom. The internal/external distinction in automatism is particularly problematic. Court renderings concerning the status of SW have been very inconsistent and often unpredictable—at times determined to be a sane automatism and at other times as an insane automatism. Courts commonly understand conscious/unconscious states as binary, or "all-or-none," conditions, often further complicated by the embrace of Freudian psychoanalytic theory. Court precedent, which differs greatly from jurisdiction to jurisdiction, may offer direction but typically refers to such renderings that are several decades old. The perplexing manner in which the courts have dealt with automatism/unconscious involuntary acts only further emphasizes the divide between the law and medicine's understanding of human cognition. Medicine is dynamically adaptable, always in the midst of rapid growth, which also adheres to currently held principles in cognitive neuroscience, which appreciates that consciousness occurs on a broad spectrum, is evanescent, and is not binary (Hobson et al., 2000). Thus, to untangle the court's conundrum concerning human behaviors, it would appear prudent that medical scientists engage attorneys in law reform in developing standards to assist the courts in their determination of voluntary versus involuntary acts based upon current cognitive neuroscience. An SW individual's responses or reactions are often perceived as not under the individual's control. It is anticipated that the court will have difficulty in assessing the meaning of "lack of control" as some individuals vulnerable to involuntary behaviors, such as sleepwalkers, can in fact control their behaviors to an extent which may limit its impact if given notice that it may happen. For instance, though an individual clearly aware of their vulnerability toward sexsomnia cannot control their behavior in the midst of such an event, they can still engage in thoughtful behaviors prior to falling asleep. Such behaviors may include notifying prospective bedpartners of their vulnerability, taking precautions to avoid conditions known to exacerbate their condition (i.e., insufficient sleep, certain medications, problematic stress/anxiety), maintaining effective therapy for OSA assuming they have this condition, and especially avoiding co-sleeping with individuals to whom they have no committed romantic partnership, to name but a few examples. To address this concern, it has been proposed that the voluntary act requirement consist of three parts: (1) voluntary acts, (2) involuntary acts, and (3) semi-voluntary acts. Here, a violent SW act, such as sexsomnia, would be considered a semi-voluntary act as the episode itself would be involuntary but would have the potential to be dangerous again. Those who acted semi-voluntarily would appear to have a relatively greater control over their behavior, unlike those who are a "true" involuntary (Denno, 2002; Schenck & Mahowald, 1995). The main purpose of a semi-voluntary category is to avoid an unqualified acquittal and to prevent the courts from labeling sleepwalkers as insane individuals who are vulnerable to recurrent acts but have no evidence of a psychiatric disease that would have made them eligible for institutionalization under the insanity provision.

Acknowledgments

The authors would like to express their deepest gratitude to Shaddi Kamiabipour, JD, Senior Deputy District Attorney, Office of the District Attorney, Orange County, CA, and to Susan Elizabeth Reese, JD, Susan Elizabeth Reese LLC, criminal defense attorney, Newport, OR, for their enthusiastic encouragement, erudite legal insights, useful critiques, and invaluable assistance to facilitate the expert medical witness's journey through the legal system.

Notes

The following highly pertinent article was published since the original submission of this chapter, which found that Disorders of Arousal from NREM sleep were the cause of the ten homicides and four attempted homicides that were reviewed:

Castelnovo, A., Schraemli, M., Schenck, C. H., & Manconi, M. (2024). The parasomnia defense in sleep-related homicide: A systematic review and a critical analysis of the medical literature. *Sleep Medicine Reviews, 74*, 101898. https://doi.org/10.1016/j.smrv.2024.101898. Epub 2024 Jan 14. PMID: 38364685.

References

American Academy of Sleep Medicine. (2023). *International classification of sleep disorders* (3rd ed., text revision).

American Bar Association. (2019, September 9). *How courts work.* https://www.americanbar.org/groups/public_education/resources/law_related_education_network/how_courts_work/court_role/

American Bar Association. (2021, December 30). *How courts work.* https://www.americanbar.org/groups/public_education/resources/law_related_education_network/how_courts_work/

Azevedo, F. A. C., Carvalho, L. R. B., Grinberg, L. T., Farfel, J. M., Ferretti, R. E. L., Leite, R. E. P., Filho, W. J., Lent, R., & Herculano-Houzel, S. (2009). Equal numbers of neuronal and nonneuronal cells make the human brain an isometrically scaled-up primate brain. *Journal of Comparative Neurology, 513*, 532–541.

Baron, J., & Auckley, D. (2005). Gunshot wound to the head: An unusual complication of sleep apnea and bilevel positive airway pressure. *Sleep and Breathing, 8*, 161–164.

Barsky, A. E. (2012). *Clinicians in court: A guide to subpoenas, depositions, testifying, everything else you need to know* (2nd ed.). Guilford Press.

Bell, B. D. (2011). Psychomotor epilepsy. In J. S. Kreutzer, J. DeLuca, & B. Caplan (Eds.), *Encyclopedia of clinical neuropsychology* (pp. 2073–2074). Springer.

Bhat, S., Chokroverty, S., Kabak, B., Yang, Q. R., & Rosen, D. (2012). Dream-enacting behavior in non-rapid eye movement sleep. *Sleep Medicine, 13*(4), 445–446.

Boursoulian, L. J., Schenck, C. H., Mahowald, M. W., & Lagrange, A. H. (2012). Differentiating parasomnias from nocturnal seizures. *Journal of Clinical Sleep Medicine, 8*(1), 108–112.

Broughton, R., Billings, R., Cartwright, R., Doucette, D., Edmeads, J., Edwardh, M., Ervin, F., Orchard, B., Hill, R., & Turrell, G. (1994). Homicidal somnambulism: A case report. *Sleep, 17*, 253–264.

Bušková, J., Piorecký, M., & Měrková, R. (2022). Sexsomnia can be triggered by sleep-related head jerks. *Sleep Medicine, 92*, 12–14.

Carrillo-Solano, M., Leu-Semenescu, S., Golmard, J. L., Groos, E., & Arnulf, I. (2016). Sleepiness in sleepwalking and sleep terrors: A higher sleep pressure? *Sleep Medicine, 26*, 54–59.

Castelnovo, A., Amacker, J., Maiolo, M., Amato, N., Pereno, M., Riccardi, S., Danani, A., Ulzega, S., & Manconi, M. (2022). High-density EEG power topography and connectivity during confusional arousal. *Cortex, 155*, 62–74.

Castelnovo, A., Loddo, G., Provini, F., & Manconi, M. (2021). Frequent, complex and vivid dream-like/hallucinatory experiences during NREM sleep parasomnia episodes. *Sleep Medicine, 82*, 61–64.

Castelnovo, A., Siclari, F., Spaggiari, S., Borth, D., Manconi, M., Arnulf, I., & Schenck, C.H (2024). Conscious experiences during non-rapid eye movement sleep parasomnias. *Neuroscience and Biobehavioral Reviews, 167*(105919). https://doi.org/10.1016/j.neubiorev.2024.105919

Chung, S. A., Yegneswaran, B., Natarajan, A., Trajanovic, N., & Shapiro, C. M. (2010). Frequency of sexsomnia in sleep clinic patients. *Sleep, 33*, Abstract, 0673.

Cicolin, A., Tribolo, A., Giordano, A., Chiarot, E., Peila, E., Terreni, A., Bucca, C., & Mutani, R. (2011). Sexual behaviors during sleep associated with polysomnographically confirmed parasomnia overlap disorder. *Sleep Medicine, 12*(5), 523–528.

Contreras, J. B., Richardson, J., & Kotagal, S. (2019). Sexsomnia in an adolescent. *Journal of Clinical Sleep Medicine, 15*(3), 505–507.

Cramer Bornemann, M. A., & Mahowald, M. W. (2021). Criminal culpability for sleep-related violence. In M. Kryger, T. Roth, & W. C. Dement (Eds.), *Principles and practice of sleep medicine* (7th ed., pp. 709–716). Elsevier.

Cramer Bornemann, M. A., Mahowald, M. W., & Schenck, C. H. (2014). Sexsomnia and sleep forensics: The interface between sleep-related behaviors and the law. *Sleep, 37*, Abstract 0602.

Cramer Bornemann, M. A., Schenck, C. H., & Mahowald, M. W. (2019). A review of sleep-related violence: The demographics of sleep forensics referrals to a single center. *Chest, 155*(5), 1059–1066.

Danish, N., Khawaja, I. S., & Schenck, C. H. (2018). Violent parasomnia with recurrent biting and surgical interventions: Case report and differential diagnosis. *Journal of Clinical Sleep Medicine, 14*(5), 889–891.

Daubert v. Merrell Dow Pharmaceuticals, Inc., 43 F.3d 1311 (9th Cir. 1995).

Denno, D. W. (2002). Crime and consciousness: Science and involuntary acts. *Minnesota Law Review, 87*, 269–399.

Dubessy, A. L., Leu-Semenescu, S., Attali, V., Maranci, J. B., & Arnulf, I. (2017). Sexsomnia: A specialized non-REM parasomnia? *Sleep, 40*(2), Article zsw043. https://doi.org/10.1093/sleep/zsw043

Dumitrascu, O., Schenck, C. H., Applebee, G., & Attarian, H. (2013). Parasomnia overlap disorder: A distinct pathophysiologic entity or a variant of rapid eye movement sleep behavior disorder? A case series. *Sleep Medicine, 14*(11), 1217–1220.

Fernandez, J. D., & Soca, R. (2021). Sexsomnia in active duty military: A series of four cases. *Military Medicine, 188*(1–2), e436–e439. https://doi.org/10.1093/milmed/usab126

Fitzgerald, P. J. (1961). Voluntary and involuntary acts. In A. G. Guest (Ed.), *Oxford essays in jurisprudence* (pp. 1–28). Oxford University Press.

Freeman, J. M., & Nelson, K. B. (2004). Expert medical testimony. Responsibilities of medical societies. *Neurology, 63*, 1557–1558.

Friedman, L. M. (2019). *A history of American law* (4th ed.). Oxford University Press.

Frye v. United States, 293 F.1013 (D.C. Cir. 1923).

Goldrich, M. S. (2004). *Report of the Council on Ethical and Judicial Affairs* (CEJA Report 12-A-04). American Medical Association.

Haba-Rubio, J., Frauscher, B., Marques-Vidal, P., Toriel, J., Tobback, N., Andries, D., Preisig, M., Vollenweider, P., Postuma, R., & Heinzer, R. (2018). Prevalence and determinants of rapid eye movement sleep behavior disorder in the general population. *Sleep, 41*(2), Article zsx197. https://doi.org/10.1093/sleep/zsx197

Hobson, J. A., Pace-Schott, E. F., & Stickgold, R. (2000). Dreaming and the brain: Toward a cognitive neuroscience of conscious states. *Behavioral Brain Sciences, 23*, 793–842.

Ingravallo, F., Schenck, C. H., D'Aloja, E., & Puligheddu, M. (2018). Firing a loaded gun during sleep in an elderly man with a "perfect storm" of risk factors including severe obstructive sleep apnea. *Sleep & Breathing, 22*(1), 51–54.

Iranzo, A., & Santamaria, J. (2005). Severe obstructive apnea/hypopnea mimicking REM sleep behavior disorder. *Sleep, 28*(2), 2013–2016.

Irfan, M., & Schenck, C. H. (2018). Sleep-related orgasms in a 57-year-old woman: A case report. *Journal of Clinical Sleep Medicine, 14*(1), 141–144.

Jensen, P. J. (2003). Frye versus Daubert: Practically the same? *Minnesota Law Review, 87*(5), 1579–1620.

Khawaja, I. S., Hurwitz, T. D., & Schenck, C. H. (2017). Sleep-related abnormal sexual behaviors (sexsomnia) successfully treated with a mandibular advancement device: A case report. *Journal of Clinical Sleep Medicine, 13*(4), 627–628.

Kim, D. S., Foster, B. E., Scott, J. A., Rizzo, M. M., Collen, J. F., & Soca, R. (2021). A rare presentation of sexsomnia in a military service member. *Journal of Clinical Sleep Medicine, 17*(1), 107–109.

Kumar, V., Grbach, V. X., & Castriotta, R. J. (2020). Resolution of sexsomnia with paroxetine. *Journal of Clinical Sleep Medicine, 16*(7), 1213–1214.

Lateef, O., Wyatt, J., & Cartwright, R. (2005). A case of violent non-REM parasomnias that resolved with treatment of obstructive sleep apnea. *Chest, 128,* Abstract 461S.

Lavergne, G. (1997). *A sniper in the tower: The Charles Whitman murders.* University of North Texas Press.

LeDoux, J. (1998). *The emotional brain: The mysterious underpinnings of emotional life.* Simon and Schuster.

Lopez, R., Lefevre, L., Barateau, L., Micoulaud-Franchi, J. A., Dauvilliers, Y., & Schenck, C. H. (2022). A series of 8 cases of sleep-related psychogenic dissociative disorders and proposed updated diagnostic criteria. *Journal of Clinical Sleep Medicine, 18*(2), 563–573.

Mackay, R. D. (2015). An anatomy of automatism. *Medicine, Science, and the Law, 55*(3), 150–155.

Mahowald, M. W., Cramer Bornemann, M. A., & Schenck, C. H. (2011). State dissociation, human behavior, and consciousness. *Current Topics in Medicinal Chemistry, 11*(19), 2392–2402.

Mahowald, M. W., & Schenck, C. H. (1994). REM sleep behavior disorder. In M. H. Kryger, W. Dement, & T. Roth (Eds.), *Principles and practice of sleep medicine* (2nd ed., pp. 574–588). Saunders.

Mahowald, M. W., & Schenck, C. H. (2001). Evolving concepts of human state dissociation. *Archives Italiennes de Biologie, 139,* 269–300.

Martynowicz, H., Smardz, J., Wieczorek, T., Mazur, G., Poreba, R., Skomro, R., Zietek, M., Wojakowska, J., Michalek, M., & Wieckiewicz, M. (2018). The co-occurrence of sexsomnia, sleep bruxism and other sleep disorders. *Journal of Clinical Medicine, 7*(9), Article 233. https://doi.org/10.3390/jcm7090233

Meira, E., Cruz, M., & Soca, R. (2016). Sexsomnia and REM-predominant obstructive sleep apnea effectively treated with a mandibular advancement device. *Sleep Science, 9*(3), 140–141.

Miller, C., & Miller, D. W., Jr. (2014). Medicine is not science. *European Journal for Person Centered Healthcare, 2*(2), 144–153.

Mioč, M., Antelmi, E., Filardi, M., Pizza, F., Ingravallo, F., Nobili, L., Tassinari, C. A., Schenck, C. H., & Plazzi, G. (2018). Sexsomnia: A diagnostic challenge, a case report. *Sleep Medicine, 43,* 1–3.

Pillmann, F. (2009). Complex dream-enacting behavior in sleepwalking. *Psychosomatic Medicine, 71*(2), 231–234.

Muza, R., Lawrence, M., & Drakatos, P. (2016). The reality of sexsomnia. *Current Opinion in Pulmonary Medicine, 22,* 576–582.

Pirzada, A., Almeneessier, A. S., & BaHamman, A.S. (2019). Abnormal sexual behavior during sleep: Sexsomnia and more. *Sleep and Vigilance.* https://doi.org/10.1007/s41782-019-00057-5

Riha, R. L., Dodds, S., Kotoulas, S. C., & Morrison, I. (2023). A case-control study of sexualised behaviour in sleep: A strong association with psychiatric comorbidity and relationship difficulties. *Sleep Medicine, 103,* 33–40.

Rocha, A. L., & Arnulf, I. (2020). NREM parasomnia as a dream enacting behavior. *Sleep Medicine, 75,* 103–105.

Rossi, J., Gales, A., Attali, V., Leu-Semenescu, S., Dodet, P., Groos, E., & Arnulf I. (2023). Do the EEG and behavioral criteria of NREM arousal disorders apply to sexsomnia? *Sleep, 46*(7). https://doi.org/10.1093/sleep/zsad056

Schenck, C. H., Arnulf, I., & Mahowald, M. W. (2007). Sleep and sex: What can go wrong? A review of the literature on sleep related disorders and abnormal sexual behaviors and experiences. *Sleep, 30*(6), 683–702.

Schenck, C. H. (2015) Update on sexsomnia, sleep related sexual seizures, and forensic implications. *NeuroQuantology, 13*(4), 518–541.

Schenck, C. H., Cramer Bornemann, M., Kaplish, N., & Eiser, A. S. (2021). Sleep-related (psychogenic) dissociative disorders as parasomnias associated with a psychiatric disorder: Update on reported cases. *Journal of Clinical Sleep Medicine, 17*(4), 803–810.

Schenck, C. H., Lee, S. A., Cramer Bornemann, M. A., & Mahowald, M. W. (2009). Potentially lethal behaviors associated with rapid eye movement sleep behavior disorder (RBD): Review of the literature and forensic implications. *Journal of Forensic Science, 54*(6), 1475–1484.

Schenck, C. H., & Mahowald, M. W. (1995). A polysomnographically documented case of adult somnambulism with long-distance automobile driving and frequent nocturnal violence: Parasomnia with continuing danger as a noninsane automatism? *Sleep, 18*(9), 765–772.

Schenck, C. H., & Mahowald, M. W. (2002). REM sleep behavior disorder: Clinical, developmental, and neuroscience perspectives 16 years after its formal identification in *SLEEP*. *Sleep, 25*(2), 120–138.

Schenck, C. H., Milner, D. M., Hurwitz, T. D., Bundlie, S. R., & Mahowald, M. W. (1989). A polysomnographic and clinical report on sleep-related injury in 100 adult patients. *American Journal of Psychiatry, 146*(9), 1166–1173.

Shapiro, C. M., Trajanovic, N. N., & Fedoroff, J. P. (2003). Sexsomnia—A new parasomnia? *Canadian Journal of Psychiatry, 48*(5), 311–317.

Shroder, O., & Mather, N. J. (1976). Forensic psychiatry. In F. E. Camps (Ed.), *Gradwohl's legal medicine* (p. 505). A. John Wright & Sons.

Siclari, F., Khatami, R., Urbaniok, F., Nobili, L., Mahowald, M. W., Schenk, C. H., Cramer Bornemann, M. A., & Bassetti, C. L. (2010). Violence in sleep. *Brain, 133*, 3494–3509.

Smith, J. Q., & MacQueen, G. R. (2017). Going, going, but not quite gone: Trials continue to decline in federal and state courts. Does it matter? *Judicature, 101*(4), 26–39.

Soca, R., Keenan, J. C., & Schenck, C. H. (2016). Parasomnia overlap disorder with sexual behaviors during sleep in a patient with obstructive sleep apnea. *Journal of Clinical Sleep Medicine, 12*(8), 1189–1191.

Szűcs, A., Kamondi, A., Zoller, R., Barcs, G., Szabó, P., & Purebl, G. (2014). Violent somnambulism: A parasomnia of young men with stereotyped dream-like experiences. *Medical Hypotheses, 83*(1), 47–52.

Toscanini, A. C., Marques, J. H., Hasan, R., & Schenck, C. H. (2021). Sexsomnia: Case based classification and discussion of psychosocial implications. *Sleep Science, 14*(2), 175–180.

Uguccioni, G., Golmard, J.-L., de Fontréaux, A. N., Leu-Semenescu, S., Brion, A., & Arnulf, I. (2013). Fight or flight? Dream content during sleepwalking/sleep terrors vs. rapid eye movement sleep behavior disorder. *Sleep Medicine, 14*(5), 391–398.

van Mierlo, P., Hermans, L. W. A., Arnulf, I., Pijpers, A., Overeem, S., & van Gilst, M. M. (2022). Validation of the Dutch translation of the Paris Arousal Disorders Severity Scale for non-REM parasomnias in a 1-year and 1-month version. *Journal of Clinical Sleep Medicine, 18*(4), 1135–1143.

Voges, B. R., Schmitt, F. C., House, P. M., Stodieck, S. R., & Schenck, C. H. (2019). Complex sexual behaviors during sleep as a manifestation of epilepsy: A case series. *Sleep, 42*(3), Article zsy233. https://doi.org/10.1093/sleep/zsy233

Yeh, S. B., & Schenck, C. H. (2016). Sexsomnia: A case of sleep masturbation documented by video-polysomnography in a young adult male with sleepwalking. *Sleep Science, 9*(2), 65–68.

INDEX

For the benefit of digital users, indexed terms that span two pages (e.g., 52–53) may, on occasion, appear on only one of those pages.

Tables, figures, and boxes are indicated by an italic *t*, *f*, and *b* following the page number.